Aminoff's Neurology and General Medicine

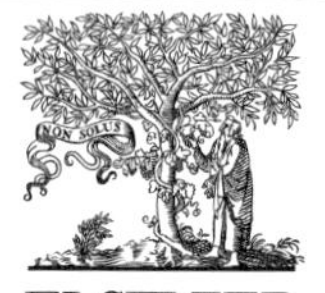

science &
technology books

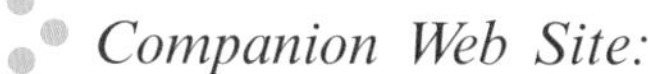

Companion Web Site:

http://booksite.elsevier.com/9780124077102

Aminoff's Neurology and General Medicine, fifth edition

Michael J. Aminoff and S. Andrew Josephson

Please visit the Companion Site for this volume to

- View figures from the book available as both Power Point slides and .jpeg files

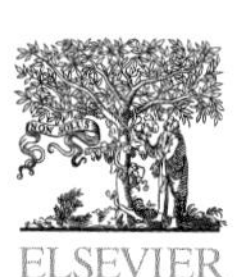

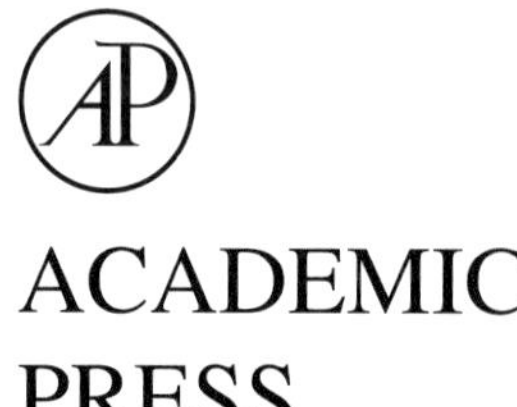

ACADEMIC
PRESS

Aminoff's Neurology and General Medicine

FIFTH EDITION

Michael J. Aminoff, MD, DSc, FRCP
Distinguished Professor, Department of Neurology,
School of Medicine, University of California,
San Francisco, California

S. Andrew Josephson, MD
Associate Professor, Department of Neurology,
C. Castro Franceschi and G. K. Mitchell Distinguished Professorship,
School of Medicine, University of California,
San Francisco, California

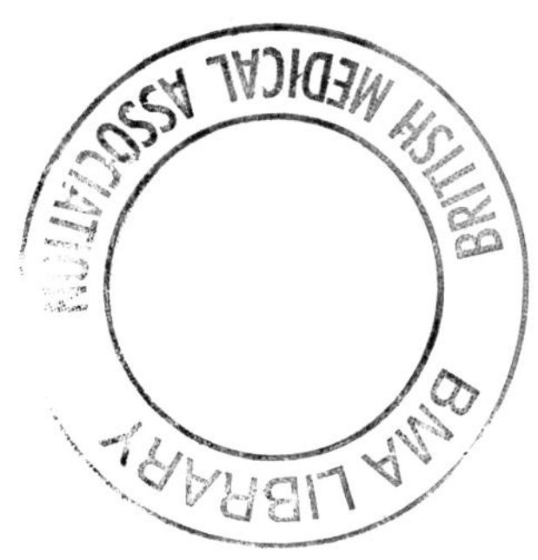

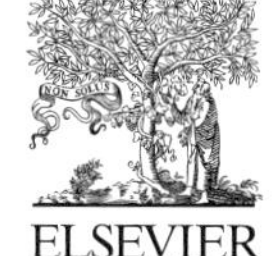

Amsterdam • Boston • Heidelberg • London • New York • Oxford
Paris • San Diego • San Francisco • Singapore • Sydney • Tokyo

Academic Press is an imprint of Elsevier

Academic Press is an imprint of Elsevier
32 Jamestown Road, London NW1 7BY, UK
225 Wyman Street, Waltham, MA 02451, USA
525 B Street, Suite 1800, San Diego, CA 92101-4495, USA

Fifth edition 2014

British Library Cataloguing-in-Publication Data
A catalogue record for this book is available from the British Library

Library of Congress Cataloging-in-Publication Data
A catalog record for this book is available from the Library of Congress

ISBN: 978-0-12-407710-2

For information on all Academic Press publications
visit our website at www.store.elsevier.com

Typeset by MPS Limited, Chennai, India
www.adi-mps.com

Printed and bound in China

14 15 16 17 18 10 9 8 7 6 5 4 3 2 1

This book is dedicated to
the memory of
Abraham S. Aminoff,
my father and friend.

It is also dedicated to my wife, Jan,
and our three children,
Alexandra, Jonathan, and Anthony.

Michael J. Aminoff

This book is dedicated to
my loving family,
whose unending caring and support
has made my work and life so incredibly gratifying

S. Andrew Josephson

Contributors

GARY M. ABRAMS, MD
Professor, Department of Neurology, School of Medicine, University of California, San Francisco, California
Chapter 20: Sex Hormone, Pituitary, Parathyroid, and Adrenal Disorders and the Nervous System

GREGORY W. ALBERS, MD
Professor, Department of Neurology and Neurological Sciences, Stanford University School of Medicine, Stanford, California
Chapter 11: Stroke as a Complication of General Medical Disorders

JAMES J. P. ALIX, PhD, MRCP
Research Fellow, Department of Neurology, Sheffield Institute for Translational Neuroscience, University of Sheffield, Sheffield, England
Chapter 18: Thyroid Disease and the Nervous System

MICHAEL J. AMINOFF, MD, DSc, FRCP
Distinguished Professor, Department of Neurology, School of Medicine, University of California, San Francisco, California
Chapter 8: Postural Hypotension and Syncope
Chapter 16: Neurologic Dysfunction and Kidney Disease
Chapter 30: Sexual Dysfunction in Patients with Neurologic Disorders
Chapter 31: Pregnancy and Disorders of the Nervous System
Chapter 35: Neurotoxin Exposure in the Workplace
Chapter 57: Seizures and General Medical Disorders
Chapter 58: Movement Disorders Associated with General Medical Diseases
Chapter 59: Neuromuscular Complications of General Medical Disorders
Chapter 62: Care at the End of Life

ADIL E. BHARUCHA, MD
Professor, Department of Medicine, Mayo Clinic College of Medicine, Rochester, Minnesota
Chapter 14: Disturbances of Gastrointestinal Motility and the Nervous System

AMIT BATLA, MD, DM (Neurology)
Fellow, Education Unit, UCL Institute of Neurology, Queen Square, London, UK
Chapter 29: Lower Urinary Tract Dysfunction and the Nervous System

CAROLYN M. BENSON, MD
Resident Surgeon, Department of Clinical Neurological Sciences, London Health Sciences Center, London, Ontario, Canada
Chapter 9: Neurologic Complications of Cardiac Arrest

JOHN P. BETJEMANN, MD
Assistant Professor, Department of Neurology, School of Medicine, University of California, San Francisco, California
Chapter 54: Preoperative and Postoperative Care of Patients with Neurologic Disorders

JARED R. BROSCH, MD
Assistant Professor, Department of Neurology, Indiana University School of Medicine, Indianapolis, Indiana
Chapter 6: Neurologic Manifestations of Infective Endocarditis

MICHAEL CAMILLERI, MD
Professor, Departments of Medicine, Pharmacology and Physiology, Mayo Clinic College of Medicine, Rochester, Minnesota
Chapter 14: Disturbances of Gastrointestinal Motility and the Nervous System

ROBERT CHEN, MA, MBBChir, MSc, FRCP(C)
Professor, Division of Neurology, Department of Medicine, University of Toronto, Toronto, Ontario, Canada; Senior Scientist, Toronto Western Research Institute, Toronto, Ontario, Canada
Chapter 1: Breathing and the Nervous System

CHADWICK W. CHRISTINE, MD
Associate Professor, Department of Neurology, School of Medicine, University of California, San Francisco, California
Chapter 58: Movement Disorders Associated with General Medical Diseases

G.A.B. DAVIES-JONES, MD, FRCP
Senior Lecturer in Medicine, University of Sheffield Medical School, Sheffield, England
Chapter 25: Neurologic Manifestations of Hematologic Disorders

LISA M. DeANGELIS, MD
Professor, Department of Neurology, Weill Cornell Medical College, New York, New York
Chapter 28: Neurologic Complications of Chemotherapy and Radiation Therapy

MARIEL B. DEUTSCH, MD
Fellow, Department of Neurology, Memorial Sloan-Kettering Cancer Center, New York, New York
Chapter 28: Neurologic Complications of Chemotherapy and Radiation Therapy

PRIYA S. DHAWAN, MD
Resident Physician, Department of Neurology, Mayo Clinic, Scottsdale, Arizona
Chapter 15: Neurologic Manifestations of Nutritional Disorders

WILLIAM P. DILLON, MD
Elizabeth Guillaumin Professor, Department of Radiology and Biomedical Imaging, School of Medicine, University of California, San Francisco, California
Chapter 53: Neurologic Complications of Imaging Procedures

VANJA C. DOUGLAS, MD
Assistant Professor, Department of Neurology, School of Medicine, University of California, San Francisco, California
Chapter 61: Dementia and Systemic Disease

CHRISTOPHER F. DOWD, MD
Professor, Department Radiology and Biomedical Imaging, School of Medicine, University of California, San Francisco, California
Chapter 53: Neurologic Complications of Imaging Procedures

ADRÉ J. DU PLESSIS, MBChB, MPH
Professor, Department of Pediatrics, School of Medicine and Health Sciences, George Washington University, Washington, DC
Chapter 4: Neurologic Complications of Congenital Heart Disease and Cardiac Surgery in Children

ERIC R. EGGENBERGER, DO, MSEpi
Professor, Department of Neurology and Ophthalmology, Michigan State University, East Lansing, Michigan
Chapter 24: Neuro-ophthalmology in Medicine

JOSEPH M. FURMAN, MD, PhD
Professor, Departments of Otolaryngology and Neurology, University of Pittsburgh School of Medicine, Pittsburgh, Pennsylvania
Chapter 23: Otoneurologic Manifestations of Otologic and Systemic Disease

DOUGLAS J. GELB, MD, PhD
Professor, Department of Neurology, University of Michigan Medical School, Ann Arbor, Michigan
Chapter 37: Abnormalities of Thermal Regulation and the Nervous System

PAUL GEORGE, PhD, MD
Instructor, Department of Neurology, Stanford University, Stanford, California
Chapter 11: Stroke as a Complication of General Medical Disorders

DAVID J. GLADSTONE, MD, FRCP(C), PhD
Associate Professor, Division of Neurology, Department of Medicine, University of Toronto, Toronto, Ontario, Canada
Chapter 5: Neurologic Manifestations of Acquired Cardiac Disease, Arrhythmias, and Interventional Cardiology

SIMON M. GLYNN, MD
Assistant Professor, Department of Neurology, University of Michigan Medical School, Ann Arbor, Michigan
Chapter 57: Seizures and General Medical Disorders

DOUGLAS S. GOODIN, MD
Professor, Department of Neurology, School of Medicine, University of California, San Francisco, California
Chapter 2: Neurologic Complications of Aortic Disease and Surgery

BRENT P. GOODMAN, MD
Assistant Professor, Department of Neurology, Mayo Clinic, Scottsdale, Arizona
Chapter 15: Neurologic Manifestations of Nutritional Disorders

JOHN E. GREENLEE, MD
Professor, Department of Neurology, University of Utah Health Sciences Center, Salt Lake City, Utah
Chapter 43: Nervous System Complications of Systemic Viral Infections

JOHN J. HALPERIN, MD
Professor, Departments of Neurology and Medicine, Icahn School of Medicine at Mount Sinai, New York, New York
Chapter 40: Spirochetal Infections of the Nervous System

SHELBY HARRIS, PhD
Assistant Professor, Saul R. Korey Department of Neurology, Albert Einstein College of Medicine, New York, New York
Chapter 51: Neurologic Aspects of Sleep Medicine

J. CLAUDE HEMPHILL, III, MD, MAS
Professor, Department of Neurology, School of Medicine, University of California, San Francisco, California
Chapter 60: Disorders of Consciousness in Systemic Diseases

JOHN R. HOTSON, MD
Professor (emeritus), Deparment of Neurology and Neurological Sciences, Stanford University School of Medicine, Stanford, California
Chapter 3: Neurologic Complications of Cardiac Surgery

OREST HURKO, MD
Professor (Hon), Departments of Medicine, Dentistry and Nursing, University of Dundee, Scotland, UK
Chapter 21: The Skin and Neurological Disease

CHERYL A. JAY, MD
Clinical Professor, Deparment of Neurology, School of Medicine, University of California, San Francisco, California
Chapter 20: Sex Hormone, Pituitary, Parathyroid, and Adrenal Disorders and the Nervous System

JASMIN JO, MD
Fellow, Department of Neurology, Division of Neuro-Oncology, University of Virginia, Charlottesville, Virginia
Chapter 26: Metastatic Disease and the Nervous System

S. CLAIBORNE JOHNSTON, MD, PhD
Professor, Department of Neurology, School of Medicine, University of California, San Francisco, California
Chapter 7: Neurologic Complications of Hypertension

S. ANDREW JOSEPHSON, MD
Associate Professor, Department of Neurology, C. Castro Franceschi and G. K. Mitchell Distinguished Professorship, School of Medicine, University of California, San Francisco, California
Chapter 34: Neurologic Complications of Recreational Drugs
Chapter 54: Preoperative and Postoperative Care of Patients with Neurologic Disorders
Chapter 61: Dementia and Systemic Disease

ANTHONY S. KIM, MD, MAS
Assistant Professor, Department of Neurology, School of Medicine, University of California, San Francisco, California
Chapter 7: Neurologic Complications of Hypertension

CHARLES H. KING, MD, MS
Professor, Center for Global Health and Diseases, Case Western Reserve University School of Medicine, Cleveland, Ohio
Chapter 47: Parasitic Infections of the Central Nervous System

JUSTIN A. KINSELLA, MB, BCh, PhD
Neurology Specialist Registrar, Department of Neurology, Adelaide and Meath Hospital, Dublin, Ireland
Chapter 5: Neurologic Manifestations of Acquired Cardiac Disease, Arrhythmias, and Interventional Cardiology

NERISSA U. KO, MD, MAS
Associate Professor, Deparment of Neurology, School of Medicine, University of California, San Francisco, California
Chapter 10: Cardiac Manifestations of Acute Neurologic Lesions

ALLAN KRUMHOLZ, MD
Professor, Department of Neurology, University of Maryland School of Medicine, Baltimore, Maryland
Chapter 49: Sarcoidosis of the Nervous System

JEFFREY S. KUTCHER, MD
Associate Professor, Department of Neurology, University of Michigan Medical School, Ann Arbor, Michigan
Chapter 38: Postconcussion Syndrome

JOHN M. LEONARD, MD
Professor, Department of Medicine, Division of Infectious Diseases, Vanderbilt University School of Medicine, Nashville, Tennessee
Chapter 41: Tuberculosis of the Central Nervous System

CATHERINE LIMPEROPOULOS, PhD
Associate Professor, Department of Diagnostic Imaging and Radiology, George Washington University School of Medicine, Washington, DC
Chapter 4: Neurologic Complications of Congenital Heart Disease and Cardiac Surgery in Children

EDWARD M. MANNO, MD
Head, Neurological Intensive Care Unit, Neurological Institute, Cleveland Clinic, Cleveland, Ohio
Chapter 56: Neurologic Complications in Critically Ill Patients

FRANK L. MASTAGLIA, MD
Professor, Centre for Neuromuscular and Neurological Disorders, University of Western Australia School of Medicine, Nedlands, Western Australia, Australia
Chapter 32: Drug-Induced Disorders of the Nervous System

ANDREW A. McCALL, MD
Assistant Professor, Department of Otolaryngology, University of Pittsburgh School of Medicine, Pittsburgh, Pennsylvania
Chapter 23: Otoneurologic Manifestations of Otologic and Systemic Disease

ROBERT O. MESSING, MD
Professor, Division of Pharmacology/Toxicology, College of Pharmacy, University of Texas at Austin, Austin, Texas
Chapter 33: Alcohol and the Nervous System

RENEE MONDERER, MD
Assistant Professor, Saul R. Korey Department of Neurology, Albert Einstein College of Medicine, New York, New York
Chapter 51: Neurologic Aspects of Sleep Medicine

JOHN A. MORREN, MD
Neuromuscular Center, Neurological Institute, Cleveland Clinic, Cleveland, Ohio
Chapter 56: Neurologic Complications in Critically Ill Patients

KEVIN D.J. O'CONNOR, MB, BCh, BAO, BMSc
Australian Neuromuscular Research Institute, QEII Medical Centre, Nedlands, Western Australia, Australia
Chapter 32: Drug-Induced Disorders of the Nervous System

PRAMOD K. PAL, MBBS, MD, DM
Professor, Deparment of Neurology, National Institute of Mental Health & Neurosciences, Bangalore, Karnataka, India
Chapter 1: Breathing and the Nervous System

JALESH N. PANICKER, MD MRCP
Honorary Senior Lecturer, Department of Uro-Neurology, UCL Institute of Neurology, Queen Square, London, UK
Chapter 29: Lower Urinary Tract Dysfunction and the Nervous System

JACK M. PARENT, MD
Professor, Department of Neurology, University of Michigan Medical School, Ann Arbor, Michigan
Chapter 57: Seizures and General Medical Disorders

ROY A. PATCHELL, MD
Director, Neuro-Oncology Department, Capital Institute for Neurosciences, Pennington, New Jersey
Chapter 45: Neurologic Complications of Organ Transplantation and Immunosuppressive Agents

MICHAEL J. PELUSO, MD, MPhil, MHS
Resident Physician, Department of Medicine, Brigham and Women's Hospital, Boston, Massachusetts
Chapter 44: HIV and Other Retroviral Infections of the Nervous System

JOHN R. PERFECT, MD
Professor, Department of Medicine, Division of Infectious Diseases, Duke University School of Medicine, Durham, North Carolina
Chapter 46: Fungal Infections of the Central Nervous System

RONALD F. PFEIFFER, MD
Professor, Department of Neurology, University of Tennessee, Health Science Center, Memphis, Tennessee
Chapter 13: Other Neurologic Disorders Associated with Gastrointestinal Disease

ANN NOELLE PONCELET, MD
Professor, Department of Neurology, School of Medicine, University of California, San Francisco, California
Chapter 22: Neurologic Disorders Associated with Bone and Joint Disease

JEROME B. POSNER, MD
Professor, Department of Neurology, Weill Cornell Medical College, New York, New York
Chapter 27: Paraneoplastic Syndromes Involving the Nervous System

JOHN H. PULA, MD
Clinician Educator, Department of Neurology, NorthShore University HealthSystem, University of Chicago Pritzker School of Medicine, Evanston, Illinois
Chapter 24: Neuro-ophthalmology in Medicine

ALEJANDRO A. RABINSTEIN, MD
Professor, Divisions of Critical Care and Cerebrovascular Neurology, Department of Neurology, Mayo Clinic, Rochester, Minnesota
Chapter 55: Neurologic Disorders and Anesthesia

JEFFREY W. RALPH, MD
Associate Professor, Department of Neurology, School of Medicine, University of California, San Francisco, California
Chapter 59: Neuromuscular Complications of General Medical Disorders

VICTOR I. REUS, MD
Professor, Department of Psychiatry, School of Medicine, University of California, San Francisco, California
Chapter 52: Functional Neurologic Symptom Disorders

JACK E. RIGGS, MD
Professor, Department of Neurology, West Virginia University School of Medicine, Morgantown, West Virginia
Chapter 17: Neurologic Complications of Electrolyte Disturbances

KAREN L. ROOS, MD
John and Nancy Nelson Professor, Department of Neurology, Indiana University School of Medicine, Indianapolis, Indiana
Chapter 39: Acute Bacterial Infections of the Central Nervous System

ANDREW P. ROSE-INNES, MD
Clinician, Neurology Division, The Oregon Clinic, Portland, Oregon
Chapter 22: Neurologic Disorders Associated with Bone and Joint Disease

RICHARD ROSENBAUM, MD
Affiliate Professor, Department of Neurology, School of Medicine, Oregon Health & Science University, Portland, Oregon
Chapter 50: Connective Tissue Diseases, Vasculitis, and the Nervous System

THOMAS D. SABIN, MD
Professor, Department of Neurology, Tufts University School of Medicine, Boston, Massachusetts
Chapter 42: Neurologic Complications of Leprosy

ROBERT A. SALATA, MD
Professor, Department of Medicine, Case Western Reserve University School of Medicine, Cleveland, Ohio
Chapter 47: Parasitic Infections of the Central Nervous System

EDSEL MAURICE T. SALVANA, MD
Associate Professor, Section of Infectious Diseases, Department of Medicine, Philippine General Hospital, University of the Philippines Manila, Manila, Philippines
Chapter 47: Parasitic Infections of the Central Nervous System

DAVID SCHIFF, MD
Professor, Department of Neurology, Division of Neuro-Oncology, University of Virginia, Charlottesville, Virginia
Chapter 26: Metastatic Disease and the Nervous System

HYMAN M. SCHIPPER, MD, PhD, FRCP(C)
Professor, Department of Neurology and Neurosurgery and Department of Medicine (Geriatrics), McGill University Faculty of Medicine, Montreal, Quebec, Canada
Chapter 20: Sex Hormone, Pituitary, Parathyroid, and Adrenal Disorders and the Nervous System

PAMELA J. SHAW, MD, FRCP, DBE
Professor, Department of Neurology, Sheffield Institute for Translational Neuroscience, University of Sheffield, Sheffield, England
Chapter 18: Thyroid Disease and the Nervous System

SERENA SPUDICH, MD, MA
Associate Professor, Department of Neurology, Yale University School of Medicine, New Haven, Connecticut
Chapter 44: HIV and Other Retroviral Infections of the Nervous System

BARNEY J. STERN, MD
Professor, Department of Neurology, University of Maryland, Baltimore, Maryland
Chapter 49: Sarcoidosis of the Nervous System

JON D. SUSSMAN, MB, ChB, PhD, FRCP
Lecturer in Medicine, University of Manchester, Manchester, England
Chapter 25: Neurologic Manifestations of Hematologic Disorders

THOMAS R. SWIFT, MD
Professor, Department of Neurology, Medical College of Georgia, Augusta, Georgia
Chapter 42: Neurologic Complications of Leprosy

MICHAEL THORPY, MD
Professor, Saul R. Korey Department of Neurology, Albert Einstein College of Medicine, New York, New York
Chapter 51: Neurologic Aspects of Sleep Medicine

CORY TOTH, MD, FRCP(C)
Associate Professor, Department of Clinical Neurosciences and the Hotchkiss Brain Institute, University of Calgary, Calgary, Alberta, Canada
Chapter 19: Diabetes and the Nervous System

ALEX C. TSELIS, MD, PhD
Professor, Department of Neurology, Wayne State University School of Medicine, Detroit, Michigan
Chapter 48: Neurologic Complications of Vaccination

DAVID B. VODUŠEK, MD, PhD
Professor, Department of Neurology, Medical School, University of Ljubljana, Ljubljana, Slovenia
Chapter 30: Sexual Dysfunction in Patients with Neurologic Disorders

KARIN WEISSENBORN, MD
Associate Professor, Department of Neurology, Hannover Medical School, Hannover, Germany
Chapter 12: Hepatic and Pancreatic Encephalopathy

LINDA S. WILLIAMS, MD
Senior Investigator, VA Center for Healthcare Information and Communication, and Professor, Department of Neurology, Indiana University School of Medicine, Indianapolis, Indiana
Chapter 6: Neurologic Manifestations of Infective Endocarditis

MARC D. WINKELMAN, MD
Associate Professor, Department of Neurology, Case Western Reserve University, School of Medicine, Cleveland, Ohio
Chapter 36: Neurologic Complications of Thermal and Electric Burns

G. BRYAN YOUNG, MD, FRCP(C)
Professor, Department of Clinical Neurological Sciences, University of Western Ontario, London, Ontario, Canada
Chapter 9: Neurologic Complications of Cardiac Arrest

DOUGLAS W. ZOCHODNE, MD, FRCP(C)
Professor, Department of Clinical Neurosciences and the Hotchkiss Brain Institute, University of Calgary, Calgary, Alberta, Canada
Chapter 19: Diabetes and the Nervous System

Preface to the Fifth Edition

These are exciting times. Amazing advances in imaging, genetics, immunology, pharmacology, and drug-delivery systems, and new technologic approaches in the operating room and intensive care unit have transformed the practice of medicine in the 25 years since this book was first published. Spectacular progress is continuing to occur in the medical sciences—for example, in molecular biology at the level of genes, proteins, and ion channels, and in the development of animal models of disease—and, over the next few years, will further impact clinical practice. These advances will undoubtedly lead to a new systematic approach to clinical medicine that should complement, rather than replace, the traditional approach. It has been suggested that the eventual availability of, for example, a simple genetic test or cheap imaging technique may sometimes make clinical consultation redundant. Such statements give cause for concern. Clinical consultations provide much more than a diagnostic label or a means to define a course of action. The interaction that occurs between patients and physicians during the course of the clinical encounter helps to establish a professional relationship that allows patients to receive optimal and multidimensional care. This interaction leads to suggestions about the diagnosis, determines whether ancillary studies are required and aids their interpretation in context, permits advice on treatment based on the individual clinical and psychosocial background, guides prognostication, and ensures that patients are both informed and educated about their disease. It also provides physicians with the opportunity—increasingly neglected—to think about the clinical problem posed by individual patients. It is therefore unfortunate that technologic advances—wonderful as they may be—are tending to dehumanize clinical medicine and erode clinical skills and common sense.

There are other issues that are emerging with regard to the practice of medicine. Therapeutic and management options are in some cases too unrestrained and in other instances curtailed unnecessarily by market forces and practitioners of evidence-based medicine. Physicians should practice medicine in such a way that decisions are based on the best available evidence, but the absence of evidence for an effect is not evidence for the absence of an effect. Clinical medicine is not always the exact science that some pretend it to be, and its practice remains both an art and a science. It is important that physicians keep this in mind and remain committed to the welfare of their patients rather than some abstract concept. It is my hope that these values are reflected in the pages of this volume.

The general acceptance of earlier editions of this book and the changes occurring in the field have prompted the development of this new—fifth—edition, aimed at all clinicians but especially neurologists, internists, hospitalists, and primary health-care providers. The aim remains the same as that of previous editions, namely to define both the neurologic aspects of general medical disorders and the general medical and other aspects of various neurologic diseases. The book therefore provides an account of clinical neurology from a different perspective than most other textbooks and serves as an interface between neurology and the other medical specialties. This is important because all physicians—including neurologists—must retain some expertise in general medicine to best serve the interests of their patients. Neurologic disorders are not encountered in isolation but occur in patients who often have or will develop other medical problems, and many general medical disorders have neurologic complications or manifest as diseases of the central or peripheral nervous system.

Physicians need to keep abreast of advances in the field, but the pace of change, the daunting size and complicated jargon of the medical literature, the need to optimize the use of limited resources, and the increasing administrative and bureaucratic demands on their time have made it difficult for them to do so. Changing market forces and health-care delivery systems have added to the problem. At the same time, communication among specialists or even among subspecialists within the same overall specialty is becoming increasingly stilted, even as a lack of consensus exists among physicians concerning the appropriate extent of specialist involvement in the care of patients with neurologic manifestations of disease. This underlines the need to coordinate patient care and ensure not only that neurologists have some understanding of the general medical issues relating to their patients but that internists, family practitioners, and other physicians, in turn, have some understanding of neurologic disorders.

This book, then, is aimed at both general physicians and neurologists, regardless of their level of training or experience. It is intended to serve as a guide to junior physicians who need experience to nurture their developing skills and then follow the path of lifelong learning to maintain them. More senior practitioners may also find this volume useful as a source of reference, as a means of keeping abreast of developments in the field, and thus as a guide to the evolving standards of care of patients with diseases that may already be familiar to them.

I am delighted that Dr. S. Andrew Josephson has joined me as co-editor of this new edition. He is a friend, colleague, and a board-certified neurologist who is widely recognized both nationally and internationally for his clinical expertise, encyclopedic knowledge, teaching skills, and clinical scholarship. One of his many achievements has been in helping to establish neurohospitalist medicine as a distinct branch of medicine in the United States. Preparing this new volume with him has been an especially enjoyable experience. As with earlier editions, this new one has been crafted to reflect the changing face of the subject but—at the same time—we have attempted to limit its size so that it does not become too intimidating. We have also limited the bibliography of individual chapters to references published only recently and at most within the last 25 years, whenever possible. Older references have been retained only when they involve classic papers or provide seminal descriptions of diseases, clinical phenomena, or specific treatments. More detailed reference to the older literature can be found in earlier editions of the book.

New chapters have been added and existing ones expanded to cover changes that have occurred in recent years. The volume has evolved from its original black-and-white format to a two-color work and now goes into full color. This will enhance its appearance and will, I hope, add to the utility of its illustrations. The book is published electronically as well as in a print format. The electronic version should make it more accessible, facilitate searches for specific information, and be attractive to younger readers.

This book has particular meaning to me. The first edition was published exactly a quarter-century ago, at a time when my three children were either at grade school or pre-school, and their fun and laughter helped to revitalize me when my work as an author or editor seemed a little overwhelming. Now they have gone their separate ways, and I follow their careers with enormous pleasure. Alexandra, a pediatrician, is just finishing a 3-year fellowship in pediatric rheumatology at the Children's Hospital of Seattle, and I envy her up-to-date knowledge of medicine. Jonathan is a federal defense attorney in Los Angeles and I am proud of his wish to serve those who are unable to help themselves. Anthony, our youngest and another lawyer, is an assistant district attorney in the office of the Manhattan District Attorney in New York, and I marvel at the prudent and judicious way in which he approaches his work. During the production of the second edition of *Neurology and General Medicine*, my father—a wonderful man—died unexpectedly, and I dedicated the book to him. I have continued to dedicate subsequent volumes to his memory, for I think of him often. My wife, Jan, has always given me the support, encouragement, and time that I need to complete my writing projects, and takes on many additional chores without even mentioning them in order to ease my burden. I cannot thank her enough.

Many of the authors of individual chapters have contributed to the book since the first edition appeared in 1989; others are more recent contributors. I am grateful to them for their help in making the volume an important part of the medical literature. In preparing this new edition, some authors from the last edition were replaced because they had retired or were in ill-health, and I thank them for their past contributions and wish them well. Dr. Josephson and I are grateful to all the contributors to this new edition. They were generous with their time and in sharing their knowledge, were tolerant of our requests, and worked hard to update their chapters from the last edition or—in the case of new authors—to review developments in their own particular field of interest. Some of the illustrations in the book are taken from previously published sources, as is acknowledged in the text, and we are grateful for permission to reproduce them here. Finally, we are grateful to a number of people at Elsevier, our publisher, for their help and especially to Mr. Thomas E. Stone and Ms. Kristi Anderson for their unfailing assistance in the development of this book, to Mr. Roger Borthwick for his careful copy-editing, and to Ms. Julia Haynes for seeing the volume through the production process. They were a wonderful team with whom it was a pleasure to work.

Michael J. Aminoff MD, DSc, FRCP

Preface to the First Edition

The increasing sophistication and complexity of modern medicine have led to greater specialization among practitioners and to more restricted communication between physicians in different disciplines. Perhaps, inevitably, this trend has created certain major problems. These difficulties are particularly well exemplified by the relationship between neurology and general medicine.

For non-neurologists, evaluation of patients with neurological symptoms and signs has always been difficult because of the complexity of the anatomy and physiology of the nervous system and frustrating because the therapeutic options have seemed somewhat limited. Nevertheless, a number of neurological diseases are exacerbated by, or occur as specific complications of, general medical disorders. Appropriate management of these neurological disturbances requires their early recognition and an appreciation of their prognosis. It is equally important to recognize the manner in which such neurological disorders may influence the management of the primary or coexisting medical condition, as well as the manner in which systemic complications of neurological disorders may require somewhat different management than when these complications occur in other settings.

For neurologists, who are being asked increasingly to evaluate neurological disturbances presenting in the context of other medical disorders, the difficulty is equally apparent. The general background of cases is frequently confusing, the relationship of the neurological to the other medical problems is commonly not appreciated, and the manner in which treatment needs to be "tailored" to the specific clinical context is often not clear. Furthermore, neurological disturbances may themselves be the presenting feature of general medical disorders or lead to general medical complications requiring speedy recognition and effective management.

I hope that the present volume will appeal to both neurologists and physicians in other specialties by providing a guide to the neurological aspects of general medical disorders and to some of the medical complications of certain neurological diseases. It is not intended to be a textbook of neurology, but rather a "bridge" between neurology and the other medical specialties.

It is a pleasure to acknowledge the help that I received from various people in developing this book. I am grateful to the various contributors, who devoted a great deal of time and energy to reviewing developments in their own fields of interest and showed considerable tolerance of the many demands that I made upon them. I am grateful also to Mr. Robert Hurley and Ms. Margot Otway at Churchill Livingstone for their help and advice during the preparation of this book. Finally, the support and encouragement of my wife, Jan, and of our children, Alexandra, Jonathan, and Anthony, did much to ease the burden involved in seeing this volume to its conclusion.

Michael J. Aminoff, MD, FRCP

Contents

SECTION

I

Respiratory and Cardiovascular Disorders

CHAPTER

1

Breathing and the Nervous System

PRAMOD K. PAL ■ ROBERT CHEN

Respiration involves pulmonary ventilation, gaseous exchange between lung alveoli and blood, and transport of oxygen and carbon dioxide between the blood, tissues, and interstitial fluid.

The nervous system plays a pivotal role in controlling pulmonary ventilation as it exerts both automatic and voluntary control over breathing. The anatomic pathways involve the cerebral hemispheres, pons, medulla, spinal cord, anterior horn cells, nerves, and neuromuscular junctions, as well as peripheral chemoreceptors and lung mechanoreceptors and the respiratory muscles themselves. Several central and peripheral neurologic disorders can affect respiration adversely, and hypoxia and hypercapnia resulting from respiratory dysfunction may affect the nervous system and produce neurologic complications.

CONTROL OF BREATHING

Breathing is normally an involuntary, rhythmic phenomenon that can be overridden by voluntary control. There are separate anatomic pathways for automatic and voluntary breathing, but these pathways are highly integrated (Fig. 1-1).

Aminoff's Neurology and General Medicine, Fifth Edition.

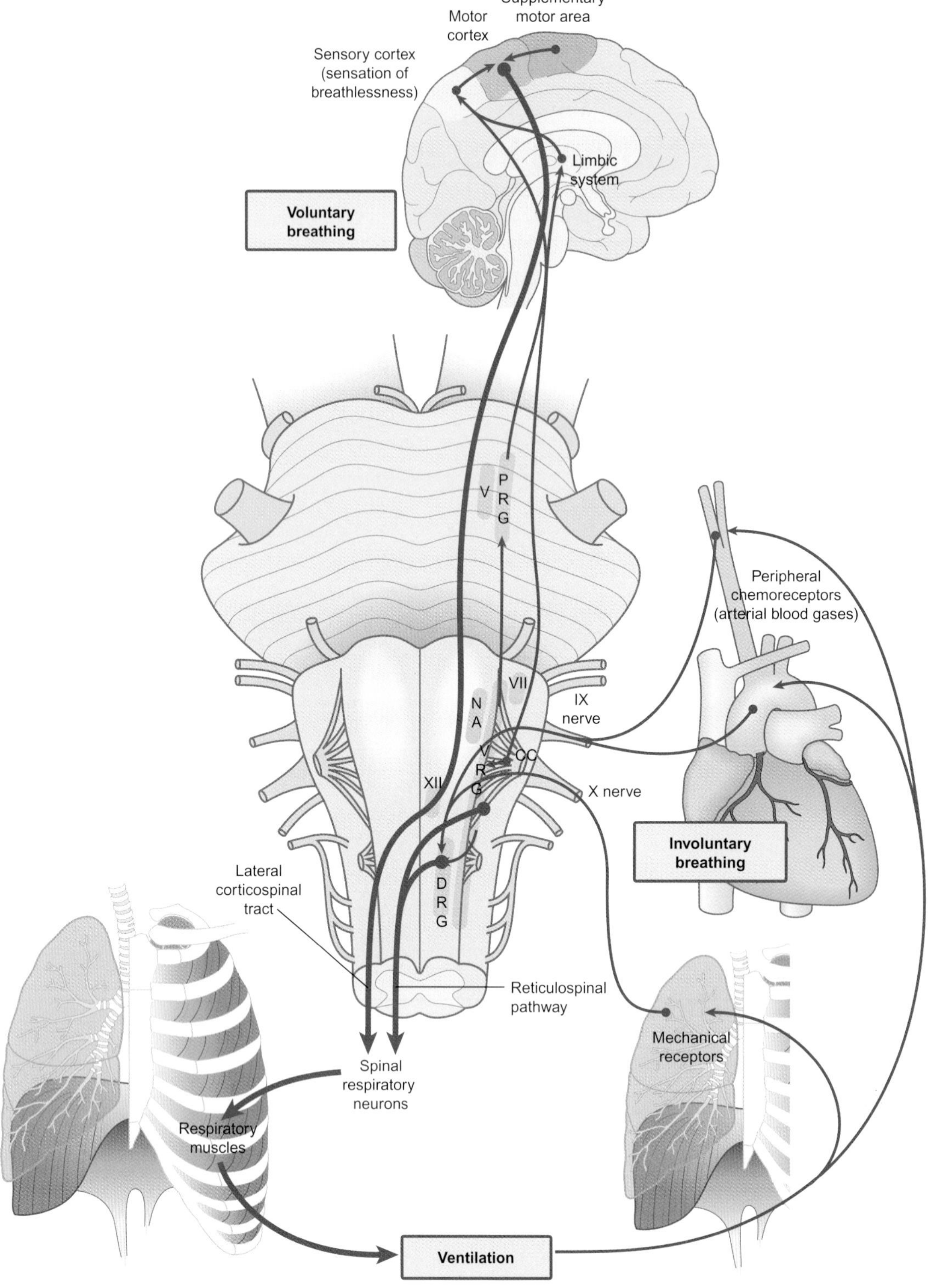

FIGURE 1-1 ■ Neural pathways controlling voluntary and involuntary breathing. The final activation of respiratory muscles occurs via the lateral corticospinal and reticulospinal pathways. CC, central chemoreceptors; DRG, dorsal respiratory group; NA, nucleus ambiguus; V, sensory nucleus of V; VRG, ventral respiratory group. (Adapted from Bolton CF, Chen R, Wijdicks EFM, et al: Neurology of Breathing. Butterworth Heinemann, Philadelphia, 2004, with permission.)

Respiratory Muscles

A number of muscles are important for respiration. The main inspiratory muscles include the diaphragm, external intercostal and scalene muscles, with accessory muscles being the sternocleidomastoid, pectoralis major and minor, serratus anterior, latissimus dorsi, and serratus posterior superior. The expiratory muscles are the internal intercostals, external oblique, internal oblique, rectus abdominis, transverse abdominis, and serratus posterior inferior. The muscles of the upper airway do not have a direct action on the chest cage but are required to keep the airway open during inspiration, regulate airway resistance, and partition airflow through nasal and oral pathways. These are the muscles of the soft palate, pharynx, larynx, trachea, nose, and mouth innervated by cranial nerves V, VII, IX, X, and XII.

Chemical Control of Breathing

Breathing is influenced by both peripheral and central chemoreceptors, and may be impaired by damage to these receptors or their neural connections. Peripheral chemoreceptors are located in the carotid and aortic bodies and are innervated by the glossopharyngeal nerve, which projects to the tractus solitarius. These receptors are primarily activated by hypoxia, and also by reduced arterial pH, increased arterial pCO_2, and hypoperfusion. Central chemoreceptors are located in the locus ceruleus and nuclei of the tractus solitarius, midline (raphe) of the ventral medulla, and ventrolateral quadrant of medulla. They respond primarily to high pCO_2 mediated through the detection of a fall in the pH of the cerebrospinal fluid (CSF), and are crucial for adequate breathing in sleep.[1] The sensation of breathlessness is probably mediated through these medullary chemoreceptors or respiratory neurons.[2,3] In congenital hypoventilation syndrome, periods of cyanosis occur during sleep due to deficiency of central chemoreception, with reduced or absent CO_2 sensitivity; mutations of the *PHOX2B* gene are sometimes responsible.[4,5] These patients, in contrast to patients with locked-in syndrome, do not experience air hunger or breathlessness with hypercapnia.[6,7]

Brainstem Respiratory Centers

There are three important brainstem respiratory centers: the pneumotaxic center or pontine respiratory group (PRG) in the dorsal lateral pons, and the dorsal (DRG) and ventral respiratory groups (VRG) in the medulla (Fig. 1-2). The PRG contains inspiratory, expiratory, and phase-spanning neurons, receives vagal afferents relating to lung volume, and modulates respiratory frequency. Its primary connections are with medullary respiratory neurons, but it also has connections with the hypothalamus, cerebral cortex, and the nucleus of tractus solitarius. PRG neurons are not essential for respiratory rhythm generation, and transection at this level produces regular breathing; vagotomy then results in slowing of the respiratory rate but not in alteration of rhythm.[8] The center is involved in modification and fine control of respiratory rhythm.[9,10] Apneusis is defined as prominent end-inspiratory pauses that can be produced by pontine transections in vagotomized animals.[11,12]

The medullary respiratory neurons generate the respiratory rhythm, and transection of the brainstem at the pontomedullary level allows rhythmic ventilator excursions to persist, whereas these movements are abolished by transection at the medullary-cervical region. The output from the medullary respiratory centers descends in the reticulospinal tract in the anterolateral funiculus of the spinal cord. DRG neurons are mainly inspiratory and are located in the ventrolateral portion of the nucleus of the tractus solitarius, primarily discharging during inspiration, and receiving pulmonary afferents via the vagus nerves. These neurons primarily project to the contralateral spinal motor neurons, and probably serve as the primary rhythmic drive to phrenic motor neurons. DRG neurons are modulated by $GABA_B$ receptors.[13]

The VRG neurons are both inspiratory and expiratory neurons, situated in a bilaterally symmetric column that extends from the caudal level of the facial nucleus to the rostral cervical spinal cord. The cell bodies are located within the nucleus ambiguus and nucleus retroambigualis and are responsible for the generation of respiratory rhythm.[14] NMDA receptors are the major mediators of VRG ventilatory drive, with modulation by non-NMDA glutamate systems.[15]

The cerebellum also influences breathing. In animals, stimulation of the fastigial nucleus produces early termination of bursting of both the inspiratory and expiratory neurons.[16] Functional imaging studies in humans have also documented activation of cerebellum along with other brainstem and basal forebrain structures during volitional breathing.[17–19]

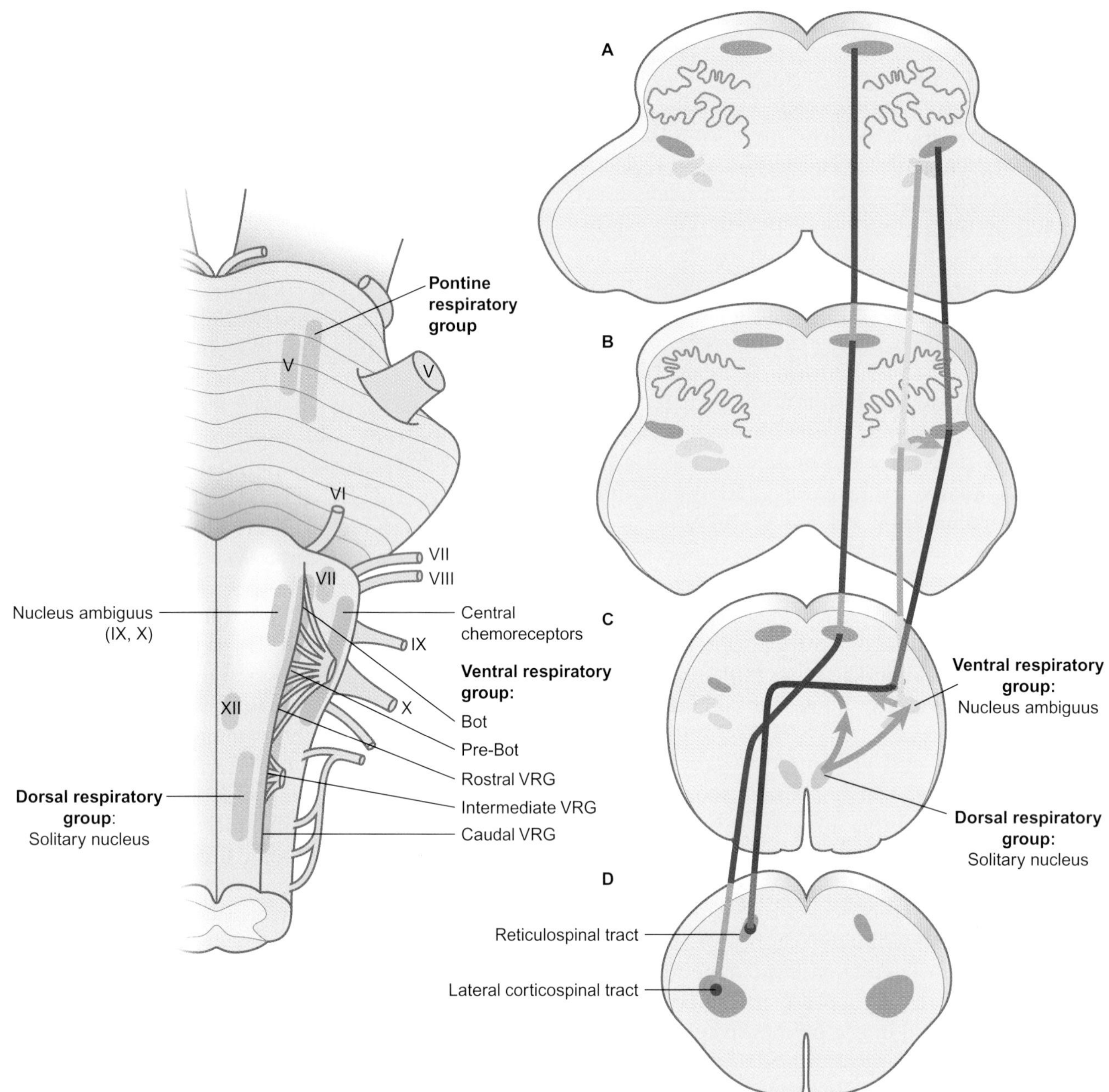

FIGURE 1-2 ■ Representation of the brainstem respiratory centers and tracts. On the left side, the nuclei are shown in light purple and the adjacent respiratory groups are orange. On the right side, the dorsal respiratory group (DRG) is located within the solitary nucleus, and the ventral respiratory group (VRG) is ventral to the nucleus ambiguus. Bot, Botzinger complex. (Adapted from Bolton CF, Chen R, Wijdicks EFM, et al: Neurology of Breathing. Butterworth Heinemann, Philadelphia, 2004, with permission.)

Voluntary Control of Breathing

Voluntary control of breathing is mediated by the descending corticospinal tract and its influence on the motor neurons innervating the diaphragm and intercostal muscles. The rate and rhythm of breathing are influenced by the forebrain, as observed during voluntary hyperventilation or breath-holding as well as during the semivoluntary or involuntary rhythmic alterations in ventilatory pattern that are required during speech, singing, laughing, and crying.

Electrophysiologic and imaging studies support the belief that specific areas of cortex are involved in different phases of voluntary breathing. The diaphragm can be activated by stimulation of the contralateral motor cortex using transcranial magnetic stimulation.[20] The diaphragm lacks significant bilateral cortical representation, consistent with the finding of attenuation of diaphragmatic excursion only on the hemiplegic side in patients with hemispheric stroke.[21] The intercostal muscles are similarly affected by hemispheric lesions. Positron emission tomographic (PET) studies have shown an increase in cerebral blood flow in the primary motor cortex bilaterally, the right supplementary motor cortex, and the ventrolateral thalamus during inspiration; the same structures, along with the cerebellum, are involved in expiration.[17,19]

The involvement of the forebrain in the regulation of breathing is further substantiated by the induction of apnea that follows stimulation of the anterior portion of the hippocampal gyrus, the ventral and medial surfaces of the temporal lobe, and the anterior portion of the insula.[8] Ictal apnea has been reported during partial seizures in a patient with encephalitis who was found to have an abnormality of the left posterior lateral temporal region on single-photon emission computed tomography.[22]

Integrated Neural Control of Breathing

The two types of control over breathing are highly integrated, as observed during speaking and singing, when automatic breathing is suppressed. Though the exact pathways of this coordination are not known, connections probably exist between the medullary respiratory centers, cerebral cortex, and extrapyramidal systems. In addition, integration occurs in the spinal cord between cortical, segmental, and breathing inputs to respiratory motor neurons.

EVALUATION OF PULMONARY FUNCTION

A detailed discussion of the evaluation of pulmonary function is beyond the scope of this chapter, and the following is a summary of an approach to evaluating patients with impaired breathing in the setting of neurologic illness.

Clinical Assessment

A detailed clinical history should be obtained including an account of any breathing or cardiac problems that presented prior to the onset of—or with a temporal relationship to—neurologic symptoms and of any antecedent illness (such as infection) that preceded onset of muscle weakness (e.g., in Guillain–Barré syndrome). The onset, distribution, character, and accompaniments of weakness may suggest the underlying cause. The history obtained from a bed-partner or caregiver is important in determining the presence of sleep-disordered breathing.

The respiratory and cardiac systems are examined to determine the respiratory rate and volume, pattern of breathing, heart rate, blood pressure, temperature, and presence of cyanosis. Bedside assessments should also include a single-breath counting exercise, observation of chest expansion, and testing of cough strength. Diaphragmatic weakness may give rise to paradoxic inward movement of the abdomen during inspiration. The presence of hypophonia, nasal intonation, dysarthria, dysphagia, and pooling of secretions suggest bulbar dysfunction. Auscultation of the chest may reveal features of bronchoconstriction, pulmonary congestion, or consolidation.

Tests of Respiratory Functions

Arterial Blood Gas Studies

Arterial blood gas analysis (pH, pCO_2, pO_2) is required for patients with impending respiratory failure to determine the need for ventilatory support. Overnight pulse oximetry is useful in patients with sleep-related breathing problems.[23]

Imaging

Apart from routine chest radiography, computed tomography (CT) scan of the thorax may sometimes be useful to detect small pleural effusions as well as mediastinal masses and lymphadenopathy. Evidence of unilateral phrenic nerve palsy includes the elevation of a hemidiaphragm on chest radiography, or the lack of descent of the affected diaphragm during a sniff test performed during fluoroscopy or ultrasound.

Pulmonary Function Tests

Bedside spirometry is useful to assess pulmonary function, especially in neuromuscular disorders. Forced vital capacity (FVC), forced expiratory volume in 1 second (FEV1), and maximal inspiratory force (MIF) should be measured. In neuromuscular disorders, a "restrictive" pattern of respiratory dysfunction is seen, evidenced by a normal or sometimes higher ratio of FEV1 to FVC. Maximal inspiratory force is an indicator of the strength of the respiratory muscles.

Polysomnography

Polysomnography is useful to study the abnormalities of breathing during different stages of sleep (see Chapter 51). The movements of the chest and abdomen are recorded to identify periods of apnea or hypopnea.

PATTERNS OF RESPIRATORY DYSFUNCTION

Disorders of the peripheral and central nervous system may result in respiratory insufficiency through different mechanisms. The pattern of respiratory dysfunction primarily depends on the site of the lesion rather than the underlying etiology, while prognosis depends on both of these factors. Weakness of respiratory muscles may result in a restrictive pattern of ventilatory insufficiency. Oropharyngeal and laryngeal weakness can result in an obstructive pattern, especially during sleep. Patients with neuromuscular diseases and bulbar involvement are at risk of recurrent aspiration pneumonia and acute upper airway obstruction.

Disorders of Involuntary Breathing

Disturbances of automatic breathing with intact volitional breathing lead to sleep apnea or Ondine curse; the patient can maintain respiration while awake (voluntarily), but experiences apnea or hypopnea during sleep. The underlying pathology involves the automatic ventilatory centers (VRG and DRG) and their descending connections. Typical clinical situations responsible include bilateral or unilateral medullary infarction, bulbar poliomyelitis, neurodegenerative disorders such as multiple system atrophy,[24] syringobulbia, paraneoplastic brainstem syndromes,[25] and idiopathic sleep apnea. Iatrogenic injury has been reported following bilateral cervical tractotomy performed for intractable pain, presumably as a result of damage to the descending reticulospinal tracts which activate phrenic motor neurons and the ascending spinoreticular fibers that carry afferent information to brainstem centers.[23]

Disorders of Voluntary Breathing

The relatively pure form of voluntary breathing dysfunction is observed in the "locked-in" syndrome. Patients are unable to voluntarily control breathing and cannot speak, but they have a regular ventilatory pattern, preserved response to CO_2 stimulation, and experience air hunger.[6] Midpontine lesions are usually responsible due to infarctions (most often), hemorrhage, myelinosis, or tumor, resulting in disruption of the corticospinal and corticobulbar fibers that control voluntary respiration, while sparing the medullary respiratory centers that control automatic ventilation. Disordered voluntary breathing is also observed in extrapyramidal and cerebellar disorders, as discussed later.

Central Neurogenic Hyperventilation

Although central neurogenic hyperventilation was thought to be a classic and specific manifestation of midbrain dysfunction during transtentorial herniation, it is now apparent that this pattern of respiration is more common with unilateral or bilateral hemispheric lesions and carries a poor prognosis.[8] This type of breathing can also occur with pontine or medullary lesions.[26–29] The underlying mechanism of this tachypnea is unknown, and it may be the result of either stimulation of receptors in the pulmonary interstitial space secondary to congestion of neurogenic cause (neurogenic pulmonary edema), or central stimulation of medullary chemoreceptors secondary to local lactate production from tumor or stroke.

Other causes of centrally mediated hyperventilation are anxiety, infections, and drugs. The latter either stimulate the central or peripheral chemoreceptors or directly affect the brainstem respiratory neurons.

Apraxia of Breathing

Inability to take or hold a deep breath in spite of normal motor and sensory function of bulbar muscles is known as respiratory or breathing apraxia.

This abnormality is most often found in elderly patients with cerebrovascular disease, dementia, or lesions of the nondominant hemisphere, and may be associated with frontal lobe release signs, paratonia, or other apraxias.[8]

Posthyperventilation Apnea

In normal awake persons, there is a brief period of apnea after voluntary hyperventilation that is usually less than 12 seconds in duration when it follows five deep breaths sufficient to reduce pCO_2 by 8 to 14 mmHg. It has been described in normal individuals engaged in an intellectual task.[30] Apnea lasting more than 12 seconds was found in more than three-fourths of patients with bilateral CNS disease (structural or metabolic), compared to only 1 to 2 percent of normal subjects. It is equally common in patients with unilateral or bilateral brain injury, but is significantly more common in drowsy than alert patients (95 versus 48%).[31] It is therefore likely that the degree of posthyperventilation apnea is an indicator of depressed CNS function.

Apneustic Breathing

Apneustic breathing is characterized by prominent, prolonged end-inspiratory pauses and is rare in humans. It has been reported following pontine section or vagotomy in animals and brainstem damage in humans.[32,33]

Cheyne–Stokes Breathing

Cheyne–Stokes breathing is characterized by an escalating hyperventilation followed by decremental hyperventilation and finally apnea, which recurs in cycles. In humans, cycle lengths from 40 to 100 seconds may occur. During Cheyne–Stokes breathing, analysis of arterial blood gases shows an increasing pH and a declining pCO_2 as a result of an increased respiratory drive and response to CO_2 due to bilateral disease of the cerebral hemispheres.[34] Cheyne–Stokes breathing was originally described in a patient who died of heart failure and is also a feature of cardiac dysfunction alone or in combination with CNS injury.[35] It occurs with equal frequency in patients with supratentorial and infratentorial stroke, and it is also seen in premature infants during sleep and in subjects at high altitudes.[36]

Ataxic Breathing

Ataxic or irregular breathing is usually due to medullary dysfunction and may be a terminal event in severe dysfunction of the lower brainstem. It is also seen in patients with autonomic failure from multiple system atrophy or familial dysautonomia.

Cluster Breathing

Cluster breathing is characterized by irregular groups of breaths interspersed with pauses of varying lengths. It can be seen in patients with lower medullary dysfunction or during sleep in patients with multiple system atrophy.[37]

Other Conditions

In *hiccup*, there is strong contraction of the diaphragm and intercostal muscles followed by laryngeal closure, usually during inspiration. Hiccup rarely may be persistent and disabling. Persistent hiccup is associated with lateral medullary lesions, raised intracranial pressure, metabolic encephalopathy from diverse causes such as uremia, and any irritation of the diaphragm or phrenic nerves, but in many instances no cause can be found.

Sneezing and *yawning* are normal phenomena mediated through respiratory muscles. The center for sneezing is near the nucleus ambiguus, and yawning is coordinated from brainstem sites near the paraventricular nucleus via extrapyramidal pathways. A sneezing reflex triggered by sudden exposure to bright light may be inherited in an autosomal dominant manner. Yawning may initiate temporal lobe seizures, may be associated with arm stretching of the paretic limb in capsular infarction,[38] or occur spontaneously in "locked-in" syndrome.[8]

In diaphragmatic myoclonus or flutter (Leeuwenhoek disease), there is involuntary contraction of diaphragm during sleep or wakefulness at the rate of approximately 3 Hz. Diaphragmatic contractions cause epigastric pulsations and may be associated with dyspnea, hyperventilation, hiccups, belching, and difficulty in weaning from the ventilator.[39] In the syndrome of isolated diaphragmatic tremor, there is usually no respiratory or functional disability and there is some voluntary control of the phenomenon (Fig. 1-3).[40]

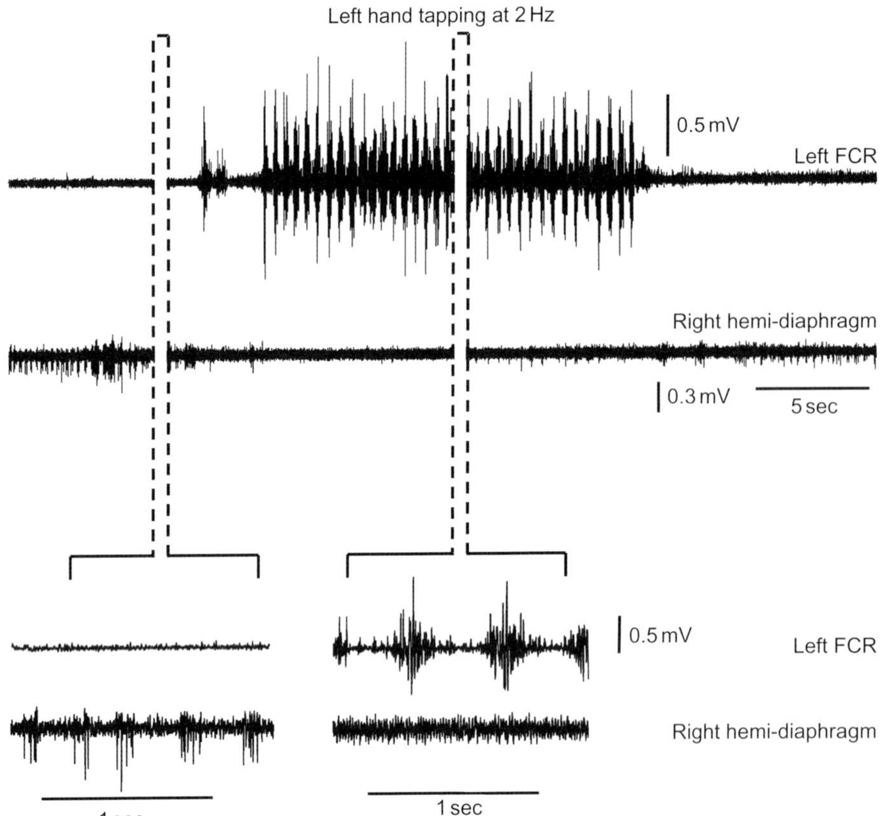

FIGURE 1-3 ■ Suppression of abnormal diaphragmatic tremor with voluntary wrist movements. The surface electromyographic (EMG) recordings from the left flexor carpi radialis (FCR) and needle EMG recordings from the right diaphragm in a 31-year-old man with isolated diaphragmatic tremor. There was rhythmic diaphragmatic EMG activity before, almost complete disappearance during, and resumption after a distracting task of left-hand metronome-guided finger tapping at 2 Hz. (From Espay AJ, Fox SH, Marras C, et al: Isolated diaphragmatic tremor: is there a spectrum in "respiratory myoclonus"? Neurology 69:689, 2007, with permission.)

RESPIRATORY DYSFUNCTION FROM NEUROLOGIC DISORDERS

Central Nervous System

Strategic lesions in the brain or spinal cord can affect breathing and such neurologic disorders can be acute or chronic.

Acute Respiratory Dysfunction

Neurogenic Pulmonary Edema

Fluid movement from the pulmonary capillary bed into the alveolar air space is governed by the Starling equation, which expresses transcapillary fluid flux as a balance between intravascular pressure and plasma osmotic force.[41] Dysfunction of the nervous system can result in increased pulmonary interstitial and alveolar fluid, leading to impaired alveolar gas exchange. This phenomenon, known as *neurogenic pulmonary edema*, may be life-threatening.

Neurogenic pulmonary edema has been reported in many conditions associated with severe brain injury such as head trauma, subarachnoid or intraparenchymal hemorrhage, ischemic stroke, multiple sclerosis, brain tumor, meningitis and encephalitis, status epilepticus, acute hydrocephalus, and spinal cord and meningeal hemorrhage.[42] In a large series of 477 cases with subarachnoid hemorrhage, 8 percent had neurogenic pulmonary edema.[43] Clinically, these patients had more severe bleeding than those without pulmonary edema, and 67 percent had increased intracranial pressure.

The exact mechanism involved is not known. Injury to the brain results in sympathetic discharges from the hypothalamus, brainstem, and spinal cord.[42,44,45] Specific anatomic regions represent so-called trigger zones for neurogenic

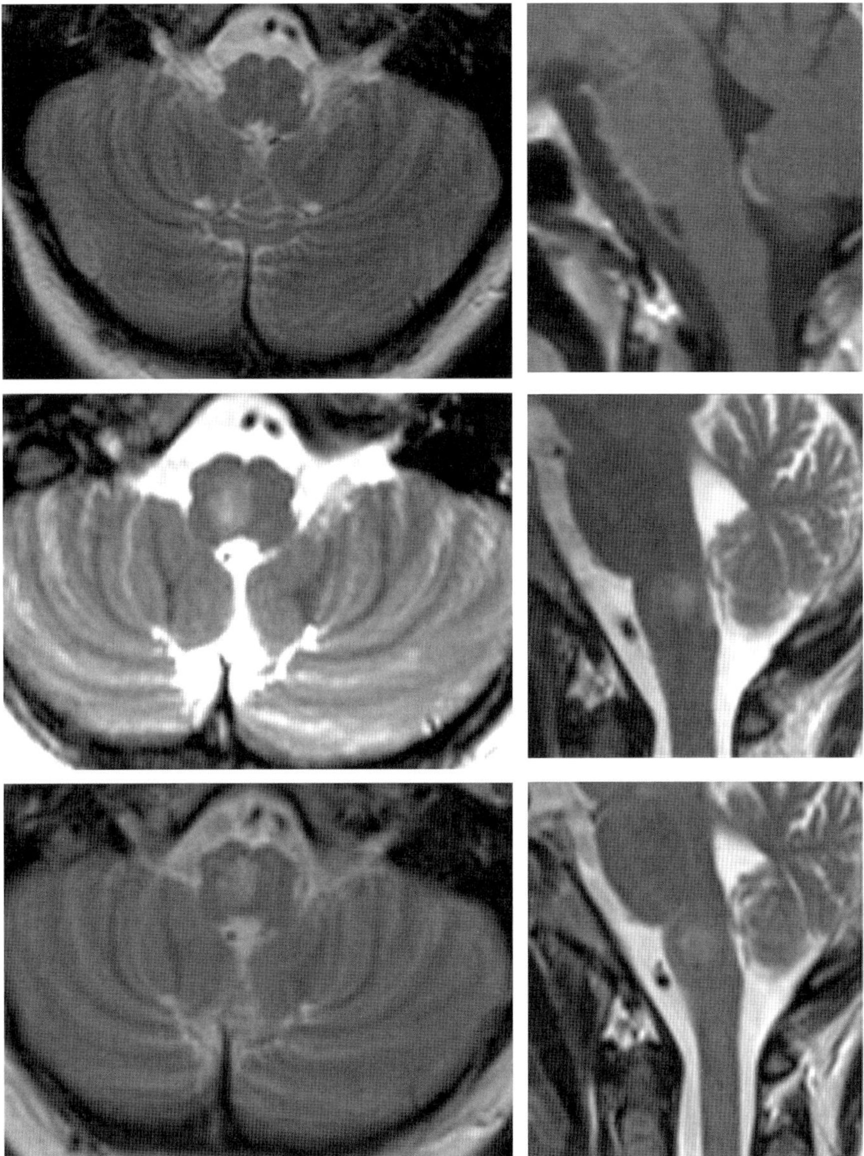

FIGURE 1-4 ■ Magnetic resonance imaging (MRI) scans (transaxial and sagittal views) at 30 days before presentation (upper panel), 4 days after presentation (middle panel), and 60 days after presentation (lower panel) in a patient with neurogenic pulmonary edema. There is a hyperintense demyelinating lesion centered at the dorsomedial rostral medulla of the day 4 image on T2-weighted MRI, best appreciated on the axial view. No such lesion was visible 30 days before (upper panel) presentation. The perilesional edema had resolved at day 60 (lower panel). (From Plummer C, Campagnaro R: Flash pulmonary edema in multiple sclerosis. J Emerg Med 44:e169, 2013, with permission.)

pulmonary edema, the most important of which are the A1 and A5 groups of neurons, nucleus of the solitary tract, the area postrema, the medial reticulated nucleus, and the dorsal motor nucleus of vagus.[45,46] Flash pulmonary edema has been reported in a young woman with multiple sclerosis who had an acute demyelinating lesion at the rostromedial medulla (Fig. 1-4).[47] Stimulation of these specific regions (directly or indirectly) following brain injury can lead to sympathetic discharges, which cause severe systemic vasoconstriction and displace blood from the systemic to pulmonary circulation. Concomitantly, there is also reduced left ventricular diastolic and systolic compliance and increased left ventricular volume and left atrial filling pressure. These cardiac changes along with intensive pulmonary vasoconstriction lead to increased pulmonary capillary pressure with endothelial injury and leakage of fluid into the interstitial space and alveoli.[42]

Increased capillary permeability may also contribute to the development of neurogenic pulmonary edema. This increased permeability is due to sympathetic microvascular stimulation causing micropores to increase in number and size, thereby allowing increased passage of fluid into alveoli as well as the release of several neurohumoral factors and inflammatory mediators such as neuropeptide Y, cytokines, fibrin and fibrin degradation products, plasma thromboplastin, and stress hormones such as corticotrophin releasing hormone, adrenocorticotrophic hormone, corticosteroids, and arginine vasopressin during CNS injury.[42,45,48,49] Thromboplastin stimulates the process of extrinsic coagulation and may contribute to fibrin embolization of pulmonary vessels, resulting in increased capillary permeability.

Trauma to Brain and Spinal Cord

Head injury may cause respiratory compromise by direct trauma to the face, pharynx, larynx, and chest and through other effects such as diffuse axonal injury resulting in reduced central voluntary drive and neurogenic pulmonary edema. The practice of hyperventilation to reduce intracranial pressure possibly results in further ischemic insults to the brain.[50,51]

Spinal cord injury can affect breathing in several ways (Table 1-1), and the degree of respiratory dysfunction depends on the severity of injury, ranging from air hunger and loss of automated breathing in complete transverse cord injuries to regular rhythmic breathing with inability to take deep breaths, hold the breath, or cough on command in partial cord injuries. In patients with lesions above C3, apnea is usually permanent. With lesions below C3, especially in the mid- or lower cervical segments, some patients may still be weaned off the ventilator successfully.[52] Delayed apnea in patients with cervical cord injury may arise secondary to manipulation of the spine in order to stabilize the fracture.[53] In chronic injury, spasticity of the respiratory muscles may compromise vital capacity and inspiratory pressure. Dyspnea and wheezing in patients with spinal cord injury can also result from vagal overactivity due to sympathetic denervation.

TABLE 1-1 ■ Mechanisms of Pulmonary Dysfunction in Patients with Spinal Cord Lesions

Injury to upper cervical cord leading to interruption of the descending respiratory control of the diaphragm and intercostal muscles
Direct injury to the anterior horn cells of the cervical and thoracic segments
Airway hyperactivity from loss of sympathetic airway innervation due to damage to sympathetic pathways in the spinal cord activating T1 to T6 ganglia
In advanced stages, spasticity of the respiratory muscles causing reduction in vital capacity and inspiratory pressure

Acute Nontraumatic High Myelopathies

Nontraumatic acute myelopathies include ischemic infarction of the spinal cord, hematomyelia, and postinfectious or immune-mediated myelopathies. The site and extent of the lesion affects respiration in a fashion similar to that described for traumatic injuries.

Multiple Sclerosis

Respiratory failure in advanced multiple sclerosis is often the cause of death.[54] Single or multiple lesions in the cervical cord and lower brainstem cause respiratory dysfunction.[55] Lesions of both corticospinal tracts or of the brainstem or upper cervical spinal cord cause paralysis of voluntary respiration, whereas those involving the dorsomedial medulla, nucleus ambiguus, and medial lemnisci result in loss of automatic respiration. Obstructive sleep apnea (OSA) may follow lesions in the medulla, and neurogenic pulmonary edema may occur with lesions in the region of nucleus tractus solitarius and the floor of the fourth ventricle.

Stroke

Respiratory compromise in stroke may be due to infarction or hemorrhage involving anatomic structures regulating breathing or as a consequence of secondary brain edema. Hemorrhagic strokes are more likely to produce early respiratory failure than ischemic strokes. Apnea, hypopnea, ataxic (irregular), tachypneic (central hyperventilation) and periodic (Cheyne–Stokes) breathing patterns have all been reported depending on the site of lesion. Although central neurogenic hyperventilation occurs with midbrain dysfunction from transtentorial herniation, it is also common with unilateral or bilateral hemispheric lesions. Ataxic breathing is more characteristic of medullary lesions and often seen terminally in patients with large stroke. Breathing abnormalities are common in pontine lesions as well as in secondary brainstem compression from expanding cerebellar hematomas. Infarction of the bilateral ventral pons results in the "locked-in" syndrome, where voluntary breathing is paralyzed (and the patient is unable to speak) due to interruption of the corticospinal and corticobulbar pathways; a normally functioning pontine tegmentum, cerebral hemispheres, and medulla results in preserved consciousness and regular automatic ventilation. In contrast, in sleep apnea (Ondine curse), automatic breathing is disturbed with preserved voluntary breathing in patients with bilateral or unilateral medullary infarctions. In focal hemispheric stroke, there may be contralateral dysfunction of chest wall movements.

Apart from anatomic lesions causing respiratory dysfunction, secondary factors following stroke increase the incidence of respiratory failure, such as oropharyngeal hypotonia due to reduced consciousness, impaired swallowing, and aspiration pneumonia.

The need for mechanical ventilation in patients with either brainstem or cerebral hemispheric stroke usually indicates a severe lesion. However, for patients requiring prolonged ventilation and tracheostomy, the likelihood of functional recovery is better in those with brainstem or cerebellar stroke than in those with hemispheric stroke.

Brain Tumors

Brainstem tumors such as gliomas, ependymomas, medulloblastomas, and cerebellar astrocytomas are more likely to cause respiratory disturbances than tumors in the cerebral hemispheres, often presenting acutely. Postoperative ventilatory support is often required. Supratentorial gliomas and other masses may also affect respiration due to tentorial herniation.

Chronic Respiratory Dysfunction

Parkinson Disease

Patients with Parkinson disease have been reported to have restrictive, obstructive, and mixed types of pulmonary dysfunction which is more severe in advanced disease and correlates with the degree of rigidity and bradykinesia.[56–59]

Two types of abnormalities on pulmonary function tests have been described in these patients.[60,61] In Type A, also known as respiratory flutter, there is regular consecutive flow deceleration and acceleration with a "saw-tooth pattern" on the flow–volume curve resulting from flow oscillation at a frequency of 4 to 8 Hz, which may improve with levodopa. The frequency is similar to that of the limb tremor, and probably results from involuntary movement of intrinsic laryngeal muscles. The type B pattern, indicative of intermittent airway closure, consists of irregular, abrupt changes in flow, sometimes with total cessation of flow.[62]

Respiratory failure in parkinsonian patients can be a consequence of poor coordination of inspiratory and expiratory muscles related to a more generalized motor impairment. Autonomic dysfunction and sleep disturbances may also contribute to nighttime pulmonary dysfunction, which in turn can lead to further sleep disturbances.

The role of levodopa in reversing pulmonary dysfunction is controversial, and published studies yield conflicting results. Improvement in dyspnea is more likely to occur, probably due to an improvement in the "mismatch" between central respiratory motor activity and afferent input from receptors in the airway, lungs, respiratory muscles, and chest wall.[63] Respiratory dysfunction can also result from levodopa-induced dyskinesias. In advanced Parkinson disease, impaired swallowing can also result in choking and aspiration, leading to further pulmonary dysfunction.

Multiple System Atrophy

Respiratory abnormalities are a major cause of death in multiple system atrophy, a disorder which often presents with a combination of parkinsonism, autonomic dysfunction, and cerebellar signs. Sleep apneas, both OSA and central sleep apnea (CSA), occur in 15 to 30 percent of patients with multiple system atrophy.[24,64] Nocturnal stridor is common, occurring in 34 of 100 patients with clinically probable multiple system atrophy and 13 percent of 203 pathologically proven cases.[65,66] Stridor may occur at any stage of the disease and is an important cause of sudden death.[67] Its exact pathogenesis is not known. Vocal cord dysfunction may result from lower motor neuron weakness of the abducting posterior cricoarytenoid muscles due to degeneration of the nucleus ambiguus or from abnormal overactivity (dystonia) of the adductor muscles due to a defect in central control mechanisms.[23] Other respiratory abnormalities in multiple system atrophy include central neurogenic hypoventilation resulting in hypercapnic respiratory failure[68] and respiratory dysrhythmias that consist of marked irregularities in tidal and minute volumes, variation of respiratory rate,[24] cluster breathing,[37] apneustic breathing,[69] and periodic breathing.[67]

Other Neurologic Disorders

Disordered ventilation is also seen in other bradykinetic syndromes as well as in patients with chorea, tremor, and dyskinesia. In postencephalitic parkinsonism, there may be tachypnea, breath-holding spells, noisy respiration, inversion of the inspiratory-to-expiratory ratio, Cheyne–Stokes breathing, respiratory tics, spasmodic coughing, sniffing, and inability to voluntarily change the respiratory rhythm.[61] In spinocerebellar degeneration, brainstem dysfunction, mitochondrial dysfunction, and thoracic skeletal deformities may contribute to respiratory compromise. In Joubert syndrome, a congenital disorder associated with a hypoplastic posterior cerebellar vermis, episodic hyperventilation and apnea have been reported, probably due to disruption of the cerebellar control pathways for breathing.[70]

Peripheral Nervous System

Disorders of the peripheral nervous system (Table 1-2) produce alveolar hypoventilation (pCO_2 >50 mmHg), hypoxia, and finally apnea in advanced stages. Initially, patients with chronic neuromuscular disorders may not experience dyspnea, as there is decreased exercise demand due to the disease process. Mild respiratory dysfunction may present with signs of anxiety, sweating, tachycardia, and tachypnea, accompanied by a reduced single-breath count, decreased chest expansion, paradoxical inward movement of the abdomen during inspiration (suggesting diaphragmatic weakness), interrupted speech, and poor cough.

TABLE 1-2 ■ Common Disorders of the Peripheral Nervous System Causing Respiratory Failure

Anterior Horn Cell Disorders
Motor neuron disease
Spinal muscular atrophy
Poliomyelitis
Neuropathies
Guillain–Barré syndrome
Critical illness polyneuropathy
Phrenic neuropathy
Multifocal motor neuropathy with conduction block
Hereditary neuropathy
Neuromuscular Junction Disorders
Myasthenia gravis and congenital myasthenic syndrome
Lambert–Eaton myasthenic syndrome
Toxins and drugs
Myopathies
Critical illness myopathy
Muscular dystrophies
Congenital myopathies

Anterior Horn Cell Disorders

Amyotrophic Lateral Sclerosis

Respiratory failure, which usually occurs late in the disease, is the most important cause of death in amyotrophic lateral sclerosis (ALS). The pathogenesis of respiratory failure is multifactorial and includes diaphragmatic weakness from loss of anterior horn cells in the cervical spinal cord, weakness of the chest wall from loss of thoracic spinal motor neurons, bulbar disease, and loss of descending corticospinal projections to the cervical and thoracic anterior horn cells. Pulmonary function tests (especially the FVC) are useful in monitoring the course of respiratory failure in the disease.[71] Bilevel intermittent positive pressure ventilation (BiPAP) improves survival and slows decline of pulmonary function, especially in bulbar-onset forms. This treatment should be offered to patients at the onset of dyspnea, when FVC falls below 50 percent of normal or when there is a rapid decline in FVC. Rarely, some patients present initially with acute respiratory failure.[72]

The duration of symptoms such as exertional dyspnea or orthopnea varies from weeks to months; once mechanical ventilation is needed due to hypercapnea, successful weaning is unlikely. Planning in advance for respiratory failure in the terminal stages of ALS is important, and patient wishes regarding prolonged ventilation and intubation should be discussed.

Other Anterior Horn Cell Disorders

Poliomyelitis is a rare cause of acute respiratory failure in children from developing countries. Respiratory failure occurs due to involvement of the anterior horn cells of spinal cord and brainstem. In survivors of acute poliomyelitis, respiratory weakness may reappear after several years along with limb weakness, especially in those who had the illness after 10 years of age and those who presented initially with respiratory failure. Other viral infections, including West Nile virus encephalomyelitis, are now more common causes of a poliomyelitis-like illness worldwide. Respiratory insufficiency also occurs terminally in patients with spinal muscular atrophy.[73]

NEUROPATHIES

Guillain–Barré Syndrome

Acute inflammatory demyelinating polyneuropathy (AIDP), of which Guillain–Barré syndrome is the prototype, is one of the most important and common neurologic causes of respiratory dysfunction. The main cause of respiratory failure in these conditions is phrenic nerve demyelination and consequent diaphragmatic paralysis. Other contributory factors include weakness of the intercostal and other accessory muscles of respiration, autonomic dysfunction, retained respiratory secretions, and atelectasis. The French Cooperative Group reported a 43 percent incidence of respiratory insufficiency in patients with Guillain–Barré syndrome, which lasted a mean duration of 31 days.[74] Approximately one-third of patients are ready for weaning within 2 weeks, but those with axonal forms have a poorer prognosis for respiratory recovery and may therefore require earlier tracheostomy.[75] Immune therapy probably reduces the length of ventilator dependence.

Early respiratory symptoms of discomfort and agitation are accompanied by signs of reduced single-breath count, weak cough, use of accessory muscles, tachypnea, paradoxical abdominal movement, and speech interrupted by brief breaths. There may be frequent awakenings at night resulting from relaxation of voluntarily activated respiratory muscles during REM sleep, which increases demand on an already weakened diaphragm.

Indications for mechanical ventilation include a vital capacity less than 20 ml per kg, maximum inspiratory pressure below $-25\,cmH_2O$, and a maximum expiratory pressure less than $40\,cmH_2O$. Mechanical ventilation will probably be required within 36 hours if the FVC is less than 50 percent of baseline.[76] Even patients with a normal vital capacity may be at risk of imminent respiratory failure when the phrenic nerves are involved by the demyelinating process; abnormalities on phrenic nerve conduction studies and on needle electromyography of the diaphragm may predict respiratory insufficiency.[77] Patients requiring mechanical ventilation have a mortality of around 20 percent.[78]

Phrenic Nerve Mononeuropathies

The severity of symptoms in phrenic neuropathies is variable and depends on the underlying cause, such as trauma, tumor infiltration, compression, infection, radiation, or an idiopathic neuropathy. Symptoms include exertional shortness of breath, and the respiratory rate may increase when lying flat. In addition to an elevated hemidiaphragm on chest radiography, there may be pulmonary atelectasis on the paralyzed side and mediastinal shift towards the normal side. Hoover sign (uninhibited movement of the costal margin away from the midline on the side of injury) can be seen clinically, and Kienback sign (affected diaphragm moves paradoxically upward with a vigorous sniff) may be present on fluoroscopy. Phrenic nerve conduction studies and needle electromyography of the diaphragm are useful for diagnosis and prognosis.

Critical Illness Polyneuropathy

In an intensive care unit, unexplained difficulty in weaning from the ventilator may result from several neuromuscular conditions that may occur in patients with the systemic inflammatory response syndrome. This syndrome occurs in 20 to 50 percent of patients in major medical or surgical care units, and its associated damage to the peripheral nervous system is probably related to the release of inflammatory mediators such as cytokines and free radicals, as discussed in Chapter 56.

Critical illness polyneuropathy is a predominantly motor, axonal polyneuropathy that occurs in 50 to 70 percent of patients with systemic inflammatory response syndrome (see Chapter 56). The initial manifestation is often difficulty in weaning from the ventilator, despite systemic improvement. Weakness is usually equally distributed in both proximal and distal muscles groups. Severe weakness with muscle wasting is observed in one-third of patients, hypo- to areflexia in the majority, and distal sensory loss in less than one-third.[79,80] Electrophysiologic studies show reduced amplitude of compound muscle action potentials as early as 2 weeks from the onset of the systemic inflammatory response syndrome, with abnormal spontaneous activity seen in muscles; sensory nerve action potentials may be normal.[79] Phrenic nerve stimulation and diaphragmatic electromyography is sometimes helpful in critical illness polyneuropathy, and degeneration of the phrenic nerves and denervation atrophy of respiratory muscles may be found at autopsy.

Other Neuropathies

Respiratory failure resulting from phrenic nerve involvement has been reported in other acquired and inherited neuropathies such as diabetes mellitus,[81] chronic renal failure,[82] arsenic exposure,[83] sarcoidosis, lead toxicity, acute organophosphate poisoning, leprosy, diphtheria, multifocal motor neuropathy with conduction block,[84] infantile axonal polyneuropathy,[85] and hereditary motor and sensory neuropathy type 2C.[86]

Neuromuscular Junction Disorders

Neuromuscular junction (NMJ) disorders should be suspected in patients with respiratory muscle weakness of unclear origin. These disorders can occur at any age, and the underlying causes include autoimmune, hereditary, paraneoplastic, and toxic diseases (see Chapter 59).

Progressive respiratory muscle weakness is commonly found in generalized myasthenia gravis. During the course of the illness, 15 to 20 percent of patients will develop a myasthenic crisis, characterized by acute respiratory failure requiring mechanical ventilation, with a mortality rate of up to 5 percent.[87] The age and sex distribution of myasthenic gravis shows a bimodal pattern with an early peak (<45 years) in women, and a later peak (>55 years) for both sexes. Infections are the most common trigger for myasthenic crisis; other precipitants include initial corticosteroid therapy, neuromuscular blocking drugs such as aminoglycosides, surgery, pregnancy and delivery, and physical and emotional stresses.

Although myasthenic crisis occurs most often in generalized myasthenia gravis, it may also occur rarely in oculobulbar variants, and isolated respiratory failure may be the initial manifestation of myasthenia gravis. Antibodies against aceytlcholine receptors may not be present in patients with predominant respiratory muscle involvement. Instead, some of these patients may have muscle-specific tyrosine kinase (MuSK) receptor antibodies and have predominantly neck, shoulder, and respiratory muscle or oculobulbar weakness.[88]

Excessive administration of anticholinesterase drugs to treat myasthenia gravis sometimes leads to respiratory weakness. Miosis, sweating, abdominal cramping and diarrhea, excessive secretions, and muscle fasciculations characterize these cholinergic crises. Bronchospasm, aspiration, and excessive inspissated secretions with weak cough cause the respiratory dysfunction.

In addition to serum antibody tests, the evaluation of patients with respiratory insufficiency and suspected myasthenia gravis may include repetitive nerve conduction studies, occasionally including the phrenic nerve, and single-fiber electromyography if the diagnosis remains unclear. The edophronium (Tensilon) test may not change respiratory muscle strength and is most useful when the patient has ptosis. Phrenic nerve conduction studies may be useful to exclude iatrogenic phrenic nerve injury in post-thymectomy myasthenia gravis patients with respiratory insufficiency.

Other neuromuscular disorders that cause respiratory insufficiency include other forms of myasthenia gravis (neonatal, congenital, and juvenile), food-borne or wound botulism, and neuromuscular toxins and drugs. Isolated or predominant involvement of the respiratory muscles is not uncommon and may be the presenting feature of Lambert–Eaton myasthenic syndrome, a disorder caused by insufficient release of neurotransmitter by the nerve terminal.[89,90]

Myopathies

Muscular Dystrophies

Among the dystrophinopathies, Duchenne muscular dystrophy (DMD) is the most common cause of respiratory muscle weakness; approximately 40 to 70 percent of these patients die of respiratory failure.

Respiratory insufficiency starts at the age of 8 or 9 years and progressively increases with age and functional disability; those with more severe thoracic scoliosis have earlier onset of respiratory failure. The causes of respiratory failure include weakness of inspiratory and expiratory muscles, progressive kyphoscoliosis, recurrent respiratory tract infections, and pulmonary edema from cardiac failure. Respiratory insufficiency is less frequent in Becker than Duchenne dystrophy. Early respiratory insufficiency and death in infancy may also occur in isolated muscular dystrophy involving the diaphragm.

Respiratory involvement is common in myotonic dystrophy and results from weakness of the diaphragm and the intercostal muscles. The cause of respiratory muscle weakness is due to CNS degeneration in 20 percent of patients.[91] Other contributory factors include the concurrence of various types of neuropathy.[92,93] Alveolar hypoventilation from diaphragmatic weakness and central hypoventilation (from neuronal loss in the dorsal raphe and superior central nuclei) underlie the hypersomnia that is common in myotonic dystrophy.[92,93]

Critical Illness Myopathy

Critically ill patients may be affected by a critical illness myopathy in addition to the neurpathy discussed earlier. This includes at least three different types of muscle abnormalities: thick filament myopathy, acute necrotizing myopathy, and cachectic myopathy. Flaccid weakness of the muscles of all limbs, neck flexors, and sometimes the face is accompanied by diaphragmatic weakness and difficulty in weaning from mechanical ventilation. Differentiation of critical illness myopathy from neuropathy may be difficult and some patients, if not most, will have a combination of these two entities. Myopathic features on electrophysiologic studies, an elevated serum creatinine kinase (which is not always present in this particular myopathy), and demonstration of myopathic features with myosin loss on histopathology are supportive of critical illness myopathy.[94] Further details are provided in Chapters 56 and 59.

Other Muscle Disorders

Many patients with various limb-girdle syndromes have dyspnea on exertion, chronic cough, and recurrent respiratory infections. Those with severe diaphragmatic involvement may have chronic alveolar hypoventilation resulting in morning headaches, excessive sleepiness, fatigue, and altered mentation.[95] Although patients with facioscapulohumeral and scapuloperoneal syndromes are usually spared respiratory muscle involvement, they may develop frequent aspiration pneumonia due to weakness of pharyngeal muscles.

Congenital myopathies are usually nonprogressive or slowly progressive muscle diseases that are present at birth, but in severe cases respiratory insufficiency can occur; respiratory muscle weakness has been reported in infants with nemaline myopathy, centronuclear myopathy, and multicore myopathy.[96]

In inflammatory myopathies (e.g., polymyositis and dermatomyositis), pulmonary complications are frequently the result of weakness of respiratory muscles, interstitial lung disease, and aspiration pneumonia from weakness of pharyngeal and upper esophageal muscles.[97,98]

In acid maltase deficiency (Pompe disease), REM sleep hypopneas and respiratory failure may occur secondary to weakness of the diaphragm.[99] Respiratory muscle weakness has also been reported in corticosteroid-induced myopathy as a result of selective atrophy of type IIB fibers,[23,100] and in HIV myopathy,[101] mitochondrial myopathies,[102] and carnitine palmitoyl transferase deficiency.[103]

DISORDERS OF BREATHING ASSOCIATED WITH SLEEP

Upper Airway Obstruction

As discussed in Chapter 51, upper airway obstruction during sleep is defined as partial (obstructive sleep hypopnea) or complete (obstructive sleep apnea) obstruction to airflow proximal to the larynx for at least 10 seconds despite ongoing respiratory efforts. There may be a mixed apnea (initial lack of respiratory effort followed by increasing effort) and upper airway resistance syndrome (frequent respiratory effort-related arousals). These conditions are collectively referred to as obstructive sleep apnea/hypopnea syndrome (OSAHS).

Stridor, a harsh or strained, high-pitched inspiratory sound, results from obstruction to inspiration at the level of the vocal cords. Several neurologic causes may result in stridor including brainstem dysfunction (e.g., from Chiari malformation), paralysis of cord abduction from recurrent laryngeal neuropathy, dystonia of the vocal-cord adductor muscles, and multiple system atrophy.[67,104]

Central Sleep Apnea Syndrome

Central sleep apnea is characterized by cessation of breathing during sleep from a loss of ventilatory effort for a minimum duration of 10 seconds while the upper airway remains open. Central sleep apnea is less common than OSAHS. Esophageal pressure monitoring is the definitive technique used to differentiate central from peripheral obstructive events. However, the differentiation can usually be made by documentation of cessation of airflow associated with absence of respiratory effort measured indirectly by inductive plethysmography, strain-gauge recordings, and intercostal electromyography.

Central sleep apnea may be associated with hypercapnia or normocapnia/hypocapnia. In hypercapnic central sleep apnea, the ventilatory response to CO_2 is reduced; the disorder occurs in patients with alveolar hypoventilation caused by neuromuscular disorders, brainstem dysfunction, or in idiopathic alveolar hyoventilation syndrome.[105] Normocapnic or hypocapnic central sleep apnea may also be idiopathic or it may occur in the setting of high altitude, with Cheyne–Stokes respiration, or with partial upper airway obstruction.

Sleep Hypoventilation Syndrome

The sleep hypoventilation syndrome is characterized by both hypercapnia and hypoxemia during sleep unexplained by discrete apneas or hypopneas. A variety of neurologic disorders may cause this disorder (Table 1-3) by affecting the central respiratory centers or their efferent pathways, or due to myopathies or neuropathies affecting the diaphragm or intercostal muscles.[67,106,107] Sleep hypoventilation syndrome is initially observed in REM sleep, but eventually daytime respiratory failure occurs. Sleep hypoventilation syndrome results in frequent nighttime arousals, nocturnal dyspnea on lying flat, morning headaches, and daytime sleepiness. Chronic hypercapnia may result in blunting of respiratory chemoreceptor responses and a secondary reduction in central respiratory drive. Nocturnal hypoventilation results in erythrocytosis, pulmonary hypertension, and, in severe cases, cor pulmonale.

TABLE 1-3 ■ Neurologic Causes of Sleep Hypoventilation Syndrome

Disorders of Brainstem Respiratory Centers
Idiopathic central alveolar hypoventilation
Multiple system atrophy
Infarcts or hemorrhage
Tumors
Infections (e.g., encephalitis)
Arnold–Chiari malformation
Disorders of Spinal Efferent Pathways
High spinal cord trauma
Cervical posterior cordotomy
Multiple sclerosis
Disorders of Anterior Horn Cells and Peripheral Nerves
Poliomyelitis and postpolio syndrome
Motor neuron diseases
Generalized peripheral neuropathies
Bilateral phrenic neuropathy
Disorders of Muscle
Congenital myopathies
Muscular dystrophies (e.g., Duchenne; myotonic dystrophy)
Inflammatory myopathies
Myasthenia gravis
Disorders Restricting Chest Cage Movement
Kyphosis
Scoliosis in chronic neurodegenerative disorders (e.g., Friedreich ataxia)

Adapted with permission from: Bolton CF, Chen R, Wijdicks EFM, et al: Neurology of Breathing. Butterworth Heinemann, Philadelphia, 2004.

Respiratory Dysrhythmias

Respiratory dysrhythmias are abnormalities of the rhythm of breathing or the relationship of inspiration to expiration. They occur more frequently during sleep and include Cheyne–Stokes breathing, apneustic breathing, irregular or ataxic breathing, and cluster breathing. The clinical features of these abnormal patterns of respiration were discussed earlier. Cheyne–Stokes breathing may be associated with central sleep apnea and is often observed in patients with cardiac failure, occurring in 30 to 50 percent of patients with ejection fractions less than 40 percent.[108]

NEUROLOGIC EFFECTS OF RESPIRATORY DYSFUNCTION

Like other organs in the body, the brain is often indirectly affected by respiratory failure. Neurologic symptoms may be acute or insidious, and signs of primary lung disease may not always be apparent.

Dysfunction Related to Pulmonary Pathology

Chronic or acute hypoxia and hypercapnia, or hypocapnia, can result from diverse primary lung disorders or cardiac illness. These abnormalities can impair the function of the nervous system in several ways.

HYPOXIA

Cerebral dysfunction usually occurs with reduction of partial pressure of oxygen to less than 40 mmHg. The effects of pure hypoxia on the brain (hypoxic hypoxia) are observed in high altitude sickness. Several days after ascending rapidly (usually to altitudes of 8,000 to 12,000 feet), headache, insomnia, anorexia, nausea, vomiting, and impaired cognitive function may occur. In the more acute and severe form (usually above 10,000 feet), there is severe headache, delirium, hallucinations, ataxia, and occasionally seizures. Papilledema and retinal hemorrhages may occur, probably due to cerebral edema. Prophylactic acetazolamide and dexamethasone are sometimes useful, and dexamethasone is used to treat the disorder when it occurs.

Following cardiac arrest, patients can develop an encephalopathy primarily as a result of cerebral ischemia rather than pure hypoxia. Structural abnormalities usually do not occur in the brain in the setting of hypoxia without ischemia.[109,110]

HYPERCAPNIA

Chronic pulmonary insufficiency is one of the important causes of chronic hypercapnia (pCO_2 levels ranging from 39 to 68 mmHg). Headache, papilledema, tremulousness, asterixis, altered consciousness, and generalized slowing of the electroencephalogram can result. Raised intracranial pressure from chronic CO_2 narcosis is believed to be the underlying factor causing headache and papilledema.[55] Management strategies include discontinuation of sedative drugs, avoidance of vigorous hyperventilation, and ventilatory support.

Encephalopathy and occasionally seizures are the main symptoms of acute severe hypercapnia with CO_2 levels ranging from 75 to 110 mmHg. CO_2 narcosis results in reduced pH of the CSF and subsequent respiratory acidosis. Acute encephalopathy probably results from hydrogen ion-induced inhibition of glutamate receptors.[111]

HYPOCAPNIA

Hypocapnia may also have deleterious effects on the brain. Hyperventilation causes acute hypocapnia resulting in cerebral vasoconstriction, hypocalcemia, a shift in the oxygen–hemoglobin dissociation curve, and reduced oxygen delivery. Symptoms include lightheadedness, dizziness, faintness, paresthesias, and altered consciousness. Hypocalcemia with alkalosis may cause seizures and tetany.

Metabolic disorders such as hepatic encephalopathy, salicylate poisoning, and sepsis also may result in a respiratory alkalosis. Alkalosis results in reduced cerebral blood flow from cerebral vasoconstriction, reduced oxygen availability to tissues from shift of the oxygen–hemoglobin dissociation curve, and hypophosphatemia, which may rarely cause acute neuromuscular weakness.

Dysfunction Related to Obstructive Sleep Apnea

VASCULAR DISORDERS

Snoring is an independent risk factor for stroke, and the frequency of OSAHS has been found to be significantly higher soon after stroke or transient ischemic attack.[112–118] Hypertension, cardiac arrhythmias, increased platelet aggregation, increased blood viscosity, decreased fibrinolysis, sympathetic hyperactivity, and changes in cerebral blood flow are each potential mechanisms for stroke in patients with OSAHS.[113]

Headache

Awakening headache and cluster headache have been associated with OSAHS, and treatment with positive airway pressure has been shown to improve headache in these patients. Hypoxia or hypercapnia-induced cerebral vasodilation is the most likely mechanism of headache. Although the exact frequency of headache in OSAHS is not known, it is more frequent in OSA and snorers than those without these disorders.[119–122]

Cognitive Dysfunction and Dementia

Several studies have showed that OSAHS can result in impaired cognition, and the severity of cognitive dysfunction increases with the degree of OSAHS.[123–126] Cognitive functions affected include intelligence quotient (IQ), attention, immediate and delayed recall, verbal and visual short-term memory, and executive function. The pathogenesis may involve both chronic intermittent hypoxemia and the effects of sleep deprivation and daytime sleepiness. Although memory dysfunction is related to the number of disordered breathing events, frontal lobe dysfunction correlates best with the degree of hypoxemia.[124] Nasal continuous positive airway pressure improves many domains of cognitive dysfunction except possibly for executive function and short-term memory.[126] Although several studies have shown a correlation between OSAHS and dementia, it is unclear whether dementia is the effect or cause of OSAHS.

REFERENCES

1. Nattie E: CO_2, brainstem chemoreceptors and breathing. Prog Neurobiol 59:299, 1999.
2. Guz A: Brain, breathing and breathlessness. Respir Physiol 109:197, 1997.
3. Liotti M, Brannan S, Egan G, et al: Brain responses associated with consciousness of breathlessness (air hunger). Proc Natl Acad Sci USA 98:2035, 2001.
4. Spengler CM, Gozal D, Shea SA: Chemoreceptive mechanisms elucidated by studies of congenital central hypoventilation syndrome. Respir Physiol 129:247, 2001.
5. Rand CM, Patwari PP, Carroll MS, et al: Congenital central hypoventilation syndrome and sudden infant death syndrome: disorders of autonomic regulation. Semin Pediatr Neurol 20:44, 2013.
6. Heywood P, Murphy K, Corfield DR, et al: Control of breathing in man; insights from the 'locked-in' syndrome. Respir Physiol 106:13, 1996.
7. Shea SA, Andres LP, Shannon DC, et al: Respiratory sensations in subjects who lack a ventilatory response to CO_2. Respir Physiol 93:203, 1993.
8. Simon RP: Breathing and the nervous system. p. 1. In Aminoff MJ (ed): Neurology and General Medicine. 4th Ed. Churchill Livingstone Elsevier, Philadelphia, 2008.
9. Lumb AB: 556 pp. Nunn's Applied Respiratory Physiology. 7th Ed. Churchill Livingstone Elsevier, Oxford, 2010.
10. Bianchi AL, Pasaro R: Organization of central respiratory neurons. p. 77. In: Miller AD, Bianchi AL, Bishop BP (eds): Neural Control of the Respiratory Muscles. CRC Press, Boca Raton, FL, 1997.
11. Lumsden T: Observations on the respiratory centres in the cat. J Physiol 57:153, 1923.
12. Wang W, Fung ML, St John WM: Pontile regulation of ventilatory activity in the adult rat. J Appl Physiol 74:2801, 1993.
13. Wagner PG, Dekin MS: GABAb receptors are coupled to a barium-insensitive outward rectifying potassium conductance in premotor respiratory neurons. J Neurophysiol 69:286, 1993.
14. Richter DW, Ballanyi AL, Ramirez JM: Respiratory rhythm generation. p. 119. In: Miller AD, Bianchi AL, Bishop BP (eds): Neural Control of the Respiratory Muscles. CRC Press, Boca Raton, FL, 1997.
15. Abrahams TP, Hornby PJ, Walton DP, et al: An excitatory amino acid(s) in the ventrolateral medulla is (are) required for breathing to occur in the anesthetized cat. J Pharmacol Exp Ther 259:1388, 1991.
16. Xu F, Frazier DT: Medullary respiratory neuronal activity modulated by stimulation of the fastigial nucleus of the cerebellum. Brain Res 705:53, 1995.
17. Colebatch JG, Adams L, Murphy K, et al: Regional cerebral blood flow during volitional breathing in man. J Physiol 443:91, 1991.
18. Gozal D, Omidvar O, Kirlew KA, et al: Functional magnetic resonance imaging reveals brain regions mediating the response to resistive expiratory loads in humans. J Clin Invest 97:47, 1996.
19. Ramsay SC, Adams L, Murphy K, et al: Regional cerebral blood flow during volitional expiration in man: a comparison with volitional inspiration. J Physiol 461:85, 1993.
20. Maskill D, Murphy K, Mier A, et al: Motor cortical representation of the diaphragm in man. J Physiol 443:105, 1991.
21. Cohen E, Mier A, Heywood P, et al: Diaphragmatic movement in hemiplegic patients measured by ultrasonography. Thorax 49:890, 1994.
22. Lee HW, Hong SB, Tae WA, et al: Partial seizures manifesting as apnea only in an adult. Epilepsia 40:1828, 1999.
23. Bolton CF, Chen R, Wijdicks EFM, et al: 232 pp. Neurology of Breathing. Butterworth Heinemann, Philadelphia, 2004.

24. Munschauer FE, Loh L, Bannister R, et al: Abnormal respiration and sudden death during sleep in multiple system atrophy with autonomic failure. Neurology 40:677, 1990.
25. Kim KJ, Yun JY, Lee JY, et al: Ondine's curse in Anti-Ri antibody associated paraneoplastic brainstem syndrome. Sleep Med 14:382, 2013.
26. Dubaybo BA, Afridi I, Hussain M: Central neurogenic hyperventilation in invasive laryngeal carcinoma. Chest 99:767, 1991.
27. Shibata Y, Meguro K, Narushima K, et al: Malignant lymphoma of the central nervous system presenting with central neurogenic hyperventilation. Case report. J Neurosurg 76:696, 1992.
28. Tarulli AW, Lim C, Bui JD, et al: Central neurogenic hyperventilation: a case report and discussion of pathophysiology. Arch Neurol 62:1632, 2005.
29. Siderowf AD, Balcer LJ, Kenyon LC, et al: Central neurogenic hyperventilation in an awake patient with a pontine glioma. Neurology 46:1160, 1996.
30. Chin K, Ohi M, Fukui M, et al: Inhibitory effect of an intellectual task on breathing after voluntary hyperventilation. J Appl Physiol 81:1379, 1996.
31. Jennett S, Ashbridge K, North JB: Post-hyperventilation apnoea in patients with brain damage. J Neurol Neurosurg Psychiatry 37:288, 1974.
32. Saito Y, Hashimoto T, Iwata H, et al: Apneustic breathing in children with brainstem damage due to hypoxic-ischemic encephalopathy. Dev Med Child Neurol 41:560, 1999.
33. Mador MJ, Tobin MJ: Apneustic breathing. A characteristic feature of brainstem compression in achondroplasia? Chest 97:877, 1990.
34. Nachtmann A, Siebler M, Rose G, et al: Cheyne-Stokes respiration in ischemic stroke. Neurology 45:820, 1995.
35. Cheyne J: A case of apoplexy in which the fleshy part of the heart was converted to fat. Dublin Hosp Rev 2:216, 1818.
36. Khoo MC, Anholm JD, Ko SW, et al: Dynamics of periodic breathing and arousal during sleep at extreme altitude. Respir Physiol 103:33, 1996.
37. Lockwood AH: Shy-Drager syndrome with abnormal respirations and antidiuretic hormone release. Arch Neurol 33:292, 1976.
38. Wimalaratna HS, Capildeo R: Is yawning a brainstem phenomenon? Lancet 1:300, 1988.
39. Chen R, Remtulla H, Bolton CF: Electrophysiological study of diaphragmatic myoclonus. J Neurol Neurosurg Psychiatry 58:480, 1995.
40. Espay AJ, Fox SH, Marras C, et al: Isolated diaphragmatic tremor: is there a spectrum in "respiratory myoclonus"? Neurology 69:689, 2007.
41. Hux W: A new view of Starling's hypthesis at the microstructural level. Microvasc Res 58:281, 1999.
42. Ridenti FAS: Neurogenic pulmonary edema: a current literature review. Rev Bras Ter Intensiva 24:91, 2012.
43. Muroi C, Keller M, Pangalu A, et al: Neurogenic pulmonary edema in patients with subarachnoid hemorrhage. J Neurosurg Anesthesiol 20:188, 2008.
44. Gajic O, Manno EM: Neurogenic pulmonary edema: another multiple-hit model of acute lung injury. Crit Care Med 35:1979, 2007.
45. Sedy J, Zicha J, Kunes J, et al: Mechanisms of neurogenic pulmonary edema development. Physiol Res 57:499, 2008.
46. Baumann A, Audibert G, McDonnell J, et al: Neurogenic pulmonary edema. Acta Anaesthesiol Scand 51:447, 2007.
47. Plummer C, Campagnaro R: Flash pulmonary edema in multiple sclerosis. J Emerg Med 44:e169, 2013.
48. Hamdy O, Nishiwaki K, Yajima M, et al: Presence and quantification of neuropeptide Y in pulmonary edema fluids in rats. Exp Lung Res 26:137, 2000.
49. Quader K, Manninen PH, Lai JK: Pulmonary edema in the neuroradiology suite: a diagnostic dilemma. Can J Anaesth 48:308, 2001.
50. Diringer MN, Yundt K, Videen TO, et al: No reduction in cerebral metabolism as a result of early moderate hyperventilation following severe traumatic brain injury. J Neurosurg 92:7, 2000.
51. Imberti R, Bellinzona G, Langer M: Cerebral tissue PO_2 and $SjvO_2$ changes during moderate hyperventilation in patients with severe traumatic brain injury. J Neurosurg 96:97, 2002.
52. Roth EJ, Lu A, Primack S, et al: Ventilatory function in cervical and high thoracic spinal cord injury. Relationship to level of injury and tone. Am J Phys Med Rehabil 76:262, 1997.
53. Lu K, Lee TC, Liang CL, et al: Delayed apnea in patients with mid- to lower cervical spinal cord injury. Spine 25:1332, 2000.
54. Howard RS, Wiles CM, Hirsch NP, et al: Respiratory involvement in multiple sclerosis. Brain 115:479, 1992.
55. Carter JL, Noseworthy JH: Ventilatory dysfunction in multiple sclerosis. Clin Chest Med 15:693, 1994.
56. Izquierdo-Alonso JL, Jimenez-Jimenez FJ, Cabrera-Valdivia F, et al: Airway dysfunction in patients with Parkinson's disease. Lung 172:47, 1994.
57. Sabate M, Rodriguez M, Mendez E, et al: Obstructive and restrictive pulmonary dysfunction increases disability in Parkinson disease. Arch Phys Med Rehabil 77:29, 1996.
58. Shill H, Stacy M: Respiratory function in Parkinson's disease. Clin Neurosci 5:131, 1998.
59. Pal PK, Sathyaprabha TN, Tuhina P, et al: Pattern of subclinical pulmonary dysfunctions in Parkinson's disease and the effect of levodopa. Mov Disord 22:420, 2007.
60. Vincken W, Cosio MG: "Saw-tooth" pattern in the flow-volume loop. Chest 88:480, 1985.
61. Vincken WG, Gauthier SG, Dollfuss RE, et al: Involvement of upper-airway muscles in

extrapyramidal disorders. A cause of airflow limitation. N Engl J Med 311:438, 1984.
62. Hovestadt A, Bogaard JM, Meerwaldt JD, et al: Pulmonary function in Parkinson's disease. J Neurol Neurosurg Psychiatry 52:329, 1989.
63. Weiner P, Inzelberg R, Davidovich A, et al: Respiratory muscle performance and the perception of dyspnea in Parkinson's disease. Can J Neurol Sci 29:68, 2002.
64. Plazzi G, Corsini R, Provini F, et al: REM sleep behavior disorders in multiple system atrophy. Neurology 48:1094, 1997.
65. Wenning GK, Ben Shlomo Y, Magalhaes M, et al: Clinical features and natural history of multiple system atrophy. An analysis of 100 cases. Brain 117:835, 1994.
66. Wenning GK, Tison F, Ben Shlomo Y, et al: Multiple system atrophy: a review of 203 pathologically proven cases. Mov Disord 12:133, 1997.
67. Silber MH, Levine S: Stridor and death in multiple system atrophy. Mov Disord 15:699, 2000.
68. Isozaki E, Naito A, Horiguchi S, et al: Early diagnosis and stage classification of vocal cord abductor paralysis in patients with multiple system atrophy. J Neurol Neurosurg Psychiatry 60:399, 1996.
69. Bannister R, Gibson W, Michaels L, et al: Laryngeal abductor paralysis in multiple system atrophy. A report on three necropsied cases, with observations on the laryngeal muscles and the nuclei ambigui. Brain 104:351, 1981.
70. Maria BL, Hoang KB, Tusa RJ, et al: "Joubert syndrome" revisited: key ocular motor signs with magnetic resonance imaging correlation. J Child Neurol 12:423, 1997.
71. Lyall RA, Donaldson N, Polkey MI, et al: Respiratory muscle strength and ventilatory failure in amyotrophic lateral sclerosis. Brain 124:2000, 2001.
72. Chen R, Grand'Maison F, Strong MJ, et al: Motor neuron disease presenting as acute respiratory failure: a clinical and pathological study. J Neurol Neurosurg Psychiatry 60:455, 1996.
73. Ioos C, Leclair-Richard D, Mrad S, et al: Respiratory capacity course in patients with infantile spinal muscular atrophy. Chest 126:831, 2004.
74. Efficiency of plasma exchange in Guillain-Barré syndrome: role of replacement fluids. French Cooperative Group on Plasma Exchange in Guillain-Barré syndrome.. Ann Neurol 22:753, 1987.
75. Lawn ND, Wijdicks EF: Tracheostomy in Guillain-Barré syndrome. Muscle Nerve 22:1058, 1999.
76. Chevrolet JC, Deleamont P: Repeated vital capacity measurements as predictive parameters for mechanical ventilation need and weaning success in the Guillain-Barré syndrome. Am Rev Respir Dis 144:814, 1991.
77. Zifko U, Chen R, Remtulla H, et al: Respiratory electrophysiological studies in Guillain-Barré syndrome. J Neurol Neurosurg Psychiatry 60:191, 1996.
78. Fletcher DD, Lawn ND, Wolter TD, et al: Long-term outcome in patients with Guillain-Barré syndrome requiring mechanical ventilation. Neurology 54:2311, 2000.
79. Zifko UA, Zipko HT, Bolton CF: Clinical and electrophysiological findings in critical illness polyneuropathy. J Neurol Sci 159:186, 1998.
80. Hund EF, Fogel W, Krieger D, et al: Critical illness polyneuropathy: clinical findings and outcomes of a frequent cause of neuromuscular weaning failure. Crit Care Med 24:1328, 1996.
81. White JE, Bullock RE, Hudgson P, et al: Phrenic neuropathy in association with diabetes. Diabet Med 9:954, 1992.
82. Zifko U, Auinger M, Albrecht G, et al: Phrenic neuropathy in chronic renal failure. Thorax 50:793, 1995.
83. Bansal SK, Haldar N, Dhand UK, et al: Phrenic neuropathy in arsenic poisoning. Chest 100:878, 1991.
84. Beydoun SR, Copeland D: Bilateral phrenic neuropathy as a presenting feature of multifocal motor neuropathy with conduction block. Muscle Nerve 23:556, 2000.
85. Mohan U, Misra VP, Britto J, et al: Inherited early onset severe axonal polyneuropathy with respiratory failure and autonomic involvement. Neuromuscul Disord 11:395, 2001.
86. Dyck PJ, Litchy WJ, Minnerath S, et al: Hereditary motor and sensory neuropathy with diaphragm and vocal cord paresis. Ann Neurol 35:608, 1994.
87. Thomas CE, Mayer SA, Gungor Y, et al: Myasthenic crisis: clinical features, mortality, complications, and risk factors for prolonged intubation. Neurology 48:1253, 1997.
88. Sanders DB, El Salem K, Massey JM, et al: Clinical aspects of MuSK antibody positive seronegative MG. Neurology 60:1978, 2003.
89. Beydoun SR: Delayed diagnosis of Lambert-Eaton myasthenic syndrome in a patient presenting with recurrent refractory respiratory failure. Muscle Nerve 17:689, 1994.
90. Nicolle MW, Stewart DJ, Remtulla H, et al: Lambert-Eaton myasthenic syndrome presenting with severe respiratory failure. Muscle Nerve 19:1328, 1996.
91. Zifko UA, Hahn AF, Remtulla H, et al: Central and peripheral respiratory electrophysiological studies in myotonic dystrophy. Brain 119:1911, 1996.
92. Brunner HG, Spaans F, Smeets HJ, et al: Genetic linkage with chromosome 19 but not chromosome 17 in a family with myotonic dystrophy associated with hereditary motor and sensory neuropathy. Neurology 41:80, 1991.
93. von Giesen HJ, Stoll G, Koch MC, et al: Mixed axonal-demyelinating polyneuropathy as predominant manifestation of myotonic dystrophy. Muscle Nerve 17:701, 1994.

94. Lacomis D, Zochodne DW, Bird SJ: Critical illness myopathy. Muscle Nerve 23:1785, 2000.
95. Bolton CF: Critical illness polyneuropathy and myopathy. Crit Care Med 29:2388, 2001.
96. Zeman AZ, Dick DJ, Anderson JR, et al: Multicore myopathy presenting in adulthood with respiratory failure. Muscle Nerve 20:367, 1997.
97. Clawson K, Oddis CV: Adult respiratory distress syndrome in polymyositis patients with the anti-Jo-1 antibody. Arthritis Rheum 38:1519, 1995.
98. Lahrmann H, Grisold W, Zifko UA: Respiratory muscle involvement in dermatomyositis. Neuromusc Disord 7:453, 1997.
99. Mellies U, Ragette R, Schwake C, et al: Sleep-disordered breathing and respiratory failure in acid maltase deficiency. Neurology 57:1290, 2001.
100. Decramer M, Lacquet LM, Fagard R, et al: Corticosteroids contribute to muscle weakness in chronic airflow obstruction. Am J Respir Crit Care Med 150:11, 1994.
101. Altobellis SS, Roy TM, Joyce BW, et al: Respiratory failure and death from HIV-associated myopathy. J Ky Med Assoc 90:174, 1992.
102. Barohn RJ, Clanton T, Sahenk Z, et al: Recurrent respiratory insufficiency and depressed ventilatory drive complicating mitochondrial myopathies. Neurology 40:103, 1990.
103. Joutel A, Moulonguet A, Demaugre F, et al: Type II carnitine palmitoyl transferase deficiency complicated by acute respiratory failure. Rev Neurol (Paris) 149:797, 1993.
104. Maschka DA, Bauman NM, McCray Jr PB, et al: A classification scheme for paradoxical vocal cord motion. Laryngoscope 107:1429, 1997.
105. Bradley TD, McNicholas WT, Rutherford R, et al: Clinical and physiologic heterogeneity of the central sleep apnea syndrome. Am Rev Respir Dis 134:217, 1986.
106. Attarian H: Sleep and neuromuscular disorders. Sleep Med 1:3, 2000.
107. Sivak ED, Shefner JM, Sexton J: Neuromuscular disease and hypoventilation. Curr Opin Pulm Med 5:355, 1999.
108. Javaheri S, Parker TJ, Wexler L, et al: Occult sleep-disordered breathing in stable congestive heart failure. Ann Intern Med 122:487, 1995.
109. Miyamoto O, Auer RN: Hypoxia, hyperoxia, ischemia, and brain necrosis. Neurology 54:362, 2000.
110. Pearigen P, Gwinn R, Simon RP: The effects in vivo of hypoxia on brain injury. Brain Res 725:184, 1996.
111. Tang CM, Dichter M, Morad M: Modulation of the *N*-methyl-D-aspartate channel by extracellular H^+. Proc Natl Acad Sci USA 87:6445, 1990.
112. Placidi F, Diomedi M, Cupini LM, et al: Impairment of daytime cerebrovascular reactivity in patients with obstructive sleep apnoea syndrome. J Sleep Res 7:288, 1998.
113. Palomaki H, Partinen M, Juvela S, et al: Snoring as a risk factor for sleep-related brain infarction. Stroke 20:1311, 1989.
114. Wessendorf TE, Teschler H, Wang YM, et al: Sleep-disordered breathing among patients with first-ever stroke. J Neurol 247:41, 2000.
115. Dyken ME, Somers VK, Yamada T, et al: Investigating the relationship between stroke and obstructive sleep apnea. Stroke 27:401, 1996.
116. Bassetti C, Aldrich MS: Sleep apnea in acute cerebrovascular diseases: final report on 128 patients. Sleep 22:217, 1999.
117. Bassetti C, Aldrich MS, Chervin RD, et al: Sleep apnea in patients with transient ischemic attack and stroke: a prospective study of 59 patients. Neurology 47:1167, 1996.
118. Arzt M, Young T, Finn L, et al: Association of sleep-disordered breathing and the occurrence of stroke. Am J Respir Crit Care Med 172:1447, 2005.
119. Rains JC, Poceta JS: Sleep-related headaches. Neurol Clin 30:1285, 2012.
120. Aldrich MS, Chauncey JB: Are morning headaches part of obstructive sleep apnea syndrome? Arch Intern Med 150:1265, 1990.
121. Poceta JS, Dalessio DJ: Identification and treatment of sleep apnea in patients with chronic headache. Headache 35:586, 1995.
122. Ulfberg J, Carter N, Talback M, et al: Headache, snoring and sleep apnoea. J Neurol 243:621, 1996.
123. Bedard MA, Montplaisir J, Richer F, et al: Obstructive sleep apnea syndrome: pathogenesis of neuropsychological deficits. J Clin Exp Neuropsychol 13:950, 1991.
124. Naegele B, Thouvard V, Pepin JL, et al: Deficits of cognitive executive functions in patients with sleep apnea syndrome. Sleep 18:43, 1995.
125. Redline S, Strauss ME, Adams N, et al: Neuropsychological function in mild sleep-disordered breathing. Sleep 20:160, 1997.
126. Bedard MA, Montplaisir J, Malo J, et al: Persistent neuropsychological deficits and vigilance impairment in sleep apnea syndrome after treatment with continuous positive airways pressure (CPAP). J Clin Exp Neuropsychol 15:330, 1993.

CHAPTER

2

Neurologic Complications of Aortic Disease and Surgery

DOUGLAS S. GOODIN

The aorta is the main conduit through which the heart supplies blood to the body, including the brain, brainstem, and spinal cord. In addition, this vessel is situated close to important neural structures. In consequence, both disease of the aorta and operations on it may have profound but variable effects on nervous system function. Often the neurologic syndrome produced by aortic disease or surgery depends more on the part of the aorta involved than on the nature of the pathologic process itself. For example, either syphilis or atherosclerosis may produce symptoms of cerebral ischemia if the disease affects the aortic arch or of spinal cord ischemia if the pathologic process is in the descending thoracic aorta. Even when the nature of the pathologic process is important in determining the resultant neurologic syndrome, several diseases may result in the same pathologic process. Thus, atherosclerosis, infection, inflammation, and trauma may each result in the formation of aortic aneurysms; similarly, coarctation of the aorta may be congenital, a result of Takayasu arteritis, or a sequela of radiation exposure during childhood.

The initial focus of this chapter is on the three major areas of neurologic dysfunction resulting from aortic disease and surgery: spinal cord ischemia, cerebral ischemia, and peripheral neuropathy. Specific conditions that merit special consideration are then discussed individually. The normal anatomic relationships are also considered in order to provide insight into the pathogenesis of the resulting neurologic syndromes.[1–5]

CLINICAL NEUROLOGIC SYNDROMES DUE TO AORTIC PATHOLOGY

Aortic disease may produce a variety of neurologic syndromes. The specific syndrome depends to a large extent on the site of involvement along the aorta.

Aminoff's Neurology and General Medicine, Fifth Edition.

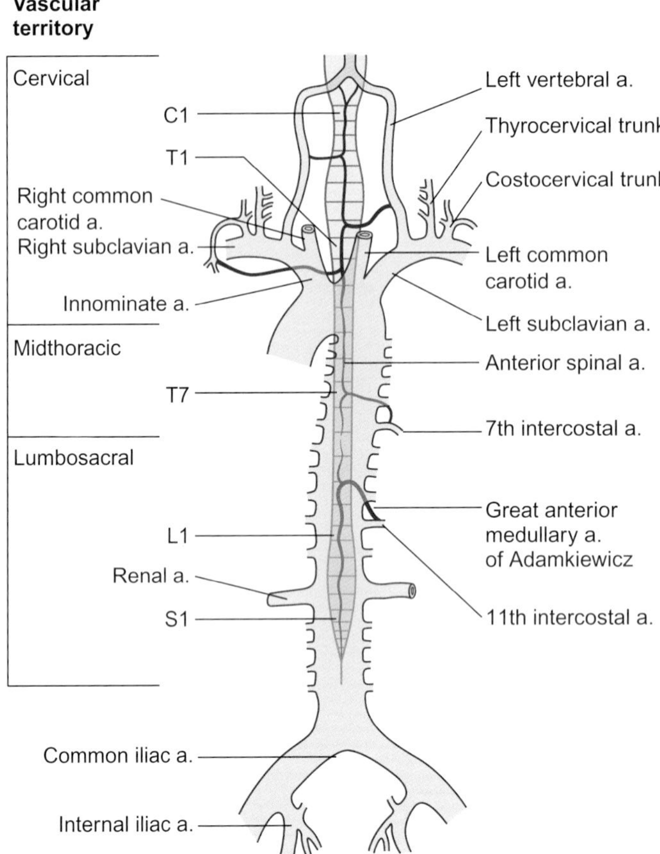

FIGURE 2-1 ▪ Extraspinal contributions to the anterior spinal arteries showing the three arterial territories. In the cervical region, an average of three arteries (derived from the vertebral arteries and the costocervical trunk) supply the anterior spinal artery. The anterior spinal artery is narrowest in the midthoracic region, often being difficult to distinguish from other small arteries on the anterior surface of the cord; occasionally it is discontinuous with the anterior spinal artery above and below. In addition, this region is often supplied by only a single small radiculomedullary vessel. The lumbosacral territory is supplied by a single large artery, the great anterior medullary artery of Adamkiewicz, which turns abruptly caudal after joining the anterior spinal artery. If it gives off an ascending branch, that branch is usually a much smaller vessel. This artery is usually the most caudal of the anterior radiculomedullary arteries, but when it follows a relatively high thoracic root, there is often a small lumbar radiculomedullary artery below. In this and subsequent illustrations, *a* indicates artery; *m*, muscle; *n*, nerve.

Spinal Cord Ischemia

Anatomy

Embryologic Development

During embryologic development, primitive blood vessels arise along the spinal nerve roots bilaterally and at each segmental level. Each of these segmental vessels then divides into anterior and posterior branches, which ramify extensively on the surfaces of the developing spinal cord. As development proceeds, most of these vessels regress and a few enlarge, so that by birth, the blood supply to the spinal cord depends on a small but highly variable number of persisting segmental vessels (Fig. 2-1). In the thoracic region, where the aorta is situated to the left of the midline, the persisting vessels entering the spinal canal are those from the left in 70 to 80 percent of cases.[1–3]

Anterior Spinal Artery

The anterior spinal artery is formed rostrally from paired branches of the intracranial vertebral arteries that descend from the level of the medulla (Fig. 2-1). These two arteries fuse to form a single anterior spinal artery that overlies the anterior longitudinal fissure of the spinal cord. This artery is joined at different levels by anterior radiculomedullary arteries, which are branches of certain segmental vessels

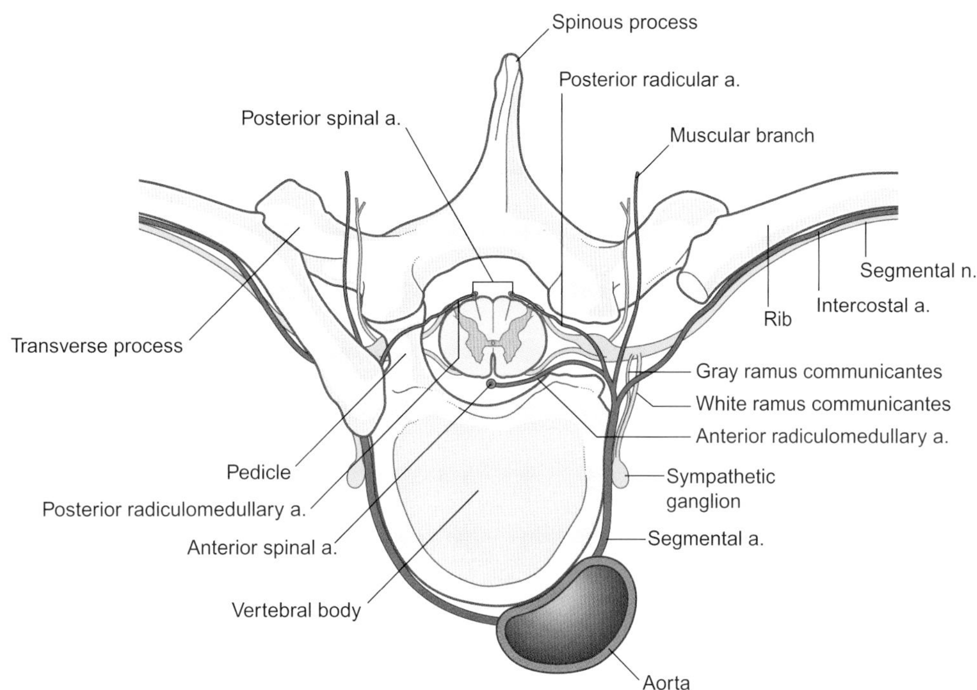

FIGURE 2-2 ■ Anatomy of the spinal cord circulation, showing the relationship of the segmental arteries and their branches to the spinal canal and cord. The left rib and the left pedicle of the vertebra have been cut away to show the underlying vascular and neural structures.

(Fig. 2-2). The number of these vessels is variable among individuals, ranging from 2 to 17, although 85 percent of individuals have between 4 and 7.[1]

The anterior spinal artery in the region that includes the cervical enlargement (C1 to T3) is particularly well supplied, receiving contributions from an average of three segmental vessels. One constant artery arises from the costocervical trunk and supplies the lower segments; the others arise from the extracranial vertebral arteries and supply the middle cervical segments. In addition, branches of the vertebral arteries have rich anastomotic connections with other neck vessels, including the occipital artery, deep cervical artery, and ascending cervical artery.

The anterior spinal artery in the midthoracic portion of the cord (T4 to T8) often receives only a single contribution from a small artery located at about T7, most often on the left.[3] The anterior spinal artery has its smallest diameter in this region, and it is sometimes—but not usually[4]—discontinuous with the vessel in more rostral or caudal regions.[1]

The anterior spinal artery in the region of the lumbar enlargement (T9 to the conus medullaris) is, as at the cervical enlargement, richly supplied, deriving its blood supply predominantly from a single large (1.0 to 1.3 mm in diameter) artery, the great anterior medullary artery of Adamkiewicz. This artery almost always accompanies a nerve root between T9 and L2, usually on the left, although rarely it may accompany a root above or below these levels. Identification of the actual location of this great vessel has become an important part of the planning and execution of operations on the aorta such as repair of thoracoabdominal aortic aneurysms. Although digital subtraction angiography has been used for this purpose, the use of contrast-enhanced magnetic resonance angiography has recently been proposed to offer a noninvasive alternative.[6] Caudally, at the conus medullaris, the anterior spinal artery anastomoses with both posterior spinal arteries.

Posterior Spinal Arteries

The paired posterior spinal arteries are formed rostrally from the intracranial portion of the vertebral arteries. They are distinct paired vessels only at their origin, however, and thereafter become intermixed with an anastomotic posterior pial arterial plexus (Fig. 2-3). This plexus is joined at different levels by a variable number (10 to 23) of posterior radiculomedullary vessels that accompany the posterior nerve roots.

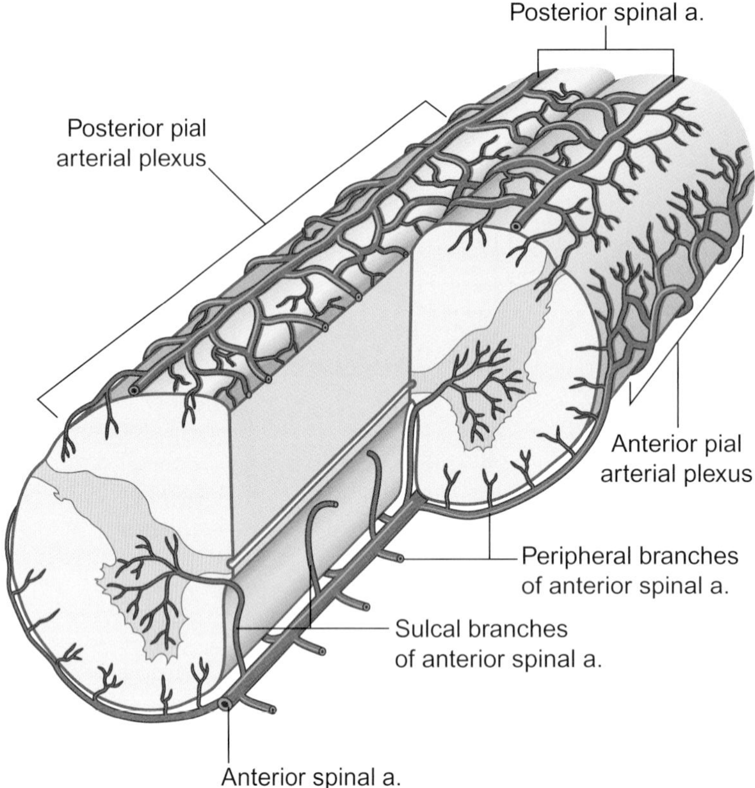

FIGURE 2-3 ■ Vascular anatomy of the spinal cord. The anterior spinal artery gives off both peripheral and sulcal branches. The sulcal branches pass posteriorly, penetrating the anterior longitudinal fissure. On reaching the anterior white commissure, they turn alternately to the right and to the left to supply the gray matter and deep white matter on each side. Occasionally two adjacent vessels pass to the same side, and on other occasions, a common stem vessel bifurcates to supply both sides. Terminal branches of these vessels overlap those from vessels above and below on the same side of the cord. The peripheral branches of the anterior spinal artery pass radially and form an anastomotic network of vessels, the anterior pial arterial plexus, which supplies the anterior and lateral white matter tracts by penetrating branches. The posterior pial arterial plexus is formed as a rich anastomotic network from the paired posterior spinal arteries. Penetrating branches from this plexus supply the posterior horns and posterior funiculi.

Intrinsic Blood Supply of the Spinal Cord

In contrast to the extreme interindividual variability in the extraspinal arteries that supply the spinal cord, the intrinsic blood supply of the cord itself is more consistent. The anterior spinal artery gives off central (sulcal) arteries that pass posteriorly, penetrating the anterior longitudinal fissure and supplying most of the central gray matter and the deep portion of the anterior white matter (Fig. 2-4). The number of these sulcal vessels is variable, with 5 to 8 vessels per centimeter in the cervical region, 2 to 6 vessels per centimeter in the thoracic region, and 5 to 12 vessels per centimeter in the lumbosacral region.

The anterior spinal artery also gives off peripheral arteries that pass radially on the anterior surface of the spinal cord to supply the white matter tracts anteriorly and laterally. These arteries form the anterior pial arterial plexus, which is often poorly anastomotic with its posterior counterpart. The posterior horns and posterior funiculi are supplied by penetrating vessels from the posterior pial arterial plexus.

Ischemic Cord Syndromes

Ischemia of the spinal cord may be produced either by the interruption of blood flow through critical feeding vessels or by aortic hypotension. The resulting neurologic syndrome depends on the location of ischemic lesions along and within the spinal cord, which depends, in turn, on the vascular anatomy discussed previously. A wide variety of pathologic disturbances of the aorta result in spinal cord ischemia. They include both iatrogenic causes, such as surgery and aortography,[7] and intrinsic aortic diseases, such as dissecting and nondissecting aneurysms,[8,9] inflammatory aortitis,[10–14] occlusive atherosclerotic

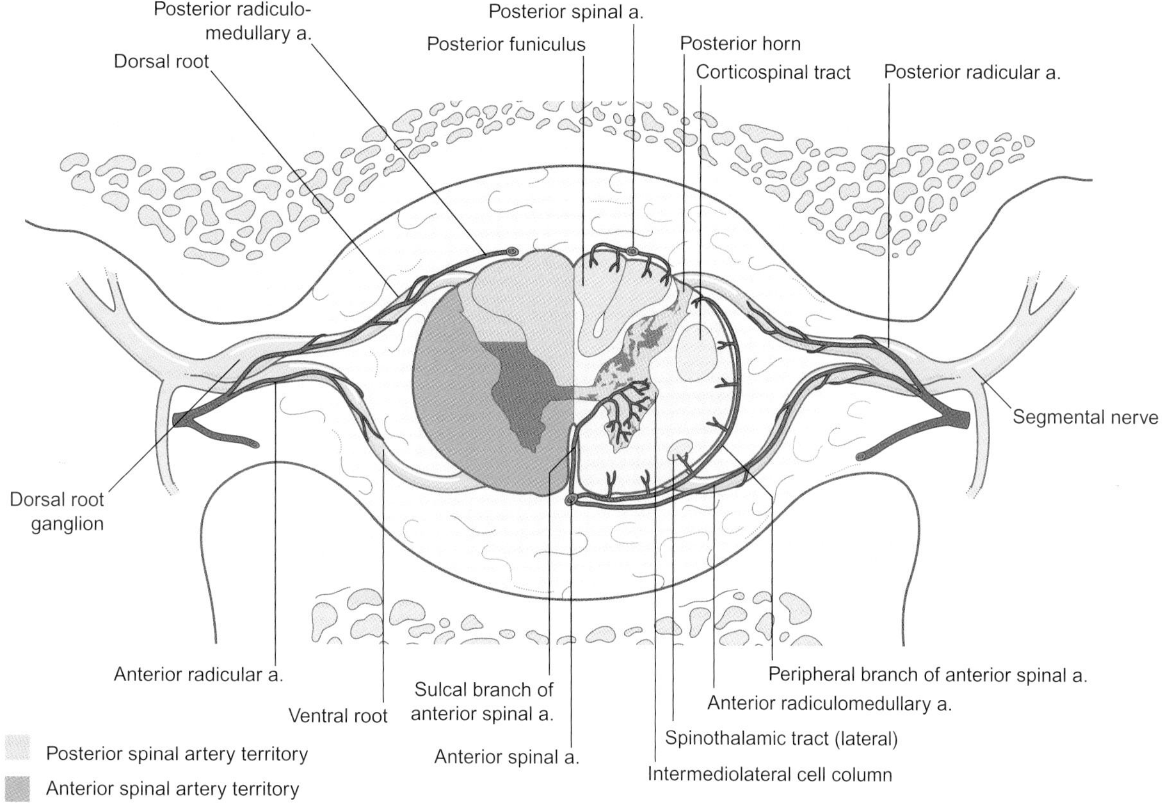

FIGURE 2-4 ■ Intrinsic blood supply of the spinal cord. The vascular territories are depicted on one side of the cord. The territory supplied by the posterior spinal arterial system is indicated. The remainder is supplied by the anterior circulation, with the darker region indicating the area supplied exclusively by the sulcal branches of the anterior spinal artery.

disease,[15,16] infective and noninfective emboli,[17] and congenital coarctation.[18] Spinal cord ischemia is a rare complication of pregnancy,[1] possibly due to aortic compression, which can occur toward the end of gestation.[19]

Some authors have suggested that the midthoracic region (T4 to T8) is particularly vulnerable to ischemia because of the sparseness of vessels feeding the anterior spinal artery in this region and its poor anastomotic connections. Others have stressed the vulnerability of the watershed areas between the three anterior spinal arterial territories. Although the concept is theoretically appealing, documentation of the selective vulnerability of these regions is not completely convincing. For example, a review of 61 case reports with respect to the distribution of ischemic myelopathies resulting from surgery on the aorta does not especially suggest that either of these areas is more vulnerable than other cord segments (Table 2-1).[1] Even when the operation was performed on the thoracic aorta (and thus the proximal clamp was placed above the midthoracic cord feeder), the lumbosacral cord segments were the site of the ischemic damage more often than the supposedly more vulnerable midthoracic segments (Table 2-1). Similarly, the watershed area between these two arterial territories (T8 to T9) does not seem particularly vulnerable. In fact, the

TABLE 2-1 ■ **Influence of Location of Aortic Surgery on the Vascular Territory of Resulting Spinal Cord Ischemia**

Vascular Territory of Ischemia	Location of Surgery: Abdominal Aorta	Location of Surgery: Thoracic Aorta
Cervical region (C1–T3)	0	0
Midthoracic region (T4–T8)	1	14
Lumbosacral region (T9–conus)	25	21

Based on 61 reported cases. (From Goodin DS: Neurologic sequelae of aortic disease and surgery. p. 23. In Aminoff MJ (ed): Neurology and General Medicine. 4th Ed. Churchill Livingstone Elsevier, Philadelphia, 2008, with permission.)

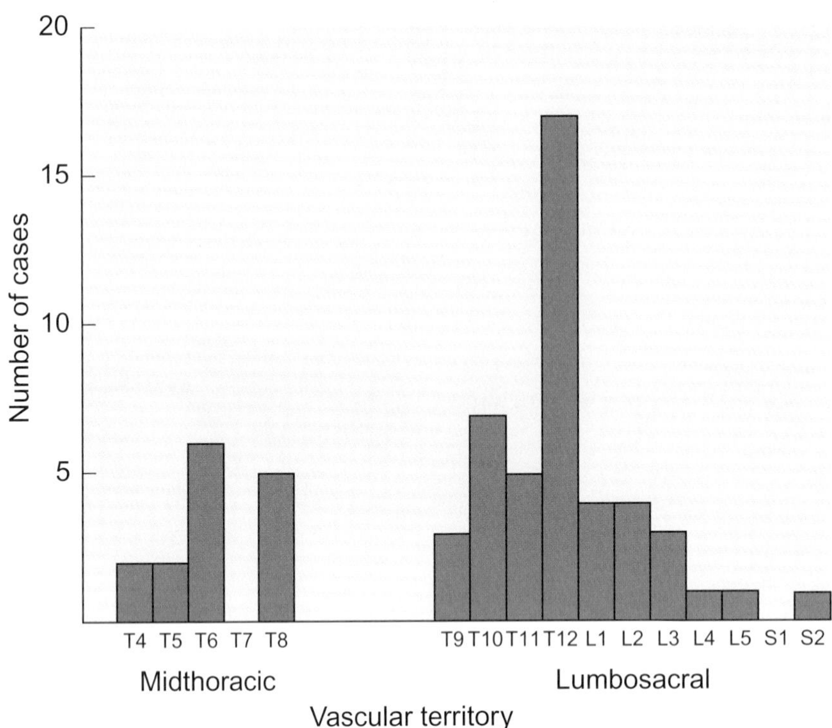

FIGURE 2-5 ■ Upper segmental level of spinal cord involvement in 61 cases of spinal cord ischemia after surgery on the aorta (based on previously published reports).

most frequently affected cord segment within each vascular territory in these 61 cases was centrally placed—T6 in the midthoracic territory and T12 in the lumbosacral territory—rather than at the borders, as might be anticipated with watershed vulnerability (Fig. 2-5).

Moreover, of the 25 cases of spinal cord infarction in an unselected autopsy series of 300 cases, two-thirds were in cervical cord segments[1]; the most commonly affected segment was C6. Such a distribution would be unexpected if either the midthoracic or the watershed area was particularly vulnerable. Perhaps relating to such observations, it has been found that, contrary to earlier reports, the anterior spinal artery is continuous along its length without interruption in all 51 cadavers studied.[4] If this observation can be generalized, it may be the case that the poorly vascularized thoracic cord, which has much less gray matter than the cervical and lumbar enlargements, actually matches its sparse blood supply with its reduced metabolic requirements.[11,20]

The site of aortic disease also plays an important role in the location of the lesion along the spinal cord. For example, distal aortic occlusion often presents with lumbosacral involvement,[1,15] whereas dissecting aneurysm of the thoracic aorta commonly presents with infarction in the midthoracic region.[1,21,22] Similarly, cord ischemia following surgery on the abdominal aorta is essentially confined to the lumbosacral territory, whereas surgery on the thoracic aorta not infrequently involves the midthoracic segments (Table 2-1). Regardless of the pathologic process affecting the aorta, however, it generally involves the suprarenal portion if there is cord ischemia[23] because the important radiculomedullary arteries usually originate above the origin of the renal arteries.

Anterior Spinal Artery Syndrome

Ischemic injury of the spinal cord at a particular segmental level may present with a complete transverse myelopathy. Within the spinal cord, however, there are certain vascular territories that can be affected selectively.[24] In particular, the territory of the anterior spinal artery, especially its sulcal branch, is prone to ischemic injury.[24] This increased vulnerability probably relates to two factors. First, the anterior circulation receives a much smaller number of feeding vessels than the posterior circulation. Second, the posterior circulation is a network of anastomotic channels[1] and therefore probably provides better collateral flow than the single and sometimes narrowed anterior artery. The relative constancy of the resulting syndrome presumably reflects the relative constancy of the intrinsic vascular anatomy of the cord.[25,26]

As mentioned earlier, the anterior spinal artery supplies blood to much of the spinal gray matter and to the tracts in the anterior and lateral white matter. Ischemia in this arterial territory therefore gives rise to a syndrome of diminished pain and temperature sensibility with preservation of vibratory and joint position sense. Weakness (either paraparesis or quadriparesis, depending on the segments involved) occurs below the level of the lesion and may be associated with other evidence of upper motor neuron involvement, such as Babinski signs, spasticity, and hyperreflexia. Bowel and bladder functions are affected, owing to interruption of suprasegmental pathways. Segmental gray matter involvement may also lead to lower motor neuron deficits and depressed tendon reflexes at the level of the lesion. Thus, a lesion in the cervical cord may produce flaccid areflexic paralysis with amyotrophy in the upper extremities, spastic paralysis in the lower extremities, and dissociated sensory loss in all limbs. In contrast, a lesion in the thoracic cord typically presents with only spastic paraplegia and dissociated sensory loss in the legs. The syndrome usually comes on abruptly, although occasionally it is more insidious and progressive. Occasionally, also, a transverse myelopathy can result from ischemia to the spinal cord.[24]

Motor Neuron Disease

On occasion, diseases of the aorta (e.g., dissecting aneurysms or atherosclerosis) that interfere with the blood supply to the anterior spinal artery result in more restricted cord ischemia, perhaps because of better anastomotic connections between the anterior and the posterior pial arterial plexuses in some individuals or because of greater vulnerability of the anterior horn cells with their greater metabolic activity. The ischemic injury in these circumstances is limited to the gray matter supplied by the sulcal branches (Fig. 2-6). Clinical impairment is then confined to the motor system and is associated with amyotrophy. When the onset is abrupt,[27] the ischemic nature of the lesion usually is apparent, but when the onset is more gradual, and especially when pyramidal signs are also present, it may mimic

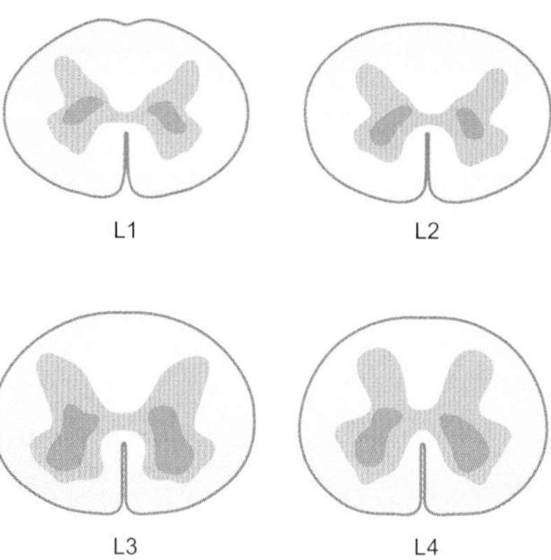

FIGURE 2-6 ▪ Area of infarction within the spinal cord over four adjacent spinal segments in a patient reported by Herrick and Mills (Herrick MK, Mills PE: Infarction of spinal cord. Two cases of selective gray matter involvement secondary to asymptomatic aortic disease. Arch Neurol 24:228, 1971). The infarction was extensive but limited to the gray matter, particularly the anterior horns.

other diseases, such as amyotrophic lateral sclerosis or spinal cord tumors.

Posterior Spinal Artery Syndrome

In contrast to the anterior spinal artery syndrome, selective ischemia of the posterior circulation, characterized by prominent loss of posterior column function with relative sparing of other functions, is rarely recognized clinically and only occasionally reported pathologically.[5,15,28] For example, in two reviews of a total of 63 cases of nonsurgical spinal cord ischemia, only 7 (9%) had posterior spinal artery patterns.[5,24] The relative infrequency of this syndrome presumably relates to the more abundant feeding vessels and better anastomotic connections in this arterial system compared to the anterior spinal artery.

Unilateral Cord Syndromes

In some cases, the area of ischemic damage can be confined to only a small portion of the spinal cord. For example, in the reviews cited previously,[5,24] 22 (35%) of the patients with nonsurgical spinal cord ischemia had unilateral syndromes involving either the anterior or posterior aspects of the spinal cord.

Intermittent Claudication

Intermittent claudication (limping) refers to a condition in which a patient experiences difficulty in walking that is brought about by use of the lower extremities. The evolution of concepts of intermittent claudication is of historical interest and is described elsewhere.[1] In brief, Charcot initially described this syndrome in 1858 and related it to occlusive peripheral vascular disease in the lower extremities. In 1906, Dejerine distinguished claudication caused by ischemia of the leg muscles from that caused by ischemia of the spinal cord. In the latter condition, the arterial pulses in the legs tend to be preserved, pain tends to be dysesthetic or paresthetic in quality and may not occur, and neurologic signs are frequently present, especially after exercise. In 1961, Blau and Logue identified another form of neurogenic claudication caused by ischemia or compression of the cauda equina and resulting from a narrowed lumbosacral canal (either congenital or due to degenerative disease). This condition is similar to that produced by ischemia of the spinal cord; however, the sensory complaints tend to have a more radicular distribution, and signs of cord involvement (e.g., Babinski signs) are not present.

The clinical distinction between various types of claudication, particularly between the two neurogenic varieties, is sometimes difficult. The cauda equina variety, however, is far more common than the spinal cord form.[1,29] Intermittent spinal cord ischemia, when it occurs, can be associated with intrinsic diseases of the aorta, such as coarctation or atherosclerotic occlusive disease although, more commonly, it is due to degenerative disease of the cervical and thoracic spine.[30] Bony erosion through vertebral bodies from an abdominal aortic aneurysm with direct compression of the spinal nerve roots has also been reported to produce intermittent neurologic symptoms.[1] The clinical details of the single reported case, however, are not sufficient to determine whether the symptoms resemble those of intermittent claudication.

Cerebral Ischemia

ANATOMY

The aortic arch gives rise to all the major vessels that provide blood to the brain, brainstem, and cervical spinal cord (Fig. 2-7). The first major branch is the innominate (brachiocephalic) artery, which subsequently divides into the right common carotid and right subclavian arteries. The latter artery subsequently gives rise to the right vertebral artery, which ascends through the foramina of the transverse processes of the upper six cervical vertebrae to join with its counterpart on the left and form the basilar artery. The basilar artery provides blood to the posterior fossa and posterior regions of the cerebral hemispheres. The second major branch of the aortic arch is the left common carotid artery, and the third is the left subclavian artery, which, in turn, gives rise to the left vertebral artery.

STROKES AND TRANSIENT ISCHEMIC ATTACKS

Diseases of the aortic arch, such as atherosclerosis, aneurysms, and aortitis as well as surgery on this segment of the aorta, may give rise to symptoms of cerebrovascular insufficiency, such as strokes or transient ischemic attacks (TIAs).[11,22,31–33] A young woman has even been reported with a stroke secondary to an occlusion of the aorta that was associated with the use of birth control pills and recurrent venous thromboses.[1] Cerebral ischemia is produced either by occlusion of a major vessel or by embolization of atheromatous or other material to more distal arteries. The resulting neurologic syndromes are not specific for any disease process but depend on the location and duration of the vascular occlusion.

Atherosclerosis

Atherosclerosis of the aortic arch and its branches, compared with atherosclerosis at the origin of the internal carotid artery, is an infrequent cause of stroke or TIAs, probably for two reasons. First, atherosclerosis is much less common in this location than at the carotid bifurcation (Table 2-2). Second, the anastomotic connections between the major vessels in the neck are extensive, and an occlusion at their origin from the aortic arch is therefore less likely to be associated with symptoms of ischemia than a more peripheral obstruction.

Transient Emboligenic Aortoarteritis

Transient emboligenic aortoarteritis has been reported by Wickremasinghe and colleagues to be a cause of stroke in young patients. They described 10 patients (aged 16 to 36 years), all of whom had presented with pathologically verified thromboembolic strokes, and 3 of whom had a history of TIAs preceding the event by as much as 4 years.[34] All these patients had both active and healed inflammatory lesions of the central elastic arteries, such as the

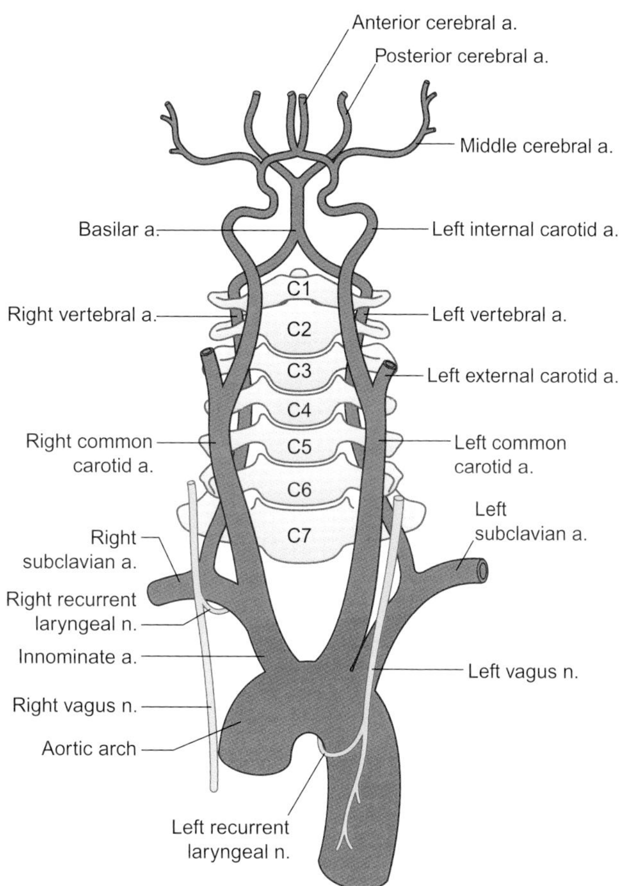

FIGURE 2-7 ■ Vascular anatomy of the aortic arch and its branches.

TABLE 2-2 ■ Distribution of Atherosclerosis in the Aorta and Its Branches

Location	Number of Lesions
External carotid artery	9
Internal carotid artery	256
Common carotid artery	16
Innominate artery	16
Subclavian artery	29
Vertebral artery	55
Aortoiliac region	952
Femoropopliteal region	772

Based on data from Crawford ES, DeBakey ME, Cooley DA, et al: Surgical considerations of aneurysms and atherosclerotic occlusive lesions of the aorta and major arteries. Postgrad Med 29:151, 1961.

aorta, innominate, common carotid, and proximal subclavian arteries. Active lesions were small (200 to 300 μm in diameter) and associated with a mural thrombus on the intimal surface. Healed lesions usually were associated with fibrous plaques but not with a mural thrombus. More peripheral arteries supplying the brain were normal. This condition seems to be distinct from segmental aortitis of the Takayasu type. Clinically it is an acute, intermittent disorder with an approximately equal sex incidence, whereas Takayasu disease is more chronic and has a strong female predominance. The systemic symptoms of Takayasu disease are absent, and occlusion of the central arteries does not occur in this condition.

Subclavian (Cerebral) Steal

Disease of the aortic arch may result in occlusion of either the innominate artery or the left subclavian artery proximal to the origin of the vertebral artery. This, in turn, may result in the reversal of the usual cephalad direction of blood flow in the ipsilateral vertebral artery (Fig. 2-8), depending on individual variations in the collateral circulation, and may result in ischemia in the posterior cerebral circulation.[35] In some patients, this is particularly evident when the metabolic demand (and therefore the

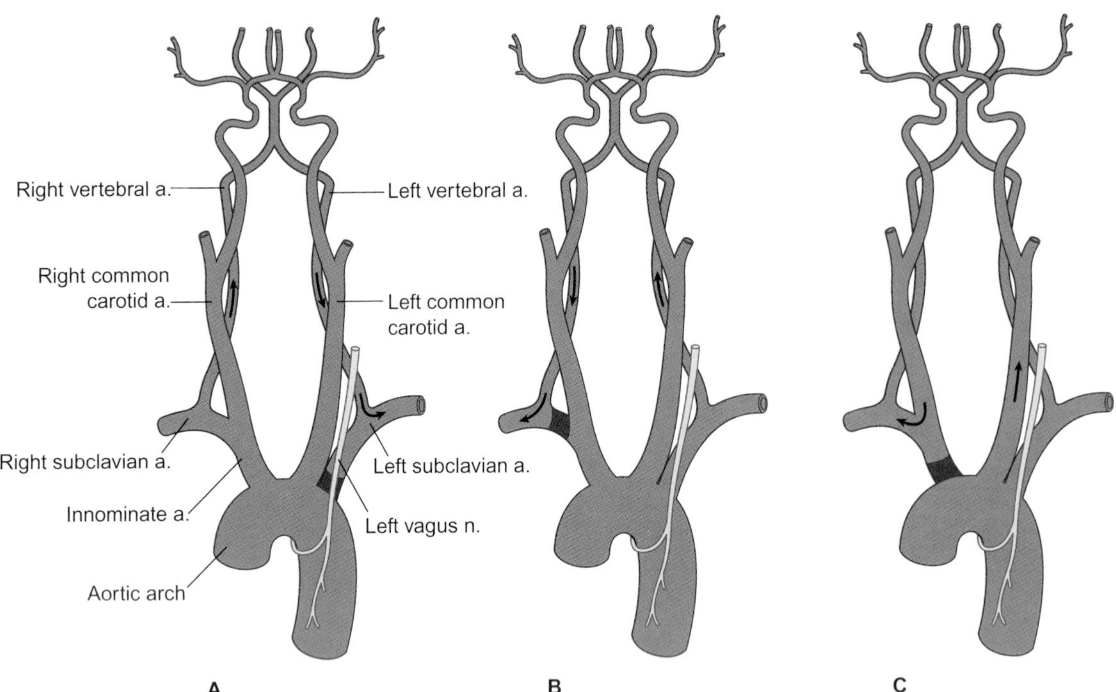

FIGURE 2-8 ■ Mechanisms producing subclavian steal syndrome in diseases of the aortic arch and its branches. **A**, Obstruction of the left subclavian artery at its origin, resulting in reversal of blood flow in the left vertebral artery. **B**, Obstruction of the right subclavian artery distal to the takeoff of the right common carotid artery, resulting in reversal of blood flow in the right vertebral artery. **C**, Obstruction of the innominate artery at its origin, producing reversal of blood flow in the right common carotid artery.

blood flow) of the affected arm is increased during exercise. If the innominate artery is blocked proximally, it may also cause a reversal of blood flow in the right common carotid artery, resulting in anterior circulation ischemia (Fig. 2-8).

Killen and colleagues reviewed the clinical features of a series of patients with demonstrated reversals of arterial blood flow in a vertebral artery (i.e., with flow from the vertebral artery into the ipsilateral subclavian artery).[36] The left subclavian artery was affected more than twice as often as the right subclavian and innominate arteries combined, probably as a result of the more frequent involvement of this artery by atherosclerosis (Table 2-2). Men were affected three times as often as women, probably reflecting the greater prevalence of atherosclerosis in men. Of the 87 patients in this series with symptoms that were adequately described, 75 (86%) had symptoms referable to the central nervous system (CNS). These symptoms were usually transient, lasting seconds to a few minutes, although the deficits were sometimes permanent. The neurologic manifestations of steal were varied but most frequently included motor difficulties, vertigo, visual deficits, or syncope. Ischemic symptoms in the arms occurred in only a few patients, and precipitation of CNS symptoms by exercise of the arm ipsilateral to the occlusion was uncommon. Although reconstructive surgery relieved symptoms in most patients in this series,[36] it was the frequent failure of surgery to correct such nonspecific symptoms that led to a reassessment of the importance of cerebral steal.[37] Thus, when noninvasive techniques such as Doppler ultrasonography have been used to define the direction of blood flow in the great vessels in a large spectrum of patients with vascular disease, the majority (50 to 75%) of patients with documented subclavian steal are found to be asymptomatic, even when the steal is bilateral.[1,35] When symptoms do occur, they are suggestive of transient vertebrobasilar insufficiency in only 7 to 37 percent of patients with steal; the occurrence of infarcts in this vascular territory is distinctly rare.[1] For this reason, a review of the topic led to the conclusion that subclavian steal is actually a marker of generalized atherosclerotic disease and that it is rarely a cause for symptoms of cerebral ischemia.[37]

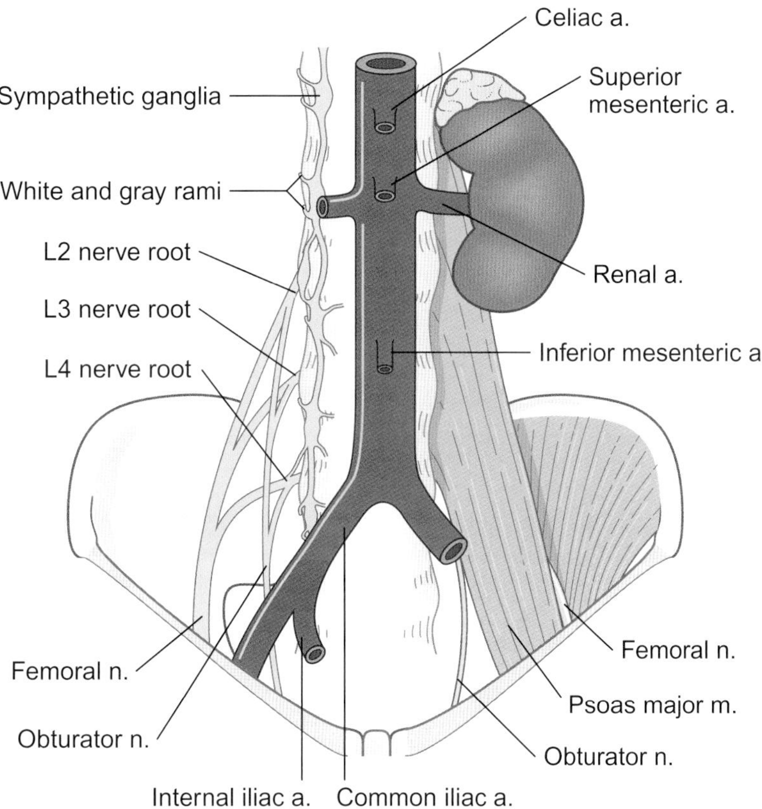

FIGURE 2-9 ■ Anatomy of the abdominal aorta showing its relationship to the femoral and obturator nerves, which form within the psoas muscle from branches of the L2, L3, and L4 segmental nerves.

Nevertheless, a related syndrome, the coronary subclavian steal syndrome, seems well documented.[38–41] This syndrome consists of angina (with or without posterior circulation symptoms such as vertigo) induced by upper limb exercise. It follows a coronary artery bypass graft using the left internal mammary artery in the setting of a hemodynamically significant subclavian stenosis.[38–41]

Peripheral Neuropathy

The peripheral nervous system is sometimes affected by aortic disease or surgery. The syndromes produced may be the presenting manifestations of aortic disease and may mimic less life-threatening conditions.

Mononeuropathies

Left Recurrent Laryngeal Nerve

The left recurrent laryngeal nerve descends in the neck as part of the vagus nerve and wraps around the aortic arch just distal to the ligamentum arteriosum (Fig. 2-7) before reascending in the neck to innervate all the laryngeal muscles on the left side except the cricothyroideus. It may be compressed by disease of the aortic arch, such as dissecting and nondissecting aneurysms or aneurysmal dilatation proximal to a coarctation of the aorta.[37] The resulting hoarse, low-pitched voice may be one of the earliest presenting symptoms of these conditions, although it is often overshadowed by other symptoms or signs, such as chest pain, shortness of breath, congestive heart failure, or hypertension.[42]

Femoral Nerve

The femoral nerve arises from the nerve roots of L2, L3, and L4. It forms within the belly of the psoas muscle and then exits on its lateral aspect to innervate the quadriceps femoris, iliacus, pectineus, and sartorius muscles and the skin of the anterior thigh and medial aspect of the leg. The nerve is located considerably lateral to the aorta (Fig. 2-9) and hence is rarely involved by direct compression. It

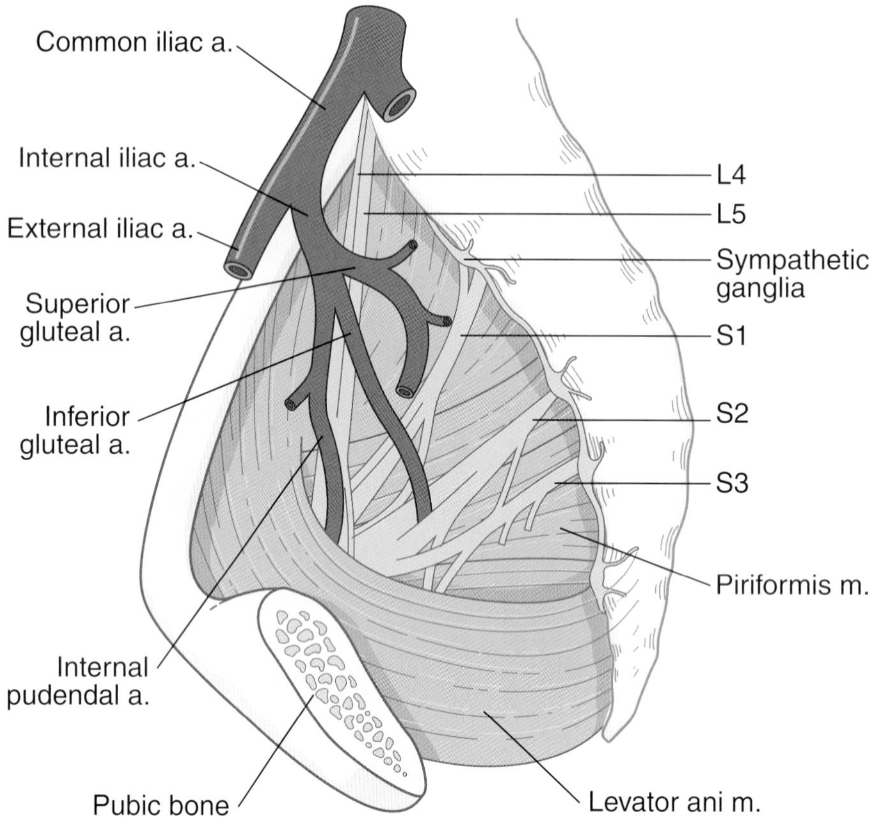

FIGURE 2-10 ■ Anatomy of the terminal branches of the aorta in relationship to the nerve roots that subsequently join to form the sciatic nerve. Aneurysmal dilatation of the abdominal aorta often includes dilatation of these branch vessels, which can compress the nerve roots, particularly the L4, L5, S1, and S2 nerve roots, which lie directly underneath.

may, however, be compressed by a hematoma from a ruptured aortic aneurysm into the psoas muscle and thereby signal a life-threatening condition that requires an urgent operation.[43]

The femoral nerve may also be injured as a consequence of aortic surgery. The mechanism of injury in such cases is presumed to be ischemic and related to poor collateral blood supply to the intrapelvic portions of the femoral nerves.

Obturator Nerve

The obturator nerve also forms within the belly of the psoas muscle by the union of fibers from the L2, L3, and L4 segments, but, in contrast to the femoral nerve, exits medially from this muscle (Fig. 2-9). It innervates the adductors of the leg and the skin on the medial aspect of the thigh. It too is lateral to the aorta and not usually involved by direct compression. Like the femoral nerve (and often together with it), the obturator nerve may be compressed by a hematoma in the psoas muscle.

Radiculopathies

Nerve roots, particularly L4, L5, S1, and S2, which lie almost directly underneath the terminal aorta and iliac arteries (Fig. 2-10), may be directly compressed by an aortic aneurysm in this region. The syndromes produced are typical of radicular disease, with unilateral radiating pain and a radicular pattern to the sensory and motor findings.

Radiculopathies may also be produced by erosion of one or more vertebral bodies by an aortic aneurysm, with consequent compression of the nerve roots in the cauda equina or at the root exit zones. The syndrome produced is not necessarily associated with back pain; it may result in multisegmental involvement on one side or even in paraplegia.[44,45]

Polyneuropathies

Ischemic Monomelic Neuropathy

Ischemic monomelic neuropathy was described in detail by Wilbourn and co-workers, who reported 3 patients (and alluded to another 11) who had a distal "polyneuropathy" in one limb after sudden occlusion of a major vessel.[46] One of their patients had a saddle embolus to the distal aorta that occluded the right common iliac artery, another had a superficial femoral artery occlusion after placement of an intra-aortic balloon pump, and the third had upper-extremity involvement. The syndrome consists of a predominantly sensory neuropathy with a distal gradient. It affects all sensory modalities and is associated with a constant, deep, causalgia-like pain. The symptoms persist for months, even after revascularization or without evidence of ongoing ischemia. The results of nerve conduction studies and needle electromyography suggest an axonal neuropathy. There is no evidence of ischemic muscle injury, such as induration, muscle tenderness, or elevated serum creatine kinase levels. Most recent reports of this condition seem to be as a complication of vascular access for dialysis,[47,48] and the syndrome appears to be quite rare as a manifestation of aortic disease.

Autonomic Neuropathies

Anatomy

The autonomic nerves, particularly the lower thoracic and lumbar sympathetic fibers that lie close to the aorta and its branches, may be injured by disease of or surgery on the aorta. The preganglionic efferent sympathetic nerve fibers originate in the intermediolateral cell column in the spinal cord (Fig. 2-4) and exit segmentally between T1 and L2 with the ventral roots.[49] The sympathetic fibers part company with the segmental nerves through the white rami communicantes (Fig. 2-2), which enter the paravertebral sympathetic ganglia and trunks to form bilateral sympathetic chains; these chains are situated lateral to and parallel with the vertebral column (Fig. 2-11). Some of these fibers synapse on postganglionic neurons in the ganglia of their segmental origin, whereas others ascend or descend in the trunk to different segmental levels before making such synapses. In the lumbosacral and cervical segments, where there are no white rami (i.e., below L2 or above T1), the segmental ganglia receive preganglionic contributions only from cord segments either above them (lumbosacral ganglia) or below them (cervical ganglia).[49] The postganglionic fibers rejoin the segmental nerves through the gray rami communicantes (Fig. 2-2) to provide vasomotor, sudomotor, and pilomotor innervation throughout the body.

Some of the preganglionic fibers, in contrast, do not synapse in the paravertebral ganglia but pass through them to form splanchnic nerves, which then unite in a series of prevertebral ganglia and plexuses (many of which overlie the thoracic and abdominal aorta). These structures, in turn, provide sympathetic innervation to the viscera. The plexus that overlies the aorta in the region of its bifurcation, the superior hypogastric plexus (Fig. 2-11), is responsible (via the inferior hypogastric and other pelvic plexuses) for sympathetic innervation of the pelvic organs, including the prostate, prostatic urethra, bladder, epididymis, vas deferens, seminal vesicles, and penis in men (Fig. 2-12) and the uterus, bladder, fallopian tubes, vagina, and clitoris in women. This plexus is formed by the union of the third and fourth lumbar splanchnic nerves with fibers from the more rostral inferior mesenteric plexus. Its segmental contribution usually derives from T11 to L2.

The visceral afferent fibers accompany the efferent autonomic fibers and pass uninterrupted back through the trunk, ganglia, and white rami to reach their nerve cells of origin in the dorsal root.

Postsympathectomy Neuralgia

Operations on the distal aorta to treat symptomatic aortic disease from atherosclerosis or other causes frequently include intentional sympathectomy as part of the effort to improve blood flow to the legs. This is usually done by dividing the sympathetic chain below the last white ramus at L2, thereby depriving the lower lumbar and sacral ganglia of their preganglionic innervation. Such an operation is often followed by a distinctive pain syndrome, termed *postsympathectomy neuralgia.* The syndrome occurs typically in patients in whom the sympathetic chain is interrupted at L3 by removal of the segmental ganglion. The pain is characterized as deep, boring, nonrhythmic, and nonradiating; onset is abrupt but delayed usually for several days. It is

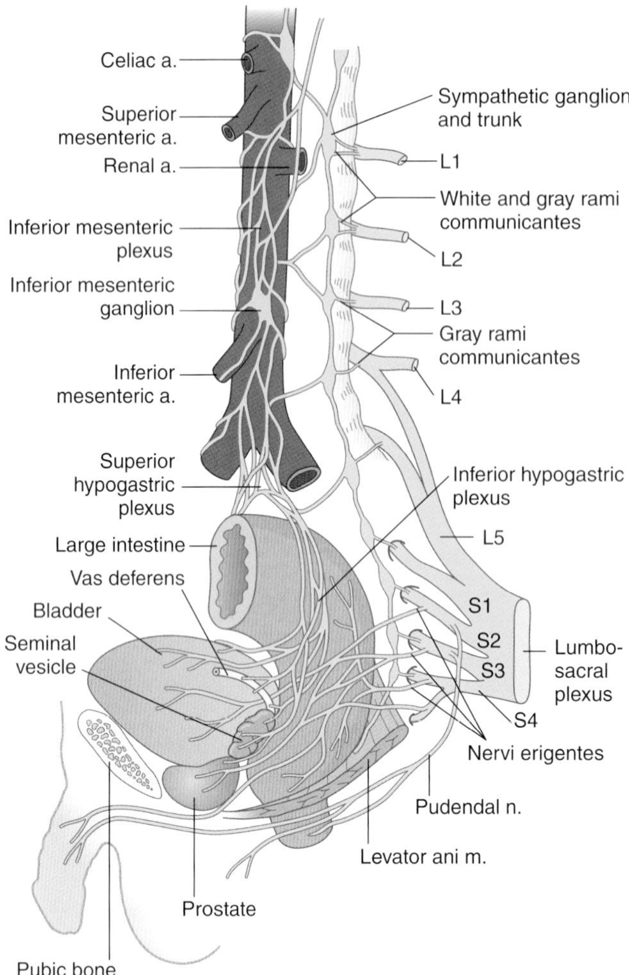

FIGURE 2-11 ■ Anatomy of the terminal aorta and pelvis in the male in relationship to the sympathetic and parasympathetic nerves in the region.

located predominantly in the thigh, either medially or laterally, and is associated with tenderness in the area of pain. The course is self-limited, with an average duration of 3 weeks.

Disorders of Sexual Function

Normal male sexual function has two distinct components. The first, erection, is a response mediated predominantly through the parasympathetic nervous system by the pelvic splanchnic nerves (nervi erigentes) arising from segments S2, S3, and S4 (Fig. 2-12). Activation of these nerves causes vasodilatation and engorgement of the penile musculature and sinuses. The blood supply to the penis is provided by the internal pudendal artery via the internal iliac artery (Fig. 2-10). The sympathetic nervous system, however, must have at least a modifying influence on erection because bilateral sympathectomy may disturb it. By contrast, unilateral sympathectomy seems not to affect sexual function.[50] The second component, ejaculation, can be divided into two phases. The first phase, expulsion of seminal fluid into the prostatic urethra, is a response mediated predominantly by the sympathetic nervous system through the superior hypogastric plexus.The second phase, emission, is produced by the clonic contraction of penile musculature (bulbocavernosus and ischiocavernosus) innervated by somatic (pudendal) nerves (Fig. 2-12).

Male sexual function may be disturbed by aortic disease or surgery.[1,51–55] Female sexual function has not been as well studied in these circumstances, although it seems to be affected to a similar degree as in men.[53] Because the superior hypogastric

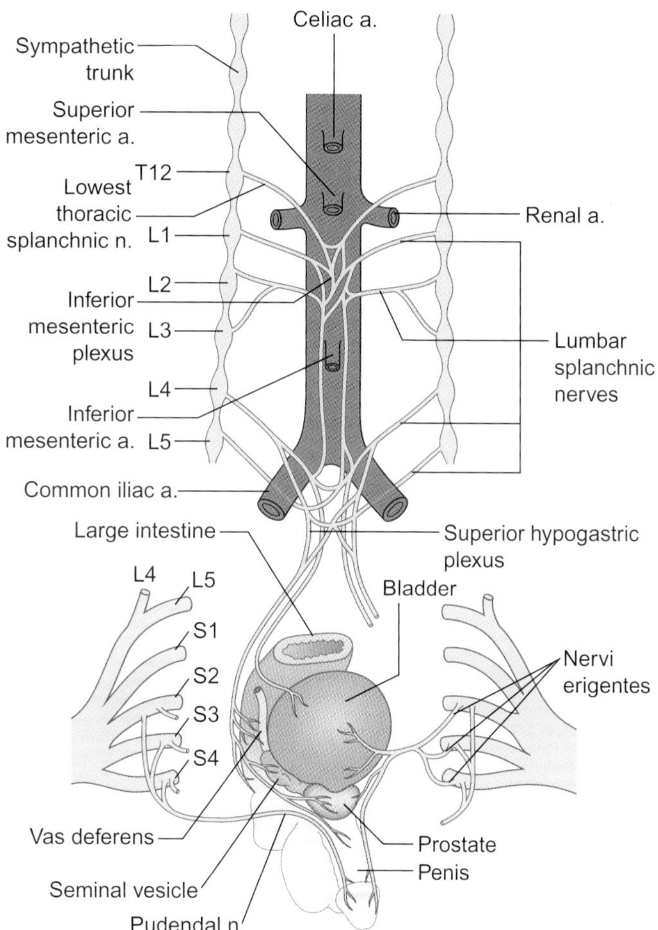

FIGURE 2-12 ■ Distribution of sympathetic *(left)* and parasympathetic *(right)* nerves to the pelvic viscera and sexual organs in the male.

plexus lies close to the aortic bifurcation (Fig. 2-11), most preoperative and postoperative sexual disturbances occur with disease of this portion of the aorta, and most involve ejaculation (Table 2-3). The pelvic splanchnic nerves are not situated near the aorta (Fig. 2-11) and usually are not affected by aortic disease or surgery. Disturbances in erection, however, do occur, possibly because of sympathetic dysfunction, a reduction in blood flow to the internal pudendal artery and penis, or cavernovenous leakage.[51,52] To determine whether blood flow or sympathetic function was more important in this regard, Ohshiro and Kosaki examined the outcome of (1) terminal aortic operations either done traditionally or designed to spare the superior hypogastric plexus and (2) operations that did or did not preserve blood flow in the internal iliac arteries.[56] Their results indicated that preservation of the hypogastric plexus appeared to be more important for maintenance of normal erection and ejaculation than was preservation of blood flow in the internal iliac arteries (Table 2-4). Other authors have also found that modification of operative technique to spare the superior hypogastric plexus considerably improves postoperative sexual function.[1]

Despite the importance of operative technique in preserving sexual function, preservation of blood flow is probably also important. Thus, Nevelsteen and colleagues reported a clear relationship between the occurrence of preoperative impotence and the adequacy of blood flow through the internal iliac arteries.[51] In this study, however, no special attempt was made to improve blood flow in the internal iliac artery during surgery, so that it is unclear whether a different operative approach

TABLE 2-3 ■ Male Sexual Dysfunction in Patients with Disease of or Surgery on the Aorta

Patient Status		Sexual Function	
Preoperative Status (All Patients)	**Number of Patients**	**Normal (%)**	**Abnormal (%)**
Iliac occlusion	22	82	18
Terminal aortic occlusion	10	40	60
Abdominal aortic aneurysm	12	83	17
Postoperative Status*		**Impaired Ejaculation (%)**	**Impaired Erection (%)**
Iliac occlusion	18	28	17
Terminal aortic occlusion	4	75	25
Abdominal aortic aneurysm	10	70	30

*All patients had normal preoperative sexual function.
Based on data from Ohshiro T, Takahashi A, Kosaki G: Sexual function in patients with aortoiliac vascular disorders. Int Surg 67:49, 1982.

TABLE 2-4 ■ Influence of Blood Flow and Sympathetic Function on Male Sexual Function after Abdominal Aortic Operations

		Postoperative Sexual Disturbance	
Parameter	**Number of Patients**	**Ejaculation (%)**	**Erection (%)**
Internal Iliac Blood Flow			
Bilaterally good	29	31	21
Unilaterally good	12	42	8
Bilaterally poor	4	50	25
Type of Surgery			
Classic	32	47	25
Nerve sparing	13	8	8

Based on data from Ohshiro T, Kosaki G: Sexual function after aortoiliac vascular reconstruction. J Cardiovasc Surg 25:47, 1984.

might have been beneficial in restoring postoperative sexual function.

AORTIC DISEASES AND SURGERY

Certain conditions affecting the aorta merit special consideration because of the variety of nervous system syndromes that each can produce.

Aortitis

Injury to the aorta by a variety of infectious, toxic, allergic, or idiopathic causes may produce similar inflammatory pathologic changes in the elastic media (Table 2-5).[10–14] Such aortic damage may lead to neurologic syndromes either primarily through direct involvement of important branch arteries by the pathologic process or secondarily through the development of aneurysms, aortic stenosis, or atherosclerosis. The neurologic syndromes produced either primarily or secondarily by aortitis depend on both the nature and the location of the resulting aortic lesion.

SYPHILITIC AORTITIS

During the prepenicillin era, syphilis was a common cause of aortitis,[1,11,57] although by the 1950s its occurrence had markedly declined.[57] A report in 1958 on the relative occurrence of atherosclerotic and syphilitic thoracic aortic aneurysms showed cases of syphilis outnumbering atherosclerosis by a ratio of 1.3:1.[1] A similar report published in 1982 gave this ratio as 0.13:1.[1] The pathologic process in syphilitic aortitis is almost always in the thoracic aorta,[1,12,57] in contrast to the distribution of atherosclerosis, which is more prevalent in the abdominal aorta (Table 2-2). The aortitis is accompanied by aneurysmal dilatation of the aorta in approximately 40 percent of cases. Rarely, it presents with multiple arterial occlusions and mimics Takayasu arteritis, although patients are generally older than those with Takayasu arteritis and are usually men.

TAKAYASU ARTERITIS

Takayasu arteritis is an idiopathic inflammatory condition affecting the large arteries, particularly the aorta and its branches.[1,31,58,59] The pathogenesis seems to involve cell-mediated autoimmunity, although the responsible antigen is unknown. The onset of disease is typically between the ages of 15 and 30 years, and the condition seems most prevalent in Asian and Hispanic populations.[1,31,58,59] More than 85 percent of affected individuals are women. In the early (prepulseless) phase, the

TABLE 2-5 ■ Causes of Aortitis

Stenosing Aortitis
Takayasu arteritis
Postradiation during infancy
Nonstenosing Aortitis
Syphilis
Mycobacterial infections
Other bacterial infections (e.g., *Salmonella* or *Staphylococcus*)
Human immunodeficiency virus infection
Mycotic aneurysms
Rheumatic fever
Rheumatoid arthritis
Giant cell arteritis
Collagen vascular and other diseases*
Ankylosing spondylitis
Relapsing polychondritis
Reiter syndrome
Behçet disease
Cogan syndrome

*Systemic lupus erythematosus, scleroderma, psoriasis, Crohn disease, and ulcerative colitis.

disease may be characterized by systemic symptoms such as fever, night sweats, weight loss, myalgia, arthralgia, arthritis, and chest pain. In some patients, however, the systemic symptoms are either inconspicuous or absent. The later (pulseless) phase of the disease is characterized by occlusion of the major vessels of the aortic arch, producing symptoms such as Takayasu retinopathy, hypertension (secondary to renal artery stenosis, coarctation, or both), aortic regurgitation, and aortic aneurysms. Symptoms of cerebral ischemia can occur; however, they are typically reported in only a few patients.[58] Nevertheless, a report from South Africa on 272 patients who were diagnosed with Takayasu arteritis, based on the criteria of the American College of Rheumatology, found that 20 percent of the cohort had symptoms of cerebrovascular disease, including TIAs and stroke.[58] In addition, 32 percent of this cohort experienced intermittent claudication of either upper or lower limbs.[58] Seizures and headaches have also been reported but are uncommon. Involvement along the aorta is typically diffuse, although some patients (perhaps as many as 20%) present with symptoms related to more restricted aortic involvement.[11,58,59] The disorder is discussed further in Chapter 50.

Giant Cell Arteritis

Giant cell arteritis (GCA) seems to be a particularly important cause of aortitis in the elderly[1,11,12,60]; although it typically affects medium-sized vessels, as many as one-fourth or more of affected individuals have large-artery involvement.[61] For example, in one series of eight consecutive patients with aortitis, GCA seemed to be its basis in many.[11] Thus, four had definite GCA diagnosed based on their age at onset, the new onset of headaches, and an elevation in erythrocyte sedimentation rate. However, all these patients were older than 57 years, each of the eight had an elevation of some serum inflammatory marker (e.g., increase in C-reactive protein levels, erythrocyte sedimentation rate, or fibrinogen levels), and three had symptoms of polymyalgia rheumatica. In another series of 45 patients undergoing aortic resection and who had microscopic evidence of active noninfectious aortitis, the majority had either unclassifiable aortitis (47%) or GCA (31%), two entities that were histopathologically indistinguishable.[60] The presenting symptoms in patients with GCA or unclassified aortitis are generally nonspecific and include exhaustion, night sweats, weight loss, chest and back pain, headache, fevers of unknown origin, TIAs, and arm claudication.[12,60] Typically, all segments of the aorta (ascending aorta, arch, and descending aorta) are involved in the inflammatory process, although involvement can be more restricted.[11,12] Between 10 and 20 percent of patients with unclassified aortitis or GCA will subsequently develop either dissecting or, more commonly, nondissecting aortic aneurysms.[60,61]

Aortic Aneurysms

Nondissecting Aneurysms

Nondissecting aortic aneurysms can be caused by any pathologic process that weakens the arterial wall, such as inflammation, infection, or atherosclerosis.[1,11,35,42,62,63] In the past, syphilis was an important cause,[64] but at present almost all these aneurysms are caused by atherosclerosis. As a result,

TABLE 2-6 ■ Distribution and Nature of Aortic Aneurysms

Site	Number of Cases
Nondissecting Aneurysms	
Aortic arch	56
Descending thoracic aorta	116
Thoracoabdominal aorta	25
Abdominal aorta	829
Dissecting Aneurysms	
Thoracic aorta	62

Based on data from Crawford ES, DeBakey ME, Cooley DA, et al: Surgical considerations of aneurysms and atherosclerotic occlusive lesions of the aorta and major arteries. Postgrad Med 29:151, 1961.

the distribution of aortic aneurysms essentially parallels the distribution of atherosclerosis within the aorta, with most occurring in the abdominal aorta (Tables 2-2 and 2-6). In a study from Sweden, it was found that the incidence of ruptured abdominal aortic aneurysms in men (but not women) had increased by more than 100 percent between 1971 to 1986 and 2000 to 2004.[65] The reason for this increased incidence is unclear, and it is unknown whether a similar increase has occurred in other parts of the world. Moreover, early experience with the untreated abdominal aortic aneurysms revealed a grave prognosis , with 80 percent of patients dying of rupture within 12 months of the onset of symptoms.[1] Nevertheless, despite the apparently alarming nature of these statistics, a study published in 2012 of 634 patients with abdominal aortic aneurisms reported that the 1- and 3-year survival rates were 98.2 percent and 90.9 percent, respectively.[66] The basis for this marked shift in natural history is unclear.

Disturbances of neurologic function in aortic aneurysms are uncommon, but when they occur, they are variable and depend in part on the location and extent of the lesion. Abdominal aneurysms may result in sexual dysfunction, compressive neuropathies,[1,42–45,51–53] or, rarely, spinal cord ischemic syndromes, including intermittent claudication, asymmetric paraparesis, and paraplegia[62]; descending thoracic aneurysms may produce spinal cord ischemia, and aortic arch aneurysms may result in cerebral ischemia or recurrent laryngeal nerve dysfunction.[1,34,40,41] Most commonly, neurologic symptoms are produced by either rupture or direct compression. Even when aneurysms result in paraplegia, the neurologic deficit is often caused by bony erosion through the vertebral bodies and direct compression of the spinal cord or cauda equina rather than by ischemia.[43–45]

Dissecting Aortic Aneurysms

Dissecting aortic aneurysms, in contrast to nondissecting aortic aneurysms, predominantly involve the thoracic aorta, either at the beginning of the ascending segment (type A) or immediately distal to the left subclavian artery at the aortic isthmus (type B).[1,8,22,67] Their etiology has not been established. Atherosclerosis is probably not a major factor because atherosclerosis is seldom found in the region of the intimal tear because the distribution of these aneurysms along the aorta is unlike that of atherosclerosis and because atherosclerosis is only infrequently present.[1,68,69] Nevertheless, hypertension probably is a factor as it is present in the large majority of patients with either type A or type B dissections.[68–70] Moreover, dissecting aortic aneurysms have been associated with cystic medial necrosis, a degenerative condition focally affecting the arterial media, which may itself be related to hypertension. This condition is increased in patients with Marfan syndrome, as are dissecting aneurysms. Most aneurysms, however, do not occur in patients with Marfan syndrome or other identifiable collagen disorders, and the pathophysiology remains unknown.[68,69] It has been estimated that 60 percent of thoracic aortic aneurysms involve the aortic root or ascending aorta, 10 percent the arch, 40 percent the descending thoracic aorta, and 10 percent the thoracoabdominal aorta.[71] More than 95 percent of thoracic aortic aneurysms are asymptomatic and their prevalence (prior to rupture or dissection) has been estimated to be greater than 0.16 to 0.34 percent.[71] There may be a familial tendency for their occurrence and, for larger aneurysms (>6 mm), the 5-year survival may be as low as 50 percent.[71] Neurologic involvement from dissecting aneurysms (due to the cut-off of important arteries by the dissection or by embolization) is well described but uncommon. It occurs more frequently with type A than type B dissections, and it usually involves either spinal or cerebral ischemia.[68,69] Neurologic involvement may also occur during surgery to repair the aneurysm. Patients with aortic dissection usually present with acute chest or back pain, which generally leads to the proper diagnosis.[68,69] On occasion, however, pain is absent, and the neurologic syndrome is the presenting feature.[45,72] Moreover, the neurologic deficit produced by the dissecting aneurysm is sometimes only transient, lasting for several hours, and thereby mimicking other transient disturbances of neurologic function.

Traumatic Aortic Injury

Brutal deceleration injuries to the chest, especially from motor vehicle accidents, may result in traumatic rupture of the thoracic aorta, often just distal to the left subclavian artery at the aortic isthmus (i.e., the slight constriction of the aorta at the point where the ductus arteriosus attaches).[73] Many of these patients die immediately, but some present with an acute paraplegia.[74] Still others have a chronic aortic aneurysm that may present years later with acute spinal cord ischemia or other neurologic symptoms. Some patients with traumatic aortic injury have a less critical condition (e.g., limited intimal flaps) and may not warrant immediate surgical treatment.[75] Nevertheless, they will still need to be monitored closely for signs of progression that would prompt urgent intervention.[75]

Coarctation of the Aorta

Coarctation of the aorta, a relatively common congenital condition,[76] typically results in constriction of the thoracic aorta just distal to the origin of the left subclavian artery. Less commonly, it occurs as part of Takayasu arteritis, and this condition should be suspected if the location of the coarctation is atypical.[1,57] It may also follow radiation exposure during infancy; in these cases, the pathologic process is focal and limited to the segment of aorta that was in the field of irradiation. Coarctation can result in a variety of neurologic symptoms (Table 2-7).[18,77] Cerebral infarcts probably result from embolization of thrombotic material in the dilated aorta proximal to the obstruction.

Subarachnoid hemorrhage from ruptured saccular aneurysms can occur with coarctation. In the general population, aneurysmal hemorrhage has an annual incidence of approximately 8 per 100,000 and rarely occurs before the age of 20 years.[1] Accordingly, the reported occurrence of ruptured aneurysms in 2.5 percent of patients with coarctation of the aorta suggests an association of these two disorders,[77] although the coincidental occurrence of the two conditions cannot be completely excluded.[1]

TABLE 2-7 ■ Neurologic Sequelae of Coarctation of the Aorta*

Sequela	Incidence (%)
Ruptured intracerebral aneurysms	2.5
Ischemic stroke during childhood	1.0
Neurogenic intermittent claudication†	7.5
Headache	25.0
Episodic loss of consciousness	3.0
Intracerebral hemorrhage‡	<1.0
Spinal cord compression‡	<1.0

*Based on a review of 200 patients with coarctation of the aorta. (Tyler and Clark: Neurologic complications in patients with coarctation of aorta. Neurology 8:712, 1958.)
†Patients with exercise-induced motor or sensory disturbances in the lower extremities.
‡These complications were not found in the series reported by Tyler and Clark but have been reported by others, as described elsewhere.[1]

Headache is a common accompaniment of coarctation, perhaps as a result of secondary hypertension, but, again, the incidental occurrence of two unrelated conditions cannot be excluded.

Episodic loss of consciousness may also occur in patients with coarctation of the aorta. It may result either from syncope due to associated cardiac abnormalities or from seizures. It is unclear, however, whether seizures unrelated to cerebrovascular disease are more prevalent in these patients than in the general population.

Neurogenic intermittent claudication can result from aortic coarctation. In patients with coarctation of the aorta, blood flow to the legs is often provided by collateral connections between the spinal arteries and the distal aorta. In these situations, the blood flow through the radiculomedullary and intercostal arteries distal to the obstruction is reversed, and the exercise-related spinal ischemia may be related to "steal" by the increased metabolic demands (and thus increased blood flow) of the legs rather than aortic hypotension distal to the coarctation (Fig. 2-13). These collaterals are sometimes so extensive that they cause spinal cord compression and mimic

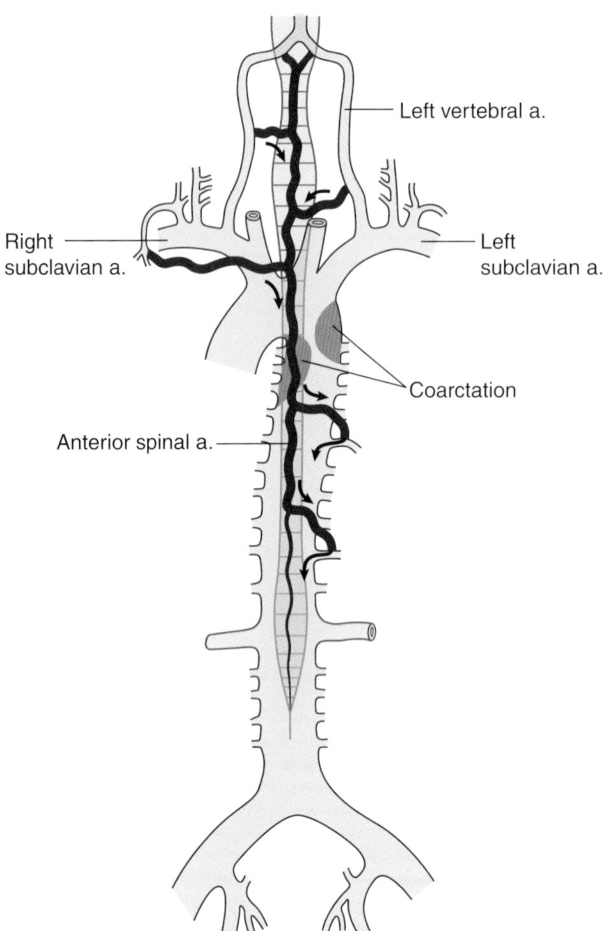

FIGURE 2-13 ■ Mechanism of steal in coarctation of the aorta. Obstruction of the aorta at the isthmus causes dilatation of the anterior spinal artery and reversal of blood flow in anterior radiculomedullary arteries distal to the obstruction. In this circumstance, the blood flow to the lower extremities is provided by these (and other) collaterals, and use of the lower extremities may cause shunting of blood from the spinal circulation to the legs, which, in turn, sometimes results in spinal cord ischemia.

(clinically and radiologically) vascular malformations of the spinal cord.[1] Spinal cord injury can rarely follow surgical repair of a coarctation, and this complication may be delayed by several months following the repair.[78]

Surgery and other Procedures

Aortic Surgery

As with diseases of the aorta, the risks of aortic surgery depend in part on the site of operation. Thus, operations on the aortic arch may produce cerebral ischemia either by intraoperative occlusion of major vessels or by embolization of material such as calcified plaque loosened during surgery.[1,32–34] Operations on the suprarenal aorta may result in spinal ischemia,[7,79] whereas operations on the distal aorta may result in sexual dysfunction or ischemia of the femoral nerve.[51–54]

The major complication of all aortic operations, however, is intraoperative spinal cord ischemia with resultant paraplegia or paraparesis. The occurrence of this complication varies with the location of the surgery and the nature of the pathologic process affecting the aorta (Table 2-8). Thus, operations on dissecting or nondissecting aortic aneurysms that are entirely abdominal are associated with a lower incidence of this complication than operations on aneurysms confined to the thoracic aorta. Surgery on aneurysms involving the entire abdominal and thoracic aorta carries the highest risk of producing

TABLE 2-8 ■ Spinal Cord Ischemia During Surgery and Procedures on the Aorta

Diagnosis	Number of Patients	Percentage With Spinal Cord Damage
Nondissecting aortic aneurysm		
Abdominal	1,724	0.46
Thoracic	585	6.3
Thoracoabdominal	102	21.6
Dissecting aortic aneurysm	102	30.4
Abdominal aortic occlusion	1,089	0
Coarctation of aorta	12,532	0.41
Aortography	17,949	0.01

From Goodin DS: Neurologic sequelae of aortic disease and surgery. p. 23. In Aminoff MJ (ed): Neurology and General Medicine. 4th Ed. Churchill Livingstone Elsevier, Philadelphia, 2008, with permission.

cord ischemia.[79] Operations on the distal aorta for occlusive disease only rarely result in spinal ischemia, especially when confined to the infrarenal portion.[1,23] This variability presumably occurs because important feeding arteries to the spinal circulation are more likely to be ligated during surgery, included within the segment of the aorta that is cross-clamped, or subjected to distal hypotension when the aortic lesion is above the level of origin of the renal arteries.

Operations on the thoracic aorta for coarctation are much less frequently complicated by spinal ischemia than thoracic operations done for other reasons.[18,80] There are probably at least two reasons for this difference. First, the former patients are younger, and the extent of overall arterial disease is therefore less. Second, as mentioned earlier, the flow in the radiculomedullary vessels below the coarctation is frequently reversed, so obstruction of blood flow in them (either by ligation or cross-clamping the aorta above and below their origin) may actually result in an increased blood supply to the spinal cord.

Aortography and other Procedures on the Aorta

Aortography may be associated with either spinal or cerebral ischemia, depending on the portion of the aorta visualized. This complication, however, is distinctly rare (Table 2-8). Paraplegia may also occur during intra-aortic balloon assistance after myocardial revascularization.[81]

Intraoperative Adjuncts to Avoid Spinal Cord Ischemia

Several adjuncts are commonly used during surgery in an attempt to avoid spinal cord injury. They include the use of hypothermia and maintenance of mild intraoperative hypertension in addition to thiopental anesthesia and/or the administration of naltrexone and intraoperative corticosteroids, all of which are thought to reduce the metabolic requirements of the spinal cord or otherwise enhance tolerance to ischemia. In addition, many authors have reported that minimization of cross-clamp time results in a lower incidence of spinal ischemia.

Other adjunctive methods such as the reattachment of intercostal arteries, the use of shunts to maintain distal perfusion pressure, and the use of cerebrospinal fluid drainage have not proved consistently effective at preventing cord ischemia,[2,82–85] although the more recent experience with such adjunctive techniques has been quite favorable.[2,84–87] Part of the difficulty with these procedures may relate to the extreme variability of the blood supply to the spinal cord. For example, if a crucial spinal artery leaves the aorta within the cross-clamped section, the preservation of distal blood flow is irrelevant. Furthermore, because the important intercostal arteries are few and unpredictably situated, the random reattachment of a few intercostal arteries may be fruitless. Spinal cord ischemia can also be delayed and occur hours to days following the aortic operation.[87] In these circumstances, the maintenance of mild hypertension coupled with the use of supplemental oxygen and cerebrospinal fluid drainage may mitigate the consequences.[87]

There has been considerable interest in the use of somatosensory evoked potentials (SEPs) and motor evoked potentials (MEPs) for assessing spinal cord function during operations on the aorta.[88–94] The combined use of SEPs and MEPs may ultimately prove better than either technique alone,[93] and, indeed, the most recent reports with both techniques have been encouraging.[21,32,92–94] An approach that seems particularly valuable is the use of intraoperative MEPs or SEPs to identify those vessels that perfuse the spinal cord and therefore need reattachment, should not be sacrificed, or should not be included within the aortic cross-clamp.[21,90,93] Another approach that has been reported to be useful is the use of intraoperative MEPs to monitor patients and to quickly increase both the distal aortic pressure and the mean arterial pressure in response to a drop in MEP amplitude.[92] Nevertheless, although these reports are encouraging, the best method of monitoring intraoperative spinal cord function and how best to use the information to alter the operative technique so that postoperative spinal cord function is maintained are yet to be determined.

REFERENCES

1. Goodin DS: Neurologic sequelae of aortic disease and surgery. p. 23. In Aminoff MJ (ed): Neurology and General Medicine. 4th Ed. Churchill Livingstone Elsevier, Philadelphia, 2008.
2. Griepp RB, Ergin MA, Galla JD, et al: Looking for the artery of Adamkiewicz: a quest to minimize paraplegia after operations for aneurysms of the descending thoracic and thoracoabdominal aorta. J Thorac Cardiovasc Surg 112:1202, 1996.
3. Milen MT, Bloom DA, Culligan J, et al: Albert Adamkiewicz (1850–1921): His artery and its significance for the retroperitoneal surgeon. World J Urol 17:168, 1999.
4. Biglioli P, Roberto M, Cannata A, et al: Upper and lower spinal cord blood supply: the continuity of the anterior spinal artery and the relevance of the lumbar arteries. J Thorac Cardiovasc Surg 127:1188, 2004.
5. Novy A, Carruzzo A, Maeder P, et al: Spinal cord ischemia: clinical and imaging patterns, pathogenesis, and outcomes in 27 patients. Arch Neurol 63:1113, 2006.
6. Nijenhuis RJ, Jacobs MJ, van Engelshoven JMA, et al: MR angiograph of the Adamkiewicz artery and anterior radiculomedullary vein: postmortem validation. AJNR Am J Neuroradiol 17:573, 2006.
7. Acher C, Wynn M: Outcomes in open repair of the thoracic and thoracoabdominal aorta. J Vasc Surg 52(suppl):3S, 2010.
8. Sandbridge L, Kern JA: Acute Descending aortic dissections: Management of visceral, spinal cord, and extremity malperfusion. Semin Thorac Cardiovasc Surg 17:256, 2005.
9. Wong SSN, Roche-Nagle G, Oreopoulos G: Acute thrombosis of an abdominal aortic aneurysm presenting as cauda equina syndrome. J Vasc Surg 57:218, 2013.
10. Katabathina VS, Restrepo CS: Infectious and noninfectious aortitis: cross-sectional imaging findings. Semin Ultrasound CT MR 33:207, 2012.
11. Scheel AK, Meller J, Vosshenrich R, et al: Diagnosis and follow up of aortitis in the elderly. Ann Rheum Dis 63:1507, 2004.
12. Tavora F, Burke A: Review of isolated ascending aortitis: differential diagnosis, including syphilitic, Takayasu's and giant cell aortitis. Pathology 38:302, 2006.
13. Park BS, Min HK, Kang DK, et al: Stanford type A aortic dissection secondary to infectious aortitis: a case report. J Korean Med Sci 28:485, 2013.
14. Lopes RJ, Almeida J, Dias PJ, et al: Infectious thoracic aortitis: a literature review. Clin Cardiol 32:488, 2009.
15. Nedeltchev K, Loher TJ, Stepper F, et al: Long-term outcome of acute spinal cord ischemia syndrome. Stroke 35:560, 2004.
16. Cowan KN, Lawlor DK: Sudden onset of paraplegia from acute aortic occlusion: a review of 2 cases and their unique presentation. Am J Emerg Med 24:479, 2006.
17. Surowiec SM, Isiklar H, Sreeram S, et al: Acute occlusion of the abdominal aorta. Am J Surg 176:193, 1998.
18. Rao PS: Coarctation of the aorta. Curr Cardiol Rep 7:425, 2005.
19. Chen GY, Kuo CD, Yang MJ, et al: Return of autonomic nervous activity after delivery: role of aortocaval compression. Br J Anaesth 82:932, 1999.
20. Duggal N, Lach B: Selective vulnerability of the lumbosacral spinal cord after cardiac arrest and hypotension. Stroke 33:116, 2002.
21. Jacobs MJ, Elenbaas TW, Schurink GW, et al: Assessment of spinal cord integrity during thoracoabdominal aortic aneurysm repair. Ann Thorac Surg 74:S1864, 2002.
22. Ohmi M, Shibuya T, Kawamoto S, et al: Spinal cord ischemia complicated with acute aortic dissection and intramural hematoma; report of two cases. Kyobu Geka 56:473, 2003.
23. Webb TH, Williams GM: Thoracoabdominal aneurysm repair. Cardiovasc Surg 7:573, 1999.
24. Kumral E, Polat F, Güllüoglu C, et al: Spinal ischaemic stroke: clinical and radiological findings and short-term outcome. Eur J Neurol 18:232, 2011.
25. Hakimi KN, Massagli TL: Anterior spinal artery syndrome in two children with genetic thrombotic disorders. J Spinal Cord Med 28:69, 2005.
26. Ogun SA, Adefuye B, Kolapo KB, et al: Anterior spinal artery syndrome complicating aortic dissecting aneurysm: case report. East Afr Med J 81:549, 2004.
27. Duc S, Delleci C, Barandon L, et al: Complications arising after thoracic aortic surgery: A case report on an unusual spinal cord infarction. Physiopathological and clinical considerations. Ann Phys Rehabil Med 56:51, 2013.
28. Blanc R, Hosseini H, Le Guerinel C, et al: Posterior cervical spinal cord infarction complicating the treatment of an intracranial dural arteriovenous fistula embolization. Case report. J Neurosurg Spine 5:79, 2006.

29. Truumees E: Spinal stenosis: pathophysiology, clinical and radiologic classification. Instr Course Lect 54:287, 2005.
30. Kikuchi S, Watanabe E, Hasue M: Spinal intermittent claudication due to cervical and thoracic degenerative disease. Spine 21:313, 1996.
31. Mwipatayi BP, Jeffery PC, Beningfield SJ, et al: Takayasu arteritis: clinical features and management: report of 272 cases. Aust N Z J Surg 75:110, 2005.
32. Erlich M, Grabenwoger M, Luckner D, et al: Operative management of aortic arch aneurysm using profound hypothermia and circulatory arrest. J Cardiovasc Surg 37:63, 1996.
33. Okita T, Ando M, Minatoya K, et al: Predictive factors for mortality and cerebral complications in arteriosclerotic aneurysm of the aortic arch. Ann Thorac Surg 33:72, 1999.
34. Wickremasinghe HR, Peiris JB, Thenabadu PN, et al: Transient emboligenic aortoarteritis. Arch Neurol 35:416, 1978.
35. Aseem WM, Makaroun MS: Bilateral subclavian steal syndrome through different paths and different sites. Angiology 50:149, 1999.
36. Killen DA, Foster JH, Walter Jr GG, et al: The subclavian steal syndrome. J Thorac Cardiovasc Surg 51:539, 1966.
37. Taylor SL, Selman WR, Ratcheson RA: Steal affecting the central nervous system. Neurosurgery 50:670, 2002.
38. Tuseth V, Hegland Ø, Fjetland L, et al: Reversed flow in internal mammary artery conduit and vertebral artery with left subclavian artery occlusion causing angina and vertigo: the coronary–subclavian steal syndrome. Int J Cardiol 79:311, 2001.
39. Takach TJ, Reul GJ, Cooley DA, et al: Myocardial thievery: the coronary-subclavian steal syndrome. Ann Thorac Surg 81:386, 2006.
40. Tan CS, Fintelmann F, Joe J, et al: Coronary-subclavian steal syndrome in a hemodialysis patient, a case report and review of literature. Semin Dial 26:E42, 2013.
41. Lee SI, Pyun SB, Jang DH: Dysphagia and hoarseness associated with painless aortic dissection: a rare case of cardiovocal syndrome. Dysphagia 21:129, 2006.
42. Sterpetti AV, Blair EA, Schultz RD, et al: Sealed rupture of abdominal aortic aneurysms. J Vasc Surg 11:430, 1990.
43. Tsubota H, Nakamura T: Chronic contained rupture of an abdominal aortic aneurysm manifesting as lower extremity neuropathy. J Vasc Surg 55:548, 2012.
44. Caynak B, Onan B, Sanisoglu I, et al: Vertebral erosion due to chronic contained rupture of an abdominal aortic aneurysm. J Vasc Surg 48:1342, 2008.
45. Shields RE, Aaron JO, Postel G, et al: A fatal illness presenting as an S1 radiculopathy. Vascular causes of lumbar radicular pain. J Ky Med Assoc 95:268, 1997.
46. Wilbourn AJ, Furlan AJ, Hulley W, et al: Ischemic monomelic neuropathy. Neurology 33:447, 1983.
47. Wodicka R, Isaacs J: Ischemic monomelic neuropathy. J Hand Surg Am 35:842, 2010.
48. Han JS, Park MY, Choi SJ, et al: Ischemic monomelic neuropathy: a rare complication after vascular access formation. Korean J Int Med 28:251, 2013.
49. Afifi AK, Bergman RA: Functional Neuroanatomy. 2nd Ed. McGraw-Hill, New York, 1998.
50. Nemes R, Surlin V, Chiutu L, et al: Retroperitoneoscopic lumbar sympathectomy: prospective study upon a series of 50 consecutive patients. Surg Endosc 25:3066, 2011.
51. Nevelsteen A, Beyens G, Duchateau J, et al: Aortofemoral reconstruction and sexual function: a prospective study. Eur J Vasc Surg 4:247, 1990.
52. Cormio L, Edgre J, Lepäntalo M, et al: Aortofemoral surgery and sexual function. Eur J Vasc Endovasc Surg 11:453, 1996.
53. Hultgren R, Sjögren B, Söderberg M, et al: Sexual function in women suffering from aortoiliac occlusive disease. Eur J Vasc Endovasc Surg 17:306, 1999.
54. Pettersson M, Mattsson E, Bergbom I: Prospective follow-up of sexual function after elective repair of abdominal aortic aneurysms using open and endovascular techniques. J Vasc Surg 50:492, 2009.
55. Eidt JF: Invited commentary. J Vasc Surg 50:499, 2009.
56. Ohshiro T, Kosaki G: Sexual function after aortoiliac vascular reconstruction. J Cardiovasc Surg 25:47, 1984.
57. Paulo N, Cascarejo J, Vouga L: Syphilitic aneurysm of the ascending aorta. Interact Cardiovasc Thorac Surg 14:223, 2012.
58. Rizzi R, Bruno S, Stellacci C, et al: Takayasu's arteritis: a cell-mediated large-vessel vasculitis. Int J Clin Lab Res 29:8, 1999.
59. Isobe M: Takayasu arteritis revisited: current diagnosis and treatment. Int J Cardiol 168:3, 2013.
60. Miller DV, Isotalo PA, Weyand CM, et al: Surgical pathology of non-infectious ascending aortitis: a study of 45 cases with an emphasis on an isolated variant. Am J Surg Pathol 30:1150, 2006.
61. Bongartz T, Matteson EL: Large vessel involvement in giant cell arteritis. Curr Opin Rheumatol 18:10, 2006.
62. Roquer J, Martí N, Cano A, et al: Spinal cord ischemia indicating aneurysm of the abdominal aorta: report of three cases. Neurologia 10:201, 1995.
63. Oderich GS, Panneton JM, Bower TC, et al: Infected aortic aneurysms: aggressive presentation, complicated early outcome, but durable results. J Vasc Surg 34:901, 2001.
64. Brindley P, Schwab EH: Aneurysms of the aorta, with a summary of pathological findings in 100 cases at autopsy. Tex State J Med 25:757, 1930.
65. Acosta S, Ögren M, Bengtsson H, et al: Increasing incidence of ruptured abdominal aortic aneurysms: a population-based study. J Vasc Surg 44:237, 2006.
66. Mell M, White JJ, Hill BB, et al: No increased mortality with early aortic aneurysm disease. J Vasc Surg 56:1246, 2012.
67. Ayala IAL, Chen YF: Acute aortic dissection: An update. Kaohsiung J Med Sci 28:299, 2012.

68. Xu SD, Huang FJ, Yang JF, et al: Endovascular repair of acute type B aortic dissection: Early and mid-term results. J Vasc Surg 43:1090, 2006.
69. Tsai TT, Evangelista A, Nienaber CA, et al: Long-term survival in patients presenting with type A acute aortic dissection: insights from the international registry of acute aortic dissection (IRAD). Circulation 114(suppl 1):350, 2006.
70. Sandbridge L, Kern JA: Acute descending aortic dissections: management of visceral, spinal cord, and extremity malperfusion. Semin Thorac Cardiovasc Surg 17:256, 2005.
71. Kuzmik GA, Sang AX, Eleferiades JA, et al: Natural history of thoracic aortic aneurysms. J Vasc Surg 56:565, 2012.
72. Colak N, Nazli Y, Alpay MF, et al: Painless aortic dissection presenting as paraplegia. Tex Heart Inst J 39:273, 2012.
73. Mosquera VX, Marini M, Muñiz J, et al: Blunt traumatic aortic injuries of the ascending aorta and aortic arch: a clinical multicentre study. Injury 44:1191, 2013.
74. Naude GP, Back M, Perry MO, et al: Blunt disruption of the abdominal aorta: report of a case and review of the literature. J Vasc Surg 25:931, 1997.
75. Kidane B, Abramowitz D, Harris JR, et al: Natural history of minimal aortic injury following blunt thoracic aortic trauma. Can J Surg 55:377, 2012.
76. Bozzani A, Arici V, Ragni F: Thoracic aorta coarctation in the adults: open surgery is still the gold standard. Vasc Endovasc Surg 47:216, 2013.
77. Tyler HR, Clark DB: Neurologic complications in patients with coarctation of aorta. Neurology 8:712, 1958.
78. Wilder MJ, Ng PP, Dailey AT: Delayed onset of anterior spinal artery syndrome after repair of aortic coarctation. Spine 37:E1476, 2012.
79. Cambria RP, Clouse D, Davison JK, et al: Thoracoabdominal aneurysm repair: Results with 337 operations performed over a 15-year interval. Ann Surg 236:471, 2002.
80. Sandrio S, Karck M, Gorenflo M, et al: Results of using cardiopulmonary bypass for spinal cord protection during surgical repair of complex aortic coarctation. Cardiol Young, in press, 2013.
81. Ussia GP, Marasini M, Pongiglione G: Paraplegia following percutaneous balloon angioplasty of aortic coarctation: a case report. Catheter Cardiovasc Interv 54:510, 2001.
82. Kumagai H, Isaka M, Sugawara Y, et al: Intra-aortic injection of propofol prevents spinal cord injury during aortic surgery. Eur J Cardiothorac Surg 29:714, 2006.
83. Patel HJ, Shillingford MS, Mihalik S, et al: Resection of the descending thoracic aorta. Ann Thorac Surg 82:90, 2006.
84. Safi HJ, Mille III CC: Spinal cord protection in descending thoracic and thoracoabdominal aortic repair. Ann Thorac Surg 67:1937, 1999.
85. Coselli JS, LeMaire SA: Left heart bypass reduces paraplegia rates after thoracoabdominal aortic aneurysm repair. Ann Thorac Surg 67:1931, 1999.
86. Becker DA, McGarvey ML, Rojvirat C, et al: Predictors of outcome in patients with spinal cord ischemia after open aortic repair. Neurocrit Care 18:70, 2013.
87. Yanase Y, Kawaharada N, Maeda T, et al: Treatment of delayed neurological deficits after surgical repair of thoracic aortic aneurysm. Ann Thorac Cardiovasc Surg 18:271, 2012.
88. Ogino H, Sasaki H, Minatoya K, et al: Combined use of Adamkiewicz artery demonstration and motor evoked potentials in descending thoracoabdominal repair. Ann Thorac Surg 82:592, 2006.
89. MacDonald DB: Intraoperative motor evoked potential monitoring: overview and update. J Clin Monit Comput 20:347, 2006.
90. Svensson LG, Patel V, Robinson MF, et al: Influence of preservation or perfusion of intraoperatively identified spinal cord blood supply on spinal motor evoked potentials and paraplegia after aortic surgery. J Vasc Surg 13:355, 1991.
91. Reuter DG, Tacker WA, Badylak SF, et al: Correlation of motor-evoked potential response to ischemic spinal cord damage. J Thorac Cardiovasc Surg 104:262, 1992.
92. Jacobs MJHM, Meylaerts SA, de Haan P, et al: Strategies to prevent neurologic deficit based on motor-evoked potentials in type I and II thoracoabdominal aortic aneurysm repair. J Vasc Surg 29:48, 1999.
93. Guerit JM, Witdoeckt C, Verhelst R, et al: Sensitivity, specificity, and surgical impact of somatosensory evoked potentials in descending aorta surgery. Ann Thorac Surg 67:1943, 1999.
94. Galla JD, Ergin MA, Lansman SL, et al: Use of somatosensory evoked potentials for thoracic and thoracoabdominal aortic resections. Ann Thorac Surg 67:1947, 1999.

CHAPTER

3

Neurologic Complications of Cardiac Surgery

JOHN R. HOTSON

Neurologic complications of cardiac surgery have the potential to nullify or limit surgical benefits. The probability of these complications has increased as coronary artery bypass graft surgery (CABG) has been used for treating ischemic heart disease in older patients, patients with multiple comorbid conditions, and patients in heart transplantation programs. In spite of the increased use of catheter-based coronary revascularization, more than 400,000 people per year receive CABG in the United States and well over a million people per year worldwide.[1,2] A substantial number of patients will experience a postoperative adverse cerebral outcome such as focal stroke, global encephalopathy, or long-term loss of cognitive performance following heart surgery.[3,4] Prevention of perioperative neurologic complications after cardiac surgery therefore remains an important medical problem.

EXTRACORPOREAL CIRCULATION

Cardiopulmonary bypass was first used successfully in cardiac surgery in 1953 and was the pivotal development that led to modern cardiac surgery.[1] Its early use in humans resulted in frequent complications, which restricted its employment to seriously ill patients with progressive heart failure. The safety of extracorporeal circulation subsequently increased, but it remains a potential cause of neurologic complications. In an attempt to decrease adverse side effects, cardiac surgery without cardiopulmonary bypass ("off-pump") was developed and compared to surgery with extracorporeal circulation ("on-pump"). Off-pump surgery has not proven superior to on-pump surgery and the latter technique continues to be used in 80 percent of cardiac surgeries in the United States.[5]

Technique

Open heart surgery with cardiopulmonary bypass requires cannulation of the ascending aorta and vena cava or right atrium with drainage of venous blood to a reservoir. The venous blood is pumped through a membrane oxygenator and routed via an arterial filter to a cannula in the aortic arch (Fig. 3-1).[6] Clamping the aorta and insertion of the aortic cannula can dislodge atheromatous material in a severely diseased aorta, thereby leading to cerebral embolization. High-velocity or turbulent blood flow from the end of the cannula may also dislodge emboli.[7] Intraoperative identification of aortic atheroma is possible with transesophageal echocardiography or the more sensitive epiaortic ultrasound technique (Fig. 3-2).[8] Such imaging demonstrates atherosclerotic plaque in 25 to 50 percent of patients undergoing CABG and may alter surgical management. The frequency of such aortic disease

Aminoff's Neurology and General Medicine, Fifth Edition.

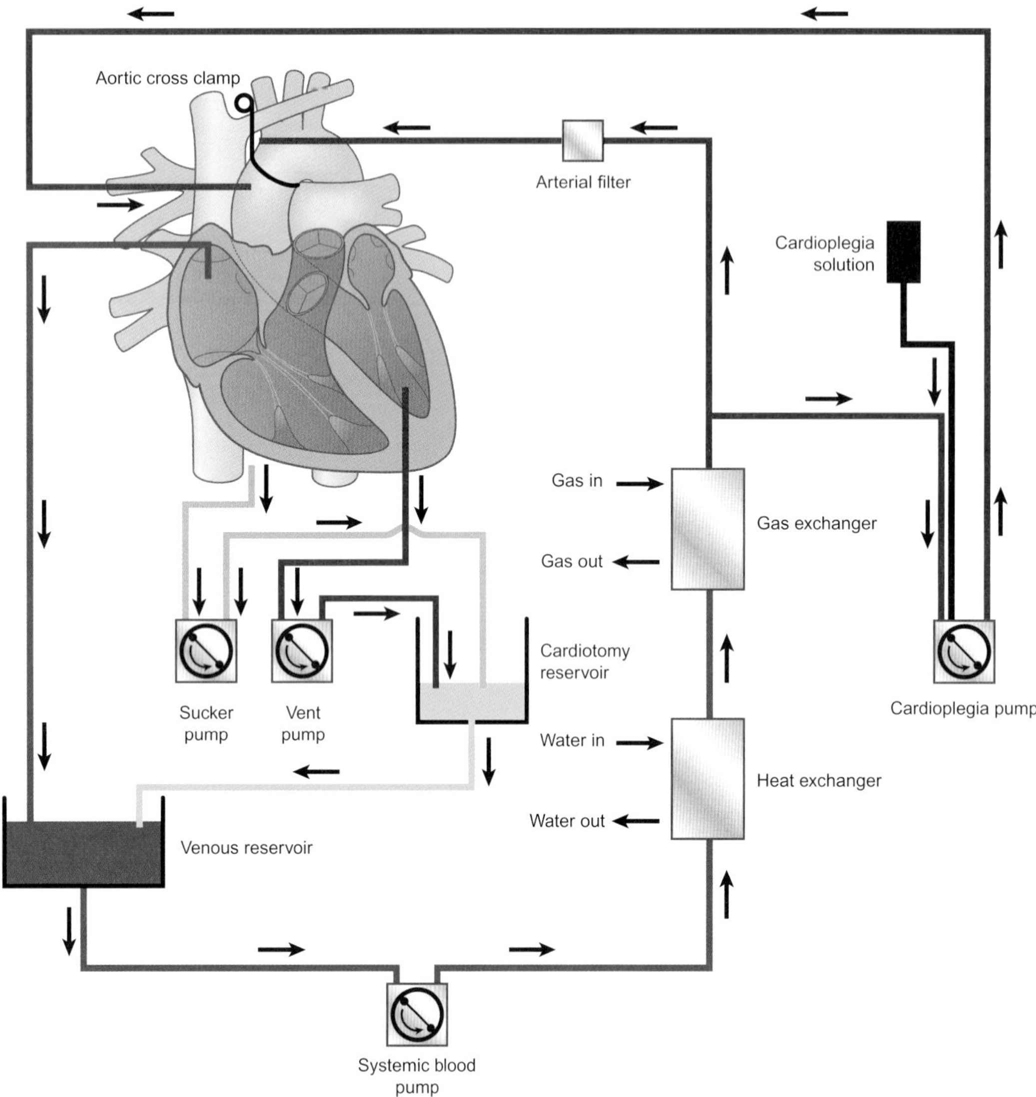

FIGURE 3-1 ■ Schematic of an extracorporeal circulation circuit used in cardiopulmonary bypass surgery. (Modified from Machin D, Allsage C: Principles of cardiopulmonary bypass. Contin Educ Anaesth Crit Care Pain 6:176, 2006 with permission from Oxford University Press.)

increases with age and is particularly prominent in patients older than 70 years.[9,10]

A secondary venous-to-arterial circuit is initiated by blood suctioned from the pericardial surgical field (Fig. 3-1). This cardiotomy suction blood contains fat and debris that could form cerebral emboli if directly reinfused into the arterial circulation. Therefore, the blood is directed to a cardiotomy reservoir where it is filtered and processed in order to remove embolic material before being reintroduced to the circulation.[8,11]

Extracorporeal circulation is used in association with systemic heparinization and hemodilution. When blood is exposed to the nonbiocompatible surfaces of the bypass circuits, a prothrombotic system inflammatory response is induced. Anticoagulation is used to prevent thrombus formation. Hemodilution is thought to improve microcirculatory flow by reducing blood viscosity. Excessive hemodilution is avoided because it reduces the oxygen-carrying capacity of blood and increases postoperative adverse outcomes.[6–8,11]

The optimal mean arterial pressure and body temperature for cardiac surgery remain unclear. In many centers, an attempt is made to maintain the mean arterial pressure above 50 mmHg; others

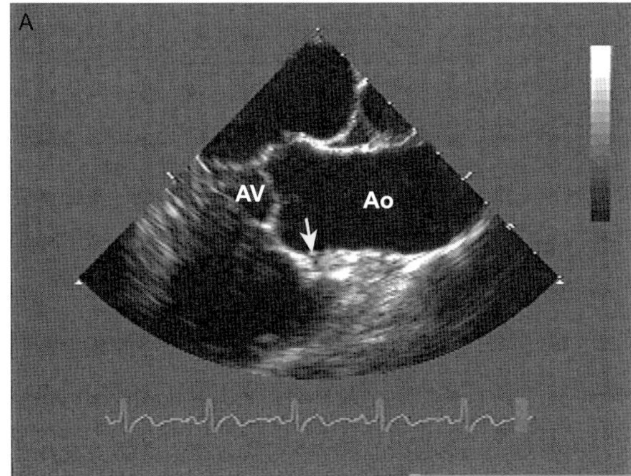

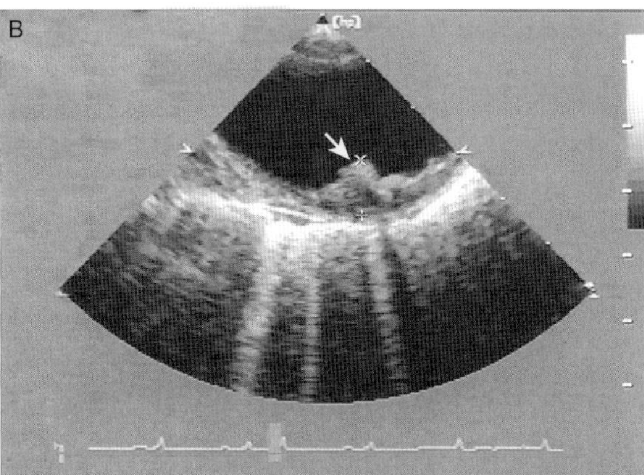

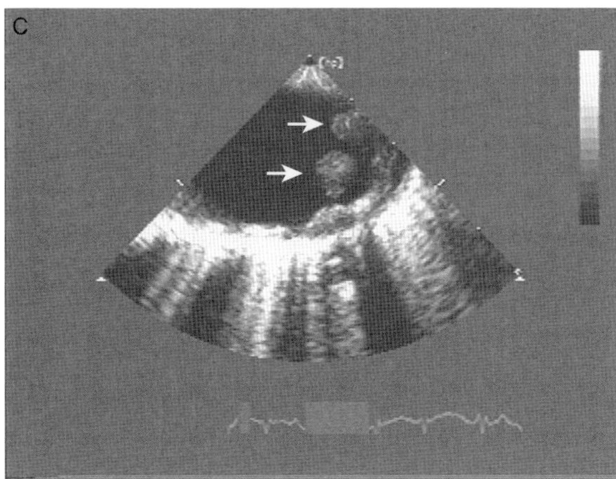

FIGURE 3-2 ▪ Transesophageal echocardiography of the aorta. **A**, Normal aorta (Ao), also illustrating the aortic valve (AV) and the takeoff of the right coronary artery (*arrow*). **B**, Atherosclerotic plaque protruding into the aorta (*arrow*). **C**, Two large thrombi (*arrows*) associated with atherosclerotic plaque. (Modified from Di Tullio MR, Homma S. Atherosclerotic disease of the proximal aorta. p. 741. In Mohr JP, Wolf PA, Grotta JC, et al (eds): Stroke. 5th Ed. Elsevier, Philadelphia, 2011, with permission from Elsevier.)

aim it above 70 mmHg in patients with prominent risk factors for cerebrovascular disease. The majority of cardiac bypass procedures use hypothermia for neuroprotection of the brain, but a meta-analysis of 19 randomized controlled trials comparing hypothermic cardiac surgery with normothermic surgery did not identify a clear advantage of either approach.[12] It is still recommended, however, to use slow rewarming rates and to avoid temperatures above 37°C in order to reduce postoperative neurocognitive impairment.[7,8,11]

NEUROLOGIC SEQUELAE OF CARDIAC SURGERY

Acute Brain Disorders

Stroke, encephalopathy, coma, and seizures are the major acute brain disorders complicating cardiac surgery.[13] Stroke has decreased in frequency over the past two decades to less than 2 percent of patients undergoing CABG.[14] Clinically silent stroke detected by magnetic resonance imaging (MRI) is probably more frequent.[15] Stroke incidence increases with the number of preoperative stroke risk factors. Stroke after cardiac surgery leads to an approximately five- to sixfold increase in hospital mortality, prolongs length of stay in the intensive care unit, and typically requires inpatient rehabilitation or nursing home placement. The majority of stroke patients who survive to hospital discharge are substantially disabled.[16] Stroke occurs more frequently when valvular heart surgery is combined with coronary artery bypass graft operations due to the additional risk of cerebral macroemboli with operations that require opening a heart chamber and removal or repair of diseased heart valves.[3,17–19]

Ischemic stroke after cardiac surgery is most often the result of emboli or hypoperfusion.[4,20] Diffusion-weighted brain MRI has identified watershed infarction as the cause of stroke after cardiac surgery and cardiopulmonary bypass in approximately half of stroke patients.[21] Watershed infarction occurs at border zones between the major cerebral arteries and typically is associated with arterial hypoperfusion. More prolonged cardiopulmonary bypass time increases the risk of watershed stroke, and bilateral watershed stroke has a particularly poor outcome.[21]

Intracranial hemorrhage is an infrequent cause of stroke, but its rapid identification is important to allow for urgent medical or surgical treatment. Hematomas may be located in the brain parenchyma itself or in the subdural or epidural space. Intracranial hemorrhage during cardiopulmonary bypass may be related to reduced platelet adhesion and coagulation factors.[20,22]

Repair of severe aortic stenosis causes a rapid increase in brain perfusion pressure and rarely can cause focal neurologic signs with MRI evidence of vasogenic brain edema without acute infarction. Both the focal neurologic deficits and brain edema may be reversible.[23]

Encephalopathy, reflecting a diffuse brain disorder, occurs in greater than 8 percent of adults following heart surgery.[24] Its prevalence is even greater in patients older than 65 to 70 years and in patients with known preexisting cerebrovascular disease.[25] These encephalopathic patients may be slow to emerge from anesthesia, can be agitated, and may have fluctuating impairment of cognitive and perceptual function. Hallucinations may be present and occasionally there are bilateral Babinski signs. Improvement often occurs during the first postoperative week. Some of these encephalopathic patients have multiple, acute, small ischemic brain lesions detected with MRI, suggesting multiple emboli.[26] However, in many patients the cause of encephalopathy cannot be defined clinically. CABG without the use of cardiopulmonary bypass results in less frequent postoperative delirium, whereas prolonged operating time increases its frequency.[24]

Electrolyte dysfunction can also lead to neurologic compromise following cardiac surgery. Postoperative hyponatremic encephalopathy is important to recognize and reverse because it can lead to brain edema, particularly in younger women. A hypoglycemic encephalopathy is a risk in patients who are under "tight" insulin control for diabetes.[27] A hypernatremic hyperosmolar state is a rare cause of encephalopathy after cardiac surgery.[28,29]

Persistent coma after uncomplicated cardiac surgery is infrequent, occurring in less than 1 percent of patients.[30] It may be due to global anoxia-ischemia, massive stroke, or multiple brain infarctions.[31] When anoxia-ischemia is the cause of coma, myoclonus, at times accompanied by seizures, may be prominent and poorly responsive to anticonvulsant therapy. The outcome in these comatose patients is usually extremely poor, with only a rare patient making a meaningful recovery.[32] The benefit of postoperative therapeutic hypothermia in patients who are comatose immediately after heart surgery is unknown.[33]

Seizures may accompany coma, encephalopathy, or delirium, or they may occur independently after cardiac surgery. They occur in approximately 1 percent of patients, usually early in the postoperative period and often within the first 24 hours.[30,34] Some early seizures have been associated temporally with high-dose tranexamic acid, a drug that decreases postoperative bleeding.[34] Tonic-clonic or focal motor seizures are clinically apparent, but focal seizures with dyscognitive features in an encephalopathic patient may be difficult to recognize clinically and require electroencephalography to make the diagnosis. Choreoathetosis after heart surgery, a complication that occurs mainly in children, sometimes is mistaken for a seizure disorder.[35] Nonconvulsive status epilepticus may occur with stroke complicating cardiac surgery and can contribute to a prolonged confusional state that is treatable with anticonvulsant drugs; therefore, electroencephalographic evaluation of patients with a persistent encephalopathy can be valuable.[36]

Peripheral Nerve Disorders

The brachial plexus and phrenic nerves are the most frequent peripheral nerves injured during cardiac surgery. Brachial plexopathy after median sternotomy has been reported to occur in 1.5 to over 5 percent of patients.[37–39] Most frequently, the lower trunk of the brachial plexus is involved, which may mimic an ulnar neuropathy. The intrinsic hand muscles are often most severely impaired, but—unlike an ulnar neuropathy—the triceps reflex may be decreased in the affected arm. Sensory loss in the hand is sometimes present, pain is prominent in some patients, and a minority of patients have a Horner syndrome. Injuries of the upper brachial plexus also occur but are less frequent. Although not life-threatening and usually reversible in 1 to 3 months, a brachial plexus injury may produce permanent disability in some cases, particularly if it affects the dominant hand or produces intractable causalgia.

These brachial plexus injuries may be due to torsional traction or compression during the open heart surgery. Intraoperative electrophysiologic monitoring of sensory nerve conduction in the upper extremity reveals significant disturbances during sternal retraction in many patients. This technique can detect disorders of the brachial plexus during surgery, predict postoperative nerve injury, and identify intraoperative factors that predispose to brachial plexus injury.[38,40,41] Brachial plexus injuries may be reduced by minimizing the opening of the sternal retractor, placing the retractor in the most caudal location, and minimizing asymmetric traction.[38]

Unilateral phrenic nerve injuries with hemidiaphragmatic paralysis occur in over 10 percent of patients during open heart surgery. The location of the phrenic nerve adjacent to the pericardium makes it particularly vulnerable to injury from manipulation and ischemia as well as from hypothermia associated with topical cold cardioplegia. Unilateral phrenic nerve injury causes atelectasis and inspiratory muscle weakness, predisposing to postoperative respiratory complications. Phrenic nerve involvement in patients with preoperative chronic obstructive pulmonary disease adds to postoperative morbidity. In most patients, however, morbidity is low and some recovery is usually evident by about 6 months. Occasionally, there may be a more protracted course consistent with axonal injury and regeneration. Severe, bilateral phrenic nerve injury is a rare complication of heart surgery and leads to prolonged mechanical ventilation.[38,39]

Mononeuropathies resulting from compression or trauma during surgery may involve the spinal accessory, facial, lateral femoral cutaneous, fibular (peroneal), radial, recurrent laryngeal, saphenous, long thoracic, and ulnar nerves.[29,38,39,42–46] Ischemia to the cochlea-auditory nerve can result in severe hearing loss.[47] A recurrent laryngeal nerve injury with vocal cord paralysis may cause only hoarseness when mild, but aspiration when severe or bilateral. Injury to the saphenous nerve when a saphenous vein is harvested for CABG may cause hyperesthesia, decreased sensation and pain along the medial lower leg.[38] A persistent fibular (peroneal) neuropathy causes a disabling foot drop and may be due to positioning in the operating room. Most mononeuropathies are transient. This reversibility, usually within 4 to 8 weeks, may reflect focal selective injury to myelin, with relative sparing of nerve axons.[48] Awareness of possible intraoperative compression sites helps to prevent these complications.

Diffuse paralysis as a result of the Guillain–Barré syndrome may follow otherwise uncomplicated cardiac surgery as well as other surgical procedures.[49] Persistent paralysis also occurs after cardiac surgery in critically ill patients who require days of vecuronium to facilitate mechanical respiration.[50] If heart surgery is complicated by sepsis and multiorgan failure lasting for more than a week, a critical illness polyneuropathy and myopathy may develop, with difficulty in weaning from the ventilator.[51]

Neuro-ophthalmologic Disorders

Visual disorders associated with cardiac surgery may involve the retina, optic nerves, or retrochiasmal visual systems. Retinal disorders include multifocal areas of retinal nonperfusion, which occur in 44 to 100 percent of patients. Cotton wool spots have been reported in 17.3 percent of patients and retinal emboli visualized in 2.6 percent.[52,53] These retinal disorders are infrequently associated with reduced visual acuity.

An anterior ischemic optic neuropathy is an uncommon, disabling complication, occurring in 0.1 percent or fewer patients after heart surgery.[54,55] There is infarction of the optic nerve head and optic disc swelling, with a painless and usually permanent decrease in visual acuity. On visual field testing, a monocular altitudinal, arcuate, or central scotoma may be seen. A retrobulbar or posterior ischemic optic neuropathy due to infarct of the intraorbital nerve is even less common, producing acute blindness without optic disc swelling, accompanied by impaired pupillary reactions.[56] Both the anterior and posterior ischemic optic neuropathies may produce unilateral or bilateral blindness.[54,55]

Homonymous visual field defects occur with focal ischemic injury to the visual cortex or retrochiasmal visual pathways. An occasional patient is found to be cortically blind after heart surgery, usually from bilateral ischemia of the occipital cortex. Retinal and pupillary examinations are both normal in such patients and some will deny any visual impairment. At least partial recovery from cortical blindness is possible.[39]

Horner syndrome occurs in association with injuries to the lower brachial plexus and may result from concomitant injury to the preganglionic sympathetic fibers that travel through the eighth cervical and first thoracic ventral roots. It also develops in the postoperative period in hypertensive and diabetic patients, presumably due to ischemic injury to sympathetic fibers.[57]

Gaze deviation, gaze paralysis, and dysconjugate gaze may occur in postoperative patients who have a brainstem or large hemispheric stroke involving eye movement systems. Intermittent gaze deviation with nystagmoid movements raises concern for postoperative focal seizures.[58]

Pituitary apoplexy resulting from acute hemorrhage or infarction of a pituitary adenoma is a rare complication of cardiopulmonary bypass.[59] The pituitary tumor is usually not recognized prior to surgery and is particularly susceptible to the ischemic and hemorrhagic risks associated with cardiopulmonary bypass. Patients awake from surgery with headache, ptosis, ophthalmoplegia, and visual impairment from compression of the adjacent cranial nerves and the anterior visual pathways. Transsphenoidal surgical decompression has been used safely in some patients. Infarction of a normal pituitary during CABG also may occur and leads to panhypopituitarism.[60]

Visual hallucinations occurring solely on eye closure have been reported following cardiovascular surgery.[61] Patients are otherwise fully alert and lucid and can stop the hallucinations simply by opening their eyes. Atropine or lidocaine toxicity as well as focal seizures with dyscognitive features have been associated with such hallucinations.

NEUROCOGNITIVE DECLINE

Neuropsychologic studies of cognitive function before and after cardiac surgery have identified both a transient early and a subsequent late decline in cognitive function occurring after heart surgery.[4] The early postoperative changes in cognition are typically reversible. Neuropsychologic test results obtained 3 weeks, 4 months, and 1 year after patients had CABG are similar to those of nonsurgical subjects receiving percutaneous coronary intervention and healthy control subjects.[62] Also, older subjects may show a reversible decline in neuropsychologic testing shortly after non-cardiac surgery and anesthesia.[63] The postsurgical transient cognitive decline may relate to the vulnerability of an aging brain.

A late decline in cognitive function occurs in the interval from 3 to 5 years after CABG. Early investigators proposed that diffuse brain microemboli during cardiopulmonary bypass injured a neuronal reserve that is needed to limit cognitive decline and prevent dementia with aging.[64]

Current evidence does not support the proposal that cardiopulmonary bypass is a defined risk factor for the late cognitive decline. Cognitive function 5 years after patients were randomly assigned to undergo either coronary surgery or angioplasty is similar.[65] Performing coronary artery surgery without cardiopulmonary bypass decreases the microemboli to the brain. However, changes in cognitive performance from baseline to 3 years showed no significant difference between patients receiving on-pump CABG and patients receiving off-pump surgery as well as in two control groups, nonsurgical patients with coronary artery disease and patients without cardiovascular risk factors.[66] The neuropsychologic testing was repeated in the same four types of patient groups 6 years after CABG, when all three groups with coronary artery disease showed a similar cognitive decline that was greater than the control group without coronary artery disease.[67] In another study comparing patients receiving on-pump and off-pump CABG, cognitive performance was similar at 5 years postsurgery.[68] Therefore the present evidence indicates that cardiopulmonary bypass is not the main risk factor for progressive late cognitive decline.

A slow accumulation of ischemic brain damage due to vascular risk factors is an alternative explanation for the late decline in neurocognitive performance with coronary artery disease. Elderly subjects with asymptomatic subcortical ischemic lesions on brain imaging who have not had heart surgery have a greater decline in cognitive function over a period of 3 to 4 years than individuals without ischemic lesions.[69,70] An increase in subcortical ischemic lesions and the decline in cognitive function progress together.[71] Patients prior to CABG typically have vascular risk factors and many have MRI evidence of brain infarctions that increase the risk of subsequent cognitive decline. One study of a small number of patients with vascular risk factors and without baseline impaired cognition showed no late decline in cognitive performance after 3 to 5 years. These patients also had very good control of vascular risk factors over the interval of neuropsychologic testing.[72] The possibility of slowing cognitive decline is another reason to stress good medical control of vascular risk factors in patients with CABG.[72]

RISK FACTORS FOR STROKE

Several preoperative factors place a patient at a higher risk of neurologic complications (Table 3-1). Older age is associated with an increased frequency

TABLE 3-1 ■ Risk Factors for Cerebral Ischemia During Cardiac Surgery

Preoperative
Older age[14,81]
Hypertension[14,18]
Diabetes mellitus[14,18]
Smoking[14,81]
History of cerebrovascular disease[14,18]
Atheromatous aorta[17]
Peripheral vascular disease[14,18]
Previous cardiac surgery[14,18]
Intraoperative
Prolonged cardiopulmonary bypass[17,18]
Combined coronary artery bypass and valvular surgeries[3,81]
Large hemodynamic fluctuations[82]
Aorta cannulation and manipulation[5]
Postoperative
Atrial fibrillation[14,81]

of neurologic and cognitive disorders following CABG.[3,18,24] An older, multicenter, prospective study of 5,000 patients found that the occurrence of stroke was 1 percent in patients younger than 50 years of age, almost 2 percent in patients aged 50 to 59 years, approaching 4 percent in patients aged 60 to 69 years, and greater than 5 percent in patients older than 70 years. More recent studies indicate a decreasing stroke incidence in CABG patients, including octogenarians.[14,73]

As previously noted, dislodgement of atheroma during instrumentation and manipulation of the aorta is an important risk factor for stroke.[10,74–76] A preoperative history of hypertension, diabetes mellitus, smoking, stroke, and markers of vascular disease are also risk factors for stroke following CABG. Cardiac surgery within 3 months of a stroke may carry a risk of worsening preoperative neurologic deficits, although this increased risk may be mitigated by a thorough stroke workup that identifies and treats the etiology of the stroke.[77]

The greater the number of preoperative risk factors, the higher is the probability of a perioperative stroke. For example, a 65- to 75-year-old patient with a history of stroke and hypertension has a risk of postoperative stroke that is three times greater than that of a patient of the same age without a history of stroke or hypertension. A patient older than 75 years with a history of stroke and hypertension has a probability of postoperative stroke that is approximately 13 times greater than a patient younger than 65 years with no previous stroke or history of hypertension. Stroke risk stratification systems may identify patients prior to CABG who are at high risk of a perioperative stroke.[78]

Intraoperative factors also influence the frequency of stroke. Individuals who require CABG combined with left-sided intracardiac procedures have a relatively high rate of stroke.[18,19] Patients who require cardiopulmonary bypass lasting more than 2 hours have a higher number of cerebral emboli detected by transcranial Doppler ultrasound monitoring and also a higher frequency of stroke.[17,18,79–81] A large fluctuation in hemodynamic parameters during surgery, such as in blood pressure, has been associated with postoperative stroke and encephalopathy.[82] The risk from intraoperative hypotension during cardiopulmonary bypass, with a mean arterial pressure below 40 to 50 mmHg, remains unclear.

Atrial fibrillation occurs in approximately one-third of continuously monitored patients following cardiac surgery and is a risk factor for stroke. Its initial occurrence is most common during the first 3 postoperative days, and 20 percent of patients have more than one episode. Advancing age and withdrawal of β-adrenergic receptor blocking agents or angiotensin-converting enzyme inhibitors increases the risk of postoperative atrial fibrillation.[5,81,83,84]

PREVENTION OF NEUROLOGIC COMPLICATIONS

Evidence-based intraoperative guidelines for heart surgery have recently been published with an aim of minimizing the risk of brain ischemia.[7,8,11] There are inconsistencies between the published practice guidelines that may reflect differences in expert opinion of the published evidence. One set of guidelines with an emphasis on brain protection is summarized in Table 3-2. There is currently insufficient evidence to guide firmly any modification of these practice guidelines in patients at high risk of brain ischemia.[7]

Perioperative preventive measures have been updated in the 2011 American College of Cardiology/American Heart Association (ACC/AHA) guidelines

TABLE 3-2 ■ Evidence-Based Cardiopulmonary Bypass Practices that May Improve Neurologic Outcome[8]

Practice	Class/Level of Evidence*	Mechanism
Arterial filtration	Class I/Level A	Minimize emboli
Intraoperative aorta imaging	Class I/Level B Class IIb/Level B	Identify aortic plaque Reduce emboli
Minimize direct reinfusion of pericardial suction blood	Class I/Level B	Reduce emboli and prothrombotic systemic inflammatory response
Process and filter pericardial suction blood before reinfusion	Class IIb/Level B	
Alpha-stat pH management‡	Class 1/Level A	Maintain metabolic coupled cerebral blood flow
Limit arterial line temperature to 37°C during rewarming	Class IIa/Level B	Avoid brain hyperthermia
Reduce blood contact with nonbiocompatible surface of CPB circuits	Class IIa/Level B	Reduce prothrombotic systemic inflammatory response
Maintain normal perioperative glucose levels	Class I/Level B	Avoid hyperglycemia
Reduce hemodilution	Class I/Level A	Avoid very low hematocrit

*Class I–Procedure or treatment should be performed. Class IIa–Reasonable to perform procedure or treatment; additional focused studies needed. Class IIb–Consider procedure or treatment; additional broad studies needed. Level A–Recommendation derived from multiple randomized studies. Level B–Recommendation derived from single randomized or multiple nonrandomized studies.
‡Other sources maintain such a recommendation is "premature."[1]

for CABG.[5] The administration of a preoperative β-blocking drug and reinstituting it as soon as possible after surgery is recommended to reduce the incidence of atrial fibrillation. The guidelines also recommend pre- and postoperative aspirin and statin therapy. Early postoperative use of aspirin decreases ischemic complications of multiple organs including the brain.[85] The ACC/AHA guidelines also recommend the routine use of epiaortic ultrasound scanning to identify aortic atherosclerosis and reduce embolic events such as stroke. Detection of severely diseased ascending aorta may alter surgical strategy such as choosing to use "off-pump" surgery and avoiding manipulation of the ascending aorta. Delaying heart surgery for 4 or more weeks after a recent stroke has been recommended if the cardiac condition allows such a delay.[86]

The optimal management of co-existing carotid stenosis in patients needing CABG is unclear. Carotid endarterectomy for patients with severe (70 to 99%) internal carotid stenosis that has been neurologically symptomatic in the past 6 months is of established benefit independent of cardiac surgery.[87] Performing a carotid endarterectomy before or simultaneous with CABG in such patients is recommended in the 2011 ACC/AHA guidelines.[5] CABG can be performed without endarterectomy in asymptomatic individuals with unilateral carotid stenosis because the carotid procedure does not reduce stroke or mortality in these individuals. The guidelines also state that endarterectomy may be considered in selected asymptomatic subjects with bilateral severe carotid stenosis or with unilateral severe stenosis and contralateral carotid occlusion. Carotid stenting is an alternative procedure when a contraindication to carotid endarterctomy exists.[5,88]

CARDIAC TRANSPLANTATION

Cardiac transplantation is an established treatment for selected patients with progressive heart failure. Survival rate at 1 year post-transplant is greater than 80 percent, at 5 years greater than 70 percent, and at 10 years greater than 50 percent. The annual number of heart transplantations worldwide is approximately 4,000. Heart recipients 60 or more years of age have increased in frequency and comprised one-fourth of the heart transplantations from 2006 to 2011.[89] Neurologic sequelae occurring either in the perioperative period or as a late complication, however, may negate an otherwise successful heart transplantation. The early identification of treatable complications offers the best opportunity to prevent severe disability.

The perioperative neurologic sequelae from cardiac transplantation are similar to the complications associated with valvular or bypass graft surgery, discussed previously, except that neurologic complications occur more frequently in transplant recipients.[90] Postoperative encephalopathy, stroke, headaches, psychosis, seizures, and peripheral nerve disorders are the most common problems.[91,92]

Vascular headaches accompanied by nausea and vomiting may occur in the first week after transplantation.[93] The headaches are associated with a rapid shift from low preoperative to high postoperative mean arterial pressures. Similar headaches may rarely precede an intraparenchymal hemorrhage. These vascular headaches respond to β-adrenergic receptor blocking agents.

Seizures occur in approximately 2 percent of cardiac transplant patients, usually during the perioperative period, but also occur as a side effect of cyclosporine and other immunosuppressive agents or as a late complication of a brain infection or tumor.[91,92] Seizures in the perioperative period may not require long-term anticonvulsant therapy. When anticonvulsant drugs are indicated, phenytoin, phenobarbital, and carbamazepine are often avoided because they induce the hepatic metabolism of cyclosporine, tacrolimus, and sirolimus. When these antiepileptic agents are used, immunosuppressive dosing may need to be adjusted. Levatiracetam and gabapentin have negligible hepatic enzyme–inducing effects and few drug interactions, and therefore may be preferred anticonvulsants. Pregabalin, a newer antiepileptic drug, can also be considered.[94]

Psychotic behavior with hallucinations, delusional thought processes, and disorganized behavior may occur during the first 2 weeks after transplantation or as a late complication. When it occurs during the postoperative period, multiple causal factors may be present, but with time such psychotic behavior usually resolves. When psychotic behavior occurs as a late complication, it is often a manifestation of an intracranial infection, most commonly viral encephalitis. A thorough neurologic evaluation is therefore indicated when a cardiac transplant recipient develops an acute late psychosis.[29]

Immunosuppression remains a cause of neurologic complications after cardiac transplantation by increasing the risk of central nervous system (CNS) opportunistic infections. These infections are typically a late complication occurring after at least a month of immunosuppression.[95] The CNS infections in three series of heart transplant recipients are listed in Table 3-3, while rarer infections, often reported as case reports, are listed in Table 3-4.[91,96–106] Pathogens may be transferred from donor to transplant recipients, reactivated, or acquired. Focal meningoencephalitis or brain abscess, meningitis, and diffuse encephalitis are common presentations; the diagnosis is based on neurologic examination, brain imaging and, when indicated, cerebrospinal fluid studies. Details of the clinical presentation, diagnostic methods and treatment of the listed infections have been described elsewhere.[107]

TABLE 3-3 ■ Comparison of CNS Infection: 1960 to 1980 versus 1988 to 2006

	Stanford Hospital Series 1968–1980[106]	Mayo Clinic Series 1988–2006[106]	Madrid, Spain Series 1988–2006[91]
Number of Transplant Recipients	182	315	384
CNS Infected Recipients No. (% of recipients)	35 (19%)[*,‡]	8 (3%)	7 (2%)[‡]
Meningoencephalitis/Abscess Number (% infections)			
Aspergillus species	10 (28%)	1 (12%)	3 (43%)
Toxoplasma gondii	4 (11%)	0	1 (14%)
Candida albicans	1 (3%)	0	0
Klebsiella pneumoniae	1 (3%)	0	0
Mucormycosis	1 (3%)	0	0
Tuberculosis	0	0	1 (14%)
Meningitis			
Cryptococcus neoformans	5 (14%)	3 (38%)	0
Listeria monocytogenes	4 (11%)	0	2 (29%)
Coccidioides immitis	1 (3%)	0	0
Streptococcus pneumoniae	0	0	1 (14%)
Viral Encephalitis			
Cytomegalovirus	≥3 (9%)[a]	0	0
Herpes simplex	≥3 (9%)[a]	0	0
Herpes zoster	≥2 (6%)[a]	2 (25%)	0
JC virus	0	2 (25%)	0
Periorbital Neuropathies			
Mucormycosis	1 (3%)	0	0

[*]The 1968–1980 Stanford series did not include viral encephalitis cases. Therefore eight viral encephalitis cases were added from a 1968–1975 Stanford series (see Hotson J, Pedley TA: The neurological complications of cardiac transplantation. Brain 99:673, 1976).
[‡]One patient had two CNS infections.

CNS infections occurred in almost 20 percent of heart transplant recipients from 1968 to 1980, but declined to 2 to 3 percent in recipients between 1988 and 2006 (Table 3-3). The infections have

TABLE 3-4 ■ Other CNS Infections

Meningoencephalitis/Abscess
Balamuthia mandrillaris[98]
Bipolaris spicifera[105]
Cladophialophora bantiana[100]
Nocardia species[102]
Pseudallescheria boydii[97]
Rhodococcus equi[101]
Syphilis, late [99]
Trypanosoma cruzi[104]
Viral Encephalitis
Human herpesvirus-6[103]
West Nile virus[96]

changed in association with antibiotic prophylaxis and preemptive therapy, the availability of antiviral drugs, preoperative vaccination for infections such as varicella zoster, and changes in immunosuppression strategies.[95] The chronic use of prophylactic trimethoprin-sulfamethoxazole is associated with a decreased frequency of toxoplasmosis meningoencephalitis. Many *Listeria* and *Nocardia* species are also sensitive to these prophylactic drugs.[95] Antiviral drugs may prevent or treat cytomegalovirus and other herpesvirus infections and decrease the risk of encephalitis.[108]

Aspergillosis, while less frequent, is still the most common fungal infection that produces a necrotizing meningoencephalitis and single or multiple brain abscesses.[91] Cerebral aspergillosis is usually disseminated from a preceding pulmonary infection, though it may invade the brain directly from a paranasal sinus infection.[108] Antifungal prophylaxis combined with early detection and treatment of pulmonary *Aspergillus* may decrease its intracranial dissemination.[95,109,110] Aspergillosis also causes an invasive necrosis of intracranial vessels that may lead to hemorrhagic infarction. Therefore, focal hemorrhage on brain imaging is suggestive of *Aspergillus* infection. Patients present with focal neurologic signs, seizures, mental status changes, and headache.[109] The diagnosis is confirmed by direct needle aspiration or biopsy of infected tissue. Cerebrospinal fluid (CSF) studies are usually nonspecific, though detection of a galactomannan antigen can be used as supportive evidence of infection, and there is interest in development of an *Aspergillus*-specific polymerase chain reaction (PCR) assay.[109,110] If the diagnosis is made late, the disease is fatal; early diagnosis and treatment in immunosuppressed patients, however, improve survival.[111] Antifungal medications that can achieve therapeutic CSF levels, such as voriconazole, together with neurosurgical management may produce the best outcome.[109,111]

Toxoplasma gondii can also cause meningoencephalitis and abscess formation following cardiac transplantation. Evidence of an active *T. gondii* infection includes seroconversion after transplantation in a previously seronegative individual or a positive polymerase chain reaction (PCR) assay of blood or CSF.[112–114] While tissue diagnosis with material aspirated from a brain abscess is diagnostic, a presumptive diagnosis based on imaging and serologic testing may lead to a therapeutic trial. Consideration of the diagnosis is mandatory because of the excellent therapeutic response to anti-*Toxoplasma* antibiotics when initiated early. Toxoplasmosis may in addition cause an inflammatory myopathy in association with multisystem infection that is also responsive to treatment.[115,116]

Cryptococcus neoformans and *Listeria monocytogenes* remain important treatable causes of meningitis after cardiac transplantation.[91,106] The typical presenting symptom of cryptoccocal meningitis is a subacute headache with a normal neurologic examination. The white blood count in the CSF varies but is usually moderately elevated with predominantly mononuclear cells. CSF cryptococcal antigen is typically present in the serum or CSF, and CSF cultures are positive.[106] Symptoms from infection with *L. monocytogenes* are more acute and may include focal neurologic signs of brainstem dysfunction or cervical myelopathy. CSF may show a prominent pleocytosis consisting of polymorphonuclear and mononuclear cells.[29]

Greater than 10 percent of heart transplant recipients develop varicella zoster virus (VZV) infection presenting with vesicular skin lesions.[91,106] A minority of these patients also develop encephalitis with a positive CSF PCR. Varicella zoster can cause brain infarction due to a large-vessel vasculopathy, deep white matter lesions from a small-vessel vasculopathy, or a ventriculitis with periventricular necrosis.[117] Herpes simplex may also cause encephalitis, but the clinical presentation is distinct in immunosuppressed individuals. Herpes simplex produces an acute necrotizing focal encephalitis in the immunocompetent individual, but a more diffuse and slowly progressive encephalitis in heart transplant recipients.[29]

Immunosuppression for cardiac transplantation combined with Epstein–Barr virus infection can lead to uncontrolled B-cell proliferation. This post-transplantation lymphoproliferative disorder may occur any time after transplantation and evolve into systemic malignant lymphoma, including involvement of the brain. Post-transplantation lymphoproliferative disorder may involve multiple organs or a single organ. The CNS can be the only site of malignant lymphoproliferation.[118,119] Epstein–Barr virus PCR may determine viral load in the blood or CSF, providing evidence of active infection. Lymphoproliferative disorders, however, can also occur unrelated to Epstein–Barr virus. The diagnosis is based on histopathologic examination of tissue.[120] Post-transplantation lymphoproliferative disorder may regress with reduction of immunosuppressive therapy. Surgical treatment or localized radiotherapy can be effective when the disorder is restricted to a single organ. More extensive disease may require the addition of chemotherapy regimens.[119,120]

Immunosuppressive agents may also be directly neurotoxic. Prior to the use of calcineurin inhibitors, high-dose prednisone in combination with azathioprine was common. The main side effects of the prednisone were weakness of the proximal lower extremities, osteoporosis with lower thoracic and lumbosacral compression fractures, or psychiatric complications.[121] With the use of the calcineurin inhibitors cyclosporine and tacrolimus, it has been possible to lower the dose of prednisone, thereby reducing its side effects. Cyclosporine and tacrolimus themselves, however, may have neurotoxic side effects, including prominent postural tremor, headache, a lowered seizure threshold, paresthesias, mental confusion, acute mania, weakness, ataxia, dysarthria, akinetic mutism, visual hallucinations, and cortical blindness.[122]

Brain imaging may reveal a calcineurin inhibitor–induced posterior leukoencephalopathy, though other brain structures may also be involved. T2-weighted MRI studies suggest that the onset of the posterior leukoencephalopathy is due to vasogenic brain edema. Calcineurin inhibitors are strong vasoconstrictors that may damage microvasculature and break down the blood–brain barrier. The induced vasogenic edema is often reversible, as are, typically, the adverse effects and MRI findings when the leukoencephalopathy is identified early and the calcineurin inhibitor dose is reduced.[122,123] Calcineurin inhibitor–induced posterior leukoencephalopathy, however, may cause residual neurologic impairment, stressing the importance of early diagnosis and treatment.[124] The newer immunosuppressive agents mycophenolate mofetil, sirolimus, and everolimus have fewer reported neurotoxic effects and may be used in combination with calcineurin inhibitors to reduce neurotoxicity.[123,125,126]

Cyclosporine also induces gout and has chronic nephrotoxicity. When gout is treated with colchicine, a peripheral neuromuscular disorder may result that improves when the colchicine is stopped.[127]

The monoclonal anti-CD3 antibody OKT3 has been used to prevent and treat graft rejection following cardiac transplantation. Aseptic meningitis with fever, headache, seizures, and a variable encephalopathy is reported to occur in 5 percent of patients. This aseptic meningitis may occur during the course of OKT3 therapy or in the weeks immediately following its administration. The aseptic meningitis and encephalopathy resolve within days of onset.[122]

REFERENCES

1. Oakes DA, Mora Mangano CT: Cardiopulmonary bypass in 2009: achieving and circulating best practices. Anesth Analg 108:1368, 2009.
2. Roger VL, Go AS, Lloyd-Jones DM, et al: Heart disease and stroke statistics–2012 update: a report from the American Heart Association. Circulation 125:e205, 2012.
3. McKhann GM, Grega MA, Borowicz Jr LM, et al: Stroke and encephalopathy after cardiac surgery: An update. Stroke 37:562, 2006.
4. Selnes OA, Gottesman RF, Grega MA, et al: Cognitive and neurologic outcomes after coronary-artery bypass surgery. N Engl J Med 366:250, 2012.
5. Hillis LD, Smith PK, Anderson JL, et al: 2011 ACCF/AHA guideline for coronary artery bypass graft surgery. Circulation 124:e652, 2011.
6. Hammon JW: Extracorporeal circulation. p. 349. In Cohn L (ed): Cardiac Surgery in the Adult. McGraw-Hill, New York, 2008.
7. Hogue Jr HW, Palin CA, Arrowsmith JE: Cardiopulmonary bypass management and neurologic outcomes: an evidence-based appraisal of current practices. Anesth Analg 103:21, 2006.

8. Shann SH, Likowsky DS, Murkin JM, et al: An evidence-based review of the practice of cardiopulmonary bypass in adults: a focus on neurologic injury, glycemic control, hemodilution, and the inflammatory response. J Thorac Cardiovasc Surg 132:283, 2006.
9. Gaudino M, Glieca F, Alessandrini F, et al: Individualized surgical strategy for the reduction of stroke risk in patients undergoing coronary artery bypass grafting. Ann Thorac Surg 67:1246, 1999.
10. Hangler HB, Nagele G, Danzmayr M, et al: Modification of surgical technique for ascending aortic atherosclerosis: impact on stroke reduction in coronary artery bypass grafting. J Thorac Cardiovasc Surg 126:391, 2003.
11. Murphy GS, Hessel II EA, Groom RC: Optimal perfusion during cardioppulmonary bypass: an evidence based approach. Anesth Analg 108:1395, 2009.
12. Rees K, Beranek-Stanley M, Burke M, et al: Hypothermia to reduce neurological damage following coronary artery bypass surgery. Cochrane Database Syst Rev:CD002138, 2001.
13. Roach GW, Kanchuger M, Mangano CM, et al: Adverse cerebral outcomes after coronary artery bypass surgery. N Engl J Med 335:1857, 1996.
14. Tarakji KG, Sabik 3rd JF, Bhudia SK, et al: Temporal onset, risk factors, and outcomes associated with stroke after coronary artery bypass grafting. JAMA 305:381, 2011.
15. Floyd TF, Shah PN, Price CC, et al: Clinically silent cerebral ischemic events after cardiac surgery: their incidence, regional vascular occurrence, and procedural dependence. Ann Thorac Surg 81:2160, 2006.
16. Salazar J, Wityk R, Grega M, et al: Stroke after cardiac surgery: short and long term outcomes. Ann Thorac Surg 72:1195, 2001.
17. Hogue Jr CW, Murphy SF, Schechtman KB, et al: Risk factors for early or delayed stroke after cardiac surgery. Circulation 100:642, 1999.
18. Bucerius J, Gummert JF, Borger MA, et al: Stroke after cardiac surgery: a risk factor analysis of 16,184 consecutive adult patients. Ann Thorac Surg 75:472, 2003.
19. Boeken U, Litmathe J, Feindt P, et al: Neurological complications after cardiac surgery: risk factors and correlation to the surgical procedure. Thorac Cardiovasc Surg 53:33, 2005.
20. Likosky D, Marrin C, Caplan L: Determination of etiologic mechanisms of strokes secondary to coronary artery bypass graft surgery. Stroke 34:2830, 2003.
21. Gottesman R, Sherman P, Grega M: Watershed strokes after cardiac surgery: diagnosis, etiology, and outcome. Stroke 37:2306, 2006.
22. Nakajima M, Tsuchiya K, Kanemaru K, et al: Subdural hemorrhagic injury after open heart surgery. Ann Thorac Surg 76:614, 2003.
23. Mehall J, Leach J, Merrill W: Posterior reversible encephalopathy syndrome with nontransplant cardiac surgery. J Thorac Cardiovasc Surg 130:1473, 2005.
24. Bucerius J, Gummert J, Borger M, et al: Predictors of delirium after cardiac surgery: effect of beating-heart (off pump) surgery. J Thorac Cardiovasc Surg 127:57, 2004.
25. Rolfson D, McElhaney J, Rockwood K, et al: Incidence and risk factors for delirium and other adverse outcomes in older adults after coronary artery bypass graft surgery. Can J Cardiol 15:771, 1999.
26. Wityk R, Goldsborough M, Hillis A, et al: Diffusion-weighted and perfusion-weighted brain magnetic resonance imaging in patients with neurologic complications after cardiac surgery. Arch Neurol 58:571, 2001.
27. Stamou SC, Nussbaum M, Carew JD, et al: Hypoglycemia with intensive insulin therapy after cardiac surgery: predisposing factors and association with mortality. J Thorac Cardiovasc Surg 142:166, 2011.
28. Hiramatsu Y, Sakakibara Y, Mitsui T, et al: Clinical features of hypernatremic hyperosmolar delirium following open heart surgery. Nippon Kyobu Geka Gakkai Zasshi 39:1945, 1991.
29. Hotson J: Neurological complications of cardiac surgery. p. 45. In Aminoff MJ (ed): Neurology and General Medicine. 4th Ed. Churchill Livingstone Elsevier, Philadelphia, 2008.
30. Carrascal Y, Guerrero A, Maroto L, et al: Neurological complications after cardiopulmonary bypass: an update. Eur Neurol 41:128, 1999.
31. Rodriguez RA, Bussiere M, Bourke M, et al: Predictors of duration of unconsciousness in patients with coma after cardiac surgery. J Cardiothorac Vasc Anesth 25:961, 2011.
32. Wijdicks EF, Parisi JE, Sharbrough FW: Prognostic value of myoclonus status in comatose survivors of cardiac arrest. Ann Neurol 35:239, 1994.
33. Chakravarthy M: Therapeutic hypothermia after cardiac arrest in cardiac surgery: a meaningful pursuit? Ann Card Anaesth 12:101, 2009.
34. Murkin J, Falter F, Granton J: High-dose tranexamic acid is associated with nonischemic clinical seizures in cardiac surgical patients. Anesth Analg 10:350, 2010.
35. Passari M, Romito S, Avesani M: Late-onset choreoathetotic syndrome following heart surgery. Neurol Sci 31:95, 2010.
36. Rittenberger J, Popescu A, Brenner R: Frequency and timing of nonconvulsive status epilepticus in comatose post-cardiac arrest subjects treated with hypothermia. Neurocrit Care 16:114, 2012.
37. Mateen F, van de Beek D, Kremers WK, et al: Neuromuscular diseases after cardiac transplantation. J Heart Lung Transplant 28:226, 2009.
38. Sharma AD, Parmley CL, Sreeram G, et al: Peripheral nerve injuries during cardiac surgery: risk factors, diagnosis, prognosis, and prevention. Anesth Analg 91:1359, 2000.
39. Grocott HP, Clark JA, Homi HM, et al: "Other" neurologic complications after cardiac surgery. Semin Cardiothorac Vasc Anesth 8:213, 2004.

40. Jellish WS, Blakeman B, Warf P, et al: Hands-up positioning during asymmetric sternal retraction for internal mammary artery harvest: a possible method to reduce brachial plexus injury. Anesth Analg 84:260, 1997.
41. Canbaz S, Turgut N, Halici U, et al: Brachial plexus injury during open heart surgery - controlled prospective study. Thorac Cardiovasc Surg 53:295, 2005.
42. Marini SG, Rook JL, Green RF, et al: Spinal accessory nerve palsy: an unusual complication of coronary artery bypass. Arch Phys Med Rehabil 72:247, 1991.
43. Parsonnet V, Karasakalides A, Gielchinsky I, et al: Meralgia paresthetica after coronary bypass surgery. J Thorac Cardiovasc Surg 101:219, 1991.
44. Tewari P, Aggarwal SK: Combined left-sided recurrent laryngeal and phrenic nerve palsy after coronary artery operation. Ann Thorac Surg 61:1721, 1996.
45. Itagaki T, Kikura M, Sato S: Incidence and risk factors of postoperative vocal cord paralysis in 987 patients after cardiovascular surgery. Ann Thorac Surg 83:2147, 2007.
46. Durmaz B, Kirazli Y, Atamaz F: Isolated spinal accessory nerve palsy after coronary artery bypass: an unusual complication. Am J Phys Med Rehabil 86:865, 2007.
47. Walsted A, Andreassen UK, Berthelsen PG, et al: Hearing loss after cardiopulmonary bypass surgery. Eur Arch Otorhinolaryngol 257:124, 2000.
48. Burns T: Neuropathy caused by compression, entrapment or physical injury. p. 1391. In: Dyck P, Thomas P (eds): Peripheral Neuropathy. Elsevier Saunders, Philadelphia, 2005.
49. Hogan JC, Briggs TP, Oldershaw PJ: Guillain-Barré syndrome following cardiopulmonary bypass. Int J Cardiol 35:427, 1992.
50. Segredo V, Caldwell JE, Matthay MA, et al: Persistent paralysis in critically ill patients after long-term administration of vecuronium. N Engl J Med 327:524, 1992.
51. Latronico N, Bolton CF: Critical illness polyneuropathy and myopathy: a major cause of muscle weakness and paralysis. Lancet Neurol 10:931, 2011.
52. Blauth CI, Smith PL, Arnold JV, et al: Influence of oxygenator type on the prevalence and extent of microembolic retinal ischemia during cardiopulmonary bypass. Assessment by digital image analysis. J Thorac Cardiovasc Surg 99:61, 1990.
53. Nenekidis I, Pournaras CJ, Tsironi E, et al: Vision impairment during cardiac surgery and extracorporeal circulation: current understanding and the need for further investigation. Acta Ophthalmol 90:e168, 2012.
54. Kalyani SD, Miller NR, Dong LM, et al: Incidence of and risk factors for perioperative optic neuropathy after cardiac surgery. Ann Thorac Surg 78:34, 2004.
55. Nuttall GA, Garrity JA, Dearani JA, et al: Risk factors for ischemic optic neuropathy after cardiopulmonary bypass: a matched case/control study. Anesth Analg 93:1410, 2001.
56. Buono LM, Foroozan R: Perioperative posterior ischemic optic neuropathy: review of the literature. Surv Ophthalmol 50:15, 2005.
57. Barbut D, Gold JP, Heinemann MD, et al: Horner's syndrome after coronary artery bypass surgery. Neurology 46:181, 1996.
58. Tusa R, Kaplan P, Hain T, et al: Ipsiversive eye deviation and epileptic nystagmus. Neurology 40:662, 1990.
59. Pliam M, Cohen M, Cheng L, et al: Pituitary adenomas complicating cardiac surgery: summary and review of 11 cases. J Cardiac Surg 10:125, 1995.
60. Davies JS, Scanlon MF: Hypopituitarism after coronary artery bypass grafting. BMJ 316:682, 1998.
61. Eissa A, Baker R, Knight J: Closed-eye hallucinations after coronary artery bypass. J Cardiothorac Vasc Anesth 19:217, 2005.
62. Sweet JJ, Finnin E, Wolfe PL, et al: Absence of cognitive decline one year after coronary bypass surgery: comparison to nonsurgical and healthy controls. Ann Thorac Surg 85:1571, 2008.
63. Price CC, Garvan CW, Monk TG: Type and severity of cognitive decline in older adults after noncardiac surgery. Anesthesiology 108:8, 2008.
64. Brown W, Moody D, Tytell M, et al: Microembolic brain injuries from cardiac surgery: are they seeds of future Alzheimer's disease? Ann NY Acad Sci 826:386, 1997.
65. Hlatky MA, Bacon C, Boothroyd D, et al: Cognitive function 5 years after randomization to coronary angioplasty or coronary artery bypass graft surgery. Circulation 96(suppl II):11, 1997.
66. Selnes OA, Grega MA, Bailey MM, et al: Neurocognitive outcomes 3 years after coronary artery bypass graft surgery: a controlled study. Ann Thorac Surg 84:1885, 2007.
67. Selnes OA, Grega MA, Bailey MM, et al: Do management strategies for coronary artery disease influence 6-year cognitive outcomes? Ann Thorac Surg 88:445, 2009.
68. Hernandez Jr F, Brown JR, Likosky DS, et al: Neurocognitive outcomes of off-pump versus on-pump coronary artery bypass: a prospective randomized controlled trial. Ann Thorac Surg 84:1897, 2007.
69. Vermeer SE, Longstreth Jr WT, Koudstaal PJ: Silent brain infarcts: a systematic review. Lancet Neurol 6:611, 2007.
70. Vermeer SE, Prins ND, den Heijer T, et al: Silent brain infarcts and the risk of dementia and cognitive decline. N Engl J Med 348:1215, 2003.
71. van Dijk EJ, Prins ND, Vrooman HA, et al: Progression of cerebral small vessel disease in relation to risk factors and cognitive consequences: Rotterdam scan study. Stroke 39:2712, 2008.
72. Mullges W, Babin-Ebell J, Reents W, et al: Cognitive performance after coronary artery bypass grafting: a follow-up study. Neurology 59:741, 2002.
73. Maganti M, Rao V, Brister S, et al: Decreasing mortality for coronary artery bypass surgery in octogenarians. Can J Cardiol 25:e32, 2009.

74. Katz ES, Tunik PA, Rusinek H, et al: Protruding aortic atheromas predict stroke in elderly patients undergoing cardiopulmonary bypass: experience with intraoperative transesophageal echocardiography. J Am Coll Cardiol 20:70, 1992.
75. van der Linden J, Hadjinikolaou L, Bergman P, et al: Postoperative stroke in cardiac surgery is related to the location and extent of atherosclerotic disease in the ascending aorta. J Am Coll Cardiol 38:131, 2001.
76. Mackensen GB, Ti LK, Phillips-Bute BG, et al: Cerebral embolization during cardiac surgery: impact of aortic atheroma burden. Br J Anaesth 91:656, 2003.
77. Rorick MB, Furlan AJ: Risk of cardiac surgery in patients with prior stroke. Neurology 40:835, 1990.
78. McKhann GM, Grega MA, Borowicz Jr LM, et al: Encephalopathy and stroke after coronary artery bypass grafting: incidence, consequences, and prediction. Arch Neurol 59:1422, 2002.
79. Barbut D, Lo Y, Gold JP, et al: Impact of embolization during coronary artery bypass grafting on outcome and length of stay. Ann Thorac Surg 63:998, 1997.
80. Libman RB, Wirkowski E, Neystat M, et al: Stroke associated with cardiac surgery. Arch Neurol 54:83, 1997.
81. Almassi G, Sommers T, Moritz T, et al: Stroke in cardiac surgical patients: determinants and outcome. Ann Thorac Surg 68:391, 1999.
82. Ganushchak YM, Fransen EJ, Visser C, et al: Neurological complications after coronary artery bypass grafting related to the performance of cardiopulmonary bypass. Chest 125:2196, 2004.
83. Almassi GH, Schowalter T, Nicolosi AC, et al: Atrial fibrillation after cardiac surgery: a major morbid event? Ann Surg 226:501, 1997.
84. Mathew J, Fontes M, Tudor I, et al: A multicenter risk index for atrial fibrillation after cardiac surgery. JAMA 291:1720, 2004.
85. Mangano DT: Aspirin and mortality from coronary bypass surgery. N Engl J Med 347:1309, 2002.
86. Eagle KA, Guyton RA, Davidoff R, et al: ACC/AHA 2004 guideline update for coronary artery bypass surgery. Circulation 110:e340, 2004.
87. Chaturvedi S, Bruno A, Feasby T, et al: Carotid endarterectomy—an evidence-based review. Neurology 65:794, 2005.
88. Van der Heyden J, Van Neerven D, Sonker U, et al: Carotid artery stenting and cardiac surgery in symptomatic patients. JACC Cardiovasc Interv 4:1190, 2011.
89. Stehlik J, Edwards LB, Kucheryavaya AY, et al: The registry of the international society for heart and lung transplantation: 29th official adult heart transplant report—2012. J Heart Lung Transplant 31:1052, 2012.
90. Inque K, Luth JU, Pottkamper KM, et al: Incidence and risk factors of perioperative cerebral operations: heart transplantation compared to coronary artery bypass grafting and valve surgery. J Cardiovasc Surg 39:201, 1998.
91. Muñoz P, Valerio M, Palomo J: Infectious and noninfectious neurologic complications in heart transplant recipients. Medicine (Baltimore) 89:166, 2010.
92. Perez-Miralles F, Sanchez-Manso JC, Almenar-Bonet L, et al: Incidence of and risk factors for neurologic complications after heart transplantation. Transplant Proc 37:4067, 2005.
93. Sila C: Spectrum of neurologic events following cardiac transplantation. Stroke 20:1586, 1989.
94. Shepard P, St. Louis E: Seizure treatment in transplant patients. Curr Treat Options Neurol 14:332, 2012.
95. Fishman J: Infections in solid-organ transplant recipients. N Engl J Med 257:2601, 2007.
96. Bragin-Sanchez D, Chang PP: West Nile virus encephalitis infection in a heart transplant recipient: a case report. J Heart Lung Transplant 24:621, 2005.
97. Castiglioni B, Sutton DA, Rinaldi MG, et al: *Pseudallescheria boydii* (anamorph *Scedosporium apiospermum*) infection in solid organ transplant recipients in a tertiary medical center and review of the literature. Medicine (Baltimore) 81:333, 2002.
98. Center for Disease Control and Prevention: Notes from the field: transplant-transmitted *Balamuthia mandrillaris*—Arizona, 2010. MMWR Morb Mortal Wkly Rep 59:1182, 2010.
99. Farr M, Rubin AI, Mangurian C, et al: Late syphilis in a cardiac transplant patient. J Heart Lung Transplant 25:358, 2006.
100. Keyser A, Schmid FX, Linde HJ, et al: Disseminated *Cladophialophora bantiana* infection in a heart transplant recipient. J Heart Lung Transplant 21:503, 2002.
101. Kohl O, Tillmanns HH: Cerebral infection with *Rhodococcus equi* in a heart transplant recipient. J Heart Lung Transplant 21:1147, 2002.
102. Lopez FA, Johnson F, Novosad DM, et al: Successful management of disseminated *Nocardia transvalensis* infection in a heart transplant recipient after development of sulfonamide resistance: case report and review. J Heart Lung Transplant 22:492, 2003.
103. Nash PJ, Avery RK, Tang WH, et al: Encephalitis owing to human herpesvirus-6 after cardiac transplant. Am J Transplant 4:1200, 2004.
104. Pittella JE: Central nervous system involvement in Chagas disease: a hundred-year-old history. Trans R Soc Trop Med Hyg 103:973, 2009.
105. Rosow L, Jiang J, Deuel T, et al: Cerebral phaeohyphomycosis caused by *Bipolaris spicifera* after heart transplantation. Transpl Infect Dis 13:419, 2011.
106. van de Beek D, Patel R, Daly R, et al: Central nervous system infections in heart transplant recipients. Arch Neurol 64:1715, 2006.
107. Scheld M, Whitley R, Marra C: Infections of the Central Nervous System. Lippincott, Williams and Wilkins, Philadelphia, 2004.
108. Andrews PA, Emery VC, Newstead C: Summary of the British Transplantation Society guidelines for the

prevention and management of CMV disease after solid organ transplantation. Transplantation 92:1181, 2011.

109. Kourkoumpetis TK, Desalermos A, Muhammed M, et al: Central nervous system aspergillosis: a series of 14 cases from a general hospital and review of 123 cases from the literature. Medicine (Baltimore) 91:328, 2012.
110. De Pauw B, Walsh TJ, Donnelly JP, et al: Revised definitions of invasive fungal disease from the European Organization for Research and Treatment of Cancer. Clin Infect Dis 46:1813, 2008.
111. Schwartz S, Ruhnke M, Ribaud P, et al: Improved outcome in central nervous system aspergillosis, using voriconazole treatment. Blood 106:2641, 2005.
112. Fernandez-Sabe N, Cervera C, Farinas MC, et al: Risk factors, clinical features, and outcomes of toxoplasmosis in solid-organ transplant recipients: a matched case-control study. Clin Infect Dis 54:355, 2012.
113. Cibickova L, Horacek J, Prasil P, et al: Cerebral toxoplasmosis in an allogeneic peripheral stem cell transplant recipient: case report and review of literature. Transpl Infect Dis 9:332, 2007.
114. Abdel Razek AA, Watcharakorn A, Castillo M: Parasitic diseases of the central nervous system. Neuroimaging Clin N Am 21:815, 2011.
115. Cuturic M, Hayat GR, Vogler CA, et al: Toxoplasmic polymyositis revisited: case report and review of literature. Neuromuscul Disord 7:390, 1997.
116. Plonquet A, Bassez G, Authier FJ, et al: Toxoplasmic myositis as a presenting manifestation of idiopathic CD4 lymphocytopenia. Muscle Nerve 27:761, 2003.
117. Kleinschmidt-DeMasters BK, Amlie-Lefond C, Gilden DH: The patterns of varicella zoster virus encephalitis. Hum Pathol 27:927, 1996.
118. Castellano-Sanchez AA, Li S, Qian J, et al: Primary central nervous system posttransplant lymphoproliferative disorders. Am J Clin Pathol 121:246, 2004.
119. Everly MJ, Bloom RD, Tsai DE, et al: Posttransplant lymphoproliferative disorder. Ann Pharmacother 41:1850, 2007.
120. American Society of Transplantation: Epstein–Barr virus and lymphoproliferative disorders after transplantation. Am J Transplant 4(suppl 10):59, 2004.
121. Patchell RA: Neurological complications of organ transplantation. Ann Neurol 36:688, 1994.
122. Wijdicks EF: Neurotoxicity of immunosuppressive drugs. Liver Transpl 7:937, 2001.
123. Senzolo M, Burra CF: P: Neurologic complications after solid organ transplantation. Transplant Int 22:269, 2009.
124. Burnett MM, Hess CP, Roberts JP, et al: Presentation of reversible posterior leukoencephalopathy syndrome in patients on calcineurin inhibitors. Clin Neurol Neurosurg 112:886, 2010.
125. Bodkin CL, Eidelman BH: Sirolimus-induced posterior reversible encephalopathy. Neurology 68:2039, 2007.
126. van de Beek D, Kremers WK, Kushwaha SS, et al: No major neurologic complications with sirolimus use in heart transplant recipients. Mayo Clin Proc 84:330, 2009.
127. Rana SS, Giuliani MJ, Oddis CV, et al: Acute onset of colchicine myoneuropathy in cardiac transplant recipients: case studies of three patients. Clin Neurol Neurosurg 99:266, 1997.

CHAPTER

4

Neurologic Complications of Congenital Heart Disease and Cardiac Surgery in Children

CATHERINE LIMPEROPOULOS ■ ADRÉ J. DU PLESSIS

In recent decades, major advances in intraoperative and critical care support have dramatically reduced mortality in infants and children with congenital heart disease. At the same time, neurologic morbidity, often characterized by lifelong neurodevelopmental problems, has become increasingly recognized among survivors. Neurologists have become important members of the acute and long-term care teams of these children.

Of the 30,000 infants born with heart defects in the United States each year, approximately half require some form of surgical intervention within the first year of life.[1] There have been major changes in the clinical profile of neurologic injury in children with congenital heart disease since the late 1960s. In earlier years, the neurologic complications were mostly mediated by chronic hypoxia and polycythemia in cyanotic children, uncorrected right-to-left shunts, and the effects of repeated palliative heart operations.[2,3] Advances in surgical technique and intensive care management have allowed for the anatomic correction of many heart lesions in early infancy, resulting in major decreases in mortality of congenital heart disease. More infants with critical congenital heart disease and profound hemodynamic disturbances in the newborn period are now rescued, only to manifest later the neurologic consequences of this early-life morbidity. The same surgical support techniques responsible for advancing survival have paradoxically been associated with an incidence of neurologic complications that approaches 25 percent in some centers.[4] Consequently, mechanisms of brain injury during cardiac surgery have been the focus of intense investigation over the past two decades. Understanding these intraoperative mechanisms has been advanced through animal experimental models and several large clinical trials, as well as through intraoperative cerebral monitoring and perioperative magnetic resonance imaging (MRI).[5–11]

It is being recognized increasingly that both acquired and developmental brain disturbances in infants with congenital heart disease may have their origin prior to surgical intervention, in many cases during the fetal period.[12–18] It is expected that these mechanisms will receive increased attention as the role of fetal imaging and fetal interventions expands.[19,20]

This chapter reviews the preoperative, intraoperative, and postoperative neurologic abnormalities in children with congenital heart disease. It is important to recognize that the manifestations of

Aminoff's Neurology and General Medicine, Fifth Edition.

neurologic dysfunction in many of these patients may result from cumulative insults occurring across these high-risk periods.

NEUROLOGIC ABNORMALITIES BEFORE CARDIAC SURGERY

Recent studies have demonstrated a high prevalence of neurologic abnormalities prior to cardiac surgery in infants, in some studies exceeding 50 percent. These clinical abnormalities include microcephaly, hypotonia, behavioral dysregulation, and feeding difficulties, which are often accompanied by abnormal electrophysiologic studies.[7,12,13,21] These preoperative abnormalities are increasingly recognized as significant predictors of longer-term neurodevelopmental sequelae following surgery.[13,21–23]

Preoperative Neurologic Disorders of Fetal Onset

Cerebral Dysgenesis

The prevalence of brain dysgenesis in children with congenital heart disease approaches 30 percent in some autopsy studies.[24,25] The risk of cerebral dysgenesis appears related to the specific underlying cardiac lesion. For example, infants with hypoplastic left heart syndrome may be at particular risk of associated developmental brain lesions, which range in severity from microdysgenesis to gross malformations including agenesis of the corpus callosum, holoprosencephaly, and immature cortical mantle.[25] The relationship between cardiac and brain dysgenesis has been more clearly defined through advances in neuroimaging. These cerebral abnormalities may present with seizures, alterations in level of consciousness, and abnormalities in motor tone in the newborn period, or they may remain clinically occult until later infancy and childhood, when they present with developmental delay, epilepsy, and cerebral palsy.

An unresolved question in this population is whether cerebral dysgenetic lesions are a consequence of primary genetic abnormalities or secondary to cerebral oxygen and substrate restriction, or both. More recent advances in quantitative MRI techniques have demonstrated subtle disturbances in cerebral development and maturation. Several studies have suggested that fetal heart anomalies may result in dysmaturity at the cellular, metabolic, and micro- and macrostructural levels in the absence of gross lesions detected by conventional MRI.[25–29]

Several studies using Doppler flow patterns in the fetal middle cerebral artery have demonstrated evidence of cerebral vasodilation (the "brain sparing" effect), especially in fetuses with hypoplastic left heart syndrome.[16,30–32] This compensatory mechanism may be limited in its ability to maintain adequate oxygen/substrate delivery as evidenced by the increased rate of impaired brain growth in these patients.[33]

Chromosomal Disorders

A number of chromosomal disorders have a phenotype that includes both cardiac and neurologic malformations, including trisomies 11, 18, and 21. The most common neurologic manifestation in children with trisomy 21 (Down syndrome) is cognitive dysfunction. Epilepsy develops in approximately 5 percent of these children, and congenital heart defects, most commonly endocardial cushion defects, are present in 40 percent of children with Down syndrome. Gross structural brain alterations in Down syndrome include a narrow superior temporal gyrus and a disproportionately small cerebellum and brainstem.[24] Trisomy 13 is associated with ventricular septal defects and patent ductus arteriosus; the associated cerebral dysgenesis in this syndrome is often severe, with holoprosencephaly and agenesis of the corpus callosum being the most common lesions. The most common cardiac lesions in infants with trisomy 18 are ventricular septal defects and patent ductus arteriosus, with neuronal migration defects being the most common form of brain dysgenesis.[34]

The phenotypic spectrum of specific chromosome 22 deletions, particularly in the 22q11 region, includes a variety of cardiac malformations and neurologic features.[35] Recent population-based data suggest that at least 700 infants with chromosome 22 deletion syndromes are born annually in the United States.[36] The acronym *CATCH 22* (*c*ardiac defect, *a*bnormal facies, *t*hymic hypoplasia, *c*left palate, *h*ypocalcemia, and chromosome *22*q11 deletions) has been used to designate this group of related syndromes. The two most common, DiGeorge and velocardiofacial (or Shprintzen) syndromes, have neurologic and cognitive manifestations in association with structural cardiac defects.[37] The fundamental problem in DiGeorge syndrome is a developmental defect of the third and fourth pharyngeal pouches, manifesting with thymic and parathyroid hypoplasia along with conotruncal cardiac malformations, which include an interrupted aortic arch (type B), truncus arteriosus, and tetralogy of Fallot.

A common neurologic presentation in both the DiGeorge and the velocardiofacial syndromes is hypocalcemic seizures due to hypoparathyroidism. In addition to the usual cardiac lesions (i.e., ventricular septal defect or tetralogy of Fallot), the velocardiofacial syndrome is associated with cleft palate or velopharyngeal insufficiency and a typical facial appearance, including a broad, prominent nose and retrognathia, along with microcephaly in up to 40 percent of cases. Neuroimaging and autopsy studies may demonstrate a small posterior fossa and vermis, small cystic lesions adjacent to the frontal horns of the lateral ventricles, dysgenesis of the corpus callosum, and abnormal cortical gyrification patterns.[38,39] Delayed opercular development and disproportionately enlarged sylvian fissures with white matter abnormalities might underlie some of the developmental problems in these children.[40,41] The mean intelligence quotient (IQ) in this syndrome is around 70, with mild to moderate cognitive problems present in up to 50 percent of patients.[37,41]

In recent years, a high rate of autism spectrum disorders and attention deficit/hyperactivity disorder has been described in this group of patients.[42,43] Psychiatric disorders occur in up to 22 percent of those with 22q11 deletion syndromes.[38,39] A peculiar and inappropriately blunt effect may be evident during childhood, often evolving to frank psychosis during adolescence and adulthood.[44] Altered prefrontal cortex-amygdala circuitry, reduced cerebellar and thalamic volumes, and increased basal ganglia and corpus callosal volumes, as shown by quantitative neuroimaging studies, may underlie disrupted emotional processing and form the neurobiologic substrate for the psychiatric disturbances in these children.[41,45–47]

Preoperative Neurologic Injury of Postnatal Onset

Infants with congenital heart disease are at increased risk of acquired antenatal or perinatal brain injury. During fetal life, congenital heart lesions may be associated with changes in cerebrovascular blood flow distribution and resistance. Fetuses with hypoplastic left heart syndrome, whose cerebral perfusion is supplied retrograde through the ductus arteriosus, may be at particular risk.[16,17] Preoperative MRI studies have demonstrated that brain injury is common in infants with critical congenital heart disease including following invasive diagnostic procedures (e.g., balloon-atrial septostomy).[48,49] Preoperative findings detected by MRI include intracranial hemorrhage, cerebral venous thrombosis, thromboembolic stroke, dilatation of the ventricles and subarachnoid spaces suggestive of cerebral atrophy, periventricular leukomalacia, and gray matter injury.[14,15,17,50] Elevated preoperative brain lactate levels have been found by magnetic resonance spectroscopy in over half of newborns with congenital heart disease.[14,20,50] Lower oxyhemoglobin saturation and longer delay to surgical correction are risk factors for MRI-detected brain injury.[51]

Complex corrective operations are now being performed in ever smaller and less mature newborn infants. Intraventricular/periventricular hemorrhage (IVH-PVH) is a common neurologic complication in these newborns. The risk of IVH-PVH is related to the severity of the vascular insult and, inversely, to the infant's gestational age. Prematurity predisposes to IVH-PVH because of the structural and physiologic vulnerability of the immature periventricular germinal matrix. The hemodynamic instability commonly seen in more severe forms of congenital heart disease predisposes to the systemic hypotension and fluctuations in blood pressure that trigger IVH-PVH. The incidence of IVH-PVH in term infants with congenital heart disease is substantially higher than in term infants overall. Around 25 percent of infants with hypoplastic left heart syndrome are found to have intracranial hemorrhage at autopsy.[52] Infants with coarctation of the aorta are at additional risk of intracranial hemorrhage because of associated intracranial vascular malformations and hypertension.

The preoperative detection of intraventricular hemorrhage in infants with congenital heart disease creates a major management dilemma as the risk of extending such hemorrhage is increased by cardiopulmonary bypass and other aspects of cardiac surgery. Cardiopulmonary bypass requires anticoagulation to prevent clot formation in the bypass circuit and has been associated with enhanced systemic fibrinolytic activity.[53] More complex operations also require periods of decreased perfusion to approach the cardiac defect. To further complicate decision-making, intracranial hemorrhage occurs more commonly in infants with the more critical cardiac lesions that are in greatest need of early surgical repair. Small hemorrhagic or ischemic lesions in the preoperative period are probably not exacerbated by cardiac surgery or cardiopulmonary bypass.

There are no prospectively tested protocols for managing preoperative intracranial hemorrhage in infants requiring cardiac surgery. At our center, preoperative cranial ultrasonography is performed to exclude IVH-PVH in all premature infants with a birth weight of less than 1,500 g as well as in newborn infants with preoperative neurologic dysfunction, coagulation disturbances, or hemodynamic instability causing significant metabolic acidosis. In those infants with IVH-PVH, surgical planning is based on the severity of the cardiac illness (which may directly affect the risk of hemorrhage extension), the likely complexity of surgery, and the severity of preoperative IVH-PVH. Minor subependymal hemorrhage carries a low risk of extension and should not delay cardiac surgery.[54,55] However, in infants with hemorrhage into the ventricles or the parenchyma, we delay cardiopulmonary bypass for at least 7 days if the cardiac condition permits.

NEUROLOGIC INJURY DURING CARDIAC SURGERY

Acute neurologic dysfunction in the early postoperative period probably relates to intraoperative hypoxic-ischemic/reperfusion injury. However, the risk of cerebrovascular injury extends into the postoperative period, when cardiorespiratory instability, together with cerebral autoregulatory dysfunction, predisposes to further cerebral hypoxic-ischemic injury. Despite advances facilitated by deep hypothermia and various pharmacologic agents, persistent neurologic morbidity in the postoperative period remains a risk.[3,56]

The precise onset and evolution of hypoxic-ischemic/reperfusion injury may be difficult to establish. The mechanisms of both parenchymal and vascular hypoxic-ischemic/reperfusion injury are known to evolve over time. During the early posthypoxic-ischemic period, cells that have sustained an insult may be at particular risk of irreversible injury due to subsequent disturbances in oxygen supply. It is therefore difficult in some cases to ascribe with any certainty hypoxic-ischemic/reperfusion injury to one of the preoperative, intraoperative, or postoperative periods. In many cases the injury is likely multifactorial and cumulative.

Mechanisms of Intraoperative Brain Injury

There are multiple interrelated mechanisms by which brain injury may occur during cardiac surgery. Hypoxic-ischemic/reperfusion injury is probably the principal mechanism since laminar cortical necrosis and periventricular white matter injury are often seen at autopsy.[52,57,58] Animal models of deep hypothermic circulatory arrest have demonstrated selective neuronal necrosis in a distribution that corresponds closely to that seen after normothermic hypoxic-ischemic/reperfusion injury. Neuropathologic studies of infants after deep hypothermic cardiac surgery suggest that cerebral white matter lesions tend to be more prevalent and severe than gray matter lesions.[57]

Changes in cerebral perfusion and metabolism during cardiac surgery are complex, interrelated, and often extreme. When these changes exceed the brain's ability to maintain a balance between cerebral oxygen or substrate supply and utilization, a hypoxic-ischemic/reperfusion insult is triggered. Factors determining intraoperative cerebral oxygen availability may be categorized as extrinsic, related to the extracorporeal circulation (e.g., loss of pulsatility, low or no pump flow, hypothermia, and emboli), or intrinsic (e.g., disturbances in autoregulation of cerebral blood flow). During deep hypothermic cardiac surgery, cerebral oxygen delivery may also be impaired by focal or multifocal vaso-occlusive phenomena generated by the bypass circuit or by global hypoperfusion due to the excessive attenuation of bypass flow rate.[3,56]

Focal or Multifocal Hypoxic-Ischemic Injury

The relatively small intravascular volume of the young infant compared with the large blood volume required to "prime" the cardiopulmonary bypass circuit results in an increased exposure to insults related to the bypass. These include both embolic and inflammatory disturbances, the latter due to the extensive interface between blood and artificial surfaces.[3,56,59,60]

The replacement of bubble oxygenators with membrane devices has decreased, but not eradicated, the embolic "load" of bypass circuits. Both gaseous and particulate emboli may enter the bypass circuit directly from the surgical field. Because the circuit delivers oxygenated blood directly to the aorta, circulating emboli circumvent the normal pulmonary filtration bed and enter the systemic (and cerebral) arterial circulation directly. In addition to emboli, cerebral capillary-bed aneurysmal dilatations have been observed.[59]

Cardiopulmonary bypass activates a host of inflammatory cascades that can cause diffuse vascular injury, resulting in a postperfusion syndrome that in severe cases is associated with multiple organ failure. Pathways triggered include those involving eicosanoids, complement, and kallikrein. These pathways activate free radical generation, cause antioxidant depletion, and upregulate adhesion molecules on neutrophils and endothelial cells.[61,62] These activated neutrophils appear to be potent mediators of cerebral reperfusion injury. Although hypothermia delays and modifies the effect of these processes, it does not completely prevent them.[63]

Global Hypoxic-Ischemic Injury

Several techniques used during neonatal cardiac surgery may jeopardize global cerebral oxygen by altering cerebral perfusion, arterial oxygen content, and tissue oxygen delivery. Under deep hypothermic conditions, cerebral oxygen availability may be limited by cold-induced increases in cerebral vascular resistance, impairment of cerebral pressure–flow autoregulation, and increased oxygen-hemoglobin affinity.[64,65] The normal response to periods of decreased perfusion pressure involves cerebral oxygen delivery being maintained by an initial vasodilatory response followed by an increase in oxygen extraction.[66] However, both of these compensatory responses are compromised at deep hypothermia.[67]

To approach these often small cardiac defects, the bypass flow rate must be decreased and even arrested for periods, depending on the complexity of the lesion. Although there are general guidelines for "safe periods" of deep hypothermic circulatory arrest at various temperatures, these remain controversial and unpredictable in the individual patient. In addition, the safety of low-flow bypass compared with hypothermic circulatory arrest is controversial. Low-flow bypass prolongs exposure to bypass-related embolic phenomena, as well as increasing the risk of incomplete ischemia. Conversely, deep hypothermic circulatory arrest allows more rapid completion of the intracardiac phases of the repair and reduces the exposure to bypass perfusion; however, the infant is exposed to periods of complete ischemia.[3,56] Deleterious effects of deep hypothermic circulatory arrest on neurologic outcome have been reported in several studies.[68–71] In a major clinical trial randomizing infants to a strategy of predominant hypothermic circulatory arrest or low-flow bypass, infants exposed to the former were at significantly greater risk of perioperative and 1-year neurologic sequelae.[7,8] At age 4 years, the deep hypothermic circulatory arrest group had significantly worse behavior, speech, and language function, but no difference in mean intelligence score.[9] At 8-year follow-up, those assigned to deep hypothermic circulatory arrest scored worse on motor and speech domains, whereas those assigned to low-flow bypass had worse impulsivity and behavior.[10] The long-term follow-up of this large cohort has provided important insights into the evolution of neurodevelopmental outcomes in this complex population over time.[72] Although it is now generally accepted that prolonged periods of uninterrupted deep hypothermic circulatory arrest may have adverse neurologic effects, shorter durations of deep hypothermic circulatory arrest have not consistently been associated with adverse outcomes.[73–75] Available data suggest that the relationship between duration of deep hypothermic circulatory arrest and neurodevelopmental sequelae is not linear, with the risk of brain injury increasing significantly after about 40 minutes.[68,76]

In addition to flow rate, a number of other factors associated with cardiopulmonary bypass may affect cerebral perfusion and predispose to hypoxic-ischemic/reperfusion injury. Most centers in the United States use nonpulsatile bypass devices as well as hemodilution in order to reduce the magnitude of red blood cell trauma. Deep hypothermia is widely used in part to suppress oxygen consumption during surgery. In addition to their intended beneficial effects, these techniques all have potential adverse effects on cerebral oxygen delivery. The nonpulsatile perfusion of cardiopulmonary bypass, particularly at low flow rates, may fail to maintain perfusion in distal capillary beds.[77] Furthermore, nonpulsatile blood flow may disrupt autoregulation.[78] Hemodilution is also used during bypass to reduce rheologic injury to circulating red cells; however, because the concentration of oxygenated hemoglobin is the major determinant of oxygen-carrying capacity, this technique may limit cerebral oxygen delivery. In animal studies, extreme hemodilution (to hematocrit levels less than 10%) is associated with neurologic injury, whereas hematocrit levels above 30 percent improved cerebral recovery after deep hypothermic circulatory arrest.[52] These experimental results were confirmed by a randomized clinical trial in which infants randomized to a hematocrit of 20 percent during cardiac surgery had significantly worse developmental scores at 1 year than those randomized to a hematocrit of around 30 percent.[6]

Another important intraoperative factor is the management of acid-base status during cardiopulmonary bypass. In a randomized, single-center trial, infants undergoing cardiac operations were assigned to an alpha-stat versus pH-stat strategy of managing acid-base status during deep hypothermic cardiopulmonary bypass.[11] The use of pH-stat management was associated with lower overall early postoperative morbidity although treatment assignment had no effect on neurodevelopmental outcomes at 1, 2, and 4 years of age.[11,79] Despite these equivocal findings, many centers are currently using pH-stat management during core cooling.

After repair of the cardiac defect, bypass flow rates are increased using rewarmed and highly oxygenated blood in order to reactivate cellular enzyme function and oxygen utilization. During this period of reperfusion, a number of factors may predispose to free radical injury.[3,56] Several studies have suggested a delay in the recovery of mitochondrial function, possibly mediated by nitric oxide, which is generated in abundance during the bypass.[80,81] The combination of highly oxygenated reperfusion along with persistent mitochondrial dysfunction may serve as a major source of oxygen free radicals.[72,82] Excessively rapid rewarming after deep hypothermia may be particularly deleterious; hyperthermia is a trigger for glutamate release, predisposing to excitotoxicity as well as further stressing the recovering cerebral metabolism.[83,84]

NEUROLOGIC ABNORMALITIES IN THE POSTOPERATIVE PERIOD

Mechanisms of Postoperative Brain Injury

During the postoperative period, a variety of factors may predispose an infant to further brain injury. Cerebral perfusion pressure may be compromised by a combination of decreased cardiac output and elevated central venous pressure resulting from postoperative cardiac dysfunction. In addition to these systemic circulatory factors, intrinsic cerebrovascular disturbances may include elevated cerebral vascular resistance, decreased cerebral blood flow, and impaired vasoregulation, especially following deep hypothermic circulatory arrest.[2,56,64,85,86]

Studies suggest a recent decrease in this acute neurologic morbidity following surgery.[87] These postoperative insults may injure the neuraxis at any level; this review focuses on the more common clinical issues confronting the neurologist.

Manifestations of Postoperative Neurologic Dysfunction

Delayed Recovery of Consciousness

Prolonged impairment of mental status after cardiac surgery, anesthesia, and postoperative sedation is a common reason for neurologic consultation. The evaluation should follow the usual approach for assessing impaired consciousness in any patient. Common etiologies which should be excluded include postoperative hepatic or renal impairment, which may directly alter the mental state or do so in the setting of impaired metabolism or excretion of sedating drugs. Prolonged use of neuromuscular blocking agents in the preoperative or postoperative period may delay the recovery of motor function and, if severe, may mimic impaired consciousness; this condition may be excluded at the bedside with a peripheral nerve stimulator or formal nerve conduction studies. Postoperative seizures are a common complication of cardiac surgery, and a prolonged postictal state should be considered in the evaluation of a depressed postoperative mental state.[7] A precise cause of an impaired postoperative mental status is not established quickly in most cases, however, and many of these children ultimately demonstrate features suggestive of hypoxic-ischemic/reperfusion injury.

Postoperative Seizures

Seizures early in the postoperative period are among the most common neurologic complications after open heart surgery, occurring in up to 19 percent of survivors of neonatal cardiac surgery[88]; in some high-risk subgroups this number may reach up to 50 percent. Clinical seizures are reported less frequently than those without typical motor correlates that are only detected by continuous electroencephalographic (EEG) monitoring.[7,89] Some seizures have a readily identifiable cause, such as hypoglycemia, hypocalcemia, and cerebral dysgenesis. Postoperative seizures may also result from hypoxic-ischemic/reperfusion injury due to either generalized cerebral hypoperfusion (e.g., cardiac arrest) or focal vasoocclusive insults. More commonly, however, the etiology of the seizures remains unknown.

Although these cryptogenic seizures, commonly referred to as *postpump seizures*, are often assumed to relate to hypoxic-ischemic/reperfusion injury, their etiology is likely multifactorial with risk factors that include the use and duration of deep hypothermic circulatory arrest, younger age at surgery, the type of heart defect (e.g., aortic arch obstruction), and genetic susceptibility.[7,88,90] Postpump seizures differ in several respects from other forms of posthypoxic seizures. They typically develop later than, for instance, those occurring after perinatal asphyxia. The prognosis of postpump seizures is significantly better than that of asphyxial seizures, in which up to 50 percent of survivors are neurologically disabled.[8,91] Both the delayed onset and more favorable outcome may be due to the partial protective effect of hypothermia at the time of the intraoperative insult.

The clinical course of postpump seizures is fairly typical, with onset between 24 and 48 hours after surgery. This is followed by several days during which serial seizures occur, often evolving to status epilepticus; following this period, the tendency toward further seizures wanes rapidly. The clinical manifestations of these electrographic seizures are often subtle even in the absence of sedating and paralyzing drugs; they may even be confined to paroxysmal autonomic changes. When evident, convulsive activity is usually focal or multifocal.

The therapeutic approach to seizures should first involve excluding reversible etiologies such as hypoglycemia, hypomagnesemia, and hypocalcemia. Repeated seizures and status epilepticus should be treated by rapid achievement of therapeutic anticonvulsant levels by an intravenous route. Most postpump seizures are controlled by lorazepam, followed by phenobarbital or phenytoin. Potential cardiotoxicity due to these agents in children recovering from cardiac surgery should be monitored carefully, particularly during treatment initiation. The short window of susceptibility to postpump seizures often allows early withdrawal of anticonvulsants.

Prospective studies have demonstrated a significant correlation between postoperative seizures and the risk of perioperative and 1-year neurologic sequelae, as well as abnormal MRI studies.[7,8,88,92] The longer-term impact of postpump seizures maybe less than previously suspected.[11,93,112] The development of subsequent epilepsy is rare; however, West syndrome (infantile spasms, mental retardation, and epilepsy) has been described following a course of intractable postpump seizures.[93]

When postoperative seizures have an identified cause, the long-term outcome is related to etiology. For instance, cerebral dysgenesis, which is increased in patients with congenital heart disease, carries a poor long-term outcome, commonly featuring the development of epilepsy.[88] Infants with seizures due to postoperative stroke have a 20 to 30 percent risk of subsequent epilepsy.[94]

Periventricular White Matter Injury

Preoperative brain MRI in neonates with congenital cardiac disease identifies white matter injury in around 30 percent, especially in those with single ventricle physiology.[50,51,95] Postoperative brain MRI studies have shown a prevalence of white matter injury in excess of 50 percent.[50,95] The precise onset of these postoperative lesions remains unclear, and these MRI features appear to be transient in many cases.[50] Reported risk factors for development of these MRI lesions include prolonged exposure to cardiopulmonary bypass (with or without deep hypothermic cardiac arrest), inflammatory mechanisms which are activated by cardiopulmonary bypass, and early postoperative hypotension (especially diastolic) and hypoxemia.[96,97] In a recent study, the development of new white matter injury on postoperative MRI was not confined to those patients undergoing cardiopulmonary bypass; however, among those who did undergo bypass, increased duration led to more severe white mater injury.[98] White matter injury has also been associated with a lower brain maturation score, the presence of preoperative white matter injury, the use of deep hypothermic circulatory arrest, and specific cardiac diagnoses including single ventricle physiology and aortic arch obstruction.[98,99]

Although significant decreases in brain *N*-acetylaspartate (a neuronal-axonal marker) were described on magnetic resonance spectroscopy, more recent data have demonstrated improved postoperative cerebral oxidative metabolism as evidenced by lactate-to-choline ratios.[14,100,101] The long-term significance of these acute structural and metabolic disturbances in these children remains uncertain.

Stroke

The incidence of stroke in children ranges from 2.5 to 8 per 100,000.[128] Congenital heart disease is a leading cause of childhood stroke, being present in 25 to 30 percent of cases.[102–104] In autopsy studies, almost 20 percent of children with congenital heart disease have evidence of infarct.

Stroke associated with heart disease may be related to a number of mechanisms including: (1) cardioembolic (i.e., a probable intracardiac embolic source); (2) paradoxical (i.e., a cardiac anatomy that permits an embolus of systemic venous origin access to the cerebral circulation); or (3) venous (e.g., cerebral vein thrombosis due to central venous hypertension and venous stasis).

Risk factors for cardiogenic stroke include the elements of Virchow triad—altered vascular surface, stasis, and hypercoagulability—as well as the presence of paradoxical embolic pathways. In earlier studies, the risk of stroke was related mainly to the effects of long-standing heart defects such as chronic hypoxia and polycythemia as well as uncorrected paradoxical pathways leading to right-to-left shunting. The trend toward earlier corrective surgery has shifted the focus to intraoperative and postoperative mechanisms for stroke.

Cardiopulmonary bypass may predispose to cerebral vascular occlusion since embolic material (particulate or gaseous) generated during bypass avoids filtration by the pulmonary bed and gains direct entry to the systemic arterial circulation.[59] The extensive interface between circulating blood and the artificial surface of the bypass circuit may trigger an inflammatory response, which then activates complex physiologic cascades, including endothelium–leukocyte interactions.[57] This process further enhances the risk of ischemic injury during the intraoperative and postoperative periods. Advances in bypass technique, including refinements in membrane oxygenators, in-line arterial filters, and anticoagulation, have reduced the incidence of macroembolization and large-vessel occlusion compared with earlier autopsy studies. The impact of these advances on the incidence of microembolization and small-vessel disease is unclear.

In the postoperative period, factors predisposing to stroke include stasis (intracardiac and extracardiac), altered vascular surfaces (native or prosthetic), and, in some situations, a procoagulant shift in humoral clotting systems.[105] Intracardiac stasis may result from localized areas of low flow or global ventricular dysfunction.[106] Transient or sustained elevations of right heart and central venous pressure predispose to local thrombosis in the right atrium and central veins. Prosthetic material in such areas of disturbed flow increases the likelihood of thrombus formation, and the presence of a right-to-left shunt (native or iatrogenic) can lead to paradoxical embolization. Elevated right atrial pressure transmitted to the cerebral venous circulation also predisposes to venous thrombosis, particularly in the dural venous sinuses. Elevated systemic venous pressure may lead to a protein-losing enteropathy, liver impairment, and pleural effusions, which all are factors that may disturb the humoral coagulant systems.[105,107] A number of the aforementioned stroke risk factors may be present after the Fontan operation. In one study, a 2.6 percent incidence of stroke was found in a retrospective review of 645 patients after the Fontan operation; this risk extended over 3 years after the procedure.[106] In another study, a 20 percent incidence of thromboembolic complications was found after the Fontan procedure.[108]

Strokes originating during or immediately following cardiac surgery may escape clinical recognition for several days because of the effects of postoperative sedating and paralyzing agents. In young infants, stroke often presents with focal seizures or changes in mental status, with focal motor deficits being subtle. In older infancy and childhood, stroke usually presents with acute focal motor deficits, language disturbance, or visual dysfunction.

The therapeutic approach to stroke in the child with heart disease includes both "rescue" and preventive strategies. Experience with rescue therapies remains mainly confined to adult and experimental stroke where therapies aim to salvage potentially viable brain by revascularization with thrombolytic therapy or to curtail injurious biochemical cascades. Consistent and universally accepted guidelines for both primary and secondary stroke prophylaxis in children are lacking. Current guidelines are largely empiric, anecdotal, and derived from experience in adults. Established indications for primary stroke prophylaxis in children include prosthetic heart valves, dilated cardiomyopathy, or intracardiac thrombus.

The decision regarding whether and when to initiate secondary stroke prophylaxis with antithrombotic agents should aim to balance the risk of recurrent cerebral embolization and secondary hemorrhage into an area of cerebral infarction. Embolus recurrence risks after cardioembolic stroke are unknown in children. In adults following myocardial infarction, this risk is highest in the early poststroke period.

Cardioembolic strokes are particularly prone to hemorrhagic transformation in the early poststroke period; hemorrhagic transformation occurs (often asymptomatically) in 20 to 40 percent of adult cardioembolic strokes. The risk of significant clinical deterioration following hemorrhagic transformation is greatest in patients taking full-dose anticoagulation. Although it is difficult to predict which infarcts will undergo hemorrhagic transformation, most will do so early, within 48 hours after stroke onset. Large infarcts, particularly those involving greater than 30 percent of a cerebral hemisphere, are at higher risk of hemorrhagic transformation. Uncontrolled systemic hypertension and stroke caused by septic emboli and cerebral venous sinus thrombosis are additional risk factors for hemorrhagic infarction.

The many neurologic manifestations of infective endocarditis include meningitis, brain abscess, and seizures (see Chapter 6). However, septic embolism and hemorrhage are the most common complications. Even with appropriate antibiotics, neurologic complications occur in one-third of children with infective endocarditis; in one-half of these cases, the complications are embolic in origin.[109] Cerebrovascular complications carry the highest mortality rate (up to 80 to 90%) of all complications of infective endocarditis, primarily due to intracranial hemorrhage. The high risk of cerebral hemorrhage in this population contraindicates anticoagulant therapy. In cases of cardiogenic stroke, the possibility of septic embolism should be considered prior to initiating anticoagulant therapy.

MOVEMENT DISORDERS

Reports of serious postoperative movement disorders were published in the early 1960s and with the emergence of deep hypothermic cardiac surgery.[110,111] Choreoathetosis was the most frequent complication of cardiac surgery, reaching 19 percent in early reports, although the incidence seems to be decreasing substantially.[72,112] Other rarer postoperative movement disorders include oculogyric crises and parkinsonism. These movement disorders are often dramatic in clinical presentation, frequently intractable, and, in severe cases, are associated with substantial mortality.

Postoperative movement disorders have a typical clinical course. Involuntary movements occur on day 2 to 7; during the preceding days of the postoperative period, neurologic recovery appears to be uncomplicated. A subacute delirium featuring marked irritability, insomnia, confusion, and disorientation usually precedes the emergence of involuntary movements, which typically start in the distal extremities and orofacial muscles, progressing proximally to involve the girdle muscles and trunk. In severe cases, violent ballismus may develop. The abnormal movements are present during wakefulness, peak with distress, and resolve during sleep. Oculomotor and oromotor apraxia are common, with loss of voluntary gaze, expressive language, and ability to feed. The movements often intensify over a 1-week period, followed by a 1- to 2-week period during which the abnormal movements are relatively constant. Recovery is highly variable in duration, and the long-term outcome of these postoperative movement disorders depends largely on their initial severity. Mild cases tend to resolve within weeks to months, whereas severe cases have a mortality rate approaching 40 percent and are associated with a high incidence of persistent dyskinesia (47%) and long-term neurodevelopmental deficits including diffuse hypotonia and pervasive deficits in memory, attention, and language.[110,112]

The diagnosis of postoperative hyperkinetic syndromes is clinical; neuroimaging studies are useful only for excluding other disorders. Changes seen on computed tomography (CT), MRI, and single-photon emission CT are nonspecific, seldom focal, and most commonly consist of diffuse cerebral atrophy in patients with movement disorders.[110] The electroencephalogram is usually normal or diffusely slow, with no ictal changes associated with the involuntary movements. Descriptions of neuropathologic findings at autopsy are limited and inconsistent, ranging from normal to showing extensive neuronal loss and gliosis, particularly in the globus pallidus externa.[113] Typical features of infarction are characteristically absent.

Risk factors for the development of these involuntary movements include cyanotic congenital heart disease, particularly with systemic-to-pulmonary collaterals from the head and neck; age at surgery older than 9 months; excessively short cooling periods prior to attenuation of intraoperative blood flow; an alpha-stat pH management strategy; deep hypothermia and extracorporeal circulation; and preexisting developmental delay.[114–116] Postoperative dyskinesias have been reported after prolonged use of fentanyl and midazolam, although these are usually mild and transient.[117]

Once manifest, these involuntary movements are very refractory to treatment and generally respond poorly to a wide variety of antidyskinetic medications including dopamine receptor blockers (e.g., phenothiazines, butyrophenones), dopamine-depleting agents (e.g., reserpine, tetrabenazine), dopamine agonists (e.g., levodopa, pramipexole), GABAergic agents (benzodiazepines, barbiturates, baclofen), and a variety of other drugs such as valproic acid, carbamazepine, phenytoin, diphenhydramine, and chloral hydrate. In general, successful movement control is achieved only at the expense of excessive sedation.

The management of postoperative movement disorders should therefore focus on the often severe agitation and insomnia that accompanies them. Decreasing the level of external (e.g., noise, light) and internal (e.g., pain) stimuli is useful in limiting the intensity of the involuntary movements. Judicious use of sedation should aim to restore a fragmented sleep-wakefulness cycle which contributes to delirium. Oromotor dyskinesia is often severe enough to impair feeding and predispose to aspiration; nasogastric or even gastrostomy tube feedings may be necessary to meet the high caloric demands of the constant involuntary movements.

Spinal Cord Injury

Spinal cord injury is a relatively rare complication following pediatric cardiac surgery and usually occurs after aortic coarctation repair (0.4 to 1.5%).[118] Intraoperative spinal cord injury is often mediated by hypoxic-ischemic/reperfusion injury to watershed territories, most commonly in the lower thoracic cord, where transverse infarction results in postoperative paraplegia. An additional watershed zone runs between the territories of the anterior and posterior spinal circulations; ischemia in this region results in predominant anterior spinal cord involvement.

Brachial Plexus and Peripheral Nerve Injury

Prolonged immobility during and following cardiac catheterization and surgery predisposes peripheral nerves to pressure and traction injury. Pressure palsies may occur at any dependent site, but most commonly involve the fibular (peroneal) and ulnar nerves.

Brachial plexus injury is not uncommon following cardiac catheterization.[119,120] Injury to the lower plexus results from prolonged traction during the extreme and sustained arm abduction required for some procedures. Symptoms usually resolve gradually and completely. The insertion of indwelling central venous catheters during cardiac catheterization through the internal jugular vein may injure the upper brachial plexus through direct physical trauma or extravasation of blood into the plexus.

Phrenic nerve injury can result from hypothermic injury due to ice packed around the heart or, alternatively, from direct intraoperative transection. Postoperative phrenic nerve injury has also been described after malposition of chest tubes.[121] Phrenic nerve injury presents with diaphragmatic palsy and prolonged postoperative ventilator dependence. Nerve conduction studies and electromyography can confirm the diagnosis. Most phrenic nerve injuries resolve spontaneously, but occasionally diaphragmatic plication (more likely in infants than children) or, in rare instances, diaphragmatic pacing is required.

Adequate postoperative ventilation is commonly facilitated by the use of neuromuscular blocking agents. Prolonged use of nondepolarizing agents, especially vecuronium and pancuronium, has been associated with prolonged neuromuscular dysfunction, and concomitant use of corticosteroids may increase the risk. The neuropathologic spectrum of these conditions is highly variable, ranging from necrotizing myopathy to an axonal motor neuropathy with variable sensory involvement (see Chapters 56 and 59).

REFERENCES

1. Rudolph AM: Congenital Diseases of the Heart; Clinical-Physiologic Considerations in Diagnosis and Management. Year Book Medical Publishers, Chicago, 2001.
2. du Plessis AJ: Neurologic complications of cardiac disease in the newborn. Clin Perinatol 24:807, 1997.
3. du Plessis AJ: Cerebral hemodynamics and metabolism during infant cardiac surgery. Mechanisms of injury and strategies for protection. J Child Neurol 12:285, 1997.
4. Ferry PC: Neurologic sequelae of open-heart surgery in children. An 'irritating question' Am J Dis Child 144:369, 1990.
5. Shin'oka T, Shum-Tim D, Jonas RA, et al: Higher hematocrit improves cerebral outcome after deep hypothermic circulatory arrest. J Thorac Cardiovasc Surg 112:1610, 1996.
6. Jonas RA, Wypij D, Roth SJ, et al: The influence of hemodilution on outcome after hypothermic cardiopulmonary bypass: results of a randomized trial in infants. J Thorac Cardiovasc Surg 126:1765, 2003.
7. Newburger JW, Jonas RA, Wernovsky G, et al: A comparison of the perioperative neurologic effects of hypothermic circulatory arrest versus low-flow cardiopulmonary bypass in infant heart surgery. N Engl J Med 329:1057, 1993.
8. Bellinger DC, Jonas RA, Rappaport LA, et al: Developmental and neurologic status of children after heart surgery with hypothermic circulatory arrest or low-flow cardiopulmonary bypass. N Engl J Med 332:549, 1995.
9. Bellinger DC, Wypij D, Kuban KC, et al: Developmental and neurological status of children at 4 years of age after heart surgery with hypothermic circulatory arrest or low-flow cardiopulmonary bypass. Circulation 100:526, 1999.
10. Bellinger DC, Wypij D, du Plessis AJ, et al: Neurodevelopmental status at eight years in children with dextro-transposition of the great arteries: the Boston Circulatory Arrest Trial. J Thorac Cardiovasc Surg 126:1385, 2003.
11. du Plessis AJ, Jonas RA, Wypij D, et al: Perioperative effects of alpha-stat versus pH-stat strategies for deep hypothermic cardiopulmonary bypass in infants. J Thorac Cardiovasc Surg 114:991, 1997.
12. Limperopoulos C, Majnemer A, Shevell MI, et al: Neurologic status of newborns with congenital heart defects before open heart surgery. Pediatrics 103:402, 1999.
13. Limperopoulos C, Majnemer A, Shevell MI, et al: Neurodevelopmental status of newborns and infants with congenital heart defects before and after open heart surgery. J Pediatr 137:638, 2000.
14. Miller SP, McQuillen PS, Vigneron DB, et al: Preoperative brain injury in newborns with transposition of the great arteries. Ann Thorac Surg 77:1698, 2004.
15. Tavani F, Zimmerman RA, Clancy RR, et al: Incidental intracranial hemorrhage after uncomplicated birth: MRI before and after neonatal heart surgery. Neuroradiology 45:253, 2003.
16. Kaltman JR, Di H, Tian Z, et al: Impact of congenital heart disease on cerebrovascular blood flow dynamics in the fetus. Ultrasound Obstet Gynecol 25:32, 2005.
17. Licht DJ, Wang J, Silvestre DW, et al: Preoperative cerebral blood flow is diminished in neonates with severe congenital heart defects. J Thorac Cardiovasc Surg 128:841, 2004.
18. Te Pas AB, van Wezel-Meijler G, Bokenkamp-Gramann R, et al: Preoperative cranial ultrasound findings in infants with major congenital heart disease. Acta Paediatr 94:1597, 2005.
19. Tworetzky W, Marshall AC: Fetal interventions for cardiac defects. Pediatr Clin North Am 51:1503, 2004.
20. Tworetzky W, Wilkins-Haug L, Jennings RW, et al: Balloon dilation of severe aortic stenosis in the fetus: potential for prevention of hypoplastic left heart syndrome: candidate selection, technique, and results of successful intervention. Circulation 110:2125, 2004.
21. Robertson CM, Joffe AR, Sauve RS, et al: Outcomes from an interprovincial program of newborn open heart surgery. J Pediatr 144:86, 2004.
22. Limperopoulos C, Majnemer A, Shevell MI, et al: Predictors of developmental disabilities after open heart surgery in young children with congenital heart defects. J Pediatr 141:51, 2002.
23. Majnemer A, Limperopoulos C, Shevell M, et al: Long-term neuromotor outcome at school entry of infants with congenital heart defects requiring open-heart surgery. J Pediatr 148:72, 2006.
24. Miller G, Vogel H: Structural evidence of injury or malformation in the brains of children with congenital heart disease. Semin Pediatr Neurol 6:20, 1999.
25. Glauser T, Rorke L, Weinberg P, et al: Congenital brain anomalies associated with the hypoplastic left heart syndrome. Pediatrics 85:984, 1990.
26. Limperopoulos C, Tworetzky W, McElhinney DB, et al: Brain volume and metabolism in fetuses with congenital heart disease: evaluation with quantitative magnetic resonance imaging and spectroscopy. Circulation 121:26, 2010.
27. Clouchoux C, du Plessis AJ, Bouyssi-Kobar M, et al: Delayed cortical development in fetuses with complex congenital heart disease. Cereb Cortex 23:2932, 2013.
28. Miller SP, McQuillen PS, Hamrick S, et al: Abnormal brain development in newborns with congenital heart disease. N Engl J Med 357:1928, 2007.
29. Licht DJ, Shera DM, Clancy RR, et al: Brain maturation is delayed in infants with complex congenital heart defects. J Thorac Cardiovasc Surg 137:529, 2009.

30. Berg C, Gembruch O, Gembruch U, et al: Doppler indices of the middle cerebral artery in fetuses with cardiac defects theoretically associated with impaired cerebral oxygen delivery in utero: is there a brain-sparing effect? Ultrasound Obstet Gynecol 34:666, 2009.
31. Szwast A, Tian Z, McCann M, et al: Comparative analysis of cerebrovascular resistance in fetuses with single-ventricle congenital heart disease. Ultrasound Obstet Gynecol 40:62, 2012.
32. Yamamoto Y, Khoo NS, Brooks PA, et al: Severe left heart obstruction with retrograde arch flow importantly influences fetal cerebral and placental blood flow. Ultrasound Obstet Gynecol 42:294, 2013.
33. Shillingford AJ, Ittenbach RF, Marino BS, et al: Aortic morphometry and microcephaly in hypoplastic left heart syndrome. Cardiol Young 17:189, 2007.
34. Eskedal L, Hagemo P, Eskild A, et al: A population-based study of extra-cardiac anomalies in children with congenital cardiac malformations. Cardiol Young 14:600, 2004.
35. Derbent M, Bikmaz YE, Yilmaz Z, et al: Variable phenotype and associations in chromosome 22q11.2 microdeletion. Am J Med Genet A 140:659, 2006.
36. Botto LD, May K, Fernhoff PM, et al: A population-based study of the 22q11.2 deletion: phenotype, incidence, and contribution to major birth defects in the population. Pediatrics 112:101, 2003.
37. Moss E, Wang P, McDonald-McGinn D, et al: Characteristic cognitive profile in patients with a 22q11.2 deletion: verbal IQ exceeds nonverbal IQ. Am J Hum Genet 57:A20, 1995.
38. Bingham PM, Lynch D, McDonald-McGinn D, et al: Polymicrogyria in chromosome 22 deletion syndrome. Neurology 51:1500, 1998.
39. Mitnick R, Bello J, Shprintzen R: Brain anomalies in velo-cardiofacial syndrome. Am J Med Genet 54:100, 1994.
40. Barnea-Goraly N, Menon V, Krasnow B, et al: Investigation of white matter structure in velocardiofacial syndrome: a diffusion tensor imaging study. Am J Psychiatry 160:1863, 2003.
41. Zinkstok J, van Amelsvoort T: Neuropsychological profile and neuroimaging in patients with 22q11.2 deletion syndrome: a review. Child Neuropsychol 11:21, 2005.
42. Lajiness-O'Neill R, Beaulieu I, Asamoah A, et al: The neuropsychological phenotype of velocardiofacial syndrome (VCFS): relationship to psychopathology. Arch Clin Neuropsychol 21:175, 2006.
43. Vorstman JA, Morcus ME, Duijff SN, et al: The 22q11.2 deletion in children: high rate of autistic disorders and early onset of psychotic symptoms. J Am Acad Child Adolesc Psychiatry 45:1104, 2006.
44. Shprintzen R, Goldberg R, Golding-Kushner K, et al: Late-onset psychosis in the velo-cardio-facial syndrome. Am J Med Genet 42:141, 1992.
45. Campbell LE, Daly E, Toal F, et al: Brain and behaviour in children with 22q11.2 deletion syndrome: a volumetric and voxel-based morphometry MRI study. Brain 129:1218, 2006.
46. Bish JP, Nguyen V, Ding L, et al: Thalamic reductions in children with chromosome 22q11.2 deletion syndrome. Neuroreport 15:1413, 2004.
47. Kates WR, Miller AM, Abdulsabur N, et al: Temporal lobe anatomy and psychiatric symptoms in velocardiofacial syndrome (22q11.2 deletion syndrome). J Am Acad Child Adolesc Psychiatry 45:587, 2006.
48. Cheng TO: That balloon atrial septostomy is associated with preoperative stroke in neonates with transposition of the great arteries is another powerful argument in favor of therapeutic closure of every patent foramen ovale. Am J Cardiol 98:277, 2006.
49. McQuillen PS, Hamrick SE, Perez MJ, et al: Balloon atrial septostomy is associated with preoperative stroke in neonates with transposition of the great arteries. Circulation 113:280, 2006.
50. Mahle WT, Tavani F, Zimmerman RA, et al: An MRI study of neurological injury before and after congenital heart surgery. Circulation 106:I109, 2002.
51. Petit CJ, Rome JJ, Wernovsky G, et al: Preoperative brain injury in transposition of the great arteries is associated with oxygenation and time to surgery, not balloon atrial septostomy. Circulation 119:709, 2009.
52. Glauser T, Rorke L, Weinberg P, et al: Acquired neuropathologic lesions associated with the hypoplastic left heart syndrome. Pediatrics 85:991, 1990.
53. Giuliani R, Szwarcer E, Aquino E, et al: Fibrin-dependent fibrinolytic activity during extracorporeal circulation. Thromb Res 61:369, 1991.
54. Rudack D, Baumgart S, Gross G: Subependymal (grade 1) intracranial hemorrhage in neonates on extracorporeal membrane oxygenation. Clin Pediatr 33:583, 1994.
55. von Allmen D, Babcock D, Matsumoto J, et al: The predictive value of head ultrasound in the ECMO candidate. J Pediatr Surg 27:36, 1992.
56. du Plessis AJ, Johnston MV: The pursuit of effective neuroprotection during infant cardiac surgery. Semin Pediatr Neurol 6:55, 1999.
57. Kinney HC, Panigrahy A, Newburger JW, et al: Hypoxic-ischemic brain injury in infants with congenital heart disease dying after cardiac surgery. Acta Neuropathol (Berl) 110:563, 2005.
58. Beca J, Gunn JK, Coleman L, et al: New white matter brain injury after infant heart surgery is associated with diagnostic group and the use of circulatory arrest.. Circulation 127:971, 2013.
59. Moody D, Bell M, Challa V, et al: Brain microemboli during cardiac surgery or aortography. Ann Neurol 28:477, 1990.
60. Casey L: Role of cytokines in the pathogenesis of cardiopulmonary-induced multisystem organ failure. Ann Thorac Surg 56:S92, 1993.

61. Pesonen EJ, Korpela R, Peltola K, et al: Regional generation of free oxygen radicals during cardiopulmonary bypass in children. J Thorac Cardiovasc Surg 110:768, 1995.
62. Pyles LA, Fortney JE, Kudlak JJ, et al: Plasma antioxidant depletion after cardiopulmonary bypass in operations for congenital heart disease. J Thorac Cardiovasc Surg 110:165, 1995.
63. Le Deist F, Menasche P, Kucharski C, et al: Hypothermia during cardiopulmonary bypass delays but does not prevent neutrophil-endothelial cell adhesion. A clinical study. Circulation 92:II354, 1995.
64. Greeley W, Ungerleider R, Smith L, et al: The effects of deep hypothermic cardiopulmonary bypass and total circulatory arrest on cerebral blood flow in infants and children. J Thorac Cardiovasc Surg 97:737, 1989.
65. Coetzee A, Swanepoel C: The oxyhemoglobin dissociation curve before, during and after cardiac surgery. Scand J Clin Lab Invest Suppl 203:149, 1990.
66. Powers W: Hemodynamics and metabolism in ischemic cerebrovascular disease. Neurol Clin 10:31, 1992.
67. Dexter F, Hindman B: Theoretical analysis of cerebral venous blood hemoglobin oxygen saturation as an index of cerebral oxygenation during hypothermic cardiopulmonary bypass. Anesthesiol 83:405, 1995.
68. Forbess JM, Visconti KJ, Hancock-Friesen C, et al: Neurodevelopmental outcome after congenital heart surgery: results from an institutional registry. Circulation 106:I95, 2002.
69. Kern JH, Hinton VJ, Nereo NE, et al: Early developmental outcome after the Norwood procedure for hypoplastic left heart syndrome. Pediatrics 102:1148, 1998.
70. Uzark K, Lincoln A, Lamberti JJ, et al: Neurodevelopmental outcomes in children with Fontan repair of functional single ventricle. Pediatrics 101:630, 1998.
71. Wernovsky G, Stiles KM, Gauvreau K, et al: Cognitive development after the Fontan operation. Circulation 102:883, 2000.
72. McGrath E, Wypij D, Rappaport LA, et al: Prediction of IQ and achievement at age 8 years from neurodevelopmental status at age 1 year in children with D-transposition of the great arteries. Pediatrics 114:e572, 2004.
73. Kirshbom PM, Flynn TB, Clancy RR, et al: Late neurodevelopmental outcome after repair of total anomalous pulmonary venous connection. J Thorac Cardiovasc Surg 129:1091, 2005.
74. Mahle WT, Clancy RR, Moss EM, et al: Neurodevelopmental outcome and lifestyle assessment in school-aged and adolescent children with hypoplastic left heart syndrome. Pediatrics 105:1082, 2000.
75. Wernovsky G, Wypij D, Jonas RA, et al: Postoperative course and hemodynamic profile after the arterial switch operation in neonates and infants: a comparison of low-flow cardiopulmonary bypass and circulatory arrest. Circulation 92:2226, 1995.
76. Wypij D, Newburger JW, Rappaport LA, et al: The effect of duration of deep hypothermic circulatory arrest in infant heart surgery on late neurodevelopment: the Boston circulatory arrest trial. J Thorac Cardiovasc Surg 126:1397, 2003.
77. Sorensen H, Husum B, Waaben J, et al: Brain microvascular function during cardiopulmonary bypass. J Thorac Cardiovasc Surg 94:727, 1987.
78. Lundar T, Lindegaard K, Froysaker T, et al: Dissociation between cerebral autoregulation and carbon dioxide reactivity during nonpulsatile cardiopulmonary bypass. Ann Thorac Surg 40:582, 1985.
79. Bellinger DC, Wypij D, du Plessis AJ, et al: Developmental and neurologic effects of alpha-stat versus pH-stat strategies for deep hypothermic cardiopulmonary bypass in infants. J Thorac Cardiovasc Surg 121:374, 2001.
80. du Plessis A, Newburger J, Jonas R, et al: Cerebral oxygen supply and utilization during infant cardiac surgery. Ann Neurol 37:488, 1995.
81. Ruvolo G, Greco E, Speziale G, et al: Nitric oxide formation during cardiopulmonary bypass. Ann Thorac Surg 57:1055, 1994.
82. Dugan LL, Sensi SL, Canzoniero LM, et al: Mitochondrial production of reactive oxygen species in cortical neurons following exposure to *N*-methyl-D-aspartate. J Neurosci 15:6377, 1995.
83. Nathan HJ, Polls T: The management of temperature during hypothermic cardiopulmonary bypass: 2. Effect of prolonged hypothermia. Can J Anaesth 42:672, 1995.
84. Ginsberg M, Sternau L, Globus M-T, et al: Therapeutic modulation of brain temperature: relevance to ischemic brain injury. Cerebrovasc Brain Metab Rev 4:189, 1992.
85. Astudillo R, van der Linden J, Ekroth R, et al: Absent diastolic cerebral blood flow velocity after circulatory arrest but not after low flow in infants. Ann Thorac Surg 56:515, 1993.
86. Jonassen A, Quaegebeur J, Young W: Cerebral blood flow velocity in pediatric patients is reduced after cardiopulmonary bypass with profound hypothermia. J Thorac Cardiovasc Surg 110:934, 1995.
87. Menache CC, du Plessis AJ, Wessel DL, et al: Current incidence of acute neurologic complications after open-heart operations in children. Ann Thorac Surg 73:1752, 2002.
88. Clancy RR, McGaurn SA, Wernovsky G, et al: Risk of seizures in survivors of newborn heart surgery using deep hypothermic circulatory arrest. Pediatrics 111:592, 2003.
89. Clancy RR, Sharif U, Ichord R, et al: Electrographic neonatal seizures after infant heart surgery. Epilepsia 46:84, 2005.
90. Gaynor JW, Jarvik GP, Bernbaum J, et al: The relationship of postoperative electrographic seizures

to neurodevelopmental outcome at 1 year of age after neonatal and infant cardiac surgery. J Thorac Cardiovasc Surg 131:181, 2006.

91. Mizrahi EM, Clancy RR: Neonatal seizures: early-onset seizure syndromes and their consequences for development. Ment Retard Dev Disabil Res Rev 6:229, 2000.
92. Rappaport LA, Wypij D, Bellinger DC, et al: Relation of seizures after cardiac surgery in early infancy to neurodevelopmental outcome. Boston Circulatory Arrest Study Group. Circulation 97:773, 1998.
93. du Plessis A, Kramer U, Jonas R, et al: West syndrome following deep hypothermic cardiac surgery. Pediatr Neurol 11:246, 1994.
94. Yang J, Park Y, Hartlage P: Seizures associated with stroke in childhood. Pediatr Neurol 12:136, 1995.
95. McQuillen PS, Barkovich AJ, Hamrick SE, et al: Temporal and anatomic risk profile of brain injury with neonatal repair of congenital heart defects. Stroke 38:736, 2007.
96. Gaynor JW: Periventricular leukomalacia following neonatal and infant cardiac surgery. Semin Thorac Cardiovasc Surg Pediatr Card Surg Annu 7:133, 2004.
97. Galli KK, Zimmerman RA, Jarvik GP, et al: Periventricular leukomalacia is common after neonatal cardiac surgery. J Thorac Cardiovasc Surg 127:692, 2004.
98. Beca J, Gunn JK, Coleman L, et al: New white matter brain injury after infant heart surgery is associated with diagnostic group and the use of circulatory arrest. Circulation 127:971, 2013.
99. Childs AM, Ramenghi LA, Cornette L, et al: Cerebral maturation in premature infants: quantitative assessment using MR imaging. AJNR Am J Neuroradiol 22:1577, 2001.
100. Ashwal S, Holshouser B, Schell R, et al: Proton magnetic resonance spectroscopy in the evaluation of children with congenital heart disease and acute central nervous system injury. J Thorac Cardiovasc Surg 112:403, 1996.
101. Ashwal S, Holshouser BA, del Rio MJ, et al: Serial proton magnetic resonance spectroscopy of the brain in children undergoing cardiac surgery. Pediatr Neurol 29:99, 2003.
102. deVeber G: Arterial ischemic strokes in infants and children: an overview of current approaches. Semin Thromb Hemost 29:567, 2003.
103. Hutchison JS, Ichord R, Guerguerian AM, et al: Cerebrovascular disorders. Semin Pediatr Neurol 11:139, 2004.
104. Barker PC, Nowak C, King K, et al: Risk factors for cerebrovascular events following Fontan palliation in patients with a functional single ventricle. Am J Cardiol 96:587, 2005.
105. Cromme-Dijkhuis A, Henkens C, Bijleveld C, et al: Coagulation factor abnormalities as possible thrombotic risk factors after Fontan operations. Lancet 336:1087, 1990.
106. du Plessis A, Chang A, Wessel D, et al: Cerebrovascular accidents following the Fontan procedure. Pediatr Neurol 12:230, 1995.
107. Hess J, Kruizinga A, Bijleveld C, et al: Protein-losing enteropathy after Fontan operation. J Thorac Cardiovasc Surg 88:606, 1984.
108. Rosenthal DN, Friedman AH, Kleinman CS, et al: Thromboembolic complications after Fontan operations. Circulation 92(suppl II):287, 1995.
109. Saiman L, Prince A, Gersony W: Pediatric infective endocarditis in the modern era. J Pediatr 122:847, 1993.
110. Wong PC, Barlow CF, Hickey PR, et al: Factors associated with choreoathetosis after cardiopulmonary bypass in children with congenital heart disease. Circulation 86:118, 1992.
111. Curless RG, Katz DA, Perryman RA, et al: Choreoathetosis after surgery for congenital heart disease. J Pediatr 124:737, 1994.
112. du Plessis AJ, Bellinger DC, Gauvreau K, et al: Neurologic outcome of choreoathetoid encephalopathy after cardiac surgery. Pediatr Neurol 27:9, 2002.
113. Kupsky WJ, Drozd MA, Barlow CF: Selective injury of the globus pallidus in children with post-cardiac surgery choreic syndrome. Dev Med Child Neurol 37:135, 1995.
114. Deleon GA, Radkowski MA, Crawford SE, et al: Persistent respiratory failure due to low cervical cord infarction in newborn babies. J Child Neurol 10:200, 1995.
115. Levin DA, Seay AR, Fullerton DA, et al: Profound hypothermia with alpha-stat pH management during open-heart surgery is associated with choreoathetosis. Pediatr Cardiol 26:34, 2005.
116. Hamrick SE, Gremmels DB, Keet CA, et al: Neurodevelopmental outcome of infants supported with extracorporeal membrane oxygenation after cardiac surgery. Pediatrics 111:e671, 2003.
117. Petzinger G, Mayer SA, Przedborski S: Fentanyl-induced dyskinesias. Mov Disord 10:679, 1995.
118. Christenson JT, Sierra J, Didier D, et al: Repair of aortic coarctation using temporary ascending to descending aortic bypass in children with poor collateral circulation. Cardiol Young 14:39, 2004.
119. Souza Neto EP, Durand PG, Sassolas F, et al: Brachial plexus injury during cardiac catheterisation in children. Report of two cases. Acta Anaesthesiol Scand 42:876, 1998.
120. Liu XY, Wong V, Leung M: Neurologic complications due to catheterization. Pediatr Neurol 24:270, 2001.
121. Hwang MS, Chu JJ, Su WJ: Diaphragmatic paralysis caused by malposition of chest tube placement after pediatric cardiac surgery. Int J Cardiol 99:129, 2005.

CHAPTER

5

Neurologic Manifestations of Acquired Cardiac Disease, Arrhythmias, and Interventional Cardiology

JUSTIN A. KINSELLA ■ DAVID J. GLADSTONE

The neurologic manifestations of acquired cardiac disease include: (1) the sudden onset of a focal neurologic deficit due to occlusion of a cerebral or retinal artery by an embolus that has developed within the heart (cardiogenic embolism); (2) transient, self-limited episodes of generalized cerebral ischemia that occur as a consequence of brief failures of cardiac output, due to rhythm disturbances or outflow obstruction, resulting in presyncope or syncope; and (3) the complications of invasive techniques for the investigation or management of cardiac disease. Exceptions to these categorizations include atrial fibrillation (AF), an arrhythmia that is associated with embolus formation rather than syncope, and chronic sinoatrial disorder, which predisposes to both syncopal and embolic disturbances.

CARDIOGENIC EMBOLISM

Clinical Features

Ischemic stroke or transient ischemic attack (TIA) has been classified into six major etiologic categories, which have implications for treatment and prognosis.[1] These categories are cardioembolism, large-artery atherosclerosis, small-artery occlusion, stroke of other determined etiology, stroke of undetermined etiology, and events of multiple possible etiologies.

Cardiogenic brain embolism accounts for approximately 20 to 25 percent of ischemic strokes.[2] The most common cardiac cause of ischemic stroke is AF, which accounts for at least one-sixth of all strokes (the proportion is greater if it includes subclinical AF detected by prolonged cardiac rhythm monitoring).[3] Other cardiac causes of stroke are listed in Table 5-1.

In a recent study in 1,008 young stroke patients aged between 15 and 49, it was found that 20 percent had a cardioembolic source for their stroke.[4] In another study, cardioembolism was responsible in 19 percent, with the top three diagnoses in this group being paradoxical embolism and prosthetic or rheumatic valve disease.[5] However, the reported incidence of stroke secondary to a cardioembolic source varies between studies. A French study of 296 patients attributed less than 9 percent to a cardiac cause.[6] An Italian hospital-based study of 394 consecutive young adults with ischemic stroke found the figure was 34 percent.[7] Of the 133 considered to be of cardiac origin, 23 had a probable cause including recent myocardial infarction, AF, valvulopathy,

Aminoff's Neurology and General Medicine, Fifth Edition.

TABLE 5-1 ■ Established and Putative Cardiac Causes of Stroke

Arrhythmias
Atrial fibrillation
Atrial flutter
Sick-sinus syndrome
Valvular heart disease
Prosthetic
Rheumatic
Mitral valve prolapse
Calcific aortic stenosis
Aortic sclerosis
Mitral annular calcification
Myocardial infarction (acute and chronic)
Left ventricular dysfunction
Cardiomyopathy
Congestive heart failure
Other echocardiographic abnormalities
Patent foramen ovale with atrial septal aneurysm
Left atrial thrombus
Spontaneous left atrial echo contrast
Cardiac tumors
Endocarditis
Infective
Marantic (nonbacterial thrombotic)
Iatrogenic causes
Cardiac surgery
Cardiac catheterization
Percutaneous coronary interventions
Thrombolytic therapy for acute myocardial infarction
Cardioversion for atrial fibrillation/flutter

patent foramen ovale (PFO) with deep vein thrombosis (DVT), and atrial myxoma. A total of 110 additional patients had various possible causes including PFO with right-to-left shunt, atrial septal aneurysm (ASA), and PFO plus ASA. Comparison of etiologic factors showed that only two cardiac sources—valvular heart disease and mitral valve prolapse—were encountered more frequently in the younger age group.[8]

Features suggesting cardioembolism are usually derived from analyses of clinical presentations and neuroimaging features of acute ischemic strokes (Table 5-2).[9–11] The anterior circulation is affected four times more frequently than the posterior in cardioembolic stroke. Although the posterior circulation is less commonly affected, studies of the mechanism of infarction in specific posterior circulation territories (e.g., posterior inferior cerebellar artery, superior cerebellar artery) implicate cardiogenic embolism in 50 percent of cases.[12]

A meta-analysis showed that the 3-month risk of recurrent stroke was 12 percent when the etiology was cardioembolism, compared to 19 percent for large-vessel atherosclerosis, 3 percent for small-vessel disease, and 9 percent for unknown cause.[13] In a population-based study of first stroke, patients with cardioembolic stroke had the lowest 2-year survival rate (55%) and were three times more likely to die than those with small-artery occlusion.[14]

Investigations

The first neurologic investigation for suspected stroke is usually a noncontrast computed tomography (CT) scan of the brain to exclude intracranial hemorrhage. In patients at high risk of cardioembolism, infarcts are more likely to involve a large territory and the combination of both superficial and deep structures. Isolated deep small infarcts (lacunes) are unlikely to be from a cardiac source.

The potential for embolic infarcts to develop hemorrhagic transformation remains a concern, especially when antithrombotic or thrombolytic therapy is considered.[15] Hemorrhagic infarction was seen on initial CT scans of 6 percent of patients in a series of 244 cases of cardioembolic stroke; none of these patients was anticoagulated at the time.[9] With magnetic resonance imaging (MRI) gradient echo (GE) sequences, nearly 21 percent of these patients show signs of hemorrhage up to 60 hours after symptom onset.[16] Nearly 50 percent of those treated with t-PA have signs of hemorrhagic conversion on sensitive MRI sequences, but most of these patients are asymptomatic and the amount of hemorrhage is inconsequential. Larger infarcts are more liable to demonstrate hemorrhagic transformation,[17] as are those occurring in older patients.[17]

Because of concerns regarding complications of acute stroke treatment with thrombolytic or anticoagulation therapy, early markers predicting increased risk of hemorrhagic transformation have been investigated. The only independent predictor identified in a study of 150 consecutive patients was focal hypodensity on CT in the first 5 hours after stroke onset.[17] In another study, the main predictors for hemorrhagic transformation were t-PA treatment, increasing severity of neurologic deficits on admission, and large-territory infarction.[16]

TABLE 5-2 ■ Clinical Features Suggesting Cardioembolic Stroke

Cortical signs (e.g., aphasia, neglect, visual field defect)
Isolated global aphasia or Wernicke aphasia (without hemiparesis)
Impaired consciousness at stroke onset
Sudden onset, reaching maximal deficit within 5 minutes of onset
Rapid dramatic neurologic recovery
Strokes in different vascular territories
Evidence of systemic embolism
Atrial fibrillation, valvular heart disease

MRI with diffusion-weighted imaging (DWI) sequences can detect early infarction with high sensitivity.[18] The pattern of DWI abnormalities can help determine the most likely etiology. A pattern of acute lesions in more than one vascular territory (bilateral lesions or lesions in the carotid and vertebrobasilar territories) is highly suggestive of a shower from a proximal cardiogenic source.

Conventional catheter-based digital subtraction angiography (DSA) remains the gold standard for assessing structural abnormalities of the extra- and intracranial circulation but is rarely used since the advent of CT and MR angiographic techniques. Use of DSA requires recognition of associated risks; a single-center study reported no stroke or permanent neurologic deficit in any of 1,715 patients undergoing DSA although 1 patient experienced a TIA during the procedure.[19] Another study reported incidence of permanent neurologic deficit ranging from 0.3 to 5.7 percent.[20] The characteristic angiographic appearance of an embolic occlusion is a proximal, meniscus-like filling defect in an artery that is otherwise normal and lacks evidence of atherosclerotic change. Emboli tend to fragment, and distal branch occlusions can be seen.

Echocardiography plays an important role in the structural evaluation of the heart. Transthoracic echocardiography (TTE) is noninvasive but has limitations that can be overcome by transesophageal echocardiography (TEE), in which the patient is usually mildly sedated and topical anesthetic is applied to the posterior pharynx. The technique employed (TEE or TTE) depends on the area of the heart to be visualized. TTE images the left ventricle well, but TEE is required for better assessment of the left atrium and its appendage.[21] TEE is also better for visualizing the interatrial septum for the presence of a PFO and for visualizing the aortic arch, another common source of proximal embolism. TEE is the most sensitive and specific test for detecting a cardiac source of embolism and, for patients with AF, it may assist in risk stratification and guide the choice of cardioversion.[3]

TTE has an overall yield of less than 1 percent in patients without clinical evidence of cardiac disease, increasing to 13 percent in those with cardiac disease. The corresponding figures for TEE are less than 2 percent and 19 percent.[22] There is fair evidence to recommend echocardiography in patients with stroke and clinical evidence of heart disease (grade B recommendation). Because the yield from TEE is higher than that for TTE, controversy arises as to whether this should be the first test or whether a sequential approach with TTE followed by TEE should be employed.[23]

Contrast-enhanced cardiac MRI is another noninvasive technique that allows for structural imaging of the heart. It is more sensitive than TTE and comparable to TEE for the detection of cardiac thrombi.[24]

Transcranial Doppler (TCD) ultrasonography can also be useful in the acute stroke setting for detecting acute intracranial vascular obstruction (e.g., due to an occlusive embolus in the middle cerebral artery) and permits recanalization to be monitored following treatment with thrombolysis. TCD can also be used to detect right-to-left cardiac shunts due to PFO by identifying microbubbles reaching the middle cerebral arteries, especially following the Valsalva maneuver; contrast-enhanced TCD ultrasonography has shown near-perfect correlation with contrast-enhanced TEE for the detection and quantification of such shunts.[25]

Clinicians must balance extensive investigation against its impact on patient management, usually the justification for lifelong anticoagulant therapy and its consequent risks. In several situations, there are no established guidelines for management of these potential sources of emboli.

Causes

ATRIAL FIBRILLATION AND FLUTTER

AF is the most common serious arrhythmia and is a major risk factor for stroke and death. It accounts for nearly one-half of all cardiac causes of stroke and about one-quarter of strokes in the elderly.[3]

Strokes associated with AF tend to be more severe than strokes due to other etiologies, and the 30-day mortality is approximately 25 percent.

The prevalence of AF is age dependent, ranging from 0.1 percent among adults younger than 55 years to 9 percent in those 80 years or older.[26] The population prevalence of AF is increasing due to an aging population.[26] AF typically occurs in patients with underlying cardiac disease (e.g,. hypertension, valvular heart disease, congestive heart failure, coronary disease, cardiomyopathy, mitral valve prolapse, mitral annular calcification, and cardiac tumors), but may also occur as "lone AF" in young patients who have no cardiac disease. AF may be paroxysmal (defined as a self-terminating episode lasting less than 7 days), recurrent (two or more episodes), persistent (more than 7 days), or permanent (cardioversion failed or not attempted). Reversible or temporary causes include alcohol, surgery, hyperthyroidism, acute myocardial infarction, pulmonary embolism, and pericarditis, among others.[3]

The average annual risk of stroke in individuals with AF is 5 percent and is heavily dependent on age and the presence of additional risk factors (Table 5-3). The most important predictor of stroke risk in patients with AF is a history of thromboembolism (i.e., previous TIA, stroke, or systemic arterial embolism). Other independent risk factors for stroke in patients with AF are increasing age, hypertension, congestive heart failure, and diabetes mellitus. Other factors that have been associated with increased stroke risk in some studies include female sex, systolic hypertension, and left ventricular dysfunction.[3] Commonly used risk stratification tools are the $CHADS_2$ scale and the CHA_2DS_2-VASC scale, which predict the risk of stroke in patients with AF based on the presence of additional risk factors.[26,27] The $CHADS_2$ scale ranges from 0 (low stroke risk, 1.9% per year) to 6 (high stroke risk, 18.2% per year) points. Online calculators are available that show the estimated annual stroke risk for patients without anticoagulant therapy and the risk reduction afforded by aspirin.

Echocardiographic features that have been used for risk stratification in patients with AF include left ventricular systolic dysfunction, atrial thrombus, dense spontaneous echo contrast or reduced blood flow velocity within the left atrium or left atrial appendage on TEE, and aortic arch atheroma.[28] Left atrial size was previously considered not to predict the risk of thromboembolism, although a large observational study found that left atrial diameter

TABLE 5-3 ■ Two-Year Stroke Risk for Patients with Atrial Fibrillation Stratified by Additional Risk Factors

	No Antithrombotic Therapy (%)	Aspirin (%)	Warfarin (%)
Low Risk	2	1.5	1
1. Age <65 years 2. No hypertension 3. No LV dysfunction 4. No previous TIA/stroke/systemic embolism			
Medium Risk	4	3	2
1. Age 65–75 years 2. No hypertension 3. No LV dysfunction 4. No previous TIA/stroke/systemic embolism			
High Risk	12	9	4
1. Age <75 years and hypertension or LV dysfunction or 2. Age >75 years without risk factors			
Very High Risk	20	16	7
1. Age >75 years and hypertension or LV dysfunction or 2. Any age and previous TIA/stroke/systemic embolism			

Reproduced with permission from McAlister F, Laupacis A, Man-Son-Hing M, et al: University of Ottawa Atrial Fibrillation Decision Aid 1996; available at: www.canadianstrokenetwork.ca (accessed August 30, 2006).
LV, left ventricular; TIA, transient ischemic attack.

measured on TTE was a predictor of all-cause mortality and of ischemic stroke (the latter in women only).[29] TEE is the method of choice for evaluating the left atrial appendage, the site at which most thrombi form, as well as the left atrium. In a prospective study of patients with AF considered on clinical grounds to be at high risk, stroke occurred at a rate of 18 percent per year in those with dense spontaneous echo contrast who were treated with low-dose warfarin (international normalized ratio [INR] 1.2 to 1.5) plus aspirin compared to 4.5 percent for those on monotherapy with dose-adjusted warfarin with a goal INR of 2.0 to 3.0. The prevalence of thrombus in the left atrial appendage was similar initially in the two treatment groups (10 to 12%) when TEE was performed more than 2 weeks after study entry, but atrial thrombus was present in 6 percent of those on warfarin compared to 18 percent of those on combination therapy. Absence of thrombus predicted a low rate of ischemic events (2.3% per year), and the presence of thrombus predicted a high rate (18%).[30]

The risk of stroke in AF is significantly reduced by anticoagulation.[31] A meta-analysis showed that warfarin reduced stroke risk by 62 percent overall compared with placebo.[32] Absolute risk reductions were higher for secondary prevention (8.4% per year) than primary prevention (2.7%). These percentages translate into numbers needed to treat (NNT) of 12 and 37, respectively. Although more intracranial hemorrhages (ICHs) occurred in the warfarin group (0.3% per year) compared to the placebo group (0.1%), this was not statistically significant. Major extracranial hemorrhage occurred in 0.6 percent per year of patients on placebo, with a relative risk for those on warfarin of 2.4 (absolute risk increase, 0.3% per year). The total number of patients in six trials that assessed dose-adjusted warfarin to placebo was 2,900, with an average follow-up of 1.7 years.[32] The risk reduction with warfarin was based on intention-to-treat analyses; the on-treatment analysis showed a relative risk reduction in stroke of more than 80 percent.

Adjusted-dose warfarin was also compared to aspirin in five trials including 2,837 individuals. Excluding one study because the range of the INR was wide (2.0 to 4.5), the relative risk reduction for warfarin compared to aspirin was 46 percent. Patients with AF at high risk of stroke generally still benefit from anticoagulation even after sinus rhythm has been restored.[33]

The use of aspirin compared to placebo has also been addressed in several trials.[32] The prescribed dose of aspirin has ranged from 25 to 1,200 mg daily, with more than 3,000 patients studied; average follow-up was 1.5 years. In patients receiving placebo, the stroke incidence was 5.2 percent per year for primary prevention and 12.9 percent for secondary prevention; aspirin reduced stroke risk by 22 percent, resulting in numbers needed to treat of 67 and 40, respectively. All-cause mortality was not reduced. Aspirin's benefit in these patients may be to prevent nondisabling stroke that is not of cardioembolic origin. Therefore, published guidelines strongly recommend warfarin rather than aspirin for stroke prevention in individuals with AF who are at high risk.[34]

In practice, despite the clear benefit of warfarin for stroke prevention in patients with AF, this medication is frequently underutilized.[35,36] Warfarin is a difficult medication for patients because of the inconvenience of INR monitoring, drug and food interactions, and bleeding risks. Physicians also frequently overestimate the bleeding risks but underestimate the benefits of warfarin compared with aspirin.[37,38]

Individual patient preferences, knowledge, and attitudes affect compliance with long-term anticoagulation therapy. Among AF patients taking warfarin in one study, about one-half did not know that AF was a risk factor for stroke and could not state why they were taking warfarin; ethnic differences in knowledge about their diagnosis and treatment were also identified.[39] Methods to encourage compliance with appropriate antithrombotic prophylaxis include use of a patient decision aid. Home INR finger-stick devices for self-monitoring may increase the time that patients spend in the therapeutic INR range.[40]

Bleeding is the major concern with anticoagulant therapy. The average risk of major bleeding in clinical trials is 1.3 percent per year with warfarin compared to 1 percent with aspirin or placebo.[41] The Stroke Prevention in Atrial Fibrillation study had a higher rate of major bleeding at 2.3 percent on warfarin and 1.1 percent per year on aspirin.[41] Rates of ICH were 0.9 percent and 0.3 percent per year, respectively. Age older than 75 years increased the risk of major hemorrhage to 4.2 percent per year, and only in this age group was intensity of anticoagulation predictive of risk.

With the exception of some patients with lone AF, all patients with AF (regardless of whether paroxysmal, persistent, or permanent) require some form of antithrombotic therapy, unless contraindicated. It remains necessary to individualize management strategies for specific patients, taking into account compliance, risk of bleeding complications, and other medical conditions. Risk stratification is essential to determine optimal treatment with warfarin or aspirin. Many schemes have been devised for identifying patients with AF unassociated with valvular heart disease who are at high, moderate, or low risk of stroke. According to the American Heart Association guidelines, high-risk factors are previous stroke, TIA, or systemic embolism; mitral stenosis; and prosthetic heart valves.[3] Moderate risk factors include age older than 75 years; hypertension; heart failure; left ventricular ejection fraction less than 35 percent; and diabetes. Warfarin is recommended for patients with any high-risk factor or more than one moderate-risk factor. This means that all patients with a previous ischemic stroke or TIA are considered at high risk and require anticoagulation for secondary stroke prevention unless contraindicated. Warfarin or aspirin (81 to 325 mg) is recommended for those with only one moderate-risk factor. Aspirin alone (81 to 325 mg) is considered sufficient for patients without any of these risk factors.

For most patients receiving warfarin for AF (excluding mechanical heart valves), the target INR is 2.5 (range 2.0 to 3.0). The INR should be monitored closely; usually weekly initially and then monthly once stable. Stroke risk increases exponentially as the intensity of anticoagulation declines below 2.0.[42]

In addition to protecting against stroke, antithrombotics can attenuate stroke severity. Patients taking warfarin at the time of stroke have, on average, less-disabling strokes compared to individuals taking aspirin or no antithrombotic therapy, and stroke severity is negatively correlated with INR at stroke onset.[43] Table 5-4 gives a summary of the indications for warfarin in secondary stroke prevention for patients with selected cardiac conditions.

Dual antiplatelet therapy (aspirin plus clopidogrel) was investigated in a randomized trial and found to be inferior to warfarin for stroke prevention in AF, but associated with a similar rate of adverse bleeding events compared to warfarin; the combination was superior to aspirin alone and therefore could be considered in some high-risk patients in whom warfarin is contraindicated.[44]

TABLE 5-4 ■ Summary of Indications for Warfarin in Secondary Stroke Prevention for Patients with Selected Cardiac Conditions

Strong or Moderate Indication for Warfarin
Mechanical heart valve
Atrial fibrillation
Atrial flutter
Cardioversion in atrial fibrillation or flutter
Bioprosthetic heart valve
Rheumatic mitral valve disease
Acute myocardial infarction and left ventricular thrombus
Possible/Uncertain Indication for Warfarin
Mitral annular calcification associated with mitral regurgitation
Warfarin Usually Not Indicated
Dilated cardiomyopathy
Left ventricular dysfunction
Patent foramen ovale associated with atrial septal aneurysm
Isolated patent foramen ovale
Isolated mitral valve prolapse
Isolated mitral annular calcification
Isolated aortic valve disease

The only class I evidence in support of warfarin for stroke prevention exists for atrial fibrillation and mechanical heart valves. Treatment recommendations are expected to change over time as new evidence emerges; the reader is advised to consult published guidelines for more detailed information.

If warfarin therapy needs to be interrupted for surgical procedures, temporary discontinuation for up to 1 week is usually considered reasonable for patients without mechanical heart valves. However, since this practice is associated with increased stroke risk, it must be individualized. Bridging heparin therapy may be substituted in high-risk patients during periods of warfarin interruption.[45]

A major development in AF treatment has been the recent arrival of a new generation of oral anticoagulant drugs that have emerged as alternatives to warfarin: the direct thrombin inhibitor dabigatran and the factor Xa inhibitors rivaroxaban and apixaban.[46] There have been four pivotal phase III randomized controlled trials testing these new agents in patients with non-valvular AF. All three agents appear to be at least as effective as warfarin for stroke prevention and are associated with a lower incidence of intracranial hemorrhage.[47–50] In contrast to warfarin, these drugs have a rapid onset of action, short half-life, fewer drug interactions, lack of food interactions, and do not require INR monitoring. Regular patient follow-up is still necessary to monitor adherence and renal function. No specific antidotes to these drugs are available yet to reverse bleeding. Contraindications to the use of these agents include severe renal failure and mechanical heart valves. If the outcomes of the new anticoagulants prove to be as good in real-world practice as in clinical trials, these agents represent a major therapeutic advance. Other new anticoagulants are under investigation.

In addition to medical therapy for stroke prevention in AF, interventional techniques are being investigated. These include percutaneously implanted left atrial appendage occlusive devices and surgical resection of the left atrial appendage, given that 91 percent of thrombi are localized at that site.[51] Carotid artery endovascular devices to filter emboli are also under investigation.[52]

It is clear that cardioversion of AF to sinus rhythm (either pharmacologic or electric) does not reduce the risk of stroke and therefore does not obviate the need for continued anticoagulation therapy for stroke prevention.[53]

AF occurring in the postoperative setting following cardiac surgery is fairly common and usually self-limited. Anticoagulation is reasonable if AF persists for more than 48 hours, but it may not need to be continued long-term if sinus rhythm is restored. Similarly, other conditions associated with transient AF (e.g., alcohol, thyrotoxicosis) usually do not need long-term antithrombotic prophylaxis.[3]

In patients with atrial flutter, the risk of thromboembolism is less than that of AF but higher than for patients in sinus rhythm. These patients often eventually develop AF. For practical purposes, the antithrombotic treatment recommendations are similar to those for AF.

Brief subclinical AF or atrial tachyarrhythmias are emerging risk factors for stroke, as demonstrated by pacemaker studies. For example, one study monitored 2,580 patients without known AF in whom a pacemaker or defibrillator had been implanted.[54] Subclinical episodes of high atrial rate (>190 beats per minute for >6 minutes) were found in 10.1 percent within 3 months of monitoring, and this finding was a significant independent predictor of clinical AF and ischemic stroke or systemic embolism during follow-up.

In patients with ischemic stroke presenting in sinus rhythm, Holter monitoring for 24 to 72 hours detects paroxysmal AF in about 5 percent of patients. However, AF can be difficult to detect because it is frequently intermittent and asymptomatic. There is increasing evidence that prolonged electrocardiographic (ECG) monitoring, through external or implanted recording devices, can improve the detection of occult paroxysmal AF in patients with strokes of undetermined etiology[55]; several studies show a rate of detection of 5 to 20 percent.

Cardioversion in Atrial Fibrillation or Flutter

Cardioversion (electric or pharmacologic) undertaken to convert AF back to sinus rhythm is associated with an increased risk of thromboembolism.[56] It is therefore recommended that warfarin (INR 2.0 to 3.0) be given for at least 3 weeks prior to elective cardioversion of patients who have been in AF for 2 days or more or when the duration of AF is unknown; warfarin should be continued until normal sinus rhythm has been maintained for 4 weeks.

For patients requiring immediate cardioversion, intravenous heparin is recommended concurrently followed by warfarin for at least 4 weeks. Alternatively, TEE prior to cardioversion can be performed; if no left atrial appendage thrombus is detected, cardioversion can occur as soon as the patient is anticoagulated and continue for at least 4 weeks. If a left atrial thrombus is detected on TEE, warfarin is recommended for at least 3 weeks prior to cardioversion and may need to be continued for a longer duration afterward.

The recommendations for cardioversion in atrial flutter are the same as for AF.[3] Atrial flutter has been studied less extensively than AF. The total incidence of acute and chronic events was found to be 7 percent over an average period of 26 months.[57] Prior TEE is not an adequate predictor of those at risk; a total of 3 of 41 patients who had no left atrial clot developed ischemic neurologic syndromes within 48 hours of elective cardioversion.[56]

Chronic Sinoatrial Disorder (Sick Sinus Syndrome)

Similar to atrioventricular block, chronic sinoatrial disease (sick sinus syndrome) usually presents with syncope and dizziness; however, those with sinoatrial disorder have a much higher rate of systemic emboli than patients with atrioventricular block, and this rate is not mitigated by pacemaker insertion. There is no significant difference in death from any cause between treatment with single-lead atrial pacing (AAIR) and dual-chamber pacing (DDDR). Single-lead atrial pacing is associated with a higher incidence of paroxysmal AF and a twofold increased risk of pacemaker reoperation.[58]

A Cochrane review concluded that physiologic (primarily dual-chamber) pacing had a statistically significant benefit in preventing the development of AF compared with ventricular pacing.[59] Patients with the "brady-tachy" form of the disorder are at higher risk of developing AF and stroke, and warfarin treatment should be considered for these patients.

Cardiomyopathies

A new definition and classification scheme for cardiomyopathy was proposed in 2006 and updated in 2008.[60,61] Cardiomyopathies are defined as a heterogeneous group of diseases of the myocardium associated with mechanical or electric dysfunction (or both) that usually, but not invariably, exhibit inappropriate ventricular hypertrophy or dilatation and are due to a variety of causes that frequently are genetic.[60] Specifically excluded are those diseases of the myocardium secondary to congenital or valvular heart disease, systemic hypertension, or atherosclerotic coronary disease.

The cardiomyopathies are divided into two major groups based on predominant organ involvement.[62] The primary cardiomyopathies are those solely or predominantly confined to heart muscle; genetic, mixed, and acquired forms are recognized. Both hypertrophic and dilated cardiomyopathies are considered primary diseases. Also included are the ion-channel disorders, in which there is a primary electric disturbance without structural cardiac pathology; these disorders are further considered in the section devoted to syncope.

Secondary cardiomyopathies involve skeletal or smooth muscle in addition to cardiac muscle. Neuromuscular or neurologic causes include Friedreich ataxia, Duchenne or Becker muscular dystrophy, Emery–Dreifuss muscular dystrophy, neurofibromatosis, and tuberous sclerosis.[63,64] The secondary cardiomyopathy classification does not include infective processes, such as Chagas disease or infection with human immunodeficiency virus.

In North America, the most common cardiomyopathy is hypertrophic cardiomyopathy, which is an autosomal dominant disease affecting 1 in 500 persons.[62] The disorder is a major cause of sudden cardiac death in athletes but is compatible with survival until old age.[65,66] Mortality rates have been estimated at around 1 percent for persons age 16 to 65, 4 percent over the next decade, and 5 percent for those older than 75 years. Stroke risk in hypertrophic cardiomyopathy was studied in a group of 900 patients.[67] Stroke occurred in 44 patients over a period of 7 years, with an annual incidence of 0.8 percent. In patients with hypertrophic cardiomyopathy, left ventricular outflow tract obstruction at rest predicts the development of heart failure and death.[68]

There are considerable geographic variations in the causes of cardiomyopathy. In Latin America, American trypanosomiasis (Chagas disease) is common. Cardioembolic stroke has been increasingly well documented as a complication, and most are in the anterior circulation. In Chagas cardiomyopathy, the apical region of the left ventricle is the typical site for formation of thrombosis or aneurysm. Echocardiography reveals an apical aneurysm in around one-third of patients and a mural thrombus in about 10 percent. Left ventricular diastolic dysfunction is present in nearly one-half of patients. The ECG is abnormal in two-thirds, including right bundle branch block, left anterior fascicular block, and AF. Oral anticoagulation has been recommended for all individuals with Chagas disease and risk factors for cardioembolism.[69]

In Africa, the major cardiomyopathy is the dilated type, but peripartum cardiomyopathy is ubiquitous with an incidence between 1 in 100 and 1 in 1,000.[70] Regional variations include endomyocardial fibrosis restricted to the tropical regions of East, Central, and West Africa.[70] The incidence of human immunodeficiency virus–associated cardiac disease, including cardiomyopathy, is increasing, in contrast to developing countries where the availability of antiretroviral therapy has reduced the incidence of myocarditis.[71]

In young adults, arrhythmogenic right ventricular dysplasia with cardiomyopathy is another rare hereditary disorder causing sudden death. In a study of the natural history in 130 patients, age at onset of symptoms averaged 32 years.[72]

Patients with dilated cardiomyopathy have a higher incidence of embolic events including systemic embolism and stroke secondary to ventricular mural thrombi, and therefore warfarin or antiplatelet therapy should be considered for secondary stroke prevention.[34]

Myocardial Infarction and Left Ventricular Dysfunction

Patients with coronary artery disease have an increased stroke risk, particularly within the first month after myocardial infarction (MI).[73] Mechanisms include embolism from left ventricular mural thrombus and the development of AF (which occurs in up to 20% of patients following MI).[74]

A community-based study of 2,160 patients hospitalized between 1979 and 1998 found stroke risk during the 30 days after a first MI to be increased 44-fold, and it remained two to three times higher than expected during the subsequent 3 years.[73] Of note, the 20-year duration of the study enabled the conclusion to be drawn that acute MI treatment with thrombolysis did not reduce stroke risk.[73] Overall, stroke risk following MI is approximately 1 percent during the first month and about 2 percent at 1 year.[75] For a non-ST elevation acute coronary syndrome, the early stroke risk is only 0.7 percent at 3 months.[76] In large randomized trials of aspirin versus the combination of aspirin and clopidogrel in patients with MI or acute coronary syndrome, the stroke rate ranged between 0.9 and 1.7 percent.[74]

In a meta-analysis, predictors of stroke following MI included advanced age, diabetes, hypertension, previous stroke or MI, anterior MI, AF, heart failure, and nonwhite race.[75] Left ventricular thrombus develops in about one-third of individuals in the first 2 weeks following an anterior MI, posing an increased risk of embolization which is reduced by anticoagulation.

The current recommendation, in the absence of thrombolytic therapy, is that after acute MI, heparin should be initiated and followed by warfarin for 3 months in patients considered to be at increased risk of embolism. High-risk patients are those with severe left ventricular dysfunction, congestive heart failure, a history of pulmonary or systemic embolism, echocardiographic evidence of mural thrombosis, or the presence of AF. Because of the increased frequency of mural thrombus in anterior as opposed to inferior myocardial infarctions, patients with an anterior Q-wave infarction should also receive heparin followed by warfarin.[77]

In patients with TIA or ischemic stroke related to an acute MI in which left ventricular mural thrombus is identified, oral anticoagulation is recommended for at least 3 months and up to 1 year (goal INR, 2.0 to 3.0), perhaps in addition to aspirin for coronary artery disease (up to 162 mg/day).[34]

Stroke risk is inversely proportional to left ventricular ejection fraction. In a study of 2,231 patients with left ventricular dysfunction following acute MI, those with an ejection fraction less than 29 percent had a stroke risk that was nearly double that of patients with ejection fraction exceeding 35 percent; the annual stroke rate was 1.5 percent overall.[78]

Congestive heart failure carries a two- to threefold increase in the relative risk of stroke. Among patients enrolled into heart failure trials, the overall annual stroke risk ranged between 1.3 and 3.5 percent; most patients were taking aspirin or warfarin in these trials.[79] In the absence of clinically overt heart failure or MI, the presence of asymptomatic left ventricular systolic dysfunction is also an independent risk factor for stroke.

The WARCEF Trial compared warfarin (target INR, 2.0 to 3.5) versus aspirin (325 mg per day) in 2,305 patients with reduced left ventricular ejection fraction (35% or less) who were in sinus rhythm and followed for up to 6 years. There was no significant overall difference between groups in the composite primary outcome of ischemic stroke, intracerebral hemorrhage, or death from any cause. A reduced risk of ischemic stroke with warfarin was offset by an increased risk of major hemorrhage.[80] Similarly, in a meta-analysis of four randomized trials comprising 4,187 patients with heart failure in sinus rhythm, warfarin was found to reduce ischemic stroke risk compared to aspirin by 0.74 percent per year but increased major bleeding by 0.99 percent per year.[81] There is therefore no convincing evidence that warfarin is superior to aspirin in stroke prevention for patients with reduced left ventricular ejection fraction.

Rheumatic Heart Disease

There is a well-established association between stroke and rheumatic heart disease (especially mitral valve stenosis), particularly in the setting of atrial fibrillation and atrial thrombus.[3] Current Class I recommendations strongly favor the use of long-term warfarin (target INR, 2.0 to 3.0) in patients with rheumatic mitral valve disease who have a history of systemic embolism or who develop AF, either chronic or paroxysmal.[3] It is also recommended that warfarin be given to patients in normal sinus rhythm if the left atrial diameter is in excess of 5.5 cm, regardless of a history of embolism.

ATRIAL MYXOMA

Atrial myxomas have long been recognized as an uncommon cause of cerebral embolism. A French hospital reviewed experience with 112 cases collected over a period of 40 years.[82] Women outnumbered men nearly 2 to 1, and ages ranged from 5 to 84 years. The presenting symptoms were cardiac (67%), constitutional (34%), and embolic (29%). Younger and male patients were more likely to experience embolic events. A literature review identified ischemic stroke as the most common neurologic manifestation.[83] Syncope, psychiatric symptoms, headache, and seizures also occur. A rare delayed complication is that of multiple cerebral aneurysm formation.[84]

MARANTIC (NONBACTERIAL THROMBOTIC) ENDOCARDITIS

There are several causes of marantic (nonbacterial thrombotic) endocarditis, a condition characterized by platelet aggregates or vegetations on previously undamaged heart valves (most often aortic and mitral) without evidence of bacteremia. It is a rare condition often associated with hypercoagulable states or advanced malignancies such as adenocarcinomas.[85]

The widespread availability of echocardiography has facilitated recognition of this disorder in patients with cancer. A prospective study of 200 unselected ambulatory patients with solid tumors found vegetations in 19 percent compared to 2 percent in controls. Vegetations were seen in 50 percent of patients with pancreatic cancer, 28 percent of those with lung cancer, and 19 percent of patients with lymphoma. Only two patients had cerebral events.[86] Brain MRI typically shows numerous lesions of various sizes in multiple arterial territories.

At one cancer center, 96 stroke patients were assessed, and TTE was performed in two-thirds.[87] An embolic mechanism was thought to be causative in over half; the heart was implicated in 14 patients, but nonbacterial thrombotic endocarditis in only 3. Stroke of embolic origin carried a dismal prognosis with life expectancy of just over 2 months; treatment had no apparent influence on outcome.

OTHER ECHOCARDIOGRAPHIC ABNORMALITIES LINKED TO STROKE

Patent Foramen Ovale and Atrial Septal Aneurysm

A PFO is present in about one-quarter of adults and represents a potential mechanism for cardiogenic embolism.[88] Case-control studies of adults younger than 55 years with cryptogenic stroke found a five-fold increase in the prevalence of PFO compared to control subjects without stroke.[89]

In a French prospective study of individuals with stroke and an isolated PFO, the 4-year stroke recurrence risk was 2.3 percent. For those with both PFO and ASA, the rate was 15.2 percent. In the "control group" with neither PFO nor ASA, the rate was 4.2 percent; all patients were taking aspirin.[90] In another study, the presence of a PFO (with or without ASA) did not significantly increase the stroke recurrence rate over a 2-year follow-up compared with a control group of stroke patients with no such lesions; furthermore, recurrence rate did not differ between patients taking aspirin or warfarin or in those with large or small PFO.[91]

The optimal management of patients with PFO has been controversial. Treatment options include antiplatelet therapy, anticoagulation, percutaneous device closure, or surgical closure. For patients with cryptogenic stroke and isolated PFO, antiplatelet therapy is usually recommended.[92] For patients with PFO and ASA, antiplatelets, anticoagulation, or PFO closure may be considered, although recent trial data have helped clarify this choice.[93]

Three large randomized controlled trials involving 2,303 patients have compared PFO device closure with medical therapy for secondary stroke prevention in patients with cryptogenic stroke and PFO (with or without ASA).[94–96] These trials showed no significant overall benefit of PFO closure on the primary study outcomes, refuting many prior nonrandomized studies that had supported PFO closure. In addition, there was no benefit to anticoagulation compared with antiplatelet treatment for the prevention of further stroke. The stroke event rate in the medical therapy control groups in these trials was low, at approximately 1 to 3 percent per year. Further research is necessary to determine whether specific higher-risk subgroups can be identified that derive significant benefit from closure, but for now there seems to be no clear benefit to closure in stroke patients with PFO.

Left Atrial Spontaneous Echo Contrast

Left atrial spontaneous echo contrast ("smoke") may be detected by TEE and is thought to represent stasis of blood within the atrium. The finding may indicate a predisposition to thrombus formation, and is most commonly encountered in patients with either AF or mitral stenosis. Left atrial spontaneous echo contrast is highly associated with previous stroke or peripheral embolism in this context.[97]

Mitral Annular Calcification

Mitral annular calcification has been suggested as a potential source of calcific or thrombotic emboli to the cerebral and retinal circulations; however, it is not clear whether the finding is an independent risk factor for stroke. The Framingham study documented a doubled stroke risk in those with mitral annular calcification compared to those without, but it is unclear whether this relationship is causal or a marker for other risk factors such as AF and generalized atherosclerotic disease, including carotid stenosis and calcified aortic plaque.[98,99]

Mitral Valve Prolapse

Mitral valve prolapse is the most frequent valvular disease in adults, with a prevalence of about 2 percent.[100] Stroke risk is increased with older age and the presence of coexistent cardiac conditions including AF, mitral valve thickening, left atrial enlargement, and mitral regurgitation.[101] In the Framingham cohort, no significant difference was found in the prevalence of stroke or TIA in those with or without mitral valve prolapse.[102]

Treatment guidelines recommend no antithrombotic therapy for primary stroke prevention in individuals with mitral valve prolapse, and long-term antiplatelet therapy for secondary prevention following ischemic stroke or TIA.[34,102]

Aortic Valve Sclerosis and Stenosis

Systemic embolism in patients with aortic valve disease is uncommon in the absence of AF or other risk factors. Aortic sclerosis (valve thickening without outflow obstruction) is a common finding in the elderly and is associated with generalized atherosclerotic vascular disease and increased cardiovascular mortality.[103]

A prospective study of patients with echocardiographically documented aortic valve calcification showed no statistically significant difference in stroke risk in patients with calcification without stenosis (8%) compared to those with calcification and stenosis (5%) or control subjects (5%).[104] Aortic valve disease is not associated with the presence of silent brain infarcts on neuroimaging. Another, larger study with a mean follow-up of 5 years showed that stroke risk was 12 percent in those with stenosis and 8 percent in those with sclerosis compared to 6 percent in those with a normal aortic valve. After adjusting for other variables, there was no statistically significant increase in stroke risk in those with aortic sclerosis.[103]

Acute Medical Treatment of Cardiogenic Embolism

The landmark study comparing acute ischemic stroke treatment with intravenous tissue plasminogen activator (t-PA) to placebo within 3 hours of stroke onset showed improved clinical outcomes at 3 months for all stroke subtypes.[105] Cardioembolism accounted for 28 percent of the patients in this study. Prompt assessment and treatment are required as the odds of a favorable outcome decline rapidly with increasing time from stroke onset to t-PA administration. A pooled analysis of thrombolytic trials supports the extension of the therapeutic time window to 4.5 hours from stroke onset.[106,107]

Specific inclusion and exclusion criteria aim to minimize the risk of intracerebral hemorrhage, the major complication of t-PA.[108] This risk increases if the treatment window is extended. Patients with CT evidence of hemorrhage on initial CT scan should not receive t-PA. The dose of t-PA for stroke thrombolysis (0.9 mg/kg) is lower than that for acute MI. Patients treated with t-PA cannot receive anticoagulation or antiplatelet therapy for the first 24 hours after infusion; subsequently, long-term anticoagulation for secondary stroke prevention may be considered.

Other interventional approaches to achieve recanalization include direct clot lysis via a microcatheter (i.e., intra-arterial thrombolysis) and mechanical clot disruption or embolectomy, but the availability of such procedures is limited to specialized centers.

Mechanical clot retrieval devices continue to be developed and may have a role in the acute treatment of patients in whom thrombolysis is contraindicated (e.g., recent cardiac surgery, high INR).[109,110]

The optimal timing for initiation of anticoagulation following cardioembolic stroke is not clear. Anticoagulation is usually delayed for about 7 days in those with large infarcts, but is started earlier in patients with smaller infarctions.[34] It is delayed also in patients with uncontrolled hypertension. Decisions must be individualized, balancing the risk of recurrent events with that of hemorrhagic transformation of the initial infarct.

SYNCOPE

Transient, self-limited interruptions of cardiac output result in generalized cerebral ischemia, a condition that is termed syncope when it results in a loss of consciousness.[111] Syncope is discussed in further detail in Chapter 8 but is considered here with regard to its occurrence in patients with acquired cardiac disease and arrhythmias.

Patients with a ventricular arrhythmia (fibrillation or tachycardia) experience syncope after around 9 seconds. Patients report feeling distant, dazed, or as if they are "fading out" before loss of consciousness. Motor activity is common, with generalized tonic contraction of axial muscles followed or accompanied by irregular jerking of the extremities, generalized rigidity without clonic activity, or irregular facial movement or eyelid flutter without tonic activity; witnesses may have difficulty in distinguishing such events from seizures. During the recovery phase, tonic flexion of the trunk may occur and patients remain dazed or confused for up to 30 seconds or more after restoration of the circulation.

Stokes Adams attacks are sudden, relatively brief (10 to 30 seconds) episodes of loss of consciousness that may feature motor activity and are typically caused by complete third-degree atrioventricular block, which can be seen on the ECG during an attack. The pulse during an episode is markedly slowed. Although coronary artery disease is a common etiology in older individuals, young individuals with congenital heart block may also experience these attacks.

Videometric analysis of syncope lasting on average 12 seconds induced in 42 healthy volunteers showed that myoclonic activity occurred in 90 percent. Head turns, oral automatisms, and writhing movements were common. Upward eye deviation was also common, and eyes remained open in three-quarters of the subjects. Visual hallucinations occurred in 60 percent and were associated with auditory hallucinations in 36 percent, although never with intelligible speech.[112] Focal neurologic symptoms are rare with cardiac arrhythmia except in the presence of preexisting atherosclerotic disease of the cerebral vasculature.

The clinical spectrum of abnormalities that occur with generalized cerebral hypoperfusion is broad, ranging from nonspecific "dizziness" to a variety of sensory disturbances, including paresthesias and alterations of vision, to loss of consciousness, sometimes with convulsive features.

A collaborative study between cardiologists and neurologists identified historical criteria to identify seizure patients among those presenting with presumed syncope: waking with a lacerated tongue, loss of consciousness with emotional stress, head turning to one side during loss of consciousness, and postictal confusion or abnormal behavior were more typical of seizure.[113] Seizures may themselves may cause arrhythmias, providing a further diagnostic challenge in patients with arrhythmias and convulsive-like movements.[114]

Syncope is especially common in the elderly, who show a high recurrence rate. Of the many causes of syncope, it is important to identify those of cardiac origin because mortality is significantly increased in this group of patients. A cardiac basis, in various studies, ranges from 1 to 8 percent for organic heart disease and 4 to 38 percent for arrhythmias.[111] In addition to common structural causes, aortic tract outflow stenosis or intermittent obstruction to outflow may occur, for example, by a mobile thrombus or tumor in the left atrium; echocardiography is the test of choice. In the case of arrhythmias, the primary objective is to document a relevant abnormality during an episode via extended cardiac telemetry.

Previously, no cause for syncope was found in about one-third of patients, but diagnostic yields as high as 76 percent have been achieved, for example, in a study of patients presenting to an emergency department.[115] Among the 650 patients, 69 (11%) were considered to have a cardiac cause, and arrhythmias were most prominent (44 patients). The 18-month mortality in the cardiac group, noncardiac group, and group without identified cause was 26, 6, and 7 percent, respectively.

A relatively common disorder predisposing to paroxysmal supraventricular tachycardia is the Wolff–Parkinson–White syndrome, which is usually sporadic with a prevalence of up to 1 in 1,000 persons.[116] AF may develop, and "dizziness," syncope, and, rarely, sudden death may occur. The characteristic ECG hallmarks are a short PR interval and a slowly rising prolonged QRS complex.

Patients with an apparently structurally normal heart present a particular challenge and raise the possibility of disorders of the conducting tissues.[117] The long QT syndrome is seen throughout the world; acquired forms, often drug related, are more common than genetic. Exertion or emotion may trigger events. The characteristic feature, as the name implies, is a prolonged QT interval (corrected for heart rate) on a standard ECG. The disorder predisposes to polymorphic ventricular tachycardia, which in turn predisposes to syncope and sudden death.[60,61]

A short QT interval syndrome has also been identified.[118] Especially affected are the young, including infants. It is a rare condition and predisposes to paroxysmal AF and episodes of ventricular fibrillation, which may lead to syncope and sudden death. It has been suggested that this short QT syndrome may be responsible for some cases of sudden infant death.[119]

Sudden death in males from Southeastern Asia attributable to ventricular fibrillation has been recognized for more than 25 years.[120] It is known as SUNDS (sudden unexplained nocturnal death syndrome) and has been linked to the Brugada syndrome, which is phenotypically, genetically, and functionally the same.[121] However, the Brugada syndrome, also characterized by sudden death due to malignant arrhythmias, has been described also in Europe and in women. The baseline ECG may be abnormal and show ST elevation in leads V1, V2, and V3 together with the presence of a right bundle branch block pattern. This ECG pattern may be concealed and require unmasking by the use of sodium channel blockers.

Another disorder, but one in which the resting ECG may be unremarkable (or show sinus bradycardia and prominent U waves), is catecholamine-induced polymorphic ventricular tachycardia.[122] This is a disorder of childhood, with an average age at symptom onset of 8 years, in which syncope or events indistinguishable from seizures are triggered by exercise or emotional stress.

Evaluation of syncope requires attention to family history including unexplained sudden deaths, age of onset, note of apparent epileptic disorders, relation of events to exertion and distress, and effects of postural change. In the presence of an apparently normal heart, evaluation of the standard ECG may suggest a cause. In the context of a normal ECG or with intermittent events, prolonged cardiac recordings may be required in order to capture an episode. With daily events, a Holter monitor may suffice. More prolonged recording techniques are available, as are sophisticated electrophysiologic studies.[123]

INTERVENTIONAL PROCEDURES

Coronary Catheterization

Coronary angiography carries a small (0.2%) risk of central nervous system complications. An unexplained observation is the preponderance of embolic events within the posterior circulation, regardless of the route of catheterization.[124] For patients experiencing an iatrogenic ischemic stroke in the context of coronary catheterization, thrombolytic therapy and clot retrieval are potential treatment options that should be considered.[125]

Percutaneous Transluminal Coronary Angioplasty and Stenting

Percutaneous transluminal coronary angioplasty was found to have an overall mortality of 0.1 percent in a large series of more than 12,000 patients. Of the 121 who died, low-output failure was the most common cause (66% of deaths), but stroke was responsible for 4 percent.[126] Another study showed that in the presence of peripheral vascular disease, the risk of any major complication (stroke included) was higher (12%).[127]

Angioplasty has also been compared to coronary stenting, and stroke rate (0.2%) was found to be equal in the two groups.[128] To prevent stent thrombosis, an antithrombotic regimen is required; the addition of clopidogrel to aspirin reduces stroke incidence both before and after percutaneous coronary intervention.[129] In a study of more than 18,000 patients with non–ST-segment elevation acute coronary syndromes, the 6-month stroke risk was 1.3 percent (1.1% for those not undergoing coronary artery bypass graft surgery) and the

6-month mortality in these patients with stroke was 27 percent.[130] Independent predictors of stroke risk included coronary bypass surgery (especially when performed early), previous stroke, diabetes, and older age.

In a study of 12,407 percutaneous coronary interventions (1990 to 1999), the periprocedural risk of stroke and TIA was 0.38 and 0.12 percent, respectively.[131] More than 90 percent of patients in this study underwent balloon angioplasty, and nearly half also underwent coronary stenting. Independent predictors of stroke were advanced age, use of an intra-aortic balloon pump, and need for saphenous vein graft intervention.[131]

Primary angioplasty, compared to thrombolysis, has been noted to decrease the risk of stroke significantly.[132] In a review of 23 randomized trials involving more than 7,000 patients with acute MI and ST-segment elevation who were randomly assigned to either primary percutaneous transluminal coronary angioplasty or thrombolysis, the overall stroke rate was 1 percent with angioplasty compared to 2 percent with thrombolysis.[133]

Thrombolytic Therapy for Acute Myocardial Infarction

Concern that thrombolytic therapy for MI would result in an increase in stroke was not substantiated by the results of an initial large Italian trial of nearly 12,000 patients. An excess of stroke was evident only during the first day after randomization to streptokinase; after this period, patients in the control group had more stroke and TIA events. The study did not include head CT scan results.[134] Comparison of four thrombolytic strategies confirmed a slight excess of hemorrhagic stroke in those receiving t-PA and in those receiving combined thrombolytic agents on the order of 2 to 3 per 1,000 treated.[135] In the four groups, stroke risk rate ranged from a low of 1.22 percent in those treated with streptokinase and subcutaneous heparin to 1.64 percent in those treated with intravenous heparin and both t-PA and streptokinase. These percentages are equal to or less than those documented in large prethrombolytic studies of acute MI.

The risk of ICH following thrombolytic therapy has been linked to the intensity of heparin anticoagulation and timing of partial thromboplastin time monitoring. Recent trials have used reduced-dose heparin regimens and 3-hour partial thromboplastin time monitoring, leading to decreased rates of ICH.[136]

When ICH does occur, it is likely to be large in size, supratentorial in location, and more often lobar than deep. Mass effect is common, and blood may extend into the ventricles or subarachnoid space. Of 244 cases, symptoms emerged within 8 hours of treatment in 55, after 30 hours in 58, and between these times in the remainder.[134] A small percentage (3%) of hemorrhages were subdural. Syncope within 48 hours of treatment, or facial or head trauma within 2 weeks of treatment were disproportionately noted in these ICH patients, but numbers were small.[137]

A review of risk factors in 150 patients with documented ICH after thrombolysis identified four independent predictors: age older than 65 years, body weight less than 70 kg, hypertension on hospital admission, and administration of alteplase. These same risk factors for ICH were identified in the GUSTO-I trial; additional predictors included a history of cerebrovascular disease or hypertension and elevated systolic or diastolic blood pressure on admission.[138]

If ICH is suspected, immediate noncontrast head CT scan and discontinuation or reversal of thrombolytic or antithrombotic therapy are recommended. Neurosurgical consultation should be considered.[139]

ACKNOWLEDGMENTS

Part of this chapter was authored by Colin Lambert, BM, FRCP, in earlier editions of this book.

REFERENCES

1. Goldstein LB, Jones MR, Matchar DB, et al: Improving the reliability of stroke subgroup classification using the Trial of ORG 10172 in Acute Stroke Treatment (TOAST) criteria. Stroke 32:1091, 2001.
2. Murtagh B, Smalling RW: Cardioembolic stroke. Curr Atheroscler Rep 8:310, 2006.
3. Fuster V, Rydén LE, Cannom DS, et al: 2011 ACCF/AHA/HRS focused updates incorporated into the ACC/AHA/ESC 2006 guidelines for the management of patients with atrial fibrillation: a report of the American College of Cardiology Foundation/American Heart Association Task Force on practice guidelines. Circulation 123:e269, 2011.
4. Putaala J, Metso AJ, Metso TM, et al: Analysis of 1008 consecutive patients aged 15 to 49 with first-ever ischemic stroke: the Helsinki young stroke registry. Stroke 40:1195, 2009.

5. Adams Jr HP, Kappelle LJ, Biller J, et al: Ischemic stroke in young adults. Experience in 329 patients enrolled in the Iowa Registry of stroke in young adults. Arch Neurol 52:491, 1995.
6. Ducrocq X, Lacour JC, Debouverie M, et al: Cerebral ischemic accidents in young subjects. A prospective study of 296 patients aged 16 to 45 years. Rev Neurol (Paris) 155:575, 1999.
7. Rasura M, Spalloni A, Ferrari M, et al: A case series of young stroke in Rome. Eur J Neurol 13:146, 2006.
8. Giovannoni G, Fritz VU: Transient ischemic attacks in younger and older patients. A comparative study of 798 patients in South Africa. Stroke 24:947, 1993.
9. Kittner SJ, Sharkness CM, Sloan MA, et al: Features on initial computed tomography scan of infarcts with a cardiac source of embolism in the NINDS Stroke Data Bank. Stroke 23:1748, 1992.
10. Kittner SJ, Sharkness CM, Sloan MA, et al: Infarcts with a cardiac source of embolism in the NINDS Stroke Data Bank: neurologic examination. Neurology 42:299, 1992.
11. Arboix A, Garcia-Eroles L, Massons JB, et al: Atrial fibrillation and stroke: clinical presentation of cardioembolic versus atherothrombotic infarction. Int J Cardiol 73:33, 2000.
12. Kase CS, Norrving B, Levine SR, et al: Cerebellar infarction. Clinical and anatomic observations in 66 cases. Stroke 24:76, 1993.
13. Lovett JK, Coull AJ, Rothwell PM: Early risk of recurrence by subtype of ischemic stroke in population-based incidence studies. Neurology 62:569, 2004.
14. Kolominsky-Rabas PL, Weber M, Gefeller O, et al: Epidemiology of ischemic stroke subtypes according to TOAST criteria: incidence, recurrence, and long-term survival in ischemic stroke subtypes: a population-based study. Stroke 32:2735, 2001.
15. Khatri R, McKinney AM, Swenson B, et al: Blood-brain barrier, reperfusion injury, and hemorrhagic transformation in acute ischemic stroke. Neurology 79(suppl 1):S52, 2012.
16. Kablau M, Kreisel SH, Sauer T, et al: Predictors and early outcome of hemorrhagic transformation after acute ischemic stroke. Cerebrovasc Dis 32:334, 2011.
17. Toni D, Fiorelli M, Bastianello S, et al: Hemorrhagic transformation of brain infarct: predictability in the first 5 hours from stroke onset and influence on clinical outcome. Neurology 46:341, 1996.
18. Gonzalez RG, Schaefer PW, Buonanno FS, et al: Diffusion-weighted MR imaging: diagnostic accuracy in patients imaged within 6 hours of stroke symptom onset. Radiology 210:155, 1999.
19. Thiex R, Norbash AM, Frerichs KU: The safety of dedicated-team catheter-based diagnostic cerebral angiography in the era of advanced noninvasive imaging. Am J Neuroradiol 31:230, 2010.
20. Connors III JJ, Sacks D, Furlan AJ, et al: Training, competency, and credentialing standards for diagnostic cervicocerebral angiography, carotid stenting, and cerebrovascular intervention: a joint statement from the American Academy of Neurology, the American Association of Neurological Surgeons, the American Society of Interventional and Therapeutic Neuroradiology, the American Society of Neuroradiology, the Congress of Neurological Surgeons, the AANS/CNS Cerebrovascular Section, and the Society of Interventional Radiology. Neurology 64:190, 2005.
21. Agmon Y, Khandheria BK, Gentile F, et al: Echocardiographic assessment of the left atrial appendage. J Am Coll Cardiol 34:1867, 1999.
22. Kapral MK, Silver FL: Preventive health care, 1999 update: 2. Echocardiography for the detection of a cardiac source of embolus in patients with stroke. Canadian task force on preventive health care. CMAJ 161:989, 1999.
23. Thompson CR: Echocardiography in stroke: which probe when? CMAJ 161:981, 1999.
24. Edelman RR: Contrast-enhanced MR imaging of the heart: overview of the literature. Radiology 232:653, 2004.
25. Belvis R, Leta RG, Marti-Fabregas J, et al: Almost perfect concordance between simultaneous transcranial Doppler and transesophageal echocardiography in the quantification of right-to-left shunts. J Neuroimaging 16:133, 2006.
26. Gage BF, Waterman AD, Shannon W, et al: Validation of clinical classification schemes for predicting stroke: results from the National Registry of Atrial Fibrillation. JAMA 285:2864, 2001.
27. Lip GY, Nieuwlaat R, Pisters R, et al: Refining clinical risk stratification for predicting stroke and thromboembolism in atrial fibrillation using a novel risk factor-based approach: The Euro Heart Survey on Atrial Fibrillation. Chest 137:263, 2010.
28. Echocardiographic predictors of stroke in patients with atrial fibrillation: a prospective study of 1066 patients from 3 clinical trials. Arch Intern Med 158:1316, 1998.
29. Bouzas-Mosquera A, Broullón FJ, Álvarez-García N, et al: Left atrial size and risk for all-cause mortality and ischemic stroke. CMAJ 183:E657, 2011.
30. Transesophageal echocardiographic correlates of thromboembolism in high-risk patients with nonvalvular atrial fibrillation. The Stroke Prevention in Atrial Fibrillation Investigators Committee on Echocardiography. Ann Intern Med 128:639, 1998.
31. Saxena R, Koudstaal P: Anticoagulants versus antiplatelet therapy for preventing stroke in patients with nonrheumatic atrial fibrillation and a history of stroke or transient ischemic attack. Cochrane Database Syst Rev 4:CD000187, 2004.
32. Hart RG, Benavente O, McBride R, et al: Antithrombotic therapy to prevent stroke in patients with atrial fibrillation: a meta-analysis. Ann Intern Med 131:492, 1999.
33. Wyse DG, Waldo AL, DiMarco JP, et al: A comparison of rate control and rhythm control in patients with atrial fibrillation. N Engl J Med 347:1825, 2002.

34. Furie KL, Kasner SE, Adams RJ, et al: Guidelines for the prevention of stroke in patients with stroke or transient ischemic attack: a guideline for healthcare professionals from the American Heart Association/American Stroke Association. Stroke 42:227, 2011.
35. Paciaroni M, Agnelli G, Caso V, et al: Atrial fibrillation in patients with first-ever stroke: frequency, antithrombotic treatment before the event and effect on clinical outcome. J Thromb Haemost 3:1218, 2005.
36. Waldo AL, Becker RC, Tapson VF, et al: Hospitalized patients with atrial fibrillation and a high risk of stroke are not being provided with adequate anticoagulation. J Am Coll Cardiol 46:1729, 2005.
37. Bungard TJ, Ghali WA, McAlister FA, et al: Physicians' perceptions of the benefits and risks of warfarin for patients with nonvalvular atrial fibrillation. CMAJ 165:301, 2001.
38. Choudhry NK, Anderson GM, Laupacis A, et al: Impact of adverse events on prescribing warfarin in patients with atrial fibrillation: matched pair analysis. BMJ 332:141, 2006.
39. Lip GY, Kamath S, Jafri M, et al: Ethnic differences in patient perceptions of atrial fibrillation and anticoagulation therapy: the West Birmingham Atrial Fibrillation Project. Stroke 33:238, 2002.
40. Bloomfield HE, Krause A, Greer N, et al: Meta-analysis: effect of patient self-testing and self-management of long-term anticoagulation on major clinical outcomes. Ann Intern Med 154:472, 2011.
41. Bleeding during antithrombotic therapy in patients with atrial fibrillation. The Stroke Prevention in Atrial Fibrillation Investigators. Arch Intern Med 156:409, 1996.
42. Hylek EM, Skates SJ, Sheehan MA, et al: An analysis of the lowest effective intensity of prophylactic anticoagulation for patients with nonrheumatic atrial fibrillation. N Engl J Med 335:540, 1996.
43. O'Donnell M, Oczkowski W, Fang J, et al: Preadmission antithrombotic treatment and stroke severity in patients with atrial fibrillation and acute ischaemic stroke: an observational study. Lancet Neurol 5:749, 2006.
44. Connolly S, Pogue J, Hart R, et al: Clopidogrel plus aspirin versus oral anticoagulation for atrial fibrillation in the Atrial fibrillation clopidogrel trial with irbesartan for prevention of vascular events (ACTIVE W): a randomised controlled trial. Lancet 367:1903, 2006.
45. Douketis JD, Spyropoulos AC, Spencer FA, et al: Perioperative management of antithrombotic therapy: antithrombotic therapy and prevention of thrombosis, 9th ed: American College of Chest Physicians Evidence-Based Clinical Practice Guidelines. Chest 141(suppl):e326S, 2012.
46. Alberts MJ, Eikelboom JW, Hankey GJ: Antithrombotic therapy for stroke prevention in non-valvular atrial fibrillation. Lancet Neurol 11:1066, 2012.
47. Connolly SJ, Ezekowitz MD, Yusuf S, et al: Dabigatran versus warfarin in patients with atrial fibrillation. N Engl J Med 361:1139, 2009.
48. Patel MR, Mahaffey KW, Garg J, et al: Rivaroxaban versus warfarin in nonvalvular atrial fibrillation. N Engl J Med 365:883, 2011.
49. Granger CB, Alexander JH, McMurray JJ, et al: Apixaban versus warfarin in patients with atrial fibrillation. N Engl J Med 365:981, 2011.
50. Connolly SJ, Eikelboom J, Joyner C, et al: Apixaban in patients with atrial fibrillation. N Engl J Med 364:806, 2011.
51. Nageh T, Meier B: Intracardiac devices for stroke prevention. Prev Cardiol 9:42, 2006.
52. Mousa AY, Campbell JE, Aburahma AF, et al: Current update of cerebral embolic protection devices. J Vasc Surg 56:1429, 2012.
53. Mead GE, Elder AT, Flapan AD, et al: Electrical cardioversion for atrial fibrillation and flutter. Cochrane Database Syst Rev:CD002903, 2005.
54. Healey JS, Connolly SJ, Gold MR, et al: Subclinical atrial fibrillation and the risk of stroke. N Engl J Med 366:120, 2012.
55. Seet RC, Friedman PA, Rabinstein AA: Prolonged rhythm monitoring for the detection of occult paroxysmal atrial fibrillation in ischemic stroke of unknown cause. Circulation 124:477, 2011.
56. Mehta D, Baruch L: Thromboembolism following cardioversion of "common" atrial flutter. Risk factors and limitations of transesophageal echocardiography. Chest 110:1001, 1996.
57. Seidl K, Hauer B, Schwick NG, et al: Risk of thromboembolic events in patients with atrial flutter. Am J Cardiol 82:580, 1998.
58. Nielsen JC, Thomsen PE, Højberg S, et al: A comparison of single-lead atrial pacing with dual-chamber pacing in sick sinus syndrome. Eur Heart J 32:686, 2011.
59. Dretzke J, Toff WD, Lip GY, et al: Dual chamber versus single chamber ventricular pacemakers for sick sinus syndrome and atrioventricular block. Cochrane Database Syst Rev:CD003710, 2004.
60. Maron BJ, Towbin JA, Thiene G, et al: Contemporary definitions and classification of the cardiomyopathies: an American Heart Association Scientific Statement from the Council on Clinical Cardiology, Heart Failure and Transplantation Committee; Quality of Care and Outcomes Research and Functional Genomics and Translational Biology Interdisciplinary Working Groups; and Council on Epidemiology and Prevention. Circulation 113:1807, 2006.
61. Elliott P, Andersson B, Arbustini E, et al: Classification of the cardiomyopathies: a position statement from the European Society of Cardiology Working Group on Myocardial and Pericardial Diseases. Eur Heart J 29:270, 2008.
62. Maron BJ, Maron MS: Hypertrophic cardiomyopathy. Lancet 381:242, 2013.

63. Groh WJ: Arrhythmias in the muscular dystrophies. Heart Rhythm 9:1890, 2012.
64. Yilmaz A, Sechtem U: Cardiac involvement in muscular dystrophy: advances in diagnosis and therapy. Heart 98:420, 2012.
65. Maron BJ, Casey SA, Haas TS, et al: Hypertrophic cardiomyopathy with longevity to 90 years or older. Am J Cardiol 109:1341, 2012.
66. Maron BJ: Sudden death in young athletes. N Engl J Med 349:1064, 2003.
67. Maron BJ, Olivotto I, Bellone P, et al: Clinical profile of stroke in 900 patients with hypertrophic cardiomyopathy. J Am Coll Cardiol 39:301, 2002.
68. Maron MS, Olivotto I, Betocchi S, et al: Effect of left ventricular outflow tract obstruction on clinical outcome in hypertrophic cardiomyopathy. N Engl J Med 348:295, 2003.
69. Carod-Artal FJ, Vargas AP, Horan TA, et al: Chagasic cardiomyopathy is independently associated with ischemic stroke in Chagas disease. Stroke 36:965, 2005.
70. Sliwa K, Damasceno A, Mayosi BM: Epidemiology and etiology of cardiomyopathy in Africa. Circulation 112:3577, 2005.
71. Ntsekhe M, Mayosi BM: Cardiac manifestations of HIV infection: an African perspective. Nat Clin Pract Cardiovasc Med 6:120, 2009.
72. Hulot JS, Jouven X, Empana JP, et al: Natural history and risk stratification of arrhythmogenic right ventricular dysplasia/cardiomyopathy. Circulation 110:1879, 2004.
73. Witt BJ, Brown Jr RD, Jacobsen SJ, et al: A community-based study of stroke incidence after myocardial infarction. Ann Intern Med 143:785, 2005.
74. Dutta M, Hanna E, Das P, et al: Incidence and prevention of ischemic stroke following myocardial infarction: review of current literature. Cerebrovasc Dis 22:331, 2006.
75. Witt BJ, Ballman KV, Brown Jr RD, et al: The incidence of stroke after myocardial infarction: a meta-analysis. Am J Med 119:354, 2006.
76. Kassem-Moussa H, Mahaffey KW, Graffagnino C, et al: Incidence and characteristics of stroke during 90-day follow-up in patients stabilized after an acute coronary syndrome. Am Heart J 148:439, 2004.
77. Cairns JA, Theroux P, Lewis Jr HD, et al: Antithrombotic agents in coronary artery disease. Chest 114:611S, 1998.
78. Loh E, Sutton MS, Wun CC, et al: Ventricular dysfunction and the risk of stroke after myocardial infarction. N Engl J Med 336:251, 1997.
79. Pullicino PM, Halperin JL, Thompson JL: Stroke in patients with heart failure and reduced left ventricular ejection fraction. Neurology 54:288, 2000.
80. Homma S, Thompson JL, Pullicino PM, et al: Warfarin and aspirin in patients with heart failure and sinus rhythm. N Engl J Med 366:1859, 2012.
81. Liew AY, Eikelboom JW, Connolly SJ, et al: Efficacy and safety of warfarin vs. antiplatelet therapy in patients with systolic heart failure and sinus rhythm: a systematic review and meta-analysis of randomized controlled trials. Int J Stroke 2013 in press.
82. Pinede L, Duhaut P, Loire R: Clinical presentation of left atrial cardiac myxoma. A series of 112 consecutive cases. Medicine (Baltimore) 80:159, 2001.
83. Ekinci EI, Donnan GA: Neurological manifestations of cardiac myxoma: a review of the literature and report of cases. Intern Med J 34:243, 2004.
84. Jean WC, Walski-Easton SM, Nussbaum ES: Multiple intracranial aneurysms as delayed complications of an atrial myxoma: case report. Neurosurgery 49:200, 2001.
85. Mazokopakis EE, Syros PK, Starakis IK: Nonbacterial thrombotic endocarditis (marantic endocarditis) in cancer patients. Cardiovasc Hematol Disord Drug Targets 10:84, 2010.
86. Edoute Y, Haim N, Rinkevich D, et al: Cardiac valvular vegetations in cancer patients: a prospective echocardiographic study of 200 patients. Am J Med 102:252, 1997.
87. Cestari DM, Weine DM, Panageas KS, et al: Stroke in patients with cancer: incidence and etiology. Neurology 62:2025, 2004.
88. Kizer JR, Devereux RB: Clinical practice. Patent foramen ovale in young adults with unexplained stroke. N Engl J Med 353:2361, 2005.
89. Overell JR, Bone I, Lees KR: Interatrial septal abnormalities and stroke: a meta-analysis of case-control studies. Neurology 55:1172, 2000.
90. Mas JL, Arquizan C, Lamy C, et al: Recurrent cerebrovascular events associated with patent foramen ovale, atrial septal aneurysm, or both. N Engl J Med 345:1740, 2001.
91. Homma S, Sacco RL, Di Tullio MR, et al: Effect of medical treatment in stroke patients with patent foramen ovale: Patent Foramen Ovale in Cryptogenic Stroke Study. Circulation 105:2625, 2002.
92. Messe SR, Silverman IE, Kizer JR, et al: Practice parameter: recurrent stroke with patent foramen ovale and atrial septal aneurysm: report of the quality standards subcommittee of the American Academy of Neurology. Neurology 62:1042, 2004.
93. Tobis J, Shenoda M: Percutaneous treatment of patent foramen ovale and atrial septal defects. J Am Coll Cardiol 60:1722, 2012.
94. Furlan AJ, Reisman M, Massaro J, et al: Closure or medical therapy for cryptogenic stroke with patent foramen ovale. N Engl J Med 15:991, 2012.
95. Carroll JD, Saver JL, Thaler DE, et al: Closure of patent foramen ovale versus medical therapy after cryptogenic stroke. N Engl J Med 368:1092, 2013.
96. Meier B, Kalesan B, Mattle HP, et al: Percutaneous closure of patent foramen ovale in cryptogenic embolism. N Engl J Med 368:1083, 2013.
97. Chimowitz MI, DeGeorgia MA, Poole RM, et al: Left atrial spontaneous echo contrast is highly associated with previous stroke in patients with atrial fibrillation or mitral stenosis. Stroke 24:1015, 1993.

98. Benjamin EJ, Plehn JF, D'Agostino RB, et al: Mitral annular calcification and the risk of stroke in an elderly cohort. N Engl J Med 327:374, 1992.
99. Allison MA, Cheung P, Criqui MH, et al: Mitral and aortic annular calcification are highly associated with systemic calcified atherosclerosis. Circulation 113:861, 2006.
100. Freed LA, Levy D, Levine RA, et al: Prevalence and clinical outcome of mitral-valve prolapse. N Engl J Med 341:1, 1999.
101. Avierinos JF, Brown RD, Foley DA, et al: Cerebral ischemic events after diagnosis of mitral valve prolapse: a community-based study of incidence and predictive factors. Stroke 34:1339, 2003.
102. Whitlock RP, Sun JC, Fremes SE, et al: Antithrombotic and thrombolytic therapy for valvular disease: antithrombotic therapy and prevention of thrombosis, 9th ed: American College of Chest Physicians Evidence-Based Clinical Practice Guidelines. Chest 141:e576S, 2012.
103. Otto CM, Lind BK, Kitzman DW, et al: Association of aortic-valve sclerosis with cardiovascular mortality and morbidity in the elderly. N Engl J Med 341:142, 1999.
104. Boon A, Lodder J, Cheriex E, et al: Risk of stroke in a cohort of 815 patients with calcification of the aortic valve with or without stenosis. Stroke 27:847, 1996.
105. The National Institute of Neurological Disorders Stroke rt-PA Stroke Study Group Tissue plasminogen activator for acute ischemic stroke. N Engl J Med 333:1581, 1995.
106. Hacke W, Kaste M, Bluhmki E, et al: Thrombolysis with alteplase 3 to 4.5 hours after acute ischemic stroke. N Engl J Med 359:1317, 2008.
107. Lees KR, Bluhmki E, von Kummer R, et al: Time to treatment with intravenous alteplase and outcome in stroke: an updated pooled analysis of ECASS, ATLANTIS, NINDS, and EPITHET trials. Lancet 375:1695, 2010.
108. Jauch EC, Saver JL, Adams Jr HP, et al: Guidelines for the early management of patients with acute ischemic stroke: a guideline for healthcare professionals from the American Heart Association/American Stroke Association. Stroke 44:870, 2013.
109. Saver JL, Jahan R, Levy EI, et al: Solitaire flow restoration device versus the Merci Retriever in patients with acute ischaemic stroke (SWIFT): a randomised, parallel-group, non-inferiority trial. Lancet 380:1241, 2012.
110. Nogueira RG, Lutsep HL, Gupta R, et al: Trevo versus Merci retrievers for thrombectomy revascularisation of large vessel occlusions in acute ischaemic stroke (TREVO 2): a randomised trial. Lancet 380:1231, 2012.
111. Kapoor WN: Syncope. N Engl J Med 343:1856, 2000.
112. Lempert T, Bauer M, Schmidt D: Syncope: a videometric analysis of 56 episodes of transient cerebral hypoxia. Ann Neurol 36:233, 1994.
113. Sheldon R, Rose S, Ritchie D, et al: Historical criteria that distinguish syncope from seizures. J Am Coll Cardiol 40:142, 2002.
114. Rocamora R, Kurthen M, Lickfett L, et al: Cardiac asystole in epilepsy: clinical and neurophysiologic features. Epilepsia 44:179, 2003.
115. Sarasin FP, Louis-Simonet M, Carballo D, et al: Prospective evaluation of patients with syncope: a population-based study. Am J Med 111:177, 2001.
116. Al-Khatib SM, Pritchett EL: Clinical features of Wolff-Parkinson-White syndrome. Am Heart J 138:403, 1999.
117. Goldschlager N, Epstein AE, Grubb BP, et al: Etiologic considerations in the patient with syncope and an apparently normal heart. Arch Intern Med 163:151, 2003.
118. Brugada R, Hong K, Cordeiro JM, et al: Short QT syndrome. CMAJ 173:1349, 2005.
119. Wolpert C, Schimpf R, Veltmann C, et al: Clinical characteristics and treatment of short QT syndrome. Expert Rev Cardiovasc Ther 3:611, 2005.
120. Gaw AC, Lee B, Gervacio-Domingo G, et al: Unraveling the enigma of bangungut: is sudden unexplained nocturnal death syndrome (SUNDS) in the Philippines a disease allelic to the Brugada syndrome? Philipp J Intern Med 49:165, 2011.
121. Hong K, Berruezo-Sanchez A, Poungvarin N, et al: Phenotypic characterization of a large European family with Brugada syndrome displaying a sudden unexpected death syndrome mutation in SCN5A. J Cardiovasc Electrophysiol 15:64, 2004.
122. Leenhardt A, Lucet V, Denjoy I, et al: Catecholaminergic polymorphic ventricular tachycardia in children. A 7-year follow-up of 21 patients. Circulation 91:1512, 1995.
123. Strickberger SA, Benson DW, Biaggioni I, et al: AHA/ACCF scientific statement on the evaluation of syncope: from the American Heart Association Councils on Clinical Cardiology, Cardiovascular Nursing, Cardiovascular Disease in the Young, and Stroke, and the Quality of Care and Outcomes Research Interdisciplinary Working Group; and the American College of Cardiology Foundation: in collaboration with the Heart Rhythm Society: endorsed by the American Autonomic Society. Circulation 113:316, 2006.
124. Keilson GR, Schwartz WJ, Recht LD: The preponderance of posterior circulatory events is independent of the route of cardiac catheterization. Stroke 23:1358, 1992.
125. Serry R, Tsimikas S, Imbesi SG, et al: Treatment of ischemic stroke complicating cardiac catheterization with systemic thrombolytic therapy. Catheter Cardiovasc Interv 66:364, 2005.
126. Malenka DJ, O'Rourke D, Miller MA, et al: Cause of in-hospital death in 12,232 consecutive patients undergoing percutaneous transluminal coronary angioplasty.

The Northern New England Cardiovascular Disease Study Group. Am Heart J 137:632, 1999.

127. Weaver WD, Simes RJ, Betriu A, et al: Comparison of primary coronary angioplasty and intravenous thrombolytic therapy for acute myocardial infarction: a quantitative review. JAMA 278:2093, 1997.

128. Grines CL, Cox DA, Stone GW, et al: Coronary angioplasty with or without stent implantation for acute myocardial infarction. Stent Primary Angioplasty in Myocardial Infarction Study Group. N Engl J Med 341:1949, 1999.

129. Sabatine MS, Cannon CP, Gibson CM, et al: Effect of clopidogrel pretreatment before percutaneous coronary intervention in patients with ST-elevation myocardial infarction treated with fibrinolytics: the PCI-CLARITY study. JAMA 294:1224, 2005.

130. Cronin L, Mehta SR, Zhao F, et al: Stroke in relation to cardiac procedures in patients with non-ST-elevation acute coronary syndrome: a study involving >18000 patients. Circulation 104:269, 2001.

131. Fuchs S, Stabile E, Kinnaird TD, et al: Stroke complicating percutaneous coronary interventions: incidence, predictors, and prognostic implications. Circulation 106:86, 2002.

132. Cucherat M, Bonnefoy E, Tremeau G: Primary angioplasty versus intravenous thrombolysis for acute myocardial infarction. Cochrane Database Syst Rev:CD001560, 2003.

133. Keeley EC, Boura JA, Grines CL: Primary angioplasty versus intravenous thrombolytic therapy for acute myocardial infarction: a quantitative review of 23 randomised trials. Lancet 361:13, 2003.

134. Maggioni AP, Franzosi MG, Farina ML, et al: Cerebrovascular events after myocardial infarction: analysis of the GISSI trial. Gruppo Italiano per lo Studio della Streptochinasi nell'Infarto Miocardico (GISSI). BMJ 302:1428, 1991.

135. The GUSTO Investigators: An international randomized trial comparing four thrombolytic strategies for acute myocardial infarction. N Engl J Med 329:673, 1993.

136. Giugliano RP, McCabe CH, Antman EM, et al: Lower-dose heparin with fibrinolysis is associated with lower rates of intracranial hemorrhage. Am Heart J 141:742, 2001.

137. Gebel JM, Sila CA, Sloan MA, et al: Thrombolysis-related intracranial hemorrhage: a radiographic analysis of 244 cases from the GUSTO-1 trial with clinical correlation. Global Utilization of Streptokinase and Tissue Plasminogen Activator for Occluded Coronary Arteries. Stroke 29:563, 1998.

138. Gore JM, Granger CB, Simoons ML, et al: Stroke after thrombolysis. Mortality and functional outcomes in the GUSTO-I trial. Global Use of Strategies to Open Occluded Coronary Arteries. Circulation 92:2811, 1995.

139. Mahaffey KW, Granger CB, Sloan MA, et al: Neurosurgical evacuation of intracranial hemorrhage after thrombolytic therapy for acute myocardial infarction: experience from the GUSTO-I trial. Global Utilization of Streptokinase and tissue-plasminogen activator (tPA) for Occluded Coronary Arteries. Am Heart J 138:493, 1999.

CHAPTER

6

Neurologic Manifestations of Infective Endocarditis

LINDA S. WILLIAMS ■ JARED R. BROSCH

The relationship between infection of the heart valves and arterial embolization was first recognized by Rudolf Virchow in the mid-1800s and the classic clinical triad of fever, heart murmur, and hemiplegia was described 30 years later by Osler in his Gulstonian Lectures of 1885.[1] The understanding of infective endocarditis (IE) has evolved since these early descriptions to a concept of the disease occurring with different predisposing conditions, different propensities for sites of valve infection, different infecting organisms, and different treatments; however, the proportion of patients with IE and neurologic manifestations has remained relatively constant. Neurologic complications are frequent and are often associated with increased morbidity and mortality in IE. Although the key to treating neurologic complications is appropriate antibiotic therapy, the presence of neurologic manifestations often alters the medical or surgical treatment of IE.

EPIDEMIOLOGY OF NEUROLOGIC COMPLICATIONS

Neurologic events have long been recognized as frequent and severe complications of IE.[1] A large prospective cohort study conducted in 25 countries from 2000 to 2005, the International Collaboration on Endocarditis, provides evidence regarding IE and its various complications.[2] The overall frequency of neurologic complications of IE has remained relatively constant at approximately 15 to 30 percent (Table 6-1).[1–10] Nevertheless, because of the high overall incidence of stroke in the general population, IE is an unusual cause of stroke. Neurologic complications of IE can be divided into three major types: ischemic stroke, hemorrhagic stroke, and direct cerebral infection. Ischemic stroke is by far the most common, accounting for 50 to 75 percent of all neurologic complications. Primary hemorrhage,

Aminoff's Neurology and General Medicine, Fifth Edition.

TABLE 6-1 ■ Common Neurologic Complications in Patients with Infective Endocarditis

Series	*n*	Ischemic Stroke	Hemorrhage	Primary Infection	All Neurologic Complications*
Heiro et al., 2000[4]	218	13 (6%)	4 (2%)	10 (5%)	55 (25%)
Hoen et al., 2002[5]	390	60 (15%)	21 (5%)	NR	NR
Durante et al., 2003[6‡]	94	20 (21%)	NR	NR	NR
Thuny et al., 2005[7‡]	384	76 (20%)	NR	NR	NR
Miro et al., 2005[8§]	1348	NR	NR	NR	210 (16%)
Heiro et al., 2006[3]	326	27 (8%)	6 (2%)	15 (5%)	86 (26%)
Murdoch 2009[2**]	2781	462 (17%)	NR	NR	NR
Leone et al, 2012[9**]	1082	160 (15%)	NR	NR	NR

NR, not reported. (The numbers in parentheses represent the percentage of patients with the indicated complication.)
*These complications include some not listed in this table.
‡Includes both cerebral embolism prior to antibiotic treatment and after treatment.
§Includes cerebral embolism, hemorrhage, and infection.
**Ischemic and hemorrhagic stroke not distinguished.

usually intraparenchymal or subarachnoid, is less common, reported in less than 10 percent of patients.[1,3–5,11–17] Secondary hemorrhagic transformation of an ischemic stroke, however, is estimated to occur in 20 to 40 percent of ischemic strokes from IE. Cerebral infections may manifest, without previous clinical evidence of ischemic or hemorrhagic stroke, in less than 10 percent of cases; typical infectious complications include cerebritis, meningitis, and microabscesses or macroabscesses. Other neurologic symptoms, including seizures, headache, mental status changes, and neuropsychologic abnormalities, sometimes occur but are usually secondary to one of the three major complications. Rarely, endocarditis has been associated with spinal cord infarction or abscess, discitis, retinal ischemia, and ischemic cranial and peripheral neuropathies.

PATHOPHYSIOLOGY OF NEUROLOGIC COMPLICATIONS

Almost all the neurologic complications of IE have embolization as their primary cause (Fig. 6-1). Although cerebral emboli are probably not more common than extracerebral emboli,[15] they are more often symptomatic and thus typically reported more frequently; they are also associated with an increased morbidity and mortality compared to other systemic emboli. Cerebral emboli most often affect the middle cerebral artery (MCA) territory and may be septic or nonseptic. Cerebral emboli may present as stroke, but in many cases (36 to 48% in recent studies) are subclinical with only MRI evidence of infarction.[18–20] Therefore, neuroimaging should be considered in all patients with IE, regardless of neurologic symptoms. Septic emboli may also lead to hemorrhagic stroke through the development of arteritis or mycotic aneurysm; to cerebral microabscess or macroabscess (Fig. 6-2), usually through seeding ischemic tissue; and to cerebritis or meningitis by seeding the meninges.

Most primary intracerebral hemorrhages in IE result from septic embolism followed by septic necrosis and rupture of the vessel wall; less commonly, they result from rupture of mycotic aneurysms.[2,12,21–23] In one study, it was found that 10 of 16 patients with IE and intracerebral bleeding had pyogenic arteritis, in 5 of whom rupture occurred without evidence of concomitant mycotic aneurysm; 13 of the 16 had either septic emboli or arteritis, or both.[22] Intracerebral hemorrhage may also occur owing to a secondary hemorrhage into an ischemic infarct (Fig. 6-3). In one histopathologic series of 17 patients, brain hemorrhage was due to secondary transformation of ischemic infarction in 24 percent of cases, necrotic arteritis in 24 percent, mycotic aneurysm in 12 percent, and other causes in 11 percent; in 29 percent it was of unknown etiology.[21]

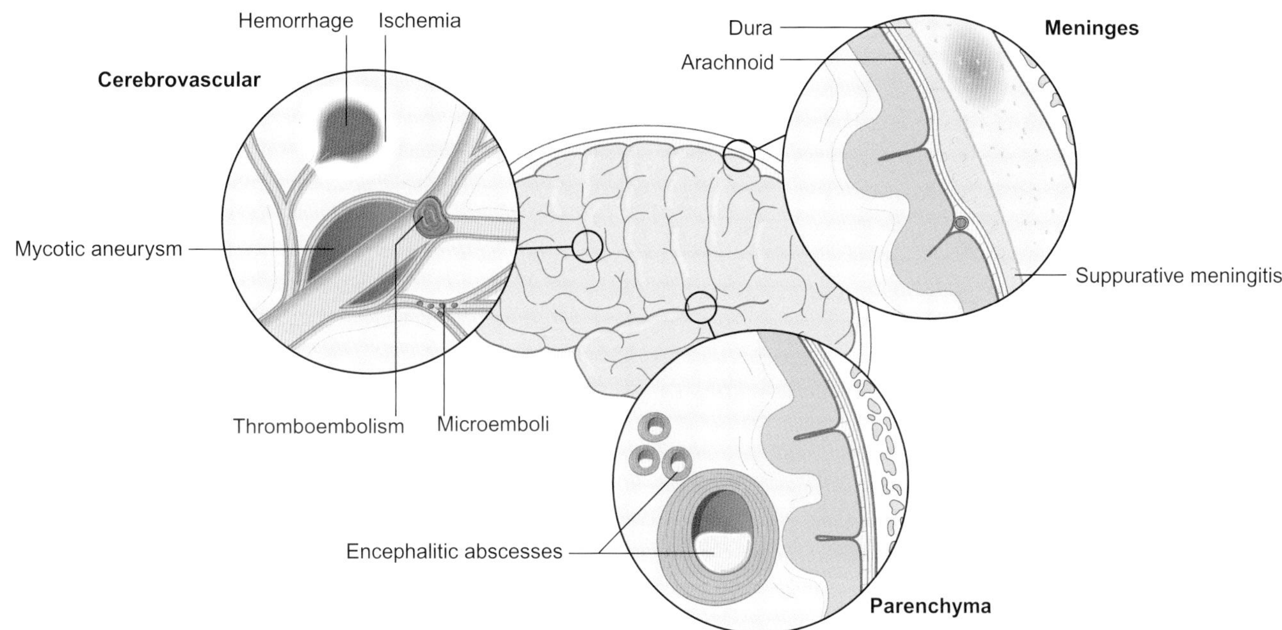

Figure 6-1 ▪ Embolization to various cerebral structures is responsible for most of the neurologic complications of IE. Emboli that lodge in the lumen of cerebral vessels may lead to ischemic stroke and can lead to arteritis or mycotic aneurysm formation with resultant vessel rupture and cerebral hemorrhage. Emboli to the meninges may produce meningitis, and emboli to the brain parenchyma, especially when associated with cerebral ischemia, may result in meningoencephalitis or abscess. (From Solenski NJ, Haley EC Jr: Neurologic complications of infective endocarditis. p. 331. In Roos KL (ed): Central Nervous System Infectious Diseases and Therapy. Marcel Dekker, New York, 1997, with permission.)

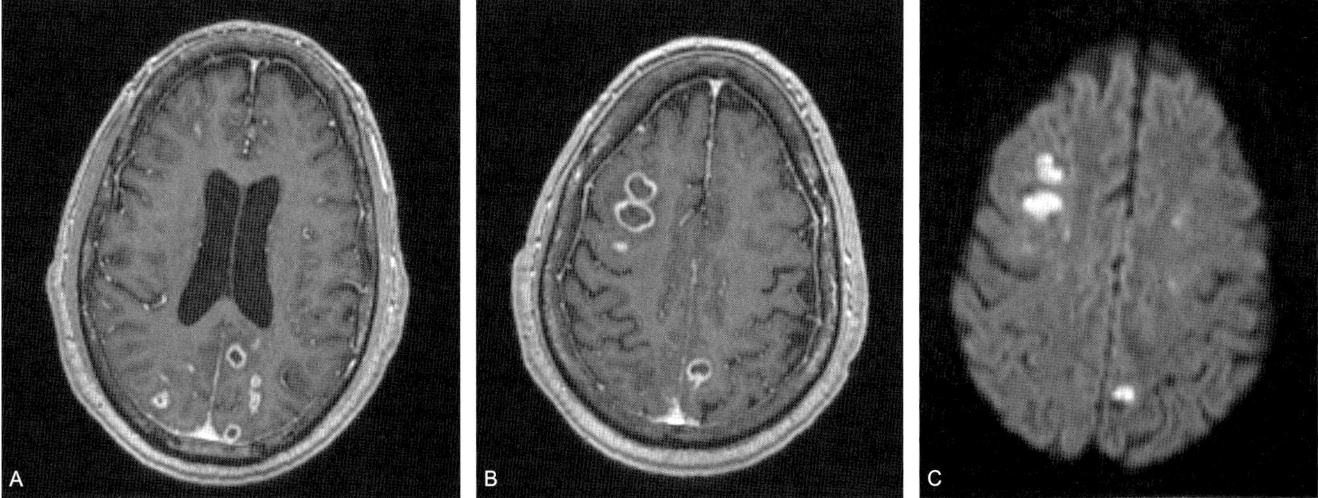

Figure 6-2 ▪ This patient presented with fever, new cardiac murmur, mental status changes, and right hemiparesis. **A** and **B**, Contrast-enhanced axial T1-weighted magnetic resonance imaging (MRI) shows multiple ring-enhancing lesions suggesting septic microembolization. **C**, Axial diffusion-weighted imaging (DWI) sequences show restricted diffusion associated with the lesions.

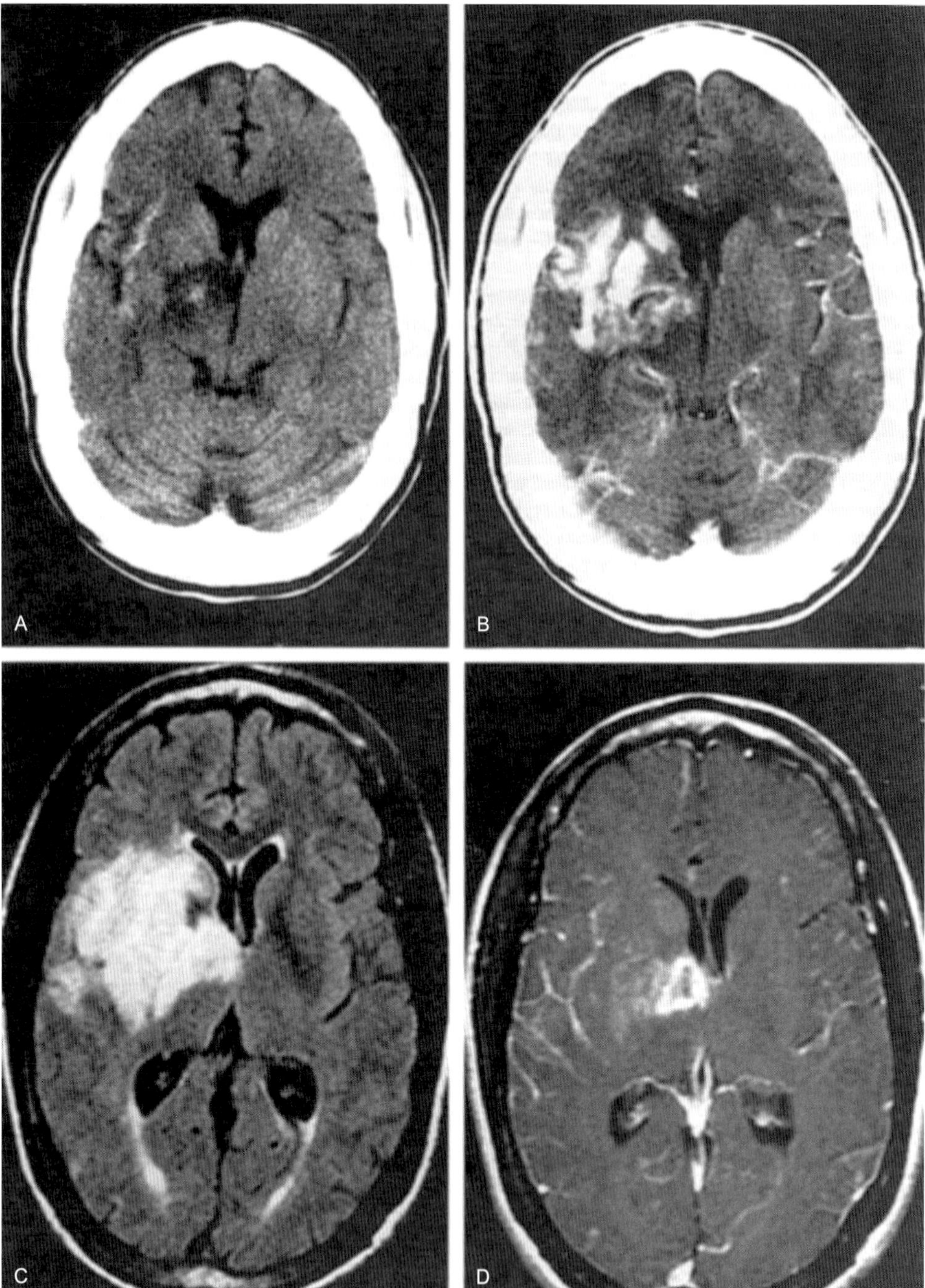

Figure 6-3 ■ This patient presented with left hemiparesis and mitral valve endocarditis. **A**, Noncontrast head CT showed a focal low-density lesion in the right internal capsule and lentiform nucleus with a central area of hemorrhage (increased density) and cortical hemorrhage in the insula. **B**, With contrast, large confluent areas of enhancement representing leaky blood–brain barrier can be seen in the right caudate and lentiform nuclei, the insula, and the temporal cortex. **C**, Fluid-attenuated inversion recovery (FLAIR) MRI 2 days after the head CT showed diffuse increased signal in the regions of CT enhancement and the right thalamus. **D**, After gadolinium, ring-like enhancement in the area of a previous infarct can be seen, representing possible secondary infection. This pattern is sometimes referred to as a "septic infarction." This enhancement pattern resolved with antibiotic treatment and without development of a macroabscess.

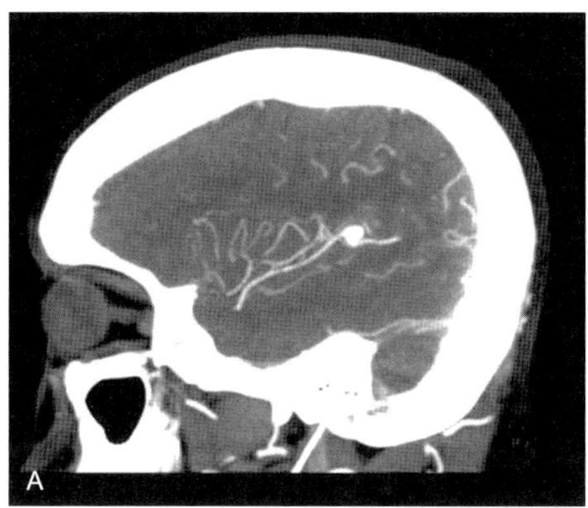

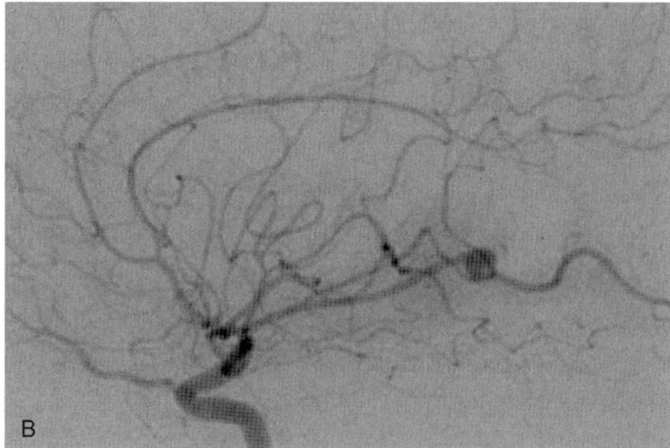

Figure 6-4 ■ This patient presented with fever, new systolic murmur, sudden headache, and altered mental status without focal neurologic deficits. Noncontrast head CT showed a small subarachnoid hemorrhage (not shown). Sagittal CTA (**A**) demonstrated a mycotic aneurysm in the distal MCA, confirmed by conventional angiography (**B**). This aneurysm enlarged despite adequate antibiotic therapy, and the patient subsequently underwent successful clipping.

Mycotic aneurysm formation has been related to (1) septic embolization to the arterial lumen, producing intraluminal wall necrosis and outward extension of infection, and (2) septic embolization to the adventitial layer of the artery, resulting in destruction of the adventitia and muscularis layers and subsequent aneurysmal dilatation. Mycotic aneurysms are usually small, located at distal arterial bifurcations, rather than around the circle of Willis, and can be single or multiple. Branches of the MCA are the most common location for mycotic aneurysms (Fig. 6-4).

Brain macroabscesses account for less than 1 percent of all neurologic complications of IE and may occur secondary to ischemic infarction from a septic embolus or to extension of infection from adjacent arteritis or mycotic aneurysm. Brain microabscesses are more common than macroabscesses, are often associated with *Staphylococcus aureus* infections, and usually occur in cases with multiple ischemic infarctions from distal migration of septic embolic fragments. Meningoencephalitis is usually a result of direct embolization to meningeal vessels, with subsequent parenchymal or cerebrospinal fluid (CSF) invasion of the infecting organism. Aseptic meningitis may also occur with subarachnoid hemorrhage due to a necrotic arteritis or ruptured mycotic aneurysm.

RISK FACTORS FOR NEUROLOGIC COMPLICATIONS

A variety of clinical and laboratory features have been associated with an increased risk of neurologic complications from IE (Table 6-2).

Site of Infection

Neurologic complications are probably more common with left-sided IE than with right-sided valve involvement.[4,11,16,24–29] A Finnish study spanning more than 20 years found that as the proportion of intravenous drug use–associated IE increased, the proportion with tricuspid valve involvement also increased.[3] Cerebral embolization in right-sided endocarditis may occur through a patent foramen ovale or a pulmonary arteriovenous fistula (Fig. 6-5).[27–29] Most reports comparing native and prosthetic valve endocarditis indicate no significant difference in the proportion of patients with neurologic complications. Among those with prosthetic

TABLE 6-2 ■ Suggested Risk Factors for Embolization in Infective Endocarditis

Risk Factor	Proposed Mechanism
Mitral valve infection	Increased valve mobility and left-sided position predispose to systemic embolization
"Virulent" organism	More rapid endothelial invasion leads to more friable, unstable valve surface
Acuteness of infection	More rapid endothelial invasion leads to more friable, unstable valve surface
Valvular vegetations	Increasing vegetation size and vegetation mobility may predispose to embolism
Hematologic factors	Increased endothelial cell activity, platelet aggregability, and antiphospholipid antibodies may be associated with increased risk of embolization

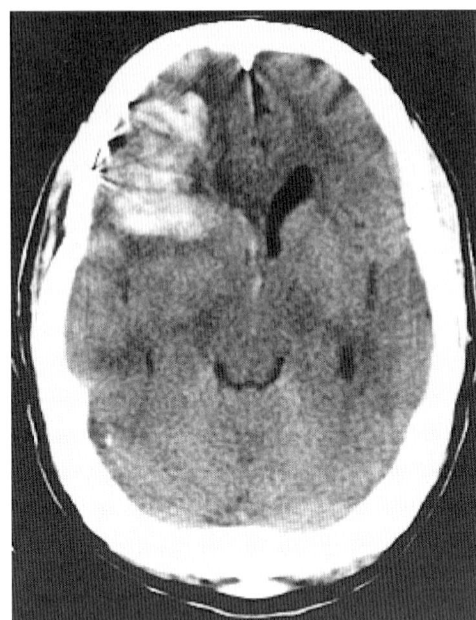

Figure 6-5 ▪ This patient had tricuspid valve endocarditis secondary to intravenous drug abuse. Initially, the patient had no neurologic symptoms but left the hospital against medical advice after completing 6 days of antibiotic therapy. He returned 2 days later with a decreased level of consciousness and a right gaze preference. A toxicology screen was positive for cocaine. Noncontrast axial head CT at that time showed an approximately 3- × 4-cm hemorrhage in the right frontal lobe with intraventricular extension and subfalcial herniation. Cerebral angiography did not show a mycotic aneurysm. Echocardiography showed a large patent foramen ovale with right-to-left shunting and vegetations on the tricuspid valve. This case underscores several clinical points: (1) neurologic complications of endocarditis are more common during uncontrolled infection; (2) neurologically asymptomatic patients may have silent cerebral emboli, particularly in the nondominant hemisphere; and (3) patients with right-sided endocarditis may develop cerebral embolization via a right-to-left shunt.

valve endocarditis, however, mechanical valves may be associated with complications more often than bioprosthetic valves.[30]

Infecting Organism

Streptococci, staphylococci, and enterococci are the three most prevalent infecting organisms. Despite one United States population-based study reporting viridans group streptococci as the most common infecting organism,[31] most recent studies show that staphylococcal infection is the most common responsbile pathogen.[2,3,5,9,32] There is a growing prevalence of antibiotic resistance among these organisms, especially viridans group streptococci and methacillin- and vancomycin-resistant *S. aureus*.[33,34] This changing resistance pattern is reflected in updated treatment guidelines.[35–38]

It is unclear whether antibiotic susceptibility changes affect the risk of embolic complications, although infections that take longer to control might theoretically have an increased risk of embolization. Even after adjusting for other factors, *S. aureus*,[7–9,20] and *Streptococcus bovis*[7] are independently associated with embolism.[39] In prosthetic valve endocarditis, *Staphylococcus epidermidis* may be associated with more neurologic complications than *S. aureus*.[40] The virulence of the organism, the availability of effective antimicrobial therapy, and the potential development of large, friable vegetations all contribute to the propensity for embolization.

Acuteness of Infection

There is a higher risk of neurologic complications with acute endocarditis than with subacute endocarditis, probably relating to the specific typical etiologic agents noted in acute disease (*S. aureus* and β-hemolytic streptococci) and the potential for large vegetations or valve damage acutely. The risk of cerebral embolization is highest in the first 1 to 2 weeks of infection, with most patients either presenting with a neurologic complication or experiencing an acute event in the first 48 hours after diagnosis.[6,7,12,16,29,41] Similarly, the risk of embolization decreases as the duration of effective antibiotic treatment increases, with most events occurring in the first 2 weeks of therapy.[7,29,41]

Valvular Vegetations

Valvular vegetations are detected by two-dimensional echocardiography in 50 to 80 percent of patients with IE and by transesophageal echocardiography (TEE) in more than 90 percent of cases.[3,10,42–44] Because of its increased sensitivity and ability to evaluate the more posteriorly located aortic valve, TEE appears to be cost-effective as the initial study when clinical suspicion of IE is high.[45,46] Although the findings in some clinical series have suggested no significant difference in the development of neurologic complications between patients with and without vegetations,[11,41,47–50] others have linked the presence of vegetations, increased vegetation size, or vegetation mobility to an increased risk of embolization.[6,25,26,28,51–53] A prospective study of 384 patients with IE, all of whom underwent TEE, found that vegetation length greater than 10 mm and vegetation mobility increased the risk of embolism; vegetation length greater than 15 mm independently increased 1-year mortality.[7] The significance of changes in vegetations on serial echocardiography remains unclear; some investigators report that morphologic changes in size or consistency are not associated with complications,[54] whereas others have found that an increase in vegetation size during antibiotic treatment is associated with more complications.[29,55,56] A final echocardiographic variable that may be related to complications is the presence of spontaneous echo contrast imaging, possibly as a marker of increased spontaneous platelet aggregation.[57] Current recommendations suggest that repeat echocardiography may be useful if clinical changes that suggest treatment failure occur during antibiotic therapy and that it should be performed urgently for unexplained progression of heart failure, new heart murmurs, or the development of atrioventricular block.[38]

Hematologic Risk Factors

In addition to spontaneous echo contrast, some reports associate coagulation system activation and embolic events.[6,58–61] In a series of 91 patients with IE, antiphospholipid antibodies were present in 62 percent of patients with embolic events compared to 23 percent of those without such events, and were also correlated significantly with other markers of endothelial cell activation, thrombin generation, and impaired fibrinolysis.[59] Antiphospholipid antibodies have also been reported to decrease after successful treatment of IE. Soluble adhesion molecules have also been reported to independently increase the risk of embolism.[6,60,61] At present, however, these hematologic studies do not clearly aid in risk prediction for patients with IE.

ISCHEMIC AND HEMORRHAGIC STROKE

Ischemic stroke secondary to embolization of friable valvular material is the most common neurologic complication of IE. Ischemic stroke is the presenting symptom of IE in up to 20 percent of cases and is most common in the acute stage of the infection, that is, before antibiotic treatment is begun or during the first several days of treatment (median time, 4 to 10 days).[11,12,16] Because of this clustering of symptoms in the acute phase, transient focal neurologic symptoms in a febrile patient, especially in the presence of a regurgitant murmur, should always raise suspicion of IE.

TABLE 6-3 ■ Causes of Intracerebral Hemorrhage in Infective Endocarditis

Primary Intracerebral Hemorrhage
Arterial rupture secondary to arteritis
Rupture of a mycotic aneurysm
Secondary Intracerebral Hemorrhage
Hemorrhagic conversion of ischemic stroke
Anticoagulation
Hematologic disorder
Disseminated intravascular coagulopathy
Thrombocytopenia
Vitamin K deficiency
Preexisting central nervous system lesion (e.g., aneurysm, arteriovenous malformation)

Intracerebral hemorrhage in IE may be primary or secondary to ischemic stroke or other pharmacologic or hematologic conditions (Table 6-3). Of the primary hemorrhages, intraparenchymal and subarachnoid hemorrhage are most common. Secondary transformation of an ischemic stroke is the most common form of intracerebral hemorrhage in IE, accounting for 24 to 56 percent of all hemorrhages.[21,22] In one series, only 8 cases of subarachnoid hemorrhage occurred among 489 patients with IE; in 6 of these, no cause for the hemorrhage was identified by autopsy or angiography.[62] The prevalence of asymptomatic mycotic aneurysms in patients with IE is not known, but seems to be low.[21]

As discussed, in at least 40 percent of patients septic embolization is the first event leading to intracerebral hemorrhage.[21,63] Depending on the location of the embolus, arteritis with secondary vessel rupture or development of a mycotic aneurysm may occur. Other conditions that sometimes accompany IE may also predispose to bleeding, including disseminated intravascular coagulation, thrombocytopenia, and vitamin K deficiency. Although mycotic aneurysms are most commonly found in the intracranial vessels, rarely these aneurysms may involve the extracranial carotid, thoracic, or abdominal vessels.[64,65]

Clinical Presentation

In accordance with their embolic etiology, the majority of ischemic strokes involve the cortex rather than subcortical brain tissue. In one series, 62 percent of strokes affected the cerebral or cerebellar cortex (with or without additional subcortical involvement), and only 16 percent were exclusively subcortical.[12] In addition to the more typical isolated cerebral hemispheric or brainstem syndromes, multiple microemboli are clinically manifest in at least 10 percent of cases, and in more than 50 percent of cases a shower of emboli are found on neuroimaging.[15,19,20,66,67] Patients with multiple microemboli can present with nonlocalizing symptoms, including diminished level of consciousness, encephalopathy, or psychosis.

Clinical worsening of ischemic stroke may result from a variety of mechanisms, including development of cerebral edema, recurrent embolization, secondary hemorrhage into the ischemic area, and development of cerebral abscesses. Cerebral edema may occur regardless of ischemic stroke mechanism, is more likely to be symptomatic in larger strokes and in younger patients, and is typically maximal between 3 and 5 days after stroke. Recurrent embolization should be suspected when new focal deficits develop; this complication is most likely to occur early in the course of treatment or when infection is uncontrolled. Hemorrhagic transformation of an ischemic stroke occurs in 18 to 42 percent of all patients and has been reported to be more common in cardioembolic strokes.[68] In an autopsy series of patients with neurologic complications of IE, hemorrhagic transformation of an ischemic infarct occurred in 9 of 16 patients.[22] Hemorrhagic transformation of an ischemic stroke is often asymptomatic, although development of a large intra-infarct hematoma is more likely to be symptomatic than is the development of petechial hemorrhage.[68] The term "septic infarction" has been used when, several days to weeks following an ischemic stroke, a cerebral abscess develops within the infarcted tissue.[67]

As with ischemic stroke, intracerebral hemorrhage usually presents with focal neurologic disturbances, but nonlocalizing symptoms, such as headache and decreased level of consciousness, may also predominate. Seizures may occur at the onset of the hemorrhage or later in its course. When subarachnoid hemorrhage occurs, either from rupture of an arteritic vessel or from a mycotic aneurysm, meningismus may be a prominent feature. Headaches may be more diffuse and subacute than is typical with ruptured saccular aneurysms.[62]

Seizures

Although seizures may occur in patients with IE from toxic or metabolic disturbances (e.g., hypoxia, antibiotic toxicity), most often seizures are secondary to ischemic or hemorrhagic stroke. Older series suggest that approximately 10 percent of patients with endocarditis have seizures at some point. Seizures that are secondary to stroke are usually focal in nature, with or without secondary generalization, whereas seizures due to metabolic or toxic factors are more often primarily generalized. The development of seizures during antibiotic treatment often signifies clinical worsening from recurrent stroke, hemorrhagic transformation, or abscess formation. Therefore, the new onset of seizures in a patient with IE should always prompt an urgent neuroimaging study. Rarely, seizures are secondary to antibiotic therapy, with imipenem being a commonly used antibiotic having the greatest seizure proclivity.

Evaluation of Patients

Brain Imaging

All patients with acute focal neurologic deficits should undergo either a noncontrast computed tomography (CT) scan of the head or brain magnetic resonance imaging (MRI). Noncontrast CT may be done more quickly than MRI in most settings. If IE is known or suspected, head CT with and without contrast may be useful; areas of increased contrast enhancement allow possible cerebral abscesses or mycotic aneurysms to be distinguished from areas of ischemia. However, brain MRI is the most sensitive modality for detecting the multiplicity of neurologic lesions seen in IE, especially small, multiple emboli (Fig. 6-2).[18–20,67] In one series, multiple lesions were found in 10 of 12 patients studied, with embolic branch infarction, multiple emboli and microabscesses, and hemorrhagic stroke being the most common findings.[67] MRI findings have been categorized into four patterns: (1) embolic infarction, (2) multiple patchy infarctions (nonenhancing), (3) small nodular or ring-enhancing white matter lesions (probably microabscesses), and (4) hemorrhagic infarctions (intracerebral or subarachnoid).[69] Multiple cerebral microbleeds, detected best on MRI, have also been described as a feature strongly associated with the presence of IE.[70] Hemorrhagic transformation of ischemic infarcts is most often patchy and may follow the contour of the gyri, but may also appear as a homogeneous hematoma within an infarct. A clue to the presence of an underlying mycotic aneurysm may be a focal area of cortical enhancement adjacent to an area of hemorrhage.

Vascular Imaging

Based on evidence that subarachnoid hemorrhage can occur without preceding symptoms in more than 50 percent of patients with mycotic aneurysm, some have advocated that all patients with IE should undergo noninvasive vascular imaging with MR angiography (MRA) or CT angiography (CTA) for aneurysm screening. Guidelines suggest screening for mycotic aneurysms in patients with endocarditis and neurologic deficits, including severe headache, erythrocytes or xanthochromia in the CSF, confusion, seizure, or focal neurologic signs.[36,38] In patients with intracranial hemorrhage or those in whom noninvasive imaging suggests aneurysm formation, conventional cerebral angiography should be performed.[71] Since mycotic aneurysms tend to be small and—unlike saccular aneurysms—occur distally rather than at more proximal arterial branch points, conventional cerebral angiography is probably more sensitive for aneurysm detection than noninvasive modalities. Vascular imaging in IE has not been associated with a survival benefit, largely owing to the low prevalence of mycotic aneurysms and the low risk of their rupture in patients with adequate antibiotic therapy.[72]

Patients with ischemic or hemorrhagic stroke who require long-term anticoagulation for mechanical valves or treatment of systemic thromboembolism may also benefit from repeat noninvasive angiography to exclude a mycotic aneurysm, even if initial studies performed at the time of presentation are negative. Patients with known mycotic aneurysms require serial monitoring of aneurysm size to ensure adequate response to therapy; CTA and MRA are likely adequate for this purpose.[73]

Cerebrospinal Fluid Examination

CSF examination was once part of the standard evaluation of patients with IE and neurologic symptoms, but it does not often change management decisions for patients today. The interpretation of CSF findings in IE with acute stroke is complicated by the tendency for patients with stroke unrelated to endocarditis also to have mild to moderate increases in CSF white blood cells, red blood cells, or protein concentration. In one large series, CSF was abnormal in around 70 percent of patients with IE; of these, around one-third had a purulent profile, one-fourth were aseptic, and one-tenth were hemorrhagic in character. With the exception of purulent CSF in patients with meningismus, the CSF pattern did not correlate with neurologic symptoms. For these reasons, CSF examination does not usually aid in the diagnosis or management of patients with neurologic symptoms and IE.

Echocardiography and Stroke

The diagnosis of IE depends on the documentation of a responsible organism on serial blood cultures and, in part, on the presence of valvular abnormalities on echocardiography.[38] Echocardiography is also important in assessing valvular function and excluding conditions such as valve thrombosis or abscess formation that would change clinical management. TEE is more sensitive to mitral and aortic valve pathology and has been reported to change patient management in as many as one-third of cases.[74] TEE may be especially important in older patients with IE, who, in one large study, commonly had vegetations seen only on TEE.[10] Whether serial echocardiography provides data that reliably predict risk of subsequent stroke or otherwise influence neurologic management is not known.

Treatment of Ischemic Stroke

Antibiotic Therapy

The cornerstone of treatment of IE is appropriate antibiotic therapy directed at the infecting organism. Numerous studies have shown that the risk of either initial or recurrent thromboembolism decreases sharply after the first few days of adequate antibiotic therapy.[11–14,29,43] In 2007, the International Collaboration on Endocarditis published a large prospective cohort study that showed that the risk of stroke after 1 week of therapy declined to 1 to 3 percent, depending on the responsible organism.[75] It is therefore critical to ensure that antibiotics are begun promptly and empirically, immediately after drawing initial blood for cultures (preferably three sets from separate sites) in febrile patients with stroke in whom IE is being considered. As effective long-term antimicrobial therapy will be required, the isolation and susceptibility testing of the pathogen are of critical importance. Involvement of a specialist in infectious diseases is recommended. Thorough discussion of a current approach to diagnosis and antimicrobial treatment in various clinical scenarios can be found in the American, European, and British guideline statements, including the appropriate conditions for which antibiotic prophylaxis for the prevention of IE should be considered.[35–38,76] IE with or without accompanying valve infection is also an emerging complication of implantable cardiac devices; in this setting, device removal is also typically required.[77]

Thrombolysis

Acute use of tissue plasminogen activator in patients with ischemic stroke and IE is generally felt to be inadvisable due to an increased bleeding risk. However, case reports differ in their reported outcome of thrombolysis and IE.[78–80] Due to the probability of positive publication bias and the known risk of hemorrhagic conversion in patients with IE, the use of thrombolytics in patients with stroke resulting from IE should generally be undertaken only with caution. More recently, reports of successful endovascular interventions have emerged, suggesting an alternative approach to acute stroke management in IE.[81]

Antiplatelet and Anticoagulant Therapy

In animal models of IE, aspirin or aspirin plus ticlopidine has been found to reduce vegetation weight, echocardiographic evidence of vegetation growth, bacterial titer of vegetations, or systemic emboli rates.[82–84] Although a pilot study in humans confirmed this finding,[85] a larger randomized controlled trial found no reduction of embolic events in patients treated with 325 mg aspirin compared to those given placebo, and there was a nonsignificant trend toward increased bleeding in the aspirin-treated group.[86] Therefore, routine use of antiplatelet therapy for the purpose of decreasing embolic risk in patients with acute IE is not recommended.[38] Several studies have also looked at the impact of prior antiplatelet therapy on outcomes after IE. One study showed that antiplatelet use in the 6 months prior to IE decreased the risk of symptomatic emboli.[87] Other studies have shown mixed results, with one study showing a decreased need for valve replacement and another finding no overall mortality benefit.[88,89]

Anticoagulation in patients with IE remains a controversial and complicated topic.[90–92] Hemorrhagic complications are clearly more common in anticoagulated patients, but patients with mechanical prosthetic valves may require long-term anticoagulation, and the decision as to whether and for how long to withhold anticoagulants in these patients is complex, depending on the type of valve involved.

Anticoagulation in Native Valve Endocarditis

There is an increased risk of hemorrhagic complications in patients with native valve endocarditis and ischemic stroke who are treated with anticoagulation, and the risk of recurrent embolism is low in those patients receiving appropriate antibiotic therapy. Accordingly, there appears to be little benefit for stroke risk reduction to anticoagulate these patients routinely.[91] An important consideration is whether, prior to the development of endocarditis, these patients were being anticoagulated for a specific indication such as clotting disorders, atrial fibrillation, or pulmonary embolism. In these cases, a review of MRI sequences, looking for occult hemorrhage, and of noninvasive angiography should be part of a risk-to-benefit analysis before anticoagulants are stopped. When anticoagulation is deemed to be necessary, switching from oral to intravenous medications is recommended for optimal control of anticoagulation.[92] Whether lower-level anticoagulation (e.g., for prevention of deep venous thrombosis) is safe in patients with stroke and IE is unknown. Because other strategies, such as the use of sequential compression devices, may be equally efficacious, a conservative approach is to use these nonpharmacologic methods primarily.

Anticoagulation in Prosthetic Valve Endocarditis

Patients with bioprosthetic valves typically do not receive long-term anticoagulant therapy, and they have a lower risk of stroke in IE than patients with mechanical valves[30,40]; thus, the same approach as outlined for native valve endocarditis is recommended. Patients with mechanical prostheses who have endocarditis and stroke, however, present more difficult management dilemmas. Most studies indicate that the proportions of patients with native and prosthetic valves having endocarditis with cerebral embolism are similar.[11,12] Therefore, initiating anticoagulation in a previously nonanticoagulated patient with IE and a prosthetic valve appears unwarranted.

If a patient with a mechanical valve is receiving long-term anticoagulant therapy and develops a cerebral embolus as a complication of IE, the decision as to whether to continue anticoagulation or temporarily withhold it depends on several factors. Because larger strokes, especially those secondary to emboli, may be more likely to develop secondary hemorrhagic complications,[72] some authors favor temporarily withholding anticoagulation for several days, especially when *S. aureus* is the infecting organism.[93,94] Other factors, including hemorrhage on CT scan, presence of mycotic aneurysm, uncontrolled infection or infection with *S. aureus*, history of bleeding diathesis, and possibly advanced patient age, also argue against the use of anticoagulants in patients with neurologic complications of mechanical valve endocarditis.[95] Whether anticoagulation should be avoided on a long-term basis or discontinued just temporarily depends on the indication for anticoagulation and the patient's specific clinical situation.[12,96] When temporary discontinuation of anticoagulation is being considered, determination of the type of mechanical valve and consultation with a cardiologist or cardiothoracic surgeon concerning the risk of valve thrombosis will help guide the decision. If anticoagulation continues, converting to the most controllable and reversible (i.e., intravenous) form of therapy along with frequent monitoring of anticoagulation parameters (activated partial thromboplastin time or international normalized ratio [INR]) are recommended.[93,95]

Surgical Treatment

Valve replacement is not recommended therapy for preventing initial or recurrent stroke. Typically, surgery is recommended for patients with acute or refractory congestive heart failure, perivalvular abscess, unstable valve prosthesis, continued embolism, infection with a pathogen resistant to effective antimicrobial agents, or inability to clear the infection.[25,53] A study involving more than 4,000 patients with IE showed that adjusted in-hospital and 1-year mortality (including adjustment for the presence of stroke) was significantly lower in patients with congestive heart failure undergoing surgery than in those managed medically.[97] In a subgroup of patients with the greatest indications, early surgery was associated with significant decreases in mortality.[98] Surgery is required in almost half of patients with prosthetic valve endocarditis, but in-hospital mortality remains high and is increased by the presence of stroke and other neurologic complications.[99]

If surgery is required, the timing of the procedure in the setting of stroke is controversial. Early surgery is associated with greatest benefit in reducing embolization since the risk is greatest in the first 2 weeks of the infection. The first 72 to 120 hours after stroke, however, is the period of maximal risk of cerebral edema and disruption of cerebral autoregulation. Thus, most authors recommend delaying cardiac surgery for at least 2 weeks after ischemic stroke and 4 weeks after hemorrhagic stroke if possible, as mortality rates for patients in the first postoperative week are as high as 31 percent.[100] The Society of Thoracic Surgeons has a practice guideline for the surgical management of endocarditis,[71] and practice may be shifting toward more rapid surgical interventions in those with specific risk factors including congestive heart failure, uncontrolled infection, valve abscess, or high embolic risk since, even in models adjusting for bias introduced by selection for treatment, early surgery appears to confer a survival benefit in these situations.[101,102]

Treatment of Hemorrhagic Stroke

Intraparenchymal Hemorrhage

The mainstay of treatment for either primary or secondary intracerebral hemorrhage in patients with IE is the same as that for cerebral emboli: effective treatment of the underlying infectious organism. This is especially true for patients with pyogenic arteritis, but is also critical for the treatment of mycotic aneurysms. Some patients with intracerebral hemorrhage and progressive neurologic deterioration, either from expanding hematoma or from edema, may benefit from surgical evacuation of the clot, but no firm guidelines exist. Similarly, although recombinant factor VIIa was used successfully to reduce hematoma growth in one trial (and unsuccessfully in another), no data are available for its use in patients with IE and cerebral hemorrhage.[103] Patients with mechanical valves often will have their anticoagulant discontinued temporarily or converted to an intravenous form. All patients with IE and hemorrhage should have close neurologic monitoring in an intensive care setting since deterioration from recurrent hemorrhage or edema is not uncommon.

Mycotic Aneurysms

The natural history of mycotic aneurysms is that approximately one-third resolve completely with 6 to 8 weeks of antibiotic treatment, one-third remain unchanged in size, and the remaining one-third are equally divided among those that increase and those that decrease in size.[21,73,104,105] Because of their propensity to resolve with antibiotic therapy, the evaluation and treatment of mycotic aneurysms are controversial. Aspects of care that remain unclear are whether serial angiography is necessary to follow mycotic aneurysms and the indications for surgical repair.

Some authors recommend serial angiography of mycotic aneurysms every 2 weeks during antibiotic treatment.[63,106] If an aneurysm enlarges, surgical treatment to prevent rupture may be advocated.[106,107] The need for ongoing or subsequent long-term anticoagulation is another factor that may suggest the need for angiographic surveillance and surgical treatment. Since at least half of mycotic aneurysms persist after adequate antibiotic treatment and since new aneurysms can appear, it seems reasonable to at least repeat angiography, with either conventional or noninvasive techniques, at the conclusion of antibiotic therapy (usually 4 to 6 weeks). Late hemorrhage from a ruptured mycotic aneurysm in patients who have completed adequate antibiotic therapy is rare, occurring in none of 122 patients with a mean 40-month follow-up[63]; therefore continued surveillance of a stable aneurysm following antibiotic treatment is probably unnecessary.

Once an aneurysm is discovered, controversy also exists regarding treatment. Asymptomatic aneurysms are often treated medically, with surgical intervention reserved for those that enlarge.[106,107] Although symptomatic aneurysms may also resolve with antibiotic treatment, some authors favor surgical treatment of any ruptured mycotic aneurysm in addition to antibiotic therapy.[106,107] This recommendation is usually based on the fear of recurrent bleeding (which is low) and the associated increased morbidity and mortality with rerupture. Aneurysm accessibility and number are other features that influence the decision for surgical treatment; single aneurysms in a peripheral location are more likely to be treated surgically. More proximal aneurysms may be successfully treated endovascularly, although the management and outcomes in these cases are highly individualized.[108–111]

Because mycotic aneurysms often lack a defined neck amenable to clipping, other surgical techniques, including wrapping, trapping, excision, or endovascular therapy, may be necessary. Because mycotic aneurysms are often small and difficult to locate at the time of surgery, techniques including stereoscopic brain-surface imaging with MRA and stereotactic angiographic localization are sometimes used intraoperatively.[112–113]

CEREBRAL INFECTION

Cerebral infection, most commonly abscess or meningitis, has been reported as a complication of IE in 6 to 31 percent of patients, although these cases typically represent less than 10 percent of patients with endocarditis and neurologic complications (Table 6-1). These infections most typically occur after cerebral embolism; infection arising without clinical evidence of prior embolization is unusual. Encephalitis has also been reported, although the usual pathology in these cases is multiple emboli with microabscess formation.

Meningitis accounts for 4 to 7 percent of all neurologic manifestations of IE and is more common with either *S. aureus* or *S. pneumoniae* infections. When meningitis is associated with involvement of the cerebral cortex, evidenced by gyral enhancement on MRI, the terms "cerebritis" and "meningoencephalitis" are used. Rarely, cerebritis leads to the development of a parameningeal abscess in the cerebral cortex. Meningitis typically results from septic emboli to the meningeal vessels with subsequent CSF colonization. Less commonly, meningitis is nonseptic, resulting from sterile inflammation of the meninges due to blood products or circulating immune complexes released into the CSF.

Cerebral abscesses are rare, accounting for approximately 2 percent of all neurologic complications in

IE.[114] Small "microabscesses," often defined as abscesses smaller than 1 cm, are more common than "macroabscesses." Cerebral abscesses usually develop as the result of septic emboli and are not necessarily preceded by clinical symptoms. Radiographically, infarction-related abscesses are usually small and multiple and demonstrate areas of nodular or ringlike enhancement in an area of prior ischemic stroke.[67,69]

Clinical Presentation

Although the clinical diagnosis of meningitis is infrequent in IE, symptoms of meningitis occur in more than 40 percent of patients with endocarditis.[27] In addition to meningismus, headache, encephalopathy, cranial neuropathies, seizures, and increased intracranial pressure may occur. These symptoms may be subtle, especially in the elderly, and when associated with fever, elevated peripheral white blood cell count, and regurgitant murmur should prompt an urgent evaluation for IE.

Evaluation

All patients with known or suspected IE and neurologic symptoms, whether focal or nonfocal, should undergo imaging with noncontrast head CT prior to lumbar puncture because multiple embolic strokes, intracerebral hemorrhage, and abscess may all cause significant compartmental increases in intracranial pressure, thus increasing the risk of cerebral herniation. Lumbar puncture should not be perfomed in any patient with a focal lesion and evidence of mass effect on neuroimaging studies. Because patients with endocarditis have a propensity toward hematologic abnormalities, coagulation tests and a platelet count are important prior to lumbar puncture.

Treatment of Cerebral Infection

As for any type of meningitis, the goal of treatment is adequate antibiotic therapy to which the infecting organism is sensitive with good CSF penetration. Both microabscesses and macroabscesses usually respond to antibiotic treatment, although macroabscesses may occasionally produce significant mass effect and thus require stereotactic aspiration or surgical drainage.

OTHER NEUROLOGIC COMPLICATIONS

Other extracerebral neurologic complications may rarely occur. Although cerebral and systemic emboli appear to occur with similar frequency,[15] cerebral neurologic complications predominate over extracerebral complications, probably because the brain receives more blood flow than peripheral neurologic tissues and because cerebral complications are more likely to be symptomatic.

Mononeuropathy simplex or multiplex has been reported in as many as 1 percent of patients with IE. Both peripheral and cranial nerves may be involved, and *S. viridans* appears to be an especially common infectious organism in these cases. Discitis, occasionally with associated epidural abscess or osteomyelitis, is more common with *S. aureus* infection. Other rare sites of embolization include the spinal cord and the retina.

SUGGESTED MANAGEMENT ALGORITHM

The management of neurologic complications of IE is not standardized and substantial variations in care may be necessary based on individual patient characteristics. Nonetheless, it is helpful to consider a treatment algorithm that includes pathways for the major neurologic manifestations of the disease (Fig. 6-6). This algorithm differs from some proposed previously in that cerebral angiography is not suggested for all patients with ischemic stroke, lumbar puncture is not recommended for all patients with neurologic complications, and serial vascular imaging every 2 weeks is optional.[95,106] The two keys to managing patients, regardless of neurologic complications, are (1) a high level of suspicion of the possibility of IE and (2) prompt initiation of appropriate antibiotic therapy after obtaining multiple sets of blood cultures.

PROGNOSIS

Among patients with IE, short-term mortality is increased in those with neurologic complications compared to those without them.[3,11,15,16] Estimates of in-hospital mortality range from 16 to 58 percent compared with 14 to 20 percent for patients without neurologic complications. Mortality is higher in infections with more virulent organisms, with several large cohort studies showing an association between

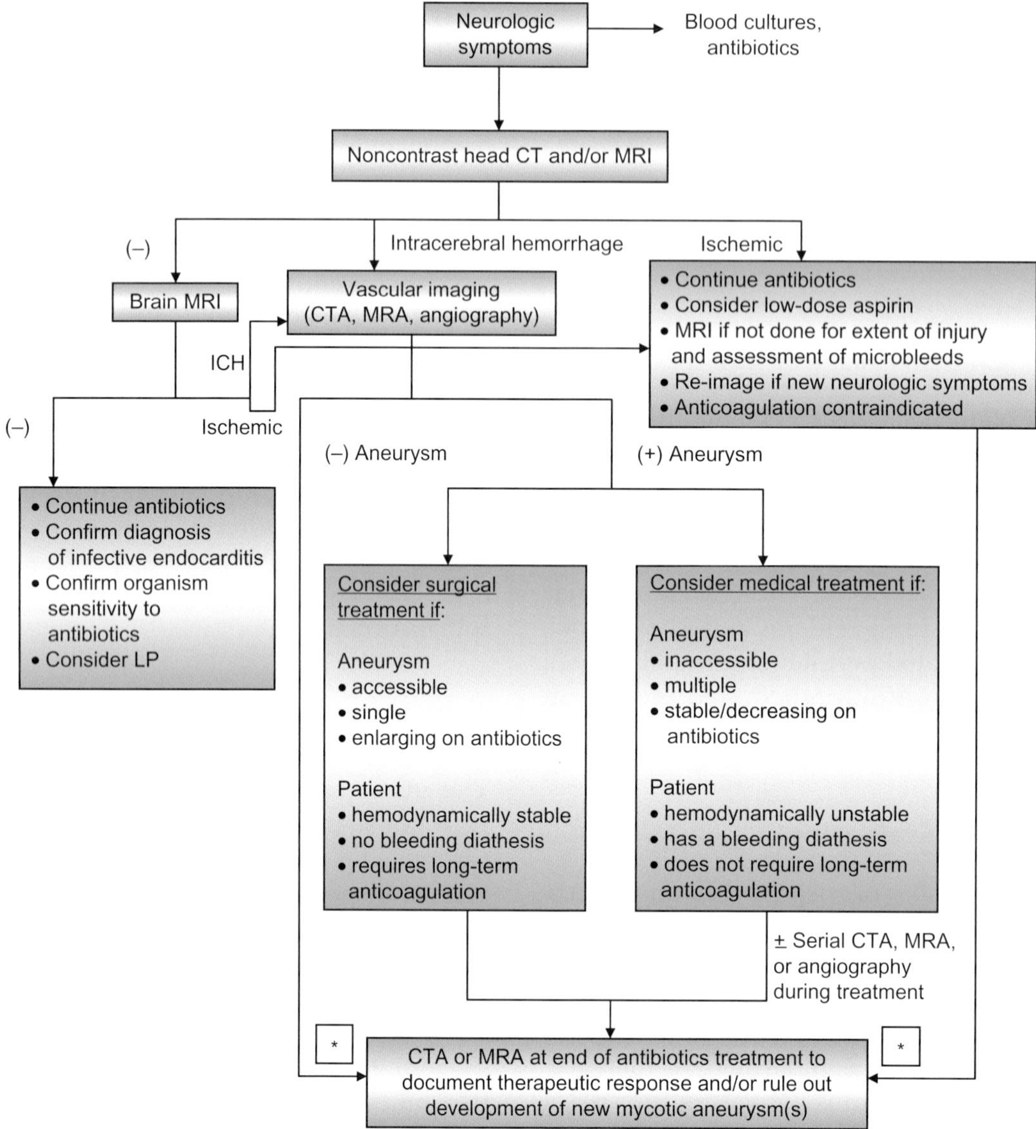

Figure 6-6 ■ Suggested management algorithm for patients with focal neurologic deficits and known or suspected IE. Factors favoring either surgical or medical treatment of mycotic aneurysms are presented; management of these cases is highly individualized. Repeat angiography at the conclusion of medical therapy is suggested for all patients with known mycotic aneurysms and may be considered either for patients with intracerebral hemorrhage and a negative initial angiogram or for patients with ischemic stroke who require long-term anticoagulation. CTA, computed tomography angiography; ICH, intracerebral hemorrhage; LP, lumbar puncture; MRA, magnetic resonance angiography.

S. aureus infection and mortality.[7,8,32,115] Intracerebral hemorrhage appears to confer added risk, with reported mortality of 40 to 90 percent.[21,115] Although rare, rupture of a mycotic aneurysm is associated with even higher mortality.[107] Mortality in patients with unruptured mycotic aneurysms appears no different from the aggregate mortality rate in all patients with neurologic manifestations of endocarditis.

Longer-term mortality after IE may be less related to neurologic events. A multicenter, prospective study of 384 patients with IE found that increasing age, female gender, serum creatinine greater than 2.0 mg/L, moderate to severe congestive heart failure, infection with *S. aureus*, increased medical comorbidities, and vegetation length greater than 15 mm were all independently associated with 1-year mortality.[7] Another study found that heart failure was the only independent predictor of mortality after the first year post-infection.[116]

The risk of recurrent neurologic events, either embolic or hemorrhagic, is quite low.[12,13,63] Recurrent ischemia has been documented in less than 0.5 percent of cases per day[12] and recurrent hemorrhage in less than 1 percent of all cases.[63] Elimination of recurrent events appears to depend more on effective antibiotic treatment than on any other specific therapy.[29,40,41,117]

CONCLUDING COMMENTS

Although IE has evolved with regard to frequency of involvement of different valves and prevalence and susceptibility of infecting organisms, the proportion of patients with neurologic manifestations and the type of neurologic complications remain remarkably consistent. Most neurologic complications are caused by embolization of friable valvular material resulting in either ischemic or hemorrhagic stroke. A high index of suspicion for IE as the cause of stroke is critical because common treatments for acute stroke, such as thrombolysis or anticoagulation, are often contraindicated in patients with native valve endocarditis and ischemic stroke. Although many clinical decisions in patients with neurologic manifestations of IE must be individualized, it is clear that the cornerstone of prevention and treatment of all neurologic complications is rapid delivery of appropriate antibiotic therapy.

ACKNOWLEDGMENTS

Dr. Williams is supported by grants from the Department of Veterans Affairs, Health Services Research and Development and the VA Quality Enhancement Research Initiative. Images were provided by Dr. Juan Tejada, Indiana University Department of Radiology, Division of Neuroradiology.

REFERENCES

1. Williams LS, Allen BL: Neurologic manifestations of infective endocarditis. p. 97. In Aminoff MJ (ed): Neurology and General Medicine. 4th Ed. Churchill Livingstone Elsevier, Philadelphia, 2008.
2. Murdoch DR, Corey GR, Hoen B, et al: Clinical presentation, etiology, and outcome of infective endocarditis in the 21st century: the International Collaboration on Endocarditis-Prospective Cohort Study. Arch Intern Med 169:463, 2009.
3. Heiro M, Helenius H, Makila S, et al: Infective endocarditis in a Finnish teaching hospital: a study on 326 episodes treated during 1980–2004. Heart 92:1457, 2006.
4. Heiro M, Nikoskelainen J, Engblom E, et al: Neurologic manifestations of infective endocarditis: a 17-year experience in a teaching hospital in Finland. Arch Intern Med 160:2781, 2000.
5. Hoen B, Alla F, Selton-Suty C, et al: Changing profile of infective endocarditis: results of a 1-year survey in France. JAMA 288:75, 2002.
6. Durante ME, Adinolfi LE, Tripodi MF, et al: Risk factors for "major" embolic events in hospitalized patients with infective endocarditis. Am Heart J 146:311, 2003.
7. Thuny F, Di SG, Belliard O, et al: Risk of embolism and death in infective endocarditis: prognostic value of echocardiography: a prospective multicenter study. Circulation 112:69, 2005.
8. Miro JM, Anguera I, Cabell CH, et al: *Staphylococcus aureus* native valve infective endocarditis: report of 566 episodes from the International Collaboration on Endocarditis Merged Database. Clin Infect Dis 41:507, 2005.
9. Leone S, Ravasio V, Durante-Mangoni E, et al: Epidemiology, characteristics, and outcome of infective endocarditis in Italy: the Italian Study on Endocarditis. Infection 40:527, 2012.
10. Durante-Mangoni E, Bradley S, Selton-Suty C, et al: Current features of infective endocarditis in elderly patients: results of the International Collaboration on Endocarditis Prospective Cohort Study. Arch Intern Med 168:2095, 2008.
11. Salgado AV, Furlan AJ, Keys TF, et al: Neurologic complications of endocarditis: a 12-year experience. Neurology 39:173, 1989.
12. Hart RG, Foster JW, Luther MF, et al: Stroke in infective endocarditis. Stroke 21:695, 1990.
13. Paschalis C, Pugsley W, John R, et al: Rate of cerebral embolic events in relation to antibiotic and anticoagulant therapy in patients with bacterial endocarditis. Eur Neurol 30:87, 1990.
14. Matsushita K, Kuriyama Y, Sawada T, et al: Hemorrhagic and ischemic cerebrovascular complications of active infective endocarditis of native valve. Eur Neurol 33:267, 1993.
15. Millaire A, Leroy O, Gaday V, et al: Incidence and prognosis of embolic events and metastatic infections in infective endocarditis. Eur Heart J 18:677, 1997.
16. Roder BL, Wandall DA, Espersen F, et al: Neurologic manifestations in *Staphylococcus aureus* endocarditis: a review of 260 bacteremic cases in nondrug addicts. Am J Med 102:379, 1997.

17. Stagaman DJ, Presti C, Rees C, et al: Septic pulmonary arteriovenous fistula. An unusual conduit for systemic embolization in right-sided valvular endocarditis. Chest 97:1484, 1990.
18. Cooper H, Thompson E, Laureno R, et al: Subclinical brain embolization in left-sided infective endocarditis. Circulation 120:585, 2009.
19. Grabowski M, Hryniewiecki T, Janas J, et al: Clinically overt and silent cerebral embolism in the course of infective endocarditis. J Neurol 258:1133, 2011.
20. Snygg-Martin U, Gustafsson L, Rosengren L, et al: Cerebrovascular complications in patients with left-sided infective endocarditis are common: a prospective study using magnetic resonance imaging and neurochemical brain damage markers. Clin Infect Dis 47:23, 2008.
21. Hart RG, Kagan-Hallet K, Joerns SE: Mechanisms of intracranial hemorrhage in infective endocarditis. Stroke 18:1048, 1987.
22. Masuda J, Yutani C, Waki R, et al: Histopathological analysis of the mechanisms of intracranial hemorrhage complicating infective endocarditis. Stroke 23:843, 1992.
23. Cerebral Embolism Task Force: Cardiogenic brain embolism. The second report of the Cerebral Embolism Task Force. Arch Neurol 46:727, 1989.
24. Cabell CH, Pond KK, Peterson GE, et al: The risk of stroke and death in patients with aortic and mitral valve endocarditis. Am Heart J 142:75, 2001.
25. Di SG, Habib G, Pergola V, et al: Echocardiography predicts embolic events in infective endocarditis. J Am Coll Cardiol 37:1069, 2001.
26. Macarie C, Iliuta L, Savulescu C, et al: Echocardiographic predictors of embolic events in infective endocarditis. Kardiol Pol 60:535, 2004.
27. Kanter MC, Hart RG: Neurologic complications of infective endocarditis. Neurology 41:1015, 1991.
28. Rohmann S, Erbel R, Gorge G, et al: Clinical relevance of vegetation localization by transoesophageal echocardiography in infective endocarditis. Eur Heart J 13:446, 1992.
29. Vilacosta I, Graupner C, San Roman JA, et al: Risk of embolization after institution of antibiotic therapy for infective endocarditis. J Am Coll Cardiol 39:1489, 2002.
30. Keyser DL, Biller J, Coffman TT, et al: Neurologic complications of late prosthetic valve endocarditis. Stroke 21:472, 1990.
31. Tleyjeh I, Steckelberg JM, Murad H, et al: Temporal trends in infective endocarditis. JAMA 293:3022, 2005.
32. Cabell CH, Jollis JG, Peterson GE, et al: Changing patient characteristics and the effect on mortality in endocarditis. Arch Intern Med 162:90, 2002.
33. Gordon KA, Beach ML, Biedenbach DJ, et al: Antimicrobial susceptibility patterns of beta-hemolytic and viridans group streptococci: report from the SENTRY Antimicrobial Surveillance Program (1997–2000). Diagn Microbiol Infect Dis 43:157, 2002.
34. Salgado CD, Farr BM, Calfee DP: Community-acquired methicillin-resistant *Staphylococcus aureus*: a meta-analysis of prevalence and risk factors. Clin Infect Dis 36:131, 2003.
35. Nishimura RA, Carabello BA, Faxon DP, et al: ACC/AHA 2008 Guideline update on valvular heart disease: focused update on infective endocarditis: a report of the American College of Cardiology/American Heart Association Task Force on Practice Guidelines: endorsed by the Society of Cardiovascular Anesthesiologists, Society for Cardiovascular Angiography and Interventions, and Society of Thoracic Surgeons. Circulation 118:887, 2008.
36. Habib G, Hoen B, Tornos P, et al: Guidelines on the prevention, diagnosis, and treatment of infective endocarditis (new version 2009): the Task Force on the Prevention, Diagnosis, and Treatment of Infective Endocarditis of the European Society of Cardiology (ESC). Endorsed by the European Society of Clinical Microbiology and Infectious Diseases (ESCMID) and the International Society of Chemotherapy (ISC) for Infection and Cancer. Eur Heart J 30:2369, 2009.
37. Gould FK, Denning DW, Elliott TS, et al: Guidelines for the diagnosis and antibiotic treatment of endocarditis in adults: a report of the Working Party of the British Society for Antimicrobial Chemotherapy. J Antimicrob Chemother 67:269, 2012.
38. Baddour LM, Wilson WR, Bayer AS, et al: Infective endocarditis: diagnosis, antimicrobial therapy, and management of complications: a statement for healthcare professionals from the Committee on Rheumatic Fever, Endocarditis, and Kawasaki Disease, Council on Cardiovascular Disease in the Young, and the Councils on Clinical Cardiology, Stroke, and Cardiovascular Surgery and Anesthesia, American Heart Association: endorsed by the Infectious Diseases Society of America. Circulation 111:e394, 2005.
39. Kupferwasser I, Darius H, Muller AM, et al: Clinical and morphological characteristics in *Streptococcus bovis* endocarditis: a comparison with other causative microorganisms in 177 cases. Heart 80:276, 1998.
40. Davenport J, Hart RG: Prosthetic valve endocarditis 1976–1987. Antibiotics, anticoagulation, and stroke. Stroke 21:993, 1990.
41. Steckelberg JM, Murphy JG, Ballard D, et al: Emboli in infective endocarditis: the prognostic value of echocardiography. Ann Intern Med 114:635, 1991.
42. Schulz R, Werner GS, Fuchs JB, et al: Clinical outcome and echocardiographic findings of native and prosthetic valve endocarditis in the 1990's. Eur Heart J 17:281, 1996.
43. Mugge A, Daniel WG, Frank G, et al: Echocardiography in infective endocarditis: reassessment of prognostic implications of vegetation size determined by the transthoracic and the transesophageal approach. J Am Coll Cardiol 14:631, 1989.

44. Erbel R, Rohmann S, Drexler M, et al: Improved diagnostic value of echocardiography in patients with infective endocarditis by transoesophageal approach. A prospective study. Eur Heart J 9:43, 1988.
45. Reynolds HR, Jagen MA, Tunick PA, et al: Sensitivity of transthoracic versus transesophageal echocardiography for the detection of native valve vegetations in the modern era. J Am Soc Echocardiogr 16:67, 2003.
46. Heidenreich PA, Masoudi FA, Maini B, et al: Echocardiography in patients with suspected endocarditis: a cost-effectiveness analysis. Am J Med 107:198, 1999.
47. Weng MC, Chang FY, Young TG, et al: Analysis of 109 cases of infective endocarditis in a tertiary care hospital. Zhonghua Yi Xue Za Zhi (Taipei) 58:18, 1996.
48. Jung HO, Seung KB, Kang DH, et al: A clinical consideration of systemic embolism complicated to infective endocarditis in Korea. Korean J Intern Med 9:80, 1994.
49. Heinle S, Wilderman N, Harrison JK, et al: Value of transthoracic echocardiography in predicting embolic events in active infective endocarditis. Duke Endocarditis Service. Am J Cardiol 74:799, 1994.
50. De CS, Magni G, Beni S, et al: Role of transthoracic and transesophageal echocardiography in predicting embolic events in patients with active infective endocarditis involving native cardiac valves. Am J Cardiol 80:1030, 1997.
51. Lancellotti P, Galiuto L, Albert A, et al: Relative value of clinical and transesophageal echocardiographic variables for risk stratification in patients with infective endocarditis. Clin Cardiol 21:572, 1998.
52. Deprele C, Berthelot P, Lemetayer F, et al: Risk factors for systemic emboli in infective endocarditis. Clin Microbiol Infect 10:46, 2004.
53. Sanfilippo AJ, Picard MH, Newell JB, et al: Echocardiographic assessment of patients with infectious endocarditis: prediction of risk for complications. J Am Coll Cardiol 18:1191, 1991.
54. Vuille C, Nidorf M, Weyman AE, et al: Natural history of vegetations during successful medical treatment of endocarditis. Am Heart J 128:1200, 1994.
55. Rohmann S, Erbel R, Darius H, et al: Prediction of rapid versus prolonged healing of infective endocarditis by monitoring vegetation size. J Am Soc Echocardiogr 4:465, 1991.
56. Rohmann S, Erhel R, Darius H, et al: Effect of antibiotic treatment on vegetation size and complication rate in infective endocarditis. Clin Cardiol 20:132, 1997.
57. Rohmann S, Erbel R, Darius H, et al: Spontaneous echo contrast imaging in infective endocarditis: a predictor of complications? Int J Card Imaging 8:197, 1992.
58. Taha TH, Durrant S, Crick J, et al: Hemostatic studies in patients with infective endocarditis: a report on nine consecutive cases with evidence of coagulopathy. Heart Vessels 6:102, 1991.
59. Kupferwasser LI, Hafner G, Mohr-Kahaly S, et al: The presence of infection-related antiphospholipid antibodies in infective endocarditis determines a major risk factor for embolic events. J Am Coll Cardiol 33:1365, 1999.
60. Lydakis C, Apostolakis S, Lydataki N, et al: Stroke-complicated endocarditis with positive lupus anticoagulant–a case report. Angiology 56:503, 2005.
61. Korkmaz S, Ileri M, Hisar I, et al: Increased levels of soluble adhesion molecules, E-selectin and P-selectin, in patients with infective endocarditis and embolic events. Eur Heart J 22:874, 2001.
62. Chukwudelunzu FE, Brown Jr RD, Wijdicks EF, et al: Subarachnoid haemorrhage associated with infectious endocarditis: case report and literature review. Eur J Neurol 9:423, 2002.
63. Salgado AV, Furlan AJ, Keys TF: Mycotic aneurysm, subarachnoid hemorrhage, and indications for cerebral angiography in infective endocarditis. Stroke 18:1057, 1987.
64. Jebara VA, Acar C, Dervanian P, et al: Mycotic aneurysms of the carotid arteries–case report and review of the literature. J Vasc Surg 14:215, 1991.
65. Heyd J, Yinnon AM: Mycotic aneurysm of the external carotid artery. J Cardiovasc Surg (Torino) 35:329, 1994.
66. Cooper HA, Thompson EC, Laureno R, et al: Subclinical brain embolization in left-sided infective endocarditis: results from the evaluation by MRI of the brains of patients with left-sided intracardiac solid masses (EMBOLISM) pilot study. Circulation 120:585, 2009.
67. Bakshi R, Wright PD, Kinkel PR, et al: Cranial magnetic resonance imaging findings in bacterial endocarditis: the neuroimaging spectrum of septic brain embolization demonstrated in twelve patients. J Neuroimaging 9:78, 1999.
68. Moulin T, Crepin-Leblond T, Chopard JL, et al: Hemorrhagic infarcts. Eur Neurol 34:64, 1994.
69. Kim SJ, Lee JY, Kim TH, et al: Imaging of the neurological complications of infective endocarditis. Neuroradiology 40:109, 1998.
70. Klein I, Iung B, Labreuche J, et al: Cerebral microbleeds are frequent in infective endocarditis: a case-control study. Stroke 40:3461, 2009.
71. Byrne JG, Rezai K, Sanchez JA, et al: Surgical management of endocarditis: The Society of Thoracic Surgeons Clinical Practice Guideline. Ann Thorac Surg 91:2012, 2011.
72. van der Meulen JH, Weststrate W, van GJ, et al: Is cerebral angiography indicated in infective endocarditis? Stroke 23:1662, 1992.
73. Ahmadi J, Tung H, Giannotta SL, et al: Monitoring of infectious intracranial aneurysms by sequential computed tomographic/magnetic resonance imaging studies. Neurosurgery 32:45, 1993.
74. Ellis CJ, Waite ST, Coverdale HA, et al: Transoesophageal echocardiography in patients with prosthetic heart valves and systemic emboli: is it a useful investigation? N Z Med J 108:376, 1995.

75. Dickerman S, Abrutyn E, Barsic B, et al: The relationship between the initiation of antimicrobial therapy and the incidence of stroke in infective endocarditis: an analysis from the ICE prospective Corhort Study (ICE-PCS). Am Heart J 154:1086, 2007.
76. Wilson W, Taubert KA, Gewitz MH, et al: Prevention of infective endocarditis: guidelines from the American Heart Association: a guideline from the American Heart Association Rheumatic Fever, Endocarditis and Kawasaki Disease Committee, Council on Cardiovascular Disease in the Young, and the Council on Clinical Cardiology, Council on Cardiovascular Surgery and Anesthesia, and the Quality of Care and Outcomes Research Interdisciplinary Working Group. Circulation 116:1736, 2007.
77. Athan E, Chu VH, Tattevin P, et al: Clinical characteristics and outcome of infective endocarditis involving implantable cardiac devices. JAMA 307:1727, 2012.
78. Sontineni S, Mooss A, Andukuri V, et al: Effectiveness of thrombolytic therapy in acute embolic stroke due to infective endocarditis. Stroke Res Treat 2010:1, 2010.
79. Tan M, Armstrong D, Birken C, et al: Bacterial endocarditis in a child presenting with acute arterial ischemic stroke: should thrombolytic therapy be absolutely contraindicated? Dev Med Child Neurol 51:151, 2009.
80. Bhuva P, Kuo S-H, Hemphill J, et al: Intracranial hemorrhage following thrombolytic use for stroke caused by infective endocarditis. Neurocrit Care 12:79, 2010.
81. Dababneh H, Hedna V, Ford J, et al: Endovascular intervention for acute stroke due to infective endocarditis. Neurosurg Focus 32:E1, 2012.
82. Nicolau DP, Freeman CD, Nightingale CH, et al: Reduction of bacterial titers by low-dose aspirin in experimental aortic valve endocarditis. Infect Immun 61:1593, 1993.
83. Nicolau DP, Tessier PR, Nightingale CH: Beneficial effect of combination antiplatelet therapy on the development of experimental *Staphylococcus aureus* endocarditis. Int J Antimicrob Agents 11:159, 1999.
84. Kupferwasser LI, Yeaman MR, Shapiro SM, et al: Acetylsalicylic acid reduces vegetation bacterial density, hematogenous bacterial dissemination, and frequency of embolic events in experimental *Staphylococcus aureus* endocarditis through antiplatelet and antibacterial effects. Circulation 99:2791, 1999.
85. Taha TH, Durrant SS, Mazeika PK, et al: Aspirin to prevent growth of vegetations and cerebral emboli in infective endocarditis. J Intern Med 231:543, 1992.
86. Chan KL, Dumesnil JG, Cujec B, et al: A randomized trial of aspirin on the risk of embolic events in patients with infective endocarditis. J Am Coll Cardiol 42:775, 2003.
87. Anavekar N, Tleyjeh I, Anavekar N, et al: Impact of prior antiplatelet therapy on risk of embolism in infective endocarditis. Clin Infect Dis 44:1180, 2007.
88. Eisen D, Corey G, McBryde E, et al: Reduced valve replacement surgery and complication rate in *Staphylococcus aureus* endocarditis patients receiving acetylsalicylic acid. J Infect 58:332, 2009.
89. Snygg-Martin U, Rasmussen R, Hassager C, et al: The relationship between cerebrovascular complications and previously established use of antiplatelet therapy in left-sided infective endocarditis. Scand J Infec Dis 43:899, 2011.
90. Molina CA, Selim MH: Anticoagulation in patients with stroke with infective endocarditis: the sword of Damocles. Stroke 42:1799, 2011.
91. Sila C: Anticoagulation should not be used in most patients with stroke with infective endocarditis. Stroke 42:1797, 2011.
92. Rasmussen RV: Anticoagulation in patients with stroke with infective endocarditis is safe. Stroke 42:1795, 2011.
93. Delahaye JP, Poncet P, Malquarti V, et al: Cerebrovascular accidents in infective endocarditis: role of anticoagulation. Eur Heart J 11:1074, 1990.
94. Tornos P, Almirante B, Mirabet S, et al: Infective endocarditis due to *Staphylococcus aureus*: deleterious effect of anticoagulant therapy. Arch Intern Med 159:473, 1999.
95. Solenski NJ, Haley Jr EC: Neurological complications of infective endocarditis. In Roos KL (ed): Central Nervous System Infectious Diseases and Therapy. Marcel Dekker, New York, 1997.
96. Salgado AV: Central nervous system complications of infective endocarditis. Stroke 22:1461, 1991.
97. Kiefer T, Park L, Tribouilloy C, et al: Association between valvular surgery and mortality among patients with infective endocarditis complicated by heart failure. JAMA 306:2239, 2011.
98. Cabell CH, Abrutyn E, Fowler Jr VG, et al: Use of surgery in patients with native valve infective endocarditis: results from the International Collaboration on Endocarditis Merged Database. Am Heart J 150:1092, 2005.
99. Wang A, Athan E, Pappas P, et al: Contemporary clinical profile and outcome of prosthetic valve endocarditis. JAMA 297:1354, 2007.
100. Yeates A, Mundy J, Griffin R, et al: Early and mid-term outcomes following surgical management of infective endocarditis with associated cerebral complications: a single centre experience. Heart Lung Circ 19:523, 2010.
101. Lalani T, Cabell CH, Benjamin D, et al: Analysis of the impact of early surgery on in-hospital mortality of native valve endocarditis: use of propensity score and instrumental variable methods to adjust for treatment-selection bias. Circulation 121:1005, 2010.
102. Kim DH, Kang DH, Lee MZ, et al: Impact of early surgery on embolic events in patients with infective endocarditis. Circulation 122:S17, 2010.

103. Mayer SA, Brun NC, Begtrup K, et al: Recombinant activated factor VII for acute intracerebral hemorrhage. N Engl J Med 352:777, 2005.
104. Brust JC, Dickinson PC, Hughes JE, et al: The diagnosis and treatment of cerebral mycotic aneurysms. Ann Neurol 27:238, 1990.
105. Corr P, Wright M, Handler LC: Endocarditis-related cerebral aneurysms: radiologic changes with treatment. AJNR Am J Neuroradiol 16:745, 1995.
106. Barrow DL, Prats AR: Infectious intracranial aneurysms: comparison of groups with and without endocarditis. Neurosurgery 27:562, 1990.
107. Monsuez JJ, Vittecoq D, Rosenbaum A, et al: Prognosis of ruptured intracranial mycotic aneurysms: a review of 12 cases. Eur Heart J 10:821, 1989.
108. Scotti G, Li MH, Righi C, et al: Endovascular treatment of bacterial intracranial aneurysms. Neuroradiology 38:186, 1996.
109. Frizzell RT, Vitek JJ, Hill DL, et al: Treatment of a bacterial (mycotic) intracranial aneurysm using an endovascular approach. Neurosurgery 32:852, 1993.
110. Chapot R, Houdart E, Saint-Maurice JP, et al: Endovascular treatment of cerebral mycotic aneurysms. Radiology 222:389, 2002.
111. Sugg RM, Weir R, Vollmer DG, et al: Cerebral mycotic aneurysms treated with a neuroform stent: technical case report. Neurosurgery 58:E381, 2006.
112. Kato Y, Yamaguchi S, Sano H, et al: Stereoscopic synthesized brain-surface imaging with MR angiography for localization of a peripheral mycotic aneurysm: case report. Minim Invasive Neurosurg 39:113, 1996.
113. Cunha e Sá M, Sisti M, Solomon R: Stereotactic angiographic localization as an adjunct to surgery of cerebral mycotic aneurysms: case report and review of the literature. Acta Neurochir (Wien) 139:625, 1997.
114. Tunkel AR, Kaye D: Neurologic complications of infective endocarditis. Neurol Clin 11:419, 1993.
115. Chu VH, Cabell CH, Benjamin Jr DK, et al: Early predictors of in-hospital death in infective endocarditis. Circulation 109:1745, 2004.
116. Heiro M, Helenius H, Hurme S, et al: Long-term outcome of infective endocarditis: a study on patients surviving over one year after the initial episode treated in a Finnish teaching hospital during 25 years. BMC Infect Dis 8:49, 2008.
117. Ruttmann E, Willeit J, Ulmer H, et al: Neurological outcome of septic cardioembolic stroke after infective endocarditis. Stroke 37:2094, 2006.

CHAPTER

7

Neurologic Complications of Hypertension

ANTHONY S. KIM ■ S. CLAIBORNE JOHNSTON

Blood pressure was first measured in 1707 by an English divinity student, Stephan Hales, using a glass tube attached directly into the arteries of animals. Methods of measurement improved slowly over the next 200 years, with Nikolai Korotkoff describing the modern cuff-and-stethoscope technique in 1905. Hypertension was recognized as an indicator of poor prognosis by Theodore Janeway, who published a case series of 7,872 hypertensive patients gathered between 1903 and 1912, in which hypertension was defined as a systolic blood pressure greater than 160 mmHg. He found a mean survival of 4 to 5 years after the development of symptoms of hypertension, with stroke being an important cause of death. A tolerable oral agent to treat hypertension was not available until 1957, when chlorothiazide was shown to reduce blood pressure in patients with essential hypertension and rapidly became the most commonly prescribed medication.

Both acute hypertension and chronic hypertension produce neurologic disease. Acute hypertension is associated with hypertensive encephalopathy, an uncommon presentation since the widespread identification and treatment of hypertension. Chronic hypertension is associated with stroke, which is its most important neurologic complication. All stroke subtypes are linked to hypertension, including ischemic infarction, intraparenchymal hemorrhage, and aneurysmal subarachnoid hemorrhage. Chronic hypertension is also associated with dementia.

EPIDEMIOLOGY

Both systolic and diastolic blood pressures are distributed approximately normally in the population. For convenience, physicians have defined pathologic states such as hypertension based on specific blood pressure thresholds, typically a systolic blood pressure of 140 mmHg or greater or a diastolic blood pressure of 90 mmHg or greater, or both. Thus defined, hypertension is common, affecting approximately 78 million adults in the United States.[1] The number of hypertensive adults worldwide is expected to reach 1.54 billion by 2025.[2] In the Framingham study, individuals who were

Aminoff's Neurology and General Medicine, Fifth Edition.

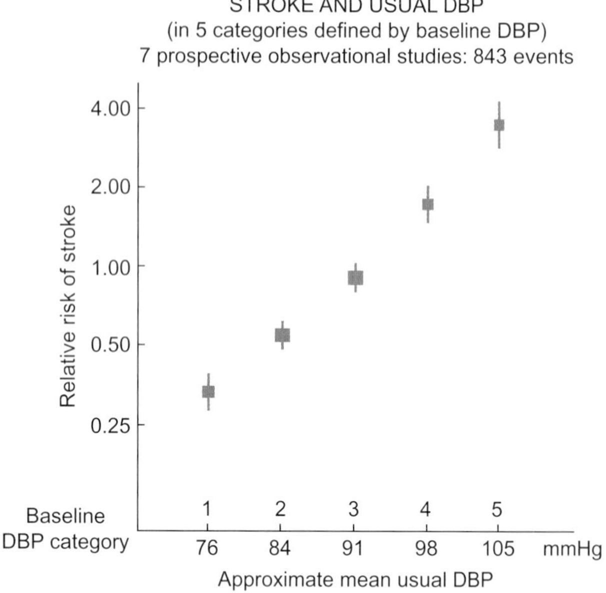

FIGURE 7-1 ■ Relative risks of stroke. Estimates of the usual diastolic blood pressure (DBP) in each baseline DBP category are taken from mean DBP values 4 years after baseline in the Framingham study. Solid squares represent disease risks in each category relative to risk in the whole study population; sizes of squares are proportional to the number of events in each DBP category; and 95 percent confidence intervals for estimates of relative risk are denoted by vertical lines. (From MacMahon S, Peto R, Cutler J, et al: Blood pressure, stroke, and coronary heart disease. Lancet 335:764, 1990, with permission.)

normotensive at age 55 had an approximately 90 percent lifetime risk of developing hypertension.[3]

Despite the frequent division of blood pressure into diagnostic categories such as hypertension and normotension, there is no obvious threshold at which higher blood pressure begins affecting the risk of complications, and even patients with diastolic blood pressures of 80 to 90 mmHg are at increased risk of stroke compared with those with blood pressures of 70 to 80 mmHg (Fig. 7-1).[4] Reflecting a growing awareness of the continuous risk associated with blood pressure, blood pressures in the range of 120–140/80–90 mmHg, once considered to be "normal," are now labeled as "prehypertensive."[5]

PATHOPHYSIOLOGY

In the brain, the primary pathophysiologic process of hypertension is related to increases in vasomotor tone and peripheral arterial resistance. Acute elevation in blood pressure results in constriction of small arteries in the brain in a compensatory response termed *autoregulation*. Blood flow to the brain is maintained at a relatively constant level over a range of pressures. At high pressures, vasoconstriction is thought to be protective by reducing pressure at smaller, more distal vessels. Acute severe hypertension overwhelms normal autoregulation at a mean arterial pressure of approximately 150 mmHg, with increased cerebral blood flow occurring above this pressure threshold. Vasoconstriction in acute hypertension is patchy, and some small vessels are exposed to high pressures, which may lead to endothelial injury and focal breakdown of the blood–brain barrier.[6] Acute hypertensive encephalopathy is a fulminant presentation of this process. Fibrinoid necrosis of small vessels may also occur, lowering the threshold for future ischemic and hemorrhagic events.

Chronic hypertension results in cerebral vascular remodeling. The media hypertrophies, and the lumen becomes narrowed.[7] These changes are protective, with reduction in wall tension and shifting of the autoregulation curve to allow compensation at higher blood pressures.[8] However, vascular remodeling is accompanied by endothelial dysfunction, with impaired relaxation and poor compensation for hypoperfusion. The result is greater susceptibility to ischemic injury due to reduced collateral flow.[6]

Hypertension also predisposes to atherosclerosis. Hypertension is proinflammatory and is accompanied by increased plasma oxygen free radicals.[9] Free radicals induce vascular smooth muscle cell proliferation and may oxidize low-density lipoproteins, which in turn promotes macrophage activation and monocyte extravasation. Angiotensin II is elevated in many hypertensive patients and may play a direct role in atherogenesis independent of its effects on blood pressure.[10] It directly stimulates smooth muscle cell growth, hypertrophy, and lipoxygenase activity, with resultant inflammation and low-density lipoprotein oxidation,[9] thus accelerating atherosclerosis.

EVALUATION AND TREATMENT

The gold standard of blood pressure measurement is auscultation using a mercury sphygmomanometer. Newer devices can provide accurate readings but require calibration. Blood pressure should be measured in the seated position after a 5-minute rest with the patient's feet resting on the floor and the arm supported at heart level during the measurement. Accurate readings depend on the use of an appropriate-sized cuff with the bladder covering at least 80 percent of the arm. The classification of blood pressure into specific diagnostic categories is based on the average of two or more readings on each of two or more office visits.[11] A complete history and physical examination with basic laboratory measurements are essential to evaluate for identifiable causes of hypertension and assess risk. Several patient characteristics may suggest an identifiable cause of hypertension including young age, severe hypertension, hypertension that is refractory to multiple interventions, and physical or laboratory findings suggestive of endocrinologic disorders, such as truncal obesity or hypokalemia. Abdominal bruits or decreased femoral pulses may also be an indicator of renovascular disease or coarctation of the aorta.[12]

Lifestyle modification is recommended as an initial therapy for patients with blood pressure of 120/80 mmHg or higher.[5] Effective lifestyle interventions include weight loss, limited alcohol intake, aerobic physical activity, adequate potassium intake, reduction in sodium intake, and dietary regimens such as the Dietary Approaches to Stop Hypertension (DASH) eating plan.[13] Antihypertensive medications are recommended in addition to lifestyle measures for patients with blood pressure of 140/90 mmHg or higher, with a lower threshold of 130/80 mmHg or higher in those with diabetes and chronic kidney disease.

For patients without a history of cardiovascular disease or other compelling indication, initiating therapy with a thiazide diuretic such as chlorthalidone is generally recommended. In a trial involving more than 33,000 participants, therapy with chlorthalidone was either equivalent or superior to lisinopril and amlodipine for the primary prevention of cardiovascular end-points, with a particular benefit for African Americans in terms of both safety and efficacy.[14] When the blood pressure is 160/100 mmHg or higher, initiating therapy with two-drug combinations is generally recommended.[15]

There are many benefits to treating hypertension, including a reduction in myocardial infarctions, congestive heart failure, retinopathy, renal failure, and overall mortality. The focus of the remainder of this chapter is on specific neurologic complications of hypertension and the unique aspects of treatment that they necessitate.

STROKE

Of all the identified modifiable risk factors for stroke, hypertension appears to be the most important, owing to its high prevalence and its associated three- to fivefold increase in stroke risk.[15] Based on epidemiologic data, approximately 50 percent of strokes could be prevented if hypertension were eliminated (Table 7-1).[16] Even small reductions in blood pressure result in large reductions in stroke risk. For example, in a meta-analysis of 37,000 hypertensive subjects from 14 studies, a reduction of 5 to 6 mmHg in diastolic blood pressure with active treatment was associated with a 42 percent reduction in stroke risk.[17] The benefits of blood pressure reduction on stroke risk extend similarly to the elderly with isolated elevations in systolic blood

TABLE 7-1 ■ Estimated Impact of Modifiable Risk Factors on Stroke in the United States*

Risk Factor	Percentage Exposed	Relative Risk	Population-Attributable Risk (%)	Projected Number of Strokes Preventable
Hypertension	56	2.7	49	370,000
Cigarette smoking	27	1.5	12	92,000
Atrial fibrillation	4	3.6	9	71,000
Heavy alcohol consumption	7	1.7	5	35,000

Adapted from Gorelick PB: Stroke prevention: an opportunity for efficient utilization of health care resources during the coming decade. Stroke 25:220, 1994.

*Relative risks are from the Framingham study. Population-attributable risk is the expected decrease in stroke rates if the risk factor were eliminated. Projected number of strokes preventable is based on an estimated 750,000 strokes per year.

pressure. In one trial of 4,736 subjects aged 60 years or more, a 36 percent reduction in stroke was seen with a 12-mmHg decline in systolic pressure, a finding confirmed in other large randomized trials.[18,19] The best available data suggest that benefits of treating blood pressure in the oldest old (>85 years) are comparable to those seen in younger individuals.[20]

The burden of stroke has generally declined in the developed world.[21] Although these historic trends are not entirely explained by better control of blood pressure, the rates of decline have roughly paralleled the increased use of antihypertensive medications. However, hypertension remains the leading risk factor for death globally,[22] and the developing world continues to bear a disproportionate, substantial, and increasing burden of disease from stroke (Fig. 7-2).[23,24]

Hypertension contributes to each of the major intermediate causes of both ischemic and hemorrhagic stroke including carotid stenosis, intracranial atherosclerosis, small-vessel arteriosclerosis, and both macroscopic and microscopic aneurysms. Each of these conditions is considered separately in this chapter.

In the acute phase of cerebral ischemia, hypertension may play a compensatory role in maintaining cerebral perfusion to viable but threatened areas of the brain.[25] Loss of normal cerebral autoregulation has been demonstrated in areas of ischemic brain. When autoregulation is lost, blood flow to the brain becomes directly proportional to mean arterial pressure and therefore, in theory, pharmacologic increases in blood pressure could have salutatory effects in preserving hypoperfused regions of the brain.[26] In some small studies, rapid pharmacologic reductions in blood pressure have predicted worse outcomes, and there are numerous anecdotal reports of the recrudescence of stroke symptoms after a decrease in blood pressure.[27,28] Therefore, most stroke guidelines recommend withholding or reducing pharmacologic treatments of blood pressure in acute ischemic stroke in the absence of acute end-organ injury or administration of thrombolytics, unless the blood pressure exceeds 220/120 mmHg.[29]

There is overwhelming evidence to support the use of pharmacologic interventions to lower blood pressure for secondary stroke prevention.

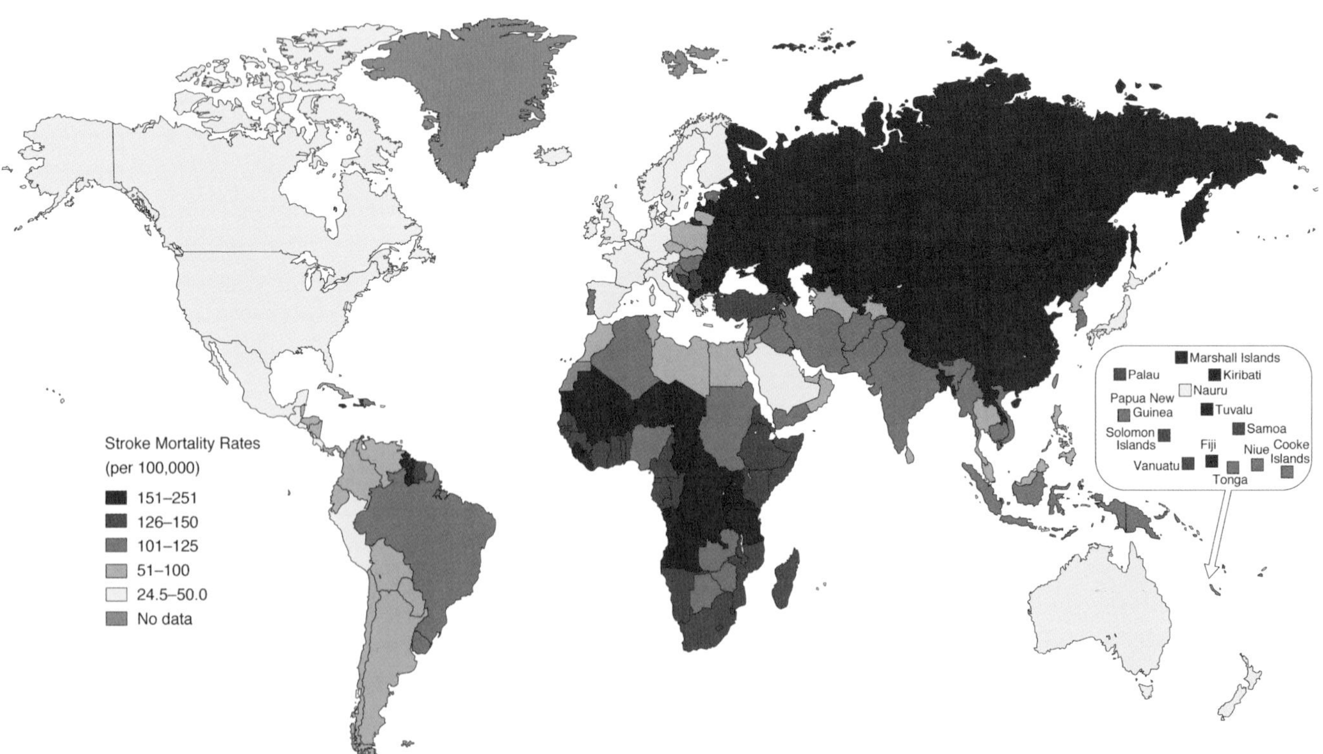

FIGURE 7-2 ▪ Age-adjusted and sex-adjusted stroke mortality rates, 2000. (From Johnston SC, Mendis S, Mathers CD: Global variation in stroke burden and mortality: estimates from monitoring, surveillance, and modeling. Lancet Neurol 8:345, 2009. Copyright 2009, with permission.)

In 6,105 subjects with a history of stroke, one study demonstrated a 43 percent relative risk reduction for secondary stroke prevention when subjects were randomized to the combination of the angiotensin-converting enzyme (ACE) inhibitor perindopril and the thiazide diuretic indapamide.[30] Combination therapy with the ACE inhibitor and thiazide, which resulted in a mean blood pressure reduction of 12.3/5 mmHg, produced a substantially more robust benefit for stroke prevention than monotherapy with ramipril (relative risk reduction, 5%), which produced only a 4.9/2.8-mmHg average reduction in blood pressure (*P* for heterogeneity between treatments <0.001). Combination therapy with an ACE inhibitor and a thiazide diuretic is now commonly recommended for secondary stroke prevention, with benefits appearing to be similar regardless of whether measured blood pressure is above or below the traditional cut points for hypertension.[31] Although other studies have supported the finding that therapy with renin-angiotensin system antagonists and diuretics provides especially strong benefits for stroke prevention, particularly when compared with β-blockers,[32] the degree of hypertension control that is achieved is usually the best predictor of protection against recurrent stroke. Therefore, response to therapy and other comorbidities, such as heart failure, diabetes, asthma, and arrhythmia, should be considered when deciding on an appropriate antihypertensive drug regimen.[5] The Scandinavian Acute Stroke Trial (SCAST) of 2,029 patients suggested no benefit (hazard ratio for vascular death, MI, or stroke = 1.09) and possible harm (adjusted hazard ratio for 6-month functional outcome = 1.17) with acute blood pressure lowering with candesartan for 7 days after stroke,[33] though starting antihypertensive therapy before hospital discharge may improve initial patient adherence.[31,34]

CEREBRAL ANEURYSMS

Cerebral aneurysms are focal dilatations of blood vessels. Subarachnoid hemorrhage, an important form of hemorrhagic stroke, occurs when a cerebral aneurysm ruptures (Fig. 7-3). Hypertension is associated with cerebral aneurysm formation and with subarachnoid hemorrhage. In a large sample of Medicare patients, hypertension was listed as a secondary diagnosis in 43 percent of patients admitted with unruptured aneurysms and in 34 percent of hospitalized control subjects.[35] In a meta-analysis, the risk of subarachnoid hemorrhage was 2.8 times greater in those with a history of hypertension.[36]

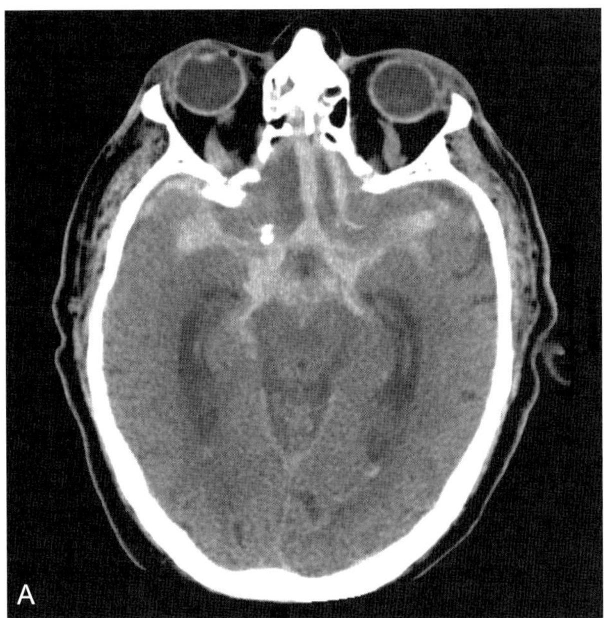

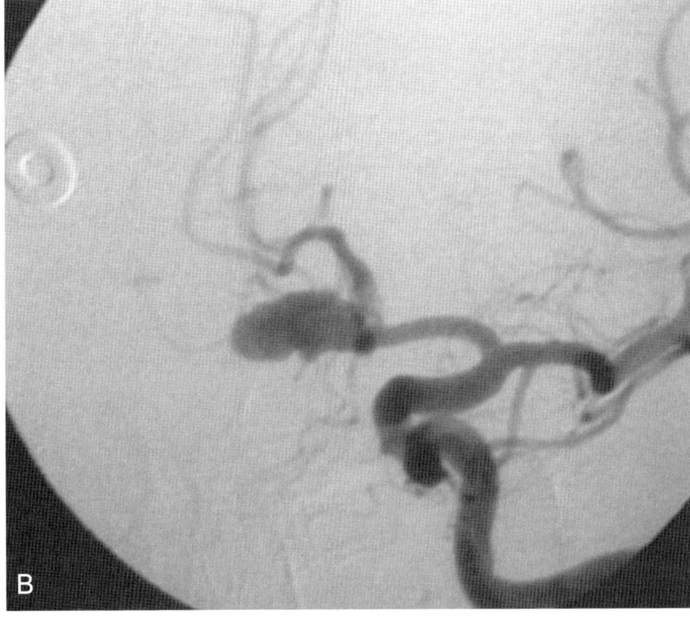

FIGURE 7-3 ■ A ruptured anterior communicating artery aneurysm producing acute subarachnoid hemorrhage. **A**, Head computed tomography (CT) shows a large amount of blood at the base of the brain and a small amount of intraventricular blood. **B**, Angiogram reveals a complex saccular aneurysm.

The cause of the development and rupture of cerebral aneurysms is probably multifactorial. Epidemiologic studies have found several environmental risk factors for subarachnoid hemorrhage other than hypertension. Cigarette smoking increases the risk of subarachnoid hemorrhage by 100 percent or more,[36] perhaps by increasing the release of proteolytic enzymes that affect blood-vessel integrity.[37] Heavy alcohol consumption increases subarachnoid hemorrhage risk with a pooled odds ratio of 1.5 in case control studies and a relative risk of 4.7 in cohort studies.[36] Alcohol-induced hypertension, relative anticoagulation, or increased cerebral blood flow may be responsible.[37] Oral contraceptives are associated with a small but significant excess risk of subarachnoid hemorrhage, with a relative risk of 1.4 in current and past users.[38]

Genetic factors are also important to aneurysm formation and subarachnoid hemorrhage. The risk of subarachnoid hemorrhage is three to seven times greater in patients with an affected first-degree relative,[39,40] and the prevalence of unruptured aneurysms is probably at least twice as high when a family history of aneurysm is present.[41] Females are nearly twice as likely as males to have an aneurysm or to present with subarachnoid hemorrhage. African Americans have twice the rate of subarachnoid hemorrhage as whites. Polycystic kidney disease, Ehlers–Danlos syndrome type 4, and α_1-antitrypsin deficiency are also associated with increased risk.[42]

Unruptured Cerebral Aneurysms

Estimates of the prevalence of unruptured aneurysms vary widely. A meta-analysis of 68 studies estimated that overall prevalence would be 3.2 percent in a population without comorbidities, with a mean age of 50 years, and consisting of 50 percent males.[43] In a prior meta-analysis, approximately 90 percent of aneurysms were less than 10 mm in diameter, and 70 percent were less than 6 mm.[44] Based on these estimates, 11 million American adults have an unruptured aneurysm. These aneurysms are being detected more frequently as imaging technology improves and as imaging studies are applied more frequently.[45] The annual cost for unruptured aneurysms in the United States was estimated at $522 million in the 1980s and is significantly greater now.[46]

Unruptured aneurysms are often asymptomatic, discovered incidentally in the work-up for an unrelated problem. Some aneurysms produce symptoms by compressing neighboring structures. Presentation with a new cranial neuropathy is considered a worrisome sign of imminent rupture and often prompts urgent treatment. New headaches are also a presenting sign of unruptured aneurysm. Although migraine may simply represent an unrelated occurrence that prompts head imaging, some headaches may be due to the aneurysm itself. A sudden, severe "thunderclap" headache may herald rapid aneurysm growth or a small leak without evidence of subarachnoid hemorrhage.[47]

Catheter angiography remains the gold standard for detection of aneurysms. Magnetic resonance (MR) angiography is approximately 85 percent sensitive for detecting aneurysms larger than 3 mm, with 85 percent specificity.[48] Head computed tomography (CT) does not reliably detect unruptured aneurysms, though CT angiography may be useful to identify certain aneurysms, particularly those that are larger than 3 mm.[49]

Prognosis of unruptured aneurysms, as reflected in the rate of rupture, is a subject of controversy. In the largest prospective cohort study, 1,692 subjects with unruptured aneurysms who did not undergo surgery or endovascular treatment were followed prospectively for an average of 4.1 years.[50] The size of the aneurysm ($\geq$7 mm in maximum diameter) and location at the basilar tip or posterior communicating artery were independent predictors of hemorrhage. Among 1,077 subjects with no history of subarachnoid hemorrhage, the annual risk of hemorrhage for an aneurysm less than 7 mm in diameter in the anterior circulation was essentially 0 percent; it was 0.5 percent when the aneurysm was located in the posterior circulation.[50]

The standard of care for treatment of aneurysms has historically been surgical clipping, in which a metal clip is placed over the neck of the aneurysm, isolating it from the circulation. Coil embolization is an alternative therapy that involves packing platinum coils into an aneurysm through a microcatheter in an angiographic endovascular procedure. This approach has been widely applied and appears to be a generally safer approach when technically feasible.[51]

Whether a given aneurysm requires treatment depends on the anticipated rupture rate and procedural risks. For asymptomatic aneurysms smaller than 7 mm with no history of subarachnoid hemorrhage, treatment may not be justified, particularly when in the anterior circulation, given the risks of surgery and endovascular therapy.[52] Treatment of unruptured aneurysms appears to be cost-effective when they are larger or symptomatic or when there is a history of subarachnoid hemorrhage from a different aneurysm.[52]

Controlling or eliminating risk factors, such as hypertension, smoking, and alcohol abuse, may reduce rupture rates, but this has not been systematically studied.

Subarachnoid Hemorrhage

Subarachnoid hemorrhage accounts for approximately 5 percent of all strokes, but it tends to occur at a younger age than other stroke subtypes, with median age at death being 59 years for subarachnoid hemorrhage, 73 years for intracerebral hemorrhage, and 81 years for ischemic stroke.[53] Subarachnoid hemorrhage accounts for nearly one-third of the years of potential life lost before age 65 due to stroke. Case fatality rates approach 50 percent, and another 10 to 20 percent remain disabled and dependent at follow-up.[54] Approximately 30,000 Americans present with subarachnoid hemorrhage each year, with total costs estimated at well over $5.6 billion.[55]

Presentation with subarachnoid hemorrhage generally involves the sudden onset of severe headache, sometimes accompanied by neck pain. Alteration of consciousness occurs in a minority of patients, but it may be severe enough to produce coma or sudden death outside the hospital. Head CT often shows blood surrounding the base of the brain. Intraventricular and intraparenchymal hemorrhage may be present and can provide clues as to the location of the ruptured aneurysm. Lumbar puncture may rarely show signs of hemorrhage when there is no evidence of it on head CT. Blood in the spinal fluid that does not clear is suggestive of subarachnoid hemorrhage. Xanthochromia is present in nearly all cases and may persist for more than 3 weeks, but its appearance is delayed by more than 12 hours in 10 percent of cases. Angiography is required for the characterization of the aneurysm and to plan treatment.

Prognosis depends on the ability to treat the underlying aneurysm and on the patient's condition at presentation. Recurrent hemorrhage occurs in more than 4 percent of untreated patients during the first day and then in 1 to 2 percent per day for the next 2 weeks and is associated with even greater fatality and morbidity than primary rupture.[39] Regardless of treatment and recurrent hemorrhage, the level of consciousness at presentation is the major predictor of mortality (Table 7-2).[56] The World Federation of Neurological Surgeons developed a Universal Subarachnoid Hemorrhage Grading Scale, similar to the older Hunt and Hess scale, which has been widely adopted but offers little advantage over determinations based on level of consciousness alone.[57]

To reduce the risk of recurrent hemorrhage, ruptured aneurysms should be identified rapidly and repaired with surgical clipping or endovascular coil embolization as early as feasible.[58] Hydrocephalus from obstruction of the cerebral aqueduct or the meninges by blood clot may require external

TABLE 7-2 ■ Overall Outcome after Subarachnoid Hemorrhage by Consciousness Level on Admission*

Consciousness Level	Good Recovery		Moderately Disabled		Severely Disabled		Vegetative Survival		Dead		Totals	
	Number	Percent	Number	Percent	Number	Percent	Number	Percent	Number	Percent	Number	Percent
Alert	1,279	74.3	130	7.5	70	4.1	18	1.0	225	13.1	1,722	100.0
Drowsy	608	53.5	125	11.0	71	6.3	19	1.7	313	27.6	1,136	100.0
Stuporous	105	30.2	48	13.8	28	8.0	15	4.3	152	43.7	348	100.0
Comatose	35	11.1	17	5.4	25	7.9	11	3.5	227	72.1	315	100.0
Totals	2,027	57.6	320	9.1	194	5.5	63	1.8	917	26.0	3,521	100.0

From Kassell NF, Torner JC, Haley EC, et al: The International Cooperative Study on the timing of aneurysm surgery. J Neurosurg 73:18, 1990, with permission.
*Percentages are of row totals. Relationship between admission level of consciousness and outcome: $\chi^2 = 720.5$; $P < 0.001$.

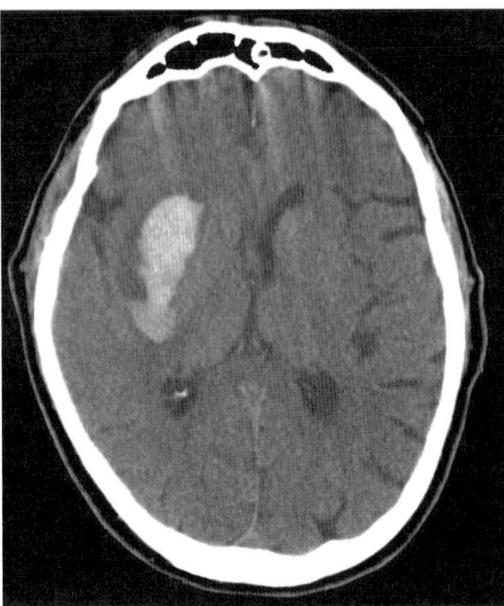

FIGURE 7-4 ■ Head CT of an acute basal ganglia intracerebral hemorrhage with mass effect compressing the ventricles.

drainage. Vasospasm is a common complication that produces cerebral ischemia due to blood-vessel constriction in areas exposed to subarachnoid blood. It becomes symptomatic in one-third of cases, usually 3 to 14 days after hemorrhage, and results in cerebral infarction or death in 15 to 20 percent.[58] Transcranial Doppler ultrasonography can detect vasospasm before it becomes symptomatic.[59] Oral nimodipine, a calcium-channel antagonist, reduces poor outcomes from vasospasm and is generally given for the first 21 days after the initial bleed. Hypertension induced with pressors and hydration with intravenous fluids may reduce the risk of infarction, but these measures have never been studied in trials. They should not be used in patients with untreated aneurysms because of the risk of precipitating further episodes of bleeding. Vasodilatation through angioplasty or intra-arterial verapamil (or other vasodilators) immediately reverses angiographic vasospasm in many cases, but clinical benefits have not been definitely demonstrated.

INTRACEREBRAL HEMORRHAGE

Bleeding directly into the substance of the brain is termed *intraparenchymal* or *intracerebral hemorrhage* (Fig. 7-4). It may occur as a complication of ischemic stroke, termed *hemorrhagic conversion*, or as the primary injury without preceding ischemia. Hypertension is the most important identified risk factor for intracerebral hemorrhage. More than 70 percent of patients with intracerebral hemorrhage have a history of hypertension, and the risk of hemorrhagic stroke is elevated 9.5-fold in the highest compared with the lowest quintile of systolic blood pressure.[60]

Intracranial hemorrhage is responsible for 10 to 15 percent of all stroke deaths but for more than one-third of the years of life lost before age 65 due to the younger age distribution of intracerebral hemorrhage.[53] Case fatality rates are high, with 35 to 50 percent dead at 1 month and only 20 percent returning to independence at 6 months.[61] In the United States, an estimated 37,000 cases of intracerebral hemorrhage occur each year, with the total estimated cost of care exceeding $6 billion annually.[55]

Other risk factors for intracerebral hemorrhage include age, race, substance abuse, anticoagulation, platelet dysfunction, and vascular and structural anomalies. Rates of intracerebral hemorrhage increase with age. African Americans have rates that are 40 percent higher than those of whites, with larger differences at younger ages.[62] Cocaine and amphetamine use is associated with increased risk, particularly acutely, possibly because of transient severe hypertension.[60] Abnormalities in clotting may account for an increased incidence of intracerebral hemorrhage with heavy alcohol use. Excessive anticoagulation and antiplatelet therapy also increase the risk of intracerebral hemorrhage.[63,64] Thrombolytic agents used for ischemic stroke and myocardial infarction cause intracerebral hemorrhage in some cases. It may also occur with severe thrombocytopenia and platelet dysfunction.

Intracerebral hemorrhage may result from and occur in brain tumors, such as glioblastoma multiforme and in metastatic melanoma, choriocarcinoma, renal cell carcinoma, and bronchogenic carcinoma. Cerebral amyloid angiopathy, a vasculopathy common in the elderly, is associated with lobar hemorrhages, often centered at the gray-white junction. Other punctate hemorrhages may be apparent on gradient-echo MR images (Fig. 7-5), supporting the diagnosis. Arteriovenous malformations, abnormal complexes of arteries and veins in brain parenchyma, account for 5 percent of intracerebral hemorrhages.[60] Cavernous malformations are dense collections of thin-walled vascular

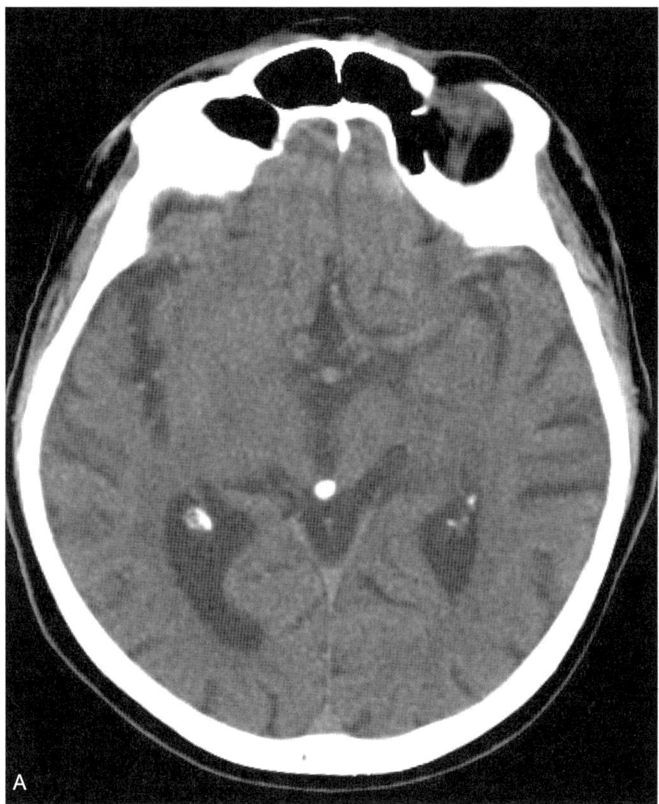

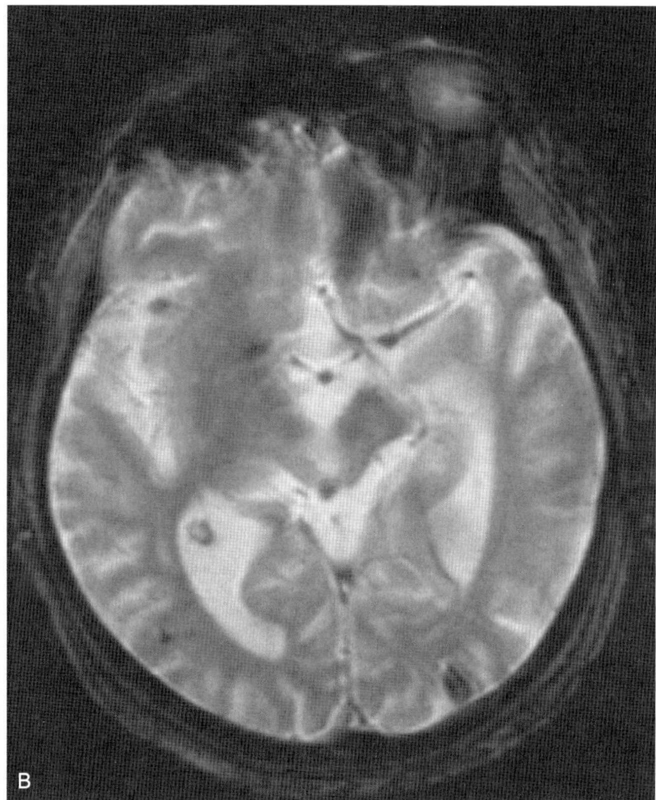

FIGURE 7-5 ■ Imaging findings of amyloid angiopathy, with no evidence of hemorrhage on CT (**A**) but multiple punctate areas of susceptibility at the gray-white junction on T2-weighted multiplanar gradient-recalled (MPGR) magnetic resonance imaging (MRI) (**B**), suggesting prior hemorrhage.

channels and appear to be the cause of intracerebral hemorrhage in 5 percent of autopsies[64]; they are not apparent on angiography but have a "popcorn" appearance on MR images, with a hyperintense core surrounded by hypointense hemosiderin from previous small hemorrhages (Fig. 7-6). Aneurysms may produce intracerebral hemorrhages when blood is directed into the brain, and these rarely are mistaken for primary hypertensive hemorrhages.

Primary hypertensive intracerebral hemorrhage was thought to be caused by chronic vascular injury, resulting in formation of microscopic aneurysms, first characterized by Charcot and Bouchard in 1868. Advances in pathologic tissue preparation have raised doubts about the frequency and importance of microscopic aneurysms, which may actually represent complex vascular coils.[65] More recently, fibrinoid necrosis of small arteries has been proposed as the initial step in intracerebral hemorrhage.[66] Brain injury occurs because of compression of surrounding tissue and from the direct toxic effects of blood. Mass effect from the hematoma may lead to uncal, subfalcine, tonsillar, or transtentorial herniation, depending on location, and death may ensue.

Clinical presentation depends on the location and size of the hemorrhage (Table 7-3). Nearly all intracerebral hemorrhage is characterized by the sudden onset of neurologic deficits, progressing over minutes and accompanied by headache, often with alteration of consciousness. Deterioration due to surrounding edema, hydrocephalus, or continuing or recurrent hemorrhage often occurs within the first 24 hours but may be delayed by days.

Prognosis is multifactorial. Hemorrhage volume, most easily measured by halving the product of the length, width, and depth on axial head CT images, is a powerful predictor of mortality, with 80 percent 30-day mortality in those with volumes greater than 60 ml, and 22 percent mortality in hemorrhages less than 30 ml.[67] Mortality is much greater in those with intraventricular extension of blood.[68]

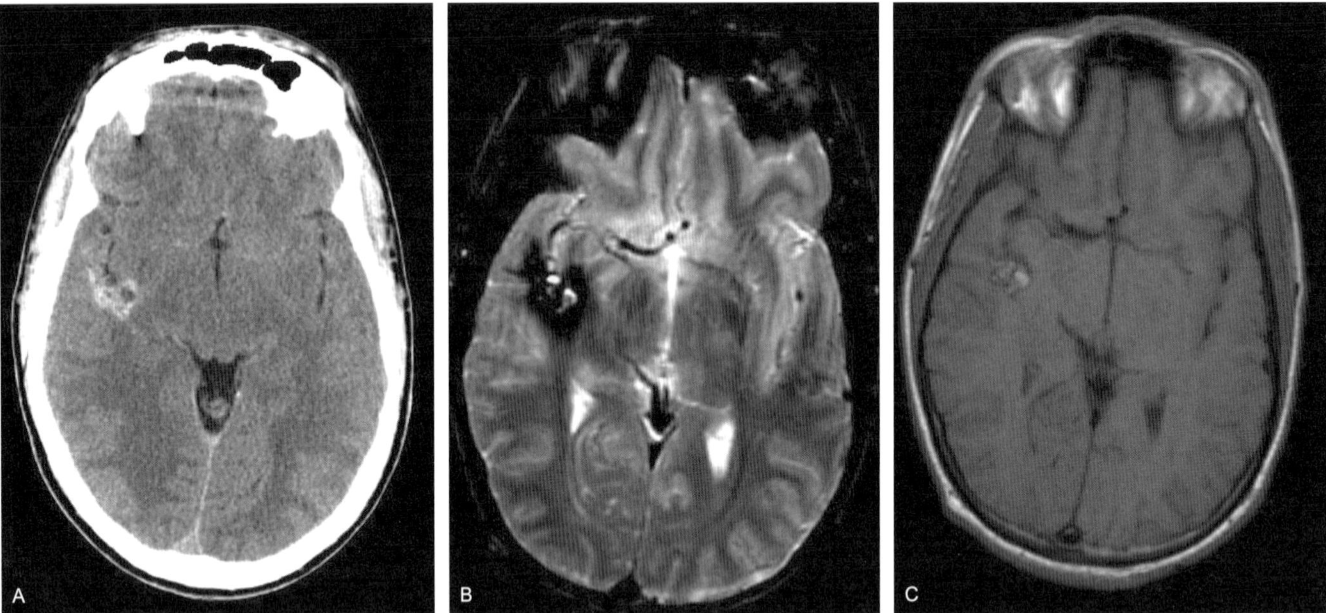

FIGURE 7-6 ■ A cavernous malformation with a small amount of acute, intracerebral hemorrhage surrounding it on CT (**A**). T2-weighted MRI (**B**) shows a lesion with a focal area of high signal intensity surrounded by a thick rim of hypointense hemisiderin. T1-weighted MRI (**C**) showing the typical "popcorn" appearance. The high signal intensity represents methemoglobin.

Hydrocephalus due to intraventricular extension or cerebrospinal fluid (CSF) outflow obstruction predicts in-hospital mortality: 51 percent of those with and 2 percent of those without hydrocephalus died in one series.[69] Lower Glasgow Coma Scale scores, greater age, location, and blood pressure or pulse pressure are other independent predictors of mortality. Simple multivariable prediction models have been developed and validated.[70,71]

Urgent head CT is required in patients with suspected intracerebral hemorrhage. MRI is as sensitive as CT for detecting hemorrhage and is more sensitive for detecting an underlying structural etiology, but the rapidity, availability, and ease of interpretation of CT favor its initial use. Contrast-enhanced head CT scan may show evidence of persistent hemorrhage at the time of presentation, a sign associated with poor prognosis.[72] Vascular imaging is required

TABLE 7-3 ■ Clinical Presentation of Intracerebral Hemorrhage

Location	Occurrence	Clinical Signs	Nonhypertensive	Mortality
Putamen	28–42%	Motor and sensory deficit; depressed consciousness	10%	20%
Thalamus	10–26%	Sensory and motor deficit; depressed consciousness; homonymous hemianopia	10%	40%
Subcortical white matter (lobar)	19–30%	Higher incidence of seizures; coma unlikely; other symptoms depend on involved lobe	65%	20%
Cerebellum	8–15%	Ataxia, cranial neuropathies; ± depressed consciousness	15%	Coma 75% Other 17%
Brainstem	4–11%	Coma, decerebrate posturing, pinpoint reactive pupils, cranial neuropathies	30%	85%

Adapted from Thrift AG, Donnan GA, McNeil JJ: Epidemiology of intracerebral hemorrhage. Epidemiol Rev 17:361, 1995.

whenever aneurysmal subarachnoid hemorrhage is possible, such as in cases with a large amount of subarachnoid blood, and should be considered for all patients without a clear etiology who would be surgical candidates. Early MRI may be indicated if a structural etiology is suspected, but findings are often obscured by the hemorrhage, and a scan delayed by 4 to 8 weeks may provide more useful information if urgent diagnosis is unnecessary. MRI is useful in diagnosing cavernous malformations and may suggest cerebral amyloid angiopathy.

Treatment is generally supportive, although surgical intervention is indicated in some cases. Severe hypertension is common after intracerebral hemorrhage, in part because it is a response to elevated intracranial pressure and brain injury. In patients with a systolic blood pressure of 150 to 220 mmHg, acute lowering of systolic blood pressure to 140 mmHg is probably safe. Current consensus guidelines suggest treating with antihypertensive medications for systolic blood pressure greater than 180 mmHg or mean arterial pressure greater than 130 mmHg, though clinical trials to determine optimal blood pressure control after intracerebral hemorrhage are ongoing.[61] Increased intracranial pressure may lead to coma and is treated with extraventricular drainage, osmotherapy, or hyperventilation.

Surgical evacuation of primary intracerebral hemorrhages is commonly performed when there is posterior fossa hemorrhage with a risk of brainstem compression or when there is evolving neurologic deterioration in patients with lobar hemorrhages and other prognostic signs are favorable. A large, international trial randomized 1,033 subjects with supratentorial hemorrhage to receive early surgical evacuation of the hematoma or initial conservative treatment followed by surgical evacuation only if it was necessitated by neurologic deterioration. There was a favorable outcome at 6 months in 26 percent of those allocated to early surgery as compared with 24 percent in those allocated to initial conservative treatment ($P = 0.89$). In subgroup analysis, it appeared that early surgery was more effective than conservative therapy when the hematoma was 1 cm or less from the cortical surface. Additional trials will be needed to resolve the issue of early surgical benefit for superficial hematomas.[73]

After the acute period, aggressive treatment of hypertension is indicated. In addition to reducing cardiovascular disease and ischemic stroke, one study has shown that treating hypertension reduces the risk of intracerebral hemorrhage by more than 50 percent.[74]

LACUNAR INFARCT

The term *lacune* was first introduced in 1843 by M. Durand-Fardel to describe small, subcortical areas lacking gray and white matter. These lesions were attributed to infarct and associated with particular clinical presentations by Marie and Ferrand more than 50 years later. In the 1950s, Miller Fisher reintroduced the term into modern neurology.[75] In a rapid succession of articles, he described the clinical and pathologic presentation, recognized the importance of hypertension as an etiology, and developed a theory of pathogenesis that survives today.

Less than 2 cm in diameter, lacunes are small infarcts that result from occlusion of small penetrating branches arising from large arteries (Fig. 7-7). There is general agreement about the definition of lacune, but much argument about the interrelationship between lacunar infarcts, lacunar strokes (symptomatic lacunes), lacunar syndromes (symptom complexes often associated with lacunar strokes), and lacunar disease (lacunes due to intrinsic small-vessel changes). Arguments arise from imperfect correlations between these entities. First, not all lacunes produce lacunar strokes because some are silent. Second, lacunar syndromes are sometimes associated with large-vessel strokes. Third, lacunes are produced by intrinsic small-vessel disease and by other etiologies.

More than 50 percent of lacunes are located in the basal ganglia and thalamus, with the remainder in the internal capsule, pons, cerebellum, and subcortical white matter. Approximately 20 to 30 percent of ischemic strokes are due to lacunes. In a recent study, 23 percent of randomly selected subjects 65 years or older had a lacune on MR scanning, and 89 percent of those with a lacune denied a history of stroke or transient ischemic attack.[76] These "silent" lacunes were associated with impairment in cognitive and functional tasks, suggesting that the overall clinical burden of lacunes may be greater than previously suspected.

Hypertension is the most important risk factor for development of lacunes in multivariable models.[76,77] However, the strength of the association may be no greater for lacunes than for other forms

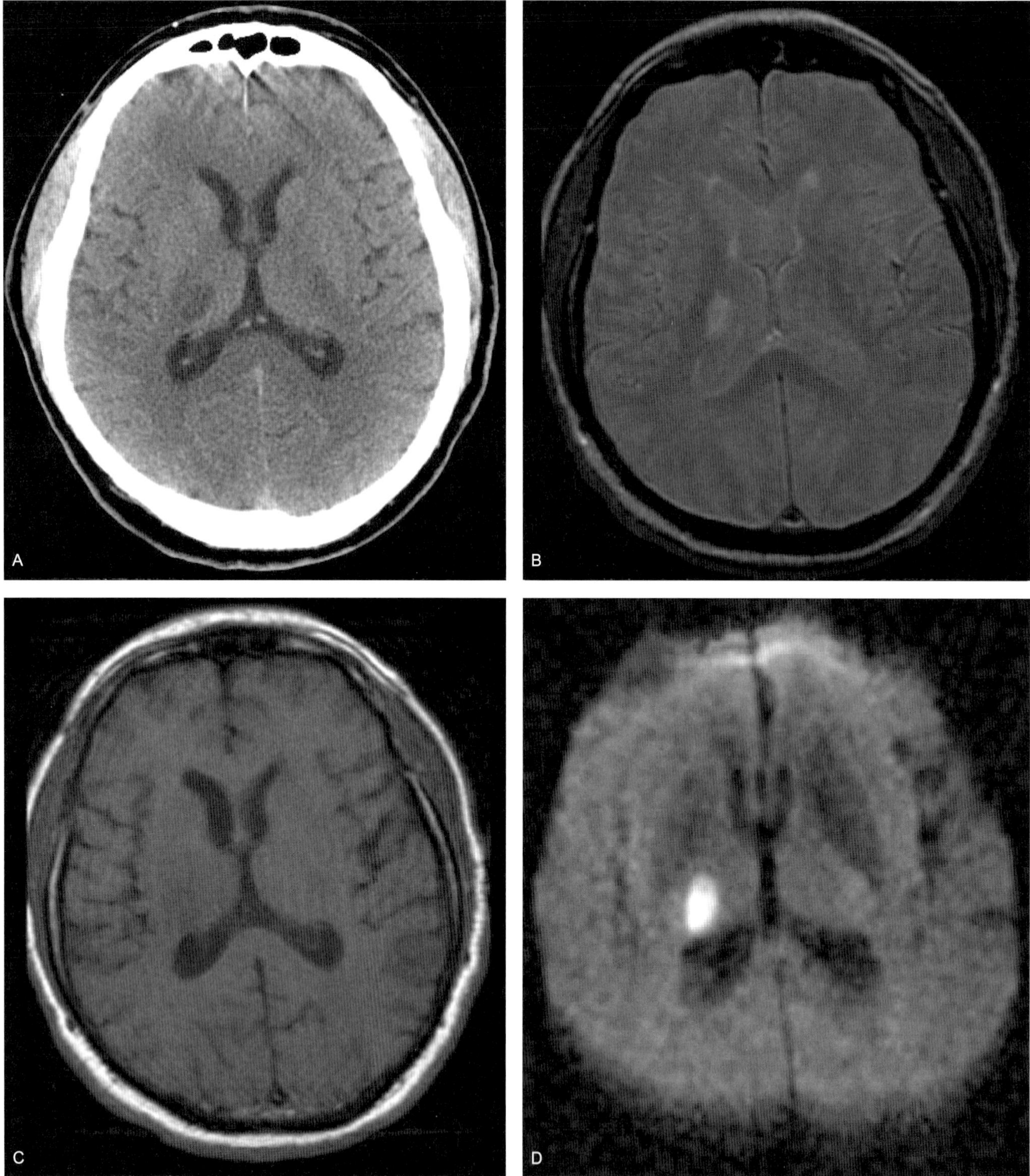

FIGURE 7-7 ■ An acute right thalamocapsular lacunar stroke producing a left sensorimotor syndrome. The lesion was hypodense on noncontrast head CT (**A**). With MRI, it was hyperintense on T2-weighted images (**B**), inconspicuous on T1-weighted images (**C**), and hyperintense on diffusion-weighted images (**D**).

of ischemic stroke,[78] and hypertension is not always present.[79] Elevation in the level of serum creatinine is independently associated with lacunar infarction, perhaps because it is a marker for chronic end-organ damage from hypertension.[76]

Diabetes mellitus is a risk factor for symptomatic lacunes, approximately doubling the risk. However, the influence of diabetes on lacunar stroke does not appear to differ from its effect on other ischemic stroke subtypes.[78] This is also true for cigarette smoking, which doubles the risk of all ischemic strokes, including lacunes. Carotid artery stenosis is associated with an increased risk of lacunar stroke, with more than twice the risk of a symptomatic lacune above a 50 percent or greater stenosis.[76] Cardiac disease is less common in patients with lacunes (20%) than in those with other ischemic stroke types (47%).[78]

The etiology of lacunes has been argued bitterly. Some have suggested that the vast majority of lacunes are due to changes within small penetrating vessels, primarily because of chronic hypertension,[80] but others have argued that emboli to small vessels and intracranial atherosclerosis are responsible for a significant number of lesions.[79] Fisher produced much of the data supporting an intrinsic small-vessel disease mechanism. He found degenerative changes in small vessels that he termed lipohyalinosis and fibrinoid degeneration, characterized by layers of connective tissue within the vascular media, obstructing the lumen.[81] These changes were proximal to infarcts in some cases. Atherosclerosis at the origin appeared responsible for other infarcts. Fisher recognized that emboli may be responsible for some lacunes.[81] Animal models have shown that particles may embolize to small penetrating arteries, producing lacunes.[82] The etiology of lacunes is likely multifactorial. Intrinsic small-vessel disease may predominate, but emboli and intracranial atherosclerosis almost certainly account for a significant minority of cases.

Several classic presentations of lacunar strokes have been described, termed the lacunar syndromes. Pure motor hemiparesis is the most common, accounting for 45 percent of cases. Motor functions involving face, arm, and leg are impaired, but other neurologic functions are spared. The appearance is different from that with cortical strokes, in which deficits in sensation or cognition often accompany motor changes. Pure motor hemiparesis is not always due to a lacune, with 10 to 20 percent of cases attributed to a cortical stroke. When a lacune is responsible, it is most often located in the posterior limb of the internal capsule or in the basis pontis, but any other site along the path of corticospinal fibers can produce the syndrome.

Sensorimotor syndrome is the second most common lacunar syndrome, accounting for 20 percent of cases.[78] Weakness and numbness are present in varying degrees, usually involving the face, arm, and leg. The syndrome is most commonly produced by a lacune involving the lateral thalamus and internal capsule, but 13 percent of cases are not due to lacunes.[78]

Ataxic hemiparesis accounts for 10 to 18 percent of lacunar syndromes.[78,83] In the affected limbs, pyramidal weakness is combined with elements normally attributed to cerebellar ataxia. Intention tremor, exaggerated rebound, and irregular rapid alternating movements are superimposed on ipsilateral weakness. The findings are highly suggestive of a lacunar stroke, with 95 percent attributable to lacunes.[78] Infarct locations are identical to those that cause pure motor hemiparesis.

Among patients with lacunar syndromes, 7 percent have a pure sensory stroke, characterized by impaired sensation without other accompanying neurologic deficits.[78,83] When the face, arm, and leg are involved, the lesion is nearly always a lacune in the contralateral thalamus. A lesion in the medial lemnicus in the midbrain or rostral pons may occasionally produce an identical syndrome. Pain and dysesthesia in the affected region may accompany the lesion acutely or may be delayed by weeks to months.

Many other lacunar syndromes have been described, including clumsy-hand dysarthria, hemiballism, and pure motor hemiparesis combined with various eye movement abnormalities.[81] Although lacunes occur more commonly in certain regions of the brain, they can occur anywhere, producing a multiplicity of potential syndromes.[79] Even signs generally attributed to cortical lesions may be produced by lacunes, including aphasia, abulia, confusion, and neglect.

Prognosis for recovery after a lacunar stroke is generally more favorable than for ischemic strokes due to occlusion of major vessels,[84] although symptoms may occasionally worsen in the first few days after symptom onset. Recurrent stroke and mortality rates are also lower than for other stroke subtypes.[85]

Lacunar syndromes may be produced by cortical strokes or even by small hemorrhages. Also, some lacunes may be associated with carotid disease or intracranial atherosclerosis, and knowledge of this could alter treatment decisions. Therefore, diagnostic imaging has been recommended for all those presenting with lacunar syndromes. An immediate head CT scan will rule out hemorrhage as an etiology but may not distinguish lacunes from large-vessel infarctions. MRI provides more definitive confirmation, and MR or CT angiography may suggest intracranial atherosclerosis. For lacunar strokes in the internal carotid distribution, carotid artery imaging should be performed because a stenosis proximal to the lacune would generally be considered symptomatic.

In the National Institute of Neurological Disorders and Stroke trial of tissue plasminogen activator, the drug was effective in the subgroup of patients judged to have small-vessel occlusive strokes prior to randomization.[84] In fact, absolute differences in favorable outcomes were greater for small-vessel strokes than for large-vessel occlusive and cardioembolic strokes, and differences in two indices reached statistical significance despite small numbers. Furthermore, the correlation between lacunar stroke and lacunar syndrome is so poor that a diagnosis of nonthrombotic small-vessel occlusion cannot be made with accuracy. Therefore, the current American Heart Association guidelines do not recommend avoiding tissue plasminogen activator in lacunar syndromes.[29] Other acute treatment for lacunar strokes is supportive.

Aspirin reduces the risk of subsequent ischemic stroke, regardless of etiology. Clopidogrel and the combination of dipyridamole/aspirin are alternatives for secondary prevention in those who cannot tolerate aspirin, although the incremental improvement in efficacy compared to aspirin is small.[86] Long-term use of aspirin and clopidogrel together to prevent recurrent stroke is generally not recommended. Among the 7,599 high-risk patients with recent stroke or transient ischemic attack in one trial, combination antiplatelet therapy did not reduce the rate of recurrent ischemic events compared to aspirin alone, but led to an increase in the rate of bleeding complications.[87] For lacunar stroke in particular, the risk of recurrent stroke among 3,020 patients with recent lacunar infarct was not significantly reduced with combination of aspirin and clopidogrel compared to aspirin alone.[88] Importantly though, there is emerging evidence to support the shorter-term (90-day) use of the combination of aspirin and clopidogrel over aspirin alone in patients with transient ischemic attack or minor stroke.[89,90]

Anticoagulation with warfarin is generally indicated in patients with ischemic stroke where atrial fibrillation is identified. Control of hypertension reduces subsequent ischemic stroke risk, and risk reduction may be even greater for lacunes. Treatment of isolated systolic hypertension in elderly patients halved the risk of lacunar stroke, a more dramatic effect than that seen for other ischemic strokes.[74]

PERIVENTRICULAR WHITE MATTER DISEASE

With improvements in head imaging, changes in the white matter surrounding the lateral ventricles are frequently recognized in the elderly, a finding termed *leukoaraiosis*. Head CT shows a periventricular mantle of hypodensity, often most profound at the frontal and occipital horns, which is hyperintense on T2-weighted MRI (Fig. 7-8). Age is the most important risk factor, with 96 percent of those older than 65 years showing at least some evidence of such change.[91] Clinically, the changes are most frequently associated with insidious declines in cognitive and motor performance, particularly on tests that depend on reaction time and speed.[91,92]

The white matter lesions have been related to several distinct pathologic processes, including hypoperfusion injury, cerebral amyloid angiopathy, dilated perivascular spaces, axonal loss, astrocytic gliosis, and loss of ependymal integrity with resulting cerebrospinal fluid extravasation. Lesions contiguous with the ventricles show fewer histologic and molecular markers of ischemia than lesions in the deep subcortical areas, where they resemble areas of "incomplete" infarction on pathologic examination.[93] Loss of vasomotor reactivity and autoregulation due to small-vessel vasculopathy is hypothesized to be a frequent cause of the ischemic changes.[94] Leukoaraiosis may be an important clinical indicator of end-organ injury from hypertension, integrating information about cumulative exposure to high blood pressure as well as susceptibility to injury. Individuals with white matter lesions in the brain are at high risk of incident stroke and other clinical cardiovascular events.[95] White matter burden is also one of the strongest predictors of incident brain infarction defined by serial brain MRI.[96]

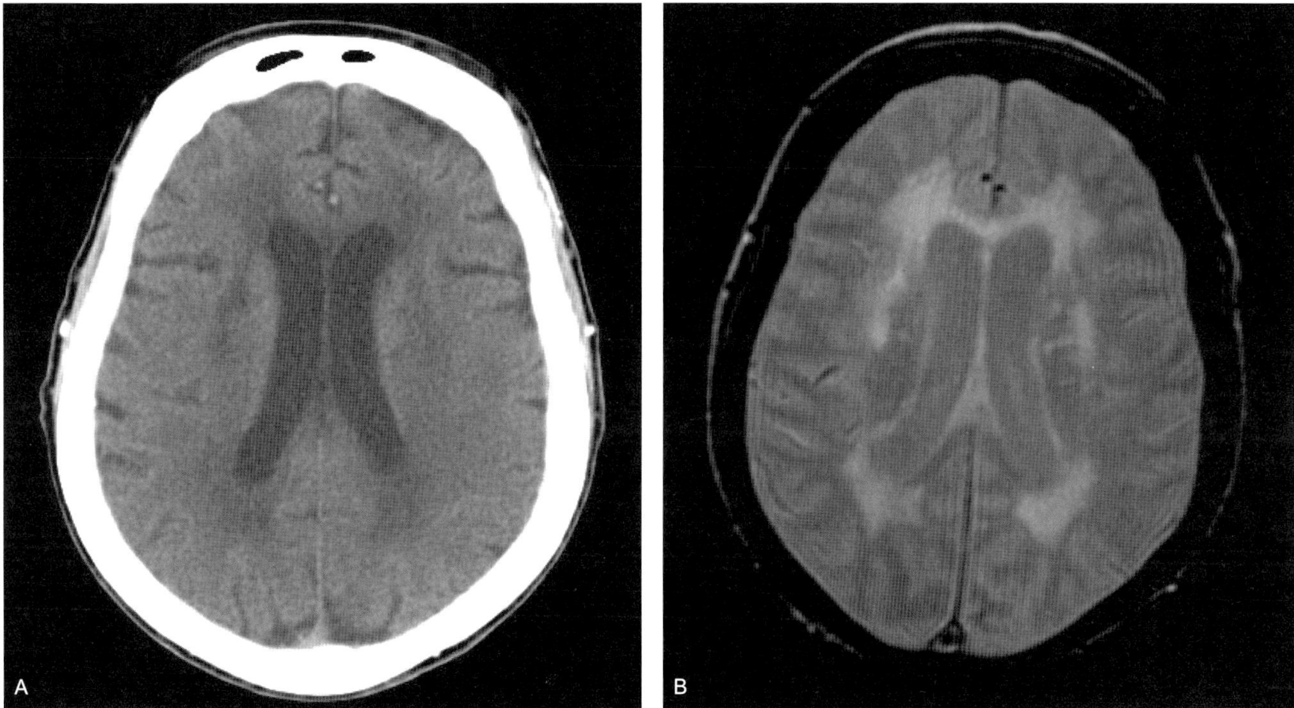

FIGURE 7-8 ■ Imaging findings of periventricular white matter disease, with hypodensity on head CT (**A**) and T2-weighted hyperintensities on MRI (**B**).

CADASIL

Cerebral autosomal-dominant arteriopathy with subcortical infarcts and leukoencephalopathy (CADASIL) is a dementing illness caused by mutations in the *NOTCH3* gene, which encodes a transmembrane receptor protein of unclear function and is characterized by a stepwise decline in cognitive and motor functions.[97] Onset is early, beginning at 30 to 50 years of age, and it is often preceded by migraines with aura. Hypertension and diabetes are not associated. Head imaging shows multiple lacunes superimposed on periventricular white matter disease.[98] Degeneration of vascular smooth muscle cells and granular deposits characterize vessels in the brain and in other regions. Involvement of the dermis allows confirmation by skin biopsy though molecular genetic tests are now available. No treatment is available.

CAROTID ARTERY STENOSIS

The first comprehensive description of carotid occlusion and stroke is attributed to Hunt, who in 1914 described a patient with decreased carotid pulsation contralateral to a hemiparesis. Autopsy confirmed a hemispheric infarct and showed patent intracranial vessels. With the advent of angiography and surgical exploration, internal carotid artery occlusion with recent thrombus was confirmed in the 1940s.

The precise contribution of internal carotid artery stenosis to the incidence of stroke is unclear because it is difficult to definitively attribute a stroke to the stenosis. The Stroke Data Bank of the National Institute of Neurological Disorders and Stroke classified 69 of 1,273 ischemic stroke cases as atherothrombotic and 41 as embolic due to severe carotid stenosis or occlusion.[99,100] Based on these numbers, approximately 9 percent of ischemic strokes are due to internal carotid stenosis or occlusion. In one study, 34 percent of randomly selected subjects aged 45 to 64 years had evidence of carotid plaque on ultrasonography.[101] An asymptomatic carotid stenosis of more than 60 percent is found in approximately 5 percent of 65-year-olds and increases with age.[102]

Hypertension is an important risk factor for carotid stenosis. In the Framingham study, systolic hypertension was a powerful predictor of subsequent carotid stenosis, with twice the odds for each 20-mmHg increase in systolic blood pressure.[103] Systolic blood pressure is also a predictor of progression in patients with asymptomatic stenoses.[104] Cigarette smoking, high serum cholesterol level, and increased homocysteine are other risk factors for carotid stenosis.[103]

Internal carotid artery stenosis is produced by atherosclerosis just distal to the common carotid bifurcation. The pathophysiology of carotid artery stenosis is complex. Hypertension induces vascular remodeling, resulting in medial thickening, luminal narrowing, and impaired smooth muscle relaxation.[7] These changes are concentrated in areas of nonlaminar flow, such as the common carotid bifurcation. Atherosclerotic plaques are thought to develop in these areas as a response to injury produced by hypertension, blood-flow abnormalities, lipids, and possibly infection.[9] This initiating injury induces endothelial cell expression of cell adhesion molecules that mediate local extravasation of mononuclear cells, resulting in inflammation of vessel walls, with foamy, lipid-laden macrophages and T lymphocytes. Chronic injury leads to intimal hyperplasia and formation of complex plaques that may include a lipid core. When a plaque ruptures into the vessel lumen, thrombosis is induced, which may produce local occlusion, distal embolus, or, after organization, progressive luminal stenosis. Shear forces associated with a severe stenosis may induce platelet activation and thrombus formation without plaque rupture.

Clinically, symptomatic patients present with large-vessel ischemic strokes or transient ischemic attacks in the distribution of the ophthalmic, middle, or anterior cerebral artery. Transient monocular blindness (amaurosis fugax), weakness, numbness, aphasia, or neglect may occur, depending on the affected region of the anterior circulation. Borderzone ischemia due to distal hypoperfusion in the anterior and middle cerebral artery territories presents with proximal upper and lower extremity weakness and numbness ("man-in-the-barrel" syndrome) and may indicate a critical stenosis or occlusion with inadequate collateral blood flow. Artery-to-artery emboli classically appear as cortical wedge-shaped infarcts, indistinguishable from emboli from other sources. Lacunar infarcts, often attributed to intrinsic small-vessel disease, probably represent embolic events from carotid artery stenoses in some instances because endarterectomy appears to reduce the risk of ipsilateral lacune.[105]

A cervical bruit may be a sign of carotid stenosis, but it is absent in 25 to 40 percent of cases later confirmed to have stenosis exceeding 70 percent and is present in 25 to 40 percent of those without a severe stenosis.[106] Therefore, carotid imaging studies are generally indicated for patients with anterior circulation ischemic strokes or transient ischemic attacks.

Carotid Doppler ultrasonography, neck MR angiography, CT angiography, or catheter angiography is required for the determination of whether an internal carotid stenosis is present. Catheter angiography is considered the gold standard but carries a small procedural risk. Therefore, it is generally preferable to obtain noninvasive imaging first. Carotid Doppler ultrasonography is widely available and is usually less expensive. CT angiography may be helpful to quickly exclude significant internal carotid artery stenosis at initial presentation.[107] MR angiography provides three-dimensional views and can be extended to include the intracranial vasculature. When the findings on one of these noninvasive imaging studies are positive, a second noninvasive study confirming the degree of stenosis may obviate the need for catheter angiography.

From the societal perspective, screening patients for asymptomatic carotid stenosis does not appear to be cost-effective.[102] Because of the limited benefit of surgery and the costs of carotid ultrasonography, the pretest probability of finding a stenosis must be greater than 40 percent before it is cost-effective to screen those without symptoms. Carotid ultrasonography probably is not cost-effective even in asymptomatic elderly patients with bruits because the pretest probability of finding a high-grade stenosis is only approximately 15 percent, given the 5 percent prevalence of a high-grade stenosis in those older than 65 years and a threefold increased likelihood of stenosis in those with a bruit.[106]

Aspirin has been shown to reduce risk of stroke and myocardial infarction in patients with ischemic stroke or transient ischemic attack, with a risk reduction of about 20 percent.[108] Some clinicians use anticoagulation with heparin to treat symptomatic carotid stenosis in the acute setting, but there are no reliable data supporting this approach. Based on results in coronary artery disease, a process with similar pathophysiology, and on overall risk reduction of ischemic stroke, treatment with cholesterol-lowering agents may be of benefit even in those without hypercholesterolemia.

Urgent surgical removal of the obstructing plaque by endarterectomy is the established standard of

TABLE 7-4 ■ Yearly Ipsilateral Stroke Rates with Carotid Artery Stenosis Based on 5-Year Follow-up

	Endarterectomy*	Medical Therapy	*P* Value	NNT 5-year†
Symptomatic stenosis				
NASCET ≥70%	2.6%	5.2%	<0.001	8
50–69%	3.1%	4.4%	0.045	15
30–49%	3.0%	3.7%	0.16	
ECST‡ ≥60%	1.8%	4.0%	<0.001	9
40–60%	2.8%	1.6%	NS	
Asymptomatic stenosis				
ACAS ≥60%	1.0%	2.2%	0.004	17

*Includes any perioperative stroke or death.
†NNT with surgery to prevent one ipsilateral stroke in 5 years.
‡Degree of stenosis converted to NASCET criteria (diameter at narrowest/diameter in most proximal normal internal carotid artery). End-point included perioperative death or major strokes and was calculated based on mean 6-year follow-up.
ACAS, Asymptomatic Carotid Atherosclerosis Study; ECST, European Carotid Surgery Trial; NASCET, North American Symptomatic Carotid Endarterectomy Trial; NNT, number needed to treat; NS, not significant.

therapy for symptomatic patients with carotid artery stenosis of at least 70 percent (Table 7-4).[109,110] Endarterectomy also reduces recurrent stroke rates in patients with symptomatic carotid stenoses of 50 to 69 percent, but the number needed to treat (NNT) to prevent one recurrent stroke is considerably higher in this group when compared to those with stenoses exceeding 70 percent (~15.4 to prevent one stroke over 5 years in those with 50 to 69 percent stenosis versus ~5.8 to prevent one stroke over 2 years in those with 70 to 99 percent stenosis).[105] Endarterectomy is not beneficial in patients with stenosis less than 50 percent and is generally impractical in those with carotid artery occlusion. The risk of stroke with medical therapy is greater in those with cerebral events than ocular events, with plaque surface irregularity consistent with ulceration, with a symptomatic event within 2 weeks of presentation, and with greater degrees of stenosis.[111] The risk of surgery is greater in females, in those with severe hypertension, and in those with peripheral vascular disease. These prognostic factors may be useful in fine-tuning patient selection for endarterectomy.

For patients with asymptomatic carotid artery stenosis, endarterectomy also prevents stroke when there is stenosis of at least 60 percent as assessed by carotid ultrasonography, but again the number needed to treat to prevent one stroke over 5 years remains large (~20), and therefore current guidelines recommend consideration of endarterectomy for asymptomatic stenosis for patients with a surgical risk less than 3 percent and life expectancy of at least 5 years.[31,112]

Endovascular angioplasty and stenting are an alternative approach to treatment of carotid stenosis, and stenting has been shown to be not inferior to endarterectomy in patients with both symptomatic and asymptomatic stenoses who have comorbidities associated with high surgical risk during endarterectomy.[113] A large-scale trial comparing endarterectomy and stenting in more representative patient populations showed comparable long-term outcomes, though there was an increased risk of periprocedural stroke in the endovascular group and a higher risk of myocardial infarction in the surgical group.[114]

INTRACRANIAL ATHEROSCLEROSIS

Atherosclerosis involving the large intracranial vessels causes about 8 percent of ischemic strokes.[115] African Americans, Hispanics, and Asians have a higher prevalence of intracranial atherosclerosis, and a relatively lower prevalence of extracranial carotid artery stenosis compared with whites.[115,116] Extracranial carotid atherosclerosis is associated with a higher prevalence of peripheral vascular and coronary artery disease, but intracranial atherosclerosis is not.[115] Given racial and risk factor distribution differences, it seems appropriate to consider intracranial atherosclerosis an entity distinct from carotid artery disease rather than as an additional manifestation of widespread atherosclerotic changes.

Hypertension is an important risk factor for intracranial atherosclerosis, with a two- to threefold higher risk of disease in those with a history of hypertension.[117] Smoking may be the most important risk factor, with a 50 percent increase in odds of disease for every 10 years of smoking. Diabetics have about three times the risk of developing intracranial atherosclerosis. Hypercholesterolemia also increases risk, but probably to a lesser degree. The relative contribution of these factors to intracranial atherosclerosis as opposed to other stroke subtypes is unclear. The distribution of known risk factors probably accounts for some of the racial differences.[115]

There are intriguing differences in the pathophysiology of intracranial atherosclerosis and other forms of vascular disease. Intracranial arteries are less susceptible to hypercholesterolemia than are extracranial arteries,[118] and atherosclerotic plaque rupture appears to be less common.[119] Release of endothelial adhesion molecules is greater with intracranial atherosclerosis than in other ischemic stroke subtypes, suggesting that inflammation is particularly important in its pathogenesis.[120]

Clinical presentation is characterized by large-vessel or penetrating artery ischemia. The middle cerebral artery is most commonly involved, followed in order by the basilar, intracranial internal carotid, anterior cerebral, and posterior cerebral arteries.[115] Thrombosis at the site of the stenosis may lead to hypoperfusion in the entire distal territory or artery-to-artery embolus indistinguishable from events caused by extracranial carotid artery stenosis or cardiac embolus. Basilar thrombosis may result from underlying atherosclerosis in the basilar or vertebral arteries or after cardiac embolus; it is a life-threatening, often delayed diagnosis characterized by coma, quadriplegia, and cranial nerve findings. Involvement of the origin of penetrating small vessels may produce lacunar infarctions. Presentation with transient ischemic attack prior to infarction is more common with intracranial atherosclerosis than with other stroke subtypes.

Intracranial MR or CT angiography may reveal narrowing or occlusion of large vessels. Time-of-flight MR angiography is prone to artifacts and may suggest a stenosis where none is present, and sensitivity is low for medium-sized and smaller vessels. CT angiography offers a true luminal image, but involves use of ionizing radiation. Transcranial Doppler ultrasonography shows increased blood-flow velocities in large stenotic vessels. Its sensitivity and specificity are also low, so it may be most useful as an adjunct. Catheter angiography is the gold standard for establishing the diagnosis, but it is associated with an approximately 1 percent stroke risk. Given the risk of angiography, it is justified only if results will alter treatment decisions.

Prognosis in symptomatic patients is poor but can be improved with aggressive medical therapy. Stenoses generally become more severe with time, but regression in some segments may occur. In the largest randomized trial of treatment for symptomatic intracranial atherosclerosis, the Warfarin-Aspirin Symptomatic Intracranial Disease (WASID) trial, 569 subjects were randomized to aspirin (1,300 mg/day) or warfarin (target international normalized ratio, or INR, of 2.0 to 3.0).[121] The trial was stopped early because of safety concerns among subjects randomized to warfarin, and there was no significant difference in the primary end-point of stroke, brain hemorrhage, or vascular death ($P = 0.83$). The 2-year rates of ischemic stroke were 19.7 percent in the aspirin group and 17.2 percent in the warfarin group ($P = 0.29$), indicating that intracranial atherosclerosis confers a high-risk for recurrent stroke. In a subsequent study, intracranial angioplasty and stenting was compared to an aggressive medical regimen. This trial was also stopped early because the aggressive medical therapy group, which included rosuvastatin and a combination of aspirin and clopidogrel for 90 days, had a significantly lower 30-day stroke or death rate (5.8 percent) than the endovascular group (14.7 percent).[89] The aggressive medical therapy group's event rate was also lower than the historical event rate reported in WASID (10.7 percent), which some speculate is due to improvements in medical therapy over the last several years.

Patients with intracranial atherosclerosis also have a theoretical risk of hypoperfusion distal to the stenosis when blood pressure is lowered. Since these lesions are less commonly corrected compared with those in the carotid artery, some physicians may be less aggressive about treating hypertension in these patients. There is currently no evidence to justify higher long-term blood pressure thresholds in patients with intracranial atherosclerosis or to support the belief that lower blood pressures could increase the risk of infarction distal to a stenosis.[122] In fact, targeted blood pressure management was an important component of the aggressive medical treatment in the trial comparing it with angioplasty and stenting.[89]

AORTIC ARCH ATHEROSCLEROSIS

The aortic arch has come to be appreciated as a source of emboli to the brain.[123] An autopsy study found a 28 percent prevalence of ulcerated plaque in the aortic arch of patients with ischemic stroke compared with a 5 percent prevalence in a control population.[123] Transesophageal echocardiograms show evidence of a thickened aortic arch in 14 percent of stroke patients and 2 percent of control subjects.[124] In those with no other identified etiology, a thickened aortic arch is present in 28 percent. Aortic arch atherosclerosis is more strongly associated with peripheral vascular disease than with carotid stenosis.[125] Epidemiologic studies have been small, and only cigarette smoking has been identified as an important risk factor. Hypertension, diabetes, and hypercholesterolemia may be risk factors, but this has not been confirmed.

Strokes and transient ischemic attacks produced by aortic atherosclerosis are identical to those produced by cardiac sources of emboli. Large-vessel territories are generally affected, producing weakness and numbness in similar distributions or cortical signs, such as aphasia and neglect.

Stroke patients with atherosclerotic plaque 4 mm thick or larger in the aortic arch have a fourfold increase in the risk of recurrence after correcting for other risk factors.[125] A large study comparing the combination of aspirin and clopidogrel to warfarin to prevent recurrent stroke in patients with aortic arch disease has recently completed enrollment and when reported may provide additional information on the optimal treatment for these patients.[126] Aortic endarterectomy has been performed in some patients who have failed medical therapy, but it has not been studied systematically.

CARDIAC EMBOLUS

Hypertension increases the risk of myocardial infarction and atrial fibrillation. These diseases are associated with increased stroke risk from cardiac embolus, as discussed in Chapter 5.

DEMENTIA

There is evidence from multiple cohort studies that cardiovascular risk factors, including hypertension, are risk factors for the development of dementia and cognitive impairment.[127–129] The biologic basis for these associations remains unresolved. Although there are some data to support a direct association between hypertension and Alzheimer pathology,[130] there is increasing recognition that most individuals with dementia have a combination of neurodegenerative and vascular pathology.[131] The association between hypertension and dementia is likely to be mediated in part by the accumulation of subclinical vascular injury in the brain, including infarct and leukoaraiosis, that results in the interruption of cognitive networks. Whether this process is simply additive to the cognitive effects of Alzheimer pathology or whether there is synergism between the two processes remains unresolved.

There is currently no convincing evidence that treatment of hypertension will make a large impact on the occurrence of dementia outside its established benefits for stroke prevention. Although one large primary prevention trial using the calcium-channel blocker nitrendipine found that the risk of dementia was reduced by 50 percent in those receiving active therapy, the finding has not been confirmed in other trials.[132–134] In one trial, which included subjects exclusively with a history of stroke, active therapy with perindopril and indapamide reduced the risk of dementia overall, but the benefit was not statistically significant when the analysis was restricted to those without recurrent stroke.[135]

Although it hardly seems necessary to define additional benefits of treating hypertension, the recognition that cognitive decline may be an important manifestation of end-organ injury from hypertension has important implications for testing new treatments for cerebrovascular disease, assessing risk of stroke, and encouraging adherence to treatment.[136] If hypertension therapy is proven to prevent dementia among those without stroke, the cost–benefit ratio for more aggressive screening and therapy could also be substantially improved, an important issue given that the elderly, who are at highest risk of dementia, are also the least likely to have their hypertension adequately treated. Some have suggested that aggressive blood pressure reduction could worsen cognition, particularly among those with loss of cerebral autoregulation due to small-vessel arteriopathy.[137] Therefore, the benefits of blood pressure therapy for cognition will need better definition in order to optimize treatment regimens.

HYPERTENSIVE ENCEPHALOPATHY

Hypertensive encephalopathy is one of several forms of posterior reversible encephalopathy, a syndrome also encompassing other etiologies, including renal failure, immunosuppressive therapy, and eclampsia.[138]

The incidence of hypertensive encephalopathy is thought to have declined with greater use of antihypertensives. It tends to occur with a sudden elevation in blood pressure rather than with chronic hypertension. A number of medical conditions are known precipitants. Hyperadrenergic states may be responsible, including pheochromocytoma, tyramine ingestion with monoamine oxidase inhibitors, abrupt antihypertensive discontinuation, lower gastrointestinal irritation in paraplegic patients, and stimulant medications.[139] Structural precipitants include aortic coarctation and renal artery stenosis. Acute or chronic renal failure is another cause, probably through volume overload in addition to hypertension, and human recombinant erythropoietin may be a precipitant.[140] In patients in the postoperative period after endarterectomy, changes ipsilateral to the surgery may be identical to those seen with hypertensive encephalopathy, even in the absence of blood pressure elevation, probably because vessels compensate for chronic hypoperfusion distal to a severe stenosis and sudden return of blood flow produces relative hypertension.

Hypertensive encephalopathy is associated with vasogenic cerebral edema, particularly severe in the posterior regions of the cerebral hemispheres, which is sometimes sufficient to result in herniation. The pathophysiology linking hypertension and cerebral edema has been argued. At mean arterial pressures greater than 120 to 170 mmHg, cerebral blood flow increases linearly with blood pressure, and some have argued that this is the threshold for hypertensive encephalopathy, when a "breakthrough of autoregulation" occurs.[138,141] Angiotensin II may contribute to the formation of edema by increasing cerebrovascular permeability through oxygen free radicals.[142] A predilection toward involvement of the posterior hemispheres may be due to differential vascular innervation by the sympathetic nervous system.[141]

Hypertensive encephalopathy is a neurologic emergency that can lead to death if untreated. Diagnosis may be delayed when the connection between acute neurologic dysfunction and hypertension is not obvious. High blood pressure may be attributed to an underlying neurologic condition or agitation rather than identified as the causative agent. Headache is a common early complaint, sometimes accompanied by nausea and vomiting. Confusion with either agitation or lethargy may proceed to obtundation and coma if the process is untreated. Visual disturbance is frequent due to involvement of the retina and occipital lobes, with papilledema and subjective blurred vision, hemianopia, or cortical blindness.[138] Other cortical deficits may occur, including neglect, aphasia, and weakness. Focal or generalized seizures may complicate the course.

Head imaging should be performed to exclude hemorrhage or a structural etiology for both the encephalopathy and the hypertension. Since increased intracranial pressure can result in severe hypertension, which may be required to maintain cerebral perfusion, an urgent study is necessary. Head CT may show hypodensity in subcortical white matter, often most obvious in the occipital lobes (Fig. 7-9). MRI findings may be dramatic, with multifocal T2-weighted hyperintensities particularly apparent in fluid-attenuated inversion recovery sequences. These changes are distinguished from infarcts by sparing of the cortex and absence of reduced diffusion, as expected with vasogenic edema.[26] Because cerebral edema may be severe, lumbar puncture should be avoided.

Once a structural etiology has been excluded, treatment of hypertension must be initiated. Target blood pressures are tailored to individual patients, with the goal of returning patients to their recent baseline. For patients without a history of hypertension, normal blood pressure parameters are appropriate, but for those with chronic hypertension, an abrupt return to 140/90 mmHg may result in hypoperfusion owing to chronic vascular compensatory changes. Close observation and intravenous antihypertensives are generally indicated. Nitroprusside is a good choice because of its effectiveness, rapid onset, and ease of adjustment. It produces some cerebral vasodilation, but there is no clinical evidence that this elevates the risk of herniation. Intravenous dihydropyridine calcium-channel blocking agents and ACE inhibitors are also effective and easy to titrate and may have less-profound effects on cerebral vessels. The underlying cause of the hypertensive episode should be sought. Prognosis in treated patients is generally excellent. Neurologic deficits usually recover completely within 2 weeks.

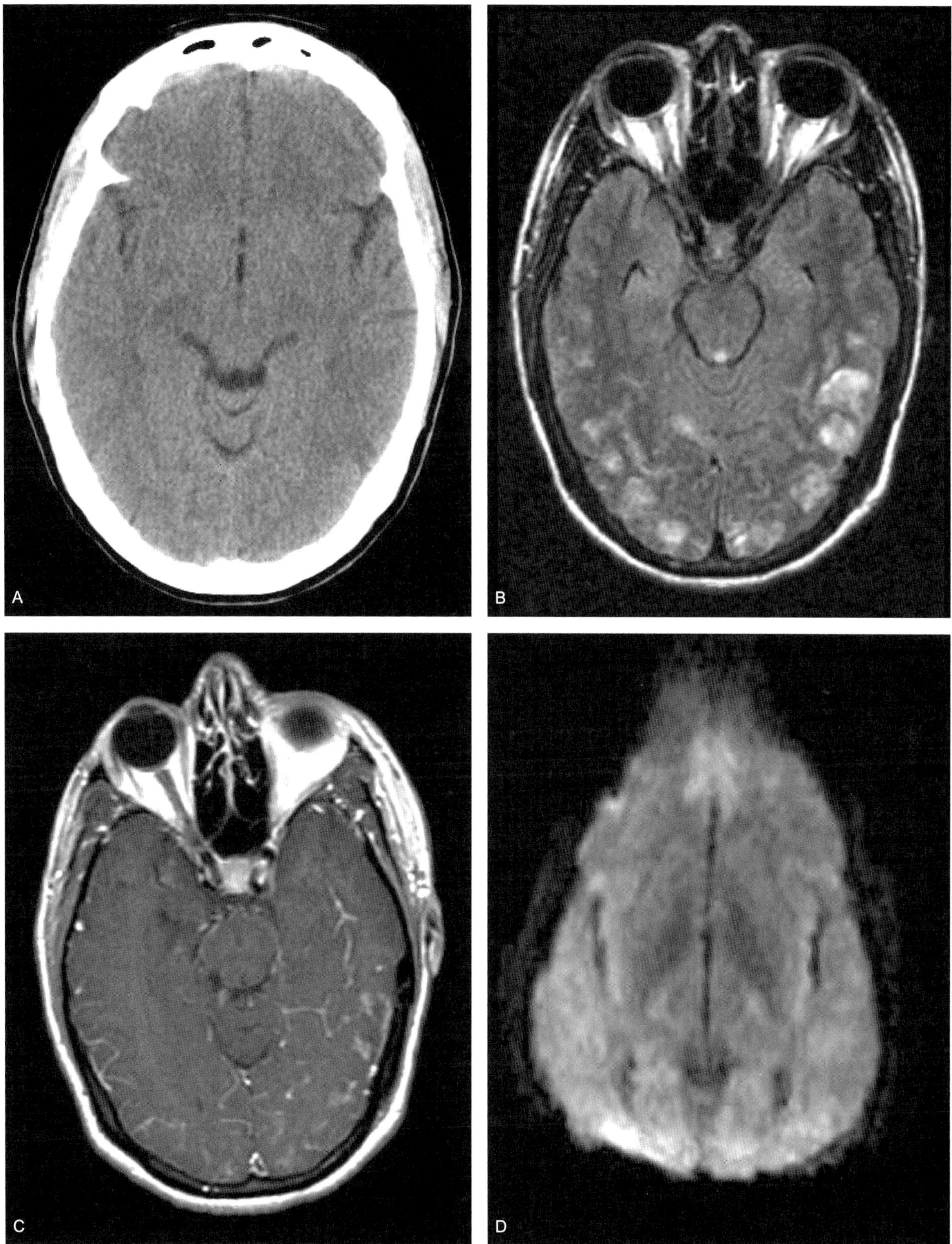

FIGURE 7-9 ■ A patient with eclampsia. Typical findings in hypertensive encephalopathy are identical and include normal or subtle hypodensity on CT (**A**), subcortical hyperintensities on MRI fluid-attenuated inversion recovery (FLAIR) (**B**), enhancement with gadolinium on T1-weighted images (**C**), and no abnormality on diffusion-weighted MRI (**D**).

ECLAMPSIA

Eclampsia is a form of posterior reversible encephalopathy. Occurring during the second half of pregnancy or the puerperium, eclampsia presents with proteinuria and clinical and imaging manifestations identical to hypertensive encephalopathy. Hypertension may not be severe, so additional effects on brain endothelial cell permeability are probably important. There is evidence of generalized endothelial cell dysfunction with abnormal vascular reactivity.[143] An underlying inflammatory response may be causative, but other potential etiologies have also been hypothesized.

Cerebral venous sinus thrombosis is another complication of pregnancy and delivery and can present with findings similar to those seen with eclampsia. MRI and venography are usually adequate to distinguish the two diseases, showing obstructed venous sinuses or ischemia with cytotoxic edema on diffusion-weighted sequences in cerebral venous sinus thrombosis.

Treatment includes delivery of the fetus and intravenous magnesium.[144] Other antihypertensive medications and anticonvulsants can also be used. Prognosis is good if treatment is initiated quickly.

IMMUNOSUPPRESSION

Several immunosuppressive agents produce a posterior reversible encephalopathy identical to hypertensive encephalopathy. Cyclosporine is the most commonly identified, and it may produce neurologic symptoms at therapeutic levels and without evident hypertension. Tacrolimus, interferon-α, cytarabine, and fludarabine have also been associated.[138] An alteration in the permeability of cerebral endothelial cells has been postulated. Lowering blood pressure and discontinuing immunosuppression generally reverses the process.

REFERENCES

1. Go AS, Mozaffarian D, Roger VL, et al: Heart disease and stroke statistics—2013 update: a report from the American Heart Association. Circulation 127:e6, 2013.
2. Kearney PM, Whelton M, Reynolds K, et al: Global burden of hypertension: analysis of worldwide data. Lancet 365:217, 2005.
3. Vasan RS, Beiser A, Seshadri S, et al: Residual lifetime risk for developing hypertension in middle-aged women and men: The Framingham Heart Study. JAMA 287:1003, 2002.
4. MacMahon S, Peto R, Cutler J, et al: Blood pressure, stroke, and coronary heart disease. Part 1, Prolonged differences in blood pressure: prospective observational studies corrected for the regression dilution bias. Lancet 335:765, 1990.
5. Chobanian AV, Bakris GL, Black HR, et al: The Seventh Report of the Joint National Committee on Prevention, Detection, Evaluation, and Treatment of High Blood Pressure: the JNC 7 report. JAMA 289:2560, 2003.
6. Johansson BB: Hypertension mechanisms causing stroke. Clin Exp Pharmacol Physiol 26:563, 1999.
7. Gibbons GH, Dzau VJ: The emerging concept of vascular remodeling. N Engl J Med 330:1431, 1994.
8. Heistad DD, Baumbach GL: Cerebral vascular changes during chronic hypertension: good guys and bad guys. J Hypertens Suppl 10:S71, 1992.
9. Ross R: Atherosclerosis—an inflammatory disease. N Engl J Med 340:115, 1999.
10. Rossi G, Rossi A, Sacchetto A, et al: Hypertensive cerebrovascular disease and the renin-angiotensin system. Stroke 26:1700, 1995.
11. Pickering TG, Hall JE, Appel LJ, et al: Recommendations for blood pressure measurement in humans and experimental animals: part 1: blood pressure measurement in humans: a statement for professionals from the Subcommittee of Professional and Public Education of the American Heart Association Council on High Blood Pressure Research. Circulation 111:697, 2005.
12. Akpunonu BE, Mulrow PJ, Hoffman EA: Secondary hypertension: evaluation and treatment. Dis Mon 42:609, 1996.
13. Appel LJ, Moore TJ, Obarzanek E, et al: A clinical trial of the effects of dietary patterns on blood pressure. DASH Collaborative Research Group. N Engl J Med 336:1117, 1997.
14. ALLHAT Officers Coordinators for the ALLHAT Collaborative Research Group: Major outcomes in high-risk hypertensive patients randomized to angiotensin-converting enzyme inhibitor or calcium channel blocker vs diuretic: the Antihypertensive and Lipid-Lowering Treatment to Prevent Heart Attack Trial (ALLHAT). JAMA 288:2981, 2002.
15. Sacco RL: Risk factors and outcomes for ischemic stroke. Neurology 45:S10, 1995.
16. Gorelick PB: Stroke prevention. An opportunity for efficient utilization of health care resources during the coming decade. Stroke 25:220, 1994.
17. Collins R, Peto R, MacMahon S, et al: Blood pressure, stroke, and coronary heart disease. Part 2, Short-term reductions in blood pressure: overview of randomised drug trials in their epidemiological context. Lancet 335:827, 1990.
18. SHEP Cooperative Research Group Prevention of stroke by antihypertensive drug treatment in older

persons with isolated systolic hypertension. Final results of the Systolic Hypertension in the Elderly Program (SHEP). SHEP Cooperative Research Group. JAMA 265:3255, 1991.

19. Staessen JA, Fagard R, Thijs L, et al: Randomised double-blind comparison of placebo and active treatment for older patients with isolated systolic hypertension. The Systolic Hypertension in Europe (Syst-Eur) Trial Investigators. Lancet 350:757, 1997.
20. Gueyffier F, Bulpitt C, Boissel JP, et al: Antihypertensive drugs in very old people: a subgroup meta-analysis of randomised controlled trials. INDANA Group. Lancet 353:793, 1999.
21. Thom TJ: Stroke mortality trends. An international perspective. Ann Epidemiol 3:509, 1993.
22. Lim SS, Vos T, Flaxman AD, et al: A comparative risk assessment of burden of disease and injury attributable to 67 risk factors and risk factor clusters in 21 regions, 1990–2010: a systematic analysis for the Global Burden of Disease Study 2010. Lancet 380:2224, 2012.
23. Wang H, Dwyer-Lindgren L, Lofgren KT, et al: Age-specific and sex-specific mortality in 187 countries, 1970–2010: a systematic analysis for the Global Burden of Disease Study 2010. Lancet 380:2071, 2012.
24. Johnston SC, Mendis S, Mathers CD: Global variation in stroke burden and mortality: estimates from monitoring, surveillance, and modelling. Lancet Neurol 8:345, 2009.
25. Meyer JS, Shimazu K, Fukuuchi Y, et al: Impaired neurogenic cerebrovascular control and dysautoregulation after stroke. Stroke 4:169, 1973.
26. Schwartz RB, Mulkern RV, Gudbjartsson H, et al: Diffusion-weighted MR imaging in hypertensive encephalopathy: clues to pathogenesis. AJNR Am J Neuroradiol 19:859, 1998.
27. Britton M, de Faire U, Helmers C: Hazards of therapy for excessive hypertension in acute stroke. Acta Med Scand 207:253, 1980.
28. Ahmed N, Nasman P, Wahlgren NG: Effect of intravenous nimodipine on blood pressure and outcome after acute stroke. Stroke 31:1250, 2000.
29. Jauch EC, Saver JL, Adams Jr HP, et al: Guidelines for the early management of patients with acute ischemic stroke: a guideline for healthcare professionals from the American Heart Association/American Stroke Association. Stroke 44:870, 2013.
30. PROGRESS Collaborative Group Randomised trial of a perindopril-based blood-pressure-lowering regimen among 6,105 individuals with previous stroke or transient ischaemic attack. Lancet 358:1033, 2001.
31. Furie KL, Kasner SE, Adams RJ, et al: Guidelines for the prevention of stroke in patients with stroke or transient ischemic attack: a guideline for healthcare professionals from the American Heart Association/ American Stroke Association. Stroke 42:227, 2011.
32. Dahlof B, Devereux RB, Kjeldsen SE, et al: Cardiovascular morbidity and mortality in the Losartan Intervention For Endpoint reduction in hypertension study (LIFE): a randomised trial against atenolol. Lancet 359:995, 2002.
33. Sandset EC, Bath PM, Boysen G, et al: The angiotensin-receptor blocker candesartan for treatment of acute stroke (SCAST): a randomised, placebo-controlled, double-blind trial. Lancet 377:741, 2011.
34. Ovbiagele B, Saver JL, Fredieu A, et al: PROTECT: a coordinated stroke treatment program to prevent recurrent thromboembolic events. Neurology 63:1217, 2004.
35. Taylor CL, Yuan Z, Selman WR, et al: Cerebral arterial aneurysm formation and rupture in 20,767 elderly patients: hypertension and other risk factors. J Neurosurg 83:812, 1995.
36. Teunissen LL, Rinkel GJ, Algra A, et al: Risk factors for subarachnoid hemorrhage: a systematic review. Stroke 27:544, 1996.
37. Longstreth Jr WT, Nelson LM, Koepsell TD, et al: Cigarette smoking, alcohol use, and subarachnoid hemorrhage. Stroke 23:1242, 1992.
38. Johnston SC, Colford Jr JM, Gress DR: Oral contraceptives and the risk of subarachnoid hemorrhage: a meta-analysis. Neurology 51:411, 1998.
39. Schievink WI: Intracranial aneurysms. N Engl J Med 336:28, 1997.
40. Broderick JP, Brown Jr RD, Sauerbeck L, et al: Greater rupture risk for familial as compared to sporadic unruptured intracranial aneurysms. Stroke 40:1952, 2009.
41. The Magnetic Resonance Angiography in Relatives of Patients with Subarachnoid Hemorrhage Study Group: Risks and benefits of screening for intracranial aneurysms in first-degree relatives of patients with sporadic subarachnoid hemorrhage. N Engl J Med 341:1344, 1999.
42. Schievink WI: Genetics and aneurysm formation. Neurosurg Clin N Am 9:485, 1998.
43. Vlak MH, Algra A, Brandenburg R, et al: Prevalence of unruptured intracranial aneurysms, with emphasis on sex, age, comorbidity, country, and time period: a systematic review and meta-analysis. Lancet Neurol 10:626, 2011.
44. Rinkel GJ, Djibuti M, Algra A, et al: Prevalence and risk of rupture of intracranial aneurysms: a systematic review. Stroke 29:251, 1998.
45. Smith-Bindman R, Miglioretti DL, Johnson E, et al: Use of diagnostic imaging studies and associated radiation exposure for patients enrolled in large integrated health care systems, 1996–2010. JAMA 307:2400, 2012.
46. Wiebers DO, Torner JC, Meissner I: Impact of unruptured intracranial aneurysms on public health in the United States. Stroke 23:1416, 1992.
47. Day JW, Raskin NH: Thunderclap headache: symptom of unruptured cerebral aneurysm. Lancet 2:1247, 1986.
48. Atlas SW, Sheppard L, Goldberg HI, et al: Intracranial aneurysms: detection and characterization with MR angiography with use of an advanced postprocessing technique in a blinded-reader study. Radiology 203:807, 1997.

49. McKinney AM, Palmer CS, Truwit CL, et al: Detection of aneurysms by 64-section multidetector CT angiography in patients acutely suspected of having an intracranial aneurysm and comparison with digital subtraction and 3D rotational angiography. AJNR Am J Neuroradiol 29:594, 2008.
50. Wiebers DO, Whisnant JP, Huston 3rd J, et al: Unruptured intracranial aneurysms: natural history, clinical outcome, and risks of surgical and endovascular treatment. Lancet 362:103, 2003.
51. Johnston SC, Wilson CB, Halbach VV, et al: Endovascular and surgical treatment of unruptured cerebral aneurysms: comparison of risks. Ann Neurol 48:11, 2000.
52. Johnston SC, Gress DR, Kahn JG: Which unruptured cerebral aneurysms should be treated? A cost-utility analysis. Neurology 52:1806, 1999.
53. Johnston SC, Selvin S, Gress DR: The burden, trends, and demographics of mortality from subarachnoid hemorrhage. Neurology 50:1413, 1998.
54. Hop JW, Rinkel GJ, Algra A, et al: Case-fatality rates and functional outcome after subarachnoid hemorrhage: a systematic review. Stroke 28:660, 1997.
55. Taylor TN, Davis PH, Torner JC, et al: Lifetime cost of stroke in the United States. Stroke 27:1459, 1996.
56. Kassell NF, Torner JC, Haley Jr EC, et al: The International Cooperative Study on the Timing of Aneurysm Surgery. Part 1: overall management results. J Neurosurg 73:18, 1990.
57. Germanson TP, Lanzino G, Kongable GL, et al: Risk classification after aneurysmal subarachnoid hemorrhage. Surg Neurol 49:155, 1998.
58. Connolly Jr ES, Rabinstein AA, Carhuapoma JR, et al: Guidelines for the management of aneurysmal subarachnoid hemorrhage: a guideline for healthcare professionals from the American Heart Association/American Stroke Association. Stroke 43:1711, 2012.
59. Grosset DG, Straiton J, McDonald I, et al: Use of transcranial Doppler sonography to predict development of a delayed ischemic deficit after subarachnoid hemorrhage. J Neurosurg 78:183, 1993.
60. Thrift AG, Donnan GA, McNeil JJ: Epidemiology of intracerebral hemorrhage. Epidemiol Rev 17:361, 1995.
61. Morgenstern LB, Hemphill JC, Anderson C, et al: Guidelines for the management of spontaneous intracerebral hemorrhage: a guideline for healthcare professionals from the American Heart Association/American Stroke Association. Stroke 41:2108, 2010.
62. Broderick JP, Brott T, Tomsick T, et al: The risk of subarachnoid and intracerebral hemorrhages in blacks as compared with whites. N Engl J Med 326:733, 1992.
63. He J, Whelton PK, Vu B, et al: Aspirin and risk of hemorrhagic stroke: a meta-analysis of randomized controlled trials. JAMA 280:1930, 1998.
64. Kase CS, Mohr JP, Caplan LR: Intracerebral hemorrhage. In: Barnett HJM, Mohr JP, Stein BM, Yatsu FM (eds): Stroke Pathophysiology, Diagnosis, and Management. 3rd Ed. Churchill Livingstone, New York, 1998.
65. MacKenzie JM: Intracerebral haemorrhage. J Clin Pathol 49:360, 1996.
66. Rosenblum WI: The importance of fibrinoid necrosis as the cause of cerebral hemorrhage in hypertension. Commentary. J Neuropathol Exp Neurol 52:11, 1993.
67. Broderick JP, Brott TG, Duldner JE, et al: Volume of intracerebral hemorrhage. A powerful and easy-to-use predictor of 30-day mortality. Stroke 24:987, 1993.
68. Tuhrim S, Horowitz DR, Sacher M, et al: Volume of ventricular blood is an important determinant of outcome in supratentorial intracerebral hemorrhage. Crit Care Med 27:617, 1999.
69. Diringer MN, Edwards DF, Zazulia AR: Hydrocephalus: a previously unrecognized predictor of poor outcome from supratentorial intracerebral hemorrhage. Stroke 29:1352, 1998.
70. Tuhrim S, Horowitz DR, Sacher M, et al: Validation and comparison of models predicting survival following intracerebral hemorrhage. Crit Care Med 23:950, 1995.
71. Hemphill 3rd JC, Bonovich DC, Besmertis L, et al: The ICH score: a simple, reliable grading scale for intracerebral hemorrhage. Stroke 32:891, 2001.
72. Becker KJ, Baxter AB, Bybee HM, et al: Extravasation of radiographic contrast is an independent predictor of death in primary intracerebral hemorrhage. Stroke 30:2025, 1999.
73. Mendelow AD, Gregson BA, Fernandes HM, et al: Early surgery versus initial conservative treatment in patients with spontaneous supratentorial intracerebral haematomas in the International Surgical Trial in Intracerebral Haemorrhage (STICH): a randomised trial. Lancet 365:387, 2005.
74. Davis BR, Vogt T, Frost PH, et al: Risk factors for stroke and type of stroke in persons with isolated systolic hypertension. Systolic Hypertension in the Elderly Program Cooperative Research Group. Stroke 29:1333, 1998.
75. Fisher CM: Lacunes: small, deep cerebral infarcts. Neurology 15:774, 1965.
76. Longstreth Jr WT, Bernick C, Manolio TA, et al: Lacunar infarcts defined by magnetic resonance imaging of 3660 elderly people: the Cardiovascular Health Study. Arch Neurol 55:1217, 1998.
77. You R, McNeil JJ, O'Malley HM, et al: Risk factors for lacunar infarction syndromes. Neurology 45:1483, 1995.
78. Gan R, Sacco RL, Kargman DE, et al: Testing the validity of the lacunar hypothesis: the Northern Manhattan Stroke Study experience. Neurology 48:1204, 1997.
79. Millikan C, Futrell N: The fallacy of the lacune hypothesis. Stroke 21:1251, 1990.

80. Caplan LR: Stroke: A Clinical Approach. Butterworth-Heineman, Newton, 1993.
81. Fisher CM: Lacunar strokes and infarcts: a review. Neurology 32:871, 1982.
82. Macdonald RL, Kowalczuk A, Johns L: Emboli enter penetrating arteries of monkey brain in relation to their size. Stroke 26:1247, 1995.
83. Chamorro A, Sacco RL, Mohr JP, et al: Clinical-computed tomographic correlations of lacunar infarction in the Stroke Data Bank. Stroke 22:175, 1991.
84. The National Institute of Neurological Disorders and Stroke rt-PA Stroke Study Group: Tissue plasminogen activator for acute ischemic stroke. N Engl J Med 333:1581, 1995.
85. Salgado AV, Ferro JM, Gouveia-Oliveira A: Long-term prognosis of first-ever lacunar strokes. A hospital-based study. Stroke 27:661, 1996.
86. CAPRIE Steering Committee CAPRIE Steering Committee: a randomised, blinded, trial of clopidogrel versus aspirin in patients at risk of ischaemic events (CAPRIE). Lancet 348:1329, 1996.
87. Diener HC, Bogousslavsky J, Brass LM, et al: Aspirin and clopidogrel compared with clopidogrel alone after recent ischaemic stroke or transient ischaemic attack in high-risk patients (MATCH): randomised, double-blind, placebo-controlled trial. Lancet 364:331, 2004.
88. Benavente OR, Hart RG, McClure LA, et al: Effects of clopidogrel added to aspirin in patients with recent lacunar stroke. N Engl J Med 367:817, 2012.
89. Chimowitz MI, Lynn MJ, Derdeyn CP, et al: Stenting versus aggressive medical therapy for intracranial arterial stenosis. N Engl J Med 365:993, 2011.
90. Wang Y, Wang Y, Zhao X, et al: Clopidogrel with aspirin in acute minor stroke or transient ischemic attack. N Engl J Med 369:11, 2013.
91. Longstreth Jr WT, Manolio TA, Arnold A, et al: Clinical correlates of white matter findings on cranial magnetic resonance imaging of 3301 elderly people. The Cardiovascular Health Study. Stroke 27:1274, 1996.
92. Longstreth Jr WT, Arnold AM, Beauchamp Jr NJ, et al: Incidence, manifestations, and predictors of worsening white matter on serial cranial magnetic resonance imaging in the elderly: the Cardiovascular Health Study. Stroke 36:56, 2005.
93. Fernando MS, Simpson JE, Matthews F, et al: White matter lesions in an unselected cohort of the elderly: molecular pathology suggests origin from chronic hypoperfusion injury. Stroke 37:1391, 2006.
94. Isaka Y, Okamoto M, Ashida K, et al: Decreased cerebrovascular dilatory capacity in subjects with asymptomatic periventricular hyperintensities. Stroke 25:375, 1994.
95. Vermeer SE, Hollander M, van Dijk EJ, et al: Silent brain infarcts and white matter lesions increase stroke risk in the general population: the Rotterdam Scan Study. Stroke 34:1126, 2003.
96. Longstreth Jr WT, Dulberg C, Manolio TA, et al: Incidence, manifestations, and predictors of brain infarcts defined by serial cranial magnetic resonance imaging in the elderly: the Cardiovascular Health Study. Stroke 33:2376, 2002.
97. Kalimo H, Viitanen M, Amberla K, et al: CADASIL: hereditary disease of arteries causing brain infarcts and dementia. Neuropathol Appl Neurobiol 25:257, 1999.
98. Chabriat H, Vahedi K, Iba-Zizen MT, et al: Clinical spectrum of CADASIL: a study of 7 families. Cerebral autosomal dominant arteriopathy with subcortical infarcts and leukoencephalopathy. Lancet 346:934, 1995.
99. Timsit SG, Sacco RL, Mohr JP, et al: Early clinical differentiation of cerebral infarction from severe atherosclerotic stenosis and cardioembolism. Stroke 23:486, 1992.
100. Timsit SG, Sacco RL, Mohr JP, et al: Brain infarction severity differs according to cardiac or arterial embolic source. Neurology 43:728, 1993.
101. Li R, Duncan BB, Metcalf PA, et al: B-mode-detected carotid artery plaque in a general population. Atherosclerosis Risk in Communities (ARIC) Study Investigators. Stroke 25:2377, 1994.
102. Lee TT, Solomon NA, Heidenreich PA, et al: Cost-effectiveness of screening for carotid stenosis in asymptomatic persons. Ann Intern Med 126:337, 1997.
103. Wilson PW, Hoeg JM, D'Agostino RB, et al: Cumulative effects of high cholesterol levels, high blood pressure, and cigarette smoking on carotid stenosis. N Engl J Med 337:516, 1997.
104. Muluk SC, Muluk VS, Sugimoto H, et al: Progression of asymptomatic carotid stenosis: a natural history study in 1004 patients. J Vasc Surg 29:208, 1999.
105. Barnett HJ, Taylor DW, Eliasziw M, et al: Benefit of carotid endarterectomy in patients with symptomatic moderate or severe stenosis. North American Symptomatic Carotid Endarterectomy Trial Collaborators. N Engl J Med 339:1415, 1998.
106. Sauve JS, Laupacis A, Ostbye T, et al: The rational clinical examination. Does this patient have a clinically important carotid bruit? JAMA 270:2843, 1993.
107. Josephson SA, Bryant SO, Mak HK, et al: Evaluation of carotid stenosis using CT angiography in the initial evaluation of stroke and TIA. Neurology 63:457, 2004.
108. Barnett HJ, Eliasziw M, Meldrum HE: Drugs and surgery in the prevention of ischemic stroke. N Engl J Med 332:238, 1995.
109. North American Symptomatic Carotid Endarterectomy Trial Collaborators: Beneficial effect of carotid endarterectomy in symptomatic patients with high-grade carotid stenosis. N Engl J Med 325:445, 1991.

110. European Carotid Surgery Trialists' Collaborative Group: MRC European Carotid Surgery Trial: interim results for symptomatic patients with severe (70–99%) or with mild (0–29%) carotid stenosis. European Carotid Surgery Trialists' Collaborative Group. Lancet 337:1235, 1991.
111. Rothwell PM, Warlow CP: Prediction of benefit from carotid endarterectomy in individual patients: a risk-modelling study. European Carotid Surgery Trialists' Collaborative Group. Lancet 353:2105, 1999.
112. Halliday A, Mansfield A, Marro J, et al: Prevention of disabling and fatal strokes by successful carotid endarterectomy in patients without recent neurological symptoms: randomised controlled trial. Lancet 363:1491, 2004.
113. Yadav JS, Wholey MH, Kuntz RE, et al: Protected carotid-artery stenting versus endarterectomy in high-risk patients. N Engl J Med 351:1493, 2004.
114. Brott TG, Hobson 2nd RW, Howard G, et al: Stenting versus endarterectomy for treatment of carotid-artery stenosis. N Engl J Med 363:11, 2010.
115. Sacco RL, Kargman DE, Gu Q, et al: Race-ethnicity and determinants of intracranial atherosclerotic cerebral infarction. The Northern Manhattan Stroke Study. Stroke 26:14, 1995.
116. Wityk RJ, Lehman D, Klag M, et al: Race and sex differences in the distribution of cerebral atherosclerosis. Stroke 27:1974, 1996.
117. Ingall TJ, Homer D, Baker Jr HL, et al: Predictors of intracranial carotid artery atherosclerosis. Duration of cigarette smoking and hypertension are more powerful than serum lipid levels. Arch Neurol 48:687, 1991.
118. Postiglione A, Napoli C: Hyperlipidaemia and atherosclerotic cerebrovascular disease. Curr Opin Lipidol 6:236, 1995.
119. Lammie GA, Sandercock PA, Dennis MS: Recently occluded intracranial and extracranial carotid arteries. Relevance of the unstable atherosclerotic plaque. Stroke 30:1319, 1999.
120. Fassbender K, Bertsch T, Mielke O, et al: Adhesion molecules in cerebrovascular diseases. Evidence for an inflammatory endothelial activation in cerebral large- and small-vessel disease. Stroke 30:1647, 1999.
121. Chimowitz MI, Lynn MJ, Howlett-Smith H, et al: Comparison of warfarin and aspirin for symptomatic intracranial arterial stenosis. N Engl J Med 352:1305, 2005.
122. Turan TN, Cotsonis G, Lynn MJ, et al: Relationship between blood pressure and stroke recurrence in patients with intracranial arterial stenosis. Circulation 115:2969, 2007.
123. Amarenco P, Duyckaerts C, Tzourio C, et al: The prevalence of ulcerated plaques in the aortic arch in patients with stroke. N Engl J Med 326:221, 1992.
124. Amarenco P, Cohen A, Tzourio C, et al: Atherosclerotic disease of the aortic arch and the risk of ischemic stroke. N Engl J Med 331:1474, 1994.
125. The French Study of Aortic Plaques in Stroke Group: Atherosclerotic disease of the aortic arch as a risk factor for recurrent ischemic stroke. N Engl J Med 334:1216, 1996.
126. Clinicaltrials.gov: Aortic Arch Related Cerebral Hazard Trial (ARCH). 2013.
127. Launer LJ, Masaki K, Petrovitch H, et al: The association between midlife blood pressure levels and late-life cognitive function. The Honolulu-Asia Aging Study. JAMA 274:1846, 1995.
128. Kivipelto M, Helkala EL, Laakso MP, et al: Apolipoprotein E epsilon4 allele, elevated midlife total cholesterol level, and high midlife systolic blood pressure are independent risk factors for late-life Alzheimer disease. Ann Intern Med 137:149, 2002.
129. Skoog I, Lernfelt B, Landahl S, et al: 15-year longitudinal study of blood pressure and dementia. Lancet 347:1141, 1996.
130. Petrovitch H, White LR, Izmirilian G, et al: Midlife blood pressure and neuritic plaques, neurofibrillary tangles, and brain weight at death: the HAAS. Honolulu-Asia Aging Study. Neurobiol Aging 21:57, 2000.
131. Langa KM, Foster NL, Larson EB: Mixed dementia: emerging concepts and therapeutic implications. JAMA 292:2901, 2004.
132. Forette F, Seux ML, Staessen JA, et al: Prevention of dementia in randomised double-blind placebo-controlled Systolic Hypertension in Europe (Syst-Eur) trial. Lancet 352:1347, 1998.
133. Di Bari M, Pahor M, Franse LV, et al: Dementia and disability outcomes in large hypertension trials: lessons learned from the Systolic Hypertension in the Elderly Program (SHEP) trial. Am J Epidemiol 153:72, 2001.
134. Prince MJ, Bird AS, Blizard RA, et al: Is the cognitive function of older patients affected by antihypertensive treatment? Results from 54 months of the Medical Research Council's trial of hypertension in older adults. BMJ 312:801, 1996.
135. Tzourio C, Anderson C, Chapman N, et al: Effects of blood pressure lowering with perindopril and indapamide therapy on dementia and cognitive decline in patients with cerebrovascular disease. Arch Intern Med 163:1069, 2003.
136. Elkins JS, Knopman DS, Yaffe K, et al: Cognitive function predicts first-time stroke and heart disease. Neurology 64:1750, 2005.
137. Birns J, Markus H, Kalra L: Blood pressure reduction for vascular risk: is there a price to be paid? Stroke 36:1308, 2005.
138. Hinchey J, Chaves C, Appignani B, et al: A reversible posterior leukoencephalopathy syndrome. N Engl J Med 334:494, 1996.
139. Pentel P: Toxicity of over-the-counter stimulants. JAMA 252:1898, 1984.

140. Delanty N, Vaughan C, Frucht S, et al: Erythropoietin-associated hypertensive posterior leukoencephalopathy. Neurology 49:686, 1997.
141. Sheth RD, Riggs JE, Bodenstenier JB, et al: Parietal occipital edema in hypertensive encephalopathy: a pathogenic mechanism. Eur Neurol 36:25, 1996.
142. Blezer EL, Nicolay K, Bar D, et al: Enalapril prevents imminent and reduces manifest cerebral edema in stroke-prone hypertensive rats. Stroke 29:1671, 1998.
143. Redman CW, Sacks GP, Sargent IL: Preeclampsia: an excessive maternal inflammatory response to pregnancy. Am J Obstet Gynecol 180:499, 1999.
144. Mabie WC: Management of acute severe hypertension and encephalopathy. Clin Obstet Gynecol 42:519, 1999.

CHAPTER

8

Postural Hypotension and Syncope

MICHAEL J. AMINOFF

When a healthy person stands up after being recumbent, approximately 500 ml of blood (or more) pools in the vessels of the legs and abdomen, causing a reduction in filling pressure of the right atrium and thus a decrease in cardiac output and systemic blood pressure. This leads to changes in baroreceptor activity and thus to changes in impulse traffic in the ninth and tenth cranial nerves. These changes affect the activity of the brainstem vasomotor center, which, in turn, influences the autonomic neurons in the intermediolateral cell columns of the thoracolumbar spinal cord, producing reflex peripheral vasoconstriction and an increase in force and rate of myocardial contraction (Figs. 8-1 and 8-2). Cardiopulmonary reflexes, subserved by vagal afferent fibers from mechanoreceptors in the heart and stretch receptors in the lungs, contribute to maintenance of the blood pressure, acting synergistically with the baroreceptor reflexes. The venoarteriolar axonal reflexes may also be important in limiting blood flow to the skin, muscle, and adipose tissues. Standing up also leads to release of norepinephrine. Venous return is aided during maintenance of the upright posture by mechanical factors, such as the tone in the leg muscles and the pumping action of these muscles during walking, and by maneuvers that increase intra-abdominal pressure. This has important therapeutic implications (see p. 164).[1] In addition, there is secretion of antidiuretic hormone (arginine vasopressin) and activation of the renin-angiotensin-aldosterone system, so that salt and water are conserved and blood volume increases. These, however, are typically longer-term rather than immediate control mechanisms.

Aminoff's Neurology and General Medicine, Fifth Edition.

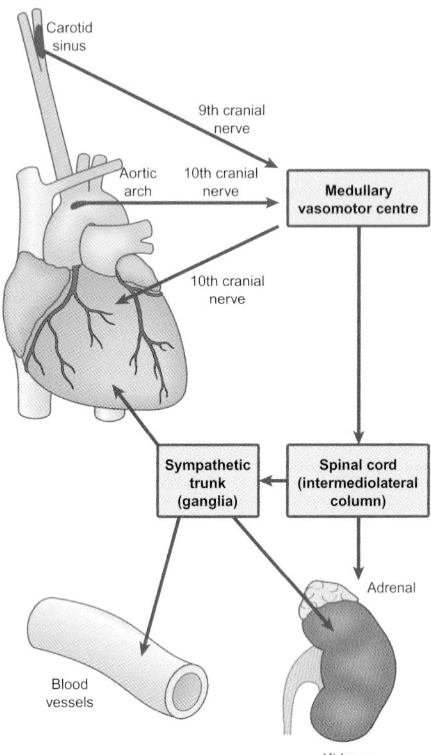

Figure 8-1 ■ Anatomy of the autonomic pathways involved in maintaining the blood pressure on standing.

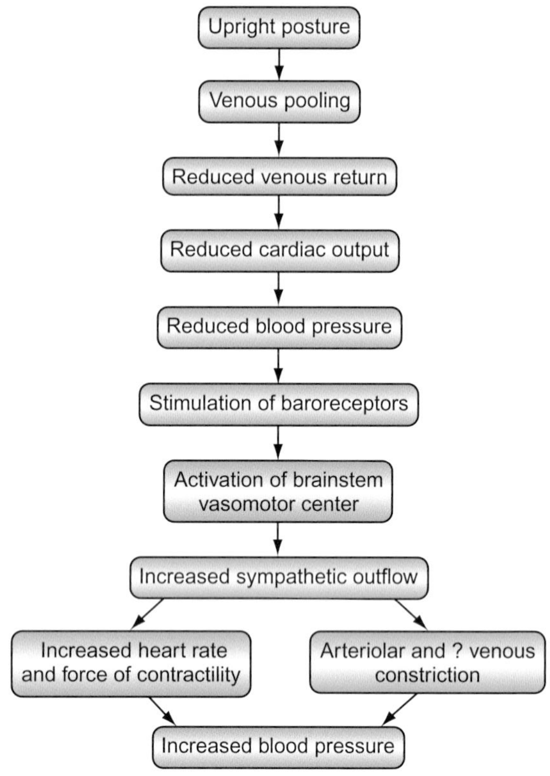

Figure 8-2 ■ Sequence of events that ensure maintenance of the blood pressure after adoption of the upright posture. Only the immediate cardiovascular changes are shown. As indicated in the text, a variety of other humoral mechanisms are also activated.

Postural hypotension is defined as a decrease of at least 20 mmHg in systolic pressure or 10 mmHg in diastolic pressure within 3 minutes of standing. It occurs when there is a failure of the autoregulatory mechanisms that maintain the blood pressure on standing. It may therefore occur with any neurologic disorder that impairs baroreceptor function, disturbs the afferent input from these receptors, directly involves the brainstem vasomotor center or its central connections, or interrupts the sympathetic outflow pathway either centrally or peripherally. It may also occur with a number of non-neurologic disorders, and it is important to consider these disorders if patients are to be managed correctly.

NON-NEUROLOGIC CAUSES OF POSTURAL HYPOTENSION

Cardiovascular Disorders

A variety of cardiac disorders may lead to postural hypotension or even syncope. Pathologic processes such as mitral valve prolapse, aortic stenosis, or hypertrophic cardiomyopathy may limit cardiac output. Cardiac outflow may also be blocked in rare instances by a thrombus or myxoma when the patient is in the upright position. Certain paroxysmal cardiac dysrhythmias (bradycardias or tachycardias) may occur with activity or on standing and produce episodic hypotension or syncope; however, disturbances of cardiac rhythm are common in asymptomatic elderly persons, and their presence must be interpreted with caution. In patients with congestive heart failure, the heart rate and level of sympathetic tone may be such that compensatory adjustments cannot be made when the patient stands, and postural hypotension therefore results.

Alterations of Effective Blood Volume

Postural hypotension can occur because of loss of effective blood volume. Normal adults can withstand the loss of 500 ml of blood or bodily fluids with few if any symptoms, but greater volume depletion may occur acutely for a variety of reasons (e.g., hemorrhage or burns) and cause a postural drop in blood pressure. Hyponatremia and Addison disease may also lead to an absolute reduction in blood volume. Postural hypotension may occur owing to venous pooling in patients with severe varicose veins or congenital absence of venous valves or because of poor peripheral resistance and reduced muscle tone in patients with paralyzed limbs. Similarly, it may occur during the late stages of pregnancy owing to obstructed venous return by the gravid uterus. Marked vasodilatation, such as occurs in the heat or with the use of certain drugs or alcohol, sometimes causes postural hypotension.

Drugs

Numerous drugs may produce postural hypotension, including those given to treat neurologic disorders (e.g., dopamine agonists and levodopa) and psychiatric disturbances (e.g., tranquilizing, sedative, hypnotic, and antidepressant agents).[2,3] Antihypertensive drugs, diuretics, and vasodilators commonly lead to postural hypotension as a side effect. Insulin may cause nonhypoglycemic postural hypotension in diabetic patients with autonomic neuropathy, possibly because of vasodilatation and reduced venous return in the absence of functioning compensatory mechanisms or because of impaired baroreceptor responses to changes in arterial pressure. Iatrogenic and toxic autonomic neuropathy is considered later.

Endocrine and Metabolic Disorders

Autonomic neuropathy, with consequent postural hypotension, is a major and common complication of diabetes. Postural hypotension may be a feature of Addison disease, hypopituitarism, myxedema, thyrotoxicosis, pheochromocytoma, carcinoid syndrome, and hypokalemia. It may also occur with anorexia nervosa. Anemia may exacerbate or cause postural hypotension.

Inadequate Postural Adjustments

Prolonged bed rest may result in postural hypotension when patients first begin standing again, but this problem is self-limited. Its cause is poorly understood, but it may be multifactorial. Carotid baroreceptor function is impaired, cardiac vagal activity is reduced, blood pooling is increased in the legs because of greater venous compliance, the total circulating blood volume and central venous pressure are reduced, and the red cell mass may decline.[4–6] Prolonged bed rest also leads to an increased incidence of cardiac dysrhythmias. In otherwise healthy subjects, vigorous exercise to the point of exhaustion may also cause a postural decline in blood pressure, possibly because of marked peripheral vasodilatation and venous pooling.

Age

Many patients older than 70 years have a decline in systolic pressure of 20 mmHg or more on standing. Several causes of reduced orthostatic tolerance with advancing age have been identified.[7] Baroreflex sensitivity declines with age and certain adrenoreceptors exhibit reduced sensitivity. Loss of preganglionic neurons also occurs with age and becomes symptomatic when approximately 50 percent of the cells are lost. Diuretics (which are commonly taken by the elderly) reduce blood volume and may lead to postural hypotension. Finally, structural, mechanical, and functional changes in the vascular system,[8] such as loss of vascular elasticity and the occurrence of varicose veins, may be contributory, as may a reduction in the skeletal muscle mass. Prolonged bed rest, intercurrent illness, and adverse reactions to medication may also be important. Postural hypotension appears not to have an impact on mortality, at least among patients discharged from an acute geriatric ward.[9]

Syncope is a common problem in the elderly. Often no precise explanation for it can be found, but postural hypotension is probably responsible in many instances. Nevertheless, it is best not to ascribe patients' symptoms to postural hypotension unless they can be reproduced by a demonstrable fall in blood pressure on standing. Many of the homeostatic mechanisms that maintain intravascular volume and blood pressure may be impaired with advancing age, as discussed earlier, so that syncope is more likely to occur. Indeed, in many elderly patients a number of factors can be found to account for syncope, and it is then difficult to determine which of these factors is responsible in any individual instance.

AUTONOMIC REGULATION OF THE HEART AND BLOOD VESSELS

The central nervous system (CNS) is important in regulating cardiovascular function. Various lower brainstem centers receive inputs from both the periphery and other central structures such as the cerebral cortex, temporal lobe, amygdala, hypothalamus, cerebellum, periaqueductal gray matter, and pontine nuclei.[10,11] The nucleus tractus solitarius is the site of termination of baroreceptor, chemoreceptor, and cardiopulmonary afferent fibers; it connects with the nucleus ambiguus and dorsal nucleus of the vagus and with neurons in the lateral reticular formation that project to the cord in the bulbospinal pathway, thereby influencing the cardiovascular system.[12,13]

The vagus nerve has a major role in regulating the heart rate responses to various maneuvers. The sympathetic nervous system is important in influencing vasomotor tone and peripheral vascular resistance, but the sympathetic outflow to different regions and structures is regulated separately. The sympathetic nervous system causes a vasoconstriction in response to the release of norepinephrine. The occurrence of vasodilatation in the limbs probably depends on reduced sympathetic activity, and, to a lesser extent, on axon reflexes and antidromic conduction, but some of the vessels in limb muscles are probably also supplied by sympathetic vasodilator cholinergic fibers.

Microneurographic studies in humans have shown that bursts of impulses occur rhythmically in sympathetic efferent vasomotor fibers to the skin and muscles and are time-locked to the pulse. This rhythmic activity depends on supraspinal mechanisms and is not seen below the level of a complete cord transection. Such sympathetic impulse traffic to vessels in the limb muscles is markedly affected by baroreceptor activity, but not by brief mental stress,[14] whereas the traffic in human cutaneous nerves is markedly increased by mental stress. High-pressure arterial baroreceptors are located primarily in the carotid sinus and aortic arch, from which afferent fibers pass to the brainstem in the glossopharyngeal and vagus nerves, respectively.

Sympathetic efferent activity is inhibited by an increase in the pressure in the carotid sinus and aortic arch, whereas a reduced pressure causes increased sympathetic activity and a peripheral vasoconstriction. The heart rate is also influenced by the baroreceptors and cardiopulmonary stretch receptors, so that a bradycardia occurs when the pressure is increased and a tachycardia when the blood pressure declines.

Change from recumbency to an erect posture causes blood to pool in the legs and lower abdomen. There is a slight fall in systolic blood pressure; this leads to baroreceptor activation, a peripheral vasoconstriction, and an increase in heart rate and contractile force. Compensatory changes in the splanchnic vasculature, constriction of venous beds, and activation of the renin-angiotensin system also occur.

The carotid baroreceptor reflexes seem to be more important in responding to the immediate changes in blood pressure that occur on standing, whereas the aortic baroreceptors assume a greater role with maintenance of the upright posture. The cardiopulmonary stretch receptors act synergistically with the baroreceptor reflexes. The venoarteriolar axon reflex, which is activated by venous distention in the legs and an associated increase in transmural venous pressure, is also important in ensuring an increase in limb vascular resistance with change to an erect posture. During activity, the baroreceptors are reset by an uncertain, probably neural, mechanism to allow the blood pressure to increase with exercise. Unmyelinated chemoreceptor afferent fibers from skeletal muscles are also activated,[15] thereby increasing blood pressure and correcting any deficiency in muscle perfusion pressure during moderate to heavy exercise. In addition, activation of mechanically sensitive muscle receptors (muscle mechanoreflex) occurs, and these exercise pressor reflexes (peripheral neural reflexes originating in skeletal muscle) contribute significantly to cardiovascular regulation during exercise.[16] At the initiation of exercise, "central command" from higher brain centers leads to an immediate increase in heart rate and output as well as in blood pressure and respiration.[17,18]

NEUROLOGIC CAUSES OF POSTURAL HYPOTENSION

Central Lesions and Spinal Injury

The autonomic consequences of spinal cord injuries depend on the level and severity of the lesion. In quadriplegic patients, the period of spinal shock that follows injury is associated with a dysautonomia in which the resting blood pressure and heart rate are typically low and postural hypotension is marked. This mandates that the patient be kept flat, without elevation of the head of the bed, and that any loss of blood volume be avoided or treated vigorously.

A few weeks after transection of the cervical cord, activity returns to the isolated spinal segment, but the brain is no longer able to control the sympathetic nervous system. Loss of regulation during postural change leads to orthostatic hypotension, whereas overactivity occurs if spinal sympathetic reflexes are activated and leads to the syndrome of *autonomic hyperreflexia*, which occurs in patients with cervical or high thoracic lesions. It is characterized by episodic hypertension, bradycardia, headache, and hyperhidrosis above the level of the lesion, with pallor and piloerection distal to it. Anxiety, confusion, nasal congestion, and facial flushing may also occur. Treatment of this syndrome thus requires avoidance of stimuli that activate spinal sympathetic reflexes (e.g., a distended bladder), elevation of the head of the bed, and, if necessary, use of short-acting antihypertensive agents such as calcium-channel blockers. In general, spinal cord transection produces postural hypotension if the lesion is above about the T6 level. Intramedullary and extramedullary tumors, transverse myelitis, and syringomyelia involving the cord above T6 may also produce dysautonomia.[19]

A variety of brainstem lesions can impair autonomic function and affect control of the blood pressure, including syringobulbia[20] and posterior fossa tumors. Chiari malformation with tonsillar herniation may lead to syncopal episodes.[21] Impairment in Wernicke encephalopathy may relate to central or peripheral involvement. The extent to which autonomic reflex function, and particularly cardiovascular regulation, is impaired in Parkinson disease is disputed. Many patients with Parkinson disease have postural hypotension from cardiac (especially left ventricular) and extra-cardiac sympathetic denervation.[22,23] In such patients, responses to the Valsalva maneuver are also abnormal.[24] Other dysautonomic symptoms, such as disturbances of bladder or gastrointestinal function, and excessive salivation, are relatively common.

The findings in certain other disorders with parkinsonian features (e.g., multiple system atrophy, olivopontocerebellar atrophy, and striatonigral degeneration) are discussed on p. 153. Postural hypotension may also occur in diffuse Lewy body disease. Mild dysautonomic features may occur late in the course of progressive supranuclear palsy, but cardiovascular reflexes are usually preserved or show only minor abnormalities of dubious significance.[24–26] A variety of dysautonomic symptoms may occur in Huntington disease,[27,28] but any abnormalities of blood pressure regulation are usually mild and subclinical, except when related to neuroleptic medication taken for chorea or behavioral disturbances. Postural hypotension or other disturbances of cardiovascular autonomic function occur occasionally in patients with multiple sclerosis,[29,30] but disturbances of bladder and bowel function are much more common dysautonomic features of that disorder. Wallenberg syndrome or bilateral brainstem strokes may lead to bradycardia and hypotension that may exacerbate the underlying neurologic problem.[31]

Root and Peripheral Nerve Lesions

Postural hypotension may occur in patients with tabes dorsalis because of interruption of circulatory reflexes. In patients with polyneuropathies, autonomic involvement is not uncommon. It is particularly frequent in diabetic neuropathy, although usually relatively mild in severity[32]; indeed, diabetes is the most common cause of autonomic neuropathy in the more developed countries.[33] Postural hypotension occurs in approximately 25 percent of patients with diabetic neuropathy. In addition to postural lightheadedness, the dysautonomia of diabetes may be manifest by impotence, postprandial bloating, early satiety, gastrointestinal motility disturbances, abnormalities of bladder control, and alterations of sweating. Cardiac vagal control is usually impaired early, before the development of postural hypotension; the quantitative sudomotor axon reflex test is commonly abnormal and indicates involvement of distal postganglionic sympathetic fibers.[34]

Other polyneuropathies associated with postural hypotension include those of alcoholism, Guillain–Barré syndrome, malignant disease, idiopathic small-fiber neuropathies, and acute porphyria. In many patients with chronic alcoholism, however, there is no excessive decline in blood pressure on standing, although the cardiovascular responses to various maneuvers are often abnormal; both sympathetic and parasympathetic functions may be abnormal, and the presence of autonomic neuropathy has been correlated with nutritional status.[35]

Primary amyloidosis and familial amyloid polyneuropathy of Portuguese type (FAP type 1) are often accompanied by dysautonomia consequent to the loss of predominantly unmyelinated and small myelinated peripheral fibers and of cells in the intermediolateral columns of the cord. Postural hypotension and impotence are early manifestations; episodic constipation and diarrhea, distal anhidrosis, impotence, urinary retention, and cardiac arrhythmias may also be conjoined. Tests of sympathetic and parasympathetic function are typically abnormal.[36]

Autonomic dysfunction with abnormal cardiovascular responses occurs in some patients with chronic renal failure on intermittent hemodialysis, but the site of autonomic involvement is unclear. Vitamin B_{12} deficiency may lead to autonomic neuropathy and postural hypotension that improves or resolves completely after vitamin supplementation.[37,38] Autonomic involvement, with impairment of sweating and cardiovascular responses, may occur in leprosy, sometimes without conspicuous features of peripheral nerve involvement.[39,40] Symptoms of autonomic impairment, including postural hypotension, may be a presenting feature of systemic autoimmune disorders.[41]

In Fabry disease, disturbed sweating, reduced saliva and tear production, impaired pupillary responses, and gastrointestinal symptoms are common, but postural hypotension does not usually occur, and postural cardiovascular reflexes are normal or only mildly abnormal.[42]

Autonomic involvement in Guillain–Barré syndrome is usually mild, but paroxysmal cardiac arrhythmias or asystole or episodic hypertension may lead to a fatal outcome.[43] Postural hypotension is common. It has a number of possible causes including inactivity and bed rest, baroreceptor deafferentation, efferent sympathetic denervation, hypovolemia, cardiac abnormalities, or some combination of these and other factors. The severity of autonomic involvement in Guillain–Barré syndrome is not related to the degree of sensory or motor disturbance, and a wide variety of autonomic abnormalities is found if patients are studied in detail. The hypertensive episodes may relate to catecholamine supersensitivity or denervation of baroreceptors. Treatment of Guillain–Barré syndrome is by supportive measures or with plasmapheresis or intravenous immunoglobulin therapy depending on disease severity. Patients with autonomic instability require close observation and management in an intensive care unit. Further aspects of treatment are given on p. 164. Curiously, postural hypotension is uncommon in chronic inflammatory demyelinating polyneuropathy, although mild impairment may be found in many patients on tests of autonomic function.[44,45]

Autonomic neuropathy of acute or subacute onset, possibly on an autoimmune basis, sometimes occurs as a monophasic disorder in isolation or with associated sensory or motor involvement. It has occurred in the context of antecedent viral infections, malignancy, Hodgkin disease, infectious mononucleosis, ulcerative colitis, and certain connective tissue diseases.[46,47] In approximately 50 percent of patients, high titers of ganglionic acetylcholine receptor (AChR) antibody are found. In patients with a paraneoplastic etiology, other autoantibodies may be present, including antineuronal nuclear antibody 1 (ANNA-1 or anti-Hu) or 2 (ANNA-2), Purkinje cell antibody 2 (PCA-2), and collapsin response-mediator protein 5 antibody (CRMP5).[48] The presence of such antibodies may suggest the likely site of an underlying primary tumor. Both sympathetic and parasympathetic fibers are usually involved, leading to marked postural hypotension accompanied by a fixed heart rate, anhidrosis or hypohidrosis, heat intolerance, sphincter disturbances, gastroparesis, ileus, and dryness of the eyes and mouth, but occasionally abnormalities are confined to postganglionic cholinergic neurons (acute cholinergic neuropathy), in which case postural hypotension does not occur. Pure adrenergic neuropathy has also been described. Autonomic function tests reflect the clinical findings. Nerve conduction study results are typically normal, but sensory abnormalities are sometimes found. Treatment is supportive; immunomodulating therapy may have a role in those with severe disease. Paraneoplastic dysautonomia may remit if the underlying malignancy is treated. The prognosis of patients with acute or subacute autonomic neuropathies is guarded: approximately one-third of patients do well, but the remainder either fail to improve or are left with a major residual deficit, including marked postural hypotension.

Autonomic involvement may occur in a variety of hereditary polyneuropathies. In familial dysautonomia, or Riley–Day syndrome, many parts of the nervous system are affected. Presentation during infancy may be with inability to suck, but episodic vomiting, recurrent pulmonary infections, hypertension, tachycardia, and diaphoresis occur, especially after 3 years of age. There may also be emotional outbursts, difficulty in swallowing, hypothermia or hyperthermia, poor flow of tears, postural hypotension, and syncope. Sensory abnormalities include impaired pain and temperature appreciation, and the tendon reflexes are depressed. The tongue is smooth and lacks fungiform papillae. Cardiac arrest may occur on tracheal intubation. Treatment is essentially supportive.[49,50] Postural hypotension usually is not a feature of the other hereditary sensory and autonomic neuropathies, whereas sudomotor function is often markedly impaired.

Autonomic symptoms or signs may occur in patients with hereditary motor and sensory neuropathy type 1, and abnormal vascular reflex responses may be present.[51] Postural hypotension is usually not a conspicuous feature of the disorder.

Iatrogenic postural hypotension is common in the elderly[52,53] and relates most often to the use of antihypertensive agents or diuretics. Iatrogenic polyneuropathies may be responsible in other instances, as reviewed elsewhere[54]; postural hypotension may be conspicuous in patients with the neuropathy caused by perhexiline maleate, cisplatin, paclitaxel (Taxol), vinca alkaloids, or amiodarone.[54]

Toxic Exposure

Autonomic dysfunction may result from occupational or other exposure to certain neurotoxins but does not usually lead to postural hypotension. Long-term occupational exposure to a mixture of organic solvents may cause subtle disturbances of peripheral parasympathetic nerves as well as sensorimotor peripheral neuropathies,[55] as reflected by cardiovascular reflex studies,[56] but other reports of autonomic involvement in this context are few. Intentional inhalation of *n*-hexane or methyl-*n*-butyl-ketone for recreational purposes may lead to a rapidly progressive neuropathy with associated postural hypotension.[54] Acrylamide neuropathy is usually accompanied by hyperhidrosis and cold, cyanotic extremities; experimental studies in animals reveal baroreceptor dysfunction, but the clinical significance of this in humans is unclear.[57] A variety of autonomic symptoms (including tachycardia, hypertension, and disturbances of sweating) may occur with thallium, arsenic, or mercury poisoning, but postural hypotension is not usually a feature. The rodenticide *N*-3-pyridylmethyl-*N′*-*p*-nitrophenyl urea (Vacor) has caused severe dysautonomia with disabling postural hypotension, as well as sensorimotor peripheral neuropathy and encephalopathic states. Symptoms reflecting autonomic dysfunction (anorexia, nausea, hyperhidrosis, and tachycardia) have been associated with cumulative exposure to moderate levels of pesticides, particularly organophosphate or organochlorine insecticides, regardless of recent exposure or history of poisoning,[58] but specific comment was not made concerning symptoms of postural hypotension.

Primary Degeneration of the Autonomic Nervous System

Postural hypotension resulting from primary degeneration of the autonomic nervous system is well described. The postural hypotension is often exacerbated postprandially, and the normal circadian rhythm is reversed so that the blood pressure is highest at night and lowest in the morning. In addition, blood pressure typically declines with activity rather than increasing as in normal subjects. Other symptoms of dysautonomia in these patients include impotence, disturbances of bladder and bowel function, impaired thermoregulatory sweating, and xerostomia. Two distinct groups of patients are now recognized. In one, primary or *pure autonomic failure* leads to idiopathic orthostatic hypotension and other evidence of dysautonomia without peripheral neuropathy or CNS involvement. In the other, autonomic failure is associated with more widespread neurologic degeneration (i.e., with evidence of *multiple system atrophy* or MSA) such that there may be clinical features of parkinsonism or striatonigral degeneration (MSA-P), and often of more widespread neurologic lesions as well. A disorder similar to olivopontocerebellar atrophy may also occur (MSA-C). The autonomic deficit may precede the somatic neurologic one, or vice versa, but within a short period there is clinical evidence of both.[59] Occasionally there is a family history of dysautonomia.

The time course and pattern of the dysautonomia reportedly differ between these two disorders. In pure autonomic failure, syncope and sudomotor dysfunction may precede the onset of constipation, bladder dysfunction, or respiratory disturbances whereas in multiple system atrophy, urinary complaints occur early and are then followed by abnormalities of sweating or by postural hypotension.[60] Patients with pure autonomic failure had a slower functional deterioration and a better prognosis.[60] The ingestion of water temporarily increases the seated blood pressure by uncertain mechanisms in patients with chronic autonomic failure.[61] This occurs earlier in pure autonomic failure than multiple system atrophy, perhaps reflecting differing lesion sites in these two disorders.

In patients of both groups, plasma renin activity is usually subnormal. There are, however, a number of reported pharmacologic differences between them. Patients with pure autonomic failure have low plasma norepinephrine levels when lying down, and these levels fail to increase appropriately on standing; they also have a lower threshold for the pressor response to infused norepinephrine. The increase in plasma norepinephrine level in response to tyramine (see p. 161) is significantly less than in normal subjects or patients with multiple system atrophy.[62] Extensive cell loss occurs in the intermediolateral cell columns of the thoracic cord, and the autonomic dysfunction has been attributed primarily to loss of these preganglionic sympathetic neurons. However, the pharmacologic studies described previously indicate that loss of postganglionic noradrenergic neurons also occurs, and norepinephrine may be depleted from sympathetic nerve endings.

By contrast, in multiple system atrophy, in which lesions are situated at multiple sites in the CNS, circulating norepinephrine levels are normal, suggesting that peripheral sympathetic neurons are intact, but plasma norepinephrine fails to increase appropriately with standing, implying that these neurons have not been activated.[62,63] There is also an exaggerated pressor response to infused norepinephrine, but only patients with idiopathic orthostatic hypotension show a shift to the left in their dose–response curve, reflecting true adrenergic receptor supersensitivity.[62]

Central catecholamine deficiency in these disorders is reflected by the levels in the cerebrospinal fluid of dihydroxyphenylacetic acid (a neuronal metabolite of dopamine), which are lower in patients with multiple system atrophy or pure autonomic failure than normal subjects, as also is dihydroxyphenylglycol, a metabolite of norepinephrine.[64]

Endogenous arginine vasopressin is a powerful vasoconstrictor; it also acts on the kidney to control urinary concentrating mechanisms. The cardiovascular responses usually associated with arginine vasopressin are reduced cardiac output, heart rate, and plasma renin activity and increased vascular resistance and blood pressure. Arginine vasopressin helps maintain arterial pressure in certain hypotensive situations such as hemorrhage or volume depletion, but increased levels of arginine vasopressin do not normally affect the blood pressure significantly because the acute vasoconstrictor effects are buffered by the baroreceptor reflex. The chronic effects of vasopressin on renal function do not produce sustained retention of sodium and water, and so produce only minimal changes in mean arterial pressure.

Vasopressin release is influenced by the plasma's osmotic pressure and by the activity of vascular stretch receptors. In normal people, plasma arginine vasopressin increases in response to standing, presumably because a decrease in venous return influences afferent activity from these stretch receptors. In patients with progressive autonomic failure or with multiple system atrophy, plasma levels similar to control values are found in the horizontal position, but the postural increase is markedly attenuated. A vulnerability has been suggested of the noradrenergic neurons of the caudal ventrolateral medulla that are involved in activating hypothalamic neurons involved in vasopressin secretion.[65] However, in multiple system atrophy, loss of vasopressin neurons occurs in the posterior region of the hypothalamic paraventricular nucleus and may contribute to sympathetic failure, whereas loss of catecholaminergic input from the brainstem to the magnocellular vasopressin neurons may contribute to impaired vasopressin secretion following orthostatic stress.[66]

Miscellaneous Disorders

Patients with Holmes–Adie syndrome may present with or develop postural hypotension or abnormalities of thermoregulatory sweating.[67–69] Postural hypotension may occur in botulism[70]; however, blurred vision, dry mouth, and constipation are much more common autonomic manifestations. In rare instances, it relates to excessive amounts of endogenous bradykinin (a vasodilator) or a congenital defect of norepinephrine release. In patients with dopamine β-hydroxylase deficiency, norepinephrine and epinephrine cannot be synthesized, and dopamine is released from central and peripheral adrenergic nerve terminals.[71,72] Severe postural hypotension is accompanied by other autonomic disturbances in association with absent norepinephrine and excessive dopamine levels in the plasma.

Orthostatic symptoms may develop in association with a significant tachycardia (an increase of 30 beats per minute or more or a heart rate of at least 120 beats per minute), but in the absence of consistent postural hypotension or an autonomic neuropathy.[73,74] The designation *postural orthostatic tachycardia syndrome* (POTS) is applied to this disorder, which is more common in women than men and tends to occur in patients between 20 and 60 years of age. Symptoms on standing include tremulousness, lightheadedness, palpitations, visual disturbances, weakness, fatigue, anxiety, hyperventilation, nausea, postprandial bloating, and sweating, and may occur cyclically. Thus, orthostatic symptoms are accompanied by symptoms of sympathetic activation.

POTS can be associated with certain other disorders, especially joint hypermobility syndrome but also diabetes, paraneoplastic syndrome, amyloidosis, sarcoidosis, alcoholism, lupus, Sjögren syndrome, and heavy metal intoxication, and it may follow pregnancy, trauma, chemotherapy (especially with vinca alkaloids), or viral infections. It may also occur in association with mitral valve prolapse or a more specific dysautonomia. Its etiology remains uncertain. Proposed mechanisms include peripheral denervation, hypovolemia or a redistributed blood volume, prolonged deconditioning, β-receptor supersensitivity, psychologic mechanisms, and impaired brainstem regulation.[74] Partial sympathetic denervation in the legs was suggested by studies of norepinephrine spill-over into the venous circulation of the limbs in response to various stimuli.[75] There is impaired peripheral vasoconstriction on the Valsalva maneuver, but cardiovagal responses are normal.[76] The optimal therapy for the disorder is not clear, but treatment may include volume repletion, a high salt diet and copious fluids, postural and psychophysiologic training, fludrocortisone, β-blocking agents, midodrine, serotonin reuptake inhibitors, and phenobarbital. Pyridostigmine is sometimes helpful, as also is methylphenidate.[77]

SYMPTOMS OF DYSAUTONOMIA

General

Postural hypotension is usually the most disabling feature of autonomic failure. It leads to symptoms on or shortly after standing; they are relieved by sitting or lying down, and do not occur in the supine position. Such symptoms reflect cerebral hypoperfusion and include faintness, lightheadedness, blurred vision, and syncope. They may be particularly troublesome after exercise or a heavy meal (particularly a meal rich in carbohydrates) or in the morning when the blood pressure tends to be at its lowest (in contrast to healthy subjects). However, in some patients, marked postural hypotension may be clinically asymptomatic or may be accompanied by symptoms not usually regarded as suggestive of postural hypotension, such as nausea, breathlessness, heaviness or weakness of the limbs, episodic confusion, falling, staggering, headache and neck pain, and generalized weakness. Constipation may precipitate syncopal attacks during straining. Symptoms may also worsen in the heat because of vasodilatation and volume loss due to sweating. The symptoms of idiopathic POTS (discussed earlier) may be mistakenly attributed to postural hypotension, but occur without a significant decrease in blood pressure. Other causes, such as hypoglycemia, cardiac arrhythmias, or transient ischemic attacks, must be excluded if symptoms develop with the patient supine.

Impotence is a common initial symptom of autonomic dysfunction in men, often preceding other symptoms by several months or years. Bladder involvement may manifest by urinary frequency, urgency, incontinence, retention, and increased residual urine; urinary infections and renal calculi may occur in some patients with urinary stasis. Bowel dysfunction may lead to constipation, fecal incontinence, and diarrhea. Thermoregulatory sweating may be impaired. Pupillary abnormalities include Horner syndrome and anisocoria. Lacrimal dysfunction may lead to inadequate or excessive production of tears. Other symptoms of dysautonomia include night blindness, nasal congestion, and, sometimes, supine hypertension. Vocal abnormalities and respiratory disturbances (especially involuntary inspiratory gasps, cluster breathing, airway obstruction, and sleep apnea) sometimes occur, especially in patients with multiple system atrophy.

Syncope

Syncope refers to a sudden, transient loss of consciousness due to diffuse cerebral hypoperfusion or hypoxia. It is usually associated with flaccidity, but a generalized increase in muscle tone sometimes occurs with continuing cerebral ischemia/hypoxia, and there may be arrhythmic transient motor activity as well. Postictal confusion is usually brief (less than 30 seconds) when it occurs at all, unlike the marked postictal confusion that often follows a convulsion. Syncope has been divided into syncope from postural hypotension, reflex (i.e., neurally mediated) syncope, and cardiac syncope (arrhythmic or associated with structural cardiac disease).[78]

Postural Hypotension

In patients with postural hypotension due to autonomic dysfunction, there is a decline in blood pressure on standing, without adequate compensatory change in total peripheral resistance or heart rate, and syncope may result. When postural hypotension occurs because of one of the non-neurologic causes discussed earlier, it may also lead to syncope if autonomically mediated compensatory mechanisms fail to limit the decline in blood pressure.

Neurally Mediated Syncope

During *vasovagal syncope*, there is an initial increase in heart rate, blood pressure, total peripheral resistance, and cardiac output, followed by peripheral vasodilatation, increased blood flow to the muscles, decreased heart rate, and a decrease in venous return to the heart. Blood pressure falls owing to failure to increase the heart rate and cardiac output sufficiently, a decrease in systemic vascular resistance, or both. The decline in heart rate and cardiac contractility constitute the cardioinhibitory response. The vasodilatation and decline in systemic vascular resistance constitute the vasodepressor response. These various phenomena have been related to Bezold–Jarisch reflexes arising from cardiac sensory receptors and subserved by vagal afferent fibers, perhaps in consequence of a decrease of central blood volume and decreased ventricular filling.[77,78] Recordings from nerve fibers reveal that impulse traffic ceases in the sympathetic outflow to skeletal muscle during syncope and gradually builds up again over the following 5 minutes or so.[14,79] Withdrawal of sympathetically mediated vasoconstriction may underlie the profound systemic vasodilatation that leads to hypotension and subsequent syncope, but other mechanisms are probably also involved in the peripheral vasodilation.[79]

Syncope of this sort may be precipitated by pain, fear, emotional reactions, injury, and surgical manipulation. It may occur in association with missed meals, heat, or crowds; it usually occurs while subjects are standing. Warning symptoms include weakness, sweating, pallor, nausea, yawning, sighing, hyperventilation, blurred vision, impaired external awareness, and dilatation of pupils. Lying down or squatting at this time may abort actual loss of consciousness.

Deglutition syncope is characterized by syncope precipitated by swallowing. In such instances, there may be associated esophageal disorders.[80] The syncope has usually been attributed to atrioventricular heart block or cardiac arrhythmia. It is presumed that the prime factor is clinical or subclinical disease of the conducting system of the heart and that disturbances of cardiac rhythm are then triggered by reflexes originating in the esophagus. A pacemaker may prevent further episodes.[80,81]

Micturition syncope occurs after urination, particularly when the patient has arisen from bed at night. It may relate to sudden release of the reflex vasoconstriction elicited by a full bladder. Assumption of the upright posture, the peripheral vasodilatation resulting from the warmth of the bed, and, particularly in elderly men, straining to micturate may also contribute to the drop in blood pressure. Occasionally, syncope occurs in response to cardiac dysrhythmia induced by a full bladder before micturition.

Carotid sinus syncope may be provoked by neck-turning or a tight collar in susceptible subjects. Certain drugs have also been shown to predispose toward it, especially propranolol, digitalis, and α-methyldopa, and it may occur during internal carotid angioplasty.[82] A hypersensitive carotid sinus reflex is defined by a slowing in heart rate of more than 50 percent or a decline in systolic pressure by more than 40 mmHg during carotid sinus massage. However, less than 50 percent of patients with carotid hypersensitivity have syncope as a result. Conversely, in many patients with syncope of unidentifiable cause, the carotid sinus syndrome may have been overlooked.

The *Valsalva maneuver* may lead to syncope, as when syncope occurs during vigorous coughing or straining at stool as a result of the reduced cardiac output and the peripheral vasodilatation caused by the high intrathoracic pressure. Cerebral perfusion may also be reduced by an increase in intracranial pressure.

Cardiac Syncope

As discussed earlier, postural hypotension may have a cardiac basis. In addition, disturbances of cardiac rhythm may lead to sudden loss of consciousness, regardless of the position of the body (Adams–Stokes attacks). Further discussion of this topic is provided in Chapter 5. Exertional syncope suggests obstructive valvular disease or a right-to-left shunt. Coronary artery disease may lead to arrhythmias that cause syncope.

Hyperventilation

Hyperventilation, with consequent hypocapnia and reduced cerebral perfusion, is a common cause of presyncopal symptoms, but actual loss of consciousness is uncommon.

EVALUATION OF AUTONOMIC FUNCTION

After neurologic, cardiologic, and metabolic causes of syncope have been excluded, a number of patients remain in whom the diagnosis is unclear. The utility of autonomic studies in these circumstances was examined by Mathias and colleagues.[83] They found that screening autonomic function tests revealed postural hypotension and confirmed chronic autonomic failure in 5 percent, and neurally mediated syncope was diagnosed in 43.5 percent based on clinical features and autonomic studies. Thus, in recurrent syncope or presyncope, autonomic studies are worthwhile as they may clarify the diagnosis. In patients with unexplained syncope, the implantable loop recorder is an important diagnostic tool that may clarify the underlying pathophysiology.[84]

Postural Change in Blood Pressure

In investigating patients with suspected autonomic dysfunction or postural hypotension, the blood pressure should be measured with the patient supine for at least 10 (preferably 20) minutes. The patient then stands up, and the blood pressure is measured again after 5 to 10 seconds, and again after 1, 2, and 5 minutes. There is normally an increase in pulse rate on standing, but the pulse rate may not change if there is already a high resting pulse or in patients with dysautonomia; furthermore, the change in heart rate may be blunted in the elderly. As for the blood pressure, there is normally a slight decline in systolic pressure, whereas diastolic pressure increases slightly. The response of the blood pressure is regarded as abnormal if systolic pressure decreases by at least 20 mmHg or diastolic pressure by 10 mmHg on standing. In some instances, postural hypotension develops only after exercise; it is therefore worthwhile to record the postactivity blood pressure if clinically feasible. It may be necessary to record the blood pressure on a number of occasions before the diagnosis of postural hypotension can be confirmed. In other instances, prolonged tilt (for up to 60 minutes) may be required to detect abnormalities.

The effect of postural change on blood pressure can be evaluated more accurately if the blood pressure is measured using an intra-arterial cannula or a noninvasive plethysmographic device with the patient resting quietly on a tilt-table; measurements are made continuously while the patient is supine and then at a 60-degree head-up tilt. The response to head-up tilt may differ from that obtained by standing because less enhancement occurs of the venous return to the heart by contraction of leg and abdominal muscles, and thus there is greater peripheral pooling of blood.

Blood pressure normally is higher in the day, declines at night, and rises prior to awakening. Patients with postural hypotension may show a circadian trend in blood pressure that is the reverse of normal subjects, with the highest pressures found at night and the lowest in the morning. Further, postural hypotension may be more severe in the morning after prolonged nocturnal recumbency due to a decline in stroke volume and cardiac output, resulting not only from nocturnal polyuria but also from a redistribution of body fluid.[85] Such temporal variation in blood pressure implies that physiologic testing should be carried out at a standard time of day, especially if comparative studies are to be performed, and potentially harmful hypertension in response to treatment should be looked for especially during the early part of the night.

Postural Change in Heart Rate

A simple, noninvasive test of autonomic function consists of evaluating the response in heart rate to change from a recumbent to a standing position.

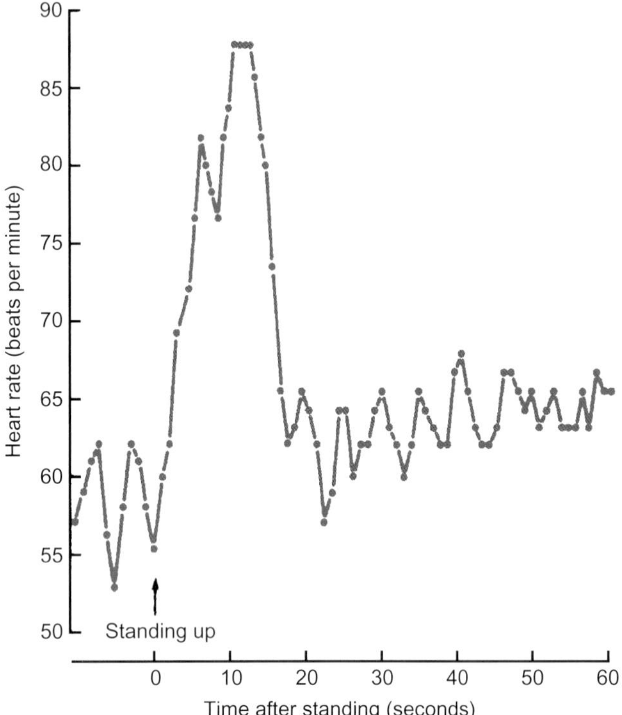

Figure 8-3 ■ Heart rate responses to standing in a normal subject. Immediately on standing, there is a rapid increase in heart rate that is maximal at approximately the fifteenth beat after standing.

There is typically a rapid increase in heart rate that is maximal at approximately the fifteenth beat after standing, with a subsequent slowing from the initial tachycardia (i.e., a relative bradycardia) that is maximal at approximately the thirtieth beat (Fig. 8-3). This response is mediated by the vagus nerve. For testing purposes, the R-R interval at beats 15 and 30 after standing can be measured to give the 30/15 ratio, as reviewed in detail elsewhere.[86] Values greater than 1.03 occur in normal subjects, whereas in diabetic patients with autonomic neuropathy (who typically show only a gradual increase in heart rate), values are 1.00 or less. Some prefer to measure the ratio of the absolute maximum to absolute minimum heart rate after standing, which may not coincide with the heart rates at beats 15 and 30.[87] This test does not depend on the resting heart rate and correlates well with the Valsalva ratio and the beat-to-beat variation in heart rate, described later. Studies suggest that the value for the 30/15 ratio declines with age in normal subjects.[86,87]

In some patients, an excessive and sustained tachycardia develops in response to standing or head-up tilt, without significant drop in blood pressure. A prolonged tilt (for up to 60 minutes) may be necessary to elicit the abnormality. The mechanisms underlying this postural tachycardia have not been clearly established.

Valsalva Maneuver

The Valsalva maneuver consists of a forced expiration maintained for at least 10 seconds (preferably 15 seconds) against a closed glottis after a full inspiration. Intrathoracic pressure should be increased by 30 to 40 mmHg. Clinically, this can be ensured by requiring the patient to blow into a mouthpiece connected to a manometer. The response can be recorded with an intra-arterial needle (Fig. 8-4), a noninvasive photoplethysmographic recording device (Finapres), or an electrocardiograph (ECG) (Fig. 8-5).

The cardiovascular response is usually divided into four stages. Stage 1 is characterized by a transient increase in blood pressure at the onset of the forced expiration, reflecting the increased intrathoracic pressure. In stage 2, there is normally a gradual decrease in systolic and diastolic pressures, pulse pressure, and stroke volume for several seconds because of a reduction in venous return to the heart, with an associated reflex tachycardia. Reflex vasoconstriction arrests the decline in blood pressure after about 5 to 7 seconds. Stage 3 occurs when the patient releases the expiratory maneuver and is characterized by a transient fall in the blood pressure because of pooling of blood and expansion of the pulmonary vascular bed with the abrupt decline in intrathoracic pressure. In stage 4, there is an overshoot of the blood pressure above baseline value as a result of the peripheral vasoconstriction, with a compensatory bradycardia.

The Valsalva maneuver is an accurate indicator of baroreceptor reflex sensitivity. Abnormalities are found in patients with dysautonomia (Fig. 8-4) and may consist of loss of the overshoot in systolic blood pressure and compensatory bradycardia in stage 4, a fall in mean blood pressure in stage 2 to less than 50 percent of the previous resting mean pressure, and loss of the tachycardia in stage 2 or a lower heart rate in stage 2 than stage 4. However, abnormalities may also be found in patients with severe congestive

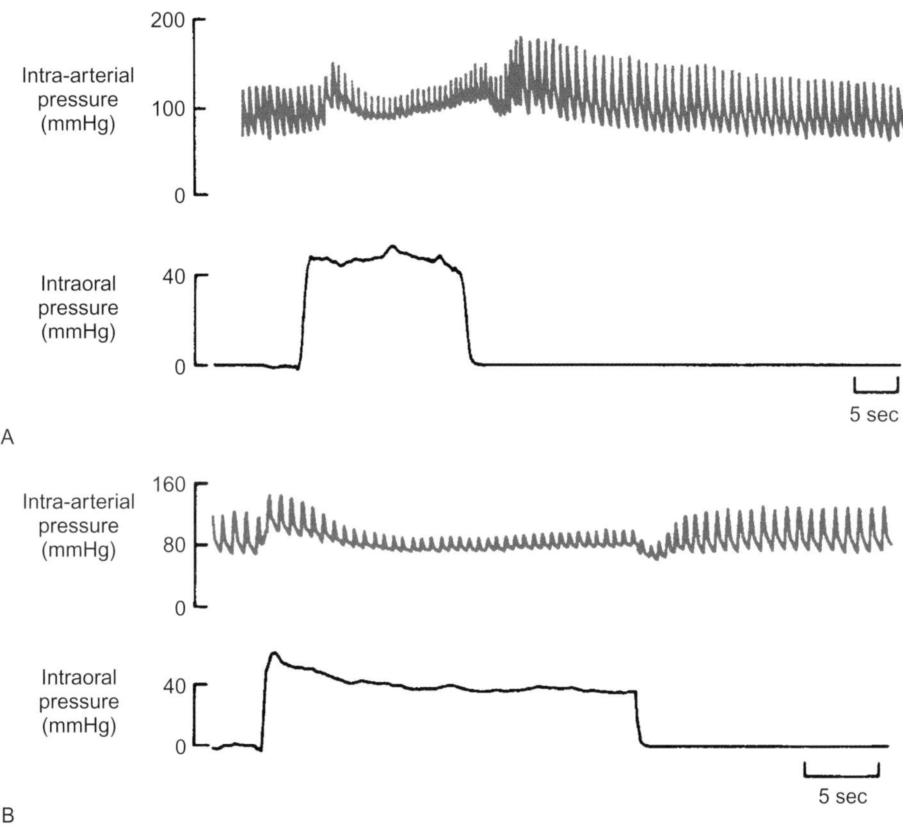

Figure 8-4 ■ Cardiovascular responses to the Valsalva maneuver, as recorded with an intra-arterial needle. **A**, Normal response. **B**, Abnormal response in a patient with multiple system atrophy. (From Aminoff MJ: Electromyography in Clinical Practice. 3rd Ed. Churchill Livingstone, New York, 1998, p. 206, with permission.)

heart failure and in those with cardiac lesions other than primary myocardial dysfunction.

If the response is recorded noninvasively using an electrocardiograph, the ratio of the shortest R-R interval (the tachycardia) during the maneuver to the longest R-R interval (bradycardia) after it is determined and expressed as the Valsalva ratio. In early studies, a value of 1.1 or less was arbitrarily defined as an abnormal response, 1.21 or greater as a normal response, and 1.11 to 1.20 as borderline. Using such criteria, the Valsalva maneuver was found to be abnormal in about 60 percent of diabetic patients with symptoms and signs suggestive of autonomic neuropathy. When more generous criteria for abnormality were used, with a lower limit for normal of 1.50, the value was abnormal in 86 percent of these patients, and such an abnormality correlated well with the presence of a significant postural drop in blood pressure. Subsequent studies have shown that age- and gender-based normal values should be used.[88,89]

Other Cardiovascular Responses

Other cardiovascular responses can also be measured noninvasively (e.g., the beat-to-beat variation in heart rate and the heart rate responses to deep breathing and sustained hand grip). Such tests of parasympathetic function appear to give abnormal results more often and earlier than tests of sympathetic efferent function (blood pressure response to change in posture and isometric exercise), at least with the dysautonomia that occurs in diabetes. Reduced cardiovascular autonomic function, as reflected by heart rate variability, is associated with an increased risk of silent myocardial ischemia and death.[90]

A particularly useful test is to measure the heart rate variation during deep breathing (Fig. 8-6). In normal subjects, there is considerable heart rate variation, which is accentuated during deep breathing. This variation is reduced or absent in diabetic patients with autonomic neuropathy. The optimal

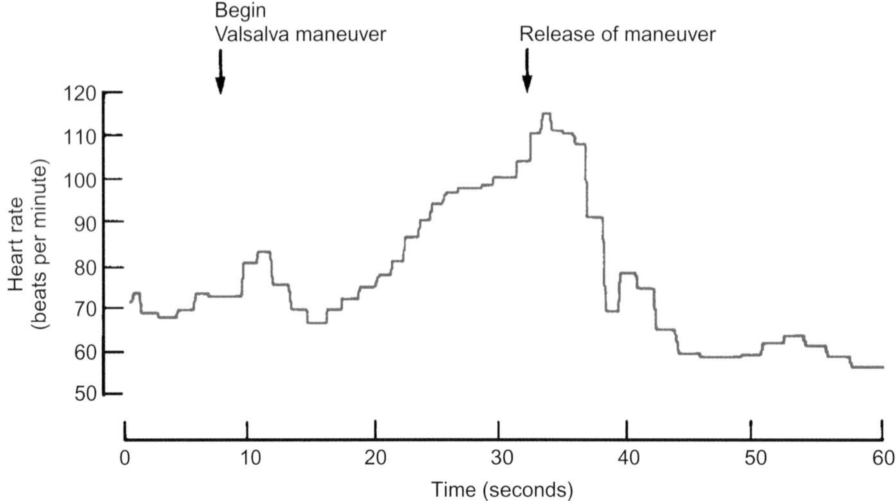

Figure 8-5 ■ Valsalva maneuver as recorded using an electrocardiograph (ECG) or heart rate monitor in a normal subject. The tachycardia that occurs during the forced expiratory maneuver is clearly evident, as is the compensatory bradycardia that occurs when the maneuver is released.

breathing rate for this test is six breaths per minute (i.e., inspiration = expiration = 5 seconds). Heart rate variation scores can be calculated by measuring the difference between the maximal and minimal heart rates in inspiration and expiration, taking the average from 10 breaths in and 10 breaths out. Normal subjects usually have a score greater than 9, and autonomic neuropathy is probably absent if scores greater than 12 are obtained; the normal range, however, is age dependent.[88,89,91] Thus, heart rate variability may decline by 3 to 5 beats per minute per decade in normal subjects.[89] The use of a single normal value regardless of age may therefore limit the utility of the test. Physical fitness, body weight and position, time of testing, and concomitant medication may affect the test results.

An increase in heart rate and blood pressure should also occur in response to startle, such as occurs with a sudden loud noise, and to mental stress, as is produced when the patient attempts to subtract 7 serially from 100 while constantly being distracted.

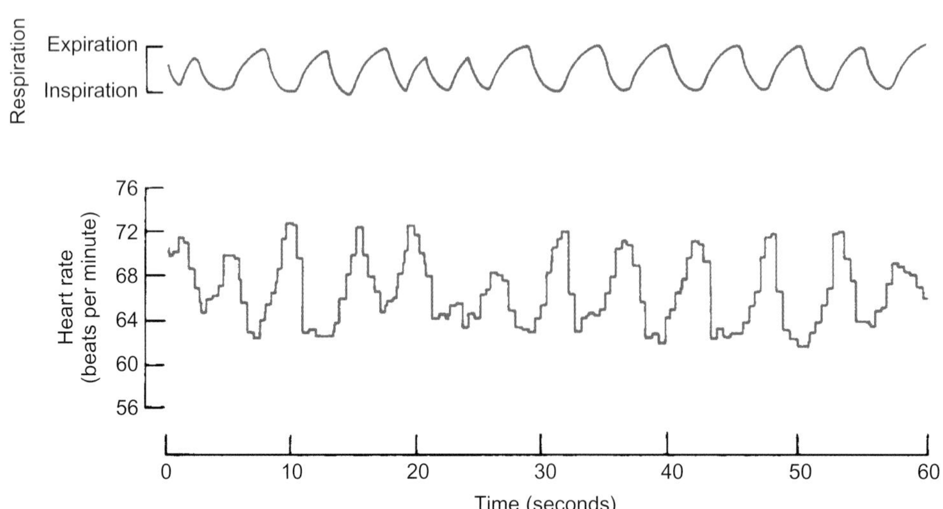

Figure 8-6 ■ Normal variation in heart rate that occurs in response to deep breathing.

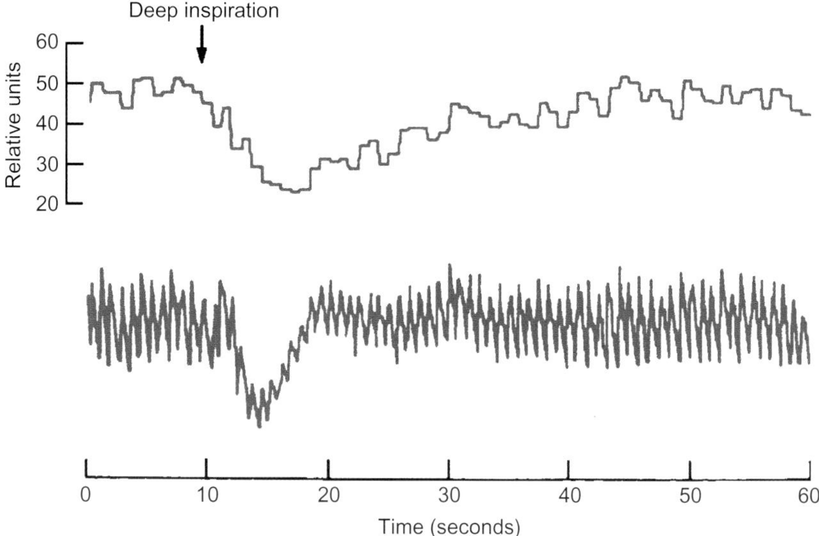

Figure 8-7 ▪ Variation in blood volume after a deep inspiration in a normal subject, measured photoplethysmographically by means of an infrared emitter and detector placed on the pad of the index finger. The bottom trace represents the sensor output after it has been amplified by the photoplethysmographic module of a computerized autonomic testing system; it is a function of the absolute blood volume in the finger. Each peak represents a heartbeat, and the amplitude of each wave reflects blood volume in the area about the sensor. The apparent shift of the direct-current signal component is due to the long time constant that is necessary so that signal information is not lost. The relative voltage, representing the amplitude of each pulse, is shown in the upper trace. It is evident in both traces that after the deep inspiration there is a reduction in digital blood flow (i.e., reduced amplitude of the waveforms in the lower trace and a corresponding decline in the upper trace).

Digital Blood Flow

Blood flow to a finger can be measured by conventional plethysmography or photoplethysmography. A sudden inspiratory gasp causes reflex digital vasoconstriction as a spinal or brainstem reflex, and this is easily measured plethysmographically (Fig. 8-7).[92] The response is impaired or absent in patients with a lesion of the cord or sympathetic efferent pathway, as in peripheral neuropathy or pure autonomic failure.[93] In entrapment neuropathy, such as carpal tunnel syndrome, the vasoconstrictor response may be abolished in fingers supplied by the affected nerve but not in those supplied by other nerves.

Mental stress (e.g., performing mental arithmetic despite distraction) or startle (as from a sudden loud noise) leads to a transient increase in sympathetic vasomotor activity and thus to a reduction in digital blood flow; this can be used to evaluate sympathetic efferent pathways. Normal subjects sometimes have no response to these tests, however, leading to false-positive results.

Cold Pressor Test

In the cold pressor test, one hand is immersed in ice water at 4°C, and this normally produces an increase in systolic pressure of 15 mmHg or more within 1 minute. The afferent pathway involves the spinothalamic tract, and if this tract is intact, the lack of a pressor response suggests a lesion centrally or in the sympathetic efferent pathway. A normal response in a patient with an abnormal Valsalva response and intact pain and temperature sensation suggests an afferent baroreceptor lesion.

Norepinephrine Infusion

The plasma norepinephrine level can be used as an index of sympathetic activity. Perhaps of greater value, the blood pressure can be measured in response to intravenous infusion of norepinephrine at several dose rates up to 20 μg/min.[62] In this way, a dose–response curve can be constructed. In normal subjects, it is usually necessary to administer 15 to 20 μg/min to increase systolic blood pressure to 40 mmHg above baseline. A similar increase in blood pressure results from doses of 5 to 10 µg/min in multiple system atrophy and less than 2.5 µg/min in patients with idiopathic orthostatic hypotension.[62]

Response to Tyramine

Tyramine, an indirectly acting sympathomimetic drug, can be used to test neuronal uptake and release of norepinephrine. Bolus injections ranging from 250 to 6,000 µg are administered and blood pressure is measured at 1-minute intervals. The amount of norepinephrine released into plasma by tyramine can be quantified by obtaining a blood sample shortly after the rise in blood pressure.[62]

Sweat Tests

Cutaneous blood vessels and sweat glands are supplied by sympathetic fibers intermingled in the same fascicles but of different size and conduction velocity.[14] Commonly used tests of sweating are messy and require application of heat, which is time-consuming. A heat cradle placed over the trunk is used to produce an increase of 1°C (from a resting level of 36.5° to 37.0°C) in the oral temperature over the course of 30 to 60 minutes, and the presence of sweat over selected regions of the trunk and limbs is detected by the change in color produced in quinizarine powder, a starch-iodide mixture, or some other indicator powder. The pattern of any impairment of sweating may be helpful in suggesting the underlying cause (Fig. 8-8).[94–96] For example, impairment is usually distal in the limbs in patients with polyneuropathies. The method does not distinguish preganglionic from postganglionic lesions.

The volume of sweat produced by axon-reflex stimulation either electrically (faradic sweat response) or with parasympathomimetic drugs under specified conditions indicates the state of sudomotor innervation in the tested limb (Fig. 8-9). After a short latent period, sweating occurs in an area that is approximately 4 to 5 cm in diameter about the site of stimulation. The reflex is subserved by sympathetic postganglionic fibers; impulses pass centripetally along these fibers until they reach a branch point and then pass distally again. The receptor involved in the reflex has not been defined. To quantify the volume of sweat, recordings are made of the humidity change of an air stream of defined flow.[94–98] Such quantitative sudomotor axon reflex testing (QSART) is a sensitive means of assessing postganglionic sympathetic function by

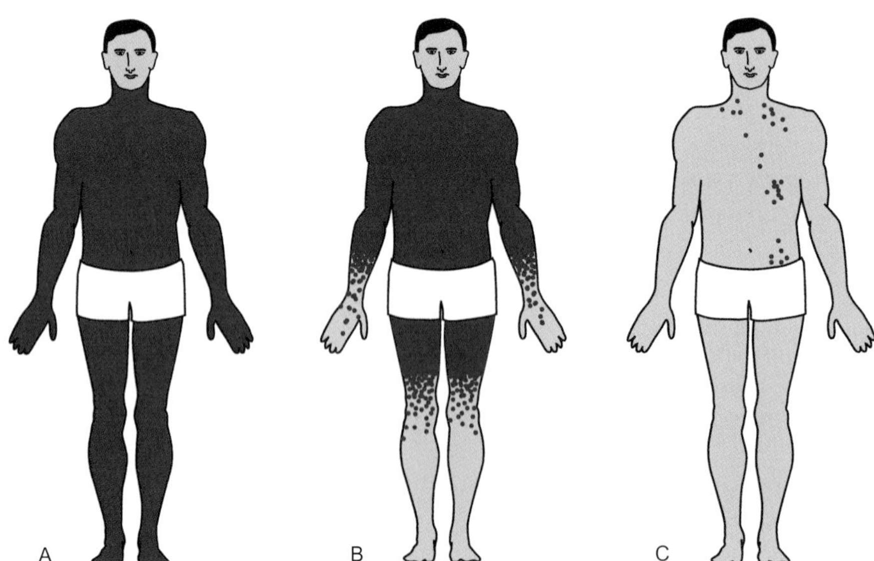

Figure 8-8 ■ Thermoregulatory sweat tests. **A**, An increase in body temperature leads normally to sweating over the entire body. An indicator powder becomes discolored (purple) by the moisture. It was not placed on the face and head, so that no discoloration is seen in these regions. **B**, In a patient with a length-dependent neuropathy involving the sudomotor fibers, sweating is absent in a stocking-and-glove-pattern. **C**, A patient with multiple system atrophy and almost complete anhidrosis, showing only small scattered areas of sweating.

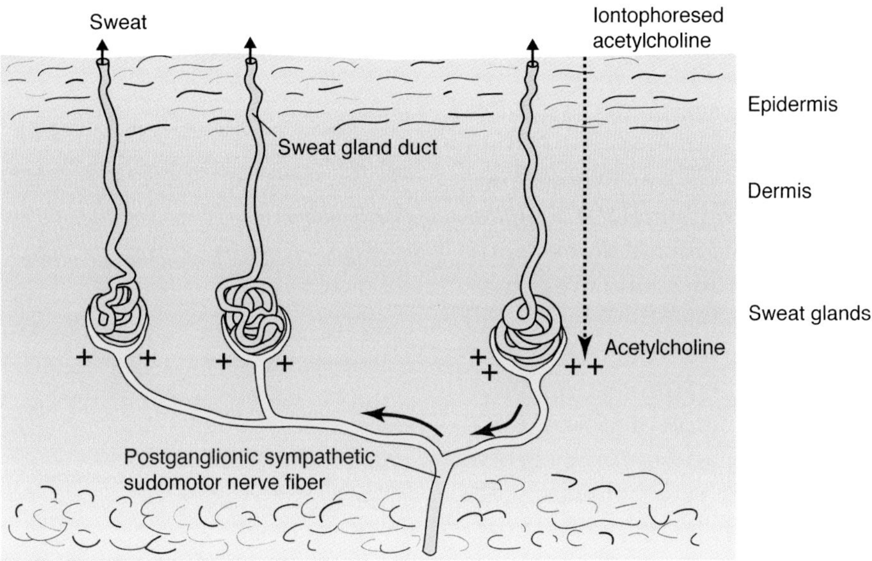

Figure 8-9 ■ Sweating induced through an axon reflex. Iontophoresed acetylcholine stimulates sweat gland production locally and—by an axon reflex—in adjacent areas.

using iontophoresed acetylcholine to stimulate the involved receptors; it yields reproducible results but requires sophisticated and expensive equipment. Yet another approach to evaluating postganglionic sympathetic sudomotor function is with the silicone mold technique, in which imprints are made of sweat droplets stimulated by iontophoresed acetylcholine.[94]

Sudomotor function can also be evaluated by measuring changes in skin resistance. With sweating, there is a reduction in skin resistance. This is the so-called *galvanic skin response*, which can be elicited by painful or emotional stimuli or by deep inspiration.

Sudomotor function has been evaluated also by recording the change in voltage measured from the skin surface after deep inspiration or startle or after electrical stimuli applied to a contralateral mixed or cutaneous nerve at the wrist or ankle (*sympathetic skin response*).[95,96,98–100] Responses are recorded from a pair of electrodes placed on the palm and dorsum of the hand or the sole and dorsum of the foot. The sympathetic skin response is simple to record, but responses tend to habituate and are affected by the recording technique and a number of other factors. The absence of a response, and not the absolute values of latency or amplitude, is regarded as significant for determining abnormality. The normal latency in the upper limb is on the order of 1.5 seconds and in the lower limb is about 2 seconds, reflecting the slow conduction velocity of postganglionic C fibers (approximately 1 m/sec) Abnormalities of the sympathetic skin response reportedly correlate well with the quantitative sudomotor axon reflex test.

Other Studies

Pupillary Responses

Pupillary constriction with 2.5 percent methacholine applied locally indicates denervation supersensitivity due to interruption of postganglionic parasympathetic fibers, as in the Holmes–Adie syndrome. Local instillation of 1:1,000 epinephrine hydrochloride (one or two drops) produces little or no response unless there is postganglionic sympathetic denervation, in which case marked pupillary dilatation occurs. A 4 percent solution of cocaine hydrochloride applied to the conjunctival sac dilates the normal pupil, but fails to do so if sympathetic innervation has been interrupted outside the CNS.

Radiologic Studies

Radiologic studies may be helpful in characterizing gastrointestinal and bladder function but are beyond the scope of this chapter.

PATIENT MANAGEMENT

The initial investigative approach to patients presenting with syncope or other symptoms suggestive of postural hypotension or autonomic dysfunction is to exclude reversible causes such as hypovolemia or certain medications (see pp. 148 to 149). The history must include a detailed account of illnesses and drug intake. An instrument (questionnaire) to assess autonomic symptoms has been developed and validated.[101] Simple laboratory investigations may include a full blood count and erythrocyte sedimentation rate as well as determination of plasma urea, electrolytes, glucose, morning and evening cortisol levels, and lying and standing catecholamine concentrations. Urinary screen for porphyrins, serum protein electrophoresis and immunophoresis, hepatic, renal, and thyroid function tests, chest radiograph, and electrocardiogram (to exclude recent cardiac infarction or cardiac ischemia, heart block, or persisting cardiac dysrhythmia) may also be performed, as may serologic tests for syphilis and nerve conduction studies. Neuroimaging studies may be helpful if a structural intracranial lesion is suspected. An echocardiogram may help when evaluating patients with suspected structural lesions of the heart predisposing to syncope. Prolonged tilt-table evaluations and invasive cardiac electrophysiologic studies may be necessary when an arrhythmia is likely. In patients with symptoms of uncertain etiology in whom general medical causes have been excluded, more detailed evaluation of autonomic function in the manner suggested earlier may be helpful.

Treatment

If a specific reversible cause, such as a metabolic or endocrinologic disturbance, can be recognized, it must be treated appropriately. The need for continuing with drugs likely to be responsible should be reviewed and, if feasible, treatment discontinued. Patients should be advised against using alcohol. Treatment with antiarrhythmic agents, cardiac pacemaker, or surgery may be indicated in patients with a cardiac cause of syncope or postural hypotension. Pacemaker therapy may also help patients with syncope due to carotid sinus hypersensitivity.

If no specific cause can be identified, treatment should be directed to the minimization of symptoms (Tables 8-1 and 8-2). The actual extent to which the blood pressure falls on standing, for example,

TABLE 8-1 ■ Management of Postural Hypotension

Treatment of Specific Underlying Cause or Aggravating Factors
Discontinue drugs that may be responsible, if feasible
Correct electrolyte/metabolic/hormonal disorders
Avoid alcohol
Eliminate conditions that favor pooling of blood or that impede venous return
Prescribe antiarrhythmic drugs, pacemaker, or surgery for selected cardiac disorders
Consider a cardiac pacemaker for carotid sinus hypersensitivity
Symptomatic Treatment
Nonpharmacologic management
Stand up gradually
Eat small meals and avoid postprandial activity
Wear waist-high elastic stockings
Elevate the head of the bed
Ingest fluid (approx. 500 ml) before arising
Eat a liberal salt diet
Pharmacologic and other treatment
Fludrocortisone
Indomethacin; ibuprofen; flurbiprofen
Dihydroergotamine; Cafergot
Sympathomimetic drugs (phenylephrine, ephedrine, amphetamines)
Midodrine
β-Blocker drugs (propranolol, pindolol)
Pyridostigmine
Cardiac pacing in selected circumstances
Other approaches
Vasopressin; desmopressin
Erythropoietin
Yohimbine
Atomoxetine
L-Dihydroxyphenylserine (Droxidopa)
Metoclopramide
Clonidine
Octreotide
Oxilofrine
Norepinephrine (by infusion pump)
Deep brain stimulation

TABLE 8-2 ■ Mechanisms Involved in the Management of Postural Hypotension by Selected Drugs

Mechanism	Medication
Reduced sodium excretion	Fludrocortisone; (? clonidine)
Sympathetic vasoconstriction	Phenylephrine; ephedrine; midodrine; L-dihydroxyphenylserine; norepinephrine; yohimbine; dihydroergotamine
β-Blocker with sympathomimetic activity	Pindolol
Enhanced ganglionic cholinergic stimulation (increased total peripheral resistance)	Pyridostigmine
Reduced vasodilatation	Prostaglandin synthetase inhibitors (e.g., indomethacin; ibuprofen; flurbiprofen)
Increased red cell mass	Erythropoietin

is of less significance than the occurrence of symptoms. Patients without symptoms generally require no treatment. Symptomatic patients with dysautonomia should avoid extreme heat, alcohol, large meals, rapid postural changes, prolonged periods of recumbency, and excessive straining (e.g., during micturition or defecation), each of which may exacerbate symptoms. Diuretics should be stopped, if possible, and salt intake liberalized.

When standing, patients often find it helpful to work the leg muscles because this aids the venous return to the heart. Symptoms may also be reduced if patients stand up gradually (e.g., by first adopting the seated position and, after a short pause, getting up from this position). Other physical maneuvers that may be helpful include standing with legs crossed, bending forward, squatting, or placing a foot on a chair, thereby slightly increasing the mean arterial pressure so that cerebral blood flow remains adequate. The underlying common mechanism is held to be an increase of thoracic blood volume by transfer from below the diaphragm to the chest.[1] Resistance exercise may increase orthostatic tolerance, plasma volume, and baroreflex gain.

Waist-high elastic stockings may be helpful in alleviating postural symptoms but are often difficult to put on (especially for elderly patients) and may be uncomfortable in hot weather. To be effective, the stockings must extend at least as high as the waist. They should not be worn at night as they may then aggravate nocturnal diuresis. Antigravity suits have been used in the past but are awkward, restrictive, impractical, and not generally available.

Many dysautonomic patients have a disturbance in the regulation of body fluids. In particular, there is defective sodium conservation, especially during recumbency at night, associated with, but not entirely due to, low aldosterone levels; there are also abnormal posture-dependent changes in urine volume (Fig. 8-10) accompanied by an alteration in the secretion of antidiuretic hormone. This leads to relative hypovolemia and postural hypotension that are worse in the morning and improve during the day. The disturbed regulation of body fluids could be due, at least in part, to diminished adrenergic activity in the renal nerves, which affects tubular reabsorption and renin release (and thus angiotensin formation). The effect of recumbency can be minimized by elevating the head of the bed by 5 to 20 degrees, which leads to reduced renal artery pressure, thereby stimulating the renin-angiotensin system and promoting sodium retention. Head-up tilt at night reduces nocturnal shifts of interstitial fluid from the legs into the circulation; furthermore, such interstitial fluid may exert hydrostatic force, opposing the tendency of blood to pool in the legs on standing. Head-up tilt at night also reduces supine hypertension. Patients are sometimes helped by drinking 500 ml water about 15 to 30 minutes before arising from bed in the morning, as this has a transient pressor effect that may diminish postural hypotension at a time when it is usually most troublesome.

If these measures are unsuccessful, the mineralocorticoid fludrocortisone can be tried. This agent seems to exert its effect in part by temporarily increasing plasma volume and also by increasing vascular sensitivity to norepinephrine and improving the vasoconstrictor response to sympathetic stimulation. Treatment is usually commenced with a daily dose of 0.1 mg, which can then be increased by 0.1 mg every 2 weeks or so until benefit occurs or there are intolerable side effects. Some patients may require as much as 1.0 mg daily, but usually a dose of 0.3 mg or less is sufficient. During treatment with fludrocortisone, a positive sodium balance should be ensured, with a sodium intake of at least 150 mEq/day. Side effects include pedal edema, weight gain, recumbent hypertension, cardiomegaly, hypokalemia,

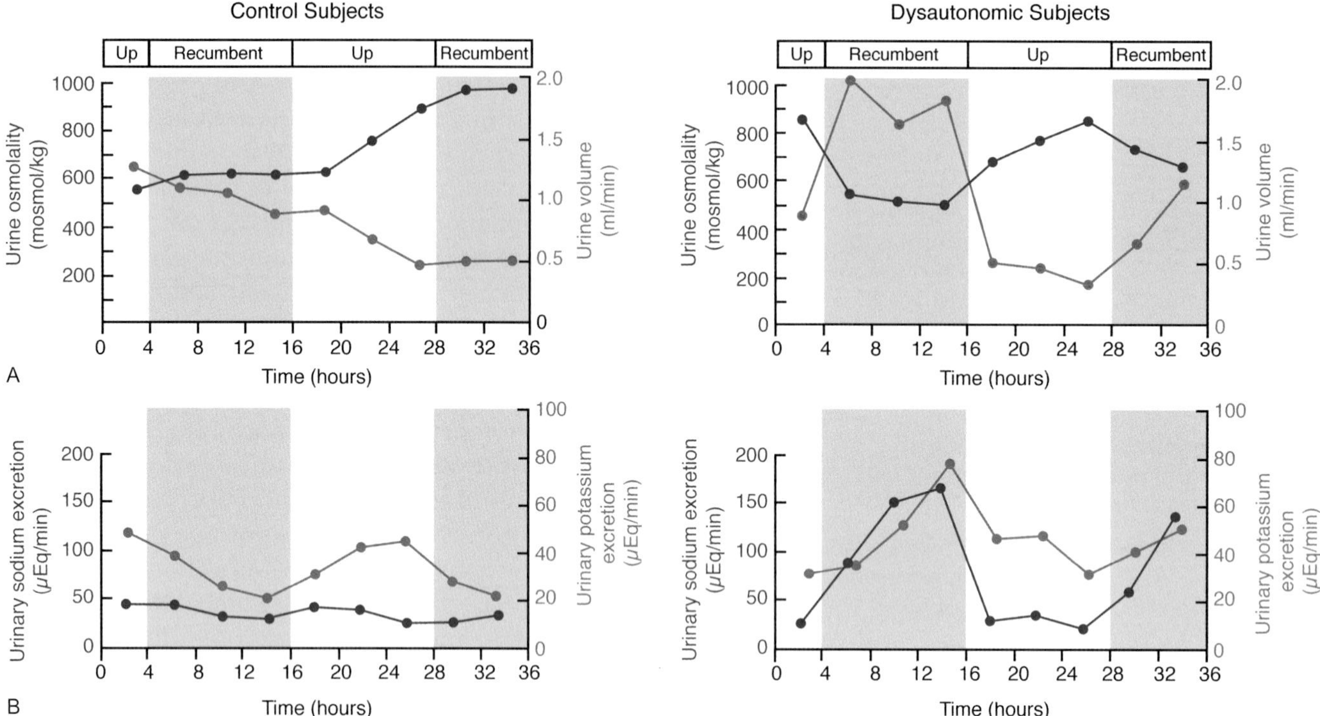

Figure 8-10 ■ Renal responses to fluid deprivation for 36 hours of five dysautonomic patients with multiple system atrophy (right panels) and four control subjects with Parkinson disease and preserved autonomic reflexes (left panels). Deprivation commenced at 6 P.M. Mean results for each successive 4-hour period are shown for urine osmolality (blue) and volume (red) in **A**, and for sodium (blue) and potassium excretion (red) in **B**. Subjects were recumbent during the night (10 P.M. to 10 A.M.; shaded area) and were up and about during the day (10 A.M. to 10 P.M.). In the control subjects, urine volume declined and osmolality increased during the period of fluid deprivation; sodium excretion was unchanged whereas potassium excretion was greater during the day than night. In the dysautonomic subjects, similar changes were seen during the day; during recumbency at night, however, a considerable increase occurred in urinary volume and sodium and potassium excretion, and urinary osmolality declined. (Data from Wilcox CS, Aminoff MJ, Penn W: Basis of nocturnal polyuria in patients with autonomic failure. J Neurol Neurosurg Psychiatry 37:677, 1974.)

and retinopathy; coexisting diabetes mellitus may also be exacerbated.

Prostaglandin synthetase inhibitors should expand plasma volume and inhibit vasodilator prostaglandin synthesis. Indomethacin (25 to 75 mg three times daily with meals) increases peripheral vascular resistance, promotes fluid retention, and may increase the sensitivity of the peripheral vasculature to norepinephrine and angiotensin II. It is said to be helpful in some patients with postural hypotension,[102] especially if they are also on fludrocortisone, but, in general, the results with it have been rather disappointing despite the theoretical advantages of its use. Ibuprofen (200 to 600 mg four times daily before meals) can also be tried and is sometimes helpful. Side effects include gastric irritation, nausea, constipation, and skin rashes. Flurbiprofen has also been used with benefit.

Dihydroergotamine is a relatively selective constrictor of peripheral veins. Its action may be mediated partially through α-adrenoreceptors, and enhanced synthesis of a vasoconstrictor prostaglandin may also be important. It is sometimes helpful for treating postural hypotension, but may cause recumbent hypertension. Although it is effective when administered intravenously, its efficacy when taken orally (5 to 10 mg three times daily) is more limited and variable. Inhaled preparations may be effective.[103] Cafergot (caffeine and ergotamine) suppositories have sometimes been helpful.[104]

Sympathomimetic drugs that either act directly to constrict blood vessels (e.g., phenylephrine) or that have an indirect action, preventing the destruction of norepinephrine at sympathetic nerve terminals (e.g., ephedrine and amphetamines), have been used to treat postural hypotension. These drugs can sometimes be helpful, but any benefit is often mild and temporary, and they may cause severe recumbent hypertension. Other side effects include nervousness, anxiety, restlessness, tachycardia, and tachyphylaxis. Midodrine is a direct α-adrenergic agonist that causes constriction of arterioles and venous vessels. It is started in a low daily dose (2.5 mg three times daily) that is built up gradually to 10 mg three times daily, depending on response and tolerance. Side effects include supine hypertension, piloerection, and pruritus.[105,106] Pyridostigmine bromide may reduce postural hypotension by enhancing ganglionic cholinergic transmission without aggravating or precipitating supine hypertension. A recent clinical trial showed that its greatest effect was on diastolic blood pressure, suggesting that improvement is due to increased total peripheral resistance.[107,108] Propranolol may help the postural hypotension associated with postural tachycardia syndrome and also reduces sodium excretion, leading to an increase in blood volume. Furthermore, it has been said to help the hypotension of both idiopathic orthostatic hypotension and multiple system atrophy; this action has been attributed to the β-blockade correcting an imbalance of α- and β-adrenoreceptor activity in the peripheral nervous system. It can be initiated at a dose of 10 mg four times daily and built up to 40 mg four times daily. Pindolol, a β-blocker with intrinsic sympathomimetic activity, may also be helpful in occasional instances; more often it produces no benefit and may lead to cardiac failure. Octreotide[102] and oxilofrine[109] have also been used, with mixed results.

A number of these and other therapies were examined in a systematic review; 36 trials (21 interventions) overall were included. The heterogeneous population and wide variety of study methods precluded meta-analysis. Most trials were of poor quality and had a high risk of bias. Changes in postural drop in blood pressure and symptoms were frequently inconsistent. Compression bandages, indomethacin, oxilofrine, potassium chloride and yohimbine improved the postural drop. Several vasoactive drugs, including midodrine and pyridostigmine, improved the standing blood pressure but the postural decline in blood pressure worsened.[110]

In patients with sympathetic efferent failure, clinical benefit, with a decline in the severity of postural hypotension and an increase in blood pressure on standing, may follow cardiac pacing to protect against vagal overactivity. However, the benefits of this approach are not clear, with benefit reported by some authors[111,112] but not others in patients with orthostatic hypotension.[113]

Vasopressin responses to upright posture are often defective in autonomic failure, and patients are hypersensitive to exogenous vasopressin. The antidiuretic, V2-receptor specific, vasopressin analogue desmopressin increases the intravascular volume.[114] Intranasal desmopressin administered once at night in patients with multiple system atrophy and nocturnal polyuria has led to an improvement in nocturia without serious adverse effects.[115] If this approach is to be used, serum sodium should be monitored, especially during the first 4 to 5 days of treatment and then at monthly intervals. The long-term therapeutic utility of vasopressin is unclear, however, and treatment with desmopressin should be limited to patients with severe, refractory disease.[116]

Recombinant erythropoietin helps the mild anemia that is common in dysautonomic patients; it increases the red cell mass, blood pressure and cerebral oxygenation, and reduces postural hypotension.[117] It is expensive, may require concomitant iron supplementation, and sometimes leads to supine hypertension, but can be tried in cases that are otherwise difficult to manage. It is given subcutaneously, with the dose and frequency of administration individualized.

There have been a variety of other investigative therapeutic approaches. Yohimbine, a centrally acting α_2-adrenoreceptor antagonist, potentiates sympathetic activity[117] and reduces the postural decline in blood pressure in dysautonomic patients,[110] but its clinical utility is not clear. Other approaches with encouraging results include the use of L-dihydroxyphenylserine (Droxidopa),[118] which is converted to norepinephrine after oral administration, or atomoxetine, which inhibits norepinephrine reuptake.[117]

The use of a dopamine receptor antagonist, metoclopramide, was suggested because dopaminergic drugs (e.g., bromocriptine) may depress the blood pressure, but evidence of efficacy is lacking.[118] In some patients with pure autonomic failure, the selective partial α-agonist clonidine may be helpful; it may reduce supine hypertension and nocturnal natriuresis.[119] It is probably most likely to help in patients with an efferent sympathetic lesion. It is started in a dose of 0.1 mg taken in the morning, and the dose is then built up gradually to 0.2 to 1 mg twice daily. Side effects include xerostomia, constipation, drowsiness, and supine hypertension;

hypotension may be exacerbated in patients with non-neurologic causes of postural hypotension. Administration of caffeine with meals may markedly reduce postprandial hypotension and is worthy of trial when symptoms are particularly troubling after meals. A possible role for deep brain stimulation of the periventricular/periaqueductal gray region has been suggested.[120,121]

Patients with vasovagal syncope require reassurance coupled with advice about ensuring adequate fluid and salt intake and about sympathetic activation techniques (such as isometric hand exercises) to increase the blood pressure[122]; sitting or lying down or sitting with head between the knees may help to abort attacks.

The effects of impaired thermoregulatory sweating may be alleviated by external temperature regulation, such as by air conditioning. High-fiber diets, bulking agents, fecal softeners, laxatives, osmotic agents (e.g., lactulose), and glycerine suppositories may reduce constipation. Depending on their nature, urinary disturbances may be helped by bladder training and timed urination, avoidance of diuretics and certain foods and beverages, physical therapy to strengthen the pelvic floor muscles, anticholinergic medications, intermittent self-catheterization or suprapubic catheterization, and measures to contain incontinence such as penile sheaths and pads. The treatment of erectile dysfunction is discussed in Chapter 30.

General Precautions in Dysautonomic Patients

Patients may show postprandial falls in blood pressure because blood is diverted to the hepatic and splanchnic beds. Vasoactive substances may also contribute to the hypotensive response. To avoid or minimize this postprandial hypotension, it is helpful to eat smaller meals and to avoid excessive activity during the immediate postprandial period.

Dysautonomic patients often have low circulating catecholamine levels and denervation supersensitivity to sympathomimetic amines. Medications containing such substances should therefore be avoided, even though they are often available without prescription in over-the-counter preparations.

Patients with dysautonomia pose special problems during anesthesia. They are unable to tolerate hemodynamic stresses normally because of impaired cardiovascular reflexes. Maintenance of fluid balance is more difficult because of the abnormal manner in which they handle salt and water, and their enhanced sensitivity to volume changes influences blood pressure control.

REFERENCES

1. Wieling W, van Lieshout JJ, van Leeuwen AM: Physical manoeuvres that reduce postural hypotension in autonomic failure. Clin Auton Res 3:57, 1993.
2. Schoenberger JA: Drug-induced orthostatic hypotension. Drug Saf 6:402, 1991.
3. Mosnaim AD, Abiola R, Wolf ME, et al: Etiology and risk factors for developing orthostatic hypotension. Am J Ther 17:86, 2010.
4. Alfrey C: Regulation of red cell volume at microgravity. Med Sci Sports Exerc 28(suppl):542, 1996.
5. Convertino VA: Conditions of reduced gravity. p. 429. In Low PA (ed): Clinical Autonomic Disorders. 2nd Ed. Lippincott-Raven, Philadelphia, 1997.
6. Craven CG, Engelke KA, Pawelczyk JA, et al: Power spectral and time-based analysis of heart rate variability following 15 days of head-down bed rest. Aviat Space Environ Med 65:1105, 1994.
7. Low PA: The effect of aging on the autonomic nervous system. p. 161. In Low PA (ed): Clinical Autonomic Disorders. 2nd Ed. Lippincott-Raven, Philadelphia, 1997.
8. Mattace-Raso FU, van der Cammen TJ, Knetsch AM, et al: Arterial stiffness as the candidate underlying mechanism for postural blood pressure changes and orthostatic hypotension in older adults: the Rotterdam Study. J Hypertens 24:339, 2006.
9. Weiss A, Beloosesky Y, Kornowski R, et al: Influence of orthostatic hypotension on mortality among patients discharged from an acute geriatric ward. J Gen Intern Med 21:602, 2006.
10. Spyer KM: Physiology of the autonomic nervous system: CNS control of the cardiovascular system. Curr Opin Neurol Neurosurg 4:528, 1991.
11. Loewy AD: Anatomy of the autonomic nervous system: an overview. p. 3. In: Loewy AD, Spyer KM (eds): Central Regulation of Autonomic Functions. Oxford University Press, New York, 1990.
12. Andersen MC, Kunze DL: Nucleus tractus solitarius: gateway to neural circulatory control. Annu Rev Physiol 56:93, 1994.
13. Dampney RA: Functional organization of central pathways regulating the cardiovascular system. Physiol Rev 74:323, 1994.
14. Wallin BG, Elam M: Microneurography and autonomic dysfunction. p. 233. In Low PA (ed): Clinical Autonomic Disorders. 2nd Ed. Lippincott-Raven, Philadelphia, 1997.

15. Sheriff DD, O'Leary DS, Scher AM, et al: Baroreflex attenuates pressor response to graded muscle ischemia in exercising dogs. Am J Physiol 258:H305, 1990.
16. Smith SA, Mitchell JH, Garry MG: The mammalian exercise pressor reflex in health and disease. Exp Physiol 91:89, 2006.
17. Williamson JW: The relevance of central command for the neural cardiovascular control of exercise. Exp Physiol 95:1043, 2010.
18. Matsukawa K: Central command: control of cardiac sympathetic and vagal efferent nerve activity and the arterial baroreflex during spontaneous motor behaviour in animals. Exp Physiol 97:20, 2012.
19. Derrey S, Maltête D, Ahtoy P, et al: Severe orthostatic hypotension and intramedullary tumor: a case report and review of the literature. Neurochirurgie 55:589, 2009.
20. Heidel KM, Benarroch EE, Gene R, et al: Cardiovascular and respiratory consequences of bilateral involvement of the medullary intermediate reticular formation in syringobulbia. Clin Auton Res 12:450, 2002.
21. Weig SG, Buckthal PE, Choi SK, et al: Recurrent syncope as the presenting symptom of Arnold-Chiari malformation. Neurology 41:1673, 1991.
22. Jain S, Goldstein DS: Cardiovascular dysautonomia in Parkinson disease: from pathophysiology to pathogenesis. Neurobiol Dis 46:572, 2012.
23. Goldstein DS, Holmes CS, Dendi R, et al: Orthostatic hypotension from sympathetic denervation in Parkinson's disease. Neurology 58:1247, 2002.
24. Holmberg B, Kallio M, Johnels B, et al: Cardiovascular reflex testing contributes to clinical evaluation and differential diagnosis of parkinsonian syndromes. Mov Disord 16:217, 2001.
25. Williams DR, Lees AJ: What features improve the accuracy of the clinical diagnosis of progressive supranuclear palsy-parkinsonism (PSP-P)? Mov Disord 25:357, 2010.
26. Gutrecht JA: Autonomic cardiovascular reflexes in progressive supranuclear palsy. J Auton Nerv Syst 39:29, 1992.
27. Aziz NA, Anguelova GV, Marinus J, et al: Autonomic symptoms in patients and pre-manifest mutation carriers of Huntington's disease. Eur J Neurol 17:1068, 2010.
28. Kobal J, Melik Z, Cankar K, et al: Autonomic dysfunction in presymptomatic and early symptomatic Huntington's disease. Acta Neurol Scand 121:392, 2010.
29. Flachenecker P: Autonomic dysfunction in Guillain-Barré syndrome and multiple sclerosis. J Neurol 254(suppl 2):II96, 2007.
30. Haensch CA, Jorg J: Autonomic dysfunction in multiple sclerosis. J Neurol 253(suppl 1):I3, 2006.
31. Norrving B, Cronqvist S: Lateral medullary infarction: prognosis in an unselected series. Neurology 41:244, 1991.
32. Low PA, Benrud-Larson LM, Sletten DM, et al: Autonomic symptoms and diabetic neuropathy: a population-based study. Diabetes Care 27:2942, 2004.
33. Freeman R: Autonomic peripheral neuropathy. Lancet 365:1259, 2005.
34. Low VA, Sandroni P, Fealey RD, et al: Detection of small-fiber neuropathy by sudomotor testing. Muscle Nerve 34:57, 2006.
35. Miralles R, Espadaler JM, Navarro X, et al: Autonomic neuropathy in chronic alcoholism: evaluation of cardiovascular, pupillary and sympathetic skin responses. Eur Neurol 35:287, 1995.
36. Bernardi L, Passino C, Porta C, et al: Widespread cardiovascular autonomic dysfunction in primary amyloidosis: does spontaneous hyperventilation have a compensatory role against postural hypotension? Heart 88:615, 2002.
37. Graber JJ, Sherman FT, Kaufmann H, et al: Vitamin B_1 responsive severe leukoencephalopathy and autonomic dysfunction in a patient with "normal" serum B_{12} levels. J Neurol Neurosurg Psychiatry 81:1369, 2010.
38. Beitzke M, Pfister P, Fortin J, et al: Autonomic dysfunction and hemodynamics in vitamin B_{12} deficiency. Auton Neurosci 97:45, 2002.
39. Oskam L, Wilder-Smith A, Sampaio EP, et al: High prevalence of vasomotor reflex impairment in newly diagnosed leprosy patients. Eur J Clin Invest 35:658, 2005.
40. Abbot NC, Beck JS, Mostofi S, et al: Sympathetic vasomotor dysfunction in leprosy patients: comparison with electrophysiological measurement and qualitative sensation testing. Neurosci Lett 206:57, 1996.
41. Koike H, Watanabe H, Sobue G: The spectrum of immune-mediated autonomic neuropathies: insights from the clinicopathological features. J Neurol Neurosurg Psychiatry 84:98, 2013.
42. Biegstraaten M, van Schaik IN, Wieling W, et al: Autonomic neuropathy in Fabry disease: a prospective study using the Autonomic Symptom Profile and cardiovascular autonomic function tests. BMC Neurol 10:38, 2010.
43. McLeod JG: Autonomic dysfunction in peripheral nerve disease. J Clin Neurophysiol 10:51, 1993.
44. Lyu RK, Tang LM, Wu YR, et al: Cardiovascular autonomic function and sympathetic skin response in chronic inflammatory demyelinating polyradiculoneuropathy. Muscle Nerve 26:669, 2002.
45. Stamboulis E, Katsaros N, Koutsis G, et al: Clinical and subclinical autonomic dysfunction in chronic inflammatory demyelinating polyradiculoneuropathy. Muscle Nerve 33:78, 2006.
46. Mori K, Iijima M, Koike H, et al: The wide spectrum of clinical manifestations in Sjogren's syndrome-associated neuropathy. Brain 128:2518, 2005.
47. Sandhu V, Allen SC: The effects of age, seropositivity and disease duration on autonomic cardiovascular reflexes in patients with rheumatoid arthritis. Int J Clin Pract 58:740, 2004.

48. Etienne M, Weimer LH: Immune-mediated autonomic neuropathies. Curr Neurol Neurosci Rep 6:57, 2006.
49. Axelrod FB: Familial dysautonomia. Muscle Nerve 29:352, 2004.
50. Axelrod FB: Familial dysautonomia: a review of the current pharmacological treatments. Expert Opin Pharmacother 6:561, 2005.
51. Stojkovic T, de Seze J, Dubourg O, et al: Autonomic and respiratory dysfunction in Charcot-Marie-Tooth disease due to Thr124Met mutation in the myelin protein zero gene. Clin Neurophysiol 114:1609, 2003.
52. Low PA: Prevalence of orthostatic hypotension. Clin Auton Res 18(suppl 1):8, 2008.
53. Poon IO, Braun U: High prevalence of orthostatic hypotension and its correlation with potentially causative medications among elderly veterans. J Clin Pharm Ther 30:173, 2005.
54. Low PA, Vernino S, Suarez G: Autonomic dysfunction in peripheral nerve disease. Muscle Nerve 27:646, 2003.
55. Aminoff MJ, Lotti M: Neurotoxic effects of workplace exposures. p. 1151. In: Baxter PJ, Aw T-C, Cockcroft A (eds): Hunter's Diseases of Occupations. 10th Ed. Hodder Arnold, London, 2010.
56. Murata K, Araki S, Yokoyama K, et al: Changes in autonomic function as determined by ECG R-R interval variability in sandal, shoe and leather workers exposed to n-hexane, xylene and toluene. Neurotoxicology 15:867, 1994.
57. Satchell PM: Baroreceptor dysfunction in acrylamide axonal neuropathy. Brain 113:167, 1990.
58. Kamel F, Engel LS, Gladen BC, et al: Neurologic symptoms in licensed pesticide applicators in the Agricultural Health Study. Hum Exp Toxicol 26:243, 2007.
59. Consensus Committee of the American Autonomic Society and the American Academy of Neurology Consensus statement on the definition of orthostatic hypotension, pure autonomic failure, and multiple system atrophy. Neurology 46:1470, 1996.
60. Mabuchi N, Hirayama M, Koike Y, et al: Progression and prognosis in pure autonomic failure (PAF): comparison with multiple system atrophy. J Neurol Neurosurg Psychiatry 76:947, 2005.
61. Young TM, Mathias CJ: The effects of water ingestion on orthostatic hypotension in two groups of chronic autonomic failure: multiple system atrophy and pure autonomic failure. J Neurol Neurosurg Psychiatry 75:1737, 2004.
62. Polinsky RJ: Clinical autonomic neuropharmacology. Neurol Clin 8:77, 1990.
63. Iodice V, Lipp A, Ahlskog JE, et al: Autopsy confirmed multiple system atrophy cases: Mayo experience and role of autonomic function tests. J Neurol Neurosurg Psychiatry 83:453, 2012.
64. Goldstein DS, Holmes C, Sharabi Y: Cerebrospinal fluid biomarkers of central catecholamine deficiency in Parkinson's disease and other synucleinopathies. Brain 135:1900, 2012.
65. Deguchi K, Sasaki I, Touge T, et al: Abnormal baroreceptor-mediated vasopressin release as possible marker in early diagnosis of multiple system atrophy. J Neurol Neurosurg Psychiatry 75:110, 2004.
66. Benarroch EE, Schmeichel AM, Sandroni P, et al: Differential involvement of hypothalamic vasopressin neurons in multiple system atrophy. Brain 129:2688, 2006.
67. Jacobson DM, Hiner BC: Asymptomatic autonomic and sweat dysfunction in patients with Adie's syndrome. J Neuroophthalmol 18:143, 1998.
68. Bacon PJ, Smith SE: Cardiovascular and sweating dysfunction in patients with Holmes-Adie syndrome. J Neurol Neurosurg Psychiatry 6:1096, 1993.
69. Emond D, Lebel M: Orthostatic hypotension and Holmes-Adie syndrome. Usefulness of the Valsalva ratio in the evaluation of baroreceptor dysfunction. J Hum Hypertens 16:661, 2002.
70. Topakian R, Heibl C, Stieglbauer K, et al: Quantitative autonomic testing in the management of botulism. J Neurol 256:803, 2009.
71. Timmers HJ, Deinum J, Wevers RA, et al: Congenital dopamine-beta-hydroxylase deficiency in humans. Ann N Y Acad Sci 1018:520, 2004.
72. Senard JM, Rouet P: Dopamine beta-hydroxylase deficiency. Orphanet J Rare Dis 1:7, 2006.
73. Mathias CJ, Low DA, Iodice V, et al: Postural tachycardia syndrome—current experience and concepts. Nat Rev Neurol 8:22, 2011.
74. Low PA, Sandroni P, Joyner M, et al: Postural tachycardia syndrome (POTS). J Cardiovasc Electrophysiol 20:352, 2009.
75. Jacob G, Costa F, Shannon JR, et al: The neuropathic postural tachycardia syndrome. N Engl J Med 343:1008, 2000.
76. Sandroni P, Novak V, Opfer-Gehrking TL, et al: Mechanism of blood pressure alterations in response to the Valsalva maneuver in postural tachycardia syndrome. Clin Auton Res 10:1, 2000.
77. Kanjwal K, Saeed B, Karabin B, et al: Use of methylphenidate in the treatment of patients suffering from refractory postural tachycardia syndrome. Am J Ther 19:2, 2012.
78. van Dijk JG, Thijs RD, Benditt DG, et al: A guide to disorders causing transient loss of consciousness: focus on syncope. Nat Rev Neurol 5:438, 2009.
79. Wallin BG, Charkoudian N: Sympathetic neural control of integrated cardiovascular function: insights from measurement of human sympathetic nerve activity. Muscle Nerve 36:595, 2007.
80. Gawrieh S, Carroll T, Hogan WJ, et al: Swallow syncope in association with Schatzki ring and hypertensive esophageal peristalsis: report of three cases and review of the literature. Dysphagia 20:273, 2005.
81. Omi W, Murata Y, Yaegashi T, et al: Swallow syncope, a case report and review of the literature. Cardiology 105:75, 2006.

82. Martinez-Fernandez E, García FB, Gonzalez-Marcos JR, et al: Clinical and electroencephalographic features of carotid sinus syncope induced by internal carotid artery angioplasty. AJNR Am J Neuroradiol 29:269, 2008.
83. Mathias CJ, Deguchi K, Schatz I: Observations on recurrent syncope and presyncope in 641 patients. Lancet 357:348, 2001.
84. Kusumoto F, Goldschlager N: Implantable cardiac arrhythmia devices—Part II: implantable cardioverter defibrillators and implantable loop recorders. Clin Cardiol 29:237, 2006.
85. Omboni S, Smit AA, van Lieshout JJ, et al: Mechanisms underlying the impairment in orthostatic tolerance after nocturnal recumbency in patients with autonomic failure. Clin Sci (Lond) 101:609, 2001.
86. Aminoff MJ: Evaluation of the autonomic nervous system. p. 455. In Aminoff MJ (ed): Aminoff's Electrodiagnosis in Clinical Neurology. 6th Ed. Elsevier, Philadelphia, 2012.
87. Ziegler D, Laux G, Dannehl K, et al: Assessment of cardiovascular autonomic function: age-related normal ranges and reproducibility of spectral analysis, vector analysis, and standard tests of heart rate variation and blood pressure responses. Diabet Med 9:166, 1992.
88. Low PA, Denq JC, Opfer-Gehrking TL, et al: Effect of age and gender on sudomotor and cardiovagal function and blood pressure response to tilt in normal subjects. Muscle Nerve 20:1561, 1997.
89. Freeman R: Assessment of cardiovascular autonomic function. Clin Neurophysiol 117:716, 2006.
90. Vinik AI, Maser RE, Mitchell BD, et al: Diabetic autonomic neuropathy. Diabetes Care 26:1553, 2003.
91. Barnett SR, Morin RJ, Kiely DK, et al: Effects of age and gender on autonomic control of blood pressure dynamics. Hypertension 33:1195, 1999.
92. Wilder-Smith EP, Fook-Chong S, Liurong L: Reflex vasoconstrictor responses of the healthy human fingertip skin. Normal range, repeatability, and influencing factors. Microvasc Res 69:101, 2005.
93. Young TM, Asahina M, Nicotra A, et al: Skin vasomotor reflex responses in two contrasting groups of autonomic failure: multiple system atrophy and pure autonomic failure. J Neurol 253:846, 2006.
94. Illigens BM, Gibbons CH: Sweat testing to evaluate autonomic function. Clin Auton Res 19:79, 2009.
95. Ravits JM: Autonomic nervous system testing. Muscle Nerve 20:919, 1997.
96. Low PA, Opfer-Gehrking TL: The autonomic laboratory. Am J Electroneurodiagnostic Technol 39:65, 1999.
97. Riedel A, Braune S, Kerum G, et al: Quantitative sudomotor axon reflex test (QSART): a new approach for testing distal sites. Muscle Nerve 22:1257, 1999.
98. Hilz MJ, Dütsch M: Quantitative studies of autonomic function. Muscle Nerve 33:6, 2006.
99. Vetrugno R, Liguori R, Cortelli P, et al: Sympathetic skin response: basic mechanisms and clinical applications. Clin Auton Res 13:256, 2003.
100. Arunodaya GR, Taly AB: Sympathetic skin response: a decade later. J Neurol Sci 129:81, 1995.
101. Suarez GA, Opfer-Gehrking TL, Offord KP, et al: The Autonomic Symptom Profile: a new instrument to assess autonomic symptoms. Neurology 52:523, 1999.
102. Lamarre-Cliche M: Drug treatment of orthostatic hypotension because of autonomic failure or neurocardiogenic syncope. Am J Cardiovasc Drugs 2:23, 2002.
103. Biaggioni I, Zygmunt D, Haile V, et al: Pressor effect of inhaled ergotamine in orthostatic hypotension. Am J Cardiol 65:89, 1990.
104. Toh V, Duncan E, Lewis N, et al: Ergotamine use in severe diabetic autonomic neuropathy. Diabet Med 23:574, 2006.
105. Jankovic J, Gilden JL, Hiner BC, et al: Neurogenic orthostatic hypotension: a double-blind, placebo-controlled study with midodrine. Am J Med 95:38, 1993.
106. Low PA, Gilden JL, Freeman R, et al: Efficacy of midodrine vs placebo in neurogenic orthostatic hypotension. JAMA 277:1046, 1997.
107. Singer W, Sandroni P, Opfer-Gehrking TL, et al: Pyridostigmine treatment trial in neurogenic orthostatic hypotension. Arch Neurol 63:513, 2006.
108. Low PA, Singer W: Management of neurogenic orthostatic hypotension: an update. Lancet Neurol 7:451, 2008.
109. Pohl K, Kriech W: Therapy of orthostatic disorders of cardiovascular regulation. Placebo controlled double-blind study with oxilofrine. Fortschr Med 109:685, 1991.
110. Logan IC, Witham MD: Efficacy of treatments for orthostatic hypotension: a systematic review. Age Ageing 41:587, 2012.
111. Kochar MS: Management of postural hypotension. Curr Hypertens Rep 2:457, 2000.
112. Kohno R, Abe H, Oginosawa Y, et al: Effects of atrial tachypacing on symptoms and blood pressure in severe orthostatic hypotension. Pacing Clin Electrophysiol 30(suppl 1):S203, 2007.
113. Sahul ZH, Trusty JM, Erickson M, et al: Pacing does not improve hypotension in patients with severe orthostatic hypotension—a prospective randomized cross-over pilot study. Clin Auton Res 14:255, 2004.
114. Hilz MJ, Marthol H, Neundörfer B: Syncope—a systematic overview of classification, pathogenesis, diagnosis and management. Fortschr Neurol Psychiatr 70:95, 2002.
115. Sakakibara R, Matsuda S, Uchiyama T, et al: The effect of intranasal desmopressin on nocturnal waking in urination in multiple system atrophy patients with nocturnal polyuria. Clin Auton Res 13:106, 2003.
116. Stumpf JL, Mitrzyk B: Management of orthostatic hypotension. Am J Hosp Pharm 51:648, 1994.

117. Shibao C, Okamoto L, Biaggioni I: Pharmacotherapy of autonomic failure. Pharmacol Ther 134:279, 2012.
118. Kaufmann H: L-dihydroxyphenylserine (Droxidopa): a new therapy for neurogenic orthostatic hypotension: the US experience. Clin Auton Res 18(suppl 1):19, 2008.
119. Shibao C, Gamboa A, Abraham R, et al: Clonidine for the treatment of supine hypertension and pressure natriuresis in autonomic failure. Hypertension 47:522, 2006.
120. Green AL, Wang S, Owen SL, et al: Controlling the heart via the brain: a potential new therapy for orthostatic hypotension. Neurosurgery 58:1176, 2006.
121. Green AL, Wang S, Owen SL, et al: The periaqueductal grey area and the cardiovascular system. Acta Neurochir Suppl 97:521, 2007.
122. Mathias CJ: Autonomic diseases: management. J Neurol Neurosurg Psychiatry 74(suppl 3):42, 2003.

CHAPTER

9

Neurologic Complications of Cardiac Arrest

CAROLYN M. BENSON ■ G. BRYAN YOUNG

INTRODUCTION

Despite advances in the management of cardiac arrest, patients continue to have high mortality, exceeding 90 percent. Following the return of spontaneous circulation, dysfunction of multiple organ systems along with a systemic inflammatory response, collectively termed the "post-arrest syndrome," can lead to substantial morbidity. The diagnosis of primary anoxic-ischemic brain injury and the prevention of secondary neurologic injury are primary goals of early management. Persistence of coma or the prediction of long-term severe neurologic deficits commonly leads to withdrawal of life support; therefore, accurate prediction of neurologic outcome early after resuscitation is important. This chapter reviews the pathophysiology of anoxic-ischemic brain injury and the neuroprotective mechanisms of therapeutic hypothermia. In addition, the clinical, biochemical, radiographic, and electrophysiologic tests used to predict neurologic outcome following cardiac arrest are reviewed, as are the ethical implications that follow prognostication.

ANOXIC-ISCHEMIC ENCEPHALOPATHY

There is a delay between the time of ischemic cell injury and the manifestation of cell death. This delay may be hours, or up to 4 days following the initial insult. During cardiac arrest, oxygen levels decline and cerebral blood flow ceases, and cells must switch to anaerobic metabolism in order to produce adenosine triphosphate (ATP). Anaerobic glycolysis leads to an accumulation of hydrogen ions, phosphate, and lactate, all of which result in intracellular acidosis. The resulting excess of hydrogen ions displaces calcium from intracellular proteins, increasing its intracellular concentration. Dysfunction of the Na^+/K^+ ATP pump and ATP-dependent channels leads to further increases in intracellular calcium. In addition, hypoxia results in the release of excitatory neurotransmitters, such as glutamate, that cause the endoplasmic reticulum to release calcium stores. This excess calcium activates intracellular proteases and leads to further release of excitatory neurotransmitters following depolarization of the cell membrane. Activation of *N*-methyl-D-aspartate (NMDA) glutamate receptors results in sodium and chloride influx, leading to hyperosmolarity that causes water influx and neuronal death.[1,2] Restoration of the circulation can lead to further glutamate release and the formation of oxygen-derived free radicals and reperfusion injury, which can cause additional damage.[3] In addition, apoptosis, due to caspase-3 activation in neurons and oligodendroglia in the cerebral

Aminoff's Neurology and General Medicine, Fifth Edition.

neocortex, hippocampus, and striatum, can contribute to cell death, at least in perinatal models of anoxia-ischemia.[4]

Different brain regions and specific neuronal populations appear more susceptible to hypoxic-ischemic injury, probably due to their location in a vascular border-zone or to higher metabolic rates requiring increased oxygen or density of various glutamate receptors on neuronal membranes. The CA1 neurons of the hippocampus are the most sensitive to ischemia, and injury commonly results in memory dysfunction. The Purkinje cells of the cerebellum, the pyramidal neurons in layers 3, 5, and 6 of the neocortex, and the reticular neurons of the thalamus are also commonly affected. In addition, three vascular border-zones are susceptible to a reduction in blood flow due to their distance from the parent vessel; these areas become clinically important in cases of severe hypotension and incomplete cardiopulmonary arrest. The cortical border-zones are the anterior border-zone between the anterior cerebral artery and the middle cerebral artery territories, and the posterior border-zone between the middle cerebral artery and posterior cerebral artery territories. Infarction of the anterior border-zone results in brachial diplegia, or "man-in-a-barrel" syndrome. Infarction of the posterior border-zone results in visual deficits including cortical blindness if bilateral.[2] The internal, or subcortical, border-zone is found at the junctions between the branches of the anterior, middle, and posterior cerebral arteries with the deep perforating vessels, including the lenticulostriate and anterior choroidal arteries.

THERAPEUTIC HYPOTHERMIA

The use of therapeutic hypothermia (TH) in patients after cardiac arrest was first reported in the 1950s, but the complication rate was high and results were inconclusive. In 2002, two landmark studies were published showing that TH improves neurologic outcomes following cardiac arrest when the initial rhythm was ventricular fibrillation (or possibly pulseless ventricular tachycardia). Bernard and colleagues randomized 77 patients to either moderate hypothermia (33°C) or normothermia. Among the hypothermia group, 49 percent survived and were able to be discharged home or to a rehabilitation facility, compared to 26 percent of controls.[5] In the second study, in which patients were randomized to mild hypothermia (32° to 34°C) or standard of care, mortality was 41 percent in the TH group and 55 percent in the control group. In addition, 55 percent of patients treated with TH had favorable neurologic outcome, defined as Cerebral Performance Category 1 (normal) or 2 (moderate disability), compared to 39 percent of controls. No significant differences were found between the groups with respect to complications, including bleeding, infection, and arrhythmias, and the number needed to treat in these trials was impressively in the single digits.[6] Follow-up studies investigating the implementation of TH at multiple centers confirmed the benefit and feasibility of TH.

There are many postulated mechanisms to explain the neurologic benefits that occur with TH, including a decrease of the extracellular levels of excitatory neurotransmitters such as glutamate and dopamine. The NMDA receptor is glycine dependent, and TH has been shown to decrease cerebral levels of glycine following ischemia, and thus to lessen glutamate-related hyperexcitability. TH reduces the proliferation of astroglial cells and their release of inflammatory cytokines and free radicals.[1] TH also results in decreased cerebral blood flow, as well as decreased metabolism and oxygen and glucose utilization. A study investigating hypothermia and brain metabolism in rats revealed that decreases in metabolism of 5 to 10 percent occur for every decline in temperature of 1°C.[7]

PROGNOSTIC DETERMINATION

Following return of spontaneous circulation, neurologists are often consulted to determine prognosis, specifically the probability of regaining consciousness and of the likely presence, severity, and extent of any persistent neurologic deficits. While prognostication with 100 percent certainty is not possible, a reasonable goal is to identify, with virtually no false positives, those patients who will have severe neurologic deficits with complete dependency at 6 months following the arrest. Much of the published literature attempts to predict which patients will have a Glasgow outcome score of 3 or less at 6 months after cardiac arrest, such an outcome includes death, vegetative state (defined as wakefulness without awareness), and severe disability with total dependency. However, a growing body of evidence suggests that some patients previously diagnosed as being in vegetative state may have some degree of preserved awareness (the "minimally conscious state") and thus this definition is being challenged.[8] To avoid this controversy, our preference is to define a poor outcome generally as severe disability with total dependency at 6 months after the arrest. As many patients and their families would likely not choose to continue aggressive measures in the face of such a dismal prognosis, withdrawal of life support often follows. It is essential that the combination of clinical, radiographic, and electrophysiologic tests used to arrive at this conclusion therefore have a false-positive rate (FPR) that is essentially zero.

The neurologic examination following stabilization of the patient should include assessment of the pupillary reaction to light, corneal reflexes, and motor response to command and noxious stimuli. As the brainstem is more resilient than the cortex to anoxic-ischemic injury, brainstem dysfunction usually implies severe cortical injury. Axial myoclonus, defined as bilateral synchronous jerks of the face, trunk, shoulders, or hips, should be noted as it portends a poor prognosis, and these movements should be distinguished from multifocal myoclonus, which is distal, asynchronous, and of no prognostic value. Patients with a purely anoxic insult, as opposed to anoxic-ischemic injury, may recover despite having symmetric myoclonus, perhaps due to a reversible synaptic injury affecting γ-aminobutyric acid type A (GABA-A)-mediated neurotransmission.[3] No neurologic prognostication should occur until a minimum of 24 hours after the arrest; in patients treated with hypothermia, it may take days to establish a prognosis because the lowered temperature affects the clinical and electrophysiologic findings.

Prognostication in the Absence of Therapeutic Hypothermia

Prognostication following cardiac arrest has largely been based on the work of Levy and colleagues, who analyzed a single cohort of 210 patients and identified factors that could accurately predict at various times the development of a poor neurologic outcome.[8] Systematic reviews on the topic have been published.[9] In 2006, the American Academy of Neurology (AAN) published practice parameters that summarized the available literature and provided an algorithm to establish prognosis.[10] After 24 hours, if a patient has absence of all brainstem reflexes, motor responses, and is apneic, ancillary testing can be used to confirm a diagnosis of brain death. In patients who remain comatose but have a less severe neurologic insult, clinical signs and electrophysiologic tests can be used to establish a poor prognosis. The clinical signs that predicted poor neurologic outcome were myoclonus status epilepticus on day 1 (FPR 0%, CI 0–8.8), absence of the pupillary light reflex or corneal reflex on day 3 (FPR 0%, CI 0–3), and best motor response of extension or worse on day 3 (FPR 0%, CI 0–3). Somatosensory evoked potentials (SSEPs) recorded between days 1 and 3 demonstrating bilaterally absent N20 responses also predicted poor outcome (FPR of 0.7%, CI 0–3.7). Serum neuron-specific enolase (NSE) levels greater than 33 μg/L on day 1 to 3 were also a negative prognosticator (FPR 0%, CI 0–3).[10] The practice parameters allow a physician to identify patients who will definitively have a poor neurologic outcome, but it is important to note that many other patients not meeting these criteria will also have a poor outcome.

Caution must be exercised when applying these prognostic criteria to patients who have undergone TH, a well-established confounder of the neurologic and electrophysiologic examination, as the practice parameters were based on literature published before its widespread adoption.

Therapeutic Hypothermia and the Neurologic Examination

In patients treated with TH, the pupillary light reflexes, corneal reflexes, motor responses, serum NSE levels, and presence of axial myoclonus have all been shown to have reduced accuracy for predicting poor neurologic outcome. Rossetti and colleagues prospectively studied a cohort of post-arrest patients undergoing TH in order to evaluate the application of established AAN practice parameters for prognostication.[11] When these patients were examined 72 hours after the arrest, they found higher FPRs for predicting mortality when using the absence of pupillary reactivity (FPR 4%), the presence of axial myoclonus (FPR 3%) and best motor response of extensor posturing or worse (FPR 24%).[11] Al Thenayan and colleagues found that motor response, specifically extensor posturing or worse, was not prognostically reliable at day 3 following TH.[12] In their prospective review, 14 patients had delayed return of the motor response as late as 6 days after cardiac arrest, and two of these patients had favorable outcomes.[12] We have also encountered a patient treated with TH who lacked motor response until day 21 after cardiac arrest.

Axial myoclonus may arise from the cerebral cortex or brainstem. The cortical form, unlike the brainstem form, has a reliable correlate on the electroencephalogram (EEG). Until recently, the presence of axial myoclonus was considered uniformly fatal based on studies in the prehypothermic era, including a series of 11 patients with postarrest axial myoclonus who all died. These patients all had severe damage to various gray matter structures in the brain and spinal cord, demonstrating the cause of death to be anoxic-ischemic insult rather than status epilepticus.[13] Six more recently published cases of good outcome despite axial myoclonus suggest that TH may modify the outcome of a small but significant number of patients who develop axial myoclonus after resuscitation from cardiac arrest.[14–16] Thus, the presence of this sign is still suggestive of a poor neurologic outcome but should not be used in isolation to prognosticate.

After cardiac arrest many patients have other confounders of the neurologic examination than hypothermia, including cardiogenic shock, metabolic acidosis, and other metabolic derangements. Organ failure, especially hepatic and renal dysfunction, may cause reversible encephalopathy and cloud the predictive power of the neurologic examination. Comatose patients require sedation for presumed pain or distress, ventilator asynchrony, or as part of many hypothermia protocols, and clearance of these drugs may be delayed due to organ dysfunction. TH itself can also result in increased serum concentrations of certain drugs, increased duration of action, and decreased clearance, including with fentanyl, midazolam, propofol, and neuromuscular blocking agents. Use of these types of drugs is indeed common in TH protocols. Samaniego and colleagues found that 83 percent of patients undergoing a hypothermia protocol after cardiac arrest were still receiving at least one sedating agent 72 hours later, in comparison to 60 percent of normothermic patients; both the corneal reflexes and motor responses became unreliable at predicting outcome at 72 hours after arrest if a patient had received a sedating drug within 12 hours of the neurologic examination, regardless of whether they had been treated with TH.[17]

Specifics of the Cardiac Arrest

Characteristics of the cardiac arrest, including anoxia time (the time from onset to initiation of cardiopulmonary resuscitation) and total arrest duration, have been explored as predictors of prognosis. A retrospective review of a cohort of 64,339 patients with in-hospital cardiac arrest identified 8,724 patients with available neurologic outcome data. The duration of resuscitation did not affect neurologic outcome: favorable outcome occurred in 81 percent of patients with a resuscitation time of less than 15 minutes, 80 percent for durations between 15 and 30 minutes, and 78 percent for resuscitation lasting greater than 30 minutes.[18] The Brain Resuscitation Clinical Trial and Study Group found that anoxia time greater than 5 minutes and total resuscitation time exceeding 20 minutes independently predicted mortality.[19] However, even in this study, the presence of prolonged anoxia time or cardiopulmonary resuscitation exceeding 20 minutes did not preclude a favorable neurologic outcome. Among 245 patients, 41 (17%) with anoxia time exceeding 5 minutes had a cerebral performance category of 1 or 2 at outcome assessment but, similarly, 48 of 311 patients (15%) with resuscitation times exceeding 20 minutes also had this favorable outcome.[19] Increased age was associated with increased mortality, but was not an independent predictor of poor neurologic outcome.[19] Although arrest features such as longer anoxia time and duration of resuscitation are associated with poorer outcomes, the false-positive rates are too high to be useful for prognostication purposes.

Electrophysiologic Tests

Electrophysiologic tests, including SSEPs and EEG, can aid in prognostication after cardiac arrest. The most common SSEP measured involves stimulation of the median nerve at the wrist and recording the response over the contralateral scalp, specifically over the primary somatosensory cortex. In a normal adult this response occurs 20 msec from the time of median nerve stimulation and is therefore called the N20 response (Fig. 9-1). During this test, additional electrodes are placed over Erb point (over the brachial plexus) and high on the posterior neck (over the dorsal columns of the spinal cord); stimulation of the median nerve results in responses at these

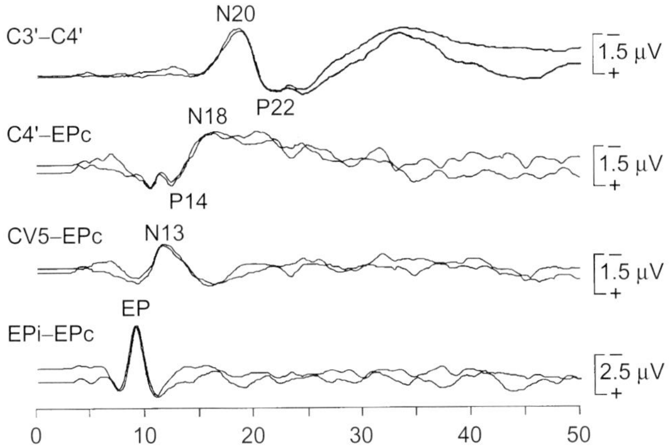

FIGURE 9-1 ■ Normal somatosensory evoked potential elicited by stimulation of the right median nerve at the wrist. Responses were recorded over the brachial plexus at ipsilateral Erb point (EPi), over the fifth cervical spine (CV5), and over the ipsilateral scalp (C4′) with contralateral Erb point (EPc) used as a reference, as well as over the contralateral scalp (C3′) referenced to the ipsilateral scalp (C4′). An N9 potential is seen over Erb point, an N13 over the cervical spine, subcortical far-field P14 and N18 potentials over the ipsilateral scalp area, and an N20 over the contralateral "hand" area (C3′) of the scalp. Loss of the N20 response bilaterally (with preserved N9 and N13 responses) portends a poor neurologic prognosis. (From Aminoff MJ, Eisen A: Somatosensory evoked potentials. p. 581. In Aminoff MJ (ed): Aminoff's Electrodiagnosis in Clinical Neurology. 6th Ed. Elsevier, Oxford, 2012, with permission.)

electrodes at approximately 9 msec and 13 msec, respectively. These N9 and N13 responses, along with the N20, examine the continuity of the nervous system from the median nerve through the brachial plexus and high cervical cord to the cortex and reduce false-positive results from conduction problems below the cranium. The AAN practice parameter found that bilaterally absent N20 responses on SSEPs accurately predicted poor outcome with an FPR of 0.7 percent when performed between day 1 and day 3 following arrest.[10] Tiainen and colleagues evaluated SSEPs in post-arrest patients randomized to TH or standard care and found that although TH resulted in delayed latencies of the waveforms, 100 percent of patients with bilaterally absent N20 responses, regardless of whether they had undergone TH, had poor neurologic outcomes.[20] Leithner and colleagues found a slightly lower predictive value in the setting of TH, identifying 1 of 36 patients who, despite bilaterally absent N20 responses after cardiac arrest, eventually regained consciousness.[21] While median nerve SSEPs can still be used to accurately predict outcome, the false-positive rate is not zero, again emphasizing that in patients who have undergone TH, no test should be used in isolation to determine prognosis.

The EEG may be used to prognosticate after cardiac arrest, but multiple confounders exist including sedation, TH, and multi-organ failure. The AAN practice parameter found that generalized suppression of the EEG to less than 20 μV, burst suppression with epileptiform bursts, and periodic complexes on a flat background were each associated with poor outcome but had insufficient accuracy (Fig. 9-2).[10] Additional EEG patterns that are often considered poor predictors include status epilepticus, alpha-pattern coma, theta-pattern coma, spindle coma, triphasic waves, a non-variant EEG, and burst suppression with nonepileptifom bursts.

EEG reactivity is defined as a change in frequency or amplitude that occurs in response to verbal or noxious stimuli, and this reactivity has been examined as a method of prognostication following cardiac arrest. Thenayan and colleagues retrospectively reviewed the EEG of 29 patients who had had a cardiac arrest and found that 17 of 18 patients who lacked EEG reactivity did not regain awareness.[22] In a prospective series of 34 patients, a nonreactive background had a positive predictive value of 100 percent; in addition, all survivors had EEG reactivity and 74 percent of these patients had a favorable neurologic outcome.[23] In an additional series, nonreactivity was found to have an FPR of 7 percent for predicting mortality following cardiac arrest.[11]

After cardiac arrest, up to 30 percent of patients may develop status epilepticus, which is associated with poor outcomes.[16] Even epileptiform activity on the initial EEG recording predicts poor outcome with an FPR of 9 percent.[16] Antiseizure medications should be administered aggressively to these patients until other criteria suggest a poor outcome.

In summary, the EEG may aid in prognostication, both for favorable and unfavorable outcomes, but must be considered in context with other established prognostic indicators as the positive predictive value is insufficient to use in isolation.

Neuroimaging

Computerized tomographic (CT) imaging performed early after cardiac arrest is usually negative,

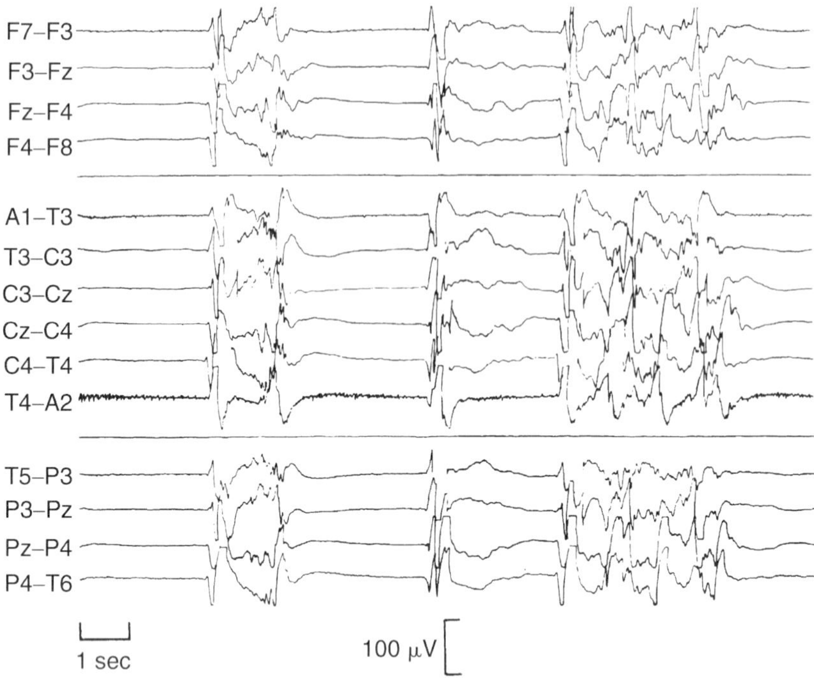

FIGURE 9-2 ■ Burst-suppression pattern recorded in the EEG of a 70-year-old man after a cardiac arrest from which he was resuscitated. (From Aminoff MJ: Electroencephalography: General principles and clinical applications. p. 37. In Aminoff MJ (ed): Aminoff's Electrodiagnosis in Clinical Neurology. 6th Ed. Elsevier, Oxford, 2012, with permission.)

although in severe cases of anoxic-ischemic injury, loss of gray-white differentiation and cerebral edema may be seen.[24] Out-of-hospital cardiac arrest has been associated with subarachnoid hemorrhage, with incidence rates ranging from 0 to 16 percent.[21] It is our current practice to perform CT imaging of the head in all patients after cardiac arrest to exclude this etiology for the arrest. Diffusion-weighted imaging or fluid-attenuated inversion recovery sequences on magnetic resonance imaging (MRI) have shown some utility in predicting poor neurologic outcomes (Fig. 9-3). Choi and colleagues found that restricted diffusion in the cortex or basal ganglia was associated with unfavorable outcome.[25] Of patients with poor outcomes, restricted diffusion was present in the cortex in 81 percent and in the basal ganglia in 77 percent; in contrast, these findings were present in only 8 percent and 23 percent, respectively, in those with a favorable outcome.[25] The median whole-brain apparent diffusion coefficient was found in one study to predict poor outcome, defined as a modified Rankin Scale score of 3 or more at 6 months after the arrest, with 100 percent specificity and 41 percent sensitivity.[26] Wijman and colleagues evaluated the predictive value of quantitative MRI measurements, using various cut-off points of the apparent diffusion coefficient and found that a value below 650×10^{-6} mm^2/sec differentiated patients with favorable outcome from those who died or were left in a vegetative state.[27] The percentage of brain parenchyma demonstrating an apparent diffusion coefficient cut-off of 400 to 450 $\times 10^{-6}$ mm^2/sec differentiated Glasgow outcome score of 1 or 2 from a score of 3.[27]

Functional MRI may offer further prognostic ability. Norton and colleagues performed resting-state functional MRI on 11 patients after cardiac arrest and found that the default mode network was preserved in all patients who regained consciousness and disrupted in those who did not recover.[28]

Biomarkers

Several biomarkers have shown potential for prognostication following cardiac arrest. The use of serum or cerebrospinal fluid (CSF) biomarkers is appealing as it does not require either patient transport or trained technicians, nor are the levels affected by sedation. NSE is a gamma isomer of enolase, an intracytoplasmic enzyme found in

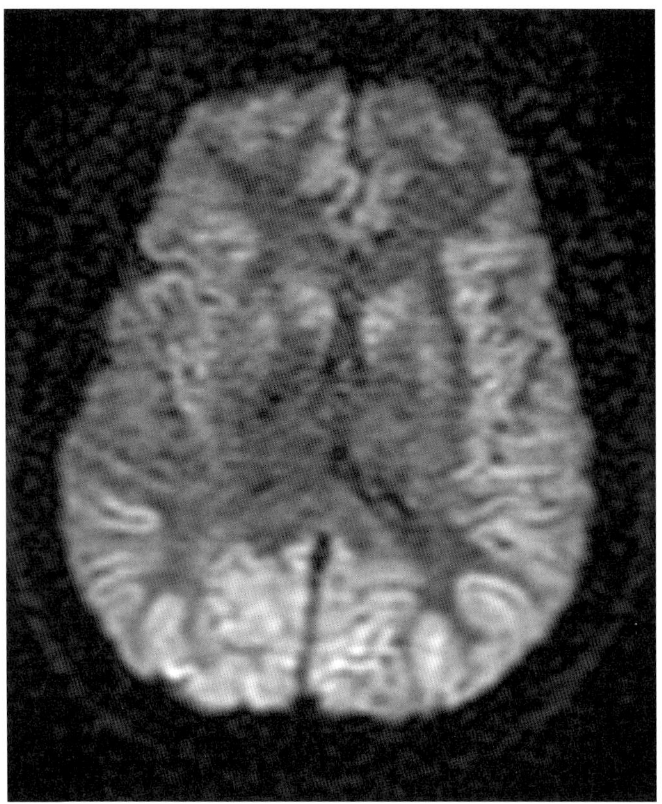

FIGURE 9-3 ■ Axial brain MRI after cardiac arrest, demonstrating extensive restricted diffusion consistent with cytotoxic edema.

neurons and neuroectodermal cells. Damage to neurons results in release of NSE into the CSF and eventually it is measurable in the serum. A prospective study of 231 patients who sustained a cardiac arrest showed that serum NSE measures at 24, 48, or 72 hours accurately predicted poor outcome with an FPR of 0 percent.[29] Based on this and other literature preceding the widespread use of TH, the AAN practice parameter recommended using a serum NSE cut-off of 33 μg/L to predict poor outcome.[10] Results from studies performed after hypothermia came into widespread use, however, have challenged the accuracy of this cut-off. Fugate and colleagues found that following TH, this recommended cut-off had an unacceptably high FPR of 29 percent for poor outcome.[30] Daubin and colleagues measured serum NSE at 24 and 72 hours after cardiac arrest and found that a serum level of 97 μg/L was needed to achieve a 100 percent positive predictive value.[31] A meta-analysis, which included studies with and without TH, found that the reported cut-off to achieve reliable prediction varied from as low as 5 μg/L to as high as 91 μg/L.[32] Currently no accepted value of NSE can definitively predict poor outcome following cardiac arrest.

S100B is a calcium-binding protein secreted by glial and Schwann cells. It may also act as a cytokine, resulting in neuronal apoptosis, and it has a biologic half-life of 2 hours. Results from a meta-analysis suggest the cut-off level for S100B to predict poor neurologic outcome varies across multiple studies, ranging from 0.7 to 5.2 μg/L.[32] Other biomarkers that require further research before they can be useful clinically for prognostication include creatine kinase BB isoenzyme, glial fibrillary acidic protein, and brain-derived neurotrophic factor. The limited number of laboratories that can provide speedy results for these biomarker studies, as well as the conflicting evidence over serum cut-off measurements that predict poor outcome with 100 percent specificity, currently limit the use of biomarkers in prognostication.

Improving Prognostication Accuracy

Since the introduction of TH, it has become increasingly difficult to identify those patients who will have poor neurologic outcomes. Ensuring the presence of at least two negative prognosticators can improve prognostic accuracy. This approach has the additional benefit of allowing for the use of some prognostic elements, such as EEG and MRI, which have good but not perfect predictive ability. Rossetti and colleagues found that the presence of at least two indicators of a bad prognosis—absent brainstem reflexes, axial myoclonus, unreactive EEG, and bilaterally absent N20 responses in the median-derived SSEP—had a positive predictive value of 100 percent for poor neurologic outcome.[16]

Most of the literature on prognosis after cardiac arrest aims to identify with accuracy those patients who will die or be left severely disabled with complete dependency. However, many patients who do not have these prognostic signs will also have a poor outcome. It is therefore also useful to consider the factors that may indicate a favorable outcome, usually defined as the ability to obey commands, indicating the return of awareness. These favorable signs include localization on motor examination, minimal or no diffusion restriction on MRI, and preserved EEG reactivity.[16] Further research is needed to clarify the effect of hypothermia on current prognostic signs and also to help differentiate those patients who will have near-complete neurologic recovery from those who will have moderate disability.

ETHICAL CONSIDERATIONS

Patients who have been resuscitated from cardiac arrest and are left with significant neurologic deficits pose several ethical challenges. Several studies have shown that physicians tend to overestimate poor outcomes and underestimate good outcomes, especially in the first days following arrest.[33–38] Some families express doubt about the accuracy and sincerity of physicians' prognostic opinions and management suggestions. Ultimately, however, what "experts" say to families, fellow physicians, and other caregivers has enormous influence. There is a need for accuracy, honesty, frankness, consideration, acknowledgement, and patience in discussions that involve possible end-of-life decisions. The principal issues include accurate prognostication and discussions with substitute decision-makers, in which autonomy of the patient is given primacy.

Accurate Prognostication

Most of this chapter has been devoted to accurate prognostication. Using the results of studies, it should be possible in most patients to arrive at some estimate of the probability that recovery of awareness will occur. In some cases, the prognosis will remain uncertain and more time and possibly more or repeated testing will be necessary.

Discussion with Substitute Decision-Makers

Patient autonomy is given the greatest priority in most North American and European cultures. After cardiac arrest, patients generally are unable to participate in discussions regarding prognosis and management, and so this responsibility falls to substitute decision-makers. In hierarchical order, this person is typically: the spouse, children older than 18 years, a parent or guardian, a sibling, or the closest next-of-kin. In some cases, the substitute decision-maker is identified in a Power of Attorney statement or similar document. In rare cases, no person can be identified and a public trustee is often then appointed.

Research indicates that there are often problems in the communication between physicians and substitute decision-makers in the critical care setting. A French study revealed that over half of substitute decision-makers did not understand either the diagnosis, prognosis, or both, after the first meeting with physicians.[39] An American study found that in half of surveyed cases, substitute decision-makers perceived a conflict with the health care team in the intensive care unit, usually related to problems with communication.[40] Often substitute decision-makers experience anxiety and depression, and these issues can interfere with comprehension and executive decision-making functions. Physicians, along with nursing staff, need to be sensitive to these issues and involve substitute decision-makers in repeated discussions while providing empathy and support.[41] Information pamphlets or visual aids, such as MRI scans, can be helpful in improving comprehension of the severity of the illness.

A good starting point for discussion is to ask substitute decision-makers about their understanding of the patient's illness—further explanation and clarification then follow. Substitute decision-makers should be forewarned if there is "bad news," and the emotional reaction acknowledged.[42] They need to understand that they are speaking for the patient and should be encouraged to help the health care team understand what the patient would want to do, given the prognosis provided. Substitute decision-makers should be asked whether there are advance directives, either written or verbally stated, which may give a clear idea of the patient's perspectives, at least at some point in the past. If there are no clear advance directives, substitute decision-makers and family members are asked to describe their understanding of the patient's values and to formulate a response for him or her.

Occasionally differences of opinion among family members arise or the substitute decision-maker cannot make a decision. Cultures also vary in their view of "futility," even if the medical team is convinced that the patient will not benefit from further life-supporting therapies. Physicians should maintain respect and understanding, while providing further meetings. Involvement of an ethicist or a member of the clergy is sometimes helpful. In rare instances the issue needs to be resolved legally, either in court or by the appointment of a special board.

REFERENCES

1. Gonzalez-Ibarra FP: Therapeutic hypothermia: critical review of the molecular mechanisms of action. Front Neurol 2:4, 2011.
2. Busl KM, Greer DM: Hypoxic-ischemic brain injury: Pathophysiology, neuropathology and mechanisms. NeuroRehabilitation 26:5, 2010.
3. Greer DM: Mechanisms of injury in hypoxic-ischemic injury: implications to therapy. Semin Neurol 26:373, 2006.
4. Hee Han B, D'Costa A, Black SA, et al: BDNF blocks caspase-3 activation in neonatal hypoxia-ischemia. Neurobiol Dis 7:38, 2000.
5. Bernard SA, Gray TW, Buist MD, et al: Treatment of comatose survivors of out-of-hopsital cardiac arrest with induced hypothermia. N Engl J Med 346:557, 2002.
6. Hypothermia after Cardiac Arrest Study Group: Mild therapeutic hypothermia to improve the neurologic outcome after cardiac arrest. N Engl J Med 346:549, 2002.
7. Hagerdal M, Harp J, Nilsson L, et al: The effect of induced hypothermia upon oxygen consumption in the rat brain. J Neurochem 24:311, 1975.
8. Levy DE, Caronna JJ, Singer BH, et al: Predicting outcome from hypoxic-ischemic coma. JAMA 253:1420, 1985.
9. Owen AM, Coleman MR, Boly M, et al: Detecting awareness in the vegetative state. Science 313:1402, 2006.
10. Wijdicks EFM, Hijdra A, Young GB, et al: Practice parameter: prediction of outcome in comatose survivors after cardiopulmonary resuscitation (an evidence-based review): report of the Quality Standards Subcommittee of the American Academy of Neurology. Neurology 67:203, 2006.
11. Rossetti AO, Oddo M, Logroscino G, et al: Prognostication after cardiac arrest and hypothermia: A prospective study. Ann Neurol 67:301, 2010.
12. Al Thenayan E, Savard M, Sharpe M, et al: Predictors of poor neurologic outcome after induced mild hypothermia following cardiac arrest. Neurology 71:1535, 2008.
13. Young GB, Gilbert JJ, Zochodne DW: The significance of myoclonic status epilepticus in postanoxic coma. Neurology 40:1843, 1990.
14. Chen CJ, Coyne PJ, Lyckhom LJ, et al: A case of inaccurate prognostication after the ARCTIC protocol. J Pain Symptom Manage 43:1120, 2012.
15. Lucas JM, Cocchi MN, Salciccioli J, et al: Neurologic recovery after hypothermia in patients with post-cardiac arrest myoclonus. Resuscitation 83:265, 2012.
16. Rossetti AO, Oddo M, Liaudet L, et al: Predictors of awakening from postanoxic status epilepticus after therapeutic hypothermia. Neurology 72:744, 2009.
17. Samaniego EA, Mlynash M, Finley Caulfield A, et al: Sedation confounds outcome prediction in cardiac arrest survivors treated with hypothermia. Neurocrit Care 15:113, 2011.
18. Goldberger ZD, Chan PS, Berg RA, et al: Duration of resuscitation efforts and survival after in-hospital cardiac arrest: an observational study. Lancet 380:14741, 2012.
19. Rogove HJ, Safar P, Sutton-Tyrrell K, et al: Old age does not negate good cerebral outcome after cardiopulmonary resuscitation: analyses from the brain resuscitation clinical trials. The Brain Resuscitation Clinical Trial I and II Study Groups. Crit Care Med 23:18, 1995.
20. Tiainen M, Kovala TT, Takkunen OS, et al: Somatosensory and brainstem auditory evoked potentials in cardiac arrest patients treated with hypothermia. Crit Care Med 33:1736, 2005.
21. Leithner C, Ploner CJ, Hasper D, et al: Does hypothermia influence the predictive value of bilateral absent N20 after cardiac arrest? Neurology 74:965, 2010.
22. Thenayan EA, Savard M, Sharpe MD, et al: Electroencephalogram for prognosis after cardiac arrest. J Crit Care 25:300, 2010.
23. Rossetti AO, Urbano LA, Delodder F, et al: Prognostic value of continuous EEG monitoring during therapeutic hypothermia after cardiac arrest. Crit Care 14:R173, 2010.
24. Metter RB, Rittenberger JC, Guyette FX, et al: Association between a quantitative CT scan measure of brain edema and outcome after cardiac arrest. Resuscitation 82:1180, 2011.
25. Choi SP, Park KN, Park HK, et al: Diffusion-weighted magnetic resonance imaging for predicting the clinical outcome of comatose survivors after cardiac arrest: a cohort study. Crit Care 14:R17, 2010.
26. Wu O, Sorensen AG, Benner T, et al: Comatose patients with cardiac arrest: predicting clinical outcome with diffusion-weighted MR imaging. Radiology 252:173, 2009.
27. Wijman CA, Mlynash M, Caulfield AF, et al: Prognostic value of brain diffusion-weighted imaging after cardiac arrest. Ann Neurol 65:394, 2009.
28. Norton L, Hutchison RM, Young GB, et al: Disruptions of functional connectivity in the default mode network of comatose patients. Neurology 78:175, 2012.
29. Zandbergen EG, Hijdra A, Koelman JH, et al: Prediction of poor outcome within the first 3 days of postanoxic coma. Neurology 66:62, 2006.
30. Fugate JE, Wijdicks EF, Mandrekar J, et al: Predictors of neurologic outcome in hypothermia after cardiac arrest. Ann Neurol 68:907, 2010.
31. Daubin C, Quentin C, Allouch S, et al: Serum neuron-specific enolase as predictor of outcome in comatose cardiac-arrest survivors: a prospective cohort study. BMC Cardiovasc Disord 11:48, 2011.
32. Shinokzaki K, Oda S, Sadahiro T, et al: S-100B and neuron-specific enolase as predictors of neurological outcome in patients after cardiac arrest and return of spontaneous circulation: a systematic review. Crit Care 13:R121, 2009.

33. Becker KJ, Baxter AB, Cohen WA, et al: Withdrawal of support in intracerebral hemorrhage may lead to self-fulfilling prophecies. Neurology 56:766, 2001.
34. Diringer MN, Edwards DF, Aiyagari V, et al: Factors associated with withdrawal of mechanical ventilation in a neurology/neurosurgery intensive care unit. Crit Care Med 29:1792, 2001.
35. Hemphill 3rd JC, Newman J, Zhao S, et al: Hospital usage of early do-not-resuscitate orders and outcome after intracerebral hemorrhage. Stroke 35:1130, 2004.
36. Kaufmann MA, Buchmann B, Scheidegger D, et al: Severe head injury: should expected outcome influence resuscitation and first-day decisions? Resuscitation 23:199, 1992.
37. Mayer SA, Kossoff SB: Withdrawal of life support in the neurological intensive care unit. Neurology 52:1602, 1999.
38. Rocker G, Cook D, Sjokvist P, et al: Level of Care Study Investigators; Canadian Critical Care Trials Group. Clinician predictions of intensive care unit mortality. Crit Care Med 32:1149, 2004.
39. Azoulay E, Chevret S, Leleu G, et al: Half the families of intensive care patients experience inadequate communication with physicians. Crit Care Med 28:3044, 2000.
40. Abott KH, Sago JG, Breen CM, et al: Families looking back: one year after discussion of withdrawal or withholding of life-sustaining support. Crit Care Med 29:197, 2001.
41. Heyland DK, Cook DJ, Rocker GM, et al: Decision making in the intensive care unit: perspectives of the substitute decision-maker. Int Care Med 29:75, 2003.
42. Ptacek JT, Ptacek JJ, Ellison NM: "I'm sorry to tell you ..." Physicians' reports of breaking bad news. J Behav Med 24:205, 2001.

CHAPTER

10

Cardiac Manifestations of Acute Neurologic Lesions

NERISSA U. KO

Cardiac abnormalities are common after acute neurologic injury. Disturbances can range in severity from transient electrocardiographic (ECG) abnormalities to profound myocardial injury and dysfunction. Evidence from animal models and clinical observations indicate that the central nervous system (CNS) is involved in the generation of cardiac arrhythmias and dysfunction even in an otherwise normal myocardium. Neurologic lesions may influence cardiovascular function and affect cardiac prognosis, and—in addition—the presence of cardiac abnormalities may be associated with poor neurologic outcomes. A better understanding of cardiac abnormalities after acute neurologic injury can improve the clinical management of patients and may also have important prognostic implications.

This chapter briefly outlines the cardiac manifestations that follow acute neurologic injury, summarizes the neurophysiology and neuroanatomy of cardiac control, and discusses the clinical implications and diagnostic and treatment recommendations for the most common cardiac complications.

HISTORICAL PERSPECTIVE

Cushing first described hemodynamic changes after acute intracerebral hemorrhage in 1903.[1] The bradycardia and hypertension in response to increased intracranial pressure (ICP), known as the "Cushing reflex," was later proved in animal models to be mediated by the CNS. Over subsequent decades, clinical observations began to identify the importance of the brain–heart interaction in patients with cerebral lesions. Cardiac abnormalities were described with various CNS diseases including seizures, trauma, ischemic stroke, and intracerebral hemorrhage (ICH), and less commonly with tumors, electroconvulsive therapy, and meningitis.[2,3] Cardiac pathology with features of subendocardial hemorrhage was described in these neurologic patients without known previous cardiac disease.[4] After World War II, patients with subarachnoid hemorrhage (SAH) were noted to have cardiac myocytolysis similar to that in pheochromocytoma.[5] An emotional- and stress-induced cardiomyopathy was then described in Japan, and subsequently reported in other populations.[6–8]

ANATOMY AND PHYSIOLOGY

The anatomy and physiology of the pathways involved in brain–heart interactions have been elucidated in both animal and human studies. The medulla has been described as the principal site

Aminoff's Neurology and General Medicine, Fifth Edition.

of vagal parasympathetic and sympathetic areas involved in cardiac control. In addition, both anatomic and physiologic evidence exists to implicate the hypothalamus in cardiac control.[9] Electrical stimulation experiments suggest a posteriorly located area of cardiovascular sympathetic control and an anterior parasympathetic control region.[10] Beattie and colleagues first described cardiac arrhythmias after hypothalamic stimulation.[11] Arrhythmias from hypothalamic stimulation were subsequently confirmed in other animal models.

Areas of the cerebral cortex with connections to the autonomic nervous system can also elicit cardiac responses. The autonomic–emotional interactions with cardiovascular function have been linked to the central nucleus of the amygdala. Stimulation of the orbitofrontal, cingulate, and temporal lobes may elicit a cardiac response, but with much less frequency than the hypothalamus and brainstem. The central autonomic network has been investigated further with modern neuroimaging. The majority of evidence suggests that the insular cortex has a pivotal role in integrating autonomic responses involved in the regulation of the cardiovascular system and is strongly associated with adverse cardiac events after neurologic injury.[12]

The Insular Cortex

The insular cortex has widespread connectivity with other areas of the brain that are known to be involved in autonomic control. Both experimental and clinical evidence strongly suggest a role for the insula in cardiovascular function. In microstimulation experiments in rats, Oppenheimer and colleagues first identified the insular cortex as a site from which lethal cardiac arrhythmias and myocardial damage could be produced, resembling changes seen in patients after stroke and in association with sudden death in patients with epilepsy.[13]

Animal models of stroke have provided further evidence for involvement of the insula in the autonomic regulation of the heart. In a rat model of cerebral ischemia, insular infarction was associated with increased renal sympathetic nerve activity, prolongation of the QT interval, and elevated norepinephrine levels.[14] Pathologically, cardiac myocytolysis was demonstrated only if the insular cortex was involved.[15] This evidence collectively supports the belief that stroke can alter cardiovascular tone by directly damaging the insular cortex or other interrelated areas and shifting the balance toward a predominance of sympathetic activation.

Although there is considerable evidence suggesting lateralization of cardiac control in animal models, the clinical impact of the laterality of insular strokes in humans has proved to be more complicated. In patients undergoing temporal lobectomy for the control of intractable seizures, stimulation of either insula resulted in alterations of blood pressure and heart rate, but bradycardia and decreased blood pressure occurred with greater frequency from the left anterior insular cortex.[16] Other observations during infusion of amyl barbital during the Wada test are of tachycardia after left carotid infusion and bradycardia with right internal carotid infusion.[17] Collectively, these observations support a greater sympathetic cardiovascular representation on the right and greater parasympathetic regulation on the left.[12]

Observational stroke studies in humans have provided conflicting results without a predominant laterality related to prognosis and outcomes. In an observational study of 62 acute stroke patients, an increased incidence of sudden death occurred among patients with right insular strokes.[18] In addition, right middle cerebral artery strokes were associated with a significantly increased incidence of supraventricular tachyarrhythmias.[19] When anterior left insular lesions were specifically isolated, there was increased cardiac sympathetic and decreased cardiac parasympathetic tone.[20] In contrast, left parietoinsular stroke was associated with an increased incidence of new-onset atrial fibrillation, often considered a parasympathetically derived abnormality.[21] In a prospective study of patients with stroke and transient ischemic attacks (TIAs), left insular strokes were an independent risk factor for adverse cardiac outcome in patients without heart disease.[22] In the Northern Manhattan Study, left parietal lobe infarction was an independent predictor of long-term cardiac death and myocardial infarction.[23] Similarly, in a secondary analysis of the North American Symptomatic Endarterectomy Trial, long-term risk of sudden death was significantly increased in patients with left brain infarction.[24] These observations highlight the complex interactions of the insular cortex and other autonomic centers of the brain.

ISCHEMIC AND HEMORRHAGIC STROKE

Clinical observations in patients with stroke have greatly advanced the understanding of interactions between the brain and heart. Cardiac abnormalities occur in a majority of patients after stroke, and can range from transient ECG findings to serious cardiac events and cardiac death.[25,26] The most common disturbances include ECG abnormalities, cardiac arrhythmias, and myocardial injury and dysfunction. Distinguishing cardiac abnormalities caused directly by stroke, however, remains difficult because the prevalence of preexisting cardiac disease is high, particularly among patients with ischemic stroke.[27,28] However, substantial evidence exists supporting the occurrence of cardiac disturbances after stroke even in the absence of significant coronary artery disease (CAD). Increasing evidence suggests that the presence of stroke should be a deemed a risk-factor equivalent contributing to absolute risk estimates for outcomes and prevention of vascular disease.[29] A meta-analysis of patients with acute stroke followed for a mean of 3.5 years revealed an annual risk of myocardial infarction of 2 percent.[30] Cardiac disturbances are the most common cause of death after stroke, accounting for up to 6 percent of unexpected deaths during the first month.[31] Understanding the mechanisms of cardiac disturbances may prevent future cardiac complications and improve survival in these patients.

The Electrocardiogram

ECG abnormalities are common, presenting in the majority of patients with acute stroke.[32] In 1947, Byer and colleagues first described marked QT prolongation with large T and U waves in the ECG of four patients with acute stroke.[33] Subsequently, Burch and colleagues described an ECG pattern after acute stroke consisting of large inverted T waves, prolonged QT intervals, and large septal U waves that has become distinctive of cerebrovascular injury (Fig. 10-1).[34] In the 17 abnormal ECGs reported in their study, the abnormalities were most frequently observed after SAH, followed by ICH and ischemic lesions. These early studies did not control for the incidence of concomitant or preexisting ischemic cardiac disease, but subsequent case-control studies suggested that repolarization abnormalities on ECGs are not present prior to the stroke event. Overall,

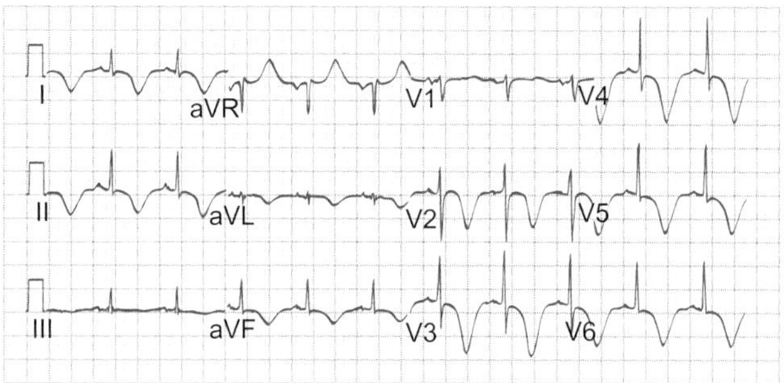

FIGURE 10-1 ■ Typical "neurogenic" electrocardiographic changes with symmetric deep T-wave inversions in a patient with acute subarachnoid hemorrhage. These abnormalities were transient and not associated with myocardial infarction. (Courtesy of Dr. Jonathan Zaroff, MD.)

there was a significantly increased incidence of ST depression, prolongation of the QT interval, T-wave inversion, and ventricular premature beats among stroke patients compared to age- and sex-matched controls. Although patients with known cardiac disease were excluded, limitations of these studies were the lack of detailed cardiac evaluations and comparison to antecedent ECG tracings that may not have completely excluded coexistent heart disease.[35]

QT Prolongation

The most common stroke-related ECG abnormality is QT prolongation, a myocardial repolarization abnormality associated with an increased risk of a characteristic life-threatening cardiac arrhythmia, known as torsade de pointes (Fig. 10-2).[36] Interestingly, congenital forms of long QT may be related to imbalance of sympathetic innervation of the heart.[37] Among acute stroke patients, prolonged QT interval is more frequently observed after hemorrhagic strokes, occurring in 45 to 71 percent of patients with SAH or ICH compared to 38 percent of those with ischemic strokes.[38–40] Ventricular tachyarrhythmias including sudden death and torsade de pointes are often preceded by QT prolongation in patients with SAH.[39,41] QT prolongation, accompanied by U waves and T-wave changes, often correlates with elevated systolic blood pressure on admission.[32,39] Assessment of common causes of these ECG changes, such as hypokalemia, hypomagnesemia, and medication toxicity, is recommended before attributing them to the underlying stroke.

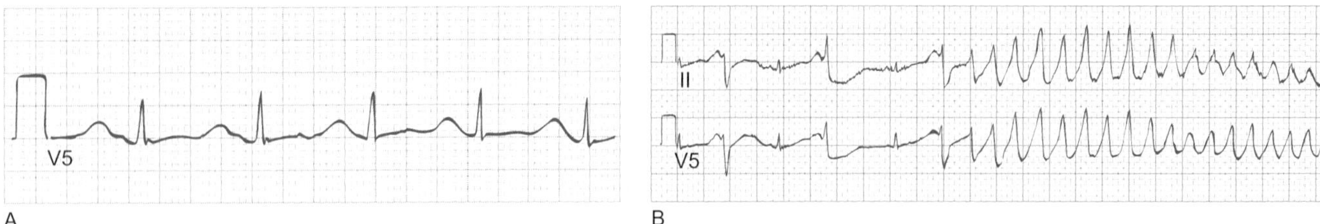

FIGURE 10-2 ■ Electrocardiographic (ECG) changes can precede pathologic arrhythmias in patients with severe neurologic injuries. **A**, Prolongation of the QT interval is common after subarachnoid hemorrhage. Electrolyte abnormalities or medications can also prolong the QT interval. **B**, Torsades de pointes is a polymorphic ventricular tachycardia associated with QT prolongation. (Courtesy of Dr. Byron Lee, MD.)

Repolarization Abnormalities

The similarities between ECG changes due to acute myocardial ischemia and infarction and those associated with stroke are most striking with the repolarization abnormalities involving the ST segment, leading many investigators to hypothesize coexisting cardiac disease as the primary cause. ST segment changes (including ST elevations) occur in 22 to 35 percent of patients with ischemic stroke, but interpretation of such findings is complicated by the increased prevalence of cardiac disease in this subgroup of stroke patients.[42] However, new T-wave abnormalities appear in approximately 15 percent of patients with acute stroke, even in the absence of electrolyte disturbances or primary ischemic heart disease. Inverted or flat T waves have also been reported in up to 55 percent of patients with SAH, the stroke subgroup with the lowest prevalence of coexistent cardiac disease.[43,44] Kono and colleagues performed detailed cardiac assessments on 12 patients with acute SAH and ST elevations on ECG. Although patients were found to have apical wall motion abnormalities on echocardiogram, there was no evidence of coronary artery stenosis or vasospasm on cardiac angiography.[45] These findings, along with the observation that stroke-induced ECG changes are evanescent, resolving over a period of days to months with little residuum, argue against myocardial ischemia or infarction as the only cause of repolarization changes on ECG.

Q Waves and U Waves

New Q waves similar in morphology to those observed in acute myocardial infarction are also common after acute stroke, reported in approximately 10 percent of patients with acute ischemic or hemorrhagic stroke.[40] To complicate matters, Q waves may be transient or proceed through the evolutionary changes seen in myocardial infarction.[32] Further cardiac evaluation may be necessary in patients with Q waves and ST segment alterations, particularly if they are over 65 years of age with coronary risk factors such as diabetes mellitus.

New U waves occur in isolation or with T waves and QT abnormalities in approximately 13 to 15 percent of patients with acute ischemic stroke and SAH.[32,46] Isolated U waves were equally distributed between ischemic and hemorrhagic strokes, but the combination of U waves and QT prolongation was more common among patients with hemorrhagic strokes.[32] There is no relationship between the presence of U waves and stroke mortality, suggesting that this ECG change should not require any specific treatment or evaluation.

Cardiac Arrhythmias

Nearly every type of cardiac arrhythmia has been reported after acute stroke, including bradycardia, supraventricular tachycardia, atrial flutter, atrial fibrillation, ectopic ventricular beats, multifocal ventricular tachycardias, torsade de pointes, ventricular flutter, and ventricular fibrillation. Most arrhythmias occur within the first week after stroke, occurring in 25 to 40 percent of patients with ischemic stroke or ICH, and 98 percent of patients with SAH.[47,48] In a prospective study, the incidence of serious arrhythmia was highest in the first 24 hours after hospital admission, and clinically symptomatic in 25 percent of events. Atrial fibrillation was the most common cardiac arrhythmia, accounting for 60 percent of the events.[49] In these studies, which did not control for preexisting cardiac disease, rhythm disturbances may have preceded the stroke event and, at least for atrial fibrillation, may have been causally related to the ischemic stroke. Not surprisingly, since the ECG is a relatively insensitive test for arrhythmia, a higher incidence of ventricular extrasystoles, followed by atrial extrasystoles, supraventricular tachycardia, and atrial fibrillation was found in a prospective study of ischemic stroke patients using cardiac telemetry monitoring.[50] Importantly, the presence of arrhythmias after stroke is significantly associated with increased mortality.[51]

In studies of hemorrhagic strokes, the incidence of ventricular arrhythmias was 10 percent after ICH. Location of hemorrhage appears to correlate with the rhythm disturbances. Yamour and colleagues reported a correlation between the occurrence of brainstem bleeds and atrial fibrillation.[40] Ventricular arrhythmias correlated with temporoparietal location, whereas sinus bradycardia and supraventricular tachycardias were seen more commonly with traumatic frontal lobe hemorrhage.

Patients with SAH have even more profound rhythm disturbances that may be related to the diffuse nature of the injury and the degree of monitoring in the intensive care unit. Stober and colleagues described multifocal ventricular ectopy (54%), asystolic intervals (27%), sinus bradycardia (23%), and atrial fibrillation (4%).[52] Because the frequency and severity of arrhythmias are significantly higher in patients studied within 48 hours of onset of SAH,[41] we recommend continuous cardiac monitoring in an intensive care setting for all patient with acute SAH.

Cardiac Injury and Dysfunction

Myocardial infarction in the setting of acute stroke is not uncommon, and often represents concomitant CAD in older patients with ischemic stroke and vascular risk factors. However, evidence from autopsy series in both ischemic and hemorrhagic stroke indicates that cardiac dysfunction may occur in the absence of underlying CAD. When myocardial tissue injury is present, suspicion for underlying cardiac disease increases, but pathologic and functional studies of the heart suggest a mechanism distinct from coronary artery–induced ischemia. Subendocardial hemorrhages were initially described in patients dying after acute strokes and seizures. Further studies suggested that these pathologic changes are secondary to excessive sympathetic stimulation. Following intracranial hemorrhage, catecholamines increase in cardiac tissue. Catecholamine-induced subendocardial lesions include scattered foci of swollen myocytes surrounded by infiltrating monocytes, interstitial hemorrhages, and myofibrillar degeneration.[5] Collectively, the characteristic pathologic changes have been called contraction band necrosis, coagulative myocytolysis, or myofibrillar degeneration (Fig. 10-3).[53] The pattern of myofibrillar necrosis localizing near cardiac nerves is identical to other lesions thought to be of sympathetic origin such as catecholamine infusion, "voodoo death," hypothalamic stimulation, or reperfusion of transiently ischemic cardiac muscle. The *Takotsubo* or *"broken heart" syndrome* is a severe cardiomyopathy associated with such major life events or stresses as the death of a loved one or intense fear. There is no evidence of CAD and survivors may recover left ventricular function completely over the following 1 to 2 weeks.[54]

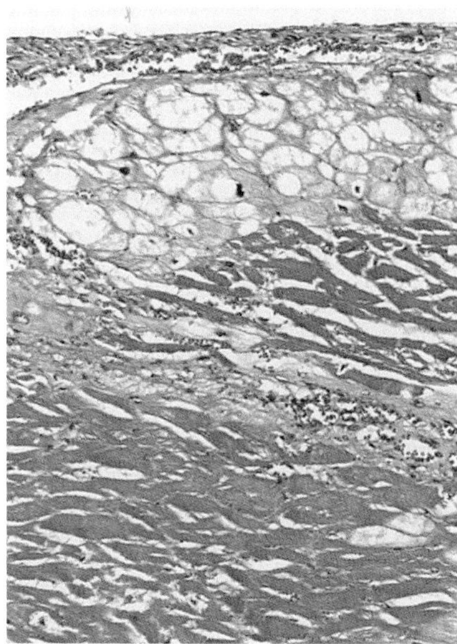

FIGURE 10-3 ■ A representative cross-section of myocardium after hematoxylin–eosin stain showing marked myocyte hypertrophy with nucleomegaly, and myocytolysis. (Courtesy of Dr. Philip Ursell, MD.)

In patients with CAD, myocardial necrosis typically follows a vascular distribution. The timing of the injury is also distinct from the necrosis seen in CAD, which typically occurs in a delayed fashion after progressive ischemia and muscle cell death. Neurogenic myocardial injury can be visible within minutes of onset, with appreciable differences observed on a cellular level. In myocytolysis, mononuclear infiltration predominates, with early calcification and myocardial cells in a hypercontracted state with contraction bands.[55]

Further evidence for a neurogenic mechanism of cardiac injury comes from studies of cardiac function after SAH, which typically affects younger patients without a history of coexistent cardiac disease. Global or regional left ventricular systolic dysfunction on echocardiogram has been described after SAH with an approximate incidence of 10 to 28 percent.[45,56,57] The severity of neurologic injury is strongly associated with the presence of left ventricular dysfunction.[58] Similarly, diastolic dysfunction is also common after SAH, is associated with the severity of neurologic injury, and may be the cause of pulmonary edema in these patients.[59] The onset of left ventricular dysfunction occurs early in the course of SAH.[60,61] In the largest study to date, a regional wall motion abnormality was most likely to be present within the first 2 days.[61] The prevalence then declined during days 3 to 8 after hemorrhage. In this same study, the authors demonstrated complete or partial resolution of left ventricular dysfunction in the majority of patients during their acute hospitalization. Thus, cardiac dysfunction appears to be reversible in most cases and normalizes over time.[62–65]

There is a well-demonstrated, unique, apical-sparing pattern of regional wall motion abnormality that differentiates SAH patients from those with the typical patterns seen in CAD. A retrospective study of patients with SAH demonstrated reversibility and both global and regional left ventricular dysfunction, most commonly affecting the anterior and anteroseptal walls and not involving the apex.[60] Younger age and anterior aneurysm position were independent predictors of this pattern.[66] This apical-sparing pattern of left ventricular dysfunction argues against an obstruction or vasospasm of coronary arteries and provides indirect evidence of a neurally mediated mechanism of injury.

Experimental and clinical studies have addressed a neurogenic catecholamine-mediated mechanism ("catecholamine hypothesis") of cardiac dysfunction.[67–69] In a cohort of patients with SAH who had echocardiograms and nuclear scans of cardiac innervation and perfusion, regions of contractile dysfunction were associated with abnormalities in myocardial sympathetic innervation while cardiac perfusion was normal. Degree of cardiac innervation was measured with a scintigraphic evaluation using [^{123}I]metaiodobenzylguanidine (MIBG),

TABLE 10-1 ■ Myocardial Injury and Dysfunction by MIBG Heart-to-Mediastinum Ratio

	(H:M) >1.57 (*n* = 19)	(H:M) <1.57 (*n* = 18)	*P*
LVEF <50%	32%	61%	0.072*
Mean LVEF	53 ± 15	51 ± 16	0.61†
RWMS >1.0	47%	83%	0.038‡
Mean RWMS	1.3 ± 0.5	1.5 ± 0.5	0.071†
cTi >1.0	16%	50%	0.038‡
Mean cTi	2.9 ± 10.2	5.3 ± 11.8	0.15†

*Chi-square test.
†Wilcoxon rank-sum.
‡Fisher exact test.
cTi, cardiac troponin I; H:M, heart-to-mediastinum ratio; LVEF, left ventricular ejection fraction; MIBG, [^{123}I]metaiodobenzylguanidine; RWMS, regional wall motion score.
From Banki NM, Kopelnik A, Dae MW, et al: Acute neurocardiogenic injury after subarachnoid hemorrhage. Circulation **112**:3314, 2005, with permission.

cardiac perfusion was measured using [^{99m}Tc] sesta-methoxyisobutylisonitrile (MIBI), and regions of myocardial dysfunction were determined by echocardiography simultaneously in the patients. Patients with functional cardiac denervation had worse regional wall motion scores (RWMS) and more troponin release than patients without evidence of cardiac denervation (Table 10-1). Figure 10-4 illustrates normal perfusion and global denervation in a patient with SAH whose echocardiogram showed global left ventricular systolic dysfunction. All study subjects had normal perfusion imaging, which excluded significant coronary artery disease and supported a neurogenic mechanism of cardiac injury.[70] In addition, data suggest that genetic polymorphisms of the adrenoceptors are associated with an increased risk of cardiac abnormalities after SAH.[71] These data support the hypothesis that cardiac dysfunction after SAH is a form of neurocardiogenic injury.

Plasma Markers

In addition to pathologic data and measurements of cardiac function, elevations in cardiac enzymes provide evidence of myocardial injury after stroke. Creatine kinase (CK) and specifically the cardiac isoenzyme CK-MB are released from damaged myocardium. Elevated serum levels occur in

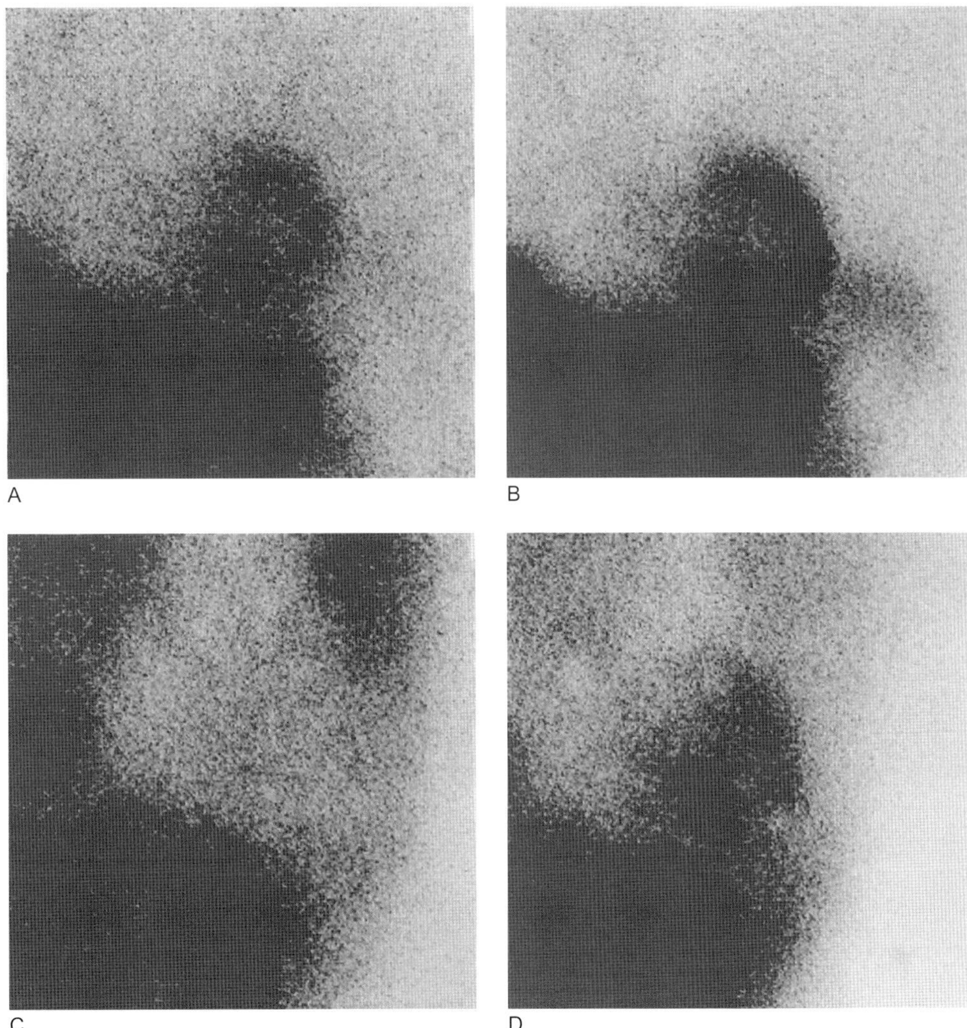

FIGURE 10-4 ■ Normal myocardial innervation (**A**) and perfusion (**B**) in a 71-year-old man with SAH. Global functional denervation (**C**) and normal perfusion, except for a nonspecific apical irregularity (**D**), in a 41-year-old woman with SAH. (From Banki NM, Kopelnik A, Dae MW, et al: Acute neurocardiogenic injury after subarachnoid hemorrhage. Circulation 112:3314, 2005, with permission.)

10 to 45 percent of stroke patients, and there is a good correlation between elevation in CK-MB and stroke-induced ECG changes or cardiac arrhythmias.[48] Unlike acute myocardial infarction, a stroke-induced increase in serum CK-MB levels occurs more slowly and peaks at a much lower value on around day 4 after stroke.

Cardiac troponin I is a specific and more sensitive marker of myocardial damage. Elevations in troponin I have been described in 20 to 25 percent of patients with SAH.[72–74] The degree of neurologic injury and female gender are strong predictors of myocardial necrosis after SAH (Table 10-2).[74] Acute troponin I elevation after SAH is associated with ECG abnormalities, left ventricular dysfunction, pulmonary edema, hypotension, and delayed cerebral ischemia from vasospasm.[75] In a meta-analysis of measurements of cardiac complications after SAH, markers for cardiac damage and dysfunction were associated with increased mortality, delayed cerebral ischemia, and poor functional outcome.[76] Among SAH survivors, there is an increased long-term mortality associated with SAH-related cardiac injury, providing more evidence for the role of cardiac injury in adverse outcomes.[77]

Serum B-type natriuretic peptide (BNP) is often used as a marker of heart failure. Elevated serum BNP levels after SAH have been independently associated with hyponatremia, delayed ischemic neurologic deficits, and a poor Glasgow Coma Scale

TABLE 10-2 ■ Determinants of Myocardial Necrosis

	Univariate			Multivariate		
Predictors	**OR**	***P***	**95% CI**	**OR**	***P***	**95% CI**
Age (per 10 year increase)	1.16	0.262	0.90–1.49	1.54	0.112	0.90–2.62
Female (vs. male)	2.98	0.019	1.20–7.43	34.96	0.009	2.47–495.01
Body surface area (per 0.2 m^2 increase)	1.03	0.847	0.78–1.36	2.20	0.025	1.11–4.39
Hunt and Hess score >2 (vs. 1–2)	8.47	<0.001	3.43–20.92	6.62	0.026	1.25–34.82
Systolic blood pressure (per 20 mmHg increase)	0.78	0.019	0.64–0.96	0.52	0.007	0.32–0.83
Heart rate (per 10 bpm increase)	1.26	0.001	1.10–1.43	1.61	0.005	1.16–2.25
Phenylephrine dose (per 50 μg/min increase)	1.17	<0.001	1.07–1.28	1.47	0.010	1.10–1.98
LVMI (per 20 g/m^2 increase)	1.23	0.083	0.97–1.55	1.74	0.032	1.05–2.89
SAH to cTi* (per 1 day increase)	0.86	0.001	0.78–0.94	0.70	0.008	0.54–0.91

*Time in days from SAH symptom onset to measurement of cardiac troponin (cTi). CI, confidence interval; LVMI, left ventricular mass index; OR, odds ratio. From Tung P, Kopelnik A, Banki N, et al: Predictors of neurocardiogenic injury after subarachnoid hemorrhage. Stroke 35:548, 2004, with permission.

score at 2 weeks.[78] In a prospective study, elevated levels were significantly correlated with systolic and diastolic dysfunction, pulmonary edema, elevated troponin I levels, and lower cardiac ejection fractions (Fig. 10-5). The predominance of cardiac abnormalities similar to heart failure suggests that although BNP is found in heart and brain, elevated levels are likely to be of cardiac origin.[79] Moreover, elevated troponin I and BNP levels are independent and strong predictors of inpatient mortality after SAH.[80] Elevated levels of BNP are also strongly and independently associated with cerebral infarction after SAH.[81] These data provide additional evidence that the degree of myocardial injury and dysfunction has significant implications for prognosis in these patients.

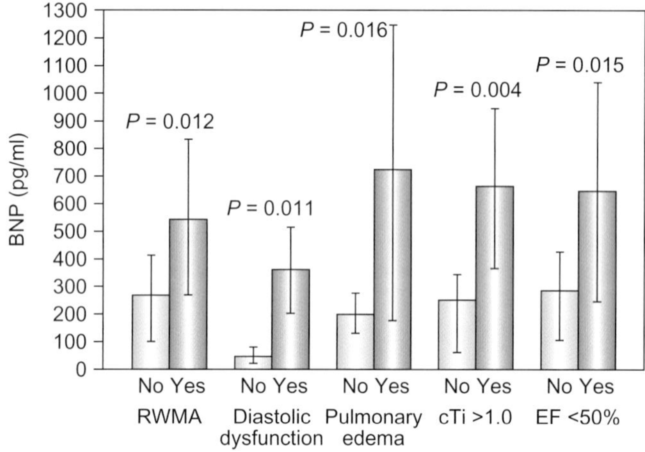

FIGURE 10-5 ■ Serum B-type natriuretic peptide (BNP) levels and cardiac outcomes. The column height indicates the mean BNP and the error bars indicate 95% confidence intervals. Probability values indicate results of Wilcoxon rank-sum tests. cTi, cardiac troponin I more than 1.0 μg/L; EF, left ventricular ejection fraction less than 50%; RWMA, regional wall motion abnormality. (From Tung PP, Olmsted E, Kopelnik A, et al: Plasma B-type natriuretic peptide levels are associated with early cardiac dysfunction after subarachnoid hemorrhage. Stroke 36:1567, 2005, with permission.)

EPILEPSY, TRAUMA, AND OTHER NEUROLOGIC INJURIES

Similar cardiac arrhythmias and ECG findings have been described in patients with epilepsy, brain tumors, head trauma, meningitis, multiple sclerosis, and spinal lesions. In all cases, a common mechanism of neurogenic cardiac injury is supported by increased sympathetic nervous system discharge, increased adrenomedullary catecholamine production, and reduced parasympathetic activity.[82] Autopsy case reports in young patients who died suddenly from seizures and brain tumors describe cardiac pathology identical to myocardial injury from excessive sympathetic activation and catecholamine infusion.[4] Epilepsy and traumatic brain injury (TBI) are well-studied models of brain–heart interactions, and will be discussed in more detail.

Clinical observations as well as experimental work suggest sympathetic activation may be important in the pathogenesis of cardiac arrhythmia and sudden unexpected death in epilepsy (SUDEP). Experimental studies in animal models of epilepsy have revealed an increase in cardiac arrhythmias that corresponded with desynchronization of firing between the vagus and sympathetic nerves, and with an increase in ictal cortical discharges.[83] Furthermore, electric stimulation studies in both animals and humans have provided direct evidence of cardiac autonomic activation from specific regions of the insula.[16]

Advances in cardiac monitoring have enabled better prospective studies of the changes in heart rate accompanying seizures to better understand the phenomenon of SUDEP. Sinus tachycardia and ECG changes are commonly associated with seizures. In studies using simultaneous ambulatory electroencephalographic (EEG)/ECG monitoring, sinus tachycardia occurring at the time of the seizure was seen in 90 percent of patients. Cardiac arrhythmias were identified in 52 percent of all seizures and most frequently comprised a marked beat-to-beat variation in the R-R interval accompanied by changes in P-wave shape. Sinus bradycardia or asystole was rare, seen in 0.5 percent.[84,85] Ambulatory ECG studies suggest that there is more sympathetic tone during seizures and that no significant cardiac disturbances occur during the interictal period.[84] However, measurements of cardiac innervation using MIBI suggest baseline dysfunction in cardiac sympathetic innervation with normal myocardial perfusion in patients with chronic temporal lobe epilepsy.[86] These results suggest an increase in parasympathetic activity during the interictal period. Increased parasympathetic activity has been described previously, affecting variation in blood pressure and heart rate after sympathetic challenge.[87]

Ictal bradycardia and asystole occurring in association with seizures were previously considered to be rare. Long-term cardiac monitoring using implantable loop recorders, however, suggests that bradyarrythmias may be more common than previously supposed. Among 20 patients with focal epilepsy monitored over a 2-year period, over one-third had ictal bradycardia, and over one-half required pacemaker insertion for clinically significant arrhythmias.[88] Epilepsy is associated with an increased mortality rate compared to the general population, and approximately half of seizure-related deaths are sudden and unexplained.[89–93] The incidence of SUDEP has been estimated at 2 cases per 100 patient years.[90] The risk of sudden unexpected death has been related to increased seizure frequency, generalized seizures, younger age, lower concentration of antiepileptic medications, use of multiple medications, and duration of epilepsy.[93–95] The etiology for sudden death in these patients remains elusive. Cardiac arrhythmia is a potentially treatable cause of sudden death, but direct evidence of increased mortality with ictal arrhythmias is lacking. Recent studies have focused on ictal bradyarrhythmias and asystole, as well as interictal heart rate variability, which may represent a high risk of sudden death.[96,97] Improvements in cardiac monitoring and early intervention with cardiac pacing could improve outcomes if arrhythmias are found to be a significant risk factor for sudden death.[98,99]

In studies of intensive cardiac monitoring after severe TBI, abnormalities in heart rate variability were correlated with elevated ICP, decreased cerebral perfusion pressure, and hospital mortality.[100,101] In TBI where a hyperdynamic cardiac state was detected, increased arterial levels of epinephrine and norepinephrine were correlated.[102] Episodic autonomic dysfunction—known as paroxysmal sympathetic hyperactivity—has been described with an incidence of 8 to 33 percent in patients with moderate to severe TBI. Heart rate and blood pressure variability is typically observed with other symptoms of dysautonomia including temperature changes, sweating, confusion, and agitation, and with dystonic posturing.[103] Risk factors for paroxysmal sympathetic hyperactivity include younger age and presence of diffuse axonal injury on imaging.[104,105] Treatment is typically supportive with opioid analgesia, benzodiazepines, or antipsychotics for sedation.[106,107] There are currently no proven treatments that have been effective in improving outcomes, but clinical trials are ongoing to determine efficacy of treatments using β-blockade and other central acting α-antagonists after TBI.[108]

CARDIAC EVALUATION

Proper evaluation of cardiac injury and dysfunction remains important for both cardiac and neurologic prognosis. Patients with ischemic stroke, in particular, are more likely to have concomitant significant CAD.[28] A strong association between cerebrovascular disease and CAD has been established in a number of clinical studies.[30] In the longitudinal Framingham Study, similar risk factors predicted both stroke and heart disease, with similar rates of cerebral and cardiac ischemic events (annual rates of 6 and 7%, respectively).[109] Coronary angiography of stroke patients showed that 40 percent had significant narrowing of their coronary arteries that was asymptomatic at the time of stroke presentation.[110] Using functional testing with thallium stress imaging, significant CAD was present in 45 to 60 percent of patients with TIA or stroke.[27] Given the higher probability of CAD, several diagnostic evaluations are recommended in the acute period for all patients with ischemic stroke including an echocardiogram and measurement of serum troponin I levels. Further functional testing with echocardiogram and continuous cardiac monitoring are often initiated to determine the risk of a cardiogenic source of embolic ischemic strokes. Exercise or pharmacologic stress test (nuclear or echocardiographic) and coronary angiogram should be obtained based on the patient's risk level and functional status.

The majority of patients with acute stroke would not be considered for acute treatments for myocardial infarction, but coronary angiography may be indicated if there is a strong clinical suspicion of plaque rupture or thrombus formation that may be safely treated endovascularly. As previously described, distinguishing cardiogenic from neurogenic causes of myocardial injury can be problematic in this patient population. Evaluation for clinical signs of heart failure, such as cardiogenic pulmonary edema and hypotension, careful analysis of the ECG, assessment of cardiac function by echocardiogram, and evaluation of myocardial necrosis by cardiac markers may help to determine the need for cardiac catheterization. The serum CK-MB levels are insensitive and should not be used for differentiation between neurogenic and cardiogenic injury. A large increase in serum troponin I levels with a significant temporal trend, along with ECG changes that correlate to the location of left ventricular systolic dysfunction on echocardiogram, may be more helpful.[111] In contrast, common "neurogenic" ECG changes, including T-wave inversion, QTc prolongation, a shorter PR interval, and the presence of U waves, may aid in differentiating neurogenic injury from myocardial infarction.

In hemorrhagic strokes, the frequency of cardiac arrhythmias is high and often correlates with ECG changes. Baseline ECG and continuous cardiac monitoring in this population are often performed in the intensive care unit. Patients with SAH pose a greater challenge when the complication of cerebral vasospasm arises. The typical management of these patients includes induced hypertension with pressors, hypervolemia, and hemodilution to improve cerebral blood flow through narrowed vasculature. The reduction of cardiac output from normally elevated levels may increase the risk of cerebral ischemia related to vasospasm, and increase the risk of cardiopulmonary complications.[112] SAH patients could potentially benefit from measurement of serum troponin I and BNP levels as well as a transthoracic echocardiogram as part of their initial management. Moreover, a close, independent relationship has been established between severity of SAH and the probability of troponin release, and could be used to anticipate greater risk of cardiac abnormalities in these patients.[74] Coronary angiography after SAH is not recommended because most patients with left ventricular dysfunction following SAH who undergo cardiac catheterization have normal epicardial coronary arteries and no evidence of coronary vasospasm.[45]

For patients with epilepsy, sudden unexpected death is the most feared complication. Growing evidence suggests that neurogenic cardiac arrhythmias may contribute to the risk of sudden death. Identifying patients at highest risk of sudden death has been challenging. In addition to clinical risk factors and promoting better compliance with medication, advanced cardiac monitoring with ambulatory ECG and long-term implantable loop recorders may help to identify patients with pathologic arrhythmias.[88] In addition, other methods for measuring cardiac autonomic input, such as heart rate variability and spectral analysis, may be useful.[113]

In patients with TBI, continuous cardiac monitoring in the intensive care unit often detects heart rate and blood pressure variability and, combined with multimodality monitoring, can correlate changes associated with elevations in ICP and cerebral perfusion pressure. Incorporating measurements of heart rate variability may also be useful for prognosis.[100]

CLINICAL MANAGEMENT

After identification of the common cardiac abnormalities, management should be initiated to prevent their detrimental effect on patient outcomes. The most common ECG changes generally do not require specific treatment, but may prompt further testing and continuous monitoring.[48] Identification of other causes or contributors to ECG changes can lead to rapid resolution. In particular, specific treatment of hypokalemia, hypomagnesemia, and medication toxicity may correct a prolonged QT interval. Antiarrhythmic (e.g., quinidine, sotalol, amiodarone) or antipsychotic drugs (e.g., haloperidol) known to affect the QT interval should be avoided in these patients, especially if their neurologic injury exacerbates underlying hereditary long QT syndrome. When repolarization abnormalities occur, it may be necessary to exclude acute myocardial infarction. Common electrolyte abnormalities such as hyperkalemia can produce tall T waves, whereas hypokalemia is the most common cause of U waves. Correction of electrolyte abnormalities may reduce the risk of arrhythmias.

Cardiac rhythm disturbances after neurologic injury can be complex, requiring cardiology consultation. The most important aim is to identify patients who may be hemodynamically unstable in the presence of an arrhythmia. This is a medical emergency and should be managed immediately by appropriate personnel in the intensive care unit, with the involvement of a cardiac team. In a stable, asymptomatic patient, identifying the type of arrhythmia can guide management. Atrial or ventricular premature contractions generally do not require specific treatment. For sinus bradycardia or tachycardia, identification and treatment of the common underlying conditions, such as fever, thyroid dysfunction, anemia, pain, sepsis, and anxiety, will often correct the rhythm disturbance.

Specific pharmacologic treatment may be required if the patient develops stable tachyarrhythmias. A trial of adenosine can terminate supraventricular tachycardia and assist in determining the underlying rhythm disturbance. Rate control with an intravenous β-blocker, calcium-channel blocker, or amiodarone can be used in patients with atrial fibrillation or flutter, most common after ischemic stroke and ICH. Stable ventricular tachyarrhythmias can also be managed with intravenous amiodarone or lidocaine. Specific treatment of torsade de pointes includes intravenous magnesium. Any arrhythmia more complex than ectopic beats or sinus bradycardia or tachycardia should prompt a cardiology consultation.

When more significant cardiac dysfunction or injury is identified by elevated serum markers or dysfunction on ECG, several steps can be taken to improve cardiac prognosis. If CAD is present, management of atherosclerosis risk factors (diabetes, hyperlipidemia, hypertension, and smoking) and treatment with antiplatelet agents and lipid-lowering agents may help both the ischemic stroke and heart disease. The β-blockers reduce the risk of vascular events after myocardial infarction, but their role in the prevention of cardiac events in other high-risk patients with stroke is unclear. Finally, revascularization by angioplasty or coronary artery bypass grafting is beneficial for patients with symptomatic CAD, but the decision to treat must balance the risk to the patient with an acute neurologic injury. The value of revascularization in patients with asymptomatic CAD is less clear.[28]

In the rare event of coronary plaque rupture in a patient with SAH, coronary angioplasty along with stenting may be considered once the aneurysm is secured and the necessary anticoagulation regimen can be tolerated safely. Although further studies are needed to determine the safety of percutaneous coronary intervention and anticoagulation after successful aneurysmal intervention, patients with unsecured aneurysms should not undergo any coronary intervention given the unacceptably high risk of rebleeding.

In patients with SAH, the presence of cardiac injury and dysfunction often directly affects management. The decision to treat a ruptured aneurysm should not be delayed because of concerns regarding cardiac injury. Because the mechanism of neurogenic cardiac injury is probably mediated by catecholamines, treatment should focus on correcting or improving the underlying neurologic process. Prevention of rebleeding with early aneurysm clipping or endovascular coiling has proved beneficial and does not appear to affect cardiac outcomes. In our patient cohort, there was no significant difference in cardiac morbidity between surgical and endovascular therapies.[114]

Management of cerebral vasospasm in the setting of significant neurocardiogenic injury is challenging and directly impacts neurologic prognosis. Permissive hypertension requiring pressors to improve cerebral blood flow often leads to increased myocardial wall stress and oxygen consumption, whereas hemodilution will decrease oxygen delivery to the myocardium, predisposing to further injury. Although most patients tolerate treatment for cerebral vasospasm, phenylephrine, the most commonly used pressor, is relatively ineffective in patients with a poor cardiac ejection fraction.[80] Other studies have also suggested the use of alternative agents such as dobutamine and milrinone, which may be more effective in this setting.[115] In those patients with diastolic dysfunction, iatrogenic hypervolemia may cause increased filling pressures, leading to pulmonary edema. Continued aggressive therapy for vasospasm is recommended, but more effective pressors and volume repletion strategies should be considered in patients with concomitant cardiogenic injury. In patients with severe neurogenic cardiac injury and evidence of heart failure who are unable to tolerate medical therapy for vasospasm, placement of an intra-aortic balloon pump to increase cerebral perfusion pressure has been successful.[62,116–118]

Given the potential role of excessive catecholamines in neurocardiogenic injury, β-blockers may have a role in providing cardioprotection if administered early in the hospital course, but supporting evidence is limited and based on small studies. Pathologic correlation suggests that β-blockade may protect myocytes from the hostile environment caused by massive levels of catecholamines released from cardiac sympathetic nerve terminals following SAH. Larger studies will help to determine the role of early administration of β-blockers in patients with cardiac dysfunction following SAH. Calcium-channel blockers targeting the calcium overload preceding contraction-band necrosis have not been well studied. There does not appear to be a significant cardiac benefit from nimodipine, the calcium-channel blocker already administered to patients with SAH for vasospasm prophylaxis.

CONCLUDING COMMENTS

Cardiac disturbances are diverse and frequent in the setting of acute neurologic injury. More importantly, the presence of cardiac abnormalities has significant impact on clinical management and affects cardiac and neurologic outcomes adversely. Understanding of the underlying pathophysiology and localization of the important autonomic regulatory centers involved in brain–heart interactions has progressed significantly in recent years. Animal models have been translated into important clinical research studies that have revealed further complexity in the brain regulation of cardiac function. Early recognition and appropriate treatment interventions have already impacted clinical management and may influence treatment for prevention and improving outcomes for both the heart and the brain.

REFERENCES

1. Cushing H: The blood pressure reaction of acute cerebral compression illustrated by cases of intracranial hemorrhage. Am J Med Sci 125:1017, 1903.
2. Banki NM, Zaroff JG: Neurogenic cardiac injury. Curr Treat Options Cardiovasc Med 5:451, 2003.
3. Katsanos AH, Korantzopoulos P, Tsivgoulis G, et al: Electrocardiographic abnormalities and cardiac arrhythmias in structural brain lesions. Int J Cardiol 167:328, 2013.
4. Oppenheimer S: Cerebrogenic cardiac arrhythmias: cortical lateralization and clinical significance. Clin Auton Res 16:6, 2006.
5. Greenhoot JH, Reichenbach DD: Cardiac injury and subarachnoid hemorrhage. A clinical, pathological, and physiological correlation. J Neurosurg 30:521, 1969.
6. Ako J, Sudhir K, Farouque HM, et al: Transient left ventricular dysfunction under severe stress: brain-heart relationship revisited. Am J Med 119:10, 2006.
7. Bybee KA, Kara T, Prasad A, et al: Systematic review: transient left ventricular apical ballooning: a syndrome that mimics ST-segment elevation myocardial infarction. Ann Intern Med 141:858, 2004.
8. Wittstein IS, Thiemann DR, Lima JA, et al: Neurohumoral features of myocardial stunning due to sudden emotional stress. N Engl J Med 352:539, 2005.
9. Calaresu FR, Ciriello J: Projections to the hypothalamus from buffer nerves and nucleus tractus solitarius in the cat. Am J Physiol 239:R130, 1980.
10. Melville KI, Blum B, Shister HE, et al: Cardiac ischemic changes and arrhythmias induced by hypothalamic stimulation. Am J Cardiol 12:781, 1963.
11. Beattie J, Brow G, Long C: Physiology and anatomical evidence for the existence of nerve tracts connecting the hypothalamus with spinal sympathetic centres. Proc R Soc Lond (Biol) 106:253, 1930.
12. Nagai M, Hoshide S, Kario K: The insular cortex and cardiovascular system: a new insight into the brain-heart axis. J Am Soc Hypertens 4:174, 2010.
13. Oppenheimer SM, Wilson JX, Guiraudon C, et al: Insular cortex stimulation produces lethal cardiac arrhythmias: a mechanism of sudden death? Brain Res 550:115, 1991.
14. Hachinski VC, Oppenheimer SM, Wilson JX, et al: Asymmetry of sympathetic consequences of experimental stroke. Arch Neurol 49:697, 1992.
15. Cechetto DF, Wilson JX, Smith KE, et al: Autonomic and myocardial changes in middle cerebral artery

occlusion: stroke models in the rat. Brain Res 502:296, 1989.

16. Oppenheimer SM, Gelb A, Girvin JP, et al: Cardiovascular effects of human insular cortex stimulation. Neurology 42:1727, 1992.
17. Zamrini EY, Meador KJ, Loring DW, et al: Unilateral cerebral inactivation produces differential left/right heart rate responses. Neurology 40:1408, 1990.
18. Tokgozoglu SL, Batur MK, Topuoglu MA, et al: Effects of stroke localization on cardiac autonomic balance and sudden death. Stroke 30:1307, 1999.
19. Lane RD, Wallace JD, Petrosky PP, et al: Supraventricular tachycardia in patients with right hemisphere strokes. Stroke 23:362, 1992.
20. Oppenheimer SM, Kedem G, Martin WM: Left-insular cortex lesions perturb cardiac autonomic tone in humans. Clin Auton Res 6:131, 1996.
21. Vingerhoets F, Bogousslavsky J, Regli F, et al: Atrial fibrillation after acute stroke. Stroke 24:26, 1993.
22. Laowattana S, Zeger SL, Lima JA, et al: Left insular stroke is associated with adverse cardiac outcome. Neurology 66:477, 2006.
23. Rincon F, Dhamoon M, Moon Y, et al: Stroke location and association with fatal cardiac outcomes: Northern Manhattan Study (NOMAS). Stroke 39:2425, 2008.
24. Algra A, Gates PC, Fox AJ, et al: Side of brain infarction and long-term risk of sudden death in patients with symptomatic carotid disease. Stroke 34:2871, 2003.
25. Hachinski VC: The clinical problem of brain and heart. Stroke 24:I1, 1993.
26. Kumar S, Selim MH, Caplan LR: Medical complications after stroke. Lancet Neurol 9:105, 2010.
27. Love BB, Grover-McKay M, Biller J, et al: Coronary artery disease and cardiac events with asymptomatic and symptomatic cerebrovascular disease. Stroke 23:939, 1992.
28. Wilterdink JL, Furie KL, Easton JD: Cardiac evaluation of stroke patients. Neurology 51:S23, 1998.
29. Dhamoon MS, Elkind MS: Inclusion of stroke as an outcome and risk equivalent in risk scores for primary and secondary prevention of vascular disease. Circulation 121:2071, 2010.
30. Touze E, Varenne O, Chatellier G, et al: Risk of myocardial infarction and vascular death after transient ischemic attack and ischemic stroke: a systematic review and meta-analysis. Stroke 36:2748, 2005.
31. Silver FL, Norris JW, Lewis AJ, et al: Early mortality following stroke: a prospective review. Stroke 15:492, 1984.
32. Goldstein DS: The electrocardiogram in stroke: relationship to pathophysiological type and comparison with prior tracings. Stroke 10:253, 1979.
33. Byer E, Ashman R, Toth LA: Electrocardiograms with large, upright T waves and QT intervals. Am Heart J 33:796, 1947.
34. Burch GE, Meyers R, Abildskov JA: A new electrocardiographic pattern observed in cerebrovascular accidents. Circulation 9:719, 1954.
35. Khechinashvili G, Asplund K: Electrocardiographic changes in patients with acute stroke: a systematic review. Cerebrovasc Dis 14:67, 2002.
36. Moss AJ: Long QT syndrome. JAMA 289:2041, 2003.
37. Jackman WM, Friday KJ, Anderson JL, et al: The long QT syndromes: a critical review, new clinical observations and a unifying hypothesis. Prog Cardiovasc Dis 31:115, 1988.
38. Dimant J, Grob D: Electrocardiographic changes and myocardial damage in patients with acute cerebrovascular accidents. Stroke 8:448, 1977.
39. Oppenheimer SM, Cechetto DF, Hachinski VC: Cerebrogenic cardiac arrhythmias. Cerebral electrocardiographic influences and their role in sudden death. Arch Neurol 47:513, 1990.
40. Yamour BJ, Sridharan MR, Rice JF, et al: Electrocardiographic changes in cerebrovascular hemorrhage. Am Heart J 99:294, 1980.
41. Di Pasquale G, Pinelli G, Andreoli A, et al: Torsade de pointes and ventricular flutter-fibrillation following spontaneous cerebral subarachnoid hemorrhage. Int J Cardiol 18:163, 1988.
42. Valeriano J, Elson J: Electrocardiographic changes in central nervous system disease. Neurol Clin 11:257, 1993.
43. Solenski NJ, Haley EC Jr, Kassell NF, et al: Medical complications of aneurysmal subarachnoid hemorrhage: a report of the multicenter, cooperative aneurysm study. Participants of the Multicenter Cooperative Aneurysm Study. Crit Care Med 23:1007, 1995.
44. Sommargren CE, Warner R, Zaroff JG, et al: Electrocardiographic abnormalities in patients with subarachnoid hemorrhage and normal adults: a comparison study. J Electrocardiol 37(suppl):42, 2004.
45. Kono T, Morita H, Kuroiwa T, et al: Left ventricular wall motion abnormalities in patients with subarachnoid hemorrhage: neurogenic stunned myocardium. J Am Coll Cardiol 24:636, 1994.
46. Sommargren CE, Zaroff JG, Banki N, et al: Electrocardiographic repolarization abnormalities in subarachnoid hemorrhage. J Electrocardiol 35(suppl):257, 2002.
47. Andreoli A, di Pasquale G, Pinelli G, et al: Subarachnoid hemorrhage: frequency and severity of cardiac arrhythmias. A survey of 70 cases studied in the acute phase. Stroke 18:558, 1987.
48. Cheung RT, Hachinski V: Cardiac effects of stroke. Curr Treat Options Cardiovasc Med 6:199, 2004.
49. Kallmunzer B, Breuer L, Kahl N, et al: Serious cardiac arrhythmias after stroke: incidence, time course, and predictors—a systematic, prospective analysis. Stroke 43:2892, 2012.
50. Rem JA, Hachinski VC, Boughner DR, et al: Value of cardiac monitoring and echocardiography in TIA and stroke patients. Stroke 16:950, 1985.

51. Wong KY, Mac Walter RS, Douglas D, et al: Long QTc predicts future cardiac death in stroke survivors. Heart 89:377, 2003.
52. Stober T, Anstatt T, Sen S, et al: Cardiac arrhythmias in subarachnoid haemorrhage. Acta Neurochir (Wien) 93:37, 1988.
53. Fineschi V, Michalodimitrakis M, D'Errico S, et al: Insight into stress-induced cardiomyopathy and sudden cardiac death due to stress. A forensic cardio-pathologist point of view. Forensic Sci Int 194:1, 2010.
54. Kawai S, Suzuki H, Yamaguchi H, et al: Ampulla cardiomyopathy ('Takotusbo' cardiomyopathy)—reversible left ventricular dysfunction: with ST segment elevation. Jpn Circ J 64:156, 2000.
55. Samuels M: Electrocardiographic manifestations of neurologic disease. Semin Neurol 4:453, 1984.
56. Kuroiwa T, Morita H, Tanabe H, et al: Significance of ST segment elevation in electrocardiograms in patients with ruptured cerebral aneurysms. Acta Neurochirurgica 133:141, 1995.
57. Zaroff J, Aronson S, Lee B, et al: The relationship between immediate outcome after cardiac surgery, homogeneous cardioplegia delivery, and ejection fraction. Chest 106:38, 1994.
58. Kothavale A, Banki NM, Kopelnik A, et al: Predictors of left ventricular regional wall motion abnormalities after subarachnoid hemorrhage. Neurocrit Care 4:199, 2006.
59. Kopelnik A, Fisher L, Miss JC, et al: Prevalence and implications of diastolic dysfunction after subarachnoid hemorrhage. Neurocrit Care 3:132, 2005.
60. Zaroff JG, Rordorf GA, Ogilvy CS, et al: Regional patterns of left ventricular systolic dysfunction after subarachnoid hemorrhage: evidence for neurally mediated cardiac injury. J Am Soc Echocardiogr 13:774, 2000.
61. Banki N, Kopelnik A, Tung P, et al: Prospective analysis of prevalence, distribution, and rate of recovery of left ventricular systolic dysfunction in patients with subarachnoid hemorrhage. J Neurosurg 105:15, 2006.
62. Donaldson JW, Pritz MB: Myocardial stunning secondary to aneurysmal subarachnoid hemorrhage. Surg Neurol 55:12, 2001.
63. Handlin LR, Kindred LH, Beauchamp GD, et al: Reversible left ventricular dysfunction after subarachnoid hemorrhage. Am Heart J 126:235, 1993.
64. Wells C, Cujec B, Johnson D, et al: Reversibility of severe left ventricular dysfunction in patients with subarachnoid hemorrhage. Am Heart J 129:409, 1995.
65. Banki N, Parmley W, Foster E, et al: Reversibility of left ventricular systolic dysfunction in humans with subarachnoid hemorrhage. Circulation 104:II, 2001.
66. Khush K, Kopelnik A, Tung P, et al: Age and aneurysm position predict patterns of left ventricular dysfunction after subarachnoid hemorrhage. J Am Soc Echocardiogr 18:168, 2005.
67. Allman FD, Herold W, Bosso FJ, et al: Time-dependent changes in norepinephrine-induced left ventricular dysfunction and histopathologic condition. J Heart Lung Transplant 17:991, 1998.
68. Mertes P, Carteaux J, Jaboin Y, et al: Estimation of myocardial interstitial norepinephrine release after brain death using cardiac microdialysis. Transplantation 57:371, 1994.
69. Yeh T Jr, Wechsler AS, Graham LJ, et al: Acute brain death alters left ventricular myocardial gene expression. J Thorac Cardiovasc Surg 117:365, 1999.
70. Banki NM, Kopelnik A, Dae MW, et al: Acute neurocardiogenic injury after subarachnoid hemorrhage. Circulation 112:3314, 2005.
71. Zaroff JG, Pawlikowska L, Miss JC, et al: Adrenoceptor polymorphisms and the risk of cardiac injury and dysfunction after subarachnoid hemorrhage. Stroke 37:1680, 2006.
72. Horowitz MB, Willet D, Keffer J: The use of cardiac troponin-I (cTnI) to determine the incidence of myocardial ischemia and injury in patients with aneurysmal and presumed aneurysmal subarachnoid hemorrhage. Acta Neurochirurgica 140:87, 1998.
73. Parekh N, Venkatesh B, Cross D, et al: Cardiac troponin I predicts myocardial dysfunction in aneurysmal subarachnoid hemorrhage. J Am Coll Cardiol 36:1328, 2000.
74. Tung P, Kopelnik A, Banki N, et al: Predictors of neurocardiogenic injury after subarachnoid hemorrhage. Stroke 35:548, 2004.
75. Naidech AM, Kreiter KT, Janjua N, et al: Cardiac troponin elevation, cardiovascular morbidity, and outcome after subarachnoid hemorrhage. Circulation 112:2851, 2005.
76. van der Bilt IA, Hasan D, Vandertop WP, et al: Impact of cardiac complications on outcome after aneurysmal subarachnoid hemorrhage: a meta-analysis. Neurology 72:635, 2009.
77. Zaroff JG, Leong J, Kim H, et al: Cardiovascular predictors of long-term outcomes after non-traumatic subarachnoid hemorrhage. Neurocrit Care 17:374, 2012.
78. McGirt MJ, Blessing R, Nimjee SM, et al: Correlation of serum brain natriuretic peptide with hyponatremia and delayed ischemic neurological deficits after subarachnoid hemorrhage. Neurosurgery 54:1369, 2004.
79. Tung PP, Olmsted E, Kopelnik A, et al: Plasma B-type natriuretic peptide levels are associated with early cardiac dysfunction after subarachnoid hemorrhage. Stroke 36:1567, 2005.
80. Yarlagadda S, Rajendran P, Miss J, et al: Cardiovascular predictors of inpatient mortality after subarachnoid hemorrhage. Neurocrit Care 5:102, 2006.
81. Taub PR, Fields JD, Wu AH, et al: Elevated BNP is associated with vasospasm-independent cerebral infarction following aneurysmal subarachnoid hemorrhage. Neurocrit Care 15:13, 2011.
82. Cheung RT, Hachinski V: Cardiology. p. 305. In Samuels MA (ed): Hospitalist Neurology. Butterworth-Heinemann, Woburn, 1999.

83. Lathers CM, Schraeder PL, Weiner FL: Synchronization of cardiac autonomic neural discharge with epileptogenic activity: the lockstep phenomenon. Electroencephalogr Clin Neurophysiol 67:247, 1987.
84. Blumhardt LD, Smith PE, Owen L: Electrocardiographic accompaniments of temporal lobe epileptic seizures. Lancet 1:1051, 1986.
85. Zijlmans M, Flanagan D, Gotman J: Heart rate changes and ECG abnormalities during epileptic seizures: prevalence and definition of an objective clinical sign. Epilepsia 43:847, 2002.
86. Druschky A, Hilz MJ, Hopp P, et al: Interictal cardiac autonomic dysfunction in temporal lobe epilepsy demonstrated by [^{123}I]metaiodobenzylguanidine-SPECT. Brain 124:2372, 2001.
87. Devinsky O, Perrine K, Theodore WH: Interictal autonomic nervous system function in patients with epilepsy. Epilepsia 35:199, 1994.
88. Rugg-Gunn FJ, Simister RJ, Squirrell M, et al: Cardiac arrhythmias in focal epilepsy: a prospective long-term study. Lancet 364:2212, 2004.
89. Devinsky O: Sudden, unexpected death in epilepsy. N Engl J Med 365:1801, 2011.
90. Shorvon S, Tomson T: Sudden unexpected death in epilepsy. Lancet 378:2028, 2011.
91. Lhatoo SD, Johnson AL, Goodridge DM, et al: Mortality in epilepsy in the first 11 to 14 years after diagnosis: multivariate analysis of a long-term, prospective, population-based cohort. Ann Neurol 49:336, 2001.
92. Nashef L, Fish DR, Sander JW, et al: Incidence of sudden unexpected death in an adult outpatient cohort with epilepsy at a tertiary referral centre. J Neurol Neurosurg Psychiatry 58:462, 1995.
93. Walczak TS, Leppik IE, D'Amelio M, et al: Incidence and risk factors in sudden unexpected death in epilepsy: a prospective cohort study. Neurology 56:519, 2001.
94. Leestma JE, Walczak T, Hughes JR, et al: A prospective study on sudden unexpected death in epilepsy. Ann Neurol 26:195, 1989.
95. Nilsson L, Farahmand BY, Persson PG, et al: Risk factors for sudden unexpected death in epilepsy: a case-control study. Lancet 353:888, 1999.
96. Nei M, Ho RT, Abou-Khalil BW, et al: EEG and ECG in sudden unexplained death in epilepsy. Epilepsia 45:338, 2004.
97. Schuele SU, Bermeo AC, Alexopoulos AV, et al: Video-electrographic and clinical features in patients with ictal asystole. Neurology 69:434, 2007.
98. Moseley BD, Ghearing GR, Munger TM, et al: The treatment of ictal asystole with cardiac pacing. Epilepsia 52:e16, 2011.
99. Strzelczyk A, Cenusa M, Bauer S, et al: Management and long-term outcome in patients presenting with ictal asystole or bradycardia. Epilepsia 52:1160, 2011.
100. Winchell RJ, Hoyt DB: Analysis of heart-rate variability: a noninvasive predictor of death and poor outcome in patients with severe head injury. J Trauma 43:927, 1997.
101. Kahraman S, Dutton RP, Hu P, et al: Heart rate and pulse pressure variability are associated with intractable intracranial hypertension after severe traumatic brain injury. J Neurosurg Anesthesiol 22:296, 2010.
102. Clifton GL, Robertson CS, Grossman RG: Cardiovascular and metabolic responses to severe head injury. Neurosurg Rev 12(suppl 1):465, 1989.
103. Perkes I, Baguley IJ, Nott MT, et al: A review of paroxysmal sympathetic hyperactivity after acquired brain injury. Ann Neurol 68:126, 2010.
104. Baguley IJ, Slewa-Younan S, Heriseanu RE, et al: The incidence of dysautonomia and its relationship with autonomic arousal following traumatic brain injury. Brain Inj 21:1175, 2007.
105. Rabinstein AA: Paroxysmal sympathetic hyperactivity in the neurological intensive care unit. Neurol Res 29:680, 2007.
106. Baguley IJ, Cameron ID, Green AM, et al: Pharmacological management of dysautonomia following traumatic brain injury. Brain Inj 18:409, 2004.
107. Rabinstein AA, Benarroch EE: Treatment of paroxysmal sympathetic hyperactivity. Curr Treat Options Neurol 10:151, 2008.
108. Hinson HE, Sheth KN: Manifestations of the hyperadrenergic state after acute brain injury. Curr Opin Crit Care 18:139, 2012.
109. Chambers BR, Norris JW: Outcome in patients with asymptomatic neck bruits. N Engl J Med 315:860, 1986.
110. Kantor HL, Krishnan SC: Cardiac problems in patients with neurologic disease. Cardiol Clin 13:179, 1995.
111. Bulsara KR, McGirt MJ, Liao L, et al: Use of the peak troponin value to differentiate myocardial infarction from reversible neurogenic left ventricular dysfunction associated with aneurysmal subarachnoid hemorrhage. J Neurosurg 98:524, 2003.
112. Mayer S, Lin J, Homma S, et al: Myocardial injury and left ventricular performance after subarachnoid hemorrhage. Stroke 30:780, 1999.
113. Ansakorpi H, Korpelainen JT, Huikuri HV, et al: Heart rate dynamics in refractory and well controlled temporal lobe epilepsy. J Neurol Neurosurg Psychiatry 72:26, 2002.
114. Miss JC, Kopelnik A, Fisher LA, et al: Cardiac injury after subarachnoid hemorrhage is independent of the type of aneurysm therapy. Neurosurgery 55:1244, 2004.
115. Naidech A, Du Y, Kreiter KT, et al: Dobutamine versus milrinone after subarachnoid hemorrhage. Neurosurgery 56:21, 2005.
116. Apostolides PJ, Greene KA, Zabramski JM, et al: Intra-aortic balloon pump counterpulsation in the management of concomitant cerebral vasospasm

and cardiac failure after subarachnoid hemorrhage: technical case report. Neurosurgery 38:1056, 1996.

117. Rosen CL, Sekhar LN, Duong DH: Use of intra-aortic balloon pump counterpulsation for refractory symptomatic vasospasm. Acta Neurochir (Wien) 142: 25, 2000.

118. Lazaridis C, Pradilla G, Nyquist PA, et al: Intra-aortic balloon pump counterpulsation in the setting of subarachnoid hemorrhage, cerebral vasospasm, and neurogenic stress cardiomyopathy. Case report and review of the literature. Neurocrit Care 13:101, 2010.

CHAPTER

11

Stroke as a Complication of General Medical Disorders

PAUL GEORGE ■ GREGORY W. ALBERS

Stroke is the fourth leading cause of death in the United States, where approximately 795,000 first or recurrent strokes occur annually.[1] Stroke is increasingly recognized as a sequela of other medical diseases, and a number of medical conditions may predispose individuals to cerebrovascular disease. In this chapter, some newly recognized risk factors are highlighted and the relationship between a number of common medical diseases and the risk of stroke is examined. The effects of hypertension and of diabetes are discussed in Chapters 7 and 19, respectively.

PROTEIN C, PROTEIN S, AND ANTITHROMBIN III DEFICIENCY

Protein C, protein S, and antithrombin III deficiencies account for 14 to 25 percent of cases of familial thrombotic disease (including systemic thrombosis), although the majority tend to be venous rather than arterial.[2] Hematologic disorders may account for as many as 8 percent of all ischemic strokes.[3] However, the combined prevalence of these disorders is 1 percent or less in the general population.[4] Deficiencies occur in either the amount (quantitative deficiency) or the molecular function (qualitative deficiency) of these coagulant proteins.

Protein C is a vitamin K-dependent factor converted to an active protease by thrombin.[3] Once in active form, it limits coagulation by proteolysis of clotting factors Va and VIIIa. Protein S acts as a cofactor for activated protein C.[3] Antithrombin III acts as a protease inhibitor of clotting factors in the coagulation cascade, except for factors Va and VIIIa, which are regulated by proteins C and S.[2] Combined, these factors help to maintain the delicate balance between vascular hemostasis and fibrinolysis.

The risk of venous thrombosis and thromboembolism in patients with inherited deficiencies of protein C, protein S, and antithrombin III has been recognized widely, although there are fewer data on arterial thrombotic events. A study by Allaart and colleagues showed that by the age of 45 years, half of subjects with heterozygous protein C deficiency had experienced venous thrombosis,[5] and a study by Pabinger and Schneider showed that

Aminoff's Neurology and General Medicine, Fifth Edition.

80 to 90 percent of subjects with protein C, protein S, or antithrombin III deficiency had some type of thrombotic event (usually venous) by the age of 50 to 60 years.[6] There are many reports of ischemic arterial strokes occurring in the setting of protein C deficiency in the absence of other risk factors.[7–10] Inherited deficiencies seem to figure more prominently in the pathogenesis of stroke in young adults and children than in the elderly. In a study of 120 young patients with stroke or transient ischemic attack (TIA) and a mean age of 38 years, protein S, protein C, and antithrombin III deficiencies were detected in 20, 3, and 3 patients, respectively.[11] A confirmed coagulation disorder was more common among patients with large-vessel disease.[11] In a retrospective study of 37 children with cryptogenic ischemic stroke, protein C deficiency or protein S deficiency was the only identified risk factor for approximately 5 percent and 14 percent, respectively.[12] In another study of 36 patients younger than 40 years examined at least 3 months after cerebral infarction of undetermined cause, protein S deficiency was found in 5 cases, protein C deficiency in 1, and antithrombin III deficiency in 1.[13] Based on these findings, the authors recommended testing for these inherited deficiencies in every young patient with cryptogenic stroke.[13]

Protein S deficiency has also been reported in a number of cases of cerebral venous sinus thrombosis, but the association of protein C and antithrombin III deficiency with cerebral venous thromboses is less well-established.[14,15]

When testing for these deficiencies, it is important to recognize that activity levels may be influenced by nongenetic factors. Acute-phase reactants may interfere with both quantitative levels and qualitative function of these anticoagulant proteins.[11] Because low levels of protein C may occur in the setting of acute stroke, any studies with abnormal results should be repeated 3 months after the acute stroke period.[3] Protein S levels may be lowered in chronic or acute illness, such as liver disease, nephrotic syndrome, and disseminated intravascular coagulation (DIC), as well as in the immediate postoperative period.[3] Low levels of protein C and S have also been reported with pregnancy and with the use of vitamin K antagonists taken for oral anticoagulation.[3] The most common causes of secondary protein C and S deficiencies are inflammatory illnesses in which the complement system is activated, leading to increased serum binding of these proteins.[16]

The interactions between antithrombin III and heparin are important to recognize when testing for antithrombin III deficiency. Heparin increases the activity of antithrombin III by approximately 100-fold.[12] Because the anticoagulant effect of heparin is mediated by antithrombin III activity, heparin resistance is a clue to potential antithrombin III deficiency. Antithrombin III levels usually normalize within 48 to 72 hours after cessation of heparin treatment.[12]

Treatment decisions in patients with any of the inherited deficiencies should be made on an individual basis because there are inadequate prospective studies to guide therapy. Some authors recommend that any patient with protein C, protein S, or antithrombin III deficiency should be considered for lifelong anticoagulation following a thrombosis; others recommend treatment only during periods of heightened thrombotic risk (e.g., bed rest, pregnancy, and postoperative periods).[4] Antithrombin III deficiency has the highest risk of recurrence of thrombotic events, and any patient with an inherited deficiency should be advised of the risks of thrombosis with oral contraceptive use, prolonged bed rest, and pregnancy.[17] Warfarin-induced skin necrosis may occur in individuals with protein C deficiency.[3]

ACTIVATED PROTEIN C RESISTANCE AND FACTOR V LEIDEN DEFICIENCY

Activated protein C resistance has been described in a number of patients with venous thromboembolic events, and some authors recognize it as the single most common cause of hereditary thrombophilia.[2,3,18] At a site of blood vessel or endothelial injury, thrombin activates platelets, leading to aggregation. Fibrinogen is converted to fibrin, which binds the aggregated platelets to form a platelet plug. In addition to its procoagulant effects, thrombin plays an anticoagulant role in a feedback mechanism by binding to thrombomodulin. Once bound to thrombomodulin, thrombin loses its procoagulant activity and then activates protein C, which—in turn—acts with protein S to inactivate factors Va and VIIIa, thereby preventing further clotting (Fig. 11-1). Activated protein C also inhibits tissue plasminogen activator inhibitor to stimulate fibrinolysis.[2]

Although there are many genetic and environmental factors that contribute to activated protein

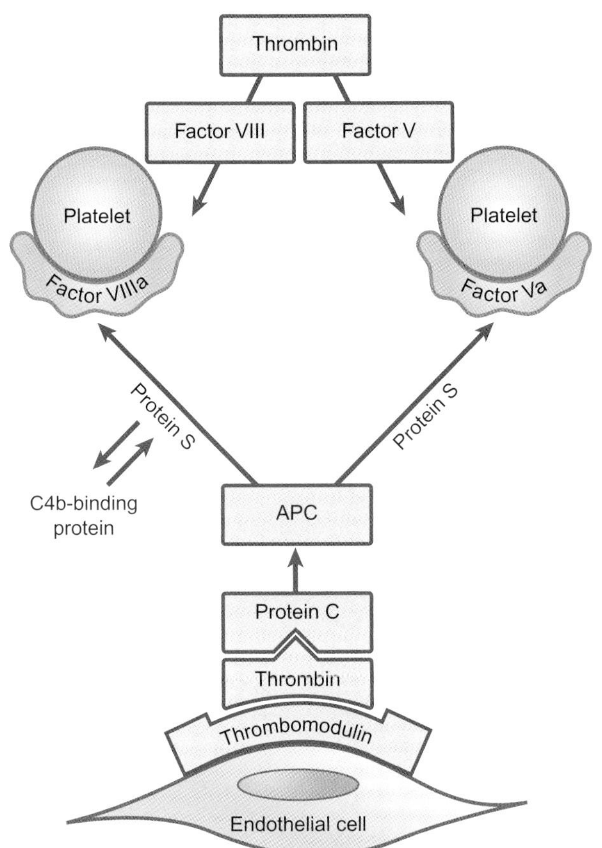

FIGURE 11-1 ■ The protein C anticoagulant pathway. Thrombin converts factor VIII and factor V to their activated forms, factor VIIIa and factor Va. A complex of thrombin with the endothelial cell receptor thrombomodulin activates protein C (APC). APC inactivates factor VIIIa and factor Va on the platelet surface, and this reaction is accelerated by APC cofactor and free protein S. (From Bauer KA: Hypercoagulability: a new cofactor in the protein C anticoagulant pathway. N Engl J Med 330:567, 1994, with permission. © 1994, Massachusetts Medical Society. All rights reserved.)

C resistance, a genetic defect in factor V is the most commonly described, accounting for 85 to 95 percent of cases in some series.[2,19] Dysfunctional factor V, referred to as factor V Leiden, is caused by a G-to-A mutation in the factor V gene.[19] This amino acid substitution renders factor V resistant to protein C–induced enzymatic cleavage, thereby negating the anticoagulant properties of activated protein C.[2] In vitro studies show that factor V Leiden is inactivated by activated protein C 10 times more slowly than normal factor V.[2]

The prevalence of the factor V Leiden mutation was found to be 4.4 percent among European subjects, although only 4 percent of these were homozygous for the mutation.[20] A study of the 15,000 men in the Physician's Health Study showed a carrier rate of approximately 6 percent.[21] There appears to be an uneven geographic distribution of the factor V Leiden mutation, which occurs more rarely in Japanese, Asian, and Middle Eastern populations than in Europeans.[2] However, it is estimated that only 6 percent of those with the genetic defect will actually develop venous thrombosis over a 30-year period.[2]

Activated protein C resistance is more of a risk for venous than arterial thrombotic events, including stroke.[9,22,23] The presence of the factor V Leiden mutation has been associated with a nearly fivefold increased risk of ischemic stroke in children.[24] Women who smoke and have the factor V mutation had an almost ninefold increased risk of stroke.[25] In a population-based study of 826 men, the risk of carotid stenosis increased linearly with a decreased response to activated protein C.[18] This association applied to those with and without the factor V Leiden mutation, suggesting that there are also hormonal and environmental factors that contribute to activated protein C resistance.

A study of the role of activated protein C resistance in 40 patients with cerebral venous thrombosis showed that 15 percent had an underlying thrombophilia of protein C deficiency, protein S deficiency, or activated protein C resistance.[17] In most of these cases, other risk factors for venous thrombosis were also present, suggesting that thrombophilia may make individuals more susceptible to thrombogenic environmental or physiologic factors. A study of 321 women with the factor V Leiden mutation showed a 50-fold increased risk of venous thrombosis in heterozygotes taking oral contraceptives and a greater than 100-fold increased risk in homozygotes using oral contraceptives.[26] Other small series have shown that between 20 and 25 percent of patients with cerebral venous thrombosis carry the factor V Leiden mutation.[27,28]

There is a limited amount of data concerning the exact risk of cerebral venous thrombosis and venous infarction with the factor V Leiden mutation, and this risk cannot confidently be extrapolated from the data on peripheral venous disease.[29–31]

Testing for activated protein C resistance and the factor V Leiden mutation following stroke should be performed in young patients without other risk factors, those with a personal or family history of thrombotic or venous occlusive disease, and patients with venous infarctions. Laboratory testing for activated protein C resistance measures the activated partial thromboplastin time in the presence and absence of activated protein C. Because anticoagulants may increase the activated partial thromboplastin time, tests should be performed only after the cessation of heparin and oral anticoagulants.[2] If activated protein C resistance is discovered, it is appropriate then to test for the factor V Leiden mutation. Initial testing for the mutation is preferable in some instances because the results are not affected by anticoagulant use or treatment.[4]

It is common to treat stroke patients with activated protein C resistance with anticoagulation. However, the decision to treat with oral anticoagulation, rather than antiplatelet therapy, is not based on prospective trials. No studies have established an adequate treatment regimen or optimal length of therapy. Some investigators advocate lifelong treatment and others opt for a short course of anticoagulants (3 to 6 months) followed by conversion to antiplatelet medications.[6]

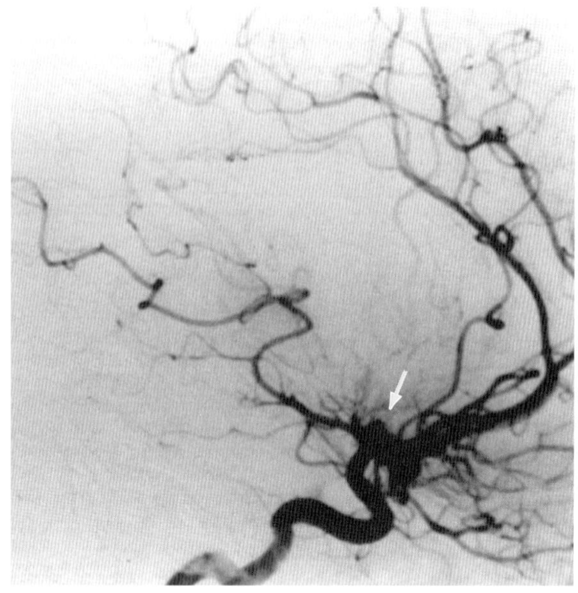

FIGURE 11-2 ■ Angiography showing a middle cerebral artery occlusion (*arrow*) in a young woman with anticardiolipin antibodies, the lupus anticoagulant, and myxomatous mitral valve thickening. (From Coull BM, Levine SR, Brey RL: The role of antiphospholipid antibodies in stroke. Neurol Clin 10:130, 1992, with permission.)

ANTIPHOSPHOLIPID ANTIBODIES: LUPUS ANTICOAGULANT AND ANTICARDIOLIPIN ANTIBODIES

The lupus anticoagulant and anticardiolipin antibodies fall under the category of antiphospholipid antibodies, and both are recognized as markers for an increased risk of thrombosis, spontaneous abortion, cerebral ischemia, and vascular dementia.[32] The presence of anticardiolipin antibodies in association with thrombotic events has been recognized increasingly in patients without evidence of connective tissue disease and is referred to as primary antiphospholipid antibody syndrome (APS).[32]

Thrombotic episodes affecting virtually every organ in the body have been reported in persons with antiphospholipid antibodies, and this association has been particularly well demonstrated for stroke and TIA (Fig. 11-2).[33] In one study, it was found that antiphospholipid antibodies were present in 46 percent of young patients with stroke,[34] and antiphospholipid antibodies may be a contributing factor in approximately 10 percent of all cerebrovascular events.[33] The presence of either the lupus anticoagulant or anticardiolipin antibodies in patients with systemic lupus erythematosus (SLE) doubles the risk of thrombotic events.[35] Increased stroke risk correlates with high anticardiolipin immunoglobulin G (IgG) titers; IgM titers appear to be less predictive.[36]

Studies have failed to show a clear association between antiphospholipid antibodies and recurrent vascular events of many types. In one large study of stroke patients regardless of age or sex, an increased risk of subsequent vascular occlusive events was not found, although the follow-up period was relatively short (2 years).[37] Other studies have demonstrated an association between stroke and antiphospholipid antibodies mainly in young women, suggesting that these individuals may be at increased risk of stroke and its recurrence.[38]

The pathophysiologic process of antiphospholipid antibody–associated thrombosis remains speculative (Fig. 11-3).[39] The lupus anticoagulant inhibits prostacyclin, which acts as a vasodilator and inhibitor of platelet aggregation, and this may be responsible.[32] Other possible mechanisms include an interference with the activation of protein C.[32,33] Because platelet membranes as well as endothelial cells are rich in phospholipids, antiphospholipid antibodies may bind to or damage these membranes, increasing the risk of thrombogenesis.[33,39] Antiphospholipid antibodies have also been associated with an increased incidence of Libman–Sacks

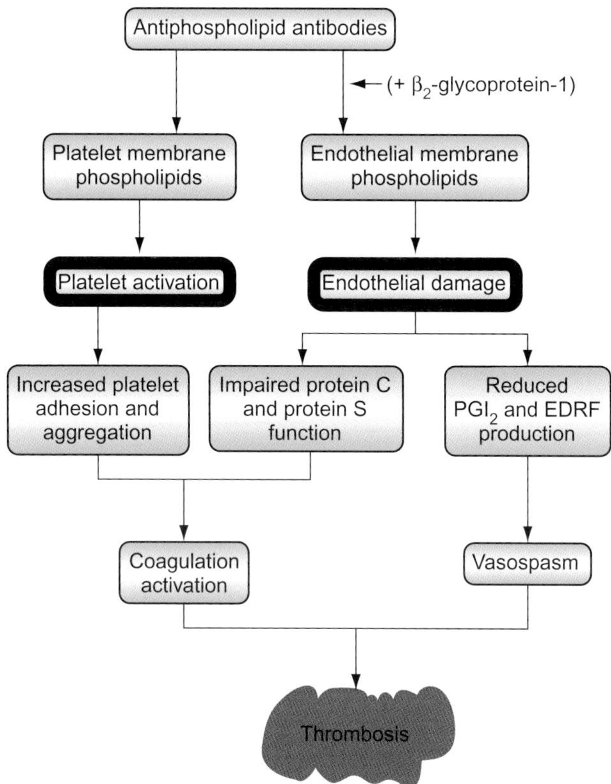

FIGURE 11-3 ▪ Proposed mechanism of antiphospholipid antibody-induced thrombosis. Antiphospholipid antibodies in a complex with β_2-glycoprotein-1 bind to platelet or endothelial membrane phospholipids, thereby causing platelet activation and endothelial damage. The ensuing platelet adhesion, aggregation, and impairment of endothelial anticoagulant function promote coagulation activation, vasospasm, and thrombosis. EDRF, endothelium-derived relaxing factor; PGI_2, prostacylin. (From Coull BM, Clark WM: Abnormalities of hemostasis in ischemic stroke. Med Clin North Am 77:86, 1993; modified from Eisenberg GM: Antiphospholipid syndrome: the reality and implications. Hosp Pract 27:121, 1992, with permission.)

endocarditis and other left-sided cardiac valvular abnormalities that are associated with an increased stroke risk.[40,41]

The presence of antiphospholipid antibodies has been found in up to 58 percent of patients with SLE.[35] Antiphospholipid antibodies have also been found in patients with a host of other connective tissue diseases, including Sjögren syndrome, Behçet syndrome, mixed connective tissue disease, rheumatoid arthritis, and autoimmune thrombocytopenic purpura.[33] Systemic infections, especially syphilis, Lyme disease, and viral infections, may also cause an elevation of antiphospholipid antibodies, but their presence in these conditions usually has little or no association with thrombotic events.[33]

The diagnosis of APS involves both clinical and laboratory criteria. Individuals younger than 55 years with one or more thrombotic events without known vascular risk factors should be screened for the presence of these antibodies.[42] Associated clinical signs include the presence of left-sided cardiac valvular lesions, spontaneous abortions, livedo reticularis, migraine headaches, and a prolonged activated partial thromboplastin time or a positive Venereal Disease Research Laboratory (VDRL) test result.[42] Because the lupus anticoagulant and anticardiolipin antibodies are probably different immunoglobulins, patients should be tested for both; they may occur independently, and it is unclear which antibody is more predictive of thrombosis. In patients with the lupus anticoagulant, the activated partial thromboplastin time is prolonged in 80 percent of cases, and mixing studies show that this prolongation is not correctable by the addition of normal sera and is thus not a consequence of a factor deficiency. One large study failed to find any difference in recurrent events with aspirin or warfarin treatment in patients with antiphospholipid antibodies and initial ischemic stroke.[37] Therefore, at present, antiplatelet agents are generally recommended in this setting, and efforts should be made to identify and treat other stroke risk factors. In patients with antiphospholipid antibodies and recurrent strokes or in those with APS and stroke, anticoagulants are often recommended.[43] Previously it was thought that higher levels of anticoagulation were necessary in these patients, but the recent literature indicates that a goal INR of 2.0 to 3.0 is effective.[44] Corticosteroids are of no benefit in these patients.

Sneddon Syndrome

Sneddon syndrome is an arteriopathy characterized by multiple strokes and livedo reticularis.[33] Affected patients may also have Raynaud phenomenon or acrocyanosis of the digits.[33] Antiphospholipid antibodies are usually prominent, and progressive cognitive decline from the arteriopathy may occur even in young persons.[33] Accordingly, any young patient presenting with progressive vascular dementia and livedo reticularis should be evaluated for the presence of antiphospholipid antibodies.

HOMOCYSTEINE

Homocysteine is an intermediate in the metabolism of the amino acid methionine. An elevated level of plasma total homocysteine increases the risk of all-cause vascular disease and is an independent risk factor for stroke.[46] Hyperhomocysteinemia can be caused by an error in metabolism of sulfur-containing amino acids, nutritional deficiencies of folate, vitamin B_{12}, or vitamin B_6, or a genetic defect in the methylenetetrahydrofolate reductase (*MTHFR*) gene. It is unclear whether elevated blood levels of homocysteine have a causative role in the pathogenesis of vascular disease or are merely a secondary effect of an underlying causal process.

A number of vascular and hematologic abnormalities are associated with elevated serum homocysteine levels. Mild hyperhomocysteinemia increases carotid artery wall thickness and plaque formation, and smooth muscle cells cultured in the presence of homocysteine show increases in both cell density and collagen production, perhaps leading to prothrombotic effects.[48,49] Other reported pathophysiologic changes include endothelial cell injury, increased platelet aggregation, and abnormalities of the clotting cascade by activation of factors V, X, and XII.[50,51]

Several studies have documented the association between hyperhomocysteinemia and cerebrovascular disease. Yoo and colleagues performed a case-control study of 78 men with ischemic stroke and 140 control subjects and found an odds ratio of 1.7 (adjusted for total cholesterol, hypertension, smoking, age, and diabetes) for stroke in patients with the highest 5 percent of homocysteine levels.[52] In a substudy of the Framingham Study, 1,947 elderly participants were followed prospectively and nonfasting homocysteine levels were measured.[53] After the investigators adjusted for other risk factors, the relative risk of stroke associated with nonfasting homocysteine levels of 14.24 to 219.84 μmol/L compared with levels of 4.13 to 9.25 μmol/L was 1.82.[53] The Rotterdam Study examined the relationship between elevated homocysteine levels in the elderly and the risk of stroke and myocardial infarction and found an increased risk of 6 to 7 percent for every 1 μmol/L increase in total plasma homocysteine.[54] In a case-control study of 80 young patients with stroke between the ages of 18 and 44 years, a 4.8-fold increased risk of ischemic stroke was found in those with postmethionine load elevations in plasma homocysteine levels.[55] A number of other studies have also shown this association in younger patients.[56,57]

Although supplementation with folate, pyridoxine (vitamin B_6), or cobalamin (vitamin B_{12}) can reduce homocysteine levels, it is unclear whether these supplements lower the risk of subsequent vascular events. A recent Cochrane review evaluated 12 randomized trials of homocyteine-lowering interventions and found no significant effect on stroke or death from any cause.[58] Therefore, at present, we do not perform routine screening of serum homocysteine levels in stroke patients and do not recommend lowering elevated homocysteine levels with folic acid and B vitamins.

LIPOPROTEIN (a)

Lipoprotein (a) is a low-density lipoprotein (LDL)–like molecule that has been linked to both coronary artery and cerebrovascular disease.[59–61] Levels are partially genetically determined and do not appear to be correlated with age, sex, blood pressure, smoking habits, or levels of total cholesterol or triglycerides.[60] A number of medical conditions have been associated with elevated lipoprotein (a) levels, particularly diabetes with poor glycemic control and renal impairment.[62] Reduced levels of lipoprotein (a) have been reported also in women taking hormone replacement therapy, although oral contraceptives seem to have little effect on levels.[62]

The lipoprotein (a) molecule is composed of two components: apolipoprotein B and apolipoprotein A, or apoA.[63] The apoA portion shares significant structural homology with plasminogen, and it has been postulated that lipoprotein (a) may compete for plasminogen-binding sites on fibrin and endothelial cells, thereby inhibiting endogenous fibrinolysis.[64] Lipoprotein (a) accumulation has been demonstrated histopathologically in coronary atherosclerotic lesions in humans, and modification of lipoprotein (a) by sulfated polysaccharides leads to cholesterol deposition in mouse macrophages, similar to the atherogenic process caused by high levels of LDL cholesterol.[45,65] Because of its fibrin-binding activity, lipoprotein (a) may help deliver cholesterol to developing thrombi or areas of endothelial injury.[63,66] However, despite these observations, it still remains unclear whether elevated lipoprotein (a) levels actually contribute to atherosclerotic plaque formation or merely reflect the presence of atherosclerotic disease.

Numerous studies have linked high serum lipoprotein (a) levels to cerebrovascular disease and stroke. Even after controlling for other risk factors, lipoprotein (a) levels higher than 30 mg/dl are an independent risk factor for ischemic stroke, even in normocholesterolemic and normolipidemic patients.[67–70]

Some studies show a reduction in lipoprotein (a) levels when diets are enriched with palm oil and polyunsaturated fatty acids.[63] Alcohol consumption has also been associated with lower serum lipoprotein (a) levels,[63] as has the use of low-dose (81 mg) aspirin.[71] A study by Guyton and colleagues showed a 36 percent reduction in elevated lipoprotein (a) levels in individuals taking a mean nightly dose of 2,000 mg extended-release niacin.[72] None of these therapies has been associated convincingly with reducing subsequent vascular events. Despite the similarity of lipoprotein (a) to other cholesterol constituents of the blood, 3-hydroxy-3-methylglutaryl coenzyme A (HMG-CoA) reductase inhibitors, bile acid sequestrants, and fibric acid derivatives seem to have little effect on lipoprotein (a) concentrations.[66] Other risk factors such as dyslipidemia, diabetes, and obesity may enhance the atherothrombotic risk attributable to lipoprotein (a). Therefore, treatable risk factors should be tightly controlled in patients with elevated lipoprotein (a).[73,74]

Screening for elevated lipoprotein (a) levels can be considered for patients younger than 55 years who experience a stroke, those with a personal or family history of premature cardiovascular disease, and patients with stroke who lack other conventional risk factors.

SICKLE CELL ANEMIA

Hematological disorders are estimated to be the causative factor for up to 8 percent of all ischemic strokes and are particularly important in the etiology of stroke in young patients.[6,12] Sickle cell anemia, in addition to causing a host of peripheral complications such as sickle cell crises, has been linked to cerebrovascular events. Strokes occur in 8 to 17 percent of patients with sickle cell anemia, although cerebral ischemic events usually do not occur in the context of a sickle cell crisis.[11]

Approximately 15 percent of homozygotes (designated HbSS) experience a cerebral ischemic event during their lifetime.[75] There are conflicting data as to whether individuals with sickle cell trait (heterozygotes, HbSA) and those with sickle C disease are at increased risk of stroke. The estimated prevalence of stroke is 1.5 to 2.0 percent in blacks with HbSA, which is essentially the same as the incidence in the overall black population.[75] However, the risk of stroke in those with sickle C disease (HbSC) has been reported as high as 2 to 5 percent, which suggests a higher risk of stroke in these patients.[45] In HbSS patients, the average age of stroke onset is relatively young, with a mean age of 7 to 9 years.[75] Approximately 8 percent of all children with sickle cell anemia experience a cerebrovascular event by the age of 15.[12] The actual risk of stroke may be significantly higher, however, because up to 24 percent of patients with HbSS have silent infarcts on neuroimaging, with no apparent clinical manifestations.[76]

Most strokes in patients with sickle cell disease are ischemic, although older individuals are also at increased risk of hemorrhagic cerebral events.[12] Thrombosis of large arteries is common although venous sinus thrombosis also occurs. Some evidence indicates that individuals with particularly severe sickle cell disease, characterized by a high number of crises and complications, are more prone to cerebrovascular events, possibly because of higher blood viscosity and greater endothelial damage.

The pathophysiologic process of stroke in patients with sickle cell anemia (discussed in Chapter 25) is still under investigation. It was initially believed that the lowered solubility of deoxygenated hemoglobin S resulted in aggregation and sickling in small vessels, but increasing evidence suggests large-vessel stenosis as the primary etiology of cerebrovascular events. In one study, cerebral angiograms performed in seven patients with sickle cell anemia and stroke revealed partial or complete occlusion of the internal carotid artery in six, with concurrent vertebral and large intracranial artery stenosis in others. Similarly, angiographic evidence of large-vessel arterial disease was found in 10 of 12 patients and 23 of 30 patients in two other studies.[45]

The vascular damage, when examined histologically, consists of segmental thickening due to intimal proliferation of fibroblasts and smooth muscle cells.[77,78] Once these vascular changes occur, vessel occlusion likely results from in situ thrombus formation or embolization.[77] Given that HbSS erythrocytes are abnormally adherent to the vascular endothelium, this cascade of events could lead to vessel thrombosis, occlusion, and subsequent stroke.[79]

Arterial narrowing and occlusion may also lead to a pattern like that of moyamoya syndrome on conventional angiography.[12] Contrast agents used during angiography may enhance intravascular sickling, so angiography should be performed with caution, but is probably safe if the hemoglobin S level is less than 20 percent.[12,75]

Conventional imaging studies such as computed tomography (CT) and MRI typically show infarcts in a watershed or border zone distribution, consistent with the large-vessel involvement of the disease.[11,79] Transcranial Doppler (TCD) ultrasonography is a useful diagnostic imaging tool because increased middle cerebral artery flow velocities indicate the presence of underlying arteriopathy and increased stroke risk in patients with sickle cell disease.[77] The risk of stroke during childhood in those with sickle cell disease is 1 percent per year, but patients with TCD evidence of high cerebral blood-flow velocities (>200 cm per second) have a stroke rate in excess of 10 percent per year.[80] A study using transcranial Doppler imaging in 190 children with sickle cell disease showed that in those with Doppler imaging evidence of vessel stenosis, 26 percent went on to sustain cerebrovascular events, compared with 0.6 percent of patients without evidence of stenosis.[81]

Once a diagnosis of stroke has been made, immediate therapy to prevent further episodes of brain ischemia should be instituted because the recurrence rate may be as high as 67 percent,[12] usually within the first 12 to 24 months after the initial event. The mainstay of preventive therapy is lowering of the percentage of hemoglobin S in the blood, most effectively carried out by exchange transfusion therapy, which effectively lowers the percentage of red blood cells that can sickle.[78] Most authors recommend maintaining the hemoglobin S level at less than 30 percent by performing exchanges every 3 to 4 weeks.[77] In 1995, the National Heart, Lung, and Blood Institute conducted a multicenter, randomized, controlled study that was stopped prematurely when a 90 percent stroke reduction was noted in patients treated with exchange transfusions.[81] The Stroke Prevention in Sickle Cell Anemia (STOP) study showed that the risk of stroke could be reduced from 10 percent per year to less than 1 percent per year with routine exchange transfusion therapy guided by TCD velocities.[82] The optimal duration of therapy is unclear. A prospective, randomized trial that investigated the effect of stopping exchange transfusions once TCD velocities had normalized was ended prematurely because 14 of the 41 patients who had stopped monthly exchange transfusions re-developed high-risk velocities and 2 had strokes (compared with no strokes in the arm with continued exchange transfusions).[83] Based on these data, it appears that exchange transfusions may be required indefinitely, although such an extensive treatment regimen should be weighed against the risks of iron overload, transfusion reactions, and donor-borne transmission of infectious diseases. Guidelines on primary prevention of ischemic stroke from the American Heart Association and American Stroke Association recommend that children with sickle cell disease be screened with TCD beginning at 2 years of age.[84]

SYSTEMIC LUPUS ERYTHEMATOSUS

SLE predisposes affected individuals to a host of neurologic disorders, including strokes, seizures, chorea, dementia, psychosis, neuropathy, and myelopathy, as discussed in Chapter 50.[85] In one study, 63 of 91 patients with SLE had central or peripheral neurologic dysfunction, with cerebrovascular events being the third most common manifestation, following seizures and delirium.[85]

Stroke occurs in 3 to 20 percent of patients with SLE. These ischemic events typically involve younger patients, with a mean age at the time of stroke of 42 years.[45,85] Elderly patients with SLE also are at high risk, perhaps due to the presence of other vascular risk factors which may act synergistically with SLE.

Although most infarcts in SLE are ischemic, intracerebral hemorrhage has been reported, usually in the setting of concurrent thrombocytopenia.[85] Subarachnoid hemorrhage in SLE is also well documented, although many published studies are from Japan, where there is an overall increased risk of hemorrhagic stroke presumably due to genetic factors.[86] The most frequent mechanism for ischemic cerebrovascular events appears to be either cardiogenic embolus or an antibody-mediated hypercoagulable state.[85] In one autopsy study, cardiac valvular disease was discovered in nearly half of the patients, with Libman–Sacks endocarditis being the most frequent valvular lesion.[45] These valvular lesions are often associated with the presence of antiphospholipid antibodies.[41] Therefore, echocardiography and laboratory testing for antiphospholipid antibodies should be performed in any patient with SLE and an unexplained stroke or TIA.

The incidence of an inflammatory cerebral vasculitis in SLE has been extremely low or zero in autopsy studies, making this an unlikely cause of stroke in patients with lupus. Fibrin-platelet occlusion of intracranial arterioles may occur, and a noninflammatory vasculopathy secondary to vessel-wall hyalinization and endothelial proliferation has been the most common cerebrovascular abnormality in other autopsy studies.[41] These lesions appear to correlate with the scattered punctate periventricular and white matter hyperintensities seen on MRI in patients with SLE.[41] The cause of the vasculopathy in SLE is unclear, although postulated mechanisms include endothelial damage by antineuronal antibodies or immune complex deposition.[41] Other pathologic findings include isolated large-vessel stenosis, arterial dissection, and fibromuscular dysplasia.[87]

Although prospective studies of stroke treatment or prevention strategies in SLE are lacking, the occurrence of multiple infarcts in some patients (up to 64% of patients with SLE and stroke in one study[85]), as well as a high recurrence rate approaching 50 percent, underscores the need for thorough evaluation and secondary prevention. In one study, patients with SLE and stroke were compared with patients with SLE without cerebrovascular events.[85] Concurrent cardiac valvular disease, coagulopathy, previous TIA or stroke, and age older than 60 years were all more common in the group with stroke.

The use of anticoagulants may reduce the risk of stroke recurrence in patients with SLE. Oral anticoagulation may be warranted in patients with SLE who have concurrent risk factors of cardiac valvular lesions or APS, although standard secondary prevention still involves antiplatelet medications. Given the absence of inflammatory vascular lesions in patients with SLE who have strokes, corticosteroids probably have no role,[41,85] although most authors recommend their use in the setting of systemic vasculitis and high anticardiolipin antibody titers.[87]

CRYOGLOBULINS

Cryoglobulins are serum proteins with temperature-dependent insolubility, precipitating below 37°C. These proteins may occur in association with a number of autoimmune disorders, including SLE. Among connective tissue disorders, SLE, rheumatoid arthritis, and Sjögren syndrome are the diseases most frequently associated with the presence of cryoglobulins (8 to 48%).[45] Most of the clinical manifestations of cryoglobulinemia are attributed to the precipitation of cryoglobulins in small vessels leading to arterial and venous occlusion.[88] Both peripheral (most commonly neuropathy) and CNS involvement occur in cryoglobulinemia.[88] Imaging studies of the brain in select patients with cryoglobulinemia show multiple small hyperintensities compatible with ischemic lesions.[89] The association of stroke with cryoglobulinemia may relate to hyperviscosity, cold agglutinization of erythrocytes, or defective clotting and platelet functions. Stroke may result when blood vessels in the nervous system are injured by mixed cryoglobulin deposition that causes an immune complex–mediated vasculitis. In support of this possibility, Serena and co-workers found evidence of vasculitis in the vasa nervorum of small vessels in the brain of a patient with vascular dementia secondary to cryoglobulinemia.[88]

Plasmapheresis has been effective in some patients with neurologic complications, presumably through lowering of cryoglobulinemia and therefore improvement of the microcirculation. Beneficial results may be obtained in some cases by minimizing cold exposure. Immunosuppressive agents have had limited success, as have cytotoxic agents, and controlled clinical trials are needed before any definitive treatment recommendations can be made.

STROKE AND MALIGNANCY

CNS lesions are present on postmortem examination in approximately 30 percent of patients with cancer. Although the most common manifestation is metastatic disease to the brain, hemorrhagic and ischemic infarcts make up a substantial percentage of these lesions. Approximately 50 percent of those with evidence of cerebrovascular disease are symptomatic, although a diffuse encephalopathy, rather than focal neurologic deficits, is the most common presenting symptom.[90]

The results of one study suggest that, at least in elderly patients with cancer, conventional stroke risk factors account for most ischemic events.[91] Other studies clearly implicate malignancy-specific causes of stroke. There is a high incidence of embolic strokes in cancer patients, due either to malignancy-related hypercoagulable states or to cardioembolism.[92] Four etiologic categories of cerebrovascular events have been described in patients with cancer: direct tumor effects, coagulation disorders, infections, and complications of therapeutic or diagnostic procedures. The cause of cerebrovascular events in patients with cancer often correlates with the type of primary tumor, the extent of metastases or disseminated malignancy, and the type of cancer therapy administered.

Direct Tumor Effects

Direct tumor effects include intratumoral hemorrhage, arterial and venous invasion by tumor mass or leptomeningeal infiltrates, and tumor emboli. Tumor emboli occur rarely and exclusively in patients with solid tumors; they are virtually impossible to distinguish from thrombogenic emboli on clinical grounds alone. These metastatic emboli typically result from heart or lung tumors: atrial myxomas may shower tumor fragments into the vasculature, and lung tumor embolism may occur at the time of thoracotomy. Tumors that demonstrate aggressive intravascular invasion such as choriocarcinoma may also cause embolic cerebrovascular events. Neoplastic aneurysms, with subsequent rupture causing hemorrhage, have been described; tumor emboli may invade an arterial wall after acute occlusion of the vessel, eventually resulting in dilatation and aneurysm formation. Cerebral venous sinus thrombosis may occur by direct tumor invasion from neuroblastoma, lung carcinoma, and lymphoma.

Coagulopathy

Disorders of coagulation affect up to 15 percent of patients with cancer.[93] A hypercoagulable state associated with malignancy was first described by Armand Trousseau in 1865, who reported a case of migratory thrombophlebitis in the setting of gastric carcinoma.[93,94] Trousseau syndrome has been linked to a broad spectrum of malignancies but is most commonly described with adenocarcinomas, particularly of the pancreas, lung, colon, and breast, and with prostate and gastric cancer as well as leukemia.[94]

A common pathologic mechanism for hypercoagulability in patients with cancer may involve exposure of tumor cell tissue factor thromboplastin to the systemic circulation.[94] This sequence of events may result in a chronic low-grade prothrombotic state that clinically resembles DIC.[94] A DIC-like clinical picture has been reported commonly in acute promyelocytic leukemia, presumably from the release of nuclear or granular fractions of tumor cells that have procoagulant activity. A number of tumor procoagulants have been identified, with tissue factor and cancer procoagulant being the best recognized.[93] Tumor cells can also activate platelets in vivo through adenosine diphosphate–dependent mechanisms.[93]

Although abnormalities of blood coagulation are reported in 60 to 92 percent of patients with cancer, these coagulopathies rarely produce clinical symptoms. When present, a coagulation disorder may manifest by either superficial or deep venous thrombosis, or arterial thrombosis.[93] Intravascular coagulation, as evidenced by small thrombotic cerebral infarcts without an identifiable embolic source, is a common cause of symptomatic cerebral infarction in patients with cancer. Whether such findings are indicative of a type of low-grade DIC or represent a separate malignancy-related coagulation disorder is unclear.

Regardless of the pathophysiology, patients tend to have a poor prognosis. These coagulation abnormalities are usually present in the setting of advanced and disseminated disease. Laboratory testing is usually not helpful because routine coagulation studies are often only mildly abnormal.[90] Laboratory analysis is further confounded by the fact that a host of other malignancy-related conditions, such as concurrent chemotherapy or liver disease, may affect normal clotting activity, and approximately 90 percent of patients with metastatic disease have abnormal coagulation parameters, with thrombocytosis and increased fibrinogen levels being the most common.[93]

Nonbacterial Thrombotic Endocarditis

A case of "thromboendocarditis" was first described by Ziegler in 1888, when fibrin deposits were found at autopsy on cardiac valves in a patient with cancer. Since then, the terms *marantic* and *cachectic endocarditis* have been used to describe the same clinical entity. Although nonbacterial thrombotic endocarditis (NBTE) may represent a continuum with intravascular coagulation and malignancy-induced DIC,

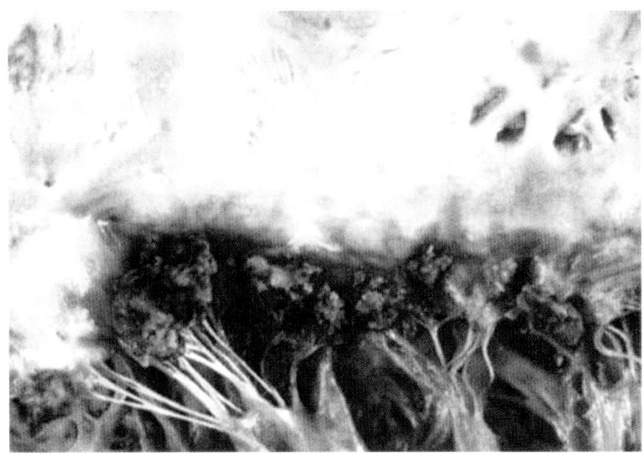

FIGURE 11-4 ■ A typical mitral valve lesion in a patient with lupus and nonbacterial thrombotic endocarditis (NBTE). (From Moder KG, Miller TD, Tazelaar HD, et al: Cardiac involvement in systemic lupus erythematosus. Mayo Clinic Proc 74:275, 1999, with permission.)

this clinical entity warrants separate consideration because it plays a prominent role in the pathogenesis of cerebrovascular disease and stroke. Although the prevalence of NBTE is relatively low in patients with cancer (approximately 1%), it is a leading cause of stroke in these patients.

Pathologically, NBTE consists of platelet-fibrin vegetations that develop on the cardiac valves, with the aortic and mitral valves (Fig. 11-4) being the most common sites of involvement.[90,93,95] These friable vegetations frequently embolize, causing infarction in brain, lung, kidney, and cardiac tissue. Symptoms of brain ischemia may occur concurrently with pulmonary embolism, myocardial infarction, or peripheral emboli, and the presence of these clinical events in multiple locations increases the probability of a cardiac embolic source.

NBTE is most frequently described with lung and gastrointestinal tumors, although it has been reported with a host of neoplasms. A review of the literature shows adenocarcinoma, particularly of the lung, pancreas, and stomach, to account for 60 to 80 percent of NBTE cases. In one series, lymphoreticular malignancies were reported in 25 percent of patients with NBTE.[95] Other, noncancerous conditions such as rheumatic heart disease, pregnancy, cirrhosis, SLE, anticardiolipin antibodies, vasculitis, severe burns, and amitriptyline overdose have all been associated with NBTE.[45] In some cases, stroke caused by NBTE is the first indication of malignancy. The possibility of an underlying malignancy should be considered in any patient lacking conventional stroke risk factors or a clear embolic source who presents with evidence of embolic cerebral infarction.

The pathogenesis of NBTE may relate to an underlying cardiac valvular abnormality that acts as a predisposing factor for the deposition of platelets and fibrin, which is facilitated by cancer-related hypercoagulability. Once valvular damage occurs, underlying exposed collagen may act as a nidus for platelet adhesion and subsequent thrombus formation. Most vegetations are multiverrucous and less than 3 mm, which accounts for the relatively low diagnostic yield of conventional echocardiography. Microscopically, the valvular lesions consist of agglutinated blood and platelet thrombi in the absence of an inflammatory reaction. Embolic fragments are primarily composed of fibrin. Systemic emboli may be found in 50 percent of patients with NBTE, with cerebral, coronary, and renal involvement being most frequent.[45]

There is a higher diagnostic yield with transesophageal echocardiography.[96] Diffusion-weighted MRI sequences of the brain may show multiple strokes of differing sizes in multiple vascular territories.[97] A new or changing cardiac murmur is rare; because of their small size, the vegetations rarely interfere with valvular function.[90] Angiography may be helpful because the presence of multiple embolic occlusions, in the absence of a clear cardiac or vascular abnormality, is suggestive of NBTE. The presence of emboli to the skin, extremities, or other end organs may also provide clues to the diagnosis.

Once a diagnosis of NBTE is made, treatment of the primary malignancy should be addressed. If there is no recognized malignancy, a thorough search should be undertaken for occult cancer as well as autoimmune and rheumatologic disease.[98] In addition to cancer therapy, attempts to control the pathologically altered coagulation mechanism that results in the valvular vegetations should be considered. Although there have been no prospective studies, a number of case series—summarized elsewhere—suggest that clinical benefit follows anticoagulation with intravenous heparin.[45] In one series of 12 patients treated with heparin, 1 patient experienced symptomatic improvement, 3 patients clinically worsened, and 4 patients worsened after discontinuation of heparin therapy. In another, a 94 percent "response rate" was noted with intravenous heparin administration, as characterized by resolution of thrombophlebitis or cessation of arterial embolic events.[45] Recent guidelines have recommended use of low molecular weight or unfractionated heparin for treatment of NBTE and evidence of emboli.[99]

Strokes Related to Cancer Therapy

The chemotherapeutic agent L-asparaginase is most frequently associated with cerebral infarction, usually from cerebral venous sinus thrombosis. Most patients make a good clinical recovery. Although the cause for sinus thrombosis is unclear, some studies have shown that L-asparaginase may cause a decreased partial thromboplastin time (PTT) and increased platelet aggregation, as well as antithrombin III and plasminogen deficiencies.[45]

A large retrospective study of almost 11,000 cancer patients treated with chemotherapy showed a relatively low incidence of stroke (0.14%), the majority occurring within 10 days of chemotherapy treatment; treatment with platinum compounds was associated with stroke more frequently than other chemotherapeutic agents.[100]

In addition to chemotherapeutic cerebrovascular complications, radiation-induced injury to the cervical and intracranial carotid arteries is a potential cause of stroke, presumably by causing accelerated arteriopathy.[90,101] The interval from radiation treatment to onset of occlusive cerebrovascular disease ranged from 6 months to 57 years in one report, although most strokes usually occurred at least 1 year after exposure.[45] The cumulative radiation dose is usually greater than 50 Gy.[90] Angiography reveals occlusion or extensive stenosis of the arteries in the previously applied radiation field, and carotid artery lesions in patients irradiated for head and neck cancers are the most common.[90] Limited data on treatment options for symptomatic carotid disease are available, but carotid stenting appears to be less technically difficult than endarterectomy.[90]

Intracerebral Hemorrhage

Intracerebral hemorrhage is most commonly reported with leukemic conditions, specifically acute promyelocytic leukemia.[90] Although the pathogenesis of the hemorrhage has been postulated to involve infiltration and rupture of vessels by leukemic nodules or damage to small vessels by hyperviscosity, most patients with intracranial hemorrhage do not have evidence of leukostasis, leukemic nodules, or perivascular leukemic infiltration on histologic examination.[90] Among the patients who do have evidence of leukemic infiltration, the peripheral white blood cell count is usually above 70,000/mm^3. In addition to leukemic conditions, malignant lymphoma and multiple myeloma may cause hemostatic deficiencies that predispose to brain hemorrhage through inhibition of fibrin formation by excess immunoglobulins.[93]

MEDICATION USE AND THE RISK OF STROKE

Oral Contraceptives

The association between oral contraceptive use and stroke was demonstrated as early as 1969, with reports of up to a sixfold increase in the risk of stroke.[102] These early studies involved oral contraceptives that contained relatively high doses of hormones, as opposed to the low-dose estrogen preparations used currently.

The World Health Organization (WHO) has performed the largest case-control study of oral contraceptive use and stroke risk. In 697 women aged 20 to 44 years with ischemic stroke, the adjusted odds ratio for stroke occurrence among women who used oral contraceptives compared with those who had never used them was 3.0 in Europeans and 2.9 in non-Europeans.[103] A history of hypertension or tobacco use increased the risk in both groups, and the risk was lower if women had had a blood pressure measurement before starting the drug. In European subjects, the odds ratio in women using drug preparations containing less than 50 μg of estrogen was 1.53, compared with 5.3 in those using higher-dose preparations. In another large population-based, case-control study performed at Northern California Kaiser Permanente Medical Centers, 408 cases of stroke occurred in over 1 million women.[104]

Migraine may increase the risk of stroke with oral contraceptives. In a pooled analysis of two population-based studies, Schwartz and associates found an adjusted odds ratio for ischemic stroke in current low-dose oral contraceptive users of 0.66 compared with women who had never used oral contraceptives, and an odds ratio of 0.95 for hemorrhagic stroke.[105] These odds ratios increased to 2.08

and 2.15 for ischemic and hemorrhagic stroke, respectively, in current oral contraceptive users who also had a history of migraine. These results should be interpreted with caution, however, because hemiplegic migraines might be miscategorized as stroke, artificially elevating the calculated stroke risk in these patients.

Overall, the data suggest that women using low doses of oral contraceptives are not at increased risk of stroke.[104,106–109] With an incidence rate of 11 cases per 100,000 women-years, even with an assumed relative risk of 2, only one additional stroke per 100,000 women-years would occur as a result of oral contraceptive use, and the benefits of the drug far outweigh the potential risks. In one of the most comprehensive reviews of the literature to date, Thorogood estimated that the use of low-dose oral contraceptives increases the risk of stroke by not more than one event per 50,000 women-years, which is considerably less than the risk of stroke due to pregnancy.[110] Gillum and colleagues found a slightly higher stroke risk in their meta-analysis of 73 studies of ischemic stroke and oral contraceptive use, finding an additional 4.1 ischemic strokes per 100,000, with a relative risk of 1.93 for low-estrogen preparations.[111] Given the seemingly additive stroke risk conferred by traditional risk factors in oral contraceptive users (such as hypertension, smoking, and diabetes), more careful consideration is required if one chooses to prescribe oral contraceptives to these "higher risk" patients.

Oral contraceptives may cause a predisposition to hypercoagulability and are associated with a higher risk of venous thromboembolic disease.[112] Women already at risk of vascular disease because of other causes, such as tobacco use, hypertension, the factor V Leiden mutation, or inherited coagulopathies, may be at even greater risk with oral contraceptives.[112] Although the effects of estrogens on the mechanisms of hemostasis are extensive, platelet function tests have provided contradictory data.[113] Estrogens have been shown to increase serum levels of a number of coagulation cascade proteins, including fibrinogen, factors II, VII, IX, X, and XII, and protein C.[113] It is appropriate to screen for underlying coagulopathies (protein C and protein S deficiency, antithrombin III deficiency, the factor V Leiden mutation) in any woman who has a stroke while taking oral contraceptives, because contraceptive use may unmask previously latent clotting abnormalities.

Postmenopausal Hormone Replacement

There have been several randomized clinical trials investigating the relationship between stroke and postmenopausal hormone replacement therapy.[114–116] These trials revealed that postmenopausal hormone therapy is not effective in reducing the risk of a recurrent stroke or death among women with established vascular disease or for prevention of a first stroke.[117] Notably, two of these studies showed an increased stroke risk in those individuals on active hormone replacement therapy, with a relative risk of 2.3 during the first 6 months in one[115] and an increase in the number of vascular events in the other, leading to its termination.[116] Therefore, long-term postmenopausal hormone replacement therapy should be discouraged in individuals at high risk of cerebrovascular events.

Cocaine

Cocaine is the street drug most commonly associated with stroke.[118] Because cocaine's principal pharmacologic effect is the blockade of presynaptic norepinephrine and dopamine reuptake, use of the drug causes a sympathomimetic response. The resultant hypertension, vasoconstriction, tachycardia, and ventricular arrhythmias all may contribute to the pathogenesis of stroke in cocaine users. Further discussion of this topic is provided in Chapter 34.

Petitti and co-workers in the Kaiser Permanente Health Care System in Northern California studied all cases of stroke in young women aged 15 to 44 years.[119] Among 347 cases of stroke, the adjusted odds ratio for women reporting the use of cocaine or amphetamines before stroke onset was 7.0. A retrospective case-control study by others failed to find a similar association.[120]

All methods of cocaine use (inhalation and intranasal, intravenous, and intramuscular) may be associated with stroke. Many cocaine-induced strokes with the inhalational form occur within 1 hour of use.[121] In a study of MRI ischemic changes in long-term cocaine users, a strong association was noted between patient age and the degree of ischemic lesions in both patients and control subjects, but the equivalent severity of ischemic lesions was seen 20 years earlier in the cocaine users, suggesting an accelerated form of arteriopathy induced by cocaine.[122]

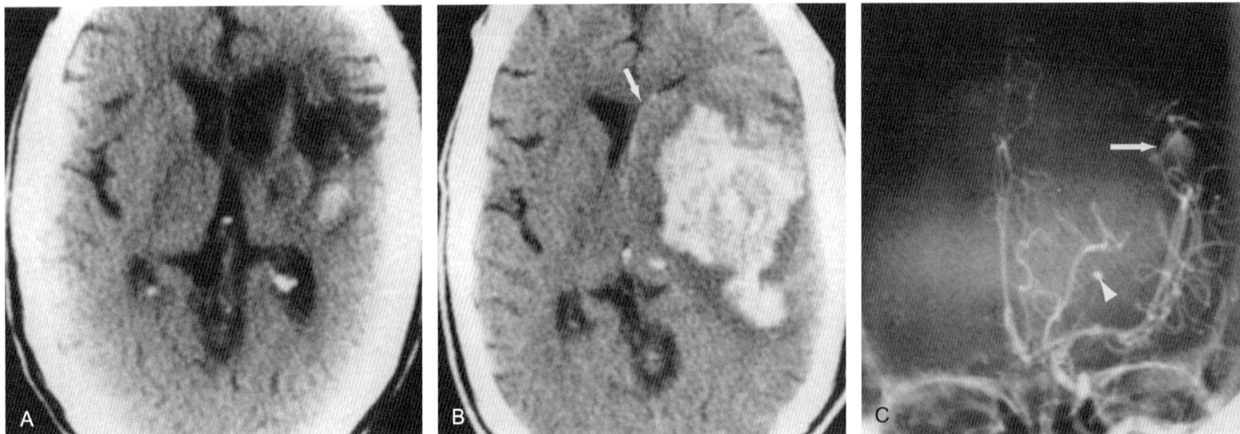

FIGURE 11-5 ■ Intraparenchymal hemorrhage due to aneurysm. **A**, Computed tomography (CT) scan obtained because of a complaint of headache in a 46-year-old chronic cocaine abuser shows a hyperintense lesion in the left frontal lobe that is probably an unruptured aneurysm. A small hemorrhage around the aneurysm is suggested. **B**, CT scan obtained 2 days later because of increasing headache and neurologic signs shows a large hematoma with intraventricular hemorrhage (*arrow*). The left lateral ventricle is markedly compressed and the midline is shifted. **C**, Angiogram shows two aneurysms, a larger one (*arrow*) in a branch of the middle cerebral artery and a smaller one (*arrowhead*) with associated vasospasm from a lenticulostriate artery. (From Brown E, Prager J, Lee HY, et al: CNS complications of cocaine abuse: prevalence, pathophysiology, and neuroradiology. AJR Am J Roentgenol 159:142, 1992, with permission.)

In addition to ischemic stroke, subarachnoid hemorrhage and intraparenchymal hemorrhage may occur immediately after cocaine use (Fig. 11-5). It remains unclear whether cocaine plays a pathogenic role in the development of vascular malformations or whether the drug facilitates bleeding from pre-existing vascular abnormalities.

Besides its direct effects of blood pressure elevation and vasoconstriction, cocaine may predispose users to cardiac arrhythmias and resultant embolic cerebrovascular events.[123] Cocaine use is associated with an increased risk of myocardial infarction and resultant left ventricular akinesis.

Amphetamines

Amphetamines have also been causally linked to stroke (Fig. 11-6) in a number of studies, as discussed in Chapter 34.[124–126] Methamphetamine, the most common illicitly used type of amphetamine, can be injected, smoked, or inhaled. Similar to cocaine, the presumed pathophysiologic process of stroke involves elevated blood pressure or vasculopathy.[126,127] The drug 3,4-methylenedioxymethamphetamine, more commonly known as "ecstasy," has also been implicated as the cause of stroke in isolated case reports.[128] Although both ischemic and hemorrhagic strokes have been reported in the literature, a higher incidence of hemorrhagic events was found in one small study, which would be consistent with a presumed hypertensive pathophysiologic process.[124] Despite an apparent causative role in some stroke

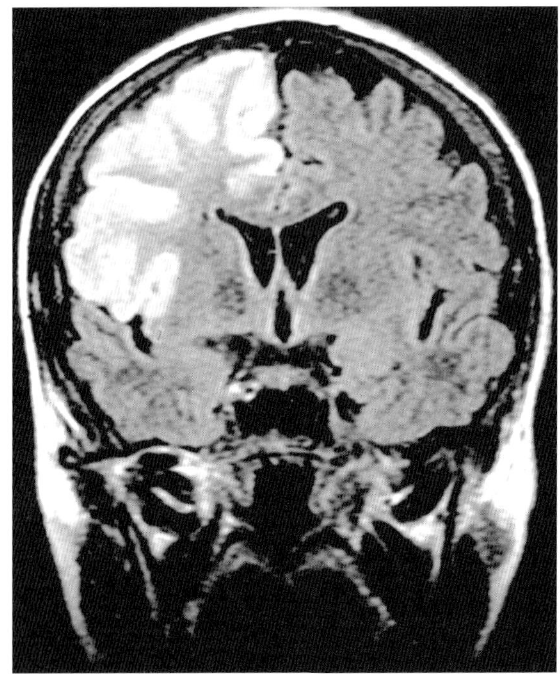

FIGURE 11-6 ■ Magnetic resonance image (MRI) of a 41-year-old woman, showing a large right parietal infarct that occurred in the setting of acute methamphetamine use. The patient had no other risk factors for stroke.

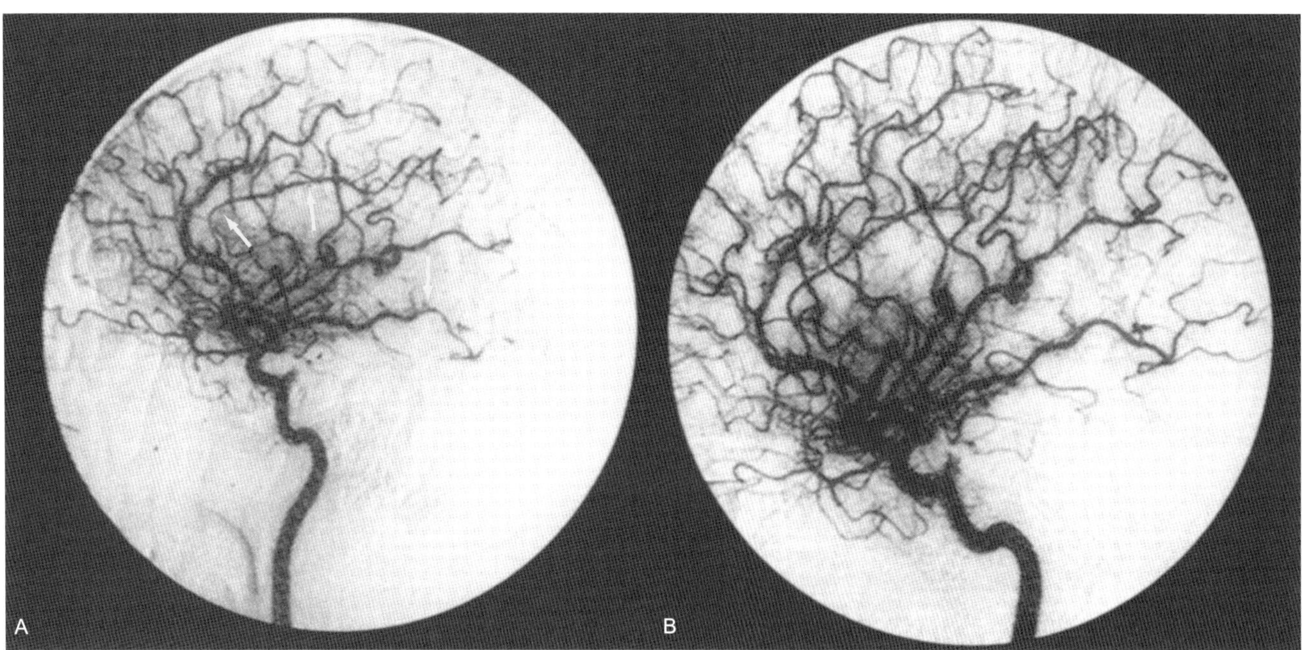

FIGURE 11-7 ▪ Carotid angiograms in a patient after excessive use of sumatriptan and Midrin. **A**, Angiogram showing segmental arterial narrowing (*arrows*) at the time of stroke. **B**, Normalized angiogram taken 39 days later. (Modified from Meschia JF, Malkoff MD, Biller J: Reversible segmental cerebral arterial vasospasm and cerebral infarction: possible association with excessive use of sumatriptan and Midrin. Arch Neurol 55:713, 1998, with permission.)

cases, amphetamine derivatives have been shown to increase the rate and extent of motor recovery in patients with stroke undergoing physical therapy and may exert a neurofacilitatory role in functional recovery from stroke.[129]

Triptans

Stroke may occur in the context of triptan administration for the treatment of migraine. Such agents act as scrotonin agonists at the 5-hydroxytryptamine type 1 receptor and induce potent vasoconstriction of human intracranial arteries in vitro[130] and possibly in vivo.[131] Cases have been reported of arterial or venous infarction after sumatriptan administration, sometimes with segmental arterial narrowing in multiple intracerebral vessels (Fig. 11-7).[130,132,133] Other serotonergic drugs have also been associated with cerebral vasoconstriction and stroke.[134] However, because of the long-recognized association between complicated migraine headaches and ischemic stroke, sumatriptan use cannot be implicated definitively as the sole causative factor. A retrospective study by Hall and associates of 63,575 migraine patients showed no increased risk of stroke in the 13,664 individuals prescribed triptans.[135] Another retrospective study of 140,000 migraineurs failed to show an increased risk of stroke in triptan users, although migraineurs were 67 percent more likely to suffer a stroke than nonmigraineurs.[136]

The large number of triptan users compared with the limited number of cases of triptan-related stroke in the literature suggests that the risk (if any) of cerebrovascular events with the use of this medication is extremely small. Nonetheless, sumatriptan should be used with caution in patients with a history of stroke and should not be used in patients with a history of complicated migraine (migraine with neurologic deficits) or of coronary artery disease.

Alcohol

The relationship between alcohol intake and stroke is complex. There is strong evidence that heavy alcohol use and chronic alcoholism increase the risk of stroke, although mild to moderate alcohol consumption has been associated with a decreased risk.[137] In a cohort of 15,000 men and women in Sweden, an elevated risk of ischemic stroke was found in men (but not women) who were intoxicated or reported episodes of "binge drinking" a few times per year.[138] Alcohol has long been recognized for its broad range of effects on the CNS, as discussed in Chapter 33. In response to a series of studies from the 1970s and 1980s, the World Health Organization and the Stroke Council elevated alcohol to the status of a "less well-documented" risk factor for stroke.[139]

The association between alcohol and stroke risk appears much stronger for intracerebral and subarachnoid hemorrhage than for ischemic stroke. A study of 8,000 men in the Honolulu Heart Program showed that compared with nondrinkers, the risk of hemorrhagic stroke more than doubled for light drinkers and nearly tripled for those considered to be heavy drinkers. In a review of the epidemiologic data, a positive linear association was found between moderate alcohol intake (<60 g of alcohol per day, with one drink containing approximately 12 g of alcohol) and the risk of both intracerebral and subarachnoid hemorrhage in diverse populations.[45] A reduction in alcohol consumption may be accompanied by a reduction in the risk of subsequent hemorrhagic stroke.

A number of studies have shown that mild to moderate consumption of alcohol may reduce the risk of stroke.[140,141] In a study of a multiethnic population in northern Manhattan, Sacco and colleagues found that moderate consumption of up to two drinks per day was significantly protective for ischemic stroke after adjustment for other concurrent risk factors.[140] This study again provides evidence of a J-shaped curve, with an increased risk of ischemic stroke among those consuming seven or more drinks per day (Fig. 11-8). These associations held for both men and women and varying ethnicities, including whites, blacks, and Hispanics. No differential protective effect was found among the types of alcohol consumed. Similarly, a meta-analysis of 35 studies investigating the relationship between alcohol use and stroke showed that compared with nondrinkers, those consuming greater than five drinks per day had a 69 percent increase in ischemic stroke risk. Consumption of less than one drink per day was associated with a reduced risk (relative risk, 0.80), while consumption of one to two drinks per day conferred the lowest risk reduction (0.72).[142]

Several pathophysiologic relationships may exist between alcohol and stroke. Alcohol may induce cardiac arrhythmias and cause a cardiomyopathy with global akinesis, thereby predisposing to the formation of cardiac emboli. Alcohol has also been linked to hypertension, increased platelet aggregation, and activity of the clotting cascade.[45] Acute increases in systolic blood pressure and alterations in cerebral arterial tone may serve as mechanisms triggering hemorrhagic strokes along with a decrease in the production of circulating clotting factors by the liver.[143]

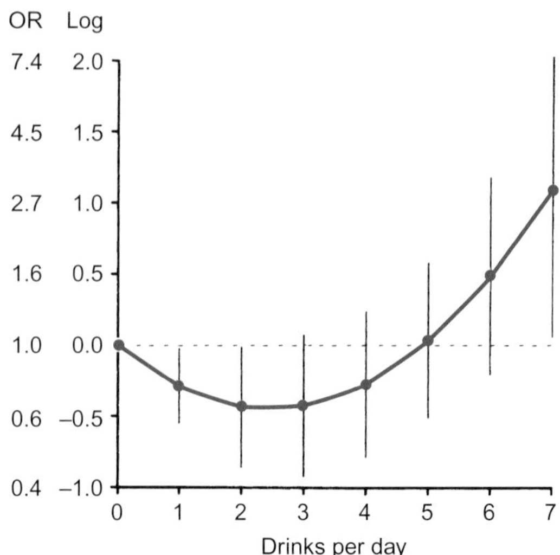

FIGURE 11-8 ■ Relationship between alcohol and the risk of ischemic stroke. OR denotes odds ratio for ischemic stroke. (From Sacco RL, Elkind M, Boden-Albala B, et al: The protective effect of moderate alcohol consumption on ischemic stroke. JAMA 281:57, 1999, with permission. © 1999, American Medical Association.)

GENETICS AND STROKE

Multiple single-gene disorders associated with stroke as well as genetic risk factors for stroke have been discovered. Over 190 mutations in the *NOTCH3* gene have been associated with cerebral autosomal dominant arteriopathy with subcortical infarcts and leukoencephalopathy (CADASIL).[144] This syndrome generally begins with migraines and progresses to involve ischemic insults to the deep gray nuclei and subcortical white matter. Over time, psychiatric disturbances and apathy are common, and patients develop dementia.[145] Strokes are believed to be caused by degeneration of the smooth muscle component of small arteries and arterioles leading to recurrent lacunar and small-vessel infarcts (Fig. 11-9).[146] Granular osmiophilic material in arterial walls of the brain and systemic organs is the key pathologic feature of CADASIL.[147] Cerebral

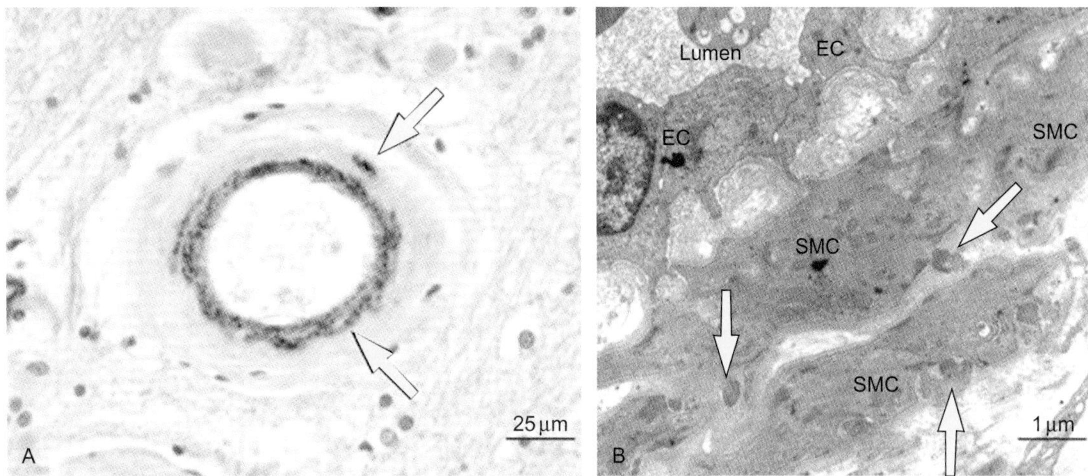

FIGURE 11-9 ■ Examples of vascular changes in CADASIL. **A**, A small white matter artery stained for NOTCH3 demonstrates a thickened wall and the aggregations of NOTCH3 around degenerated smooth muscle cells (*arrows*). **B**, An electron micrograph with multiple granular osmiophilic deposits (*arrows*) in the smooth muscle cells' basement membrane. (From Chabriat H, Joutel A, Dichgans M: CADASIL. Lancet Neurol 8:643, 2009, with permission.)

autosomal recessive arteriopathy with subcortical infarcts and leukoencephalopathy (CARASIL) is similar and results from a mutation of the *HTRA1* gene on chromosome 10q which plays a role in TGF-β signaling. Disinhibition of TGF-β signaling may lead to arteriopathy and hypertensive disease.[148] The phenotype is similar to CADASIL but also classically includes spinal abnormalities and alopecia.[146,148] Retinal vasculopathy with cerebral leukodystrophy (*TREX1* on chromosome 3p) and *COL4A1* gene mutations are also single-gene disorders linked to small-vessel disease.[146,149]

Fabry disease, a lysosomal storage disease, is an X-linked recessive disorder resulting from deficient or absent α-galactosidase A activity. Approximately half of male and one-third of female patients who experience stroke present prior to being diagnosed with Fabry disease.[150] Dolichoectasia, neuropathic pain, and white matter changes are other neurologic manifestations that can accompany systemic skin changes, renal failure, and cardiomyopathy.[144,150]

Mitochondrial encephalomyopathy, lactic acidosis and stroke-like episodes (MELAS) is a mitochondrial genetic disorder that results in ischemic lesions which do not correspond to typical vascular territories. The clinical presentation is heterogeneous and includes seizures, migraines, short stature, deafness, muscle weakness, and gastrointestinal symptoms in addition to infarctions.[151] Roughly 80 percent of patients have a common A to G substitution at nucleotide 3243 in the mitochondrial genome.[152]

Sickle cell disease and the relationship between homocysteine and stroke were discussed earlier. Sickle cell disease results from a substitution of valine for glutamic acid in the β-hemoglobin chain. Homocystinuria, a rare genetic disorder caused by homozygosity of the defective *MTHFR* gene, causes premature atherosclerosis as well as stroke.[51] Heterozygosity for the defective gene has been reported in 30 to 41 percent of the general population, and it is not an independent risk factor for cerebrovascular disease.[153]

Although single-gene disorders are important, they represent a small percentage (~5%) of strokes,[146] and more complex genetic interactions have proven difficult to elucidate with large genome studies. Recently, genome-wide association studies (GWAS) have been performed to further evaluate genetic risk factors for stroke.[146] The first GWAS results, released in 2007, failed to identify a single locus associated with increased stroke risk.[154] The Cohorts for Heart and Aging Research in Genomic Epidemiology (CHARGE) studied four prospective cohorts and identified one single nucleotide polymorphism on chromosome 12p13 that carries an increased risk of stroke, which was replicated in several cohort studies but not in other case-control studies.[144,155] Currently, 15,000 patients with ischemic stroke are being evaluated by GWAS in the

International Stroke Genetic Consortium and the NINDS Stroke Genetic Network (SiGN) in order to identify other genes associated with stroke.[152]

Pharmacogenetics are another area of development that will continue to influence stroke treatment. In the future, pharmacogenetics will help improve treatment efficacy as well as reduce side effects of medications. *CYP2C19* variants lead to unpredictable rates of clopidogrel metabolism, and *ABCB1* gene variations result in decreased concentrations of the active drug.[144] Variations in *CYP2C9* and *VKORC1* genes affect warfarin kinetics.[156] Avoidance of serious side effects through evaluation of a patient's genome may also prove to be a powerful tool as demonstrated by studies showing an increased risk of myopathy or mylagias with simvastatin use in patients with the *SLCO1B1*5* allele.[157,158]

REFERENCES

1. Go AS, Mozaffarian D, Roger VL, et al: Heart disease and stroke statistics—2013 Update: a report from the American Heart Association. Circulation 127:143, 2013.
2. Perry DJ, Pasi KJ: Resistance to activated protein C and factor V Leiden. QJM 90:379, 1997.
3. Markus HS, Hambley H: Neurology and the blood: haematological abnormalities in ischaemic stroke. J Neurol Neurosurg Psychiatry 64:150, 1998.
4. Nichols WL, Heit JA: Activated protein C resistance and thrombosis. Mayo Clin Proc 71:897, 1996.
5. Allaart CF, Poort SR, Rosendaal FR, et al: Increased risk of venous thrombosis in carriers of hereditary protein C deficiency defect. Lancet 341:134, 1993.
6. Pabinger I, Schneider B: Thrombotic risk in hereditary antithrombin III, protein C, or protein S deficiency: a cooperative, retrospective study. Gesellschaft fur Thrombose- und Hämostaseforschung (GTH) Study Group on Natural Inhibitors. Arterioscler Thromb Vasc Biol 16:742, 1996.
7. Kohler J, Kasper J, Witt I, et al: Ischemic stroke due to protein C deficiency. Stroke 21:1077, 1990.
8. Camerlingo M, Finazzi G, Casto L, et al: Inherited protein C deficiency and nonhemorrhagic arterial stroke in young adults. Neurology 41:1371, 1991.
9. Simioni P, de Ronde H, Prandoni P, et al: Ischemic stroke in young patients with activated protein C resistance: a report of three cases belonging to three different kindreds. Stroke 26:885, 1995.
10. van Kuijck MA, Rotteveel JJ, van Oostrom CG, et al: Neurological complications in children with protein C deficiency. Neuropediatrics 25:16, 1994.
11. Coull BM, Clark WM: Abnormalities of hemostasis in ischemic stroke. Med Clin North Am 77:77, 1993.
12. Tatlisumak T, Fisher M: Hematologic disorders associated with ischemic stroke. J Neurol Sci 140:1, 1996.
13. Barinagarrementeria F, Santos J, Ruiz-Sandoval J, et al: Prothrombotic states as triggering of cerebral infarction in patients with patent foramen ovale. Neurology 50:A155, 1998.
14. Heistinger M, Rumpl E, Illiasch H, et al: Cerebral sinus thrombosis in a patient with hereditary protein S deficiency: case report and review of the literature. Ann Hematol 64:105, 1992.
15. Confavreux C, Brunet P, Petiot P, et al: Congenital protein C deficiency and superior sagittal sinus thrombosis causing isolated intracranial hypertension. J Neurol Neurosurg Psychiatry 57:655, 1994.
16. Ganesan V, McShane MA, Liesner R, et al: Inherited prothrombotic states and ischaemic stroke in childhood. J Neurol Neurosurg Psychiatry 65:508, 1998.
17. Deschiens MA, Conard J, Horellou MH, et al: Coagulation studies, factor V Leiden, and anticardiolipin antibodies in 40 cases of cerebral venous thrombosis. Stroke 27:1724, 1996.
18. Dahlback B, Carlsson M, Svensson PJ: Familial thrombophilia due to a previously unrecognized mechanism characterized by poor anticoagulant response to activated protein C: prediction of a cofactor to activated protein C. Proc Natl Acad Sci USA 90:1004, 1993.
19. Bertina RM, Koeleman BP, Koster T, et al: Mutation in blood coagulation factor V associated with resistance to activated protein C. Nature 369:64, 1994.
20. Thomas DP, Roberts HR: Hypercoagulability in venous and arterial thrombosis. Ann Intern Med 126:638, 1997.
21. Ridker PM, Hennekens CH, Lindpaintner K, et al: Mutation in the gene coding for coagulation factor V and the risk of myocardial infarction, stroke, and venous thrombosis in apparently healthy men. N Engl J Med 332:912, 1995.
22. Soare AM, Popa C: Deficiencies of proteins C, S and antithrombin and activated protein C resistance—their involvement in the occurrence of arterial thromboses. J Med Life 3:412, 2010.
23. Halbmayer WM, Haushofer A, Schon R, et al: The prevalence of poor anticoagulant response to activated protein C (APC resistance) among patients suffering from stroke or venous thrombosis and among healthy subjects. Blood Coagul Fibrinolysis 5:51, 1994.
24. Kenet G, Sadetzki S, Murad H, et al: Factor V Leiden and antiphospholipid antibodies are significant risk factors for ischemic stroke in children. Stroke 31:1283, 2000.
25. Lalouschek W, Schillinger M, Hsieh K, et al: Matched case-control study on factor V Leiden and the prothrombin gene 20210A mutation in patients with ischemic stroke/transient ischemic attack up to the age of 60 years. Stroke 36:1405, 2006.
26. Bloemenkamp KW, Rosendaal FR, Helmerhorst FM, et al: Enhancement by factor V Leiden mutation of

risk of deep-vein thrombosis associated with oral contraceptives containing a third-generation progestagen. Lancet 346:1593, 1995.

27. Weih M, Vetter B, Ziemer S, et al: Increased rate of factor V Leiden mutation in patients with cerebral venous thrombosis. J Neurol 245:149, 1998.
28. Zuber M, Toulon P, Marnet L, et al: Factor V Leiden mutation in cerebral venous thrombosis. Stroke 27:1721, 1996.
29. Pugliese D, Nicoletti G, Andreula C, et al: Combined protein C deficiency and protein C activated resistance as a cause of caval, peripheral, and cerebral venous thrombosis: a case report. Angiology 49:399, 1998.
30. Martinelli I, Landi G, Merati G, et al: Factor V gene mutation is a risk factor for cerebral venous thrombosis. Thromb Haemost 75:393, 1996.
31. Dulli DA, Luzzio CC, Williams EC, et al: Cerebral venous thrombosis and activated protein C resistance. Stroke 27:1731, 1996.
32. Vrethem M, Ernerudh J, Lindstrom F, et al: Cerebral ischemia associated with anticardiolipin antibodies. Acta Neurol Scand 85:412, 1992.
33. Coull BM, Levine SR, Brey RL: The role of antiphospholipid antibodies in stroke. Neurol Clin 10:125, 1992.
34. Brey RL, Hart RG, Sherman DG, et al: Antiphospholipid antibodies and cerebral ischemia in young people. Neurology 40:1190, 1990.
35. Love PE, Santoro SA: Antiphospholipid antibodies: anticardiolipin and the lupus anticoagulant in systemic lupus erythematosus (SLE) and in non-SLE disorders. Prevalence and clinical significance. Ann Intern Med 112:682, 1990.
36. Levine SR, Deegan MJ, Futrell N, et al: Cerebrovascular and neurologic disease associated with antiphospholipid antibodies: 48 cases. Neurology 40:1181, 1990.
37. Levine SR, Brey RL, Tilley BC, APASS Investigators Antiphospholipid antibodies and subsequent thrombo-occlusive events in patients with ischemic stroke. JAMA 291:576, 2004.
38. Brey RL, Stallworth CL, McGlasson DL, et al: Antiphospholipid antibodies and stroke in young women. Stroke 33:2396, 2002.
39. Giannakopoulos B, Krilis SA: Mechanisms of disease: the pathogenesis of the antiphospholipid syndrome. N Engl J Med 368:1033, 2013.
40. Nihoyannopoulos P, Gomez PM, Joshi J, et al: Cardiac abnormalities in systemic lupus erythematosus: association with raised anticardiolipin antibodies. Circulation 82:369, 1990.
41. Ware AE, Mongey AB: Lupus and cerebrovascular accidents. Lupus 6:420, 1997.
42. Harris EN, Pierangeli S: Antiphospholipid antibodies and cerebral lupus. Ann N Y Acad Sci 823:270, 1997.
43. Sacco RL, Adams R, Albers G, et al: Guidelines for prevention of stroke in patients with ischemic stroke or transient ischemic attack: a statement for healthcare professionals from the American Heart Association/American Stroke Association Council on Stroke: co-sponsored by the Council on Cardiovascular Radiology and Intervention: the American Academy of Neurology affirms the value of this guideline. Stroke 37:577, 2006.
44. Finazzi G, Marchioli R, Brancaccio V, et al: A randomized clinical trial of high-intensity warfarin vs. conventional antithrombotic therapy for the prevention of recurrent thrombosis in patients with the antiphospholipid syndrome (WAPS). J Thromb Haemost 3:848, 2005.
45. Delio PR, Albers GW: Stroke as a complication of general medical disorders. p. 1157. In Aminoff MJ (ed): Neurology and General Medicine. 4th Ed. Churchill Livingstone Elsevier, Philadelphia, 2008.
46. Giles WH, Croft JB, Greenlund KJ, et al: Total homocyst(e)ine concentration and the likelihood of nonfatal stroke: results from the Third National Health and Nutrition Examination Survey, 1988–1994. Stroke 29:2473, 1998.
47. Kark JD, Selhub J, Bostom A, et al: Plasma homocysteine and all-cause mortality in diabetes. Lancet 353:1936, 1999.
48. McQuillan BM, Beilby JP, Nidorf M, et al: Hyperhomocysteinemia but not the C677T mutation of methylenetetrahydrofolate reductase is an independent risk determinant of carotid wall thickening: the Perth Carotid Ultrasound Disease Assessment Study (CUDAS). Circulation 99:2383, 1999.
49. Majors A, Ehrhart LA, Pezacka EH: Homocysteine as a risk factor for vascular disease: enhanced collagen production and accumulation by smooth muscle cells. Arterioscler Thromb Vasc Biol 17:2074, 1997.
50. Lentz SR: Mechanisms of thrombosis in hyperhomocysteinemia. Curr Opin Hematol 5:343, 1998.
51. Stein JH, McBride PE: Hyperhomocysteinemia and atherosclerotic vascular disease: pathophysiology, screening, and treatment. Arch Intern Med 158:1301, 1998.
52. Yoo JH, Chung CS, Kang SS: Relation of plasma homocyst(e)ine to cerebral infarction and cerebral atherosclerosis. Stroke 29:2478, 1998.
53. Bostom AG, Rosenberg IH, Silbershatz H, et al: Nonfasting plasma total homocysteine levels and stroke incidence in elderly persons: the Framingham Study. Ann Intern Med 131:352, 1999.
54. Bots ML, Launer LJ, Lindemans J, et al: Homocysteine and short-term risk of myocardial infarction and stroke in the elderly: the Rotterdam Study. Arch Intern Med 159:38, 1999.
55. Kristensen B, Malm J, Nilsson TK, et al: Hyperhomocysteinemia and hypofibrinolysis in young adults with ischemic stroke. Stroke 30:974, 1999.
56. Perry IJ, Refsum H, Morris RW, et al: Prospective study of serum total homocysteine concentration and risk of

stroke in middle-aged British men. Lancet 346:1395, 1995.
57. Graham IM, Daly LE, Refsum HM, et al: Plasma homocysteine as a risk factor for vascular disease: the European Concerted Action Project. JAMA 277:1775, 1997.
58. Martí-Carvajal AJ, Solà I, Lathyris D, et al: Homocysteine lowering interventions for preventing cardiovascular events. Cochrane Database Syst Rev 4:6612, 2009.
59. Valentine RJ, Grayburn PA, Vega GL, et al: Lp(a) lipoprotein is an independent, discriminating risk factor for premature peripheral atherosclerosis among white men. Arch Intern Med 154:801, 1994.
60. Shintani S, Kikuchi S, Hamaguchi H, et al: High serum lipoprotein(a) levels are an independent risk factor for cerebral infarction. Stroke 24:965, 1993.
61. Jovicic A, Ivanisevic V, Ivanovic I: Lipoprotein(a) in patients with carotid atherosclerosis and ischemic cerebrovascular disorders. Atherosclerosis 98:59, 1993.
62. Lip GY, Jones AF: Lipoprotein (a) and vascular disease: thrombogenesis and atherogenesis. QJM 88:529, 1995.
63. Enkhmaa B, Anuurad E, Zhang W, et al: Lipoprotein(a): genotype-phenotype relationship and impact on atherogenic risk. Metab Syndr Relat Disord 9:411, 2011.
64. Ridker PM, Stampfer MJ, Hennekens CH: Plasma concentration of lipoprotein(a) and the risk of future stroke. JAMA 273:1269, 1995.
65. Nagayama M, Shinohara Y, Nagayama T: Lipoprotein(a) and ischemic cerebrovascular disease in young adults. Stroke 25:74, 1994.
66. Scott J: Lipoprotein. BMJ 303:663, 1991.
67. Pedro-Botet J, Senti M, Nogues X, et al: Lipoprotein and apolipoprotein profile in men with ischemic stroke: role of lipoprotein(a), triglyceride-rich lipoproteins, and apolipoprotein E polymorphism. Stroke 23:1556, 1992.
68. Ohira T, Schreiner PJ, Morrisett JD, et al: Lipoprotein (a) and incident ischemic stroke: the Atherosclerosis Risk in Communities (ARIC) study. Stroke 37:1407, 2006.
69. Kargman DE, Tuck C, Berglund L, et al: Lipid and lipoprotein levels remain stable in acute ischemic stroke: the Northern Manhattan Stroke Study. Atherosclerosis 139:391, 1998.
70. Erquo S, Kaptoge S, Perry P, et al: Lipoprotein (a) concentration and the risk of coronary heart disease, stroke, and nonvascular mortality. JAMA 302:412, 2009.
71. Akaike M, Azuma H, Kagawa A, et al: Effect of aspirin treatment on serum concentrations of lipoprotein (a) in patients with atherosclerotic diseases. Clin Chem 48:1454, 2002.
72. Guyton JR, Goldberg AC, Kreisberg RA, et al: Effectiveness of once-nightly dosing of extended release niacin alone and in combination for hypercholesterolemia. Am J Cardiol 82:737, 1998.
73. Zamboni M, Facchinetti R, Armellini F, et al: Effects of visceral fat and weight loss on lipoprotein(a) concentration in subjects with obesity. Obes Res 5:332, 1997.
74. Hopkins PN, Wu LL, Hunt SC, et al: Lipoprotein(a) interactions with lipid and non-lipid risk factors in early familial coronary artery disease. Arterioscler Thromb Vasc Biol 17:2783, 1997.
75. Hart RG, Kanter MC: Hematologic disorders and ischemic stroke: a selective review. Stroke 21:1111, 1990.
76. Glauser TA, Siegel MJ, Lee BC, et al: Accuracy of neurologic examination and history in detecting evidence of MRI-diagnosed cerebral infarctions in children with sickle cell hemoglobinopathy. J Child Neurol 10:88, 1995.
77. Ohene-Frempong K: Stroke in sickle cell disease: demographic, clinical, and therapeutic considerations. Semin Hematol 28:213, 1991.
78. Duncan GW: Ischemic stroke in sickle cell disease: a review. Tenn Med 90:498, 1997.
79. Francis RB: Large-vessel occlusion in sickle cell disease: pathogenesis, clinical consequences, and therapeutic implications. Med Hypotheses 35:88, 1991.
80. Adams RJ, McKie VC, Carl EM, et al: Long-term stroke risk in children with sickle cell disease screened with transcranial Doppler. Ann Neurol 42:699, 1997.
81. Adams R, McKie V, Nichols F, et al: The use of transcranial ultrasonography to predict stroke in sickle cell disease. N Engl J Med 326:605, 1992.
82. Adams RJ, McKie VC, Hsu L, et al: Prevention of a first stroke by transfusions in children with sickle cell anemia and abnormal results on transcranial Doppler ultrasonography. N Engl J Med 339:5, 1998.
83. Adams RJ, Brambilla D: Discontinuing prophylactic transfusions used to prevent stroke in sickle cell disease. N Engl J Med 353:2769, 2005.
84. Goldstein L, Adams R, Alberts M, et al: AHA/ASA Guideline: primary prevention of ischemic stroke. Stroke 37:1583, 2006.
85. Futrell N, Schultz LR, Millikan C: Central nervous system disease in patients with systemic lupus erythematosus. Neurology 42:1649, 1992.
86. Nagayama Y, Okamoto S, Konishi T, et al: Cerebral berry aneurysms and systemic lupus erythematosus. Neuroradiology 33:466, 1991.
87. Mitsias P, Levine SR: Large cerebral vessel occlusive disease in systemic lupus erythematosus. Neurology 44:385, 1994.
88. Serena M, Biscaro R, Moretto G, et al: Peripheral and central nervous system involvement in essential mixed cryoglobulinemia: a case report. Clin Neuropathol 10:177, 1991.
89. Origgi L, Vanoli M, Carbone A, et al: Central nervous system involvement in patients with HCV-related cryoglobulinemia. Am J Med Sci 315:208, 1998.
90. Rogers LR: Cerebrovascular complications in cancer patients. Neurol Clin 9:889, 1991.

91. Chaturvedi S, Ansell J, Recht L: Should cerebral ischemic events in cancer patients be considered a manifestation of hypercoagulability? Stroke 25:1215, 1994.
92. Cestari DM, Weine DM, Panageas KS, et al: Stroke in patients with cancer: incidence and etiology. Neurology 62:2025, 2004.
93. Goad KE, Gralnick HR: Coagulation disorders in cancer. Hematol Oncol Clin North Am 10:457, 1996.
94. Callander N, Rapaport SI: Trousseau's syndrome. West J Med 158:364, 1993.
95. Glass JP: The diagnosis and treatment of stroke in a patient with cancer: nonbacterial thrombotic endocarditis (NBTE): a case report and review. Clin Neurol Neurosurg 95:315, 1993.
96. Dutta T, Karas MG, Segal AZ, et al: Yield of transesophageal echocardiography for nonbacterial thrombotic endocarditis and other cardiac sources of embolism in cancer patients with cerebral ischemia. Am J Cardiol 97:894, 2006.
97. Singhal AB, Topcuoglu MA, Buonanno FS: Acute ischemic stroke patterns in infective and nonbacterial thrombotic endocarditis: a diffusion-weighted magnetic resonance imaging study. Stroke 33:1267, 2002.
98. Eiken PW, Edwards WD, Tazelaar HD, et al: Surgical pathology of nonbacterial thrombotic endocarditis in 30 patients, 1985–2000. Mayo Clin Proc 76:1204, 2001.
99. Whitlock RP, Sun JC, Fremes SE, et al: Antithrombotic and thrombolytic therapy for valvular disease: Antithrombotic Therapy and Prevention of Thrombosis, 9th ed: American College of Chest Physicians Evidence-Based Clinical Practice Guidelines. Chest 141:e576S, 2012.
100. Li SH, Chen WH, Tang Y, et al: Incidence of ischemic stroke post-chemotherapy: a retrospective review of 10,963 patients. Clin Neurol Neurosurg 108:150, 2006.
101. Dorresteijn LD, Kappelle AC, Scholz NM, et al: Increased carotid wall thickening after radiotherapy on the neck. Eur J Cancer 41:1026, 2005.
102. Thorogood M: Stroke and steroid hormonal contraception. Contraception 57:157, 1998.
103. Poulter NR, Chang CL, Farley TM, et al: Ischaemic stroke and combined oral contraceptives: results of an international, multicentre, case-control study. WHO Collaborative Study of Cardiovascular Disease and Steroid Hormone Contraception. Lancet 348:498, 1996.
104. Petitti DB, Sidney S, Bernstein A, et al: Stroke in users of low-dose oral contraceptives. N Engl J Med 335:8, 1996.
105. Schwartz SM, Petitti DB, Siscovick DS, et al: Stroke and use of low-dose oral contraceptives in young women: a pooled analysis of two US studies. Stroke 29:2277, 1998.
106. Hannaford PC, Croft PR, Kay CR: Oral contraception and stroke: evidence from the Royal College of General Practitioners' Oral Contraception Study. Stroke 25:935, 1994.
107. Lidegaard O: Oral contraception and risk of a cerebral thromboembolic attack: results of a case-control study. BMJ 306:956, 1993.
108. Schwartz SM, Siscovick DS, Longstreth WT Jr, et al: Use of low-dose oral contraceptives and stroke in young women. Ann Intern Med 127:596, 1997.
109. Chan WS, Ray J, Wai EK, et al: Risk of stroke in women exposed to low-dose oral contraceptives: a critical evaluation of the evidence. Arch Intern Med 164:741, 2004.
110. Thorogood M: Risk of stroke in users of oral contraceptives. JAMA 281:1255, 1999.
111. Gillum LA, Mamidipudi AK, Johnston SC: Ischemic stroke risk with oral contraceptives: a meta-analysis. JAMA 284:72, 2000.
112. Poulter NR, Chang CL, Farley TM, et al: Effect on stroke of different progestagens in low oestrogen dose oral contraceptives. WHO Collaborative Study of Cardiovascular Disease and Steroid Hormone Contraception. Lancet 354:301, 1999.
113. Wessler S: Estrogen-associated thromboembolism. Ann Epidemiol 2:439, 1992.
114. Hulley S, Grady D, Bush T, The HERS Research Group. Randomized trial of estrogen plus progestin for secondary prevention of coronary heart disease in postmenopausal women. JAMA 280:605, 1998.
115. Kernan WN, Brass LM, Viscoli CM, et al: Estrogen after ischemic stroke: clinical basis and design of the Women's Estrogen for Stroke Trial. J Stroke Cerebrovasc Dis 7:85, 1998.
116. Writing Group for the Women's Health Initiative Investigators. Risk and benefits of estrogen plus progestin in health postmenopausal women. JAMA 288:321, 2002.
117. Brass LM: Hormone replacement therapy and stroke: clinical trials review. Stroke 35:2644, 2004.
118. Kelly MA, Gorelick PB, Mirza D: The role of drugs in the etiology of stroke. Clin Neuropharmacol 15:249, 1992.
119. Petitti DB, Sidney S, Quesenberry C, et al: Stroke and cocaine or amphetamine use. Epidemiology 9:596, 1998.
120. Qureshi AI, Akbar MS, Czander E, et al: Crack cocaine use and stroke in young patients. Neurology 48:341, 1997.
121. Levine SR, Brust JC, Futrell N, et al: Cerebrovascular complications of the use of the "crack" form of alkaloidal cocaine. N Engl J Med 323:699, 1990.
122. Bartzokis G, Goldstein IB, Hance DB, et al: The incidence of T2-weighted MR imaging signal abnormalities in the brain of cocaine-dependent patients is age-related and region-specific. AJNR Am J Neuroradiol 20:1628, 1999.
123. Sauer CM: Recurrent embolic stroke and cocaine-related cardiomyopathy. Stroke 22:1203, 1991.

124. Yen DJ, Wang SJ, Ju TH, et al: Stroke associated with methamphetamine inhalation. Eur Neurol 34:16, 1994.
125. Lambrecht GL, Malbrain ML, Chew SL, et al: Intranasal caffeine and amphetamine causing stroke. Acta Neurol Belg 93:146, 1993.
126. Perez JA Jr, Arsura EL, Strategos S: Methamphetamine-related stroke: four cases. J Emerg Med 17:469, 1999.
127. Brust JC: Vasculitis owing to substance abuse. Neurol Clin 15:945, 1997.
128. Hanyu S, Ikeguchi K, Imai H, et al: Cerebral infarction associated with 3,4-methylenedioxymethamphetamine ("ecstasy") abuse. Eur Neurol 35:173, 1995.
129. Walker-Batson D, Smith P, Curtis S, et al: Amphetamine paired with physical therapy accelerates motor recovery after stroke; further evidence. Stroke 26:2254, 1995.
130. Cavazos JE, Caress JB, Chilukuri VR, et al: Sumatriptan-induced stroke in sagittal sinus thrombosis. Lancet 343:1105, 1994.
131. Friberg L, Olesen J, Iversen HK, et al: Migraine pain associated with middle cerebral artery dilatation: reversal by sumatriptan. Lancet 338:13, 1991.
132. Meschia JF, Malkoff MD, Biller J: Reversible segmental cerebral arterial vasospasm and cerebral infarction: possible association with excessive use of sumatriptan and Midrin. Arch Neurol 55:712, 1998.
133. Jayamaha JE, Street MK: Fatal cerebellar infarction in a migraine sufferer whilst receiving sumatriptan. Intensive Care Med 21:82, 1995.
134. Singhal AB, Caviness VS, Begleiter AF, et al: Cerebral vasoconstriction and stroke after use of serotonergic drugs. Neurology 58:130, 2002.
135. Hall GC, Brown MM, Mo J, et al: Triptans in migraine: the risks of stroke, cardiovascular disease, and death in practice. Neurology 62:563, 2004.
136. Velentgas P, Cole JA, Mo J, et al: Severe vascular events in migraine patients. Headache 44:642, 2004.
137. Hillborn M, Numminen H, Juvela S: Recent heavy drinking of alcohol and embolic stroke. Stroke 30:2307, 1999.
138. Hansagi H, Romelsjo A, Gerhardsson de Verdier M, et al: Alcohol consumption and stroke mortality: 20-year follow-up of 15,077 men and women. Stroke 26:1768, 1995.
139. Goldstein M, Barnett HJM, Orgogozo JM, et al: Report of the WHO Task Force on Stroke and Other Cerebrovascular Disorders: recommendations on stroke prevention, diagnosis, and therapy. Stroke 20:1407, 1989.
140. Sacco RL, Elkind M, Boden-Albala B, et al: The protective effect of moderate alcohol consumption on ischemic stroke. JAMA 281:53, 1999.
141. Berger K, Ajani UA, Kase CS, et al: Light-to-moderate alcohol consumption and risk of stroke among U.S. male physicians. N Engl J Med 341:1557, 1999.
142. Reynolds K, Lewis B, Nolen JD, et al: Alcohol consumption and risk of stroke: a meta-analysis. JAMA 289:579, 2003.
143. Hillbom M: Alcohol consumption and stroke: benefits and risks. Alcohol Clin Exp Res 22:352S, 1998.
144. Meschia JF, Worrall BB, Rich SS: Genetic susceptibility to ischemic stroke. Nat Rev Neurol 7:369, 2011.
145. Pescini F, Nannucci S, Bertaccini B, et al: The Cerebral Autosomal-Dominant Arteriopathy with Subcortical Infarcts and Leukoencephalopathy (CADASIL) Scale: a screening tool to select patients for NOTCH3 gene analysis. Stroke 43:2871, 2012.
146. Yamamoto Y, Craggs L, Baumann M, et al: Review: molecular genetics and patholol gy of hereditary small vessel diseases of the brain. Neuropathol Appl Neurobiol 37:94, 2011.
147. Lewandowska E, Dziewulska D, Parys M, et al: Ultrastructure of granular osmiophilic material deposits (GOM) in arterioles of CADASIL patients. Folia Neuropathol 49:174, 2011.
148. Hara K, Shiga A, Fukutake T, et al: Association of HTRA1 mutations and familial ischemic cerebral small-vessel disease. N Engl J Med 360:1729, 2009.
149. Lemmens R, Maugeri A, Niessen HWM: Novel COL4A1 mutations cause cerebral small vessel disease by haploinsufficiency. Human Molecular Genetics 22:391, 2013.
150. Germain D: Fabry disease. Orphanet J Rare Dis. 5:30, 2010.
151. Dashe FE, Boyer PJ: Case 39-1998—a 13-year-old girl with a relapsing-remitting neurological disorder. N Engl J Med 339:1914, 1998.
152. Della-Morte D, Guadagni F, Palmirotta R, et al: Genetics of ischaemic stroke, stroke-related risk factors, stroke precursors and treatment. Pharmocogenomics 13:595, 2012.
153. Lalouschek W, Aull S, Serles W, et al: Genetic and nongenetic factors influencing homocysteine levels in patients with ischemic cerebrovascular disease and in healthy control subject. J Lab Clin Med 133:575, 1999.
154. Matarín M, Brown WM, Scholz S, et al: A genome-wide genotyping study in patients with ischaemic stroke: initial analysis and data release. Lancet Neurol 6:414, 2007.
155. Ikram MA, Seshadri S, Bis JC, et al: Genomewide association studies of stroke. N Engl J Med 360:1718, 2009.
156. Wadelius M, Chen LY, Eriksson N, et al: Association of warfarin dose with genes involved in its action and metabolism. Hum Genet 121:23, 2007.
157. Voora D, Shah SH, Spasojevic I, et al: The SLCO1B1*5 genetic variant is associated with statin-induced side effects. J Am Coll Cardiol 54:1609, 2009.
158. Link E, Parish S, Armitage J, et al: SLCO1B1 variants and statin-induced myopathy—a genomewide study. N Engl J Med 359:789, 2008.

SECTION

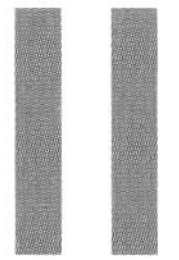

Gastrointestinal Tract and Related Disorders

CHAPTER

12

Hepatic and Pancreatic Encephalopathy

KARIN WEISSENBORN

HEPATIC ENCEPHALOPATHY

Definition

The term *hepatic encephalopathy* (HE) refers to any type of cerebral dysfunction that is due to liver insufficiency and/or portosystemic shunting and is detectable by either clinical, neuropsychologic or neurophysiologic means. Three types of HE are differentiated based on the underlying cause: type A occurs in patients with acute liver failure, type B in patients with portosystemic shunting in the absence of liver dysfunction, and type C in patients with cirrhosis. Episodic, recurrent and chronic progressive forms have been described.[1]

Clinical Features

HE is characterized by alterations of cognition, motor function, and consciousness in various combinations. The most commonly used grading system that distinguishes grades of HE (I-IV) based on degree of alteration in consciousness is the West Haven system (Table 12-1). Motor symptoms can be detected in all grades, but with increasing frequency and severity in grades II and III (Fig. 12-1). The most characteristic motor findings are extrapyramidal and cerebellar symptoms, including hypomimia, hypo- and bradykinesia, rigidity, tremor, dysarthria, dysdiadochokinesia, and ataxia. Hyperreflexia and pyramidal signs are observed predominantly in patients with grade III and IV encephalopathy. Asterixis (flapping tremor), a form of negative myoclonus, may be present in the absence of any alteration of consciousness or cognition, but is observed most frequently in patients with grade II or III disease.

Difficulties in writing and speech disturbances are some of the first symptoms of HE. In the early phases, tremulous writing, omission of single letters, reversal of order, and misspellings are common. With later stages of HE, letters become superimposed and lines of writing converge. Patients become unable to sign their names or to move the pencil from left to right. Speech, initially monotonous and slowed, becomes slurred and unintelligible with associated dysphasia in later stages of the illness.

Aminoff's Neurology and General Medicine, Fifth Edition.

Personality changes and alterations of mood may be the first symptoms of HE and are generally first observed by relatives or friends. As the disease progresses, patients may become uninhibited and bizarre due to increasing difficulties in visual perception and disorientation, illusions and hallucinations. Mood alterations including euphoria and depression are common and may exhibit rapid fluctuations.

TABLE 12-1 ■ West Haven Criteria for Grading of Clinically Overt Hepatic Encephalopathy

Grade I	Trivial lack of awareness, shortened attention span, impaired performance of addition, euphoria or anxiety
Grade II	Lethargy or apathy, minimal disorientation for time and place, inappropriate behavior
Grade III	Somnolence to semistupor but responsiveness to verbal stimuli, confusion, gross disorientation
Grade IV	Coma

From Ferenci P, Lockwood A, Mullen K, et al: Hepatic encephalopathy–definition, nomenclature, diagnosis, and quantification: final report of the working party at the 11th World Congresses of Gastroenterology, Vienna, 1998. Hepatology 35:716, 2002, with permission.

Chronic Progressive Hepatic Encephalopathy

The chronic progressive (or persistent) form of HE has predominantly been observed in patients with extensive portosystemic shunting that developed either spontaneously or after transjugular intrahepatic portosystemic stent shunting (TIPPS) or other shunting procedures. Data regarding the prevalence of this subtype of HE are sparse. Cirrhosis-related parkinsonism and hepatic myelopathy are the best-characterized manifestations of this form of HE. In a prospective study of 214 patients with cirrhosis awaiting liver transplantation, cirrhosis-related parkinsonism was found in 4 percent and hepatic myelopathy in 2 percent of patients.[2] The parkinsonian patients show hypomimia, hypokinesia, tremor, and rigidity similar to patients with idiopathic Parkinson disease (PD), but typically they do not develop the characteristic shuffling gait of PD and have predominant involvement of their upper limbs. Moreover, symptoms develop faster and are symmetric more often. Tremor occurs predominantly with action; a parkinsonian rest tremor is observed less commonly. The extrapyramidal

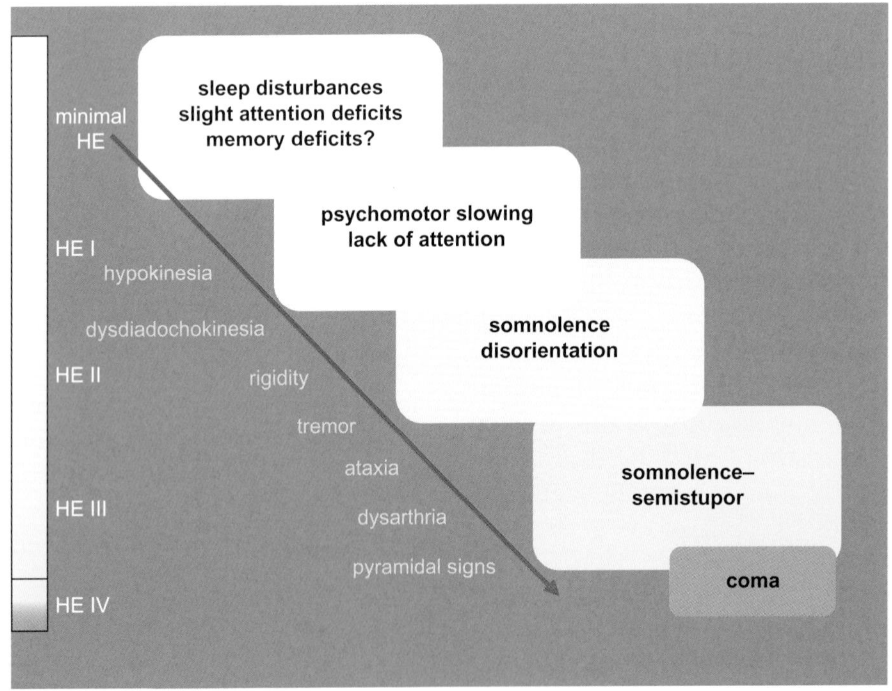

FIGURE 12-1 ■ Hepatic encephalopathy (HE) should be considered as a continuum of decreasing brain function rather than a sequence of well-defined steps of cerebral alteration. To compare different patient groups, however, grading systems such as the West Haven criteria have been developed, which subdivide patients with HE into groups depending on the extent of any alteration of consciousness. Motor symptoms of HE may be present in all grades, even in the absence of cognitive dysfunction.

symptoms may be associated with cerebellar and corticospinal deficits.

Some patients present with a combination of cirrhosis-related parkinsonism and hepatic myelopathy. The myelopathy is characterized by a rapidly progressive spastic paraparesis without accompanying sensory deficits or disturbances of bladder or bowel functions.[2,3] After only a few months of progressive disability, most patients with hepatic myelopathy either depend upon an assistive device or are confined to a wheelchair. For unknown reasons most patients with hepatic myelopathy are men, whereas cirrhosis-related parkinsonism is equally prevalent in men and women.[2,4]

Minimal Hepatic Encephalopathy

Minimal hepatic encephalopathy is considered the mildest form of HE and is defined as cerebral dysfunction detectable only by neuropsychologic or neurophysiologic means in the absence of clinically overt symptoms of encephalopathy. The concept of minimal HE was developed in the 1970s when it became obvious that some patients who were considered unimpaired clinically nevertheless had significant deficits in attention, visual perception, and motor speed and accuracy on neuropsychometric tests[5]; some only showed slowing of the electroencephalogram (EEG).[6] These observations led to this early stage of HE being added to established grading systems.[7]

The prevalence of minimal HE ranges between 30 and 60 percent of patients with HE. Variations in prevalence estimates are due to differences in methods used for diagnosis and population differences regarding underlying liver disorders.

It has been suggested that minimal and grade I HE should be merged into a new class termed "covert HE" as grade I HE may only be apparent to clinicians with experience in neurologic assessment.[8] More detailed clinical examination of HE patients yields a higher number with grade I HE and fewer with minimal HE. In one study, among patients initially thought to be clinically unimpaired, bradykinesia, tremor, and hyperactive muscle stretch reflexes were detected in about 30 percent when examined in detail, and 50 percent of these patients showed eye movement abnormalities indicating cerebellar dysfunction.[9]

Encephalopathy in Acute Liver Failure

In diagnosing acute liver failure (ALF), the presence of HE is a prerequisite in patients with jaundice, coagulopathy, and no preexisting liver disease. Thus, HE is present by definition in all patients with ALF. In contrast, clinically overt HE is prevalent in 10 to 14 percent of all cirrhotic patients, and in about 20 percent of patients with decompensated cirrhosis.[10] The risk of developing recurrent HE is 40 percent within 1 year.[11]

In contrast to HE in patients with liver cirrhosis, HE with ALF may be complicated by significant brain edema (25 to 35% in grade III; 65 to 75% in grade IV).[12] Currently there seems to be a decline in the prevalence of brain edema in patients with ALF for unclear reasons. An analysis of the case records of 3,305 patients with ALF or acute liver injury from King's College Hospital, London, between 1973 and 2008 showed that the proportion of patients with intracranial hypertension fell from 76 percent in the period from 1984 to 1988 to 20 percent in 2004 to 2008. Multivariate analysis showed an association of intracranial hypertension with younger age, female gender, and elevated international normalized ratio (INR).[13]

ALF patients usually present initially as restless, agitated, and irritable, whereas HE in patients with cirrhosis usually begins with psychomotor slowing. With increasing grade of HE, clinical presentations are more similar, as depressed consciousness predominates. Extrapyramidal symptoms are not typically observed in patients with ALF, but signs of corticospinal tract dysfunction are present.[14] Seizures are a frequent complication of ALF, but occur only rarely in patients with cirrhosis.

Diagnosis of Forms of Hepatic Encephalopathy

The diagnosis of HE can only be made after exclusion of other possible causes of brain dysfunction, as the symptoms are not specific. Hyponatremia, hypo- or hyperglycemia, uremia, diabetes mellitus, and renal dysfunction are frequent in patients with cirrhosis and may resemble HE. Other important disorders to distinguish are septic encephalopathy and Wernicke encephalopathy.[15] In a neuropathologic study of the brains of 32 patients with cirrhosis who died with HE, cerebellar lesions suggestive of Wernicke encephalopathy were observed in 50 percent; the diagnosis of Wernicke encephalopathy was made in 9 patients, whereas in only 2 patients had the diagnosis been made clinically.[16]

Due to altered coagulation, intracranial hemorrhage must be considered in the differential diagnosis of HE, and brain imaging should be obtained in all patients, usually with noncontrast computed tomography (CT). Magnetic resonance imaging (MRI) requires much more cooperation than CT, and thus is not practical in agitated patients.

Hepatic encephalopathy may occasionally present with focal neurologic symptoms such as dysphasia or hemiparesis. Of 10 observed focal presentations of HE, only 2 were due to intracranial hemorrhage.[17]

CIRRHOSIS-RELATED PARKINSONISM

In patients with cirrhosis who develop clinical signs of extrapyramidal motor dysfunction, the differential diagnosis includes acquired hepatocerebral degeneration or an independent neurodegenerative disease. The course of the disease and the symptom combination may help to differentiate between these entities.[2]

The clinical features of cirrhosis-related parkinsonism resemble those of patients with PD. As discussed earlier, however, symptoms in PD are more often asymmetric, develop more slowly, may be associated with early gait abnormalities, are not accompanied by cerebellar or corticospinal deficits, and respond well to dopaminergic drugs.

More difficult is the distinction from multiple system atrophy (MSA), which combines extrapyramidal symptoms with cerebellar and pyramidal deficits and thereby can resemble cirrhosis-related parkinsonism. MSA likewise shows rapid progression and often a poor response to dopaminergic agents. In contrast to patients with cirrhosis-related parkinsonism, however, patients with MSA characteristically show severe autonomic dysfunction and many show alterations of the basal ganglia, midbrain, and cerebellum on MRI.[18] Single-photon emission computed tomography (SPECT) in patients with cirrhosis-related parkinsonism shows a decreased binding capacity of striatal dopamine receptors and the dopamine transporter similar to the findings in MSA but different from those in PD, in which there is decreased availability of the transporter but not of the receptors.[2,19]

HEPATIC MYELOPATHY

A diagnosis of hepatic myelopathy can be based on the clinical findings of myelopathy and exclusion of other possible causes through MRI and cerebrospinal fluid analysis, both of which are normal in hepatic myelopathy.[4]

MINIMAL HEPATIC ENCEPHALOPATHY

The diagnosis of minimal HE depends on the results of neuropsychologic or neurophysiologic examinations in the setting of a normal clinical examination. Debate about the most useful method for diagnosing minimal HE is ongoing. Currently the PSE Syndrome Test, Inhibition Control Test, critical flicker frequency analysis, and automated EEG analysis are the most frequently used methods.[1,20] A combination of the number connection tests A and B and either the digit symbol test or the block design test, or both, are used as an alternative. Working groups commissioned to elaborate an expert recommendation for diagnosing minimal HE agreed on the PSE Syndrome Test as valuable, objective, and reliable. For the United States, the Repeatable Battery for the Assessment of Neuropsychological Status (RBANS) has been recommended as an alternative, because it is a valid, objective, and reliable test battery, and there are no US norms for the PSE Syndrome Test. However, the RBANS has only rarely be used for diagnosing minimal HE, and thus data regarding its suitability for this purpose are sparse.[21,22]

The PSE Syndrome Test is a battery of five paper-pencil tests: the number connection tests A and B, the digit symbol test, the serial dotting test, and the line-tracing test.[5,23] The latter is evaluated by measuring the time needed to perform the test and the number of errors that occur. Thus, six subtest results are scored compared to normative values. A sum score termed the portosystemic hepatic encephalopathy score (PHES) is generated ranging between +6 and −18 points; scores lower than −4 are considered pathologic. The PHES correlates significantly with cerebral glucose utilization at rest in patients with minimal HE.[24] It is a reliable predictor of the risk of developing overt HE as well as of mortality.[25]

The critical flicker frequency is a psychophysiologic test that has been used in the past for the assessment of central nervous system drug effects. It was recommended for diagnosing minimal HE in 2002.[26] Light pulses are presented to the subject in decreasing frequency (usually from 60 Hz downwards), and the subject has to react as soon as the impression of fused light switches to flickering light. The critical flicker frequency depends on the experimental setting—the color and luminance of the stimuli, distance between the light source and the subject's eye, visual angle, and subject age. The assessment requires intact binocular vision and absence of red-green blindness. Normative data have to be elaborated for the specific equipment used. The results correlate with the portosystemic hepatic encephalopathy score and can predict the development of overt HE.[27] Of note, scores in patients with alcoholic cirrhosis are lower than in patients with cirrhosis due to other causes.[26] The results may be affected by propofol given during endoscopy, though only temporarily.[28]

The Inhibitory Control Test (ICT) has been recommended for diagnosing minimal HE as well.[29] It is freely available online (www.hecme.tv) and is a test of attention and response inhibition. Results depend on age and education and are compared with normative values.[30,31]

The Continuous Reaction Time Test (CRT) requires a simple reaction to a series of 500-Hz tones. With developing HE, not only reaction time but especially the variability of reaction times increases. The reaction time variability is represented by the so-called CRT index, which is calculated from the 50th reaction time percentile/(90th−10th percentile). Recently it was shown that the CRT index does not depend on age or sex, and is more sensitive for cerebral dysfunction in patients with liver cirrhosis than the critical flicker frequency test.[32,33]

The EEG has been used for diagnosing HE for decades after the observation that the amount of theta and delta activity increases with increasing grade of HE. This initially is associated with an increase in amplitude and the appearance of triphasic waves, followed in later stages by a decrease in amplitude, a discontinuous pattern, and finally isoelectricity in patients with coma (Fig. 12-2).[34] Occasionally it is unaltered in spite of clinically overt HE.[35] Quantitative EEG analysis shows a decrease in the mean dominant frequency and an increase in theta and delta activity in only 15 to 30 percent of patients with cirrhosis having no clinical signs of HE, and in up to 40 percent of patients with clinically overt HE. Thus EEG appears more appropriate for serially following the progression of HE than for diagnosis.

Computerized EEG analysis continues to be refined, but diagnostic utility is limited at this time.[36]

Increased Intracranial Pressure in Acute Liver Failure

The percentage of patients with brain edema and increased intracranial pressure increases with more severe grades of HE in patients with ALF.[12] Since intubation and sedation are required in these patients, brain edema cannot always be detected by clinical examination. Repeated brain imaging may show the development of cerebral edema but is not feasible. Continuous monitoring of intracranial pressure (ICP) is recommended by some clinicians,[37] but the coagulopathy that accompanies ALF holds a significant risk of intracranial bleeding. As a result, ICP monitoring is not standard in the management of patients with ALF. Studies have shown no difference in mortality between patients who underwent or did not undergo ICP monitoring.[14,38]

Neuroimaging

Brain imaging in HE is used to exclude other possible causes of brain dysfunction such as intracranial hemorrhage or Wernicke encephalopathy. MRI, however, may not be feasible in HE patients because of lack of cooperation due to alterations of consciousness.

Although MRI of the brain in patients with cirrhosis shows characteristic symmetric signal change with predominance in the pallidum on T1-weighted sequences, these MRI findings cannot be used to diagnose HE since some patients may show signal change with no signs of HE and others may be severely affected by HE without MRI abnormalites.[9,39] These MRI changes are thought to be due to deposition of manganese in the brain and correlate with serum manganese levels in patients with cirrhosis.[40,41] It is still controversial whether the extent of MRI signal change is related to the extent of extrapyramidal symptoms; although these MRI changes fade over about 1 year following successful liver transplantation, the clinical symptoms of HE usually disappear immediately.[42–44]

Laboratory Studies

There are no laboratory parameters that can aid in making the diagnosis of HE. Plasma ammonia levels follow the clinical course in an individual patient, but there is no clear correlation between them and the degree of HE.[45] However, if plasma ammonia is

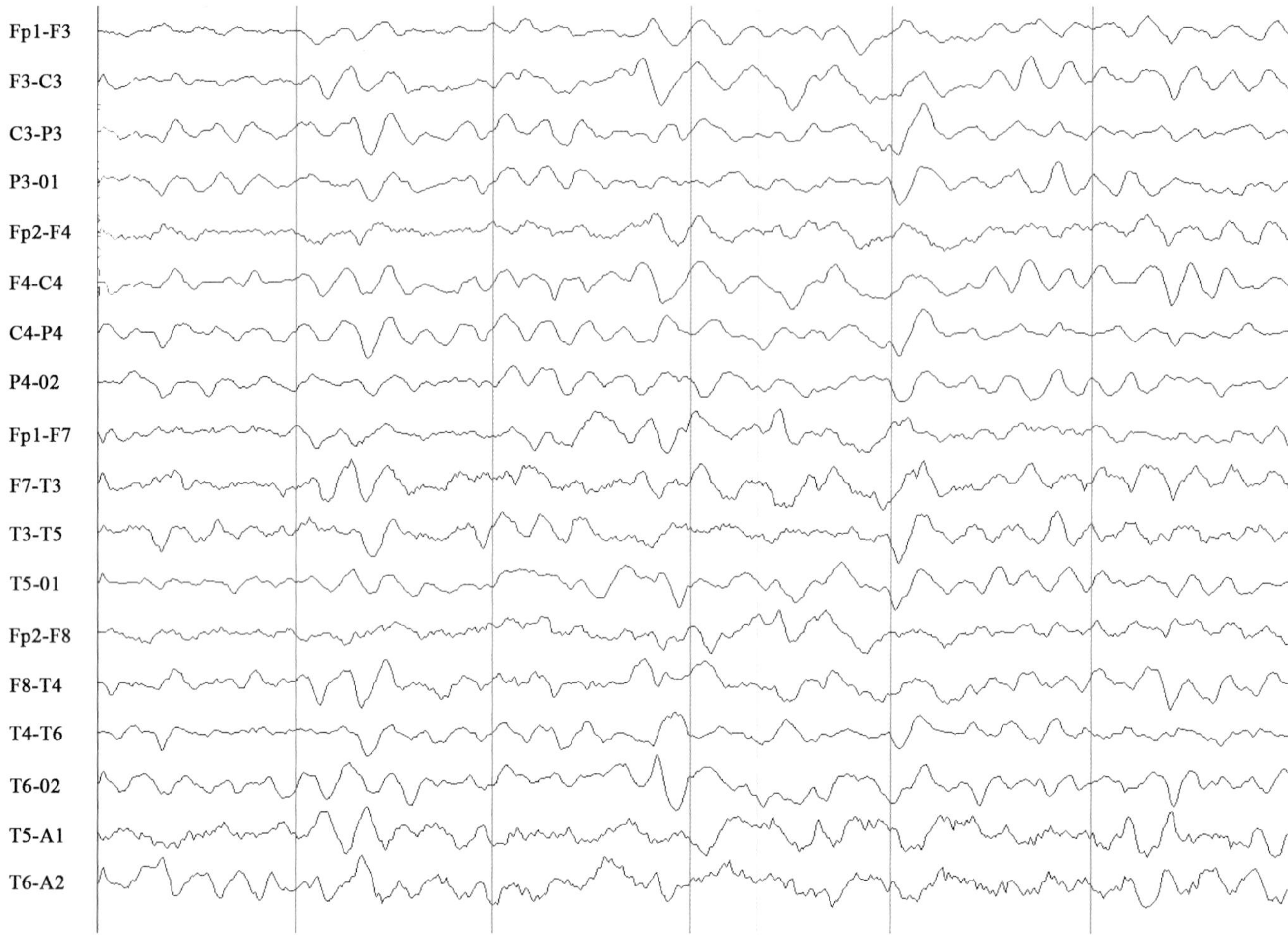

FIGURE 12-2 ▪ The EEG of a patient with hepatic encephalopathy (grade II according to the West Haven criteria). The portosystemic hepatic encephalopathy score was −17. The EEG shows diffuse slow activity (mean dominant frequency 4.49) with triphasic components. Time marker, 1 second.

normal in a patient with liver cirrhosis and severe alteration of consciousness, the diagnosis of HE should be questioned.

Pathophysiology

The pathophysiology of HE is still incompletely understood, although ammonia and inflammatory cytokines likely play a major role.[46,47] Blood ammonia levels may increase in patients with liver cirrhosis up to 300 μmol/L, but range between normal levels (up to 40 μmol/L) and 100 μmol/L in the majority of patients.[45] Although there is a correlation between plasma ammonia level and the grade of HE, there is substantial overlap, indicating that other factors besides hyperammonemia play a role in the development of HE.[45–47] Increased blood ammonia levels are accompanied by an increase in cerebral ammonia concentration; in the brain, ammonia is detoxified in astrocytes by glutamine synthesis. Increased cerebral ammonia levels induce glutamine synthase activity, glutamate uptake, and glutamine production leading to osmotic pressure and water uptake.[48] Inhibition of glutamine release from astrocytes due to a downregulation of glutamine transporters adds to cell swelling unless other osmolytes such as *myo*-inositol are released in compensation.

Astrocyte swelling is considered the key factor in the pathogenesis of HE as it triggers multiple alterations of cell function and gene expression.[49] Astrocyte swelling induces the formation of reactive oxygen and nitrogen oxide species, including nitric oxide (NO), which in turn induce further astrocyte swelling.[50–52] Part of this cycle leads to a collapse of the mitochondrial inner membrane potential, swelling of the mitochondrial matrix, defective oxidative phosphorylation, cessation of adenosine triphosphate (ATP) synthesis, and finally the generation of reactive oxygen species.[53]

HE in patients with cirrhosis is often precipitated by electrolyte disturbances, benzodiazepines, or infection. Astrocyte swelling may be induced also by inflammatory cytokines, hyponatremia, or benzodiazepines.[49] The vulnerability of the brain to these precipitating factors depends on the amount of astrocytic osmolyte depletion that has taken place prior to the insult; for example, lower *myo*-inositol levels increase the risk of developing neuropsychiatric symptoms in response to a protein load.[54]

The toxic effects of ammonia and inflammatory cytokines are amplified by intracerebral manganese deposition in patients with hepatic cirrhosis, due to impaired biliary manganese excretion.[40,41] Manganese increases ammonia toxicity in astrocyte cultures and alters dopaminergic neurotransmission.[55,56] Brain autopsy examinations show that manganese deposition causes cell loss and gliosis in the globus pallidus, caudate, putamen, and subthalamic nucleus.[57]

HE in its episodic form is not accompanied by significant neuronal alterations, but the size and number of Alzheimer type II astrocytes increases. The extent of this astrocytosis correlates with the severity of HE and blood ammonia levels.[58] Neuronal cell death is considerably less than would be expected considering the numerous cell death mechanisms present in this condition, such as NMDA receptor–mediated excitotoxicity, oxidative/nitrosative stress, and the presence of proinflammatory cytokines.[59] It has been hypothesized that the extent of neuronal damage in liver failure may be attenuated by compensatory mechanisms including downregulation of NMDA receptors or the presence of neuroprotective steroids such as allopregnanolone.[59] In contrast to patients with episodic HE, patients with acquired hepatocerebral degeneration show neuronal degeneration in the deep layers of cerebral cortex and subcortical white matter, particularly in the parieto-occipital cortex, basal ganglia, and cerebellum. The reason that some patients are more susceptible than others to progressive neuronal degeneration is unknown.

In patients with ALF, blood ammonia levels are increased markedly and correlate with high ICP, severity of clinical presentation, and death due to cerebral herniation.[60–63] However, ammonia-lowering strategies have not been shown to be effective in treating HE and brain edema in ALF.[64] Additional mechanisms of injury may involve proinflammatory cytokines; serum levels of tumor necrosis factor-α (TNF-α) and interleukin 6 are invariably increased in ALF patients and relate to the severity of HE.[65,66] The presence of a systemic inflammatory response syndrome (SIRS) has been identified as predictor of HE progression in patients with ALF due to acetaminophen overdose.[67] Current models explaining brain dysfunction in ALF suggest a simultaneous reaction between systemic proinflammatory cytokines and a neuroinflammatory response to the increase of cerebral ammonia, with a corresponding increase in cerebral lactate level.[68] The cause of the increased lactate level is not known—it was previously thought to be the consequence of an alteration of energy metabolism but currently is attributed to an altered astrocyte–neuron lactate shuttle, as high-energy phosphate levels are unaltered in animal models of ALF.[48]

The reasons for the development of increased ICP in ALF are still unclear. Cytotoxic cerebral edema occurs in ALF, but the occurrence of vasogenic edema is controversial.[68] Pathologic studies of patients who died with ALF have not shown evidence of a breakdown of the blood–brain barrier.[69] However, in patients with ALF and a concomitant infection or sepsis, blood–brain barrier breakdown may occur as it does in many forms of septic encephalopathy. An increase in cerebral blood flow due to an alteration of cerebrovascular autoregulation may also play a role in the development of increased ICP in ALF.

Treatment

Hepatic Encephalopathy in Cirrhosis

Most HE episodes in patients with cirrhosis are precipitated by medications such as diuretics or sedatives, excessive protein intake, gastrointestinal bleeding, or infection. Correction of these precipitating factors is the basis of any initial therapy in these patients. In addition, treatment with drugs that reduce gut ammonia production and absorption is recommended. The most frequently used medication for this purpose is lactulose. The initial dose should be 50 ml of lactulose syrup every 1 to 2 hours until at least two bowel movements are produced. Thereafter, the dose should be reduced to produce two to three bowel movements per day (30 to 60 g or 45 to 90 ml daily). A meta-analysis of lactulose trials did not support lactulose as an effective therapeutic agent for the treatment of overt HE.[70] This conclusion was reached mainly because the majority of studies did not fulfil current quality criteria, and many clinicians still recommend the use of lactulose as first-line therapy in patients with overt HE.[71]

When a patient's condition does not improve with lactulose, and concomitant disorders that might impair brain function have been excluded, lactulose should be combined with antibiotics, which also reduce gut ammonia production and absorption. In the past, the most often used antibiotics were neomycin and metronidazole. A randomized, double-blind trial comparing neomycin to placebo in episodic HE demonstrated a more rapid, though not significant, symptomatic improvement in patients treated with neomycin.[72] This trial was underpowered, limiting the conclusions to be drawn from it. The use of neomycin is limited by its unfavorable side effects, including ototoxicity and nephrotoxicity. Neomycin has been replaced by rifaximin, which has minimal side effects and good efficacy in the treatment of HE.[73]

In some countries, L-ornithine L-aspartate (LOLA) is also used for the treatment of overt HE in conjunction with lactulose. Data on its efficacy are sparse. It appears to be more effective with more severe HE (grades II to IV).[71] Branched-chain amino acids (BCAA) have also been used for treating HE but have not found general acceptance. A meta-analysis of 11 trials involving 556 patients (only 3 of whom had ALF) found an improvement with treatment in 59 percent compared to 41 percent in the control group.[74] Nevertheless the authors concluded that there was no convincing evidence of benefit because an "effect was not seen when only trials of high quality were included." Indeed the trial design, patient assessment, and the severity of HE differed significantly between these 11 trials. A recent update of this meta-analysis including three further trials, however, confirmed the beneficial effect of BCAA on HE, though limited to oral application of the drug.[75]

Prevention of Further Spells

Although lactulose is frequently used for the prevention of HE episodes, data supporting its use for this purpose are scant. A single-center, unblinded, randomized-controlled study showed less recurrence of HE with lactulose therapy than with placebo.[11] This positive effect was also observed in cirrhotic patients with gastrointestinal bleeding.[76] In one study, lactulose, probiotics, and no therapy were compared for prevention in 235 patients who had recovered from an HE episode.[77] Both lactulose and probiotics were significantly more effective than no therapy in preventing a further HE episode during a 12-month follow-up period. A positive effect of lactulose for preventing HE episodes was also shown in patients with cirrhosis without a history of overt HE, supporting its use for primary prevention.[78] Among the patients, 55 percent had minimal HE. Minimal HE responded to lactulose in 66 percent of cases, while improving spontaneously in only 25 percent.

In a double-blind, randomized, placebo-controlled trial, rifaximin was found to significantly reduce the risk of HE recurrence as well as the frequency of hospitalization for HE.[79]

The impact of branched-chain amino-acid supplementation on the recurrence of HE was studied in 116 patients who had been hospitalized for an episode of HE in the prior 2 months. Recurrence of HE was not prevented, although performance on some neuropsychologic tests was improved compared with controls.[80]

Minimal Hepatic Encephalopathy

Whether minimal HE should be treated is controversial, and data on the therapeutic effects of drugs are sparse. Since cognitive changes can impair quality of life, many physicians consider treating these patients. Minimal HE responds to lactulose.[78] A meta-analysis of 9 studies involving 434 patients showed a significant effect of lactulose on neuropsychologic test results, health-related quality of life, and the risk of progression to overt HE.[81] In a recent study, lactulose, probiotics, and LOLA each had significant and comparable beneficial effects on minimal HE and health-related quality of life compared to no therapy.[82] Rifaximin also improved cognitive function and health-related quality of life in these patients with minimal HE.[83]

Cirrhosis-Related Parkinsonism and Hepatic Myelopathy

Cirrhosis-related parkinsonism does not respond to ammonia-lowering therapies but may respond to dopaminergic drugs.[2] Liver transplantation is also sometimes helpful, but only a few cases have been reported. Patients unresponsive to lactulose may improve with rifaximin therapy.[84] Hepatic myelopathy similarly fails to respond to ammonia-lowering therapies but liver transplantation may lead to an improvement in walking ability.[2,4,85]

Hepatic Encephalopathy in Acute Liver Failure

In patients with ALF, treatment of HE and brain edema is aimed at reducing levels of plasma ammonia and systemic cytokines. A basic treatment strategy is the prophylactic use of antibiotics and antifungals along with early renal support to allow highly efficacious ammonia removal.[86] Persistent hyperammonemia above 122 µmol/L for more than 3 days is associated with an increased risk of developing brain edema, seizures, and death.[87] Drugs that are used for the reduction of plasma ammonia levels in patients with cirrhosis such as lactulose or LOLA have not shown a significant beneficial effect in ALF.[12,64] Lactulose treatment is discouraged because gaseous distension of the bowel may impede liver transplantation surgery.[12]

Hyponatremia is one of the causes of brain edema and intracranial hypertension in patients with ALF. Therefore normalization and even a slight elevation of plasma sodium levels up to 155 mEq/L (mmol/L) is recommended.[12] Intracranial pressure has been shown to decrease significantly in patients in whom serum sodium levels were maintained in a range of 145 to 155 mEq/L (mmol/L).[88]

Moderate hypothermia (32°C to 34°C) has been demonstrated to reduce plasma levels of proinflammatory cytokines and elevated intracranial pressure in patients awaiting emergency liver transplantation.[89] Whether hypothermia should become part of ALF management in all patients who develop brain edema remains unclear and is the subject of ongoing studies.[90]

Brain edema in patients with ALF is currently treated with mannitol infusion every 6 hours (1 g mannitol/kg body weight) or, in cases with ICP monitoring, in response to ICP increases above 20 to 25 mmHg; mannitol should be held if serum osmolality exceeds 320 mOsm/L or in patients with oliguric renal dysfunction.[12] ICP monitoring is often not feasible due to severe coagulopathy.

To maintain a sufficient cerebral perfusion pressure of 60 to 80 mmHg, mean arterial blood pressure should be raised in patients with hypotension to greater than 75 mmHg through repletion of intravascular volume with normal saline and the use of vasopressors (e.g., vasopressin and norepinephrine).[12] One of the most important tasks in the treatment of patients with ALF is the identification of those who will need liver transplantation; the King's College criteria are frequently used for this purpose.[91]

PANCREATIC ENCEPHALOPATHY

Definition and Clinical Features

Pancreatic encephalopathy is a controversial entity consisting of a confusional state due to acute pancreatitis. The underlying pathophysiology remains unclear. Since acute pancreatitis is accompanied by the systemic inflammatory response syndrome (SIRS), electrolyte abnormalities, hypotension, renal failure, acute respiratory distress syndrome, disseminated intravascular coagulation, and hyperglycemia, all of which can induce brain dysfunction, the delineation of a discrete disease is difficult.[92] There is some evidence that pancreatic enzymes themselves are involved in the development of a metabolic encepalopathy. The activation of phospholipase A by trypsin and bile acid likely plays a key role in the pathophysiology of pancreatic encephalopathy. Activated phospholipase A converts lecithin and cephalin into their hemolytic forms. Phospholipase A and hemolytic lecithin then may destroy the blood–brain barrier, resulting in demyelination, hemorrhage, and edema due to increased vascular permeability.[93] Neuropathologic studies of patients who died with pancreatic encephalopathy show capillary necrosis with diffuse petechial hemorrhages, encephalomalacia, and perivascular demyelination.[93,94]

Pancreatic encephalopathy usually begins within 2 weeks after the onset of acute pancreatitis, most often between the second and fifth day.[93] Clinical symptoms, which may fluctuate, include disorientation, confusion, agitation, anxiety, irritability, delirium, hallucinations, dysarthria, ataxia, akinetic mutism, rigidity, hemiparesis, hyperreflexia, and seizures. Patients may develop stupor and coma.[92–96] In a 7-year follow-up case report, recurrence of neurologic symptoms occurred with each relapse of pancreatitis, and a close relationship was found between serum amylase levels and the occurrence of neurologic symptoms.[96] Neuropsychiatric symptoms do not correlate in severity with the pancreatitis, and improvement of these symptoms may lag behind recovery from pancreatitis.[93,95,96] The mortality rate from pancreatic encephalopathy is estimated to be as high as 50 percent.[97]

Diagnosis

Pancreatic encephalopathy should be suspected in any patient with severe abdominal pain and altered consciousness. Since neither symptoms nor laboratory or imaging results are specific for the disorder, the diagnosis can only be made after exclusion of other possible causes of brain dysfunction. The EEG typically shows generalized slowing. The cerebrospinal fluid may show a mild increase in protein and glucose concentration, but is normal in most cases. In a few cases, lipase concentrations in the cerebrospinal fluid have been assessed and were slightly elevated.[93] There are only a few reports of brain MRI findings in patients with pancreatic encephalopathy and these describe predominantly diffuse or scattered white matter abnormalities.[94,98,99] Abnormalities of the pons and cerebellar peduncles have been seen on diffusion-weighted and fluid-attenuated inversion recovery (FLAIR) sequences. A case of pancreatic encephalopathy associated with pontine and extrapontine myelinolysis involving the brain and spinal cord has been described.[99]

Treatment

There are no standard recommendations for the treatment of pancreatic encephalopathy other than supportive therapy along with treatment of the underlying pancreatitis. In one study, a significant decrease was found in the frequency of pancreatic encephalopathy in patients with acute pancreatitis treated with low-molecular-weight heparin compared to a control group.[100] This effect may result from a reduction in pancreatitis-associated microvascular disturbances and hemorrhagic necrosis.

Patients with pancreatitis are also at risk of developing Wernicke encephalopathy due to hyperemesis, anorexia, and the necessity of prolonged total parenteral nutrition. Thiamine deficiency should be considered in these patients and treated prophylactically.

REFERENCES

1. Ferenci P, Lockwood A, Mullen K, et al: Hepatic encephalopathy—definition, nomenclature, diagnosis, and quantification: final report of the working party at the 11th World Congresses of Gastroenterology, Vienna, 1998. Hepatology 35:716, 2002.
2. Tryc AB, Goldbecker A, Berding G, et al: Cirrhosis-related parkinsonism: prevalence, mechanisms and response to treatments. J Hepatol 58:698, 2012.
3. Ferrara J, Jankovic J: Acquired hepatocerebral degeneration. J Neurol 256:320, 2009.
4. Weissenborn K, Tietge UJ, Bokemeyer M, et al: Liver transplantation improves hepatic myelopathy: evidence by three cases. Gastroenterology 124:346, 2003.
5. Weissenborn K, Ennen JC, Schomerus H, et al: Neuropsychological characterization of hepatic encephalopathy. J Hepatol 34:768, 2001.
6. Weissenborn K, Scholz M, Hinrichs H, et al: Neurophysiological assessment of early hepatic encephalopathy. Electroencephalogr Clin Neurophysiol 75:289, 1990.
7. Lockwood AH: "What's in a name?" Improving the care of cirrhotics. J Hepatol 32:859, 2000.
8. Bajaj JS, Cordoba J, Mullen KD, et al: International Society for Hepatic Encephalopathy and Nitrogen Metabolism (ISHEN). Review article: the design of clinical trials in hepatic encephalopathy—an International Society for Hepatic Encephalopathy and Nitrogen Metabolism (ISHEN) consensus statement. Aliment Pharmacol Ther 33:739, 2011.
9. Krieger S, Jauss M, Jansen O, et al: Neuropsychiatric profile and hyperintense globus pallidus on T1-weighted magnetic resonance images in liver cirrhosis. Gastroenterology 111:147, 1996.
10. Coltorti M, Del Vecchio-Blanco C, Caporaso N, et al: Liver cirrhosis in Italy. A multicentre study on presenting modalities and the impact on health care resources. National Project on Liver Cirrhosis Group. Ital J Gastroenterol 23:42, 1991.
11. Sharma BC, Sharma P, Agarwal A, Sarin SK: Secondary prophylaxis of hepatic encephalopathy: an open-label randomized controlled trial of lactulose versus placebo. Gastroenterology 137:885, 2009.
12. Lee WM, Larson AM, Stravitz RT: AASLD position paper: the management of acute liver failure: update 2011. www.aasld.org, 2011.
13. Bernal W, Hyyrylainen A, Gera A, et al: Lessons from look-back in acute liver failure? A single centre experience of 3,300 patients. J Hepatol 59:74, 2013.
14. Shawcross DL, Wendon JA: The neurological manifestations of acute liver failure. Neurochem Int 60:662, 2012.
15. Butterworth RF: Thiamine deficiency-related brain dysfunction in chronic liver failure. Metab Brain Dis 24:189, 2009.
16. Kril JJ, Butterworth RF: Diencephalic and cerebellar pathology in alcoholic and nonalcoholic patients with end-stage liver disease. Hepatology 26:837, 1997.
17. Cadranel JF, Lebiez E, Di Martino V, et al: Focal neurological signs in hepatic encephalopathy in cirrhotic patients: an underestimated entity? Am J Gastroenterol 96:515, 2001.

18. Mahlknecht P, Hotter A, Hussl A, et al: Significance of MRI in diagnosis and differential diagnosis of Parkinson's disease. Neurodegener Dis 7:300, 2010.
19. Isaias IU, Antonini A: Single-photon emission computed tomography in diagnosis and differential diagnosis of Parkinson's disease. Neurodegener Dis 7:319, 2010.
20. Randolph C, Hilsabeck R, Kato A, et al: International Society for Hepatic Encephalopathy and Nitrogen Metabolism (ISHEN). Neuropsychological assessment of hepatic encephalopathy: ISHEN practice guidelines. Liver Int 29:629, 2009.
21. Randolph C: The Repeatable Battery for the Assessment of Neuropsychological Status (RBANS). The Psychological Corporation, San Antonio, 1998.
22. Mooney S, Hasssanein TI, Hilsabeck RC, et al: Utility of the Repeatable Battery for the Assessment of Neuropsychological Status (RBANS) in patients with end-stage liver disease awaiting liver transplant. Arch Clin Neuropsychol 22:175, 2007.
23. Schomerus H, Weissenborn K, Hamster W, et al: PSE-Syndrom-Test. Swets Test Services. Swets & Zeitlinger, Frankfurt, 1999.
24. Lockwood AH, Weissenborn K, Bokemeyer M, et al: Correlations between cerebral glucose metabolism and neuropsychological test performance in nonalcoholic cirrhotics. Metab Brain Dis 17:29, 2002.
25. Dhiman RK, Kurmi R, Thumburu KK, et al: Diagnosis and prognostic significance of minimal hepatic encephalopathy in patients with cirrhosis of liver. Dig Dis Sci 55:2381, 2010.
26. Kircheis G, Wettstein M, Timmermann L, et al: Critical flicker frequency for quantification of low-grade hepatic encephalopathy. Hepatology 35:357, 2002.
27. Romero-Gómez M, Córdoba J, Jover R, et al: Value of the critical flicker frequency in patients with minimal hepatic encephalopathy. Hepatology 45:879, 2007.
28. Sharma P, Singh S, Sharma BC, et al: Propofol sedation during endoscopy in patients with cirrhosis, and utility of psychometric tests and critical flicker frequency in assessment of recovery from sedation. Endoscopy 43:400, 2011.
29. Bajaj JS, Saeian K, Verber MD, et al: Inhibitory control test is a simple method to diagnose minimal hepatic encephalopathy and predict development of overt hepatic encephalopathy. Am J Gastroenterol 102:754, 2007.
30. Amodio P, Ridola L, Schiff S, et al: Improving the inhibitory control task to detect minimal hepatic encephalopathy. Gastroenterology 139:510, 2010.
31. Goldbecker A, Weissenborn K, Hamidi Shahrezaei G, et al: Comparison of the most favoured methods for the diagnosis of hepatic encephalopathy in liver transplantation candidates. Gut 62:1497, 2013.
32. Lauridsen MM, Grønbæk H, Næser EB, et al: Gender and age effects on the continuous reaction times method in volunteers and patients with cirrhosis. Metab Brain Dis 27:559, 2012.
33. Lauridsen MM, Jepsen P, Vilstrup H: Critical flicker frequency and continuous reaction times for the diagnosis of minimal hepatic encephalopathy: a comparative study of 154 patients with liver disease. Metab Brain Dis 26:135, 2011.
34. Guerit JM, Amantini A, Fischer C, et al: Members of the ISHEN Commission on Neurophysiological Investigations. Neurophysiological investigations of hepatic encephalopathy: ISHEN practice guidelines. Liver Int 29:789, 2009.
35. Montagnese S, Jackson C, Morgan MY: Spatio-temporal decomposition of the electroencephalogram in patients with cirrhosis. J Hepatol 46:447, 2007.
36. Marchetti P, D'Avanzo C, Orsato R, et al: Electroencephalography in patients with cirrhosis. Gastroenterology 141:1680, 2011.
37. Frontera JA, Kalb T: Neurological management of fulminant hepatic failure. Neurocrit Care 14:318, 2011.
38. Vaquero J: Complications and use of intracranial pressure monitoring in patients with acute liver failure and severe encephalopathy. Liver Transpl 11:1581, 2005.
39. Lockwood AH, Weissenborn K, Butterworth RF: An image of the brain in patients with liver disease. Curr Opin Neurol 10:525, 1997.
40. Pomier-Layrargues G, Spahr L, Butterworth R: Increased manganese concentration in pallidum of cirrhotic patients. Lancet 345:735, 1995.
41. Rose C, Butterworth RF, Zayed J, et al: Manganese deposition in basal ganglia structures results from both portal-systemic shunting and liver dysfunction. Gastroenterology 117:640, 1999.
42. Spahr L, Burkhard PR, Grötzsch H, et al: Clinical significance of basal ganglia alterations at brain MRI and 1H MRS in cirrhosis and role in the pathogenesis of hepatic encephalopathy. Metab Brain Dis 17:399, 2002.
43. Burkhard PR, Delavelle J, Du Pasquier R, et al: Chronic parkinsonism associated with cirrhosis: a distinct subset of acquired hepatocerebral degeneration. Arch Neurol 60:521, 2003.
44. Weissenborn K, Ehrenheim C, Hori A, et al: Pallidal lesions in patients with liver cirrhosis: clinical and MRI evaluation. Metab Brain Dis 10:219, 1995.
45. Ong JP, Aggarwal A, Krieger D, et al: Correlation between ammonia levels and the severity of hepatic encephalopathy. Am J Med 114:188, 2003.
46. Shawcross DL, Olde Damink SWM, Butterworth RF, et al: Ammonia and hepatic encephalopathy: the more things change, the more they remain the same. Metab Brain Dis 20:169, 2005.
47. Butterworth RF: Pathophysiology of hepatic encephalopathy: a new look at ammonia. Metab Brain Dis 17:221, 2002.
48. Bosoi CR, Rose CF: Brain edema in acute liver failure and chronic liver disease: similarities and differences. Neurochem Int 62:446, 2013.

49. Häussinger D, Schliess F: Pathogenetic mechanisms of hepatic encephalopathy. Gut 57:1156, 2008.
50. Görg B, Qvartskhava N, Keitel V, et al: Ammonia induces RNA oxidation in cultured astrocytes and brain in vivo. Hepatology 48:567, 2008.
51. Görg B, Qvartskhava N, Bidmon H-J, et al: Oxidative stress markers in the brain of patients with cirrhosis and hepatic encephalopathy. Hepatology 52:256, 2010.
52. Schliess F, Görg B, Häussinger D: Pathogenetic interplay between osmotic and oxidative stress: the hepatic encephalopathy paradigm. Biol Chem 387:1363, 2006.
53. Norenberg MD, Rama Rao KV, Jayakumar AR: Signaling factors in the mechanism of ammonia neurotoxicity. Metab Brain Dis 24:103, 2009.
54. Shawcross DL, Balata S, Olde-Damink SW, et al: Low myo-inositol and high glutamine levels in brain are associated with neuropsychological deterioration after induced hyperammonemia. Am J Physiol 287:G503, 2004.
55. Jayakumar AR, Rama Rao KV, Kalaiselvi P, et al: Combined effects of ammonia and manganese on astrocytes in culture. Neurochem Res 29:2051, 2004.
56. Aschner M, Guilarte TR, Schneider JS, et al: Manganese: recent advances in understanding its transport and neurotoxicity. Toxicol Appl Pharmacol 221:131, 2007.
57. Butterworth RF, Spahr L, Fontaine S, Layrargues GP: Manganese toxicity, dopaminergic dysfunction and hepatic encephalopathy. Metab Brain Dis 10:259, 1995.
58. Martin H, Voss K, Hufnagl P, et al: Morphometric and densitometric investigations of protoplasmic astrocytes and neurons in human hepatic encephalopathy. Exp Pathol 32:241, 1987.
59. Butterworth RF: Neuronal cell death in hepatic encephalopathy. Metab Brain Dis 22:309, 2007.
60. Vaquero J, Chung C, Cahill ME, et al: Pathogenesis of hepatic encephalopathy in acute liver failure. Semin Liver Dis 23:259, 2003.
61. Bernal W, Hall C, Karvellas CJ, et al: Arterial ammonia and clinical risk factors for encephalopathy and intracranial hypertension in acute liver failure. Hepatology 46:1844, 2007.
62. Clemmesen JO, Larsen FS, Kondrup J, et al: Cerebral herniation in patients with acute liver failure is correlated with arterial ammonia concentration. Hepatology 29:648, 1999.
63. Tofteng F, Hauerberg J, Hansen BA, et al: Persistent arterial hyperammonemia increases the concentration of glutamine and alanine in the brain and correlates with intracranial pressure in patients with fulminant hepatic failure. J Cereb Blood Flow Metab 26:21, 2006.
64. Acharya SK, Bhatia V, Sreenivas V, et al: Efficacy of L-ornithine L-aspartate in acute liver failure: a double-blind, randomized, placebo-controlled study. Gastroenterology 136:2159, 2009.
65. Odeh M: Pathogenesis of hepatic encephalopathy: the tumour necrosis factor-alpha theory. Eur J Clin Invest 37:291, 2007.
66. Jiang W, Desjardins P, Butterworth RF: Cerebral inflammation contributes to encephalopathy and brain edema in acute liver failure: protective effect of minocycline. J Neurochem 109:485, 2009.
67. Vaquero J, Polson J, Chung C, et al: Infection and the progression of hepatic encephalopathy in acute liver failure. Gastroenterology 125:755, 2003.
68. Bemeur C, Butterworth RF: Liver-brain proinflammatory signalling in acute liver failure: role in the pathogenesis of hepatic encephalopathy and brain edema. Metab Brain Dis 28:145, 2013.
69. Kato M, Hughes RD, Keays RT, et al: Electron microscopic study of brain capillaries in cerebral edema from fulminant hepatic failure. Hepatology 15:1060, 1992.
70. Als-Nielsen B, Gluud LL, Gluud C: Non-absorbable disaccharides for hepatic encephalopathy: systematic review of randomised trials. BMJ 328:1046, 2004.
71. Morgan MY, Blei A, Grüngreiff K, et al: The treatment of hepatic encephalopathy. Metab Brain Dis 22:389, 2007.
72. Strauss E, Tramote R, Silva EP, et al: Double-blind randomized clinical trial comparing neomycin and placebo in the treatment of exogenous hepatic encephalopathy. Hepatogastroenterology 39:542, 1992.
73. Patidar KR, Bajaj JS: Antibiotics for the treatment of hepatic encephalopathy. Metab Brain Dis 28:307, 2013.
74. Als-Nielsen B, Koretz RL, Kjaergard LL, et al: Branched-chain amino acids for hepatic encephalopathy. Cochrane Database Syst Rev:CD001939, 2003.
75. Gluud LL, Dam G, Borre M, et al: Lactulose, rifaximin or branched chain amino acids for hepatic encephalopathy: what is the evidence? Metab Brain Dis 28:221, 2013.
76. Sharma P, Agrawal A, Sharma BC, et al: Prophylaxis of hepatic encephalopathy in acute variceal bleed: a randomized controlled trial of lactulose versus no lactulose. J Gastroenterol Hepatol 26:996, 2011.
77. Agrawal A, Sharma BC, Sharma P, et al: Secondary prophylaxis of hepatic encephalopathy in cirrhosis: an open-label, randomized controlled trial of lactulose, probiotics, and no therapy. Am J Gastroenterol 107:1043, 2012.
78. Sharma P, Sharma BC, Agrawal A, et al: Primary prophylaxis of overt hepatic encephalopathy in patients with cirrhosis: an open labeled randomized controlled trial of lactulose versus no lactulose. J Gastroenterol Hepatol 27:1329, 2012.
79. Bass NM, Mullen KD, Sanyal A, et al: Rifaximin treatment in hepatic encephalopathy. N Engl J Med 362:1071, 2010.
80. Les I, Doval E, García-Martínez R, et al: Effects of branched-chain amino acids supplementation in patients with cirrhosis and a previous episode of hepatic encephalopathy: a randomized study. Am J Gastroenterol 106:1081, 2011.
81. Luo M, Li L, Lu CZ, et al: Clinical efficacy and safety of lactulose for minimal hepatic encephalopathy: a meta-analysis. Eur J Gastroenterol Hepatol 23:1250, 2011.

82. Mittal VV, Sharma BC, Sharma P, et al: A randomized controlled trial comparing lactulose, probiotics, and L-ornithine L-aspartate in treatment of minimal hepatic encephalopathy. Eur J Gastroenterol Hepatol 23:725, 2011.
83. Sidhu SS, Goyal O, Mishra BP, et al: Rifaximin improves psychometric performance and health-related quality of life in patients with minimal hepatic encephalopathy (the RIME Trial). Am J Gastroenterol 106:307, 2011.
84. Kok B, Foxton MR, Clough C, et al: Rifaximin is an efficacious treatment for the parkinsonian phenotype of hepatic encephalopathy. Hepatology 58:1516, 2013.
85. Baccarani U, Zola E, Adani GL, et al: Reversal of hepatic myelopathy after liver transplantation: fifteen plus one. Liver Transpl 16:1336, 2010.
86. Ryan JM, Tranah T, Mitry RR, et al: Acute liver failure and the brain: a look through the crystal ball. Metab Brain Dis 28:7, 2013.
87. Kumar R, Shalimar Sharma H, et al: Persistent hyperammonemia is associated with complications and poor outcomes in patients with acute liver failure. Clin Gastroenterol Hepatol 10:925, 2012.
88. Murphy N, Auzinger G, Bernel W, et al: The effect of hypertonic sodium chloride on intracranial pressure in patients with acute liver failure. Hepatology 39:464, 2004.
89. Jalan R, Olde Damink SW, Deutz NE, et al: Moderate hypothermia in patients with acute liver failure and uncontrolled intracranial hypertension. Gastroenterology 127:1338, 2004.
90. Larsen F, Murphy N, Bernal W, et al: The prophylactic effect of mild hypothermia to prevent brain oedema in patients with acute liver failure: results of a multicentre randomised controlled trial. J Hepatol 54(suppl 1):S26, 2011.
91. Bernal W, Auzinger G, Dhawan A, et al: Acute liver failure. Lancet 376:190, 2010.
92. Jacewicz M, Marino CR: Diseases of the pancreas. Pancreatic encephalopathy. p. 238. In Biller J (ed): The Interface of Neurology and Internal Medicine. Lippincott Williams & Wilkins, Philadelphia, 2008.
93. Weathers AL, Lewis SL: Rare and unusual ... or are they? Less commonly diagnosed encephalopathies associated with systemic disease. Semin Neurol 29:136, 2009.
94. Chan C, Fryer J, Herkes G, et al: Fatal brain stem event complicating acute pancreatitis. J Clin Neurosci 10:351, 2003.
95. Bartha P, Shifrin E, Levy Y: Pancreatic encephalopathy—a rare complication of a common disease. Eur J Intern Med 17:382, 2006.
96. Ruggieri RM, Lupo I, Piccoli F: Pancreatic encephalopathy: a 7-year follow-up case report and review of the literature. Neurol Sci 23:203, 2002.
97. Sun GH, Yang YS, Liu QS, et al: Pancreatic encephalopathy and Wernicke encephalopathy in association with acute pancreatitis: a clinical study. World J Gastroenterol 12:4224, 2006.
98. Ohkubo T, Shiojiri T, Matsunaga T: Severe diffuse white matter lesions in a patient with pancreatic encephalopathy. J Neurology 51:476, 2004.
99. Hornik A, Rodriguez Porcel FJ, Agha C, et al: Central and extrapontine myelinolysis affecting the brain and spinal cord. An unusual presentation of pancreatic encephalopathy. Front Neurol 3:135, 2012.
100. Lu XS, Qiu F, Li YX, et al: Effect of lower-molecular weight heparin in the prevention of pancreatic encephalopathy in the patient with severe acute pancreatitis. Pancreas 39:516, 2010.

CHAPTER

13

Other Neurologic Disorders Associated with Gastrointestinal Disease

RONALD F. PFEIFFER

In recent years, the presence of gastrointestinal (GI) dysfunction in the setting of neurologic disease has received increasing attention, particularly in disorders such as Parkinson disease. Much less attention has been devoted to the occurrence of neurologic dysfunction in primary GI disease processes. The enteric nervous system (ENS), which lines virtually the entire GI tract, contains approximately the same number of neurons as the spinal cord and is capable of generating and controlling many functions entirely independently of the central nervous system (CNS).[1] It should therefore not be surprising, then, that processes that affect the GI system, including the enteric nervous system, also may affect the CNS or systems controlled by the CNS.

GASTROINTESTINAL DISORDERS

Bariatric Surgery

The growing girth of the American populace has led to immense growth in bariatric surgery for the treatment of obesity, which is typically performed after dietary and medical management has failed. Gastric restriction procedures (e.g., gastric stapling, laparoscopic banding) and gastric bypass procedures (e.g., Roux-en-Y gastric bypass) have been performed most frequently, but sleeve gastrectomy, in which approximately 75 to 85 percent of the stomach is removed along the greater curvature, is growing in popularity. Neurologic complications may occur following all of these procedures.

Neurologic complications were noted in one study in only 4.6 percent of 500 patients nearly 2 years after surgery, but other studies have suggested higher rates.[2] Peripheral neuropathy was reported in 16 percent of 435 patients after bariatric surgery, compared with only 3 percent of 126 patients undergoing cholecystectomy.[3] In a subsequent cohort drawn from a single tertiary referral center, the same group of investigators noted peripheral neuropathy in only 7 percent and did not report on the frequency of other types of neurologic complications.[4] Although peripheral nervous system disorders appear to be the

Aminoff's Neurology and General Medicine, Fifth Edition

most frequent neurologic complications, encephalopathy, myelopathy, and optic neuropathy all have been reported.[5,6]

Polyneuropathy, mononeuropathy, and radicular or plexus involvement have been described following bariatric surgery.[3] Peripheral neuropathy typically is chronic, although acute inflammatory demyelinating polyneuropathy also has been reported.[7] Carpal tunnel syndrome is the most frequent mononeuropathy, accounting for 79 percent of cases in one study.[3] Lateral femoral cutaneous neuropathy (meralgia paresthetica) develops in only 0.5 to 1.4 percent of individuals despite recent weight loss being a well-known risk factor for its development.[2,3,8]

Nutritional deficiencies (see Chapter 15) due to malabsorption are responsible for the development of neuropathy in many, though not all, instances. Deficiencies of thiamine, riboflavin, pyridoxine, vitamin B_{12}, and vitamin E have all been described.[5] Thiamine deficiency, with neuropathic beriberi as one consequence, may be particularly important.[9] Immunologic mechanisms also have been proposed as causing neuropathy in these patients.[3] Compression either during or following surgery is likely responsible for most of the mononeuropathies.

Muscle weakness has been described in 7 percent of patients.[7] Postoperative rhabdomyolysis may occur and is especially frequent in patients undergoing Roux-en-Y gastric bypass; small series suggest up to three-quarters of patients may experience this complication, which presents with muscle pain, typically in the gluteal region, accompanied by an increase in serum creatine kinase levels.[10–12] The development of surface and deep tissue pressure during surgery may be responsible.[13] The risk of rhabdomyolysis is greatest when the BMI of the patient is greater than 56 kg/m^2.[14] Osteomalacia and associated osteomalacic myopathy may develop postoperatively.[15] An acquired myotonic syndrome also has been reported.[2]

Spinal cord dysfunction is another potential complication of bariatric surgery. Symptoms may not occur until 5 to 10 years later.[16] Many of these patients are found to have low serum vitamin B_{12} or copper levels.[17]

Cortical dysfunction, bearing the characteristics of Wernicke encephalopathy, was found to complicate bariatric surgery in around one-quarter of patients in one study but was noted much less frequently in a larger prospective investigation.[2,7]

Celiac Disease

Celiac disease (CD) is characterized by a constellation of diarrhea, malabsorption, weight loss, and gaseous distension that develops as a consequence of damage to the mucosa of the small intestine, triggered by an immune-mediated response to gluten. The prevalence of CD in American and European populations has been estimated to be approximately 1 percent, but because the number of undiagnosed patients may be considerable, its prevalence is probably much higher.[18–20] Genetic factors play a role, and 90 to 95 percent of individuals with CD carry HLA-DQ2.5 or -DQ8 heterodimers.[21]

Individuals with classic CD are found to have serum antigliadin antibodies along with additional gliadin-related antibodies (e.g., anti-endomysial, antitransglutaminase). The pathology of CD extends beyond the GI tract, leading to proposals that the term *gluten sensitivity* be used for individuals displaying more widespread involvement, with the label CD reserved for those with evidence of enteropathy on small bowel biopsy.

Neurologic dysfunction has been reported in around 6 to 12 percent of patients with CD.[22,23] It is often ascribed to nutritional deficiency secondary to malabsorption, although immunologic mechanisms may be an alternative explanation in some instances.[24]

ATAXIA

Gluten ataxia has no uniquely distinguishing clinical characteristics and remains a controversial entity.[25] Gait ataxia is present in all individuals by definition; limb ataxia, dysarthria, and ocular signs are present in most. The combination of ataxia and action myoclonus has been described in some patients.[26] The mean age of onset of symptoms is 53 years.[22] Cerebellar atrophy and white matter abnormalities may be evident on magnetic resonance imaging (MRI).[27] The classic GI symptoms of CD are present in only a minority of individuals with gluten ataxia (less than 10%).[28] Evidence of classic CD is found on duodenal biopsy in 25 to 33 percent.[22,29]

In the initial reports, antigliadin antibodies (IgG, IgA, or both) were found in 41 percent of patients with sporadic idiopathic ataxia, compared with only 15 percent of those with clinically probable multiple system atrophy (MSA), 14 percent with familial ataxia, and 12 percent of normal controls.[29] More recently, 148 out of 635 (23%) patients with sporadic ataxia evaluated at the same clinic were noted to have evidence of gluten sensitivity.[30] Individuals with gluten ataxia, independent of intestinal involvement, demonstrate antitransglutaminase 6 IgG and IgA antibodies, whereas antitransglutaminase 2 IgA antibodies are present in persons with gastrointestinal disease.[31] The cerebellar damage has been attributed to a chronic, immune-mediated inflammatory process.[32] Autopsy examination in several affected individuals has demonstrated Purkinje cell loss and lymphocytic infiltration within the cerebellum as well as the posterior columns of the spinal cord.[33] Cerebellar IgA deposits containing transglutaminase 6 have also been found.[31]

Gluten ataxia sometimes responds to a gluten-free diet.[29,34] Intravenous immunoglobulin therapy reportedly ameliorates the ataxia in some patients.[35] Screening has been suggested for all individuals who present with adult-onset ataxia without any other obvious cause, but this recommendation remains controversial.

Peripheral Neuropathy

In one retrospective chart review, peripheral neuropathy accounted for 17 percent of the neurologic abnormalities in patients with CD.[36] In another study, chronic axonal sensorimotor neuropathy was identified in 23 percent.[37] Sural nerve biopsy demonstrates axonal injury in these patients.[38] The etiology of the neuropathy is uncertain; both nutritional and autoimmune mechanisms have been proposed.

As with sporadic ataxia, some studies suggest that the prevalence of CD or of antigliadin antibodies is higher in individuals with peripheral neuropathy than in the general population.[38–40] This has led to the use of the term *gluten neuropathy* for individuals with idiopathic neuropathy and serologic evidence of gluten sensitivity.[22] Improvement with a gluten-free diet has been reported by some, but other studies have failed to show improvement.[41,42]

Myopathy

CD is more prevalent in patients with inflammatory myopathies, particularly inclusion-body myositis.[43] Immunologic mechanisms probably are responsible in most instances, but in one patient with CD and a myopathy resembling inclusion-body myopathy, reversal of both clinical and pathologic abnormalities was documented upon treatment with vitamin E and institution of a gluten-free diet.[44]

Epilepsy

An association between CD and epilepsy is controversial. The reported prevalence of epilepsy in CD has ranged from 0.8 to 7.2 percent and that of CD in individuals with epilepsy from 0.8 to 8.1 percent.[45] In one large study, the presence of CD-associated antibodies did not differ between 968 patients with epilepsy and a group of 584 individuals without epilepsy.[46] A specific syndrome of epilepsy, bilateral occipital lobe calcifications, and CD has been described, largely in Italians.[47] The mechanism for such an association is obscure. Even in CD patients without calcifications, seizures originate most frequently in the occipital lobe.[45] A gluten-free diet may improve seizure control, especially when started early.[45,47]

Other Manifestations

A number of other neurologic manifestations of CD have been reported but less extensively evaluated, including migraine, learning disabilities, autonomic neuropathy, and neuromyelitis optica.[32,48–50] The significance of these associations is uncertain.

Inflammatory Bowel Disease

Two similar but distinct disease entities, ulcerative colitis and Crohn disease, are part of a group of conditions collectively labeled as inflammatory bowel disease (IBD). These two conditions share many clinical and even pathologic features, but also display important differences (Table 13-1).

TABLE 13-1 ■ Gastrointestinal Features of Inflammatory Bowel Disease

Feature	Crohn Disease	Ulcerative Colitis
Diarrhea	Common, nonbloody, less urgent	Common, bloody, urgent
Rectal Bleeding	Occasional	Very common
Weight Loss	Common	Uncommon
Abdominal Pain	Prominent	Not prominent
Stricture Formation	Common	Rare
Fistula Formation	Common	Very rare

An autoimmune etiology in genetically susceptible individuals, characterized by a dysregulated mucosal immune response to antigens normally present within the intestinal lumen, is suspected in both.

In Europe and North America, the incidence of ulcerative colitis is in the range of 3 to 15 per 100,000 persons.[51] Incidence rates of 6 to 10 per 100,000 have been reported for Crohn disease in the same regions, but in other parts of the world, such as Asia, a previously low incidence appears to be increasing.

Involvement outside the GI tract is well described in IBD.[52,53] Neurologic dysfunction is probably relatively infrequent, with wide-ranging estimates from 0.2 to 47.5 percent of patients.[54] Neurologic dysfunction may precede the appearance of GI symptoms, and both peripheral and central nervous system involvement occurs (Table 13-2).[55] Autoimmune mechanisms are primarily responsible for the development of neurologic involvement in IBD; however, nutritional deficiency, infection, and other processes may also secondarily involve the nervous system. Treatment for both Crohn disease and ulcerative colitis involves potent medications, including antitumor necrosis factor α (anti-TNF-α) agents, that can have neurologic complications.[56]

TABLE 13-2 ■ Nervous System Involvement in Inflammatory Bowel Disease

Peripheral
Generalized
Sensorimotor neuropathy
Large fiber
Small fiber
Inflammatory demyelinating neuropathy
Acute
Chronic
Focal
Mononeuropathy
Brachial plexopathy
Multifocal
Mononeuritis multiplex
Multifocal motor neuropathy
Sensorineural hearing loss
Melkersson–Rosenthal syndrome
Myopathic
Myopathy
Myasthenia
Abscess formation
Central
Cerebrovascular
Large artery
Lacunar
Venous sinus thrombosis
Demyelinating
Myelopathic
Seizures
Encephalopathy
Nutritional
Vasculitis

PERIPHERAL NEUROPATHY

Peripheral neuropathy is the most frequent neurologic complication of both Crohn disease and ulcerative colitis, and has been reported in 1.9 to 13.4 percent of IBD patients.[57–60] The etiology of peripheral nerve involvement in IBD appears to be multifactorial, including nutritional deficiency, medication side effects, and an autoimmune mechanism as part of the primary disease. Involvement may take the form of focal (e.g., mononeuropathy, cranial neuropathy, brachial plexopathy), multifocal (e.g., mononeuritis multiplex, multifocal motor neuropathy), and generalized (acute or chronic inflammatory demyelinating polyneuropathy, small- or large-fiber axonal sensorimotor neuropathy) neuropathic processes.[57,59,61–63] Carpal tunnel syndrome appears to be the most frequently occurring isolated mononeuropathy.[59] Axonal neuropathy occurs more frequently than demyelinating neuropathy.[59,63]

Two specific patterns of cranial nerve involvement have been described in IBD. Acute sensorineural hearing loss or chronic subclinical hearing impairment has been described in ulcerative colitis.[64] In contrast, Melkersson–Rosenthal syndrome, characterized by recurrent facial nerve palsy along with intermittent orofacial swelling and fissuring of the tongue, has been reported in patients with Crohn disease.[65]

DEMYELINATING DISEASE

An association between IBD, especially ulcerative colitis, and multiple sclerosis has been reported.[66] In one study examining two large populations, the odds ratio for multiple sclerosis in patients with IBD was around 1.5.[67] White matter lesions may be present on MRI in patients with IBD; whether these represent multiple sclerosis or another ischemic or demyelinating process is unclear.[68,69] The development of demyelination within the CNS as a side effect of anti-TNF-α agents has been reported.[54]

Cerebrovascular Disease

Vascular complications are rare, but well-documented, extraintestinal manifestations of IBD. A large, population-based case-control study involving over 8,000 patients with Crohn disease demonstrated an increased risk of ischemic stroke only in younger individuals (age <50 years) with the disorder.[70] Responses to both immunosuppressive therapy (e.g., corticosteroids and azathioprine) and anticoagulation have been reported, suggesting that both hypercoagulable and autoimmune processes may play a role.[71,72]

A variety of cerebrovascular events has been reported in ulcerative colitis and Crohn disease, including both large artery and lacunar infarcts.[73,74] Cerebral venous sinus thrombosis in IBD occurs more frequently in ulcerative colitis than Crohn disease; individuals with active disease are at greater risk.[75] The lateral and superior sagittal sinuses are involved most frequently. Severe iron-deficiency anemia may be a significant risk factor for thrombosis.

Myopathy

Myopathy is relatively rare in IBD, occurring in 0.5 percent of patients.[57] Symptoms may precede the appearance of GI dysfunction, but this is unusual.

Generalized inflammatory muscle disease has been described as well as focal involvement of muscle, primarily in Crohn disease. Abscess formation in the psoas or other muscles is an important potential complication; psoas muscle abscess is characterized by flank, pelvic or abdominal pain, usually associated with fever and leukocytosis, and diagnosis is confirmed by ultrasound or computerized tomography (CT). Focal myositis involving the gastrocnemius and other muscles has been reported.[76,77]

Myelopathy

Slowly progressive myelopathy may develop in the setting of IBD and accounts for around 25 percent of patients with neurologic involvement in one study.[57] It is more likely to occur in patients with Crohn disease, who may develop vitamin B_{12} deficiency as a consequence of surgical resection of the terminal ileum. Patients with Crohn disease also may develop a more acute myelopathy or cauda equina syndrome due to empyema from extension of a fistula to the epidural or subdural space.[78]

Other Manifestations

Seizures may occur as a complication of the surgical management of IBD, precipitated by fluid overload, electrolyte imbalance, hypoxia, and corticosteroid administration or withdrawal. They may occur also as a complication of cyclosporine treatment.[79] Diffuse encephalopathy and acute disseminated encephalomyelitis have also been reported.[80] Both Wernicke encephalopathy and possible selenium-induced encephalopathy have been described in individuals with Crohn disease receiving total parenteral nutrition.[81,82] Autonomic neuropathy has been reported rarely in both Crohn disease and ulcerative colitis.

Whipple Disease

Although originally described as a GI disease, with symptoms of diarrhea, weight loss, and abdominal pain, Whipple disease is a multisystem disorder that also may be characterized by joint, dermatologic, lymphatic, cardiac, pulmonary, ocular, and neurologic dysfunction.[83,84] The average age of symptom onset is approximately 50 years, and males are affected much more frequently than females.[83] Farmers are at increased risk of developing Whipple disease; one possible explanation is that the organism responsible, *Tropheryma whipplei*, is a member of the actinomycete family found in the soil.[83]

Neurologic dysfunction is the presenting feature in approximately 5 percent of persons with Whipple disease.[85] Symptoms of CNS involvement eventually develop in 10 to 43 percent of patients, and postmortem examinations demonstrate CNS lesions in over 90 percent of individuals (Table 13-3).[83,85] Cognitive changes are the most frequently observed neurologic manifestation, occurring in 71 percent of patients, often accompanied by psychiatric symptoms such as depression and personality or behavioral changes.[86] Cerebellar dysfunction with gait and balance impairment occurs in approximately 20 percent of persons; pyramidal tract abnormalities also may occur.[86] Symptoms indicative

TABLE 13-3 ■ Neurologic Features of Whipple Disease

Cognitive impairment
Psychiatric dysfunction Depression Personality change
Hypothalamic manifestations Insomnia Hypersomnia Hyperphagia Polydipsia and polyuria
Oculomasticatory myorhythmia
Oculofacial-skeletal myorhythmia
Vertical gaze impairment
Seizures
Ataxia
Peripheral neuropathy

of hypothalamic involvement, such as insomnia, hypersomnia, hyperphagia, polyuria, and polydipsia, are uncommon.[83,86] Peripheral neuropathy also has been reported.

Oculomasticatory myorhythmia, characterized by the combination of pendular convergence nystagmus and concurrent slow, rhythmic synchronous contractions of the masticatory muscles, develops in approximately 20 percent of individuals with CNS manifestations of Whipple disease.[86,87] These movements invariably are accompanied by a supranuclear vertical gaze paresis. Sometimes the muscle contractions also involve the extremities, prompting use of the term oculofacial-skeletal myorhythmia. These two movement disorders are considered by some to be pathognomonic of Whipple disease. Other ophthalmologic abnormalities, such as ptosis, internuclear ophthalmoplegia, and pupillary dysfunction, also may occur.

Prompt diagnosis of Whipple disease is important because effective treatment is available. Cerebrospinal fluid (CSF) PCR analysis appears to be a more sensitive method of diagnosis than identification of PAS-positive inclusions in macrophages in duodenal biopsy specimens, but there is some evidence that *Tropheryma whipplei* DNA may be present in healthy individuals without the disorder.[83,85] In individuals with CNS symptomatology, brain biopsy is positive in 80 percent of instances.[86] CSF analysis may show an inflammatory response that sometimes contains PAS-positive macrophages.[88] CSF PCR is positive in 80 percent of patients with Whipple disease and neurologic symptoms.[89]

The rarity of the disorder has precluded formal clinical trials, but an initial 2-week course of parenteral therapy with either a combination of penicillin G and streptomycin or with a third-generation cephalosporin (e.g., ceftriaxone) is recommended, followed by a 1-year course of oral trimethoprim-sulfamethoxazole.[83] The prolonged course of trimethoprim-sulfamethoxazole, which crosses the blood–brain barrier, is intended to treat CNS involvement. A combination of doxycycline and hydroxychloroquine, supplemented by sulfadiazine, is an alternative regimen.[90] It is important to treat the disease adequately when first identified, because CNS relapses have a poor prognosis and high mortality rate.

Malabsorption Syndromes

Malabsorption occurs through a variety of mechanisms, including diminished gastric holding capacity; hepatic, gall bladder or pancreatic disease; enterocyte dysfunction; and a reduction in intestinal absorptive surface. Abdominal distension and pain, flatulence, diarrhea, weight loss, and ascites are the classic GI features of malabsorption. Systemic involvement may be characterized by dermatologic, musculoskeletal, renal, hematologic, and neurologic dysfunction. These and other nutritional disorders are discussed further in Chapter 15.

Vitamin E Deficiency

Neurologic dysfunction in the setting of vitamin E deficiency can be genetic in origin, due to a mutation in the α-tocopherol transfer protein gene, with a clinical presentation that can mimic Friedreich ataxia.[91] In most instances, however, it is the consequence of fat malabsorption, which can occur in a variety of circumstances.

Neurologic symptoms and signs of vitamin E deficiency may include ataxia, dysarthria, and nystagmus. Symptoms and signs of peripheral neuropathy, including paresthesias, impaired proprioception and vibration, and hyporeflexia are common. Proximal muscle weakness from myopathy, pigmentary retinopathy, action tremor, limb dysmetria, and dystonia also have been described.[92,93]

Somatosensory evoked potentials may demonstrate abnormalities indicative of posterior column dysfunction. Diffuse white matter changes have been described in patients with vitamin E deficiency, in both the cerebrum and spinal cord; some of these patients present with upper motor neuron signs.

The appearance of symptoms of vitamin E deficiency can be strikingly delayed. In post-gastrectomy patients, it may take up to 50 months for evidence of vitamin E deficiency to appear.[94] Replacement doses of vitamin E need to be 300 mg/day or more.

Familial Hypocholesterolemia

Three distinct genetic disorders—familial hypobetalipoproteinemia, abetalipoproteinemia, and chylomicron retention disease—have been identified as causes of chronic diarrhea, malabsorption, malnutrition, growth retardation, and vitamin E deficiency. Of the three, neurologists are most familiar with abetalipoproteinemia, previously known as the Bassen–Kornzweig syndrome.

Abetalipoproteinemia is an autosomal recessive disorder due to a mutation in the microsomal triglyceride transfer protein (*MTP*) gene on chromosome 4, which leads to impaired biogenesis of chylomicrons and very-low-density lipoprotein (VLDL) along with an inability to absorb fats and fat-soluble vitamins including vitamin E. The clinical features of abetalipoproteinemia include steatorrhea, diarrhea, retinitis pigmentosa, acanthocytosis, and a variety of neurologic features. Blood lipid analysis demonstrates extremely low plasma levels of total cholesterol, VLDL, and low-density lipoproteins (LDL); apolipoprotein B, triglycerides, and chylomicrons are virtually absent.[95] Gastrointestinal symptoms are usually evident during infancy, and neurologic dysfunction may not appear until individuals are in their teens or even older.[96] Neurologic symptoms include progressive cerebellar ataxia and sometimes a sensorimotor neuropathy. Both the ataxia and the peripheral neuropathy are probably due to vitamin E deficiency. Additional neurologic abnormalities that have been described include upper motor neuron signs and both resting and postural tremor.[97,98] Treatment of neurologic dysfunction with both vitamin E and vitamin A has been advocated, but results have been mixed.[97,99]

Tropical Sprue

Tropical malabsorption may affect both indigenous residents of tropical countries and travelers visiting the tropics.[100] Secondary forms due to small intestine mucosal damage inflicted by protozoa, helminths, bacteria, and viruses may produce a malabsorption syndrome, as can a variety of other disease processes of inflammatory, autoimmune, or neoplastic origin.[100] In individuals in whom no etiology can be ascertained, the term “tropical sprue” has been applied.

Infrequently encountered in North America, tropical sprue has been reported to account for approximately 40 percent of malabsorption in children and adults in some portions of south Asia.[101] Gastrointestinal symptoms include chronic nonbloody diarrhea, bloating, weight loss, and abdominal cramping.[102] Tropical sprue typically involves the entire length of the small intestine, in contrast to celiac disease, which typically spares the terminal ileum.[102] Mucosal damage results in malabsorption of fat, carbohydrates, and multiple vitamins, including folate and vitamins A, E, and B_{12}.[100]

Neurologic symptoms are present in around two-thirds of individuals with tropical sprue.[103] Proximal muscle weakness and peripheral neuropathy are most common. Night blindness, presumably due to vitamin A deficiency, and combined system degeneration, presumably the result of vitamin B_{12} deficiency, have been described.[100] The peripheral neuropathy has been attributed to vitamin E deficiency.

Antibiotic therapy, typically with tetracycline or doxycycline for several months, and vitamin replacement therapy are the standard treatments for tropical sprue, but abnormal small intestine permeability may remain following treatment.[104]

Wernicke Encephalopathy

Wernicke encephalopathy is most closely linked to chronic alcoholism with nutritional thiamine deficiency, but can result from malabsorption of thiamine (see Chapters 15 and 33). In nonalcoholic patients, the full classic triad of neurologic features—mental status changes, ophthalmoplegia, and ataxia—develops in only 10 to 16 percent of individuals.[105]

Thiamine is absorbed primarily in the duodenum, but the stomach also plays a role.[106] As a result, Wernicke encephalopathy has been documented following bariatric surgery.[7,107] It may develop anywhere between 2 and 78 weeks following surgery, although 4 to 12 weeks postoperatively is the most frequent time frame.[107] Gastric bypass or a restrictive procedure is the most common surgery that predisposes to Wernicke encephalopathy.[108] Repeated vomiting, presumably with decreased thiamine absorption as a result, is a frequent risk factor.[108] Individuals undergoing Roux-en-Y gastric bypass have an additional risk since thiamine is predominantly absorbed in the duodenum, which is bypassed following this procedure.[109]

Wernicke encephalopathy also has been described in individuals with other causes of malabsorption. In one patient with a history of neonatal necrotizing enterocolitis and subsequent bowel resection, Wernicke encephalopathy developed later during pregnancy and was attributed to long-standing chronic malabsorption exacerbated by the pregnancy.[110]

Pellagra

Pellagra often is considered to be extinct in developed countries, but it still occurs in rare instances. It is caused by niacin deficiency, but can also develop secondary to deficiency of tryptophan, a precursor of niacin.[111] Pellagra most often is diagnosed in individuals with chronic alcoholism and inadequate nutritional intake, but also develops in malabsorption syndromes.

The classic clinical features of pellagra include the triad of dermatitis, diarrhea, and dementia, although most individuals do not have all three features. In addition to dementia, neurologic abnormalities may include headache, vertigo, myoclonus, tremor, rigidity, weakness, dysphagia, seizures, and various psychiatric symptoms.[105,112]

Pellagra may develop in persons with Crohn disease—there is niacin deficiency due to malabsorption and tryptophan wastage with increased urinary excretion of 5-hydroxyindoleacetic acid.[113,114] Pellagra has been reported in infectious colitis and with intestinal bacterial overgrowth with consequent malabsorption.[115,116]

Copper Deficiency

Copper deficiency is best recognized in Menkes disease, in which there is a genetically based inability to transport copper across the intestinal barrier due to a mutation in the *ATP7A* gene. However, impairment of intestinal copper absorption also may occur in the setting of various acquired malabsorptive processes.

Copper is absorbed in the proximal small intestine, primarily in the duodenum but also to a lesser extent in the stomach and more distal small intestine. Processes that remove or impair these absorptive sites result in eventual copper deficiency; thus, copper malabsorption has been identified in individuals who have previously undergone gastric or intestinal surgery.[117,118] Although malabsorption is the most frequent cause, copper deficiency also may follow excessive zinc ingestion.[119]

The clinical features of copper deficiency myelopathy closely mimic those of subacute combined degeneration due to vitamin B_{12} deficiency. The combination of posterior column dysfunction with sensory ataxia and associated corticospinal tract abnormalities is common to both; peripheral neuropathy also may be present, although it is not as common in copper deficiency as it is with vitamin B_{12} deficiency. Hematologic manifestations frequently are present in both; anemia and neutropenia are characteristic in copper deficiency and the anemia may be microcytic, macrocytic, or normocytic.[117] Optic neuropathy may also be present. T2 hyperintensities within the dorsal columns of the cervical spinal cord may be seen on MRI in both copper deficiency myelopathy and vitamin B_{12} deficiency.[120]

The response to copper replacement therapy is inconsistent. Although the hematologic abnormalities typically respond promptly, neurologic dysfunction may not. Progression usually is halted, but resolution of neurologic dysfunction often is incomplete.[117]

HEPATIC DISORDERS

When hepatic disease, regardless of its cause, progresses to a point that the liver becomes incapable of effectively eliminating toxic substances, neurologic dysfunction can ensue as these toxins invade the CNS. Hepatic failure most often evolves slowly, over a period of many months. However, fulminant hepatic failure, erupting over a period of days to weeks, also may occur, and neurologic symptoms predominate. The cerebral dysfunction that is due to liver insufficiency or portosystemic shunting is discussed in Chapter 12.

A predominantly axonal, length-dependent peripheral neuropathy may occur in patients with chronic liver disease. It is often subclinical or oligosymptomatic, but distal sensory loss and areflexia are sometimes found on examination, and quantitative studies may reveal abnormalities of small-fiber function. Median neuropathy at the wrist (carpal tunnel syndrome) is common. Autonomic neuropathy is also frequent, regardless of whether there is a concomitant somatic neuropathy, and tends to involve the parasympathetic (vagal) more often than sympathetic components[121]; its severity relates to the severity but not the cause of the hepatic dysfunction. The presence of vagal dysfunction in patients with well-compensated chronic liver disease indicates a substantially worse outlook for survival than otherwise.[122]

Various disorders causing hepatic dysfunction—such as alcohol-induced cirrhosis, porphyria, polyarteritis nodosa, and primary biliary cirrhosis—may independently cause peripheral nerve dysfunction. However, because the severity of neuropathy correlates with that of the liver disease regardless of its etiology, it seems likely that the peripheral neuropathy is caused by hepatocellular damage.

Patients infected with hepatitis C virus may develop various neuromuscular complications. A fulminant vasculitic syndrome and progressive mononeuropathy multiplex may occur in those with cryoglobulinemia,[123,124] but a length-dependent oligosymptomatic distal peripheral neuropathy may occur without cryoglobuminemia. Acute or chronic demyelinating neuropathies have been reported in the setting of viral hepatitis.[125,126] Muscle disease also occurs. Myalgia is common but of uncertain cause; muscle weakness is uncommon. There have been several case reports of polymyositis or dermatomyositis occurring in patients with hepatitis C. In addition, interferon therapy for hepatitis C infection may precipitate or aggravate the myopathy.[127]

Patients with primary biliary cirrhosis form a separate group in which a pure sensory neuropathy may develop, with or without xanthomatous infiltration of the nerves.[128] Autonomic involvement may also occur.[129]

Wilson Disease

Wilson disease is an autosomal recessive disorder caused by a mutation in the *ATB7P* gene on chromosome 13. More than 400 mutations have been identified and most affected patients are compound heterozygotes.[130] The most widely published prevalence rate is 30 cases per 1 million persons, although recent studies suggest that this may be an underestimate.[131]

Pathophysiology

The defective ATP7B protein cannot carry out its transport functions within the hepatocyte. As a result, copper is neither delivered for ceruloplasmin formation nor transported into the bile canaliculus for excretion. The defect in biliary excretion of copper results in a slow accumulation of copper within the liver. Eventually, the ability of the liver to store the copper is exceeded and unbound copper escapes from the liver and accumulates in other sites, including the nervous system.

Clinical Presentation

Hepatic Manifestations

Approximately 40 to 50 percent of patients with Wilson disease experience hepatic symptoms as their initial manifestation.[132] These individuals tend to present at an earlier age (average 11.4 to 15.5 years) than those with a primary neurologic or psychiatric presentation.[133] Onset of symptoms before age 6 is rare[131]; presentation with hepatic dysfunction has been reported as late as age 74.[134]

The most frequent hepatic presentation is that of slowly progressive liver failure with cirrhosis, ascites, esophageal varices, and splenomegaly. A clinical picture similar to autoimmune (chronic active) hepatitis is evident in 10 to 30 percent; acute fulminant hepatic failure occurs in approximately 5 percent.[135] The pattern of liver enzyme abnormalities in the setting of fulminant hepatic failure may provide clues to the diagnosis as hemolysis may produce disproportionate elevation of the total bilirubin.[132] The combination of an alkaline phosphatase to total bilirubin ratio of less than 4 and an aspartate aminotransferase to alanine aminotransferase ratio of greater than 2.2 is highly suggestive of Wilson disease, especially if the serum hemoglobin level also is reduced.[136]

Neurologic Manifestations

Neurologic dysfunction is the second most frequent initial clinical manifestation of Wilson disease, with estimates that range from 35 to 60 percent. The average age of symptom onset (18.9 to 20.2 years) is later than when the initial presentation is hepatic in nature, but ages from 6 to 72 years have been reported.[133,137,138]

Tremor is the initial symptom of neurologic involvement in around one-half of patients.[139] The tremor is typically asymmetric and may be resting, postural, kinetic, or a combination of these. Dystonia may be as frequent as tremor.[139] Chorea occurs relatively infrequently, but may be present at the time of diagnosis in around 15 percent of patients.[139] Athetosis has also been described. Parkinsonism frequently is present, with one case series finding 45 percent of patients with neurologic dysfunction having parkinsonian symptoms or signs.[140,141] Although unusual, myoclonus has also been reported.[142]

Cerebellar dysfunction develops in 25 to 50 percent of individuals with Wilson disease.[141] It may take the form of ataxia, dysarthria, kinetic tremor, or incoordination. Dysarthria in one study was evident in 91 percent of patients at diagnosis.[139] Several patterns of dysarthria have been described including a hypokinetic form with difficulty in initiating speech; reduced volume, phonation, and intonation; inadequate tongue movements; and imprecise articulation along with a tendency for speech to accelerate as it proceeds. Dysarthria of cerebellar or brainstem origin has also been described in Wilson disease. Dysphagia may develop during the course of the illness.[139] An unusual laugh, in which most of the sound is generated during inspiration, also may occur.

Gait abnormalities are another common neurologic feature, present in 45 to 75 percent of patients at diagnosis.[139] Gait impairment ranges from parkinsonian, with small shuffling steps and difficulty initiating gait, to cerebellar, with a wide-based and unsteady appearance.[132]

Psychiatric Manifestations

Psychiatric symptoms are the presenting feature in approximately 15 to 20 percent of patients with Wilson disease and may cause delays in diagnosis.[131,143] Most individuals will experience psychiatric dysfunction at some point during their illness. This may range from subtle personality changes to mania and frank psychosis. Major depression develops in around one-quarter of patients. Suicidal behavior has been described in some.

Ophthalmologic Manifestations

The ophthalmologic hallmark of the disease is the formation of Kayser–Fleischer rings within the cornea (Fig. 13-1) They are virtually always bilateral, but unilateral Kayser–Fleischer rings have been described, possibly as a consequence of reduced intraocular pressure in the eye without the ring. Because of their dark color, Kayser–Fleischer rings often can be identified easily in patients with blue eyes, but only with difficulty in brown-eyed persons without the benefit of slit lamp examination. Kayser–Fleischer rings first appear in the superior aspect of the cornea, followed by the inferior aspect; the medial and lateral portions of the ring then subsequently fill in. Because of this pattern of ring evolution, it is important to lift the eyelid during the examination so that incomplete ring formation is not overlooked.

Kayser–Fleischer rings are virtually always present in patients with neurologic or psychiatric symptoms, but they may not yet have formed in persons who present with isolated hepatic involvement.

Other Manifestations

Radiographic evidence of osteoporosis is common. Coombs-negative hemolytic anemia may present initially in 10 to 15 percent of cases.[144] Renal

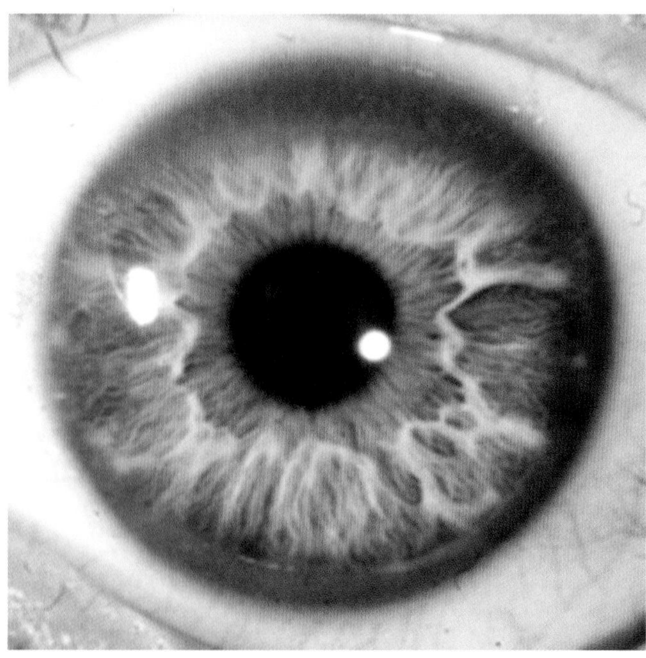

FIGURE 13-1 ■ Kayser–Fleischer ring. (Courtesy of Wayne Cornblath, MD, University of Michigan, Kellogg Eye Center, Ann Arbor, Michigan.)

impairment was the initial symptom in 8 percent of children in another study.[145] Myocardial involvement in Wilson disease is under-recognized.[146] The myocardial damage is presumably due to copper deposition within the heart. Autonomic dysfunction, most often asymptomatic and evident only upon neurophysiologic testing, has been noted in almost 40 percent of persons, predominantly those with neurologic involvement.[147] Skin changes, including hyperpigmentation of the legs and a dark complexion, may occur and be mistaken for Addison disease. Bluish discoloration of the lunulae of the nails and acanthosis nigricans have also been reported.

Diagnosis

The presence of over 400 different mutations has made genetic testing difficult. However, it has been suggested that *ATP7B* gene sequencing should now be standard practice in the diagnosis of Wilson disease.[148]

Determination of hepatic copper content via liver biopsy is currently the single most sensitive and specific test for the diagnosis. Hepatic copper elevation in Wilson disease is typically quite striking, with levels greater than 250 μg/g dry tissue, compared to normal values of 15 to 55 μg/g. In patients with neurologic or psychiatric dysfunction, liver biopsy is generally unnecessary since other tests will provide the diagnosis; it is, however, usually required in individuals presenting with hepatic dysfunction.

The visualization of Kayser–Fleischer rings is an invaluable aid in diagnosis. Slit-lamp examination by a neuroophthalmologist or experienced ophthalmologist is a vital part of the diagnostic evaluation, particularly in persons displaying neurologic or psychiatric dysfunction. Individuals with only hepatic dysfunction may not display Kayser–Fleischer rings because copper accumulation may not yet have exceeded the liver's capacity to store the excess.

Serum ceruloplasmin determination cannot be relied upon as the sole screening study in patients with possible Wilson disease. Ceruloplasmin may be normal or only slightly lower than normal in 5 to 15 percent of persons with the disease.[132,149] Since ceruloplasmin is an acute-phase reactant, it may increase and reach normal levels during pregnancy, with estrogen or steroid administration, in the setting of infections, or with various inflammatory processes including hepatitis.[132] As many as 10 to 20 percent of heterozygotes for Wilson disease have subnormal ceruloplasmin levels.[132,149]

A 24-hour urinary copper determination is probably the single best screening test in symptomatic patients. Urinary copper levels in symptomatic patients typically exceed 100 μg/day. However, in individuals with asymptomatic Wilson disease, 24-hour urinary copper excretion may be within the normal range because the ability of the liver to store the accumulating copper has not yet been exceeded.

Although serum copper levels, which measure total serum copper, are characteristically low in patients with Wilson disease, they are of little diagnostic value. Total serum copper largely reflects ceruloplasmin concentrations and is low simply because of the marked reduction in ceruloplasmin. In a patient with fulminant hepatic failure, however, serum copper levels become markedly elevated due to the sudden release of copper from tissue stores.

A variety of neuroimaging changes may occur. The most characteristic brain MRI changes include the presence of increased signal intensity in the basal ganglia on T2-weighted sequences and reduced signal intensity on T1-weighted sequences.[150] Several distinctive neuroimaging abnormalities, such as the "face of the giant panda" sign in the midbrain, the "face of the miniature panda" sign in the pons, and the "bright claustrum sign," have been described but are present in only a relatively small percentage of patients with Wilson disease, limiting their diagnostic utility.[150,151]

Measurement of the incorporation of radioactive copper (^{64}Cu) into ceruloplasmin has also been employed for diagnostic evaluation. However, difficulty obtaining the radioactive isotope limits its availability, and an overlap of values between individuals with Wilson disease and heterozygous carriers limits the procedure's specificity.[132]

CSF copper levels are elevated in persons with Wilson disease and neurologic dysfunction and decline with successful symptomatic treatment, but measurement is not performed in routine clinical practice.[152]

Treatment

Dietary restriction of copper has, in general, not been a successful treatment approach. When administered orally, zinc is absorbed by intestinal enterocytes and induces metallothionein formation, which then binds both zinc and copper and inhibits their intestinal absorption. The use of zinc as "maintenance" therapy following initial treatment of neurologically symptomatic individuals with other, more potent, decoppering agents has become common. Some investigators now even consider zinc to be first-line therapy.[153] Zinc generally is well tolerated, with very little toxicity.

Penicillamine avidly chelates copper and holds it until the complexed copper is excreted in the urine. Improvement in function following initiation of penicillamine therapy typically does not become evident for 2 to 3 months, and then may extend gradually over 1 to 2 years. Acute sensitivity reactions and a variety of other potential adverse effects may complicate chronic penicillamine therapy. Penicillamine has the propensity to produce an initial deterioration in neurologic function when initiated, perhaps in as many as 50 percent of patients.[154] The risk that penicillamine might induce irreversible neurologic deterioration following its initiation has led to a divergence in opinion as to the proper role of the drug in treatment. Some authors suggest continuing to use penicillamine but with low initial doses; others recommend treatment induction with other, ostensibly safer, medications.

Trientine is a copper-chelating agent with a mechanism of action similar to that of penicillamine but with a somewhat gentler decoppering effect that may make it less prone to trigger deterioration in neurologic function. Adverse effects from trientine are less frequent than with penicillamine.

Tetrathiomolybdate remains an experimental treatment modality, unavailable for general use. It has a distinct, dual mechanism of action that separates it from other available treatment modalities.[132] It functions both to inhibit copper absorption from the gastrointestinal tract and to complex with copper in the bloodstream, reducing the copper load both systemically and in the gut lumen.

Orthotopic liver transplantation is essentially the one effective treatment for fulminant hepatic failure in Wilson disease. Its potential utility in treating the patient with stable liver function but severe, progressive neurologic abnormalities despite optimal medical management has been considered but is not routine standard of care.

In an individual who is asymptomatic, therapy should be initiated with zinc alone. In a patient with hepatic but not neurologic or psychiatric dysfunction, introduction of both a chelating agent and zinc simultaneously may be ideal. Trientine has gained favor over penicillamine in recent years. Some might opt for zinc monotherapy in this setting.

No unequivocally clear consensus has yet developed for treating patients with established neurologic or psychiatric dysfunction. The primary choice is whether to initiate therapy with penicillamine or trientine. Both have their advocates, but a growing preference for trientine seems evident. Zinc is usually reserved for maintenance therapy following initial employment of a chelating agent.

Guidelines for the diagnosis and treatment of Wilson disease have been published by the European Association for the Study of the Liver (EASL).[155]

REFERENCES

1. Camilleri M, Barucha AE: An overview of gastrointestinal dysfunction in diseases of central and peripheral nervous systems. p. 35. In: Quigley EMM, Pfeiffer RF (eds): Neurogastroenterology. Butterworth Heinemann, Philadelphia, 2004.
2. Arbarbanel JM, Berginer VM, Osimani A, et al: Neurologic complications after gastric resection surgery for morbid obesity. Neurology 37:196, 1987.
3. Thaisetthawatkul P, Collazo-Clavell ML, Sarr MG, et al: A controlled study of peripheral neuropathy after bariatric surgery. Neurology 63:1462, 2004.
4. Thaisetthawatkul P, Collazo-Clavell ML, Sarr MG, et al: Good nutritional control may prevent polyneuropathy after bariatric surgery. Muscle Nerve 42:709, 2010.
5. Becker DA, Balcer LJ, Galetta SL: The neurological complications of nutritional deficiency following bariatric surgery. J Obes 2012:608534, 2012.
6. Frantz DJ: Neurologic complications of bariatric surgery: involvement of central, peripheral, and enteric nervous systems. Curr Gastroenterol Rep 14:367, 2012.
7. Koffman BM, Greenfield LJ, Ali I, et al: Neurologic complications after surgery for obesity. Muscle Nerve 33:166, 2006.
8. Macgregor AM, Thoburn EK: Meralgia paresthetica following bariatric surgery. Obes Surg 9:364, 1999.
9. Lin IC, Lin YL: Peripheral polyneuropathy after bariatric surgery for morbid obesity. J Family Community Med 18:162, 2011.
10. de Oliveira LD, Diniz MT, de Fátima HS Diniz M, et al: Rhabdomyolysis after bariatric surgery by Roux-en-Y gastric bypass: a prospective study. Obes Surg 19:1102, 2009.
11. Mognol P, Vignes S, Chosidow D, et al: Rhabdomyolysis after laparoscopic bariatric surgery. Obes Surg 14:91, 2004.
12. de Freitas Carvalho DA, Valezi AC, de Brito EM, et al: Rhabdomyolysis after bariatric surgery. Obes Surg 16:740, 2006.
13. Khurana RN, Baudendistel TE, Morgan EF, et al: Postoperative rhabdomyolysis following laparoscopic

gastric bypass in the morbidly obese. Arch Surg 139:73, 2004.

14. Youssef T, Abd-Elaal I, Zakaria G, et al: Bariatric surgery: rhabdomyolysis after open Roux-en-Y gastric bypass: a prospective study. Int J Surg 8:484, 2010.
15. Georgoulas TJ, Tournis S, Lyritis GP: Development of osteomalacic myopathy in a morbidly obese woman following bariatric surgery. J Musculoskelet Neuronal Interact 10:287, 2010.
16. Juhasz-Pocsine K, Rudnicki SA, Archer RL, et al: Neurologic complications of gastric bypass surgery for morbid obesity. Neurology 68:1843, 2007.
17. Gletsu-Miller N, Broderius M, Frediani JK, et al: Incidence and prevalence of copper deficiency following Roux-en-Y gastric bypass surgery. Int J Obes (Lond) 36:328, 2012.
18. Green PH, Cellier C: Celiac disease. N Engl J Med 357:1731, 2007.
19. Tjon JM, van Bergen J, Koning F: Celiac disease: how complicated can it get? Immunogenetics 62:641, 2010.
20. Vilppula A, Collin P, Mäki M, et al: Undetected coeliac disease in the elderly: a biopsy-proven population-based study. Dig Liver Dis 40:809, 2008.
21. Megiorni F, Pizzuti A: *HLA-DQA1* and *HLA-DQB1* in celiac disease predisposition: practical implications of the HLA molecular typing. J Biomed Sci 19:88, 2012.
22. Hadjivassiliou M, Sanders DS, Grünewald RA, et al: Gluten sensitivity: from gut to brain. Lancet Neurol 9:318, 2010.
23. Briani C, Zara G, Alaedini A, et al: Neurological complications of celiac disease and autoimmune mechanisms: a prospective study. J Neuroimmunol 195:171, 2008.
24. Bürk K, Farecki ML, Lamprecht G, et al: Neurological symptoms in patients with biopsy proven celiac disease. Mov Disord 24:2358, 2009.
25. Grossman G: Neurological complications of coeliac disease: what is the evidence? Pract Neurol 8:77, 2008.
26. Javed S, Safdar A, Forster A, et al: Refractory coeliac disease associated with late onset epilepsy, ataxia, tremor and progressive myoclonus with giant cortical evoked potentials – a case report and review of literature. Seizure 21:482, 2012.
27. Currie S, Hadjivassiliou M, Clark MJR, et al: Should we be "nervous" about coeliac disease? Brain abnormalities in patients with coeliac disease referred for neurological opinion. J Neurol Neurosurg Psychiatry 83:1216, 2012.
28. Hadjivassiliou M, Sanders DS, Woodroofe N, et al: Gluten ataxia. Cerebellum 7:494, 2008.
29. Hadjivassiliou M, Grünewald R, Sharrack B, et al: Gluten ataxia in perspective: epidemiology, genetic susceptibility and clinical characteristics. Brain 126:685, 2003.
30. Sapone A, Bai JC, Ciacci C, et al: Spectrum of gluten-related disorders: consensus on new nomenclature and classification. BMC Med 10:13, 2012.
31. Hadjivassiliou M, Aeschlimann P, Strigun A, et al: Autoantibodies in gluten ataxia recognize a novel neuronal transglutaminase. Ann Neurol 64:332, 2008.
32. Zelnik N, Pacht A, Obeid R, et al: Range of neurologic disorders in patients with celiac disease. Pediatrics 113:1672, 2004.
33. Hadjivassiliou M, Grünewald RA, Chattopadhyay AK, et al: Clinical, radiological, neurophysiological, and neuropathological characteristics of gluten ataxia. Lancet 352:1582, 1998.
34. Hadjivassiliou M, Davies-Jones GA, Sanders DS, et al: Dietary treatment of gluten ataxia. J Neurol Neurosurg Psychiatry 74:1221, 2003.
35. Nanri K, Okita M, Takeguchi M, et al: Intravenous immunoglobulin therapy for autoantibody-positive cerebellar ataxia. Intern Med 48:783, 2009.
36. Vaknin A, Eliakim R, Ackerman Z, et al: Neurological abnormalities associated with celiac disease. J Neurol 251:1393, 2004.
37. Luostarinen L, Himanen SL, Luostarinen M, et al: Neuromuscular and sensory disturbances in patients with well treated coeliac disease. J Neurol Neurosurg Psychiatry 74:490, 2003.
38. Chin RL, Sander HW, Brannagan TH, et al: Celiac neuropathy. Neurology 60:1581, 2003.
39. Hadjivassiliou M, Grünewald RA, Kandler RH, et al: Neuropathy associated with gluten sensitivity. J Neurol Neurosurg Psychiatry 77:1262, 2006.
40. Matà S, Renzi D, Pinto F, et al: Anti-tissue transglutaminase IgA antibodies in peripheral neuropathy and motor neuronopathy. Acta Neurol Scand 114:54, 2006.
41. Hadjivassiliou M, Kandler RH, Chattopadhyay AK, et al: Dietary treatment of gluten neuropathy. Muscle Nerve 34:762, 2006.
42. Tursi A, Giorgetti GM, Iani C, et al: Peripheral neurological disturbances, autonomic dysfunction, and antineuronal antibodies in adult celiac disease before and after a gluten-free diet. Dig Dis Sci 51:1869, 2006.
43. Selva-O'Callaghan A, Casellas F, de Torres I, et al: Celiac disease and antibodies associated with celiac disease in patients with inflammatory myopathy. Muscle Nerve 35:49, 2007.
44. Kleopa KA, Kyriacou K, Zamba-Papanicolaou E, et al: Reversible inflammatory and vacuolar myopathy with vitamin E deficiency in celiac disease. Muscle Nerve 31:260, 2005.
45. Licchetta L, Bisulli F, Di Vito L, et al: Epilepsy in coeliac disease: not just a matter of calcifications. Neurol Sci 32:1069, 2011.
46. Ranua J, Luoma K, Auvinen A, et al: Celiac disease-related antibodies in an epilepsy cohort and matched reference population. Epilepsy Behav 6:388, 2005.
47. Pfaender M, D'Souza WJ, Trost N, et al: Visual disturbances representing occipital lobe epilepsy in patients

with cerebral calcifications and coeliac disease: a case series. J Neurol Neurosurg Psychiatry 75:1623, 2004.
48. Gabrielli M, Cremonini F, Fiore G, et al: Association between migraine and celiac disease: results from a preliminary case-control and therapeutic study. Am J Gastroenterol 98:625, 2003.
49. Gibbons CH, Freeman R: Autonomic neuropathy and coeliac disease. J Neurol Neurosurg Psychiatry 76:579, 2005.
50. Jacob S, Zarei M, Kenton A, et al: Gluten sensitivity and neuromyelitis optica: two case reports. J Neurol Neurosurg Psychiatry 76:1028, 2005.
51. Pfeiffer RF, Shanahan F: Inflammatory bowel disease. p. 228. In Biller J (ed): The Interface of Neurology and Internal Medicine. Lippincott Williams & Wilkins, Philadelphia, 2008.
52. Larsen S, Bendtzen K, Nielsen OH: Extraintestinal manifestations of inflammatory bowel disease: epidemiology, diagnosis, and management. Ann Med 42:97, 2010.
53. Levine JS, Burakoff R: Extraintestinal manifestations of inflammatory bowel disease. Gastroenterol Hepatol (NY) 7:235, 2011.
54. Singh S, Kumar N, Loftus EV Jr, et al: Neurologic complications in patients with inflammatory bowel disease: increasing relevance in the era of biologics. Inflamm Bowel Dis 19:864, 2013.
55. Benavente L, Morís G: Neurologic disorders associated with inflammatory bowel disease. Eur J Neurol 18:138, 2011.
56. Nozaki K, Silver RM, Stickler DE, et al: Neurological deficits during treatment with tumor necrosis factor-alpha antagonists. Am J Med Sci 342:352, 2011.
57. Lossos A, River Y, Eliakim A, et al: Neurologic aspects of inflammatory bowel disease. Neurology 45:416, 1995.
58. Elsehety A, Bertorini TE: Neurologic and neuropsychiatric complications of Crohn's disease. South Med J 90:606, 1997.
59. Oliveira GR, Teles BCV, Brasil ÉF, et al: Peripheral neuropathy and neurological disorders in an unselected Brazilian population-based cohort of IBD patients. Inflamm Bowel Dis 14:389, 2008.
60. Sassi SB, Kallel L, Ben Romdhane S, et al: Peripheral neuropathy in inflammatory bowel disease patients: a prospective cohort study. Scand J Gastroenterol 44:1268, 2009.
61. Coert JH, Dellon AL: Neuropathy related to Crohn's disease treated by peripheral nerve decompression. Scand J Plast Reconstr Surg Hand Surg 37:243, 2003.
62. Greco F, Pavone P, Falsaperla R, et al: Peripheral neuropathy as first sign of ulcerative colitis in a child. J Clin Gastroenterol 38:115, 2004.
63. Gondim FAA, Brannagan TH III, Sander HW, et al: Peripheral neuropathy in patients with inflammatory bowel disease. Brain 128:867, 2005.
64. Kumar BN, Smith MS, Walsh RM, et al: Sensorineural hearing loss in ulcerative colitis. Clin Otolaryngol Allied Sci 25:143, 2000.
65. Ratzinger G, Sepp N, Vogetseder W, et al: Cheilitis granulomatosa and Melkersson-Rosenthal syndrome: evaluation of gastrointestinal involvement and therapeutic regimens in a series of 14 patients. J Eur Acad Dermatol Venereol 21:1065, 2007.
66. Bernstein CN, Wajda A, Blanchard JF: The clustering of other chronic inflammatory diseases in inflammatory bowel disease: a population-based study. Gastroenterology 129:827, 2005.
67. Cohen R, Robinson D Jr, Paramore C, et al: Autoimmune disease concomitance among inflammatory bowel disease patients in the United States, 2001–2002. Inflamm Bowel Dis 14:738, 2008.
68. de Lau LML, de Vries JM, van der Woude CJ, et al: Acute CNS white matter lesions in patients with inflammatory bowel disease. Inflamm Bowel Dis 15:576, 2009.
69. Alkhawajah MM, Caminero AB, Freeman HJ, et al: Multiple sclerosis and inflammatory bowel diseases: what we know and what we would need to know! Mult Scler 19:259, 2013.
70. Andersohn F, Waring M, Garbe E: Risk of ischemic stroke in patients with Crohn's disease: a population-based nested case-control study. Inflamm Bowel Dis 16:1387, 2010.
71. Druschky A, Heckmann JG, Druschky K, et al: Severe neurological complications of ulcerative colitis. J Clin Neurosci 9:84, 2002.
72. Schluter A, Krasnianski M, Krivokuca M, et al: Magnetic resonance angiography in a patient with Crohn's disease associated cerebral vasculitis. Clin Neurol Neurosurg 106:110, 2004.
73. Younes-Mhenni S, Derex L, Berruyer M, et al: Large-artery stroke in a young patient with Crohn's disease. Role of vitamin B_6 deficiency-induced hyperhomocysteinemia. J Neurol Sci 221:113, 2004.
74. Ogawa E, Sakakibara R, Yoshimatsu Y, et al: Crohn's disease and stroke in a young adult. Intern Med 50:2407, 2011.
75. Katsanos AH, Katsanos KH, Kosmidou M, et al: Cerebral sinus thrombosis in inflammatory bowel diseases. QJM 106:401, 2013.
76. Christopoulos C, Savva S, Pylarinou S, et al: Localised gastrocnemius myositis in Crohn's disease. Clin Rheumatol 22:143, 2003.
77. Berger P, Wolf R, Flierman A, et al: Myositis as the first manifestation of an exacerbation of Crohn's disease. Ned Tijdschr Geneeskd 151:1295, 2007.
78. Smith C, Kavar B: Extensive spinal epidural abscess as a complication of Crohn's disease. J Clin Neurosci 17:144, 2010.
79. Rosencrantz R, Moon A, Raynes H, et al: Cyclosporine-induced neurotoxicity during treatment of Crohn's disease: lack of correlation with previously reported risk factors. Am J Gastroenterol 96:2778, 2001.

80. Aziz M, Stivaros S, Fagbemi A, et al: Acute disseminated encephalomyelitis in conjunction with inflammatory bowel disease. Eur J Paediatr Neurol 17:208, 2013.
81. Hahn JS, Berquist W, Alcorn DM, et al: Wernicke encephalopathy and beriberi during total parenteral nutrition attributable to multivitamin infusion shortage. Pediatrics 101:E10, 1998.
82. Kawakubo K, Iida M, Matsumoto T, et al: Progressive encephalopathy in a Crohn's disease patient on long-term total parenteral nutrition: possible relationship to selenium deficiency. Postgrad Med J 70:215, 1994.
83. Dutly F, Altwegg M: Whipple's disease and "Tropheryma whippelii". Clin Microbial Rev 14:561, 2001.
84. Schneider T, Moos V, Loddenkemper C, et al: Whipple's disease: new aspects of pathogenesis and treatment. Lancet Infect Dis 8:179, 2008.
85. Peters G, du Plessis DG, Humphrey PR: Cerebral Whipple's disease with a stroke-like presentation and cerebrovascular pathology. J Neurol Neurosurg Psychiatry 73:336, 2002.
86. Louis ED, Lynch T, Kaufmann P, et al: Diagnostic guidelines in central nervous system Whipple's disease. Ann Neurol 40:561, 1996.
87. Schwartz MA, Selhorst JB, Ochs AL, et al: Oculomasticatory myorhythmia: a unique movement disorder occurring in Whipple's disease. Ann Neurol 20:677, 1986.
88. Perkin GD, Murray-Lyon I: Neurology and the gastrointestinal system. J Neurol Neurosurg Psychiatry 65:291, 1998.
89. von Herbay A, Ditton HJ, Schuhmacher F, et al: Whipple's disease: staging and monitoring by cytology and polymerase chain reaction analysis of cerebrospinal fluid. Gastroenterology 113:434, 1997.
90. Lagier JC, Fenollar F, Lepidi H, et al: Failure and relapse after treatment with trimethoprim/sulfamethoxazole in classic Whipple's disease. J Antimicrob Chemother 65:2005, 2010.
91. Di Donato I, Bianchi S, Federico A: Ataxia with vitamin E deficiency: update of molecular diagnosis. Neurol Sci 31:511, 2010.
92. Angelini L, Erba A, Mariotti C, et al: Myoclonic dystonia as unique presentation of isolated vitamin E deficiency in a young patient. Mov Disord 17:612, 2002.
93. Hammond N, Wang Y: Fat soluble vitamins. p. 449. In Biller J (ed): The Interface of Neurology and Internal Medicine. Lippincott Williams & Wilkins, Philadelphia, 2008.
94. Ueda N, Suzuki Y, Rino Y, et al: Correlation between neurological dysfunction with vitamin E deficiency and gastrectomy. J Neurol Sci 287:216, 2009.
95. Stevenson VL, Hardie RJ: Acanthocytosis and neurological disorders. J Neurol 248:87, 2001.
96. Fogel BL, Perlman S: Clinical features and molecular genetics of autosomal recessive cerebellar ataxias. Lancet Neurol 6:245, 2007.
97. Zamel R, Khan R, Pollex RL, et al: Abetalipoproteinemia: two case reports and literature review. Orphanet J Rare Dis 3:19, 2008.
98. Soejima N, Ohyagi Y, Kikuchi H, et al: An adult case of probable Bassen-Kornzweig syndrome, presenting resting tremor. Rinsho Shinkeigaku 46:702, 2006.
99. Grant CA, Berson EL: Treatable forms of retinitis pigmentosa associated with systemic neurological disorders. Int Ophthalmol Clin 41:103, 2001.
100. Ramakrishna BS, Venkataraman S, Mukhopadhya A: Tropical malabsorption. Postgrad Med J 82:779, 2006.
101. Ranjan P, Ghoshal UC, Aggarwal R, et al: Etiological spectrum of sporadic malabsorption syndrome in northern Indian adults at a tertiary hospital. Indian J Gastroenterol 23:94, 2004.
102. Batheja MJ, Leighton J, Azueta A, et al: The face of tropical sprue in 2010. Case Rep Gastroenterol 4:168, 2010.
103. Iyer GV, Taori GM, Kapadia CR, et al: Neurologic manifestations in tropical sprue. A clinical and electrodiagnostic study. Neurology 23:959, 1973.
104. Kumar S, Ghoshal UC, Jayalakshmi K, et al: Abnormal small intestinal permeability in patients with idiopathic malabsorption in tropics (tropical sprue) does not change even after successful treatment. Dig Dis Sci 56:161, 2011.
105. Weathers AL, Lewis SL: Rare and unusual...or are they? Less commonly diagnosed encephalopathies associated with systemic disease. Semin Neurol 29:136, 2009.
106. Uruha A, Shimizu T, Katoh T, et al: Wernicke's encephalopathy in a patient with peptic ulcer disease. Case Rep Med 2011:156104, 2011.
107. Singh S, Kumar A: Wernicke encephalopathy after obesity surgery: a systematic review. Neurology 68:807, 2007.
108. Aasheim ET: Wernicke encephalopathy after bariatric surgery: a systematic review. Ann Surg 248:714, 2008.
109. Iannelli A, Addeo P, Novellas S, et al: Wernicke's encephalopathy after laparoscopic Roux-en-Y gastric bypass: a misdiagnosed complication. Obes Surg 20:1594, 2010.
110. Williams NL, Wiegand S, McKenna DS: Wernicke's encephalopathy complicating pregnancy in a woman with neonatal necrotizing enterocolitis and resultant chronic constipation. Am J Perinatol 26:519, 2009.
111. Lanska DJ: Historical aspects of the major neurological vitamin deficiency disorders: the water-soluble B vitamins. Handb Clin Neurol 95:445, 2010.
112. Spivak JL, Jackson DL: Pellagra: an analysis of 18 patients and a review of the literature. Johns Hopkins Med J 140:295, 1977.
113. Zaki I, Millard L: Pellagra complicating Crohn's disease. Postgrad Med J 71:496, 1995.

114. Abu-Qurshin R, Naschitz JE, Zuckermann E, et al: Crohn's disease associated with pellagra and increased excretion of 5-hydroxyindoleacetic acid. Am J Med Sci 313:111, 1997.
115. Lu JY, Yu CL, Wu MZ: Pellagra in an immunocompetent patient with cytomegalovirus colitis. Am J Gastroenterol 96:932, 2001.
116. Wierzbicka E, Machet L, Karsenti D, et al: Pellagra and panniculitis induced by chronic bacterial colonization of the small intestine. Ann Dermatol Venereol 132:140, 2005.
117. Kumar N: Copper deficiency myelopathy (human swayback). Mayo Clin Proc 81:1371, 2006.
118. Jaiser SR, Winston GP: Copper deficiency myelopathy. J Neurol 257:869, 2010.
119. Kumar N, Gross JB Jr, Ahlskog JE: Myelopathy due to copper deficiency. Neurology 61:273, 2003.
120. Kumar N, Ahlskog JE, Klein CJ, et al: Imaging features of copper deficiency myelopathy: a study of 25 cases. Neuroradiology 48:78, 2006.
121. Thuluvath PJ, Triger DR: Autonomic neuropathy and chronic liver disease. QJM 72:737, 1989.
122. Hendrickse MT, Thuluvath PJ, Triger DR: Natural history of autonomic neuropathy in chronic liver disease. Lancet 339:1462, 1992.
123. David WS, Peine C, Schlesinger P, et al: Nonsystemic vasculitic mononeuropathy multiplex, cryoglobulinemia, and hepatitis C. Muscle Nerve 19:1596, 1996.
124. Apartis E, Leger JM, Musset L, et al: Peripheral neuropathy associated with essential mixed cryoglobulinaemia: a role for hepatitis C virus infection? J Neurol Neurosurg Psychiatry 60:661, 1996.
125. Inoue A, Tsukada N, Koh CS, et al: Chronic relapsing demyelinating polyneuropathy associated with hepatitis B infection. Neurology 37:1663, 1987.
126. Lacaille F, Zylberberg H, Hagège H, et al: Hepatitis C associated with Guillain–Barré syndrome. Liver 18:49, 1998.
127. Matsuya M, Abe T, Tosaka M, et al: The first case of polymyositis associated with interferon therapy. Intern Med 33:806, 1994.
128. Illa I, Graus F, Ferrer I, Enriquez J: Sensory neuropathy as the initial manifestation of primary biliary cirrhosis. J Neurol Neurosurg Psychiatry 52:1307, 1989.
129. Keresztes K, Istenes I, Folhoffer A, et al: Autonomic and sensory nerve dysfunction in primary biliary cirrhosis. World J Gastroenterol 10:3039, 2004.
130. Schmidt HH: Role of genotyping in Wilson's disease. J Hepatol 50:449, 2009.
131. Mak CM, Lam CW: Diagnosis of Wilson's disease: a comprehensive review. Crit Rev Clin Lab Sci 45:263, 2008.
132. Brewer GJ: Wilson's Disease: A Clinician's Guide to Recognition, Diagnosis, and Management. Kluwer, Boston, 2001.
133. Merle U, Schaefer M, Ferenci P, et al: Clinical presentation, diagnosis and long-term outcome of Wilson's disease: a cohort study. Gut 56:115, 2007.
134. Czlonkowska A, Rodo M, Gromadzka G: Late onset Wilson's disease: therapeutic implications. Mov Disord 23:896, 2008.
135. Lech T, Hydzik P, Kosowski B: Significance of copper determination in late onset of Wilson's disease. Clin Toxicol (Phila) 45:688, 2007.
136. Korman JD, Volenberg I, Balko J, et al: Screening for Wilson disease in acute liver failure: a comparison of currently available diagnostic tests. Hepatology 48:1167, 2008.
137. Strickland GT, Leu ML: Wilson's disease. Clinical and laboratory manifestations in 40 patients. Medicine (Baltimore) 54:113, 1975.
138. Ala A, Borjigin J, Rochwarger A, et al: Wilson disease in septuagenarian siblings: raising the bar for diagnosis. Hepatology 41:668, 2005.
139. Machado A, Chien HF, Deguti MM, et al: Neurological manifestations in Wilson's disease: report of 119 cases. Mov Disord 21:2192, 2006.
140. Mueller A, Reuner U, Landis B, et al: Extrapyramidal symptoms in Wilson's disease are associated with olfactory dysfunction. Mov Disord 21:1311, 2006.
141. Walshe JM, Yealland M: Wilson's disease: the problem of delayed diagnosis. J Neurol Neurosurg Psychiatry 55:692, 1992.
142. Barbosa ER, Silveira-Moriyama L, Machado AC, et al: Wilson's disease with myoclonus and white matter lesions. Parkinsonism Relat Disord 13:185, 2007.
143. Shanmugiah A, Sinha S, Taly AB, et al: Psychiatric manifestations in Wilson's disease: a cross-sectional analysis. J Neuropsychiatry Clin Neurosci 20:81, 2008.
144. Roberts EA, Schilsky ML: A practice guideline on Wilson disease. Hepatology 37:1475, 2003.
145. Zhuang XH, Mo Y, Jiang XY, et al: Analysis of renal impairment in children with Wilson's disease. World J Pediatr 4:102, 2008.
146. Factor SM, Cho S, Sternlieb I, et al: The cardiomyopathy of Wilson's disease. Myocardial alterations in nine cases. Virchows Arch A Pathol Anat Histol 397:301, 1982.
147. Meenakshi-Sundaram S, Taly AB, Kamath V, et al: Autonomic dysfunction in Wilson's disease – a clinical and electrophysiological study. Clin Auton Res 12:185, 2002.
148. Bennett J, Hahn SH: Clinical molecular diagnosis of Wilson disease. Semin Liver Dis 31:233, 2011.
149. Scheinberg IH, Sternlieb I: Wilson's Disease. WB Saunders, Philadelphia, 1984.

150. Sinha S, Taly AB, Ravishankar S, et al: Wilson's disease: cranial MRI observations and clinical correlation. Neuroradiology 48:613, 2006.
151. Das SK, Ray K: Wilson's disease: an update. Nat Clin Pract Neurol 2:482, 2006.
152. Weisner B, Hartard C, Dieu C: CSF copper concentration: a new parameter for diagnosis and monitoring therapy of Wilson's disease with cerebral manifestation. J Neurol Sci 79:229, 1987.
153. Hoogenraad TU: Paradigm shift in treatment of Wilson's disease: zinc therapy now treatment of choice. Brain Dev 28:141, 2006.
154. Walshe JM, Yealland M: Chelation treatment of neurological Wilson's disease. QJM 86:197, 1993.
155. European Association for the Study of the Liver EASL clinical practice guidelines: Wilson's disease. J Hepatol 56:671, 2012.

CHAPTER

14

Disturbances of Gastrointestinal Motility and the Nervous System

MICHAEL CAMILLERI ■ ADIL E. BHARUCHA

INTERACTIONS BETWEEN EXTRINSIC NERVOUS SYSTEM AND THE GUT

Normal motility and transit through the gastrointestinal tract result from an intricately balanced series of control mechanisms (Fig. 14-1): the electrical and contractile properties of the smooth muscle cell that result from transmembrane fluxes of ions; control by the intrinsic nervous system through chemical transmitters, such as acetylcholine, biogenic amines, gastrointestinal neuropeptides, and nitric oxide; and regulatory extrinsic pathways (sympathetic and parasympathetic nervous systems). The neuropeptides may act as circulating hormones or at the site of their release (paracrine or neurocrine functions).

In the mammalian digestive tract, the intrinsic (or enteric) nervous system (ENS) contains about 100 million neurons, approximately the number present in the spinal cord. This integrative system is organized in ganglionated plexuses (Fig. 14-2), which include the interstitial cells of Cajal (the gastrointestinal pacemakers). The ENS is separate from the autonomic nervous system. It has several components: sensory mechanoreceptors and chemoreceptors, interneurons that process sensory input and control effector (motor and sensory) units, and effector secretor or motor neurons involved in secretory or motor functions of the gut. Preprogrammed neural circuits serve to integrate motor function within and between different regions and thereby control the coordinated functions of the entire gastrointestinal tract, such as the peristaltic reflex and probably the interdigestive migrating motor complex (Fig. 14-1). The synaptic pathways in the

Aminoff's Neurology and General Medicine, Fifth Edition.

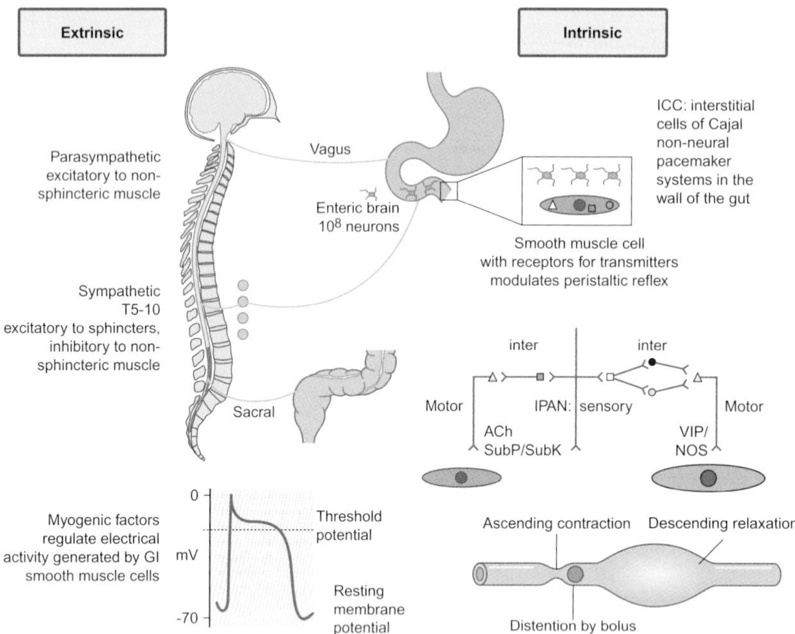

FIGURE 14-1 ■ Control of gut motility: interactions between extrinsic neural pathways and the intrinsic nervous system ("enteric brain" or enteric nervous system plexuses) modulate contractions of gastrointestinal smooth muscle. Interactions between transmitters (e.g., peptides and amines) and receptors alter muscle membrane potentials by stimulating bidirectional ion fluxes. In turn, membrane characteristics dictate whether the muscle cell contracts. (Adapted from Camilleri M, Phillips SF: Disorders of small intestinal motility. Gastroenterol Clin North Am 18:405, 1989, by permission of Mayo Foundation.)

gut wall are capable of autonomous adjustment in response to sensory input. They can also be modulated by the extrinsic nervous system, excitation by vagal and sacral (S2-4) preganglionic fibers, and inhibition by sympathetic activity.

Motor or secretory programmed circuits of the ENS are controlled by command vagal preganglionic or sympathetic postganglionic fibers. Thus, there are approximately 40,000 preganglionic vagal fibers (many of which are afferent, not efferent) at the level of the diaphragm; in contrast, 100 million neurons populate the enteric nervous system. The sympathetic supply inactivates neural circuits that generate motor activity while allowing intrinsic inhibitory innervation by the enteric nerves. Loss of the sympathetic inhibitory outflow from the intermediolateral column of the spinal cord between the fifth thoracic and upper lumbar levels ("the brake") may manifest with gut motor overactivity, including diarrhea.

The literature on this topic is extensive. Hence older citations for specific statements made in this chapter can be found in prior editions of the chapter.[1]

COMMON GASTROINTESTINAL SYMPTOMS IN NEUROLOGIC DISORDERS

Dysphagia

Dysphagia is the sensation of difficulty in swallowing. Oropharyngeal, or transfer, dysphagia is the inability to initiate a swallow or propel food from the mouth to the esophagus. The hold-up occurs in the cervical area and is generally caused by a lesion affecting any level of the swallowing pathway rather than by a process affecting the oropharyngeal mucosa. Stroke and Parkinson disease are the neurologic disorders most commonly associated with oropharyngeal dysphagia, which may also occur in brainstem diseases (e.g., bulbar polio, Arnold–Chiari malformations, tumors) or muscle diseases such as dystrophies and mitochondrial cytopathies. Esophageal dysphagia is caused by abnormal esophageal peristalsis, more typically with smooth muscle disorders (e.g., progressive systemic sclerosis).

Neuromuscular dysphagia typically results in dysphagia to both liquids and solids, and aspiration into the upper airways.

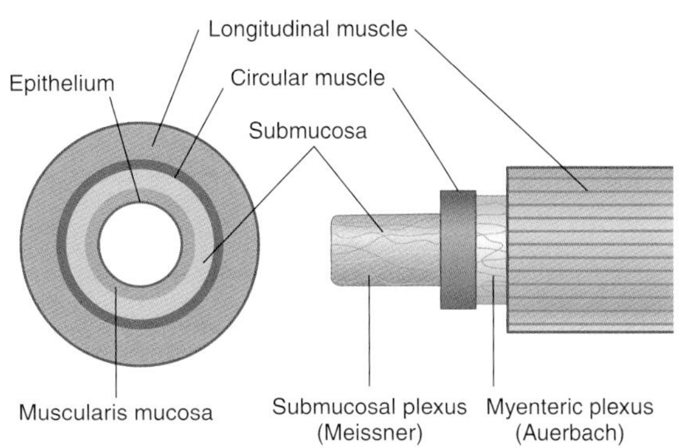

FIGURE 14-2 ▪ The enteric plexuses in the intestinal layers. The chief neural plexuses are in the submucosal and intermuscular layers.

Physical examination shows evidence of the coexisting neurologic disease, such as abnormal palatal or pharyngeal movements or a brisk jaw jerk, suggesting pseudo-bulbar palsy. Barium videofluoroscopy or a fiberoptic endoscopic evaluation of swallowing (FEES) can identify the motor and sensory disturbances, and may help stratify the risk of aspiration in patients with pharyngeal weakness.[2] Pharyngoesophageal motility studies using solid-state pressure transducers also complement the diagnosis. Re-education of the swallowing process is feasible in many patients, often in a program that incorporates speech therapy. Nutritional support and prevention of bronchial aspiration are essential for those with more severe dysphagia not responding to conservative measures. This may require a gastrostomy feeding tube. Since swallowing may improve considerably in the first 2 weeks after a stroke, long-term decisions should be delayed for that period.

Gastroparesis

Gastric motor dysfunction resulting in delayed gastric emptying is a common gastrointestinal manifestation of autonomic neuropathies such as those associated with diabetes mellitus,[3,4] surgical vagotomy (e.g., laparoscopic fundoplication), and numerous medications, most commonly narcotic analgesics, tricyclic antidepressants, and dopamine agonists. Symptoms range from vague postprandial abdominal discomfort to recurrent postprandial nausea, emesis, and bloating and pain resulting in weight loss and malnutrition. In diabetes mellitus, delayed gastric emptying is often asymptomatic. There may be a succussion splash on physical examination. It is essential to exclude gastric outlet obstruction by imaging the stomach or by endoscopy. Scintigraphic or stable isotope gastric emptying tests confirm delayed gastric emptying.[4] Gastric stasis in neurologic diseases may result from abnormal motility of the stomach or small bowel; studies of pressure profiles by manometry or solid-state pressure transducers (Fig. 14-3A) are rarely required to differentiate neuropathic from myopathic processes (Fig. 14-3B), and exclude mechanical obstruction. Gastroparesis management guidelines have been updated,[4] including the use of prokinetic agents, nutritional support, and interventions such as surgery and gastric electrical stimulation.

Chronic Intestinal Pseudo-Obstruction

Chronic intestinal pseudo-obstruction is a syndrome characterized by nausea, vomiting, early satiety, abdominal discomfort, weight loss, and altered bowel movements suggestive of intestinal obstruction in the absence of a mechanical obstruction. These symptoms are the consequence of abnormal intestinal motility, including neurologic diseases extrinsic to the gut (e.g., disorders at any level of the neural axis), dysfunction of neurons in the myenteric plexus, or degeneration or malfunction of gut smooth muscle (Table 14-1).

The patient's accompanying clinical features may suggest an underlying disease process. Such features include postural dizziness, difficulties in visual accommodation in bright lights, sweating abnormalities, recurrent urinary infections, and problems with bladder voiding that suggest an autonomic neuropathy. Urinary manifestations are more commonly the result of pelvic floor dysfunction that accompanies constipation, independent of any neurologic disease. Examination should evaluate pupillary reflexes to

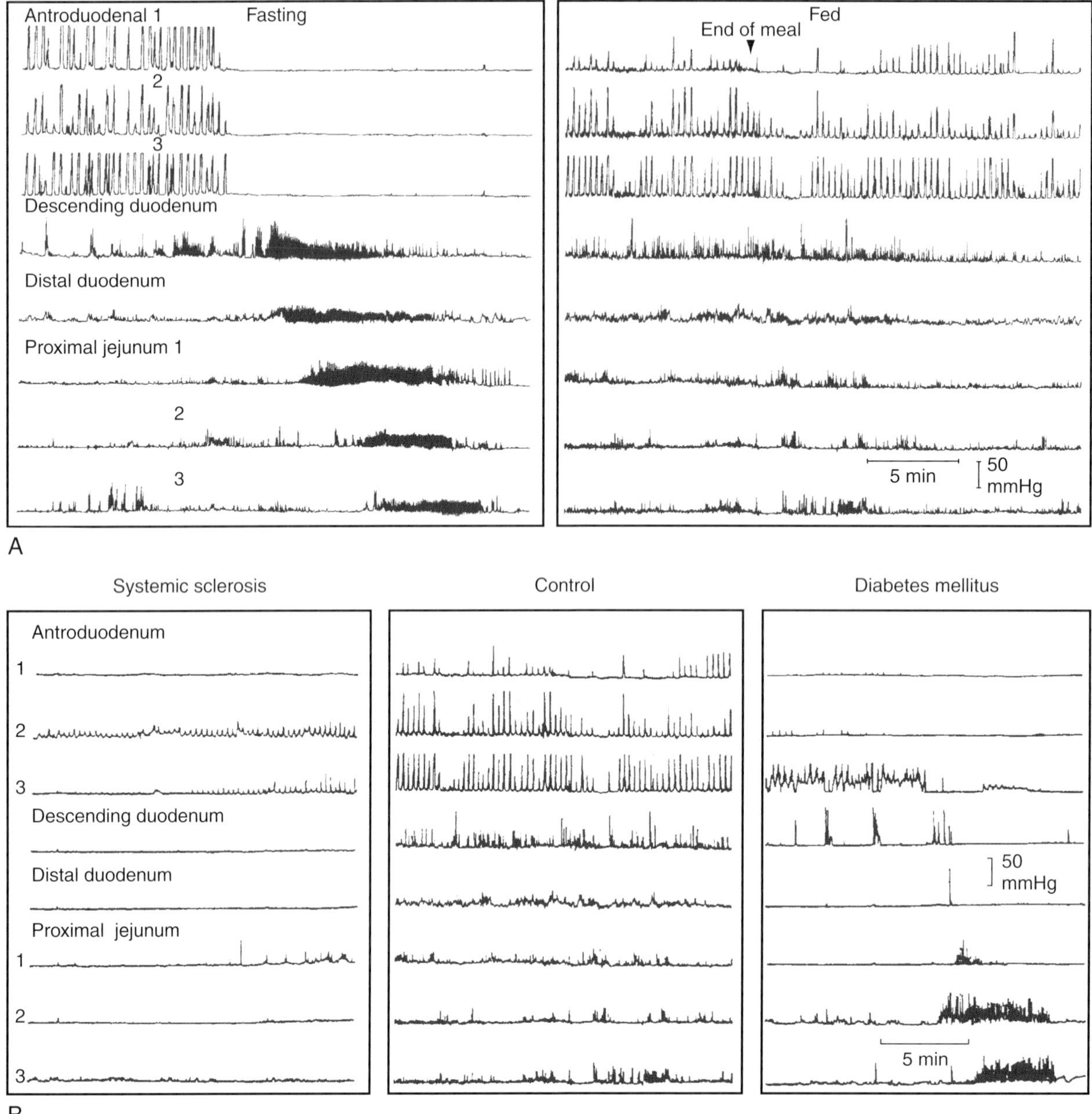

FIGURE 14-3 ■ **A**, Tracing showing normal upper gastrointestinal motility in the fasting and fed states. The fasting tracing shows phase III of the interdigestive migrating motor complex. **B**, Manometric tracings showing the myopathic pattern of intestinal pseudo-obstruction due to systemic sclerosis (*left panel*). Note the low amplitude of phasic pressure activity compared with control (*middle panel*). A manometric example of neuropathic intestinal pseudo-obstruction in diabetes mellitus shows the absence of antral contractions and persistence of cyclical fasting-type motility in the postprandial period (*right panel*). (**A** from Malagelada J-R, Camilleri M, Stanghellini V: Manometric Diagnosis of Gastrointestinal Motility Disorders. Thieme, New York, 1986, by permission of Mayo Foundation. **B** from Camilleri M: Medical treatment of chronic intestinal pseudo-obstruction. Pract Gastroenterol 15:10, 1991, with permission.)

light and accommodation, blood pressure and pulse in lying and standing positions, and abdominal distention or succussion splash.

The combination of external ophthalmoplegia, high dysphagia, peripheral neuromyopathy (e.g., increased serum creatine kinase) and acidosis (e.g., increased lactate, pyruvate) suggests mitochondrial cytopathy, a rare disorder associated with small bowel pseudo-obstruction and diverticulosis.[5] Use of narcotics, phenothiazines, dopaminergic agents, antihypertensive agents such as clonidine, and tricyclic antidepressants

TABLE 14-1 ■ Causes of Chronic Intestinal Pseudo-Obstruction

Cause	Myopathic	Neuropathic
Infiltrative	Progressive systemic sclerosis (PSS) Amyloidosis	Early PSS Amyloidosis
Familial	Familial visceral myopathies, including metabolic myopathies	Familial visceral neuropathies
General neurologic diseases	Myotonic and other dystrophies Mitochondrial cytopathies	Diabetes mellitus Porphyria Heavy metal poisoning Brainstem tumor Parkinson disease Multiple sclerosis Spinal cord transection
Infectious		Chagas disease Cytomegalovirus infection
Drug-induced		Tricyclic antidepressants Narcotic bowel syndrome
Neoplastic		Paraneoplastic (bronchial small cell carcinoma or carcinoid)
Idiopathic	Hollow visceral myopathy	Chronic intestinal pseudo-obstruction (possibly myenteric plexopathy)

having anticholinergic effects may cause intestinal dysmotility.

Plain radiographs and barium follow-through or computed tomographic (CT) or magnetic resonance (MR) enterography are often nonspecific; dilatation of the small intestine is more frequent in later stages of myopathic than neuropathic disorders. Motility studies (Fig. 14-3) help differentiate myopathic and neuropathic processes. When a neuropathic process is identified, autonomic, radiologic and serologic tests should be performed to identify the cause of the autonomic neuropathy or cerebrospinal disease (see later).

The goals of treatment of chronic intestinal pseudo-obstruction include the restoration of hydration and nutrition, stimulation of normal intestinal propulsion, and suppression of bacterial overgrowth.

Constipation

Constipation is a common complaint and may be perceived by the patient as infrequent bowel movements, excessively hard stools, the need to strain excessively during defecation, or a sense of incomplete evacuation after defecation. The need for enemas or finger evacuation to expel the stool from the lower rectum suggests a disturbance of the pelvic floor or anorectum. The coexistence of incontinence and lack of rectal sensation suggests a neuropathy and is common among patients with diabetic neuropathy. The presence of blood in the stool with constipation necessitates further tests to exclude colonic mucosal lesions such as polyps, or perianal conditions such as hemorrhoids.

Broadly, constipation in neurologic disorders may be caused by potentially reversible factors (e.g., inadequate dietary fiber intake, lack of exercise, medications), slow colonic transit or pelvic floor dysfunction (i.e., a defecatory disorder) that may be related to the neurologic disorder, or another disease (e.g., colon cancer),[6] or it may be a manifestation of functional disorder in patients who have a neurologic disease (Fig. 14-4). Many neurologic diseases (e.g., Parkinson disease, multiple sclerosis, spinal cord injury, and autonomic neuropathies) can affect colonic transit and pelvic floor functions or lead to diminished rectal sensation (e.g., due to a neuropathy or spinal cord injury).

The diagnosis and management of constipation in patients with neuromuscular disease include assessment of colonic anatomy, transit, and rectal evacuation.[6,7] Slow colonic transit occurs frequently in wheelchair- or bed-bound patients and may require, in addition, stimulant cathartics or prokinetic medications and scheduled enemas daily or on alternate days. In patients with paraplegia, computer-assisted sacral anterior root stimulation has been used to evoke sigmoid and rectal contraction coordinated with sphincter relaxation, which resembles normal defecation. This procedure reduces the time for defecation and the interval between defecations. A dorsal rhizotomy must be performed to avoid general stimulation of autonomic responses. This treatment is available at specialized centers. An alternative treatment for colonic inertia (severe neuromuscular dysfunction with absent response to food ingestion or intravenous neostigmine) may be subtotal colectomy with ileorectostomy; however, if sphincter function is deficient and cannot be rehabilitated with physical therapy, a colostomy or ileostomy may be necessary. Other surgical procedures may correct a rectal prolapse or a rectocele.

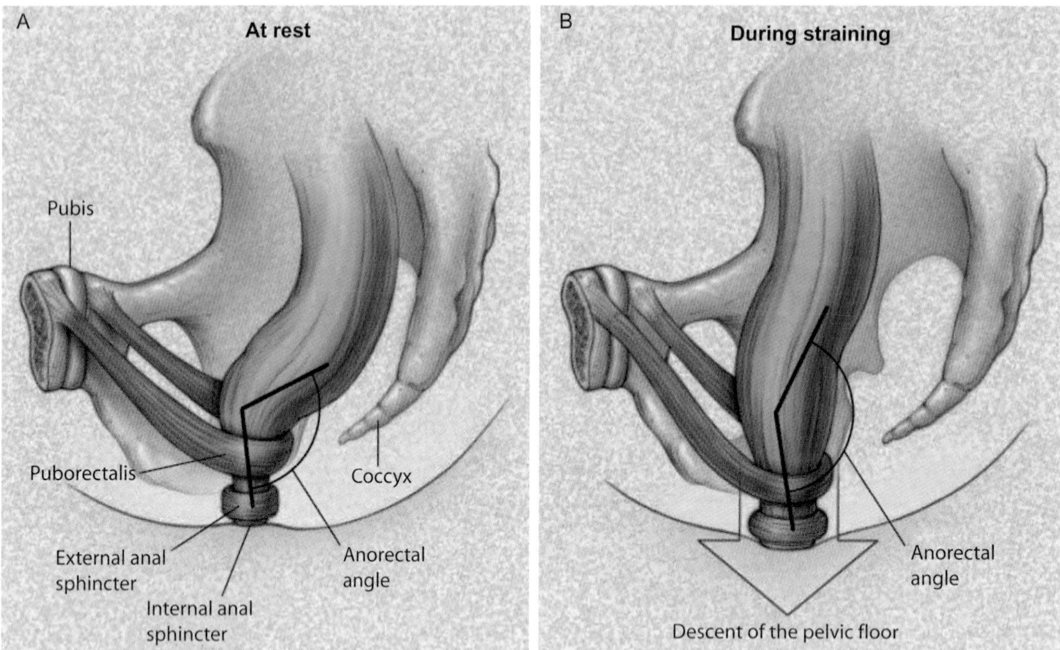

FIGURE 14-4 ■ Schema showing normal alternations of pelvic floor, rectoanal angle, and sphincters during defecation. (From Lembo T, Camilleri M: Chronic constipation. N Engl J Med 349:1360, 2003, with permission.)

Diarrhea

Diarrhea is defined as passage of abnormally liquid or unformed stools at an increased frequency, and is termed "chronic" if more than 4 weeks in duration. Acute diarrhea in neurologic patients is most frequently caused by infectious agents or medications. The differential diagnosis of chronic diarrhea is discussed in detail elsewhere.[8] In autonomic neuropathies, as in patients with diabetic neuropathy, chronic diarrhea is often multifactorial and may be associated with intake of osmotic agents (e.g., artificial sweeteners), secretion, malabsorption secondary to rapid transit (possibly due to sympathetic denervation), small bowel bacterial overgrowth, bile acid diarrhea, and high-amplitude propulsive contractions in the colon that result in urgency and sometimes incontinence of stool.[8,9]

Generally, the aid of a gastroenterologist is necessary to evaluate patients and guide diagnostic tests. Features of fat malabsorption (e.g., greasy, difficult-to-flush stools, weight loss) should prompt a 24- to 48-hour stool collection with quantitation of stool fat and, where available, total stool bile acids. The coexistence of diarrhea and neurologic manifestations may be explained by autonomic dysfunction (e.g., in diabetic neuropathy), the neurologic consequences of malabsorption (e.g., myopathy or neuropathy in celiac disease), and rare diseases with neurologic manifestations (e.g., Whipple disease). After excluding a structural cause (e.g., inflammatory bowel disease) and malabsorption, most patients with diarrhea due to disordered motility can be treated effectively with loperamide, beginning with 2 mg taken 30 minutes before meals, and titrated to control symptoms up to a maximum of 16 mg daily. Patients should be tested and treated for bacterial overgrowth. The α_2-adrenergic agonist clonidine reduces diarrhea by improving intestinal absorption, inhibiting intestinal and colonic motility, and enhancing resting anal sphincter tone; however, it aggravates postural hypotension, even when administered by transdermal patch. Other agents to be considered are oral bile acid sequestrants (e.g., cholestyramine and colesevelam) and subcutaneous octreotide.

Fecal Incontinence

Fecal incontinence may result from multiple sclerosis, Parkinson disease, multiple system atrophy, Alzheimer disease, stroke, diabetic neuropathy, and spinal cord lesions. In addition to generalized neuropathies (e.g., diabetes), obstetric trauma and stretch-induced pudendal nerve injury related to excessive straining in constipated patients are other causes of a pudendal neuropathy.[10] Incontinence occurring only at night suggests internal anal sphincter dysfunction (e.g., progressive systemic sclerosis); stress incontinence during coughing, sneezing, or laughing suggests loss of external sphincter control, typically from pudendal nerve or S2, S3, and S4 root lesions. Leakage of formed stool suggests more severe sphincter weakness than leakage of liquid stool alone.

Examination of the incontinent patient should include inspection of the anus with and without straining to detect rectal prolapse, a digital rectal examination, and proctoscopy to exclude impaction or mucosal disease. Anal examination may disclose normal (e.g., multiple sclerosis) or reduced (e.g., diabetes mellitus, scleroderma) anal resting tone. The external sphincter and puborectalis contractile responses during squeeze are reduced, and the perianal wink reflex is absent in conditions affecting the lower spinal cord or pudendal nerves. Perineal weakness is often manifested by excessive perineal descent (>4cm) on straining.

In evaluating such patients, it is important first to exclude overflow incontinence due to fecal impaction; overuse of laxatives or magnesium-containing antacids may result in reversible incontinence. If these are not identified as the cause of incontinence, further tests may be necessary: anorectal manometry, rectal sensation, ability to expel a balloon from the rectum, endoanal ultrasound or MRI to identify anal sphincter defects, and dynamic barium or MR defecography to identify rectal evacuation and anatomic abnormalities (e.g., rectocele, rectal intussusception). EMG of the anal sphincter is rarely required in patients with clinically suspected neurogenic sphincter weakness, particularly if there are features suggestive of proximal (i.e., sacral root) involvement; EMG provides evidence of denervation (fibrillation potentials), myopathic damage (small polyphasic motor unit potentials), neurogenic damage (large polyphasic motor unit potentials), or mixed injury.[11,12] Pudendal neuropathy can be diagnosed with certainty when neurogenic changes affect anterior and posterior quadrants of the anal sphincter or they are also identified in the ischiocavernosus muscle.

Medical management includes perianal hygiene, protective devices to maintain skin integrity, and restoration of regular bowel habits. Biofeedback therapy has little impact in patients with weakness of the pelvic floor muscles or poor rectal sensation. Clonidine may help some patients, if it is tolerated. A colostomy may be necessary in patients with medically refractory fecal incontinence. Before resorting to this, it is important to exclude mucosal prolapse in association with incontinence, since surgical correction of the prolapse may temporarily improve continence by permitting better function of the external sphincter.[13] More complex surgical procedures (i.e., artificial anal sphincter, dynamic graciloplasty) are not routinely performed in the United States. Sacral nerve stimulation can improve symptoms, anal pressures, and rectal sensation, even in patients with neurogenic fecal incontinence.[14]

EXTRINSIC NEUROLOGIC DISORDERS CAUSING GUT DYSMOTILITY

Certain diseases affect both intrinsic and extrinsic neural control. This review concentrates on diseases of extrinsic neural control and smooth muscle. Diseases affecting the enteric nervous system are reviewed elsewhere.

Brain Diseases

Stroke

Dysphagia may result from cranial nerve involvement and may cause malnutrition or aspiration pneumonia. Videofluoroscopy of the pharynx and upper esophagus typically shows transfer dysphagia or tracheal aspiration. Colonic pseudo-obstruction occurs rarely. Percutaneous endoscopic gastrostomy is usually the most effective method to provide nutrition without interfering with rehabilitation; feedings can be given in the forms of boluses or by infusion at night. Swallowing improves in a majority of survivors over 1 week to 3 months. The severity of the initial neurologic deficit is the strongest predictor of eventual recovery. The gastrostomy tube can be removed when oral intake is shown to be sufficient to maintain caloric requirements.

Alzheimer Disease

In a retrospective population-based study, people with Alzheimer disease, aged 65 years and older, had a higher incidence of serious upper and lower gastrointestinal (GI) events including ulceration, perforation and bleeding than a well-matched random sample of people without Alzheimer disease. The association was also present in participants without a history of GI bleeding.[15] Treatment of Alzheimer disease with the acetylcholinesterase medications, such as donepezil or rivastigmine, is associated with gastrointestinal symptoms, such as nausea, vomiting, and diarrhea. These may be dose related and may be reduced by using transdermal preparations.[16,17]

Parkinsonism

Gastrointestinal dysfunction is a prominent manifestation of Parkinson disease. Symptoms include reduced salivation, dysphagia, impaired gastric emptying, constipation, and defecatory dysfunction. Constipation may precede the development of somatic motor symptoms by several years. Patients with Parkinson disease or progressive supranuclear palsy may have oropharyngeal dysfunction with impaired swallowing. Shy–Drager syndrome, or multiple system atrophy, is considered later. Patients may have mild to moderate malnutrition; moderate dysphagia may be diagnosed by videofluoroscopy. In the absence of severe malnutrition or significant aspiration, conservative treatment with attention to the consistency of food (thickened liquids) and to adequate caloric content of meals will suffice. Feeding through a percutaneous gastrostomy is an appropriate alternative for severe dysphagia. In one study, gastric emptying of liquids was not inhibited by levodopa and a dopa decarboxylase inhibitor.[18]

Constipation is common in patients with parkinsonism and may be the result of slow colonic transit or of pelvic floor or anal sphincter dysfunction. Gastrointestinal hypomotility, generalized hypokinesia, associated autonomic dysfunction, and the effects of various anticholinergic and dopamine agonist medications may all play a role. The bioavailability of other medications can be altered considerably by the effects of parkinsonism on gut transit and delivery of medications to the small bowel for absorption.

In addition to gastrointestinal symptoms, it has been suggested that the gut is a portal of entry for prions leading to neurologic diseases such as Alzheimer and Parkinson disease and transmissible spongiform encephalopathies.[19] Neuropathologic studies have shown early accumulation of abnormal inclusions containing α-synuclein (Lewy neurites) in the enteric nervous system and dorsal motor nucleus of the vagus, in both Parkinson and incidental Lewy body disease. These findings led to the hypothesis that α-synuclein pathology progresses in a centripetal, prion-like fashion from the ENS to the dorsal motor nucleus of the vagus and then to more rostral areas of the central nervous system. Colonic biopsies may show accumulation of α-synuclein immunoreactive Lewy neurites in the submucosal plexus of patients with Parkinson disease.[20] On the other hand, α-synuclein is abundantly expressed in all nerve plexus of the human ENS, especially with increasing age, and may not, therefore, be regarded as a pathologic correlate.[21] Mucosal biopsies from the ascending colon showed signs of inflammation in patients with Parkinson disease, but there was no correlation with disease severity, duration, or presence of enteric Lewy pathology.[22]

Head Injury

Immediately following moderate to severe head injury, most patients develop transient delays in gastric emptying. The underlying mechanism is unknown, although a correlation exists between the severity of injury, increased intracranial pressure, and severity of the gastric stasis. These patients are frequently intolerant of enteral feeding and may require parenteral nutrition temporarily. Enteral nutrition can often be reintroduced within 2 to 3 weeks.

Autonomic Epilepsy and Migraine

Autonomic epilepsy and migraine are infrequent causes of upper abdominal symptoms, such as nausea and vomiting. Treatment is of the underlying neurologic disorder.

Amyotrophic Lateral Sclerosis

Patients with amyotrophic lateral sclerosis (ALS) and progressive bulbar palsy have predominant weakness of the muscles supplied by the glossopharyngeal and vagus nerves. Dysphagia is a frequent complaint, and patients may have respiratory difficulty while eating as a result of aspiration or respiratory muscle fatigue. Rarely, patients with vagal dysfunction develop chronic intestinal pseudo-obstruction.

Physical examination reveals cranial nerve palsies, muscle fasciculations, or an exaggerated jaw jerk. Videofluoroscopic barium swallow of liquids and solids is employed to evaluate swallowing, determine whether aspiration occurs, and guide decisions about the route to use for nutritional support (oral feeding or a percutaneous gastrostomy). Cervical esophagostomy or cricopharyngeal myotomy have been performed in selected cases for significant cricopharyngeal muscle dysfunction.

Postpolio Dysphagia

Patients with postpolio syndrome frequently have dysphagia and aspiration, especially if there was bulbar involvement during the initial attack. Videofluoroscopy is useful for screening and monitoring progression of disease. Attention to the position of the patient's head during swallowing and alteration of food consistency to a semisolid state can decrease the prevalence of choking and aspiration.

Brainstem Lesions

Brainstem lesions can present with isolated gastrointestinal motor dysfunction. Compression of the brainstem and lower cranial nerves can cause potentially life-threatening neurogenic dysphagia in patients with Arnold–Chiari malformations. In the absence of increased intracranial pressure, gastrointestinal symptoms in association with brain tumors typically result from distortion of the vomiting center on the floor of the fourth ventricle, with delay in gastric emptying. Although vomiting is the most common symptom, colonic and anorectal dysfunction has also been described. The presence of more widespread autonomic dysfunction, particularly if preganglionic sympathetic nerves are involved, necessitates a search for a structural lesion in the central nervous system.

Autonomic System Degenerations

Pandysautonomias or Selective Dysautonomias

Pandysautonomias are characterized by preganglionic or postganglionic lesions affecting both the sympathetic and parasympathetic nervous systems. Vomiting, paralytic ileus, constipation, and a chronic pseudo-obstruction syndrome have been reported in acute, subacute, and congenital pandysautonomia. Selective cholinergic dysautonomia may also impair upper and lower gastrointestinal motor activity. This picture usually follows a viral infection such as infectious mononucleosis[23] or influenza A.[24]

Idiopathic Orthostatic Hypotension

Idiopathic orthostatic hypotension is sometimes associated with motor dysfunction of the gut, such as esophageal dysmotility, gastric stasis, alteration in bowel movements, and fecal incontinence. Cardiovascular and sudomotor abnormalities usually precede gut involvement. The precise site of the lesion causing the gut dysmotility is unknown.

Postural Orthostatic Tachycardia Syndrome

About one-third of patients with postural orthostatic tachycardia syndrome (POTS) have gastrointestinal manifestations, including pseudo-obstruction syndrome. It is important to exclude dehydration, deconditioning, and functional gastrointestinal disorders that produce similar clinical features.

Multiple System Atrophy

In the original description of this disorder, constipation and fecal incontinence were included among its classic features. Abnormal esophageal motility was demonstrated by videofluoroscopy and by the occurrence of frequent, simultaneous, low-amplitude peristaltic waves on esophageal manometry. Fasting and postprandial antral and small bowel motility may be reduced.

Spinal Cord Lesions

Spinal Cord Injury

Dysphagia after acute cervical spinal cord injury (SCI) generally improves during the initial hospitalization.[25] Early recognition of dysphagia, which often precedes other brainstem symptoms, is important to avoid irreversible brainstem injury, to preserve nutrition and pulmonary functions, and to maximize restoration of function after surgery.

Ileus is a frequent finding soon after spinal cord injury, but it is rarely prolonged. Acalculous cholecystitis occurs in 3.7 percent of patients with acute SCI.

Bowel problems occur in 27 to 62 percent of patients with SCI, most commonly constipation, distention, abdominal pain, rectal bleeding, hemorrhoids, fecal incontinence, and autonomic hyperreflexia; gallstones occur in 17 to 31 percent of patients.[26] In the chronic phase after injury, disorders of upper gastrointestinal motility are uncommon, whereas colonic and anorectal dysfunctions are common. The latter probably result from interruption of supraspinal control of the sacral parasympathetic supply to the colon, pelvic floor, and anal sphincters. After thoracic SCI, colonic compliance and postprandial colonic motor responses may be reduced. The loss of voluntary control of defecation may be the most significant disturbance in patients who rely on reflex rectal stimulation for stool evacuation. Fecal impaction may present with anorexia and nausea. Diverticula, internal hemorrhoids, and polyps in veterans with SCI were associated with time elapsed since SCI; however, in a small study, these complications were not more prevalent than in non-SCI veterans matched for age, gender, and race/ethnicity.

Loss of control of the external anal sphincter commonly results in fecal incontinence after SCI. The usual management for irregular bowel function is a combination of laxatives, bulking agents, anal massage, manual evacuation, and scheduled enemas. Randomized, double-blind studies demonstrated the effectiveness of neostigmine, which increases cholinergic tone, combined with glycopyrrolate, an anticholinergic agent with minimal activity in the colon that reduces extracolonic side effects. Computerized stimulation of the sacral anterior roots may restore normal function to the pelvic colon and anorectal sphincters; this anterior sacral root stimulation may be combined with S2 to S4 posterior sacral rhizotomy in order to interrupt the spasticity-causing sensory nerves and avoid autonomic dysreflexia. If these measures are unavailable or ineffective and severe constipation persists, a colostomy reduces time for bowel care and avoidance or healing of decubitus ulcers.

The acute abdomen may be a significant challenge in SCI, with mortality of 9.5 percent in one series. In SCI patients, acute abdominal conditions do not present with rigidity or absent bowel sounds, but with dull or poorly localized pain, vomiting, or restlessness, with tenderness, fever, and leukocytosis in up to 50 percent of patients.[26]

Multiple Sclerosis

Severe constipation (typically slow transit) frequently accompanies urinary bladder dysfunction in patients with advanced multiple sclerosis; there may be fecal incontinence even in patients with constipation. Impaired function of the supraspinal or descending pathways that control the sacral parasympathetic outflow may impair colonic motor dysfunction or affect defecation. Motility disturbances are more frequent in the lower than in the upper gut.

Neuromyelitis Optica

Area postrema (including morphologic evidence of aquaporin-4 [AQP4] autoimmunity) may be a selective target of the disease process in neuromyelitis optica. These findings are compatible with clinical reports of nausea and vomiting preceding episodes of optic neuritis and transverse myelitis or being the heralding symptom of the disorder.[27]

Peripheral Neuropathy

Acute Peripheral Neuropathy

Autonomic dysfunction associated with certain acute viral infections may result in nausea, vomiting, abdominal cramps, constipation, or a clinical picture of pseudo-obstruction. In the Guillain–Barré syndrome, visceral involvement may include gastric distention or adynamic ileus. Persistent gastrointestinal motor disturbances may also occur in association with herpes zoster, Epstein–Barr virus infection, or botulism B. The site of the neurologic lesion is uncertain. Cytomegalovirus has been identified in the myenteric plexus in some patients with chronic intestinal pseudo-obstruction. Selective cholinergic dysautonomia (with associated gastrointestinal dysfunction) has been reported to develop within a week of the onset of infectious mononucleosis.[23] Diarrhea induced by human immunodeficiency virus (HIV) may be another manifestation of autonomic dysfunction (see later), but the data require confirmation.

Chronic Peripheral Neuropathy

Chronic peripheral neuropathy is the most commonly encountered extrinsic neurologic disorder that results in gastrointestinal motor dysfunction.

Diabetes Mellitus

Diabetic autonomic neuropathy of the gut has been studied extensively and has been reviewed elsewhere. In patients with type I diabetes mellitus seen at university medical centers, gastrointestinal symptoms, particularly constipation, are quite common. A US based study in the community showed that constipation, with or without the use of laxatives, was the only gut symptom more frequent in patients with type I diabetes mellitus than in age- and gender-matched controls. Patients with constipation tended to be taking some medications that cause the symptoms or to have bladder symptoms.[28]

Gastric emptying of digestible or nondigestible solids is abnormal in patients with diabetes mellitus and gastrointestinal symptoms ("gastroparesis"). There is a paucity of distal antral contractions during fasting and postprandially; small bowel motility may also be abnormal. These features are consistent with an "autovagotomy," or loss of the interstitial cells of Cajal (pacemaker cells).

Constipation among community diabetics was associated equally with slow transit, normal transit, or pelvic floor dysfunction.[29] Diarrhea or fecal incontinence (or both) may result from several mechanisms: dysfunction of the anorectal sphincter or abnormal rectal sensation, osmotic diarrhea from bacterial overgrowth due to small bowel stasis, rapid transit from uncoordinated small bowel motor activity, or the intake of artificial sweeteners such as sorbitol. Rarely, an associated gluten-sensitive enteropathy or pancreatic exocrine insufficiency is present.

Histopathologic studies of the vagus nerve have revealed a reduction in the number of unmyelinated axons; surviving axons are usually of small caliber. In patients with diabetic diarrhea, there are giant sympathetic neurons and dendritic swelling of the postganglionic neurons in prevertebral and paravertebral sympathetic ganglia as well as reduced fiber density in the splanchnic nerves.

Treatment of gastroparesis follows guidelines reviewed elsewhere,[4] and therapeutic options have resulted in only transient relief. Pancreas transplantation is reported to restore normal gastric emptying in patients with diabetic gastroparesis. Long-term results are not available, however, and the gastric stasis and autonomic neuropathy may not be resolved with the pancreas transplant.

Paraneoplastic Neuropathy

Autonomic neuropathy and gastrointestinal symptoms may occur in association with small cell carcinoma of the lung or pulmonary carcinoid.[1] In one series, all seven patients suffered constipation, six had gastroparesis, four had esophageal dysmotility suggestive of spasm or achalasia, and two had other evidence of autonomic neuropathy that affected bladder and blood pressure control. There are circulating IgG antibodies (e.g., ANNA-1 or anti-Hu) directed against enteric neuronal nuclei, suggesting that the enteric plexus is the major target of this paraneoplastic phenomenon. However, several patients have also had evidence of extrinsic visceral neuropathies, suggesting a more extensive neuropathologic process. The chest x-ray is frequently normal in these patients; a chest computed tomography (CT) scan is therefore indicated when the syndrome is suspected, typically in middle-aged smokers with recent onset of nausea, vomiting, or feeding intolerance. Whole-body fluorodeoxyglucose positron emission tomography (FDG-PET) or FDG-PET/computed tomography may be helpful for detecting malignancies that cannot be detected by conventional screening tests.[30] In other reports, there has not been FDG uptake in the tumor or metastases.[31]

Ganglionic receptor-binding antibodies have also been found in a subset of patients with idiopathic, paraneoplastic, or diabetic autonomic neuropathy and idiopathic gastrointestinal dysmotility; the antibody titer correlated with more severe autonomic dysfunction.[32] This autoimmune model of gastrointestinal dysmotility has been replicated in an animal model.[33]

Immunomodulatory treatment before, during, or after antineoplastic therapy may be of benefit for patients with paraneoplastic neuropathy and has been used even when the underlying malignancy cannot be identified.

Amyloid Neuropathy

Gastrointestinal disease in amyloidosis results from either mucosal infiltration or neuromuscular infiltration. In addition, an extrinsic autonomic neuropathy may also affect gut function. A retrospective series reported that 76 of 2,334 (3.2%) patients with amyloidosis had biopsy-proven amyloid involvement of the gastrointestinal tract.[34] Of these 76 patients, 79 percent had systemic amyloidosis while 21 percent had GI amyloidosis without evidence of an associated plasma cell dyscrasia or other organ involvement. Amyloid neuropathy may lead to constipation, diarrhea, and steatorrhea. Patients have uncoordinated nonpropagated contractions in the small bowel.[23] These features are similar to the intestinal myoelectric disturbances observed in animals subjected to ganglionectomy. Familial amyloidosis may also affect the gut.

Manometric studies and monitoring of the acute effects of cholinomimetic agents can distinguish between neuropathic (uncoordinated but normal-amplitude pressure activity) and myopathic (low-amplitude pressure activity) types of amyloid gastroenteropathy. These strategies may identify patients (i.e., those with the neuropathic variant) who are more likely to respond to prokinetic agents. The effects of advanced therapies for amyloidosis (autologous or allogeneic stem cell transplantation in combination with cytotoxic therapy) on gastrointestinal dysmotility are unclear.

Chronic Sensory and Autonomic Neuropathy of Unknown Cause

This is a rare, nonfamilial form of slowly progressive neuropathy that affects a number of autonomic functions. Patients may exhibit only a chronic autonomic disturbance (e.g., abnormal sudomotor, vasomotor, or gastrointestinal function) for many years before peripheral sensory symptoms develop. Autonomic dysfunction is probably responsible for functional gastrointestinal motor disorders when these develop prior to the onset of more obvious features of dysautonomia. This may account for a subset of patients with symptoms suggestive of irritable bowel syndrome.

A high nicotinic acetylcholine receptor antibody titer with postganglionic autonomic damage and evidence of somatic nerve fiber involvement suggests that such cases may have an immune etiology,[35] as is discussed later.

Some investigators have reported familial cases of intestinal pseudo-obstruction with degeneration of the myenteric plexus and evidence of sensory or motor neuropathies affecting peripheral or cranial nerves.[36]

Porphyria

Acute intermittent porphyria and hereditary coproporphyria frequently present with abdominal pain, nausea, vomiting, and constipation.[37] Porphyric polyneuropathy may lead to dilatation and impaired motor function in any part of the intestinal tract, presumably because of autonomic dysfunction. Effects of porphyria on the enteric nervous system have not been described.

Neurofibromatosis

Children with neurofibromatosis type 1 frequently have symptoms of constipation, which can be associated with enlarged rectal diameter and prolonged colonic transit time.[38]

Human Immunodeficiency Virus Infection

Neurologic disease may manifest at any phase of HIV infection. Chronic diarrhea may result from increased extrinsic parasympathetic activity to the gut[39] or damage to adrenergic fibers within the enteric plexuses. Further studies are needed to characterize these abnormalities; it is, of course, important to exclude gut infections and infestations in patients with HIV seropositivity and diarrhea.

Autoimmune Neuropathies

Autoimmune neuropathies are rare causes of gastrointestinal dysmotilities.

Antibodies to Ganglionic Acetylcholine Receptors

Antibodies that bind to or block ganglionic acetylcholine receptors have been identified in patients with various forms of autoimmune autonomic neuropathy. In one series, 9 percent of patients with idiopathic GI dysmotility had antibodies toward ganglionic acetylcholine receptors, and antibody titers were positively correlated with the severity of autonomic dysfunction, suggesting a pathogenic role.[32] Moreover, passive transfer of ganglionic AChR-specific IgG impaired autonomic synaptic transmission and caused autonomic dysfunction in mice. The antibody effect was potentially reversible, suggesting that early use of immunomodulatory therapy directed at lowering IgG levels and abrogating IgG production may be therapeutically effective in patients with autoimmune autonomic neuropathy.[40]

Antibodies to Specific Ion Channels

Autoantibodies directed against specific neural antigens, including ion channels, may be associated with gut motility disorders including esophageal dysmotility, slow transit constipation, and chronic intestinal pseudo-obstruction. Among 33 patients with ganglionitis shown on full-thickness jejunal laparoscopic biopsies, 2 patients with symptoms of irritable bowel syndrome had antibodies directed towards neuronal ion channels (one against voltage-gated potassium channels and the other against neuronal alpha3-AChR). The pathogenic role of such antibodies requires further determination.[41] Similarly, in pediatric patients with suspected neurologic autoimmunity, there was a minority (<3%) with serum positive for neuronal potassium channel complex-reactive immunoglobulin G and, among these, two of seven patients had gastrointestinal dysmotility.[42]

Similar ion channel or acetylcholine receptor antibodies were reported in 24 patients with GI motility disorders (such as achalasia, and delayed gastric emptying); 11 patients had associated malignancies.[43] The prevalence of these antibodies is not higher in community-based patients with irritable bowel syndrome or functional dyspepsia than in asymptomatic controls.[44] Antibodies against voltage-gated potassium channels (particularly CASPR2-IgG-positivity) are also associated with chronic idiopathic pain and hyperexcitability of nociceptive pathways; however, there was no association with significant gastrointestinal pain.[45]

GENERAL MUSCLE DISEASES CAUSING GUT DYSMOTILITY

At an advanced stage, progressive systemic sclerosis and amyloidosis result in an infiltrative replacement of smooth muscle cells in the digestive tract. Rarely, Duchenne or Becker muscular dystrophy[46] and polymyositis or dermatomyositis[47] have been associated with gastroparesis. There are a number of case or family reports of chronic intestinal pseudo-obstruction, sometimes in association with an external ophthalmoplegia, secondary to a mitochondrial myopathy.[5,48] Patients with myotonic dystrophy may have megacolon; anal sphincter dysfunction also occurs and is consistent with an expression of myopathy, muscular atrophy, and neural abnormalities. The myopathic nature of these disorders is reflected by the low-amplitude contractions that occur at affected levels of the gut, as studied especially in systemic sclerosis.[49] Myopathic disorders may be complicated by bacterial overgrowth and small bowel diverticula; pneumatosis cystoides intestinalis and spontaneous pneumoperitoneum sometimes occur in progressive systemic sclerosis. However, it is worth noting that the latter disorder affects the gut from the distal two-thirds of the esophagus to the anorectum; thus, it may present with dysphagia (which may also be due to reflux esophagitis and stricture), gastric stasis, chronic intestinal pseudo-obstruction, steatorrhea due to bacterial overgrowth, constipation, incontinence (particularly at night, owing to involvement of the internal anal sphincter), and rectal prolapse.[13] Other manifestations include chronic fever, recurrent acute migrant arthritis, muscle cramps, exercise intolerance, and peripheral neuropathy.[50] Skeletal muscle EMG or biopsy may be needed to establish the nature of the generalized neuromuscular disorder, as in mitochondrial myopathy.[48] Treatment includes restoration of nutrition (which may necessitate total parenteral nutrition), suppression of bacterial overgrowth, and treatment of complications such as gastroesophageal reflux (with an H_2-receptor antagonist or proton pump inhibitor) or esophageal strictures (by endoscopic dilatation). Colonic dilatation and intractable constipation may necessitate subtotal colectomy with ileorectostomy. Prokinetics are rarely effective but should at least be tried. The somatostatin analogue octreotide improves symptoms in the short term and may suppress bacterial overgrowth. However, octreotide retards postprandial small bowel transit,[51] and we use it only once per day, at least 3 hours after the last meal, to induce migrating motor activity and clear

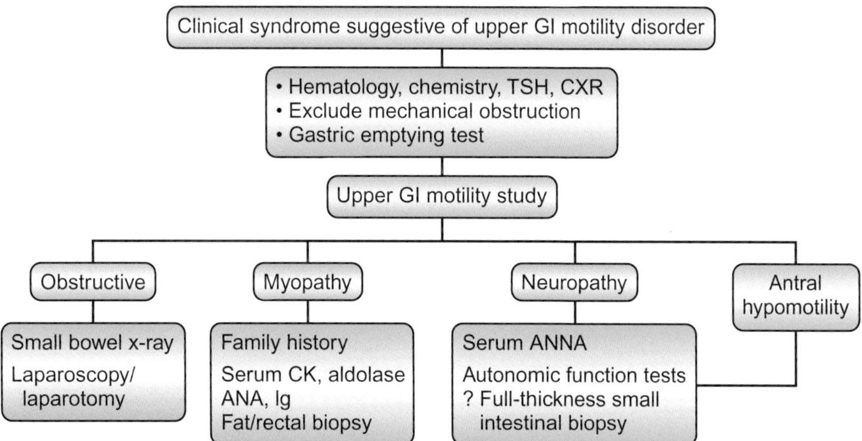

FIGURE 14-5 ■ Algorithm for the investigation of suspected gastrointestinal (GI) dysmotility. ANA, antinuclear antibodies; ANNA, antineuronal enteric antibodies; CK, creatine kinase; CXR, chest radiograph; Ig, immunoglobulin; TSH, thyroid-stimulating hormone. (From Camilleri M: Study of human gastroduodenojejunal motility: applied physiology in clinical practice. Dig Dis Sci 38:785, 1993, with permission.)

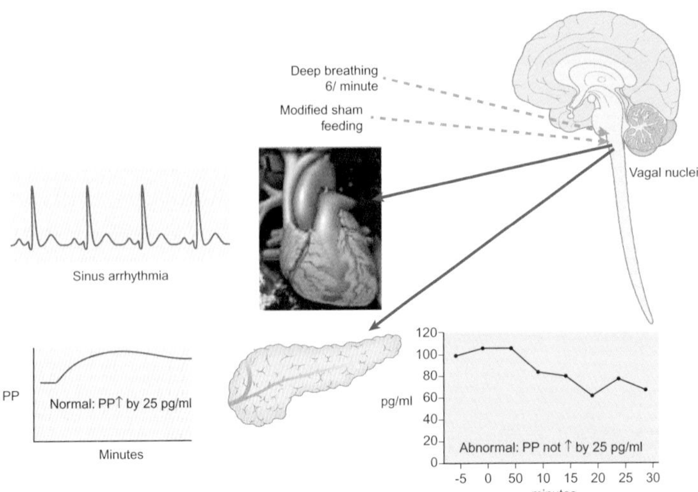

FIGURE 14-6 ■ Assessment of thoracic vagal function by documentation of sinus arrhythmia and abdominal vagal function by the plasma pancreatic polypeptide (PP) response to modified sham feeding by chewing and spitting a bacon-and-cheese toasted sandwich.

residue from the stomach and small bowel. Allogeneic stem cell transplantation has been proposed as an early treatment for mitochondrial neurogastrointestinal encephalomyopathy while patients are still relatively healthy. In two patients, post-transplant clinical follow-up showed improvement in gastrointestinal dysmotility, abdominal cramps and diarrhea.[52]

IDENTIFICATION OF EXTRINSIC NEUROLOGIC DISEASE WITH GASTROINTESTINAL SYMPTOMS OF DYSMOTILITY

Patients with lesions at virtually any level of the nervous system may have symptoms of gastrointestinal motor dysfunction. Therefore, a strategy is necessary in the diagnostic evaluation of disordered gastrointestinal function (Fig. 14-5). Here there is convergence of the paths of the neurologist and gastroenterologist. Patients should undergo further testing, particularly if they have clinical features suggestive of autonomic or peripheral nerve dysfunction or a known underlying neuromuscular disorder. It is essential to record the use of all medications that influence gut motility.

Gastrointestinal motility and transit measurements help the clinician to objectively confirm the disturbance in the motor function of the gut and distinguish between neuropathic and myopathic disorders. Tests of autonomic function (see Chapter 8) are useful for identifying the extent of involvement and localizing the anatomic level of the disturbance in extrinsic neural control. There is generally good agreement between abnormalities of abdominal vagal function, including the plasma pancreatic polypeptide response to modified sham feeding (Fig. 14-6) and cardiovagal dysfunction in patients with diabetes. When a defect of the sympathetic nervous system has been identified by conventional tests, the effect of intravenous administration of edrophonium on plasma norepinephrine levels may provide further assessment of the integrity of postganglionic sympathetic nerves, many of which supply the digestive tract.

Once visceral autonomic neuropathy is identified, further tests are needed to identify any occult causes of the neuropathy; examples include lung tumors (CT of the chest), porphyria (uroporphyrinogen-1-synthase and coproporphyrinogen oxidase in erythrocytes), and amyloidosis (special protein studies in blood and urine, fat, or a rectal biopsy specimen). Imaging of the brain and spinal cord is needed when autonomic tests indicate a central lesion, as when a thermoregulatory sweat test is abnormal, but tests of postganglionic nerves (e.g., the quantitative sudomotor axon reflex test, or plasma norepinephrine response to edrophonium) are normal.

MANAGEMENT OF GASTROINTESTINAL MOTILITY DISORDERS

The principles of management of any gastrointestinal motility disorder are restoration of hydration and nutrition by the oral, enteral, or parenteral route; suppression of bacterial overgrowth (e.g., with oral tetracycline); use of prokinetic agents or stimulant laxatives; and resection of localized disease. An update of pharmacotherapy is provided elsewhere.[4,7,53]

Pyridostigmine (usually 30 to 60 mg taken four times daily, with escalation up to maximum 360 mg per day) has been used to treat autoimmune neuropathy causing dysmotility[54] or diabetic neuropathy with constipation.[55] Oral pyridostigmine accelerates colonic transit and improves bowel function in diabetic patients with chronic constipation.

The role of surgery for motility disorders due to neurologic disease is restricted to those patients with intractable colonic or rectal symptoms, particularly incontinence. There is no good rationale for vagotomy or for partial or total gastrectomy in patients with chronic neuropathies causing gastric stasis. In patients with severe colonic inertia, subtotal colectomy with ileorectostomy is usually successful, but this treatment has been used only rarely in patients with neurologic or muscle disease. Surgery for local complications of severe constipation may be necessary, as in patients with rectal intussusception or prolapse.

A Cochrane systematic review of the management of fecal incontinence and constipation in adults with central neurologic diseases concluded that it was not possible to make any recommendations, and bowel management remains empirical.[56]

CONCLUDING COMMENTS

Gastrointestinal motor abnormalities result when extrinsic nerves are disturbed and are unable to modulate the motor functions of the digestive tract, which depend on the enteric nervous system and the automaticity of the smooth muscles. Disorders at all anatomic levels of the extrinsic neural control system and degenerations of gut smooth muscle have been reported in association with gut motor dysfunction and illustrate the important role of the nervous system in the etiology of gastrointestinal symptoms. Although much emphasis in the literature is placed on dysphagia and constipation in neurologic disorders, more recent studies have highlighted incontinence, vomiting, and abdominal distention in the symptomatology of such patients. Strategies that evaluate the physiologic functions of the digestive tract and the function of the extrinsic neural control are available and aid in the selection of rational therapies for patients, including physical and biofeedback training (e.g., for dysphagia or incontinence), prokinetic agents (for neuropathic forms of gastroparesis, intestinal pseudo-obstruction, or slow-transit colonic disorders), and nutritional support using the enteral or parenteral route. Electric or magnetic stimulation of lumbar sacral roots may alleviate certain symptoms, such as constipation in paraplegics.

REFERENCES

1. Camilleri M, Bharucha AE: Disturbances of gastrointestinal motility and the nervous system. p. 293. In Aminoff MJ (ed): Neurology and General Medicine. 4th Ed. Churchill Livingstone Elsevier, Philadelphia, 2008.
2. Aviv JE, Kim T, Sacco RL, et al: FEESST: a new bedside endoscopic test of the motor and sensory components of swallowing. Ann Otol Rhinol Laryngol 107:378, 1998.
3. Camilleri M: Clinical practice: diabetic gastroparesis. N Engl J Med 356:820, 2007.
4. Camilleri M, Parkman HP, Shafi MA, et al: Clinical guideline: management of gastroparesis. Am J Gastroenterol 108:18, 2013.
5. Mueller LA, Camilleri M, Emslie-Smith AM: Mitochondrial neurogastrointestinal encephalomyopathy: manometric and diagnostic features. Gastroenterology 116:959, 1999.
6. Lambo T, Camilleri M: Chronic constipation. N Engl J Med 349:1360, 2003.
7. Bharucha AE, Pemberton JH, Locke 3rd GR: American Gastroenterological Association technical review on constipation. Gastroenterology 144:218, 2013.
8. Camilleri M: Chronic diarrhea: a review on pathophysiology and management for the clinical gastroenterologist. Clin Gastroenterol Hepatol 2:198, 2004.
9. Choi M-G, Camilleri M, O'Brien MD, et al: A pilot study of motility and tone of the left colon in diarrhea due to functional disorders and dysautonomia. Am J Gastroenterol 92:297, 1997.
10. Bharucha A: Fecal incontinence. Gastroenterology 124:1672, 2003.
11. Bharucha AE, Fletcher JG, Harper CM, et al: Relationship between symptoms and disordered continence mechanisms in women with idiopathic fecal incontinence. Gut 54:546, 2005.
12. Bharucha AE, Daube J, Litchy W, et al: Anal sphincteric neurogenic injury in asymptomatic nulliparous women and fecal incontinence. Am J Physiol 303:G256, 2012.
13. Leighton JA, Valdovinos MA, Pemberton JH, et al: Anorectal dysfunction and rectal prolapse in progressive systemic sclerosis. Dis Colon Rectum 36:182, 1993.
14. Rosen HR, Urbarz C, Holzer B, et al: Sacral nerve stimulation as a treatment for fecal incontinence. Gastroenterology 121:536, 2001.

15. Wu JH, Guo Z, Kumar S, et al: Incidence of serious upper and lower gastrointestinal events in older adults with and without Alzheimer's disease. J Am Geriatr Soc 59:2053, 2011.
16. Farlow M, Veloso F, Moline M, et al: Safety and tolerability of donepezil 23mg in moderate to severe Alzheimer's disease. BMC Neurol 11:57, 2011.
17. Darreh-Shori T, Jelic V: Safety and tolerability of transdermal and oral rivastigmine in Alzheimer's disease and Parkinson's disease dementia. Expert Opin Drug Saf 9:167, 2010.
18. Arai E, Arai M, Uchiyama T, et al: Subthalamic deep brain stimulation can improve gastric emptying in Parkinson's disease. Brain 135:1478, 2012.
19. Da Costa Dias B, Jovanovic K, Weiss SF: Alimentary prion infections: touchdown in the intestine. Prion 5:6, 2011.
20. Cersosimo MG, Benarroch EE: Pathological correlates of gastrointestinal dysfunction in Parkinson's disease. Neurobiol Dis 46:559, 2012.
21. Böttner M, Zorenkov D, Hellwig I, et al: Expression pattern and localization of alpha-synuclein in the human enteric nervous system. Neurobiol Dis 48:474, 2012.
22. Devos D, Lebouvier T, Lardeux B, et al: Colonic inflammation in Parkinson's disease. Neurobiol Dis 50:42, 2013.
23. Vassallo M, Camilleri M, Caron BL, et al: Gastrointestinal motor dysfunction in acquired selective cholinergic dysautonomia associated with infectious mononucleosis. Gastroenterology 100:252, 1991.
24. Lukkarinen H, Peltola V: Influenza A induced acute autonomic neuropathy in an adolescent. Pediatr Neurol 43:425, 2010.
25. Wolf C, Meiners TH: Dysphagia in patients with acute cervical spinal cord injury. Spinal Cord 41:347, 2003.
26. Ebert E: Gastrointestinal involvement in spinal cord injury: a clinical perspective. J Gastrointestin Liver Dis 21:75, 2012.
27. Popescu BF, Lennon VA, Parisi JE, et al: Neuromyelitis optica unique area postrema lesions: nausea, vomiting, and pathogenic implications. Neurology 76:1229, 2011.
28. Maleki D, Locke III GR, Camilleri M, et al: Gastrointestinal symptoms among persons with diabetes in the community. Arch Intern Med 160:2808, 2000.
29. Maleki D, Camilleri M, Burton DD, et al: Pilot study of pathophysiology of constipation among community diabetics. Dig Dis Sci 43:2373, 1998.
30. Koike H, Tanaka F, Sobue G: Paraneoplastic neuropathy: wide-ranging clinicopathological manifestations. Curr Opin Neurol 24:504, 2011.
31. Block MS, Vassallo R: Lack of FDG uptake in small cell carcinoma associated with ANNA-1 positive paraneoplastic autonomic neuropathy. J Thorac Oncol 3:542, 2008.
32. Vernino S, Low PA, Fealey RD, et al: Autoantibodies to ganglionic acetylcholine receptors in autoimmune autonomic neuropathies. N Engl J Med 343:847, 2000.
33. Lennon VA, Ermilov LG, Szurszewski JH, et al: Immunization with neuronal nicotinic acetylcholine receptor induces neurologic autoimmune disease. J Clin Invest 111:907, 2003.
34. Cowan AJ, Skinner M, Seldin DC, et al: Amyloidosis of the gastrointestinal tract: a 13-year single center referral experience. Haematologica 98:141, 2013.
35. Manganelli F, Dubbioso R, Nolano M, et al: Autoimmune autonomic ganglionopathy: a possible postganglionic neuropathy. Arch Neurol 68:504, 2011.
36. Krishnamurthy S, Schuffler MD: Pathology of neuromuscular disorders of the small intestine and colon. Gastroenterology 93:610, 1987.
37. Kauppinen R: Porphyrias. Lancet 365:241, 2005.
38. Pedersen CE, Krogh K, Siggaard C, et al: Constipation in children with neurofibromatosis type 1. J Pediatr Gastroenterol Nutr 56:229, 2013.
39. Coker RJ, Horner P, Bleasdale-Barr K, et al: Increased gut parasympathetic activity and chronic diarrhoea in a patient with the acquired immunodeficiency syndrome. Clin Auton Res 2:295, 1992.
40. Vernino S, Ermilov LG, Sha L, et al: Passive transfer of autoimmune autonomic neuropathy to mice. J Neurosci 24:7037, 2004.
41. Törnblom H, Lang B, Clover L, et al: Autoantibodies in patients with gut motility disorders and enteric neuropathy. Scand J Gastroenterol 42:1289, 2007.
42. Dhamija R, Renaud DL, Pittock SJ, et al: Neuronal voltage-gated potassium channel complex autoimmunity in children. Pediatr Neurol 44:275, 2011.
43. Dhamija R, Tan KM, Pittock SJ, et al: Serologic profiles aiding the diagnosis of autoimmune gastrointestinal dysmotility. Clin Gastroenterol Hepatol 6:988, 2008.
44. Pittock SJ, Lennon VA, Dege CL, et al: Neural autoantibody evaluation in functional gastrointestinal disorders: a population-based case-control study. Dig Dis Sci 56:1452, 2011.
45. Klein CJ, Lennon VA, Aston PA, et al: Chronic pain as a manifestation of potassium channel-complex autoimmunity. Neurology 79:1136, 2012.
46. Borrelli O, Salvia G, Mancini V, et al: Evolution of gastric electrical features and gastric emptying in children with Duchenne and Becker muscular dystrophy. Am J Gastroenterol 100:695, 2005.
47. Laskin BL, Choyke P, Keenan GF, et al: Novel gastrointestinal tract manifestations in juvenile dermatomyositis. J Pediatr 135:371, 1999.
48. Lowsky R, Davidson G, Wolman S, et al: Familial visceral myopathy associated with a mitochondrial myopathy. Gut 34:279, 1993.

49. Sjolund K, Bartosik I, Lindberg G, et al: Small intestinal manometry in patients with systemic sclerosis. Eur J Gastroenterol Hepatol 17:1205, 2005.
50. Filosto M, Scarpelli M, Tonin P, et al: Pitfalls in diagnosing mitochondrial neurogastrointestinal encephalomyopathy. J Inherit Metab Dis 34:1199, 2011.
51. von der Ohe MR, Camilleri M, Thomforde GM, et al: Differential regional effects of octreotide on human gastrointestinal motor function. Gut 36:743, 1995.
52. Filosto M, Scarpelli M, Tonin P, et al: Course and management of allogeneic stem cell transplantation in patients with mitochondrial neurogastrointestinal encephalomyopathy. J Neurol 259:2699, 2012.
53. Katzka DA, Loftus Jr EV, Camilleri M: Evolving molecular targets in the treatment of nonmalignant gastrointestinal diseases. Clin Pharmacol Ther 92:306, 2012.
54. Pasha SF, Lunsford TN, Lennon VA: Autoimmune gastrointestinal dysmotility treated successfully with pyridostigmine. Gastroenterology 131:1592, 2006.
55. Bharucha AE, Low P, Camilleri M, et al: A randomised controlled study of the effect of cholinesterase inhibition on colon function in patients with diabetes mellitus and constipation. Gut 62:708, 2013.
56. Coggrave M, Wiesel PH, Norton C: Management of faecal incontinence and constipation in adults with central neurological diseases. Cochrane Database Syst Rev(2):CD002115, 2006.

CHAPTER

15

Neurologic Manifestations of Nutritional Disorders

PRIYA S. DHAWAN ■ BRENT P. GOODMAN

Maintenance of medical and neurologic health requires adequate ingestion, absorption, and storage of vitamins and minerals. Nutritional deficiencies may result from inadequate intake or malabsorption of these critical vitamins and micronutrients. Individuals at risk of deficient nutrient intake include the impoverished in developed and underdeveloped countries (where certain nutritional disorders may be endemic), individuals with eating disorders or those engaging in fad or restrictive diets, chronic alcoholics, and those with chronic medical conditions that result in malabsorption or require prolonged parenteral nutrition.

Malabsorption may result from gastrointestinal surgery, including bariatric surgery for obesity, and from chronic gastrointestinal disorders such as celiac disease, Whipple disease, bacterial overgrowth, and inflammatory bowel disease. Excessive ingestion of certain substances, including vitamins and micronutrients, may result in neurologic impairment directly (e.g., vitamin B_6 excess) or indirectly by interfering with absorption of certain other vitamins (e.g., copper deficiency induced by high zinc levels). Awareness of the characteristic clinical features of the various nutritional disorders facilitates timely recognition and treatment, and directly impacts prognosis (Table 15-1).

Aminoff's Neurology and General Medicine, Fifth Edition.

TABLE 15-1 ■ Diagnosis and Treatment of Nutritional Disorders

Vitamin	Diagnosis	Treatment
Vitamin B_{12} Deficiency	Serum cobalamin Serum methylmalonic acid Serum homocysteine	IM vitamin B_{12} 1000 μg for 5 days then once monthly or oral vitamin B_{12} 1000 μg daily
Nitrous Oxide	Serum cobalamin (rendered inactive by N_2O) Serum homocysteine	Stop nitrous oxide exposure; IM vitamin B_{12}; consider oral methionine
Folate Deficiency	Serum folate, homocysteine	Oral folate 1 mg tid initially; 1 mg daily thereafter
Copper Deficiency	Serum copper and ceruloplasmin; urinary copper	Discontinue zinc; oral copper 8 mg daily for 1 week; 6 mg daily for 1 week; 4 mg daily for 1 week; 2 mg daily thereafter
Vitamin E	Serum vitamin E; ratio serum vitamin E to sum of cholesterol and triglycerides	Vitamin E 200 mg–200 mg/kg daily oral or IM
Thiamine	Clinical diagnosis; brain MRI	Thiamine 100 mg IV followed by 50–100 mg IV or IM until nutritional status stable
Pyridoxine	Serum pyridoxal phosphate	Pyridoxine 50–100 mg daily
Niacin	Urinary excretion niacin metabolites	Nicotinic acid 25–50 mg oral or IM

IM, intramuscular; IV, intravenous.

As is true with the evaluation of all suspected neurologic disorders, the identification of nutritional deficiencies requires a careful history and examination. A meticulous review of medication history, including prescription and over-the-counter medications, is necessary since certain drugs may increase an individual's risk of developing a vitamin deficiency (e.g., H2 blockers and vitamin B_{12} deficiency), and excessive ingestion of some supplement medications may result in vitamin malabsorption (e.g., zinc-induced copper deficiency) and deficiency. Review of past medical and surgical history is critical, as gastric bypass surgery, inflammatory bowel disease, celiac disease, and other medical and surgical conditions may compromise nutritional status (Table 15-2). Knowledge of the time course over which various vitamin deficiencies may develop also is important. For example, body stores of thiamine are limited, and thiamine deficiency may develop within weeks, whereas cobalamin (vitamin B_{12}) deficiency only develops over years. The identification of a particular vitamin deficiency should prompt a thorough laboratory evaluation for other vitamin deficiencies, as multiple vitamin deficiencies often occur in the same patient.

VITAMIN B_{12} DEFICIENCY

Vitamin B_{12} (cobalamin) deficiency is a common condition, with estimated prevalence rates ranging from around 2 to 15 percent of the elderly, depending upon the population studied and diagnostic criteria used. Despite these high prevalence rates, no consensus exists on how best to diagnose and evaluate patients with suspected vitamin B_{12} deficiency.[1] Recognition of vitamin B_{12} deficiency is critical, as the hematologic and neurologic manifestations are potentially reversible only if diagnosed and treated in a timely manner.[2]

Vitamin B_{12} is a cofactor for the enzymes methionine synthase and L-methylmalonyl-coenzyme A mutase, and is required for proper red blood cell formation, normal neurologic function, and DNA synthesis.[3,4] It is necessary for the initial myelination, development, and maintenance of myelination within the central nervous system (CNS).[4] Classically, vitamin B_{12} deficiency results in a myelopathy, or "subacute combined degeneration," which results from demyelination of the posterolateral columns of the cervical and thoracic spinal cord.[5] Demyelination of cranial nerves, peripheral nerves, and brain may also occur and has been referred to as "combined-systems disease."[6] Vitamin B_{12} deficiency may result in a megaloblastic anemia, with macrocytosis, anisocytosis, hypersegmented neutrophils, leukopenia, thrombocytopenia, pancytopenia, or some combination of these abnormalities.[4]

Etiology

Vitamin B_{12} is a water-soluble vitamin that exists in several forms, all of which contain cobalt and are collectively referred to as cobalamins. Methylcobalamin and 5-deoxyadensoylcobalamin are the forms of vitamin B_{12} that are active in human metabolism.[7]

TABLE 15-2 ■ Risk Factors for Vitamin B_{12} Deficiency

Pernicious anemia
Atrophic gastritis
Achlorhydria-induced cobalamin malabsorption
Partial gastrectomy
Ileal resection
Bariatric surgery
H2 receptor antagonists
Proton pump inhibitors
Glucophage
Bacterial overgrowth
Pancreatic disease
Celiac disease
Helicobacter pylori infection
Diphyllobothrium latum infection
Nitrous oxide
Dietary restriction

Vitamin B_{12} is contained in a number of animal proteins, in fortified breakfast cereals, and in certain nutritional yeast products.[8] Daily losses of vitamin B_{12} are minimal, and even in cases of severe malabsorption, it may take 5 years or more to develop symptomatic vitamin B_{12} deficiency.[9]

Vitamin B_{12} deficiency in elderly patients most commonly results from pernicious anemia, atrophic gastritis, and achlorhydria-induced cobalamin malabsorption (Table 15-2).[10,11] The incidence of atrophic gastritis increases with age and may at least partially explain the increased frequency of vitamin B_{12} deficiency with aging.[10] Achlorhydria results in impaired extraction of the vitamin from food sources. Partial gastrectomy, bariatric surgery, and ileal resection may result in malabsorption of vitamin B_{12}, and partial gastrectomy has been associated with loss of intrinsic factor, which is necessary for its absorption. Gastroenterologic disorders such as celiac disease, Crohn disease, ileitis, pancreatic disease, and bacterial overgrowth may also result in vitamin B_{12} deficiency.[12] Certain medications, such as histamine (H2) blocking agents, proton pump inhibitors, and glucophage may also increase the risk of developing vitamin B_{12} deficiency.[13–16] Vitamin B_{12} deficiency rarely results from inadequate intake in vegans and would be expected to develop only after many years, and may not be associated with any clinical manifestations of deficiency.[12]

Nitrous oxide alters the cobalt core of cobalamin, converting it into an inactive, oxidized form.[17] Hence, nitrous oxide exposure may result in cobalamin deficiency, with most reported cases associated with low or borderline low vitamin B_{12} levels. A single exposure to nitrous oxide may be enough to precipitate neurologic impairment in an individual with unsuspected vitamin B_{12} deficiency, with time to symptom onset ranging from immediately after exposure up to around 2 months. Nitrous oxide remains one of the more commonly used anesthetic agents worldwide, and can also be obtained for abuse in the form of whipped cream canisters and as "whippets," which are small bulbs containing nitrous oxide (see Chapter 34). Surveys of medical and dental students in New Zealand and the United States revealed recreational nitrous oxide abuse in 12 and 20 percent, respectively.[18,19]

Clinical Manifestations

Neurologic signs and symptoms may be the initial manifestation of vitamin B_{12} deficiency. Paresthesias and a sensory ataxia are the most common initial symptoms.[6] Classically, a myelopathy occurs and may be accompanied by a peripheral neuropathy. The myelopathy results from posterior column and lateral corticospinal tract dysfunction, with a combination of pyramidal signs and posterior column sensory loss evident on examination. The peripheral neuropathy is typically mild and is predominantly axonal on electrodiagnostic testing.[20]

Neuropsychiatric manifestations include memory impairment, change in personality, delirium, and even psychosis.[6,21] Optic neuropathy, resulting in diminished visual acuity, centrocecal scotomas, and optic atrophy may be seen. Symptoms of orthostatic hypotension are an uncommon manifestation.[22] Other much less commonly encountered neurologic conditions attributed to vitamin B_{12} deficiency include cerebellar ataxia, orthostatic tremor, ophthalmoplegia, and vocal cord paralysis.[12,23–26] A number of constitutional symptoms may accompany these neurologic signs and symptoms, including fatigue, weight loss, fever, dyspnea, and gastrointestinal symptoms.

Diagnosis

Serum cobalamin is the initial screening test in patients with suspected vitamin B_{12} deficiency (Table 15-1). However, some patients will have normal serum cobalamin levels. In patients with borderline low serum levels, and particularly in those patients strongly suspected of vitamin B_{12} deficiency, methylmalonic acid and homocysteine levels should also be checked. Methylmalonic acid and homocysteine levels are increased, suggesting intracellular deficiency of vitamin B_{12} (although not completely specific), in as many as one-third of patients with low-normal serum cobalamin levels.

Once the diagnosis has been established, further testing may be pursued in order to determine the cause. Antibodies to intrinsic factor are seen in only 50 to 70 percent of patients with pernicious anemia, but are highly specific.[27–29] Antiparietal cell antibodies lack sensitivity and specificity and have limited utility.[29] Gastrin antibodies are 70 percent sensitive and specific for pernicious anemia.[30] Elevated serum gastrin and decreased pepsinogen I levels have been reported to be abnormal in 80 to 90 percent of patients with pernicious anemia, but their specificity is limited.[31] The Schilling test is rarely utilized today due to concerns about radiation exposure, cost, and diagnostic accuracy.[32]

Nerve conduction studies and needle electromyography (EMG) may confirm the presence of an axonal sensorimotor peripheral neuropathy.[20] Somatosensory evoked potentials may show slowing in central proprioceptive pathways.[33] Brain and spinal cord magnetic resonance imaging (MRI) studies may demonstrate signal change in subcortical white matter and in the posterolateral columns of the spinal cord.[33–36]

Treatment

Treatment involves the administration of high-dose oral, sublingual, or intramuscular cobalamin. With malabsorption, 1000 μg of cobalamin is administered intramuscularly for 5 days and monthly thereafter, although some have suggested more frequent administration after the first 5 days. There is evidence to suggest that 1000 μg of oral or sublingual cobalamin, given daily, is as effective as intramuscular administration.[37,38] Lifelong vitamin B_{12} supplementation therapy is typically necessary, unless a potentially reversible cause is identified and treated. Hematologic recovery occurs within the first 1 to 2 months and is complete. The neurologic condition should stabilize and improvement may occur over the first 6 to 12 months following the initiation of treatment. Neurologic recovery may be incomplete, particularly in those with significant neurologic deficits prior to the initiation of therapy. Methylmalonic acid and homocysteine levels should be utilized to monitor response to therapy, and typically should normalize within 10 to 14 days.

Patients with pernicious anemia should undergo endoscopy, as they are at higher risk of developing gastric and carcinoid cancers.[39] Upper endoscopy should be considered in other patients as well, including those with other gastrointestinal symptoms and those with other concomitant vitamin deficiencies.

FOLATE DEFICIENCY

The active form of folate, tetrahydrofolic acid, is essential in the transfer of one-carbon units to substrates utilized in the synthesis of purine, thymidine, and amino acids. Methyltetrahydrofolate is required for the cobalamin-dependent remethylation of homocysteine to methionine, and methylene tetrahydrofolate methylates deoxyuridylate to thymidylate.[12] Although folate deficiency might be expected to result in similar complications as vitamin B_{12} deficiency, neurologic manifestations of isolated folate deficiency are extremely uncommon.

Etiology

Folate is present in animal products, citrus fruits, and green, leafy vegetables. Normal body stores of folate range from 500 to 20,000 μg, and 50 to 100 μg are required daily. Serum folate declines within 3 weeks of diminished intake or malabsorption, and clinical signs of folate deficiency may occur within months. After ingestion, folate polyglutamates normally undergo hydrolysis to monoglutamates, which are absorbed in the proximal small intestine and ileum. Absorbed folate monoglutamates are then metabolized by the liver to 5-methyltetrahydrofolate, the principal circulating form of folate. The cellular uptake of 5-methyltetrahydrofolate is mediated by four different carrier systems: a proton-coupled folate transporter, a low-affinity high-capacity reduced folate carrier, and two high-affinity folate receptors.[40]

Folate deficiency is one of the more common nutritional disorders worldwide.[40] Risk factors include malnutrition, conditions associated with increased folate requirements (e.g., pregnancy, lactation, and chronic hemolytic anemia), gastroenterologic disorders, and certain medications (Table 15-3).[12] Gastroenterologic conditions that affect folate absorption in the small bowel include tropical sprue, celiac disease, bacterial overgrowth syndrome, inflammatory bowel disease, and pancreatic insufficiency. Gastric surgeries or medications that reduce gastric secretions may also result in folate deficiency.[41,42] A number of other medications such as methotrexate, aminopterin, pyrimethamine, trimethoprim, and triamterene inhibit dihydrofolate reductase and may also result in folate deficiency. Mechanisms by which other medications such as anticonvulsants, sulfasalazine, oral contraceptives, and antituberculous drugs affect folate levels have not been established.[12]

Eight inborn errors of folate absorption have been described, including hereditary folate malabsorption, cerebral folate transporter deficiency, glutamate formiminotransferase deficiency, severe methylenetetrahydrofolate reductase deficiency, dihydrofolate reductase deficiency, methylenetetrahydrofolate dehydrogenase 1 protein deficiency, and functional methionine synthase deficiency (due to deficiency of methionine synthase reductase or of the methionine synthase apoenzyme itself).[40] Clinical manifestations of these disorders may include megaloblastic anemia, cognitive decline, seizures, movement disorders, and peripheral neuropathy. Early identification and treatment with folate may result in clinical improvement in some forms of these disorders. Methylenetetrahydrofolate reductase deficiency is the most common of these disorders, with variable neurologic and vascular manifestations including cognitive changes, seizures, motor and gait disorders, schizophrenia, and thromboses; laboratory studies show hyperhomocysteinemia and homocystinuria.

TABLE 15-3 ■ Causes of Folate Deficiency

Malnutrition (e.g., alcoholics, premature infants, adolescents)
Increased folate requirement (e.g., pregnancy, lactation, chronic hemolytic anemia)
Dietary restriction (e.g., phenylketonuria)
Malabsorption (e.g., tropical sprue, celiac disease, bacterial overgrowth, inflammatory bowel disease, giardiasis)
States of reduced gastric secretion (e.g., gastric surgery, atrophic gastritis, H2 receptor antagonists, proton pump inhibitors, treatment of pancreatic insufficiency)
Medications that inhibit dihydrofolate reductase (e.g., aminopterin, trimethoprim, methotrexate, pyrimethamine, triamterene)
Other medications (unclear mechanism) (e.g., anticonvulsants, antituberculous drugs, sulfasalazine, oral contraceptive agents)
Inborn errors of folate metabolism (e.g., hereditary folate malabsorption, cerebral folate transporter deficiency, glutamate formiminotransferase deficiency, severe methylenetetrahydrofolate reductase deficiency, dihydrofolate reductase deficiency, methylenetetrahydrofolate dehydrogenase 1 deficiency, functional methionine synthase deficiency)

Clinical Manifestations

Maternal folate deficiency during or around the time of conception has been reported to cause more than 50 percent of neural tube defects.[43] Myeloneuropathy, peripheral neuropathy, and megaloblastic anemia have been described with folate deficiency.[44–48] These potential manifestations of folate deficiency are clinically indistinguishable from those seen with vitamin B_{12} deficiency. Some reports suggest that folate deficiency may be associated with an increased risk of peripheral vascular disease, coronary artery disease, cerebrovascular disease, and cognitive impairment.[49,50]

Diagnosis

Serum folate, erythrocyte folate, and homocysteine levels may be used to evaluate an individual with suspected folate deficiency. Results of these studies are highly dependent upon the methods and laboratories used. Serum folate levels fluctuate considerably and do not always accurately reflect tissue stores.[51] Erythrocyte folate levels may more accurately predict tissue stores, but there is considerable laboratory assay variability.[52,53] Homocysteine levels have been demonstrated to be elevated in 86 percent of patients with clinically significant folate deficiency.[54] Typically, a serum folate level of 2.5 μg/l has been utilized as the cut-off for folate deficiency[12]; however, it has been suggested that levels in the range of 2.5 to 5 ng/ml may reflect mildly compromised folate status.

Treatment

Oral administration of folic acid may be adequate, typically 1 mg three times daily for 4 weeks followed by a maintenance dose of 1 mg daily.[12] Parenteral administration of folic acid may be considered in acutely ill patients, and particularly in patients with malabsorption. Folate supplementation of at least 0.4 mg daily is recommended in women of childbearing age; higher doses are suggested for those taking anticonvulsant medications. Vitamin B_{12} levels should also be assessed in patients with suspected folate deficiency and, if low, vitamin B_{12} supplementation should be initiated immediately.

COPPER DEFICIENCY

Copper is a trace element involved in a number of metalloenzymes which are critical in the development and maintenance of nervous system structure and function. These enzymes include cytochrome *c* oxidase (used for electron transport and oxidative phosphorylation), copper/zinc superoxide dismutase (used for antioxidant defense), tyrosinase (used for melanin synthesis), dopamine β-hydroxylase (used for catecholamine synthesis), lysl oxidase (used for cross-linking collagen and elastin), and others.[55]

Copper deficiency in animals was first recognized in sheep in 1937, manifesting as an enzootic ataxia (also known as swayback), and subsequently was noted to affect other animals similarly.[56,57] Hematologic abnormalities were the first signs of acquired copper deficiency recognized in humans, with anemia, neutropenia, and sideroblastic anemia evident in some but not all patients. Neurologic manifestations of acquired copper deficiency are now increasingly recognized.

Etiology

Copper is present in a wide variety of foods, with shellfish, oysters, legumes, organ meats, chocolate, nuts, and whole-grain products being particularly rich in copper. The estimated daily requirement for copper is 0.70 mg, and the estimated total body copper content is 50 to 120 mg. Copper absorption occurs in the stomach and proximal small intestine via active and passive transport processes. The Menkes P-type ATPase (*ATP7A*) is responsible for copper efflux from enterocytes.

Malabsorption following prior gastric surgery and excessive, exogenous zinc ingestion are the most frequently identified causes of symptomatic copper deficiency (see Chapter 13). Copper deficiency may also occur in premature, low-birth-weight, and malnourished infants, and may occur as a complication of total parenteral or enteral nutrition.[58–60] Chronic gastrointestinal conditions such as celiac disease, cystic fibrosis, inflammatory bowel disease, and bacterial overgrowth may result in copper malabsorption.[61,62] Patients should be queried about the use of zinc supplements including denture creams, some of which have excessive zinc and may also induce copper deficiency.[63] It is hypothesized that excessive zinc ingestion upregulates intestinal enterocyte metallothionein production, which has a higher affinity for copper than zinc, resulting in retention of copper in intestinal enterocytes and loss of copper in the stool.[64] Some patients will not have any identifiable cause of copper deficiency.[55]

Menkes disease is a congenital disorder with clinical signs and symptoms that result from copper deficiency. This condition results from a mutation in the *ATP7A* gene, which leads to failure of intestinal copper transport across the gastrointestinal tract and subsequent copper deficiency.[55] Wilson disease is a disorder of copper toxicity that results from an impairment in biliary copper excretion (see Chapter 13).

Clinical Manifestations

Hematologic abnormalities have been well described in copper deficiency, and include primarily anemia and neutropenia.[65,66] Failure to recognize hematologic derangements as resulting from copper deficiency leads to incorrect diagnoses such as myelodysplastic syndrome, aplastic anemia, and sideroblastic anemia. Patients with copper deficiency may develop a myeloneuropathy that resembles the syndrome of subacute combined degeneration associated with vitamin B_{12} deficiency.[67] Pyramidal signs, such as brisk muscle stretch reflexes at the knees and extensor plantar responses, are typically present, along with impairment in posterior column sensory modalities. Sensory loss is characteristically severe, and frequently leads to a sensory ataxia.[68]

Neuropathic extremity pain may be reported, and distal lower limb weakness and atrophy may develop, suggesting peripheral nerve involvement.

Diagnosis

Low serum copper and ceruloplasmin levels establish the diagnosis of copper deficiency. The 24-hour urinary copper level will often be decreased, in contrast to an elevation in urinary copper seen with Wilson disease. Serum and 24-hour urine zinc levels should also be assessed. Ceruloplasmin is an acute-phase reactant and may be increased in various conditions including pregnancy, oral contraceptive use, liver disease, malignancy, hematologic disease, smoking, diabetes, uremia, and other inflammatory and infectious diseases.[12] In the presence of these conditions, copper deficiency may be masked. Serum copper and ceruloplasmin may occasionally be decreased in Wilson disease; hence laboratory evidence of copper deficiency needs to be correlated with clinical features consistent with the diagnosis.

Cervical spine MRI may show T2 hyperintensity involving the dorsal columns (Fig. 15-1). Somatosensory evoked potentials often show slowing in central proprioceptive pathways, and nerve conduction studies and needle EMG demonstrate findings consistent with an axonal sensorimotor peripheral neuropathy.[68] Brain MRI may show diffuse T2 hyperintensities involving the subcortical white matter, suggestive of demyelination.[68,69]

Treatment

Treatment of copper deficiency involves copper supplementation and discontinuation of zinc in those with excessive zinc consumption. A recommended regimen is 8 mg of orally administered elemental copper daily for 1 week, followed by 6 mg daily for the next week, 4 mg daily during the third week, and 2 mg daily thereafter.[12] Occasionally intravenous copper supplementation is necessary. Ongoing copper supplementation may not be necessary in patients with copper deficiency due to zinc excess (when zinc ingestion is discontinued) or in those with a treatable gastrointestinal condition resulting in copper malabsorption (e.g., celiac disease). Patients without an identifiable cause of copper deficiency or those with copper malabsorption due to gastric bypass surgery typically require lifelong copper supplementation.

Similar to vitamin B_{12} deficiency, the hematologic abnormalities associated with copper deficiency

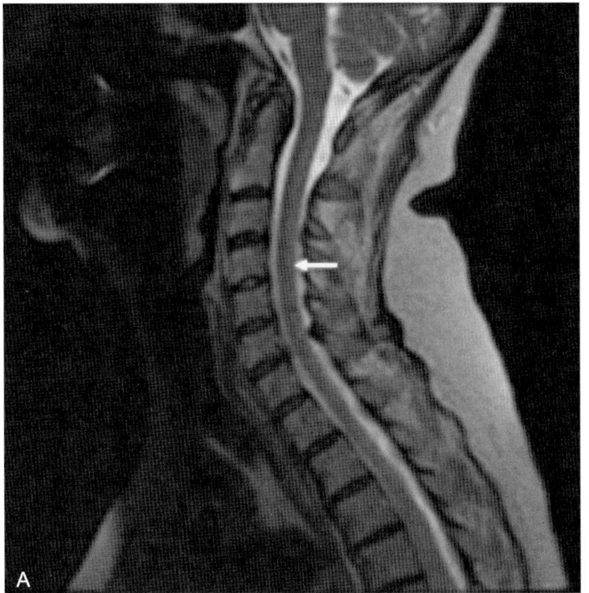

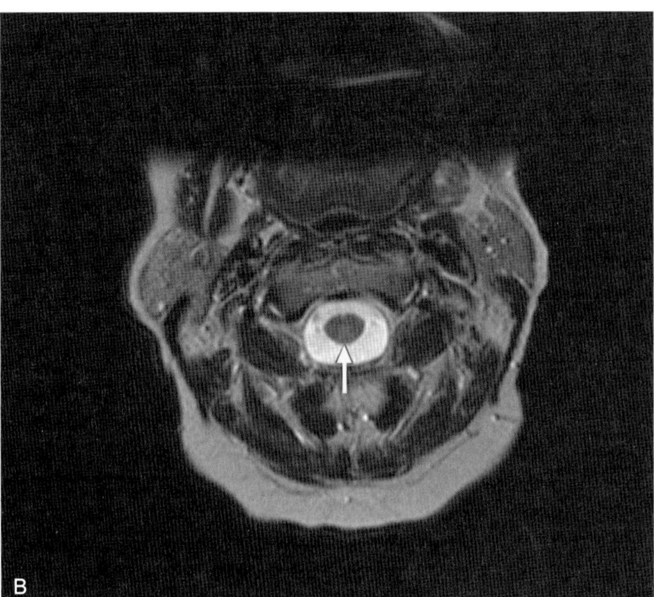

FIGURE 15-1 ■ A 60-year-old woman with copper deficiency in the setting of long-standing excessive use of zinc-containing denture cream. Sagittal (**A**) and axial (**B**) T2-weighted cervical spine magnetic resonance imaging (MRI) sequences demonstrate hyperintensity involving the posterior columns of the spinal cord.

normalize within 1 month of copper repletion. Neurologic deficits are expected to stabilize, but there may be little improvement in neurologic signs and symptoms, particularly in those with more severe neurologic impairment.

VITAMIN E DEFICIENCY

Vitamin E is a fat-soluble vitamin with important antioxidant properties, providing protection against oxidative stress and inhibiting the fatty acid peroxidation of membrane phospholipids. Vitamin E refers to a family of tocopherols and tocoretinols, of which α-tocopherol is the most abundant and active biologic form of vitamin E in the human diet.

Etiology

Nut oils, sunflower seeds, whole grains, wheat germ, and spinach are foods high in vitamin E. Vitamin E absorption requires both bile salts and pancreatic esterases. Vitamin E is incorporated into chylomicrons in intestinal enterocytes, and upon release into the circulation lipolysis ensues, resulting in the transfer of vitamin E to high-density and other lipoproteins. Alpha-tocopherol transfer protein in the liver is responsible for the incorporation of vitamin E into very-low-density lipoprotein (VLDL), which also delivers vitamin E to tissues.

Vitamin E absorption requires pancreatic and biliary secretions, and deficiency may therefore result from chronic cholestasis and pancreatic insufficiency. Chronic total parenteral nutrition with inadequate vitamin E supplementation may result in vitamin E deficiency. Other gastrointestinal disorders that result in vitamin E malabsorption include celiac disease, inflammatory bowel disease, blind loop syndrome, bacterial overgrowth, bowel irradiation, and cystic fibrosis (see Chapter 13). Genetic causes of vitamin E deficiency include ataxia with vitamin E deficiency resulting from α-tocopherol transport protein deficiency, apolipoprotein B mutations (homozygous hypobetalipoproteinemia), or a defect in the microsomal triglyceride transfer protein (abetalipoproteinemia).

Clinical Manifestations

Numerous neurologic manifestations of vitamin E deficiency have been reported including ophthalmoplegia, retinopathy, and a spinocerebellar syndrome with an associated peripheral neuropathy. The latter manifests with signs of a cerebellar ataxia, posterior column sensory loss, pyramidal signs, and sensory loss that resembles Friedreich ataxia.[70–72] A myopathy has been associated with vitamin E deficiency with pathologic features of inflammatory infiltrates and rimmed vacuoles.[73,74] Vitamin E deficiency has rarely been associated with a demyelinating neuropathy.[75,76]

Diagnosis

Low serum vitamin E levels confirm the diagnosis. Serum lipids, cholesterol, and VLDL affect serum vitamin E levels, and serum vitamin E levels should be corrected for these factors by dividing the serum vitamin E value by the sum of serum triglycerides and cholesterol. Increased stool fat and decreased serum carotene levels may also be noted in patients with fat malabsorption as the etiology.

Spine MRI studies may show T2 hyperintensity in the dorsal columns, similar to that seen with vitamin B_{12} and copper deficiency.[77] Median and tibial somatosensory evoked potentials may demonstrate slowing in central proprioceptive pathways.

Treatment

Vitamin E supplementation with dosages ranging from 200 mg/day to 200 mg/kg daily should be administered. Parenteral administration may be necessary in some conditions, particularly for those with severe malabsorption. Unless there is a reversible cause of vitamin E deficiency, lifelong supplementation may be necessary.

THIAMINE (VITAMIN B_1) DEFICIENCY

The active form of thiamine is thiamine pyrophosphate (TPP), which functions as a coenzyme in the metabolism of carbohydrates, lipids, and branched-chain amino acids. It is involved in decarboxylation of α-keto acids during adenosine triphosphate (ATP) synthesis and maintenance of reduced glutathione in erythrocytes.[78] Thiamine pyrophosphate additionally serves as a coenzyme in myelin synthesis and has been hypothesized to play a role in cholinergic and serotonergic neurotransmission through effects on sodium channel function.[79]

Etiology

Thiamine, or vitamin B_1, is a water-soluble vitamin most commonly found in unrefined cereal grains, wheat germ, yeast, soybean flour, and pork. Since it is a water-soluble vitamin, hepatic storage is minimal, and excess is excreted in the urine. Its lack of storage and short (10- to 14-day) half-life necessitate a regular dietary supply of thiamine to prevent deficiency. The recommended daily allowance ranges from 1.0 to 1.5 mg/day, but requirements increase in proportion to carbohydrate intake and metabolic rate.[80]

Thiamine is converted in the jejunum to thiamine pyrophosphate and absorbed throughout the small intestine, passing through the portal circulation prior to active and passive transport across the blood–brain barrier.[81] Clinical manifestations of deficiency occur within days of depletion or reduced stores.[82]

With thiamine supply being intake-dependent, deficiency is seen in persons with compromised nutritional status: reduced intake (e.g., alcoholism, starvation, fad dieting and dieting aids, acquired immunodeficiency syndrome, inadequate parenteral nutrition, thiaminase-containing foods), malabsorption (bariatric surgery, gastrointestinal/liver/pancreatic disease, excess antacid use), and increased losses (persistent emesis or diarrhea, renal failure/dialysis) (see Chapters 13 and 33, and Table 15-4).[83–85] Deficiency is also seen from increased thiamine requirements such as in high metabolic states including pregnancy, critical illness, hyperthyroidism, malignancy, and infection as well as with high carbohydrate intake (e.g., intravenous glucose administration, refeeding syndrome, parenteral nutrition). In these high carbohydrate states, the demand for thiamine, which is needed for glucose oxidation, exceeds replacement.[86]

In developed countries, thiamine deficiency is seen most commonly with excessive alcohol use, although the rise of fad dieting and bariatric surgery has led to an increasing incidence in nonalcoholics.[87] Inadequate intake, reduced gastrointestinal absorption, impaired conversion to active metabolites, increased demand for carbohydrate metabolism, and reduced hepatic storage of thiamine all contribute to the development of thiamine deficiency in alcoholics. Genetic polymorphisms in thiamine and alcohol metabolism may predispose to the development of a thiamine deficiency syndrome.[88]

TABLE 15-4 ■ Causes of Thiamine Deficiency

Reduced Intake
Alcoholism
Starvation
Fad dieting/dieting aids
Acquired immunodeficiency syndrome (AIDS)
Inadequate parenteral nutrition
Thiaminase-containing foods (polished rice, overbaked bread, prolonged milk pasteurization)
Malabsorption
Bariatric surgery
Gastrointestinal, hepatic, or pancreatic disease
Antacids
Increased Loss
Persistent emesis
Persistent diarrhea
Renal failure or dialysis
High Metabolic State
Pregnancy
Critical illness
Hyperthyroidism
Malignancy
Infection
Chemotherapy (e.g., ifosfamide)
Increased Carbohydrate Intake
Intravenous glucose administration
Refeeding syndrome
Parenteral nutrition

Clinical Manifestations

Thiamine is a key cofactor in carbohydrate metabolism, acting as a coenzyme in the tricarboxylic acid cycle and hexose monophosphate shunt. Deficiency results in the reduction of high-energy phosphates with corresponding lactic acid accumulation and impaired oxygen uptake. Cerebral tissue is dependent on glucose for energy and is particularly vulnerable to damage from impaired glucose metabolism. Neurotoxicity is thought to result from disruption in osmotic gradients, glutamate accumulation, and impaired blood–brain barrier permeability.[89] Animal models have shown a predilection for brainstem and cerebellar involvement.[90]

Thiamine deficiency most commonly affects the heart and both the central and peripheral nervous systems. Three well-described manifestations include beriberi (dry and wet), infantile beriberi, and Wernicke encephalopathy with Korsakoff syndrome.[91]

Beriberi

Thiamine deficiency classically presents with a painful, length-dependent sensorimotor axonal neuropathy. In malnourished individuals, concomitant deficiency of other B vitamins such as pantothenic acid and pyridoxine may also contribute to the development of a nutritional polyneuropathy.[92] Fatigue, irritability, and muscle cramps may be the earliest manifestation, presenting within days to weeks of deficiency. Symptoms can be rapidly progressive and evolve from distal sensory loss or burning dysesthesias to muscle weakness.[93] Cranial neuropathy and recurrent laryngeal nerve palsy have been described.[94] An autonomic neuropathy may additionally be present.[95]

Dry beriberi refers to the presence of polyneuropathy, while wet beriberi is used when the development of high output cardiac failure and peripheral edema predominate.[96] These two states are considered the clinical spectra of the same disease process, with the potential of one to evolve into the other.

Infantile beriberi is seen in infants with thiamine-deficient diets, including breast-fed children of thiamine-deficient mothers. The clinical spectrum is varied and may involve the development of cardiac, ophthalmologic, CNS, and systemic abnormalities. Infants can present with irritability, vomiting, diarrhea, failure to thrive, seizures, ophthalmoplegia, drowsiness, and respiratory difficulty.[97]

Wernicke Encephalopathy

Wernicke encephalopathy refers to a syndrome characterized by varying degrees of subacute gait and truncal ataxia, ocular abnormalities, and mental status changes.[98] The presentation is heterogeneous and autopsy studies suggest that many cases of Wernicke encephalopathy are undiagnosed.[99] Ataxia is caused primarily by cerebellar dysfunction and can be accompanied by other localizing abnormalities such as dysarthria and dysmetria. Vestibular dysfunction and coexisting neuropathy can contribute to the development of ataxia.[100] Ocular manifestations are many and include nystagmus, ophthalmoparesis, pupillary abnormalities, and decreased visual acuity.[101] Delirium, somnolence, impaired attention, and lack of orientation are prominent cognitive manifestations.[102] Brainstem or hypothalamic involvement in addition to comorbid autonomic neuropathy may result in fluctuations in body temperature, blood pressure, and heart rate.[103,104] Typically, the pathology involves the limbic system, including the mammillary bodies.[105]

Korsakoff Syndrome

Approximately 80 percent of patients with Wernicke encephalopathy develop residual Korsakoff syndrome, an amnestic condition characterized by severe retrograde and anterograde memory loss with subsequent confabulation.[106] The dorsal medial nucleus of the thalamus is often affected, and involvement of the limbic and frontal cortex has been implicated in the development of anterograde and retrograde amnesia respectively.[107] Memory impairment in Korsakoff syndrome is often chronic and progressive.[108]

Diagnosis

Thiamine deficiency remains a clinical diagnosis; urine and serum thiamine levels are not reflective of tissue thiamine concentrations and can often be normal.[109] Surrogate measurements can include erythrocyte thiamine diphosphate levels or the transketolase activation assay, but these must be measured prior to treatment initiation due to rapid normalization.[110] Impaired aerobic metabolism can cause elevations in lactate and subsequent anion-gap metabolic acidosis.[111] Brain MRI may show T2 hyperintensities in the paraventricular regions including the thalamus, hypothalamus, mammillary bodies, periaqueductal midbrain, pons, medulla, and cerebellum (Fig. 15-2).[112] Contrast enhancement of the mammillary bodies may be seen in Wernicke encephalopathy.[113] Development of vasogenic edema may cause diffusion-weighted abnormalities, which often resolve with treatment.[114] In some patients, brain MRI is completely normal. MR spectroscopy may show elevation in cerebral lactate but is not commonly used.[115]

Treatment

Parenteral thiamine replacement is the mainstay of treatment, but must be administered to high-risk patients prior to glucose or total parenteral nutrition infusion[116]; glucose oxidation is highly thiamine-dependent and glucose supplementation can result in an intracellular shift of already depleted thiamine stores with resultant neurotoxicity. Ongoing poor

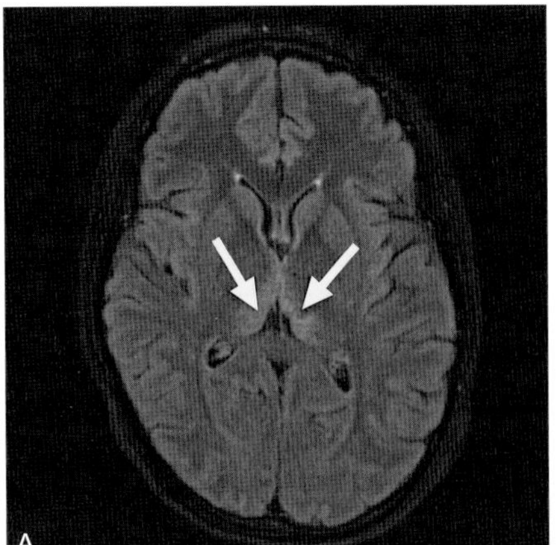

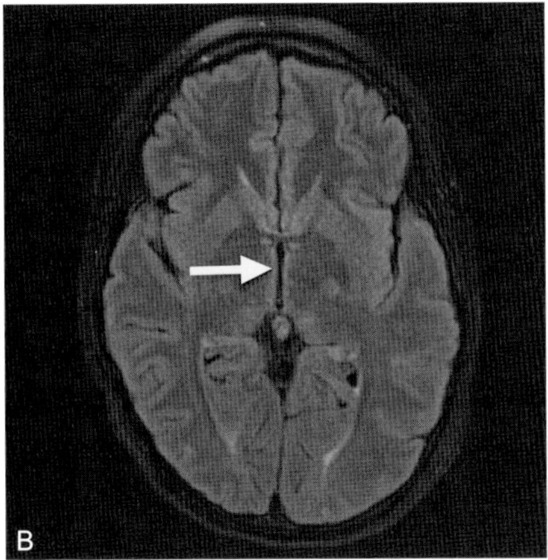

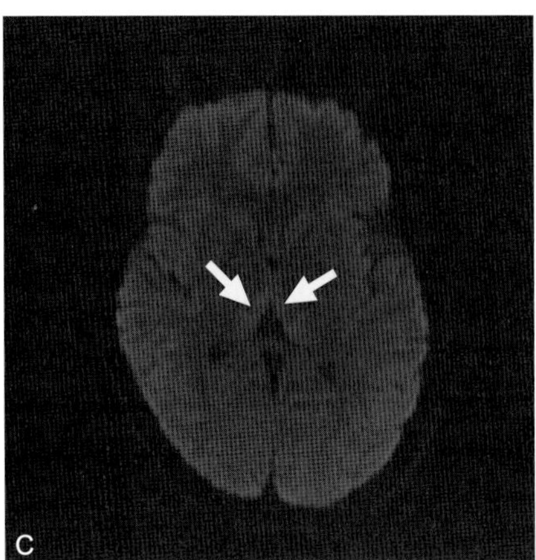

FIGURE 15-2 ■ Acute Wernicke encephalopathy resulting from malnutrition in a 22-year-old woman. Axial brain MRI fluid-attenuated inversion recovery (FLAIR) sequences demonstrate hyperintensity involving the thalamus bilaterally (**A**) and the periventricular region of the third ventricle (**B**). Axial diffusion-weighted sequences (**C**) show periventricular signal change.

nutritional status often necessitates oral maintenance therapy at 50 to 100 mg daily. Attention should be given to the possibility of an underlying cause of malnutrition or increased metabolic demand such as sepsis.[117,118]

Clinical manifestations of thiamine deficiency are partially reversible with treatment; heart failure, ocular abnormalities, and acute mental status changes often resolve quickly. Neuropathic symptoms and gait ataxia recover slowly and can persist.[119] Memory impairment from Korsakoff syndrome is often permanent.[117]

PYRIDOXINE (VITAMIN B_6) DEFICIENCY

Pyridoxine, or vitamin B_6, is a water-soluble vitamin involved in tryptophan, methionine, and γ-amminobutyric acid (GABA) metabolism. The active form of pyridoxine is pyridoxal 5′-phosphate (PLP), a coenzyme that is critical in amino acid and sphingolipid metabolism, as well as in the biosynthesis of glucose, many neurotransmitters, and heme.

Etiology

Pyridoxine is abundant in meat, fish, eggs, and dairy products and is absorbed in the small intestine. As most adult diets provide adequate pyridoxine, clinical deficiency is predominantly seen as a side effect of pyridoxine-antagonizing medications (e.g., isonicotinic acid hydrazide, hydralazine, and penicillamine).[120] The elderly, pregnant and lactating women, alcoholics, patients with sickle cell anemia, and those with chronic gastrointestinal or malabsorptive conditions are additionally susceptible to pyridoxine deficiency.[121] Genetic mutations can also result in an infantile deficiency syndrome.

Clinical Manifestations

Autosomal recessive mutations in the antiquin gene result in inactivation of pyridoxal 5′-phosphate and can manifest with pyridoxine-responsive seizures in adequately nourished neonates.[122,123] Rarely, seizures may develop in breast-feeding infants of malnourished mothers. In adults, chronic pyridoxine deficiency causes a painful sensorimotor peripheral neuropathy.[124] Patients may additionally develop a microcytic hypochromic or sideroblastic anemia.[125] A pellagra-type syndrome (with skin, gastrointestinal, and cognitive abnormalities) has also been described due to abnormal tryptophan metabolism and subsequent niacin deficiency. Conversely, ingestion of pyridoxine exceeding 100 mg per day, as seen with excessive vitamin intake, can result in a pure sensory neuropathy or dorsal root ganglionopathy.[126,127]

Diagnosis

Pyridoxine deficiency is often diagnosed clinically and confirmed through measurement of serum pyridoxal 5′-phosphate levels. An empiric diagnostic trial of pyridoxine is indicated for unexplained neonatal seizures. Elevation of pipecolic acid and α-aminoadipic semialdehyde levels are seen in infants with genetic pyridoxine-dependent seizures and can be measured in serum, urine, and cerebrospinal fluid. In adults, serum pyridoxal 5′-phosphate levels in excess of 20 to 30 nmol/L are considered indicative of adequate pyridoxine status.[128] Elevated serum homocysteine levels following a methionine load can also be seen with pyridoxine deficiency but are rarely measured.[129]

Treatment

Infantile seizures are usually responsive to high doses of pyridoxine but require years of oral maintenance therapy as seizures will recur days after treatment cessation.[123] Drug-induced neuropathy often recovers with discontinuation of the offending agent along with oral pyridoxine replacement at 50 to 100 mg/day. Excess supplementation must be avoided to prevent an associated toxic sensory neuropathy.[127] Treatment of any underlying gastrointestinal, malabsorptive, or hematologic disease is indicated.

NIACIN (VITAMIN B_3) DEFICIENCY

Etiology

Niacin, or vitamin B_3, is an end-product of tryptophan metabolism involved in carbohydrate metabolism. Niacin deficiency results in the clinical syndrome pellagra, and is seen primarily in developing countries where corn is the primary carbohydrate source since corn lacks both niacin and tryptophan.[130] Several vitamins and minerals are necessary for the conversion of tryptophan to niacin, including iron, copper, and vitamins B_2 (riboflavin) and B_6 (pyridoxine). Deficiency of vitamin B_6 may result in secondary niacin deficiency.[111] Niacin deficiency may also develop in alcoholics, with malabsorption (see Chapter 13), and in the setting of bacterial overgrowth. Hartnup syndrome may also result in pellagra due to an impairment in the conversion of tryptophan to niacin.

Clinical Manifestations

Niacin deficiency affects the skin, gastrointestinal tract, and the nervous system, but skin and gastrointestinal manifestations are frequently absent. Potential gastrointestinal manifestations include stomatitis, abdominal pain, and diarrhea. A hyperkeratotic rash, preferentially involving the face, chest, and dorsum of the hands and feet, may be seen. Potential neurologic manifestations include encephalopathy, coma, and peripheral neuropathy.

Diagnosis and Treatment

There are currently no reliable serologic studies to identify niacin deficiency. Measurement of urinary excretion of the methylated niacin metabolites N^1-methylnicotinamide and N^1-methyl-2-pyridone-5-carboxamide can assess niacin status. Oral or parenteral nicotinic acid is administered three times daily to treat the condition.

VITAMIN A DEFICIENCY

Etiology

Vitamin A refers to a collective group of fat-soluble retinoids that includes retinol, retinal, retinoic acid, and retinyl esters.[131] Vitamin A plays an important role in vision, reproduction, and cellular communication.[132] Preformed vitamin A (retinol and retinyl ester) and provitamin A carotenoids are available in the diet. Preformed vitamin A is found in animal sources (e.g., dairy products, fish, and meat), while the provitamin A carotenoids (e.g., β-carotene) are present in various plant sources. Both of these forms of vitamin A are converted intracellularly into retinal and retinoic acid, the biologically active forms of vitamin A.[131]

The various forms of vitamin A are absorbed primarily in the duodenum and stored in the liver as retinyl esters. Vitamin A deficiency may result from dietary restriction (e.g., diets lacking β-carotene, alcoholics), and may develop in conditions associated with fat malabsorption such as celiac disease, pancreatitis, cystic fibrosis, biliary atresia, and cholestatic liver disease.[111]

Clinical Manifestations

Chronic, excessive ingestion of vitamin A may lead to headache, increased intracranial pressure, nausea, dizziness, skin changes, bone and joint pain, coma, and even death.[131,133] Conversely, vitamin A deficiency can cause night blindness, corneal dryness and keratinization, white foamy spots on the cornea (Bitot spots), dysgeusia, and hyperkeratosis of the skin and respiratory, gastrointestinal, and urinary tracts.[111]

Diagnosis and Treatment

Assessment of serum vitamin A levels establishes states of vitamin A deficiency or toxicity. Oral vitamin A supplementation is used to treat vitamin A deficiency.

VITAMIN D DEFICIENCY

Vitamin D is a fat-soluble vitamin that promotes calcium absorption in the gut, thereby maintaining normal serum calcium and phosphate concentrations and enabling normal bone mineralization, bone growth, and remodeling. Vitamin D is also involved in cell growth modulation, neuromuscular and immune function, and reduction of inflammation.[134,135] There are two forms of vitamin D: vitamin D_2 or ergocalciferol (produced by plants) and vitamin D_3 or cholecalciferol (produced by sunlight conversion of 7-dehydrocholesterol in the skin).[111]

Etiology

Very few foods in the human diet contain vitamin D. Fatty fish such as tuna, salmon, mackerel and fish liver contain the highest amounts, while smaller amounts can be found in beef liver, cheese, and egg yolk. The majority of vitamin D in the American diet comes from fortified foods such as milk, some breakfast cereals, and orange juice. Most people obtain the majority of their vitamin D needs through sun exposure.

Vitamin D is absorbed passively in the small intestine then bound to lipoproteins before transport to the liver by chylomicrons. In the liver, vitamin D is hydroxylated to 25-(OH)-vitamin D, and then subsequently hydroxylated a second time to the biologically active 1,25-(OH)-vitamin D in the kidneys. Causes of vitamin D deficiency include inadequate sun exposure, dietary insufficiency, gastrectomy and gastric bypass surgery, pancreatic disease, liver disease, renal disease, and malabsorption. As is true with many other vitamin deficiencies, inflammatory bowel disease, celiac disease, extensive small intestine resection, and cholestatic liver disease may also lead to vitamin D deficiency. Phenobarbital and phenytoin inhibit vitamin D hydroxylation in the liver and can lead to deficiency. Breast-fed infants are at risk because breast milk does not have adequate levels to meet vitamin D requirements. People with dark skin are also at greater risk of developing vitamin D deficiency because melanin in the epidermis reduces the skin's ability to generate cholecalciferol.

Clinical Manifestations

Vitamin D deficiency may cause rickets in children and osteomalacia in adults due to defective bone mineralization. A proximal myopathy may develop, often associated with bone pain and osteomalacia.[136] A multitude of other medical conditions have been associated with suboptimal vitamin D levels including hypertension, diabetes mellitus, certain types of cancers, and multiple sclerosis, but more definitive, prospective studies are necessary to establish a definite link.[137–140] Excessive intake of vitamin D may lead to non-specific symptoms such as anorexia, weight loss, and polyuria, but it may increase blood levels of calcium, leading to vascular and tissue calcification and thereby cause cardiovascular and renal pathology. Sun exposure does not lead to vitamin D toxicity.

Diagnosis and Treatment

Total 25-(OH)-vitamin D is the best laboratory study to assess vitamin D body stores and can be used to monitor vitamin D deficiency. A frequently employed strategy to treat severe vitamin D deficiency is to give a loading dose of 50,000 IU of vitamin D once weekly for 2 to 3 months or 3 times weekly for 1 month. A lower dose (800 to 2000 IU daily) may be utilized in mild to moderate vitamin D deficiency.[141]

LATHYRISM

Lathyrism is one of the oldest known neurotoxic disorders, resulting from excessive consumption of *Lathyrus sativus*, a species of chickpea.[142] Lathyrism is currently restricted to areas of Bangladesh, India, and Ethiopia, and results in a nonprogressive, but irreversible, spastic paraparesis. Neurophysiologic studies suggest anterior horn cell impairment, and neuropathologic studies have demonstrated myelin loss in the corticospinal tract along with anterior horn cell involvement.[143,144] It has been suggested that lathyrism results from the toxin β-*N*-oxalyl-amino-L-alanine, an agonist of the excitatory neurotransmitter glutamate.[145]

KONZO

Konzo is a neurologic disorder confined to rural Africa, resulting from a diet of excessive cyanogen consumption from inadequately processed cassava root combined with a low protein diet.[146] Cassava root is drought tolerant and therefore may become the major or sole food source during agricultural crises. Konzo is characterized clinically by a symmetric, nonprogressive spastic paraparesis.

REFERENCES

1. Hvas AM, Nexo E: Diagnosis and treatment of vitamin B_{12} deficiency. An update. Haematologica 91:1506, 2006.
2. Beck WS: Neuropsychiatric consequences of cobalamin deficiency. Adv Intern Med 36:33, 1991.
3. Stabler SP: Vitamin B_{12}. p. 343. In: Erdman Jr JW, MacDonald IA, Ziesel SH (eds): Present Knowledge in Nutrition. 10th Ed. Wiley-Blackwell, New York, 2012.
4. Stabler SP: Vitamin B_{12} deficiency. N Engl J Med 368:149, 2013.
5. Russell JSR, Batten FE, Collier J: Subacute combined degeneration of the spinal cord. Brain 23:39, 1900.
6. Healton EB, Savage DG, Brust JC, et al: Neurologic aspects of cobalamin deficiency. Medicine (Baltimore) 70:229, 1991.
7. Institute of Medicine Food and Nutrition Board. Dietary Reference Intakes: Thiamin, Riboflavin, Niacin, Vitamin B_6, Folate, Vitamin B_{12}, Pantothenic Acid, Biotin, and Choline. National Academy Press, Washington DC, 1998.
8. Dietary Supplement Fact Sheet: Vitamin B_{12}. NIH. Web. Updated 6/24/2011. Accessed March 22, 2013. (http://ods.od.nih.gov/factsheets/vitaminb12/).
9. Green R, Kinsella LJ: Current concepts in the diagnosis of cobalamin deficiency. Neurology 45:1435, 1995.
10. Carmel R: Cobalamin, the stomach, and aging. Am J Clin Nutr 66:750, 1997.
11. Hurwitz A, Brady DA, Schall SE, et al: Gastric acidity in older adults. JAMA 27:659, 1997.
12. Kumar N: Neurologic presentations of nutritional deficiencies. Neurol Clin 28:107, 2010.
13. Marcuard SP, Albernaz L, Khanzanie PG: Omeprazole therapy causes malabsorption of cyanocobalamin (vitamin B_{12}). Ann Intern Med 120:211, 1994.
14. Koop H, Bachem MG: Serum iron, ferritin, and vitamin B-12 during prolonged omeprazole therapy. J Clin Gastroenterol 14:288, 1992.
15. Andres E, Noel E, Abdelghani MB: Vitamin B_{12} deficiency associated with chronic acid suppression therapy. Ann Pharmacother 37:1730, 2003.
16. de Jager J, Kooy A, Lehert P, et al: Long term treatment with metformin in patients with type 2 diabetes and risk of vitamin B-12 deficiency: randomised placebo controlled trial. BMJ 340:c2181, 2010.
17. Deacon R, Lumb M, Perry J, et al: Selective inactivation of vitamin B_{12} in rats by nitrous oxide. Lancet 2:1023, 1978.
18. Rosenberg H, Orkin FK, Springstead J: Abuse of nitrous oxide. Anesth Analg 58:104, 1979.
19. Ng J, O'Grady G, Petit T, et al: Nitrous oxide use in first-year students at Auckland University. Lancet 361:1349, 2003.
20. Kayser-Gatchalian MC, Neundörfer B: Peripheral neuropathy with vitamin B12 deficiency. J Neurol 214:183, 1977.
21. Lindenbaum J, Healton EB, Savage DG, et al: Neuropsychiatric disorders caused by cobalamin deficiency in the absence of anemia or macrocytosis. N Engl J Med 318:1720, 1988.
22. White WB, Reik L, Cutlip DE: Pernicious anemia seen initially as orthostatic hypotension. Arch Intern Med 141:1543, 1981.
23. Kandler RH, Davies-Jones GA: Internuclear opthalmoplegia in pernicious anaemia. BMJ 297:1583, 1988.
24. Benito-Leon J, Port-Etessam J: Shaky-leg syndrome and vitamin B_{12} deficiency. N Engl J Med 342:981, 2000.
25. Morita S, Miwa H, Kihira T, et al: Cerebellar ataxia and leukoencephalopathy associated with cobalamin deficiency. J Neurol Sci 216:183, 2003.
26. Ahn TB, Cho JW, Jeon BS: Unusual neurological presentations of vitamin B_{12} deficiency. Eur J Neurol 11:339, 2004.
27. Rothenberg SP, Kantha KR, Ficarra A: Autoantibodies to intrinsic factor: their determination and clinical usefulness. J Lab Clin Med 77:476, 1971.
28. Fairbanks VF, Lennon VA, Kokmen E, et al: Tests for pernicious anemia: serum intrinsic factor blocking antibody. Mayo Clinic Proc 58:203, 1983.
29. Carmel R: Reassessment of the relative prevalences of antibodies to gastric parietal cell and to intrinsic factor in patients with pernicious anaemia: influence of patient age and race. Clin Exp Immunol 89:74, 1992.
30. Miller A, Slingerland DW, Cardarelli J, et al: Further studies on the use of serum gastrin levels in assessing the significance of low serum B_{12} levels. Am J Hematol 31:194, 1989.

31. Carmel R: Pepsinogens and other serum markers in pernicious anemia. Am J Clin Pathol 90:442, 1988.
32. Carmel R: The disappearance of cobalamin absorption testing: a critical diagnostic loss. J Nutr 137:2481, 2007.
33. Hemmer B, Glocker FX, Schumacher M, et al: Subacute combined degeneration of the spinal cord: clinical, electrophysiological, and magnetic resonance imaging findings. J Neurol Neurosurg Psychiatry 65:822, 1998.
34. Timms SR, Cure JK, Kurent JE: Subacute combined degeneration of the spinal cord: MR findings. AJNR Am J Neuroradiol 14:1224, 1993.
35. Larner AJ, Zeman AZ, Allen CM, et al: MRI appearances in subacute combined degeneration of the spinal cord due to vitamin B_{12} deficiency. J Neurol Neurosurg Psychiatry 62:99, 1997.
36. Ravina B, Loevner LA, Bank W: MR findings in subacute combined degeneration of the spinal cord: a case of reversible cervical myelopathy. AJR Am J Roentgenol 174:863, 2000.
37. Vidal-Alaball J, Butler CC, Cannings-John R, et al: Oral vitamin B12 versus intramuscular vitamin B12 for vitamin B12 deficiency. Cochrane Database Syst Rev 3:CD004655, 2005.
38. Butler CC, Vidal-Alaball J, Cannings-John R, et al: Oral vitamin B_{12} versus intramuscular vitamin B_{12} for vitamin B_{12} deficiency: a systematic review of randomized controlled trials. Fam Pract 23:279, 2006.
39. Kokkola A, Sjoblom SM, Haapiainen R, et al: The risk of gastric carcinoma and carcinoid tumors in patients with pernicious anaemia. A prospective follow-up study. Scand J Gastroenterol 33:88, 1998.
40. Baumgartner MR: Vitamin-responsive disorders: cobalamin, folate, biotin, vitamins B_1 and E. Handb Clin Neurol 113:1799, 2013.
41. Elsborg L: Malabsorption of folic acid following partial gastrectomy. Scand J Gastroenterol 9:271, 1974.
42. Russell RM, Golner BB, Krasinski SD, et al: Effect of antacid and H2 receptor antagonists on the intestinal absorption of folic acid. J Lab Clin Med 12:458, 1988.
43. Blom HJ, Shaw GM, Den Hijer M, et al: Neural tube defects and folate: case far from closed. Nat Rev Neurosci 7:724, 2006.
44. Grant HC, Hoffbrand AV, Wells DG: Folate deficiency and neurological disease. Lancet 2:763, 1965.
45. Reynolds EH, Rothfeld P, Pincus JH: Neurological disease associated with folate deficiency. Br Med J 2:398, 1973.
46. Manzoor M, Runcie J: Folate-responsive neuropathy: report of 10 cases. BMJ 1:1176, 1976.
47. Lever EG, Elwes RD, Williams A, et al: Subacute combined degeneration of the cord due to folate deficiency: response to methyl folate treatment. J Neurol Neurosurg Psychiatry 49:1203, 1986.
48. Parry TE: Folate responsive neuropathy. Presse Med 23:131, 1994.
49. Green R, Miller JW: Folate deficiency beyond megaloblastic anemia: hyperhomocysteinemia and other manifestations of dysfunctional folate status. Semin Hematol 36:47, 1999.
50. Diaz-Arrastia R: Homocysteine and neurological disease. Arch Neurol 57:1422, 2000.
51. Eichner ER, Hillman RS: Effect of alcohol on serum folate level. J Clin Invest 52:584, 1973.
52. Lucock M, Yates Z: Measurement of red blood cell methylfolate. Lancet 360:1021, 2002.
53. Gunter EW, Bowman BA, Caudill SP, et al: Results of an international round robin for serum and whole-blood folate. Clin Chem 42:1689, 1996.
54. Savage DG, Lindenbaum J, Stabler SP, et al: Sensitivity of serum methylmalonic acid and total homocysteine determinations for diagnosing cobalamin and folate deficiencies. Am J Med 96:239, 1994.
55. Kumar N: Copper deficiency myelopathy (human swayback). Mayo Clinic Proc 81:1371, 2006.
56. Bennetts HW, Chapman FE: Copper deficiency in sheep in western Australia: a preliminary account of the aetiology of enzootic ataxia of lambs and anaemia of ewes. Aust Vet J 13:138, 1937.
57. Barlow RM: Further observations on swayback, I: transitional pathology. J Comp Pathol 73:51, 1963.
58. Wasa M, Satani M, Tanano H, et al: Copper deficiency with pancytopenia during total parenteral nutrition. JPEN J Parenter Enteral Nutr 18:190, 1994.
59. Fuhrman MP, Herrmann V, Masidonski P, et al: Pancytopenia after removal of copper from total parenteral nutrition. JPEN J Parenter Enteral Nutr 24:361, 2000.
60. Tamura H, Hirose S, Watanabe O, et al: Anemia and neutropenia due to copper deficiency in enteral nutrition. JPEN J Parenter Enteral Nutr 18:185, 1994.
61. Goodman BP, Mistry DH, Pasha SF, et al: Copper deficiency myeloneuropathy due to occult celiac disease. Neurologist 15:355, 2009.
62. Spinazzi M, De Lazzari F, Tavolato B, et al: Myelo-optico-neuropathy in copper deficiency occurring after partial gastrectomy. Do small bowel bacterial overgrowth syndrome and occult zinc ingestion tip the balance? J Neurol 254:1012, 2007.
63. Nations SP, Boyer PJ, Love LA, et al: Denture cream: an unusual source of excess zinc, leading to hypocupremia and neurologic disease. Neurology 71:639, 2008.
64. Yuzbasiyan-Gurkan V, Grider A, Nostrant T, et al: Intestinal metallothionein induction. J Lal Clin Med 120:380, 1992.
65. Halfdanarson TR, Kumar N, Li CY, et al: Hematologic manifestations of copper deficiency. A retrospective review. Eur J Haematol 80:523, 2008.
66. Willis MS, Monaghan SA, Miller ML, et al: Zinc-induced copper deficiency: a report of 3 cases initially recognized on bone marrow examination. Am J Clin Pathol 123:125, 2005.

67. Kumar N, Gross JB, Ahlskog JE: Copper deficiency myelopathy produces a clinical picture like subacute combined degeneration. Neurology 63:33, 2004.
68. Goodman BP, Bosch EP, Ross MA, et al: Clinical and electrodiagnostic findings in copper deficiency myeloneuropathy. J Neurol Neurosurg Psychiatry 80:524, 2009.
69. Kumar N, Gross JB, Ahlskog JE: Myelopathy due to copper deficiency. Neurology 61:273, 2009.
70. Harding AE: Vitamin E and the nervous system. Crit Rev Neurobiol 3:89, 1987.
71. Sokol RJ: Vitamin E deficiency and neurologic disease. Annu Rev Nutr 8:351, 1988.
72. Ben Hamida M, Belal S, Sirugo G, et al: Friedreich's ataxia phenotype not linked to chromosome 9 and associated with selective autosomal recessive vitamin E deficiency in two inbred Tunisian families. Neurology 43:2179, 1993.
73. Burck U, Goebel HH, Kuhlendahl HD, et al: Neuromyopathy and vitamin E deficiency in man. Neuropediatrics 12:267, 1981.
74. Kleopa KA, Kyriacou K, Zamba-Papanicolaou E, et al: Reversible inflammatory and vacuolar myopathy with vitamin E deficiency in celiac disease. Muscle Nerve 31:260, 2005.
75. Palmucci L, Doriguzzi C, Orsi L, et al: Neuropathy secondary to vitamin E deficiency in acquired intestinal malabsorption. Ital J Neurol Sci 9:599, 1988.
76. Puri V, Chaudry N, Tatke M, et al: Isolated vitamin E deficiency with demyelinating neuropathy. Muscle Nerve 32:230, 2005.
77. Vorgerd M, Tegenthoff M, Kuhne D, et al: Spinal MRI in progressive myeloneuropathy associated with vitamin E deficiency. Neuroradiology 38(suppl 1):S111, 1996.
78. Butterworth RF: Cerebral thiamine-dependent enzyme changes in experimental Wernicke's encephalopathy. Metab Brain Dis 1:165, 1986.
79. Bettendorff L: Thiamine in excitable tissues: reflections on a non-cofactor role. Metab Brain Dis 9:183, 1994.
80. Escott-Stump S (ed): Nutrition and Diagnosis-Related Care. 6th Ed. Lippincott Williams & Wilkins, Philadelphia, 2008.
81. Thomson AD, Cook CC, Touquet R, et al: The Royal College of Physicians report on alcohol: guidelines for managing Wernicke's encephalopathy in the accident and emergency department. Alcohol Alcohol 37:513, 2002.
82. Schenker S, Henderson GI, Hoyumpa Jr AM, et al: Hepatic and Wernicke's encephalopathies: current concepts of pathogenesis. Am J Clin Nutr 33:2719, 1980.
83. Baughman Jr FA, Papp JP: Wernicke's encephalopathy with intravenous hyperalimentation: remarks on similarities between Wernicke's encephalopathy and the phosphate depletion syndrome. Mt Sinai J Med 43:48, 1976.
84. Lonsdale D: Wernicke's encephalopathy and hyperalimentation. JAMA 239:1133, 1978.
85. Vimokesant SL, Hilker DM, Nakornchai S, et al: Effects of betel nut and fermented fish on the thiamin status of northeastern Thais. Am J Clin Nutr 28:1458, 1975.
86. Sauberlich HE, Herman YF, Stevens CO, et al: Thiamin requirement of the adult human. Am J Clin Nutr 32:2237, 1979.
87. Thomson AD: Mechanisms of vitamin deficiency in chronic alcohol misusers and the development of the Wernicke-Korsakoff syndrome. Alcohol Alcohol Suppl 35:2, 2000.
88. Sechi G, Serra A: Wernicke's encephalopathy: new clinical settings and recent advances in diagnosis and management. Lancet Neurol 6:442, 2007.
89. Hazell AS, Todd KG, Butterworth RF: Mechanisms of neuronal cell death in Wernicke's encephalopathy. Metab Brain Dis 13:97, 1998.
90. Mancall EL, McEntee WJ: Alteration in the cerebellar cortex in nutritional encephalopathy. Neurology 15:33, 1965.
91. Donnino MW, Vega J, Miller J, et al: Myths and misconceptions of Wernicke's encephalopathy: what every emergency physician should know. Ann Emerg Med 50:715, 2007.
92. Saperstein DS, Bahron RJ: Polyneuropathy caused by nutritional and vitamin deficiency. p. 2051. In: Dyck PJ, Thomas PK (eds): Peripheral Neuropathy. 4th Ed. Elsevier Saunders, Philadelphia, 2005.
93. Koike H, Ito S, Morozumi S, et al: Rapidly developing weakness mimicking Guillain–Barré syndrome in beriberi neuropathy: two case reports. Nutrition 24:776, 2008.
94. Koike H, Misu K, Hattori N, et al: Postgastrectomy polyneuropathy with thiamine deficiency. J Neurol Neurosurg Psychiatry 71:357, 2001.
95. Mellion M, Gilchrist JM, de la Monte S: Alcohol-related peripheral neuropathy: nutritional, toxic, or both? Muscle Nerve 43:309, 2011.
96. Tanphaichitr V: Overview of water soluble vitamins. p. 38. In: Shils M, Olson JA, Shike M (eds): Modern Nutrition in Health and Disease. 9th Ed. Lippincott Williams & Wilkins, Philadelphia, 1999.
97. Fattal-Valevski A, Kesler A, Sela BA, et al: Outbreak of life-threatening thiamine deficiency in infants in Israel caused by a defective soy-based formula. Pediatrics 115:e233, 2005.
98. So YT, Simon RP: Deficiency diseases of the nervous system. p. 1643. In: Bradley WG, Daroff RB, Fenichel GM (eds): Neurology in Clinical Practice. 4th Ed. Elsevier, Philadelphia, 2008.
99. Harper C: The incidence of Wernicke's encephalopathy in Australia: a neuropathological study of 131 cases. J Neurol Neurosurg Psychiatry 46:593, 1983.
100. Ghez C: Vestibular paresis: a clinical feature of Wernicke's disease. J Neurol Neurosurg Psychiatry 32:134, 1969.

101. Surges R, Beck S, Niesen WD, et al: Sudden bilateral blindness in Wernicke's encephalopathy: case report and review of the literature. J Neurol Sci 260:261, 2007.
102. Torvik A, Lindboe CF, Rogde S: Brain lesions in alcoholics. A neuropathological study with clinical correlations. J Neurol Sci 56:233, 1982.
103. Birchfield RI: Postural hypotension in Wernicke's disease. A manifestation of autonomic nervous system involvement. Am J Med 36:404, 1964.
104. Ackerman WJ: Stupor, bradycardia, hypotension and hypothermia. A presentation of Wernicke's encephalopathy with rapid response to thiamine. West J Med 121:428, 1974.
105. Suarez GA: Peripheral neuropathy associated with alcoholism, malnutrition and vitamin deficiencies. p. 2294. In Noseworthy JN (ed): Neurological Therapeutics: Principles and Practice. Informa Healthcare, Abingdon, 2006.
106. Cook CC, Hallwood PM, Thomson AD: B vitamin deficiency and neuropsychiatric syndromes in alcohol misuse. Alcohol Alcohol 33:317, 1998.
107. Kopelman MD: The Korsakoff syndrome. Br J Psychiatry 166:154, 1995.
108. Brokate B, Hildebrandt H, Eling P, et al: Frontal lobe dysfunctions in Korsakoff's syndrome and chronic alcoholism: continuity or discontinuity? Neuropsychology 17:420, 2003.
109. Lu J, Frank EL: Rapid HPLC measurement of thiamine and its phosphate esters in whole blood. Clin Chem 54:901, 2008.
110. Talwar D, Davidson H, Cooney J, et al: Vitamin B_1 status assessed by direct measurement of thiamin pyrophosphate in erythrocytes or whole blood by HPLC: comparison with erythrocyte transketolase activation assay. Clin Chem 46:704, 2000.
111. Donnino MW, Miller J, Garcia AJ, et al: Distinctive acid-base pattern in Wernicke's encephalopathy. Ann Emerg Med 50:722, 2007.
112. Victor M: MR in the diagnosis of Wernicke-Korsakoff syndrome. AJR Am J Roentgenol 155:1315, 1990.
113. Shogry ME, Curnes JT: Mamillary body enhancement on MR as the only sign of acute Wernicke encephalopathy. AJNR Am J Neuroradiol 15:172, 1994.
114. Bergui M, Bradac GB, Zhong JJ, et al: Diffusion-weighted MR in reversible Wernicke encephalopathy. Neuroradiology 43:969, 2001.
115. Rugilo CA, Uribe Roca MC, Zurru MC, et al: Proton MR spectroscopy in Wernicke encephalopathy. AJNR Am J Neuroradiol 24:952, 2003.
116. Koguchi K, Nakatsuji Y, Abe K, et al: Wernicke's encephalopathy after glucose infusion. Neurology 62:512, 2004.
117. Galvin R, Bråthen G, Ivashynka A, et al: EFNS guidelines for diagnosis, therapy and prevention of Wernicke encephalopathy. Eur J Neurol 17:1408, 2010.
118. Tanphaichitr V: Thiamin. p. 432. In: Shils ME, Olsen JA, Shike M (eds): Modern Nutrition in Health and Disease. 9th Ed. Lippincott Williams & Wilkins, Philadelphia, 1999.
119. Ohnishi A, Tsuji S, Igisu H, et al: Beriberi neuropathy. Morphometric study of sural nerve. J Neurol Sci 45:177, 1980.
120. Bhagavan HN, Brin M: Drug–vitamin B6 interaction. Curr Concepts Nutr 12:1, 1983.
121. Mackey AD, Davis SR, Gregory JFI: Vitamin B_6. p. 452. In: Shils ME, Shike M, Ross AC (eds): Modern Nutrition in Health and Disease. 10th Ed. Lippincott Williams & Wilkins, Baltimore, 2006.
122. Plecko B, Paul K, Paschke E, et al: Biochemical and molecular characterization of 18 patients with pyridoxine-dependent epilepsy and mutations of the antiquitin (ALDH7A1) gene. Hum Mutat 28:19, 2007.
123. Plecko B: Pyridoxine and pyridoxalphosphate-dependent epilepsies. Handb Clin Neurol 113:1811, 2013.
124. Goldman AL, Braman SS: Isoniazid: a review with emphasis on adverse effects. Chest 62:71, 1972.
125. Mason DY, Emerson PM: Primary acquired sideroblastic anaemia: response to treatment with pyridoxal-5-phosphate. BMJ 1:389, 1973.
126. Schaumburg H, Kaplan J, Windebank A, et al: Sensory neuropathy from pyridoxine abuse. A new megavitamin syndrome. N Engl J Med 309:445, 1983.
127. Parry GJ, Bredesen DE: Sensory neuropathy with low-dose pyridoxine. Neurology 35:1466, 1985.
128. Leklem JE: Vitamin B-6: a status report. J Nutr 120(suppl 11):1503, 1990.
129. Rimm EB, Willett WC, Hu FB, et al: Folate and vitamin B6 from diet and supplements in relation to risk of coronary heart disease among women. JAMA 279:359, 1998.
130. Bourgeois C, Cerbantes-Laurean D, Moss J: Niacin. p. 442. In: Shils ME, Shike M, Ross AC (eds): Modern Nutrition in Health and Disease. 10th Ed. Lippincott Williams & Wilkins, Baltimore, 2006.
131. Ross CA: Vitamin A. p. 778. In: Coates PM, Betz JM, Blackman MR (eds): Encyclopedia of Dietary Supplements. 2nd Ed. Informa Healthcare, London, 2010.
132. Johnson EJ, Russell RM: Beta-carotene. p. 81. In: Coates PM, Betz JM, Blackman MR (eds): Encyclopedia of Dietary Supplements. 2nd Ed. Informa Healthcare, London, 2010.
133. Solomons NW: Vitamin A. p. 157. In: Bowman B, Russell R (eds): Present Knowledge in Nutrition. 9th Ed. ILSI Press, Washington DC, 2006.
134. Holick MF: Vitamin D. p. 376. In: Shils ME, Shike M, Ross AC (eds): Modern Nutrition in Health and Disease. 10th Ed. Lippincott Williams & Wilkins, Baltimore, 2006.

135. Norman AW, Henry HH: Vitamin D. p. 198. In: Bowman B, Russell R (eds): Present Knowledge in Nutrition. 9th Ed. ILSI Press, Washington DC, 2006.
136. Russelll JA: Osteomalacic myopathy. Muscle Nerve 17:578, 1994.
137. Pittas AG, Dawson-Hughes B, Li T, et al: Vitamin D and calcium intake in relation to type 2 diabetes in women. Diabetes Care 29:650, 2006.
138. Institute of Medicine Food and Nutrition Board: Dietary Reference Intakes for Calcium and Vitamin D. National Academy Press, Washington DC, 2010.
139. Tamez H, Thadani RI: Vitamin D and hypertension: an update and review. Curr Opin Nephrol Hypertens 21:492, 2012.
140. Simon KC, Munger KL, Ascherio A: Vitamin D and multiple sclerosis: epidemiology, immunology, and genetics. Curr Opin Neurol 25:246, 2012.
141. Kennel KA, Drake MT, Hurley DL: Vitamin D deficiency in adults: when to test and how to treat. Mayo Clin Proc 85:752, 2010.
142. Spencer PS, Schaumburg HH: Lathyrism: a neurotoxic disease. Neurobehav Toxicol Teratol 5:625, 1983.
143. Drory VE, Rabey MJ, Cohn DF: Electrophysiologic features in patients with chronic neurolathyrism. Acta Neurol Scand 85:401, 1992.
144. Striefler M, Cohn DF, Hirano A, et al: The central nervous system in a case of neurolathyrism. Neurology 27:1176, 1977.
145. Spencer PS, Roy DN, Ludolph A, et al: Lathyrism: evidence for role of the neuroexcitatory aminoacid BOAA. Lancet 2:1066, 1986.
146. Nzwalo H, Cliff J: Konzo: from poverty, cassava, and cyanogen intake to toxico-nutritional neurological disease. PLoS Negl Trop Dis 5:e1051, 2011.

SECTION

III

Renal and Electrolyte Disorders

CHAPTER

16

Neurologic Dysfunction and Kidney Disease

MICHAEL J. AMINOFF

The neurologic aspects of renal disease and the neurologic complications of dialysis and renal transplantation are discussed in this chapter. The neurologic complications of renal carcinoma are not considered, but paraneoplastic complications of malignancy are considered in Chapter 27, and the neurologic consequences of radiation and chemotherapy in Chapter 28. The subject itself is complicated because many of the causes of renal failure lead to neurologic complications that also occur in uremia. Thus, collagen vascular diseases are commonly associated with encephalopathy or seizures, and diabetes with neuropathy or encephalopathy. Attention here is directed primarily to complications that are a direct consequence of the renal failure and its treatment rather than to the underlying cause of the kidney disease. In addition, however, certain hereditary disorders that affect both the nervous system and the kidneys are considered. In order to limit the size of the chapter, the bibliography has largely been restricted to references published since 1990, and particularly to those published in the last 10 to15 years. Earlier references can be found in previous editions of this book.

UREMIC ENCEPHALOPATHY

The neurologic consequences of uremia resemble other metabolic and toxic disorders of the central nervous system (CNS). Thus, the clinical features of the encephalopathy that occurs in uremic patients include an impairment of external awareness that ranges from a mild confusional state, with diminished attention and concentration, to coma. The presence of coma may indicate severe uremia or reflect a complication such as hypertensive encephalopathy, posterior reversible encephalopathy syndrome,[1–3] fluid and electrolyte disturbances, seizures, or sepsis.

Aminoff's Neurology and General Medicine, Fifth Edition.

Other causes of an encephalopathy in uremic patients include dialysis, thiamine deficiency, drug toxicity, and transplant rejection. Finally, the encephalopathy and renal impairment may both relate independently to the same underlying systemic illness, such as diabetes or connective tissue diseases. All these factors complicate clinical assessment.

In addition to an alteration in external awareness, patients with uremic encephalopathy may have seizures, dysarthria, gait ataxia, asterixis, tremor, and multifocal myoclonus. As with all metabolic encephalopathies, symptoms and signs typically fluctuate in severity over short periods of time, such as over the course of a day or from day to day.

Pathophysiology

In early studies, various pathologic changes were described in the brain of uremic patients, but these probably did not relate directly to the uremia. Thus, neuronal degeneration and necrosis of the granular cell layer of the cerebellar cortex probably related to preterminal hypoxia, and focal demyelination and necrosis to coexisting hypertensive cerebrovascular disease that led to small infarcts.[4] Glycolysis and energy utilization are reduced in the brain, probably as a consequence of a disturbance of synaptic transmission that leads to decreased neuronal interaction and thus to reduced cerebral oxygen consumption.[4]

Uremic encephalopathy almost certainly relates to a variety of metabolic abnormalities, with the accumulation of numerous metabolites, imbalance in excitatory and inhibitory neurotransmitters, and hormonal disturbances leading to cerebral dysfunction. The European Uremic Toxin Work Group has listed 90 compounds considered to be uremic toxins; 68 have a molecular weight less than 500 Da, 12 exceed 12,000 Da, and 10 have a molecular weight between 500 and 12,000 Da.[5,6] A few merit brief discussion here. Retention of urea occurs; urea clearance, even in well-dialyzed patients, amounts to only one-sixth of physiologic clearance.[6] Accumulation of guanidinosuccinic acid, methylguanidine, guanidine, and creatinine, all of which are guanidine compounds, in the serum and cerebrospinal fluid (CSF) of uremic patients, may play a role in causing uremic seizures and cognitive dysfunction.[7–9] Activation of *N*-methyl-D-aspartate (NMDA) receptors and inhibition of γ-aminobutyric acid-A ($GABA_A$) transmission may be involved, on the basis of studies in animals.[7] Guanidinosuccinic acid may inhibit transketolase, a thiamine-dependent enzyme involved in the pentose phosphate pathway and in the maintenance of myelin.[8,9] It remains unclear whether low-level aluminum overload in renal failure causes gradual deterioration in cerebral function.[10] Abnormalities of the membrane pumps for both Na^+,K^+–adenosine triphosphatase and calcium ions have been described in experimental studies in animals and may be of clinical relevance.

Hormonal changes may also be important in the pathogenesis of uremic encephalopathy. Serum concentrations of parathyroid hormone, growth hormone, prolactin, luteinizing hormone, insulin, and glucagon are elevated in uremic patients.[11] Parathyroid hormone levels increase with the severity of the encephalopathy, and alterations in brain calcium could influence neurotransmitter release, the sodium-potassium pump, intracellular enzyme activity, and intracellular metabolic processes, and thereby may affect cerebral function. Experimental studies show that the calcium content of the cerebral cortex is greatly increased in uremia, and this is unrelated to alterations in calcium concentration in the plasma or cerebrospinal fluid.[12,13] Both clinical and electroencephalographic (EEG) abnormalities, and changes in cerebral calcium concentration,[12] are improved by parathyroidectomy.

In contrast to the process in subjects with normal kidneys, the removal of uremic toxins in dialysis is achieved by a one-step, membrane-based process and is intermittent. The resulting stepwise variation in plasma concentrations of uremic toxins contrasts with the continuous function of normal kidneys.[6]

Clinical Features

The clinical features of uremic encephalopathy do not show a good correlation with any single laboratory abnormality but can sometimes be related to the rate at which renal failure develops.[13] Thus, stupor and coma are relatively common in acute renal failure, whereas symptoms may be less conspicuous and progression more insidious despite more marked laboratory abnormalities in chronic renal failure. Dialysis relieves or prevents some of the more severe features of this encephalopathy.

The most reliable early indicators of uremic encephalopathy are a waxing and waning reduction in alertness and impaired external awareness.[2] The ability to concentrate is impaired, so that patients seem preoccupied and apathetic, with a poor attention span; they become increasingly disoriented with regard to place and time and may exhibit emotional lability and sleep inversion. An impairment of higher cognitive abilities, such as of executive function, becomes evident, and patients become increasingly forgetful and apathetic. With progression, patients become more obtunded so that it may then be necessary to shout or gently shake them to engage their attention and elicit any responses, which are likely to be of variable accuracy and relevance. Delusions, illusions, and hallucinations (typically visual) often develop, and patients may become agitated and excited, with an acute delirium that eventually is replaced by stupor and a preterminal coma.

Tremulousness may be conspicuous and usually occurs before asterixis is found. A coarse postural tremor is seen in the fingers of the outstretched hands, and a kinetic tremor is also common. Asterixis is a nonspecific sign of metabolic cerebral dysfunction. An intermittent loss of postural tone produces the so-called flapping tremor of asterixis after several seconds when the upper limbs are held outstretched with the elbows and wrists hyperextended and fingers spread apart; irregular flexion-extension occurs at the wrist and of the fingers at the metacarpophalangeal joints, with flexion being the more rapid phase. There is complete electrical silence in the wrist flexors and extensors during the downward (flexor) movements, followed by electrical activity in the extensors as they restore the limb's posture. The axial structures, including the trunk or neck, may also be affected. Asterixis can also be demonstrated in the lower limbs, and flapping may even be elicited in the face by forceful eyelid closure, strong retraction of the corners of the mouth, pursing of the lips, or protrusion of the tongue, provided that some degree of voluntary muscle control persists.[4] In obtunded or comatose patients, or others in whom voluntary effort is limited, asterixis can still be elicited, but at the hip joints.[7] With the patient lying supine, the examiner grasps both ankles of the supine patient and moves the feet upward toward the patient's body, flexing and abducting the thighs: irregular abduction–adduction movements at the hips indicate asterixis.

Spontaneous and stimulus-sensitive myoclonus is common in uremia and in other metabolic encephalopathies and reflects increased cerebral excitability. The myoclonus is typically multifocal, irregular, and asymmetric; it may be precipitated by voluntary movement (action myoclonus). The myoclonic jerks may be especially conspicuous in the facial and proximal limb muscles. Uremic myoclonus in humans resembles the reticular reflex form of postanoxic action myoclonus. It is usually not associated with EEG spike discharges, although such discharges have sometimes been encountered with the myoclonus. The myoclonus may respond to clonazepam. Multifocal myoclonus is sometimes so intense that muscles appear to be fasciculating (*uremic twitching*).[4] Tetany may occur.

Seizures are common. They are usually generalized convulsions, may be multiple, and are often multifactorial in etiology. In acute renal failure, convulsions commonly occur several days after onset, during the anuric or oliguric phase. In chronic renal failure, they tend to occur with advanced disease, often developing preterminally; they may relate to the uremia itself or to electrolyte disturbances, medications (such as penicillin, aminophylline, or isoniazid), or an associated reversible posterior leukoencephalopathy syndrome (characterized by vasogenic white-matter edema predominantly localized to the posterior cerebral hemispheres on imaging studies, as shown in Fig. 16-1). Their incidence has declined, perhaps because of more effective treatment of renal failure and its complications. Seizures also occur in patients undergoing hemodialysis as part of the *dialysis dysequilibrium syndrome* (discussed later). Focal seizures sometimes occur. Occasionally patients develop nonconvulsive status epilepticus that may not be recognized unless an EEG is obtained.[14,15]

During the early stages of uremia, patients may be clumsy or have an unsteady gait. Paratonia (*gegenhalten*), a variable, velocity-dependent resistance to passive movement, especially rapid movement, is common, and grasp and palmomental reflexes may be present, presumably as a result of a depression of frontal lobe function. As uremia advances, extensor muscle tone increases and may be asymmetric; opisthotonos or decorticate posturing of the limbs may eventually occur. Motor deficits may include transient or alternating hemiparesis that shifts sides during the course of the illness, flaccid quadriparesis related to hyperkalemia, or distal weakness from uremic neuropathy. The tendon reflexes are generally brisk unless a significant peripheral neuropathy is present and may be asymmetric; Babinski signs are often present.

Encephalopathy may occur in uremic patients for reasons other than uremia, such as in relation

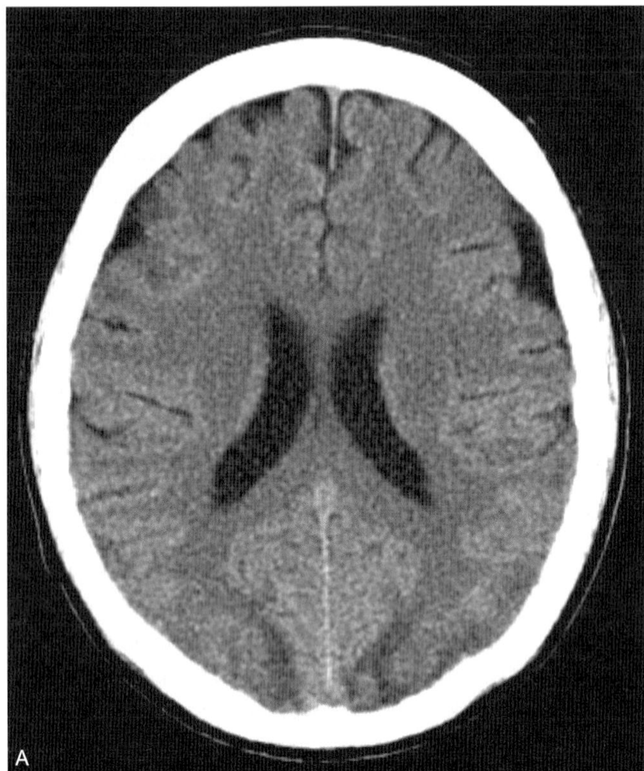

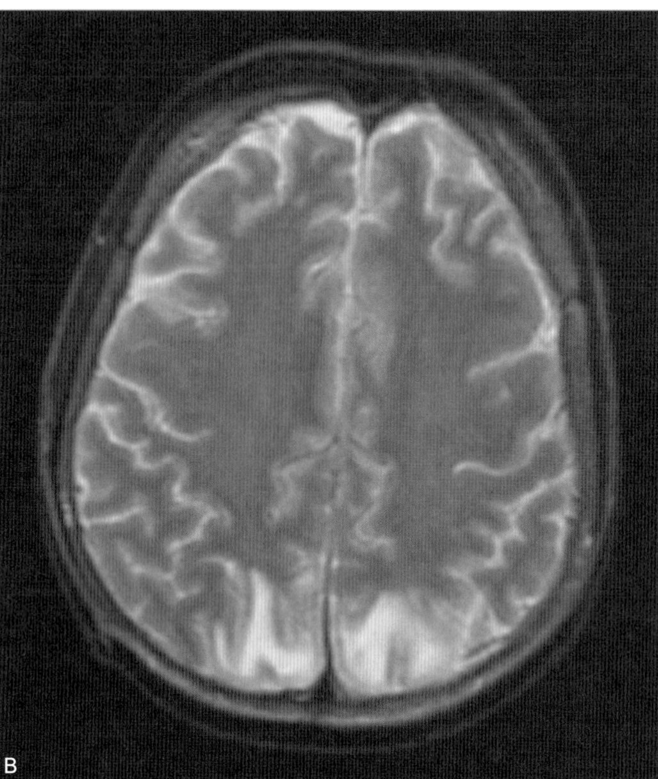

FIGURE 16-1 ■ Imaging findings of a patient with seizures who was diagnosed with posterior reversible encephalopathy syndrome. **A**, Axial computed tomography (CT) scan demonstrates bilateral low-density involvement of the occipital lobes. **B**, Axial T2-weighted magnetic resonance imaging (MRI) shows high signal intensity lesions without mass effect involving white matter bilaterally in the occipital lobes. (Courtesy of William P. Dillon, MD, University of California, San Francisco.)

to dialysis, thiamine deficiency, electrolyte imbalance, medication-related toxicity, and graft rejection. These disorders are considered in later sections of this chapter.

Investigations

Laboratory studies provide evidence of impaired renal function but are of limited utility in monitoring the course of the encephalopathy. Furthermore, abnormal renal function tests do not exclude other causes of encephalopathy. An underlying structural lesion must be excluded in uremic patients who have had seizures, especially when focal or multiple seizures have occurred.

The CSF is commonly abnormal, with a pleocytosis that is unrelated to the degree of azotemia and an increased protein content that sometimes exceeds 100 mg/dl. In the older literature, summarized by Raskin,[4] up to 30 percent of uremic patients were found to have neck stiffness and Kernig sign, and in this context the finding of abnormal CSF may lead to the erroneous conclusion that the patient has a meningitic or encephalitic illness.

The EEG is diffusely slowed, with an excess of intermittent or continuous theta and delta waves that may show a frontal emphasis, perhaps reflecting a decreased cerebral metabolic rate. Triphasic waves are often present, with an anterior predominance (Fig. 16-2). Bilateral spike-wave complexes may be present either in the resting EEG or with photic stimulation. The EEG becomes increasingly slowed with progression of the encephalopathy, so that delta activity becomes more continuous; the findings correlate best with the level of retained nitrogenous compounds, although no clear relationship exists between the EEG and a specific laboratory abnormality. Similarly, there are delays of visual, auditory, and somatosensory evoked cerebral potentials.[16] Event-related potentials reveal abnormalities even in asymptomatic patients, with an increase in P3 latency.[11] In a study involving transcranial magnetic stimulation, 36 patients with end-stage renal disease

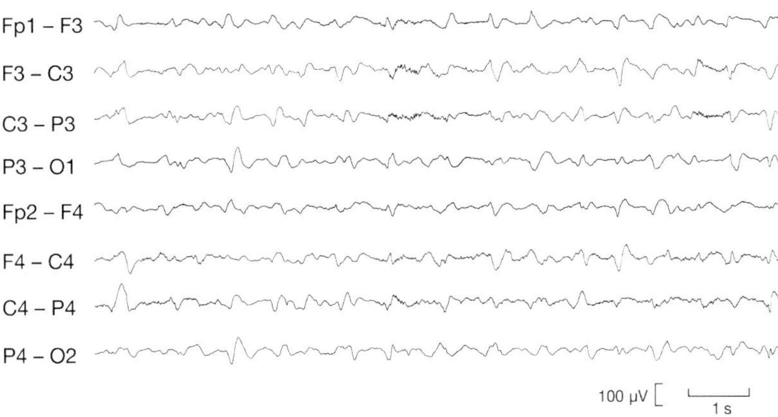

FIGURE 16-2 ■ Electroencephalogram (EEG) showing a diffusely slowed background with triphasic waves in a patient with uremic encephalopathy.

were evaluated at different stages of the disease and under different treatment.[16] Patients on conservative treatment showed a significant reduction of short-interval intracortical inhibition that could be reversed by hemodialysis, peritoneal dialysis, or renal transplantation. After hemodialysis, intracortical facilitation increased, and this was inversely correlated with the decline in plasma osmolarity induced by the dialytic procedure. In other words, patients showed alterations in cortical excitability that were reversed by treatment of the renal disease.

Cerebral imaging studies are of limited help except in excluding other, structural causes of the encephalopathy. They may reveal a reversible, predominantly posterior leukoencephalopathy, with subcortical edema without infarction.[2,3] There may be multiple areas of symmetric edema in the basal ganglia, brainstem, or cerebellum, with—in severe cases—focal infarcts, sometimes hemorrhagic.[1]

Treatment of Uremic Convulsions

Treatment involves correction of renal failure and related metabolic abnormalities. In patients who have had seizures, anticonvulsant medication may be required, especially when the convulsions are of uncertain cause. If status epilepticus occurs, it is managed as in other circumstances.

Various considerations make anticonvulsant therapy difficult to manage in uremia. As discussed in Chapter 57 and also reviewed elsewhere,[17] plasma protein binding and renal excretion are reduced, and dialysis may remove drugs from the circulation. Phenytoin is often used in this context; reduced protein binding leads to a greater volume of distribution and lower serum concentrations, but the proportion of unbound (active) phenytoin increases and maintains the benefit of a given dose. Free phenytoin rather than total plasma levels are used to monitor treatment; the optimal therapeutic range is 1 to 2 μg/ml. The total daily dose generally need not be changed, but it is probably best taken divided rather than in a single dose. Dialysis does not remove phenytoin from the circulation to any significant extent.[18] Plasma phenobarbital levels are unaffected by renal insufficiency. Lower doses of phenobarbital are used for long-term maintenance therapy, however, because the drug may accumulate; additional doses may be required after dialysis. Primidone and its metabolites may also accumulate, causing toxicity in uremic patients.

Valproic acid is helpful for treating myoclonic seizures and generalized convulsions in uremic patients. Protein binding decreases, but the free fraction remains constant.[18] Dialysis does not necessitate additional doses.

Serum carbamazepine levels are unchanged, and dosing does not need alteration.[18] Impaired renal function leads to decreased clearance of felbamate, gabapentin, topiramate, levetiracetam, vigabatrin, pregabalin, and oxcarbazepine. Gabapentin, pregabalin, and topiramate are excreted mainly by the kidneys,[19–21] and the daily dose will need to be reduced in uremic patients; dosing of zonisamide may also need reduction.[22] Hemodialysis necessitates additional doses of levetiracetam (typically 250 to 500 mg)[23] and gabapentin (200 to 300 mg); supplemental doses of topiramate [21] and pregabalin[20] after hemodialysis may also be required. Extra doses of zonisamide may not be necessary if this drug is given in a single daily dose after dialysis sessions.[24] Tiagabine and lamotrigine pharmacokinetics show little change even in severe uremia, and dosage adjustment is usually unnecessary.[25,26]

UREMIC NEUROPATHY

Polyneuropathy

Peripheral nerve function becomes impaired at glomerular filtration rates of less than 12 ml/min, with clinical deficits developing at rates of about 6 ml/min.[11] More than 50 percent of patients with end-stage renal disease have clinical (neuropathic symptoms or signs) or electrophysiologic abnormalities, the exact number depending on the series and diagnostic criteria utilized.

Pathophysiology

Because uremic neuropathy improves with dialysis, uremic neuropathy has been attributed to the accumulation of dialyzable metabolites. Hemodialysis regimes sufficient to control urea or creatinine may nevertheless fail to prevent the development of neuropathy, and this observation led to the "middle molecule" hypothesis. In particular, the lower prevalence of neuropathy in patients on peritoneal dialysis than on hemodialysis suggested that the responsible substance was better dialyzed by the peritoneum, and it was proposed that these substances might be in the middle-molecule range (500 to 12,000 Da), which is poorly cleared by hemodialysis membranes. The adoption of dialysis strategies to improve the clearance of middle molecules reduced the rates of severe neuropathy.[4,27]

The identity of the responsible neurotoxin has remained elusive. Some evidence exists for the neurotoxicity of parathyroid hormone, as was discussed earlier. Parathyroid hormone prolongs motor conduction velocities in dogs perhaps through accumulation of calcium in peripheral nerves; parathyroidectomy of three dogs with chronic renal failure was associated with reversal of the motor conduction abnormalities and calcium content of nerve despite an additional period of renal failure.[28] Studies in uremic patients of the effect of parathyroid hormone on peripheral nerves, however, have yielded both supporting and conflicting results.

On the basis of the published literature, Bostock and colleagues have emphasized that for a substance to be accepted as a uremic neurotoxin, it must satisfy certain criteria, namely, (1) it must be an identifiable chemical; (2) its concentration in the blood should be increased in patients with uremia; (3) a direct relationship should exist between its blood level and neurologic dysfunction; (4) it should be neurotoxic in animals at appropriate blood levels; (5) its removal from the blood should abolish neurologic dysfunction; and (6) dialysis should remove the substance from the body, but more slowly than it removes urea.[29] If these criteria are accepted, the middle molecule hypothesis cannot be accepted at this time because no identifiable chemical with established neurotoxicity has been demonstrated, with a clear relationship between its blood level and neurologic dysfunction, except for parathyroid hormone, which is not dialyzable. These authors proposed instead that mild hyperkalemia was responsible. It is known that hyperkalemia typically recurs within a few hours of a dialysis session as a result of re-equilibration between intracellular and extracellular fluid compartments.[30] Prolonged hyperkalemia may disrupt normal ionic gradients and activate Ca^{++}-mediated processes that are damaging to axons.[27,29]

Motor[31] and sensory nerve excitability[32] has been studied in relation to changes in serum levels of potential neurotoxins, including calcium and potassium ions, urea, uric acid, and certain middle molecules. Predialysis measures of nerve excitability were abnormal, consistent with axonal depolarization, and correlated strongly with serum potassium levels, suggesting that hyperkalemic depolarization may underlie the development of uremic neuropathy. The severity of symptoms also correlated with excitability abnormalities. Most nerve excitability parameters were normalized by hemodialysis.[31,32] The findings support the belief that hyperkalemia is primarily responsible for uremic depolarization and probably contributes to the development of neuropathy. There is no evidence of significant Na^+/K^+ pump dysfunction,[33] despite earlier suggestions to the contrary.

If hyperkalemia does indeed have a role in mediating these abnormalities, measures of dialysis adequacy based solely on blood urea or creatinine concentrations may be inadequate for determining whether dialysis will prevent neurotoxicity. Monitoring the serum potassium level and ensuring that it is maintained within normal limits between periods of dialysis may be more relevant in this regard.

CLINICAL FEATURES

Uremic neuropathy is more common in men than women and in adults than children. It is characterized by a length-dependent, symmetric, mixed sensorimotor polyneuropathy of axonal type that resembles other axonal metabolic-toxic neuropathies. Its clinical manifestations, severity, and rate of progression are variable. As with uremic encephalopathy, its severity correlates poorly with biochemical abnormalities in the blood, but neuropathy is more likely to develop in chronic or severe renal failure.

Initial symptoms commonly consist of dysesthesias distally in the legs; muscle cramps may also be troublesome. The restless legs syndrome often develops before or with the clinical onset of neuropathy, and its occurrence may therefore indicate incipient peripheral nerve involvement. As with many other neuropathies, the earliest clinical signs are of impaired vibration appreciation and depressed or absent tendon reflexes distally in the legs, indicating involvement of large-diameter myelinated fibers. Progression is typically insidious over many months but occasionally is rapid, leading early to severe disability.[34,35] Thus, a more progressive, predominantly motor subacute neuropathy may occur in uremic patients with diabetes and lead to severe weakness over a few weeks or months; nerve conduction studies typically demonstrate features of an axonal neuropathy[35] but may show demyelination features,[34] and the neuropathy may respond to transplantation[43] or to a switch from conventional to high-flux hemodialysis.[35] The course may be arrested at any time despite continuing or worsening renal failure. It is hard to predict the likely clinical course in individual patients. Most patients are left with distal motor and sensory deficits, but some become severely disabled with a flaccid quadriparesis or paraparesis. Severe neuropathy has become less prevalent with the introduction of dialysis and transplantation techniques but remains common.

Histopathologic examination of nerve biopsy specimens confirms that the neuropathy is a length-dependent axonal degeneration accompanied by secondary demyelination, although in some cases the demyelination seems the predominant finding; damaged endoneural blood capillaries may also be found and support an ischemic theory as one mechanism in the pathogenesis of uremic neuropathy. Nerve conduction studies also support an axonal process, with reduced conduction velocities and response amplitudes; abnormalities are common even in clinically unaffected nerves. The amplitude of the sensory nerve action potential is affected particularly, especially that of the sural nerve. Large fibers are affected more often than small fibers,[36] but in occasional patients a predominantly small-fiber neuropathy occurs. The findings on nerve conduction studies may improve after effective treatment of the underlying renal failure, sometimes very rapidly, but this is not always the case[37]; sensory nerve conduction velocities in the median, ulnar, and sural nerves may be the most sensitive electrophysiologic indices of the beneficial effect of hemodialysis. Needle electromyography (EMG) may reveal evidence of denervation, particularly in the distal muscles of the legs. Abnormalities of late responses (F waves and H reflexes) are frequent and may be helpful early in the course of renal failure, when standard nerve conduction study results are sometimes normal.[38]

Laaksonen and colleagues examined the clinical severity of uremic neuropathy in 21 patients, using a modified version of the neuropathy symptom score combined with results of electrophysiologic studies.[39] They found that 81 percent of uremic patients were diagnosed with neuropathy: the neuropathy was asymptomatic in 19 percent, associated with nondisabling symptoms in 48 percent, and accompanied by disabling symptoms in 14 percent.

TREATMENT

Uremic polyneuropathy may stabilize or even show some improvement with dialysis, but mild progression is not uncommon and recovery from severe neuropathy is unlikely.[37,40] Renal transplantation improves uremic neuropathy, sometimes very rapidly and with a negative correlation between electrophysiologic change and serum creatinine and *myo*-inositol concentrations, suggesting that metabolic factors may underlie the rapid improvement; in other instances, improvement is more gradual over a number of months, is characterized electrophysiologically by improvement in motor and sensory conduction velocities, and is often incomplete, perhaps because the main reason for improvement is segmental remyelination, with some fibers remaining degenerate in severe neuropathies.

Autonomic Neuropathy

Uremic patients may develop postural hypotension, impaired sweating, impotence, gastrointestinal disturbances, and other dysautonomic symptoms, which progress in some patients—but not all—despite continuing hemodialysis. The dysautonomia correlates with the presence or severity of peripheral neuropathy in many but not all patients and may be corrected by renal transplantation. The mechanism underlying the development of uremic autonomic neuropathy is unknown. In patients with diabetic renal failure, dysautonomia may relate also to the diabetes. Studies of both cardiovagal and sympathetic function (discussed in Chapter 8) have revealed objective evidence of dysautonomia[41–44] that may be subclinical.

Intradialytic hypotension is a frequent complication of hemodialysis and has been shown to relate to impaired autonomic function[42,44] regardless of whether a peripheral neuropathy is present[42]; however, there is no agreement on this point, and some investigators have found that hypotension-prone patients are not distinguished by impaired predialytic or intradialytic control of the blood pressure.[45] Midodrine may have a role in the therapy of patients with intradialytic hypotension.[46]

Dialysis may not benefit autonomic neuropathy.[47] However, Vita and colleagues found that when patients were switched from acetate to bicarbonate dialysis, all the patients in a small series eventually showed a reversal of autonomic damage.[48] After renal transplantation, autonomic function may improve or normalize but at a variable rate. Specific treatments, such as sildenafil for impotence, may be helpful. [49]

RESTLESS LEGS SYNDROME

Development of the restless legs syndrome may indicate incipient peripheral nerve involvement or may occur as an isolated disorder. Patients develop an irresistible urge to move the legs that is worse at night and during periods of inactivity. They complain of curious sensations—often described as creeping, crawling, prickling, or itchy feelings—in the lower limbs, and these tend to be worse in the evening or when the limbs are not in motion. Such sensations are experienced most commonly in the legs but occasionally occur in the thighs or feet; the upper limbs are also sometimes involved. The disorder may occur in nondialyzed patients with chronic renal failure.[50] When it occurs in uremic patients undergoing hemodialysis, it has been related to low hemoglobin levels, high serum phosphorus levels, high anxiety levels, and a great degree of emotion-oriented coping.[51] Treatment of restless legs syndrome is with clonazepam, dopamine agonists, levodopa, certain anticonvulsants, or opioids (propoxyphene or codeine) taken at bedtime.[52] In addition, coexisting anemia and hyperphosphatemia should be corrected. Successful renal transplantation may ameliorate or eliminate symptoms within a few weeks.[53,54]

UREMIC MYOPATHY

Proximal muscle weakness, atrophy, and muscle fatigue are common in uremic patients, and the progression of the underlying myopathy parallels the decline in renal function.[55] Muscle involvement is more common in patients undergoing chronic hemodialysis. Onset is insidious. The hip girdle is affected more than the shoulder girdle. The primary systemic disease responsible for the renal failure—or its treatment, such as with steroids—may lead to a myopathy. Other causal factors include malnutrition, anemia, accumulation of toxins (including aluminum and iron), endocrine disorders (such as secondary hyperparathyroidism), hypercalcemia, hypophosphatemia, vitamin D deficiency, carnitine deficiency, hyper- and hypokalemia, and physical inactivity. Calciphylaxis in end-stage kidney disease is a rare cause of painful ischemic myopathy; vascular calcification and occlusion of small and medium-sized arteries is responsible. Dialysis-associated systemic fibrosis may cause a myopathy.[56] Myopathy may relate to β_2-microglobulin–associated amyloidosis.[57]

Treatment is of the underlying cause of the muscle weakness. Hemodialysis patients treated with vitamin D have been found to have greater muscle size and power than those not receiving vitamin supplementation.[58] Renal transplantation is sometimes indicated.[11,57]

STROKE

Chronic kidney disease is a significant risk factor for stroke and occult cerebrovascular disease.[59–61] A mildly diminished estimated glomerular filtration rate increases the risk of ischemic stroke,[62] and a severely decreased glomerular filtration rate increases that of hemorrhagic stroke compared to the general population.[62,63] The control of chronic hypertension is particularly important in reducing stroke risk in patients with chronic kidney disease. In patients with previous atherosclerotic strokes, antiplatelet agents help to reduce secondary stroke risk. Those with atrial fibrillation may benefit from anticoagulation. Statins have a lipid-lowering effect[64] but are probably not useful for stroke-risk reduction in patients on dialysis as they have little or no effect on all-cause mortality or on cardiovascular mortality or events in these circumstances[65]; they have uncertain effects in kidney transplant recipients.[65] Optimizing diabetic control, cessation of smoking, dietary salt restriction, weight reduction, and correction of coexisting anemia may be important in reducing cardiovascular and stroke risk in individual cases,[66] and carotid endarterectomy is worthwhile in selected patients. The risk of stroke is also high in patients receiving chronic hemodialysis, as is discussed in a later section.

The effect of chronic kidney disease on clinical outcomes after acute ischemic stroke has been studied and found to be an important predictor of poor clinical outcomes.[67–69] Thus, after adjusting for demographic factors, stroke risk factors, and stroke severity on admission, the estimated glomerular filtration rate was found to be an independent predictor of stroke mortality at 10 years.[70] Proteinuria independently contributes to the increased risks of neurologic deterioration, mortality, and poor functional outcome after acute stroke.[67]

OPTIC NEUROPATHY

A progressive unilateral or bilateral optic neuropathy may occur over several days, sometimes as the initial manifestation of end-stage kidney disease[71]; visual loss is accompanied by reduced pupillary response to light and by papillitis. Prompt hemodialysis and corticosteroid therapy may restore vision in some patients. The optic neuropathy may be neurotoxic, ischemic, related to side effects of medication or intracranial hypertension, or inflammatory in nature.[72]

In ischemic optic neuropathy occurring in patients on hemodialysis, coexisting hypotension and anemia are important risk factors, and treatment may require intravenous saline or blood transfusions in addition to the other measures mentioned earlier.[73] Calcific uremic arteriolopathy may also have an etiologic role.[74] Several cases of nonarteritic ischemic optic neuropathy related to hemodialysis have been reported. The optic neuropathy is produced by compromise of oxygen delivery to the optic nerve, resulting in hypoxic swelling, nerve compression in the optic canal, and ischemia of the optic nerve head.[75] Presentation is with sudden, unilateral, painless inferior visual field defect and a fixed unreactive pupil after relative hypotension. This complication must be considered when examining dialysis options, particularly in patients with other risk factors such as hypotension, anemia, and a past history of anterior ischemic optic neuropathy.[75]

NEUROLOGIC COMPLICATIONS OF NEPHROTIC SYNDROME

The nephrotic syndrome, which results from glomerular damage, is characterized by excessive proteinuria in the absence of hematuria, and is accompanied by edema, hypoalbuminemia, and hyperlipidemia. There is an increased risk of arterial or venous thromboembolism, and this may involve the cerebral circulation.[76] The causes of the responsible hypercoagulable state are not entirely clear, but alterations occur in various blood coagulation factors, platelet reactivity, and blood viscosity, and in the fibrinolytic system. Cerebral venous thrombosis—particularly involving the major intracranial venous sinuses—is a well-known complication in patients of any age, signaled by the development of headache, seizures, or clinical features of increased intracranial pressure.[77–79] Arterial thrombosis is less common but may involve a variety of peripheral arteries,[80] including the carotid artery,[81] sometimes as the initial manifestation of the nephrotic syndrome.[82] Presentation is with transient cerebral ischemic attacks or ischemic stroke. By analogy to patients without nephrotic syndrome, treatment of arterial or venous disease involves anticoagulation, typically with heparin followed by oral anticoagulation.

Posterior reversible encephalopathy syndrome (PRES) has also been associated with the nephrotic syndrome or its treatment with immunosuppressive drugs in children or adults.[83–85] The disorder is characterized by impaired consciousness, seizures, headache, and transient visual disturbances in the setting of hypertension, and is associated with cortical and subcortical edema manifest by high signal intensity on T2 weighted MRI, especially posteriorly. Fluid-attenuated inversion recovery (FLAIR) imaging improves diagnostic confidence and the conspicuousness of the T2 hyperintensities.[86] The prognosis is usually benign, with symptoms settling after several days of adequate treatment. Treatment involves the control of associated hypertension, the management of seizures, and the withdrawal of any medication that is likely to have been responsible for the disorder.

Certain neuromuscular disorders may relate to the nephrotic syndrome. There have been several case reports of the simultaneous development of nephrotic syndrome and Guillain–Barré syndrome.[87,88] In one such case, plasmapheresis and corticosteroids led to simultaneous recovery of both disorders, suggesting a common pathogenesis of the two conditions.[87] Myasthenia gravis may coexist with nephrotic syndrome,[89,90] and its temporary improvement may result from antibody elimination during proteinuria in nephrotic syndrome.[89]

NEUROLOGIC COMPLICATIONS OF DIALYSIS

Dialysis has been associated with subtle *cognitive alterations*, possibly reflecting an early manifestation of dialysis dementia at a reversible stage. More commonly, psychologic studies have shown significant improvement in short-term memory both after onset of maintenance dialysis and when comparisons are made between the day before and after an individual dialysis treatment session; attentional functions also seem to improve after dialysis. *Subdural hematoma* (Fig. 16-3) may occur in patients on maintenance hemodialysis; it has a 20-times higher incidence than in the general population and is associated with high mortality.[91] The symptoms of the subdural hematoma may be attributed erroneously to dysequilibrium syndrome or dialysis dementia.[92] Its occurrence may relate to anticoagulation used to maintain the patency of the conduit for hemodialysis [93]; platelet function may be impaired in uremia but, in itself, is unlikely to be responsible.[91] A rare case of manganese-induced *parkinsonism* has been described in a patient on maintenance hemodialysis and was attributed to long-term ingestion of a health supplement; the clinical, laboratory, and magnetic resonance imaging (MRI) findings were abnormal, but the patient improved on edetic acid infusion therapy.[94] The occurrence of hemodialysis-related *optic neuropathy* was mentioned in an earlier section. These complications will receive no further discussion here.

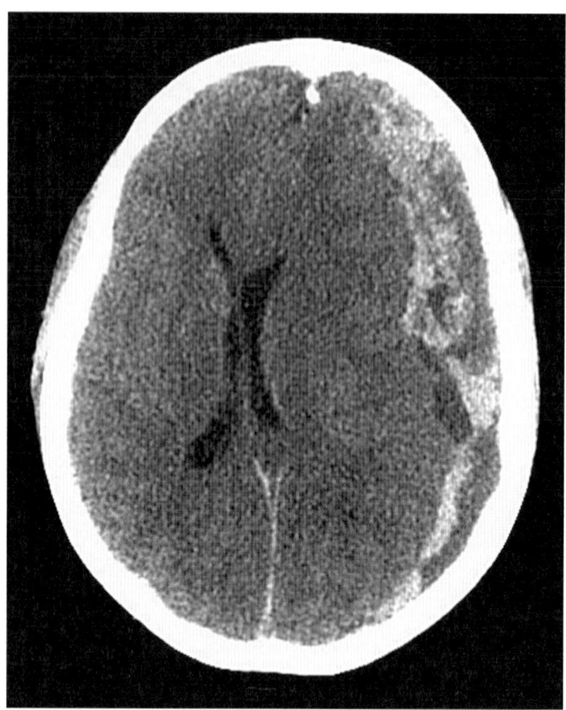

FIGURE 16-3 ■ Axial noncontrast CT scan shows a mixed-density left subdural hematoma producing marked mass effect on the left hemisphere and midline shift. The low density within the subdural hematoma is a feature of active hemorrhage. (Courtesy of William P. Dillon, MD, University of California, San Francisco.)

Muscle *cramps* are common, tending to occur toward the end of a dialysis session: their etiology is uncertain, but plasma volume contraction and hyponatremia are among the factors that have been incriminated. Headache, nausea, and vomiting may also occur during dialysis, sometimes as the initial manifestations of the dysequilibrium syndrome (discussed later).

The risk of *cerebrovascular disease* is increased in patients undergoing dialysis and seems related to accelerated cerebrovascular disease and the high incidence of malnutrition, hypertension, diabetes, and hyperlipidemia among these patients.[95,96] In one study, the high incidence of stroke resulted, at least in part, from inadequately treated hypertension.[97] Presentation may be with hypertensive encephalopathy, transient ischemic attacks, or occlusive or hemorrhagic stroke. Infarcts may show a predilection for the vertebrobasilar arterial territory.[98] Although stroke symptoms are common and are associated with cognitive and functional impairments, clinically significant stroke events are often unrecognized. [99]

The *osmotic demyelination syndrome* may occur after hemodialysis, leading clinically to convulsions, an alteration in the level of consciousness, and quadriparesis with hyperactive tendon reflexes and bilateral Babinski responses. MRI shows findings of demyelination in pontine and often extrapontine regions.[100] The effects of dialysis on uremic encephalopathy and neuropathy have already been discussed, but dialysis may cause other neurologic disturbances that merit comment.

Sleep disturbances have a high prevalence in patients with end-stage kidney disease undergoing chronic hemodialysis. They include insomnia, obstructive sleep apnea, excessive daytime sleepiness, restless legs syndrome, and various parasomnias.[101]

Entrapment Mononeuropathies

Carpal Tunnel Syndrome

It was originally believed that carpal tunnel syndrome occurred because of increased venous pressure in the distal limb when an arteriovenous shunt had been placed for hemodialysis, the increased extravascular volume within the carpal tunnel or steal being held responsible for the median nerve compression. Recent studies support an etiologic role for arteriovenous fistulas. Thus, in one study, carpal tunnel syndrome was diagnosed significantly less frequently in the contralateral wrist than that ipsilateral to the arteriovenous fistula, and a positive correlation was found between the duration of the fistula and development of carpal tunnel syndrome; in contrast to such clinical assessment, however, electrodiagnostic studies indicate no significant association between the frequency of carpal tunnel syndrome and arteriovenous fistula or its duration.[102]

The occurrence of β_2-microglobulin amyloidosis is probably more important etiologically in this context, particularly in patients on long-term hemodialysis.[103] Amyloid fibrils have been isolated from amyloid-laden tissues inside the carpal tunnel and the protein identified as β_2-microglobulin. Circulating β_2-microglobulin presumably cannot be removed by conventional hemodialysis and accumulates in tissues; the consequent formation of amyloid fibrils appears to have a relatively high affinity for the region of the carpal tunnel, leading to carpal tunnel syndrome. A significant increase in carpal tunnel width and thickness in the palmoradiocarpal ligament, correlating with duration of long-term hemodialysis, has been reported based on ultrasound examination of the wrists of hemodialysis patients.[104] The prevalence of carpal tunnel syndrome and the severity of symptoms have been improved by maneuvers to reduce the levels of β_2-microglobulin.[105] Uremic tumoral calcinosis may also be responsible in some instances.[106]

Treatment is as in other patients, with decompressive surgery if symptoms fail to respond to conservative measures.

Ulnar Nerve Lesions

A high prevalence (between 41 and 60%) of ulnar neuropathy has recently been reported in patients receiving hemodialysis for end-stage renal disease.[107] This may relate to arm positioning during hemodialysis, underlying polyneuropathy, upper-extremity vascular access, and uremic tumoral calcinosis.[107,108]

Ischemic Neuropathy

A shunt for access during chronic hemodialysis and inserted between the radial artery and cephalic vein in the upper arm was reported by Bolton and colleagues to have caused an acute distal, ischemic neuropathy in two patients; electrophysiologic evidence was present of axonal degeneration of sensory fibers with mild ischemia, and of both motor and sensory nerve fibers with more severe ischemia.[109] This has been attributed to shunting of arterial blood away from the limb distally, with the nerves being selectively affected because of their greater vulnerability to ischemia. Other cases of this so-called *ischemic monomelic neuropathy* have since been reported, and the disorder is particularly likely in diabetics with renal failure and preexisting peripheral vascular disease or neuropathy, although it may also occur in nondiabetic patients.[110] Multiple upper-limb mononeuropathies develop, leading to burning pain and to sensory and motor deficits in the forearm and hand. Motor conduction block may be detected electrophysiologically shortly after the onset of symptoms, preferentially involving the median nerve, with clinical and electrophysiologic improvement following ligation or revision of the shunt.[102] In some instances, onset is more insidious; more widespread signs of upper-extremity ischemia due to arterial steal are found distal to the fistula, such as established or impending tissue loss or nonhealing wounds.[111,112]

In addition to arterial steal and venous hypertension syndromes, other complications of arteriovenous access for hemodialysis include high-output cardiac failure, pseudoaneurysm formation, hemorrhage, noninfectious fluid collections, and access-related infections.[113]

Dialysis Dysequilibrium Syndrome

Several neurologic disturbances may arise during or after hemodialysis, including headache, nausea, anorexia, muscle cramps, irritability, restlessness, agitation, confusion, coma, and seizures; increased intracranial pressure may lead to papilledema. Such symptoms tend to occur at the beginning of a dialysis program and were particularly conspicuous in the past when patients with advanced uremia were dialyzed aggressively. Patients now enter dialysis programs at an earlier stage of renal failure and have shortened dialysis times, and this may account for the reduced incidence of the disorder, which seems more common in children and the elderly than in other age groups. Marked metabolic acidosis and the presence of other CNS disease may also be predisposing factors.[114]

Symptoms typically appear toward the end of a dialysis session, sometimes 8 to 24 hours later, and subside over several hours. When an agitated confusional state develops, it may persist for several days. Many patients manifest exophthalmos and increased intraocular pressure at the height of the syndrome, which may be helpful clinically for diagnostic purposes.[4] Headache is the most common symptom reported by patients undergoing dialysis, and migrainous episodes may be precipitated during or after hemodialysis in patients with preexisting migraine. Headache is otherwise usually diffuse and throbbing in quality. Subdural hematoma sometimes mimics the dysequilibrium syndrome and requires exclusion.[92]

Movement of water into the brain leads to cerebral edema. According to the hypothesis known as the *reverse urea effect,* a rapid reduction in blood urea level lowers the plasma osmolality, thereby producing an osmotic gradient between blood and brain.[115] Although urea is able to permeate cell membranes, this may take several hours to reach completion; accordingly, there is not enough time for urea equilibration when the blood urea level is reduced rapidly by hemodialysis. There is thus an influx of water into the cells. This results in increased intracranial pressure and cerebral edema. Alternatively or additionally, the osmotic gradient between brain and blood may not reflect simply the movement of urea; unidentified osmotically active substances ("idiogenic osmoles") are present in the brain of dialyzed uremic animals (but not dialyzed nonuremic animals) and may be responsible. It has been suggested that a decrease in cerebral intracellular pH, reflecting an increased production of organic acids that are osmotically active, is important in this regard.[114]

A number of other disorders, such as uremic encephalopathy, intracranial infection or hemorrhage, cerebral infarction, hyponatremia, hypoglycemia, and medication-related encephalopathy must be excluded before the diagnosis is made with confidence. Prophylactic measures involve the gradual reduction in blood urea level by attention to the hemodialysis technique. In patients with established dialysis dysequilibrium syndrome, mild symptoms usually clear spontaneously over several hours, and symptomatic and supportive measures are all that are required; however, it may be necessary to slow or discontinue the dialysis session. Dialysis is stopped in patients with seizures or an altered level of consciousness and, if necessary, the plasma osmolality can be raised with either hypertonic saline or mannitol. Management is otherwise supportive, and improvement can be expected over the following day.

Wernicke Encephalopathy

Thiamine is a water-soluble vitamin that passes through dialysis membranes. However, dialysis does not remove more thiamine than is normally excreted in the urine, and no consistent change occurs after hemodialysis in plasma levels of the B vitamins. Wernicke encephalopathy has occurred in patients on chronic dialysis,[116] but is relatively infrequent. It has been related to anorexia, vomiting, a diet low in thiamine-containing foods, and intravenous alimentation without thiamine supplementation; other potential causes in uremia are infections that may stress thiamine reserves and the use of repeated infusions of glucose, insulin, and bicarbonate to lower the serum potassium level.

Among patients undergoing dialysis in whom Wernicke encephalopathy develops in the absence of alcoholism or other precipitating factors and is diagnosed at autopsy, ophthalmoplegia may be evident in only occasional instances, but in other cases the full triad of ophthalmoplegia, ataxia, and an altered level of consciousness are encountered.[117] Hypothermia is common. Intravenous administration of thiamine reverses the clinical deficit. Given the reversible nature of the disorder, it is important to consider it in all patients on hemodialysis who exhibit at least one of its classic features; dialysis dysequilibrium syndrome, dialysis dementia, and uremic encephalopathy have each been diagnosed erroneously in patients who were subsequently found to have Wernicke encephalopathy.[117] Indeed, in one series of 30 consecutive patients on regular hemodialysis or peritoneal dialysis who were admitted with an alteration in mental status, 10 had an unexplained encephalopathy after initial evaluation and were eventually found to have thiamine deficiency; nine responded to thiamine supplementation and one died.[118]

Dialysis Dementia

Clinical Aspects

There has been a decline in the incidence of this progressive encephalopathy, which may occur in patients undergoing long-term dialysis. The first symptom is often a stammering hesitancy of speech that eventually progresses to speech arrest, dysarthria, and expressive aphasia. The speech disorder is intensified during and immediately after dialysis and initially may occur only at these times. Other manifestations such as tremor, myoclonus, asterixis, seizures, and dementia become apparent as the disorder advances, and hallucinations and delusional thinking round out the clinical picture. Focal neurologic abnormalities are found occasionally. Symptoms initially occur immediately after dialysis and then clear, but eventually they fail to resolve and the patient becomes increasingly demented. The EEG shows abnormal bursts of high-voltage slow activity and spikes anteriorly. The CSF is normal. The differential diagnosis includes other causes of dementia, but metabolic encephalopathy and structural lesions such as subdural hematoma,[92] normal-pressure hydrocephalus, hypertensive encephalopathy, multi-infarct dementia, and stroke require exclusion.

Pathogenesis

A clustering of cases in areas with aluminum-contaminated water was noted originally, and water-purification measures have led to a substantial reduction in the incidence of the disorder. The disorder results from accumulation of aluminum in the brain and is now rarely encountered because of elimination of aluminum in the dialysate. Phosphate retention occurs in renal failure, leading eventually to hyperparathyroidism, and reduction of the serum phosphate concentration with phosphate binders is therefore important. The substitution of phosphate binders such as calcium carbonate and calcium acetate, and of nonmineral-containing phosphate binders, for oral aluminum-containing phosphate binders has also been important in reducing the aluminum content in the brain.[119] Although parathyroid hormone increases aluminum absorption from the gut, parathyroidectomy has not affected the course of dialysis dementia.[4] The toxicity of aluminum may involve disruption of the inositol phosphate system and calcium regulation, facilitation of oxidative injury, and disruption of basic cell processes.[115] Postmortem immunochemical analysis of frontal cortex of 15 dialysis patients treated with aluminum showed changes in tau protein processing in the brain resembling those seen in Alzheimer disease, although none had signs of dialysis dementia.[120,121]

Treatment

Diazepam is initially helpful in treating the myoclonus and seizures and in improving speech, but it is less effective later. Increased dialysis time and renal transplantation have not altered the natural history.[4] In untreated patients, death usually occurs within a year of the onset of symptoms. The chelator deferoxamine can remove excess aluminum and thereby reverse acute encephalopathy, as well as the osteomalacia and anemia that may also be associated with aluminum overload. However, its introduction was associated with visual and auditory toxicity and with increased neurologic and other side effects from acute aluminum toxicity (presumably because of the rapid mobilization of stored aluminum) in occasional patients; some patients developed a rapidly progressive and fatal systemic or rhinocerebral mucormycosis.[122] Experimental studies in animals suggest that deferoxamine enhances the pathogenicity of the responsible organism and reduces the effectiveness of treatment with amphotericin.[123] Nevertheless it is the mainstay of treatment for established dialysis dementia.

Several protocols for the administration of deferoxamine have been proposed, and the National Kidney Foundation has published guidelines.[124] A baseline serum aluminum level is determined: normal levels are 6 ± 3 μg/L, but excess aluminum deposition is unlikely when values are less than 20 μg/L. If baseline levels are increased, a low-dose deferoxamine test is performed by administering 5 mg/kg 1 hour before the end of dialysis if aluminum overload (serum aluminum levels of 60 to 200 μg/L) is present or toxicity is suspected clinically. Deferoxamine can be given to symptomatic patients in a single dose of 1 to 6 g (30 to 40 mg/kg) once weekly in the last hour of a dialysis session; however, to avoid the risk of deferoxamine neurotoxicity, it is not given to patients with serum aluminum levels exceeding 120 μg/L until the level is first lowered by withdrawal of aluminum exposure. When serum levels exceed 200 μg/L, daily hemodialysis using high-flux membranes and a low dialysate aluminum concentration, and withdrawal of all aluminum-containing oral agents, is necessary; a low-dose deferoxamine test (5 mg/kg) is given after 4 to 6 weeks of such treatment (if serum levels are <200 μg/L) to determine the timing of further treatment. Further details are given elsewhere.[124] The length of treatment required is uncertain, but it may need to be for many months.[4] Many cases of dialysis dementia have been stabilized or improved by deferoxamine. The need for treatment is unclear in patients with an asymptomatic increase in aluminum levels.

COMPLICATIONS OF TRANSPLANTATION

Various neurologic complications are caused by the neurotoxicity of immunosuppressive agents, as discussed in Chapter 45. When acute rejection encephalopathy occurs, patients experience headache, confusion, and seizures, sometimes accompanied by papilledema, increased CSF pressure, and computed tomography (CT) evidence of diffuse cerebral edema. The EEG is diffusely slowed and may show focal features. Treatment of the rejection episode leads to improvement.

Femoral and Related Neuropathy

Femoral neuropathy is a common complication of renal transplantation in the iliac fossa, occurring ipsilateral to the transplant surgery with an incidence on the order of 2 percent.[125] Nerve compression typically occurs intraoperatively, for example, with prolonged use of retractors. When compression leads to neurapraxia, recovery is likely to be rapid and complete, as in most patients; severe compression or nerve ischemia leads to axonal loss, delayed recovery, and residual deficits. In patients undergoing renal transplantation involving either the internal or external iliac artery, sensory disturbances may be the sole manifestation and are not necessarily confined to the territory of the femoral nerve: in one series of 20 patients in which the internal iliac artery was used, for example, sensory complaints were in the anterior thigh in 15, lateral thigh in 3, and anterolateral thigh in 2,[126] suggestive of involvement of the lateral femoral cutaneous nerve.

The rates of malignancies among 35,765 first-time recipients of deceased or living donor kidney transplantations between 1995 and 2001 was examined by Kasiske and associates using Medicare billing claims.[127] For common tumors, such as of the colon, lung, prostate, stomach, esophagus, pancreas, ovary, and breast, cancer rates were approximately twice as high after kidney transplantation as in the general population. Melanoma, leukemia, hepatobiliary tumors, cervical, and vulvovaginal tumors were each increased about 5-fold; testicular and bladder cancers about 3-fold; kidney cancer (typically of the native kidney) 15-fold; and Kaposi sarcoma, non-Hodgkin lymphomas, and nonmelanoma skin cancers more than 20-fold. Thus, cancer screening and attention to prophylactic measures are important after kidney transplantation. The development of such neoplasms may involve the nervous system directly by metastatic spread, may lead to a paraneoplastic syndrome, or may produce secondary neurologic abnormalities as a consequence of treatment (Chapters 27 and 28).

Brain Tumors

Non-Hodgkin lymphoma constitutes more than 90 percent of lymphomas in transplant recipients. Most of these lymphomas are of the B-cell type[128] and follow B-cell proliferation related to infection with Epstein–Barr virus in patients who are chronically immunosuppressed. Extranodal involvement after organ transplantation occurs commonly and—in almost one-quarter of patients[129]—involves the CNS (Fig. 16-4). Involvement of the transplanted kidney may also occur, causing renal failure. The degree of immunosuppression, age (greater in those younger than 25 years), time since transplant (greater in the first year), race (greater in Caucasians than in African Americans), and serologic status regarding

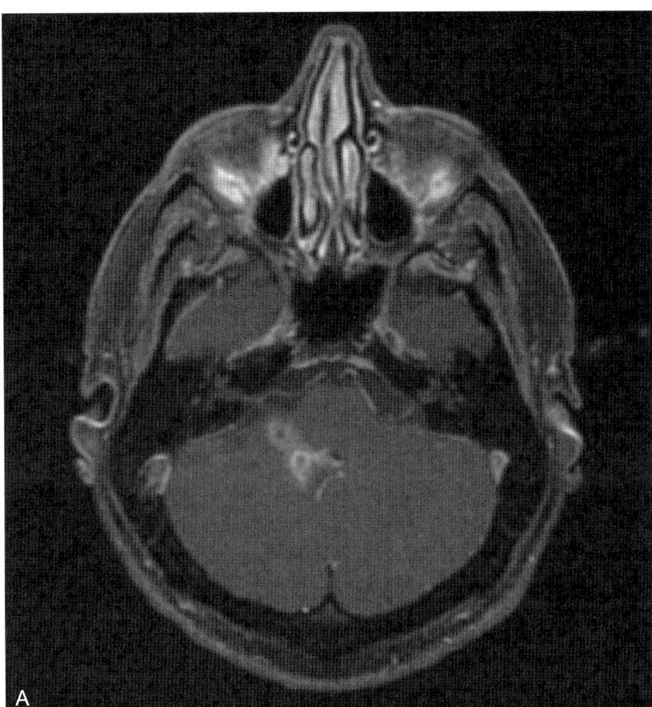

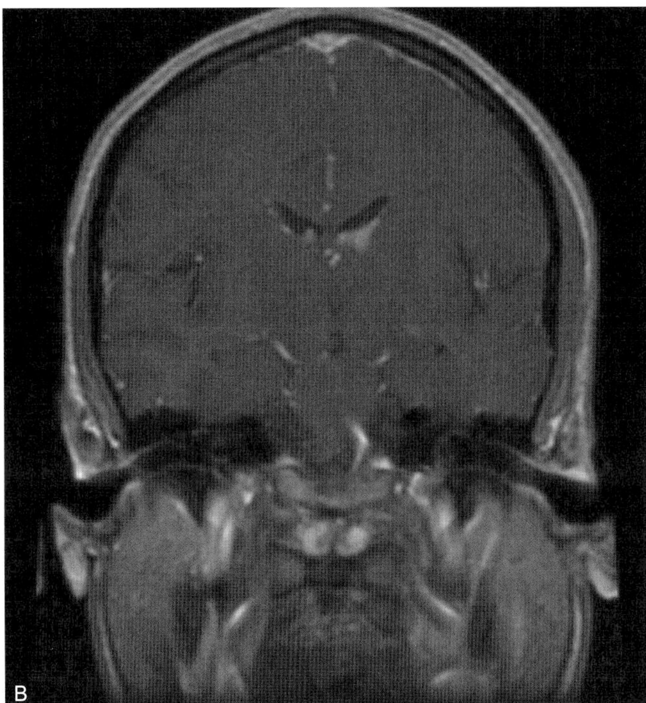

FIGURE 16-4 ■ **A**, Axial postcontrast T1-weighted MRI demonstrates an enhancing mass located in the right lateral recess of the fourth ventricle. **B**, Coronal postcontrast T1-weighted image shows an enhancing subependymal mass involving the left lateral ventricle. The findings are most consistent with CSF spread of lymphoma. (Courtesy of William P. Dillon, MD, University of California, San Francisco.)

Epstein–Barr virus infection influence the risk of disease. The development of mental status changes or new neurologic abnormalities should raise concern about the possibility of CNS involvement. Imaging studies (CT or MRI) of the head, CSF analysis for Epstein–Barr virus and cytologic examination for malignant cells, and brain biopsy generally lead to the diagnosis. MRI may underestimate the extent of the tumor.

The use of corticosteroids, which alter the imaging and histopathologic findings, may confound interpretation of imaging studies. Since the advent of modern chemotherapeutic regimens, the natural history seems to have changed in that systemic metastases outside the CNS are uncommon, and some patients may survive for much longer than in the past.[128]

The incidence of *primary CNS lymphoma* is increasing, especially among the elderly.[130] The tumor is located supratentorially in more than two-thirds of instances and typically is periventricular and involves deep subcortical structures such as the basal ganglia and corpus callosum (Fig. 16-5); subependymal spread is common. Abnormal lymphocytes may disseminate along CSF pathways and subsequently spread throughout the CNS. The eye may also be involved. As with systemic lymphoma, the high incidence of primary CNS lymphoma in transplant recipients receiving immunosuppressants indicates involvement of the immune system in its pathogenesis and, again, the Epstein–Barr virus may have a role. Presenting symptoms depend on the location of the lesion. Supratentorial lesions may cause headaches (sometimes from increased intracranial pressure or meningeal involvement), personality changes, cognitive abnormalities, blurred vision, or focal motor or other deficits. Convulsions are relatively uncommon. Cranial neuropathies, ataxic syndromes, and other signs of brainstem involvement occur with infratentorial intracranial involvement. Meningeal involvement is relatively common as the disease advances and leads to multifocal disease with cranial and spinal neuropathies, headaches, signs of meningeal irritation, and, occasionally, hydrocephalus. In rare instances of primary spinal involvement, there is weakness, sensory loss, and sphincter dysfunction, depending on the site and extent of the lesion. Spinal lesions are more often intramedullary, whereas in patients with systemic lymphoma diffuse leptomeningeal involvement or

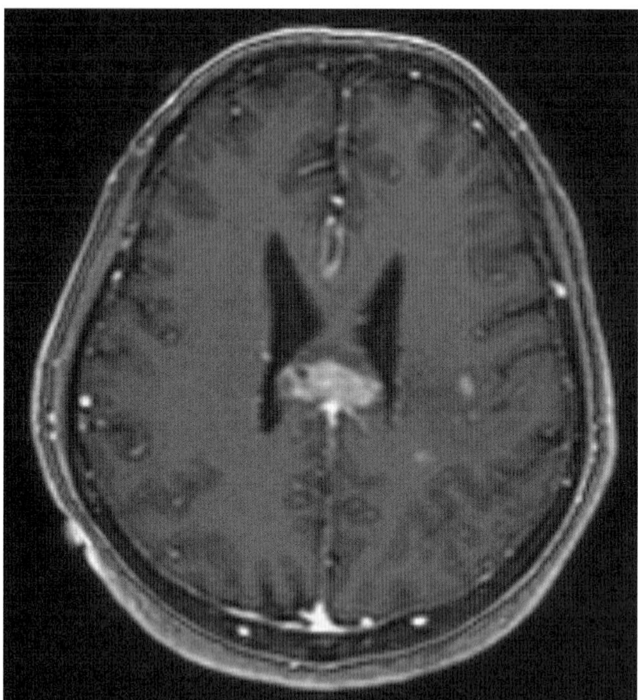

FIGURE 16-5 ■ MRI of a patient with biopsy-proven primary lymphoma of the brain. Axial postcontrast T1-weighted MRI shows an enhancing mass involving the splenium of the corpus callosum as well as two satellite nodules within the white matter of the left posterior frontal lobe. (Courtesy of William P. Dillon, MD, University of California, San Francisco.)

extradural nodules are more likely. Recurrence is usually within the brain, but systemic dissemination occurs occasionally and tends to involve extranodal organs, such as kidneys or skin.

The CSF usually shows nonspecific findings, but cytology may reveal malignant cells, especially if repeated examinations are performed. The absence of such cells does not exclude the diagnosis. CT usually shows a mass much larger than that suggested by the clinical findings; there are usually isodense, hyperdense, and hypodense areas, with contrast enhancement. On T2-weighted MRI, the mass may appear isointense to hypointense, enhances homogeneously with contrast administration, may be associated with extensive edema, is often in contact with the subarachnoid space, and typically is without necrosis.[131] One-third of these tumors are multifocal. Tumors may be missed by one imaging modality and detected by the other; both may miss meningeal disease. MRI or myelography detects spinal disease. A definitive diagnosis is made by histopathologic examination after stereotactic biopsy. Extensive resection of the tumor is usually not attempted given its deep location and often multifocal nature and because of the high surgical morbidity. The combination of whole-brain radiotherapy and methotrexate-based chemotherapy is effective but may cause severe neurotoxicity. Ongoing studies are therefore examining the use of high-dose chemotherapy with stem-cell rescue and lower-dose radiotherapy.[132]

Central Nervous System Infections

In renal transplant recipients, the risk of infections (and neoplasia), with their attendant mortality and morbidity, increases with increasing immunosuppression[133] rather than with the use of a specific immunosuppressive agent. It is important to bear this in mind when the addition of a potent immunosuppressive agent is under consideration for the treatment of acute rejection episodes. The risk of infection is also influenced by environmental exposure, by the presence of indwelling catheters that may serve as a conduit for infection, and by whether peritoneal dialysis rather than hemodialysis was utilized prior to transplantation (as the former is associated with a higher risk of infection). Other factors that bear on the issue are coexisting diseases such as diabetes that render patients more prone to infection, poor nutritional status, metabolic abnormalities such as uremia, and infection with immunomodulating viruses such as Epstein–Barr and human immunodeficiency virus.

CNS infections are an important consideration in transplant recipients. When acute meningitis occurs, it is usually caused by *Listeria monocytogenes*, whereas subacute or chronic meningitis is commonly caused by *Cryptococcus neoformans*, although systemic infection with *M. tuberculosis*, *L. monocytogenes*, *H. capsulatum*, *N. asteroides*, and certain other organisms may have a similar presentation.[134] Signs of meningeal irritation may be subtle or absent because of the anti-inflammatory effects of immunosuppressants.[134] Fever, headache, and impairment of consciousness may also be due to CNS lymphoma, which must therefore be distinguished, as described earlier. The presence of unexplained fever and headache in transplant recipients mandates brain imaging by CT scan or MRI and examination of the CSF. Brain abscesses (Fig. 16-6) are well described in transplant recipients and, in most instances, the primary source of infection is the lung. CT of the chest is therefore important, especially when chest

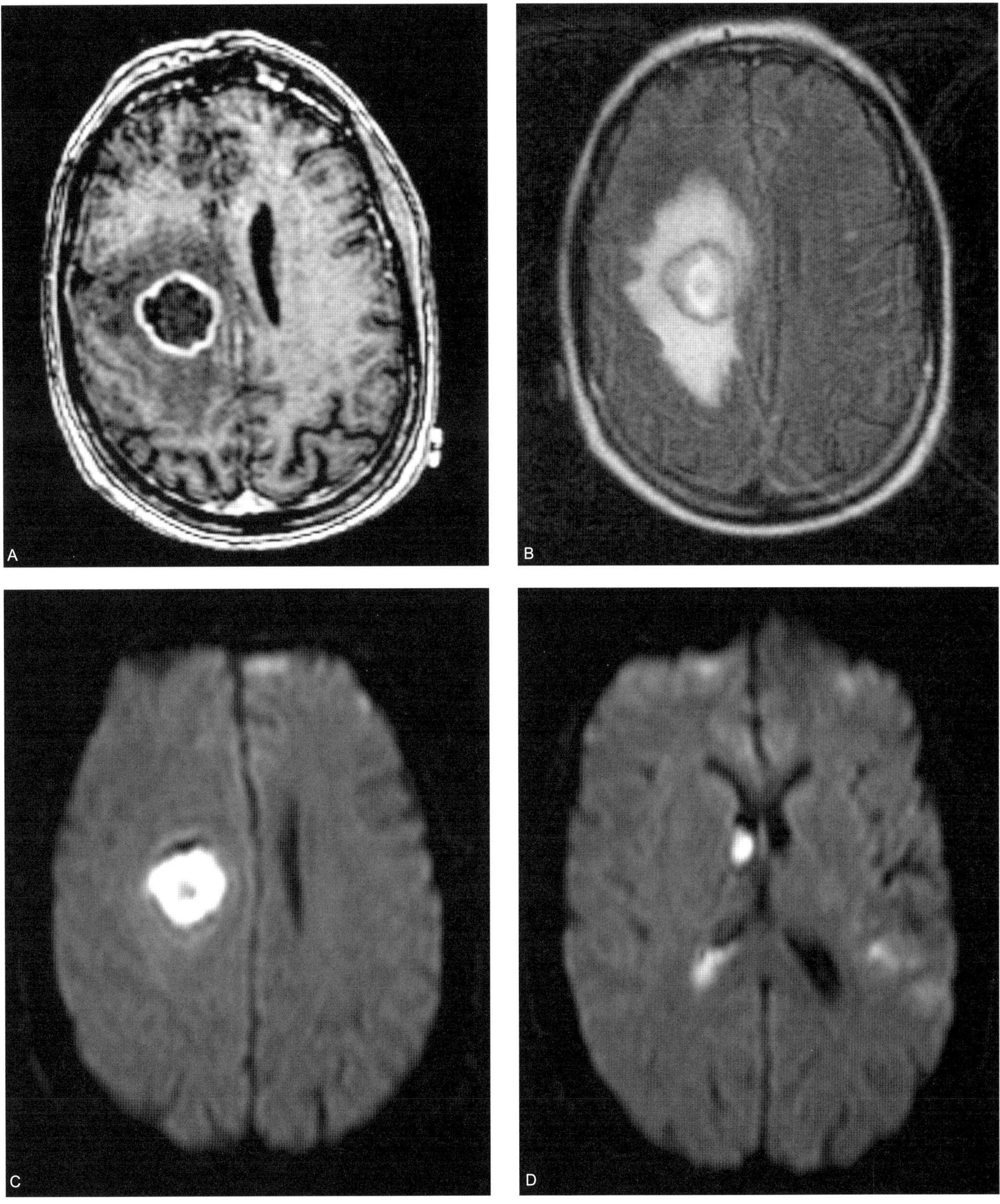

FIGURE 16-6 ■ Brain abscess. **A**, Axial postcontrast T1-weighted image demonstrates a ring-enhancing mass lesion in the right frontal lobe with surrounding vasogenic edema. **B**, Axial T2-weighted fluid-attenuated inversion recovery (FLAIR) image demonstrates a mass surrounded by a zone of increased signal intensity consistent with vasogenic edema. The mass itself consists of several layers of abnormal signal. Within the center of the mass, a zone of lower signal is seen, surrounded by alternating zones of higher and lower signal. The capsule of the mass shows low signal and is the area that enhances with contrast material (see **A**). **C**, Axial diffusion-weighted image. The central portion of the mass shows high signal, consistent with restricted diffusion. The appearance of a ring-enhancing mass containing material with restricted diffusion is most consistent with a cerebral abscess. **D**, Axial diffusion-weighted image at the level of the lateral ventricles shows abnormal high-signal layering within the right lateral ventricle and in the sulci of the left hemisphere, consistent with both meningeal and intraventricular extension of abscess material. (Courtesy of William P. Dillon, MD, University of California, San Francisco.)

radiographs are normal or unhelpful, for diagnostic purposes in differentiating fungal brain abscess from brain tumor in transplant recipients. *Aspergillus* has a predilection for dissemination to the brain and accounts for most fungal brain abscesses; such fungal infections usually lead to multiple brain abscesses and have a poor prognosis. Abscess may also result from *L. monocytogenes*, *Toxoplasma gondii, or N. asteroides*. With *Listeria* infection, abscesses are also commonly multiple, with a high mortality.[138] The clinical presentation is often with neurologic deficits or seizures of abrupt onset or with a worsening confusional state.[139] The CT scan may show poorly circumscribed, low-absorption areas with minimal or no contrast enhancement and little mass effect. MRI shows ring-enhancing lesions with surrounding edema; distinction from tumor is sometimes difficult, but diffusion-weighted imaging is helpful in this regard. The CSF may be unrevealing. Brain biopsy is sometimes the only reliable way to establish a diagnosis. Treatment is discussed in later chapters.

Progressive multifocal leukoencephalopathy (Fig. 16-7) due to JC virus infection has been described in transplant recipients and leads to cognitive changes, seizures, and focal neurologic deficits. In one reported case, immunosuppression was discontinued and the patient returned to hemodialysis; his neurologic symptoms and imaging abnormalities gradually resolved completely.[135] Similar clinical deficits may relate to other viral infections, such as herpes simplex or Epstein–Barr virus, or may reflect toxicity of immunosuppressants such as cyclosporine or tacrolimus.

West Nile virus infection manifests similarly in transplant recipients as in other patients, but neurologic damage tends to be especially severe.[136]

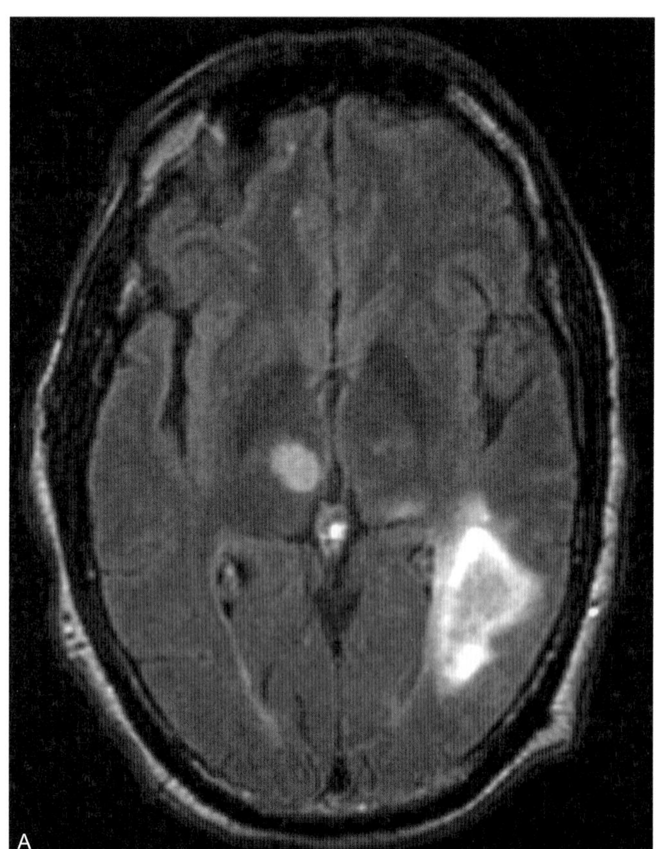

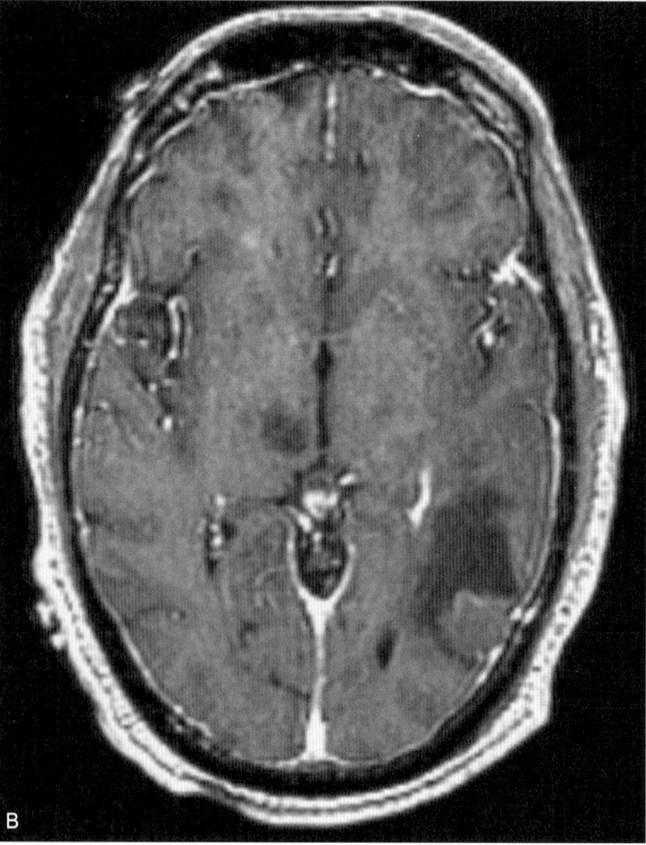

FIGURE 16-7 ■ **A**, An immunosuppressed patient with alteration of mental status. Axial T2-weighted fluid-attenuated inversion recovery MRI demonstrates several discrete areas of T2 prolongation involving the right and left thalamus and the left posterior frontotemporal area. Despite the large size of the lesion, no mass effect is present. **B**, Axial postcontrast T1-weighted image demonstrates well-circumscribed low-intensity lesions without contrast enhancement. Subsequent brain biopsy confirmed the diagnosis of progressive multifocal leukoencephalopathy. (Courtesy of William P. Dillon, MD, University of California, San Francisco.)

HEREDITARY DISORDERS OF THE NERVOUS SYSTEM AND KIDNEYS

Various uncommon inherited disorders affect both the kidneys and the nervous system, meriting brief discussion here.

Fabry Disease

Fabry disease is an X-linked lysosomal storage disease resulting from deficiency of ceramide trihexosidase (α-galactosidase), which catalyzes the hydrolytic cleavage of the terminal galactose from globotriaosylceramide. It relates to mutations of the α-galactosidase A (GLA) gene at Xq22. It leads to a small-fiber neuropathy, with severe neuropathic or limb pain and dysautonomic symptoms,[137] accompanied by evidence of other organ involvement from glycosphingolipid accumulation, including in the kidneys.[138] Renal involvement leads to polyuria and polydipsia; progressive renal failure typically develops in adulthood. Kidney function is worse in patients with undetectable α-galactosidase activity compared to those with some residual activity. Cerebrovascular involvement is associated with transient ischemic attacks and strokes; the vertebrobasilar circulation was symptomatic in 67 percent of hemizygotes and 60 percent of the heterozygotes in one meta-analysis, and elongated, ectatic, tortuous vertebral and basilar arteries were the most common angiographic and pathologic findings.[139] The MRI may show white matter lesions in affected males and in female carriers. A fatal outcome is common in middle life from uremia or cerebrovascular disease. Management involves the administration of enzyme replacement therapy with agalsidase alfa or agalsidase beta.[140] This may help to reduce neuropathic pain and improve sensory threshold, but its effect on CNS manifestations is unclear.[141] Treatment of neuropathic pain with gabapentin, carbamazepine, or amitriptyline may be helpful. Nonsteroidal anti-inflammatory agents are usually ineffective, and narcotics are best avoided.

von Hippel–Lindau Disease

In autosomal-dominantly inherited von Hippel–Lindau disease, the responsible gene maps to chromosome 3p25 and is a tumor suppressor gene. Renal cysts and cancers occur in patients with CNS and retinal hemangioblastomas (often bilateral), and sometimes with pancreatic cysts and pheochromocytoma. The CNS hemangioblastomas commonly involve the cerebellar hemispheres and may be asymptomatic; spine and brainstem lesions are also well described (Fig. 16-8). A variety of visual complications may occur, mandating the need for regular ophthalmologic screening. Monitoring for the development of renal lesions by CT scan and ultrasound, and for CNS lesions by gadolinium-enhanced MRI of the entire neuraxis, also is important. Treatment is surgical or by radiation therapy.

Polycystic Kidney Disease

At least two different genetic loci for autosomal-dominant polycystic kidney disease have been identified. The renal manifestations of this disorder include hypertension, urinary tract infection, polyuria, hematuria, nephrolithiasis, pain in the flank, and progressive

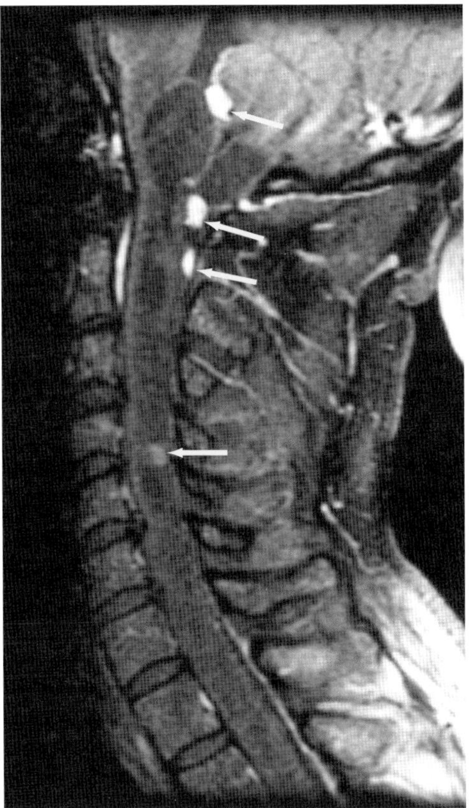

FIGURE 16-8 ▪ Sagittal postcontrast T1-weighted image through the cervical spinal cord and lower cerebellum demonstrating several intensely enhancing pial-based hemangioblastomas *(arrows)* associated with nonenhancing cysts. (Courtesy of William P. Dillon, MD, University of California, San Francisco.)

renal failure. Hypertension also may occur in relation to the kidney disease. Intracranial arterial aneurysms, sometimes multiple and unrelated to the occurrence of hypertension, are associated, and rupture may lead to subarachnoid or intracerebral hemorrhage. In a retrospective study of 77 patients from 64 families with ruptured (71 instances) or unruptured (6) aneurysms, mean age at the time of rupture was 39.5 years (range, 15 to 69 years), renal function was normal in half of the patients, and 11 percent were on renal replacement therapy. The ruptured aneurysm was usually located on the middle cerebral artery; in 31 percent of the patients, additional intact aneurysms were found. On long-term follow-up, 27 (38%) were left with severe disability. Five patients bled from another aneurysm 2 days to 14 years after initial rupture.[142] Treatment of ruptured aneurysms is as for aneurysmal subarachnoid hemorrhage occurring for other reasons, involving emergency CT scanning, four-vessel angiography, and surgery or endovascular treatment. Screening by MR angiography or high-resolution CT angiography at periodic intervals for the presence of aneurysms is probably worthwhile, at least in high-risk patients, such as those with previous aneurysmal rupture or a positive family history of an intracerebral bleed, but no clear guidelines exist for the frequency with which this should be undertaken. The value of widespread screening for intracranial aneurysms in patients with polycystic kidneys has otherwise been questioned because most intracranial aneurysms detected by presymptomatic screening in this population are small, and follow-up studies do not suggest an increased risk of growth and rupture, compared to intracranial aneurysms in the general population.[143]

REFERENCES

1. Port JD, Beauchamp Jr NJ: Reversible intracerebral pathologic entities mediated by vascular autoregulatory dysfunction. Radiographics 18:353, 1998.
2. Arnoldus EP, Van Laar T: A reversible posterior leukoencephalopathy syndrome. N Engl J Med 334:1745, 1996.
3. Hinchey J, Chaves C, Appignani B, et al: A reversible posterior leukoencephalopathy syndrome. N Engl J Med 334:494, 1996.
4. Raskin NH: Neurological complications of renal failure. p. 293. In Aminoff MJ (ed): Neurology and General Medicine. 3rd Ed. Churchill Livingstone, New York, 2001.
5. Vanholder R, Glorieux G, De Smet R, et al: New insights in uremic toxins. Kidney Int Suppl 84:S6, 2003.
6. Yavuz A, Tetta C, Ersoy FF, et al: Uremic toxins: a new focus on an old subject. Semin Dial 18:203, 2005.
7. Pan JC, Pei YQ, An L, et al: Epileptiform activity and hippocampal damage produced by intrahippocampal injection of guanidinosuccinic acid in rat. Neurosci Lett 209:12, 1996.
8. D'Hooge R, Pei YQ, Manil J, et al: The uremic guanidino compound guanidinosuccinic acid induces behavioral convulsions and concomitant epileptiform electrocorticographic discharges in mice. Brain Res 598:316, 1992.
9. De Deyn PP, Vanholder R, Eloot S, et al: Guanidino compounds as uremic (neuro)toxins. Semin Dial 22:340, 2009.
10. Kerr DN, Ward MK, Ellis HA, et al: Aluminium intoxication in renal disease. Ciba Found Symp 169:123, 1992.
11. Brouns R, De Deyn PP: Neurological complications in renal failure: a review. Clin Neurol Neurosurg 107:1, 2004.
12. Smogorzewski MJ: Central nervous dysfunction in uremia. Am J Kidney Dis 38(suppl 1):S122, 2001.
13. Burn DJ, Bates D: Neurology and the kidney. J Neurol Neurosurg Psychiatry 65:810, 1998.
14. Tanimu DZ, Obeid T, Awada A: Absence status: an overlooked cause of acute confusion in hemodialysis patients. J Nephrol 11:146, 1998.
15. Saurina A, Vera M, Pou M, et al: Nonconvulsive status epilepticus in dialysis patients. Am J Kidney Dis 39:440, 2002.
16. Battaglia F, Quartarone A, Bagnato S, et al: Brain dysfunction in uremia: a question of cortical hyperexcitability? Clin Neurophysiol 116:1507, 2005.
17. Aminoff MJ, Parent JM: Comorbidity in adults. p. 2007. In: Engel Jr J, Pedley TA (eds): Epilepsy: A Comprehensive Textbook. 2nd Ed. Lippincott-Raven, Philadelphia, 2008.
18. Lauer RM, Flaherty JF, Gambertoglio JG: Neuropsychiatric drugs. p. 207. In: Schrier RW, Gambertoglio JG (eds): Handbook of Drug Therapy in Liver and Kidney Disease. Little, Brown, Boston, 1991.
19. Blum RA, Comstock TJ, Sica DA, et al: Pharmacokinetics of gabapentin in subjects with various degrees of renal function. Clin Pharmacol Ther 56:154, 1994.
20. Randinitis EJ, Posvar EL, Alvey CW, et al: Pharmacokinetics of pregabalin in subjects with various degrees of renal function. J Clin Pharmacol 43:277, 2003.
21. Langtry HD, Gillis JC, Davis R: Topiramate: a review of its pharmacodynamic and pharmacokinetic properties and clinical efficacy in the management of epilepsy. Drugs 54:752, 1997.
22. Leppik IE: Zonisamide: chemistry, mechanism of action, and pharmacokinetics. Seizure 135:S5, 2004.
23. Dooley M, Plosker GL: Levetiracetam: a review of its adjunctive use in the management of partial onset seizures. Drugs 60:871, 2000.

24. Ijiri Y, Inoue T, Fukuda F, et al: Dialyzability of the antiepileptic drug zonisamide in patients undergoing hemodialysis. Epilepsia 45:924, 2004.
25. Cato A, Gustavson LE, Qian J, et al: Effect of renal impairment on the pharmacokinetics and tolerability of tiagabine. Epilepsia 39:43, 1998.
26. Wootton R, Soul-Lawton J, Rolan PE, et al: Comparison of the pharmacokinetics of lamotrigine in patients with chronic renal failure and healthy volunteers. Br J Clin Pharmacol 43:23, 1997.
27. Krishnan AV, Kiernan MC: Uremic neuropathy: clinical features and new pathophysiological insights. Muscle Nerve 35:273, 2007.
28. Akmal M, Massry SG: Role of parathyroid hormone in the decreased motor nerve conduction velocity of chronic renal failure. Proc Soc Exp Biol Med 195:202, 1990.
29. Bostock H, Walters RJL, Andersen KV, et al: Has potassium been prematurely discarded as a contributing factor to the development of uraemic neuropathy? Nephrol Dial Transplant 19:1054, 2004.
30. Blumberg A, Roser HW, Zehnder C, et al: Plasma potassium in patients with terminal renal failure during and after haemodialysis: relationship with dialytic potassium removal and total body potassium. Nephrol Dial Transplant 12:1629, 1997.
31. Krishnan AV, Phoon RKS, Pussell BA, et al: Altered motor nerve excitability in end-stage kidney disease. Brain 128:2164, 2005.
32. Krishnan AV, Phoon RK, Pussell BA, et al: Sensory nerve excitability and neuropathy in end stage kidney disease. J Neurol Neurosurg Psychiatry 77:548, 2006.
33. Krishnan AV, Phoon RK, Pussell BA, et al: Ischaemia induces paradoxical changes in axonal excitability in end-stage kidney disease. Brain 129:1585, 2006.
34. Ropper AH: Accelerated neuropathy of renal failure. Arch Neurol 50:536, 1993.
35. Bolton CF, McKeown MJ, Chen R, et al: Subacute uremic and diabetic polyneuropathy. Muscle Nerve 20:59, 1997.
36. Angus-Leppan H, Burke D: The function of large and small nerve fibers in renal failure. Muscle Nerve 15:288, 1992.
37. Ogura T, Makinodan A, Kubo T, et al: Electrophysiological course of uraemic neuropathy in haemodialysis patients. Postgrad Med J 77:451, 2001.
38. Van den Neucker K, Vanderstraeten G, Vanholder R: Peripheral motor and sensory nerve conduction studies in haemodialysis patients: a study of 54 patients. Electromyogr Clin Neurophysiol 38:467, 1998.
39. Laaksonen S, Metsarinne K, Voipio-Pulkki LM, et al: Neurophysiologic parameters and symptoms in chronic renal failure. Muscle Nerve 25:884, 2002.
40. Bazzi C, Pagani C, Sorgato G, et al: Uremic polyneuropathy: a clinical and electrophysiological study in 135 short- and long-term hemodialyzed patients. Clin Nephrol 35:176, 1991.
41. Wang SJ, Liao KK, Liou HH, et al: Sympathetic skin response and R-R interval variation in chronic uremic patients. Muscle Nerve 17:411, 1994.
42. Chang MH, Chou KJ: The role of autonomic neuropathy in the genesis of intradialytic hypotension. Am J Nephrol 21:357, 2001.
43. Vita G, Bellinghieri G, Trusso A, et al: Uremic autonomic neuropathy studied by spectral analysis of heart rate. Kidney Int 56:232, 1999.
44. Sato M, Horigome I, Chiba S, et al: Autonomic insufficiency as a factor contributing to dialysis-induced hypotension. Nephrol Dial Transplant 16:1657, 2001.
45. Ligtenberg G, Blankestijn PJ, Boomsma F, et al: No change in automatic function tests during uncomplicated haemodialysis. Nephrol Dial Transplant 11:651, 1996.
46. Prakash S, Garg AX, Heidenheim AP, et al: Midodrine appears to be safe and effective for dialysis-induced hypotension: a systematic review. Nephrol Dial Transplant 19:2553, 2004.
47. Vita G, Savica V, Puglisi RM, et al: The course of autonomic neural function in chronic uraemic patients during haemodialysis treatment. Nephrol Dial Transplant 7:1022, 1992.
48. Vita G, Savica V, Milone S, et al: Uremic autonomic neuropathy: recovery following bicarbonate hemodialysis. Clin Nephrol 45:56, 1996.
49. Krishnan AV, Kiernan MC: Neurological complications of chronic kidney disease. Nat Rev Neurol 5:542, 2009.
50. Merlino G, Lorenzut S, Gigli GL, et al: A case-control study on restless legs syndrome in nondialyzed patients with chronic renal failure. Mov Disord 25:1019, 2010.
51. Takaki J, Nishi T, Nangaku M, et al: Clinical and psychological aspects of restless legs syndrome in uremic patients on hemodialysis. Am J Kidney Dis 41:833, 2003.
52. Earley CJ: Restless legs syndrome. N Engl J Med 348:2103, 2003.
53. Winkelmann J, Stautner A, Samtleben W, et al: Long-term course of restless legs syndrome in dialysis patients after kidney transplantation. Mov Disord 17:1072, 2002.
54. Kavanagh D, Siddiqui S, Geddes CC: Restless legs syndrome in patients on dialysis. Am J Kidney Dis 43:763, 2004.
55. Lacerda G, Krummel T, Hirsch E: Neurologic presentations of renal diseases. Neurol Clin 28:45, 2010.
56. Levine JM, Taylor RA, Elman LB, et al: Involvement of skeletal muscle in dialysis-associated systemic fibrosis (nephrogenic fibrosing dermopathy). Muscle Nerve 30:569, 2004.
57. Al-Hayk K, Bertorini TE: Neuromuscular complications in uremics: a review. Neurologist 13:188, 2007.
58. Gordon PL, Sakkas GK, Doyle JW, et al: Relationship between vitamin D and muscle size and strength in patients on hemodialysis. J Ren Nutr 17:397, 2007.

59. Nickolas TL, Khatri M, Boden-Albala B, et al: The association between kidney disease and cardiovascular risk in a multiethnic cohort: findings from the Northern Manhattan Study (NOMAS). Stroke 39:2876, 2008.
60. Ovbiagele B: Impairment in glomerular filtration rate or glomerular filtration barrier and occurrence of stroke. Arch Neurol 65:934, 2008.
61. Khella SL: New insights into stroke in chronic kidney disease. Adv Chronic Kidney Dis 15:338, 2008.
62. Holzmann MJ, Aastveit A, Hammar N, et al: Renal dysfunction increases the risk of ischemic and hemorrhagic stroke in the general population. Ann Med 44:607, 2012.
63. Bos MJ, Koudstaal PJ, Hofman A, et al: Decreased glomerular filtration rate is a risk factor for hemorrhagic but not for ischemic stroke: the Rotterdam Study. Stroke 38:3127, 2007.
64. Upadhyay A, Earley A, Lamont JL, et al: Lipid-lowering therapy in persons with chronic kidney disease: a systematic review and meta-analysis. Ann Intern Med 157:251, 2012.
65. Palmer SC, Craig JC, Navaneethan SD, et al: Benefits and harms of statin therapy for persons with chronic kidney disease: a systematic review and meta-analysis. Ann Intern Med 157:263, 2012.
66. Karohl C, Raggi P: Approach to cardiovascular disease prevention in patients with chronic kidney disease. Curr Treat Options Cardiovasc Med 14:391, 2012.
67. Kumai Y, Kamouchi M, Hata J, et al: Proteinuria and clinical outcomes after ischemic stroke. Neurology 78:1909, 2012.
68. MacWalter RS, Wong SY, Wong KY, et al: Does renal dysfunction predict mortality after acute stroke? A 7-year follow-up study. Stroke 33:1630, 2002.
69. Yahalom G, Schwartz R, Schwammenthal Y, et al: Chronic kidney disease and clinical outcome in patients with acute stroke. Stroke 40:1296, 2009.
70. Tsagalis G, Akrivos T, Alevizaki M, et al: Renal dysfunction in acute stroke: an independent predictor of long-term all combined vascular events and overall mortality. Nephrol Dial Transplant 24:194, 2009.
71. Seo JW, Jeon DH, Kang Y, et al: A case of end-stage renal disease initially manifested with visual loss caused by uremic optic neuropathy. Hemodial Int 15:395, 2011.
72. Winkelmayer WC, Eigner M, Berger O, et al: Optic neuropathy in uremia: an interdisciplinary emergency. Am J Kidney Dis 37:E23, 2001.
73. Basile C, Addabbo G, Montanaro A: Anterior ischemic optic neuropathy and dialysis: role of hypotension and anemia. J Nephrol 14:420, 2001.
74. Korzets A, Marashek I, Schwartz A, et al: Ischemic optic neuropathy in dialyzed patients: a previously unrecognized manifestation of calcific uremic arteriolopathy. Am J Kidney Dis 44:e93, 2004.
75. Bartlett S, Cai A, Cairns H: Non-arteritic ischaemic optic neuropathy after first return to haemodialysis. BMJ Case Rep Jul 15, 2011.
76. Singhal R, Brimble KS: Thromboembolic complications in the nephrotic syndrome: pathophysiology and clinical management. Thromb Res 118:397, 2006.
77. Fluss J, Geary D, de Veber G: Cerebral sinovenous thrombosis and idiopathic nephrotic syndrome in childhood: report of four new cases and review of the literature. Eur J Pediatr 165:709, 2006.
78. Komaba H, Kadoguchi H, Igaki N, et al: Early detection and successful treatment of cerebral venous thrombosis associated with minimal change nephrotic syndrome. Clin Nephrol 68:179, 2007.
79. Xu H, Chen K, Lin D, et al: Cerebral venous sinus thrombosis in adult nephrotic syndrome. Clin Nephrol 74:144, 2010.
80. Schwartz JC, Wyrzykowski AD, Dente CJ, et al: The nephrotic syndrome: an unusual case of multiple embolic events. Vasc Endovascular Surg 43:207, 2009.
81. Laksomya T, Chanchairujira T, Parichatikanond P, et al: Arterial occlusion in nephrotic syndrome: report of four cases in Siriraj hospital. J Med Assoc Thai 92(suppl 2):S119, 2009.
82. Nandish SS, Khardori R, Elamin EM: Transient ischemic attack and nephrotic syndrome: case report and review of literature. Am J Med Sci 332:32, 2006.
83. de Oliveira RA, Fechine LM, Neto FC, et al: Posterior reversible encephalopathy syndrome (PRES) induced by cyclosporine use in a patient with collapsing focal glomeruloesclerosis. Int Urol Nephrol 40:1095, 2008.
84. Kabicek P, Sulek S, Seidl Z, et al: Posterior reversible encephalopathy syndrome (PRES) in 5-year-old girl with nephrotic syndrome. Neuro Endocrinol Lett 31:297, 2010.
85. Sakai N, Kawasaki Y, Imaizumi T, et al: Two patients with focal segmental glomerulosclerosis complicated by cyclosporine-induced reversible posterior leukoencephalopathy syndrome. Clin Nephrol 73:482, 2010.
86. Casey SO, Sampaio RC, Michel E, et al: Posterior reversible encephalopathy syndrome: utility of fluid-attenuated inversion recovery MR imaging in the detection of cortical and subcortical lesions. AJNR Am J Neuroradiol 21:1199, 2000.
87. Souayah N, Cros D, Stein TD, et al: Relapsing Guillain Barré syndrome and nephrotic syndrome secondary to focal segmental glomerulosclerosis. J Neurol Sci 270:184, 2008.
88. Kitamura H, Nakano T, Kakihara M, et al: A case of Guillain-Barré syndrome developed minimal change nephrotic syndrome simultaneously. Am J Nephrol 18:151, 1998.
89. Almsaddi M, Bertorini TE, Bastnagel W: Remission of myasthenia gravis caused by proteinuria in nephrotic syndrome. Muscle Nerve 20:1583, 1997.

90. Ogawa M, Tsukahara T, Saisho H: Nephrotic syndrome with acute renal failure and cerebral infarction in a patient with myasthenia gravis. Am J Nephrol 19:622, 1999.
91. Power A, Hamady M, Singh S, et al: High but stable incidence of subdural haematoma in haemodialysis–a single-centre study. Nephrol Dial Transplant 25:2272, 2010.
92. Sengul G, Tuzun Y, Kadioglu HH, et al: Acute interhemispheric subdural hematoma due to hemodialysis: case report. Surg Neurol 64(suppl 2):S113, 2005.
93. Sood P, Sinson GP, Cohen EP: Subdural hematomas in chronic dialysis patients: significant and increasing. Clin J Am Soc Nephrol 2:956, 2007.
94. Ohtake T, Negishi K, Okamoto K, et al: Manganese-induced parkinsonism in a patient undergoing maintenance hemodialysis. Am J Kidney Dis 46:749, 2005.
95. Seliger SL, Gillen DL, Tirschwell D, et al: Risk factors for incident stroke among patients with end-stage renal disease. J Am Soc Nephrol 14:2623, 2003.
96. Seliger SL, Gillen DL, Longstreth Jr WT, et al: Elevated risk of stroke among patients with end-stage renal disease. Kidney Int 64:603, 2003.
97. Iseki K, Fukiyama K: Predictors of stroke in patients receiving chronic hemodialysis. Kidney Int 50:1672, 1996.
98. Toyoda K, Fujii K, Fujimi S, et al: Stroke in patients on maintenance hemodialysis: a 22-year single-center study. Am J Kidney Dis 45:1058, 2005.
99. Kurella Tamura M, Meyer JB, et al: Prevalence and significance of stroke symptoms among patients receiving maintenance dialysis. Neurology 79:981, 2012.
100. Tarhan NC, Agildere AM, Benli US, et al: Osmotic demyelination syndrome in end-stage renal disease after recent hemodialysis: MRI of the brain. AJR Am J Roentgenol 182:809, 2004.
101. Merlino G, Piani A, Dolso P, et al: Sleep disorders in patients with end-stage renal disease undergoing dialysis therapy. Nephrol Dial Transplant 21:184, 2006.
102. Gousheh J, Iranpour A: Association between carpal tunnel syndrome and arteriovenous fistula in hemodialysis patients. Plast Reconstr Surg 116:508, 2005.
103. Gejyo F, Narita I: Current clinical and pathogenetic understanding of beta2-m amyloidosis in long-term haemodialysis patients. Nephrology 8(suppl):S45, 2003.
104. Takahashi T, Kato A, Ikegaya N, et al: Ultrasound changes of the carpal tunnel in patients receiving long-term hemodialysis: a cross-sectional and longitudinal study. Clin Nephrol 57:230, 2002.
105. Kuchle C, Fricke H, Held E, et al: High-flux hemodialysis postpones clinical manifestation of dialysis-related amyloidosis. Am J Nephrol 16:484, 1996.
106. Cofan F, Garcia S, Combalia A, et al: Carpal tunnel syndrome secondary to uraemic tumoral calcinosis. Rheumatology (Oxford) 41:701, 2002.
107. Nardin R, Chapman KM, Raynor EM: Prevalence of ulnar neuropathy in patients receiving hemodialysis. Arch Neurol 62:271, 2005.
108. Garcia S, Cofan F, Combalia A, et al: Compression of the ulnar nerve in Guyon's canal by uremic tumoral calcinosis. Arch Orthop Trauma Surg 120:228, 2000.
109. Bolton CF, Driedger AA, Lindsay RM: Ischaemic neuropathy in uraemic patients caused by bovine arteriovenous shunt. J Neurol Neurosurg Psychiatry 42:810, 1979.
110. Rogers NM, Lawton PD: Ischaemic monomelic neuropathy in a non-diabetic patient following creation of an upper limb arteriovenous fistula. Nephrol Dial Transplant 22:933, 2007.
111. Redfern AB, Zimmerman NB: Neurologic and ischemic complications of upper extremity vascular access for dialysis. J Hand Surg (Am) 20:199, 1995.
112. Lazarides MK, Staramos DN, Kopadis G, et al: Onset of arterial 'steal' following proximal angioaccess: immediate and delayed types. Nephrol Dial Transplant 18:2387, 2003.
113. Padberg Jr FT, Calligaro KD, Sidawy AN: Complications of arteriovenous hemodialysis access: recognition and management. J Vasc Surg 48(suppl):55S, 2008.
114. Arieff AI: Dialysis disequilibrium syndrome: current concepts on pathogenesis and prevention. Kidney Int 45:629, 1994.
115. Patel N, Dalal P, Panesar M: Dialysis disequilibrium syndrome: a narrative review. Semin Dial 21:493, 2008.
116. Ueda K, Takada D, Mii A, et al: Severe thiamine deficiency resulted in Wernicke's encephalopathy in a chronic dialysis patient. Clin Exp Nephrol 10:290, 2006.
117. Ihara M, Ito T, Yanagihara C, et al: Wernicke's encephalopathy associated with hemodialysis: report of two cases and review of the literature. Clin Neurol Neurosurg 101:118, 1999.
118. Hung SC, Hung SH, Tarng DC, et al: Thiamine deficiency and unexplained encephalopathy in hemodialysis and peritoneal dialysis patients. Am J Kidney Dis 38:941, 2001.
119. Salusky IB, Foley J, Nelson P, et al: Aluminum accumulation during treatment with aluminum hydroxide and dialysis in children and young adults with chronic renal disease. N Engl J Med 324:527, 1991.
120. Harrington CR, Wischik CM, McArthur FK, et al: Alzheimer's-disease-like changes in tau protein processing: association with aluminium accumulation in brains of renal dialysis patients. Lancet 343:993, 1994.
121. Yokel RA: The toxicology of aluminum in the brain: a review. Neurotoxicology 21:813, 2000.
122. Boelaert JR, Fenves AZ, Coburn JW: Desferoxamine therapy and mucormycosis in dialysis patients: report of an international registry. Am J Kidney Dis 18:660, 1991.
123. Boelaert JR, Van Cutsem J, de Locht M, et al: Deferoxamine augments growth and pathogenicity

of Rhizopus, while hydroxypyridinone chelators have no effect. Kidney Int 45:667, 1994.

124. National Kidney Foundation: K/DOQI clinical practice guidelines for bone metabolism and disease in chronic kidney disease. Am J Kidney Dis 42(suppl 3):S1, 2003.

125. Sharma KR, Cross J, Santiago F, et al: Incidence of acute femoral neuropathy following renal transplantation. Arch Neurol 59:541, 2002.

126. Murata Y, Sakamoto K, Hayashi R, et al: Sensory disturbance of the thigh after renal transplantation. J Urol 165:770, 2001.

127. Kasiske BL, Snyder JJ, Gilbertson DT, et al: Cancer after kidney transplantation in the United States. Am J Transplant 4:905, 2004.

128. Miller DC, Hochberg FH, Harris NL, et al: Pathology with clinical correlations of primary central nervous system non-Hodgkin's lymphoma: the Massachusetts General Hospital experience 1958–1989. Cancer 74:1383, 1994.

129. Penn I, Porat G: Central nervous system lymphomas in organ allograft recipients. Transplantation 59:240, 1995.

130. Ahsan H, Neugut AI, Bruce JN: Trends in incidence of primary malignant brain tumors in USA, 1981–1990. Int J Epidemiol 24:1078, 1995.

131. Buhring U, Herrlinger U, Krings T, et al: MRI features of primary central nervous system lymphomas at presentation. Neurology 57:393, 2001.

132. Graber JJ, Omuro A: Primary central nervous system lymphoma: is there still a role for radiotherapy? Curr Opin Neurol 24:633, 2011.

133. Jamil B, Nicholls K, Becker GJ, et al: Impact of acute rejection therapy on infections and malignancies in renal transplant recipients. Transplantation 68:1597, 1999.

134. Fishman JA, Rubin PH: Infection in organ-transplant recipients. N Engl J Med 338:1741, 1998.

135. Crowder CD, Gyure KA, Drachenberg CB: Successful outcome of progressive multifocal leukoencephalopathy in a renal transplant patient. Am J Transplant 5:1151, 2005.

136. Kleinschmidt-DeMasters BK, Marder BA, Levi ME, et al: Naturally acquired West Nile virus encephalomyelitis in transplant recipients: clinical, laboratory, diagnostic, and neuropathological features. Arch Neurol 61:1210, 2004.

137. Biegstraaten M, Hollak CE, Bakkers M, et al: Small fiber neuropathy in Fabry disease. Mol Genet Metab 106:135, 2012.

138. Najafian B, Mauer M, Hopkin RJ, et al: Renal complications of Fabry disease in children. Pediatr Nephrol 28:679, 2013.

139. Mitsias P, Levine SR: Cerebrovascular complications of Fabry's disease. Ann Neurol 40:8, 1996.

140. Deegan PB: Fabry disease, enzyme replacement therapy and the significance of antibody responses. J Inherit Metab Dis 35:227, 2012.

141. Toyooka K: Fabry disease. Curr Opin Neurol 24:463, 2011.

142. Chauveau D, Pirson Y, Verellen-Dumoulin C, et al: Intracranial aneurysms in autosomal dominant polycystic kidney disease. Kidney Int 45:1140, 1994.

143. Irazabal MV, Huston 3rd J, Kubly V, et al: Extended follow-up of unruptured intracranial aneurysms detected by presymptomatic screening in patients with autosomal dominant polycystic kidney disease. Clin J Am Soc Nephrol 6:1274, 2011.

CHAPTER

17

Neurologic Complications of Electrolyte Disturbances

JACK E. RIGGS

Electrolyte disturbances occur frequently in clinical practice and are associated with a variety of characteristic central or peripheral (including muscle) neurologic manifestations. Since electrolyte disturbances are usually secondary processes, effective management requires prompt identification and treatment of the underlying primary disorder in addition to correction of the electrolyte abnormality. Moreover, the neurologic consequences of electrolyte disorders are usually functional rather than structural. Consequently, the neurologic manifestations of electrolyte disturbances are often reversible, particularly if corrected and effectively managed at an early stage. The neurologic manifestations of abnormalities of serum sodium, potassium, calcium, and magnesium are reviewed.

SODIUM

Extracellular fluid volume is directly dependent on total body sodium, the principal osmotic component of that fluid compartment. Consequently, most patients with hyponatremia are also hypoosmolar, and those with hypernatremia are hyperosmolar. The symptomatic neurologic manifestations of serum sodium abnormalities typically involve the central, rather than the peripheral, nervous system and generally are the consequence of hypoosmolarity in hyponatremia and hyperosmolarity in hypernatremia. Because of the brain's ability to adapt effectively to changes in serum osmolarity, the propensity of hyponatremia or hypernatremia to produce neurologic symptoms generally depends on the rapidity with which the sodium disturbance develops.

Hyponatremia

Hyponatremia with normal osmolarity (pseudohyponatremia) is relatively infrequent and usually occurs in the setting of hyperlipidemia or hyperproteinemia. Hyponatremia with hyperosmolarity usually occurs in the setting of hyperglycemia. Hyponatremia is most often associated with hypoosmolarity and is classified into three categories that are dependent on whether the extracellular fluid volume is decreased, normal, or increased. *Hypo-osmolar hyponatremia with hypovolemia* results from excessive renal sodium loss (e.g., from diuretic usage, mineralocorticoid deficiency, salt-losing nephropathy, or osmotic diuresis) or extrarenal sodium loss (e.g., from vomiting, diarrhea, or third-space losses). *Hypo-osmolar hyponatremia with normovolemia* (no edema) results from conditions such as

Aminoff's Neurology and General Medicine, Fifth Edition.

the syndrome of inappropriate secretion of antidiuretic hormone (SIADH), glucocorticoid deficiency, hypothyroidism, and stress, or in response to various drugs, including carbamazepine and many psychotropic agents. *Hypo-osmolar hyponatremia with excess extracellular fluid* (edema) occurs in conditions such as cirrhosis, cardiac failure, nephrotic syndrome, and acute or chronic renal failure. The separation of hypo-osmolar hyponatremia into these three categories based on the extracellular fluid volume status has therapeutic implications. In normovolemic and hypervolemic hypo-osmolar hyponatremia, the fundamental principle of therapy is water restriction, whereas in hypovolemic hypo-osmolar hyponatremia the basis of therapy is replacement of water and sodium (generally with isotonic saline or lactated Ringer solution).[1]

Among hospitalized patients, hyponatremia is the most common electrolyte abnormality encountered and is associated with a significant increased risk of death, although this increased mortality likely reflects the seriousness of underlying disorders rather than the hyponatremia itself.[2–7]

Neurologic symptoms related to hyponatremia are seen much more frequently in patients with acute, rather than chronic, hyponatremia. For example, a serum sodium concentration of 130 mEq/L might produce neurologic symptoms if it developed rapidly, whereas a serum sodium concentration of 115 mEq/L might be asymptomatic if it developed very slowly. An alteration in mental status is the most common neurologic manifestation of hyponatremia and ranges from mild confusion to coma; patients with underlying neurodegenerative disorders and those of advanced age are particularly susceptible to delirium from even small changes in serum sodium. This hyponatremic encephalopathy may be associated with nonspecific generalized slowing on the electroencephalogram. As the level of serum sodium decreases, the risk of seizures increases.[8] The occurrence of convulsions in the setting of acute hyponatremia (typically with a serum sodium concentration less than 120 mEq/L) can be ominous and portend a mortality rate exceeding 50 percent. The occurrence of seizures in patients with acute hyponatremia represents a medical emergency and necessitates rapid, but only partial, correction of the serum sodium concentration. Control of hyponatremic seizures can obtained by the judicious use of 3 percent saline (4 to 6 ml/kg) in an attempt to raise the serum sodium concentration by small 3 to 5 mEq/L increments; careful monitoring with frequent sodium measurements is required to avoid rapid correction.[9] Occasionally, focal neurologic signs and symptoms are seen in the setting of hyponatremia and include hemiparesis, monoparesis, ataxia, nystagmus, tremor, rigidity, aphasia, and unilateral corticospinal tract signs. These focal abnormalities can represent aggravation of an underlying structural lesion and often remit with resolution of the hyponatremia. Such focal deficits therefore require neuroimaging even if they fully resolve with sodium correction. Although occasional muscle twitches and fasciculations may be seen in acute hyponatremia, muscle symptoms other than cramps are not common. The central nervous system (CNS) manifestations of acute hyponatremia are related to cerebral edema, but understanding is incomplete regarding the factors that mitigate hyponatremic osmotic brain swelling and reduction in the brain's intracellular organic osmolytes.[10–13]

The use or restriction of fluids can have profound effects on the eventual outcome of patients with hyponatremia and neurologic symptoms and therefore any specific treatment approach should be implemented carefully.

Subarachnoid Hemorrhage and Other Intracranial Diseases

Hyponatremia frequently develops in patients with subarachnoid hemorrhage and has often been attributed to SIADH. Clinicians typically manage all forms of SIADH by instituting some degree of fluid restriction. In an insightful retrospective study of 134 consecutive patients from the Netherlands, 44 patients developed hyponatremia between the second and tenth days following subarachnoid hemorrhage.[14] Hyponatremia was defined as a serum sodium level below 135 mEq/L on at least two consecutive days. Of the 44 hyponatremic patients, 25 fulfilled the laboratory criteria for SIADH. Cerebral infarction, defined as a focal neurologic deficit with or without computed tomography (CT) confirmation or deterioration in the level of consciousness with CT confirmation of ischemic changes, occurred in 46 of the 134 patients. Of the cerebral infarcts, 27 occurred in the 44 hyponatremic patients (61.4%), but only 19 occurred in the 90 normonatremic patients (21.1%). Of the 44 hyponatremic patients, 26 were fluid-restricted; of these, 21 developed infarcts (80.8%). Of the 18 hyponatremic patients who were not fluid-restricted, only 6 developed infarcts (33.3%). Of the 25 patients who fulfilled the laboratory criteria for SIADH, 17 were fluid-restricted; of these, 15 developed infarcts (88.2%). Thus, fluid restriction in hyponatremia following subarachnoid hemorrhage, particularly in those thought to have SIADH, appears to markedly increase the risk of cerebral infarction.

Understanding has been gained of the basis for this risk in fluid restriction in patients with subarachnoid hemorrhage and other intracranial disorders. Care should be taken to carefully distinguish between SIADH and cerebral salt wasting.[15] Because absence of hypovolemia is considered one of the criteria for making the diagnosis of SIADH,[16] the finding of decreased blood volume in patients with hyponatremia and intracranial disease suggests that these patients do not have SIADH. In a prospective study of 21 patients with aneurysmal subarachnoid hemorrhage, plasma volume decreased by more than 10 percent in 11 of the patients.[17] Serum sodium decreased in 9 of the 21 patients. Plasma volume decreased by more than 10 percent in 6 of 9 patients with hyponatremia, and a similar decrease occurred in 5 of 12 patients with normal serum sodium. Eight of the 9 patients with hyponatremia had a negative sodium balance, whereas only 4 of the 12 patients with normal serum sodium had a negative sodium balance. Finally, 10 of the 12 patients with a negative sodium balance had a decrease in plasma volume exceeding 10 percent. Hyponatremia following aneurysmal subarachnoid hemorrhage appears frequently to be related to cerebral salt-wasting[17,18] and not SIADH. Fluid restriction instituted to correct hyponatremia attributed to presumed SIADH in patients with subarachnoid hemorrhage may exacerbate an already volume-depleted state and subject patients to a greater risk of ischemic cerebral damage from vasospasm. Therefore, patients with subarachnoid hemorrhage and hyponatremia are typically treated instead with oral or intravenous sodium repletion in an attempt to restore or maintain normovolemia.

Central Pontine Myelinolysis (Osmotic Myelinolysis)

The history of the recognition and pathogenesis of central pontine myelinolysis has been summarized elsewhere.[1] Central pontine myelinolysis was recognized as a distinct clinical entity in 1959 in four cases, occurring on a background of alcoholism and malnutrition. Its pathologic features involve a symmetric noninflammatory demyelination in the base of the pons with relative sparing of neurons and axons. The classic clinical presentation includes pseudobulbar palsy and spastic quadriparesis. Following the original description, many additional cases were reported in rapid succession, suggesting that central pontine myelinolysis is not a rare disorder. Many cases were not associated with alcoholism or malnutrition. It may, for example, occur in subjects with extensive burns. By 1964, the relatively high frequency of subclinical lesions (Fig. 17-1) was noted, and this was validated by many subsequent reports.

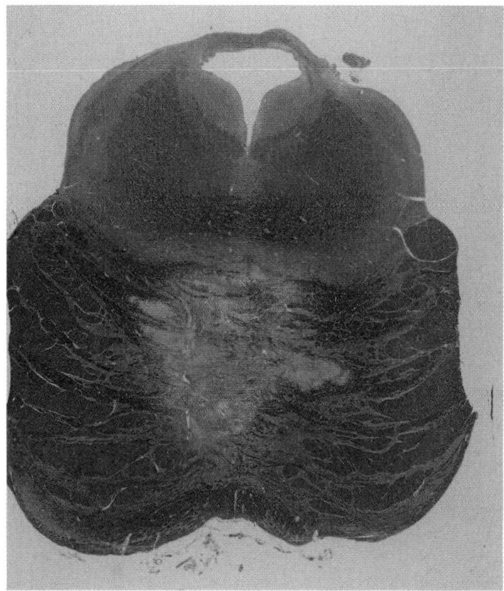

FIGURE 17-1 ■ Macrosection of the pons demonstrating central demyelination, an incidental finding of subclinical central pontine myelinolysis in a patient with a history of electrolyte abnormalities and diuretic use (Luxol fast blue).

In 1963, Aleu and Terry suggested that central pontine myelinolysis is related to some recently introduced factors. Also in 1963, the initial suggestion that an electrolyte imbalance was a contributing factor in the pathogenesis of central pontine myelinolysis was first made. It was subsequently observed that acute cases of central pontine myelinolysis (i.e., acute quadriparesis) developed only in hospitalized patients who were being hydrated. From an analysis of 12 acute cases in 1980, Leslie and associates noted that there had been a recent rapid rise of serum sodium in each patient, suggesting that central pontine myelinolysis was an iatrogenic disorder that in most cases was caused by too rapid correction of serum sodium. The factors that led to the appearance of this disorder during the 1950s were the introduction of diuretics, the liberal use of intravenous fluids, and the ability to rapidly measure serum electrolytes.[1] Prospective magnetic resonance imaging (MRI) studies have demonstrated the development of characteristic pontine lesions in patients treated for hyponatremia in whom the rate of correction of the hyponatremia was rapid.[19] In one retrospective study of published reports of patients with central pontine myelinolysis in whom initial values of sodium and potassium were given, all patients who developed the disorder were also hypokalemic initially; this observation is of unclear significance.[20] Patients who develop hyponatremia following liver transplantation may be particularly vulnerable to central pontine myelinolysis if their hyponatremia is corrected rapidly.[21]

Sterns and colleagues, in a review of their experience, noted neurologic complications in eight patients whose serum sodium had been corrected by more than 12 mEq/L per day.[22] Conversely, patients with hyponatremia that was corrected more slowly made uncomplicated recoveries. In a review of the literature, those authors found 80 patients with severe hyponatremia (less than 106 mEq/L). Of these 80 patients, enough detail was reported in 51 to determine a maximal rate of correction of serum sodium. In 39 of 51 patients who were corrected rapidly (greater than 12 mEq/L per day), 22 (58%) had some type of neurologic complication. Of these 22 patients, 14 (64%) were suspected of having central pontine myelinolysis. Of the 13 patients who were corrected slowly (less than 12 mEq/L per day), none experienced a neurologic complication.

Because chronic hyponatremia is less likely to produce neurologic symptoms, and rapid correction of chronic hyponatremia is more likely to produce neurologic injury in experimental models,[1] a judicious approach to the correction of chronic hyponatremia is urged, especially in cases where the sodium has been chronically depressed.[23] There is no justification for using hypertonic saline to treat asymptomatic hyponatremia, or to rapidly correct hyponatremia to levels above 120 to 125 mEq/L in significantly symptomatic hyponatremia.

Animal models of central pontine myelinolysis have been developed in the dog and the rat.[24] In both animals, demyelination follows rapid correction of sustained, vasopressin-induced hyponatremia with hypertonic saline. The label *osmotic myelinolysis* has been suggested in preference to

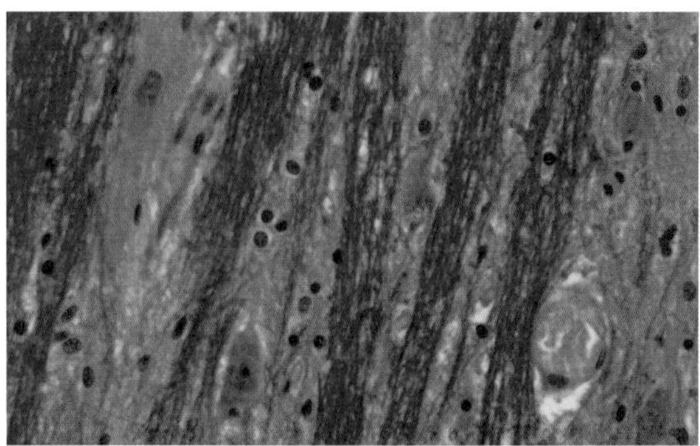

FIGURE 17-2 ■ Gray and white matter bundles in normal human pons. Note that most oligodendrocytes (*small cells with dark nuclei*) are within gray matter rather than within the white matter bundles (hematoxylin and eosin, 640 ×).

central pontine myelinolysis because of the well-recognized occurrence of extrapontine myelinolysis.[25] This myelinolysis occurs in areas of the brain characterized by an extensive admixture and apposition of gray and white matter.[26] Although the pathogenesis of osmotic myelinolysis remains undefined, the topography of oligodendrocytes may play a role. Oligodendrocytes in these vulnerable areas are predominantly located within adjacent gray matter rather than within the white matter bundles (Fig. 17-2). Because gray matter is much more vascular than white matter, oligodendrocytes in this location may be more vulnerable to serum osmotic shifts.[26]

The rapid re-induction of hyponatremia has been associated with a reduction in neurologic signs and symptoms suggestive of osmotic myelinolysis in rats[27] and in a single human case[28] in which a rapid increase in serum sodium occurred during the treatment of chronic hyponatremia; it is unclear if this strategy should be employed routinely. Corticosteroids, *myo*-inositol, immunoglobulin, and thyrotrophin-releasing hormone have all been suggested as possible treatments of or preventive measures for the osmotic demyelination syndrome with little evidence to recommend such therapies.[29,30] The lack of proven treatment for this disorder further emphasizes the need to avoid its occurrence by slow correction of hyponatremia.

Hypernatremia

Symptoms due to hypernatremia are usually referable to the CNS and most often are seen with serum sodium concentrations above 160 mEq/L.[1,31] Hypernatremia is most frequently encountered in the very young or very old. In infants, fluid loss due to gastroenteritis is a common cause. In the elderly, dehydration resulting from an inability to obtain water because of debilitation is the most frequent cause. Diabetes insipidus rarely presents with severe hypernatremia unless the patient is also denied access to water. Structural lesions (e.g., gliomas and metastatic tumors) in the hypothalamic thirst center are an uncommon cause of hypernatremia in patients with neurologic disease.

Alteration of mental status is a frequent manifestation of hypernatremia and ranges from lethargy to coma. Pathologic studies suggest that osmotic forces present during the development of hypernatremia, particularly when acute, may produce shrinkage of brain parenchyma. This may result in parenchymal hemorrhages or tearing of bridging veins, producing subdural hematomas or subarachnoid hemorrhage. An initial mortality rate of 20 percent and an incidence of permanent brain damage of more than 33 percent have been noted in children with severe hypernatremia.[1] Seizures may occur in the setting of hypernatremia and paradoxically may be more frequent during rehydration.[1] These hypernatremic seizures may be related to either focal hemorrhages that occur during the development of hypernatremia or cerebral edema that may develop during rehydration. Rigidity, tremor, myoclonus, asterixis, and chorea have also been associated with hypernatremia. Transient thalamic signal changes on MRI have been seen with severe hypernatremia.[32] Neuromuscular manifestations of hypernatremia are much less frequent. Rhabdomyolysis and episodic muscle weakness have been reported.[33,34] Treatment of symptomatic hypernatremia typically involves administration of hypotonic fluids to correct the free water deficit, using caution to avoid rapid correction.

POTASSIUM

In contrast to sodium, the neurologic manifestations of potassium disturbance, whether hypokalemia or hyperkalemia, rarely involve the CNS. About 98 percent of total body potassium is located intracellularly, and 60 percent of intracellular potassium is within muscle. This distribution may, in part, account for the predominance of muscle symptoms associated with either hypokalemia or hyperkalemia.

Hypokalemia

Hypokalemia is the most frequent electrolyte disorder encountered in clinical practice and is produced by a variety of mechanisms, including inadequate potassium intake or excessive renal or gastrointestinal potassium loss. Neurologic symptoms of hypokalemia are typically muscular.[35,36] Serum potassium concentrations of 3.0 to 3.5 mEq/L may be associated with mild muscle weakness, myalgia, and ease of fatigue. Serum potassium concentrations of 2.5 to 3.0 mEq/L are associated with the development of clinically significant muscle weakness, particularly of the proximal limb muscles, and with muscle cramps. The cranial musculature is characteristically spared in hypokalemia-induced muscle weakness. When the serum potassium level falls below 2.5 mEq/L, and usually below 2.0 mEq/L, structural muscle damage, including rhabdomyolysis and myoglobinuria, may occur.[37]

Tetany occurs in some patients with hypokalemia, particularly when associated with alkalosis. Hypokalemia may mask the tetany of hypocalcemia. Paradoxically, tetany may occur during the treatment of hypokalemia in patients who are also hypocalcemic.

Cerebral symptoms in hypokalemia are distinctly unusual. Reference to symptoms such as lethargy, apathy, drowsiness, confusion, irritability, delirium, and coma in hypokalemia are rare[1] and suggest that an associated acid-base disturbance or other electrolyte abnormality may have been responsible for these encephalopathic symptoms. Brain concussion has been shown to lead to a mild transient hypokalemia.[38]

Hyperkalemia

The cardiac toxicity of hyperkalemia essentially precludes the appearance of significant neurologic manifestations. Most patients develop serious cardiac abnormalities, such as ventricular fibrillation or asystole, before the appearance of neurologic symptoms.[39,40]

Chronic potassium homeostasis is dependent on renal mechanisms. Acute potassium regulation is dependent on extrarenal hormonal mechanisms primarily involving insulin, aldosterone, and epinephrine. Clinically important etiologies of hyperkalemia include renal failure, adrenal insufficiency (Addison disease), and acidosis with or without insulin deficiency. Cerebral symptoms due to hyperkalemia must be uncommon, since they do not occur in hyperkalemic periodic paralysis.[41] The cerebral symptoms (nervousness and lethargy) that frequently occur in Addison disease are more likely related to the associated hyponatremia or acidosis than the elevated potassium. The most frequent neurologic manifestation of hyperkalemia is the development of mild muscle weakness, which occurs most often in the setting of chronic adrenal insufficiency. However, profound muscle weakness with hyperkalemia is reported only rarely.[42]

CALCIUM

Plasma calcium stabilizes excitable membranes in muscle and nervous tissue. Disorders of calcium would therefore be expected to produce neurologic manifestations. The coordinated interactions of parathyroid hormone, cholecalciferol, and probably calcitonin regulate intestinal calcium absorption, renal calcium reabsorption, and bone resorption to control closely plasma calcium concentration.[43]

Hypercalcemia

Malignant neoplasms and hyperparathyroidism account for 70 to 80 percent of cases of hypercalcemia.[44] The neoplasms most frequently associated with hypercalcemia are breast cancer, lung cancer, and multiple myeloma. Although most instances of hypercalcemia in the setting of malignancy are due to osteolytic skeletal metastases, some carcinomas, particularly of the lung, are associated with hypercalcemia due to elevated levels of parathyroid hormone. Single adenomas of the parathyroid gland account for 75 percent of cases of primary hyperparathyroidism. Because patients with malignant neoplasms often have several mechanisms for neurologic injury, the incidence of neurologic manifestations in hyperparathyroidism (which is at least 40%) represents a reasonable incidence of the neurologic disorders associated with hypercalcemia.[45]

Alterations in mental status are common in hypercalcemia (particularly with serum calcium concentrations of more than 14 mg/dl) and generally consist of progressive lethargy, confusion, and ultimately coma. These reversible symptoms are directly related to the degree of hypercalcemia and require immediate therapy. Headache, elevated cerebrospinal fluid protein, and, rarely, convulsions also occur in patients with hypercalcemia.[1,44,45] Hyperparathyroidism has also been associated rarely with other CNS disturbances including ataxia, internuclear ophthalmoplegia, corticospinal tract dysfunction, dysarthria, and dysphagia.[1] Hypercalcemia has also been associated with apnea in children[46] as well as with the posterior reversible encephalopathy syndrome, a radiographic diagnosis due to many etiologies that can present with seizures, altered mental status, or focal neurologic deficits.[47]

Hypercalcemia produces reduced neuromuscular excitability and may cause muscle weakness. Easy fatigability and muscle weakness are more common in hyperparathyroidism than in other hypercalcemic conditions. The clinical features of hyperparathyroid myopathy include proximal, though seldom disabling, muscle weakness and wasting with preserved or even brisk reflexes and mild nonspecific myopathic features on electromyography and muscle biopsy, as discussed in Chapter 59. The pathogenesis of hyperparathyroid myopathy remains undefined, although hypercalcemia, vitamin D deficiency, chronic phosphate deficiency, or neuropathic influences may play a role. Hyperparathyroid myopathy is similar to the vitamin D deficiency myopathy that can occur with uremia, phenytoin therapy, and osteomalacia. Neuropathy is not a common feature of hypercalcemia, but carpal tunnel syndrome has occasionally been associated with hyperparathyroidism.[1]

Hypocalcemia

Hypocalcemia is relatively rare except in neonates and individuals with renal failure. Severe acute hypocalcemia is most frequently iatrogenic, following thyroid or parathyroid surgery. Hypocalcemia is also a common complication of acute pancreatitis and is frequent in patients in the intensive care unit with a variety of conditions.[48] The neurologic manifestations of hypoparathyroidism resulting from primary, secondary, or pseudohypoparathyroidism (parathyroid hormone–resistant syndromes) largely reflect hypocalcemia. The most common CNS manifestations of hypocalcemia are seizures (which may be focal or generalized) and alterations of mental status. The latter symptoms include irritability, anxiety, agitation, confusion, delirium, delusions, hallucinations, psychosis, depression, mental dullness, mental retardation, and dementia. Chorea and parkinsonism are seen with increased frequency in patients with chronic hypocalcemia; although a causal relationship has not been established, the regularity with which calcification of the basal ganglia is seen in patients with chronic hypoparathyroidism seems more than coincidental, and some may have quite prominent associated movement disorders (discussed in Chapter 58).[49] Less frequent CNS manifestations of hypoparathyroidism are pseudotumor cerebri and myelopathy due to vertebral lamina overgrowth.

Tetany is the most frequently recognized symptom of hypocalcemia referable to the peripheral nervous system.[44] Tetany originates in the peripheral nerve axon and is due to spontaneous, irregular, repetitive nerve action potentials. When the ionized calcium concentration reaches a low enough level, the peripheral nerve membrane may spontaneously discharge at the normal resting membrane potential. Latent tetany may be unmasked clinically by hyperventilation or ischemia (Trousseau test). The first symptom of tetany is tingling that initially occurs periorally and distally in the limbs and then spreads proximally. This is followed by a feeling of muscle spasm that has an initial distribution similar to that of the early sensory complaints and becomes increasingly severe as it spreads proximally. Finally, muscles may go into tonic spasms, commencing distally (carpopedal spasm). Laryngeal stridor may ultimately develop.[50] Opisthotonos may occur if spasms involve the trunk.

Elevated serum creatine kinase levels have been reported in patients with hypoparathyroidism, although clinical and morphologic evidence of myopathy has been scant. Hypoparathyroidism has been associated with the mitochondrial disorder Kearns–Sayre syndrome as well as with muscle phosphorylase deficiency (perhaps related to failure of calcium to activate phosphorylase kinase).

MAGNESIUM

Less than 2 percent of total body magnesium is located within the extracellular fluid compartment. Although magnesium has an intracellular-extracellular distribution similar to that of potassium, most of the intracellular magnesium is bound and not exchangeable with the extracellular fluid. Intracellular free magnesium is rigidly regulated despite wide variations in extracellular magnesium concentrations. The teleological basis for this situation relates to the critical role of magnesium in intracellular metabolism. Magnesium is required for activation of a wide range of intracellular enzymes. Additionally, extracellular magnesium exerts significant effects on synaptic transmission in the central and peripheral nervous system.[1,51]

Hypomagnesemia

Because magnesium is predominantly an intracellular electrolyte, the finding of hypomagnesemia does not always accurately reflect magnesium depletion. Important mechanisms of hypomagnesemia and magnesium depletion include decreased intake (as in starvation), decreased intestinal absorption (as in malabsorption syndromes such as nontropical sprue), and increased renal loss (as with diuretic usage, chronic alcoholism, diabetic acidosis, and renal tubular acidosis).

The neurologic manifestations of hypomagnesemia are essentially hyperirritability with agitation, confusion, seizures, tremor, myoclonus, hyperreflexia, Chvostek sign, and tetany.[52,53] These signs and symptoms typically occur with serum magnesium concentrations of less than 0.8 mEq/L. Occasionally, even focal neurologic signs may be seen in patients with hypomagnesemia.[54] When convulsions occur in patients with hypomagnesemia, parenteral administration of magnesium salts is required. However, renal function should be assessed before parenteral magnesium is administered as those with renal failure may not be able to excrete magnesium adequately. When magnesium is given, it should be given by slow intravenous bolus, and calcium gluconate should be available to counteract transient hypermagnesemia, which may rarely cause apnea as a result of respiratory muscle paralysis. The neurologic manifestations of hypomagnesemia are similar to those of hypocalcemia, which is not surprising, since hypocalcemia often accompanies hypomagnesemia. The hypocalcemia or hypomagnesemia is produced or exaggerated in some instances by a hypomagnesemia-induced decrease in parathyroid hormone or end-organ resistance to the action of parathyroid hormone. This leads to an important therapeutic point—it is necessary to evaluate magnesium in a hypocalcemic patient who fails to respond to calcium supplementation. Conversely, in magnesium-deficient patients who are normocalcemic but have symptoms suggestive of hypocalcemia, calcium may still be responsible for the symptoms, since apparently normocalcemic hypomagnesemic patients may have decreased serum ionized calcium concentrations.

Hypomagnesemia develops frequently with cisplatin use. In that setting, only patients who are also hypocalcemic develop tetany with carpopedal spasm. Muscle weakness develops in some patients with hypomagnesemia, although coexistent hypokalemia or hypophosphatemia may contribute. Chronic hypomagnesemia has been associated with a cardioskeletal mitochondrial myopathy.[55]

Hypermagnesemia

Symptomatic hypermagnesemia is uncommon in clinical practice and is typically encountered in the setting of excessive magnesium intake in conjunction with impaired renal function. Unsuspected symptomatic hypermagnesemia may occur more frequently in the elderly.[56] In contrast to hypomagnesemia, the neurologic manifestations of hypermagnesemia are characterized by nervous system depression. Loss of deep tendon reflexes is an early sign of hypermagnesemia and occurs at serum magnesium concentrations of 5 to 6 mEq/L. This loss of reflexes may be utilized in obstetrics to titrate magnesium sulfate infusions used in the treatment of preeclampisa. At serum magnesium concentrations of 8 to 10 mEq/L, CNS depression is said to occur, with lethargy and confusion being the most common reported neurologic manifestations. However, in human subjects in whom the serum magnesium concentration was increased to 15 mEq/L, no CNS depression occurred, although there was slowing of the electroencephalogram, leading to the conclusion that clinical CNS effects of hypermagnesemia are likely rare.[1] The predominant neurologic manifestation of severe hypermagnesemia is muscular paralysis. Untreated, this weakness, which can involve respiratory muscles, may result in respiratory insufficiency with subsequent hypoxia, hypercapnia, coma, and ultimately death. The flaccid muscle weakness of hypermagnesemia is due to a blockade of neuromuscular transmission, which may not resolve until magnesium levels return to normal through renal excretion or with the aid of hemodialysis.

REFERENCES

1. Riggs JE: Neurologic manifestations of electrolyte disturbances. Neurol Clin 20:227, 2002.
2. Upadhyay A, Jaber BL, Madias NE: Incidence and prevalence of hyponatremia. Am J Med 119(7A):S30, 2006.
3. Gill G, Huda B, Boyd A, et al: Characteristics and mortality of severe hyponatremia – a hospital-based study. Clin Endocrinol 65:246, 2006.
4. Asadollahi K, Beeching N, Gill G: Hyponatremia as a risk factor for hospital mortality. QJM 99:877, 2006.
5. Whelan B, Bennett K, O'Riordan D, et al: Serum sodium as a risk factor for in-hospital mortality in acute unselected general medical patients. QJM 102:175, 2009.
6. Walker SS, Mount DB, Curhan GC: Mortality after hospitalization with mild, moderate, and severe hyponatremia. Am J Med 122:857, 2009.
7. Wald R, Jaber BL, Price LL, et al: Impact of hospital-associated hyponatremia on selected outcomes. Arch Intern Med 170:294, 2010.
8. Halawa I, Andersson T, Tomson T: Hyponatremia and risk of seizures: a retrospective cross-sectional study. Epilepsia 52:410, 2011.
9. Sarnaik AP, Meert K, Hackbarth R, et al: Management of hyponatremic seizures in children with hypertonic saline: a safe and effective strategy. Crit Care Med 19:758, 1991.
10. Verbalis JG, Gullans SR: Hyponatremia causes large sustained reductions in brain content of multiple organic osmolytes in rats. Brain Res 567:274, 1991.
11. Lien Y-HH, Shapiro JI, Chan L: Study of brain electrolytes and organic osmolytes during correction of chronic hyponatremia: implications for the pathogenesis of central pontine myelinolysis. J Clin Invest 88:303, 1991.
12. Massieu L, Montiel T, Robles G, et al: Brain amino acids during hyponatremia in vivo: clinical observations and experimental studies. Neurochem Res 29:73, 2004.
13. Sterns RH, Silver SM: Brain volume regulation in response to hypo-osmolality and its correction. Am J Med 119(512) 2006.
14. Wijdicks EFM, Vermeulen M, Hijdra A, et al: Hyponatremia and cerebral infarction in patients with ruptured intracranial aneurysms: is fluid restriction harmful? Ann Neurol 17:137, 1985.
15. Nathan BR: Cerebral correlates of hyponatremia. Neurocrit Care 6:72, 2007.

16. Palmer BF: Hyponatremia in patients with central nervous system disease: SIADH versus CSW. Trends Endocrinol Metab 14:182, 2003.
17. Wijdicks EFM, Vermeulen M, ten Haaf JA, et al: Volume depletion and natriuresis in patients with a ruptured intracranial aneurysm. Ann Neurol 18:211, 1985.
18. Sherlock M, O'Sullivan E, Agha A, et al: The incidence and pathophysiology of hyponatraemia after subarachnoid hemorrhage. Clin Endocrinol 64:250, 2006.
19. Brunner JE, Redmond JM, Haggar AM, et al: Central pontine myelinolysis and pontine lesions after rapid correction of hyponatremia: a prospective magnetic resonance imaging study. Ann Neurol 27:61, 1990.
20. Lohr JW: Osmotic demyelination syndrome following correction of hyponatremia: association with hypokalemia. Am J Med 96:408, 1994.
21. Abbasoglu O, Goldstein RM, Vodapally MS, et al: Liver transplantation in hyponatremic patients with emphasis on central pontine myelinolysis. Clin Transplant 12:263, 1998.
22. Sterns RH, Riggs JE, Schochet SS: Osmotic demyelination syndrome following correction of hyponatremia. N Engl J Med 314:1535, 1986.
23. Soupart A, Decaux G: Therapeutic recommendations for management of severe hyponatremia: current concepts on pathogenesis and prevention of neurologic complications. Clin Nephrol 46:149, 1996.
24. Verbalis JG, Martinez AJ, Drutarosky MD: Neurological and neuropathological sequelae of correction of chronic hyponatremia. Kidney Int 39:1274, 1991.
25. Martin RJ: Central pontine and extrapontine myelinolysis: the osmotic demyelination syndromes. J Neurol Neurosurg Psychiatry 75(22) 2004.
26. Riggs JE, Schochet SS: Osmotic stress, osmotic myelinolysis, and oligodendroctye topography. Arch Pathol Lab Med 113:1386, 1989.
27. Soupart A, Penninckx R, Stenuit A, et al: Reinduction of hyponatremia improves survival in rats with myelinolysis-related neurologic symptoms. J Neuropathol Exp Neurol 55:594, 1996.
28. Soupart A, Ngassa M, Decaux G: Therapeutic relowering of the serum sodium in a patient after excessive correction of hyponatremia. Clin Nephrol 51:383, 1999.
29. Sugimura Y, Murase T, Takefuji S, et al: Protective effect of dexamethasome on osmotic-induced demyelination in rats. Exp Neurol 192:178, 2005.
30. Silver SM, Schroeder BM, Sterns RH, et al: Myoinositol administration improves survival and reduces myelinolysis after rapid correction of chronic hyponatremia in rats. J Neuropathol Exp Neurol 65:37, 2006.
31. Bichet DG, Mallie J-P: Hypernatremia and the poluric disorders. p. 241. In: DuBose T, Hamm L (eds): Acid-Base and Electrolyte Disorders: A Companion to Brenner & Rector's The Kidney. WB Saunders, New York, 2002.
32. Hartfield DS, Loewy JA, Yager JY: Transient thalamic changes on MRI in a child with hypernatremia. Pediatr Neurol 20:60, 1999.
33. Kung AWC, Pun KK, Lam KSL, et al: Rhabdomyolysis associated with cranial diabetes insipidus. Postgrad Med J 67:912, 1991.
34. Abramovici MI, Singhal PC, Trachtman H: Hypernatremia and rhabdomyolysis. J Med 23:17, 1992.
35. Krishna GG, Steigerwalt SP, Pikus R, et al: Hypokalemic states. p. 659. In Narins RG (ed): Clinical Disorders of Fluid and Electrolyte Metabolism. 5th Ed. McGraw-Hill, New York, 1994.
36. Kone BC: Hypokalemia. p. 381. In: DuBose TD, Hamm LL (eds): Acid-Base and Electrolyte Disorders: A Companion to Brenner & Rector's The Kidney. WB Saunders, New York, 2002.
37. Singhal PC, Abramovici M, Venkatesan J, et al: Hypokalemia and rhabdomyolysis. Miner Electrolyte Metab 17:335, 1991.
38. Lazar L, Erez I, Gutermacher M, et al: Brain concussion produces transient hypokalemia in children. J Pediatr Surg 32:88, 1994.
39. DeFronzo RA, Smith JD: Clinical disorders of hyperkalemia. p. 697. In Narins RG (ed): Clinical Disorders of Fluid and Electrolyte Metabolism. 5th Ed. McGraw-Hill, New York, 1994.
40. Weiner ID, Wingo CS: Hyperkalemia. p. 395. In: DuBose TD, Hamm LL (eds): Acid-Base and Electrolyte Disorders: A Companion to Brenner & Rector's The Kidney. WB Saunders, New York, 2002.
41. Riggs JE: The periodic paralyses. Neurol Clin 6:485, 1988.
42. Freeman SJ, Fale AD: Muscular paralysis and ventilatory failure caused by hyperkalemia. Br J Anaesth 70:226, 1993.
43. Bourdeau JE, Attie MF: Calcium metabolism. p. 243. In Narins RG (ed): Clinical Disorders of Fluid and Electrolyte Metabolism. 5th Ed. McGraw-Hill, New York, 1994.
44. Benabe JE, Martinez-Maldonado M: Disorders of calcium metabolism. p. 1009. In Narins RG (ed): Clinical Disorders of Fluid and Electrolyte Metabolism. 5th Ed. McGraw-Hill, New York, 1994.
45. Tonner DR, Schlechte JA: Neurologic complications of thyroid and parathyroid disease. Med Clin North Am 77:251, 1993.
46. Kooh S-W, Binet A: Hypercalcemia in infants presenting with apnea. Can Med Assoc J 143:509, 1990.
47. Kim JH, Kim MJ, Kang JK, et al: Vasogenic edema in a case of hypercalcemia-induced posterior reversible encephalopathy. Eur Neurol 53:160, 2005.
48. Cooper MS, Gittoes NJL: Diagnosis and management of hypocalcemia. BMJ 336:1298, 2008.
49. Cheek JC, Riggs JE, Lilly RL: Extensive brain calcification and progressive dysarthria and dysphagia

associated with chronic hypoparathyroidism. Arch Neurol 47:1038, 1990.

50. Sharief N, Matthew DJ, Dillon MJ: Hypocalcemic stridor in children, how often is it missed? Clin Pediatr 30:51, 1991.
51. Agus ZS, Massry SG: Hypomagnesemia and hypermagnesemia. p. 1099. In Narins RG (ed): Clinical Disorders of Fluid and Electrolyte Metabolism. 5th Ed. McGraw-Hill, New York, 1994.
52. Langley WF, Mann D: Central nervous system magnesium deficiency. Arch Intern Med 151:593, 1991.
53. Galland L: Magnesium, stress and neuropsychiatric disorders. Magnes Trace Elem 10:287, 1991–1992.
54. Leicher CR, Mezoff AG, Hyams JS: Focal cerebral deficits in severe hypomagnesemia. Pediatr Neurol 7:380, 1991.
55. Riggs JE, Klingberg WG, Flink EB, et al: Cardioskeletal mitochondrial myopathy associated with chronic hypomagnesemia. Neurology 42:128, 1992.
56. Clark BA, Brown RS: Unsuspected morbid hypermagnesemia in elderly patients. Am J Nephrol 12:336, 1992.

SECTION

IV

Endocrine Disorders

CHAPTER

18

Thyroid Disease and the Nervous System

JAMES J.P. ALIX ■ PAMELA J. SHAW

Disorders of the thyroid gland are common and are frequently accompanied by neurologic complications. One study of unselected general medical, geriatric, and psychiatric inpatients showed that 1 to 2 percent of patients had some form of thyroid disease.[1] Neurologists should be aware of the common and the more unusual neurologic complications of thyroid disease, since they may be the presenting feature of the thyroid disorder and because they are usually readily corrected with appropriate treatment.

NEUROLOGIC COMPLICATIONS OF HYPOTHYROIDISM

Hypothyroidism is a common disorder, with data from the National Health and Nutrition Examination Survey indicating that 1 in 300 persons in the United States has hypothyroidism.[2] The commonest causes of hypothyroidism are autoimmune destruction, thyroidectomy, and radioiodine ablation of the gland. Fewer than 10 percent of

Aminoff's Neurology and General Medicine, Fifth Edition.

cases of hypothyroidism are secondary to pituitary or hypothalamic disease.

Neurologic complications are common in patients with hypothyroidism, and all levels of the nervous system may be involved. The neurologic complications of hypothyroidism may be grouped into the following categories: (1) congenital hypothyroidism; (2) encephalopathy that may result in coma or a seizure disorder; (3) psychologic changes; (4) sleep disorders; (5) cerebellar ataxia; (6) cranial nerve lesions; (7) myopathy; (8) peripheral nerve disorders; and (9) miscellaneous conditions.

Neurologic Features of Congenital Hypothyroidism

Congenital hypothyroidism (CH), previously called cretinism, is the commonest treatable cause of neonatal encephalopathy, with data from neonatal screening programs revealing an incidence of 1:3,000 to 1:4,000.[3] It occurs secondary to dysgenesis of the thyroid gland or to severe maternal deficiency of dietary iodine. A study of endemic CH in western China and central Java revealed the following neurologic complications as common: developmental delay, pyramidal signs in a proximal distribution, and extrapyramidal signs.[4] Many patients had a characteristic gait, reflecting dysfunction of both the pyramidal and the extrapyramidal motor systems, in combination with laxity and deformity of the joints. Other common clinical features included strabismus, deafness, ataxia, and primitive reflexes. Imaging of the brain showed basal ganglia calcification in one-third of patients. In addition, recent evidence suggests that CH leads to reduced hippocampal volume even when treated[5]; in this study population, psychometric testing revealed that patients with CH scored below age-matched controls in verbal memory. Similarly, reduced IQ scores have also been reported in children with CH.[6] Learning impairment and changes in hippocampal CA1 pyramidal cell excitability have been reported in hypothyroid mice.[7,8]

Adult patients with CH typically manifest physical signs of spasticity affecting the trunk and proximal limb-girdle musculature, with relative sparing of the distal extremities.[9] Magnetic resonance imaging (MRI) of the brain in three patients showed abnormalities in the globus pallidus and substantia nigra, with increased signal on T1-weighted images and hypointensity on T2-weighted images. Only a modest degree of cerebral atrophy was reported, and the authors suggested that the main insult to the CNS may involve processes such as dendritic arborization and synaptogenesis, which are not evident on MRI.

Studies have shown that, in the developing brain, thyroid hormone has important effects on the regulation of neurofilament gene expression[10] and on several genes encoding mitochondrial proteins.[11] Hypothyroidism increases AMP hydrolysis in the hippocampal and cortical synaptosomes of rats and influences synaptic function throughout cortical development.[12] Thyroid hormone also regulates the timing of appearance and regional distribution of laminin, an extracellular matrix protein that provides key guidance signals to migrating neurons within the CNS. Disruption in the expression of laminin may play a role in the derangement of neuronal migration observed in the brain of patients with congenital hypothyroidism.[13]

A detailed consideration of the inborn errors of thyroid gland development and thyroid hormone synthesis responsible for permanent congenital hypothyroidism is beyond the scope of this chapter, and interested readers are directed to recent reviews.[14,15] Primary CH is due to abnormal development of the thyroid gland in 85 percent of instances.[16] A group of patients with CH poorly responsive to treatment and featuring additional signs of choreoathetosis, muscular hypotonia, and pulmonary problems were found to have mutations to Thyroid Transcription Factor 1.[17] Mutations to genes coding proteins required for thyroid hormone synthesis cause 10 to 15 percent of permanent primary CH; thyroid peroxidase is the protein most commonly affected.[18] Furthermore, mutations in a transmembrane thyroid hormone transporter, MCT-8, result in abnormal levels of circulating iodothyronines as well as global developmental delay, central hypotonia, spastic quadriplegia, dystonic movements, rotatory nystagmus, and impaired gaze and hearing in affected males.[19] Heterozygous females have a milder thyroid phenotype and no neurologic abnormalities.

Encephalopathy, Coma, and Seizures

Slowness, impairment of attention and concentration, somnolence, and lethargy are common symptoms in hypothyroidism. Occasionally, a life-threatening encephalopathy (myxedema coma) develops in patients with chronic, untreated hypothyroidism. A high index of suspicion is required to diagnose myxedema coma, particularly in the elderly, in whom features of hypothyroidism may be difficult to distinguish from depression or dementia.

In the compensated hypothyroid state, physiologic adaptations include a shift of the vascular pool away from the periphery to the central core to sustain normal body temperature.[20] In chronic hypothyroidism, these adaptations tend to produce a degree of diastolic hypertension, as well as a decrease in blood volume of up to 20 percent. Many organ systems and metabolic pathways are profoundly altered by chronic deficiency of thyroid hormone. Alterations in myocardial biochemistry produce impairment of cardiac contractility, the ventilatory response to hypercapnia is abnormal, hyponatremia may result from a reduction in free water clearance, and suppression of bone marrow function may result in normochromic normocytic anemia and an impaired white blood cell response to infection. Reduction in insulin clearance and decreased gluconeogenesis may produce a tendency to hypoglycemia, and patients are predisposed to toxic drug effects owing to reduced plasma clearance of all drugs. The corticosteroid response to stress is also likely to be impaired, even when basal serum cortisol levels are normal.[20]

The majority of patients who develop myxedema coma are elderly and have a history suggestive of gradual deterioration. Three key clinical features are universally present in myxedema coma: a depression of consciousness, a precipitating illness or event, and defective temperature control. Common precipitating factors include infection, trauma, stroke, hypothermia, hypoglycemia, carbon dioxide narcosis, and administration of certain drugs.[20] The body temperature is subnormal in many cases, but relative hypothermia may also occur, with the patient having an inappropriately normal temperature in the presence of sepsis. Most patients have clinical signs in keeping with long-standing hypothyroidism. Seizures occur in approximately 20 percent of cases; focal neurologic signs are not usually observed unless there has been a concomitant cerebrovascular event.

The pathophysiology is not fully understood but centers on the effects of low intracellular triiodothyronine (T3), particularly on the heart, which leads to decreased inotropism and chronotropism.[21] Laboratory investigations are often abnormal but seldom show diagnostic abnormalities. In critically ill patients, it may be difficult to distinguish between severe hypothyroidism and the euthyroid sick syndrome, and it may be necessary to measure levels of free circulating thyroid hormone. The electrocardiogram typically shows sinus bradycardia, with low voltage and prolongation of the QT interval. Chest radiography may reveal a pleural or pericardial effusion. The patient may have a mild normocytic normochromic anemia. Hyponatremia may be present, and the serum cholesterol level is sometimes elevated. Serum creatine kinase (CK) and lactate dehydrogenase levels are often raised. Lumbar puncture may reveal an elevated opening pressure, and the cerebrospinal fluid (CSF) protein concentration is often raised. The electroencephalogram (EEG) is commonly abnormal; in keeping with a metabolically induced encephalopathy, the frequency of the posterior dominant rhythm decreases, often into the theta range, and triphasic waves may be present.

The key to the successful treatment of myxedema coma is early recognition and the rapid institution of appropriate therapeutic measures, usually in the intensive care unit (ICU). Hypothyroid coma has a high mortality rate, and treatment should not be delayed for confirmatory laboratory data. Besides the use of intravenous thyroxine, it should include broad-spectrum antibiotics to cover any underlying infection and stress doses of glucocorticoids until specific laboratory results become available. Patients may not mount an appropriate leukocyte response or fever even in the presence of severe infection. The main principles of management also include correction of electrolyte and blood sugar abnormalities, passive rewarming, control of seizures, and respiratory and circulatory support. Different specific treatment regimens are advocated, with some authors preferring thyroxine (T4) monotherapy at a loading dose of 200 to 300 μg intravenously followed by 100 μg intravenously for maintenance. When stable, oral replacement at a dose of 1.6 μg/kg can be used with dose adjustment guided by thyroid-stimulating hormone (TSH) and free T4 levels.[22]

Early recognition and improved ICU care have improved outcomes over the last two decades, but mortality remains at around 20 percent[22]; factors associated with poor outcome include hypotension and bradycardia at presentation, sepsis, reduced

Glascow Coma Scale score, the need for mechanical ventilation, and hypothermia unresponsive to treatment.[23]

Neuropathologic studies of patients with myxedema coma have been few and usually have shown only the presence of cerebral edema with or without diffuse neuronal changes.

There is a relatively high incidence of seizures in hypothyroidism. Approximately 20 percent of patients with untreated hypothyroidism will develop seizures or syncopal episodes. Drop attacks (sudden repeated falls without warning symptoms and without loss of consciousness) also occur and resolve with therapy.[24] Patients with severe hypothyroidism may also present with convulsive or nonconvulsive status epilepticus.[25] Clinicians should be alert to the possibility of underlying hypothyroidism when the recovery time of the patient following a seizure is unusually prolonged.

Mental Changes

Hypothyroidism may be associated with mood disorders, in particular, depression.[26] Treatment of the hypothyroidism usually resolves the affective problem, although the response of individuals to treatment may be modulated by common polymorphisms of thyroid hormone transporters and deiodinases.[26] The colorful term *myxedema madness* has been used to describe the florid mental-state changes that may occur in hypothyroid patients, including irritability, paranoia, hallucinations, delirium, and psychosis. These symptoms are typically reversible but often take longer than physical symptoms to resolve; in some cases a degree of cognitive impairment may persist, particularly if treatment is delayed, perhaps due to irreversible damage secondary to chronic metabolic changes.[27]

Several investigators have reported an increase in the incidence of hypothyroidism in patients with various major psychiatric illnesses. An association between hypothyroidism and bipolar affective disorder has been reported, particularly in patients with a "rapid cycling" form of the illness.[28] Up to 50 percent of these patients have positive antithyroid antibody titers. Clinical and subclinical hypothyroidism in depression and bipolar disorder may adversely affect or delay the response to treatment.[29] Many patients with depression, even when viewed as chemically euthyroid, have alterations in their thyroid function, including slight elevation of the serum thyroxine, blunting of the TSH response to thyrotropin-releasing hormone (TRH) stimulation, and detectable titers of antithyroid antibodies.[30] These changes are generally reversed following alleviation of the depression. Depressed patients with hypothyroidism may also manifest different symptoms than patients with low mood and no concurrent hypothyroidism.[31] One study reported an increase in anxiety symptoms in patients with hypothyroidism but a decrease in core and biologic symptoms.[31] Hypothyroidism is also a reversible cause of cognitive impairment, most commonly manifesting as psychomotor slowing, memory impairment, visuospatial problems, and reduced constructional dexterity.[32]

More subtle neuropsychologic abnormalities have also been documented in hypothyroid patients and may include impairment of learning, word fluency, and some aspect of attention, visual scanning, and motor speed.[33] Treatment of the hypothyroidism may result in some cognitive improvement. Mood and neuropsychologic function may improve more satisfactorily in hypothyroid patients treated with a combination of thyroxine plus triiodothyronine, rather than thyroxine alone.[34]

Disorders of Sleep

Both obstructive and central sleep apnea may occur in patients with hypothyroidism.[33] Obstructive sleep apnea (OSA) appears to be far more common and epidemiologic studies suggest that while the prevalence of hypothyroidism among subjects with OSA is low ($<3\%$), OSA occurs in over 50 percent of subjects with hypothyroidism.[35] The combination of hypothyroidism and OSA appears to increase the risk of cognitive impairment.[36] Factors contributing to the development of obstructive sleep apnea are likely to include narrowing of the upper airway due to deposition of mucopolysaccharides and extravasation of protein into the tissues of the tongue and nasopharynx, as well as hypertrophy of the genioglossus. Centrally there appears to be reduced chemosensitivity to hypercapnia.[37]

Thyroid hormone replacement therapy usually results in improvement in ventilatory drive following normalization of TSH.[38] Improvement in airway dimensions may require a longer period of euthyroidism (up to 12 months), and only at this stage will nocturnal snoring decrease.[39] In some patients, additional measures such as nasal continuous positive airway pressure may be required.

Cerebellar Ataxia

Reference to unsteadiness of gait may be found in the earliest clinical descriptions of hypothyroidism. Several studies have indicated that approximately 5 to 10 percent of patients with hypothyroidism develop significant ataxia of gait.[40] Typical clinical features include a broad-based ataxic gait, impaired tandem gait, incoordination of the limbs, and, more rarely, cerebellar dysarthria. Rapid and complete or almost complete resolution of the cerebellar features usually occurs following achievement of euthyroidism.

The pathophysiologic basis of cerebellar dysfunction in hypothyroidism remains unknown. The rapid resolution of the ataxia with thyroid replacement therapy in most patients suggests a reversible metabolic factor. Selim and Drachman reported six patients with Hashimoto autoimmune thyroiditis who developed clinical ataxia while euthyroid (three were on oral replacement with L-thyroxine); all had midline cerebellar atrophy on MRI, and alternate causes were excluded. The authors postulated an immune-mediated mechanism of cerebellar degeneration in a subset of patients and suggested that immune suppression may be a therapeutic option for this group.[41] Many patients have had coexisting medical problems, including cerebrovascular disease and alcoholism. Pathologic reports are few, but depletion of Purkinje cells may occur.

Cranial Nerve Disorders

Primary thyroid failure may be associated with pituitary enlargement resulting from hyperplasia due to lack of negative feedback from circulating thyroid hormones. In one recent study, pituitary enlargement on MRI was found in 37 of 53 (70%) patients with primary hypothyroidism.[42] A reduction in pituitary size following treatment occurred in 85 percent of these patients. Visual evoked potentials may be abnormal in hypothyroid patients, but severe visual field loss and blindness are rare. The association between pituitary gland enlargement and primary hypothyroidism should be kept in mind when pituitary hyperplasia is detected on neuroimaging, so that unnecessary invasive interventions are avoided.

Some patients with hypothyroidism develop pseudotumor cerebri (intracranial hypertension) resulting in headache and papilledema after the initiation of thyroxine replacement therapy.[43] An atypical facial pain syndrome may also occur.

Hearing impairment and tinnitus commonly occur in patients with hypothyroidism. Estimations of reduced auditory acuity based on pure-tone audiometry vary but indicate that over half of patients suffer hearing impairment[44] that may originate from the cochlea, central auditory pathways, or the retrocochlear region.[45] Overall, the hearing loss associated with hypothyroidism is thought to be sensorineural in nature and may improve when the hypothyroidism is treated.[44]

Dysphonia in patients with hypothyroidism appears to arise from local myxedematous changes in the larynx rather than from cranial nerve dysfunction.

Hypothyroid Myopathy

Clinical Features

Muscle involvement is common in clinical and subclinical hypothyroidism, with more than 60 percent of patients reported to have an elevated serum CK level.[46] The level of increase correlates with the severity of hypothyroidism and corrects when thyroid function normalizes with treatment. Symptomatic muscle disease is less common. Clinical evidence of hypothyroid myopathy occurs in 30 to 80 percent of patients.[47] A study of clinical and electrophysiologic features prior to commencement of thyroxine therapy revealed that 45 percent of patients with hypothyroidism had decreased or absent deep tendon reflexes, 30 percent had clinical muscle weakness, 15 percent had neuropathy, and 8 percent had evidence of myopathy on electromyography (EMG).[48]

The major clinical features of hypothyroid myopathy include weakness, cramps, aching or painful muscles, sluggish movements and reflexes, and myoedema (mounding of the muscle on direct percussion). There may be a discernible increase in muscle bulk that is most obvious in the tongue, arms, and legs. The degree of weakness is usually relatively mild and tends to involve the pelvic- and shoulder-girdle muscles. The gait tends to be slow and clumsy. Occasionally, patients have been described with more severe myopathic symptoms, including the development of rhabdomyolysis and renal failure[49] or, very rarely, respiratory insufficiency, which may respond to hormone replacement.[50] Muscle pain, particularly during and after exertion, is a prominent feature,[51] and hypothyroidism should be considered in patients presenting with musculoskeletal pains of uncertain cause.

Muscle pain, stiffness, cramps, and delayed relaxation of the tendon reflexes in adult hypothyroidism is sometimes referred to as Hoffmann syndrome. Kocher–Debré–Sémélaigne syndrome is the unusual association of muscle hypertrophy with childhood hypothyroidism. The patient may have the typical clinical features of CH, with the added feature of generalized muscular hypertrophy so that the child has an athletic, almost herculean appearance.

A delay in the relaxation of muscle (pseudomyotonia) is commonly observed during assessment of the tendon reflexes in hypothyroid patients. All phases of the tendon reflex are delayed, although slowing of the relaxation phase is most apparent clinically. Pseudomyotonia differs from true myotonia in that there is reduction in the speed of both the contraction and relaxation phases, and this slowness is not increased after rest or relieved by repeated muscle contractions. EMG does not show the characteristic "dive-bomber" effect seen in true myotonia. In the pseudomyotonia of hypothyroidism, there is a continuous burst of action potentials that begins and terminates abruptly, with firing at a constant rate. Percussion of the muscle commonly causes a slow prolonged mounding effect (myoedema). This event, unlike myotonia, is electrically silent and has been attributed to derangement of intracellular calcium homeostasis.

The differential diagnosis of hypothyroid myopathy includes other causes of painful stiff muscles, such as polymyalgia rheumatica and polymyositis.[52] Attention has been directed to the frequency of neuromuscular symptoms in patients with subclinical hypothyroidism, and the suggestion has been made that such patients should be treated early not only to prevent progression to frank hypothyroidism but also to improve neuromuscular dysfunction.[53]

Investigations

The majority of patients with hypothyroidism have an elevated serum CK level, even when the myopathic features are not clinically obvious. In symptomatic patients, the serum CK level may rise to more than 10 times the upper limit of normal.[54] Due to the patchy nature of the myopathy, neurophysiologic assessment may show no significant abnormalities. However, in up to 30 percent of patients with hypothyroidism, "myopathic" short-duration, low-amplitude, polyphasic motor unit potentials are seen on EMG.[47]

Pathology

In many cases of hypothyroidism, pathologic changes in muscle are subtle and nonspecific. Light microscopy may reveal increased central nuclear counts, type I fiber predominance, or type II fiber atrophy; common abnormalities on electron microscopy are the accumulation of glycogen and lipids, abnormal and increased numbers of mitochondria in perinuclear and subsarcolemmal regions, dilated sarcoplasmic reticulum, and focal myofibrillar degeneration.[55] There may be vacuolation in many large fibers, and crescents of material containing acid mucopolysaccharides may be found beneath the sarcolemmal sheath. Often these changes resolve with thyroxine replacement therapy.

Pathophysiology

Thyroid hormone is intimately linked to carbohydrate metabolism and mitochondrial function and, possibly, to the function of the sarcoplasmic reticulum and intrinsic contractile properties of muscle.[40] However, the structure–function relationships are still incompletely understood, although it is assumed that underlying biochemical changes in hypothyroidism lead to prolongation of the contraction and relaxation phases of muscle activity. Magnetic resonance spectroscopy of hypothyroid muscle shows a low intracellular pH in resting muscle and delayed glycogen breakdown in exercising muscle.[56] In addition, mitochondrial oxidative capacity is reduced in hypothyroidism.[57] Low levels of the mitochondrial transcription factor A (h-mtTFA), a proposed thyroid hormone target, occur in hypothyroid myopathy, and abnormal h-mtTFA turnover may be implicated in mitochondrial alterations in the condition.[58] The decreased responsiveness to adrenergic stimulation and alterations in muscle carbohydrate metabolism may contribute to the impaired ischemic lactate production, weakness, exertional pain, and fatigue occurring in hypothyroidism. Hypothyroidism is associated with changes in myosin, lactate dehydrogenase, and myofibrillar ATPase activity.[40] These changes may underlie the observed slowing of muscle contraction and relaxation. Both protein synthesis and breakdown are reduced in hypothyroidism, resulting in net protein catabolism.

Treatment and Prognosis

The only effective therapy for hypothyroid myopathy is to restore the patient to the euthyroid state. Most patients respond to thyroxine therapy with complete clinical and biochemical recovery; however, some patients require prolonged therapy with thyroxine before they recover from their muscle disorder and some may never regain full function. Serum CK levels correct rapidly with thyroxine replacement therapy.[46] Some patients may develop increased muscle pain and weakness after starting thyroxine replacement, and the short-term addition of corticosteroid therapy may be helpful if this problem arises.

Peripheral Neuropathy

Hypothyroidism may be complicated by the development of entrapment mononeuropathies or a more diffuse peripheral neuropathy.

Entrapment Neuropathy

Evidence of entrapment neuropathy is found in around 35 percent of patients with hypothyroidism.[59] The most common mononeuropathy is carpal tunnel syndrome involving compression of the median nerve at the wrist from deposition of acid mucopolysaccharides in the nerve and surrounding tissues. Surgical decompression for the median nerve entrapment is not usually required in patients with underlying hypothyroidism, as symptoms gradually resolve once euthyroidism is achieved.[60]

Diffuse Peripheral Neuropathy

The peripheral neuropathy of hypothyroidism is usually a relatively mild, predominantly sensory axonal peripheral neuropathy.[47] The symptoms of peripheral neuropathy in patients with hypothyroidism may be masked by more intrusive symptoms. Perhaps for this reason, the reported incidence of peripheral neuropathy has varied widely, ranging from 15 to 60 percent.[61] Skin biopsy studies indicate that damage to small-diameter nerve fibers also occurs; indeed, a minority of patients may have only small-fiber involvement.[61] In patients with a generalized large-fiber neuropathy, severity appears to correlate with the duration of the disease rather than the severity of the biochemical disorder.[40] Multifocal motor neuropathy associated with elevated titers of IgM antibodies against GM1 and responsive to intravenous immunoglobulin therapy has been described in association with Hashimoto thyroiditis.[62]

The pathologic changes described in hypothyroid neuropathy include axonal degeneration, segmental demyelination and deposition of mucopolysaccharides in the endoneurial interstitium and perineurial sheath. Opinions have varied as to whether axonal degeneration or demyelination is the primary pathologic process, but most reports favor a primary axonal pathology.

Miscellaneous Associated Conditions

Myasthenia Gravis

An association between hypothyroidism and myasthenia gravis has been reported, although this is less common than the association with hyperthyroidism. The myasthenic symptoms can appear before, with, or after the development of hypothyroidism, and the severity of the myasthenia may or may not improve following treatment of the hypothyroidism.

Giant Cell Arteritis and Polymyalgia Rheumatica

An association of giant cell arteritis and polymyalgia rheumatica with hypothyroidism has long been appreciated. Clinicians managing such patients should be careful not to misinterpret the musculoskeletal symptoms of hypothyroidism as an exacerbation of previously diagnosed polymyalgia rheumatica.

Hypothyroidism and Anticonvulsant Therapy

Subclinical hypothyroidism may occur in children with epilepsy treated with valproate or carbamazepine therapy.[63] Rare cases of central hypothyroidism believed to be secondary to treatment with oxcarbazepine have been reported.[64] Phenytoin may also impact thyroid function, either by inducing hypothyroidism or by worsening preexisting hypothyroidism.[65] Hypothyroidism also increases the risk of phenytoin toxicity.

NEUROLOGIC COMPLICATIONS OF HYPERTHYROIDISM AND GRAVES DISEASE

There are several potential underlying causes of hyperthyroidism including: (1) Graves disease, (2) excess release of stored hormone during subacute thyroiditis or following thyroid irradiation, (3) uncontrolled hormone formation in single or multinodular goiters (Plummer disease), (4) ingestion of excess thyroid hormone, (5) rare TSH-secreting pituitary tumors, and (6) drug-induced disease. Graves disease is the commonest cause of thyrotoxicosis and occurs with a female-to-male preponderance of 7:1. The neurologic complications of hyperthyroidism are diverse.

Hyperthyroid Myopathy

Clinical Features

Muscle weakness and wasting in patients with thyrotoxicosis were observed in early classic descriptions of the condition. A degree of predominantly proximal muscle weakness probably occurs in almost every patient with hyperthyroidism. The muscle weakness may not always be sufficiently severe for the affected individual to be aware of it. Men appear to develop symptomatic myopathy more commonly than women. The thyroid overactivity can be relatively mild and of long duration, or may be present for only a few weeks before the onset of weakness. A prospective cohort study of patients with newly diagnosed thyroid dysfunction found that 67 percent of hyperthyroid patients had neuromuscular complaints, and 62 percent had objective muscle weakness.[47] In addition, myalgia and elevated serum CK levels have been reported in hyperthyroid patients after commencement of therapy, suggesting that relative hypothyroidism may also contribute to musculoskeletal complaints in previously hyperthyroid patients.[66]

Individuals with thyrotoxic myopathy characteristically complain of difficulty with activities involving use of the shoulder- and pelvic-girdle muscles, such as climbing stairs, rising from a low chair, or performing tasks that involve raising the arms above the head. Muscle pain and stiffness are common associated symptoms, and occasionally patients report severe muscle cramps. Symptomatic weakness of the bulbar musculature resulting in dysphagia and dysarthria is very uncommon in hyperthyroidism and usually follows the development of limb weakness, although there are reports of isolated bulbar dysfunction (sometimes of acute onset) attributed to hyperthyroid myopathy.[67] Bulbar symptoms in hyperthyroid patients may not be due to bulbar myopathy but may have another cause. A large goiter or thymic hyperplasia may physically compress the esophagus, leading to mechanical dysphagia, or compress the recurrent laryngeal nerve, leading to dysphonia. Involvement of the respiratory muscles occurs rarely but may necessitate ventilatory support. Muscle wasting is commonly found on examination of patients and most notably affects proximal girdle muscles such as the deltoid, supraspinatus, and quadriceps muscles. Some patients, especially males, show gluteal muscle wasting, and in some patients winging of the scapula is noticeable. The presence of tremor may create the appearance of muscle fasciculations; this disappears if the limb is relaxed. The tendon reflexes are normal or hyperactive, with shortening of the relaxation phase. Other features of thyrotoxicosis may not be obvious or may be masked, for example, if the patient is on β-blocker therapy.

These neuromuscular features may resemble the progressive muscular atrophy variant of motor neuron disease. The severity of the muscle weakness may be marked, but most patients retain the ability to walk. Acute thyrotoxic myopathy is rare and some have doubted its existence, suggesting that most of the described cases had myasthenia gravis superimposed on the hyperthyroid state. Patients present with muscle weakness progressing rapidly over a few days; weakness may be profound, bulbar muscles are often affected, and the patient may develop respiratory failure. The tendon reflexes may be reduced or absent. Some patients develop an associated encephalopathic state.

In contrast to hypothyroid myopathy, the serum CK level in hyperthyroid myopathy is usually normal or reduced, although rhabdomyolysis and elevation of the serum CK level may occur.[68] EMG abnormalities are found in most patients with thyrotoxicosis and include the typical features of myopathy.

Physiologic and Biochemical Changes in Skeletal Muscle

Skeletal muscle is a major target organ of the thyroid hormones so it is not surprising that the biochemistry, electrophysiology, and even structure of skeletal muscle can be profoundly affected by an excess of thyroid hormone. A detailed examination of this literature is beyond the scope of this review, and more detailed consideration of the subject can be found elsewhere.[69]

Hyperthyroidism affects both the physiologic and the biochemical properties of skeletal muscle with a preferential effect on type I (slow) muscle fibers, shifting their characteristics towards those resembling fast muscle fibers.[70] The speed of muscle contraction is enhanced and its duration is reduced. This effect underlies the clinical observation that the duration of muscle contraction after a deep tendon is struck with a tendon hammer is briefer than normal in the hyperthyroid state and prolonged in the hypothyroid state. The expression of isotypes of the myosin heavy chain is altered in hyperthyroidism to favor expression of MHC type IIX associated with fast-fiber characteristics, with this isoform replacing MHC type I associated with slow-fiber characteristics. These changes reverse on treatment.[71]

The pattern of glycogen utilization and lactate production in muscle is also altered in hyperthyroidism. Using magnetic resonance spectroscopy, Erkintalo and associates found that skeletal muscle was less efficient in hyperthyroidism, requiring more energy to function.[72] At rest, the concentration of phosphocreatine was reduced in thyrotoxic patients compared with controls; at the onset of exercise, the magnitude of glycolysis activation was significantly larger in those with thyrotoxicity, resulting in a marked decrease in pH. The energy cost of exercise was significantly higher in thyrotoxic patients, with greater activation of both anaerobic and aerobic pathways throughout 3 minutes of exercise. The authors concluded that muscle requires more energy to function in the hyperthyroid than euthyroid state. Evidence that in hyperthyroidism the mitochondrial transport chain is uncoupled supports this finding.[73]

Pathology

There is no pathognomonic pathologic finding in hyperthyroid myopathy. Biopsy may be needed on occasion to exclude other pathologic processes. Microscopic examination may show no abnormality or varying degrees of fiber atrophy, fatty infiltration, and nerve terminal damage, with clubbing of the motor end-plate and swelling of terminal axons.[40] Most patients show an increase in mitochondrial size and number in muscle fibers. In addition, features of an inflammatory myositis with a marked endomysial mononuclear cell infiltrate have been reported in a patient with biochemically proven hyperthyroidism and symptoms and signs of hyperthyroid myopathy.[74]

Treatment and Prognosis

Nørrelund and associates undertook a serial study of muscle mass assessed by computed tomography (CT) and isometric muscle strength in patients with thyrotoxicosis before and after treatment.[75] They concluded that in thyrotoxic patients muscle mass is reduced by approximately 20 percent and muscle strength by about 40 percent and that 5 to 9 months will elapse before normal muscle mass and power are restored following treatment. Mean resolution of muscle weakness in one series was 3.6 months in hyperthyroid patients compared to 6.9 months in the hypothyroid group.[47] Dysphagia and dysarthria due to hyperthyroid myopathy also typically resolve after treatment.

Periodic Paralysis

Hypokalemic periodic paralysis as a complication of hyperthyroidism is relatively common in Asian populations, with a reported incidence of about 1.9 percent in those with thyrotoxicosis.[76] The disorder is rare in other ethnic groups but the effects of globalization on population mobility mean that it is now seen more often in other parts of the world. Periodic paralysis may occur in association with hyperthyroidism of any cause, but is most commonly seen in patients with Graves disease.

Clinical Features

Except for concomitant features of thyrotoxicosis, the clinical picture of thyrotoxic periodic paralysis (TPP) is identical to that seen in familial hypokalemic periodic paralysis (FHPP). Males are affected much more commonly than females. Affected individuals develop recurrent attacks of flaccid weakness, which may be asymmetric and affect the lower more than the upper limbs, and the proximal more than the distal muscles. The attacks may be heralded by prodromal symptoms of muscle aching, stiffness, or cramps. The weakness usually develops rapidly and varies in severity from mild weakness to total paralysis. The muscles most vigorously used before an attack tend to be most severely affected. Bulbar, ocular, and respiratory muscles tend to be spared, although there have been occasional reports of respiratory compromise. Cardiac dysrhythmias occasionally accompany the paralytic attacks. Usually, the tendon reflexes are depressed or absent during an attack, but in some patients they remain normal. Weakness usually resolves within 24 hours, but in the wake of severe attacks weakness and muscle pain may persist for several days. Patients may be able to abort impending attacks by mild exercise.

Attacks may occur with or without a triggering factor; recognized precipitants include high carbohydrate intake, strenuous physical activity followed by a period of rest, trauma, cold exposure, infection, menses, and drugs, including amiodarone and corticosteroids.[77] A seasonal pattern of attacks has been recognized, with episodes being more common in the summer months. There is also a characteristic diurnal pattern, with attacks frequently developing during the night while patients are in bed.

The cardinal biochemical abnormality during an attack of TPP is hypokalemia resulting from an intracellular shift in potassium. Although the serum potassium decreases during the attack, it may not always decline below the normal range. Urinary excretion of potassium is reduced with a low potassium–creatinine ratio. The neuromuscular symptoms resolve over a period of hours as potassium moves back to the extracellular space.

Between attacks, a long exercise test may prove a useful diagnostic aid. In this test, a preexercise compound muscle action potential (CMAP) is recorded from a selected muscle. After this, the patient performs maximal voluntary muscle contractions for 5 minutes, with relaxation for 3 to 4 seconds every 15 seconds or so to avoid muscle ischemia. The CMAP is then recorded every 2 minutes until the amplitude of the elicited potential stabilizes. The test is interpreted as positive if the decrement exceeds 40 percent.[78]

The most consistent ultrastructural finding in muscles from patients with thyrotoxic periodic paralysis is a proliferation and focal dilatation of the sarcoplasmic reticulum and transverse tubular system, resulting in the appearance of vacuoles. The vacuoles are characteristically seen in paralyzed muscles and are less apparent between attacks.

Physiology and Pathophysiology

Attacks of weakness in TPP are clinically similar to those of FHPP, a channelopathy caused by inherited defects to genes encoding sodium and calcium channels in skeletal muscle. This phenotypic similarity led investigators to postulate that TPP might also be a channelopathy, albeit one that manifests only in the presence of excess thyroid hormone. It is thought that TPP patients have a genetic predisposition to the disease unmasked by independently occurring hyperthyroidism.

Gene sequencing in cohorts of largely Asian TPP patients has revealed no mutations in FHPP-causing genes, or in components of the sodium-potassium ATPase (Na^+,K^+-ATPase) pump.[79] Recently six different mutations to an inwardly rectifying potassium channel, Kir2.6, expressed strongly in skeletal muscle, were found in 33 percent of an unrelated cohort of TPP patients from the United States, Brazil, and France, 25 percent of a Singaporean cohort, but none of 31 patients from Thailand.[80] The mutations discovered all had effects upon the stability of the muscle cell membrane, altering its excitability. The gene for Kir2.6 is transcriptionally regulated by thyroid hormone and levels of the channel are increased in hyperthyroidism, explaining why it is only in this circumstance that the mutation becomes manifest. A susceptibility locus has been identified near the gene for Kir2.1, which is also highly expressed in skeletal muscle and can associate with other K^+ channels, including Kir2.6[81]; incorporation of Kir2.6 into the channel heterotetramer reduces the abundance of Kir2-type channels on the plasma membrane with consequences for membrane excitability.[82]

Mutations in potassium channels appear to combine with other factors to produce the clinical phenotype. Thyroid hormones increase the activity of the Na^+,K^+-ATPase, which drives K^+ into cells; catecholamines have a similar effect.[83] The Na^+,K^+-ATPase pump is also stimulated by insulin, hence attacks may be precipitated by carbohydrate-rich meals and exercise. In addition, testosterone appears to drive the Na^+,K^+-ATPase pump, while estogren and progesterone reduce activity, perhaps explaining the male preponderance.[84] Interestingly, men with TPP have higher levels of testosterone than men with a sole diagnosis of thyrotoxicosis.[85] These effects on the Na^+,K^+-ATPase pump sum together to increase the intracellular K^+ concentration and as the efflux usually permitted by outwardly rectifying K^+ channels is reduced, a paradoxic depolarization occurs inactivating Na^+ channels. As a result the hypokalemia seen in attacks of weakness in TPP is not due to loss of potassium, but rather to the shift of extracellular potassium into cells driven by the Na^+,K^+-ATPase pump, which has direct implications for treatment.

Treatment

First, emergency treatments of the attack of weakness, hypokalemia, and any complications are required. TPP patients presenting with severe weakness are treated with potassium chloride to speed recovery. Urgent assessment of cardiac and respiratory involvement must be carried out and appropriate supportive management and monitoring instituted pending recovery. Potassium chloride may be administered orally or intravenously until weakness resolves. Mid-attack, TPP patients do not have a potassium deficit but rather an intracellular shift of their potassium. There is therefore a risk of rebound hyperkalemia on recovery as the potassium shift reverses. In one study patients given potassium recovered twice as fast as untreated patients, but 70 percent experienced rebound hyperkalemia.[86] In practice this is rarely of clinical importance but most authorities recommend giving lower doses of potassium (<50 mEq total). Potassium chloride does not always abort an attack of weakness in TPP. In cases of refractory weakness, propranolol administered intravenously or orally may be effective.[87]

Patients should also be educated about TPP and its precipitants in order to prevent further attacks. They should avoid food and drink with high salt or carbohydrate content as well as alcohol. Formal exercise is best halted until the patient is euthyroid. Propranolol (40 mg daily) reduces the likelihood of further attacks until the euthyroid state is regained. Finally, definitive treatment of the hyperthyroidism and return of the patient to the euthyroid state stop further attacks of weakness altogether although, depending upon the underlying cause, it may take months for the euthyroid state to be achieved.

Myasthenia Gravis

A long-recognized association exists between thyroid disease and myasthenia gravis. There is no evidence that thyroid dysfunction causes myasthenia gravis, and the coexistence of the two conditions probably reflects an underlying predisposition to autoimmune disease. A study of over 2,000 patients with myasthenia gravis reported hyperthyroidism in 5 percent of patients (2% had hypothyroidism).[88] Hyperthyroidism was diagnosed before or concurrent with the onset of myasthenia in 73.8 percent and after myasthenia in 18.3 percent; the exact time was unknown in 7.9 percent. Patients who were hyperthyroid were more likely to have ocular myasthenia (63%). In general, there are few unusual characteristics of either condition in terms of clinical features or management when the two occur in the same patient. However, Marinó and colleagues, in a study of 129 patients with myasthenia gravis, of whom 56 had autoimmune thyroid disease (25 with autoimmune thyroiditis and 31 with Graves disease), concluded that myasthenia associated with autoimmune thyroid disease has a mild clinical expression, with preferential ocular involvement, a lower frequency of thymic disease, and less likelihood of detectable acetylcholine receptor antibodies in the serum.[89]

While control of the myasthenia may deteriorate with departure from the euthyroid state, treatment of the thyroid disorder does not have a predictable effect on the myasthenia. Dramatic increases in the severity of myasthenia have been reported following treatment of the thyroid disease, but this is uncommon. In some patients, an improvement in myasthenic weakness occurs after treatment of hyperthyroidism.

Peripheral Neuropathy

Peripheral neuropathy is rarely associated with hyperthyroidism, in contrast to its relatively common association with hypothyroidism. As a result, the pathophysiologic basis of any peripheral nerve dysfunction in hyperthyroidism is unclear, although one report has described a severe subacute motor axonal neuropathy induced by T3 hyperthyroidism and reversible on control of the hyperthyroid state.[90]

Mononeuropathies associated with hyperthyroidism are also relatively rare. Up to 5 percent of patients may have clinical and neurophysiologic features of carpal tunnel syndrome, the symptoms of which often resolve once control of the thyroid disease is achieved.[91]

A rare acute thyrotoxic peripheral neuropathy resembling Guillain–Barré syndrome and causing paraplegia was first described by Charcot and termed Basedow paraplegia by Joffroy. The syndrome is acute in onset and presents as a flaccid, areflexic paraplegia with upper limbs much less affected than the lower limbs. There is sensory involvement in some cases and sphincter function is typically preserved. Electrophysiologic examination reveals a mixed sensorimotor peripheral neuropathy with demyelinating and axonal features; ultrastructural analysis in one case with sural nerve biopsy demonstrated axonal loss and myelin damage.[92] Treatment resulted in a largely full recovery.

Corticospinal Tract Dysfunction

Signs of corticospinal tract dysfunction may be associated with thyrotoxicosis. Clinical features include spasticity and weakness, particularly affecting the lower limbs, as well as hyperreflexia, clonus at the ankles and knees, and extensor plantar responses. Occasionally, patients with upper motor neuron signs in the limbs also have had sensory abnormalities, including impaired vibration sensation and proprioception, upper motor neuron bladder disturbance, and urinary incontinence. A clinical picture similar to that of motor neuron disease has also been reported in patients with untreated hyperthyroidism.[93] Treatment of the hyperthyroid state usually results in complete or near-complete recovery of the upper motor neuron signs.

A neurophysiologic correlate of these observations has been documented through studies on central motor conduction using transcranial magnetic stimulation of the motor cortex.[94] The mean central motor conduction time was significantly prolonged in the hyperthyroid group compared with a control group. Further histopathologic and neurochemical studies are required to define the pathophysiologic basis of corticospinal tract dysfunction in thyrotoxicosis.

Movement Disorders

Chorea

Chorea is an unusual complication of hyperthyroidism and its association with the condition is not universally accepted. Some authors suggest that it is simply an exaggeration of the fidgetiness seen in thyrotoxicosis whereas others believe that hyperthyroidism unmasks preexisting and subclinical basal ganglia dysfunction. The problem appears to be more common in women, and the underlying cause of the hyperthyroidism is most commonly Graves disease. Choreiform movements typically involve the limbs, with the face, neck, or tongue affected in some cases. There are case reports of hemichorea and bilateral ballism associated with thyrotoxicosis.[95,96] The chorea usually resolves once hyperthyroidism has been controlled, but there are reports of it persisting long after euthyroidism has been achieved.[95]

The pathophysiologic basis of hyperthyroid chorea is unknown. Given that most cases occur in autoimmune hyperthyroidism, many have assumed that the associated chorea also has an autoimmune basis. It has been suggested that chorea may be mediated by the sympathetic nervous system because β-blockers may help in controlling symptoms. A disruption of striatial dopamine receptors may have some role and dopamine receptor antagonists, such as haloperidol, have been effective in the treatment of hyperthyroid chorea.[97] Cases in which chorea develops when a patient is hyperthyroid, resolves on treatment, and then recurs when the patient once more becomes hyperthyroid due to, for instance, poor compliance, lend support to the idea that the chorea is a direct effect of high levels of thyroid hormone on the function of the basal ganglia. This contention is supported by a single case report of chorea associated with iatrogenic hyperthyroidism due to overtreatment of hypothyroidism in an elderly woman.[98]

Tremor

Tremor is almost invariably seen in hyperthyroidism, so is best considered a feature of the hyperthyroid state rather than a neurologic complication. The tremor seen in thyrotoxicosis can be considered an exaggerated physiologic tremor.[99] It is postural, persists on movement (but is not present at rest), and has a frequency of 8 to 12 Hz. The tremor most commonly affects the outstretched hands and the tongue, but the lips and facial muscles may also be affected. Therapy with β-blockers provides relief, suggesting that increased β-adrenergic activity is likely to be responsible.

Other Movement Disorders

Case reports have described several other movement disorders in patients with hyperthyroidism including platysmal myoclonus and paroxysmal kinesogenic dyskinesia.[100,101]

Thyroid-Associated Ophthalmopathy

Graves disease is an autoimmune condition in which antibodies to thyrotropin receptors are generated and bind to their antigen on follicular cells in the thyroid gland, inducing them to produce and release excess thyroid hormone, which causes hyperthyroidism. It is associated with two main extrathyroid complications: thyroid dermopathy (also known as pretibial myxedema) and thyroid-associated ophthalmopathy. Thyroid-associated ophthalmopathy, sometimes called Graves ophthalmopathy, is a potentially disfiguring and sight-threatening complication most commonly occurring in patients with hyperthyroidism due to Graves disease, or who have a past history of hyperthyroid Graves disease. While present in around 50 percent of patients, only 3 to 5 percent of those with Graves disease have severe, sight-threatening ophthalmopathy requiring aggressive therapeutic intervention.[102] Graves ophthalmopathy is generally managed by ophthalmologists. Patients do, however, present to neurologists with complaints of visual loss or diplopia, and a summary focusing on these neurologic presentations and diagnosis therefore follows. More detailed descriptions can be found elsewhere.[103]

Clinical Features

Symptoms and signs of Graves ophthalmopathy are usually bilateral and begin within 18 months of the onset of Graves hyperthyroidism. Ophthalmopathy in Graves disease may uncommonly appear to be unilateral (5 to 14%), although in these cases orbital imaging usually identifies subclinical involvement of the clinically unaffected eye. The onset of ophthalmopathy may precede the development of hyperthyroidism and may also develop some years after Graves disease has been diagnosed and treated.[104] Whether Graves ophthalmopathy may be induced or existing eye disease worsened by radioiodine treatment for hyperthyroidism remains contentious.[105,106] Smoking is clearly an independent and modifiable risk factor, and the more cigarettes smoked, the greater is the risk.[107] Patients with Graves hyperthyroidism who smoke carry a 7.7-fold increased risk for development of ophthalmopathy. The group at most risk appears to be patients treated with radioiodine who also smoke.[108]

The majority of ocular symptoms and signs in Graves ophthalmopathy are the result of an increase in the amount of cushioning fat within the orbit and an enlargement of the extraocular muscles. Patients complain of a sensation of grittiness in the eyes, photophobia, and pressure or pain behind the eyes. The commonest features of Graves ophthalmopathy are periorbital and conjunctival edema and erythema (secondary to compression of orbital veins and resultant venous stasis), retraction of the upper eyelid (due to overactive sympathetic activity), and proptosis due to the increased volume of orbital contents (Fig. 18-1). If proptosis is severe, ptosis may occur. Proptosis is defined as measured exophthalmos greater than 2 mm above the upper normal limit. It is found in approximately 20 to 30 percent of patients with Graves disease. Proptosis serves to decompress the orbit—visual loss due to compressive optic neuropathy occurs more often in those with little or no compensatory proptosis. Apart from any cosmetic problems associated with proptosis, failure of the eyelids to close completely may result in sight-threatening exposure keratopathy.

Extraocular muscle involvement leading to ophthalmoparesis is clinically apparent in 10 to 15 percent of patients with Graves hyperthyroidism. Orbital imaging demonstrates enlargement

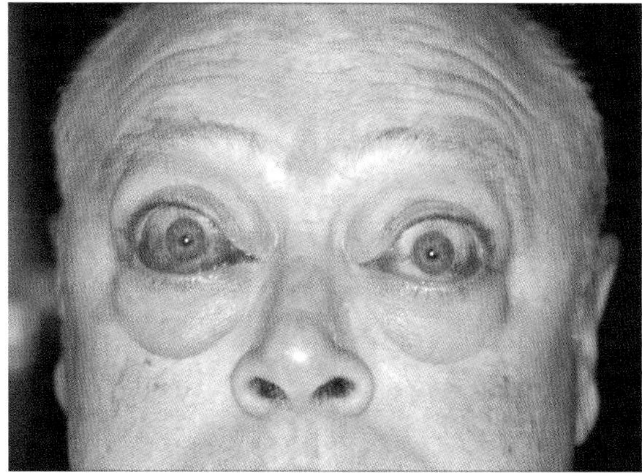

FIGURE 18-1 ▪ Fifty-year-old man with thyroid eye disease, showing periorbital edema, conjunctival injection, proptosis, and eyelid retraction. (Courtesy of Jonathan Horton, MD, PhD.)

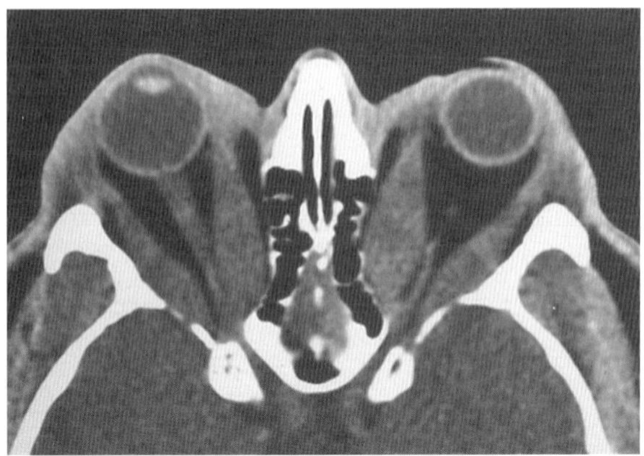

FIGURE 18-2 ■ Axial computed tomographic scan of the patient in Fig. 18-1, showing massive enlargement of the horizontal rectus muscles and soft tissue edema in each orbit, causing compression of the optic nerves. (Courtesy of Jonathan Horton, MD, PhD.)

of the extraocular muscles in 60 to 98 percent of these patients (Fig. 18-2). Patients may complain of blurred vision with binocular gaze, diplopia that may be continuous or intermittent, or a pulling sensation on attempted upgaze. For reasons that are not understood, there is preferential involvement of the inferior and medial rectus muscles.

Optic nerve compression occurs in fewer than 5 percent of patients with Graves disease.[109] It results from apical crowding of the orbit due to enlargement of the extraocular muscles and excess orbital connective tissue. Early recognition is important to prevent loss of vision. A recent review highlighted the fact that dysthyroid optic neuropathy may not be accompanied by proptosis and orbital inflammation and that the most useful diagnostic criteria are optic disc swelling, impaired color vision, and radiologic evidence of optic nerve compression.[110]

Diagnostic Tools

Diagnosis is largely clinical based on clinical features, with orbital imaging used to confirm the diagnosis and exclude other entities, especially in apparently unilateral cases. As levels of antithyrotropin antibody correlate with disease severity, these should be measured and thyroid function tests performed. In patients with Graves orbitopathy, MRI is the imaging modality of choice and can reveal disease activity through interstitial edema within the extraocular muscles.[111] The presence of such observations, rather than the fibrotic changes associated with end-stage disease, may direct treatments towards immunomodulatory therapies. MRI may also be used to assess response to such interventions. By contrast, CT is suited to the assessment of bony periorbital structures and is thus the technique of choice for planning of CT-guided orbital decompression surgery.[111] Amplitude reduction on pattern electroretinogram may be a sensitive measure for demonstrating early impairment of optic nerve function, as may measurements of visual evoked potentials.[112]

Pathogenesis

Although significant progress has been made in understanding the pathogenesis of Graves ophthalmopathy, there remain a number of contentious issues and unanswered questions.[103] Environmental and immunogenetic factors are both likely to play a role. It is widely accepted that antithyrotropin antibodies are pathogenic in Graves ophthalmopathy and that their target within the eye is orbital fibroblasts, which express the thyrotropin receptor to a greater extent than do orbital fibroblasts in unaffected subjects.[113] Interaction of these pathogenic antibodies with thyrotropin receptors triggers an inflammatory cascade within the orbit, resulting in the expansion of orbital adipose tissue. Antithyrotropin antibodies are not the only pathogenic antibodies in Graves ophthalmopathy. The best supported of several additional candidates are antibodies to insulin-like growth factor-1. It seems likely that many of the other antibodies detected in Graves ophthalmopathy will turn out to be secondary markers of the orbital immune-mediated reaction rather than pathogenic effectors.

Treatment

A consensus statement on the management of thyroid-associated ophthalmopathy was released in 2008 and has been addressed in review articles.[103,114] In summary, there is currently no recommended preventive therapy and the condition is usually only treated when symptoms are severe or vision is threatened. In ophthalmopathy where there is evidence of active inflammation, corticosteroids and orbital radiotherapy may be used. Sight-threatening keratopathy due to proptosis and optic neuropathy due to apical crowding are treated surgically with orbital decompression. Some authorities use a 3-month course of corticosteroids starting immediately after radioiodine treatment to prevent development or exacerbation of Graves ophthalmopathy. Whether such treatment is effective remains unclear, and the literature is contradictory.[115,116] Treatment of dysthyroid strabismus is surgical once Graves disease has burnt out and the ophthalmoparesis is stable. Prism glasses are an alternative in those preferring not to undergo surgery. During the active phase of the disease, botulinum toxin may also be used to improve strabismus. A number of new immunomodulatory therapies have been suggested for use in Graves ophthalmopathy.[103]

Encephalopathy

Florid thyrotoxic encephalopathy, sometimes referred to as "thyroid storm," is seen less often now that active monitoring and treatment of hyperthyroidism is undertaken. Its clinical features and treatment have been well reviewed.[117] Thyroid storm is thought to make up 1 to 2 percent of thyroid-related admissions to hospital. Precipitating factors include radioactive iodine therapy, surgery (either thyroid or nonthyroid), trauma, pregnancy, and intercurrent illness. While there is no consensus definition of what constitutes thyroid storm, four groups of symptoms dominate the clinical picture—fever, tachycardia, CNS dysfunction, and gastrointestinal symptoms. Fever is high and associated with profound sweating. Patients may develop supraventricular tachyarrythmias including atrial fibrillation with consequent cardiac failure or embolic stroke. Diarrhea and vomiting are common, and patients may develop jaundice. Biochemically, thyroid storm may be indistinguishable from uncomplicated thyrotoxicosis, making its diagnosis a clinical one. CNS symptoms may be prominent. Affected individuals are commonly confused or agitated and may present with frank psychosis.[118] The patient's level of consciousness may deteriorate, with the development of coma sometimes associated with seizures, bulbar weakness, and corticospinal tract signs.[40] Status epilepticus has been reported.[119]

The mortality of thyroid storm remains over 10 percent, so patients should be managed in an intensive care unit.[120] Successful treatment depends on early recognition and aggressive intervention. Treatment is aimed at: (1) reducing production and secretion of thyroid hormones by the thyroid gland, for which antithyroid medication and sometimes iodine are used; (2) reducing the effects of the excess thyroid hormone on target organs in the periphery using β-blockade; (3) reversing systemic problems such as fever and cardiovascular compromise; and (4) treating any precipitating factor such as systemic infection. Administration of corticosteroids is suggested in recognition of adrenal axis dysfunction.[121] Plasmapheresis has been employed occasionally to reduce levels of thyroid hormone.[122]

Seizures

Seizures are a relatively frequent complication of metabolic encephalopathy in general, but are not commonly seen as a complication of thyrotoxicosis. A retrospective analysis of over 3,000 patients diagnosed with hyperthyroidism revealed that only 0.2 percent experienced seizures not attributable to other causes.[123] In these instances, generalized tonic-clonic events were most common. The cause of the hyperthyroidism appears not to be important, and seizures have even been reported in the context of hypothyroidism overtreated with thyroxine.[124] The etiology of thyrotoxic seizures is unknown.

A range of nonspecific EEG abnormalities may be seen in patients with hyperthyroidism, including generalized slow activity and an excess of fast activity.[123] EEG changes usually improve when the thyrotoxic state is controlled.

Mental and Psychiatric Disorders

Minor mental disturbances are almost uniformly found in patients presenting with untreated hyperthyroidism. Complaints of insomnia and impairment of concentration and attention are common. Patients' relatives frequently describe irritability, emotional lability, and capricious behavior. Several types of more serious neuropsychologic disturbances have been described, which usually resolve with successful treatment of the hyperthyroidism.[125] Agitated delirium, presenting with confusion, restlessness, hyperkinesia, and an apathetic state with lethargy and depression may occur in thyrotoxic patients. Both psychosis and affective disorders have been described, and there is a significant overlap between symptoms of hyperthyroidism and of depression-anxiety.[126,127] Engum and associates, in contrast, assessed the thyroid status and self-rating of depression and anxiety of 589 adults and found no significant association between thyroid dysfunction and the presence of a depressive or anxiety disorder.[128] It is important to be alert to the possible psychiatric manifestations of thyroid dysfunction and to reassess patients once they become euthyroid.

Stroke

The association between thyroid disease and stroke has been thoroughly reviewed elsewhere.[129] Atrial fibrillation may develop in 10 to 15 percent of patients with hyperthyroidism and it has been suggested that 10 to 40 percent of patients with thyrotoxic atrial fibrillation have embolic events, the majority of which are cerebral.[130] Whether thyrotoxic patients in atrial fibrillation have a higher embolic risk than euthyroid patients with chronic atrial fibrillation is uncertain. Sheu and associates followed over 3,000 young hyperthyroid patients (aged 18 to 44 years) for 5 years and compared the incidence of ischemic stroke with a large cohort of euthyroid controls.[131] Although the absolute risk of stroke in both groups was small (1.0% of hyperthyroid patients vs. 0.6% of controls), after controlling for confounders such as atrial fibrillation, age, hypertension, and diabetes, an increased risk of ischemic stroke was found in the hyperthyroid patients.

Evidence for associations between hyperthyroidism and rarer causes of stroke is sparse. The possible link between moyamoya syndrome and hyperthyroidism continues, and recent studies have demonstrated elevated thyroid function and thyroid antibodies in moyamoya patients relative to control subjects.[132]

Hashimoto Encephalopathy

Hashimoto encephalopathy (HE) is a relatively rare condition arising as a complication of Hashimoto thyroiditis. In Hashimoto thyroiditis, an antibody-mediated attack on the thyroid gland eventually brings about hypothyroidism although there may be an initial, transient hyperthyroidism and a period of intervening euthyroidism. HE typically occurs in patients with Hashimoto thyroiditis who are hypothyroid or euthyroid but it can, less often, occur in hyperthyroid patients. For this reason, HE is not believed to be a consequence of the patient's thyroid status. Numerous case studies of HE exist as well as a few small case series.[133–135] The rarity of the disorder and the absence of consensus diagnostic criteria mean that qualifying clinical features and even the existence of HE as an entity are ongoing subjects of debate.

Clinical Features

Clinical features of HE include relapsing episodes of encephalopathy, seizures, and sometimes superimposed stroke-like neurologic deficits. The encephalopathy ranges from confusion to coma with an acute or subacute onset, but it may also present insidiously as gradual cognitive decline; in adults it may be confused with dementia, and in children it can manifest as a falling-off of school performance.[136,137] Seizures in HE may be focal or generalized, and status epilepticus can occur.[138,139] Patients have high levels of antithyroid antibodies and the episodes are responsive to treatment with corticosteroids.

Patients with HE are usually euthyroid but may be hypothyroid. Cases of encephalopathy with antithyroid antibodies, an abnormal EEG, and hyperthyroidism have also been reported and are termed *thyrotoxic Hashimoto thyroiditis.*[140] Women are affected by HE more than men—81 percent in one series of 85 adult patients.[135] The typical age of onset is around 40 years but the condition has been reported in children as young as 9 years of age.[141] The encephalopathy is generally accepted as essential for a diagnosis of HE to be contemplated but there is less agreement about associated features. Cases of HE featuring aphasia, ataxia, myoclonus, tremor, headache, psychosis, and visual hallucinations have all been reported.

Pathophysiology

The presence of antithyroid antibodies is a prerequisite for the diagnosis of HE, but it remains unclear whether these antibodies are pathogenetic effectors or simply proxy markers of the disease. The fact that antithyroid antibodies are associated with diverse and unrelated conditions and are found in a proportion of the healthy population argues against a direct role. Few reports have found HE-specific CNS epitopes to which antithyroid antibodies bind. Antithyroid peroxidase antibodies were found to bind to cerebellar astrocytes in HE but not Hashimoto thyroiditis, although the significance of this finding is unclear.[142] The presence of lymphocytic infiltration of CNS vessels has been reported,[143] implying that the disorder invokes a vasculitic process, but the largely favorable outcome of this rare condition means that few cases come to autopsy when the condition is active.[143]

Diagnosis

Differential Diagnosis

The lack of clear diagnostic criteria and the variety of neurologic symptoms and signs reported in addition to encephalopathy mean that HE should be considered in the differential diagnosis of all cases of encephalopathy in which an alternative explanation is not quickly evident. Although HE is rare, it is treatable; thyroid antibodies therefore should be checked as part of the standard laboratory evaluation of encephalopathy. In a series of 20 patients with a final diagnosis of HE, all were initially given another diagnosis including dementia, encephalitis, stroke, Creutzfeld–Jacob disease, and migraine.[133]

Antithyroid Antibodies

Antibodies directed against thyroid antigens are a defining feature of HE. Despite this, there is little consensus about which antithyroid antibodies are associated with HE and whether they have a role in pathogenesis. Antithyroid peroxidase (anti-TPO) antibodies are raised in almost all cases of HE. They are also raised in other nonthyroid autoimmune disorders and in some healthy controls. Antibodies against thyroglobulin (anti-TG) are often found in cases of HE but less commonly than are anti-TPO antibodies. Anti-TG antibodies are also found in a proportion of healthy subjects without thyroid disease. Anti-α-enolase antibodies have also been found in the serum of some patients with HE.[144]

Other Diagnostic Tests

Cerebrospinal Fluid

The most common finding in HE is a raised protein concentration although a mild pleocytosis and, independently, oligoclonal bands (not present in serum) or an elevated IgG index are also common.

Imaging

Although CT of the brain is typically normal, MRI in HE has shown diffuse white matter abnormalities in up to half of patients, and these may resolve with treatment. A variety of other abnormalities have been reported in individual cases, but no HE-defining abnormality has been identified.[133] The few reports of single photon emission computed tomography in HE document focal hypoperfusion, generalized hypoperfusion, or no abnormalities at all. Cerebral angiography is generally normal, showing no evidence of large-vessel vasculopathy.

Electroencephalography

Most patients have an abnormal EEG.[135] Generalized slowing is the commonest abnormality, but triphasic waves and periodic complexes have also been reported. No HE-specific EEG features have been identified.

Treatment

There is reasonable evidence that the vast majority of episodes of HE respond to treatment with corticosteroids. Of the 85 cases in one series, 98 percent responded to corticosteroids alone, whereas only 67 percent of those treated solely with levothyroxine improved.[135] Plasmapheresis has also been effective, including in cases resistant to corticosteroids.[145] Treated, the prognosis of HE is generally good. It is therefore sensible to consider a trial of corticosteroids in an encephalopathic patient with antithyroid antibodies and no other obvious underlying cause, once CNS infection has been excluded.

MISCELLANEOUS ASSOCIATIONS BETWEEN NEUROLOGIC DISORDERS AND THYROID DYSFUNCTION

Endocrine Dysfunction in Long-Term Survivors of Primary Brain Tumors

Endocrine dysfunction, including hypothyroidism, is a frequent and often overlooked long-term complication of radiotherapy for primary brain tumors, with a significant impact on the well-being of patients. In one case series, 26 percent of patients had evidence of hypothalamic hypothyroidism. Hypothalamic hypogonadism in males and hyperprolactinemia and oligomenorrhea in female patients were also reported.[146] Endocrine function should therefore be evaluated periodically in long-term survivors of primary brain tumors treated with radiotherapy.

Multiple Sclerosis and Thyroid Disease

A controlled prospective study evaluating the prevalence of thyroid disease in patients with multiple sclerosis found that thyroid disorders were at least three times more common in women with multiple sclerosis than in female control subjects, mainly due to an increase in the prevalence of hypothyroidism.[147] Recent reports have also documented thyroid-related complications in patients treated with alemtuzumab, which alters the immune response from the Th1 phenotype, suppressing disease activity in multiple sclerosis but permitting the generation of antibody-mediated thyroid disease.[148,149]

Recurrent Laryngeal Nerve Palsy

Both malignant disease of the thyroid gland and thyroidectomy may be associated with hoarseness and other bulbar symptoms due to damage of the recurrent laryngeal nerve.[150,151] Invasion of the recurrent laryngeal nerve by thyroid carcinoma can be accurately predicted by the finding of effaced fatty tissue on MR imaging.[150]

REFERENCES

1. Attia J, Margetts P, Guyatt G: Diagnosis of thyroid disease in hospitalized patients: a systematic review. Arch Intern Med 159:658, 1999.
2. Gaitonde DY, Rowley KD, Sweeney LB: Hypothyroidism: an update. Am Fam Physician 86:244, 2012.
3. Klett M: Epidemiology of congenital hypothyroidism. Exp Clin Endocrinol Diabetes 105(Suppl 4):19, 1997.
4. Halpern JP, Boyages SC, Maberly GF, et al: The neurology of endemic cretinism. A study of two endemias. Brain 114:825, 1991.
5. Wheeler SM, Willoughby KA, McAndrews MP, et al: Hippocampal size and memory functioning in children and adolescents with congenital hypothyroidism. J Clin Endocrinol Metab 96:E1427, 2011.
6. LaFranchi SH, Austin J: How should we be treating children with congenital hypothyroidism? J Pediatr Endocrinol Metab 20:559, 2007.
7. Chen C, Zhou Z, Zhong M, et al: Thyroid hormone promotes neuronal differentiation of embryonic neural stem cells by inhibiting STAT3 signaling through TRα1. Stem Cells Dev 21:2667, 2012.
8. Sánchez-Alonso JL, Sánchez-Aguilera A, Vicente-Torres MA, et al: Intrinsic excitability is altered by hypothyroidism in the developing hippocampal CA1 pyramidal cells. Neuroscience 207:37, 2012.
9. Ma T, Lian ZC, Qi SP, et al: Magnetic resonance imaging of brain and the neuromotor disorder in endemic cretinism. Ann Neurol 34:91, 1993.
10. Ghosh S, Rahaman SO, Sarkar PK: Regulation of neurofilament gene expression by thyroid hormone in the developing rat brain. Neuroreport 10:2361, 1999.
11. Vega-Núñez E, Menéndez-Hurtado A, Garesse R, et al: Thyroid hormone-regulated brain mitochondrial genes revealed by differential cDNA cloning. J Clin Invest 96:893, 1995.
12. Bruno AN, Ricachenevsky FK, Pochmann D, et al: Hypothyroidism changes adenine nucleotide hydrolysis in synaptosomes from hippocampus and cerebral cortex of rats in different phases of development. Int J Dev Neurosci 23:37, 2005.
13. Farwell AP, Dubord-Tomasetti SA: Thyroid hormone regulates the expression of laminin in the developing rat cerebellum. Endocrinology 140:4221, 1999.
14. Djemli A, Van Vliet G, Delvin EE: Congenital hypothyroidism: from paracelsus to molecular diagnosis. Clin Biochem 39:511, 2006.
15. Rastogi MV, LaFranchi SH: Congenital hypothyroidism. Orphanet J Rare Dis 5:17, 2010.
16. Macchia PE, Lapi P, Krude H, et al: PAX8 mutations associated with congenital hypothyroidism caused by thyroid dysgenesis. Nat Genet 19:83, 1998.
17. Krude H, Schutz B, Biebermann H, et al: Choreoathetosis, hypothyroidism, and pulmonary alterations due to human NKX2-1 haploinsufficiency. J Clin Invest 109:475, 2002.
18. Bakker B, Bikker H, Vulsma T, et al: Two decades of screening for congenital hypothyroidism in The Netherlands: TPO gene mutations in total iodide organification defects (an update). J Clin Endocrinol Metab 85:3708, 2000.
19. Dumitrescu AM, Liao XH, Best TB, et al: A novel syndrome combining thyroid and neurological abnormalities is associated with mutations in a monocarboxylate transporter gene. Am J Hum Genet 74:168, 2004.
20. Nicoloff JT, LoPresti JS: Myxedema coma. A form of decompensated hypothyroidism. Endocrinol Metab Clin North Am 22:279, 1993.
21. Mathew V, Misgar RA, Ghosh S, et al: Myxedema coma: a new look into an old crisis. J Thyroid Res 2011: 493462, 2011.
22. Kwaku MP, Burman KD: Myxedema coma. J Intensive Care Med 22:224, 2007.
23. Dutta P, Bhansali A, Masoodi SR, et al: Predictors of outcome in myxoedema coma: a study from a tertiary care centre. Crit Care 12:R1, 2008.
24. Kramer U, Achiron A: Drop attacks induced by hypothyroidism. Acta Neurol Scand 88:410, 1993.
25. Rocco M, Pro S, Alessandri E, et al: Nonconvulsive status epilepticus induced by acute hypothyroidism in a critically ill patient. Intensive Care Med 37:553, 2011.

26. Bunevicius R, Prange Jr AJ: Thyroid disease and mental disorders: cause and effect or only comorbidity? Curr Opin Psychiatry 23:363, 2010.
27. Azzopardi L, Murfin C, Sharda A, et al: Myxoedema madness. BMJ Case Rep 2010.
28. Kilzieh N, Akiskal HS: Rapid-cycling bipolar disorder. An overview of research and clinical experience. Psychiatr Clin North Am 22:585, 1999.
29. Cole DP, Thase ME, Mallinger AG, et al: Slower treatment response in bipolar depression predicted by lower pretreatment thyroid function. Am J Psychiatry 159:116, 2002.
30. Heinrich TW, Grahm G: Hypothyroidism presenting as psychosis: myxedema madness revisited. Prim Care Companion J Clin Psychiatry 5:260, 2003.
31. Mowla A, Kalantarhormozi MR, Khazraee S: Clinical characteristics of patients with major depressive disorder with and without hypothyroidism: a comparative study. J Psychiatr Pract 17:67, 2011.
32. Dugbartey AT: Neurocognitive aspects of hypothyroidism. Arch Intern Med 158:1413, 1998.
33. Osterweil D, Syndulko K, Cohen SN, et al: Cognitive function in non-demented older adults with hypothyroidism. J Am Geriatr Soc 40:325, 1992.
34. Bunevicius R, Kazanavicius G, Zalinkevicius R, et al: Effects of thyroxine as compared with thyroxine plus triiodothyronine in patients with hypothyroidism. N Engl J Med 340:424, 1999.
35. Rosenow F, McCarthy V, Caruso AC: Sleep apnoea in endocrine diseases. J Sleep Res 7:3, 1998.
36. Lal C, Strange C, Bachman D: Neurocognitive impairment in obstructive sleep apnea. Chest 141:1601, 2012.
37. Duranti R, Gheri RG, Gorini M, et al: Control of breathing in patients with severe hypothyroidism. Am J Med 95:29, 1993.
38. Jha A, Sharma SK, Tandon N, et al: Thyroxine replacement therapy reverses sleep-disordered breathing in patients with primary hypothyroidism. Sleep Med 7:55, 2006.
39. Lin CC, Tsan KW, Chen PJ: The relationship between sleep apnea syndrome and hypothyroidism. Chest 102:1663, 1992.
40. Burness CE, Shaw PJ: Thyroid disease and the nervous system. p. 357. In Aminof MJ (ed): Neurology and General Medicine. 4th Ed. Elsevier Churchill Livingstone, Philadelphia, 2008.
41. Selim M, Drachman DA: Ataxia associated with Hashimoto's disease: progressive non-familial adult onset cerebellar degeneration with autoimmune thyroiditis. J Neurol Neurosurg Psychiatry 71:81, 2001.
42. Khawaja NM, Taher BM, Barham ME, et al: Pituitary enlargement in patients with primary hypothyroidism. Endocr Pract 12:29, 2006.
43. Raghavan S, DiMartino-Nardi J, Saenger P, et al: Pseudotumor cerebri in an infant after L-thyroxine therapy for transient neonatal hypothyroidism. J Pediatr 130:478, 1997.
44. Malik V, Shukla GK, Bhatia N: Hearing profile in hypothyroidism. Indian J Otolaryngol Head Neck Surg 54:285, 2002.
45. Santos KT, Dias NH, Mazeto GM, et al: Audiologic evaluation in patients with acquired hypothyroidism. Braz J Otorhinolaryngol 76:478, 2010.
46. Hekimsoy Z, Oktem IK: Serum creatine kinase levels in overt and subclinical hypothyroidism. Endocr Res 31:171, 2005.
47. Duyff RF, Van den Bosch J, Laman DM, et al: Neuromuscular findings in thyroid dysfunction: a prospective clinical and electrodiagnostic study. J Neurol Neurosurg Psychiatry 68:750, 2000.
48. Eslamian F, Bahrami A, Aghamohammadzadeh N, et al: Electrophysiologic changes in patients with untreated primary hypothyroidism. J Clin Neurophysiol 28:323, 2011.
49. Barahona MJ, Mauri A, Sucunza NP, et al: Hypothyroidism as a cause of rhabdomyolysis. Endocr J 49:621, 2002.
50. Novik V, Pérez ME, Anwandter G: Global respiratory failure as the presentation form of hypothyroidism. Report of one case. Rev Med Chil 132:81, 2004.
51. Lochmüller H, Reimers CD, Fischer P, et al: Exercise-induced myalgia in hypothyroidism. Clin Invest 71:999, 1993.
52. Madariaga MG: Polymyositis-like syndrome in hypothyroidism: review of cases reported over the past twenty-five years. Thyroid 12:331, 2002.
53. Monzani F, Caraccio N, Del Guerra P, et al: Neuromuscular symptoms and dysfunction in subclinical hypothyroid patients: beneficial effect of L-T4 replacement therapy. Clin Endocrinol (Oxf) 51:237, 1999.
54. Scott KR, Simmons Z, Boyer PJ: Hypothyroid myopathy with a strikingly elevated serum creatine kinase level. Muscle Nerve 26:141, 2002.
55. Pavlu J, Carey MP, Winer JB: Hypothyroidism and nemaline myopathy in an adult. J Neurol Neurosurg Psychiatry 77:708, 2006.
56. Taylor DJ, Rajagopalan B, Radda GK: Cellular energetics in hypothyroid muscle. Eur J Clin Invest 22:358, 1992.
57. Zoll J, Ventura-Clapier R, Serrurier B, et al: Response of mitochondrial function to hypothyroidism in normal and regenerated rat skeletal muscle. J Muscle Res Cell Motil 22:141, 2001.
58. Siciliano G, Monzani F, Manca ML, et al: Human mitochondrial transcription factor A reduction and mitochondrial dysfunction in Hashimoto's hypothyroid myopathy. Mol Med 8:326, 2002.
59. Khedr EM, El Toony LF, Tarkhan MN, et al: Peripheral and central nervous system alterations in hypothyroidism: electrophysiological findings. Neuropsychobiology 41:88, 2000.
60. Kececi H, Degirmenci Y: Hormone replacement therapy in hypothyroidism and nerve conduction study. Neurophysiol Clin 36:79, 2006.

61. Nebuchennykh M, Løseth S, Mellgren SI: Aspects of peripheral nerve involvement in patients with treated hypothyroidism. Eur J Neurol 17:67, 2010.
62. Toscano A, Rodolico C, Benvenga S, et al: Multifocal motor neuropathy and asymptomatic Hashimoto's thyroiditis: first report of an association. Neuromuscul Disord 12:566, 2002.
63. Eiris-Punal J, Del Rio-Garma M, Del Rio-Garma MC, et al: Long-term treatment of children with epilepsy with valproate or carbamazepine may cause subclinical hypothyroidism. Epilepsia 40:1761, 1999.
64. Miller J, Carney P: Central hypothyroidism with oxcarbazepine therapy. Pediatr Neurol 34:242, 2006.
65. Betteridge T, Fink J: Phenytoin toxicity and thyroid dysfunction. N Z Med J 122:102, 2009.
66. Shaheen D, Kim CS: Myositis associated with the decline of thyroid hormone levels in thyrotoxicosis: a syndrome? Thyroid 19:1413, 2009.
67. Lleo A, Sanahuja J, Serrano C, et al: Acute bulbar weakness: thyrotoxicosis or myasthenia gravis? Ann Neurol 46:434, 1999.
68. Lichtstein DM, Arteaga RB: Rhabdomyolysis associated with hyperthyroidism. Am J Med Sci 332:103, 2006.
69. Brennan MD, Powell C, Kaufman KR, et al: The impact of overt and subclinical hyperthyroidism on skeletal muscle. Thyroid 16:375, 2006.
70. Levine JA, Nygren J, Short KR, et al: Effect of hyperthyroidism on spontaneous physical activity and energy expenditure in rats. J Appl Physiol 94:165, 2003.
71. Brennan MD, Coenen-Schimke JM, Bigelow ML, et al: Changes in skeletal muscle protein metabolism and myosin heavy chain isoform messenger ribonucleic acid abundance after treatment of hyperthyroidism. J Clin Endocrinol Metab 91:4650, 2006.
72. Erkintalo M, Bendahan D, Mattei JP, et al: Reduced metabolic efficiency of skeletal muscle energetics in hyperthyroid patients evidenced quantitatively by in vivo phosphorus-31 magnetic resonance spectroscopy. Metabolism 47:769, 1998.
73. Lebon V, Dufour S, Petersen KF, et al: Effect of triiodothyronine on mitochondrial energy coupling in human skeletal muscle. J Clin Invest 108:733, 2001.
74. Hardiman O, Molloy F, Brett F, et al: Inflammatory myopathy in thyrotoxicosis. Neurology 48:339, 1997.
75. Nørrelund H, Hove KY, Brems-Dalgaard E, et al: Muscle mass and function in thyrotoxic patients before and during medical treatment. Clin Endocrinol (Oxf) 51:693, 1999.
76. Hsieh CH, Kuo SW, Pei D, et al: Thyrotoxic periodic paralysis: an overview. Ann Saudi Med 24:418, 2004.
77. Wongraoprasert S, Buranasupkajorn P, Sridama V, et al: Thyrotoxic periodic paralysis induced by pulse methylprednisolone. Intern Med 46:1431, 2007.
78. Tsai MH, Chang WN, Lu CH, et al: Exercise test in the inter-attack period of thyrotoxic periodic paralysis: a useful diagnostic tool. Acta Neurol Taiwan 15:259, 2006.
79. Kung AW, Lau KS, Cheung WM, et al: Thyrotoxic periodic paralysis and polymorphisms of sodium-potassium ATPase genes. Clin Endocrinol (Oxf) 64:158, 2006.
80. Ryan DP, da Silva MR, Soong TW, et al: Mutations in potassium channel Kir2.6 cause susceptibility to thyrotoxic hypokalemic periodic paralysis. Cell 140:88, 2010.
81. Cheung CL, Lau KS, Ho AY, et al: Genome-wide association study identifies a susceptibility locus for thyrotoxic periodic paralysis at 17q24.3. Nat Genet 44:1026, 2012.
82. Dassau L, Conti LR, Radeke CM, et al: Kir2.6 regulates the surface expression of Kir2.x inward rectifier potassium channels. J Biol Chem 286:9526, 2011.
83. Falhammar H, Thoren M, Calissendorff J: Thyrotoxic periodic paralysis: clinical and molecular aspects. Endocrine 43:274, 2013.
84. Magsino Jr CH, Ryan AJ Jr: Thyrotoxic periodic paralysis. South Med J 93:996, 2000.
85. Li W, Changsheng C, Jiangfang F, et al: Effects of sex steroid hormones, thyroid hormone levels, and insulin regulation on thyrotoxic periodic paralysis in Chinese men. Endocrine 38:386, 2010.
86. Lu KC, Hsu YJ, Chiu JS, et al: Effects of potassium supplementation on the recovery of thyrotoxic periodic paralysis. Am J Emerg Med 22:544, 2004.
87. Kung AW: Clinical review: thyrotoxic periodic paralysis: a diagnostic challenge. J Clin Endocrinol Metab 91:2490, 2006.
88. Huang X, Liu WB, Men LN, et al: Clinical features of myasthenia gravis in southern China: a retrospective review of 2,154 cases over 22 years. Neurol Sci 34:911, 2013.
89. Marinó M, Ricciardi R, Pinchera A, et al: Mild clinical expression of myasthenia gravis associated with autoimmune thyroid diseases. J Clin Endocrinol Metab 82:438, 1997.
90. Caparros-Lefebvre D, Benabdallah S, Bertagna X, et al: Subacute motor neuropathy induced by T3 hyperthyroidism. Ann Med Interne (Paris) 154:475, 2003.
91. Roquer J, Cano JF: Carpal tunnel syndrome and hyperthyroidism. A prospective study. Acta Neurol Scand 88:149, 1993.
92. Pandit L, Shankar SK, Gayathri N, et al: Acute thyrotoxic neuropathy–Basedow's paraplegia revisited. J Neurol Sci 155:211, 1998.
93. Patial RK, Kumar V, Kumari R: Motor neurone disease like picture in hyperthyroidism. Indian J Med Sci 49:114, 1995.

94. Ozata M, Ozkardes A, Dolu H, et al: Evaluation of central motor conduction in hypothyroid and hyperthyroid patients. J Endocrinol Invest 19:670, 1996.
95. Baba M, Terada A, Hishida R, et al: Persistent hemichorea associated with thyrotoxicosis. Intern Med 31:1144, 1992.
96. Ristic AJ, Svetel M, Dragasevic N, et al: Bilateral chorea-ballism associated with hyperthyroidism. Mov Disord 19:982, 2004.
97. Yu JH, Weng YM: Acute chorea as a presentation of Graves disease: case report and review. Am J Emerg Med 27:369, 2009.
98. Isaacs JD, Rakshi J, Baker R, et al: Chorea associated with thyroxine replacement therapy. Mov Disord 20:1656, 2005.
99. Milanov I, Sheinkova G: Clinical and electromyographic examination of tremor in patients with thyrotoxicosis. Int J Clin Pract 54:364, 2000.
100. Teoh HL, Lim EC: Platysmal myoclonus in subclinical hyperthyroidism. Mov Disord 20:1064, 2005.
101. Puri V, Chaudhry N: Paroxysmal kinesigenic dyskinesia manifestation of hyperthyroidism. Neurol India 52:102, 2004.
102. Wiersinga WM, Bartalena L: Epidemiology and prevention of Graves' ophthalmopathy. Thyroid 12:855, 2002.
103. Bahn RS: Graves' ophthalmopathy. N Engl J Med 362:726, 2010.
104. Bartley GB, Fatourechi V, Kadrmas EF, et al: Clinical features of Graves' ophthalmopathy in an incidence cohort. Am J Ophthalmol 121:284, 1996.
105. Bartalena L, Marcocci C, Bogazzi F, et al: Relation between therapy for hyperthyroidism and the course of Graves' ophthalmopathy. N Engl J Med 338:73, 1998.
106. Tallstedt L, Lundell G, Torring O, et al: Occurrence of ophthalmopathy after treatment for Graves' hyperthyroidism. The Thyroid Study Group. N Engl J Med 326:1733, 1992.
107. Prummel MF, Wiersinga WM: Smoking and risk of Graves' disease. JAMA 269:479, 1993.
108. Traisk F, Tallstedt L, Abraham-Nordling M, et al: Thyroid-associated ophthalmopathy after treatment for Graves' hyperthyroidism with antithyroid drugs or iodine-131. J Clin Endocrinol Metab 94:3700, 2009.
109. Cascone P, Rinna C, Reale G, et al: Compression and stretching in Graves orbitopathy: emergency orbital decompression techniques. J Craniofac Surg 23:1430, 2012.
110. McKeag D, Lane C, Lazarus JH, et al: Clinical features of dysthyroid optic neuropathy: a European Group on Graves' Orbitopathy (EUGOGO) survey. Br J Ophthalmol 91:455, 2007.
111. Kirsch E, von Arx G, Hammer B: Imaging in Graves' orbitopathy. Orbit 28:219, 2009.
112. Genovesi-Ebert F, Di Bartolo E, Lepri A, et al: Standardized echography, pattern electroretinography and visual-evoked potential and automated perimetry in the early diagnosis of Graves' neuropathy. Ophthalmologica 212(Suppl 1):101, 1998.
113. Bahn RS, Dutton CM, Natt N, et al: Thyrotropin receptor expression in Graves' orbital adipose/connective tissues: potential autoantigen in Graves' ophthalmopathy. J Clin Endocrinol Metab 83:998, 1998.
114. Bartalena L, Baldeschi L, Dickinson AJ, et al: Consensus statement of the European Group on Graves' Orbitopathy (EUGOGO) on management of Graves' orbitopathy. Thyroid 18:333, 2008.
115. Lai A, Sassi L, Compri E, et al: Lower dose prednisone prevents radioiodine-associated exacerbation of initially mild or absent Graves' orbitopathy: a retrospective cohort study. J Clin Endocrinol Metab 95:1333, 2010.
116. Vannucchi G, Campi I, Covelli D, et al: Graves' orbitopathy activation after radioactive iodine therapy with and without steroid prophylaxis. J Clin Endocrinol Metab 94:3381, 2009.
117. Sarlis NJ, Gourgiotis L: Thyroid emergencies. Rev Endocr Metab Disord 4:129, 2003.
118. Snabboon T, Khemkha A, Chaiyaumporn C, et al: Psychosis as the first presentation of hyperthyroidism. Intern Emerg Med 4:359, 2009.
119. Lee TG, Ha CK, Lim BH: Thyroid storm presenting as status epilepticus and stroke. Postgrad Med J 73:61, 1997.
120. Akamizu T, Satoh T, Isozaki O, et al: Diagnostic criteria, clinical features, and incidence of thyroid storm based on nationwide surveys. Thyroid 22:661, 2012.
121. Carroll R, Matfin G: Endocrine and metabolic emergencies: thyroid storm. Ther Adv Endocrinol Metab 1:139, 2010.
122. Muller C, Perrin P, Faller B, et al: Role of plasma exchange in the thyroid storm. Ther Apher Dial 15:522, 2011.
123. Song TJ, Kim SJ, Kim GS, et al: The prevalence of thyrotoxicosis-related seizures. Thyroid 20:955, 2010.
124. Aydin A, Cemeroglu AP, Baklan B: Thyroxine-induced hypermotor seizure. Seizure 13:61, 2004.
125. Brownlie BE, Rae AM, Walshe JW, et al: Psychoses associated with thyrotoxicosis – 'thyrotoxic psychosis.' A report of 18 cases, with statistical analysis of incidence. Eur J Endocrinol 142:438, 2000.
126. Larisch R, Kley K, Nikolaus S, et al: Depression and anxiety in different thyroid function states. Horm Metab Res 36:650, 2004.
127. Demet MM, Ozmen B, Deveci A, et al: Depression and anxiety in hyperthyroidism. Arch Med Res 33:552, 2002.
128. Engum A, Bjøro T, Mykletun A, et al: An association between depression, anxiety and thyroid function—a

clinical fact or an artefact? Acta Psychiatr Scand 106:27, 2002.

129. Squizzato A, Gerdes VE, Brandjes DP, et al: Thyroid diseases and cerebrovascular disease. Stroke 36:2302, 2005.
130. Parmar MS: Thyrotoxic atrial fibrillation. Med Gen Med 7:74, 2005.
131. Sheu JJ, Kang JH, Lin HC: Hyperthyroidism and risk of ischemic stroke in young adults: a 5-year follow-up study. Stroke 41:961, 2010.
132. Li H, Zhang ZS, Dong ZN, et al: Increased thyroid function and elevated thyroid autoantibodies in pediatric patients with moyamoya disease: a case-control study. Stroke 42:1138, 2011.
133. Castillo P, Woodruff B, Caselli R, et al: Steroid-responsive encephalopathy associated with autoimmune thyroiditis. Arch Neurol 63:197, 2006.
134. Shaw PJ, Walls TJ, Newman PK, et al: Hashimoto's encephalopathy: a steroid-responsive disorder associated with high anti-thyroid antibody titers–report of 5 cases. Neurology 41:228, 1991.
135. Chong JY, Rowland LP, Utiger RD: Hashimoto encephalopathy: syndrome or myth? Arch Neurol 60:164, 2003.
136. Spiegel J, Hellwig D, Becker G, et al: Progressive dementia caused by Hashimoto's encephalopathy–report of two cases. Eur J Neurol 11:711, 2004.
137. Vasconcellos E, Pina-Garza JE, Fakhoury T, et al: Pediatric manifestations of Hashimoto's encephalopathy. Pediatr Neurol 20:394, 1999.
138. Ferlazzo E, Raffaele M, Mazzu I, et al: Recurrent status epilepticus as the main feature of Hashimoto's encephalopathy. Epilepsy Behav 8:328, 2006.
139. Tsai MH, Lee LH, Chen SD, et al: Complex partial status epilepticus as a manifestation of Hashimoto's encephalopathy. Seizure 16:713, 2007.
140. Barker R, Zajicek J, Wilkinson I: Thyrotoxic Hashimoto's encephalopathy. J Neurol Neurosurg Psychiatry 60:234, 1996.
141. Alink J, de Vries TW: Unexplained seizures, confusion or hallucinations: think Hashimoto encephalopathy. Acta Paediatr 97:451, 2008.
142. Blanchin S, Coffin C, Viader F, et al: Anti-thyroperoxidase antibodies from patients with Hashimoto's encephalopathy bind to cerebellar astrocytes. J Neuroimmunol 192:13, 2007.
143. Duffey P, Yee S, Reid IN, et al: Hashimoto's encephalopathy: postmortem findings after fatal status epilepticus. Neurology 61:1124, 2003.
144. Yoneda M, Fujii A, Ito A, et al: High prevalence of serum autoantibodies against the amino terminal of alpha-enolase in Hashimoto's encephalopathy. J Neuroimmunol 185:195, 2007.
145. Nieuwenhuis L, Santens P, Vanwalleghem P, et al: Subacute Hashimoto's encephalopathy, treated with plasmapheresis. Acta Neurol Belg 104:80, 2004.
146. Arlt W, Hove U, Müller B, et al: Frequent and frequently overlooked: treatment-induced endocrine dysfunction in adult long-term survivors of primary brain tumors. Neurology 49:498, 1997.
147. Karni A, Abramsky O: Association of MS with thyroid disorders. Neurology 53:883, 1999.
148. Cohen JA, Coles AJ, Arnold DL, et al: Alemtuzumab versus interferon beta 1a as first-line treatment for patients with relapsing-remitting multiple sclerosis: a randomised controlled phase 3 trial. Lancet 380:1819, 2012.
149. Coles AJ, Wing M, Smith S, et al: Pulsed monoclonal antibody treatment and autoimmune thyroid disease in multiple sclerosis. Lancet 354:1691, 1999.
150. Takashima S, Takayama F, Wang J, et al: Using MR imaging to predict invasion of the recurrent laryngeal nerve by thyroid carcinoma. AJR Am J Roentgenol 180:837, 2003.
151. Chiang FY, Wang LF, Huang YF, et al: Recurrent laryngeal nerve palsy after thyroidectomy with routine identification of the recurrent laryngeal nerve. Surgery 137:342, 2005.

CHAPTER

19

Diabetes and the Nervous System

DOUGLAS W. ZOCHODNE ■ CORY TOTH

Both type 1 and type 2 diabetes mellitus commonly target the nervous system. In the peripheral nervous system, complications include polyneuropathies and focal neuropathies. In the central nervous system, diabetes may be associated with cognitive decline, leukoencephalopathy, and a heightened risk of both stroke and dementia. Acute changes in glycemia are also associated with neurologic signs and symptoms. This chapter summarizes the acute and chronic neurologic complications of diabetes mellitus that clinicians should keep in mind when caring for patients with this disorder.

ACUTE NEUROLOGIC FEATURES

Diabetic Ketoacidosis

Diabetic ketoacidosis (DKA) in patients with type 1 diabetes is a medical emergency that may present with neurologic signs and symptoms.[1,2] Anorexia, lethargy, thirst, polyuria, vague abdominal pain, and Kussmaul respiration are followed by confusion and a decreased level of consciousness. Rarely, a primary CNS infection, such as bacterial meningitis, accompanies diabetic ketoacidosis. Cerebral edema complicates diabetic ketoacidosis and may present with headache, papilledema, and bilateral abducens neuropathies; it may develop on presentation or during correction of the metabolic disorder. Secondary complications include cerebral infarction, cerebral venous sinus thrombosis, and compression neuropathies.

Nonketotic Hyperosmolar Syndrome

Neurologic symptoms and signs may also herald a nonketotic hyperosmolar syndrome, which is defined as a blood glucose level exceeding 33 mmol/L (600 mg/dl) and a plasma osmolarity greater than 320 mOsm/L, without accompanying acidosis or ketonemia.[1] Polyuria, polydipsia, thirst, fatigue, and generalized weakness are common, and neurologic signs include a decreased level of consciousness, hemiplegia, aphasia, brainstem

Aminoff's Neurology and General Medicine, Fifth Edition.

abnormalities, dystonia, chorea, and seizures. Seizures are often focal and can include tonic, movement-induced, or continuous forms (e.g., epilepsia partialis continua). Unusual neurologic features are visual symptoms, hallucinations, hemichorea, tonic eye deviation, nystagmus, abnormal pupil reactivity, and meningeal signs. The correction of hyperglycemia may be more effective than using antiepileptic agents in the treatment of seizures.

Hypoglycemia

Hypoglycemia most often presents with altered neurologic function.[1] In diabetic subjects, hypoglycemia may occur in the setting of insulin use. A high index of suspicion is required as patients may present with focal neurologic signs or seizures that mimic stroke. Hypoglycemia is defined as a plasma glucose concentration less than 2.7 mmol/L (50 mg/dl), a level which is typically associated with a decline in cognitive function. Premonitory systemic symptoms include anxiety, tachycardia, perspiration, nausea, and tremor, but these signs may be absent in patients taking β-adrenergic–blocking medications or in patients with autonomic neuropathy. Early neurologic symptoms include decreased attention and concentration, drowsiness, poor memory, disorientation, clumsiness, and tremor. Patients may progress to experience seizures and loss of consciousness. Seizures may be focal or generalized and may lead to status epilepticus. Rapid detection through expectant testing and early treatment are essential as severe untreated hypoglycemia is associated with diffuse cortical, basal ganglia, and dentate gyrus damage, leading to permanent disability.

PERIPHERAL NEUROPATHIES

A length-dependent polyneuropathy related to diabetes is typically a chronic, symmetric disorder that targets the distal terminals of axons first. Focal or localized neuropathies of a single plexus or nerve, also known as mononeuropathies, are also common in patients with diabetes and develop from mechanical compression, ischemia, or other, less well-defined causes. Autonomic neuropathy is the other major category of peripheral nervous system dysfunction in these patients.

Diabetic Polyneuropathy

Diabetic polyneuropathy is the most common form of peripheral neuropathy. With detailed evaluation, approximately 50 percent of both type 1 and type 2 diabetic subjects have the disorder. Symptomatic polyneuropathy may occur in approximately 15 percent of these patients.[3] Lower prevalence numbers have been derived from studies only of hospitalized patients, or studies using exclusively clinical signs of polyneuropathy. Sensory forms predominate, with or without lesser degrees of motor involvement. Positive sensory symptoms are common and include prickling, tingling, "pins and needles," burning, crawling, itching, electric, sharp, jabbing, and tight sensations in the legs, feet, hands, and fingers. Warm stimuli may be inappropriately perceived as cold, and cold stimuli as warm or hot. Nocturnal burning of the feet accompanies allodynia, defined as the generation of discomfort from normally innocuous stimuli. Many of these symptoms are associated with severe pain, which may become intractable.

Symptoms are generally symmetric and initially confined to the toes, with later spread to more proximal parts of the feet, legs, and fingers (Fig. 19-1). The involvement of the longest sensory axon terminals in the skin results in this "stocking and glove" pattern of sensory symptoms and loss. Negative symptoms include loss of sensation to light touch, pinprick, and temperature. In more severe forms, dense loss of these sensations predisposes patients to the development of foot ulcers. Additional factors that promote foot ulceration include loss of sweating, abnormal foot architecture from muscle wasting, and delayed healing from both macrovascular (atherosclerosis) and microvascular disease.

Motor weakness is less common in early diabetic polyneuropathy but may eventually lead to distal weakness of foot and toe dorsiflexion, predisposing patients to falls. Weakness is accompanied by wasting of the intrinsic foot muscles. Symptoms from concurrent abnormalities of the autonomic nervous system are common and include erectile dysfunction in men, distal loss of sweating, orthostatic symptoms such as "dizziness," and bowel and bladder dysfunction.

A detailed neurologic examination is essential to the evaluation of diabetic polyneuropathy, providing a low-cost, direct evaluation. While some variation in findings, especially in those patients with very early disease, is expected, the examination

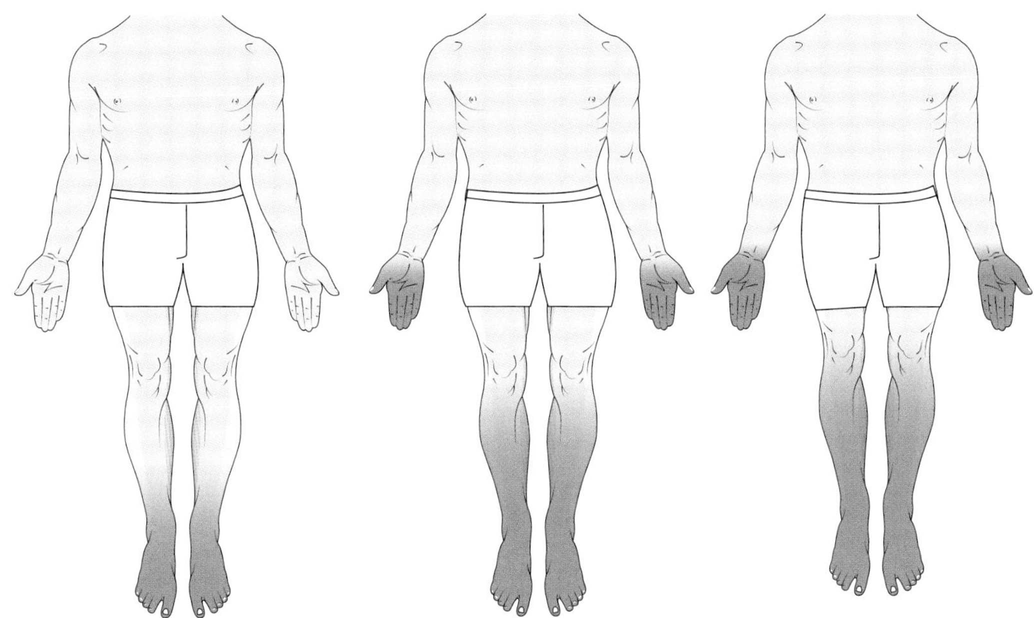

FIGURE 19-1 ■ Illustration of progressive "stocking and glove" sensory changes in a patient with progressive diabetic polyneuropathy. Sensory symptoms and signs begin in the distal territories of sensory nerves in the toes before fingers with a gradual spread proximally. (From Zochodne DW, Kline G, Smith EE, et al: Diabetic Neurology. Informa Healthcare, New York, 2010, with permission.)

remains the gold standard for diagnosis and is not replaced by quantitative methods or electrophysiologic evaluation, which are considered ancillary tests.

On sensory examination, there is distal loss of sensation to light touch, pinprick, cold, and vibration with a 128-Hz tuning fork. Some patients with denser sensory loss are unable to distinguish sharp (pinprick) from dull (analgesia) or to feel light touch at all (anesthesia). The Semmes–Weinstein (10 g) monofilament test is a useful adjunct to the neurologic examination; the filament is pressed against the skin over the dorsum of the great toe or other selected areas of the foot until it bows into a C shape for 1 second, and the patient is asked whether the stimulus is felt. The Rydel–Seiffer tuning fork provides semiquantitative information regarding vibratory sensory perception. Vibratory loss may involve the distal toes, the foot below the ankle, or more extensive territories, depending on its severity. Testing for proprioceptive abnormalities in the toes is often normal except in severe cases.

Distal motor wasting, for example, in the extensor digitorum brevis muscle, and associated weakness especially involving foot and toe dorsiflexion usually accompany more severe sensory loss. Patients may have foot ulcers or, less commonly, a destructive arthropathy from repetitive injury, known as a Charcot joint. Loss of the muscle stretch reflex at the ankle is common in early diabetic polyneuropathy; severe forms lead to loss of all deep tendon reflexes. The feet may be dry from loss of sweating. Patients with concurrent atherosclerosis have loss of distal pulses and sometimes femoral bruits. Orthostatic vital signs should be assessed; in patients with involvement of the autonomic nervous system, a decline of over 20 mmHg in the systolic blood pressure or of 10 mmHg in diastolic pressure indicates postural hypotension.[4]

Diabetic polyneuropathy has been divided into subcategories depending on whether large- or small-fiber involvement occurs. In large-fiber polyneuropathy, there is more prominent loss of sensation to light touch, vibration, and proprioception, and patients may have accompanying ataxia of gait. In small-fiber polyneuropathy, pinprick and thermal appreciation are impaired, and autonomic dysfunction is common, as is neuropathic pain, especially at night. Neuropathic pain can accompany other forms of diabetic polyneuropathy as well.[5]

Several scales have been developed to grade the severity of diabetic polyneuropathy for clinical trials. The San Antonio criteria are divided as follows: class I is polyneuropathy without signs or symptoms but with abnormalities on electrophysiologic testing, autonomic testing, or quantitative sensory testing (QST); class II includes signs, symptoms, or both.[6] Other scales, not reviewed here, include the Modified Toronto Neuropathy Scale, the Utah Neuropathy Scale, the Michigan Neuropathy Scale, and the Mayo Clinic diabetic polyneuropathy classification.[7–9]

Testing

In patients with established diabetes mellitus and typical symptoms of polyneuropathy, extensive additional testing may not be required. Exclusion of other causes of sensory polyneuropathy can be accomplished through judicious screening for hypothyroidism, vitamin B_{12} deficiency, monoclonal gammopathy, and ethanol abuse. Table 19-1 details an extensive list of alternative diagnoses that may resemble diabetic polyneuropathy.

Electrophysiologic testing is recommended for patients with unexpectedly severe or atypical forms of polyneuropathy including motor-predominant disease, rapidly progressive symptoms, asymmetric signs, or when another neuromuscular condition is suspected. It is important to choose a laboratory with appropriate certification, training, and experience in performing these techniques. Two major components are usually performed: nerve conduction studies and needle electromyography (EMG). In patients with only sensory symptoms and findings, nerve conduction studies alone may be sufficient. Initial changes include reductions in the amplitude and conduction velocity of the sural sensory nerve action potential (SNAP) recorded from behind the ankle.[10] Slowing of conduction velocity in fibular (peroneal) motor nerve axons detected by recording over the extensor digitorum brevis is an additional early abnormality. In severe neuropathy, there may be widespread loss of sensory nerve action potentials and diffuse mild-to-moderate conduction velocity slowing in multiple motor and sensory nerve territories (Fig. 19-2). In some patients with severe involvement, these findings may resemble the changes expected in a demyelinating polyneuropathy such as chronic inflammatory demyelinating polyneuropathy, but there are usually much more striking electrophysiologic features of primary demyelination in chronic inflammatory demyelinating polyneuropathy such as motor conduction block or dispersion of compound muscle action potentials.

TABLE 19-1 ■ Differential Diagnosis of Diabetic Polyneuropathy

Vitamin Deficiency
B vitamin deficiency (e.g., vitamin B_1 or B_{12})
Vitamin E deficiency
Infectious and Inflammatory
Human immunodeficiency virus (HIV) infection
Leprosy
Lyme disease
Hepatitis C infection
Guillain–Barré syndrome
Chronic inflammatory demyelinating polyneuropathy
Anti-MAG neuropathy, Lewis–Sumner syndrome, distal demyelinating sensory neuropathy
Neuropathies associated with monoclonal gammopathies
Primary biliary cirrhosis
Endocrine
Hypothyroidism
Acromegaly (with diabetes)
Drugs and Toxins
Antibiotics (e.g., metronidazole, isoniazid, nitrofurantoin)
Antineoplastic agents (e.g., vincristine, vinblastine, cisplatinum)
Ethanol (often in association with thiamine deficiency)
Organophosphate poisoning
Pyridoxine
Antiretroviral therapies
Interferon-α
Anti-TNF-α treatment for inflammatory disorders
Sinemet (via vitamin B_{12} deficiency)
Metformin (via vitamin B_{12} deficiency)
Metabolic
Hepatic cirrhosis
Renal failure
Critical illness (sepsis and multiorgan failure)
Acquired amyloidosis
Bariatric surgery
Congenital/Inherited
Charcot–Marie–Tooth disease (multiple subtypes)
Hereditary susceptibility to pressure palsies
Hereditary amyloidosis
Hereditary sensory and autonomic neuropathies
Vascular
Necrotizing vasculitis (confined to peripheral nerves or in association with systemic vasculitis)
Severe peripheral vascular disease
Cryoglobulinemia (with or without hepatitis C infection)
Neoplastic
Paraneoplastic neuropathies (anti-Hu, anti-Ma, others)
Leptomeningeal carcinomatosis, lymphomatosis, gliomatosis
Angioendotheliosis
Primary intraneural lymphoma

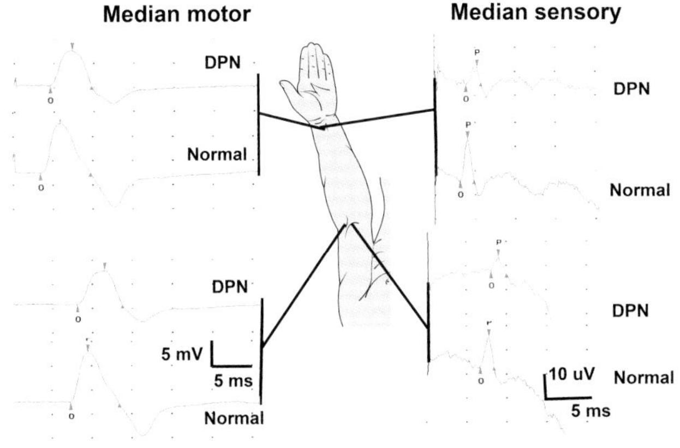

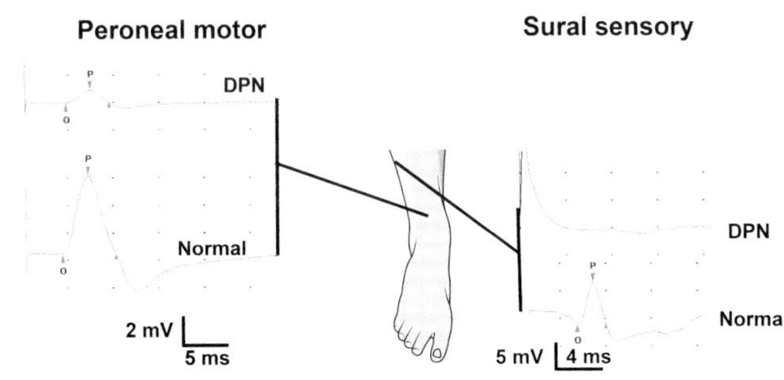

FIGURE 19-2 ■ Examples of nerve conduction abnormalities in a patient with moderately severe diabetic polyneuropathy (DPN) compared with waveforms in a normal subject. Note the decreased amplitude and prolonged latency of compound muscle action potentials and sensory nerve action potentials (the sural sensory nerve action potential is absent). Lines indicate nerve stimulation sites (recording site for the median motor nerve is the abductor pollicis brevis; for the median sensory nerve, the index finger; for the fibular (peroneal) motor nerve, the extensor digitorum brevis; and for the sural nerve, behind the lateral ankle). (From Zochodne DW, Kline G, Smith EE, et al: Diabetic Neurology. Informa Healthcare, New York, 2010, with permission.)

Loss of motor axons in more advanced diabetic polyneuropathy is detected by a decline or loss of compound muscle action potentials, initially in the lower and then the upper limbs. In these patients, needle EMG may detect abnormal spontaneous activity, including fibrillation potentials and positive sharp waves, in denervated muscles. In the setting of partial loss of motor axons, remaining fibers will sprout and innervate adjacent denervated muscle fibers; when activated, the motor unit action potentials recorded from these partially denervated muscles are enlarged but reduced in number, indicative of cycles of chronic denervation and reinnervation. Electrophysiologic testing is also valuable in identifying superimposed entrapment, or compression neuropathies, which are discussed below.

To reproducibly detect or track sensory changes, quantitative sensory testing (QST) using a computer interface may be used. While its chief utility is currently for clinical trials, it may offer early detection should better therapy for diabetic polyneuropathy emerge. QST equipment is available from several manufacturers and most use calibrated electronic interfaces to measure thermal thresholds (warm, cold), pain, touch-pressure, and vibration. As expected, these thresholds in the feet are raised in patients with diabetic polyneuropathy.

Specific testing of the autonomic nervous system is available for evaluating coexisting autonomic neuropathy (see Chapter 8). In some patients with diabetes mellitus, prominent and apparently selective autonomic damage occurs without polyneuropathy, as discussed later. Since postganglionic autonomic axons are unmyelinated, autonomic function testing may detect small-fiber forms of diabetic polyneuropathy.

Two additional forms of testing, not in routine clinical use for diabetic polyneuropathy, also evaluate small-fiber involvement. These include skin biopsy, using a 3-mm punch to count the number of epidermal axons, and corneal confocal microscopy, which is a noninvasive measure of unmyelinated axons in the cornea.[11,12]

Biopsy of the sural nerve is not indicated for the routine evaluation of diabetic polyneuropathy and should be reserved for the diagnosis of unusual or progressive neuropathies that are atypical and suspected to be from another cause. In diabetes, sural nerve biopsies show loss of myelinated and unmyelinated axons that can accompany microvascular basement membrane thickening, endothelial cell reduplication, or vessel occlusion.[13] These biopsies typically leave the patient with a sensory deficit and therefore should be considered judiciously.[14]

Cerebrospinal fluid (CSF) examination is not routinely indicated for typical diabetic polyneuropathy, although when performed it may show an elevated CSF protein concentration without pleocytosis. Imaging studies are used to exclude spinal cord disease, spinal stenosis, or other central disorders whose symptoms may occasionally resemble diabetic polyneuropathy.

Differential Diagnosis

A number of neurologic disorders may resemble diabetic polyneuropathy. Other polyneuropathies with prominent sensory involvement are listed in Table 19-1. As diabetes mellitus is very common, a detailed neurologic examination is essential to exclude other syndromes in these patients; for example, spinal cord disease may present with limb tingling and numbness, but other signs of upper motor neuron dysfunction are usually present on examination. Lesions at the cervicomedullary junction may cause sensory symptoms that begin in one limb and then progressively involve all four limbs. "Pseudoneuropathy" is a term used to describe the combination of lower limb sensory symptoms from spinal stenosis with upper limb tingling caused by carpal tunnel syndrome. It is important to identify patients with chronic inflammatory demyelinating polyneuropathy because they may respond to immunomodulatory therapies.

Pathogenesis

A number of mechanisms have been proposed to play a role in the pathogenesis of diabetic peripheral neuropathy, all with limited definitive evidence usually explored in rat and mouse models of diabetes. Excessive flux of polyols (sugar alcohols), especially sorbitol, through the aldose reductase pathway is one such proposed mechanism.[15] Aldose reductase inhibitors or protein kinase C inhibitors that interrupt this pathway have unfortunately been shown to have limited clinical benefit.[16] Free radical oxidative stress and mitochondrial dysfunction along with impaired antioxidant defenses likely contribute to neuronal damage.[17,18] Diabetic microangiopathy may lead to ischemic damage of neurons and axons, although this mechanism may occur later in the illness rather than serving as a primary trigger.[19–21] Trophic mechanisms that support neurons are also impaired in diabetes.[22] To date, clinical trials with nerve growth factor, neurotrophin-3, and brain-derived neurotrophic factor have all been disappointing.[23] An intriguing alternative is insulin itself, an important growth factor which is neurotrophic; its receptors are widely expressed in most neurons of the peripheral nervous system.[24] Intranasal insulin can access the CSF and through this route can reverse experimental diabetic neuropathy.[25,26]

Treatment

Despite extensive experimental work, no therapy is currently available to arrest or reverse diabetic polyneuropathy. Tight control of hyperglycemia helps to reduce the incidence of polyneuropathy and its progression.[27,28] Aldose reductase inhibitors have been tested extensively as a means of reversing sorbitol accumulation in peripheral nerves and associated metabolic abnormalities, but their overall impact has been disappointing.[16] Daily foot inspection for injuries and early ulceration is recommended. Treatment for neuropathic pain associated with diabetic polyneuropathy is available and is discussed later.

Focal Mononeuropathies

Focal neuropathies involving single peripheral nerves are common in diabetes. Many of these mononeuropathies develop at sites of entrapment or compression, but others are of uncertain origin or may develop from nerve trunk ischemia.

Carpal Tunnel Syndrome

Carpal tunnel syndrome arises from compression of the median nerve at the wrist beneath the transverse carpal ligament, often following repetitive use of the wrist. It is characterized by tingling, pain, and numbness in the thumb, index, and middle fingers, especially at night or on awakening. Asymptomatic carpal tunnel syndrome (electrophysiologic diagnosis) can be detected in 20 to 30 percent of diabetics, but symptomatic carpal tunnel syndrome is present in only 6 percent.[3,29] Carpal tunnel syndrome is the most common entrapment neuropathy in diabetic and nondiabetic patients. Women are more susceptible than men, and the dominant hand is more commonly involved that the nondominant hand.

Tinel sign (tapping over the median nerve at the wrist evokes positive sensory symptoms that resemble the patient's symptoms distal to the wrist) and Phalen sign (reproduction of tingling by having both wrists flexed and held against each other for 1 minute) may be present, but are nonspecific and insensitive. In mild carpal tunnel syndrome, clinical signs may be absent. Later, sensory loss may occur in the median nerve territory. In more severe carpal tunnel syndrome, weakness and wasting of the abductor pollicis brevis (thenar muscles) develops.

Electrophysiologic testing helps to distinguish carpal tunnel syndrome from radiculopathy or other upper limb neuropathies by identifying selective slowing of the conduction of median nerve fibers across the carpal tunnel. Carpal tunnel syndrome may improve with a change in activity and the nocturnal use of wrist splints. Decompression by sectioning the transverse carpal ligament is the only curative procedure. Since diabetes delays nerve regeneration, recovery in diabetics, particularly those with poor glycemic control, may be less robust than in nondiabetics.[30]

Ulnar Neuropathy at the Elbow

Ulnar neuropathy at the elbow presents with pain and sensory symptoms in the medial half of the ring finger and fifth digits, sometimes radiating into the palm as far proximal as the wrist. Sensory loss involves these fingers as well as the medial volar and dorsal hand to the wrist. There may be wasting and weakness of intrinsic ulnar-innervated hand muscles, especially in the first dorsal interosseus muscle, making it difficult for the patient to abduct or adduct the fingers. Manipulation of the ulnar nerve at the elbow may generate tingling that radiates into the hand and reproduces symptoms. Ethanol use and previous elbow trauma or fractures are predisposing factors. The disorder is commonly caused by the patient leaning on the medial elbow, compressing the nerve. The prevalence of ulnar nerve entrapment in patients with diabetes mellitus is estimated to be approximately 2 percent.[29]

Electrophysiologic studies identify slowing of ulnar motor and sensory conduction across the elbow, loss of ulnar sensory nerve action potentials and compound motor action potentials, and sometimes conduction block across the elbow. EMG demonstrates evidence of denervation in affected muscles. Changes in elbow position or protecting the nerve with padding can reverse ulnar neuropathy. There are no controlled clinical trials specifically in diabetic patients to show that surgical decompression improves long-term outcome; however, current clinical practice suggests decompression is a reasonable approach when the lesion is symptomatic, involves motor axons, and is progressive despite conservative measures.

Meralgia Paresthetica

Meralgia paresthetica is an entrapment neuropathy involving the lateral femoral cutaneous nerve of the thigh as it passes under the inguinal ligament. Symptoms are numbness, tingling, prickling, and sometimes pain over the lateral thigh that may be relieved by sitting. Bilateral involvement may occur. Examination findings include loss of sensation to light touch and pinprick over the lateral thigh. The extent of findings may vary from a small patch to most of the lateral thigh from just below the inguinal area to the knee. Hip flexion and knee extension muscle power are preserved, as is the quadriceps stretch reflex. In some patients, a compressive lesion such as an enlarged lymph node, inguinal hernia, or scar from a previous hernia repair is present. Additional risk factors are abdominal obesity, pregnancy, and the wearing of low-riding belts. The differential diagnosis includes diabetic lumbosacral plexopathy (distinguished by weakness and wasting along with loss of the quadriceps reflex), plexopathy secondary to a retroperitoneal lesion, or an L3 or L4 radiculopathy associated with back pain, weakness, positive straight leg raising sign, and loss of the quadriceps reflex. There is no evidence to support benefit from surgical decompression at the inguinal ligament; however, some patients may choose to undergo decompression if weight loss, local anaesthetic, or corticosteroid injections are unhelpful and the pain is intractable. Conservative management of pain and limiting activities that provoke symptoms may allow spontaneous recovery over time.

Intercostal or Truncal Radicular Neuropathies

Intercostal neuropathies involve the thorax and abdominal wall and may be ischemic in origin. Patients may present with severe thoracic or abdominal wall pain mistaken for an intra-abdominal or thoracic emergency. Differential diagnoses include herpes zoster without rash or radiculopathy from a segmental structural lesion. Several contiguous territories may be involved unilaterally or bilaterally.[31] Symptoms other than pain include tingling, pricking, lancinating, aching (especially at night), radiation around the chest or abdomen causing a feeling of constriction, and allodynia. Patients may occasionally have asymmetric weakness of the abdominal muscles when sitting up (asymmetric bulging). Men are affected more often than women. Imaging of the spinal cord and roots by magnetic resonance imaging (MRI) with gadolinium should be performed to exclude nerve root compression when a structural lesion is suspected. In some patients, EMG may detect signs of denervation in weak thoracic intercostal or abdominal muscles; such changes commonly are more extensive and may involve the paraspinal muscles at multiple levels. Pain may be severe enough to require treatment, but usually reaches a maximum after several weeks, continues for some months, and then gradually resolves completely. Sensory loss may also slowly resolve with time.

Oculomotor Neuropathy

Oculomotor neuropathy develops in older patients with diabetes, particularly if they are also hypertensive. Symptoms usually involve sudden diplopia and ptosis, with aching pain around or behind the eye. The eye is deviated laterally. The underlying pathology is a vascular lesion that spares the more peripheral pupillomotor fibers, so that the pupil is not involved. A single pathologic study of a patient with oculomotor palsy noted demyelination in the center of the oculomotor nerve within the cavernous sinus.[32] Imaging should include MRI of the brainstem and the course of the oculomotor nerve; MR angiography is indicated to search for evidence of an aneurysm compressing cranial nerve III, although in these cases the pupil is typically involved. Computed tomography (CT) angiography may also be used to exclude aneurysm but there is a risk of contrast nephropathy from the contrast load. Although no specific treatment is available for this neuropathy, spontaneous resolution usually occurs over approximately 3 months. An eye patch prevents diplopia but interrupts binocular depth vision so patients should refrain from driving.

Diabetic Lumbosacral Plexopathy

Diabetic lumbosacral plexopathy (also known as diabetic amyotrophy, radiculoplexus neuropathy, Bruns–Garland syndrome, and proximal diabetic neuropathy) usually develops in patients with type 2 diabetes mellitus, especially in men.[33,34] It may emerge early in the course of diabetes or following the onset of insulin therapy. Patients without diabetes rarely can develop a similar syndrome. Symptoms are severe and disabling, with impairment in standing and walking. The subacute onset of unilateral intense deep boring or aching muscle pain is typical, sometimes worse at night, located within the muscles of the thigh and often radiating to the back and perineum. These symptoms are followed by weakness and wasting of the proximal thigh muscles including the quadriceps, iliopsoas, hip adductor muscles, and occasionally the anterior tibial muscles (with associated foot drop). Sensory loss and tingling are less prominent. The condition can be distinguished from a femoral neuropathy by the pattern of muscle involvement, which typically includes the medial adductor muscles innervated by the obturator nerve and the iliopsoas muscle innervated directly by the lumbar plexus. Over the months, a slow recovery of muscle power occurs. In some patients, contralateral symptoms may emerge a few weeks after onset. Variations of diabetic lumbosacral plexopathy include symmetric involvement, more prominent foot drop, or apparent worsening of polyneuropathy.

The pathophysiologic mechanism for this form of focal neuropathy is uncertain but may include occlusive changes in microvessels supplying the lumbosacral roots or plexus, or a localized form of vasculitis.[32] Perivascular inflammation, epineurial inflammation, microvessel occlusion, and iron deposition (indicative of intraneural bleeding) accompany loss of axons in biopsies of the sural nerve or cutaneous nerves of the thigh.[35,36] Imaging studies of the lumbar spinal cord and the lumbosacral plexus, usually with MRI, help to exclude a retroperitoneal compressive plexus lesion.

Electrophysiologic studies in diabetic lumbosacral plexopathy show reduction of compound muscle action potential amplitudes recorded over the quadriceps muscle and EMG evidence of denervation in weak muscles. No therapy has been shown to arrest or reverse the motor deficit. Despite the inflammatory changes seen on pathology, the response to immunosuppressive therapy is unproven. Preliminary data suggest that an intravenous course of corticosteroids may shorten the duration of pain but not disability. Patients require intensive pain management that may include opioid use. Physiotherapy and occupational therapy are essential to recovery, and knee bracing helps to prevent falls from leg buckling in the setting of quadriceps weakness.

Other Focal Neuropathies

Other focal neuropathies described in diabetic patients are less common. Bell palsy, presenting with unilateral facial weakness, may be more common in diabetics.[37] Abducens palsy presents with lateral gaze weakness and is seen in older diabetic patients; other causes include compression, trauma, and hypertension. Trochlear palsy presents with diplopia and difficulty looking down and inward due to weakness of the superior oblique muscle; the patient tilts the head to the side opposite the palsy in order to reduce diplopia.

Autonomic Neuropathy

Autonomic neuropathy in diabetes may target one or more components of the autonomic nervous system.

Cardiovascular abnormalities include loss of reflexes such as heart-rate variability in various circumstances including at rest, with the Valsalva maneuver, and following standing. In severe disease, patients may have a fixed, mildly elevated heart rate that resembles a transplanted heart without innervation. More commonly, partial denervation of the heart may contribute to abnormal contractility and arrhythmias. For example, prolonged QTc intervals in patients with type I diabetes may predict an increased risk of mortality.[38] Postural hypotension, from loss of sympathetic control of resistance arterioles, is defined as a decline of systolic pressure of 20 mmHg or more after 1 minute of standing, with associated orthostatic dizziness or fainting; it occurs in 3 to 6 percent of diabetics and may be a late feature of diabetic autonomic neuropathy.[39] Some patients may also have abnormal tachycardia with standing (postural orthostatic tachycardia syndrome), as discussed in Chapter 8.

Treatment includes stopping or reducing doses of medications that can cause postural hypotension (e.g., tricyclic antidepressants, antihypertensive medications, and other vasodilators); arising from bed or chair slowly; sleeping with the head of bed raised 20 degrees; avoiding prolonged standing; eliminating early morning or postprandial exercise; avoiding prolonged heat exposure, hot baths, or showers; increasing salt and fluid intake; and limiting alcohol intake. Medications used to treat postural hypotension include fludrocortisone, midodrine, and desmopressin (Chapter 8).

The Ewing battery is a set of cardiovascular autonomic tests that includes heart-rate response to the Valsalva maneuver, standing, and to deep breathing, as well as blood-pressure response to standing up and sustained handgrip.[4] Radioiodinated metaiodobenzylguanidine (MIBG) is an injectable marker of sympathetic terminals found in cardiac muscle; loss of uptake in the inferior, posterior and apical portions of the heart occurs in diabetes, indicating sympathetic denervation or dysfunction.

Sexual dysfunction is common in diabetic men. Erectile dysfunction, defined as the inability to achieve or maintain an erection sufficient for sexual intercourse, may occur in over 40 percent.[40] Direct vascular factors, such as atherosclerosis, typically cause erectile dysfunction, but other causes should be excluded including psychologic factors, Peyronie disease, problems with the sexual partner, and medications (e.g., sedatives, antidepressants, and antihypertensives). The additional loss of ejaculation suggests more severe autonomic involvement. Testing includes duplex ultrasonography and nocturnal measurements of penile tumescence. Treatment for erectile dysfunction includes phosphodiesterase-5 inhibitors (e.g., sildenafil, tadalafil), apomorphine, intracavernosal and intraurethral treatments (e.g., prostaglandin E1, thymoxamine), vacuum devices, and penile prostheses, as is discussed in Chapter 30.

Gastrointestinal neuropathy is associated with abdominal pain, weight loss, early satiety, postprandial fullness, heartburn, nausea (rarely vomiting), dysphagia, fecal incontinence, diarrhea (which may be nocturnal), and constipation.[41] Esophageal transit and gastric emptying are slowed, a change directly linked to elevated glucose levels. Similarly, small intestine dysmotility develops and may accompany an increased risk of cholelithiasis and cholecystitis. Colonic dysfunction leads to constipation and diarrhea that may be alternating and may be associated with abdominal pain. Anorectal dysfunction with incontinence develops from abnormal internal or external sphincter function, loss of sensitivity, and disrupted anorectal reflexes. A superimposed history of obstetric trauma may particularly predispose diabetic women to this complication. Exclusion of other gastrointestinal problems that can occur in patients with diabetes is important, including esophageal candidiasis, gastric bezoar, *Helicobacter pylori* infection, anorectal disorders, celiac disease, hemorrhoids, impaired sphincter tone, rectal prolapse, local tumors, ulcers, rectal intussusception, and fecal impaction.

Gastric and intestinal motility studies are carried out using radiography or scintigraphy, manometry, pH recordings, and endoscopy or colonoscopy. Anorectal dysfunction is studied through manometry, ultrasonography, proctoscopy, and sigmoidoscopy. High fiber, low fat diets may facilitate gastric emptying. Pharmacologic treatments of slowed gastric emptying include prokinetic agents (e.g., domperidone, metoclopramide, erythromycin). Cisapride has been withdrawn from the market in many countries because of an increased risk of cardiac arrhythmia and death. For intractable impaired gastric emptying, a temporary or permanent jejunostomy may rarely be required. For diarrhea, opioids (e.g., loperamide, codeine), cholestyramine, fiber, and bulking agents may be useful. Biofeedback may help with fecal incontinence.[41,42]

Bladder neuropathy leads to loss of bladder sensitivity and later detrusor muscle weakness, both of which contribute to incomplete bladder emptying, recurrent infection, and eventual overflow incontinence (see Chapter 29). In late disease, an end-stage, insensitive, non-contractile atonic bladder can result. Symptoms of bladder neuropathy include urgency, nocturia, and incontinence. Other urologic problems such as bladder tumor, infection, urethral stricture, or prostatic hypertrophy should be excluded. Urodynamic studies may be helpful, including urinary tract imaging (e.g., intravenous pyelography), cystography, uroflowmetry, and postvoid ultrasonography to test for residual urine. Pharmacotherapy may include parasympathomimetics and α-adrenergic blockade to relieve sphincter hypertonicity. End-stage dysfunction may require intermittent self-catheterization.[41,42]

Sudomotor neuropathy, or abnormalities of sweating, can cause stocking and glove distribution anhidrosis, a risk factor for skin ulceration in the feet. Generalized loss of sweating increases heat intolerance. Diabetic subjects may experience inappropriate truncal sweating or gustatory sweating (facial and truncal sweating induced by eating certain foods). Thermoregulatory sweat testing (TST) examines the geographic distribution of sweating; quantitative sudomotor axon reflex testing (QSART) can quantify sweat output using a dehumidified sweat capsule; in diabetes, output may be reduced, absent, excessive, or "hung up" (persistent). The sympathetic skin response is an electrophysiologic surrogate for sweat gland activation. Other measures of sweat output include an analysis of sweat droplet numbers (numbers of functioning sweat glands) and size,[43] skin biopsy to analyze sweat gland innervation,[44] and novel rapid sweat indicator methods.[45] For patients with hypohidrosis or anhidrosis, caution regarding heat exposure should be advised. Moisturizers may be applied to dry feet and hands.

Autonomic neuropathy may cause small pupils, with sluggish or absent pupillary reflexes accompanied by light intolerance. Pupils may be examined by pupillography to measure pupillary diameter, latency to contraction, and velocity of contraction and dilatation.

Patients with diabetes may also have hypoglycemic unawareness because autonomic responses (e.g., sweating, tachycardia) and counterregulatory hormones such as epinephrine fail to increase. Patients may not recognize their impairment and thus fail to take adequate protective measures.[41,42]

CENTRAL NERVOUS SYSTEM COMPLICATIONS

Cognitive Dysfunction

A complication of diabetes mellitus that is frequently overlooked or under-reported is cognitive decline, which was first reported almost a century ago and can occur with type 1 or type 2 diabetes.[46–49] An elevated risk of dementia, cerebral atrophy, and presence of white matter abnormalities have been shown in multiple studies. Cognitive dysfunction may be apparent during childhood[50,51] or in late stages of life[52] when neurodegeneration may predominate.[47,50–52] Patients with diabetes also have an increased risk of development of Alzheimer disease (AD) as compared with subjects without diabetes.[53] A substantial number of AD patients have either glucose intolerance or diabetes.[54]

Children with type 1 diabetes have lower intelligence scores, lowered mental efficiency, and poor school performance compared to children without diabetes.[50] The younger the age of onset of the diabetes, the greater the cognitive impact.[55] Once present, early-onset cognitive dysfunction persists into adulthood, associated with impaired cognitive performance and significant cerebral atrophy.[56,57] Chronic hyperglycemia may possibly accelerate neurodegeneration.[58] Thus, some reports have speculated on the association between acute hypoglycemic episodes and cognitive impairment; a large meta-analysis failed to demonstrate such an association.[59,60] A longer duration of diabetes also appears to increase cognitive dysfunction.[61]

In type 2 diabetes mellitus, there are several other confounding factors that may influence cognition such as obesity, dyslipidemia, hypertension, and stroke.[62–64] Patients with prediabetes or impaired glucose tolerance may also have cognitive impairment to a lesser degree.[65,66] Another important comorbidity is depression in some patients with diabetes, although its impact appears to be less than the impact of diabetes itself.[67,68]

Particular domains of cognition may be impacted more than others in diabetes, including attention and executive function, processing speed, perception, and memory.[69] Language and visuospatial abilities tend to be preserved.[70] In both cross-sectional and longitudinal studies, there is mild-to-moderate impairment of working memory in patients with type 2 diabetes.[71,72] Mental flexibility and planning is also impaired in these patients, along with verbal memory.[73–75]

Many patients with type 2 diabetes have mild cognitive impairment rather than frank dementia.[76,77] However, like all patients with mild cognitive impairment, there is an increased risk of developing dementia.[78] Diabetes has been shown to be a risk factor for vascular dementia and AD.[79–81] Despite limitations of intensive glycemic management, hyperinsulinemia may be the basis of this increased risk.[72]

Changes present in the diabetic brain over time can be described pathologically as diabetic leukoencephalopathy.[46,82] The main hallmarks include cerebral atrophy and periventricular, subcortical white matter abnormalities (Fig. 19-3).[82,83]

Studies examining cognitive function in diabetic females or males demonstrate similar patterns of cognitive impairment.[84,85] Longer durations of diabetes and poor glycemic control are associated with greater microvascular end-organ complications and greater cognitive dysfunction that parallel elevated glycosylated hemoglobin (HbA1c) levels.[27,74,86–89] It is possible that cognitive dysfunction is partially reversible with improvements in glycemic control,[90,91] although optimal target levels have not yet been established.[90,91]

Stroke

Diabetes mellitus is a prominent risk factor for cerebral infarction.[92] Diabetes contributes to atherosclerosis of the cerebral arteries and alters cerebral blood flow.[93,94] It has been associated with both small-vessel lacunar infarction and large-vessel stroke.[92,95] Patients with vascular dementia have a greater prevalence of diabetes than other patients with dementia.[96] Vascular dementia is the second most common cause worldwide of dementia after AD, and its prevalence varies by country, with higher rates in Japan and Russia.[97] Men have higher rates of vascular dementia than women, in contrast to female-dominated AD populations, and the proportion of patients with vascular dementia increases further in the oldest old.[98,99] The effects of type 2 diabetes and hypertension likely act as additive factors contributing to cognitive decline, although cross-sectional studies have shown mixed results.[74,100,101]

Alzheimer Disease

In addition to its relatsionship with vascular dementia, diabetes is associated with an increased risk of AD.[102,103] Reduced glucose tolerance, insulin resistance, and hyperinsulinemia lead to poor memory and are associated with hippocampal atrophy, one of the hallmark features of AD.[72,104] In addition, diabetes mellitus is associated with neuropathologic markers of AD, including beta amyloid and tau accumulation.[71] Alterations in insulin metabolism may be associated with cognitive decline and dementia due to changes in synaptic plasticity[105] and the metabolism of cerebral amyloid and tau.[105,106] Even prior to the onset of mild cognitive impairment, insulin resistance is associated with a reduction in cerebral glucose metabolic rates and more subtle cognitive impairment.[107]

There is a possible genetic link between type 2 diabetes and the development of cognitive impairment and dementia. The apolipoprotein E gene (particularly the ε4 allelic variant), which has been linked with AD, is also associated with atherosclerotic risk factors and a higher risk of vascular dementia in patients with diabetes.[108] Patients with type 2 diabetes who also carry the ε4 allele have a twofold increased risk of dementia when compared to patients without diabetes who have this allele.[109,110] Serial MRI of the brain has identified progressive cerebral atrophy in patients with this allele.[111]

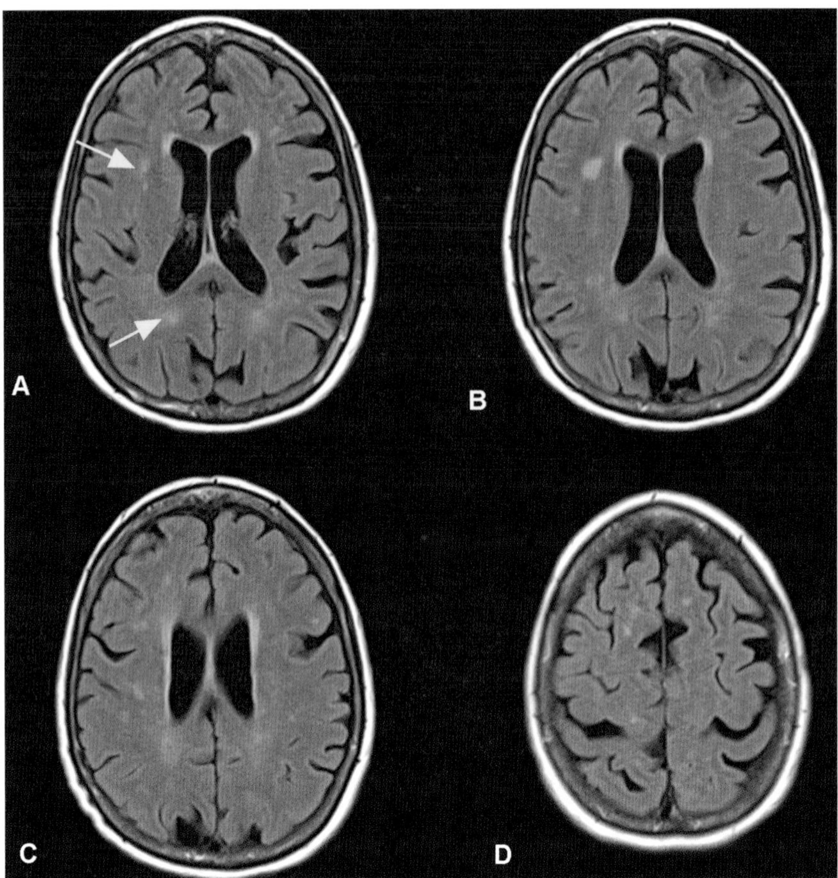

FIGURE 19-3 ■ Magnetic resonance imaging (MRI) of the brain from a 62-year-old woman with type 2 diabetes mellitus for 12 years, who presented with mild ataxia of gait and polyneuropathy. These axial T2-weighted fluid-attenuated inversion recovery (FLAIR) sequences progress from caudal to rostral cuts (**A** to **D**) and show nonenhancing bilateral white matter hyperintensities (arrows in **A**), also termed diabetic leukoencephalopathy.

Mechanisms of Cerebral Dysfunction

Pathogenic synergy exists with diabetic leukoencephalopathy and AD in apolipoprotein processing, impairment in corticosteroid regulation, and disruption of insulin signaling.[112,113] The advanced glycation end-product pathway renders additional toxicity due to oxidative stress and reduced nitric oxide bioavailability.[114] As these advanced glycation end-products propagate during aging and with diabetes, there is upregulation of their receptor, RAGE, which is a ubiquitous multi-ligand transmembrane receptor of the immunoglobulin superfamily of cell surface molecules.[114,115] Signaling through this pathway initiates protein kinases including proinflammatory gene activation and secondary immune responses.[116] A central transcription factor targeted by RAGE signaling that may be contributing to the pathogenesis of diabetic leukoencephalopathy is nuclear factor κB.[117–119] Abnormally high RAGE expression occurs in animal models of diabetes within gray matter including the hippocampus and cortex, as well as in white matter regions such as the corpus callosum and internal capsule.[46]

The human AD brain also has demonstrated attenuation of the insulin signaling pathway.[120] Intranasal insulin has been shown to potentially aid cognitive deficits in patients with AD in small trials following successful animal data.[48,121–123] Hyperinsulinemia's impact upon the brain includes downregulation of insulin signaling pathways and inactivation of glycogen synthase kinase 3, which normally prevents tau hyperphosphorylation.[48,124,125] Hyperinsulinemia or insulin resistance also promotes amyloidosis through release of intracellular Aβ from neurons in culture and enhancement of cerebral Aβ clearance.[126–128] Peripheral insulin increases measurable Aβ levels in cerebrospinal fluid,[129] potentially leading to insulin-induced acceleration of AD processes.[129–130] Insulin signaling also influences neuronal senescence and life span, which is a currently active area of research.[131]

NEUROPATHIC PAIN

Neuropathic pain can develop in the setting of diabetic polyneuropathy or mononeuropathies and is typically described as nocturnal burning discomfort, allodynia, electric-like jolts, or deep aching pain.

Pathophysiology

Altered excitability of axons as well as cell bodies of sensory ganglia contributes to the pathophysiology of neuropathic pain, explaining why some patients may have prominent pain despite only mild loss of nerve fibers. Changes in the distributions of sodium or calcium channels that promote abnormal ectopic discharges may initiate this pain cascade. Specific channels include upregulated calcium channels ($Ca_v3.2$ T-type), and sodium channels ($Na_v1.3$, $Na_v1.9$ and $Na_v1.7$).[1,132–134] Other molecular mechanisms of neuropathic pain in diabetes have been investigated. A bradykinin B1 receptor (BKB1-R) antagonist reversed thermal hyperalgesia in an animal model of type 1 diabetes.[135] Painful experimental diabetic neuropathy has been associated with changes in the expression of the VR1 (vanilloid, *TRPV1*) receptor; rises in the tetrameric membrane-expressed version of this receptor in diabetes have been through protein kinase C–mediated phosphorylation. Protein kinase C has been linked to the development of pain models of diabetic neuropathy; its inhibition attenuates hyperalgesia in diabetic rats whereas its activation increases thermal hyperalgesia.[136,137]

Changes at the level of the dorsal horn of the spinal cord may also be implicated in the development of neuropathic pain.[138] Animals with early induced diabetes show rises in spinal COX-2 protein and activity that accompany abnormalities in pain behavior.[139] These findings and others indicate that diabetic polyneuropathy is associated with multilevel changes in the neuraxis that promote pain.

Treatment

The current literature regarding analgesic therapy for diabetic polyneuropathy has been reviewed elsewhere, with evidence supporting the use of tricyclic antidepressants, gabapentin, pregabalin, duloxetine, opioids, and tramadol.[140,141] Opioids and gabapentin may have synergistic actions.[142]

Several guidelines for the treatment of neuropathic pain have been published, including specific recommendations highlighted by the American Academy of Neurology and other professional organizations.[143] Based on class I evidence, pregabalin has been determined to lessen the pain of peripheral diabetic neuropathy and improve quality of life and sleep (recommendation level A). Gabapentin and sodium valproate were classified as probably effective and given a level B recommendation. Other agents deemed probably effective (level B) included amitriptyline, venlafaxine, duloxetine, dextromethorphan, morphine sulfate, tramadol, oxycodone, capsaicin, isorbide dinitrate, and percutaneous electric stimulation. In contrast, topiramate, desipramine, imipramine, fluoxetine, alpha lipoic acid, or the combination of nortriptyline and fluphenazine had insufficient evidence for or against their use. Oxcarbazepine, lamotrigine, lacosamide, clonidine, pentoxifylline and mexiletine were found to have evidence against their effectiveness (negative level B recommendation). Other guidelines have provided similar recommendations, excepting a higher rating for duloxetine in more broad evaluations of all forms of neuropathic pain.[144,145] A small single-center randomized control trial of the cannabinoid nabilone, not discussed in the guidelines above, found that it improved neuropathic pain symptoms and quality of life.[146]

It should be noted that recommended therapy may change with time and approvals vary with jurisdiction. The following suggestions are not based on specific FDA approval in the United States. Gabapentin can be initiated in low doses such as 300 mg at bedtime and increased to a maximum of 3,600 mg daily. It does not alter the metabolism of other drugs, but requires dose reduction in renal failure. Side effects include dizziness, fatigue, and cognitive dysfunction with initial use or higher doses, as well as lower limb edema. Pregabalin is started at 75 mg at bedtime, and titrated upwards using a twice daily dosing schedule to a maximum of 600 mg daily; its side effects are similar to those of gabapentin.

Serotonin and norepinephrine reuptake inhibitors include venlafaxine, which is initiated at

37.5 mg per day and increased weekly to a maximum of 225 mg daily. Side effects include nausea, dizziness, drowsiness, hyperhidrosis, hypertension, and constipation. Duloxetine is started at 30 mg daily and titrated upwards to a maximum of 120 mg daily, although 60 mg daily often provides optimal outcomes. Adverse effects include hepatotoxicity, nausea, dry mouth, constipation, somnolence, hyperhidrosis, and decreased appetite. Amitriptyline is a tricyclic antidepressant that is started at 10 to 25 mg at bedtime and increased to 100 to 150 mg. Side effects include next-day drowsiness, lethargy, dry mouth, constipation, and bladder retention. Amitriptyline may help with prominent nocturnal pain but requires caution in patients with cardiac disease or urinary retention.

Opioids are an important therapy for neuropathic pain. Tramadol is initiated at 37.5 mg every 3 to 6 hours to a maximum of 300–400 mg daily. Controlled-release oxycodone is divided into twice daily dosing up to 100 mg daily. Long-acting morphine sulfate (30 to 60 mg twice daily) may be helpful when there is severe underlying systemic disease such as renal failure or cardiac disease. Adverse opioid reactions are cognitive dysfunction, somnolence, respiratory depression, constipation, pruritus, dizziness, nausea, vomiting, rebound headache syndrome, risk of addiction, and withdrawal syndrome.

Local agents that can be used include lidocaine patches and capsacin. Some patients find these to be acceptable alternatives to oral medications.

REFERENCES

1. Zochodne DW, Kline G, Smith EE, et al: Diabetic Neurology. Informa Healthcare, New York, 2010.
2. Freeby M, Ebner S: Ketoacidosis and hyperglycemic hyperosmolar state. p. 159. In: Biessels GJ, Luchsinger JA (eds): Diabetes and the Brain. Humana Press, New York, 2010.
3. Dyck PJ, Kratz KM, Karnes JL, et al: The prevalence by staged severity of various types of diabetic neuropathy, retinopathy, and nephropathy in a population-based cohort: The Rochester Diabetic Neuropathy Study. Neurology 43:817, 1993.
4. Ewing DJ: Recent advances in the non-invasive investigation of diabetic autonomic neuropathy. p. 667. In Bannister R (ed): Autonomic Failure. Oxford University Press, Oxford, 1988.
5. Malik RA, Veves A, Walker D, et al: Sural nerve fibre pathology in diabetic patients with mild neuropathy: relationship to pain, quantitative sensory testing and peripheral nerve electrophysiology. Acta Neuropathol 101:367, 2001.
6. Anonymous: Report and recommendations of the San Antonio conference on diabetic neuropathy. Consensus statement. Diabetes 37:1000, 1988.
7. Bril V, Tomioka S, Buchanan RA, et al: Reliability and validity of the modified Toronto Clinical Neuropathy Score in diabetic sensorimotor polyneuropathy. Diabet Med 26:240, 2009.
8. Singleton JR, Bixby B, Russell JW, et al: The Utah Early Neuropathy Scale: a sensitive clinical scale for early sensory predominant neuropathy. J Peripher Nerv Syst 13:218, 2008.
9. Feldman EL, Stevens MJ, Thomas PK, et al: A practical two-step quantitative clinical and electrophysiological assessment for the diagnosis and staging of diabetic neuropathy. Diabetes Care 17:1281, 1994.
10. Bril V: Electrophysiologic testing. p. 177. In: Gries FA, Cameron NE, Low PA (eds): Textbook of Diabetic Neuropathy. Thieme, New York, 2003.
11. Lauria G, Cornblath DR, Johansson O, et al: EFNS guidelines on the use of skin biopsy in the diagnosis of peripheral neuropathy. Eur J Neurol 12:747, 2005.
12. Tavakoli M, Quattrini C, Abbott C, et al: Corneal confocal microscopy: a novel noninvasive test to diagnose and stratify the severity of human diabetic neuropathy. Diabetes Care 33:1792, 2010.
13. Malik RA, Newrick PG, Sharma AK, et al: Microangiopathy in human diabetic neuropathy: relationship between capillary abnormalities and the severity of neuropathy. Diabetologia 32:92, 1989.
14. Theriault M, Dort J, Sutherland G, et al: A prospective quantitative study of sensory deficits after whole sural nerve biopsies in diabetic and nondiabetic patients. Surgical approach and the role of collateral sprouting. Neurology 50:480, 1998.
15. Greene DA, Lattimer SA, Sima AA: Sorbitol, phosphoinositides, and sodium-potassium-ATPase in the pathogenesis of diabetic complications. N Engl J Med 316:599, 1987.
16. Chalk C, Benstead TJ, Moore F: Aldose reductase inhibitors for the treatment of diabetic polyneuropathy. Cochrane Database Syst Rev:CD004572, 2007.
17. Zherebitskaya E, Akude E, Smith DR, et al: Development of selective axonopathy in adult sensory neurons isolated from diabetic rats: role of glucose-induced oxidative stress. Diabetes 58:1356, 2009.
18. Huang TJ, Sayers NM, Verkhratsky A, et al: Neurotrophin-3 prevents mitochondrial dysfunction in sensory neurons of streptozotocin-diabetic rats. Exp Neurol 194:279, 2005.
19. Dyck PJ, Hansen S, Karnes J, et al: Capillary number and percentage closed in human diabetic sural nerve. Proc Natl Acad Sci USA 82:2513, 1985.
20. Theriault M, Dort J, Sutherland G, et al: Local human sural nerve blood flow in diabetic and other polyneuropathies. Brain 120:1131, 1997.

21. Zochodne DW, Nguyen C: Increased peripheral nerve microvessels in early experimental diabetic neuropathy: quantitative studies of nerve and dorsal root ganglia. J Neurol Sci 166:40, 1999.
22. Brewster WJ, Fernyhough P, Diemel LT, et al: Diabetic neuropathy, nerve growth factor and other neurotrophic factors. Trends Neurosci 17:321, 1994.
23. Apfel SC, Schwartz S, Adornato BT, et al: Efficacy and safety of recombinant human nerve growth factor in patients with diabetic polyneuropathy: A randomized controlled trial. rhNGF Clinical Investigator Group. JAMA 284:2215, 2000.
24. Sugimoto K, Murakawa Y, Sima AA: Expression and localization of insulin receptor in rat dorsal root ganglion and spinal cord. J Peripher Nerv Syst 7:44, 2002.
25. Francis G, Martinez J, Liu W, et al: Intranasal insulin ameliorates experimental diabetic neuropathy. Diabetes 58:934, 2009.
26. Brussee V, Cunningham FA, Zochodne DW: Direct insulin signaling of neurons reverses diabetic neuropathy. Diabetes 53:1824, 2004.
27. Diabetes Control & Complications Trial Research Group: The effect of intensive treatment of diabetes on the development and progression of long-term complications in insulin-dependent diabetes mellitus. N Engl J Med 329:977, 1993.
28. Anonymous: The effect of intensive diabetes therapy on measures of autonomic nervous system function in the Diabetes Control and Complications Trial (DCCT). Diabetologia 41:416, 1998.
29. Wilbourn AJ: Diabetic entrapment and compression neuropathies. p. 481. In: Dyck PJ, Thomas PK (eds): Diabetic Neuropathy. 2nd Ed. WB Saunders, Toronto, 1999.
30. Kennedy JM, Zochodne DW: The regenerative deficit of peripheral nerves in experimental diabetes: its extent, timing and possible mechanisms. Brain 123:2118, 2000.
31. Stewart J: Diabetic truncal neuropathy: topography of the sensory deficit. Ann Neurol 25:233, 1989.
32. Raff MC, Sangalang V, Asbury AK: Ischemic mononeuropathy multiplex in association with diabetes mellitus. Neurology 18:284, 1968.
33. Barohn RJ, Sahenk Z, Warmolts JR, et al: The Bruns-Garland syndrome (diabetic amyotrophy). Revisited 100 years later. Arch Neurol 48:1130, 1991.
34. Dyck PJ, Windebank AJ: Diabetic and nondiabetic lumbosacral radiculoplexus neuropathies: new insights into pathophysiology and treatment. Muscle Nerve 25:477, 2002.
35. Dyck PJ, Norell JE, Dyck PJ: Microvasculitis and ischemia in diabetic lumbosacral radiculoplexus neuropathy. Neurology 53:2113, 1999.
36. Said G, Elgrably F, Lacroix C, et al: Painful proximal diabetic neuropathy: inflammatory nerve lesions and spontaneous favorable outcome. Ann Neurol 41:762, 1997.
37. Morris AM, Deeks SL, Hill MD, et al: Annualized incidence and spectrum of illness from an outbreak investigation of Bell's palsy. Neuroepidemiology 21:255, 2002.
38. Veglio M, Sivieri R, Chinaglia A, et al: QT interval prolongation and mortality in type 1 diabetic patients: a 5-year cohort prospective study. Neuropathy Study Group of the Italian Society of the Study of Diabetes, Piemonte Affiliate. Diabetes Care 23:1381, 2000.
39. Neil HA, Thompson AV, John S, et al: Diabetic autonomic neuropathy: the prevalence of impaired heart rate variability in a geographically defined population. Diabet Med 6:20, 1989.
40. Bacon CG, Hu FB, Giovannucci E, et al: Association of type and duration of diabetes with erectile dysfunction in a large cohort of men. Diabetes Care 25:1458, 2002.
41. Gries FA, Cameron NE, Low PA, et al: Textbook of Diabetic Neuropathy. Thieme, New York, 2003.
42. Low PA (ed): Clinical Autonomic Disorders. 2nd Ed. Lippincott-Raven, Philadelphia, 1997.
43. Kennedy WR, Sakuta M, Sutherland D, et al: Quantitation of the sweating deficiency in diabetes mellitus. Ann Neurol 15:482, 1984.
44. Gibbons CH, Illigens BM, Wang N, et al: Quantification of sweat gland innervation: a clinical-pathologic correlation. Neurology 72:1479, 2009.
45. Quattrini C, Jeziorska M, Tavakoli M, et al: The Neuropad test: a visual indicator test for human diabetic neuropathy. Diabetologia 51:1046, 2008.
46. Toth C, Schmidt AM, Tuor UI, et al: Diabetes, leukoencephalopathy and rage. Neurobiol Dis 23:443, 2006.
47. Biessels GJ, Deary IJ, Ryan CM: Cognition and diabetes: a lifespan perspective. Lancet Neurol 7:184, 2008.
48. Francis GJ, Martinez JA, Liu WQ, et al: Intranasal insulin prevents cognitive decline, cerebral atrophy and white matter changes in murine type I diabetic encephalopathy. Brain 131:3311, 2008.
49. Miles WR, Root HF: Psychologic tests applied to diabetic patients. Arch Intern Med 30:767, 1922.
50. Schoenle EJ, Schoenle D, Molinari L, et al: Impaired intellectual development in children with Type I diabetes: association with HbA(1c), age at diagnosis and sex. Diabetologia 45:108, 2002.
51. Northam EA, Anderson PJ, Jacobs R, et al: Neuropsychological profiles of children with type 1 diabetes 6 years after disease onset. Diabetes Care 24:1541, 2001.
52. Awad N, Gagnon M, Messier C: The relationship between impaired glucose tolerance, type 2 diabetes, and cognitive function. J Clin Exp Neuropsychol 26:1044, 2004.
53. Biessels GJ, Staekenborg S, Brunner E, et al: Risk of dementia in diabetes mellitus: a systematic review. Lancet Neurol 5:64, 2006.

54. Janson J, Laedtke T, Parisi JE, et al: Increased risk of type 2 diabetes in Alzheimer disease. Diabetes 53:474, 2004.
55. Dahlquist G, Kallen B: School performance in children with type 1 diabetes–a population-based register study. Diabetologia 50:957, 2007.
56. Ryan CM: Why is cognitive dysfunction associated with the development of diabetes early in life? The diathesis hypothesis. Pediatr Diabetes 7:289, 2006.
57. Ferguson SC, Blane A, Wardlaw J, et al: Influence of an early-onset age of type 1 diabetes on cerebral structure and cognitive function. Diabetes Care 28:1431, 2005.
58. Perantie DC, Wu J, Koller JM, et al: Regional brain volume differences associated with hyperglycemia and severe hypoglycemia in youth with type 1 diabetes. Diabetes Care 30:2331, 2007.
59. Gold AE, Deary IJ, Jones RW, et al: Severe deterioration in cognitive function and personality in five patients with long-standing diabetes: a complication of diabetes or a consequence of treatment? Diabet Med 11:499, 1994.
60. Jacobson AM, Musen G, Ryan CM, et al: Long-term effect of diabetes and its treatment on cognitive function. N Engl J Med 356:1842, 2007.
61. Spauwen PJ, Kohler S, Verhey FR, et al: Effects of type 2 diabetes on 12-year cognitive change: results from the Maastricht Aging Study. Diabetes Care 36:1554, 2013.
62. Knopman D, Boland LL, Mosley T, et al: Cardiovascular risk factors and cognitive decline in middle-aged adults. Neurology 56:42, 2001.
63. Atiea JA, Moses JL, Sinclair AJ: Neuropsychological function in older subjects with non-insulin-dependent diabetes mellitus. Diabet Med 12:679, 1995.
64. Kalmijn S, Foley D, White L, et al: Metabolic cardiovascular syndrome and risk of dementia in Japanese-American elderly men. The Honolulu-Asia aging study. Arterioscler Thromb Vasc Biol 20:2255, 2000.
65. Reaven GM: Banting lecture 1988. Role of insulin resistance in human disease. Diabetes 37:1595, 1988.
66. Kalmijn S, Feskens EJ, Launer LJ, et al: Glucose intolerance, hyperinsulinaemia and cognitive function in a general population of elderly men. Diabetologia 38:1096, 1995.
67. Saczynski JS, Beiser A, Seshadri S, et al: Depressive symptoms and risk of dementia: the Framingham Heart Study. Neurology 75:35, 2010.
68. Koekkoek PS, Rutten GE, Ruis C, et al: Mild depressive symptoms do not influence cognitive functioning in patients with type 2 diabetes. Psychoneuroendocrinology 38:376, 2013.
69. Lezak MD, Howieson DB, Loring DW: Neuropsychological Assessment. Oxford University Press, New York, 2004.
70. Perlmuter LC, Tun P, Sizer N, et al: Age and diabetes related changes in verbal fluency. Exp Aging Res 13:9, 1987.
71. Petrovitch H, White LR, Izmirilian G, et al: Midlife blood pressure and neuritic plaques, neurofibrillary tangles, and brain weight at death: the HAAS. Honolulu-Asia aging Study. Neurobiol Aging 21:57, 2000.
72. Luchsinger JA, Tang MX, Shea S, et al: Hyperinsulinemia and risk of Alzheimer disease. Neurology 63:1187, 2004.
73. Reaven GM, Thompson LW, Nahum D, et al: Relationship between hyperglycemia and cognitive function in older NIDDM patients. Diabetes Care 13:16, 1990.
74. Gregg EW, Yaffe K, Cauley JA, et al: Is diabetes associated with cognitive impairment and cognitive decline among older women? Study of Osteoporotic Fractures Research Group. Arch Intern Med 160:174, 2000.
75. Cosway R, Strachan MW, Dougall A, et al: Cognitive function and information processing in type 2 diabetes. Diabet Med 18:803, 2001.
76. Petersen RC, Smith GE, Waring SC, et al: Mild cognitive impairment: clinical characterization and outcome. Arch Neurol 56:303, 1999.
77. Ritchie K, Artero S, Touchon J: Classification criteria for mild cognitive impairment: a population-based validation study. Neurology 56:37, 2001.
78. Petersen RC, Stevens JC, Ganguli M, et al: Practice parameter: early detection of dementia: mild cognitive impairment (an evidence-based review). Report of the Quality Standards Subcommittee of the American Academy of Neurology. Neurology 56:1133, 2001.
79. Luchsinger JA, Tang MX, Stern Y, et al: Diabetes mellitus and risk of Alzheimer's disease and dementia with stroke in a multiethnic cohort. Am J Epidemiol 154:635, 2001.
80. Leibson CL, Rocca WA, Hanson VA, et al: The risk of dementia among persons with diabetes mellitus: a population-based cohort study. Ann N Y Acad Sci 826:422, 1997.
81. Ott A, Stolk RP, van Harskamp F, et al: Diabetes mellitus and the risk of dementia: The Rotterdam Study. Neurology 53:1937, 1999.
82. de Bresser J, Tiehuis AM, van den Berg E, et al: Progression of cerebral atrophy and white matter hyperintensities in patients with type 2 diabetes. Diabetes Care 33:1309, 2010.
83. van Elderen SG, de Roos A, de Craen AJ, et al: Progression of brain atrophy and cognitive decline in diabetes mellitus: a 3-year follow-up. Neurology 75:997, 2010.
84. Mooradian AD: Diabetic complications of the central nervous system. Endocr Rev 9:346, 1988.
85. Soininen H, Puranen M, Helkala EL, et al: Diabetes mellitus and brain atrophy: a computed tomography study in an elderly population. Neurobiol Aging 13:717, 1992.

86. Wong TY, Klein R, Islam FM, et al: Diabetic retinopathy in a multi-ethnic cohort in the United States. Am J Ophthalmol 141:446, 2006.
87. Brands AM, Biessels GJ, de Haan EH, et al: The effects of type 1 diabetes on cognitive performance: a meta-analysis. Diabetes Care 28:726, 2005.
88. Elias PK, Elias MF, D'Agostino RB, et al: NIDDM and blood pressure as risk factors for poor cognitive performance. The Framingham Study. Diabetes Care 20:1388, 1997.
89. Perlmuter LC, Hakami MK, Hodgson-Harrington C, et al: Decreased cognitive function in aging non-insulin-dependent diabetic patients. Am J Med 77:1043, 1984.
90. Gradman TJ, Laws A, Thompson LW, et al: Verbal learning and/or memory improves with glycemic control in older subjects with non-insulin-dependent diabetes mellitus. J Am Geriatr Soc 41:1305, 1993.
91. Ryan CM, Freed MI, Rood JA, et al: Improving metabolic control leads to better working memory in adults with type 2 diabetes. Diabetes Care 29:345, 2006.
92. Stegmayr B, Asplund K: Diabetes as a risk factor for stroke. A population perspective. Diabetologia 38:1061, 1995.
93. Kameyama M, Fushimi H, Udaka F: Diabetes mellitus and cerebral vascular disease. Diabetes Res Clin Pract 24(suppl):S205, 1994.
94. Gispen WH, Biessels GJ: Cognition and synaptic plasticity in diabetes mellitus. Trends Neurosci 23:542, 2000.
95. Lodder J, Boiten J: Incidence, natural history, and risk factors in lacunar infarction. Adv Neurol 62:213, 1993.
96. Landin K, Blennow K, Wallin A, et al: Low blood pressure and blood glucose levels in Alzheimer's disease. Evidence for a hypometabolic disorder? J InternMed 233:357, 1993.
97. Ikeda M, Hokoishi K, Maki N, et al: Increased prevalence of vascular dementia in Japan: a community-based epidemiological study. Neurology 57:839, 2001.
98. Jorm AF, Korten AE, Henderson AS: The prevalence of dementia: a quantitative integration of the literature. Acta Psychiatr Scand 76:465, 1987.
99. Jellinger KA, Attems J: Prevalence and pathology of vascular dementia in the oldest-old. J Alzheimers Dis 21:1283, 2010.
100. Hassing LB, Hofer SM, Nilsson SE, et al: Comorbid type 2 diabetes mellitus and hypertension exacerbates cognitive decline: evidence from a longitudinal study. Age Ageing 33:355, 2004.
101. Luchsinger JA, Reitz C, Honig LS, et al: Aggregation of vascular risk factors and risk of incident Alzheimer disease. Neurology 65:545, 2005.
102. Verdelho A, Madureira S, Moleiro C, et al: White matter changes and diabetes predict cognitive decline in the elderly: the LADIS study. Neurology 75:160, 2010.
103. Feinkohl I, Keller M, Robertson CM, et al: Clinical and subclinical macrovascular disease as predictors of cognitive decline in older patients with type 2 diabetes: the Edinburgh Type 2 Diabetes Study. Diabetes Care 36:2779, 2013.
104. Convit A, Wolf OT, Tarshish C, et al: Reduced glucose tolerance is associated with poor memory performance and hippocampal atrophy among normal elderly. Proc Natl Acad Sci USA 100:2019, 2003.
105. Chiu SL, Chen CM, Cline HT: Insulin receptor signaling regulates synapse number, dendritic plasticity, and circuit function in vivo. Neuron 58:708, 2008.
106. Biessels GJ, Kappelle LJ: Increased risk of Alzheimer's disease in Type II diabetes: insulin resistance of the brain or insulin-induced amyloid pathology? Biochem Soc Trans 33:1041, 2005.
107. Baker LD, Cross DJ, Minoshima S, et al: Insulin resistance and Alzheimer-like reductions in regional cerebral glucose metabolism for cognitively normal adults with prediabetes or early type 2 diabetes. Arch Neurol 68:51, 2011.
108. Peila R, Rodriguez BL, Launer LJ: Type 2 diabetes, APOE gene, and the risk for dementia and related pathologies: The Honolulu-Asia Aging Study. Diabetes 51:1256, 2002.
109. Strittmatter WJ, Saunders AM, Schmechel D, et al: Apolipoprotein E: high-avidity binding to beta-amyloid and increased frequency of type 4 allele in late-onset familial Alzheimer disease. Proc Natl Acad Sci USA 90:1977, 1993.
110. Xu WL, Qiu CX, Wahlin A, et al: Diabetes mellitus and risk of dementia in the Kungsholmen project: a 6-year follow-up study. Neurology 63:1181, 2004.
111. Vemuri P, Wiste HJ, Weigand SD, et al: Serial MRI and CSF biomarkers in normal aging, MCI, and AD. Neurology 75:143, 2010.
112. Stranahan AM, Arumugam TV, Cutler RG, et al: Diabetes impairs hippocampal function through glucocorticoid-mediated effects on new and mature neurons. Nat Neurosci 11:309, 2008.
113. Zhao WQ, Townsend M: Insulin resistance and amyloidogenesis as common molecular foundation for type 2 diabetes and Alzheimer's disease. Biochim Biophys Acta 1792:482, 2009.
114. Brownlee M: The pathobiology of diabetic complications: a unifying mechanism. Diabetes 54:1615, 2005.
115. Wautier JL, Guillausseau PJ: Advanced glycation end products, their receptors and diabetic angiopathy. Diabetes Metab 27:535, 2001.
116. Yan SF, Ramasamy R, Schmidt AM: Receptor for AGE (RAGE) and its ligands-cast into leading roles in diabetes and the inflammatory response. J Mol Med (Berl) 87:235, 2009.
117. Bierhaus A, Schiekofer S, Schwaninger M, et al: Diabetes-associated sustained activation of the

transcription factor nuclear factor-kappaB. Diabetes 50:2792, 2001.

118. Perkins ND: The Rel/NF-kappa B family: friend and foe. Trends Biochem Sci 25:434, 2000.
119. Baeuerle PA, Baltimore D: NF-kappa B: ten years after. Cell 87:13, 1996.
120. Frolich L, Blum-Degen D, Bernstein HG, et al: Brain insulin and insulin receptors in aging and sporadic Alzheimer's disease. J Neural Transm 105:423, 1998.
121. Benedict C, Hallschmid M, Schmitz K, et al: Intranasal insulin improves memory in humans: superiority of insulin aspart. Neuropsychopharmacology 32:239, 2007.
122. Craft S, Baker LD, Montine TJ, et al: Intranasal insulin therapy for Alzheimer disease and amnestic mild cognitive impairment: a pilot clinical trial. Arch Neurol 69:29, 2012.
123. Shemesh E, Rudich A, Harman-Boehm I, et al: Effect of intranasal insulin on cognitive function: a systematic review. J Clin Endocrinol Metab 97:366, 2012.
124. Cross DA, Alessi DR, Cohen P, et al: Inhibition of glycogen synthase kinase-3 by insulin mediated by protein kinase B. Nature 378:785, 1995.
125. Park CR: Cognitive effects of insulin in the central nervous system. Neurosci Biobehav Rev 25:311, 2001.
126. Su Y, Ryder J, Li B, et al: Lithium, a common drug for bipolar disorder treatment, regulates amyloid-beta precursor protein processing. Biochemistry 43:6899, 2004.
127. Ho L, Qin W, Pompl PN, et al: Diet-induced insulin resistance promotes amyloidosis in a transgenic mouse model of Alzheimer's disease. FASEB J 18:902, 2004.
128. Gasparini L, Gouras GK, Wang R, et al: Stimulation of beta-amyloid precursor protein trafficking by insulin reduces intraneuronal beta-amyloid and requires mitogen-activated protein kinase signaling. J Neurosci 21:2561, 2001.
129. Watson GS, Peskind ER, Asthana S, et al: Insulin increases CSF Abeta42 levels in normal older adults. Neurology 60:1899, 2003.
130. Pardridge WM, Kang YS, Buciak JL, et al: Human insulin receptor monoclonal antibody undergoes high affinity binding to human brain capillaries in vitro and rapid transcytosis through the blood-brain barrier in vivo in the primate. Pharm Res 12:807, 1995.
131. Cohen E, Dillin A: The insulin paradox: aging, proteotoxicity and neurodegeneration. Nat Rev Neurosci 9:759, 2008.
132. Jagodic MM, Pathirathna S, Nelson MT, et al: Cell-specific alterations of T-type calcium current in painful diabetic neuropathy enhance excitability of sensory neurons. J Neurosci 27:3305, 2007.
133. Hong S, Morrow TJ, Paulson PE, et al: Early painful diabetic neuropathy is associated with differential changes in tetrodotoxin-sensitive and -resistant sodium channels in dorsal root ganglion neurons in the rat. J Biol Chem 279:29341, 2004.
134. Craner MJ, Klein JP, Renganathan M, et al: Changes of sodium channel expression in experimental painful diabetic neuropathy. Ann Neurol 52:786, 2002.
135. Gabra BH, Benrezzak O, Pheng LH, et al: Inhibition of type 1 diabetic hyperalgesia in streptozotocin-induced Wistar versus spontaneous gene-prone BB/Worchester rats: efficacy of a selective bradykinin B1 receptor antagonist. J Neuropathol Exp Neurol 64:782, 2005.
136. Ahlgren SC, Levine JD: Protein kinase C inhibitors decrease hyperalgesia and C-fiber hyperexcitability in the streptozotocin-diabetic rat. J Neurophysiol 72:684, 1994.
137. Ohsawa M, Kamei J: Possible involvement of spinal protein kinase C in thermal allodynia and hyperalgesia in diabetic mice. Eur J Pharmacol 372:221, 1999.
138. Calcutt NA: Potential mechanisms of neuropathic pain in diabetes. Int Rev Neurobiol 50:205, 2002.
139. Ramos KM, Jiang Y, Svensson CI, et al: Pathogenesis of spinally mediated hyperalgesia in diabetes. Diabetes 56:1569, 2007.
140. Zochodne DW: Diabetes mellitus and the peripheral nervous system: manifestations and mechanisms. Muscle Nerve 36:144, 2007.
141. Vinik A: Clinical review: use of antiepileptic drugs in the treatment of chronic painful diabetic neuropathy. J Clin Endocrinol Metab 90:4936, 2005.
142. Gilron I, Bailey JM, Tu D, et al: Morphine, gabapentin, or their combination for neuropathic pain. N Engl J Med 352:1324, 2005.
143. Bril V, England J, Franklin GM, et al: Evidence-based guideline: treatment of painful diabetic neuropathy: report of the American Academy of Neurology, the American Association of Neuromuscular and Electrodiagnostic Medicine, and the American Academy of Physical Medicine and Rehabilitation. Neurology 76:1758, 2011.
144. Attal N, Cruccu G, Haanpaa M, et al: EFNS guidelines on pharmacological treatment of neuropathic pain. Eur J Neurol 13:1153, 2006.
145. Dworkin RH, O'Connor AB, Audette J, et al: Recommendations for the pharmacological management of neuropathic pain: an overview and literature update. Mayo Clin Proc 85:S3, 2010.
146. Toth C, Mawani S, Brady S, et al: An enriched-enrolment, randomized withdrawal, flexible-dose, double-blind, placebo-controlled, parallel assignment efficacy study of nabilone as adjuvant in the treatment of diabetic peripheral neuropathic pain. Pain 153:2073, 2012.

CHAPTER

20

Sex Hormone, Pituitary, Parathyroid, and Adrenal Disorders and the Nervous System

HYMAN M. SCHIPPER ■ CHERYL A. JAY ■ GARY M. ABRAMS

The most common endocrine disorders causing neurologic disease are thyroid disease and diabetes mellitus, which are addressed in Chapters 18 and 19. Nevertheless, sex hormone, pituitary, parathyroid, and adrenal disorders may have important neurologic implications or consequences and are therefore reviewed here, with emphasis on features relevant to neurologic practice.

SEX HORMONES AND THE NERVOUS SYSTEM

The effects of sex steroids on neurologic function in health and disease constitute a rich and rapidly expanding area of basic and clinical neuroscience. Sex steroids exert both organizational and activational effects within the nervous system. Organizational effects refer to the irreversible differentiation of neural circuitry resulting from exposure to sex steroids during critical periods of brain development and are discussed in the previous edition of this book.[1] The activational effects of sex steroids encompass a myriad of largely reversible neurophysiologic influences exerted by gonadal hormones on the mature nervous system. Such interactions are essential for regulation of the brain–pituitary–gonadal axis (Fig. 20-1) and the establishment of normal patterns of sexual, aggressive, cognitive, and autonomic behaviors. Furthermore, by impacting the metabolism and release of various

Aminoff's Neurology and General Medicine, Fifth Edition.

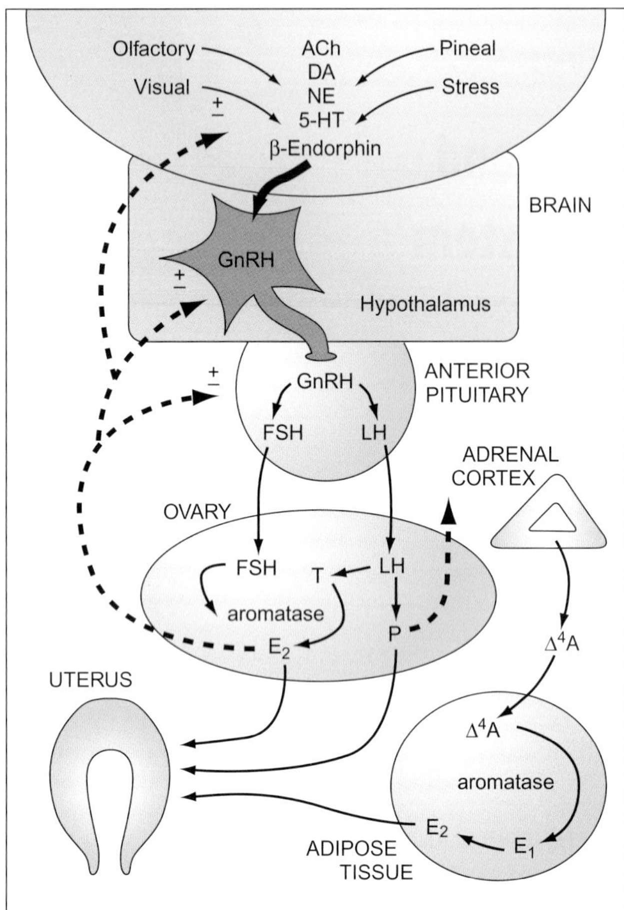

Figure 20-1 ▪ The brain–pituitary–ovarian axis. Δ^4A, delta-4-androstenedione; ACh, acetylcholine; DA, dopamine; E_1, estrone; E_2, estradiol; FSH, follicle-stimulating hormone; GnRH, gonadotropin-releasing hormone; 5-HT, 5-hydroxytryptamine (serotonin); LH, luteinizing hormone; NE, norepinephrine; P, progesterone; T, testosterone.

central neurotransmitters and neuromodulators, hormonal fluctuations associated with (1) specific phases of the menstrual cycle, (2) pregnancy, (3) the menopause, and (4) exposure to exogenous sex hormones may induce or modify a host of neurologic and neuropsychiatric disorders.[2]

Migraine

Although no gender difference in its prevalence is apparent before puberty, migraine is three times as common in adult women (18%) as in men (6%).[3] Approximately 60 percent of women with migraine experience perimenstrual exacerbations of their headaches (catamenial migraine). The late luteal-phase decline in plasma estradiol (but not progesterone) appears to play an important role in the precipitation of catamenial migraine.[1] The frequency or severity (or both) of migraine attacks often diminishes with gestation, particularly in patients whose headaches are linked to the menstrual cycle. The absence of rhythmic estrogen "withdrawal" characteristic of the pregnant state is believed to be responsible for the reduction in migraine activity. Indeed, many women whose headaches are attenuated by pregnancy experience relapses at the time of parturition, when sex hormone levels fall precipitously. In some women, breastfeeding appears to protect against migraine recurrence.[4] Occasionally, migraine arises for the first time or appears to worsen during gestation[5] or the perimenopausal period.[6] A first approach to the management of gestational migraine should be nonpharmacologic (e.g., relaxation training, biofeedback), especially during the first trimester when risks of teratogenicity and embryotoxicity are greatest. For severe attacks, acetaminophen with codeine or nonsteroidal anti-inflammatory drugs (NSAIDs) may have to be used. Further discussion is provided in Chapter 31. For status migrainosus in pregnancy, chlorpromazine, meperidine, morphine, or prednisone may need to be administered.[7] Perimenopausal migraine often responds to standard estrogen replacement therapy, but this must be weighed against the risk of developing breast cancer in individual patients. Fluoxetine and venlafaxine may be beneficial in women with perimenopausal migraine and comorbid hot flashes.[8]

An association between migraine and "the pill" is frequently encountered in clinical practice. Women often exhibit new-onset or exacerbation of migraine while taking oral contraceptives. Attacks tend to manifest during the first few cycles (particularly on placebo days in accord with the estrogen withdrawal hypothesis) and usually, but not invariably, resolve on discontinuation of the medication. A qualitative change in the pattern of migraine is noted in some patients. For example, a migraineur may develop a focal prodrome for the first time while taking oral contraceptives. Women in this category may be at high risk of infarction in regions reflecting the distribution of their auras. Amelioration of migraine after exposure to oral contraceptives is sometimes observed, perhaps related at least in part to psychologic factors.

The pathophysiology of estrogen-related migraine is incompletely understood. Estrogens may act directly on vascular smooth muscle as well as modulate the activity of vasoactive substances at the neurovascular junction. In addition, by altering central prostaglandin, serotonin, opioid, or prolactin metabolism,[9] premenstrual changes in circulating estrogens may activate vasoregulatory elements in the brainstem or hypothalamus, which, in turn, may trigger symptomatic alterations in cerebrovascular tone.[1]

First-line therapy for menstrual migraine should include the standard pharmacologic, dietary, and psychologic modalities employed in the general migraine population. Sumatriptan and related serotonin 5-HT_{1D} (presynaptic autoinhibitory) receptor agonists are equally effective for noncatamenial and menstrual migraine.[10] Refractory cases of severe catamenial migraine may benefit from late luteal-phase therapy with prostaglandin inhibitors (e.g., naproxen, 250 to 500 mg orally twice daily) and mild diuretics.[1] Various hormonal interventions in catamenial migraine have been largely unsuccessful and often complicated by unpleasant side effects. Oral contraceptives usually exacerbate migraine and probably should not be used in the treatment of this disorder. The use of estrogen implants has yielded contradictory results.[1] The risk–benefit ratio accruing to long-term estrogen therapy must be carefully assessed before such treatment can be advocated for this relatively benign condition. The antiestrogen tamoxifen may either alleviate[11] or precipitate[12] catamenial migraine. The beneficial effect of tamoxifen may be due to inhibition of calcium uptake or prostaglandin E synthesis in these subjects.[11] In several reports, danazol (200 mg twice daily for 25 days), a testosterone derivative used in the management of endometriosis, aborted or ameliorated premenstrual migraine for the duration of treatment; catamenial headaches resumed on its discontinuation.[1] Continuous bromocriptine therapy (2.5 mg three times daily) resulted in a 72 percent decline in headache frequency in a study involving 24 women with menstrual migraine.[13] In addition to migraine, menstruation, pregnancy and menopause may also influence cluster headache, other autonomic cephalalgias, and hemicrania continua.[14]

Stroke

"The pill" has been implicated as a significant risk factor in thromboembolic cerebral infarction, subarachnoid hemorrhage, and cerebral venous thrombosis. In 1969, American and British case-control studies revealed, respectively, a 19- and 6-fold increased risk of ischemic stroke in young women related to the use of oral contraceptives. Hypertension, migraine, and age older than 35 years were associated, but independent, risk factors for cerebral infarction in patients taking oral contraceptives.[1] Cigarette smoking by women on "the pill" was found to increase further the likelihood of hemorrhagic but not thromboembolic stroke. Ingestion of lower-dose (30 μg) estrogen preparations appears to be responsible for a decline in rates of thromboembolic disease among users of oral contraceptives.[15] In a population-based case-control study, the odds ratio of ischemic stroke in current users of low-dose estrogen contraceptives (20 to 35 μg) was only 1.18 in comparison with former users or women who were never exposed to oral contraceptives.[16] However, the risk of stroke remains unacceptably high in low-dose oral contraceptive users if they smoke and are older than the age of 35.[17] Recent evidence suggests that exposure to ultralow-dose oral contraceptives (containing <25 μg ethinyl estradiol) may not enhance stroke risk when used in normotensive nonsmokers.[18] Although less often implicated than estrogens, progestins may contribute to the danger of cerebral infarction by promoting hypertension, hypercoagulability, and adverse serum lipoprotein levels.[19,20]

Ischemic strokes in users of oral contraceptives have been localized to the carotid (usually the middle cerebral artery or its deep penetrating branches) and vertebrobasilar distributions. There is usually no radiologic or pathologic evidence of disseminated vascular disease in young women with oral contraceptive–related stroke. Cerebral thromboembolism resulting from estrogen-induced hypercoagulability is a likely etiology for such strokes. Estrogen increases plasma levels of fibrinogen and clotting factors VII, VIII, IX, X, and XII. The steroid also enhances platelet aggregation and suppresses antithrombin III activity and the fibrinolytic system. A host of estrogen-regulated genes may impact the risk of ischemic stroke, either positively or negatively.[21] Certain inherited prothrombotic conditions (e.g., G20210A prothrombin, factor V Leiden, or methylenetetrahydrofolate reductase C677T polymorphism) augment the risk of ischemic stroke substantially if present in oral contraceptive users.[22] Sex hormone–induced hypercoagulability is thought to play an important role in the pathogenesis of cerebral venous thrombosis complicating pregnancy, the puerperium, and use of hormonal contraceptives.[1]

Increased levels of endogenous free estradiol may be an indicator of atherothrombotic stroke risk in older postmenopausal women, particularly in those with greater central adiposity. Dyslipidemia, insulin resistance, and inflammation are potential mediators of this association.[23] Data concerning the impact of hormone replacement therapy (HRT) on stroke incidence and severity are conflicting, with reports of neutral, increased, and decreased stroke risk accruing from this intervention. In some observational studies, HRT-related stroke risk was significantly modified by the presence or absence of associated factors such as hypertension or smoking.[24] Importantly, several large randomized controlled studies indicated that HRT with conjugated equine estrogen or 17β-estradiol, alone or combined with medroxyprogesterone acetate, does not protect against stroke (or coronary artery disease) in women with established vascular disease and may actually worsen outcomes in this high-risk population.[25,26] In healthy women without prior cerebrovascular history enrolled in the Women's Health Initiative study, an increased risk of ischemic but not fatal or hemorrhagic stroke was again attributed to 17β-estradiol replacement therapy.[27] The risk of ischemic stroke in women receiving HRT does not appear to be modified by age of hormone initiation or by temporal proximity to menopause.[28] In a large, nested case-control study, the use of transdermal HRT containing low doses of estrogen did not seem to increase the risk of stroke in women aged 50 to 79 years.[29] Interestingly, men with the common ESR1 c.454-397CC variant of the estrogen receptor-alpha (*ESR*a) gene may be more prone to ischemic stroke than men bearing other *ESR*a genotypes after adjusting for age, hypertension, diabetes, blood lipid levels, and smoking status.[30]

In a study by the Royal College of General Practitioners, the relative risks of subarachnoid hemorrhage in former users, current users, or subjects who had never used moderate- to high-dose oral contraceptives were 4.5, 3.2, and 4.0, respectively.[1] The odds ratio for hemorrhagic stroke in current users of low-dose estrogen contraceptives (20 to 35 μg) in comparison with former users or nonusers is negligible (1.14). As in the case of ischemic stroke, cigarette smoking and age older than 35 years substantially increase the risk of subarachnoid hemorrhage in users of oral contraceptives.[16] Female sex hormones may predispose to bleeding from both aneurysms and arteriovenous malformations, although the pathophysiologic mechanisms underlying these phenomena remain controversial. By analogy to their effects on endometrial spiral arteries, fluctuating sex hormone levels may compromise the integrity of cerebral arterial walls, rendering them more susceptible to rupture. During pregnancy, hemodynamic changes may facilitate engorgement and bleeding from cerebral arteriovenous malformations. In addition, sex hormones may exert direct trophic influences on these malformations analogous to their effects on other highly vascularized lesions such as spider angiomas, gingival epulis, and meningiomas (discussed later). Rarely, subarachnoid hemorrhage is secondary to cyclic bleeding from hormone-sensitive ectopic endometriomas of the spinal canal.[1]

Epilepsy

Normal reproductive processes may be disrupted by seizure disorders and their therapies. Abnormal limbic discharges may be responsible for the hyposexuality and increased prevalence of hypogonadotropic hypogonadism and polycystic ovary syndrome noted in patients with temporal lobe epilepsy.

As discussed in Chapter 31, anticonvulsant therapy in women of childbearing age may result in failure of oral contraceptives and in teratogenicity. Phenytoin, phenobarbital, primidone, ethosuximide, and carbamazepine have been implicated in oral contraceptive failure.[31] These anticonvulsants induce the hepatic cytochrome P450 microsomal enzyme system, which, in turn, accelerates catabolism of endogenous and exogenous sex hormones. In addition, the anticonvulsants augment the synthesis of sex hormone–binding globulins, resulting in reduced levels of circulating free (active) hormone. Anticonvulsants may also promote the clearance of sex hormones by influencing sulfate conjugation and glucuronidation of the latter in the gut wall and liver.[1] Oral contraceptive failure does not occur with valproic acid, which may actually inhibit cytochrome P450 enzymes, causing elevations in plasma steroid concentrations. Valproic acid, however, may cause hyperandrogenism and polycystic ovaries.[32] Of the newer antiepileptic medications, lamotrigine, gabapentin, vigabatrin, levetiracetam, zonisamide and clobazam do not induce the hepatic P450 microsomal enzyme system, and oral contraceptive failure is less likely to occur with concomitant use of these drugs.[31,33,34] Topiramate and felbamate have modest effects on sex hormone pharmacokinetics and may affect contraceptive efficacy.[35] Although breakthrough bleeding has been reported with tiagabine, the impact of this drug on ovarian hormone metabolism is believed to be minimal.[36]

The course of epilepsy and its management may be greatly influenced by specific phases of the reproductive cycle and exposure to steroid contraceptives. A variety of seizure disorders have been documented to worsen around the time of ovulation or premenstrually (catamenial epilepsy) and during pregnancy. In a large study, an increased risk of epilepsy (RR 1.67, 95% CI 1.12–2.51) was associated with menstrual irregularity at ages 18 to 22 years.[37] Curiously, left-sided temporal lobe seizures appear more likely to cluster at the onset of menses than right-sided temporal seizures, which tend to occur more randomly throughout the cycle.[38] Data amassed from human and animal studies indicate that estrogens and progestins have epileptogenic and anticonvulsant properties, respectively. Estrogen augments glutamatergic and suppresses GABAergic neurotransmission, favoring epileptogenesis, whereas progesterone has the opposite effects.[2] Conceivably, a rising estrogen–progesterone ratio during the late luteal phase triggers catamenial seizure activity. Furthermore, the markedly elevated estrogen–progesterone ratio characteristic of the polycystic ovary syndrome may, in part, contribute to the relatively frequent association of this reproductive disorder with temporal lobe epilepsy. Exposure to oral contraceptives consisting of estrogen–progestin combinations does not appear to worsen seizure control significantly.[31] Management strategies for catamenial epilepsy include (1) premenstrual or periovulatory supplementation of anticonvulsant doses or addition of an adjunctive antiepileptic drug such as clobazam; (2) cyclic administration of acetazolamide, a mild diuretic with weak antiepileptic activity; and (3) progesterone supplementation by mouth or suppository.[39,40] Of note, the magnitude of perimenstrual seizure exacerbation may predict the response rate to progestin therapy.[41]

With respect to gestational epilepsy, factors such as maternal sleep deprivation, stress, and inadequate anticonvulsant levels are probably more important than direct hormonal epileptogenesis. During pregnancy, serum levels of phenytoin, phenobarbital, and valproic acid may decrease by 30 to 40 percent of pregestational levels, with a lesser decline in carbamazepine. Primidone levels are reportedly stable during pregnancy, but the concentration of primidone-derived phenobarbital is reduced. Decreased drug compliance, bioavailability, and protein binding, as well as an increased volume of distribution and metabolic clearance, are factors contributing to the fall in anticonvulsant levels during pregnancy.[39] The influences of the menstrual cycle and of oral contraceptive preparations on anticonvulsant disposition appear to be of minor clinical significance.[1,39]

Movement Disorders

Chorea

Pregnancy and steroid contraceptive therapy have infrequently been complicated by the acute or subacute development of choreiform movements of the face and extremities associated with limb hypotonia and pendular reflexes. Fever, dysarthria, and neuropsychiatric symptoms may complete the clinical picture. Gestational and oral contraceptive–related chorea have a close association with previous rheumatic fever and Sydenham chorea.[42] Oral contraceptives may elicit chorea in patients with a history of congenital cyanotic heart disease and Henoch–Schönlein purpura and exacerbate dyskinesias in chorea-acanthocytosis.[1,43] Pharmacologic, epidemiologic, and pathologic evidence suggests that altered hormonal patterns characteristic of pregnancy and ingestion of oral contraceptives may unmask latent chorea by modulating dopaminergic neurotransmission in basal ganglia previously damaged by rheumatic or hypoxic encephalopathy. In most cases, chorea gravidarum and oral contraceptive–related dyskinesias resolve completely by the end of pregnancy or after discontinuation of the medication, respectively. As many as 20 percent of women experience recurrences of chorea with subsequent pregnancies. Patients with chorea gravidarum are at increased risk of later developing oral contraceptive–related dyskinesias, and vice versa.

In patients with suspected chorea gravidarum, appropriate clinical and laboratory investigations may be required to exclude other causes of chorea, such as acute rheumatic fever, systemic lupus erythematosus, hyperthyroidism, and Wilson disease. Chorea gravidarum is usually self-limited, and abortion or premature delivery is rarely indicated. Judicious use of neuroleptics or other medications may afford symptomatic relief in severe cases. Women with a history of gestational or oral contraceptive–induced chorea should probably minimize further exposure to any estrogen-containing medications.

Parkinsonism

There are anecdotal reports in the early clinical literature of motor deterioration in idiopathic and neuroleptic-induced parkinsonism after exposure to exogenous estrogen. Furthermore, premenopausal women were reportedly more susceptible to drug-induced parkinsonism than men of similar age. These observations argued for a potentially antidopaminergic role of estrogen in this condition. Yet, in two studies of premenopausal women with idiopathic Parkinson disease, motor symptoms were noted to worsen premenstrually when estrogen titers were falling, favoring a stimulatory influence of estrogen on striatal dopamine.[1,44] Data from several studies suggest that postmenopausal estrogen replacement is beneficial in women with Parkinson disease.[45,46] In other studies, postmenopausal estrogen therapy either had no significant dopaminergic effect[47] or was associated with worsening motor scores.[48] Epidemiologic studies suggested that early menopause (natural or surgical) may be a risk factor for the development of Parkinson disease[49,50] and that the latter may be offset by postmenopausal estrogen replacement.[51] However, a large prospective study disclosed no evidence of a beneficial effect of exogenous or endogenous estrogens on the risk of developing Parkinson disease.[52] In an Italian case-control study, exposure to oral contraceptives emerged as a risk factor for the disease with an adjusted OR of 3.27 (95% CI, 1.24–8.59; $P = 0.01$).[53] In a Swedish population, polymorphisms of the estrogen receptor–beta gene (an important mediator of estrogenic effects on the nigrostriatal pathway), although not associated with an overall risk of contracting Parkinson disease, might have impacted the age of symptom onset.[54]

Wilson Disease

Wilson disease is an inborn error of copper metabolism that is characterized by hepatic cirrhosis and degenerative changes in the basal ganglia. Patients exhibit decreased serum ceruloplasmin levels, increased plasma levels of nonceruloplasmin copper, and reduced biliary excretion of the heavy metal. Movement disorders, seizures, and psychosis result from the toxic effects of excessive copper deposition in neural tissues. In normal individuals, serum ceruloplasmin and copper levels increase during pregnancy and after administration of estrogen or estrogen–progestogen contraceptives. The rise in ceruloplasmin resulting from exposure to oral contraceptives is responsible for the green-tinged serum occasionally noted in these women. In patients with Wilson disease, increased serum ceruloplasmin levels occur during pregnancy and after treatment with exogenous estrogens. Effects on serum copper, however, are inconsistent. Normalization of serum ceruloplasmin levels by estrogen administration has no therapeutic benefit, and such exposure sometimes leads to neurologic deterioration. Exposure to hormonal contraceptives may yield "falsely normal" ceruloplasmin levels in patients with Wilson disease, resulting in a delay in diagnosis.[1] Whether sex hormones similarly raise blood ceruloplasmin concentrations in other conditions featuring low levels of the protein, such as hypoceruloplasminemia and acquired copper deficiency,[55] remains to be determined.

Other Movement Disorders

A broad spectrum of movement disturbances appear to be influenced by changes in the sex steroid milieu. Included are cases of posthypoxic and hereditary myoclonus, dominantly inherited myoclonic dystonia, tardive dyskinesia, a pyramidal-extrapyramidal syndrome, hemiballismus, ill-defined tremors and drop attacks, familial episodic ataxia, Gilles de la Tourette's syndrome, and the neuroleptic malignant syndrome.[56,57]

Nervous System Neoplasms

Meningiomas

Meningiomas occur more frequently in women than men and are rarely diagnosed before puberty or during the senium, corresponding to the time of maximal gonadal activity. They are more common in patients with hormone-dependent breast carcinoma and in obese women, perhaps because of higher circulating estrogen levels derived from the aromatization of androstenedione to estrone in adipocytes. Meningiomas have been documented clinically and radiologically to undergo relatively rapid expansion during pregnancy, followed by spontaneous regression postpartum.[58] Some women suffer exacerbations of symptoms in the luteal phase of the menstrual cycle. These fluctuations in tumor size have been attributed to steroid-induced fluid retention by the lesion, increased vascular engorgement of the tumor, and direct trophic effects of gonadal hormones on meningioma cells.[59] A large Finnish study found an increase in the incidence of meningioma in women receiving HRT,[60] but this should not influence the practice of HRT as the overall frequency of meningiomas in this population remains low.[61]

Numerous investigators have demonstrated the presence of progestin- and, to a lesser extent, estrogen- and androgen-binding proteins in a significant number of human meningioma specimens. These observations suggest that progestins and possibly other gonadal steroids may directly modify the growth and differentiation of these tumors. The presence of progestin receptors may indicate a more favorable prognosis because progesterone receptor–negative meningiomas have been associated with a greater tendency for brain invasiveness, higher mitotic indices and necrosis,[62] and shorter disease-free intervals.[63] In an early study, the antiestrogen tamoxifen did not appreciably affect tumor size or neurologic status in patients with inoperable meningiomas.[1] By contrast, the antiprogestin RU486 has been reported to induce stabilization or regression of meningiomas in a cohort of patients, suggesting that antiprogesterone therapy may be useful in the management of these tumors.[64] However, the effects of progestins and RU486 on meningioma growth in vitro are contradictory,[65] and patients chronically treated with RU486 may require glucocorticoid replacement to counteract its antiglucocorticoid effects.[66]

Gliomas

There are anecdotal reports of astrocytomas enlarging during pregnancy, only to shrink spontaneously in the puerperium. As in the case of meningiomas, certain human gliomas may selectively bind estrogens, progestins, and androgens. Some may also contain enzymes (e.g., 17β-oxidoreductase and aromatase) that catalyze steroid hormone interconversions.[67,68] The origin of putative steroid receptors in glial cell tumors is obscure, although significant numbers of normal astrocytes in certain brain regions possess estrogen receptors.[69–71] Astroglial tumors predominantly express estrogen receptor–beta, and expression levels reportedly decline with increasing histologic grade of malignancy.[72] High-dose tamoxifen therapy may result in clinical and radiologic stabilization of astrocytomas and glioblastoma multiforme in some patients.[73–75] These benefits are more likely to be due to the inhibitory effects of tamoxifen on protein kinase C[73,74] or its role as a radiosensitizer[76] than to any accruing antiestrogenic activity. Human oligodendrogliomas have also been reported to contain sex steroid receptors and could theoretically be subject to hormonal manipulations.[77]

Other Tumors

Acoustic neuromas, pituitary adenomas, and breast cancer metastases to the nervous system may also be responsive to sex hormones.[78] Sex steroid receptors have also been reported in hemangioblastomas, anaplastic ependymomas, malignant lymphomas, and primitive neuroectodermal tumors, suggesting that the natural history of these neoplasms may be influenced by sex hormones and their antagonists.[79,80]

Multiple Sclerosis

Multiple sclerosis (MS) is an immune-mediated demyelinating disorder of the central nervous system (CNS) that often occurs during the reproductive years. An association between specific *ESR1* gene polymorphisms and MS has been reported in some studies[81,82] but not others[83] and may be population dependent.

Initial epidemiologic studies indicated that the overall effect of one or more pregnancies on MS-related morbidity is nil.[84] As discussed in Chapter 31, subsequent studies involving larger patient cohorts have amply demonstrated a tendency for MS exacerbation during the first 3 postpartum months that is counterbalanced by significant suppression of disease activity in the third trimester.[85] Indeed, the approximately 70 percent reduction in the relapse rate of MS in the third trimester is more robust than that accruing from interferon-beta, glatiramer acetate, or intravenous immunoglobulin therapy.[86] Immunomodulation that is necessary to prevent rejection of the semiallogenic fetus is probably responsible for the dampening of third-trimester disease activity in MS and other immune-mediated conditions. Factors that have been implicated in gestational immunosuppression include estradiol, progesterone, human chorionic gonadotropin, human placental lactogen, cortisol, 1,25-dihydroxyvitamin D_3, α-fetoprotein, pregnancy-associated glycoprotein, "blocking antibodies," immune complexes, and interleukin-10.[1,86] If necessary, intravenous steroids can be used for MS attacks in pregnancy. Interferon-beta should be discontinued 3 months before planned conception and should not be used during pregnancy or while breast-feeding.[86] In one study, none of 14 pregnant women with relapsing-remitting MS who received prophylactic intravenous immunoglobulins immediately postpartum exhibited disease relapse in the first 6 months after delivery.[87]

Earlier age at puberty may be a predisposing factor for MS in girls but not boys.[88] Although the risk of developing MS does not appear to be impacted by oral contraceptive use, the latter may delay the onset of the disease.[89] Finally, there are pilot studies reporting potentially beneficial effects of oral estriol in women with MS and transdermal testosterone in men with the disease.[90]

Alzheimer Disease

Alzheimer disease is a common dementing illness characterized by progressive neuronal degeneration, gliosis, marked depletion of acetylcholine and other neurotransmitter disturbances, and the accumulation of senile (amyloid) plaques and neurofibrillary tangles in discrete regions of the basal forebrain, hippocampus, and association cortex.[91] By the turn of the millenium, there were promising reports suggesting that estrogens play an important role in normal human cognition, have a salutary effect on the manifestations of Alzheimer disease, and may even protect against the development of this neurodegenerative disorder in women.[92] Fundamental research indicated that estrogens exert trophic influences on cholinergic neurons of the rodent basal forebrain, induce dendritic spines (synapses) and functional *N*-methyl-D-aspartate receptors (important for memory) in adult rat hippocampus,[93] and induce massive neuritic growth in rodent hypothalamic explants.[94] In addition, estrogens were shown to manifest antioxidant properties, reduce the deposition of fibrillar β-amyloid, modulate apolipoprotein E expression, suppress inflammatory responses implicated in neuritic plaque formation,[95–97] and increase cerebral blood flow and glucose utilization (which are deficient in subjects with Alzheimer disease).[95,96] There was also accumulating evidence that estrogens improve cognitive behaviors in rats and monkeys; that psychometric performance in women is influenced by menstrual cycle phase; that cross-gender hormone therapy affects cognition in transsexual men and women; and that estrogen replacement therapy augments verbal memory scores in normal menopausal women.[95,98–100] Moreover, early clinical studies suggested that estrogen replacement therapy may improve cognitive performance, especially language function, verbal memory, and attention, in menopausal women with Alzheimer disease,[95,98,100,101] and enhance the likelihood of a beneficial response to acetylcholinesterase inhibitors in affected women.[102] In several case-controlled studies,[103–105] in initial prospective studies,[106,107] and in a meta-analysis of 12 observational studies,[108] postmenopausal estrogen replacement therapy appeared to be associated with a significantly decreased risk of developing Alzheimer disease. There was also some indication that postmenopausal estrogen replacement therapy protected against the development of dementia in women with Parkinson disease[109] and that androgen (testosterone)[110,111] or estrogen[112] treatment conferred some cognitive benefits in elderly men with Alzheimer disease or mild cognitive impairment.

The results of other large, randomized, placebo-controlled prospective trials evaluating the potential benefits of sex hormone replacement therapy in preventing the dementia of Alzheimer disease have been disappointing. In a substudy of the Heart and Estrogen/Progestin Replacement Study (HERS), age-adjusted cognitive function scores were no different in women with coronary artery disease who received estrogen and progestin than in placebo-treated controls.[113] Surprisingly, in the Women's Health Initiative Memory Study (WHIMS) involving over 6,000 participants, the hazard ratios for development of dementia were 1.49 for women randomized to receive 0.625 mg conjugated equine estrogen and 2.05 for those receiving 0.625 mg estrogen plus 2.5 mg medroxyprogesterone acetate relative to placebo-treated controls.[114] Of note, certain polymorphisms of the follicle-stimulating hormone receptor may confer protection against the disease in women (but not men).[115]

The third Canadian Consensus Conference for the Diagnosis and Treatment of Dementia (2006) recommended against the use of estrogen/progestin replacement therapy for reducing the risk of dementia in postmenopausal women.[116] It was also concluded that there is insufficient evidence for or against prescription of androgen replacement for cognitive dysfunction in elderly men. Since these recommendations were published, it has been hypothesized that there may be a critical perimenopausal "window" during which HRT may protect against the development of Alzheimer disease.[117,118] Importantly, the purportedly salutary influences of estrogen on cognition and hippocampal volumes may be offset in aging women bearing one or two copies of the apolipoprotein E ε4 allele.[119] Regarding androgens, a prospective study in 2010 indicated that higher serum levels of bioavailable testosterone in late life predicts a diminished risk of developing Alzheimer disease in men,[120] perhaps due to androgen-induced down-modulation of brain β-amyloid deposition.[121] Prospective clinical trials amply powered to determine the efficacy of androgen treatment in forestalling dementia in men (and possibly women) may be warranted.[122] Several insightful analyses of the risks and benefits of sex hormones in the management of Alzheimer disease are available.[123,124]

Neuropsychiatric Disorders

The Porphyrias

The porphyrias are characterized by the excessive production of porphyrins and porphyrin precursors resulting from specific enzymatic defects in the heme biosynthetic pathway. Neurologic manifestations, when present, include seizures, neuropsychiatric symptoms, and sensorimotor and autonomic neuropathies. Estradiol and other steroids with a 5β configuration induce the enzyme δ-aminolevulinic acid synthase and may thereby precipitate porphyric crises. Oral contraceptives increase urinary excretion of this enzyme in normal individuals, and it has been suggested that asymptomatic relatives of patients with porphyria should avoid "the pill." In many women with acute intermittent porphyria, cyclic attacks of variable severity occur during the late luteal phase or, less commonly, at ovulation. Paradoxically, some patients exhibit prolonged remissions after suppression of ovarian cyclicity with oral contraceptives.

Although acute treatment with gonadotropin-releasing hormone (GnRH) agonists, such as D-His or leuprolide, stimulates the pituitary–ovarian axis, chronic administration of these agents downregulates gonadotrope GnRH receptors, resulting in long-term suppression of pituitary–ovarian function. In the first reported case, D-His administration (5 μg subcutaneously daily) yielded complete remission of severe premenstrual acute intermittent porphyria for the duration (8 months) of therapy.[1] Similar benefits were observed in subsequent cases of catamenial acute intermittent porphyria[125] and hereditary coproporphyria[126] in response to GnRH analogue therapy. Side effects of long-term GnRH treatment include hot flashes, diminished breast size, and bone demineralization.[126] GnRH analogues, unlike sex steroids, do not appear to induce porphyrin accumulation in chick embryo hepatic cell culture and provide a rational approach to the management of catamenial porphyria.

Premenstrual Syndrome

The premenstrual syndrome (or premenstrual dysphoric disorder) occurs in approximately 30 percent of women during their reproductive years. Common neuropsychiatric symptoms include headache, fatigue, depression, irritability, increased thirst or appetite, and craving for sweet or salty foods. Symptoms typically begin toward the end of the luteal phase of the cycle and usually, but not invariably, resolve with the onset of flow. The pathophysiology of this disorder remains obscure. An increased luteal-phase estrogen–progesterone ratio, hyperprolactinemia, disturbances of the renin–angiotensin–aldosterone axis, hypothyroidism, and abnormal secretion of opioid peptides are among the causes considered for this enigmatic condition.

Numerous hormonal and nonhormonal therapies—including natural progesterone, oral contraceptives, bromocriptine, GnRH agonists, diuretics, prostaglandin inhibitors, vitamin B_6, and lithium—are prescribed for the management of premenstrual syndrome. The efficacy of these treatments remains uncertain. In a double-blind crossover trial, induction of "artificial menopause" with a GnRH agonist (D-Trp-Pro-NEt-Gn-RH, 50 μg per day subcutaneously) relieved both physical and neuropsychiatric symptoms in eight women with rigorously defined premenstrual syndrome.[1] Although the authors reported no side effects (except for hot flashes in one patient), prolonged hypoestrogenemia resulting from the long-term use of these agents may predispose to osteoporosis. Such therapy should probably be reserved for patients with incapacitating symptoms, and low-dose estrogen replacement may have to be considered when the duration of treatment exceeds several months. In a recent study, continuous daily administration of levonorgestrel 90 μg/ethinyl estradiol 20 μg was reportedly well-tolerated and possibly useful in controlling physical, psychologic and behavioral symptoms of the premenstrual syndrome.[127]

Depression and Psychosis

Depression and other major affective disorders may surface in relation to the menstrual cycle, the puerperium, and menopause. Approximately 15 percent of women experience postpartum depression whereas 50 to 80 percent report milder dysphoria ("maternal blues").[128] In patients with postmenopausal depression, mood elevation and anxiolysis often occur promptly in response to estrogen replacement. Paradoxically, oral contraceptives may precipitate depression in susceptible individuals.[1,129] Estrogen has also been implicated in the pathogenesis of anorexia nervosa because of the high preponderance of this condition in women and the potent anorexic effects of estrogen in animals.[130]

Psychotic disorders characterized by extreme agitation, hallucinations, paranoid delusions, incoherent speech, and mood lability may arise during the postpartum period[131] or may recur consistently during the late luteal phase of the cycle. Such disorders may be refractory to conventional therapies (neuroleptics, lithium, electroconvulsive treatment) but may respond well to specific hormonal interventions, including the use of oral contraceptives, intramuscular progesterone, and danazol. "Menopause" induced by GnRH analogues may also be of considerable benefit in the management of cyclical psychosis.

Sleep Disorders

Estrogen and progestin replacement may shorten mean sleep latencies, extend the duration of rapid-eye-movement sleep periods, and diminish nocturnal movement arousals, thereby improving sleep in hypogonadal women.[132] The GABA-active metabolites allopregnanolone and pregnanolone may mediate the reduction in vigilance during wakefulness observed after the administration of progesterone to healthy men.[133] Progestins may also provide stimulatory drive to brainstem respiratory centers in subjects with central sleep apnea and thereby improve hypoventilation. The hypocapnic apnea threshold is lower in women than men, and testosterone administration increases this threshold in premenopausal women.[134] In one case, obstructive sleep apnea resolved in a nonobese woman after removal of a benign testosterone-producing ovarian tumor.[135] In a study involving 33 postmenopausal women, estrogen plus progesterone decreased the prevalence of nocturnal arousals, breathing irregularities, periodic limb movements, hot flashes and bruxism.[136]

Intracranial Hypertension

Progesterone suppresses post-traumatic cerebral edema and intracranial hypertension in rodents. This progestational effect has been attributed to reduction in blood–brain barrier permeability and inhibition of cerebrospinal fluid production by the choroid plexus. Estrogens, by contrast, appear to enhance cerebral endothelial cell permeability and post-traumatic brain edema in female rats. Estrogenic attenuation of the blood–brain barrier may also play a role in the pathogenesis of pseudotumor cerebri (benign intracranial hypertension) in humans and explain the robust female predilection for this disorder.[137]

Neuromuscular Diseases

Catamenial Sciatica

Ectopic endometrial tissue (endometriosis) is hormone sensitive and undergoes epithelial sloughing and hemorrhaging at the time of menses. Ectopic endometrial tissue may destroy lumbar vertebrae, producing back pain, invade the lumbosacral plexus in the retroperitoneal space, and implant within the sheath of the sciatic nerve. In this last instance, radicular pain in the distribution of the nerve usually begins 2 to 3 days before the onset of menses and may continue for a variable duration after cessation of flow (catamenial sciatica). In addition to pain, there is often numbness, weakness, and loss of ankle reflexes. In contrast to far more common discogenic radiculopathy, endometriotic sciatica is less likely to respond to bed rest, and the imaging findings are usually unimpressive. There may be evidence of endometriosis elsewhere, and surgical exploration of the sciatic nerve may be required for diagnosis. In positive cases, the nerve appears blue and a dark, hemorrhagic fluid is expressed after incision of the sheath. Biopsy specimens reveal characteristic glandular elements. Symptoms of catamenial sciatica may show dramatic improvement with standard therapy for endometriosis, including danazol, progestins, GnRH agonist, and in refractory cases, bilateral oophorectomy.[1,138]

Other Neuromuscular Disorders

Endogenous and administered sex hormones (mainly estrogens) may influence the natural history of Bell palsy, recurrent brachial plexopathy, and the carpal tunnel syndrome. Abnormally high estrogen levels have been reported in male patients with amyotrophic lateral sclerosis, Kugelberg–Welander disease, bulbospinal muscular atrophy (Kennedy syndrome), Duchenne muscular dystrophy, and the Crow–Fukase syndrome (polyneuropathy, organomegaly, endocrinopathy, M-protein, and skin changes [POEMS syndrome], usually associated with plasma cell dyscrasias). It is unclear whether hyperestrogenemia plays any significant role in the pathogenesis of these neuromuscular disorders. In an anecdotal report, high-dose testosterone therapy yielded considerable symptomatic improvement in a patient with bulbospinal muscular atrophy.[139] The authors conjectured that the testosterone therapy may have ameliorated some toxic gain of function ascribed to the mutated androgen receptor in this condition. Finally, Mastrogiacomo and co-workers have hypothesized that dysfunction of testicular peritubular myoid cells and corpus cavernosum smooth muscle contributes to the hypergonadotropic hypogonadism and impotence that complicate myotonic dystrophy in men.[140]

PITUITARY GLAND

The endocrine and nervous systems interact in intricate ways, and disorders in one system may cause dysfunction of the other in diverse ways. For example, small anterior pituitary tumors produce symptoms principally as the result of hormonal excess, but large tumors cause symptoms of either hypersecretion or hyposecretion as well as dysfunction of adjacent cranial nerves or cerebral structures.[141] The protean clinical features of hormonal excess and deficiency states include both central and peripheral nervous system dysfunction.[142,143]

The complex anatomy of the sellar region influences the clinical features of pituitary disorders.[144,145] The pituitary gland, or hypophysis, sits in a bony depression in the posterior sphenoid bone called the sella turcica, bounded anteriorly by the tuberculum sellae and anterior clinoid process and posteriorly by the dorsum sellae. Dural reflections border the pituitary superiorly and laterally. The diaphragma sellae forms the roof of the sella turcica and lies beneath the optic chiasm. Adjacent bilaterally is the cavernous sinus, through which passes the internal carotid artery and cranial nerves III, IV, V (upper two divisions), and VI. In addition the cavernous sinus serves to drain the ophthalmic and middle and inferior cerebral veins.

The anterior pituitary, or adenohypophysis, derives embryologically from Rathke pouch, of ectodermal origin, and has blood supplied by the hypophyseal-portal system. Hormones secreted by the anterior pituitary include prolactin, growth hormone (GH), adrenocorticotropic hormone (ACTH), thyrotropin (TSH), luteinizing hormone (LH), and follicle-stimulating hormone (FSH). The hypothalamus controls anterior pituitary hormone secretions through various hypophysiotropic substances, most of which are peptides (Table 20-1).[145] The hypophyseal-portal system provides the basis for feedback loops that regulate the hypothalamic–pituitary axis.

TABLE 20-1 ■ Anterior Pituitary and Hypothalamic Hormones

Pituitary Hormone	Hypothalamic Factor
Prolactin	Dopamine (inhibitory)
Growth hormone (GH)	Growth hormone–releasing hormone (GHRH) Somatastatin (inhibitory)
Adrenocorticotropin (ACTH)	Corticotropin-releasing hormone (CRH)
Thyrotropin (TSH)	Thyrotropin-releasing hormone (TRH)
Luteinizing hormone (LH) and follicle-stimulating hormone (FSH)	Gonadotropin-releasing hormone (GnRH)

The posterior pituitary, known also as the neurohypophysis or pars nervosa, derives from a neuroectodermal extension of diencephalon that fuses with Rathke pouch. Also of neuroectodermal origin is the infundibulum linking the pituitary to the hypothalamus at the median eminence, which also forms the floor of the third ventricle. The inferior hypophyseal artery, a branch of the intracavernous carotid, supplies the neurohypophysis. Neurohypophyseal hormones include oxytocin and antidiuretic hormone (ADH), or arginine vasopressin.

The juxtaposition of the pituitary gland to hypothalamus, third ventricle, intracavernous carotid arteries, and cranial nerves related to vision, extraocular movements, and mid- and upper facial sensation accounts for many of the neurologic manifestations of lesions in and around the sella. Endocrine disturbances arising from excess or insufficient secretion of one or more pituitary hormones may also cause neurologic as well as systemic symptoms and signs, and laboratory abnormalities. Improved neuroimaging techniques have greatly facilitated assessment of sellar and parasellar lesions.[144] A detailed discussion of the increasingly complex array of stimulation and inhibition studies used to assess the integrity of specific elements of the hypothalamic–pituitary axis is provided elsewhere.[145] However, a basic understanding of pituitary hormone physiology is essential to evaluating patients with mass lesions in and around the gland and it is reviewed here after a discussion of the neurologic symptoms and signs resulting from these lesions.

Sellar and Parasellar Lesions

Pituitary adenomas are the most common mass in the sellar region and account for up to 25 percent of intracranial neoplasms.[144–146] Previous classification schemes based on histologic staining properties have given way to categorization based on hormone secretion.[141,144–147] Pituitary adenomas are also classified by size. Microadenomas (Fig. 20-2A), lesions that are 10 mm or smaller, typically spare adjacent neural or vascular structures and generally come to medical attention during evaluation for symptoms and signs of hormone oversecretion. Lesions larger than 10 mm, known as macroadenomas (Fig. 20-2B), also may present with manifestations of hormone excess or may impair normal glandular

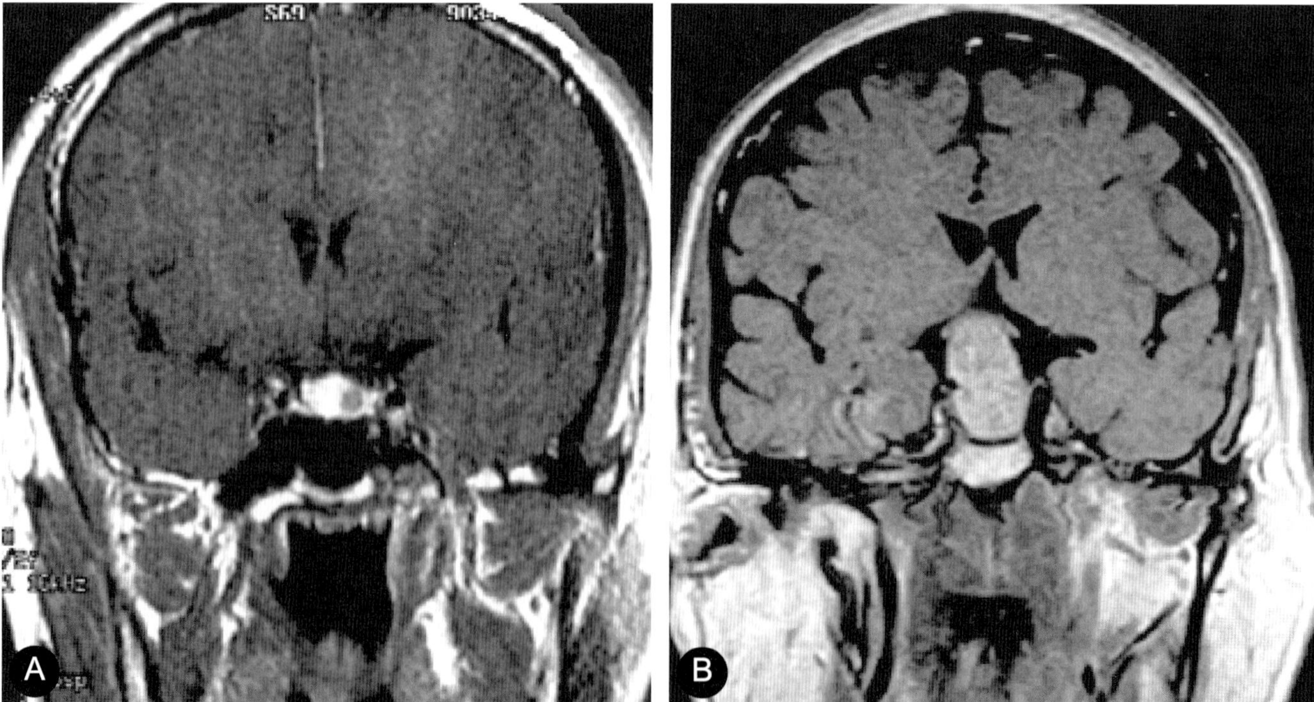

Figure 20-2 ■ Neuroimaging of pituitary adenoma. **A**, Microadenoma. Gadolinium-enhanced T1-weighted magnetic resonance imaging (MRI) shows a small focus of decreased enhancement compatible with microadenoma in a young woman with galactorrhea-amenorrhea. **B**, Macroadenoma. Large sellar lesion, subsequently shown to be a nonsecretory adenoma, in a gadolinium-enhanced T1-weighted MRI obtained in a middle-aged man with progressive visual loss.

function, resulting in hypopituitarism. When macroadenomas compress adjacent neural or vascular structures, neurologic dysfunction, such as headache, visual loss, ophthalmoparesis, and facial sensory symptoms, may develop.[141,144–147] Adenoma size does not correlate with headache, which may have features similar to migraine or trigeminal autonomic cephalgia.[148] Macroadenomas extending superiorly may compress the optic chiasm, nerves, or tracts. Bitemporal hemianopia is the classic consequence, although monocular visual loss or junctional scotoma also may occur. Because adenomas grow slowly, patients may not appreciate visual deficits until they are quite advanced. Third ventricular extension occasionally causes acute or chronic hydrocephalus. Lateral extension, with subsequent cavernous sinus involvement, disturbs extraocular motility and sensation in the upper and middle face. Very large lesions involving inferior frontal or medial temporal lobes are rare but may cause cognitive impairment, behavioral changes, or seizures. A few pituitary tumors extend inferiorly, causing epistaxis or cerebrospinal fluid (CSF) rhinorrhea.

Pituitary adenomas account for 90 percent of masses in the sellar region, with other pituitary tumors, nonpituitary neoplasms, metastases, infectious and inflammatory disorders, vascular lesions, and cysts accounting for the rest (Table 20-2).[144,149] Craniopharyngiomas arise from epithelial cell rests of Rathke pouch. Among malignant lesions, pituitary carcinomas are quite rare, and metastases to the pituitary are recognized more frequently at autopsy than during life.[144]

Among more common disorders, primary empty sella is often associated with an incompetent diaphragma sellae, which allows arachnoid and CSF to herniate into the sella.[150] Typically an incidental finding on neuroimaging studies, primary empty sella syndrome is not usually associated with endocrinopathy. Secondary empty sella occurs after spontaneous or treatment-induced regression of pituitary disease. Other important non-neoplastic sellar lesions include granulomatous processes, such as tuberculosis or sarcoidosis, and vascular lesions such as aneurysms of the intracavernous carotid artery.

Magnetic resonance imaging (MRI) before and after gadolinium enhancement, with high-resolution thin sections in the sagittal and coronal planes, is the test of choice for pituitary-region imaging. On T1-weighted images, high signal intensity in the posterior pituitary is referred to as the "bright spot"

TABLE 20-2 ■ Differential Diagnosis of Sellar Masses
Neoplasms
Pituitary origin
Anterior: pituitary adenoma or carcinoma
Posterior: granular cell tumor, stalk or posterior lobe astrocytoma
Nonpituitary origin
Craniopharyngioma
Germ cell tumor
Meningioma
Glioma (hypothalamic, optic nerve or chiasm)
Skull base: chordoma, giant cell tumor, chondroma, fibrous dysplasia
Others
Lipoma
Hemangioblastoma
Sarcoma
Schwannoma
Paraganglioma
Esthesioneuroblastoma
Metastatic
Carcinoma
Melanoma
Hematopoietic malignancies
Vascular Lesions
Intracavernous carotid aneurysm
Cavernous sinus thrombosis
Pituitary apoplexy
Cysts
Rathke cleft cyst
Arachnoid cyst
Epidermoid
Dermoid
Inflammatory Disorders
Granulomatous: sarcoidosis, tuberculosis, syphilitic gumma, giant cell granuloma
Pituitary abscess
Lymphocytic hypophysitis
Histiocytosis
Mucocele
Empty Sella Syndrome
Pituitary Hypertrophy
Puberty (in girls)
Pregnancy
Chronic primary hypothyroidism

and is believed to represent ADH in neurosecretory vessels.[144] Pituitary adenomas typically enhance less intensely than normal glandular tissue (Fig. 20-2A). In patients who cannot undergo MRI, precontrast and postcontrast computed tomography (CT) images through the area can be obtained. A consequence of modern neuroimaging is detection of the asymptomatic pituitary mass, the so-called pituitary "incidentaloma."[145,151]

Anterior Pituitary

Prolactin

Prolactin acts on mammary tissue to promote lactation and inhibit cyclic gonadotropin secretion.[145] Hypothalamic control of prolactin secretion occurs primarily by inhibition, and thus pituitary stalk disruption from lesions other than prolactinomas may elevate serum prolactin levels, although rarely above 200 µg/L (normal <25 µg/L).[145,152] Dopamine is the major inhibitory factor. Accordingly, neuroleptics and other dopamine antagonists can cause mild hyperprolactinemia, although the risk may be lower for some atypical antipsychotics; dopaminergic drugs are therefore used therapeutically to lower prolactin levels.[145–147,152,153] Prolactin-releasing factors are less well understood, although thyrotropin-releasing factor (TRH) plays a role. Consequently, in primary hypothyroidism, when TRH is elevated, the resulting hyperprolactinemia and pituitary enlargement may cause diagnostic confusion with prolactinoma.[147,152] The differential diagnosis of hyperprolactinemia (Table 20-3) also includes pregnancy, lactation, and chest wall stimulation.[145,147,152] Serum prolactin may be modestly increased in the first hour after a generalized tonic-clonic or complex partial seizure and, when measured at 10 to 20 minutes after a suspected event, is sometimes a useful adjunct for the differentiation of generalized tonic-clonic epileptic from nonepileptic seizures.[154]

Amenorrhea-galactorrhea in women and impotence and decreased libido in men should prompt consideration of hyperprolactinemia.[145] In the absence of venipuncture stress, an elevated serum prolactin level establishes the diagnosis, and further evaluation should include medication history and laboratory screening for chronic kidney disease and hypothyroidism.[152] Prolactinomas account for approximately 40 percent of hormonally active pituitary adenomas.[144,147,152] Prolactin levels exceeding 250 µg/L suggest prolactinoma, with levels above 500 µg/L diagnostic of macroprolactinoma.[152] Values lower than this may be seen with any type of macroadenoma due to stalk compression or as a consequence of the "hook effect," whereby the radioimmunoassay used to determine serum prolactin returns a falsely low value in severe hyperprolactinemia.[145,147,151,152] Performing the assay with diluted serum samples reveals the true, markedly elevated prolactin level and should be requested when prolactin levels are not markedly elevated in a patient with a macroadenoma.

TABLE 20-3 ■ Differential Diagnosis of Hyperprolactinemia

Physiologic
Pregnancy, lactation
Metabolic
Primary hypothyroidism, chronic kidney disease, cirrhosis
Drugs
Dopamine antagonists: neuroleptics, antiemetics, L-methyldopa, reserpine
Antidepressants: tricylics, monoamine oxidase inhibitors
Estrogens
Others: verapamil, benzodiazepines, opiates
Neurogenic
Chest wall injury, herpes zoster, breast stimulation, spinal cord lesion
Pituitary Disease
Prolactinoma, other pituitary adenomas or tumors, stalk section, granulomatous infiltration
Hypothalamic/Stalk Disease
Neoplastic, vascular, inflammatory, post-irradiation, severe head trauma
Others
Seizures, stress, macroprolactinemia, idiopathic

Amenorrhea-galactorrhea and infertility bring women to early medical attention, and thus microprolactinomas predominate. Symptoms of hypogonadism in men—impotence, loss of libido, and infertility—may not as reliably trigger measurement of serum prolactin level. Consequently macroprolactinomas are more common in men, classically presenting with headache or visual impairment. Medical therapy with dopamine agonists decreases prolactin levels, reverses hypogonadism, and shrinks approximately 75 percent of macroprolactinomas and an even higher percentage of microprolactinomas.[147,152,155] Cabergoline is better tolerated and more effective than bromocriptine, and is thus the preferred drug. Surgery is typically reserved for patients with acute visual impairment or who do not improve or tolerate therapy with dopaminergic agents. As is the case for medical therapy, surgical outcomes are better for patients with microadenomas than macroadenomas.[155] Trans-sphenoidal approaches are favored, although large, invasive tumors may require bifrontal craniotomy.[152] Regardless of whether the treatment plans include medication, surgery, or both, patients require monitoring with serial clinical assessment, prolactin levels, visual field testing, and neuroimaging.[147,152,155] Radiation therapy is used primarily when medical and surgical approaches have been unsuccessful.[152,155,156] Whether stereotactic radiosurgery is safer or more effective than conventional radiotherapy remains to be determined.[155,156]

Growth Hormone

Secretion of GH, a 191-amino-acid polypeptide, is regulated by stimulatory (GH-releasing hormone) and inhibitory (somatostatin) hypothalamic factors.[145,157] Secretory dynamics are complex; factors that influence pulsatile GH secretion include age, nutritional state, and sleep.[145] GH stimulates skeletal growth and exerts a variety of metabolic effects, including glucose intolerance.[145,157] The action of GH is mediated by its receptors in liver, bone, and fat, as well as by induction of insulin-like growth factor I (IGF-I).

Excessive circulating GH before epiphysial fusion in children leads to gigantism. In adults, sustained GH excess causes acromegaly, which results from pituitary hypersecretion in nearly all cases.[156,157] Coarsened facial features and enlargement of hands and feet may only be recognized in retrospect and are an infrequent presenting complaint. The diverse systemic manifestations include hyperhidrosis, reproductive dysfunction, skin tags, colonic polyps, arthropathy, hypertension, hyperlipidemia, diabetes, and sleep apnea.[147,156–159] Neurologic symptoms include proximal weakness and compression of neural structures by bony and soft tissue overgrowth causing, for example, carpal tunnel syndrome.[143,147,156–159] Macroadenomas are identified in most cases, and symptoms of an expanding sellar mass may bring patients to clinical attention. The pulsatile nature of GH secretion limits the diagnostic utility of random GH determination, hence elevated serum IGF-1 level establishes the biochemical diagnosis of acromegaly.[147,156–158] Autonomous GH secretion may be demonstrated by lack of appropriate GH suppression during an oral glucose tolerance test. Other important diagnostic tests include neuroimaging studies, visual field testing, serum prolactin level, and evaluation for panhypopituitarism and complications of acromegaly, in particular cardiovascular and bony disease, and colonic polyps.[156–159]

Cosmetic disfigurement and chronic pain impair quality of life, and patients with untreated acromegaly risk premature death from diabetes, hypertension, cardiovascular disease, and colon cancer.[147,156–159] Normalizing GH and IGF-1 is the therapeutic goal, and decreases long-term mortality.[157–159] Trans-sphenoidal resection is the primary treatment of choice for microadenomas and macroadenomas.[147,156–158] Options for adjunctive medical therapy include the somatostatin analogues octreotide or lanreotide, the GH receptor antagonist pegvisomant, and the dopamine agonists cabergoline or bromocriptine. Medical therapy is usually used after surgery to control GH and IGF-1 levels, or, in selected cases, to shrink large tumors before planned surgery or when surgery is not possible.[147,156–158] Conventional radiotherapy, stereotactic radiosurgery, or repeat surgical resection may be necessary if GH levels remain elevated.

Adrenocorticotropic Hormone and Cushing Disease

ACTH is a 39-amino-acid peptide derived from proopiomelanocortin, a precursor molecule that also gives rise to β-endorphin and β-lipotropin. Corticotropin-releasing hormone (CRH), secreted by the hypothalamus, controls ACTH release. ACTH stimulates adrenal steroidogenesis in a circadian pattern. ACTH and cortisol levels are highest in the morning and lowest in late evening; psychologic or physiologic stress also activates the pituitary–adrenal axis.

Cushing disease is due to ACTH hypersecretion from a pituitary adenoma and is a common cause of endogenous hypercortisolism.[147,156,160,161] Clinical features include central obesity, dorsocervical fat pad ("buffalo hump"), hypertension, bruising, purple abdominal striae, thin skin, facial plethora, hyperpigmentation, acne, hirsutism, osteoporosis, menstrual disorders, impotence, decreased libido, and infections.[160,161] Laboratory findings include hypokalemia, hyperglycemia, and peripheral leukocytosis. Neurologic manifestations include myopathy, headache, neuropsychiatric disturbances including particularly mood disorders and cognitive impairment, and less commonly spinal epidural lipomatosis with resulting radiculopathy or myelopathy.[142,143,147,156,160–162]

Diagnosis depends on demonstrating endogenous hypercortisolism and then localizing the source of excess ACTH secretion to the pituitary. Recommended screening tests include urinary free cortisol, late-night salivary cortisol, or either the 1-mg overnight or longer low-dose (2 mg/day for 48 hours) dexamethasone suppression test.[161] Pregnancy, depression, alcoholism, morbid obesity, glucocorticoid resistance, and poorly controlled diabetes mellitus can cause hypercortisolism without Cushing syndrome, as can stress (including hospitalization or intense exercise), and malnutrition.[160,161] A second screening test and in some instances, dexamethasone-CRH or midnight serum cortisol testing are recommended for subsequent evaluation.[161] Dexamethasone testing can be confounded by agents that alter steroid clearance, including some antiepileptic drugs.[160,161] Distinguishing pituitary from ectopic ACTH secretion can be difficult, and inferior petrosal sinus sampling aids diagnosis in centers experienced in its use. Brainstem infarctions or hemorrhages are rare but serious complications of this procedure.[163] Most tumors in Cushing disease are microadenomas and, in up to half of patients, not apparent on MRI.[156]

Trans-sphenoidal surgery is the treatment of choice, with remission rates of 65 to 95 percent for microadenomas and recurrence rates of 10 to 20 percent at 10 years.[147,164] Remission rates are lower for macroadenomas, which recur earlier and more frequently than smaller tumors. Transient or permanent adrenal insufficiency frequently develops postoperatively. Among options available for patients with persistent hypercortisolism after surgery are repeat surgery, conventional radiotherapy or stereotactic radiosurgery, and medical therapy.[164,166] Ketoconazole, metyrapone, mitotane, and etomidate inhibit adrenal steroidogenesis. Agents which target the pituitary include the somatostatin analogues octreotide and lanreotide and the dopamine agonists cabergoline and bromocriptine.[164] Bilateral total adrenalectomy can be performed laparoscopically and is another treatment option; however, it obligates permanent adrenal replacement therapy and carries the risk of Nelson syndrome, in which an ACTH-secreting pituitary adenoma enlarges rapidly due to loss of corticosteroid inhibition.[156,160,164]

Thyroid-Stimulating Hormone

Pituitary adenomas secreting TSH cause hyperthyroidism and are rare, with an estimated incidence of one case per million.[165] Clinical manifestations are those of hyperthyroidism (Chapter 18), with goiter in most cases, as well as features referable to an enlarging pituitary mass, as most are macroadenomas. Concomitant prolactin or GH hypersecretion occurs in some patients and hence galactorrhea-amenorrhea or features of acromegaly may coexist. TSH is inappropriately normal or elevated for the high peripheral thyroid hormone levels, distinguishing these lesions from Graves disease or toxic goiter. Individuals with thyroid hormone resistance have elevated laboratory studies suggesting central hyperthyroidism, but generally lack clinical manifestations of hyperthyroidism. For TSH-secreting pituitary tumors, surgical resection is the preferred primary therapy.[165] If thyroid hormones remain elevated postoperatively, radiotherapy, radiosurgery, or somatostatin analogues may be used as adjunctive therapy. Thyroidectomy or antithyroid drugs such as methimazole or propylthiouracil risk increasing tumor growth by interfering with feedback inhibition.

Clinically Nonfunctioning Pituitary Adenomas

Most pituitary tumors that are unaccompanied by clinical evidence of hormonal hypersecretion are gonadotroph cell adenomas, which inefficiently secrete gonadotropins or discordantly secrete their α, FSH-β, or LH-β subunits.[145,147,156,166] With the paucity of endocrine symptoms, most are macroadenomas or are detected as incidental findings on neuroimaging obtained for other indications. Presenting features are those of a large pituitary mass: headache, visual dysfunction, and hypopituitarism due to compression of normal pituitary or the portal system.[166] Serum prolactin, assessment of anterior pituitary function, and visual field testing should accompany neuroimaging studies. Surgery is the primary therapy of choice for patients with macroadenoma, with additional radiotherapy for significant residual tumor or recurrence.[156,166] Patients with nonsecreting microadenomas should be monitored with serial MRI scans and can often be managed conservatively.

The clinical and therapeutic features of pituitary adenomas are summarized in Table 20-4.

Pituitary Apoplexy

Headache and visual loss, variably accompanied by oculomotor dysfunction, nausea, vomiting, altered mentation, and meningismus, constitute the classic clinical features of pituitary apoplexy, caused by pituitary hemorrhage or infarction.[144,167,168] The presenting syndrome may be fulminant, resembling subarachnoid hemorrhage, but subacute or even asymptomatic forms have been recognized increasingly.[168] Headache, visual loss (frequently decreased acuity or bitemporal hemianopia), and diplopia are common, and most patients have impairment of at least one anterior pituitary hormone. Acute adrenal insufficiency may be fatal, hence empiric corticosteroid replacement should be given to all patients with pituitary apoplexy. Hypogonadism and hypothyroidism are common, as is hyponatremia.

Pituitary apoplexy often occurs in adenomas, including those that have been clinically silent, and the risk of symptomatic apoplexy is higher in patients with macroadenomas. Although most cases develop without obvious cause, reported precipitating factors include anticoagulation, trauma, dynamic hormone testing of pituitary function, radiation, and dopamine agonist treatment or its cessation. Sheehan syndrome refers to ischemic pituitary necrosis after postpartum hemorrhage and hypotension.[169]

The differential diagnosis of pituitary apoplexy includes subarachnoid hemorrhage, bacterial

TABLE 20-4 ■ Diagnosis and Management of Pituitary Adenomas

Type of Adenoma	Presenting Symptoms	Predominant Tumor Type	Primary Therapy	Adjunctive Therapy	Comments
Prolactin-secreting	Children: delayed puberty Women: amenorrhea-galactorrhea, infertility Men: headache, visual loss, impotence	Women: microadenoma Men: macroadenoma	Dopamine agonists	Surgery, radiotherapy, radiosurgery	Most common pituitary adenoma
GH-secreting	Children: gigantism Adults: acromegaly	Macroadenoma	Surgery	Somatostatin analogues, GH receptor antagonist, dopamine agonists, radiotherapy, radiosurgery	Increased mortality improves with treatment
ACTH-secreting	Central obesity, hypertension, purple striae, bruising, osteoporosis, cognitive and mood changes, myopathy	Microadenoma	Surgery	Steroidogenesis inhibitors, somatostatin analogues, dopamine agonists, radiotherapy, radiosurgery	Untreated disease associated with increased mortality
TSH-secreting	Hyperthyroidism, goiter	Macroadenoma	Surgery	Somatostatin analogues, radiotherapy, radiosurgery	Rare
Nonsecreting	Headache, visual loss, hypopituitarism Incidental finding on CT or MRI obtained for other indications (usually microadenoma)	Macroadenoma	Surgery (serial imaging for microadenomas)	Radiotherapy, radiosurgery	Most secrete gonadotroph subunits

ACTH, adrenocorticotropic hormone; GH, growth hormone; TSH, thyrotropin.

meningitis, cavernous sinus thrombosis, and upper brainstem infarction or hemorrhage. Sellar MRI is the neuroimaging study of choice, although CT may be diagnostic when MRI is unavailable or contraindicated. CSF shows nonspecific abnormalities.[167] Trans-sphenoidal decompression should be undertaken in patients with significant visual field deficit, loss of visual acuity, or deteriorating mental status.[168] Surgery may also help to preserve pituitary function. Once the acute illness has resolved, patients should be monitored for hypopituitarism, with hormone replacement instituted as needed.

Posterior Pituitary

Magnocellular neurons of the hypothalamic supraoptic and paraventricular nuclei synthesize precursor polypeptides, which ultimately are cleaved to form the posterior pituitary hormones oxytocin and ADH.[170] Oxytocin mediates the "let-down" reflex of milk expulsion in response to suckling. ADH facilitates tubular water resorption, thus controlling renal free water clearance and, in concert with hypothalamic thirst mechanisms, regulates water balance and osmolality. Deficient or inappropriate ADH secretion may complicate cerebral disorders or their treatment and lead to neurologic disturbances.[171]

Diabetes Insipidus

Diabetes insipidus is characterized by excessive renal water loss due to ADH deficiency. Awake patients present with thirst, polydipsia, and polyuria. ADH hyposecretion leads to central diabetes insipidus, and deficient renal response to adequate circulating ADH levels causes nephrogenic diabetes insipidus.[170–173] Both types of diabetes insipidus have congenital and acquired forms (Table 20-5) and must be distinguished from excessive water drinking, in which polyuria is appropriate to water intake. Awake patients with diabetes insipidus can often increase their fluid intake sufficiently to compensate for urinary losses. Patients who cannot maintain adequate water intake to balance polyuria develop hypernatremia, volume contraction, and encephalopathy. Brain shrinkage in severe hypertonic encephalopathy may lead to intracerebral hemorrhage.

TABLE 20-5 ■ Causes of Diabetes Insipidus

Central Causes
Acquired
Trauma and neurosurgery
Parasellar pathology
Neoplasms
Granulomatous disorders
Vascular lesions
Autoimmune: lymphocytic hypophysitis, autoimmune hypothalamic disease
Cerebral infection
Hypoxic-ischemic brain injury
Stroke
Pregnancy
Idiopathic
Congenital/Familial
Septo-optic dysplasia
Laurence–Moon–Biedl syndrome
Wolfram syndrome
ADH mutations
Nephrogenic Causes
Acquired
Metabolic
Hypercalcemia
Hypokalemia
Drugs
Lithium
Antibiotics: demeclocycline, amphotericin B, foscarnet
Others: colchicine, loop diuretics
Chronic renal parenchymal disease
Autoimmune
Amyloidosis
Sickle cell anemia
Post-obstructive uropathy
Congenital/Familial
ADH receptor mutations
Aquaporin-2 mutations

ADH, antidiuretic hormone.

Common acquired causes of central diabetes insipidus include trauma, cerebral hypoxia-ischemia, and neoplastic, granulomatous, and inflammatory disorders of the sellar region.[172,173] Transient diabetes insipidus is not uncommon after head trauma or neurosurgery.[171] Most acquired nephrogenic causes are metabolic or toxic, including hypokalemia, hypercalcemia, and lithium.[170,172] Diagnosis depends on demonstrating an inability to appropriately concentrate urine and is suggested by passage of large amounts of dilute urine. However, polyuria alone is not sufficient to make the diagnosis. In critically ill patients with increased intracranial pressure, for example, polyuria may reflect osmotic diuresis from mannitol therapy, rather than diabetes insipidus. Low urine osmolality in the presence of polyuria and hypertonicity in serum indicates inability to concentrate urine in severe diabetes insipidus, but the diagnosis can be challenging in milder disease.[172,173] Water deprivation tests, monitoring urine and serum osmolality in the presence of dehydration, are sometimes necessary, but are not without risk, especially in children.[170] The response, after water deprivation, to exogenously administered desmopressin, an ADH analogue, indicates whether the diabetes insipidus is central or nephrogenic.[172]

For both the central and nephrogenic disorders, correcting the water deficit is an important therapeutic goal. Desmopressin can be given parenterally, intranasally, or orally and is the treatment of choice for central diabetes insipidus.[170,172] In the nephrogenic disorder, the underlying cause should be eliminated; in addition, thiazide diuretics, which enhance sodium excretion, should be prescribed and an adequate fluid intake assured.[170]

Syndrome of Inappropriate Antidiuretic Hormone Secretion

Diagnosis of the syndrome of inappropriate antidiuretic hormone secretion (SIADH) depends on the demonstration of decreased effective plasma osmolality, increased urinary osmolality, increased urinary sodium excretion (with normal salt and water intake), euvolemia, normal adrenal and thyroid function, and absence of recent diuretic therapy.[170,171,174,175] Neurologic manifestations of SIADH are those of hyponatremia including encephalopathy and seizures, when the electrolyte disturbance is severe or acute.[175] Milder degrees of hyponatremia impair performance on tests of attention and may predispose patients to falls and fractures.[176] Neurologic causes of SIADH include head trauma, neurosurgery, brain tumor, CNS infection, stroke, hydrocephalus, and acute intermittent porphyria. Ectopic ADH production may occur from systemic malignancies or in association with pulmonary disease. Among the many drugs associated with SIADH are carbamazepine, antidepressants, neuroleptics, antineoplastic agents, and thiazide diuretics. The causes of SIADH are summarized in Table 20-6.

TABLE 20-6 ■ Causes of the Syndrome of Inappropriate ADH Secretion

Neurologic Disease
Head trauma or neurosurgery
Stroke
Cerebral infection: meningitis, encephalitis, brain abscess
Brain tumors
Others: hydrocephalus, delirium tremens, acute intermittent porphyria, Guillain–Barré syndrome
Pulmonary Disease
Infection: pneumonia, tuberculosis, empyema
Acute respiratory failure
Others: asthma, cystic fibrosis, pneumothorax, positive-pressure ventilation
Drugs
Psychotropic agents: antipsychotics, antidepressants
Chemotherapy: vinca alkaloids, cyclophosphamide, ifosfamide
Hormones: vasopressin, desmopressin, oxytocin
Others: carbamazepine, clofibrate, amiloride, thiazides
Neoplastic Ectopic ADH Production
Carcinoma: nasopharyngeal, bronchogenic, duodenal, pancreatic, endometrial, prostatic
Others: thymoma, lymphoma, mesothelioma, Ewing sarcoma
Other
Surgery
AIDS
Prolonged exercise

ADH, antidiuretic hormone; AIDS, acquired immunodeficiency syndrome.

Osmotic demyelination syndrome, a rare but often devastating cerebral disorder associated with rapid correction of hyponatremia of any cause, has helped inform the optimal management of SIADH and other hyponatremic states.[174,175,177] Fluid restriction and treatment of the underlying cause are mainstays of therapy, but patient adherence with the former is usually poor. Hypertonic saline and diuretics such as furosemide may be necessary for patients with seizures or those who are otherwise severely symptomatic. Demeclocycline, which induces nephrogenic diabetes insipidus, is occasionally used. Vasopressin receptor antagonists (the "vaptans") are under investigation as a potential treatment for SIADH.[170,174,175,177]

Cerebral salt wasting, occurring in the setting of intracranial disease, is defined as hyponatremia resulting from renal sodium loss. It causes hypovolemia, in contrast to the euvolemia of SIADH, from which it must be distinguished.[175,177,178] Rational management consists of water and sodium repletion, rather than fluid restriction, as is standard in SIADH. There are a number of unsettled issues relating to cerebral salt wasting including the difficulty of accurately determining volume status, the frequency with which the syndrome occurs, the necessity for the presence of coexisting cerebral disease, and whether it properly should be renamed renal salt wasting.[177,178]

Hypopituitarism

Hypothalamic and intrinsic pituitary disorders may lead to impaired secretion of anterior or posterior pituitary hormones (Table 20-7).[179,180] Because prolactin, unlike other anterior pituitary hormones, is primarily regulated by inhibition, large mass lesions or other processes that disrupt the pituitary stalk can elevate prolactin levels. Prolactin levels in the resulting "stalk syndrome" will be elevated, but not to levels seen with prolactinomas. Pituitary adenomas, even when large, usually spare posterior pituitary function. Thus, the triad of diabetes insipidus, hyperprolactinemia, and deficiency of one or more anterior pituitary hormones suggests hypothalamic dysfunction or disruption of the hypothalamic-pituitary stalk.

Hypopituitarism spans a broad clinical spectrum from the acute crisis of pituitary apoplexy to the indolent and easily missed fatigue, decreased sexual interest and function, loss of body hair, and cold intolerance of a nonsecreting adenoma that has grown large enough to cause deficiencies of multiple hormones. GH deficiency causes growth failure in children and accelerated atherosclerosis and osteoporosis in adults.[180] Hypoadrenalism due to ACTH deficiency is usually less severe than in intrinsic adrenal disease, owing to preserved mineralocorticoid secretion. Gonadotropin deficiency causes loss of libido and impotence. Thyroid dysfunction resulting from TSH deficiency is generally less severe than primary hypothyroidism. Neuropsychiatric abnormalities and myopathic weakness are features of hypothyroidism and hypocortisolism.[142,143]

Pituitary tumors or the consequences of their treatment account for some cases of hypopituitarism.[179,180] Hypopituitarism occurs in up to one-third of patients after traumatic brain injury and nearly half of subarachnoid hemorrhage survivors.[181]

TABLE 20-7 ■ Differential Diagnosis of Hypopituitarism

Neoplasm
Pituitary macroadenoma
Other sellar region tumors: craniopharyngioma, meningioma, glioma, chondroma, chordoma, metastases
Trauma
Head injury or neurosurgery
Radiotherapy
Stalk section
Vascular
Pituitary hemorrhage or infarction
Subarachnoid hemorrhage
Stroke
Inflammatory
Infection: meningitis, encephalitis, abscess
Granulomatous disorders
Lymphocytic hypophysitis
Other autoimmune disorders
Infiltrative
Hemochromatosis
Amyloidosis
Empty Sella Syndrome
Developmental
Septo-optic dysplasia
Pituitary aplasia

PARATHYROID GLANDS

The two pairs of parathyroid glands lie behind the thyroid, secreting parathyroid hormone (PTH). PTH increases serum calcium through direct effects on kidney and bone as well as by indirect effects on gastrointestinal absorption. PTH secretion, in turn, is regulated by ionized calcium concentration in extracellular fluid.[182,183] The C cells of the thyroid secrete calcitonin, which inhibits bone resorption, thus opposing PTH activity and lowering serum calcium levels. Vitamin D and its metabolites also influence absorption of calcium and other minerals and are sometimes used to treat parathyroid disorders.

Primary Hyperparathyroidism

Primary hyperparathyroidism most commonly results from PTH oversecretion by a solitary parathyroid adenoma and is a common cause of hypercalcemia.[184] Primary hyperparathyroidism is not rare, and the diagnosis is frequently made in patients with few or no symptoms. The classic triad of nephrolithiasis, osteitis, and peptic ulcer disease ("stones, bones, and abdominal groans") characteristic of advanced primary hyperparathyroidism, is rarely seen today.

Common symptoms include fatigue and subjective weakness, although diverse central and peripheral nervous system syndromes have been reported.[142,143,182–188] Neuropsychiatric syndromes include impaired memory, personality changes, affective disorders, delirium, and psychosis. Elderly patients may be particularly vulnerable. The degree of hypercalcemia does not always correlate with clinical severity, although neurologic manifestations typically improve with treatment of the endocrine disorder. Parkinsonism and a syndrome resembling motor neuron disease, reversing with parathyroid surgery, have been described.[186,187] Myelopathy has been reported from compression by "brown tumors" seen in osteitis fibrosa cystica or on a presumed metabolic basis with normal spine MRI.[188] Neuromuscular symptoms include proximal weakness, muscle pain and stiffness, and paresthesias and typically respond to parathyroidectomy.[142]

Hypercalcemia, usually with concomitant hypophosphatemia, and elevated levels of immunoreactive PTH suggest the diagnosis. Distinguishing malignancy-associated hypercalcemia, with or without ectopic PTH secretion, from primary hyperparathyroidism can be challenging. Parathyroidectomy relieves symptoms and normalizes serum calcium levels in mild as well as severe disease. In patients with mild symptoms or those who are not surgical candidates, bisphosphonates are an option.[182–184]

Hypoparathyroidism

Hypoparathyroidism results from decreased PTH secretion, causing hypocalcemia.[189] PTH deficiency occurs most commonly after thyroidectomy or other neck surgery, including parathyroidectomy. Hypoparathyroidism may also develop as a feature of autoimmune endocrinopathies and inherited disorders such as Kearns–Sayre syndrome and DiGeorge syndrome. Other causes include glandular destruction from infiltrative processes or radiation. Severe magnesium depletion impairs both PTH secretion and its peripheral action. PTH resistance, referred to as pseudohypoparathyroidism, may develop as a consequence of circulating antagonists, abnormal receptors, or defects in receptor-linked enzyme activity.[190]

Diverse central and peripheral nervous system disorders may occur, primarily owing to hypocalcemia.[142,143,189–192] Dementia and psychosis have been described, with varying degrees of improvement after correction of serum calcium concentration. Seizures, usually generalized, may occur and, because their response to antiepileptic drugs is often unsatisfactory, are best managed by correction of serum calcium. Intracranial calcification, most commonly in the basal ganglia and cerebellum, develops in many hypoparathyroid patients, most of whom are asymptomatic.[192] Diverse extrapyramidal syndromes, with or without associated intracranial calcification, have been described including parkinsonism, choreoathetosis, hemiballismus, and torticollis. Further discussion is provided in Chapter 58. Tetany is the classic peripheral nervous system manifestation of hypocalcemia and may be difficult to distinguish from seizures. Findings on examination include Trousseau and Chvostek signs and carpopedal spasm. Clinically significant autonomic dysfunction is rare; the electrocardiogram may demonstrate a prolonged QT interval. Less common neurologic syndromes include myopathy, peripheral neuropathy, sensorineural hearing loss, and pseudotumor cerebri.

ADRENAL GLANDS

The paired adrenal glands, situated atop the kidneys, consist of the medulla, derived from neuroectoderm, and the cortex, derived from mesoderm. Their distinct embryologic origins parallel their different endocrine functions. Adrenal medullary chromaffin cells secrete catecholamines, principally epinephrine, regulated by cholinergic preganglionic sympathetic neurons. Adrenal cortical cells secrete sex hormones, corticosteroids, and mineralocorticoids regulated by the hormones ACTH and angiotensin II. This complex neural, endocrine, and metabolic integration allows the adrenal gland to fulfill its critical role in coordinating energy homeostasis and stress responses.

Adrenal Cortex

Primary Aldosteronism

Aldosterone, the major mineralocorticoid in humans, promotes sodium retention and potassium excretion and is primarily controlled by the renin-angiotensin system.[193] In primary aldosteronism, hormone production is inappropriately elevated, most commonly from bilateral adrenal hyperplasia or an aldosterone-secreting adenoma.[194] The resulting volume expansion causes hypertension, which may be treatment-resistant. Hypokalemic alkalosis is a useful clue to the diagnosis when present and when severe can lead to muscle weakness, paresthesias, tetany, or paralysis.[194] Activity-dependent conduction block, responsive to potassium replacement, was observed in a patient with primary aldosteronism, weakness, and severe hypokalemia.[195]

Cushing Syndrome

Although Cushing disease refers specifically to excess circulating corticosteroids induced by an ACTH-secreting pituitary adenoma, Cushing syndrome is a more general term for hypercortisolism and its associated clinical features, regardless of whether steroid excess is exogenous or endogenous. Corticosteroid treatment for neurologic disorders is usually parenteral or oral, and clinicians are familiar with the importance of monitoring for medical and neurologic complications. Topical or inhaled corticosteroids occasionally may also cause symptomatic hypercortisolism.[161]

In patients with suspected Cushing syndrome who are not taking corticosteroids, diagnosis is directed toward demonstrating hypercortisolism and defining the source of corticosteroid excess beginning with the same screening tests as for Cushing disease, followed by additional confirmatory blood tests and imaging.[161,196] ACTH-dependent causes of hypercortisolism are the most common endogenous form and include Cushing disease. Adrenal lesions such as hyperplasia, adenoma, or carcinoma account for many of the ACTH-independent forms. The differential diagnosis of hypercortisolism is outlined in Table 20-8. Treatment depends on the specific underlying cause and may include steroidogenic inhibitors.

TABLE 20-8 ■ Differential Diagnosis of Hypercortisolism

Non-Cushing Hypercortisolemia
Obesity
Major depression
Alcoholism
Pregnancy
Glucocorticoid resistance
Diabetes mellitus
Others (usually without clinical features of Cushing syndrome): acute illness, malnutrition, elevated cortisol-binding globulin
Exogenous
Corticosteroid or ACTH administration
Endogenous
ACTH-Dependent
Pituitary ACTH production (Cushing disease)
Ectopic ACTH production: carcinoid or other neuroendocrine tumors
Ectopic CRH syndrome
ACTH-Independent
Adrenal adenoma or carcinoma
Adrenal macronodular hyperplasia
McCune–Albright syndrome

ACTH, adrenocorticotropic hormone; CRH, corticotropin-releasing hormone.

Adrenal Insufficiency

With exogenous corticosteroids responsible for many cases of hypercortisolism, it is not surprising that rapid withdrawal of these agents is a common cause of adrenal insufficiency.[197] Acute adrenal failure may be fatal and should be considered in patients with unexplained hypotension. When adrenal insufficiency develops more gradually, systemic manifestations include fatigue, weight loss, loss of libido, hypotension, nausea, vomiting, dry skin, loss of axillary and pubic hair, and limb pain.[198] The low specificity of these symptoms and lower frequency of more specific symptoms such as salt craving and hyperpigmentation mean that diagnosis of adrenal insufficiency is often delayed. Cerebral symptoms include apathy, depression, confusion, and, occasionally, paranoia and psychosis.[199] Myalgias, myopathic weakness, cramping, and hyperkalemic periodic paralysis may develop occasionally.[143,200,201]

Primary adrenal insufficiency, or Addison disease, results from glandular dysfunction or destruction, acutely or chronically, by hemorrhage, infection, autoimmune disorders, surgery, metastases, steroidogenesis inhibitors, or hereditary disorders.[199,202,203]

Inherited causes with their own neurologic features include adrenomyeloneuropathy and

TABLE 20-9 ■ Causes of Adrenal Insufficiency

Primary (Addison Disease)
Autoimmune adrenalitis
Infection: meningococcemia, tuberculosis, cytomegalovirus
Metastases
Adrenal infarction or hemorrhage
Adrenoleukodystrophy and other inherited disorders
Drugs: steroidogenesis inhibitors
Secondary
Corticosteroid administration
Pituitary disease or surgery

adrenoleukodystrophy, which are X-linked disorders characterized by accumulation of very-long-chain fatty acids.[204] Adrenal disease may antedate neurologic symptoms or occur in isolation, and the diagnosis should be considered in young men with Addison disease.

Secondary adrenal insufficiency results from ACTH deficiency, due to hypothalamic or pituitary lesions, surgery, or suppression of the hypothalamic–pituitary–adrenal axis by exogenous corticosteroids.[197,203] The differential diagnosis of adrenal insufficiency is outlined in Table 20-9.

The synthetic corticotropin stimulation test usually constitutes the initial step in evaluating suspected adrenal insufficiency. Steroid replacement is lifesaving in acute adrenal failure and relieves symptoms in chronic states.

Adrenal Medulla

Pheochromocytoma and Neuroendocrine Tumors

Pheochromocytoma is a rare catecholamine-secreting tumor that arises from adrenal chromaffin cells.[205] Most are sporadic, but pheochromocytomas also occur as a part of inherited disorders, including neurofibromatosis type 1 and von Hippel–Lindau disease.[206] Extra-adrenal chromaffin cell tumors ("paragangliomas") are typically nonsecretory when they occur in the head and neck and occasionally cause cranial neuropathies. More commonly, paragangliomas occur along the sympathetic chain and secrete catecholamines, with clinical features similar to pheochromocytoma. A classic cause of secondary hypertension, these tumors also present with paroxysmal headache, diaphoresis, anxiety, tremor, dizziness, or flushing, in varying combinations. They may also present acutely, with ischemic or hemorrhagic stroke, reversible cerebral vasoconstriction syndrome, seizure, or delirium.[205] Included in the extensive differential diagnosis are anxiety disorders, panic attacks, migraine, hyperthyroidism, menopausal symptoms, effects of sympathomimetic drugs, and dysautonomia. Recommended initial testing for pheochromocytoma or paraganglioma is measurement of urine or plasma fractionated metanephrines, with phlebotomy performed supine and with additional restrictions on antecedent smoking, caffeine intake, and exercise.[206] CT or MRI, increasingly supplemented with functional imaging, localize the tumor, which is usually managed surgically.

Other neuroendocrine tumors may cause neurologic symptoms related to secretion of other biogenic amines or peptides.[206] Flushing, which may raise concern for dysautonomia, is a feature of carcinoid tumors—neoplasms of the gastrointestinal tract or lung which secrete serotonin, dopamine, prostaglandins, and other molecules. Pancreatic neuroendocrine tumors may secrete insulin, causing hypoglycemic symptoms, GHRH, causing acromegaly, or ACTH, causing Cushing syndrome.

ACKNOWLEDGMENTS

Dr. Schipper thanks Jonathan Liber and Deena Rogozinsky for assistance with computer surveillance of the literature.

REFERENCES

1. Schipper HM: Sex hormones and the nervous system. p. 409. In Aminoff MJ (ed): Neurology and General Medicine. 4th Ed. Churchill Livingstone Elsevier, Philadelphia, 2008.
2. Finocchi C, Ferrari M: Female reproductive steroids and neuronal excitability. Neurol Sci 32(suppl 1):S31, 2011.
3. Silberstein S, Merriam G: Sex hormones and headache 1999 (menstrual migraine). Neurology 53:S3, 1999.
4. Nappi RE, Albani F, Sances G, et al: Headaches during pregnancy. Curr Pain Headache Rep 15:289, 2011.
5. Chancellor AM, Wroe SJ, Cull RE: Migraine occurring for the first time in pregnancy. Headache 30:224, 1990.

6. Hauser L: Migraines and perimenopause: helping women in midlife manage and treat migraine. Nurs Womens Health 16:247, 2012.
7. Silberstein SD: Migraine and pregnancy. Neurol Clin 15:209, 1997.
8. MacGregor EA: Perimenopausal migraine in women with vasomotor symptoms. Maturitas 71:79, 2012.
9. Marcus DA: Interrelationships of neurochemicals, estrogen, and recurring headache. Pain 62:129, 1995.
10. Loder E, Rizzoli P, Golub J: Hormonal management of migraine associated with menses and the menopause: a clinical review. Headache 47:329, 2007.
11. O'Dea JPK, Davis EH: Tamoxifen in the treatment of menstrual migraine. Neurology 40:1470, 1990.
12. Mathew P, Fung F: Recapitulation of menstrual migraine with tamoxifen. Lancet 353:467, 1999.
13. Herzog AG: Continuous bromocriptine therapy in menstrual migraine. Neurology 48:101, 1997.
14. Lieba-Samal D, Wober C: Sex hormones and primary headaches other than migraine. Curr Pain Headache Rep 15:407, 2011.
15. Lidegaard O: Oral contraception and risk of a cerebral thromboembolic attack: results of a case-control study. BMJ 306:956, 1993.
16. Petitti DB, Sidney S, Bernstein A, et al: Stroke in users of low-dose oral contraceptives. N Engl J Med 335:8, 1996.
17. Carr BR, Ory H: Estrogen and progestin components of oral contraceptives: relationship to vascular disease. Contraception 55:267, 1997.
18. Calhoun A: Combined hormonal contraceptives: is it time to reassess their role in migraine? Headache 52:648, 2012.
19. Meade TW, Berra A: Hormone replacement therapy and cardiovascular disease. Br Med Bull 48:276, 1992.
20. Stubblefield PG: The effects on hemostasis of oral contraceptives containing desogestrel. Am J Obstet Gynecol 168:1047, 1993.
21. Mendelsohn MR, Karas RH: The protective effects of estrogen on the cardiovascular system. N Engl J Med 240:1801, 1999.
22. Allais G, Gabellari IC, Mana O, et al: Migraine and stroke: the role of oral contraceptives. Neurol Sci 29(suppl 1):S12, 2008.
23. Lee JS, Yaffe K, Lui LY, et al: Prospective study of endogenous circulating estradiol and risk of stroke in older women. Arch Neurol 67:195, 2010.
24. Bushnell CD: Hormone replacement therapy and stroke: the current state of knowledge and directions for future research. Semin Neurol 26:123, 2006.
25. Viscoli CM, Brass LM, Kernan WN, et al: A clinical trial of estrogen replacement therapy after ischemic stroke. N Engl J Med 345:1243, 2001.
26. Simon JA, Hsia J, Cauley JA, et al: Postmenopausal hormone therapy and risk of stroke: the heart and estrogen-progestin replacement study (HERS). Circulation 103:638, 2001.
27. Wassertheil-Smoller S, Hendrix SL, Limacher M, et al: Effect of estrogen plus progestin on stroke in postmenopausal women. The Women's Health Initiative: a randomized trial. JAMA 289:2673, 2003.
28. Henderson VW, Lobo RA: Hormone therapy and the risk of stroke: perspectives 10 years after the Women's Health Initiative trials. Climacteric 15:229, 2012.
29. Renoux C, Dell'aniello S, Garbe E, et al: Transdermal and oral hormone replacement therapy and the risk of stroke: a nested case-control study. BMJ 340:c2519, 2010.
30. Shearman AM, Cooper JA, Kotwinski PJ, et al: Estrogen receptor alpha gene variation and the risk of stroke. Stroke 36:2281, 2005.
31. Zupanc ML: Antiepileptic drugs and hormonal contraceptives in adolescent women with epilepsy. Neurology 66(suppl 3):S37, 2006.
32. Herzog A: Menstrual disorders in women with epilepsy. Neurology 66(suppl 3):S23, 2006.
33. Guberman A: Hormonal contraception and epilepsy. Neurology 53:S38, 1999.
34. Crawford PM: Managing epilepsy in women of childbearing age. Drug Safety 32:293, 2009.
35. Saano V, Glue P, Banfield CR, et al: Effects of felbamate on the pharmacokinetics of a low-dose combination oral contraceptive. Clin Pharmacol Ther 58:523, 1995.
36. Mengel HB, Houston A, Back DJ: An evaluation of the interaction between tiagabine and oral contraceptives in female volunteers. J Pharm Med 4:141, 1994.
37. Dworetzky BA, Townsend MK, Pennell PB, et al: Female reproductive factors and risk of seizure or epilepsy: data from the Nurses' Health Study II. Epilepsia 53:e1, 2012.
38. Quigg M, Smithson SD, Fowler KM, et al: Laterality and location influence catamenial seizure expression in women with partial epilepsy. Neurology 73:223, 2009.
39. Herzog AG: Progesterone therapy in women with epilepsy: a 3-year follow-up. Neurology 52:1917, 1999.
40. Zahn C: Catamenial epilepsy: clinical aspects. Neurology 53:S34, 1999.
41. Herzog AG, Fowler KM, Smithson SD, et al: Progesterone vs placebo therapy for women with epilepsy: a randomized clinical trial. Neurology 78:1959, 2012.
42. Maia DP, Fonseca PG, Camargos ST, et al: Pregnancy in patients with Sydenham's chorea. Parkinsonism Relat Disord 18:458, 2012.
43. Munhoz RP, Kowacs PA, Soria MG, et al: Catamenial and oral contraceptive-induced exacerbation of chorea in chorea-acanthocytosis: case report. Mov Disord 24:2166, 2009.
44. Thulin PC, Carter JH, Nichols MD: Menstrual-cycle related changes in Parkinson's disease. Neurology 46:A376, 1996.

45. Blanchet PJ, Fang J, Hyland K, et al: Short-term effects of high-dose 17β-estradiol in postmenopausal PD patients: a crossover study. Neurology 53:91, 1999.
46. Saunders-Pullman R, Gordon-Elliott J, Parides M, et al: The effect of estrogen replacement on early Parkinson's disease. Neurology 52:1417, 1999.
47. Strijks E, Kremer JA, Horstink MW: Effects of female sex steroids on Parkinson's disease in postmenopausal women. Clin Neuropharmacol 22:93, 1999.
48. Weiner WJ, Shulman LM, Singer C, et al: Menopause and estrogen replacement therapy in Parkinson's disease. Neurology 46:A376, 1996.
49. Benedetti MD, Maraganore DM, Bower JH, et al: Hysterectomy, menopause, and estrogen use preceding Parkinson's disease: an exploratory case-control study. Mov Disord 16:830, 2001.
50. Ragonese P, D'Amelio M, Salemi G, et al: Risk of Parkinson's disease in women. Neurology 62:2010, 2004.
51. Currie LJ, Harrison MB, Trugman JM, et al: Postmenopausal estrogen use affects risk for Parkinson's disease. Arch Neurol 61:886, 2004.
52. Simon KC, Chen H, Gao X, et al: Reproductive factors, exogenous estrogen use, and risk of Parkinson's disease. Mov Disord 24:1359, 2009.
53. Nicoletti A, Nicoletti G, Arabia G, et al: Reproductive factors and Parkinson's disease: a multicenter case-control study. Mov Disord 26:2563, 2011.
54. Westberg L, Hakansson A, Melke J, et al: Association between estrogen receptor beta gene and age of onset of Parkinson's disease. Psychoneuroendocrinology 29:993, 2004.
55. Henri-Bhargava A, Melmed C, Glikstein R, et al: Neurological impairment due to vitamin E and copper deficiencies in celiac disease. Neurology 71:860, 2008.
56. Schwabe MJ, Konkol RJ: Menstrual cycle-related fluctuations of tics in Tourette syndrome. Pediatr Neurol 8:43, 1992.
57. Mizuta E, Yamasaki S, Nakatake M, et al: Neuroleptic malignant syndrome in a parkinsonian woman during the premenstrual period. Neurology 43:1048, 1993.
58. Haddad G, Haddad F, Worseley K, et al: Brain tumours and pregnancy. Can J Neurol Sci 18:231, 1991.
59. Wahab M, Al-Azzawi F: Meningioma and hormonal influences. Climacteric 6:285, 2003.
60. Korhonen K, Auvinen A, Lyytinen H, et al: A nationwide cohort study on the incidence of meningioma in women using postmenopausal hormone therapy in Finland. Am J Epidemiol 175:309, 2012.
61. Pines A: Hormone therapy and brain tumors. Climacteric 14:215, 2011.
62. Hilbig A, Barbosa-Coutinho LM: Meningiomas and hormonal receptors: immunohistochemical study in typical and non-typical tumors. Arq Neuropsiquiatr 56:193, 1998.
63. Hsu DW, Efird JT, Hedley-Whyte ET: Progesterone and estrogen receptors in meningiomas: prognostic considerations. J Neurosurg 86:113, 1997.
64. Lamberts SWJ, Tanghe HLJ, Avezaat CJJ, et al: Mifepristone (RU 486) treatment of meningiomas. J Neurol Neurosurg Psychiatry 55:486, 1992.
65. Adams EF, Schrell UMH, Fahlbusch R, et al: Hormonal dependency of cerebral meningiomas. Part 2. In vitro effect of steroids, bromocriptine, and epidermal growth factor on growth of meningiomas. J Neurosurg 73:750, 1990.
66. Lamberts SW, Koper JW, de Jong FH: The endocrine effects of long-term treatment with mifepristone (RU 486). J Clin Endocrinol Metab 73:187, 1991.
67. von Schoultz E, Bixo M, Backstrom T, et al: Sex steroids in human brain tumors and breast cancer. Cancer 65:949, 1990.
68. Chung YG, Kim HK, Lee HK, et al: Expression of androgen receptors in astrocytoma. J Korean Med Sci 11:517, 1996.
69. Donahue JE, Stopa EG, Chorsky RL, et al: Cells containing immunoreactive estrogen receptor-alpha in the human basal forebrain. Brain Res 856:142, 2000.
70. Langub Jr MC, Watson Jr RE: Estrogen receptor-immunoreactive glia, endothelia, and ependyma in guinea pig preoptic area and median eminence: electron microscopy. Endocrinology 130:364, 1992.
71. Mydlarski M, Brawer JR, Schipper HM: The peroxidase-positive subcortical glial system. p. 191. In Schipper HM (ed): Astrocytes in Brain Aging and Neurodegeneration. Landes, Austin, TX, 1998.
72. Batistatou A, Stefanou D, Goussia A, et al: Estrogen receptor beta (ERβ) is expressed in brain astrocytic tumors and declines with dedifferentiation of the neoplasm. J Cancer Res Clin Oncol 130:405, 2004.
73. Couldwell WT, Hinton DR, Surnock AA, et al: Treatment of recurrent malignant gliomas with chronic oral high-dose tamoxifen. Clin Cancer Res 2:619, 1996.
74. Pollack IF, DaRosso RC, Robertson PL, et al: A phase I study of high-dose tamoxifen for the treatment of refractory malignant gliomas of childhood. Clin Cancer Res 3:1109, 1997.
75. Mastronardi L, Puzzilli F, Ruggeri A: Tamoxifen as a potential treatment of glioma. Anticancer Drugs 9:581, 1998.
76. Donson AM, Weil MD, Foreman NK: Tamoxifen radiosensitization in human glioblastoma cell lines. J Neurosurg 90:533, 1999.
77. Verzat C, Courriere P, Hollande E: Heterotransplantation of a human oligoastrocytoma into nude mice: difference in tumour growth between males and females. Neuropathol Appl Neurobiol 18:37, 1992.
78. Pors H, von Eyben FE, Sorensen OS, et al: Long-term remission of multiple brain metastases with tamoxifen. J Neurooncol 10:173, 1991.

79. Kirby M, Zsarnovszky A, Belcher SM: Estrogen receptor expression in a primitive neuroectodermal tumor cell line from the cerebral cortex: estrogen stimulates rapid ERK1/2 activation and receptor-dependent cell migration. Biochem Biophys Res Commun 319:753, 2004.
80. Frantzen C, Kruizinga RC, van Asselt SJ, et al: Pregnancy-related hemangioblastoma progression and complications in von Hippel-Lindau disease. Neurology 79:793, 2012.
81. Mattila KM, Luomala M, Lehtimaki T, et al: Interaction between ESRI and HLA-DR2 may contribute to the development of MS in women. Neurology 56:1246, 2001.
82. Niino M, Kiruchi S, Fukazawa T, et al: Estrogen receptor gene polymorphism in Japanese patients with multiple sclerosis. J Neurol Sci 179:70, 2000.
83. Savettieri G, Citadella R, Valentino P, et al: Lack of association of estrogen receptor 1 gene polymorphisms and multiple sclerosis in southern Italy in humans. Neurosci Lett 327:115, 2002.
84. Sweeney WJ: Pregnancy and multiple sclerosis. Am J Obstet Gynecol 66:124, 1995.
85. Confavreux C, Hutchinson M, Hours MM, et al: Rate of pregnancy-related relapse in multiple sclerosis. N Engl J Med 339:285, 1998.
86. Hutchinson M: Pregnancy and multiple sclerosis. MS Management 6:3, 1999.
87. Orvieto R, Achiron R, Rotstein Z, et al: Pregnancy and multiple sclerosis: a 2-year experience. Eur J Obstet Gynecol Reprod Biol 82:191, 1999.
88. Ramagopalan SV, Valdar W, Criscuoli M, Canadian Collaborative Study Group Age of puberty and the risk of multiple sclerosis: a population based study. Eur J Neurol 16:342, 2009.
89. Alonso A, Clark CJ: Oral contraceptives and the risk of multiple sclerosis: a review of the epidemiologic evidence. J Neurol Sci 286:73, 2009.
90. Gold SM, Voskuhl RR: Estrogen and testosterone therapies in multiple sclerosis. Prog Brain Res 175:239, 2009.
91. Selkoe DJ: The molecular pathology of Alzheimer's disease. Neuron 6:487, 1991.
92. Schipper HM: Sex hormones and the nervous system. p. 365. In Aminoff MJ (ed): Neurology and General Medicine. 3rd Ed. Churchill Livingstone, New York, 2001.
93. Gazzaley AH, Weiland NG, McEwen BS, et al: Differential regulation of NMDAR1 mRNA and protein by estradiol in the rat hippocampus. J Neurosci 16:6830, 1996.
94. Toran-Allerand CD: The estrogen/neurotrophin connection during neural development: is co-localization of estrogen receptors with the neurotrophins and their receptors biologically relevant? Dev Neurosci 18:36, 1996.
95. Henderson VW: Estrogen, cognition, and a woman's risk of Alzheimer's disease. Am J Med 103:11S, 1997.
96. Solerte SB, Fioravanti M, Racchi M, et al: Menopause and estrogen deficiency as a risk factor in dementing illness: hypothesis on the biological basis. Maturitas 31:95, 1999.
97. Sapolsky RM: Is this relevant to the human? p. 305. In Sapolsky RM (ed): Stress, the Aging Brain, and the Mechanisms of Neuron Death. MIT Press, Cambridge, 1992.
98. Honjo H, Tanaka K, Kashiwagi T, et al: Senile dementia—Alzheimer's type and estrogen. Horm Metab Res 27:204, 1995.
99. Sherwin BB: Estrogen, the brain, and memory. Menopause 3:97, 1996.
100. Wickelgren I: Estrogen stakes claim to cognition. Science 276:675, 1997.
101. Van Duijn CM: Hormone replacement therapy and Alzheimer's disease. Maturitas 31:201, 1999.
102. Schneider LS, Farlow MR, Henderson VW, et al: Effects of estrogen replacement therapy on response to tacrine in patients with Alzheimer's disease. Neurology 46:1580, 1996.
103. Henderson VW, Paganini-Hill A, Emanuel CK, et al: Estrogen replacement therapy in older women. Arch Neurol 51:896, 1994.
104. Paganini-Hill A, Henderson VW: Estrogen deficiency and risk of Alzheimer's disease in women. Am J Epidemiol 140:256, 1994.
105. Waring SC, Rocca WA, Petersen RC, et al: Postmenopausal estrogen replacement therapy and risk of AD: a population-based study. Neurology 52:965, 1999.
106. Tang MX, Jacobs D, Stern Y, et al: Effect of oestrogen during menopause on risk and age at onset of Alzheimer's disease. Lancet 348:429, 1996.
107. Kawas C, Resnick S, Morrison A, et al: A prospective study of estrogen replacement therapy and the risk of developing Alzheimer's disease: the Baltimore longitudinal study of aging. Neurology 48:1517, 1997.
108. Massoud F, Yaffe K, Sano M: Estrogen. p. 523. In: Qizilbash N, Schneider LS, Chui H (eds): Evidence-Based Dementia Practice. Blackwell, Oxford, 2002.
109. Marder K, Tang M-X, Alfaro B, et al: Postmenopausal estrogen use and Parkinson's disease with and without dementia. Neurology 50:1141, 1998.
110. Tan RS, Pu SJ: A pilot study on the effects of testosterone in hypogonadal aging men with Alzheimer's disease. Aging Male 6:13, 2003.
111. Cherrier MM, Matsumoto AM, Amory JK, et al: Testosterone improves spatial memory in men with Alzheimer disease and mild cognitive impairment. Neurology 64:2063, 2005.
112. Sherwin BB, Chertkow H, Schipper H, et al: A randomized controlled trial of estrogen treatment in men with mild cognitive impairment. Neurobiol Aging 32:1808, 2011.
113. Cauley JA, Black DM, Barrett-Connor E, et al: Effects of hormone replacement therapy on clinical features

and height loss: the Heart and Estrogen/Progestin Replacement Study (HERS). Am J Med 110:442, 2001.

114. Shumaker S, Legault C, Kuller L, et al: Conjugated equine estrogens and incidence of probable dementia and mild cognitive impairment in postmenopausal women: Women's Health Initiative Memory Study. JAMA 291:2947, 2004.
115. Corbo RM, Gambina G, Broggio E, et al: Influence of variation in the follicle-stimulating hormone receptor gene (FSHR) and age at menopause on the development of Alzheimer's disease in women. Dement Geriatr Cogn Disord 32:63, 2011.
116. Patterson C, Feightner J, Garcia A, et al: Primary prevention of dementia. Alzheimers Dement 3:348, 2007.
117. Craig MC, Murphy DG: Estrogen therapy and Alzheimer's dementia. Ann New York Acad Sci 1205:245, 2010.
118. Shao H, Breitner JC, Whitmer RA, et al: Hormone therapy and Alzheimer disease dementia: new findings from the Cache County Study. Neurology 79:1846, 2012.
119. Schipper HM: Apolipoprotein E: implications for AD neurobiology, epidemiology and risk assessment. Neurobiol Aging 32:778, 2011.
120. Chu LW, Tam S, Wong RL, et al: Bioavailable testosterone predicts a lower risk of Alzheimer's disease in older men. J Alzheimers Dis 21:1335, 2010.
121. Rosario ER, Pike CJ: Androgen regulation of beta-amyloid protein and the risk of Alzheimer's disease. Brain Res Rev 57:444, 2008.
122. Cherrier MM: Testosterone effects on cognition in health and disease. Front Horm Res 37:150, 2009.
123. Carroll JC, Rosario ER: The potential use of hormone-based therapeutics for the treatment of Alzheimer's disease. Curr Alzheimer Res 9:18, 2012.
124. Barron AM, Pike CJ: Sex hormones, aging, and Alzheimer's disease. Front Biosci 4:976, 2012.
125. De Block CE, Leeuw IH, Gaal LE: Premenstrual attacks of acute intermittent porphyria: hormonal and metabolic aspects—a case report. Eur J Endocrinol 141:50, 1999.
126. Yamamori I, Asai M, Tanaka E, et al: Prevention of premenstrual exacerbation of hereditary coproporphyria by gonadotropin-releasing hormone analogue. Intern Med 38:365, 1999.
127. Halbreich U, Freeman EW, Rapkin AJ, et al: Continuous oral levonorgestrel/ethinyl estradiol for treating premenstrual dysphoric disorder. Contraception 85:19, 2012.
128. Workman JL, Barha CK, Galea LA: Endocrine substrates of cognitive and affective changes during pregnancy and postpartum. Behav Neurosci 126:54, 2012.
129. Studd J, Nappi RE: Reproductive depression. Gynecol Endocrinol 28(suppl 1):42, 2012.
130. Young JK: Estrogen and the etiology of anorexia nervosa. Neurosci Behav Rev 15:327, 1991.
131. Vinogradov S, Csernansky JG: Postpartum psychosis with abnormal movements: dopamine supersensitivity unmasked by withdrawal of endogenous estrogen? J Clin Psychiatry 51:365, 1990.
132. Polo-Kantola P, Erkkola R, Irjala K, et al: Effect of short-term transdermal estrogen replacement therapy on sleep: a randomized, double-blind crossover trial in postmenopausal women. Fertil Steril 71:873, 1999.
133. Friess E, Tagaya H, Trachsel L, et al: Progesterone-induced changes in sleep in male subjects. Am J Physiol 272:E885, 1997.
134. Zhou XS, Rowley JA, Demirovic F, et al: Effect of testosterone on the apneic threshold in women during NREM sleep. J Appl Physiol 94:101, 2003.
135. Dexter DD, Dovre EJ: Obstructive sleep apnea due to endogenous testosterone production in a woman. Mayo Clin Proc 73:246, 1998.
136. Hachul H, Bittencourt LR, Andersen ML, et al: Effects of hormone therapy with estrogen and/or progesterone on sleep pattern in postmenopausal women. Int J Gynaecol Obstet 103:207, 2008.
137. Ziylan YZ, Lefauconnier JM, Bernard G, et al: Blood-brain barrier permeability: regional alterations after acute and chronic administration of ethinyl estradiol. Neurosci Lett 118:181, 1990.
138. Floyd 2nd JR, Keeler ER, Euscher ED, et al: Cyclic sciatica from extrapelvic endometriosis affecting the sciatic nerve. J Neurosurg Spine 14:281, 2011.
139. Goldenberg JN, Bradley WG: Testosterone therapy and the pathogenesis of Kennedy's disease (X-linked bulbospinal muscular atrophy). J Neurol Sci 135:158, 1996.
140. Mastrogiacomo I, Bonanni G, Menegazzo E, et al: Clinical and hormonal aspects of male hypogonadism in myotonic dystrophy. Ital J Neurol Sci 17:59, 1996.
141. Mete O, Asa SL: Clinicopathological correlations in pituitary adenomas. Brain Pathol 22:443, 2012.
142. Douglas M: Neurology of endocrine disease. Clin Med 10:387, 2010.
143. Alshekhlee A, Kaminski HJ, Ruff RL: Neuromuscular manifestations of endocrine disorders. Neurol Clin 20:35, 2002.
144. Lucas JW, Zada G: Imaging of the pituitary and parasellar region. Semin Neurol 32:320, 2012.
145. Melmed S, Kleinberg D, Ho K: Pituitary physiology and diagnostic evaluation. p. 175. In: Melmed S, Polonsky KS, Larsen PR (eds): Williams Textbook of Endocrinology. 12th Ed. Elsevier Saunders, Philadelphia, 2011.
146. Asa SL, Ezzat S: The pathogenesis of pituitary tumors. Annu Rev Pathol Mech Dis 4:97, 2009.
147. Lleva RR, Inzucchi SE: Diagnosis and management of pituitary adenomas. Curr Opin Oncol 23:53, 2011.
148. Levy MJ: The association of pituitary tumors and headache. Curr Neurol Neurosci Rep 11:164, 2011.

149. Abele TA, Yetkin ZF, Raisanen JM, et al: Non-pituitary origin sellar tumours mimicking pituitary macroadenomas. Clin Radiol 67:821, 2012.
150. Guitelman M, Basavilbaso NG, Vitale M, et al: Primary empty sella (PES): a review of 175 cases. Pituitary 16:270, 2013.
151. Freda PU, Beckers AM, Katznelson L, et al: Pituitary incidentaloma: an Endocrine Society clinical practice guideline. J Clin Endocrinol Metab 96:894, 2011.
152. Melmed S, Casanueva FF, Hoffman AR, et al: Diagnosis and treatment of hyperprolactinemia: an Endocrine Society clinical practice guideline. J Clin Endocrinol Metab 96:273, 2011.
153. Cookson J, Hodgson R, Wildgust HJ: Prolactin, hyperprolactinaemia and antipsychotic treatment: a review and lessons for treatment of early psychosis. J Psychopharmacol 26(suppl):42, 2012.
154. Chen DK, So Y, Fisher RS: Use of serum prolactin in diagnosing epileptic seizures: report of the Therapeutics and Technology Assessment Subcommittee of the American Academy of Neurology. Neurology 65:668, 2005.
155. Mann WA: Treatment for prolactinomas and hyperprolactinaemia: a lifetime approach. Eur J Clin Invest 41:334, 2011.
156. Platta CS, MacKay C, Welsh JS: Pituitary adenoma: a radiotherapeutic perspective. Am J Clin Oncol 33:408, 2010.
157. Melmed S: Acromegaly. N Engl J Med 355:2558, 2006.
158. Katznelson L, Atkinson JL, Cook DM, et al: American Association of Clinical Endocrinologists medical guidelines for clinical practice for the diagnosis and treatment of acromegaly—2011 update. Endocr Pract 17(suppl 4):1, 2011.
159. Melmed S, Casanueva FF, Klibanski A, et al: A consensus on the diagnosis and treatment of acromegaly complications. Pituitary 16:294, 2013.
160. Bertagna X, Guignat L, Groussin L, et al: Cushing's disease. Best Pract Res Clin Endocrinol Metab 23:607, 2009.
161. Nieman LK, Biller BM, Findling JW, et al: The diagnosis of Cushing's syndrome: an Endocrine Society clinical practice guideline. J Clin Endocrinol Metab 93:1526, 2008.
162. Fassett DR, Schmidt MH: Spinal epidural lipomatosis: a review of its causes and recommendations for treatment. Neurosurg Focus 16:E11, 2004.
163. Deipolyi A, Karaosmanoglu A, Habito C, et al: The role of bilateral inferior petrosal sinus sampling in the diagnostic evaluation of Cushing syndrome. Diagn Interv Radiol 18:132, 2012.
164. Biller BM, Grossman AB, Stewart PM, et al: Treatment of adrenocorticotropin-dependent Cushing's syndrome: a consensus statement. J Clin Endocrinol Metab 93:2454, 2008.
165. Beck-Peccoz P, Persani L, Mannavola D, et al: TSH-secreting adenomas. Best Pract Res Clin Endocrinol Metab 23:597, 2009.
166. Jaffe CA: Clinically non-functioning pituitary adenomas. Pituitary 9:317, 2006.
167. Murad-Kejbou S, Eggenberger E: Pituitary apoplexy: evaluation, management, and prognosis. Curr Opin Ophthalmol 20:456, 2009.
168. Rajasekaran S, Vanderpump M, Baldeweg S, et al: UK guidelines for the management of pituitary apoplexy. Clin Endocrinol 74:9, 2011.
169. Tessnow AH, Wilson JD: The changing face of Sheehan's syndrome. Am J Med Sci 340:402, 2010.
170. Robinson AG, Verbalis JG: Posterior pituitary. p. 291. In: Melmed S, Polonsky KS, Larsen PR (eds): Williams Textbook of Endocrinology. 12th Ed. Elsevier Saunders, Philadelphia, 2011.
171. Hannon MJ, Finucane FM, Sherlock M, et al: Disorders of water homeostasis in neurosurgical patients. J Clin Endocrinol Metab 97:1423, 2012.
172. Fenske W, Allolio B: Current state and future perspectives in the diagnosis of diabetes insipidus: a clinical review. J Clin Endocrinol Metab 97:3426, 2012.
173. Bellastella A, Bizzarro A, Colella C, et al: Subclinical diabetes insipidus. Best Pract Res Clin Endocrinol Metab 26:471, 2012.
174. Esposito P, Piotti G, Bianzina S, et al: The syndrome of inappropriate antidiuresis: pathophysiology, clinical management and new therapeutic options. Nephron Clin Pract 119:c62, 2011.
175. Ellison DH, Berl T: The syndrome of inappropriate antidiuresis. N Engl J Med 356:2064, 2007.
176. Gankam Kengne G, Andres C, Sattar L, et al: Mild hyponatremia and the risk of fracture in the ambulatory elderly. QJM 101:583, 2008.
177. King JD, Rosner MH: Osmotic demyelination syndrome. Am J Med Sci 339:561, 2010.
178. Maesaka JK, Imbriano LJ, Ali NM, et al: Is it cerebral or renal salt wasting? Kidney Int 76:934, 2009.
179. Schneider HJ, Aimaretti G, Kreitschmann-Andermahr I, et al: Hypopituitarism. Lancet 369:1461, 2007.
180. Fernandez-Rodriguez E, Bernabeu I, Andujar-Plata P, et al: Subclinical hypopituitarism. Best Pract Res Clin Endocrinol Metab 26:461, 2012.
181. Schneider HJ, Kreitschmann-Andermahr I, Ghigo E, et al: Hypothalamopituitary dysfunction following traumatic brain injury and aneurysmal subarachnoid hemorrhage: a systematic review. JAMA 298:1429, 2007.
182. Fraser WD: Hyperparathyroidism. Lancet 374:145, 2009.
183. Pyram R, Mahajan G, Gliwa A: Primary hyperparathyroidism: skeletal and nonskeletal effects, diagnosis and management. Maturitas 70:246, 2011.
184. Marcocci C, Cetani F: Clinical practice: primary hyperparathyroidism. N Engl J Med 365:2389, 2011.
185. Roman S, Sosa JA: Psychiatric and cognitive aspects of primary hyperparathyroidism. Curr Opin Oncol 19:1, 2007.

186. Kovacs CS, Howse DC, Yendt ER: Reversible parkinsonism induced by hypercalcemia and primary hyperparathyroidism. Arch Intern Med 153:1134, 1993.
187. Carvalho AA, Vieira A, Simplicio H, et al: Primary hyperparathyroidism simulating motor neuron disease: case report. Arq Neuropsiquiatr 63:160, 2005.
188. Fargen KM, Lin CS, Jeung JA, et al: Vertebral brown tumors causing neurologic compromise. World Neurosurg 79:208e1, 2013.
189. Cusano NE, Rubin MR, Sliney J, et al: Mini-review: new therapeutic options in hypoparathyroidism. Endocrine 41:410, 2012.
190. Mantovani G: Clinical review: pseudohypoparathyroidism: diagnosis and treatment. J Clin Endocrinol Metab 96:3020, 2011.
191. Bhadada SK, Bhansali A, Upreti V, et al: Spectrum of neurological manifestations of idiopathic hypoparathyroidism and pseudohypoparathyroidism. Neurol India 59:586, 2011.
192. Goswami R, Sharma R, Sreenivas V, et al: Prevalence and progression of basal ganglia calcification and its pathogenic mechanism in patients with idiopathic hypoparathyroidism. Clin Endocrinol 77:200, 2012.
193. Sukor N: Primary aldosteronism: from bench to bedside. Endocrine 41:31, 2012.
194. Carey RM: Primary aldosteronism. J Surg Oncol 106:575, 2012.
195. Krishnan AV, Colebatch JG, Kiernan MC: Hypokalemic weakness in hyperaldosteronism: activity-dependent conduction block. Neurology 65:1309, 2005.
196. Boscaro M, Arnaldi G: Approach to the patient with possible Cushing's syndrome. J Clin Endocrinol Metab 94:3121, 2009.
197. Reimondo G, Bovio S, Allasino B, et al: Secondary hypoadrenalism. Pituitary 11:147, 2008.
198. Bleicken B, Hahner S, Ventz M, et al: Delayed diagnosis of adrenal insufficiency is common: a cross-sectional study in 216 patients. Am J Med Sci 339:525, 2010.
199. Anglin RE, Rosebush PI, Mazurek MF: The neuropsychiatric profile of Addison's disease: revisiting a forgotten phenomenon. J Neuropsychiatry Clin Neurosci 18:450, 2006.
200. Kinoshita H, Mizutani S, Sei K, et al: Musculoskeletal symptoms and neurological investigations in adrenocortical insufficiency: a case report and literature review. J Musculoskelet Neuronal Interact 10:281, 2010.
201. Sathi N, Makkuni D, Mitchell WS, et al: Musculoskeletal aspects of hypoadrenalism: just a load of aches and pains? Clin Rheumatol 28:631, 2009.
202. Neary N, Nieman L: Adrenal insufficiency: etiology, diagnosis, and treatment. Curr Opin Endocrinol Diabetes Obes 17:217, 2010.
203. Li-Ng M, Kennedy L: Adrenal insufficiency. J Surg Oncol 106:595, 2012.
204. Engelen M, Kemp S, de Visser M, et al: X-linked adrenoleukodystrophy (X-ALD): clinical presentation and guidelines for diagnosis, follow-up and management. Orphanet J Rare Dis 7:51, 2012.
205. Anderson NE, Chung K, Willoughby E, et al: Neurologic manifestations of phaeochromocytomas and secretory paragangliomas: a reappraisal. J Neurol Neurosurg Psychiatry 84:452, 2013.
206. Vinik AI, Woltering EA, Warner RR, et al: NANETS consensus guidelines for the diagnosis of neuroendocrine tumors. Pancreas 39:713, 2010.

SECTION

V

Cutaneous Disorders

CHAPTER

21

The Skin and Neurologic Disease

OREST HURKO

This chapter provides an overview of disorders with both neurologic and cutaneous manifestations. Because the emphasis is on diagnosis, the presentation is organized around familiar neurologic syndromes rather than pathologic entities. This approach is complementary to those based on traditional pathophysiologic categories, such as phakomatoses or autoimmune and infectious disorders. Patients present to the neurologist with signs and symptoms, not with biopsies.

Usually a disease cannot be related to either a single cutaneous sign or a single neurologic syndrome. To minimize repetition while aiming for a comprehensive presentation, the text is limited to important representative diseases. Each is described only once, grouped with its most characteristic clinical presentation where possible. Secondary manifestations are mentioned in passing or in tables. Details are necessarily limited, but are supplemented with more comprehensive tables and, where applicable, annotation with the code number in the continuously updated Online Mendelian Inheritance in Man (OMIM).[1] The discussion is limited to disorders that permit survival to adulthood.

TUMORS

Earlier classifications of neurocutaneous disorders described phakomatoses, a label originally applied to two autosomal dominant disorders associated with tumors: neurofibromatosis type I and

Aminoff's Neurology and General Medicine, Fifth Edition.

tuberous sclerosis.[2] However, this category gradually expanded to encompass a wide variety of other neurologic disorders, including Sturge–Weber syndrome, which is not associated with tumors, and von Hippel–Lindau syndrome, associated with tumors but not with cutaneous lesions. Phakomatosis has outlived its utility as a diagnostic category.

Numerous disorders are associated with tumors, cutaneous manifestations and neurologic disease. In many cases the tumors themselves are responsible for the cutaneous or neurologic symptoms, but in others they are independent manifestations of a more complex syndrome.

Neurofibromatosis Type I

Neurofibromatosis type I (NF1; von Recklinghausen disease), an autosomal dominant disorder (OMIM 162200), is characterized by café-au-lait spots, fibromatous dermal tumors, and Lisch nodules of the iris as well as neoplasms of both the peripheral and the central nervous system (CNS). The earlier designation as peripheral neurofibromatosis (strictly speaking, a misnomer) served to distinguish this disorder from the genetically and clinically distinct central neurofibromatosis,[3] now neurofibromatosis type 2 (NF2; OMIM 101000).

NF1 is the most common single-gene disorder of the nervous system, affecting 1 in 3,500 individuals. It results from heterozygosity for a mutant form of a large gene on chromosome 17q11.2 that encodes a cytoplasmic protein with multiple regulatory functions.[4] The NIH consensus criteria permit unequivocal diagnosis of NF1 even without demonstration of the genetic mutation, by clinical observation of at least two of the following: (1) the presence of six or more café-au-lait macules with a diameter of ≥5 mm in children younger than 6 years and ≥15 mm in older people (Fig. 21-1); (2) two or more neurofibromas of any type or one plexiform neurofibroma; (3) axillary or inguinal region freckling; (4) optic pathway glioma; (5) two or more Lisch nodules (whitish tumors of the iris); (6) dysplasia of the sphenoid bone or thinning of the cortex of long bones with or without pseudoarthrosis; and/or (7) a first-degree relative exhibiting these changes.

The familiar café-au-lait spots are present at birth, as are plexiform neurofibromas and focal bone dysplasias, but axillary freckling, optic gliomas, Lisch nodules, and neurofibromas appear later in childhood. Of these, axillary freckling is the most diagnostically reliable, being present in all individuals with NF1 by the end of puberty. Café-au-lait spots alone are not diagnostic of NF1 because fewer than five spots are found frequently in individuals who are well. Café-au-lait spots as an isolated trait can be transmitted as an autosomal dominant (OMIM 114030) or as occasional features in other heritable disorders including tuberous sclerosis, the microcephalic disorders Nijmegen breakage syndrome (ataxia telangiectasia variant VI, OMIM 251260), X-linked Russell–Silver syndrome (OMIM 312780), Turcot mismatch repair cancer syndrome (OMIM 276300; polyposis coli, rhabdomyosarcomas, medulloblastomas, ependymomas and other gliomas), the rare Westerhof growth retardation syndrome (OMIM 154000), and perhaps most famously in McCune–Albright polyostotic fibrous dysplasia (OMIM 174800). The old clinical pearl that the rough border of McCune–Albright café-au-lait spots distinguishes them from the smooth borders seen in NF1 is not reliable.

Malignant neoplasms or benign tumors of the nervous system occur in 45 percent of individuals with NF1.[5] Optic nerve gliomas develop in 15 percent. However, neurologic involvement most often results from benign neurofibromas in the root entry zone of peripheral nerves, causing radiculopathy or compression of the spinal cord. Plexiform neurofibromas, which can be nodular or diffuse, arise from nerve trunks. Diffuse plexiform neurofibromas are usually congenital and undergo transformation in about 4 percent of cases into malignant peripheral nerve sheath tumors that are severely painful, tender, and hard. The more common dermal neurofibromas are usually innocent, permitting conservative management in asymptomatic people. The incidence of non-neural tumors is also increased modestly, especially rhabdomyosarcomas of the urogenital tract and myelogenous leukemia.

In addition, there are neurologic sequelae not related to tumors. The most significant of these are poorly characterized T2 hyperintensities in the centrum semiovale (unidentified bright objects), the density of which correlates with mild cognitive impairment.[6–9]

Neurofibromatosis Type II

This genetically distinct autosomal dominant disorder (OMIM 101000; also known as NF2, bilateral acoustic neurofibromatosis, or BANF) is

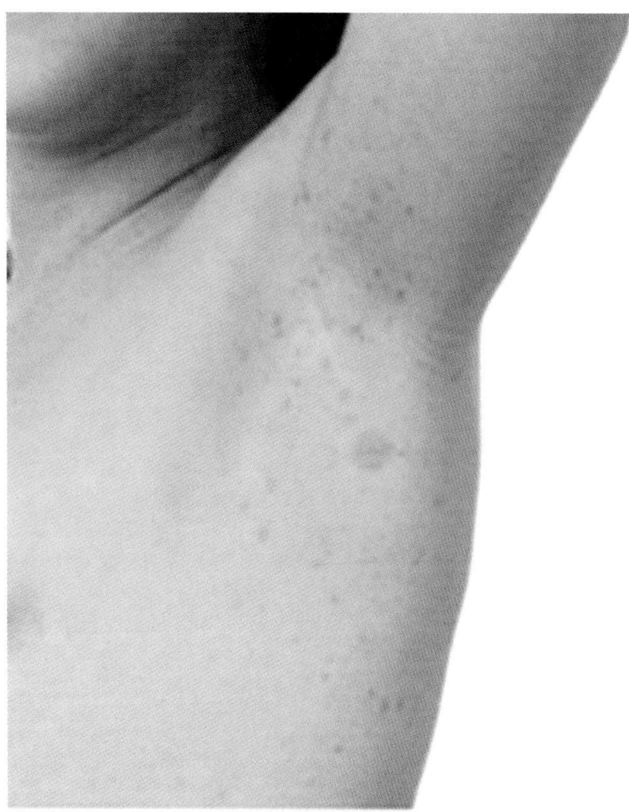

FIGURE 21-1 ■ Neurofibromatosis type 1: axillary freckling—a cluster of freckle-sized café- au-lait macules. (From Kurlemann G: Neurocutaneous syndromes. Handb Clin Neurol 108:513, 2012, with permission.)

characterized by tumors of the eighth cranial nerve in the cerebellopontine angle, meningiomas, and schwannomas of the dorsal roots of the spinal cord.[10,11] It is less common than NF1 by an order of magnitude, affecting 1 in 25,000 live births in association with heterozygosity for a mutant form of merlin, a critical regulator of cell–cell adhesion, transmembrane signaling, the actin cytoskeleton, and resultant inhibition of proliferation. It is encoded on chromosome 8. Other mutations of this gene result in a clinically related but distinct mendelian disorder, congenital cutaneous schwannomatosis (OMIM 162091) or in some familial predispositions to meningiomas (OMIM 607174). Typically, NF2 presents in young adults, but hearing loss has been reported as early as age 6. Proposed diagnostic criteria for definite NF2 are bilateral vestibular schwannomas; or a family history of NF2 in one or more first-degree relatives plus (1) unilateral vestibular schwannomas at age less than 30 years, or (2) any two of the following: meningioma, glioma, schwannoma, or juvenile posterior subcapsular lenticular opacities/juvenile cortical cataract.[2] Bilateral acoustic neuromas occur in less than 5 percent of most series. The cutaneous manifestations are also distinct from that of NF1.[12] Café-au-lait spots are present in about 40 percent of individuals, but only about 1 percent have six, the minimum seen in NF1. There are three types of cutaneous tumors: (1) discrete well-circumscribed, slightly raised, roughened areas of skin often pigmented and accompanied by excess hair, which are seen in about one-half of affected individuals; (2) subcutaneous well-circumscribed, nodular tumors located on peripheral nerves seen in about one-third; and (3) violaceous papillary skin neurofibromas, similar to those seen in NF1, in about one-fifth. One-third of NF2 patients have no cutaneous lesions.

Tuberous Sclerosis

This autosomal dominant neurocutaneous disorder was originally described as a phakomatosis, as had been NF1.[3] It is characterized by hamartomas in multiple organ systems, including the brain, skin, heart, kidneys, and lung.[13] The characteristic brain lesions, named tubers because of their fancied resemblance to potatoes, are benign, but some 5 to 15 percent of affected individuals also develop malignant brain neoplasms, most frequently subependymal giant cell astrocytomas. These often develop at the foramen of Monro or elsewhere on the wall of the lateral ventricle or the retina. More frequent neurologic presentations are learning difficulties, behavioral problems, autism or epilepsy, often the severe West syndrome.[14] The characteristic skin lesions are pale "ash leaf spots," present in 90 percent of affected individuals.[15] These are difficult to spot on light-skinned individuals unless examined with an ultraviolet Wood light (Fig. 21-2). Such an examination will also facilitate the recognition of smaller confetti-like hypopigmented patches that are present in about one-third of patients, but only rarely in normal individuals. In addition to these flat hypopigmented lesions and occasional café-au-lait spots, there are three kinds of distinctive raised cutaneous lesions: shagreen patches (Fig. 21-3), periungual fibromas (Fig. 21-4), and facial angiofibromas. The latter can be mistaken for acne on casual inspection. There are also systemic manifestations: usually asymptomatic cardiac rhabdomyomas, present at birth and

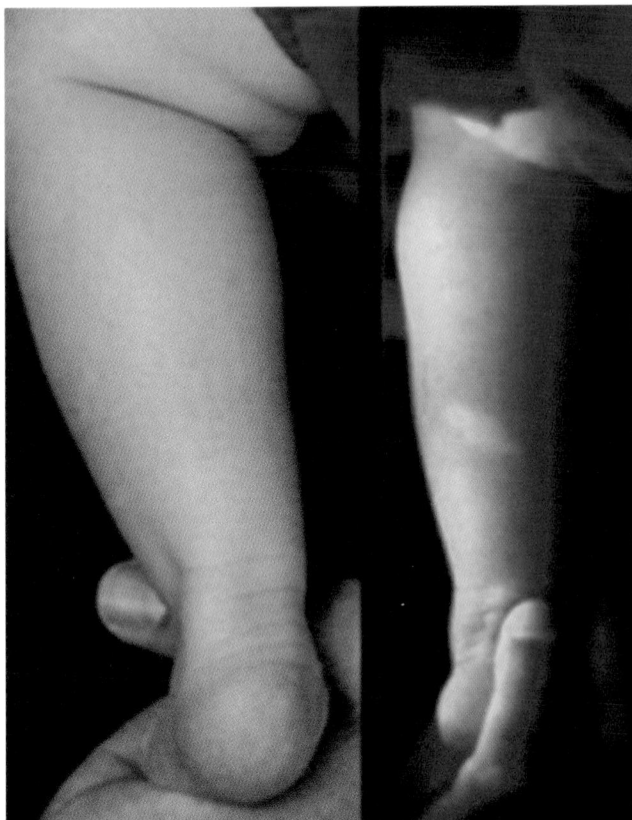

FIGURE 21-2 ■ Tuberous sclerosis: ash leaf spot in Wood light. (From Kurlemann G: Neurocutaneous syndromes. Handb Clin Neurol 108:513, 2012, with permission.)

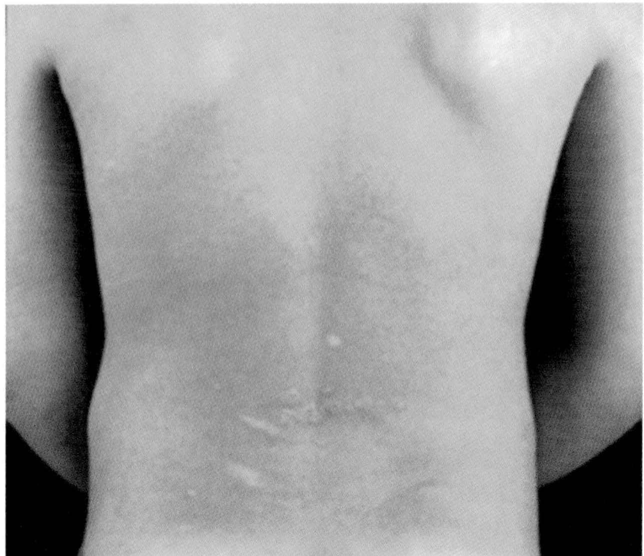

FIGURE 21-3 ■ Tuberous sclerosis: ash leaf spot and shagreen patch. (From Kurlemann G: Neurocutaneous syndromes. Handb Clin Neurol 108:513, 2012, with permission.)

regressing in childhood, but sometimes associated with arrhythmias; renal cysts, angiolipomas and carcinomas; and pulmonary lymphangioleiomyomas.

Tuberous sclerosis (TSc) can result from mutation of either of two genes. About 70 percent of cases (TSc 2, OMIM 613254) result from heterozygous mutation of tuberin encoded on chromosome 16p13.3, the remainder (TSc 1, OMIM 191100) from mutations of the gene encoding hamartin on chromosome 9q34.13. Unlike the case for the phenotypically distinct NF1 and NF2, each of which results from disruption of either of two independent, non-interacting proteins, TSc 1 and TSc 2 are practically indistinguishable clinically.[16] This is as would be predicted by the known interaction of hamartin and tuberin to form a single complex, the activity of which is disrupted by mutation of either subunit. This complex regulates the activity of the downstream pathway of the mammalian target of rapamycin (mTOR), which is disrupted by mutation in another neurocutaneous disorder, the Cowden multiple hamartoma syndrome (OMIM 158350).

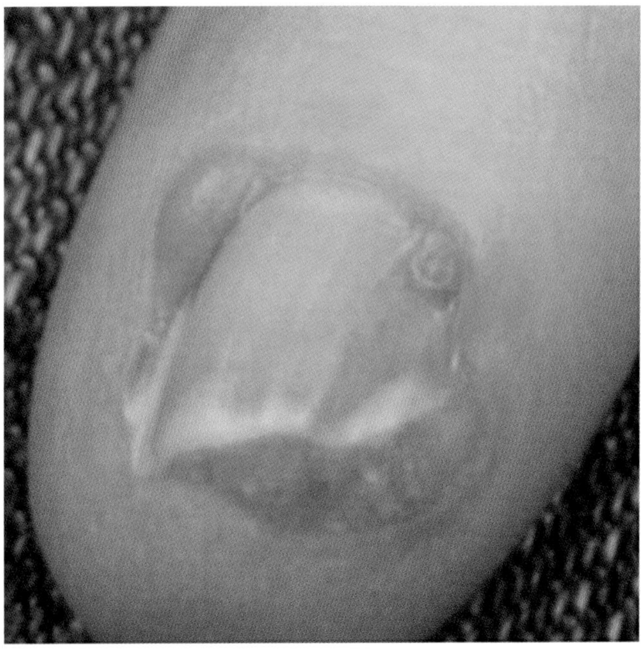

FIGURE 21-4 ■ Tuberous sclerosis: nail-fold fibroma. (From Kurlemann G: Neurocutaneous syndromes. Handb Clin Neurol 108:513, 2012.)

Melanoma

In most instances, involvement of the nervous system by melanoma is by metastasis from a primary cutaneous lesion first to a local regional lymph node, then to the lung whence it metastasizes further to brain, bone or liver.[17] Unlike the usual solitary brain metastases from more common primaries such as lung, breast, and kidney, brain metastases of melanoma are characteristically multiple.[18,19] The other two types of primary cutaneous neoplasms, the more common basal cell carcinoma and the more invasive squamous cell carcinoma, do not metastasize to the brain.

Furthermore, tumors of the nervous system (including gliomas, medulloblastomas, ependymomas, meningiomas, and acoustic neurilemmomas) have an increased likelihood as secondary tumors in patients with cutaneous melanoma as well as in their family members. The molecular bases underlying these associations are only partially understood.

An increased incidence of cutaneous melanomas is seen in a more complex heritable neurocutaneous syndrome, xeroderma pigmentosa (OMIM 610651). This autosomal recessive disorder is characterized by increased sensitivity to sunlight as well as widespread neurologic involvement. Signs include microcephaly, mental retardation, ataxia, ventriculomegaly, cerebellar atrophy, basal ganglia calcification, and disordered central and peripheral myelination.

In addition to those syndromes in which melanoma originates in the skin, there is also the rare neurocutaneous melanosis (OMIM 249400), in which there is a primary melanoma of the CNS in over 50 percent of cases, but no malignant melanoma in the periphery. In this disorder there are large multiple pigmented skin nevi (>20 cm) (Fig. 21-5), as well as cranial nerve palsies from histologically benign melanocytic invasion of the meninges, Dandy Walker malformation, and suprasellar calcifications. Death usually occurs in childhood.[20]

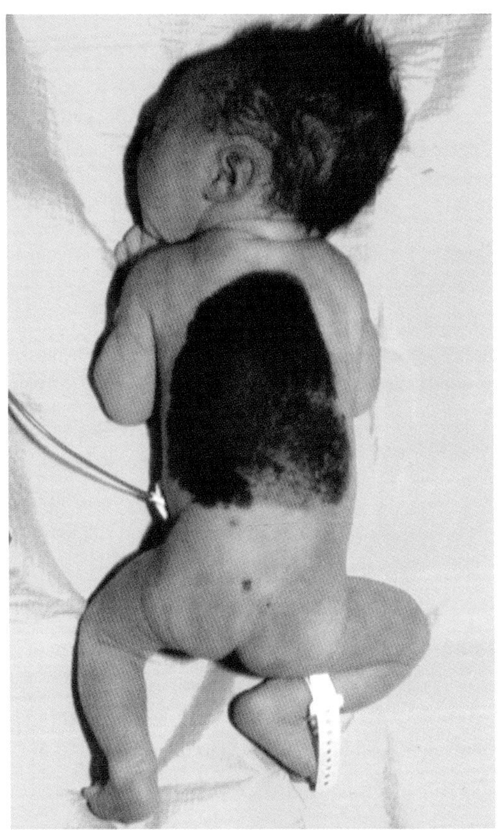

FIGURE 21-5 ■ Neurocutaneous melanosis. (From Jones, K: Smith's Recognizable Patterns of Human Malformation. Saunders, Philadelphia, 2005, with permission.)

STROKE

A number of neurocutaneous disorders are associated with either ischemic or hemorrhagic stroke, or both. The underlying mechanisms range from intrinsic vascular disease to cardiac or paradoxical embolization and to coagulopathies or platelet disorders, as summarized in Table 21-1.

Fabry Disease

Fabry disease is an X-linked neurocutaneous disorder (OMIM 301500) characterized by stroke, peripheral neuropathy, and progressive renal and cardiac failure. These sequelae occur both in hemizygous males as well as in heterozygous females, albeit later and with less severity.[21] A pathognomonic whorl-like corneal dystrophy is seen with equal severity in both sexes. Affected males are easily recognized by a purpuric skin rash: discrete angiokeratoma, most prevalent between the knees and nipples. Females, having two X chromosomes, are twice as likely to have the pathogenic mutation of α-galactosidase (also commonly known as ceramide trihexosidase). Nevertheless, affected female heterozygotes frequently remain undiagnosed because they rarely have the characteristic cutaneous lesions, even though they can have severe neurologic, cardiac and renal manifestations.[22]

Stroke is a late manifestation of the vascular deposition of lipid in Fabry disease.[23] It was underappreciated until renal transplantation and, now, enzyme-replacement therapy, prolonged survival.[24] A painful small-fiber neuropathy with autonomic dysfunction and episodic severely painful abdominal crises, reminiscent of those of the hepatic

TABLE 21-1 ■ Ischemic or Hemorrhagic Stroke with Cutaneous Manifestations

Disease	Cutaneous Lesions	Neurologic Features
Antiphospholipid syndrome	Livedo reticularis	Ischemic stroke, chorea, neuropsychiatric symptoms, relapsing-remitting central vasculitis, myelopathy
Behçet disease	Erythema nodosum, genital and oral aphthous ulcers	Brainstem meningoencephalitis, dural sinus thrombosis, ischemic stroke, peripheral neuropathy (rare)
Bone fragility with contractures, arterial rupture, and deafness (OMIM 612394)	Ecchymoses, blistering of fingers, toes, pinnae	Cerebral hemorrhage, developmental delay
Cerebral cavernous malformations; CCM (OMIM 116860 & 603284)	Angiomas, hyperkeratotic cutaneous vascular lesions	Small, localized intracranial hemorrhages
Diabetes mellitus	Necrobiosis lipoidica diabeticorum, poorly healing ulcers	Lacunar stroke, peripheral neuropathy, retinopathy, metabolic coma
Endocarditis	Petechiae, Janeway lesions, Osler nodes, splinter hemorrhages	Septic embolic strokes
Fabry disease (OMIM 301500)	Angiokeratoma starting at the umbilicus and knees, spreading to buttocks and scrotum	Ischemic stroke, seizures, peripheral neuropathy, autonomic dysfunction, acral paresthesias, painful crises
Factor XIII subunit A deficiency (OMIM 613225)	Ecchymoses	Intracranial hemorrhage
Glanzmann thrombasthenia (OMIM 273800)	Easy bruisability, purpura	Intracranial hemorrhage
Hemolytic-uremic syndrome (OMIM 235400)	Erythematous necrotic skin lesions	Seizures, coma, hemiparesis, cognitive defects, visual defects, dysphasia
Hereditary hemorrhagic telangiectasia of Osler–Weber–Rendu (OMIM 187300, 600376, 601101, 610655)	Telangiectasia	Ischemic and hemorrhagic stroke
Homocystinuria due to cystathionine β-synthase deficiency (OMIM 236200)	Malar flush, livedo reticularis, hypopigmentation	Ischemic stroke, seizures, mental retardation, psychiatric disorders, depression, personality disorder
Familial hypercholesterolemia (OMIM 143890)	Xanthomas, xanthelasma	Ischemic thromboembolic stroke
Hereditary neurocutaneous angiomas (OMIM 106070)	Large irregular flat hemangiomas	Spinal angiomas and cerebral thin-walled angiomas
Hyper-IgE recurrent infection syndrome, autosomal recessive (OMIM 243700)	Severe eczema, atopic dermatitis, recurrent skin abscesses	Ischemic infarctions, subarachnoid hemorrhage
Malignant atrophic papulosis (OMIM 602248)	Multiple asymptomatic papules with atrophic white centers surrounded by telangiectatic lesions	Ischemic infarctions
Prothrombin deficiency, congenital (OMIM 613679)	Ecchymoses, easy bruising	Intracranial hemorrhage
Pseudoxanthoma elasticum (OMIM 264800)	Pseudoxanthoma, multiple papules, peau d'orange, angioid streaks, subcutaneous calcification usually in blood vessels	Stroke, retinopathy
Pseudoxanthoma elasticum, forme fruste (OMIM 177850)	Small, yellow papules, peau d'orange, elastosis perforans serpiginosa	Cerebral hemorrhage, retinopathy
Schimke-type immuno-osseous dysplasia (OMIM 242900)	Hyperpigmented macules	Moyamoya, cerebral infarctions

(Continued)

TABLE 21-1 ■ (Continued)

Disease	Cutaneous Lesions	Neurologic Features
Systemic lupus erythematosus	Photosensitivity, malar rash, telangiectasia, discoid lupus, patchy alopecia, mucosal ulcers, angioneurotic edema, Raynaud phenomenon, subcutaneous nodules, palpable purpura, gangrene, erythema multiforme	Ischemic and hemorrhagic stroke, encephalopathy, chorea, peripheral neuropathies
Takayasu arteritis	Palpable purpura	Ischemic stroke
Thrombophilia due to protein C deficiency, autosomal dominant (OMIM 176860)	Warfarin-induced skin necrosis	Cerebral thrombosis
Thrombocytopenia–absent radius syndrome (OMIM 274000)	Nevus flammeus on forehead, dysseborrheic dermatitis	Intracranial hemorrhage, absent corpus callosum, spina bifida

porphyrias, occurs early in the disease. Other early manifestations are small infarctions in the retina and kidneys. The latter lead to renal failure, which had previously caused death of affected hemizygotes by the third decade.

Although Fabry disease is also referred to as angiokeratoma diffusum, these skin lesions are not pathognomonic. They are also manifestations of other mendelian neurocutaneous disorders associated with mental retardation: aspartylglucosaminuria (OMIM 208400; seizures), fucosidosis (OMIM 230000; seizures and peripheral neuropathy), lysosomal beta A mannosidosis (OMIM 248510), Ramon syndrome (OMIM 266270; a posterior cerebral leukoencephalopathy), Kanzaki disease (OMIM 609242), and Bannayan–Riley–Ruvalcaba syndrome (OMIM 153480; megaencephaly, meningioma, pseudopapilledema).

Hereditary Hemorrhagic Telangiectasia

Hereditary hemorrhagic telangiectasia (HHT), an autosomal dominant disorder also known eponymously as Osler–Weber–Rendu syndrome,[25] is a vascular dysplasia that gives rise to hemorrhagic and ischemic strokes. These arise from a diverse set of peripheral as well as central vascular abnormalities,[26] ranging from ischemic strokes and brain abscesses from paradoxical emboli passing through pulmonary venous malformations to intracerebral vessels, and subarachnoid hemorrhages from cerebral arteriovenous malformations. It is important to search for previously unsuspected pulmonary arteriovenous malformations before assuming local vascular pathology as a cause of stroke, because these pulmonary lesions can be effectively obliterated by embolization. The mucocutaneous telangiectasias for which the disorder is named are most often found on the tongue, lips, palate, fingers, face, conjunctiva, trunk, nail beds, and fingertips. Similar systemic vascular malformations are responsible for frequently problematic recurrent epistaxis, hepatic cirrhosis, and gastrointestinal hemorrhage later in life. Depending on the vascular anatomy, there may be either a polycythemia or an anemia.

This disorder is genetically heterogeneous. HHT type 1 (OMIM 187300) results from heterozygosity for a mutation of the gene on chromosome 9q34.11 encoding endoglin, a homodimeric membrane glycoprotein expressed mostly on the vascular endothelium, a component of the transforming growth factor–beta receptor complex; and HHT type 2 (OMIM 600376), from heterozygosity for mutation of the gene on chromosome 12q13.13 encoding activin receptor–like kinase 1. HHT type 3 (OMIM 601101) has been mapped to chromosome 5q31.3-q32) and HHT type 4 (OMIM 610655) to chromosome 7p14. The genes mutated in the latter two entities have not yet been identified.

Homocystinuria

Homocystinuria is a feature of several different neurologic disorders, only one of which, homocystinuria due to cystathionine β-synthase deficiency (OMIM 236200), is associated either with cutaneous lesions or with stroke. In this disorder cutaneous hypopigmentation, malar flush, and livedo reticularis are not as striking as the Marfan-like disproportionate tall stature and ectopia lentis, which provide the most evident clues to diagnosis. Neurologic features include ischemic thromboembolic strokes in about 25 percent of homozygotes, as well as mild mental retardation, seizures, and a variety of psychiatric disturbances that include personality disorders and depression.[27] Diagnosis is critical, because over half of affected individuals respond to simple treatment with pyridoxine, vitamin B_6.[28] Furthermore, even pyridoxine non-responders benefit from dietary modification to reduce methionine and increase cysteine as well as supplementation with betaine.

The classic syndrome associated with homozygosity for mutations in the gene cystathionine β-synthetase is rare, but heterozygotes—encountered more commonly—are also at greater risk of ischemic stroke than the general population.[29] Lacking the characteristic cutaneous or systemic signs, these individuals can only be detected by biochemical or genetic screening. As is always the case with rare autosomal recessive disorders, the vast majority of heterozygotes will not have an affected homozygous relative to prompt suspicion of the diagnosis.

Endocarditis

Septic emboli leading to ischemic or hemorrhagic stroke or intracranial hemorrhage from rupture of mycotic aneurysms occur in 40 percent of individuals with bacterial endocarditis.[30,31] In developed countries, acute endocarditis commonly occurs because of unhygienic self-administration of intravenous drugs; infections of surgically implanted artificial cardiac valves are another important cause. In the developing world, secondary infection of unrepaired congenital valvular abnormalities or those damaged by rheumatic fever are also an important cause of infective endocarditis.

The classic cutaneous findings associated with infective endocarditis are subungual splinter hemorrhages, Janeway lesions, and Osler nodes. Splinter hemorrhages (1- to 3-mm, red to reddish-brown, longitudinal hemorrhages appearing under the nail plate) are commonly seen also as a response to repetitive trauma in otherwise healthy individuals, such as manual laborers or elderly individuals using walkers.[32] In addition they have been reported as occasional findings in antiphospholipid syndrome, another neurocutaneous syndrome associated with stroke.[33]

The more diagnostic Janeway lesions are nontender, large, irregular, flat macules that appear on the palms or the soles, frequently on the planar surface of a toe.[34] These are culture-positive sites of septic emboli. In contrast, Osler nodes are tender, purple, slightly raised nodules ranging in size from 1 to 10mm. These are typically seen on the tips or sides of toes or fingers. Unlike the Janeway lesions, they are sites of vasculitis, not embolization. Both of these lesions can appear on the thenar or hypothenar eminences.

The presence or absence of neurologic complications dictates the optimal timing of surgery for both native and prosthetic valve endocarditis, as do cardiac function and the control of the infection. In the absence of embolic events or rapidly deteriorating cardiac function, cardiac surgery is best delayed for 1 or 2 weeks of antibiotic treatment before subjecting the patient to the risks of surgery, not the least of which is cardiac bypass and attendant anticoagulation. However, if there is a stroke or transient ischemic attack, and intracranial hemorrhage has been excluded by scanning, surgery is recommended without delay.

Antiphospholipid Syndrome

The twin hallmarks of antiphospholipid antibody syndrome are either a thrombotic event, such as a stroke, or a complication of pregnancy seen in association with high titers of certain antibodies. Sometimes misleadingly referred to as lupus anticoagulants, these are thought to induce hypercoagulability by neutralizing anionic phospholipids on endothelial cells and platelets.[35] This syndrome can be seen either as a primary abnormality or in the setting of a number of different neurocutaneous disorders: primary inflammatory diseases such as systemic lupus erythematosus, systemic sclerosis, Behçet disease, Sjögren syndrome and rheumatoid arthritis, or infections such as syphilis, Lyme borreliosis, and human immunodeficiency virus (HIV) infection and acquired immunodeficiency syndrome (AIDS). In some instances, antiphospholipid syndrome has been shown to be a familial trait (OMIM 107320).

Cutaneous manifestations may be the initial clinical manifestation of the antiphospholipid syndrome.[36–38] These include livedo reticularis, most commonly on the lower extremities; acrocyanosis, a Raynaud-like phenomenon; necrotizing vasculitis, with cutaneous ulceration and necrosis; erythematous macules; purpura, ecchymoses, and subungual splinter hemorrhages; and rarely, Degos malignant atrophic papulosis. The combination of livedo reticularis with multiple strokes has been designated as Sneddon syndrome. Antiphospholipid antibodies are associated with several neurologic syndromes,[39] including stroke,[40] transverse myelitis, and chorea. Many of these might be plausibly attributed to focal ischemia.

Takayasu Arteritis

Stroke in a young woman of Asian descent should prompt consideration of Takayasu arteritis (aortic arch syndrome or pulseless disease).[41,42] The cutaneous manifestation is erythema nodosa, which occurs at an early phase in the disease. Fever and synovitis also develop prior to the large-vessel vasculopathy that defines the disorder. Neurologic involvement results from ischemic stroke from inflammation or stenosis of a proximal carotid or vertebral artery. Such strokes occur in about 20 percent of affected individuals. More commonly, involvement of the subclavian arteries leads to claudication and pulse asymmetries or frank loss of palpable pulses in the upper extremities.

The etiology of this disorder appears to be autoimmune, with modest associations both to HLA-B52 and to elevations of serum levels of certain matrix metalloproteinases. The latter normalize after clinical improvement resulting from treatment with immunosuppressants.

MENINGITIS AND MENINGOENCEPHALITIS

A large number of disorders can present both dermatologic abnormalities and meningitis or meningoencephalitis, which can be acute, subacute, relapsing-remitting, or chronic. A few characteristic disorders are presented in detail, the others in Table 21-2.

Meningococcal Meningitis

Meningococcal meningitis is a fulminant disorder with a high mortality rate and serious sequelae (sensorineural hearing loss, seizures, motor deficits, hydrocephalus, cognitive abnormalities, and behavioral problems) in treated survivors.[43] Fever, headache, and meningeal irritation develop over the course of 24 hours. The distinguishing feature of meningococcal disease is the concomitant evolution of a rapidly evolving petechial rash, usually over the trunk and lower extremities, but which can also develop on the face, mucous membranes, and arms (Fig. 21-6). These cutaneous lesions can coalesce or develop into vesicles or bullae. In contrast, the cutaneous lesion associated with meningitis from infection with *Haemophilus influenzae*, previously the most common type of bacterial meningitis in children, is typically a solitary indurated area on the face, neck, upper chest, or arm. The meningococcal rash must also be distinguished from that of other disorders in Table 21-2, notably Rocky Mountain spotted fever.

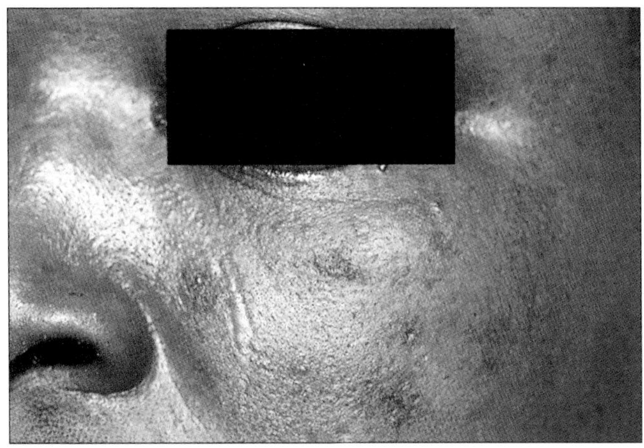

FIGURE 21-6 ■ Early cutaneous lesions of meningococcemia. (From Tyring S, Lupi O, Hengge U: Tropical Dermatology. Courtesy of Dr. Luc Van Kaer. Churchill Livingstone, New York, 2005, with permission.)

In the 10 to 30 percent of cases of meningococcemia that develop too rapidly to seed the choroid plexus and meninges, the prognosis is even worse than in those cases with meningitis. Early treatment at the first recognition of the short febrile prodome and rash is critical. Although most cases of meningococcemia, either with or without meningitis, occur in children, young adults in cramped quarters, including college students and military recruits, are also at risk.

The incidence of some meningococcal infections has been reduced significantly by the introduction of a vaccine,[44] as has the incidence of the other two most common types of acute bacterial meningitis, resulting from infection with *Haemophilus influenzae* or *Streptococcus pneumoniae*. However, the currently available meningococcal vaccine is only effective against the C serotype of the causative organism, *Neisseria meningitidis*, a serotype that has nearly been eliminated in developed countries. Furthermore,

TABLE 21-2 ■ Meningitis with Cutaneous Manifestations

Disorder	Cutaneous Lesions	Neurologic Features
Adams–Oliver aplasia cutis congenita type III (OMIM 614814)	Scalp defect at the vertex, cutis marmorata telangiectatica, hemangioma	Acute bacterial meningitis from skull defect
AIDS	Seborrhea, herpes zoster, tinea corporis, *S aureus* infection, molluscum contagiosum, Kaposi sarcoma, cryptococcosis	Transient meningitis during seroconversion
Amyloidosis V (Meretoja, Finnish) (OMIM 105120)	Cutis laxa	Cranial and peripheral neuropathies
Behçet disease	Erythema nodosum, genital and oral aphthous ulcers, papules, purpura, pustules, dermatographia, pyoderma	Chronic or recurrent meningitis, meningoencephalitis, dural sinus thrombosis
Blastomycosis	Hyperplastic granulomatous microabscesses	Rarely, chronic meningitis or cerebral abscess
Brill–Zinser epidemic typhus	Macular rash	Meningoencephalitis
Chagas disease	Romana sign, inflammation of lacrimal glands, erythema multiforme	Encephalitis
Coccidiomycosis	Erythema nodosum, draining sinus, subcutaneous cellulitis	Meningitis common
Cryptococcosis	Macules and nodules (in 10–15% of cases)	Chronic meningitis
Haemophilus influenzae infection	Typically a single indurated area on face, neck, upper chest, or arm	Acute purulent meningitis
Histiocytic reticulosis (autosomal recessive) (OMIM 267700)	Purpura, jaundice, erythroderma	Chronic aseptic meningitis, neuropathy
Leptospirosis	Scleral conjunctival injection, maculopapular rash of trunk (in 50% of cases), jaundice	Subacute meningitis
Leukemia	Erythema nodosum, Sweet syndrome (acute febrile neutrophilic dermatosis–painful raised red plaques, commonly on face and extremities)	Meningeal leukemia is common form of relapse, especially in acute lymphocytic leukemia
Listeriosis	Generalized erythematous papules or petechiae in infants; veterinarians with tender red papules on hands	Subacute meningitis
Lyme borreliosis	Target lesion	Early aseptic meningitis, polyneuropathy, delayed demyelinating disease
Lymphoma	Erythema nodosum	Subacute meningitis, cerebral or vertebral metastases
Lymphoma, cutaneous (T cell)	Scaly erythematous patches, leonine facies, poikiloderma, hypopigmented and hyperpigmented patches with atrophy and telangiectasia	Subacute meningitis, vertebral metastases
Meningococcemia	Petechiae, usually on extremities and trunk; initially can mimic a viral exanthem	Fulminant meningitis
Murine typhus	Axillary rash, macular rash of upper abdomen, shoulders, chest	Headache, encephalopathy, and nuchal rigidity without meningitis
Neurocutaneous melanosis	Melanosis; large multiple pigmented skin nevi (>20 cm), no malignant melanoma other than CNS; primary CNS melanoma in over 50% of cases	Meningeal enhancement secondary to melanosis of pia-arachnoid, cranial nerve palsies, Dandy–Walker malformation, suprasellar calcification
Reticulosis, familial histiocytic	Purpura, jaundice, erythroderma	Chronic meningitis, peripheral neuropathy

(Continued)

TABLE 21-2 ■ (Continued)

Disorder	Cutaneous Lesions	Neurologic Features
Rocky Mountain spotted fever	Progressive rash begins on the fourth day of fever with pink macules on wrists, ankles, forearms; after 6–18 hours, on palms and soles, then centrally after 1–3 days; after 2–4 days, non-blanching petechiae	Vasculitic meningoencephalitis, choreoathetosis, deafness, hemiplegia
Sarcoidosis	Dry skin, hypohidrosis, cicatricial alopecia; *acute*: erythema nodosum, vesicles, maculopapular rash; *chronic*: lupus pernio, plaques, scars, keloids	Chronic meningitis with cranial neuropathies, peripheral neuropathy, proximal myopathy, hypothalamic involvement
Sjögren syndrome	Purpura, Raynaud phenomenon, xerostomia, candidiasis	Aseptic meningitis, sensory neuronopathy, dural sinus thrombosis
Syphilis	*Primary*: chancre. *Secondary*: maculopapular non-pruritic scaling rash (acral), patchy alopecia, condyloma lata, mucous patches, erythema multiforme, hyperpigmentation on healing, split papules, palm and sole lesions	Aseptic meningitis, late meningovascular syphilis, tabes dorsalis
Tuberculosis	Cutaneous tuberculosis is rare; primary tuberculous chancre; warty tuberculous verrucosa cutis from reinfection, postprimary lupus vulgaris, scrofuloderma, erythema nodosum, erythema multiforme	Chronic meningitis, Pott disease of vertebrae, CNS tuberculomas
Varicella zoster (chickenpox)	Vesicles with oral lesions	Meningitis with cerebellar ataxia
Vogt–Koyanagi–Harada	Vitiligo-type macules, poliosis and alopecia in convalescent third phase	Meningoencephalitis in first phase of illness, preceding uveitis
Yersinia pestis (bubonic plague)	Erythema multiforme, bubos then petechiae and ecchymoses	Meningitis can complicate all three types: bubonic, bubonic-septicemic, pneumonic

even this vaccine is not available in the poor countries of the "meningitis belt" in Africa. Worldwide, meningococcal infections remain one of the leading causes of meningitis in children.[45] New vaccines are being developed for *Neisseria* serogroups A and B, but there are other serotypes of *Neisseria* for which development is required.[46]

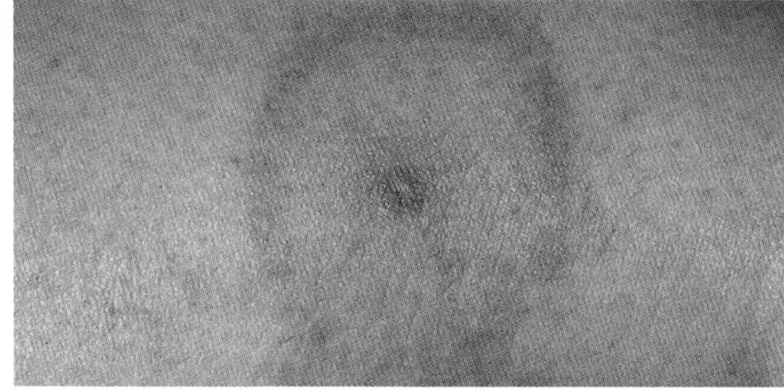

FIGURE 21-7 ■ Large 5-cm targetoid patch with central clearing, bright-red expanding border and central bite inflammation, characteristic of the erythema migrans rash of Lyme disease. (From Habif T, Campbell J, Chapman MS, et al: Dermatology DDX Deck. Saunders, Philadelphia, 2006, with permission.)

Lyme Borreliosis

The characteristic "target lesion" (*erythema chronicum migrans*) that spreads centrifugally from the site of a prolonged bite by a tick infected with the spirochete *Borrelia burgdorferi* is pathognomonic of early-stage Lyme disease.[47,48] This cutaneous lesion first develops within a few days to weeks after the infecting bite by the tiny tick, *Ixodes dammini*. The characteristic cutaneous lesion is so named because of the fancied resemblance to a target. The erythematous circumference of the lesion advances over the course of days to weeks up to a diameter of 5 cm, leaving behind a trailing central area of clearing and a persistent erythematous papule at the very center, the site of the original tick bite (Fig. 21-7). This lesion develops in about 85 percent of infected individuals, facilitating clinical diagnosis for the subsequent syndrome of migratory arthralgias and later neurologic dysfunction. However, a high degree of clinical suspicion and the use of a serologic test are necessary for diagnosis in the substantial minority of patients that do not develop the characteristic target lesion.

Although neurologic signs can develop while the erythema migrans is still present, typically they do not appear until the cutaneous signs have resolved, after 6 to 12 months of migratory arthralgia that occasionally evolves into arthritis with an effusion in a large joint. The most common neurologic syndrome, affecting about 70 percent of untreated individuals, is a mild aseptic meningitis, with a mononeuritis multiplex or typical cranial nerve palsies.[49] The latter include unilateral or bilateral facial palsies or lesions of the oculomotor, trigeminal, abducens or eighth cranial nerve. Alternatively there may be a painful radiculopathy or plexitis. Other lesions reported less frequently include a myositis, patchy demyelination mimicking multiple sclerosis, or myelopathy with radiculopathies that could be mistaken for amyotrophic lateral sclerosis.[50] Some untreated patients later develop an indolent diffuse encephalopathy.[51] Further discussion is provided in Chapter 40.

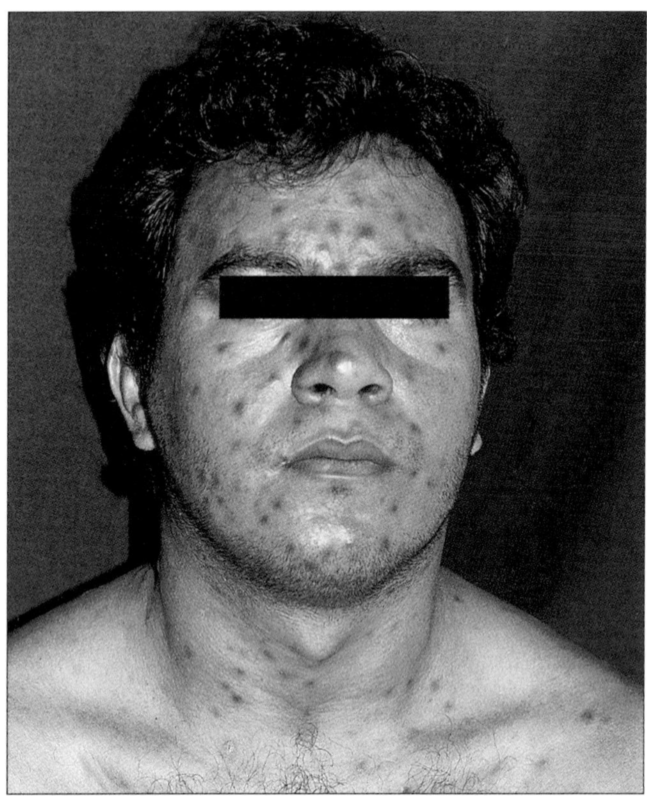

FIGURE 21-8 ■ Secondary syphilis: disseminated papular lesions. (From Tyring S, Lupi O, Hengge U: Tropical Dermatology. Courtesy of Dr. Luc Van Kaer. Churchill Livingstone, New York, 2005, with permission.)

Syphilis

As in Lyme borreliosis, dermatologic and neurologic manifestations are also temporally discordant in syphilis,[54] which is related to infection with *Treponema pallidum*. The cutaneous manifestations are limited to the painless, indurated, rubbery genital chancre of primary syphilis in the days after infection, and the flat copper-colored lesions of the palms and soles, patchy alopecia, and mucous membrane patches seen in secondary syphilis, 2 to 4 months later (Figs 21-8 and 21-9). Secondary syphilis is associated with a mild meningitis, sometimes with involvement of cranial nerves, typically the optic, facial or acoustic.

In contrast, cutaneous lesions will have resolved by the time of meningovascular syphilis, peaking 4 to 7 years after infection, and the neurologic manifestations of late-stage syphilis, namely the dementia (general paresis of the insane) and tabes dorsalis (Chapter 40). Thus the only exception to the temporal discordance of cutaneous and neurologic manifestations is their invariable association in secondary syphilis, in prenatal syphilis, and the rare occurrence of cutaneous nodules in late syphilis.

Fortunately, the late stages of syphilis have become quite rare. There had also been a period of diminishing prevalence of primary and secondary syphilis, although a 10-fold increase in incidence to 20 per 100,000 has occurred recently in the United States and to 360 per 100,000 in parts of Africa.[55] Much of this increase has occurred in association with HIV-AIDS,[56] which has also contributed to an altered natural history, including an occasional novel presentation that mimics that of herpes simplex encephalitis (but is responsive to treatment with penicillin), with focal lesions in the temporal lobe and status epilepticus or periodic lateralized discharges in the electroencephalogram.

Careful studies have also brought to light previously under-recognized syndromes of otologic syphilis,[57] characterized by early sensorineural hearing loss and occasionally by vestibular dysfunction as well; and of ocular syphilis, mostly an early posterior uveitis affecting the choroid, retina, and pigmentary

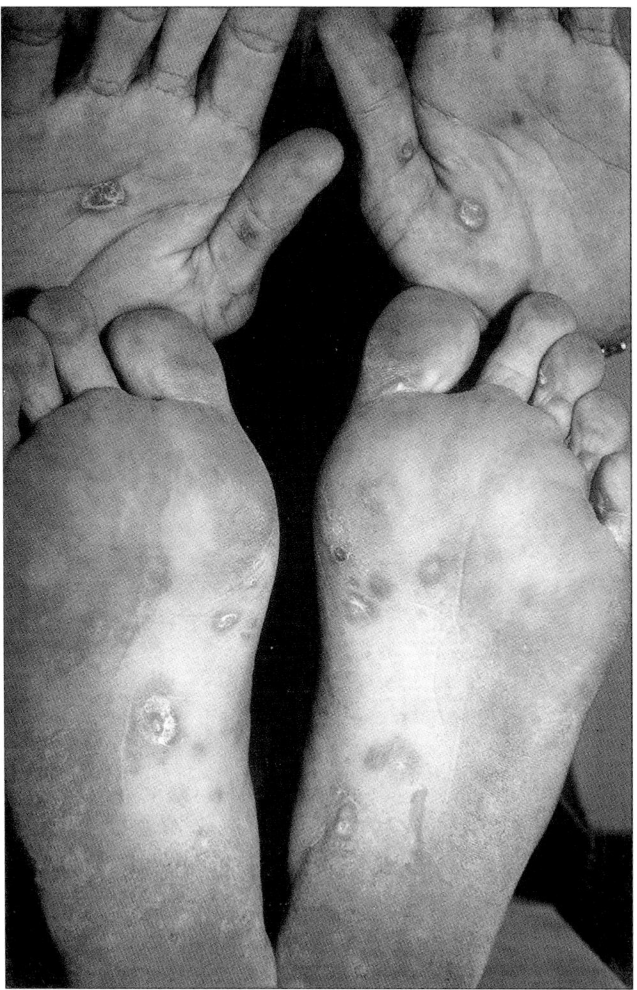

FIGURE 21-9 ▪ Secondary syphilis: hyperkeratotic lesions on palms and soles. (From Tyring S, Lupi O, Hengge U: Tropical Dermatology. Courtesy of Dr. Luc Van Kaer. Churchill Livingstone, New York, 2005, with permission.)

retinal epithelium. Involvement of the uveal tract also characterizes several other neurocutaneous disorders. Uveomeningitis is an occasional presentation of sarcoid, Behçet disease, and systemic lupus erythematosus, described in the following sections. It is also typical of the rare Vogt–Koyanagi–Harada syndrome,[58] in which a prodromal meningoencephalitis precedes uveitis as well as the characteristic dermatologic findings of leukoderma with symmetric patches of vitiligo (involving the head, neck, shoulders, and eyelids), alopecia, and poliosis.

Sarcoidosis

Both the cutaneous and neurologic manifestations of sarcoidosis (discussed in Chapter 49) are notoriously variable, complicating early diagnosis.[52,53] Indeed, only 20 to 30 percent of patients with sarcoid have cutaneous lesions, and only 5 to 10 percent have neurologic manifestations. The most typical neurologic presentation is that of a mild aseptic meningitis, with or without cranial nerve palsies. Typically these are unilateral or bilateral facial nerve palsies, but optic, auditory or vestibular neuropathies may occur as well. Neurosarcoidosis is the initial presentation of sarcoid in about 50 percent of cases, prompting a large and difficult differential. A wide variety of other neurologic manifestations also occur (Chapter 49).

The cutaneous manifestations of sarcoid are more frequent but are also highly variable. There can be acute lesions such as erythema nodosum, vesicles, and maculopapular rash. These annular lesions, papules, or nodules are either skin-colored, violaceous, or brownish-red, often appearing on the face. Chronic lesions include lupus pernio (large, bluish red, dusty, violaceous infiltrated nodules and plaques, which generally appear on the cheeks, ears, fingers, and nose), plaque, scars, and keloids. The rare angiolupoid form of sarcoidosis consists of orange-red or reddish-brown soft, well-demarcated lesions.

Behçet Disease

This poorly understood inflammatory disease is characterized by a triad of recurrent oral and genital ulceration and uveitis,[59] most commonly seen in populations along the old "Silk Road." The majority of patients have additional cutaneous abnormalities including papillopustular lesions, erythema nodosum, and a pathergy reaction (pustulation at the site of trauma).[60] The classic triad forms the basis of the current criteria for diagnosis,[61] which is entirely clinical: recurrent oral ulceration (at least three times in a year) plus two of the following: (1) recurrent genital ulceration; (2) ocular lesions (uveitis, retinal vasculitis or cells in the vitreous); and (3) skin lesions (erythema nodosum, pseudofolliculitis).[62] Other common manifestations are arthritis, present in up to half of individuals; subcutaneous thrombophlebitis in about a quarter; and, in Japan, gastrointestinal lesions that affect about one-third. In contrast, neurologic complications affect only 10 percent or less of patients with Behçet disease,[63] either as parenchymal or neurovascular disease.

These two categories are not mutually exclusive; both parenchymal and neurovascular disease can affect a substantial minority of these patients.[64–66] The pathology of the parenchymal disease is a "perivasculitis" rather than a vasculitis. There are infiltrates of polymorphonuclear leukocytes, eosinophils, lymphocytes and macrophages without infiltration of blood vessel walls or necrosis of endothelial cells. The typical MRI picture of brainstem meningoencephalitis is that of a unilateral T2-enhancing lesion of the upper brainstem. Less frequent manifestations of parenchymal disease are seizures, transverse myelopathy, diffuse encephalopathy, or, much less commonly, an optic neuropathy. In some instances, the MRI appearance may resemble that of a glioma. Movement disorders and peripheral neuropathy are rare. Although venous occlusion is common, stroke resulting from arterial occlusions is rare, occurring in about 1 percent. Intracranial venous sinus thrombosis presents as increased intracranial pressure, a presentation that also sometimes occurs in the absence of radiographically demonstrable sinus or venous occlusion.[67]

This disorder usually presents in young men, aged 20 to 40 years, but women are also affected, albeit less often. Most patients respond to treatment with corticosteroids, although about 20 percent are left with significant residual neurologic impairment and 10 percent succumb within a decade of diagnosis. Some practitioners supplement treatment of sinus thrombosis with anticoagulants after ruling out a pulmonary aneurysm, whereas others find corticosteroid treatment to be adequate. The course may be monophasic, relapsing remitting, or, most ominously, progressive.

INTERMITTENT ENCEPHALOPATHIES

Intermittent nonfocal impairment of the CNS culminating in psychiatric disturbance, confusion, delirium, stupor, or coma may result from trauma, infection, inflammation, and a wide variety of metabolic insults, some with cutaneous manifestations, as summarized in Table 21-3. Indeed, two of the most common—diabetic coma and intoxication with alcohol—are associated with cutaneous manifestations well known to most practicing physicians. The focus of this section is therefore on less common and perhaps less well-known neurocutaneous intermittent encephalopathies.

Systemic Lupus Erythematosus

Cutaneous abnormalities (malar, discoid or photosensitive rash; Fig. 21-10) are present in at least 80 percent of these patients, with malar rash topping the list of the 17 classification criteria published by the Systemic Lupus International Collaborating Clinics, of which 4 are necessary for diagnosis.[68] The others are features readily recognizable as immunologic abnormalities: serologic findings in the blood; arthritis; serositis of pleura or pericardium; glomerulonephritis or proteinuria; and hemolytic anemia, lymphopenia, or thrombocytopenia. Rounding out the list are the nonspecific neurologic symptoms, including psychosis, which can be a presenting feature before the development of signs more typically associated with autoimmune disease.[69] Because lupus typically presents between the ages of 15 and 25, which is also the peak age of onset of schizophrenia, a disorder considerably more prevalent than lupus, many patients are hospitalized in psychiatric wards before the true nature of their disease is recognized, often by appreciation of cutaneous abnormalities.

Although common, psychiatric signs and symptoms of a diffuse encephalopathy are but one of many less common but not infrequent manifestations of CNS lupus,[70] others being seizures[71]; aseptic meningitis; stroke (most commonly ischemic, either embolic from marantic endocarditis or mural cardiac thrombi after myocardial infarction, or from carotid atherosclerosis); chorea[72];

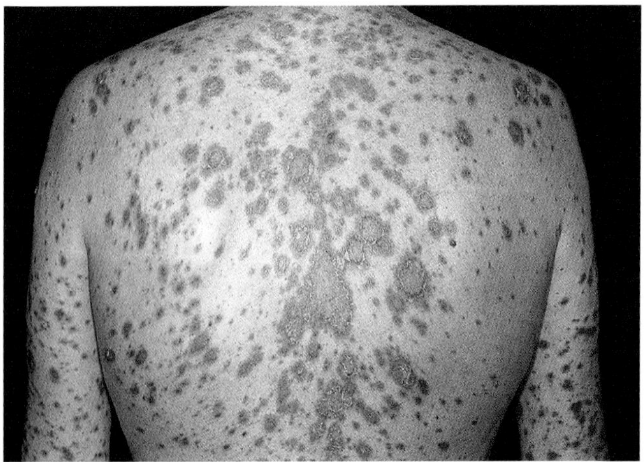

FIGURE 21-10 ■ Systemic lupus erythematosus. (From Callen J, Jorizzo J, Bolognia J, et al: Dermatological Signs of Internal Disease. Saunders, Philadelphia, 2009, with permission.)

TABLE 21-3 ■ Intermittent Encephalopathy with Cutaneous Manifestations

Disorder	Cutaneous Lesions	Neurologic Features
Alcoholism	Telangiectasia	Intoxication, delirium tremens, neuropathy, Wernicke–Korsakoff syndrome, Marchiafava–Bignami syndrome
Coproporphyria (OMIM 121300)	Photosensitivity	Peripheral neuropathy, crises of abdominal pain and mental changes
Ethylmalonic encephalopathy (OMIM 602473)	Petechiae	Pyramidal and extrapyramidal signs, ataxia, seizures, hyperintense lesions in basal ganglia on MRI
Diabetes mellitus	Poorly healing skin ulcers, necrobiosis lipoidica diabeticorum	Diabetic ketoacidosis, nonketotic hyperglycemic coma, insulin-induced hypoglycemic coma, lacunar stroke, neuropathy, retinopathy
Hemolytic-uremic syndrome, 1–6 (OMIM 235400, 612922–612926)	Purpura	Coma, seizures, hemiparesis, visual disturbances
Holocarboxylase synthetase deficiency (OMIM 253270)	Skin rash	Irritability, lethargy, coma, seizures, hypotonia, developmental delay, hypertonia
Hydroxykynureninuria (OMIM 236800)	Light-sensitive rash	Intermittent, nonprogressive, ataxic encephalopathy
Letterer–Siwe disease (OMIM 246400)	Diffuse papulovesicular rash, scaly petechial dermatitis, intertriginous denudation, seborrhea, stomatitis	Encephalopathy
Methylmalonic aciduria and homocystinuria, CBLF type (OMIM 277380)	Reticulated pigmentation and rashes	Encephalopathy, hypotonia, lethargy, developmental delay, ataxia
Murine typhus	Macular rash	Headache, encephalopathy, and nuchal rigidity
Propionic acidemia (OMIM 606054)	Dermatitis acidemica	Acute encephalopathy, axial hypotonia, limb hypertonia, psychomotor retardation, cerebral atrophy, dystonia, cerebellar hemorrhage, ischemic stroke of basal ganglia
Shaken baby syndrome	Ecchymoses, purpura	Subdural hematomas, subarachnoid hemorrhage, parenchymal lacerations
Systemic lupus erythematosus	Photosensitivity, malar rash, telangiectasia, discoid lupus, patchy alopecia, mucosal ulcers, angioneurotic edema, Raynaud phenomenon, subcutaneous nodules, palpable purpura, gangrene, erythema multiforme	Encephalopathy, ischemic and hemorrhagic stroke, chorea, multifocal demyelination, peripheral neuropathies
Thrombotic thrombocytopenic purpura	Purpura	Rapidly evolving encephalopathy
Variegate porphyria (OMIM 176200)	Photosensitivity, blistering, skin fragility with chronic scarring of sun-exposed areas and postinflammatory hyperpigmentation	Crises with neuropsychiatric symptoms, abdominal pain, motor neuropathy

relapsing-remitting disease resembling multiple sclerosis; and movement disorders. In addition, there is the more localized posterior reversible encephalopathy syndrome (PRES), presenting with headaches, seizures, altered mental status, cortical blindness, vomiting, and focal neurologic deficits.[73] Although occurring with other autoimmune disorders, this rare encephalopathy is encountered most commonly in association with systemic lupus. Systematic clinical trials have yet to be performed, but a favorable clinical response seems to follow control of blood pressure and seizures and elimination of immunosuppressive drugs. The peripheral nervous system is also a frequent site of involvement with compressive neuropathies, most commonly carpal tunnel syndrome, affecting about 30 percent of patients, and a distal symmetric axonal neuropathy, sometimes with dysautonomia, about 20 percent. In

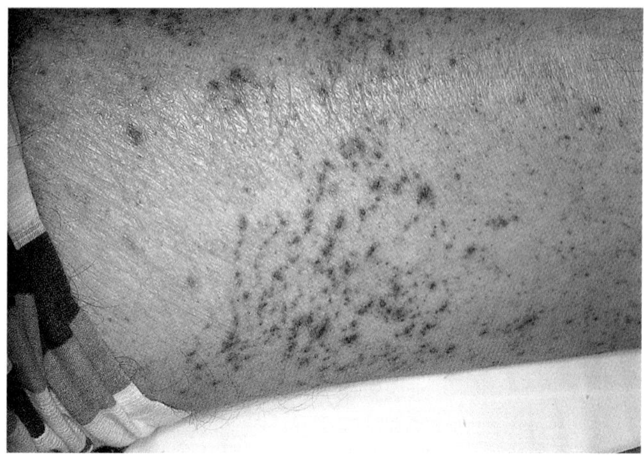

FIGURE 21-11 ▪ Small petechiae in an individual with thrombocytopenia. (From Callen J, Jorizzo J, Bolognia J, et al: Dermatological Signs of Internal Disease. Saunders, Philadelphia, 2009, with permission.)

about 1 percent or less, acute or chronic demyelinating neuropathies, mononeuritis multiplex, or cranial mononeuropathies occur.

Thrombotic Thrombocytopenic Purpura

Thrombotic thrombocytopenic purpura (TTP) (Fig. 21-11) is a fulminant disorder that may be lethal if untreated.[74] Its clinical hallmark is rapid progression through confusion and obtundation to coma in the setting of thrombocytopenia resulting in cutaneous purpura, fever, Coombs-negative hemolytic anemia with fragmentation of erythrocytes, and renal failure.[75] Unlike lupus, this is not a vasculitis but a manifestation of pathologic aggregations of platelets. The adult-onset form is triggered by endothelial injury in various clinical settings: HIV-AIDS, pregnancy, metastatic cancer, or high-dose chemotherapy, or as a drug reaction. Most frequently there is an autoantibody-mediated depletion of an enzyme (a disintegrin and metalloproteinase with a thrombospondin type 1 motif, member 13, or ADAMTS13, also known as von Willebrand factor–cleaving protease or VWFCP) that cleaves very high molecular weight complexes of von Willebrand factor, which can cause platelet adhesion and thrombosis.[76] There is also a rare congenital familial TTP that is an autosomal recessive disorder (OMIM 274150) resulting from homozygosity for mutations of the ADAMTS13 gene encoded on chromosome 9q34.2. The congenital form, also known as Schulman–Upshaw syndrome, is associated with neonatal jaundice and a propensity to recurrences that require treatment with fresh frozen plasma.

Either form can be treated with plasmapheresis and exchange transfusion to remove the uncleaved high molecular weight complexes of von Willebrand factor and to replenish ADAMTS13.[77] When needed, prophylaxis to prevent relapse of the acquired forms with autoantibodies to ADAMTS13 can also be obtained with corticosteroids, cyclosporine, or rituximab, an antibody directed at CD20, a cell-surface antigen of antibody-secreting B lymphocytes.[78] Prompt recognition and treatment of this formerly lethal disorder results in recovery without residual neurologic or renal dysfunction, but mortality is still estimated at 10 to 20 percent.

The disorder must be distinguished from the similar hemolytic-uremic syndrome, of which there are several heritable susceptibility syndromes (OMIM 235400, 612922–612926). This disease occurs in children under age 3, usually after a prodromal diarrheal illness resulting from serotoxin-producing *E. coli*, and is not always associated with encephalopathy. Six genes have been identified that confer susceptibility to this less-threatening disorder, all of them related to the complement system, a quite distinct mechanism from that underlying TTP.

Porphyria

The porphyrias are a family of genetically unrelated disorders resulting from mutations that disrupt heme metabolism. Clinically they can be divided into the hepatic porphyrias, which have neurologic but no cutaneous manifestations, and the cutaneous porphyrias, in which the opposite is true.[79] Thus, none are neurocutaneous disorders, with the exception of variegate porphyria (OMIM 176200; heterozygous mutation of the protoporphyrinogen oxidase gene on chromosome 1q23.3, encoding the penultimate enzyme in the heme biosynthetic pathway) and coproporphyria (OMIM 121300; heterozygous mutation of the coproporphyrinogen oxidase gene on chromosome 3q11.2-q12.1). In both of these disorders, there is increased photosensitivity of the skin, and in variegate porphyria, fragility of the skin with blistering and chronic scarring of sun-exposed areas, followed by postinflammatory hyperpigmentation. In both, certain drugs induce a delirious encephalopathic crisis with psychotic symptoms, as well as neuropathic abdominal pain, constipation, and vomiting. In addition to the peripherally mediated abdominal crises there is a severe interictal peripheral neuropathy, which in variegate porphyria includes bulbar involvement as well as symmetric motor impairment in the extremities.[80]

Both of these disorders violate the general rule of thumb that hereditary enzyme deficiencies are recessive disorders. In both, heterozygosity for a single mutant allele is sufficient to give rise to the disease phenotype, accounting for the unusual pattern of dominant inheritance for a metabolic disorder.

DEMENTIA

Certain neurocutaneous disorders lead to a progressive loss of cognitive ability. Two important examples are described in greater detail in the following paragraphs.

HIV-AIDS

Cognitive impairment, ranging in severity from mild HIV-1–associated neurocognitive disorder (HAND) to a severe progressive dementia,[85] as well as a peripheral neuropathy[86] continue to be significant neurologic manifestations of HIV-AIDS, despite the availability of combination antiretroviral therapy. The incidence of severe AIDS-related dementia has decreased, as have a number of adventitious infections of the nervous system in AIDS patients, including progressive multifocal encephalopathy, tuberculosis, toxoplasmosis, and infection with cytomegalovirus.[87] However, the incidence of milder cognitive impairment persists, for reasons not yet understood. These and other neurologic aspects of HIV-AIDS are discussed in Chapter 44. Cutaneous manifestations have always been a hallmark of HIV-AIDS, affecting an estimated 85 percent of patients.[88] A major clue in the early history of our understanding of AIDS was the high frequency of an unusual rapidly growing cutaneous tumor, atypical Kaposi sarcoma, in young homosexual men. Cutaneous herpes zoster or, more rarely, disseminated cryptococcal infection with cutaneous lesions resembling molluscum contagiosum may also be AIDS-defining events in HIV-positive individuals. The most common cutaneous manifestation, however, is seborrheic dermatitis, a chronic inflammation of the scalp and face, and, less commonly, intertriginous areas such as axillae and groin. Other cutaneous manifestations are virally mediated verruca vulgaris and molluscum contagiosum, recurrent staphylococcal infections, and tinea corporis.

Cockayne Syndrome

Cockayne syndrome (OMIM 216400) is an autosomal recessive disorder of “cachectic dwarfism” and significant cutaneous and neurologic abnormalities, with progressive dementia and multiple systemic abnormalities, that usually results in death in early adolescence, but with occasional survival to young adulthood. Other CNS abnormalities include microcephaly, calcifications of the basal ganglia, patchy subcortical demyelination, normal pressure hydrocephalus, sensorineural hearing loss, pigmentary retinopathy, optic atrophy, ataxia, nystagmus and peripheral neuropathy.[81]

The syndrome is a consequence of homozygosity for mutations in a DNA-repairing enzyme, excision-repair cross-complementing, group 8 (ERCC8) on chromosome 5q12.1 (Cockayne syndrome A, OMIM 216400) or ERCC6 on chromosome 10q11.23 (Cockayne syndrome B, OMIM 133540) The resulting deficit confers increased sensitivity to ultraviolet irradiation, but not to x-irradiation. In a striking contrast with ataxia telangiectasia and xeroderma pigmentosa,[82–84] other neurocutaneous disorders resulting from defects in DNA repair, there is no increased susceptibility to infections or malignancy.

SEIZURE DISORDERS

A great many neurocutaneous syndromes are associated with seizures.Three syndromes frequently included by some authors under a broadened definition of phakomatosis are discussed here in greater detail.

Sturge–Weber Syndrome

The characteristic feature of the Sturge–Weber syndrome (OMIM 185300) is the congenital port wine stain (Fig. 21-12), typically in the distribution of one of the branches of the trigeminal nerve. If this cutaneous lesion overlies the first division, there is a 75 percent chance that there will be a corresponding

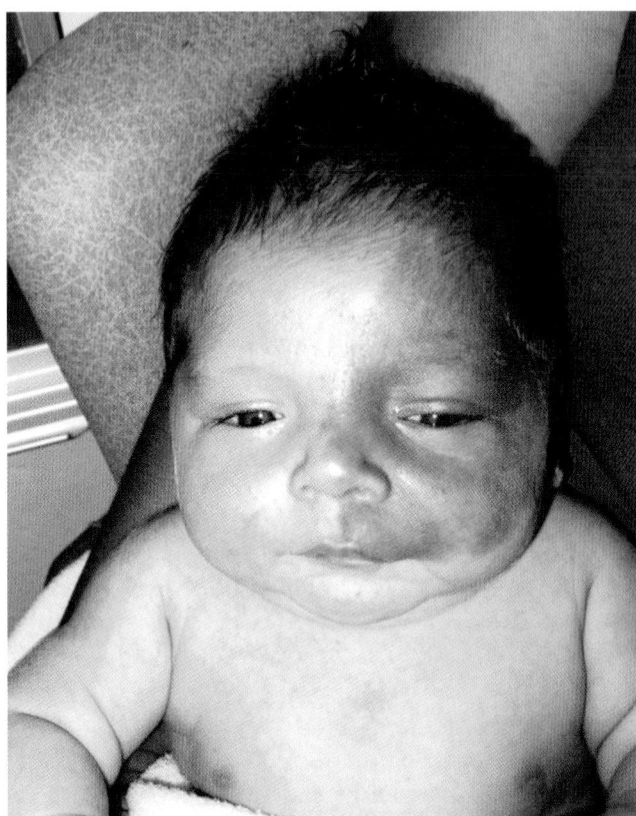

FIGURE 21-12 ■ Sturge–Weber syndrome: port-wine stain. (From Jones K: Smith's Recognizable Patterns of Human Malformation. Saunders, Philadelphia, 2005, with permission.)

leptomeningeal venous malformation overlying focal deep cortical calcifications This is often visible on skull radiographs as a "tram sign," the two tracks of which follow the contours of the calcified gyri.[89]

Sturge–Weber syndrome is believed to result from somatic mosaicism for a mutation in an as-yet unidentified gene, vertical transmission from parent to child never having been observed. The most common neurologic manifestation is epilepsy, typically partial complex seizures. The age of onset of seizures varies from birth to young adulthood. Often these seizures cannot be managed satisfactorily with anticonvulsants and therefore lead to consideration of surgery.

Unlike the classic phakomatoses with which it has occasionally been classified, Sturge–Weber syndrome is not associated with tumors of the nervous system or elsewhere. However, clinically significant neurologic involvement accompanies epilepsy in a significant proportion of affected individuals. Developmental delay and requirement for special education are typical of many patients with Sturge–Weber syndrome, but not for those who do not experience seizures. In contrast, the majority of individuals in both groups experience behavioral and emotional disturbances, as well as impediments to gainful employment, albeit to a greater degree in those with seizures. The major non-neurologic sequela is glaucoma, with onset as early as birth and as late as the fifth decade.

Incontinentia Pigmenti (Bloch–Sulzberger Disease)

Incontinentia pigmenti (OMIM 308300) is an X-linked dominant disorder that is lethal *in utero* to males, and is therefore only seen in those living female heterozygotes who preferentially inactivate the X chromosome bearing the mutant NEMO gene on Xp28 (a regulatory kinase of an inhibitor of the kappa light polypeptide gene enhancer in B cells) by lyonization. There is selective loss of cells expressing the X chromosome with the mutant gene at the time of birth, a process that continues until completion in young adulthood, at which time only cells expressing the normal X chromosome remain. This gradual elimination of cells expressing the mutant gene appears to be temporally correlated with the course of the characteristic cutaneous disorder, which occurs in four stages: (1) within hours to days of birth, lines of erythema develop into inflammatory vesicles that last from weeks to months; (2) these lesions then develop into verrucous, wart-like patches that persist for months; (3) hyperpigmentation develops, very gradually becoming pale and finally disappearing by age 20 years; and (4) dermal scarring develops in the final stage (Figs 21-13 and 21-14). Hair loss may affect the scalp and other parts of the body, and there may be lined or pitted nails and toenails.

Seizures are the most common neurologic manifestation, occurring in about 70 percent of affected women, followed by various motor impairments (40%), cognitive impairment (30%), and microcephaly (7%). Structural abnormalities detectable by brain scanning include focal atrophy, infarcts and lesions of the corpus callosum.[90]

Classic Bloch–Sulzberger disease, as described above, had previously been called incontinentia pigmenti type II (IP2), IP1 being a term erroneously assigned by earlier investigators to some cases of hypomelanosis of Ito (OMIM 300337), which

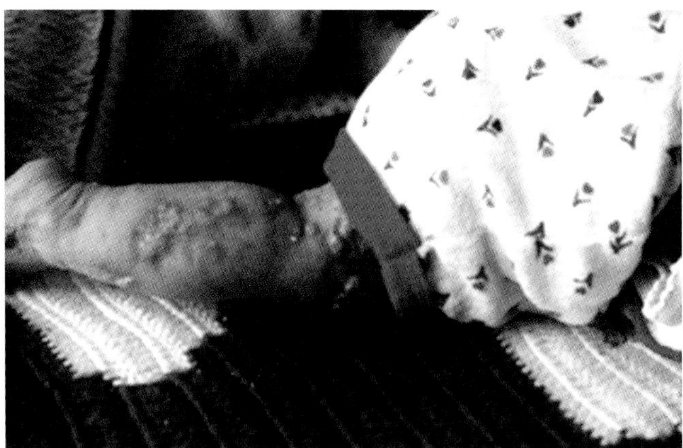

FIGURE 21-13 ▪ Incontinentia pigmenti (Bloch–Sulzberger) stage 3: the beginning of hyperpigmentation. (From Kurlemann G: Neurocutaneous syndromes. Handb Clin Neurol 108:513, 2012, with permission.)

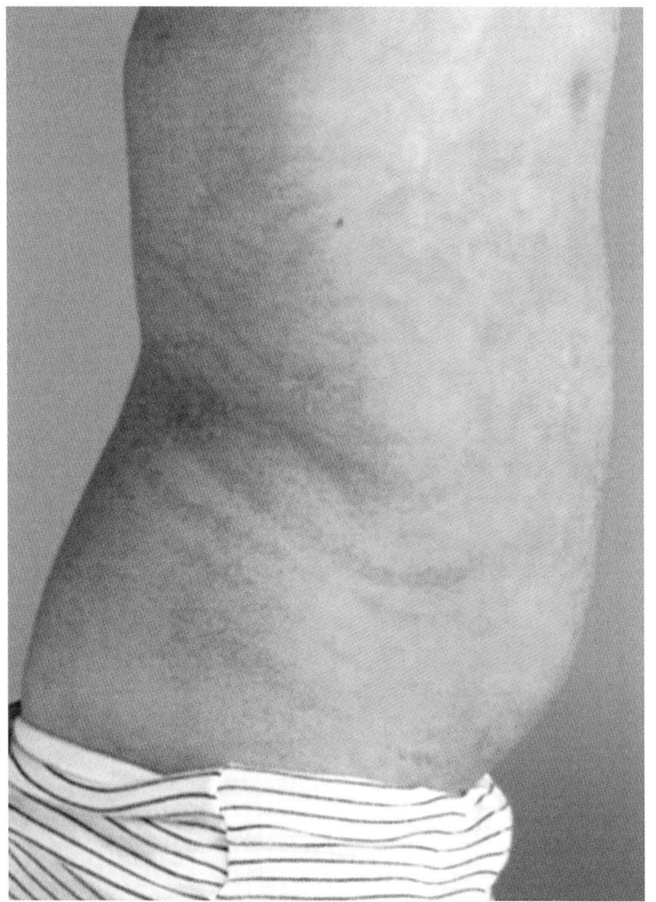

FIGURE 21-14 ▪ Incontinentia pigmenti (Bloch–Sulzberger) stage 4: hypopigmentation on the trunk. (From Kurlemann G: Neurocutaneous syndromes. Handb Clin Neurol 108:513, 2012, with permission.)

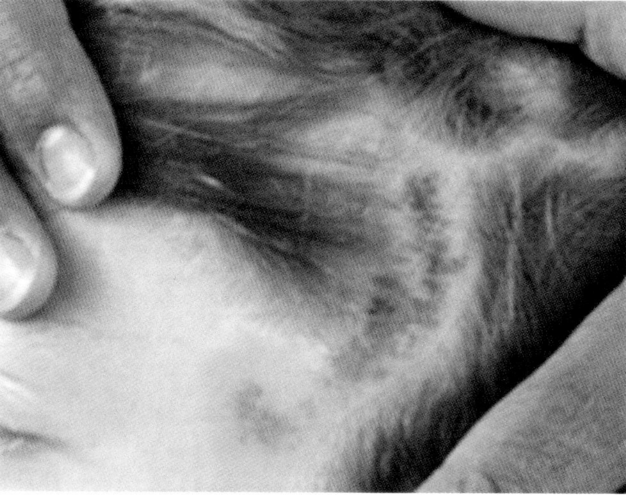

FIGURE 21-15 ▪ Linear nevus sebaceous above the left eye near the hairline in Schimmelpenning–Feuerstein–Mims syndrome. (From Kurlemann G: Neurocutaneous syndromes. Handb Clin Neurol 108:513, 2012, with permission.)

does not represent a distinct entity but is rather a manifestation of many different states of mosaicism. The hypopigmented skin lesions in hypomelanosis have been described as the "negative pattern" of the hyperpigmented lesions of incontinentia pigmenti. Neurologic abnormalities, typically seizures, are quite variable but can include severe mental retardation. The most prominent neuroanatomic abnormalities are histologically benign cortical heterotopias. It is best that the IP1/IP2 terminology be discarded, these disorders being both clinically and genetically distinct.

Linear Sebaceous Nevus Syndrome

Another dominant-lethal neurocutaneous syndrome associated with epilepsy that survives only by somatic mosaicism is the linear sebaceous nevus syndrome (OMIM 163200), also known as the Schimmelpenning–Feuerstein–Mims syndrome (Fig. 21-15). The characteristic sebaceous nevi typically present in the first year of life and persist through adulthood, and are often the site of secondary lesions such as basal cell carcinomas, hemangiomas, hypopigmentation, trichoblastoma, syringocystadenoma papilliferum, and central giant cell granuloma. Neurologic involvement (most commonly seizures, but also mental retardation, ophthalmoplegia, hemimegencephaly, attention deficit disorder) is only present in about 7 percent of individuals, who can present with any of a large variety of systemic abnormalities including coarctation of the aorta, horseshoe kidney, phosphaturia, osteopenia with fractures, and short stature. This disorder results from a mutation in either of two RAS genes: KRAS (V-Ki-Ras2 kirsten rat sarcoma viral oncogene homolog gene on chromosome 12p12.1) or HRAS (V-Ha-Ras Harvey rat sarcoma viral oncogene homolog gene on chromosome 11p15.5).

ATAXIA

Neurocutaneous disorders in which ataxia is a prominent feature are listed in Table 21-4. Four

TABLE 21-4 ■ Ataxia with Cutaneous Manifestations

Disorder	Cutaneous Lesions	Neurologic Features
Acrodermatitis enteropathica, zinc-deficiency type (OMIM 201100)	Bullous, pustular dermatitis of extremities; oral, anal, and genital areas dermatitis; impaired wound healing	Lethargy; ataxia; tremors; emotional lability
Angiomatosis, diffuse corticomeningeal, of Divry & van Bogaert (OMIM 206570)	Cutis marmorata; telangiectasia	Seizures; dementia; ataxia; dysarthria; pseudobulbar symptoms; emotional lability
Ataxia-telangiectasia (OMIM 208900)	Cutaneous telangiectasia; café-au-lait spots; progeric and sclerodermatous changes	Hyporeflexia; dysarthria; ataxia; choreoathetosis; seizures; oculomotor abnormalities
Biotinidase deficiency (OMIM 253260)	Seborrheic dermatitis; skin infections	Seizures; ataxia; developmental delay
Celiac disease; CD (OMIM 212750)	Dermatitis herpetiformis; follicular keratosis	Peripheral neuropathy; ataxia; anxiety; depression; cerebral calcification
Cerebrotendinous xanthomatosis (OMIM 213700)	Tuberous xanthoma; xanthelasma	Dementia; spasticity; ataxia; pseudobulbar palsy; psychiatric symptoms; leukoencephalopathy
Cowden disease (OMIM 158350)	Multiple facial papules; acral keratosis; palmoplantar keratosis; multiple skin tags; facial trichilemmomas; subcutaneous lipomas	Mild to moderate mental retardation; Lhermitte–Duclos disease; appendicular ataxia; cerebellar gangliocytoma; meningioma
Dyskeratosis congenita, autosomal dominant, 3 (OMIM 613990)	Reticular pigmentation pattern; leukoplakia; dry skin	Speech delay; learning difficulties; intracranial calcifications; ataxia; cerebellar hypoplasia
Flynn–Aird disease (OMIM 136300)	Skin atrophy, chronic ulceration	Seizures; dementia; ataxia; peripheral neuropathy
Hartnup disorder (OMIM 234500)	Photosensitive dermatitis	Intermittent ataxia; seizures; hypertonia; hyperreflexia; emotional instability; psychosis
Hemophagocytic lymphohistiocytosis (OMIM 267700 & 603553)	Purpuric rashes	Seizures; meningitis; encephalitis; ataxia; coma; increased intracranial pressure; delayed psychomotor development
Hydroxykynureninuria (OMIM 236800)	Light-sensitive rash	Intermittent nonprogressive ataxic encephalopathy
Neuroblastoma (OMIM 256700)	Bluish skin nodules	Paraneoplastic opsoclonus, myoclonus, and/or ataxia; spinal cord compression
PHACE association (OMIM 606519)	Hemangioma, facial, plaque-like	Developmental delay; Dandy–Walker malformation; seizures; migraine headaches (ipsilateral to facial hemangioma); cerebral infarction
Plasminogen deficiency, type I (OMIM 217090)	Juvenile colloid milium; small papules on sun-exposed areas	Dandy–Walker malformation; macrocephaly; adult onset of symptoms has been reported
Refsum disease (OMIM 266500)	Ichthyosis	Ataxia; peripheral neuropathy; retinitis pigmentosa; sensorineural deafness; anosmia
Renal tubulopathy, diabetes mellitus, and cerebellar ataxia (OMIM 560000)	Mottled pigmentation of photoexposed areas; episodic cold-triggered erythrocyanosis of toes and fingers	Myoclonic jerks; ataxia; hypotonia; psychomotor regression
Revesz syndrome (OMIM 268130)	Fine, reticulate skin pigmentation (trunk, palm, and soles)	Psychomotor retardation; cerebellar hypoplasia; ataxia; cerebral calcifications; hypertonia; progressive neurologic deterioration
Spinocerebellar ataxia 34 (OMIM 133190)	Erythrokeratodermia; papulosquamous erythematous plaques; hyperkeratosis	Spinocerebellar ataxia; mild spasticity; dysarthria

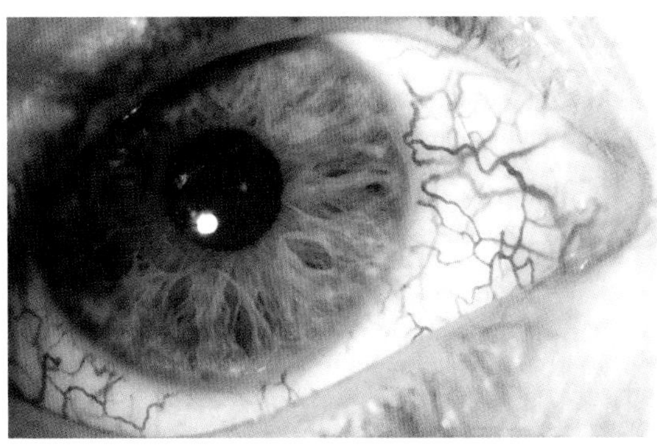

FIGURE 21-16 ■ Ataxia-telangiectasia: bulbar conjunctiva. (From Jones K: Smith's Recognizable Patterns of Human Malformation. Saunders, Philadelphia, 2005, with permission.)

representative disorders are described in the following paragraphs.

Ataxia Telangiectasia

Also known as Louis-Bar syndrome (OMIM 208900), the cardinal features of this autosomal recessive disorder are cerebellar ataxia, cutaneous telangiectases, immune defects, and a predisposition to malignancy (Fig. 21-16).[83,84] The invariable, progressive neurologic disorder, chiefly ataxia, begins at birth, often initially causing diagnostic confusion because the characteristic oculocutaneous telangiectasias do not appear until 3 to 5 years of age. The ataxia is initially truncal and only later appendicular. It is associated with a characteristic oculomotor apraxia.[91] A large-fiber neuropathy becomes evident in late childhood and spinal muscular atrophy evolves in early adulthood. About 10 percent of individuals also develop a more complex movement disorder, with choreoathetosis that can be severe.

Major issues in clinical management include a strong predisposition to malignancy (chiefly leukemia and lymphoma, but also others), as well as impairment of both humoral and cellular immunity, often manifested by frequent sinopulmonary infections. A marked hypersensitivity to ionizing radiation is a fundamental feature of this disorder: the need to minimize exposure requires significant modification of radiotherapeutic dosages and the use of radiologic monitoring.

Affected individuals are homozygous for mutation of the ataxia-telangiectasia mutated (ATM) gene, consisting of 66 exons encoding a phosphatidylinositol 3-kinase that repairs certain types of DNA damage, on chromosome 11q22.3. As such, it fits the classic definition of an autosomal recessive disorder. However, heterozygotes for ATM mutations, who cannot be identified by routine clinical examination and who vastly outnumber manifesting homozygotes, have a significantly increased sensitivity to radiation as well as increased propensity to certain types of malignancy. As such, they represent a larger concern to public health than do the rare, unfortunate homozygotes.

Cerebrotendinous Xanthomatosis

The dermatologic manifestations of this lipid storage disorder (OMIM 2137000) are tuberous xanthomata and xanthelasma, similar to the characteristic deposits of cholesterol and cholestanol in multiple other tissues, particularly in the Achilles tendon, for which deposits the disorder is named. The progressive neurologic disorder begins in puberty with ataxia and progresses to involve the spinal cord and brainstem.[92,93] These cardinal features correlate with focal lipid deposits, visible on either CT or MRI scans, in the cerebellar white matter and the cerebral peduncles as well as the brainstem and basal ganglia.[94,95] Unlike in ataxia telangiectasia, a progressive dementia may develop as well as psychotic symptoms such as delusions and hallucinations. Systemic symptoms include cataracts, respiratory complaints, bony fragility, and myocardial infarction even though plasma cholesterol levels are either normal or only modestly elevated.

This autosomal recessive disorder results from the lack of functional sterol 27-hydroxylase, an enzyme involved in the synthesis of bile acids, resulting from mutations in the *CYP27A1* gene on chromosome 2q35. This metabolic abnormality leads to decreased synthesis of bile acids and a compensatory increase in the activity of the rate-limiting enzyme in bile acid synthesis, cholesterol 7α-hydroxylase, and accumulation of 7α-hydroxylated bile acid precursors, including a precursor to cholestanol that readily crosses the blood–brain barrier. This complex biochemistry can be ameliorated by treatment with cholic acid, chenodeoxycholic acid, and statins, which reduce xanthomata and improve central neurologic symptoms, but not the axonal peripheral neuropathy which is part of this systemic disorder.

Classic Refsum Disease

This is a complex neurocutaneous disorder in which progressive ataxia is part of an invariable tetrad that also includes peripheral neuropathy, retinitis pigmentosa, and elevated protein in acellular cerebrospinal fluid (OMIM 266500). In most cases, there is also progressive hearing loss. The classic dermatologic abnormality of ichthyosis is less common, as are cardiac abnormalities and a skeletal abnormality, multiple epiphyseal dysplasia. Classic Refsum disease is to be distinguished from the genetically and clinically distinct infantile Refsum disease, which is one of a heterogeneous group of peroxisomal biogenesis disorders that include Zellweger syndrome and neonatal adrenoleukodystrophy.

Classic Refsum disease is a treatable autosomal recessive disorder. Affected individuals are homozygous for inactivating mutations in the gene encoding phytanoyl-CoA hydroxylase on chromosome 10p13. As a result, there is impaired degradation of phytanic acid, an unusual branched-chain fatty acid derived exclusively from dietary sources. Restriction of foods containing chlorophyll and phytols leads to reduction of blood levels of phytanic acid and some amelioration of clinical signs. Plasmapheresis may allow modest liberalization of the diet.[96]

Hartnup Disease and Related Disorders

Unlike the previously described neurocutaneous ataxias, which are progressive when treatment is unavailable, Hartnup disease (OMIM 234500) is an intermittent ataxia, associated with a light-sensitive, pellagra-like skin rash and emotional instability. The characteristic rash is symmetric, hyperkeratotic, hyperpigmented and desquamated in exposed areas.[97]

It results from homozygosity for mutations that alter the activity of system B(0) neutral amino acid transporter 1, also referred to as solute carrier family 6 (neurotransmitter transporter), member 19 (SLC6A19), an amino acid transporter present in the intestinal brush border and renal cortical proximal tubules, but not in the skin or the nervous system.[98] For this reason, signs and symptoms can be attributed to low plasma levels of neutral amino acids, principally tryptophan and methionine, resulting from aminoaciduria and selective intestinal malabsorption. The frequency of Hartnup disease is similar to that of phenylketonuria, i.e., 1 in about 14,000 live births. Unlike phenylketonuria, however, Hartnup disease has no ill effects on the fetus because placental transport of amino acids is not affected. Indeed, despite this significant frequency, the full-blown classic disorder is now rarely seen in the United States because most diets supply sufficient levels of neutral amino acids to at least partially compensate for intestinal and renal losses.

A similar rash occurs in two other neurocutaneous disorders in which tryptophan metabolism is implicated. *Pellagra*, rarely seen in the developed world, results from dietary deficiency of a B vitamin, niacin, which can be taken directly in the diet or synthesized from dietary tryptophan, both of which are in short supply in a corn-based diet. This chronic wasting disease is characterized by a triad of dermatitis, dementia, and diarrhea.

Hydroxykynureninuria (OMIM 236800) is an autosomal recessive disorder resulting from deficiency of kynureninase, an enzyme apparently required for the synthesis of niacin from tryptophan. Its neurologic phenotype is intermediate between that of pellagra and Hartnup disease. In addition to the characteristic light-sensitive rash, there is a nonprogressive ataxic encephalopathy that can reversibly worsen under the stress of a viral infection, on occasion leading to coma and death.

MYELOPATHY

Transverse or compressive myelopathies may be rare presentations of a number of neurocutaneous syndromes. Two, in which myelopathy is a common presentation, are described here.

Rheumatoid Arthritis

Subcutaneous nodules at sites of trauma, such as extensor surfaces of forearms, posterior scalp, and ears are characteristic manifestations of rheumatoid arthritis. In addition, there may be painful papules of the finger pulp, bright red "liver palms," or a vivid washable yellow discoloration of the skin from inspissated sweat.

The most feared neurologic abnormality in rheumatoid arthritis is not from intrinsic inflammation of the nervous system but a potentially life-threatening compressive high cervical myelopathy resulting from localized pachymeningitis[99] or arthritis with laxity of the atlantoaxial joint, present in about half of individuals with advanced rheumatoid arthritis. This can cause either horizontal atlantoaxial instability[100] or vertical translation of the dens with a normal atlantoaxial interval.[101] Repeated microtrauma to the craniocervical junction may give rise to a gradually progressive, high cervical myelopathy. However, moderately severe trauma from a fall or an otherwise minor motor vehicle accident can result in catastrophic, lethal, spinal cord compression.

The high frequency of these potentially preventable complications requires screening with lateral radiographs of the cervical spine in the neutral position and in flexion to assess the atlantoaxial interval even in neurologically asymptomatic individuals in order to assess the potential for catastrophic subluxation. MRI of the craniocervical junction is useful for two purposes: (1) detection of an altered intraparenchymal signal indicating injury from milder repetitive compression due to minor subluxation of the atlanto-axial joint; and (2) for detection of an inflammatory pannus around the dens, which can further compromise the subarachnoid space. Neurosurgical intervention is warranted if there is a high degree of instability or evidence of myelopathy. Anatomy dictates the required intervention: a high degree of positional instability requires fusion; obliteration of the subarachnoid space without significant instability requires decompression.

Other neurologic complications of rheumatoid arthritis are discussed in detail in Chapter 50.

Sjögren Syndrome

Sjögren syndrome is characterized by autoimmune involvement of lacrimal and salivary glands, causing dry eyes and dry mouth (the sicca syndrome), but also by more widespread systemic and neurologic manifestations. Cutaneous involvement, when present, is palpable purpura, a classic sign of cutaneous vasculitis. Both the central and the peripheral nervous system are frequently also affected,[102] as discussed in Chapter 50. The classic peripheral neurologic manifestation is a ganglionitis or a distal small-fiber axonal sensory neuropathy,[103] but there may be multiple cranial neuropathies and mononeuritis multiplex as well.[104] Although less frequent, the most common CNS presentation is a focal, transverse myelopathy with a T2 bright MRI lesion that spans several segments.[105] This may mistakenly be attributed to multiple sclerosis, as may various other presentations of Sjögren syndrome including focal cerebral or brainstem lesions associated with perivenular inflammation, more often in the white matter than gray.[106] Recognition of the sicca syndrome and cutaneous manifestations may therefore be critical in suggesting the correct diagnosis.

PERIPHERAL NEUROPATHY

Various entrapment neuropathies, mononeuropathies, plexopathies, distal symmetric and cranial neuropathies with cutaneous manifestations are listed in Table 21-5. Three disorders in which peripheral nerve involvement is either the principal or only neurologic manifestation are described in this section.

Leprosy

Leprosy is also known as Hansen disease in honor of the Norwegian physician who discovered the causative organism, *Mycobacterium leprae*, in 1873. The disorder is discussed in detail in Chapter 42. Until the 1980s leprosy was perhaps the most common peripheral neuropathy and neurocutaneous disorder worldwide, affecting in excess of 10 million individuals and permanently disfiguring millions.[107] A steady decline in its incidence has followed the introduction of multidrug therapy. The majority of cases are in the tropics, with about 50 percent of the cases in India, and high numbers in a periequatorial belt that includes Brazil, Madagascar, and Myanmar. About 250,000 new cases are diagnosed annually.[108] Armadillos, the only other species to harbor the obligate intracellular bacillus, *Mycobacterium leprae*, are still hunted for food in the American Southwest and can be a source of exposure to this infectious agent.

The neuropathy typically presents with characteristic skin lesions and a hypesthetic mononeuritis multiplex with palpably thickened nerves. The distribution of the mononeuritis is influenced by the organism's proclivity for endoneural invasion in the cool exposed face and extremities, as discussed in detail in Chapter 42. In addition to commonly affected superficial cutaneous nerves, there is frequent motor involvement in the distribution of the ulnar nerve and sensory involvement of the posterior tibial nerve.[109]

Although all lepromatous neuropathy is a consequence of local mycobacterial invasion, the cutaneous manifestations depend on the strength of the host's immune response. A vigorous response leads to tuberculoid, or paucibacillary leprosy with granuloma formation, anesthetic patches of skin adjacent

TABLE 21-5 ■ Peripheral Neuropathy with Cutaneous Manifestations

Disorder	Cutaneous Manifestations
AIDS	Seborrheic dermatitis, verruca vulgaris, molluscum contagiosum, Kaposi sarcoma
Alcoholism	Telangiectasias, malar rash, psoriasis and discoid eczema, exacerbation of rosacea, porphyria cutanea tarda, acne
Amyloidosis (primary)	Purpura in skin folds or flat surfaces or eyelids, papules, sometimes alopecia, rarely bullae on skin or oral mucosa
Angioedema, hereditary, type I (OMIM 106100)	Erythema marginatum
Arsenic poisoning	Dry scaly desquamation, linear hyperpigmentation of nails, Mees lines
Brachydactyly mental retardation syndrome (OMIM 600430)	Eczema
Cardiofaciocutaneous syndrome (OMIM 115150)	Severe atopic dermatitis, ichthyosis, hyperkeratosis (especially extensor surfaces), cavernous hemangiomas, keratosis pilaris, multiple palmar creases, multiple lentigines
Celiac disease (OMIM 212750)	Dermatitis herpetiformis, follicular keratosis
Cerebral dysgenesis, neuropathy, ichthyosis, and palmoplantar keratoderma syndrome (OMIM 609528)	Palmoplantar keratoderma, ichthyosis
Cerebrotendinous xanthomatosis (OMIM 213700)	Tuberous xanthoma, xanthelasma
Chediak–Higashi (OMIM 214500)	Partial albinism, silvery blond hair
Coenzyme Q10 deficiency, primary, 2; (OMIM 614651)	Hypopigmentation, malar flush, livedo reticularis
Coproporphyria, hereditary (OMIM 121300)	Photosensitivity
Cronkhite–Canada gastrointestinal hamartomatous polyposis (OMIM 175500)	Alopecia, skin hyperpigmentation, onychodystrophy
Diabetes mellitus	Necrobiosis lipoidica diabeticorum, poorly healing ulcers
Diphtheria (cutaneous)	Jungle sore
Fabry disease (OMIM 610651)	Angiokeratoma
Flynn–Aird disease (OMIM 136300)	Skin atrophy, hyperkeratosis, chronic ulceration
Fucosidosis (OMIM 230000)	Angiokeratoma; thin, dry skin; anhidrosis
Hemochromatosis (OMIM 235200)	Bronze pigmentation, telangiectasias
Histiocytic reticulosis	Purpura, jaundice, erythroderma
Hyperoxaluria, primary, Type I (OMIM 259900)	Livedo reticularis, calcinosis cutis metastatica, acrocyanosis
Impaired long-chain fatty acid oxidation	Congenital ichthyosis, ichthyosiform erythroderma
Kanzaki disease (OMIM 609242)	Angiokeratoma corporis diffusum, hyperkeratosis, dry skin, diffuse maculopapular eruption, telangiectasia on lips and oral mucosa
Leprosy	Hypopigmentation and hyperpigmentation, leonine facies, erythema nodosum leprosum, Lucio phenomenon
Linear sebaceous nevi of Jadassohn (OMIM 163200, Schimmelpenning–Feuerstein–Mims syndrome)	Sebaceous and epithelial nevi, linear nevus sebaceous
Lyme disease	Target lesions
Neurocutaneous melanosis (OMIM 249400)	Large multiple pigmented skin nevi (>20 cm), no malignant melanoma other than CNS
Pellagra	Erythematous photosensitive rash, erythema, vesicles, glossitis, malar and supraorbital hyperpigmentation, rhagades

(Continued)

TABLE 21-5 ■ Peripheral Neuropathy with Cutaneous Manifestations

Disorder	Cutaneous Manifestations
Peripheral demyelinating neuropathy, central dysmyelination, Waardenburg syndrome, and Hirschsprung disease (OMIM 609136)	Hypopigmented skin patches
Phenylketonuria (OMIM 261600)	Pale pigmentation, dry skin, eczema, scleroderma
POEMS syndrome	Hyperpigmentation, thickening, verrucous angiomas, hirsutism, Raynaud phenomenon
Poikiloderma-spastic paraplegia	Poikiloderma: delicate, smooth, wasted skin
Refsum disease (classic) (OMIM 266500)	Ichthyosis
Sarcoidosis	Hypohidrosis, cicatricial alopecia; *acute*: erythema nodosum, vesicles, maculopapular rash; *chronic*: lupus pernio, plaques, scars, keloids
Sjögren syndrome	Purpura, Raynaud phenomenon, xerostomia, candidiasis
Spastic paraplegia 23 (OMIM 270750)	Patchy vitiligo, hyperpigmentation of exposed areas, lentigines
Stiff skin syndrome (OMIM 184900)	Thick, indurated skin over entire body
Systemic lupus erythematosus	Photosensitivity, malar rash, discoid lupus
Thallium intoxication	Hair loss
Trichorrhexis nodosa	Ichthyosis, flexural eczema, photosensitivity, short wooly hair
Vitamin B_{12} deficiency	Black nail pigmentation (nail bed and matrix), oral aphthae
Werner syndrome (pangeria) (OMIM 277700)	Scleroderma-like skin, graying hair and baldness, leg ulcers, progressive scalp alopecia, sparse body hair, telangiectasia, mottled pigmentation; loss of subcutaneous fat, subcutaneous calcification
Xeroderma pigmentosum (OMIM 610651)	Photosensitivity, early-onset skin cancer, atrophy, telangiectasia, actinic keratosis, angioma, keratoacanthomas

to thickened peripheral nerves, and severe destruction of nerve. At the other end of the spectrum is lepromatous leprosy with widespread nodular cutaneous lesions (e.g., leonine facies) (Fig. 21-17) containing large quantities of *M. leprae*, leading to a more insidious destruction of nerves, in which there is an absence of a cell-mediated immune response. Most patients lie along a spectrum between these two extremes, depending in part on their complement of susceptibility genes, which have been mapped to a half dozen gene loci, but not yet fully characterized.

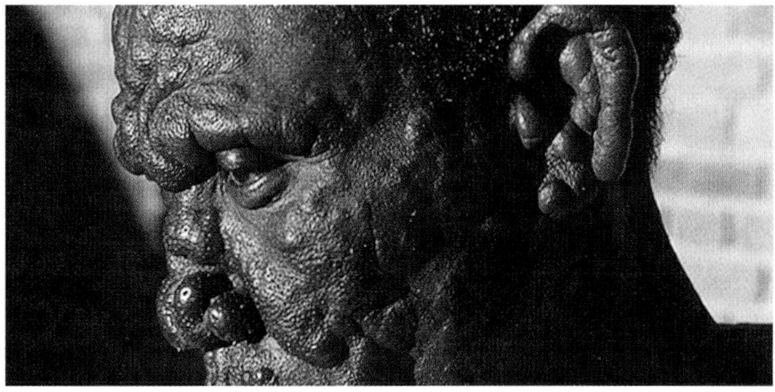

FIGURE 21-17 ■ Infiltrated nodules of the forehead and face resulting in the leonine facies of lepromatous leprosy. (From Peters W, Pasvol G: Atlas of Tropical Medicine and Parasitology. 6th Ed. Mosby, St Louis, 2007, with permission.)

Although the fully developed neurocutaneous syndrome is easily diagnosed in endemic areas even by individuals who are not medically trained, the long incubation period provides ample opportunity for transmission before the disease is evident. Furthermore, clinically evident nerve damage and disfigurement are irreversible. Recent development of an inexpensive diagnostic test by the Brazilian firm OrangeLife gives hope that presymptomatic leprosy can be diagnosed and treated, possibly as a final step to the goal of the World Health

Organization of complete eradication of this neurocutaneous disorder.

Systemic Sclerosis

This disorder is often commonly referred to as scleroderma, which is the name more properly applied to its characteristic cutaneous manifestation—a thickening of the skin—that can also occur as an isolated syndrome independent of the systemic and neurologic manifestations of systemic sclerosis.[110] Another cutaneous feature of systemic sclerosis is a diffuse hyperpigmentation. Various peripheral neuropathies are by far the most common manifestations of systemic sclerosis,[111] the most common being carpal tunnel syndrome, which occurs in about a quarter of patients, and cranial neuropathies, especially trigeminal neuralgia. Less commonly there are symmetric axonal neuropathies, often with autonomic involvement, as well as mononeuritis multiplex and plexopathies. In contrast to the frequent involvement of the peripheral nerves, the links between systemic sclerosis and pathology of the CNS are much more tenuous,[112] apart from asymptomatic calcification of the basal ganglia, which occurs in about one-third of affected individuals.[113]

Systemic Vasculitis

The classic neurocutaneous presentation of palpable purpura[114] and mononeuritis multiplex[115] occurs in several types of systemic vasculitis, a heterogeneous and partially overlapping group of neurocutaneous disorders that include classic polyarteritis nodosa,[116] Churg–Strauss allergic angiitis and granulomatosis,[117] and Wegener granulomatosis.[118] All three of these disorders affect small and medium-sized arteries, the first two as prime examples of a larger class of systemic necrotizing vasculitis. Occlusion of small arteries results in mononeuritis, an abrupt, painful ischemic infarction of the segment of a peripheral nerve in which perfusion is compromised. These three disorders differ histopathologically and clinically. They are discussed in detail in Chapter 50. In order of frequency, classic polyarteritis nodosa affects kidneys, joints, peripheral nervous system, skin, gastrointestinal tract, and the CNS, but never the lungs. During the course of the disease, peripheral nerve involvement is seen in over half of cases, though rarely as one of the presenting signs. In less than a quarter of cases, the necrotizing vasculitis of polyarteritis nodosa extends into the CNS.

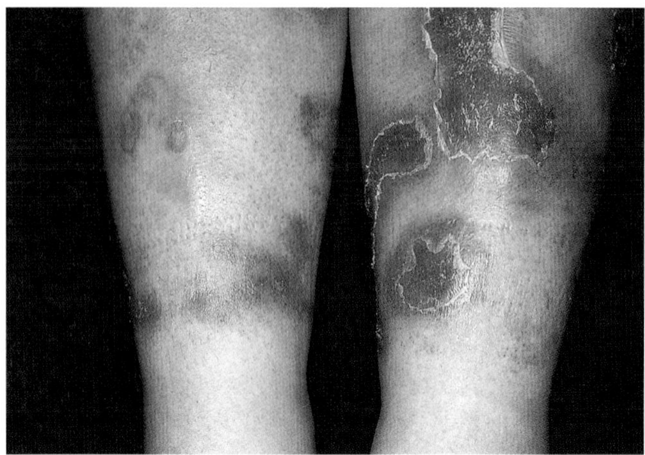

FIGURE 21-18 ▪ Cutaneous small-vessel vasculitis was the first evidence of recurrence in this patient with Wegener's granulomatosis. (From Callen J, Jorizzo J, Bolognia J, et al: Dermatological Signs of Internal Disease. Saunders, Philadelphia, 2009, with permission.)

In contrast, the lungs are affected in Churg–Strauss syndrome, a granulomatous disorder closely associated with asthma, and in Wegener granulomatosis, a distinct disorder of granulomatous vasculitis of the upper and lower respiratory tract. In Wegener granulomatosis, renal involvement dominates the clinical picture in about 75 percent of patients, cutaneous manifestations occur in about 50 percent, and neurologic manifestations in about 25 percent. Palpable purpura, the signature lesion of cutaneous vasculitis (Fig. 21-18), may be prominent, as may vesicles, papules, ulcers, and subcutaneous nodules. Nervous system involvement is usually peripheral, with a mononeuritis multiplex similar to that of polyarteritis nodosa being a frequent feature, but with a much lower frequency of CNS vasculitis.

Untreated, all three disorders are lethal. Treatment is based on corticosteroids and cyclophosphamide, except in the 20 percent of cases of polyarteritis nodosa with demonstrable blood levels of hepatitis B surface antigen, thought to be the inciting antigen for the pathophysiologic cascade initiated by deposition of immune complexes in the walls of blood vessels that attract the necrotizing leukocytic infiltrate. In such cases, there may be response to treatment with interferon-alpha and plasma exchange.

Different patterns of cutaneous and neurologic manifestations—sometimes including mononeuritis

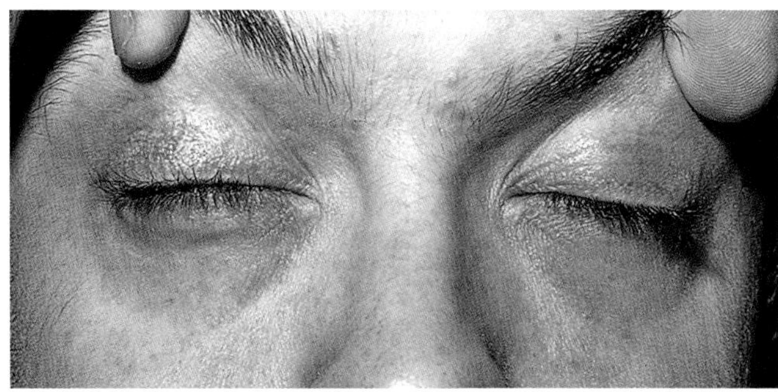

FIGURE 21-19 ■ Characteristic heliotrope rash of dermatomyositis on the eyelids. (From Habif T, Campbell J, Chapman MS, et al: Dermatology DDX Deck. Saunders, Philadelphia, 2006, with permission.)

multiplex as a minor feature—occur in other disorders classified as vasculitis: notably Behçet disease and the vasculitis associated with certain connective tissue disorders, most notably systemic lupus erythematosus. Other vasculitic disorders, such as giant cell arteritis, with no cutaneous manifestations, or the primary cutaneous vasculitides, which by definition have no neurologic or systemic manifestations, are not neurocutaneous syndromes and are not discussed here.

MYOPATHY

Dermatomyositis

Dermatomyositis is not "polymyositis with a rash" but a distinct vasculitis that can be diagnosed unequivocally by considering either the cutaneous[119] or muscle pathology[120] on its own. Unlike polymyositis, it commonly affects children and adults. Photosensitivity either precedes or accompanies muscle weakness, facilitating diagnosis. This manifests as an erythematous rash over sun-exposed areas: the malar region, the "shawl" of the neck and shoulders, and the exposed anterior "V" of the chest as well as over the knuckles, malleoli or other joints. Typically there is a distinctive heliotrope rash of the eyelids (Fig. 21-19). In about two-thirds of childhood cases, there is also subcutaneous calcification. These skin lesions may be the only clinically evident manifestation, especially when the muscle involvement is unusually mild. More typically, proximal limb-girdle weakness develops subacutely over weeks to months, often involving pharyngeal muscles and neck extensors, but with sparing of facial and extraocular muscles. The muscles may be tender. Muscle histology demonstrates a microangiopathy.

Dermatomyositis is associated with malignancy in about 15 percent of cases, more often in adults than in children. This is most often in the ovary, breast, or colon or a melanoma, but occasionally the lung or some other site is involved. Alternatively, it is occasionally seen in association with systemic sclerosis, with a rare Mendelian disorder (Barraquer–Simons syndrome, OMIM 608709) or as an isolated neurocutaneous syndrome.

REFERENCES

1. McKusick VA, Antonarakis SE, Francomano CA, et al: Online Mendelian Inheritance in Man: a catalog of human genes and genetic disorders [online]. Available at: <www.ncbi.nlm.nih.gov/omim>.
2. Kurlemann G: Neurocutaneous syndromes. Handb Clin Neurol 108:513, 2012.
3. Gutmann DH, Aylsworth A, Carey JC, et al: The diagnostic evaluation and multidisciplinary management of neurofibromatosis 1 and neurofibromatosis 2. JAMA 278:51, 1997.
4. Gutmann DH, Parada LF, Silva AJ, et al: Neurofibromatosis type 1: modeling CNS dysfunction. J Neurosci 32:14087, 2012.
5. Matsui I, Tanimura M, Kobayashi N, et al: Neurofibromatosis and childhood cancer. Cancer 72:2746, 1993.
6. Ferner RE, Hughes RA, Weinman J: Intellectual impairment in neurofibromatosis 1. Neurol Sci 138:125, 1996.
7. DiMario Jr FJ, Ramsby G: Magnetic resonance imaging lesion analysis in neurofibromatosis type 1. Arch Neurol 55:500, 1998.
8. Denckla MB, Hofman K, Mazzocco MM, et al: Relationship between T2-weighted hyperintensities (unidentified bright objects) and lower IQs in children with neurofibromatosis-1. Am J Med Genet 67:98, 1996.
9. Ferner RE, Chaudhuri Bingham J, et al: MRI in neurofibromatosis 1. The nature and evolution of increased intensity T2 weighted lesions and their relationship to intellectual impairment. J Neurol Neurosurg Psychiatry 56:492, 1993.
10. Hoa M, Slattery 3rd WH: Neurofibromatosis 2. Otolaryngol Clin North Am 45:315, 2012.
11. Mautner VF, Lindenau M, Baser ME, et al: The neuroimaging and clinical spectrum of neurofibromatosis 2. Neurosurgery 38:880, 1996.
12. Evans DGR, Huson SM, Donnai D, et al: A clinical study of type 2 neurofibromatosis. QJM 84:603, 1992.
13. Borkowska J, Schwartz RA, Kotulska K, et al: Tuberous sclerosis complex: tumors and tumorigenesis. Int J Dermatol 50:13, 2011.

14. Fallah A, Guyatt GH, Snead 3rd OC: Predictors of seizure outcomes in children with tuberous sclerosis complex and intractable epilepsy undergoing resective epilepsy surgery: an individual participant data meta-analysis. PLoS One 8:e53565, 2013.
15. Webb DW, Clarke A, Fryer A, et al: The cutaneous features of tuberous sclerosis: a population study. Br J Dermatol 35:1, 1996.
16. Jones AC, Daniells CE, Snell RG, et al: Molecular genetic and phenotypic analysis reveals differences between TSC1 and TSC2 associated familial and sporadic tuberous sclerosis. Hum Mol Genet 6:2155, 1997.
17. Habif TP: Clinical Dermatology. 5th Ed. Mosby/Elsevier, St. Louis, 2010.
18. Gibney GT, Forsyth PA, Sondak VK: Melanoma in the brain: biology and therapeutic options. Melanoma Res 22:177, 2012.
19. Carlino MS, Fogarty GB, Long GV: Treatment of melanoma brain metastases: a new paradigm. Cancer J 18:208, 2012.
20. Ramaswamy V, Delaney H, Haque S, et al: Spectrum of central nervous system abnormalities in neurocutaneous melanocytosis. Dev Med Child Neurol 54:563, 2012.
21. Germain DP: Fabry disease. Orphanet J Rare Dis 5:30, 2010.
22. Hasholt L, Sorensen SA, Wandall A, et al: A Fabry's disease heterozygote with a new mutation: biochemical, ultrastructural, and clinical investigations. J Med Genet 27:303, 1990.
23. Viana-Baptista M: Stroke and Fabry disease. J Neurol 259:1019, 2012.
24. Pisani A, Visciano B, Roux GD, et al: Enzyme replacement therapy in patients with Fabry disease: state of the art and review of the literature. Mol Genet Metab 107:267, 2012.
25. McDonald J, Bayrak-Toydemir P, Pyeritz RE: Hereditary hemorrhagic telangiectasia: an overview of diagnosis, management, and pathogenesis. Genet Med 13:607, 2011.
26. Whitehead KJ, Smith MC, Li DY: Arteriovenous malformations and other vascular malformation syndromes. Cold Spring Harb Perspect Med 3:a006635, 2013.
27. Testai FD, Gorelick PB: Inherited metabolic disorders and stroke part 2: homocystinuria, organic acidurias, and urea cycle disorders. Arch Neurol 67:148, 2010.
28. Schiff M, Blom HJ: Treatment of inherited homocystinurias. Neuropediatrics 43:295, 2012.
29. Ding R, Lin S, Chen D: The association of cystathionine β synthase (CBS) T833C polymorphism and the risk of stroke: a meta-analysis. J Neurol Sci 312:26, 2012.
30. Weissler A, Perl L, Neuman Y, et al: Neurologic manifestations as presenting symptoms of endocarditis. Isr Med Assoc J 12:472, 2010.
31. Kiefer TL, Bashore TM: Infective endocarditis: a comprehensive overview. Cardiovasc Med 13:e105, 2012.
32. Han MJ, Bidinger JJ, Hivnor CM: Asymptomatic linear hemorrhages. Am Fam Physician 81:1375, 2010.
33. Mujic F, Lloyd M, Cuadrado MJ, et al: Prevalence and clinical significance of subungual splinter haemorrhages in patients with the antiphospholipid syndrome. Clin Exp Rheumatol 13:327, 1995.
34. Beaulieu A, Rehman HU: Clinical images: Janeway lesions. CMAJ 182:1075, 2010.
35. Miyakis S, Lockshin MD, Atsumi T, et al: International consensus statement on an update of the classification criteria for definite antiphospholipid syndrome (APS). J Thromb Haemost 4:295, 2006.
36. Gibson GE, Su WP, Pittelkow MR: Antiphospholipid syndrome and the skin. J Am Acad Dermatol 36:970, 1997.
37. Asherson RA, Francès C, Iaccarino L, et al: The antiphospholipid antibody syndrome: diagnosis, skin manifestations and current therapy. Clin Exp Rheumatol 24(suppl 40):S46, 2006.
38. Kriseman YL, Nash JW, Hsu S: Criteria for the diagnosis of antiphospholipid syndrome in patients presenting with dermatologic symptoms. J Am Acad Dermatol 57:112, 2007.
39. Muscal E, Brey RL: Antiphospholipid syndrome and the brain in pediatric and adult patients. Lupus 19:406, 2010.
40. Ruiz-Irastorza G, Khamashta MA: Stroke and antiphospholipid syndrome: the treatment debate. Rheumatology (Oxford) 44:971, 2005.
41. Wen D, Du X, Ma CS: Takayasu arteritis: diagnosis, treatment and prognosis. Int Rev Immunol 31:462, 2012.
42. Park M-C, Lee S-W, Park Y-B, et al: Clinical characteristics and outcomes of Takayasu's arteritis: analysis of 108 patients using standardized criteria for diagnosis, activity assessment, and angiographic classification. Scand J Rheumatol 34:284, 2005.
43. Sabatini C, Bosis S, Semino M, et al: Clinical presentation of meningococcal disease in childhood. J Prev Med Hyg 53:116, 2012.
44. Roos KL, Greenlee JE: Meningitis and encephalitis. Continuum (Minneap Minn) 17:1010, 2011.
45. Nadel S: Prospects for eradication of meningococcal disease. Child 97:993, 2012.
46. McIntyre PB, O'Brien KL, Greenwood B, et al: Effect of vaccines on bacterial meningitis worldwide. Lancet 380:1703, 2012.
47. Halperin JJ: Lyme disease: a multisystem infection that affects the nervous system. Continuum (Minneap Minn) 18:1338, 2012.
48. Biesiada G, Czepiel J, Leśniak MR, et al: Lyme disease: review. Arch Med Sci 8:978, 2012.
49. Ljøstad U, Mygland Å: Chronic Lyme; diagnostic and therapeutic challenges. Acta Neurol Scand Suppl 196:38, 2013.
50. Logigian EL: Peripheral nervous system Lyme borreliosis. Semin Neurol 17:25, 1997.

51. Miklossy J: Chronic or late Lyme neuroborreliosis: analysis of evidence compared to chronic or late neurosyphilis. Open Neurol J 6:146, 2012.
52. Spiegel DR, Morris K, Rayamajhi U: Neurosarcoidosis and the complexity in its differential diagnoses: a review. Innov Clin Neurosci 9:10, 2012.
53. Vargas DL, Stern BJ: Neurosarcoidosis: diagnosis and management. Semin Respir Crit Care Med 31:419, 2010.
54. Hook EW, Marra CM: Acquired syphilis in adults. N Engl J Med 326:1060, 1992.
55. Mattei PL, Beachkofsky TM, Gilson RT, et al: Syphilis: a reemerging infection. Am Fam Physician 86:433, 2012.
56. Chahine LM, Khoriaty RN, Tomford WJ, et al: The changing face of neurosyphilis. Stroke 6:136, 2011.
57. Marra C: Update on Neurosyphilis. Curr Infect Dis Rep 11:127, 2009.
58. Pan D, Hirose T: Vogt-Koyanagi-Harada syndrome: review of clinical features. Semin Ophthalmol 26:312, 2011.
59. Krause I, Weinberger A: Behçet's disease. Curr Opin Rheumatol 20:82, 2008.
60. Chang HK, Cheon KS: The clinical significance of a pathergy reaction in patients with Behçet's disease. J Korean Med Sci 17:371, 2002.
61. International Study Group for Behcet's Disease: Criteria for diagnosis of Behcet's disease. Lancet 335:1078, 1990.
62. Alpsoy E, Zouboulis CC, Ehrlich GE: Mucocutaneous lesions of Behcet's disease. Yonsei Med J 48:573, 2007.
63. Gurler A, Boyvat A, Tursen U: Clinical manifestations of Behçet's disease: an analysis of 2147 patients. Yonsei Med J 38:423, 1997.
64. Hirohata S, Kikuchi H, Sawada T, et al: Clinical characteristics of neuro-Behcet's disease in Japan: a multicenter retrospective analysis. Mod Rheumatol 22:405, 2012.
65. Al-Araji A, Kidd DP: Neuro-Behçet's disease: epidemiology, clinical characteristics, and management. Lancet Neurol 8:192, 2009.
66. Akman-Demir G, Serdaroglu P, Tasçi B, et al: Clinical patterns of neurological involvement in Behçet's disease: evaluation of 200 patients. Brain 122:2171, 1999.
67. Noel N, Hutié M, Wechsler B, et al: Pseudotumoural presentation of neuro-Behcet's disease: case series and review of literature. Rheumatology (Oxford) 51:1216, 2012.
68. Petri M, Orbai AM, Alarcón GS, et al: Derivation and validation of the Systemic Lupus International Collaborating Clinics classification criteria for systemic lupus erythematosus. Arthritis Rheum 64:2677, 2012.
69. Meszaros ZS, Perl A, Faraone SV: Psychiatric symptoms in systemic lupus erythematosus: a systematic review. J Clin Psychiatry 73:993, 2012.
70. Muscal E, Brey RL: Neurologic manifestations of systemic lupus erythematosus in children and adults. Neurol Clin 28:61, 2010.
71. Vincent A, Crino PB: Systemic and neurologic autoimmune disorders associated with seizures or epilepsy. Epilepsia 52(suppl 3):12, 2011.
72. Baizabal-Carvallo JF, Alonso-Juarez M, Koslowski M: Chorea in systemic lupus erythematosus. J Clin Rheumatol 17:69, 2011.
73. Dhillon A, Velazquez C, Siva C: Rheumatologic diseases and posterior reversible encephalopathy syndrome: two case reports and review of the literature. Rheumatol Int 32:3707, 2012.
74. Kessler CS, Khan BA, Lai-Miller K: Thrombotic thrombocytopenic purpura: a hematological emergency. J Emerg Med 43:538, 2012.
75. Osborn JD, Rodgers GM: Update on thrombotic thrombocytopenic purpura. Clin Adv Hematol Oncol 9:531, 2011.
76. Le Goff C, Cormier-Daire V: The ADAMTS(L) family and human genetic disorders. Hum Mol Genet 20:R163, 2011.
77. Rund D, Schaap T, Gillis S: Intensive plasmapheresis for severe thrombotic thrombocytopenic purpura: long-term clinical outcome. J Clin Apheresis 12:194, 1997.
78. Kiss JE: Thrombotic thrombocytopenic purpura: recognition and management. Int J Hematol 91:36, 2010.
79. Puy H, Gouya L, Deybach JC: Porphyrias. Lancet 375:924, 2010.
80. Simon NG, Herkes GK: The neurologic manifestations of the acute porphyrias. J Clin Neurosci 18:1147, 2011.
81. Weidenheim KM, Dickson DW, Rapin I: Neuropathology of Cockayne syndrome: evidence for impaired development, premature aging, and neurodegeneration. Mech Ageing Dev 130:619, 2009.
82. Dereure O, Marque M, Guillot B: Premature aging syndromes: from phenotype to gene. Ann Dermatol Venereol 135:466, 2008.
83. Knoch J, Kamenisch Y, Kubisch C, et al: Rare hereditary diseases with defects in DNA-repair. Eur J Dermatol 22:443, 2012.
84. Hoche F, Seidel K, Theis M, et al: Neurodegeneration in ataxia telangiectasia: what is new? What is evident? Neuropediatrics 43:119, 2012.
85. Tan IL, McArthur JC: HIV-associated neurological disorders: a guide to pharmacotherapy. CNS Drugs 26:123, 2012.
86. Harrison TB, Smith B: Neuromuscular manifestations of HIV/AIDS. J Clin Neuromuscul Dis 13:68, 2011.
87. Tan IL, Smith BR, von Geldern G, et al: HIV-associated opportunistic infections of the CNS. Lancet Neurol 11:605, 2012.
88. Hurko O, Provost TT: Neurology and the skin. J Neurol Neurosurg Psychiatry 66:417, 1999.

89. Lo W, Marchuk DA, Ball KL, et al: Updates and future horizons on the understanding, diagnosis, and treatment of Sturge-Weber syndrome brain involvement. Dev Med Child Neurol 54:214, 2012.
90. Minić S, Trpinac D, Obradović M: Systematic review of central nervous system anomalies in incontinentia pigmenti. Orphanet J Rare Dis 8:25, 2013.
91. Chan JW: Neuro-ophthalmic features of the neurocutaneous syndromes. Int Ophthalmol Clin 52:73, 2012.
92. Björkhem I, Hansson M: Cerebrotendinous xanthomatosis: an inborn error in bile acid synthesis with defined mutations but still a challenge. Biochem Biophys Res Commun 396:46, 2010.
93. Pilo-de-la-Fuente B, Jimenez-Escrig A, Lorenzo JR, et al: Cerebrotendinous xanthomatosis in Spain: clinical, prognostic, and genetic survey. Eur J Neurol 18:1203, 2011.
94. Dotti MT, Federico A, Signorini E, et al: Cerebrotendinous xanthomatosis (van Bogaert-Scherer-Epstein disease): CT and MR findings. AJNR Am J Neuroradiol 15:1721, 1994.
95. Sannegowda RB, Agrawal A, Hemrajani D, et al: 'Hot cross bun' sign in a case of cerebrotendinous xanthomatosis: a rare neuroimaging observation. BMJ Case Rep pii:bcr2012006641, 2013.
96. Baldwin EJ, Gibberd FB, Harley C, et al: The effectiveness of long-term dietary therapy in the treatment of adult Refsum disease. J Neurol Neurosurg Psychiatry 81:954, 2010.
97. Camargo SM, Bockenhauer D, Kleta R: Aminoacidurias: clinical and molecular aspects. Kidney Int 73:918, 2008.
98. Bröer S: The role of the neutral amino acid transporter B0AT1 (SLC6A19) in Hartnup disorder and protein nutrition. IUBMB Life 61:591, 2009.
99. Cellerini M, Gabbrielli S, Bongi SM, et al: MRI of cerebral rheumatoid pachymeningitis: report of two cases with follow-up. Neuroradiology 43:147, 2001.
100. Naranjo A, Carmona L, Gavrila D, et al: Prevalence and associated factors of anterior atlantoaxial luxation in a nation-wide sample of rheumatoid arthritis patients. Clin Exp Rheumatol 22:427, 2004.
101. Casey AT, Crockard HA, Geddes JF, et al: Vertical translocation: the enigma of the disappearing atlantodens interval in patients with myelopathy and rheumatoid arthritis. Part I. Clinical, radiological, and neuropathological features. J Neurosurg 87:856, 1997.
102. Chai J, Logigian EL: Neurological manifestations of primary Sjogren's syndrome. Curr Opin Neurol 23:509, 2010.
103. Font J, Ramos-Casals M, de la Red G, et al: Pure sensory neuropathy in primary Sjögren's syndrome. Long term prospective followup and review of the literature. J Rheumatol 30:1552, 2003.
104. Grant IA, Hunder GG, Homburger HA, et al: Peripheral neuropathy associated with sicca complex. Neurology 48:855, 1997.
105. Hermisson M, Klein R, Schmidt F, et al: Myelopathy in primary Sjögren's syndrome: diagnostic and therapeutic aspects. Acta Neurol Scand 105:450, 2002.
106. Miró J, Peña-Sagredo JL, Bercano J, et al: Prevalence of primary Sjögren's syndrome in patients with multiple sclerosis. Ann Neurol 27:582, 1990.
107. Rodrigues LC, Lockwood DN: Leprosy now: epidemiology, progress, challenges, and research gaps. Lancet Infect Dis 11:464, 2011.
108. World Health Organization: Leprosy update, 2011. Wkly Epidemiol Rec 86:389, 2011.
109. Richardus JH, Finlay KM, Croft RP, et al: Nerve function impairment at diagnosis and at completion of MDT: a retrospective cohort study of 786 patients in Bangladesh. Lepr Rev 67:297, 1996.
110. Hughes M, Herrick A: Systemic sclerosis. Br J Hosp Med (Lond) 73:509, 2012.
111. Hietaharju A, Jääskeläinen S, Kalimo H, et al: Peripheral neuromuscular manifestations of systemic sclerosis (scleroderma). Muscle Nerve 16:1204, 1993.
112. Hietaharju A, Jääskeläinen S, Hietarinta M, et al: Central nervous system involvement and psychiatric manifestations in systemic sclerosis (scleroderma): clinical and neurophysiological evaluation. Acta Neurol Scand 87:382, 1993.
113. Heron E, Hernigou A, Chatellier G, et al: Intracerebral calcification in systemic sclerosis. Stroke 30:2183, 1999.
114. Marzano AV, Vezzoli P, Berti E: Skin involvement in cutaneous and systemic vasculitis. Autoimmun Rev 12:467, 2013.
115. Collins MP: The vasculitic neuropathies: an update. Curr Opin Neurol 25:573, 2012.
116. Stone JH: Polyarteritis nodosa. JAMA 288:1632, 2002.
117. Abril A: Churg-Strauss syndrome: an update. Curr Rheumatol Rep 13:489, 2011.
118. deGroot K, Schmidt DK, Arlt AC, et al: Standardized neurologic evaluations of 128 patients with Wegener granulomatosis. Arch Neurol 58:1215, 2001.
119. Zaba LC, Fiorentino DF: Skin disease in dermatomyositis. Curr Opin Rheumatol 24:597, 2013.
120. Ernste FC, Reed AM: Idiopathic inflammatory myopathies: current trends in pathogenesis, clinical features, and up-to-date treatment recommendations. Mayo Clin Proc 88:83, 2013.

SECTION

VI

Bone and Joint Disease

CHAPTER

22

Neurologic Disorders Associated with Bone and Joint Disease

ANN NOELLE PONCELET ■ ANDREW P. ROSE-INNES

The brain, spinal cord, cranial nerves, and spinal roots share an intimate anatomic relationship to the spine and skull; as a result, disorders of the skeletal system may result in neurologic compromise. This broad group of conditions includes congenital malformations as well as degenerative, metabolic, traumatic, neoplastic, infectious, and inflammatory disorders of the bones and joints. The craniosynostoses (premature closure of the cranial sutures) are covered in major texts of pediatric neurology and are not addressed here. The neurologic complications of trauma and neoplastic involvement of bone are covered in other chapters. The neurologic complications of rheumatoid arthritis and some additional connective tissue disorders are discussed separately in Chapter 50.

DEGENERATIVE DISEASE OF THE SPINE

Degenerative disease of the spine includes changes to both the intervertebral discs and the vertebrae ("spondylosis") that in general become more common with age. The lifelong mechanical stress sustained by the highly mobile cervical spine and the somewhat less mobile, weight-bearing lumbar spine accounts for the preponderance of degeneration in these two regions. Spinal degeneration may be entirely asymptomatic or may cause back or neck pain, referred pain, radiculopathy, or myelopathy. Degenerative spinal disease is commonly found on imaging of asymptomatic older adults.[1,2]

The intervertebral discs change in composition and structure with age.[3] From the second decade onward, disc degeneration and its consequent clinical manifestations become more frequent. Concomitant degeneration of the bony elements of the spine also occurs, including "lipping" of the superior and inferior margins of the vertebral bodies, the formation of osteophytes, osteoarthritic changes of the facet joints (subluxation, osteophytosis, and cartilaginous changes), narrowing of the intervertebral disc spaces, hypertrophy of the ligamentum flavum, instability of adjacent vertebrae with spondylolisthesis (anteroposterior slippage of one vertebra on an adjacent one), and narrowing of the lateral recess and intervertebral foramina.[4]

Encroachment of bone or disc may compromise the spinal roots or the spinal cord, resulting in radiculopathy or myelopathy, respectively. Inflammatory mechanisms resulting from exposure of the normally immunologically sequestrated nucleus pulposus, in addition to simple mechanical compression, contribute to the development of radicular symptoms and signs.[5] Although plain radiography of the spine may occasionally identify a vertebral fracture or other focal bony pathologic process, it is not an adequate screening investigation for patients with neurologic compromise.[6] Spinal computed tomography (CT) provides detailed views of the bony components of the spine and, when paired with myelography, may demonstrate encroachment onto the thecal space.[7] Spinal magnetic resonance imaging (MRI) is the modality of choice for demonstrating disc and other soft tissue anatomy; MRI can clearly show compression of the roots and spinal cord and does not expose the patient to ionizing radiation.

Electromyography (EMG) provides additional, complementary information that helps to distinguish radiculopathy from more peripheral pathology, localize involvement to individual nerve roots, and suggest whether the underlying pathophysiology relates to axonal or demyelinating injury.

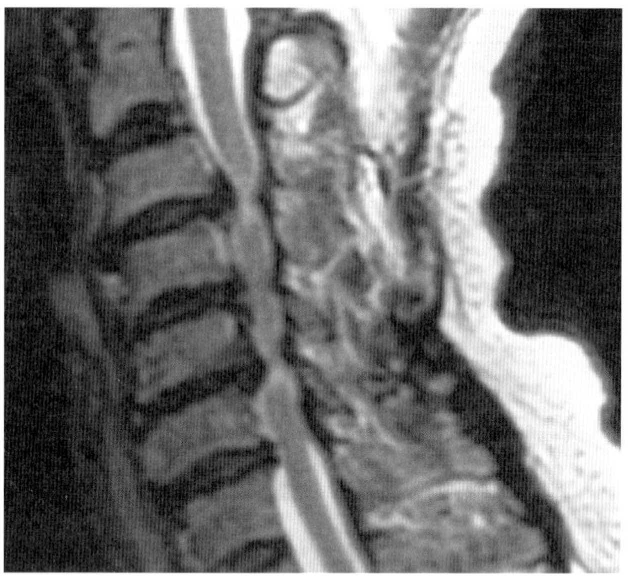

FIGURE 22-1 ■ Cervical spondylosis. Sagittal T2-weighted magnetic resonance imaging (MRI) of the cervical spine. Multilevel spondylotic disease with spinal stenosis and signal changes in the spinal cord are indicative of myelopathic injury.

Cervical Spondylosis and Disc Disease

In addition to disc degeneration and vertebral spondylosis, the contribution of a congenitally narrow spinal canal, buckling of the ligamentum flavum with neck extension, formation of compressive spondylotic "bars," and ischemic factors have all been proposed as mechanisms leading to neural injury (Figs. 22-1 and 22-2).

Several aspects of the anatomy of this region are important to appreciate: eight pairs of cervical nerve roots are arranged such that a root exits *above* its respective vertebra after leaving its segmental origin in the spinal cord. A lateral disc herniation at the C5–C6 level, for example, will tend to compromise the C6 root. This is the most common level of cervical radicular involvement, followed in order by a herniation at C6–C7 (C7 root) and at C4–C5 (C5 root).

The clinical manifestations of cervical spondylosis can include midline pain over the spine, limited range of movement, referred pain to the ipsilateral neck and arm (often made worse with coughing, straining, or particular positions of the head), and radiculomyelopathy. An acute root injury may occasionally result from rapid movement of the neck with sudden disc herniation or manifest with a less-abrupt onset more often due to progressive foraminal stenosis secondary to spondylosis. Pain tends to be a prominent early symptom, and is often sharp, radiating to a particular dermatome in association with numbness and paresthesias; weakness occurs when motor roots are involved. Corresponding motor, sensory, and reflex changes are found on examination. Single-level disease is seen in 15 to 40 percent of patients, and multilevel disease occurs in 60 to 80 percent.[8]

Cervical myelopathy tends to be a chronic, progressive process, but it may occasionally be abrupt in onset and catastrophic in severity. There are few data to indicate how often cervical spondylotic radiculopathy is eventually associated with myelopathy. Compression of the spinal cord is often heralded by difficulty in walking and may be followed by sensory loss in the lower limbs and the development of urinary frequency and nocturia. Lhermitte sign may be present. "Numb, clumsy hands" is an unusual symptom complex resulting from upper cord compression.

The natural history of cervical radiculomyelopathy is poorly documented. Good recovery of function frequently follows root injury, especially with a purely demyelinating radiculopathy, from which full recovery within weeks may be expected. Even after partial axonal injury, considerable reinnervation occurs in time. The course of untreated

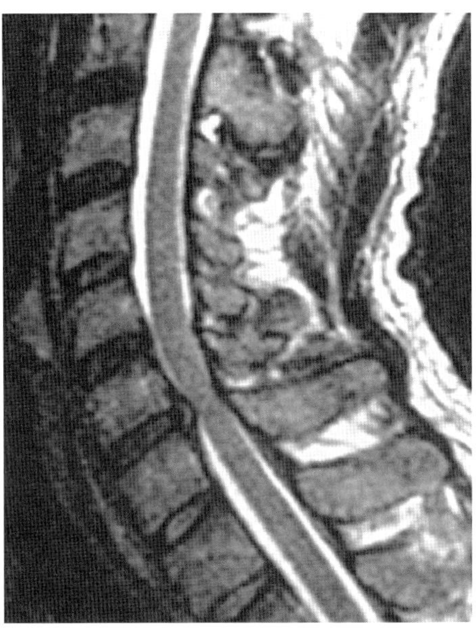

FIGURE 22-2 ■ Cervical disc disease. Sagittal T2-weighted MRI of the cervical spine. A herniated cervical disc is seen to compress the thecal sac at the C6–C7 level.

cervical myelopathy varies considerably. Slowly progressive worsening is common, but the myelopathy may remain static for years, improve with conservative measures, or progress rapidly.

Treatment of radiculopathy varies widely, and there is no universally agreed standard of care. Surgery is frequently performed for a variety of indications, despite a lack of large-scale controlled trials comparing surgical and nonsurgical outcomes.[9,10] A 2010 systematic review found only a single acceptable randomized study of surgery compared with conservative measures.[11] In view of the generally favorable prognosis for recovery of radiculopathy, it is reasonable to embark first on a trial of conservative treatment (limited rest, soft collar, analgesics, anti-inflammatory medications, muscle relaxants) in all patients except those with documented axonal radiculopathy accompanied by progressive muscle weakness.[8,12] The utility of oral corticosteroids and cervical traction is based only on anecdotal evidence and these treatment modalities are probably best avoided. The role of local corticosteroid injection is not clearly established; temporary symptomatic relief is often achieved, but it probably has little influence on the ultimate outcome and is not free of complications.[13] The most commonly performed surgery is anterior cervical discectomy and fusion. The role of disc replacement is as yet unclear. In general, surgery is indicated when clinical and electrodiagnostic findings are congruent with radiologic abnormalities, and either a progressive motor deficit or unremitting pain persists despite an adequate trial of conservative therapy. Established myelopathy is usually regarded as a firm indication for discectomy and decompressive laminectomy, with or without fusion; clinical improvement or arrest of progression usually follows, but some 15 to 20 percent of patients continue to deteriorate despite surgery.[14,15]

Lumbar Disc Disease

Around 80 percent of the adult population will have a functionally significant episode of low back pain over a lifetime; a subset of this group will have discogenic disease. Middle-aged men are most frequently affected. Disc herniation is seen less often in the elderly, probably as a consequence of a less mobile lifestyle and the gradual replacement of the disc material with fibrocartilage. Lumbar spine disease (Fig. 22-3) is frequently an asymptomatic finding on imaging, but it may produce a range of symptoms including low backache, locally referred pain, radiating radicular pain ("sciatica"), a radicular neurologic deficit, or some combination of these symptoms. The clinical onset may be spontaneous or associated with an episode of mechanical stress. A flexed posture or a transient increase in the pressure gradient across the dura (e.g., by coughing or sneezing) may exacerbate symptoms.

The site of disc pathology may be marked by local tenderness to palpation or percussion over the spinous processes. The patient may adopt a fixed posture, often tilted away from the affected side, and resist movement. Lumbosacral root or sciatic nerve involvement is suggested when passive hip flexion with the leg extended at the knee reproduces the patient's usual back or leg pain. When radiculopathy is present, the pattern of neurologic deficit will allow identification of the affected root.

Most lumbar disc pathology involves the L4–L5 and L5–S1 interspaces. Disc abnormalities at L1–L2, L2–L3, and L3–L4 are rare, accounting for less than 5 percent of patients. Lumbar disc protrusions are most often posterolateral and affect either descending or exiting nerve roots; they typically cannot result in myelopathy because the spinal cord ends above the L1–L2 interspace. The roots are posterolaterally located at the intervertebral foramen

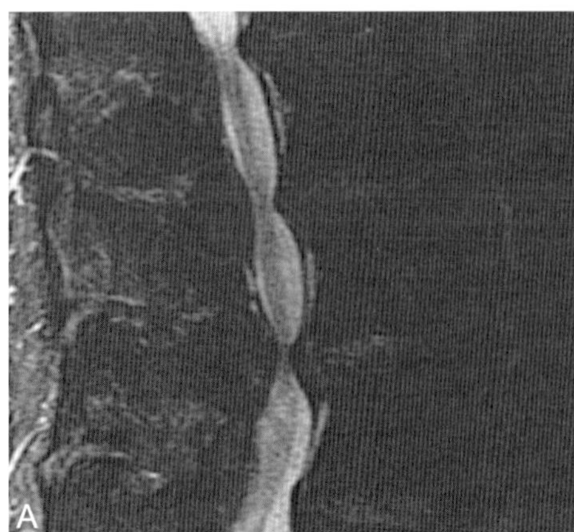

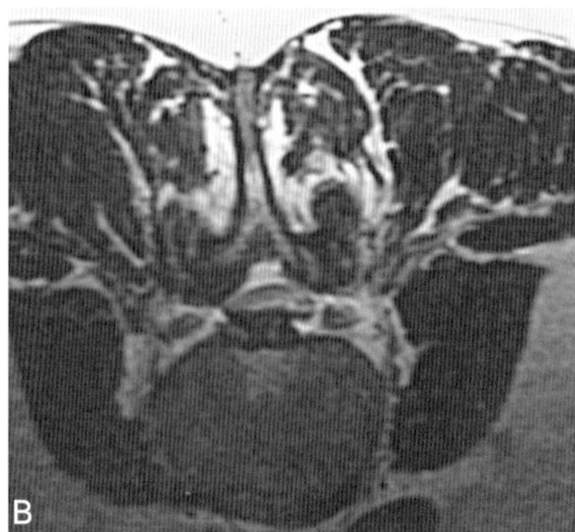

FIGURE 22-3 ■ Degenerative disease of the lumbar spine with spinal stenosis. Sagittal (**A**) and axial (**B**) T2-weighted MRI of the lumbar spine. Multilevel discogenic disease is apparent in the lumbar spine on the sagittal view. Disc material is seen compressing the anterior aspect of the thecal sac on the axial image.

and pass through this aperture in a superior position; therefore a disc protruding at the same level will tend to pass underneath the root exiting at the same interspace, often compressing the root of the segment immediately below. An L4–L5 disc, for example, will usually compromise the L5 root and leave the L4 root unaffected. There are exceptions to this rule—clinical assessment should always allow that a nerve root can be compromised at any point in its intraspinal course.

A large central disc may produce bilateral radicular signs or occasionally result in acute cauda equina syndrome characterized by flaccid paralysis, lower-limb areflexia, or urinary and fecal incontinence. Acute cauda equina syndrome is a surgical emergency and, even when managed promptly, carries a poor prognosis for neurologic recovery.[16] Chronic lumbar canal stenosis may lead to neurogenic claudication (see later).

The differential diagnosis for these symptoms is wide. For patients who present with acute (duration of less than 3 months) low back pain, the emphasis of the initial assessment is on exclusion of serious underlying pathology. Neoplastic, infectious, and traumatic causes are important to identify and require specific treatment. Otherwise, conservative measures (limited bed rest, regular graded exercise, analgesic and anti-inflammatory treatment, physical therapy, and the use of local corticosteroid injections in selected patients) without further investigation represent the most appropriate initial management.[17–19] When there is no improvement, further investigation is indicated.

The natural history of uncomplicated lumbar disc disease is usually one of eventual disc resorption with improvement of symptoms. Despite this generally good prognosis, lumbar disc surgery represents the most common elective surgical procedure involving the nervous system. The traditional approach is resection of the intervertebral disk and fusion of the vertebrae above and below. Other approaches include intervertebral disk replacement and intradiscal electrotherapy , but their role is yet to be established.[20] Surgery is indicated when a motor deficit (by clinical examination or EMG) is worsening despite conservative management. There is much debate regarding the efficacy of surgery for other patients, and few prospective data are available to help predict which patients are likely to be successfully treated.[21]

LUMBAR SPINAL STENOSIS AND NEUROGENIC CLAUDICATION

Stenosis of the lumbar spinal canal is frequently asymptomatic and found incidentally on imaging studies. Boden and colleagues found that 21 percent of asymptomatic adults older than 60 years had lumbar spinal stenosis on MRI.[1] Such narrowing may, however, be associated with symptoms including low back pain and neurogenic claudication of the cauda equina, which classically is described as discomfort and aching pain in the lower back, buttocks, and legs that is precipitated by walking and relieved by sitting.[22] Patients may experience numbness, paresthesias, or a sense of weakness in the legs, usually bilaterally and asymmetrically. Up to 11 percent of patients present with bladder and sexual dysfunction. Sitting for some time will usually relieve symptoms sufficiently to allow further walking. Relief of symptoms with flexion of the spine is the reason that it is often easier to walk up an incline than on a level surface. Neurogenic claudication is usually of gradual onset and, once established, results in symptoms that may become disabling, but tends not to be associated with progressive neurologic deficits.

The pathogenesis is incompletely understood. Venous pooling with exercise in the stenotic canal may lead to intermittent ischemic neurapraxia of the cauda equina with transient conduction failure and clinical and electrophysiologic changes.[23] The anatomic substrate is most commonly that of progressive, chronic, degenerative lumbar spine disease on a background of a congenitally narrow lumbar spinal canal.[24] Extension of the spine decreases, and flexion increases, the caliber of the spinal canal. Diagnosis requires recognition of the highly characteristic history together with radiologic evidence of lumbar spinal stenosis. Electrodiagnostic studies may show prolongation of minimum F-wave and H-reflex latencies, but are mainly useful to document associated radiculopathy.[25,26] Vascular claudication may be confused with neurogenic claudication but typically causes burning pain in the calves when walking and is usually accompanied by evidence of circulatory insufficiency in the legs. A variety of other neurologic conditions may occasionally produce pseudoclaudication: these include multiple sclerosis and spinal cord arteriovenous malformation.[27]

Many patients with lumbar spinal stenosis find that they can remain mobile within the specific constraints of their symptoms. Surgery aims to relieve symptoms and improve function. Of patients initially opting for conservative therapy, about 30 percent will eventually elect to have surgery.[28] Surgery likely benefits some patients, but the literature provides few controlled data comparing it with conservative treatment.[29,30] Decompressive laminectomy at one or several levels is typically performed with discectomy or simple foraminotomy, with or without fusion.[21] Surgery is warranted if neurogenic claudication is progressive, significantly limits activities of daily living, or becomes intolerable. Fusion is more frequently employed when there is associated spondylolisthesis.[31] Interspinous decompression with placement of a device between the spinous processes, preventing narrowing of the canal with extension, is a technique that is sometimes employed.[32,33] Medical treatment of lumbar spinal stenosis may include limited bed rest, anti-inflammatory and analgesic medication, and physical therapy. Murakami and co-workers found that lipoprostaglandin E_1 increased cauda equina blood flow and relieved symptoms in a small series.[34]

OSTEOPOROSIS

Osteoporosis is a disorder characterized by low bone mass and micro-architectural deterioration of bone tissue, leading to enhanced bone fragility and consequent increase in fracture risk. It is the most common bone disease; approximately 52 million Americans have osteoporosis or osteopenia.[35] One half of Caucasian women and around 20 percent of Caucasian men will experience an osteoporotic fracture.[36] Any neurologic disorder that impairs strength or balance leading to decreased mobility and an increased risk of falls is a risk factor for osteoporosis (Table 22-1). Patients with spinal cord injury are particularly prone to severe osteoporosis and nontraumatic fractures. Neurologic patients share common risk factors with elderly patients for osteoporosis, such as disuse and lack of exercise, being homebound, vitamin D deficiency, and poor diet. There is growing interest in "neuroskeletal research" of the central nervous system (CNS) regulation of bone remodeling.[37] Leptin is a peptide secreted by adipocytes that regulates appetite and energy metabolism by binding to a hypothalamic

TABLE 22-1 ■ Neurologic Diseases Associated with Osteoporosis and Increased Fracture Risk

Alzheimer disease	Amyotrophic lateral sclerosis
Parkinson disease	Poliomyelitis
Spinal cord injury	Muscular dystrophy
Epilepsy and anticonvulsant use	Glycogen storage diseases
Stroke and anticoagulant use (heparin)	Gaucher disease
Multiple sclerosis	Menkes steely hair syndrome
	Riley–Day syndrome

leptin receptor. Its effect on bone formation is through induction of the sympathetic nervous system. Osteoblasts in the bone marrow reside next to sympathetic neurons and express β_2-adrenergic receptors; catecholamines increase osteoblast proliferation and differentiation (bone formation) and increase bone resorption, with a resulting decrease in bone mass. There also is evidence of a circadian variation for bone remodeling.

The spine is the most frequent osteoporotic fracture site, accounting for approximately 650,000 clinically detected fractures annually. In the United States, 25 percent of women older than 70 and 50 percent of women older than 80 have evidence of vertebral fractures.[38] Low thoracic and high lumbar vertebral fractures are the most common. There is a 10-fold increased risk of a second vertebral fracture in these patients. About 25 percent of vertebral fractures occur from falls, but the majority are triggered by trivial activity such as bending, lifting a light object, or getting out of bed.

Most vertebral fractures are painless and only around 30 percent come to medical attention. Less than 10 percent result in hospital admission.[39] Symptomatic patients usually present with acute low back pain that is often localized to the site of the fracture, but can be diffuse and nonlocalizing. Radiating pain into the lower extremities is uncommon and usually does not correspond to a specific lumbar root pattern. Straining and local percussion typically increase the pain. The patient may not be able to bear weight initially, and symptoms often improve when lying down. There are typically no neurologic symptoms or signs.

Plain radiographs of the spine are the study of choice to document the presence of vertebral fracture. The most widely accepted radiologic definition of vertebral compression-fracture is a decrease of 15 to 25 percent in the anterior, central, or posterior height of a vertebral body compared with adjacent normal vertebrae or a population reference.[38] The diagnosis can be confirmed by bone scan or CT when radiographs are equivocal.

The optimal treatment of acute osteoporotic vertebral fractures without neurologic compromise is uncertain. Prolonged bed rest may accelerate the underlying osteoporosis, so analgesics, local heat alternating with cold application, and mobilization with physical therapy and hydrotherapy are recommended.[36,38] Rigid external support can prevent failed union of severe vertebral fractures when used in the first 6 months.[40] Narcotics are occasionally required for pain, and calcitonin may provide relief in the acute phase. With persistent pain, an intercostal nerve block or epidural corticosteroid injection may be helpful.[38] Vertebroplasty is a technique involving injecting polymethylmethacrylate into a fractured vertebral body; compared to conservative treatment, it shows greater pain relief, functional recovery, and health-related quality of life.[41] Asymptomatic cement leaks are a potential side effect, and uncommon severe adverse events include radiculopathy due to cement leakage and osteomyelitis. Vertebral body stenting with an expandable metallic implant is another minimally invasive technique that may help preserve vertebral body height and prevent spinal deformity with a lower cement leakage rate.[42]

Preventive treatments for osteoporosis play an increasing role in reducing the number of vertebral fractures in postmenopausal women and the elderly. Detailed recommendations for evidence-based osteoporosis prevention including exercise (weight bearing and muscle strengthening), calcium and vitamin D supplementation, bisphosphonates, hormone replacement, selective estrogen-receptor modulators, desosumab, and teriparatide are summarized elsewhere.[35,36]

The association between vertebral fractures and chronic back pain is unclear. In patients with osteoporosis and vertebral fractures, the presence and severity of back pain correlate with the number of collapsed thoracic vertebrae and the degree of kyphosis. Neurologic complications are uncommon and include myelopathy, cauda equina syndrome, and lumbosacral radiculopathy. Spinal CT or MRI reveals violation of the posterior cortex of the vertebral bodies (burst fracture) with retropulsion of bone into the spinal canal.[43] The most common location is the thoracolumbar junction. Lower-extremity symptoms may develop from 10 days to 1.5 years after the onset of acute spine pain, owing to extension of vertebral fracture.[43–45] The etiology is thought to be late collapse of the vertebral body due to disruption of the microcirculation and aseptic necrosis.[45] Severe kyphosis may be a risk factor for progression of vertebral fracture and neurologic compromise.

The best operative approach for those with neurologic deficits is not known. Goals include improvement of the deficit, correction of the deformity, and stabilization of the spine. Clinical results are mixed, ranging from marked improvement to worsening of function with significant postoperative mortality.[43–47] The approach used is often guided by presence of intervertebral instability and the degree of kyphosis.[46] Postoperative bracing potentially can reduce the rate of instrumentation failure.[44] A small group of patients treated conservatively also has been found to experience significant recovery over months.[43]

Occasionally, patients with vertebral fracture have purely radicular symptoms, with pain radiating into the lower extremity that worsens with change in position or on standing. There may be dermatomal sensory loss and weakness in muscles referable to that root. A study of seven patients with radiculopathy following osteoporotic vertebral fracture who were not operative candidates showed substantial or complete resolution of symptoms following vertebroplasty.[48]

OSTEOMALACIA

Osteomalacia is a metabolic bone disorder characterized by defective mineralization, which results in the accumulation of unmineralized matrix or osteoid in the skeleton. Normal bone mineralization requires adequate circulating levels of vitamin D metabolites, a normal supply of minerals, and optimal osteoblast function.[49] The most common cause of osteomalacia is vitamin D deficiency.[49,50] Other causes are listed in Table 22-2.[49–51] Reduced cutaneous production of vitamin D is a concern in the elderly who are institutionalized or housebound, and in postmenopausal women. Increased time indoors, sunscreen, and the use of ultraviolet-protective glass and clothing contribute to hypovitaminosis D. Dark-skinned individuals require 4 to 5 times more sun exposure than light-skinned people. Dietary sources of vitamin D are limited (wild oily fish, egg yolk, cod-liver oil, and fortified food). Malabsorption results in decreased absorption of vitamin D, increased catabolism of vitamin D metabolites, and malabsorption of calcium or phosphate. Malabsorption from gastric bypass surgery for morbid obesity is emerging as a leading cause of vitamin D deficiency in the United States.[50]

TABLE 22-2 ■ Causes of Osteomalacia

Vitamin D Deficiency
Reduced cutaneous production
Poor nutrition
Malabsorption
Abnormal Vitamin D Metabolism
Liver disease
Drugs (anticonvulsants)
Hereditary defective 25-hydroxycholecalciferol synthesis
Defective 1,25-dihydroxycholecalciferol synthesis
Renal failure
Vitamin D–dependent rickets type I (1α-hydroxylase deficiency)
Resistance to the Action of Vitamin D
Vitamin D–dependent rickets type II
Hypophosphatemia
Phosphate-binding antacids
X-linked hypophosphatemia
Oncogenic osteomalacia
Fanconi syndrome
Renal tubular acidosis
Bone Toxins
Bisphosphonates
Aluminum
Fluoride
Hypophosphatasia
Fibrogenesis Imperfecta Ossium

The prevalence of low 25(OH)D levels (<20 ng/ml) is 36 percent in healthy young adults aged 18 to 29 years, 42 percent in black women aged 15 to 49 years, 41 percent in outpatients aged 49 to 83 years, and up to 57 percent in general medicine inpatients in the United States.[49] A study of nonelderly, ambulatory primary-care patients with persistent, nonspecific musculoskeletal pain refractory to standard pharmaceutical agents demonstrated hypovitaminosis D in 93 percent.[52] Current recommendations in North America are that all adults supplement with vitamin D3 600 IU/day and that those in at-risk groups or older than 70 years should take 800 IU/day.[53]

The classic clinical features of osteomalacia include musculoskeletal pain, skeletal deformity, muscle weakness, and symptomatic hypocalcemia.[49,50] The early symptoms are vague. Bone pain is invariably present, symmetric, and especially prominent in the spine, ribs, pelvis, and lower extremities. The pain is worse with muscle strain, weight bearing, or pressure, but persists with rest. Minimal pressure with the thumb or forefinger on the sternum, ribs, pelvic girdle, or anterior tibia can reproduce the pain on physical examination; it is postulated that collagen-rich osteoid deposited on the periosteal surface of the skeleton may become swollen, putting outward pressure on the periosteal covering that is innervated with nociceptors.[49] These patients are often misdiagnosed as having fibromyalgia, chronic fatigue syndrome, or myositis and treated inappropriately with nonsteroidal anti-inflammatory drugs (NSAIDs).

Proximal myopathy is common, occurring in 73 to 97 percent of patients, and weakness is the presenting complaint in 30 percent.[54,55] The limb-girdle muscles are the most affected and result in a waddling gait, Gower sign, or inability to walk.[50] The proximal upper extremities and neck flexors are occasionally involved; distal weakness is rare, and bulbar and sphincter muscles are spared. Weakness is accompanied by myalgias and muscle atrophy, although the atrophy is often out of proportion to the degree of weakness.[50] There is no known direct effect of vitamin D on muscle, but an animal model of osteomalacia relates the degree of weakness to hypophosphatemia.[56] Deep tendon reflexes are often brisk and the combination of weakness, atrophy, and hyperreflexia can be mistaken for amyotrophic lateral sclerosis. Vitamin D deficiency may contribute to age-related muscle weakness and falls; a meta-analysis of randomized controlled trials of vitamin D supplementation for elderly ambulatory and institutionalized individuals showed a greater than 20 percent reduction in risk of falls.[57] Other studies exploring vitamin D levels and fall risk also support the role of osteomalacia-associated myopathy in elderly patients.[49]

Osteomalacia in childhood results in rickets with short stature, bowing of the legs, and widening of the metaphyses, which leads to a "rickety rosary" appearance in the ribs. Premature closure of the sagittal cranial sutures may result in craniotabes, and hydrocephalus may occur in severe cases.

Vitamin D modulates the immune system by decreasing the proliferation of proinflammatory T lymphocytes and regulating the production of cytokines. There is an association between high vitamin D levels and a reduced risk of developing multiple sclerosis, but the impact of vitamin D levels on the severity and progression of multiple sclerosis remains unclear.[58] Supplementation in this population with 1000 IU/day is recommended to reach immune-modulating serum levels of vitamin D (30 ng/ml or 75 nmol/L).

Radiologic features of osteomalacia include cortical thinning of bone, cortical striations in the metacarpals and phalanges, and osteopenia.[50] The most characteristic feature is the presence of Looser zones, which are lucent bands adjacent to the periosteum that may represent unhealed stress fractures and most commonly occur in the ribs, pubic rami, and outer borders of the scapulae. Biochemical abnormalities may be minimal and vary with the cause of osteomalacia. A classic triad is hypocalcemia, hypophosphatemia, and increased serum alkaline phosphatase. Serum 25(OH)D is the major circulating metabolite of vitamin D and reflects input from cutaneous synthesis and dietary intake. A minimum level of 20 ng/ml (50 nmol/L) is necessary to satisfy the body's vitamin D requirement, but a level of 30 to 50 ng/ml (75 to 125 nmol/L) is preferred. Despite clinical evidence of myopathy, the serum creatine kinase level is typically normal.[55] Parathyroid hormone levels may be elevated. Hypocalcemia is usually present in osteomalacia associated with renal failure, but the serum phosphate is normal or high because of reduced urinary excretion.

EMG may be normal in patients with weakness but in around 65 to 85 percent of patients shows small, short-duration, polyphasic motor unit action potentials in proximal muscles, without abnormal spontaneous activity.[55] The findings on muscle biopsy are nonspecific and most often are of type II atrophy.[55,59]

Treatment of osteomalacia includes ultraviolet irradiation (UV-B wavelength of 290 to 315 nm) and vitamin D replacement.[49] An oral dose of 50,000 IU/week of vitamin D2 for 8 weeks, with monitoring of 25(OH)D and parathyroid hormone levels, should occur in those with vitamin D deficiency.[49,50] In some cases, a second once-weekly 8-week course of 50,000 IU of vitamin D2 may be necessary to boost 25(OH)D levels into the desired range of more than 30 to 50 ng/ml (75 to 125 nmol/L). For patients prone to developing vitamin D deficiency, after correction of any deficiency, the administration of 50,000 IU every 2 weeks will maintain a vitamin D-sufficient state. An alternative to vitamin D2 is vitamin D3 1000 IU/ day. Calcium and magnesium supplements are also recommended concurrently.[49] Complications of treatment are uncommon, but include hypercalcemia, renal dysfunction, and increased long bone and hip fractures as pain improves before bone mass and strength are restored. The bone pain, symptoms of hypocalcemia, and proximal weakness often resolve completely over weeks to months with treatment, but deformities persist despite remodeling of the bone.

Hypophosphatemic osteomalacia has different neurologic complications than other causes of osteomalacia. The most common form is an X-linked syndrome with hypophosphatemia, osteomalacia, short stature, and the eventual development of new bone at various body sites associated with mutations in the *PHEX* gene.[49,60] The proximal myopathy seen with other forms of osteomalacia does not occur. Rarely, myelopathy develops as a result of intraspinal new bone formation.[61] The mid- and low thoracic spine is the predominant site of involvement, but the cervical spine may also be affected. The onset of symptoms is acute or insidious with paresis, sensory loss, and, less frequently, bladder symptoms. Symptoms can be intermittent and involve multiple levels of the spinal cord, mimicking multiple sclerosis.[61] A rare autosomal dominant form is associated with a mutation of the fibroblast growth factor 23 gene (*FGF23*). The clinical features are similar to the X-linked form but there is variable penetrance with variable age of onset and it may resolve later in life.[60] An autosomal recessive form is defined by mutations in the dentin matrix protein 1 gene (*DMP1*).[60]

CT of the spine shows enlargement of the facet joints, thickening of the laminae, and ossification within the spinal canal, resulting in severe central stenosis.[61] Surgery is difficult due to thickening of the bone and adherence of the dura to the ligamentum flavum but can result in improvement or resolution of deficit.[61] Treatment includes an oral neutral phosphate along with 1,25-dihydroxyvitamin D (calcitriol). Excess vitamin D replacement can cause hypercalcemia leading to soft tissue calcification, and serum calcium levels should therefore be measured monthly. Diuretics such as amiloride or hydrochlorothiazide enhance calcium reabsorption and can reduce the risk of nephrocalcinosis.

TABLE 22-3 ■ Inheritance of Osteopetrosis

Disease	Inheritance	Gene	Protein
Malignant (infantile) form	AR	*TCIRG1*	Subunit of V-ATPase pump
	AR	*CLCN7*	Chloride channel
	AR	*OSTMI*	Osteopetrosis-associated transmembrane protein
	AR	*RANKL*	Receptor activator for nuclear factor κB ligand
	AR	*RANK*	Receptor activator for nuclear factor κB
Intermediate form	AR	*CLCN7*	Chloride channel
	AR	*PLIKHMI*	Pleckstrin homology domain containing family M, member I
Osteopetrosis with renal tubular acidosis	AR	*CAII*	Carbonic anhydrase II
Late-onset form	AD	*CLCN7*	Chloride channel
Asymptomatic (osteopoikilosis)	AD	*LEMD3*	LEM domain-containing 3
Osteopetrosis with ectodermal dysplasia and immune defect (OLEDAID)	X	*IKBKG*	Inhibitor of kappa light polypeptide gene enhancer, kinase of
Leukocyte adhesion deficiency syndrome and osteopetrosis (LAD-III)	AR	*Kindlin-3*	Kindlin-3
	AR	*ColDAG-GEFI*	Calcium and diacylglycerol-regulated guanine nucleotide exchange factor I

AD, autosomal dominant; AR, autosomal recessive; X, X-linked.

OSTEOPETROSIS

Osteopetrosis refers to a rare group of sclerosing bone disorders characterized by a generalized increase of skeletal bone mass due to a defect in osteoclastic bone resorption.[62,63] At least 10 genes have been identified that result in a failure of osteoclast development or function (Table 22-3).[62] In osteopetrosis, the development of the marrow cavity is delayed or absent, and impaired bone modeling during longitudinal growth results in a broad cylindrical shape at the ends of the long bones. These bones become brittle, with an increased susceptibility to fracture. Radiographic features include diffuse sclerosis, bone modeling defects at the metaphyses of long bones, "bone in bone" appearance of the vertebrae and phalanges, as well as focal sclerosis of the skull base, pelvis, and vertebral endplates. The most serious complications of the osteopetroses affect the nervous system and hematopoietic system. Cranial nerves, blood vessels, and the spinal cord are compressed by either gradual occlusion or lack of growth of skull foramina.[63] The severity of osteopetrosis ranges from neonatal onset with life-threatening complications to asymptomatic.

Malignant osteopetrosis presents during infancy and is the most common form of childhood osteopetrosis. The course is severe, with only 30 percent surviving to the age of 6 years without treatment.[63] Its incidence is approximately 1 in 300,000 births. Neurologic involvement occurs frequently and includes optic atrophy with blindness, nystagmus, strabismus, trigeminal neuropathies, facial paralysis, hearing loss (78%), dysarthria, hydrocephalus, intracranial hemorrhage, cognitive dysfunction, and tetanic convulsions.[63] Hydrocephalus is due to obstruction of the venous outflow at the cranial foramina and to inadequate circulation of cerebrospinal fluid (CSF) as a consequence of thickening of the bones of the skull. Cranial nerve involvement relates to bony encroachment, and may necessitate decompression of the optic, facial, or vestibulocochlear nerves.[64] Retinal degeneration has been described in some patients and is another cause of visual loss; the most frequent sign of early damage is a change in latency of the visual evoked potential.

Non-neurologic features include short stature, dental caries, and frequent fractures. The constricted bone marrow cavity cannot support adequate hematopoiesis, resulting in hepatosplenomegaly, thrombocytopenia, anemia, and infectious complications. Clinical symptoms respond to calcitriol, which enhances bone resorption; prednisone, which improves hematologic indices; and interferon-γ1b, which reduces the number of infections and increases bone resorption as well as the size of bone marrow spaces.[62] Calcium and vitamin D supplementation can prevent tetanic seizures. Bone marrow failure is treated with transfusions of red blood cells and platelets. Allogenic hematopoietic cell transplantation is currently the only therapy capable of producing long-term benefit in children and only with mutations of the *TGIRG1* gene. Early transplant (before 3 months) has been shown to limit neurosensory defects and impaired bone growth and results in reconstitution of normal hematopoiesis and neutrophil function.[65] Significant risks include a high frequency of graft rejection, veno-occlusive disease, and severe pulmonary hypertension.

Neuropathic autosomal-recessive osteopetrosis is a rare form with nontetanic seizures, developmental delay, hypotonia, retinal atrophy, and sensorineural deafness. There is primary neurodegeneration, and brain MRI abnormalities include delayed myelination, diffuse progressive cortical and subcortical atrophy, and bilateral atrial subependydmal heterotopias.[62]

Intermediate autosomal-recessive and autosomal-dominant osteopetroses have a less severe course and do not have neurologic complications with the uncommon exception of visual and hearing loss due to cranial nerve compression.

Carbonic anhydrase II deficiency (marble brain disease) is an autosomal-recessive disorder resulting in osteopetrosis, renal tubular acidosis, and cerebral calcification.[66,67] It presents in late infancy or early childhood with developmental delay, cognitive abnormalities, short stature, failure to thrive, a large cranial vault, weakness, cranial nerve compression, and a history of multiple fractures. Patients may have apathy, global hypotonia, or muscle weakness that may be explained by acidosis and diminished blood levels of potassium from renal tubular acidosis. Rarely, episodic hypokalemic weakness occurs. More than one half of all patients develop optic atrophy associated with reduced optic canal size on imaging.[67] Other cranial nerve deficits such as facial palsy and deafness are described in earlier, but not more recent, series.[67,68]

Metabolic abnormalities include a metabolic acidosis with a persistently positive urinary anion gap without renal failure. Anemia and splenomegaly may be present. Plain radiographs show increased density in the long bones, vertebral bodies, pelvis, and skull. Cranial CT or MRI shows thickened skulls with small or absent paranasal sinuses. Symmetric brain calcifications are present involving the basal ganglia, thalamus, gray-white junction (with a frontal lobe predilection), or some combinations of these sites.[67] The amount of calcification progresses over time but does not correlate with the degree of cognitive abnormalities in these patients. The diagnosis can be made through an erythrocyte assay or by molecular probes for carbonic anhydrase II. Prenatal diagnosis requires direct carbonic anhydrase II gene sequencing. Patients are treated for acidosis with bicarbonate and Na/K citrate. Although the impact of treatment on the natural progression of the bone and neurologic features is unclear, there may be some effect in delaying the development of hearing loss and extramedullary hematopoiesis.[67]

Infantile neuroaxonal dystrophy is a rare autosomal recessive disorder with widespread accumulation of neuroaxonal spheroids in the cortex, basal ganglia, brainstem, and spinal cord, which has been reported in association with osteopetrosis.[66] It presents during the first year of life with weakness, hypotonia, rigidity, pyramidal signs, diminished pain sensation, optic atrophy, and mental impairment, accompanied by hypocalcemia, hypomagnesemia, severe anemia, thrombocytopenia, hepatosplenomegaly, jaundice, and metabolic acidosis. Neuroimaging shows agenesis of the corpus callosum and ventriculomegaly. This form of osteopetrosis is fatal within the first year of life.

PAGET DISEASE OF BONE

Paget disease is a focal disorder of bone turnover in which there is excessive bone resorption coupled with abnormal new bone formation, resulting in architecturally disorganized and mechanically weak bone.[69] It has a predilection for the axial skeleton and involves the cervical spine in 14 percent, thoracic spine in 45 percent, lumbar spine in 58 percent, and skull in 42 percent of cases.[70] The prevalence (2.5%) increases with age, and the disorder is found primarily in Caucasians.[69] There is an autosomal-dominant inheritance in up to 40 percent of patients.[69,71] The etiology is incompletely understood but probably relates to a combination of genetic susceptibility and environmental factors, although the only disease-causing gene identified to date is sequestosome 1 (*SQSTM1*), found in one-third of affected families and 9 percent of sporadic cases.[71]

Most patients with Paget disease are asymptomatic.[70] The most common presentation in symptomatic patients is local bone pain coupled with overlying skin warmth due to increased bone microvasculature. The pain is continuous and worse at rest and at night. There may be obvious deformity of the bones, and skeletal complications include osteoarthritis, fractures, and sarcomatous changes.[70]

Plain radiographs may show lytic lesions early in the disease; as the disease progresses, a chaotic, crisscross pattern with thickened cortical and trabecular bone is seen, sometimes accompanied by pseudofractures. The most sensitive metabolic marker of Paget disease is total serum alkaline phosphatase, which is elevated in 95 percent of untreated patients.[70]

Treatment depends on the location and activity of the disease.[69,70] Asymptomatic patients usually do not require treatment, and pain is the only symptom for which there is proven benefit from treatment.[69] Bisphosphonates (e.g., alendronate, ibandronate, pamidronate, risedronate, and zoledronic acid) produce a marked and prolonged inhibition of osteoclast function and are currently the first-line therapy.[69–71] These agents reduce or normalize serum total alkaline phosphatase levels.

Neurologic involvement is rare and occurs as a result of the close anatomic relationship of bone with the brain, spinal cord, cauda equina, spinal roots, and cranial nerves.[72] Compression from expanding bones or fracture is the most common cause of neurologic dysfunction. Less common causes include ossification of extradural structures, osteosarcoma, and epidural hematoma. Ischemia of the nervous system may occur occasionally due to compression of vascular structures or a vascular steal phenomenon; measurement of skeletal blood flow demonstrates that the affected bone receives up to 18 percent of cardiac output compared with 5 percent in normal bone.[73]

Other neurologic complications of cranial disease include headache, epilepsy, dementia, brainstem and cerebellar dysfunction, and cranial neuropathies. Headache is severe, frequently occipital, and worsened by coughing, sneezing, or straining. Dementia may result from direct compression of the cerebral hemispheres or from hydrocephalus.[72] Epilepsy may occur from direct compression of the cerebral cortex.

In advanced cranial disease, there is softening of the skull base that can result in an anatomic lowering of the skull onto the upper cervical vertebrae (i.e., basilar invagination), leading to obstructive hydrocephalus and compression of the cerebellum, lower cranial nerves, corticospinal tract, and upper cervical nerves. The severity ranges from asymptomatic to tonsillar herniation and death. The typical presentation is that of slowly progressive ataxia, vertigo, tinnitus, dysphagia, dysarthria, and occipital headache. Vertebrobasilar insufficiency as well as obstructed venous return may lead to cerebrovascular compromise. An unusual picture resembling amyotrophic lateral sclerosis sometimes occurs in association with cervical cord involvement.

Any of the cranial nerves may be affected with Paget disease, but the olfactory and auditory nerves are involved most commonly. Hearing loss is common, occurring in 37 percent of patients.[74] It may be neuronal, conductive, or of mixed type. The cochlea is the most common site of involvement. The optic nerve may be affected at the optic foramen by compression of the vasa nervorum; patients present with diminished vision or blindness, retinal hemorrhages, choroiditis, optic atrophy, papilledema, and angioid streaks.[72] The nerves controlling eye movements are vulnerable as they pass through the superior orbital fissure, leading to diplopia and abnormal pupillary responses. Exophthalmos from direct impingement of the extraocular muscles themselves occurs rarely. Trigeminal nerve involvement can lead to facial numbness and trigeminal neuralgia. Involvement of the facial nerve may result in hemifacial spasm or facial paresis with a frequency of 8 percent.[74]

Osteosarcoma of the skull occurs in less than 1 percent of patients with Paget disease.[75] It usually presents as a partially fluctuant and locally painful skull mass with rapid neurologic deterioration in the setting of long-standing disease. The prognosis is poor despite radiation therapy and surgery. Epidural hematomas can cause acute compression of the spinal cord or brain and are related to the increased blood flow to bone and increased risk of pathologic fractures. The prognosis in these cases is also poor, owing to excessive bleeding during surgery.

The spine is the second most common site of involvement in Paget disease and, prior to effective treatment with bisphosphonates, resulted in symptoms of spinal stenosis in 26 percent of patients.[76] Mechanisms of neurologic compromise include: (1) direct compression of the spinal cord, cauda equina, or nerve roots by enlarged vertebrae (most commonly) or expansion of facet joints; (2) pathologic fractures or subluxation; (3) ossification of extradural structures; (4) diversion of the local blood supply to highly vascular bones; and (5) pressure on vessels as they pass through the intervertebral foramina.[72] Sarcomas or epidural hematomas are rare. The onset of continuous severe spinal pain and rapid neurologic deterioration should raise concern of osteosarcoma.

Back pain occurs in 11 to 43 percent of patients with involvement of the spine.[76] Osteoarthritis is prevalent in this elderly population and can be difficult to distinguish from Paget disease as the cause of pain.[76] Other changes in the spine include thickening of the pedicles and laminae, flattening of the vertebral bodies, and encroachment of the spinal canal by osteophytes. Involved vertebrae are increased in width and reduced in height. The most commonly involved levels are the upper and lower cervical, low thoracic, and midlumbar regions. Of those with involvement of the spine demonstrated on plain radiographs, two-thirds will have evidence of spinal stenosis by CT and half of those patients will have clinical evidence of myelopathy or a cauda equina syndrome.[77] There is no association between the number of vertebrae involved and presence of symptoms.

Low back pain may respond to treatment with bisphosphonates.[76] Pain that does not respond after 3 months should be treated with nonsteroidal anti-inflammatory agents. Improvement or reversal of symptoms of spinal stenosis has been demonstrated with mithramycin, etidronate, pamidronate, and clodronate.[76] Prompt surgical decompression is appropriate for patients who do not respond to pharmacologic treatment. Preoperative assessment of bone vascularity by radionuclide bone blood flow can help direct perioperative medical therapy and prevent massive bleeding.

Extradural ossification of the ligamentum flavum and epidural fat can result in compression of the spinal cord or nerve roots and may require surgical decompression.[78] Myelopathy and cauda equina syndrome can occur without evidence of compression on neuroimaging and respond dramatically to medical therapy, suggesting that ischemia due to a vascular steal phenomenon is responsible.[79]

Serum alkaline phosphatase concentrations and urine hydroxyproline are usually increased in patients with neurologic complications, but alkaline phosphatase levels are normal in one-third of those with spinal stenosis. Plain radiographs and radionuclide scans should be obtained to localize disease activity and identify pathologic fractures. Cranial CT or MRI and CT myelography or MRI of the spine are necessary to demonstrate compression of neural structures and to exclude other causes of symptoms (Fig. 22-4). Sarcomatous transformation

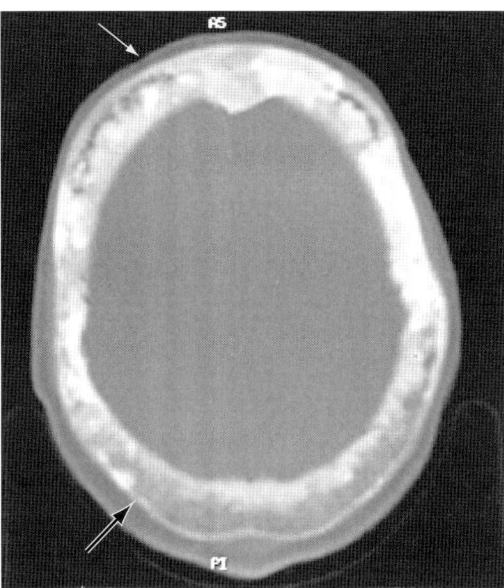

FIGURE 22-4 ■ Paget disease of bone. Axial CT scan of the head with bone windows. The closed arrow shows thickened osteosclerotic bone anteriorly. The open arrow shows thickened hypodense osteolytic bone posteriorly.

is best assessed with MRI. Patients with neurologic complications should have serum alkaline phosphatase and urinary hydroxyproline level determinations every 6 months. Clinical monitoring of neurologic function in symptomatic patients and repeat radiographs of the skull and weight-bearing long bones are recommended every 6 to 12 months in those with osteolytic lesions.

Medical and surgical management of neurologic complications depends on location, basis, and clinical course. Asymptomatic disease that affects the skull or spine should be treated with bisphosphonates.[69–71] Patients with neurologic compromise respond to etidronate and intravenous pamidronate.[72] Calcitonin is no longer recommended as the bisphosphonates are more effective with fewer treatment failures.[69–71] Rapidly progressive neurologic deterioration should be treated with intravenous bisphosphonates before surgery to minimize intraoperative bone hemorrhage.

Obstructive hydrocephalus usually requires the placement of a ventricular shunt. Hydrocephalic dementia with memory loss, gait disturbance, and urinary incontinence may improve with shunting and bisphosphonate therapy.[80,81] A case report describes a patient with confusion, hearing loss, urinary incontinence, and facial asymmetry along with imaging findings of hydrocephalus, cerebellar tonsil herniation, platybasia, basilar invagination, and increased intracranial pressure who was treated with intravenous zoledronic acid.[82] Despite pretreatment for 2 weeks with vitamin D and calcium, she became severely hypocalcemic; with replacement of calcium and shunting, her cognition returned to normal but her urinary incontinence persisted.

Bisphosphonate treatment probably results in stabilization of hearing loss.[83] Trigeminal neuralgia and hemifacial spasm are treated with carbamazepine.[72] Hemifacial spasm may also respond to alendronate or botulinum toxin injection.[74] Facial nerve paresis sometimes responds to surgical decompression, and there are older reports of benefit with suboccipital craniectomy and upper cervical laminectomy for patients with lower cranial neuropathies.[72]

Surgical treatment of spinal disease is difficult because involvement is usually at multiple levels, highly vascular bone leads to perioperative bleeding, and patients are typically in an older age group. A review of 65 surgical cases showed some degree of benefit in 85 percent but an accompanying 11 percent mortality rate.[84] Reoperation was required in 9 percent. Relapses may occur after either bisphosphonate treatment or surgical treatment,[72] and benefit may then follow by repeating or changing therapy.

Inclusion-Body Myopathy, Paget Disease, and Frontotemporal Dementia

Inclusion-body myopathy, Paget disease of bone and frontotemporal dementia (IBMPFD) is a rare autosomal-dominant disorder caused by missense mutations in the valosin-containing protein (*VCP*) gene.[85,86] There is variable penetrance of weakness (90%), osteolytic bone lesions (51%), and frontotemporal dementia (32%). The onset of the disorder is in the third and fourth decades, and over half of patients present with weakness. Clinical patterns described include: (1) proximal lower extremity weakness; (2) scapulohumeral weakness with scapular winging; (3) axial weakness with head drop and lumbar lordosis; (4) distal weakness; or (5) a mixture of these patterns. There are reports of facial or tongue weakness. The weakness is slowly progressive and is often asymmetric. Other neurologic features include sensorineural hearing loss and sensorimotor axonal neuropathy. A disorder resembling amyotrophic lateral sclerosis in some respects, with upper motor neuron findings, parkinsonism, and myotonia, is described in some families.[85] Patients die of respiratory insufficiency, cardiac failure, or complications from end-stage dementia in the fourth to sixth decades.

Laboratory findings include a serum creatine kinase level that is normal or mildly elevated. Total serum alkaline phosphatase may be elevated if pagetic involvement of bone is present. Standard motor and sensory nerve conduction studies are normal, but EMG shows myopathic units and, sometimes, abnormal spontaneous activity.[87] Patients with an amyotrophic lateral sclerosis–like phenotype may have neurogenic changes by EMG.[85] Neuropsychologic testing is helpful to assess for dementia.

Muscle biopsy shows variation in fiber size and endomysial fibrosis. Subsarcolemmal or sarcoplasmic rimmed vacuoles are present in 40 percent of patients. Electron microscopy shows ubiquitin-positive and tubulofilamentous inclusions similar to sporadic inclusion-body myopathy. A common finding is VCP and TAR DNA-binding protein 43 (TDP-43) inclusions that can co-localize with ubiquitin-positive inclusions.[86] CNS pathology includes atrophy and neuronal loss in the frontal and temporal lobes with ubiquitin-positive inclusions that are positive for TDP-43 in 55 percent of patients.[85]

VCP DNA sequencing is available to make the diagnosis but, interestingly, *VCP* mutations are also described in 2 percent of patients with familial amyotrophic lateral sclerosis. The exact pathogenesis of *VCP* mutations is not completely understood but may relate to impairment of protein degradation.[86] There is no current treatment for the myopathy and dementia in these patients other than supportive measures. Symptomatic Paget disease is treated with bisphosphonates.

VERTEBRAL OSTEOMYELITIS

Infection of the spine by a variety of pathogenic organisms is primarily a disease of older adults; men are affected twice as commonly as women, and recent observations suggest an increasing incidence.[88] Bacteria most commonly reach the spine by hematogenous spread from a distant source, but may also originate from a focus of contiguous infection or be introduced by direct penetrating trauma, surgery, epidural injections, or, rarely, lumbar puncture.[89]

The lumbar spine is most commonly affected, followed by the cervical spine. With hematogenous spread, septic emboli lodge in the metaphyseal subchondral area of the vertebra, often causing bone infarction. Infection within the vertebral body then tends to spread sequentially to involve the adjacent intervertebral disc followed by the next adjacent vertebra (spondylodiscitis). This propensity to traverse disc spaces distinguishes osteomyelitis clinically and radiographically from neoplasia, which tends to remain confined. Abscesses may form when infection extends beyond the cortex of the vertebra. An epidural abscess may cause both radicular injury and spinal cord compression. Extraspinal abscesses may track to a variety of sites (e.g., paraspinal, retroperitoneal, psoas). Chronic osteomyelitis is characterized by necrosis of bone, a predominantly mononuclear infiltrate, fibrosis, and a paucity of organisms. A sinus tract may develop occasionally between the affected bone and skin.

Osteomyelitis resulting from blood-borne bacterial seeding is almost always the result of infection by a single organism. Diabetes and chronic alcoholism are common risk factors. More than half are due to *Staphylococcus aureus* (in recent series, methicillin-susceptible isolates account for the majority) and are often associated with vascular catheters and other invasive medical procedures.[90] Causative organisms also include *Escherichia coli* and other gram-negative bacteria, *Brucella*, and fungi (e.g., candida). *Pseudomonas* and staphylococcal infections are associated with intravenous drug use. Streptococci and enterococci are frequently associated with endocarditis.[91,92] Tuberculous infection is described later. Polymicrobial ("mixed") cultures are associated with trauma and spread of contiguous infection.

Back pain, often with local tenderness, is the most frequent presenting feature. Pain is often not relieved by rest and persists at night. The spine may be held rigidly, with paraspinal muscle spasm. In many patients, back pain is preceded by a subacute prodrome of constitutional symptoms—fever, fatigue, lethargy, anorexia—for several weeks. By the time of initial presentation, however, the patient may be afebrile with few other signs of systemic infection. Neurologic deficit occurs in only approximately half the patients. Encroachment on sensory and motor roots gives rise to pain and segmental sensorimotor loss. Cauda equina syndrome may result from compression of multiple lumbosacral

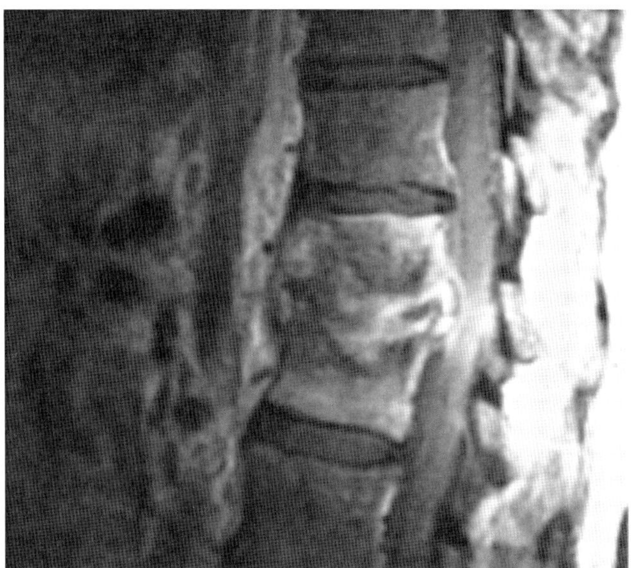

FIGURE 22-5 ▪ Osteomyelitis. Sagittal T1-weighted MRI of the lower thoracic spine, with contrast. A septic focus is seen to involve the intervertebral disc and the two adjacent vertebral bodies. An epidural abscess compresses the thecal sac.

roots. Epidural abscess formation with compression of the spinal cord may develop acutely or subacutely over several weeks and requires immediate surgical decompression.

A high index of clinical suspicion is required for the timely diagnosis of osteomyelitis and is crucial, because effective antibiotic therapy may prevent necrosis of bone and permanent skeletal abnormality. Plain radiography is frequently normal in the first 2 to 4 weeks since lytic lesions are not apparent until significant bone loss has occurred. MRI abnormalities (Fig. 22-5), in contrast, can be seen in early disease, in which vertebral body edema may be the sole imaging abnormality; other findings include spondylodiscitis, erosion of bone, and intra- and extravertebral collections.[93] Radionuclide bone scans are highly sensitive but the findings are nonspecific; this technique is particularly useful when MRI is contraindicated.[94,95]

Specimens for microbiologic culture and antibiotic sensitivity should be obtained before the institution of antibiotic therapy, although one study found that antibiotics administered prior to biopsy did not reduce culture yield.[96] Blood culture may be positive in around 30 percent of cases. Material from the focus of infection may be obtained by needle aspiration (often with CT guidance) or open biopsy, and is generally needed to confirm the diagnosis. The concurrent presence of endocarditis should always be considered.

High-dose intravenous antibiotics are used for treatment although there are no randomized, controlled trials to evaluate specific regimens or duration of therapy. Empiric treatment (usually a penicillinase-resistant penicillin or vancomycin, plus a third-generation cephalosporin) may be necessary before microbiology results return or when cultures are negative. Intravenous antibiotics should be continued for an extended period of weeks to months before switching to an oral preparation once a favorable response has been achieved. Imaging abnormalities tend to persist despite clinical measures of improvement and are not necessary to follow routinely.[97] In contrast, the erythrocyte sedimentation rate and C-reactive protein level are frequently elevated and may be useful to follow response to therapy.[98] Bed rest with external immobilization with a back brace is generally enforced until back pain has receded. With appropriate antibiotic therapy, recovery is the rule; surgery is required in 10 to 20 percent of cases, usually for drainage of large abscesses, decompression in cases of progressive neurologic deficit, fixation for spinal instability, and debridement in severe, unresponsive infection.[99,100] A systematic review found an overall mortality of 6 percent, with residual deficit seen in 32 percent of patients.[101] Osteomyelitis resulting from trauma or contiguous infection requires broad-spectrum antibiotic therapy due to its polymicrobial nature and, frequently, surgical debridement. The management of chronic osteomyelitis is difficult and controversial, usually involving complete surgical removal of the nidus of infection along with long-term antibiotic therapy.[102]

Tuberculous Osteomyelitis

First reported in detail by Sir Percivall Pott in the late eighteenth century, tuberculous involvement of bone and joint tissue accounts for 10 to 35 percent of cases of extrapulmonary tuberculosis, with the spine being the most common site. Immigrants from endemic areas to developed countries have higher rates of extrapulmonary tuberculosis. Tuberculous infection of the spine, although occasionally a presenting manifestation, is most often a late feature, representing reactivation of a focus of latent infection with hematogenous or lymphatic spread to the spine, frequently years after the initial pulmonary infection. Typically, a vertebral body in the lower thoracic or upper lumbar spine is affected, followed by spread to adjacent vertebrae, often with involvement of the intervening disc. Involvement of the intervertebral space occurs later than in bacterial osteomyelitis and may give rise to a radiologic appearance of relative disc-sparing. Destruction of cancellous bone renders the involved vertebral body liable to compression fractures and vertebral body collapse. In advanced cases, both kyphosis and scoliosis produce a striking gibbous deformity. Paravertebral collections may form at various sites including within the psoas muscle.

Back pain is common and patients may adopt a stiff-backed posture, walking with careful, short steps to avoid jarring the spine. Constitutional symptoms (lethargy, night sweats, weight loss) and systemic signs (anemia, low-grade fever) are frequent but may not be prominent. Neurologic features are present in fewer than one-half of patients. The possibility of tuberculous infection of the spine is usually an obvious consideration in patients with known pulmonary tuberculosis (particularly when treatment was incomplete), or in immunosuppressed patients.[103] In the majority of patients there is no history of tuberculosis, and a high index of clinical suspicion and appropriate (radiologic) investigations are needed for recognition; in many series, diagnosis was delayed for 12 to 18 months after presentation.

There may be few clues to the diagnosis on routine tests: erythrocyte sedimentation rate and C-reactive protein are likely to be elevated, and the peripheral white count may be normal or slightly elevated. Chest radiography is normal in half the cases, and sputum is usually negative for acid-fast bacilli.[104] Characteristic imaging findings on CT or MRI include involvement of several contiguous vertebral bodies with heterogeneous enhancement and the presence of epidural and subdural collections; the intervening discs may not be involved as is the usual case with pyogenic infections.[104]

Attempts to confirm the tuberculous nature of such lesions usually begin with a purified protein derivative (PPD) skin test, which has poor sensitivity. Biopsy (needle aspiration or open biopsy) demonstrates the characteristic caseating granulomatous histology with Langhan giant cells and acid-fast bacilli; culture may be positive.[105]

Treatment is with prolonged antituberculous drugs similar to the approach used for pulmonary tuberculosis. The duration of therapy is unclear and is judged according to clinical response. In general, 6 months of initial treatment with a regimen of first-line drugs including rifampin is sufficient in uncomplicated disease; a longer 9- to 12-month course may be needed in advanced disease or where the drug regimen does not include rifampin.[106] There is often a rapid response to treatment by clinical and laboratory measures, but radiologic changes tend to persist, suggesting that imaging need not be repeated in patients who are improving.[97,107–110] Surgery, involving debridement and possible stabilization of the spine, is sometimes required in addition to drug therapy for those patients with spinal instability or severe disease, but should not be performed routinely.[111] Spinal cord compression is a medical emergency necessitating immediate surgical decompression.

ANKYLOSING SPONDYLITIS

Ankylosing spondylitis is an HLA-B27–associated chronic inflammatory disease of joints with predilection for the sacroiliac joints and spine. HLA-B27 is present in 90 percent of Caucasian patients with the disorder.[112] Clinical manifestations typically begin in late adolescence or early adulthood. The most common symptoms are low back pain and stiffness, occurring in 90 to 95 percent of patients.[112] Pain can be severe and is often referred along the iliac crest to the greater trochanteric region or down the dorsal thigh; it may be accentuated by cough, sneeze, or a twisting motion of the back. Features that help to differentiate it from mechanical low back pain include the onset of back discomfort before the age of 40, an insidious onset, persistence for at least 3 months, associated morning stiffness, and improvement with exercise.[113] Within a few months of onset, symptoms become persistent and bilateral. Findings on physical examination include flattening of the lumbar spine and loss of the lumbar lordosis. There is limited motion of the axial skeleton, especially with hyperextension and lateral bending. Percussion over the sacroiliac joints elicits pain. Radiographs of the sacroiliac joints are used to make the diagnosis in conjunction with the examination (Fig. 22-6).

No treatment has been shown to alter the course of the illness, particularly the loss of spinal

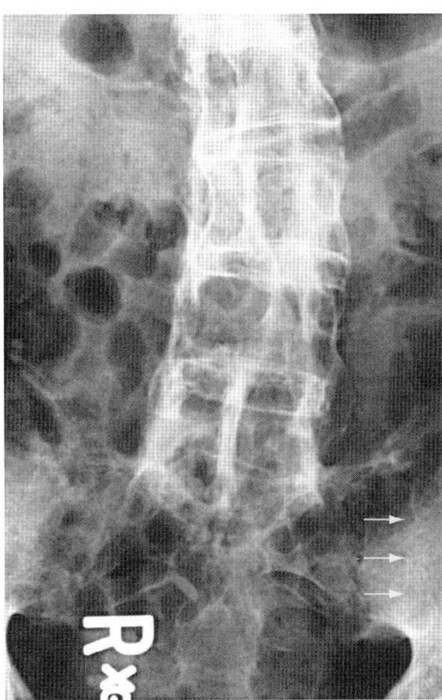

FIGURE 22-6 ■ Ankylosing spondylitis. Plain radiograph of lumbosacral spine. The characteristic "bamboo spine" with fusion of the intervertebral ligaments is evident. The arrows show fusion of the sacroiliac joint.

mobility.[112] Therapies that have evidence-based beneficial effects include physical therapy, NSAIDs, and tumor necrosis factor alpha (TNF-α) inhibitors.[114] Intensive physical therapy and exercise are important to maintain mobility, and braces, splints, and corsets should be avoided.[115] Current guidelines recommend that at least two NSAIDs be tried over 4 weeks prior to initiating treatment with a TNF-α inhibitor.[116] A detailed description of treatments for ankylosing spondylitis is summarized elsewhere.[116]

Neurologic complications are uncommon and occur in 2.1 percent of patients.[117,118] They include radiculopathy from foraminal stenosis or inflammation and myelopathy resulting from fracture-dislocation, atlantoaxial subluxation, pseudoarthritis, ossified intraspinal ligaments, or granulation tissue. Cauda equina syndrome is a late complication attributed to arachnoiditis. Sciatic nerve compression can occur secondary to inflammation of the attachment of the piriformis muscle to the sacroiliac joint, mimicking sciatica from root compression (pseudosciatica).[112]

There is a fourfold lifetime increased risk of spine fractures in patients with ankylosing spondylitis as the spine is brittle and prone to fracture.[119] The fracture often goes entirely through the vertebral body and ossified ligaments, resulting in increased instability and neurologic compromise. The most common fracture location is in the low cervical spine and in the majority of cases is caused by low-energy trauma.[119] In one series, the risk of traumatic spinal cord injury was 11.4 times greater than expected for the population at large.[120] Cervical myelopathy occurred in 84 percent of patients with traumatic spine injury compared to 48 percent of all patients with traumatic spine injury. Secondary neurologic deterioration occurred in 13.9 percent of patients, and deterioration was sometimes delayed, occurring more than 3 months after the initial fracture in some patients.[119] Delayed diagnosis was common, due to either physician misdiagnosis or patient delay in seeking care. Transfer and manipulation of these patients can be a factor in neurologic deterioration.

Surgical intervention (posterior decompression) has been described, but around 75 percent of patients have no change in their neurologic status As many as 85 percent will have a residual neurologic deficit.[112] Patients with complete paraparesis for more than 2 hours do not respond to surgical intervention.[112] Patients without surgical intervention remain unchanged in most (80%) cases, and improvement is rare (5%). Surgical complications occur frequently, including postoperative wound infections, deep vein thrombosis, pneumonia, and respiratory insufficiency. Rare fatal complications of surgery include aortic dissection, aortic pseudoaneurysm, and tracheal rupture.

Spinal stenosis with cord compression is rare. Patients may develop "radicular" pain without neurologic symptoms or signs, and this usually resolves spontaneously. The cervical spine may be involved, resulting in atlantoaxial subluxation in 2 to 21 percent of patients.[121,122] Atlanto-occipital subluxation with vertebral artery occlusion and brainstem transient ischemic attack or infarction has also been described.[121,122] Studies of the natural history of ankylosing spondylitis have demonstrated that cerebrovascular disease is a common cause of mortality in patients younger than 60 years of age, often without clear etiology; prophylactic antiplatelet therapy may be indicated.

Cauda equina syndrome occurs in rare patients, predominantly male, on average 32 years after the onset of disease.[117] In most patients, there are no inflammatory markers in the blood.[118,123] The typical presentation includes insidious onset and progression of bowel and bladder symptoms, sensory loss (often asymmetric) in an L5–S4 distribution, pain radiating into the lower limbs or the rectal area, and minimal weakness in muscles innervated by the L5–S2 segments. Bladder symptoms include decreased awareness of bladder sensation, decreased ability to empty the bladder, hesitancy, decreased force of urinary stream, urgency, and frequency. Radiography of the lumbar spine may show erosions of the lamina. Spinal MRI shows dorsal dural diverticula associated with a widened thecal sac and scalloped erosions of the laminae and spinous processes.[123] Nerve roots appear to deviate toward the diverticula and may be displaced posteriorly; they appear to be adherent to the arachnoid membrane and to each other, suggesting arachnoiditis. There is no associated gadolinium enhancement. Spinal CT typically demonstrates asymmetric, multilevel erosions that selectively involve the pedicles, laminae, and spinous processes of the lumbosacral spine.[123] Infrequently, erosion of the posterior portion of the vertebral body is found or involvement is unilateral or confined to one level. Myelography is technically difficult and can be complicated by epidural hematoma in patients with ankylosing spondylitis. CSF is normal or shows a slightly elevated protein concentration, although a case of lymphocytic pleocytosis has been described.[124] EMG shows denervation changes, often asymmetric, in the L2–S1 distribution.[118]

The pathologic findings depend on the timing of surgery or autopsy relative to the onset of neurologic symptoms.[125] Early pathologic findings include inflammation of the spinal ligaments, dura, and arachnoid. Over time, there is fibrosis and chronic arachnoiditis embedding atrophic nerve roots, with small sacral roots splayed and adherent to the dura. A CSF resorption defect has been documented and may contribute to thecal sac enlargement.[126] Compression of the nerve roots by diverticula sometimes occurs. The disease may be patchy, with some roots appearing normal.

NSAIDs result in improvement of back pain in cauda equina syndrome, but without improvement of neurologic deficits. There are several case reports of partial improvement with infliximab.[118,127] Patients may have improvement of neurologic function or halting of progression with either lumboperitoneal shunting or laminectomy, but neurologic deficits persist despite surgical intervention in more than 80 percent of patients.[112] The clinical course is slowly progressive, although patients rarely lose the ability to walk. In a meta-analysis, weakness occurred in 62 percent, sensory loss in 96 percent, loss of reflexes in 93 percent, bowel dysfunction in 80 percent, and bladder dysfunction in 95 percent of patients.[117] Any patient with longstanding ankylosing spondylitis who develops sphincter dysfunction should receive a careful neurologic assessment.

There is an unclear association between ankylosing spondylitis and multiple sclerosis. The incidence of multiple sclerosis in patients with ankylosing spondylitis is approximately 1,000 per 100,000, which is significantly greater than that of the general population (50 per 100,000).[128] Other studies have failed to demonstrate an association between the two conditions.[129] There is growing evidence of an increased incidence of autoimmune neurologic disorders including multiple sclerosis and demyelinating neuropathy in rheumatologic patients, including those with ankylosing spondylitis, treated with TNF-α inhibitors.[130,131] Multiple sclerosis is the most commonly described neurologic complication of a TNF-α inhibitor and occurs in an older age group than typical multiple sclerosis (between 36 and 65 years). There may be more CNS side effects with etanercept therapy, and peripheral nervous system side effects with infliximab.[131] The incidence of these complications in patients with ankylosing spondylitis treated with TNF-α inhibitors is unknown. It is recommended in these cases that the TNF-α inhibitor be discontinued; some, but not all, patients improve after discontinuation. The use of TNF-α inhibitors in patients with a prior history of multiple sclerosis or a CNS demyelinating disorder is best avoided. Demyelinating neuropathy should be treated with corticosteroids or intravenous immunoglobulin.

Diffuse Idiopathic Skeletal Hyperostosis

Diffuse idiopathic skeletal hyperostosis is a presumably benign, noninflammatory arthropathy with ossification of spinal longitudinal ligaments and entheses resulting in decreased mobility and ankylosis. The etiology is unknown but there is an association with obesity, adult-onset diabetes mellitus, and advanced age. Diagnosis is made by the presence of ossification of the anterior longitudinal ligament over four consecutive levels on spine radiographs. The prevalence is not well characterized but appears to be increasing in elderly Caucasian males.[119] Serious complications from cervical spine involvement are described including dysphagia, difficult endotracheal intubation, and spinal canal stenosis with myelopathy.

There is an increased incidence of traumatic vertebral fracture in these patients, and they are more likely to have multiple fractures.[119] A unique feature is fracture through the vertebral body. The cervical spine is the most common site involved (60%). Low-energy impact precedes fracture in around 70 percent of patients, and high-energy impact is recognized in around 25 percent; hyperextension is the most frequent cause. In over half of patients, there is a delay in diagnosis of the fracture and 40 percent of patients have a neurologic deficit on presentation.[119] Around 15 percent of patients will develop secondary neurologic deterioration, some due to inadequate immobilization, inconsiderate transfers, or application of a hard collar with preexisting kyphotic deformity. About half of these patients are treated with surgical posterior fixation, and the rest are managed conservatively, often with a collar or bracing for thoracic fractures. Neurologic improvement is unlikely regardless of treatment (around 6%), and overall mortality is somewhat worse in the nonsurgical group (12% compared to 7%).

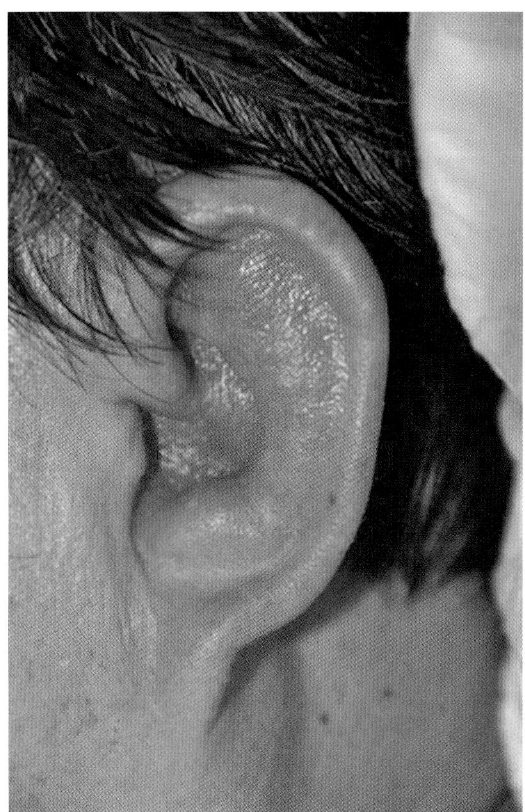

FIGURE 22-7 ▪ Relapsing polychondritis, illustrating marked auricular swelling and redness. (From Wang ZJ, Pu CQ, Wang ZJ, et al: Meningoencephalitis or meningitis in relapsing polychondritis: four case reports and a literature review. J Clin Neurosci 18:1608, 2011, with permission.)

RELAPSING POLYCHONDRITIS

Relapsing polychondritis is an uncommon, immune-mediated multisystem disorder characterized by recurrent episodes of inflammation and eventual destruction of cartilaginous tissues.[132,133] The prevalence of the disorder is 3.5 per 1 million persons, with an age range from 16 to 84 years, with peak onset in the fifth decade. There is an equal prevalence in men and women, and it has been described in all races.[133] It can affect all types of cartilage, including the ears and nose (most commonly), peripheral joints, fibrocartilage at axial sites, and the tracheobronchial tree. The eye, heart, blood vessels, and inner ear are rich in proteoglycans and can also be affected. There is a genetic association with HLA-DR4 and HLA-DR6. More than 30 percent of patients with relapsing polychondritis have an associated rheumatologic or hematologic disorder.[133] Antibodies to type II collagen are present during acute attacks, and immune-complex deposition is found in cartilage.

The clinical presentation involves the acute or subacute onset of ear pain, tenderness and swelling of the external auditory meatus, erythema, and a clear serous discharge from the ear (Fig. 22-7).[133] Ear involvement is the initial presenting symptom in 39 percent and ultimately occurs in 85 to 95 percent of patients.[134] The noncartilaginous lobule is spared. Repeated bouts of inflammation result in a floppy ear. Nasal pain, hoarseness, and difficulty in talking are also common. Nasal crusting, rhinorrhea, and epistaxis can occur, and repeated inflammation of the nasal cartilage results in a saddle nose deformity. Systemic symptoms include fever, lethargy, and weight loss. The course is typically relapsing, but over the course of the illness, progressive disability occurs in most patients. Inflammation of the trachea and larynx occurs in 50 percent of patients and may be fatal. A detailed description of the cardiovascular, joint, respiratory, and dermatologic complications is provided elsewhere.[133]

Vertigo and conductive or sensorineural hearing loss and tinnitus are common and present in 5 percent of patients at onset of the disease and in 13 to 50 percent over the course of the illness.[135] The sensorineural hearing loss is attributed to vasculitis of the vestibular or cochlear branch of the internal auditory artery. The abrupt onset of hearing loss, sometimes accompanied by vertigo, nausea, vomiting, and imbalance, can mimic a posterior circulation stroke. Ocular involvement occurs in 65 percent of patients; recurrent conjunctivitis, episcleritis, scleritis, iritis, or keratoconjuctivitis sicca is common. Rarely, chorioretinitis, retinal vasculitis, exophthalmos due to orbital pseudotumor, uveitis, and optic neuritis are seen. Extraocular palsies occur either due to direct extension of pseudotumor-like inflammation of the orbit or from vasculitic ischemia to cranial nerves III, VI, or IV.

Vasculitis occurs in 11 to 56 percent of patients with relapsing polychondritis and affects the skin, internal organs, or CNS.[136] It can affect the large arteries, resembling Takayasu arteritis, or small- to medium-sized vessels.[136,137] A combination of two systemic reviews shows that the incidence of systemic vasculitis is 18 percent, of which 21 percent have clinical features suggestive of CNS vasculitis. The prognosis in patients with systemic vasculitis is poor, with a 5-year survival rate of 45 percent.

Neurologic involvement occurs in 3 percent of patients with relapsing polychondritis but may be the presenting feature.[138] It may manifest with cranial neuropathies,[133,135] cerebral vasculitis,[135] mononeuritis multiplex,[136] sensorimotor distal symmetric neuropathy,[136] aseptic meningitis,[139,140] meningoencephalitis with limbic encephalopathy,[141] rhombencephalitis, myelitis, acute spinal cord infarction due to aortic disease, or thromboembolic strokes secondary to vasculitis, sometimes with associated anticardiolipin antibodies.[135] Cerebral aneurysms have rarely been reported.[142]

Cranial nerve abnormalities are the most frequent, with involvement of II, VI, VII, and VIII being most common. Involvement of III, IV, and XII has also been described. Vasculitic infarction is the presumed etiology. CNS involvement can be due to vasculitis or meningoencephalitis; patients present with an acute headache accompanied by encephalopathy, personality change, hallucinations, seizures, and focal or multifocal deficits such as hemiparesis, ataxia, or the clinical features of a lateral medullary syndrome.[135,143–145] An acute limbic encephalitis can present with fever, delirium, visual and auditory hallucinations, agitation, disinhibition, cognitive decline, and seizures. An association with anti-glutamate receptor ε2 antibodies has been reported.[143] CSF may show a pleocytosis and elevated protein concentration. Parkinsonism, apathy, psychosis, and dementia are also described.[143,146] Papilledema or meningeal signs can occur. Aseptic meningitis presents with headache, meningeal signs, and fever; in these cases, CSF results most often show a lymphocytic pleocytosis, but a polymorphonuclear leukocyte predominance sometimes occurs.[140] Total protein can be elevated and there are cases with a decreased CSF glucose mimicking infection.

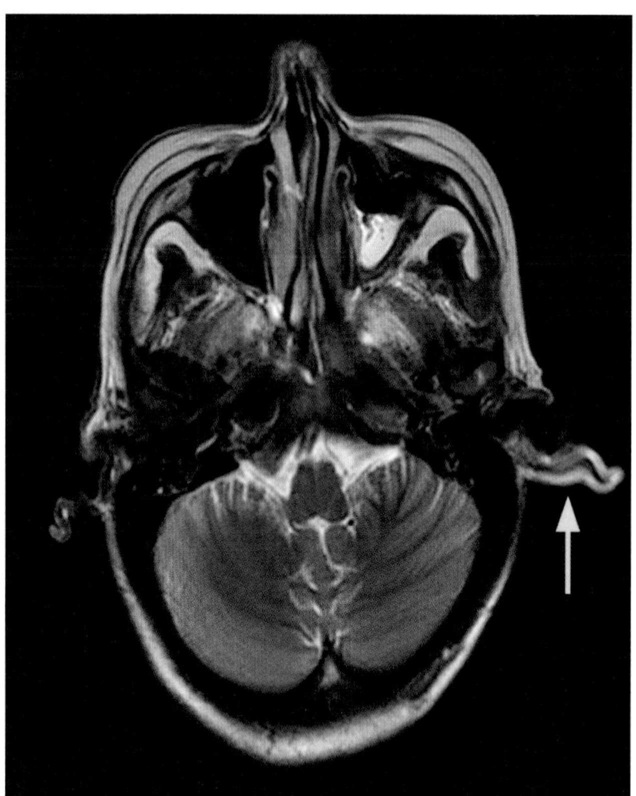

FIGURE 22-8 ▪ Relapsing polychondritis. T2-weighted MRI showing abnormal signal in the left auricle. From Wang ZJ, Pu CQ, Wang ZJ, et al: Meningoencephalitis or meningitis in relapsing polychondritis: four case reports and a literature review. J Clin Neurosci 18:1608, 2011, with permission.

With CNS vasculitis, the erythrocyte sedimentation rate is usually elevated (>100 mm/hour), and mild systemic leukocytosis may be present. The CSF is normal or shows a pleocytosis. The electroencephalogram can be normal, slow, or show focal areas of epileptiform activity. Cranial CT often shows cerebral and cerebellar atrophy or focal areas of hypodensity, but it can be normal. MRI is suggestive

TABLE 22-4 ■ Diagnostic Criteria for Relapsing Polychondritis*

Bilateral auricular chondritis
Nonerosive seronegative inflammatory arthritis
Nasal chondritis
Ocular inflammation
Respiratory tract chondritis
Audiovestibular damage

*A minimum of three criteria must be met to establish the diagnosis.

of cerebral vasculitis, with increased T2 signal in the periventricular white matter and centrum semiovale, focal lesions in the gray matter, and wedge-shaped cortical infarcts.[147] Focal occlusion of vessels on MR angiography has been described.[145] In cases of limbic encephalitis, the MRI shows increased T2 signal in one or both medial temporal lobes.[143] A clue to the diagnosis of relapsing polychondritis in some patients with neurologic presentations is increased signal on diffusion-weighted imaging of the external ears (Fig. 22-8).[139,144] Brain biopsy in these cases shows marked gliosis, perivascular cuffing, and destruction of the vascular well.

The diagnosis of relapsing polychondritis is based on clinical criteria (Table 22-4), supportive laboratory parameters, imaging, and biopsy of involved cartilaginous tissues, including the ear.[133] Nonspecific laboratory findings include an elevated erythrocyte sedimentation rate, C-reactive protein level, anemia, leukocytosis, or thrombocytosis. Esoinophilia is present in 10 percent.[133] Serum creatinine and urinalysis should be checked to assess for renal involvement. A serologic screen for associated rheumatologic disorders should occur. Type II collagen antibodies are also described in relapsing polychondritis. Evaluation of organ involvement on physical examination is critical, including the ear, nose and throat. The airway should be evaluated by radiography, pulmonary function tests, and high-resolution CT scans. Echocardiogram to evaluate the heart valves is also recommended.

The differential diagnosis includes Wegener granulomatosis. Distinguishing clinical features include involvement of the mucosa and lung parenchyma and the presence of positive cytoplasmic antineutrophil cytoplasmic antibodies, which are not seen in uncomplicated relapsing polychondritis.

Treatment of relapsing polychondritis is empiric as there are no clinical trials to guide therapy.[132,133] Mild inflammation of joints, ear, or nose can be managed with NSAIDs, dapsone, or colchicine.[132,133] If there is significant laryngotracheal, bronchial, cardiovascular, renal, or neurologic involvement, a more aggressive course is recommended.[133] Rapid response is obtained with high-dose oral or intravenous corticosteroids. Relapses occur if corticosteroids are reduced too rapidly. Corticosteroid-sparing agents may be necessary, including cyclophosphamide, azathioprine, cyclosporine, and methotrexate. TNF-α inhibitors are of particular interest since there is a massive expression of TNF-α in affected cartilaginous tissue in patients with relapsing polychondritis. A literature review of biologic agents in relapsing polychondritis showed mixed results with anti-TNFα and other agents in 43 patients; the most effective agent was infliximab followed by etanercept and rituximab.[132] There are case reports of efficacy of leflunomide, anakinra, toclizumab, abatacept, mycophenylate mofetil, and intravenous immunoglobulin in refractory cases.[132,133]

Treatment of CNS vasculitis, limbic encephalitis, meningoencephalitis, and aseptic meningitis includes high-dose corticosteroids, often with additional corticosteroid-sparing agents during the course of the illness.[143,146] A literature review of aseptic meningitis in relapsing polychondritis showed improvement with corticosteroids in most cases.[140]

REFERENCES

1. Boden SD, McCowin PR, Davis DO, et al: Abnormal magnetic-resonance scans of the cervical spine in asymptomatic subjects. A prospective investigation. J Bone Joint Surg Am 72:1178, 1990.
2. Healy JF, Healy BB, Wong WH, et al: Cervical and lumbar MRI in asymptomatic older male lifelong athletes: frequency of degenerative findings. J Comput Assist Tomogr 20:107, 1996.
3. Buckwalter JA: Aging and degeneration of the human intervertebral disc. Spine 20:1307, 1995.
4. Benoist M: Natural history of the aging spine. Eur Spine J 12(suppl 2):S86, 2003.
5. Saal JS: The role of inflammation in lumbar pain. Spine 20:1821, 1995.
6. Herzog RJ: The radiologic assessment for a lumbar disc herniation. Spine 21:19S, 1996.
7. Kaiser JA, Holland BA: Imaging of the cervical spine. Spine 23:2701, 1998.

8. Carette S, Fehlings MG: Clinical practice. Cervical radiculopathy. N Engl J Med 353:392, 2005.
9. Edwards 2nd CC, Riew KD, Anderson PA, et al: Cervical myelopathy. Current diagnostic and treatment strategies. Spine J 3:68, 2003.
10. Fouyas IP, Statham PF, Sandercock PA: Cochrane review on the role of surgery in cervical spondylotic radiculomyelopathy. Spine 27:736, 2002.
11. Nikolaidis I, Fouyas IP, Sandercock PA, et al: Surgery for cervical radiculopathy or myelopathy. Cochrane Database Syst Rev:CD001466, 2010.
12. Saal JA: Natural history and nonoperative treatment of lumbar disc herniation. Spine 21:2S, 1996.
13. Malhotra G, Abbasi A, Rhee M: Complications of transforaminal cervical epidural steroid injections. Spine 34:731, 2009.
14. Orr RD, Zdeblick TA: Cervical spondylotic myelopathy. Approaches to surgical treatment. Clin Orthop Relat Res 359:58, 1999.
15. McCormick WE, Steinmetz MP, Benzel EC: Cervical spondylotic myelopathy: make the difficult diagnosis, then refer for surgery. Cleve Clin J Med 70:899, 2003.
16. Ahn UM, Ahn NU, Buchowski JM, et al: Cauda equina syndrome secondary to lumbar disc herniation: a meta-analysis of surgical outcomes. Spine 25:1515, 2000.
17. Liddle SD, Baxter GD, Gracey JH: Exercise and chronic low back pain: what works? Pain 107:176, 2004.
18. Nelemans PJ, deBie RA, deVet HC, et al: Injection therapy for subacute and chronic benign low back pain. Spine 26:501, 2001.
19. Roelofs PD, Deyo RA, Koes BW, et al: Nonsteroidal anti-inflammatory drugs for low back pain: an updated Cochrane review. Spine 33:1766, 2008.
20. Jacobs WC, van der Gaag NA, Kruyt MC, et al: Total disc replacement for chronic discogenic low back pain: a Cochrane review. Spine 38:24, 2012.
21. Gibson JN, Waddell G: Surgery for degenerative lumbar spondylosis: updated Cochrane review. Spine 30:2312, 2005.
22. Binder DK, Schmidt MH, Weinstein PR: Lumbar spinal stenosis. Semin Neurol 22:157, 2002.
23. Goh KJ, Khalifa W, Anslow P, et al: The clinical syndrome associated with lumbar spinal stenosis. Eur Neurol 52:242, 2004.
24. Singh K, Samartzis D, Vaccaro AR, et al: Congenital lumbar spinal stenosis: a prospective, control-matched, cohort radiographic analysis. Spine J 5:615, 2005.
25. Adamova B, Vohanka S, Dusek L: Dynamic electrophysiological examination in patients with lumbar spinal stenosis: is it useful in clinical practice? Eur Spine J 14:269, 2005.
26. Bal S, Celiker R, Palaoglu S, et al: F wave studies of neurogenic intermittent claudication in lumbar spinal stenosis. Am J Phys Med Rehabil 85:135, 2006.
27. Atkinson JL, Miller GM, Krauss WE, et al: Clinical and radiographic features of dural arteriovenous fistula, a treatable cause of myelopathy. Mayo Clin Proc 76:1120, 2001.
28. Chang Y, Singer DE, Wu YA, et al: The effect of surgical and nonsurgical treatment on longitudinal outcomes of lumbar spinal stenosis over 10 years. J Am Geriatr Soc 53:785, 2005.
29. Ammendolia C, Stuber K, de Bruin LK, et al: Nonoperative treatment of lumbar spinal stenosis with neurogenic claudication: a systematic review. Spine 37:E609, 2012.
30. Mazanec DJ, Podichetty VK, Hsia A: Lumbar canal stenosis: start with nonsurgical therapy. Cleve Clin J Med 69:909, 2002.
31. Weinstein JN, Lurie JD, Tosteson TD, et al: Surgical versus nonsurgical treatment for lumbar degenerative spondylolisthesis. N Engl J Med 356:2257, 2007.
32. Anderson PA, Tribus CB, Kitchel SH: Treatment of neurogenic claudication by interspinous decompression: application of the X STOP device in patients with lumbar degenerative spondylolisthesis. J Neurosurg 4:463, 2006.
33. Kuchta J, Sobottke R, Eysel P, et al: Two-year results of interspinous spacer (X-Stop) implantation in 175 patients with neurologic intermittent claudication due to lumbar spinal stenosis. Eur Spine J 18:823, 2009.
34. Murakami M, Takahashi K, Sekikawa T, et al: Effects of intravenous lipoprostaglandin E1 on neurogenic intermittent claudication. J Spinal Dis 10:499, 1997.
35. Levis S, Theodore G: Summary of AHRQ's comparative effectiveness review of treatment to prevent fractures in men and women with low bone density or osteoporosis: update of the 2007 report. J Manag Care Pharm 18:S1, 2012.
36. National Osteoporosis Foundation: Clinician's Guide to Prevention and Treatment of Osteoporosis. National Osteoporosis Foundation, Washington DC, 2010.
37. Takeda S: Osteoporosis: a neuroskeletal disease? Int J Biochem Cell Biol 41:455, 2009.
38. Lee YL, Yip KMH: The osteoporotic spine. Clin Orthop Rel Res 323:91, 1996.
39. Sambrook P, Cooper C: Osteoporosis. Lancet 367:2010, 2006.
40. Murata K, Watanabe G, Kawaguchi S, et al: Union rates and prognostic variables of osteoporotic vertebral fractures treated with a rigid external support. J Neurosurg 17:469, 2012.
41. Anderson PA, Froyshteter AB, Tontz Jr WL: Meta-analysis of vertebral augmentation compared with conservative treatment for osteoporotic spinal fractures. J Bone Miner Res 28:372, 2012.
42. Thaler M, Lechner R, Nogler M, et al: Surgical procedure and initial radiographic results of a new augmentation technique for vertebral compression fractures. Eur Spine J 22:1608, 2013.
43. Heggeness MH: Spine fracture with neurological deficit in osteoporosis. Osteoporosis Int 3:215, 1993.
44. Nguyen HV, Ludwig S, Gelb D: Osteoporotic vertebral burst fractures with neurologic compromise. J Spinal Disord Tech 16:10, 2003.

45. Suk SI, Kim JH, Lee SM, et al: Anterior-posterior surgery versus posterior closing wedge osteotomy in posttraumatic kyphosis with neurologic compromised osteoporotic fracture. Spine 28:2170, 2003.
46. Patil S, Rawall S, Singh D, et al: Surgical patterns in osteoporotic vertebral compression fractures. Eur Spine J 22:883, 2013.
47. Shawky A, Kroeber M: Shortening spinal column reconstruction through posterior only approach for the treatment of unstable osteoporotic burst lumber fracture: a case report. Arch Orthop Trauma Surg 133:167, 2012.
48. Chung S, Lee S, Kim D, et al: Treatment of lower lumbar radiculopathy caused by osteoporotic compression fracture: the role of vertebroplasty. J Spinal Disord Tech 15:461, 2002.
49. Holick M: High prevalance of vitamin D inadequacy and implications for health. Mayo Clin Proc 81:353, 2006.
50. Bahn A, Rao A, Sudhaker R: Osteomalacia as a result of vitamin D deficiency. Endocrinol Metab Clin N Am 39:321, 2010.
51. Thabit H, Barry M, Sreenan S, et al: Proximal myopathy in lacto-vegetarian Asian patients responding to Vitamin D and calcium supplement therapy—two case reports and review of the literature. J Med Case Rep 5:178, 2011.
52. Plotnikoff G, Quigley J: Prevalence of severe hypovitaminosis D in patients with persistent, nonspecific musculoskeletal pain. Mayo Clin Proc 78:1463, 2003.
53. Boucher B: The problems of Vitamin D insufficiency in older people. Aging Dis 3:313, 2012.
54. Ruff R: Endocrine myopathies. p. 1746. In: Engel A, Banker B (eds): Myology. McGraw-Hill, New York, 1994.
55. Russell JA: Osteomalacic myopathy. Muscle Nerve 17:578, 1994.
56. Schubert L, DeLuca H: Hypophosphatemia is responsible for skeletal muscle weakness of vitamin D deficiency. Arch Biochem Biophys 500:157, 2010.
57. Bischoff-Ferrari HA, Dawson-Hughes B, Willett WC, et al: Effect of vitamin D on falls: a meta-analysis. JAMA 291:1999, 2004.
58. Mesliniene S, Ramrattan L, Giddings S, et al: Role of Vitamin D in the onset, progression and severity of multiple sclerosis. Endocr Pract 19:129, 2012.
59. Reginato AJ, Falasca GF, Pappu R, et al: Musculoskeletal manifestations of osteomalacia: report of 26 cases and literature review. Semin Arthritis Rheum 28:287, 1999.
60. Ruppe MD, Brosnan PG, Au KS, et al: Mutational analysis of PHEX, FGF23 and DMP1 in a cohort of patients with hypophosphatemic rickets. Clin Endocrinol 74:312, 2011.
61. Adams JE, Davies M: Intra-spinal new bone formation and spinal cord compression in familial hypophosphataemic vitamin D resistant osteomalacia. QJM 61:1117, 1986.
62. Stark Z, Savarirayan R: Osteopetrosis. Orphanet J Rare Dis 4:5, 2009.
63. Steward C: Neurological aspects of osteopetrosis. Neuropathol Applied Neurobiol 29:87, 2003.
64. Al-Mefty O, Fox JL, Al-Rodhan N, et al: Optic nerve decompression in osteopetrosis. J Neurosurg 68:80, 1988.
65. Peters C, Steward C: Hematopoietic cell transplantation for inherited metabolic diseases: an overview of outcomes and practice guidelines. Bone Marrow Transplant 31:229, 2003.
66. Balemans W, Van Wesenbeeck L, Van Hul W: A clinical and molecular overview of the human osteopetroses. Calcif Tissue Int 77:263, 2005.
67. Bosley T, Salih M, Alorainy I, et al: The neurology of carbonic anhydrase type II deficiency syndrome. Brain 134:3502, 2011.
68. Whyte MP: Carbonic anhydrase II deficiency. Clin Orthop Relat Res 294:52, 1993.
69. Michou L, Brown JP: Emerging strategies and therapies for treatment of Paget's disease of bone. Drug Des Devel Ther 5:225, 2011.
70. Ralston SH, Langston AL, Reid IR: Pathogenesis and management of Paget's disease of bone. Lancet 372:155, 2008.
71. Chung PY, Van Hul W: Paget's disease of bone: evidence for complex pathogenetic interactions. Semin Arthritis Rheum 41:619, 2012.
72. Poncelet A: The neurologic complications of Paget's disease. J Bone Miner Res 14(suppl 2):88, 1999.
73. Wootton R, Reeve J, Spellacy E, et al: Skeletal blood flow in Paget's disease of bone and its response to calcitonin therapy. Clin Sci Mol Med 54:69, 1978.
74. Fu KK, Ko A: The treatment with alendronate in hemifacial spasm associated with Paget's disease of bone. Clin Neurol Neurosurg 102:48, 2000.
75. Thompson JB, Patterson RH, Parsons H: Sarcomas of the calvaria: surgical experience with 14 patients. J Neurosurg 32:534, 1970.
76. Hadjipavlou AG, Gaitanis LN, Katonis PG, et al: Paget's disease of the spine and its management. Eur Spine J 10:370, 2001.
77. Hadjipavlou A, Lander P: Paget disease of the spine. J Bone Joint Surg Am 73:1376, 1991.
78. Koziarz P, Avruch L: Spinal epidural lipomatosis associated with Paget's disease of bone. Neuroradiology 44:858, 2002.
79. Yost JH, Spencer-Green G, Krant JD: Vascular steal mimicking compression myelopathy in Paget's disease of bone: rapid reversal with calcitonin and systemic steroids. J Rheumatol 20:1064, 1993.
80. Chan YP, Shui KK, Lewis RR, et al: Reversible dementia in Paget's disease. J R Soc Med 93:595, 2000.
81. Roohi F, Mann D, Kula RW: Surgical management of hydrocephalic dementia in Paget's disease of bone: the 6-year outcome of ventriculo-peritoneal shunting. Clin Neurol Neurosurg 107:325, 2005.

82. Ferraz-de-Souza B, Martin RM, Correa PH: Symptomatic intracranial hypertension and prolonged hypocalcemia following treatment of Paget's disease of the skull with zoledronic acid. J Bone Miner Metab 31:360, 2013.
83. Delmas PD, Meunier PJ: The management of Paget's disease of bone. N Engl J Med 336:558, 1997.
84. Sadar ES, Walton RJ, Gossman HH: Neurological dysfunction in Paget's disease. J Neurosurg 37:661, 1972.
85. Nalbandian A, Donkervoort S, Dec E, et al: The multiple faces of valosin-containing protein-associated diseases: inclusion body myopathy with Paget's disease of bone, frontotemporal dementia, and amyotrophic lateral sclerosis. J Mol Neurosci 45:522, 2011.
86. Weihl CC, Pestronk A, Kimonis VE: Valosin-containing protein disease: inclusion body myopathy with Paget's disease of the bone and fronto-temporal dementia. Neuromuscul Disord 19:308, 2009.
87. Kumar KR, Liang C, Needham M, et al: Axonal hyperpolarization in inclusion-body myopathy, Paget disease of the bone, and frontotemporal dementia (IBMPFD). Muscle Nerve 44:191, 2011.
88. Jensen AG, Espersen F, Skinhoj P, et al: Increasing frequency of vertebral osteomyelitis following *Staphylococcus aureus* bacteraemia in Denmark 1980–1990. J Infect 34:113, 1997.
89. Hooten WM, Mizerak A, Carns PE, et al: Discitis after lumbar epidural corticosteroid injection: a case report and analysis of the case report literature. Pain Med 7:46, 2006.
90. Priest DH, Peacock Jr JE: Hematogenous vertebral osteomyelitis due to *Staphylococcus aureus* in the adult: clinical features and therapeutic outcomes. South Med J 98:854, 2005.
91. Mulleman D, Philippe P, Senneville E, et al: Streptococcal and enterococcal spondylodiscitis (vertebral osteomyelitis). High incidence of infective endocarditis in 50 cases. J Rheumatol 33:91, 2006.
92. Pigrau C, Almirante B, Flores X, et al: Spontaneous pyogenic vertebral osteomyelitis and endocarditis: incidence, risk factors, and outcome. Am J Med 118:1287, 2005.
93. An HS, Seldomridge JA: Spinal infections: diagnostic tests and imaging studies. Clin Orthop Relat Res 444:27, 2006.
94. Concia E, Prandini N, Massari L, et al: Osteomyelitis: clinical update for practical guidelines. Nucl Med Commun 27:645, 2006.
95. Prandini N, Lazzeri E, Rossi B, et al: Nuclear medicine imaging of bone infections. Nucl Med Commun 27:633, 2006.
96. Marschall J, Bhavan KP, Olsen MA, et al: The impact of prebiopsy antibiotics on pathogen recovery in hematogenous vertebral osteomyelitis. Clin Infect Dis 52:867, 2011.
97. Le Page L, Feydy A, Rillardon L, et al: Spinal tuberculosis: a longitudinal study with clinical, laboratory, and imaging outcomes. Semin Arthritis Rheum 36:124, 2006.
98. Carragee EJ, Kim D, van der Vlugt T, et al: The clinical use of erythrocyte sedimentation rate in pyogenic vertebral osteomyelitis. Spine 22:2089, 1997.
99. Jaramillo-de la Torre JJ, Bohinski RJ, Kuntz C: Vertebral osteomyelitis. Neurosurg Clin N Am 17:339, 2006.
100. Mann S, Schutze M, Sola S, et al: Nonspecific pyogenic spondylodiscitis: clinical manifestations, surgical treatment, and outcome in 24 patients. Neurosurg Focus 17:E3, 2004.
101. Mylona E, Samarkos M, Kakalou E, et al: Pyogenic vertebral osteomyelitis: a systematic review of clinical characteristics. Semin Arthritis Rheum 39:10, 2009.
102. Swanson AN, Pappou IP, Cammisa FP, et al: Chronic infections of the spine: surgical indications and treatments. Clin Orthop Relat Res 444:100, 2006.
103. Diwakar L, Logan S, Ghaffar N, et al: Low back pain: think of tuberculosis. BMJ 333:201, 2006.
104. Abou-Raya S, Abou-Raya A: Spinal tuberculosis: overlooked? J Intern Med 260:160, 2006.
105. Colmenero JD, Ruiz-Mesa JD, Sanjuan-Jimenez R, et al: Establishing the diagnosis of tuberculous vertebral osteomyelitis. Eur Spine J 22(suppl 4):579, 2013.
106. Blumberg HM, Leonard Jr MK, Jasmer RM: Update on the treatment of tuberculosis and latent tuberculosis infection. JAMA 293:2776, 2005.
107. Cormican L, Hammal R, Messenger J, et al: Current difficulties in the diagnosis and management of spinal tuberculosis. Postgrad Med J 82:46, 2006.
108. De Backer AI, Mortele KJ, Vanschoubroeck IJ, et al: Tuberculosis of the spine: CT and MR imaging features. JBR-BTR 88:92, 2005.
109. Gouliamos AD, Kehagias DT, Lahanis S, et al: MR imaging of tuberculous vertebral osteomyelitis: pictorial review. Eur Radiol 11:575, 2001.
110. Joseffer SS, Cooper PR: Modern imaging of spinal tuberculosis. J Neurosurg Spine 2:145, 2005.
111. Jutte PC, Van Loenhout-Rooyackers JH: Routine surgery in addition to chemotherapy for treating spinal tuberculosis. Cochrane Database Syst Rev:CD004532, 2006.
112. Borenstein D: Inflammatory arthritides of the spine: surgical versus nonsurgical treatment. Clin Orthop Rel Res 443:208, 2006.
113. van der Linden S, van der Heijde D: Ankylosing spondylitis: clinical features. Rheum Dis Clin North Am 24:663, 1998.
114. Zochling J, van der Heijde D, Burgos-Vargas R, et al: ASAS/EULAR recommendations for the management of ankylosing spondylitis. Ann Rheum Dis 65:442, 2006.
115. Dagfinrud H, Kvien TK, Hagen KB: The Cochrane review of physiotherapy interventions for ankylosing spondylitis. J Rheumatol 32:1899, 2005.
116. Gensler L, Inman R, Deodhar A: The "knowns" and "unknowns" of biologic therapy in ankylosing spondylitis. Am J Med Sci 343:360, 2012.

117. Ahn N, Ahn U, Nallamshetty L, et al: Cauda equina syndrome in ankylosing spondylitis (The CES-AS syndrome): meta-analysis of outcomes after medical and surgical treatments. J Spine Dis 14:427, 2001.
118. Van Hoydonck M, de Vlam K, Westhovens R, et al: Destructive dural ectasia of dorsal and lumbar spine with cauda equina syndrome in a patient with ankylosing spondylitis. Open Rheumatol J 4:31, 2010.
119. Westerveld L, Verlaan J, Oner F: Spinal fractures in patients with anklyosing spinal disorders: a systematic review of the literature on treatment, neurological status and complications. Eur Spine J 18:145, 2009.
120. Alaranta H, Luoto S, Konttinen Y: Traumatic spinal cord injury as a complication to anklyosing spondylitis. An extended report. Clin Exp Rheumatol 20:66, 2002.
121. Ramos-Remus C, Gomez-Vargas A, Guzman-Guzman JL, et al: Frequency of atlantoaxial subluxation and neurologic involvement in patients with ankylosing spondylitis. J Rheumatol 22:2120, 1995.
122. Shim SC, Yoo D-H, Lee JK, et al: Multiple cerebellar infarction due to vertebral artery obstruction and bulbar symptoms associated with vertical subluxation and atlanto-occipital subluxation in ankylosing spondylitis. J Rheumatol 25:2464, 1998.
123. Liu C, Lin Y, Lo C, et al: Cauda equina syndrome and dural ectasia: rare manifestations in chronic ankylosing spondylitis. Br J Radiol 84:e123, 2011.
124. Lan H, Chen D, Lan J, et al: Combination of transverse myelitis and arachnoiditis in cauda equina syndrome of long-standing anklyosing spondylitis: MRI features and its role in clinical management. Clin Rheumatol 26:1963, 2007.
125. Tullous MW, Skerhut HEI, Story JL, et al: Cauda equina syndrome of long-standing ankylosing spondylitis: case report and review of the literature. J Neurosurg 73:441, 1990.
126. Confavreux C, Larbre J-P, Lejeune E, et al: Cerebrospinal fluid dynamics in the tardive cauda equina syndrome of ankylosing spondylitis. Ann Neurol 29:221, 1991.
127. Cornec D, Pensec V, Joulin S, et al: Dramatic efficacy of infliximab in cauda equina syndrome complicating anklyosing spondylitis. Arthritis Rheum 60:1657, 2009.
128. Khan MA, Kushner I: Ankylosing spondylitis and multiple sclerosis: a possible association. Arthritis Rheum 22:784, 1979.
129. Calin A: Is there an association between ankylosing spondylitis and multiple sclerosis? Ann Rheum Dis 48:971, 1989.
130. Nozaki K, Silver R, Stickler D, et al: Neurological deficits during treatment with tumor necrosis factor-alpha antagonists. Am J Med Sci 342:352, 2011.
131. Solomon A, Spain R, Kruer M, et al: Inflammatory neurological disease in patients treated with tumor necrosis factor alpha inhibitors. Mult Scler 17:1472, 2011.
132. Kemta Lekpa F, Kraus VB, Chevalier X: Biologics in relapsing polychondritis: a literature review. Semin Arthritis Rheum 41:712, 2012.
133. Lahmer T, Treiber M, von Werder A, et al: Relapsing polychondritis: an autoimmune disease with many faces. Autoimmun Rev 9:540, 2012.
134. Letko E, Zafirakis P, Baltatzis S, et al: Relapsing polychondritis: a clinical review. Semin Arthritis Rheum 31:384, 2002.
135. Trentham DE, Le CH: Relapsing polychondritis. Ann Intern Med 129:114, 1998.
136. Michet CJ: Vasculitis and relapsing polychondritis. Rheum Dis Clin North Am 16:441, 1990.
137. Yamazaki K, Suga T, Hirata K: Large vessel arteritis in relapsing polychondritis. J Laryngol Otol 115:836, 2001.
138. Nadeau SE: Neurologic manifestations of connective tissue disease. Neurol Clin 20:151, 2002.
139. Wang ZJ, Pu CQ, Wang ZJ, et al: Meningoencephalitis or meningitis in relapsing polychondritis: four case reports and a literature review. J Clin Neurosci 18:1608, 2011.
140. Yaguchi H, Tsuzaka K, Niino M, et al: Aseptic meningitis with relapsing polychondritis mimicking bacterial meningitis. Intern Med 48:1841, 2009.
141. Ota M, Mizukami K, Hayashi T, et al: Brain magnetic resonance imaging and single photon emission computerized tomography findings in a case of relapsing polychondritis showing cognitive impairment and personality changes. Prog Neuropsychopharmacol Biol Psychiatry 29:347, 2005.
142. Coumbaras M, Boulin A, Piette AM, et al: Intracranial aneurysm associated with relapsing polychondritis. Neuroradiology 43:565, 2001.
143. Kashihara K, Kawada S, Takahashi Y: Autoantibodies to glutamate receptor GluRepsilon2 in a patient with limbic encephalitis associated with relapsing polychondritis. J Neurol Sci 287:275, 2009.
144. Roux C, Guey S, Crassard I, et al: A rare cause of gait ataxia. Lancet 378:1274, 2011.
145. Topalkara K, Kaptanoglu E, Akyuz A, et al: Relapsing polychondritis with involvement of posterior inferior cerebellar artery causing acute lateral medullary syndrome. J Clin Rheumatol 9:92, 2003.
146. Defer GL, Danaila T, Constans JM, et al: Relapsing polychondritis revealed by basal ganglia lesions. Mov Disord 27:1094, 2011.
147. Massry GG, Chung SM, Selhorst JB: Optic neuropathy, headache, and diplopia with MRI suggestive of cerebral arteritis in relapsing polychonritis. J Neuroophthalmol 15:171, 1995.

SECTION

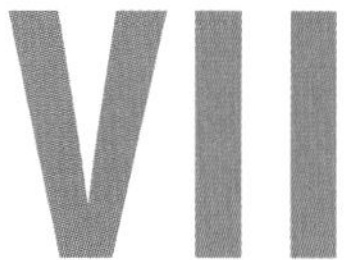

Ears, Eyes, and Related Systems

CHAPTER

23

Otoneurologic Manifestations of Otologic and Systemic Disease

JOSEPH M. FURMAN ■ ANDREW A. McCALL

NEUROLOGIC MANIFESTATIONS OF OTOLOGIC DISEASE

Complications of Middle Ear Pathology

Intracranial complications occur in 0.25 to 0.5 percent of all cases of otitis media.[1,2] The mortality rate of intracranial complications has decreased dramatically over the last century, from approximately 90 percent in the pre-antibiotic era to 10 percent now.[3–5] However, significant morbidity still exists despite this improvement in survival.[6] Diagnosis of an intracranial complication of otitis media relies heavily on an accurate history. Important elements include determining whether the patient has acute or chronic otitis media, a prior history of otologic disease or surgery, a history of head trauma or temporal bone fracture, previous antibiotic treatment, and symptoms suggesting intracranial involvement such as headache, lethargy, visual changes, fever, and nausea or vomiting.[6–8]

The differential diagnosis for a patient with otitis media and symptoms and signs of intracranial involvement is long, and potential complications are numerous, including extradural abscesses or granulation tissue, dural venous sinus thrombosis, petrous apicitis (Gradenigo syndrome; Fig. 23-1), intraparenchymal brain abscesses, subdural abscesses, otitic hydrocephalus, and meningitis (most commonly purulent).[3,7,9]

The microbiology of the intracranial complications of otitis media varies with the duration of otitis as well as the type of complication. Complications of acute otitis media usually are secondary to *Streptococcus pneumoniae* or *Haemophilus influenzae*.[3,6,7] Chronic otitis media frequently leads to complications with gram-negative bacteria, such as *Pseudomonas aeruginosa*, or anaerobes.[6,7] The most common organisms implicated in otitic meningitis include *S. pneumoniae*, *H. influenzae*, *Proteus* species, *P. aeruginosa*, and *Staphylococcus aureus*. Brain abscesses are typically polymicrobial.[10]

If an intracranial complication is suspected on the basis of the history or physical findings, further evaluation should include computerized tomography (CT) of the temporal bones to evaluate for bony erosion, congenital malformation, or fracture; contrast-enhanced magnetic resonance imaging (MRI) or CT of the head to evaluate for enhancement of the meninges, dural sinus thrombosis (Fig. 23-2), or brain abscess; and a lumbar puncture if no mass

Neurology and General Medicine, Fifth Edition.

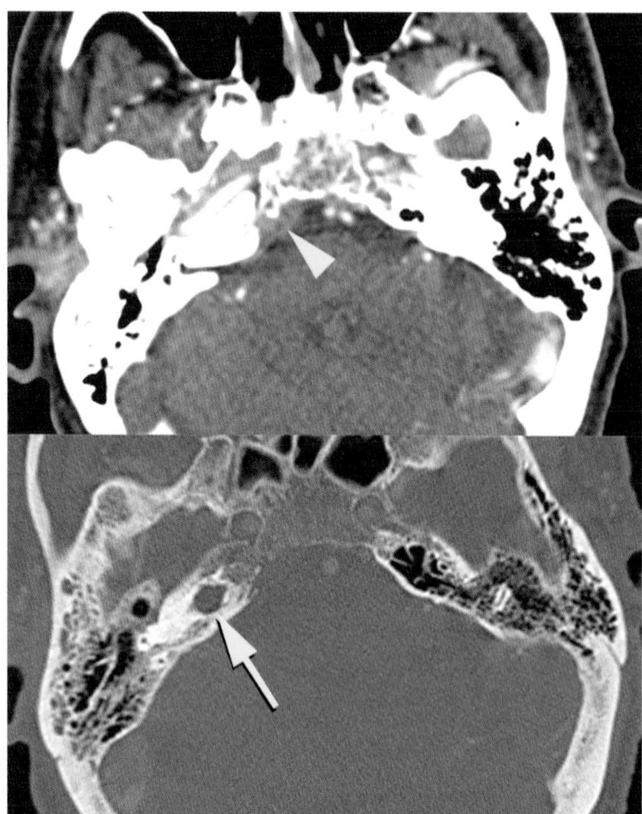

FIGURE 23-1 ■ Computed tomography (CT) scan showing right petrous apicitis. *Upper scan*: Soft tissue windowing demonstrating enhancement at the tip of the petrous apex affecting Dorello canal (*arrow head*). *Lower scan*: Bone windowing demonstrating a lytic cell in the petrous apex with loss of septation (*arrow*). (Courtesy of Hugh D. Curtin, MD, Massachusetts Eye and Ear Infirmary, Boston.)

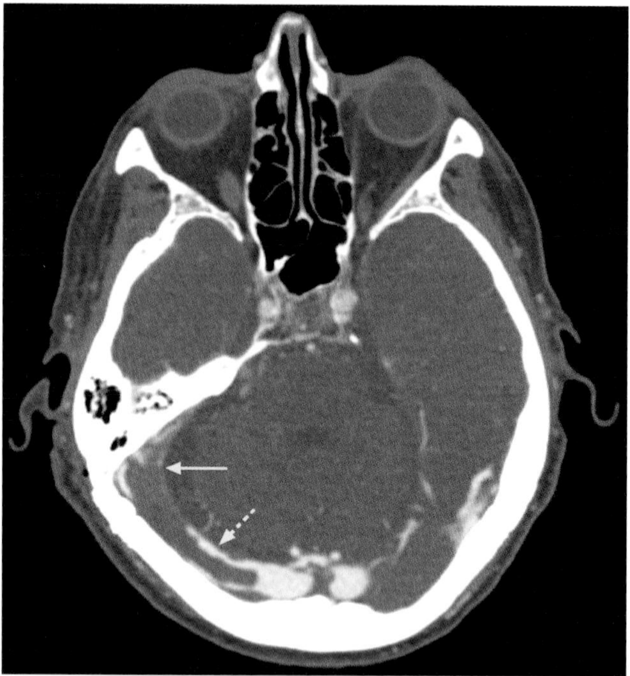

FIGURE 23-2 ■ Sigmoid sinus thrombosis. CT venography performed after retromastoid craniectomy reveals a filling defect in the right transverse (*dashed arrow*) and sigmoid (*solid arrow*) sinuses, representing subocclusive thrombus. (Courtesy of Barton F. Branstetter, MD, University of Pittsburgh.)

effect is visualized on imaging.[1,7,10] The cerebrospinal fluid (CSF) will typically show increased protein and decreased glucose concentrations along with organisms on Gram stain in bacterial meningitis; those patients given antibiotics in the days or weeks preceding the spinal tap may have more normal-appearing CSF chemistries and a negative Gram stain, but should be treated with antibiotics until cultures are negative, given the possibility of a partially treated bacterial meningitis. In otitic hydrocephalus, the opening pressure will be increased, but the other studies will be normal.

Treatment of the intracranial complications of otitis media includes medical stabilization and usually requires inpatient admission. Broad-spectrum intravenous antibiotics should be initiated empirically. Complications due to acute otitis media may be treated with a second- or third-generation cephalosporin to target the usual three pathogens: *H. influenzae*, *Moraxella catarrhalis*, and *S. pneumoniae*. Gram-negative and anaerobic coverage should be added for complications of chronic otitis media. Corticosteroids such as dexamethasone should be administered concurrently with intravenous antibiotics for otogenic meningitis in order to reduce the chance of sensorineural hearing loss and, in meningitis caused by *S. pneumoniae*, to reduce mortality.[7,11]

Labyrinthine Disorders

Meniere disease and benign paroxysmal positional vertigo are two of the most common labyrinthine disorders that cause vertigo and dysequilibrium. The pathologic correlate of Meniere disease is endolymphatic hydrops, which is usually idiopathic but may occur following inner ear trauma or infection.[12] Patients with Meniere disease typically experience episodes of unilateral tinnitus, unilateral hearing loss, unilateral ear fullness, and vertigo lasting for minutes to hours. They do not typically experience neurologic symptoms that cannot be attributable directly to the inner ear. However, some patients experience visual changes, especially blurred vision, during attacks of Meniere disease, and headaches may occur. Other patients become anxious during attacks and may experience numbness and paresthesias. The first attack of Meniere disease often prompts an evaluation in an emergency department, leading to brain imaging to exclude cerebellar hemorrhage or infarction. First-line treatment of Meniere disease consists of sodium restriction and a diuretic, typically a combination of hydrochlorothiazide and triamterene. Non-ablative procedures, such as intratympanic steroid infusion, and ablative procedures, such as intratympanic gentamicin or labyrinthectomy, are options for patients who do not respond to conservative management.[13,14]

Benign paroxysmal positional vertigo is caused by free-floating otolithic debris in the posterior semicircular canal.[12] As with Meniere disease, benign paroxysmal positional vertigo may follow inner ear trauma or infections but usually is idiopathic. Patients typically have positionally induced vertigo when rolling over in bed or looking up. The vertigo typically lasts for less than 1 minute but more generalized symptoms of dizziness and dysequilibrium may persist for several hours. Neurologic symptoms other than vertigo and transitory visual difficulties are generally absent although patients may have difficulty in walking due to their vertigo. On physical examination, the findings on Dix–Hallpike maneuvers, illustrated in Figure 23-3, are diagnostic.[15] Treatment consists of a particle repositioning maneuver (Fig. 23-4), which is highly successful and can be taught to the patient for use in future attacks. Despite the "benign" nature of benign paroxysmal positional vertigo, the initial episode often leads to emergency medical care. Since several non-benign conditions, such as posterior fossa tumors, may present with positional dizziness, a thorough neurologic evaluation of all patients with positional vertigo is warranted.

Eighth Nerve Lesions

Eighth nerve lesions leading to neurologic manifestations include auditory neuropathy and vestibular neuronitis. Auditory neuropathy is a disorder of dysfunction or dyssynchrony of the inner hair cells or cochlear nerve, leading to hearing loss and impaired speech discrimination with intact outer hair cell function.[16–18] Risk factors for auditory neuropathy include prematurity, hyperbilirubinemia, and exposure to ototoxic medications, although genetic factors have also been implicated.[19] This type of hearing loss can be associated with other neurologic diseases[16] and may be seen in up to 11 percent of children with sensorineural hearing loss.[20]

Vestibular neuronitis is an idiopathic inflammation of the vestibular portion of the eighth cranial nerve leading to acute symptoms of vertigo, nystagmus, nausea, and vomiting. Acute symptoms persist for several days and are often preceded by viral illness. In some patients, mild symptoms can last for weeks or months. Unilateral reduction in vestibular response is seen on caloric testing or vestibular evoked myogenic potentials. Possible etiologies include viral infection, immunologic causes, or vascular occlusion.[21] The superior or inferior vestibular nerve, or both, may be involved.

Cerebellopontine Angle Disorders

Cerebellopontine angle masses may cause hearing loss, tinnitus, and vertigo. The most common type of mass found in this location is a vestibular schwannoma, commonly referred to as an acoustic neuroma. Symptoms are typically of insidious onset, but sudden hearing loss or vertigo may occur. Additionally, facial numbness may be seen with large tumors due to compression of the trigeminal nerve. Facial nerve dysfunction from vestibular schwannoma is uncommon. Without treatment, lower cranial nerve involvement and brainstem compression may eventually occur (Fig. 23-5). MRI of the internal auditory canal is the typical modality used to identify these lesions. Acoustic neuromas are treated with surgical excision or stereotactic radiation; small tumors may be observed for evidence of growth. Other masses occurring in the cerebellopontine angle include meningiomas, epidermoid tumors, and metastases, which may cause similar symptoms, although the time scale of symptomatology is typically more rapid with metastatic lesions in this area.

Superior Semicircular Canal Dehiscence Syndrome

Superior semicircular canal dehiscence syndrome was first recognized in 1998 as a cause of vertigo.[22]

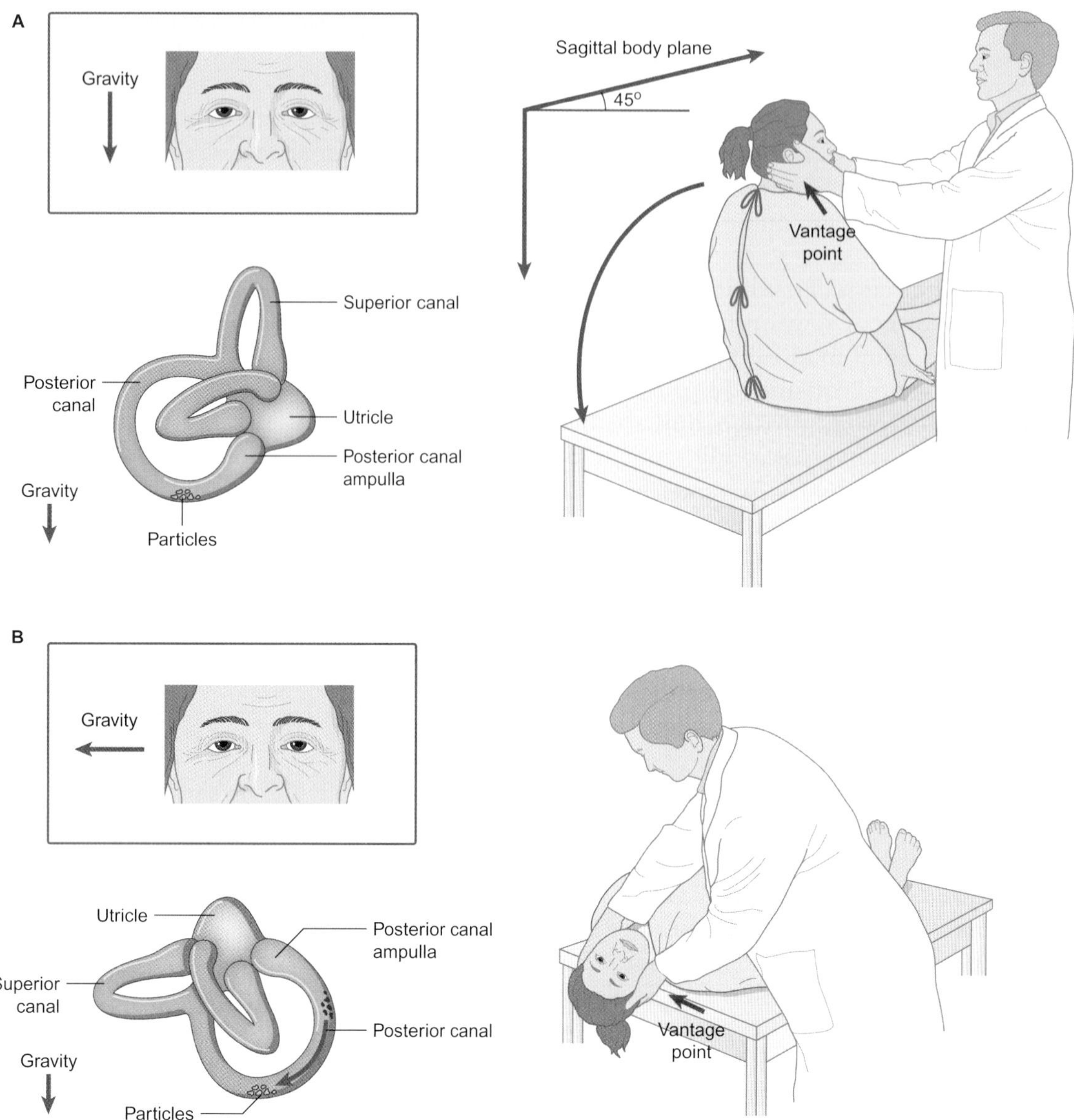

FIGURE 23-3 ▪ Dix–Hallpike Maneuver. The Dix–Hallpike test of a patient with benign paroxysmal positional vertigo affecting the right ear. **A**, The examiner stands at the patient's right side and rotates the patient's head 45 degrees to the right to align the right posterior semicircular canal with the sagittal plane of the body. **B**, The examiner moves the patient, whose eyes are open, from the seated to the supine right-ear-down position and then extends the patient's neck so that the chin is pointed slightly upward. The latency, duration, and direction of nystagmus, if present, and the latency and duration of vertigo, if present, should be noted. The arrows in the inset depict the direction of nystagmus in patients with typical benign paroxysmal positional vertigo. The presumed location in the labyrinth of the free-floating debris thought to cause the disorders is also shown. (From Furman JM, Cass SPC: Benign paroxysmal positional vertigo. N Engl J Med 341:1590, 1999, with permission.)

The disorder is caused by a defect in the bone over the superior semicircular canal, which renders the canal sound sensitive.[23] Symptoms of superior semicircular canal dehiscence syndrome include vertigo induced by sound or pressure (such as during a Valsalva maneuver), hearing loss, and autophony. Systemic neurologic symptoms are absent. Noncontrast CT scan of the temporal bone demonstrates the absence of bone over the superior semicircular canal. Treatment consists of surgically plugging the superior canal in patients with bothersome vestibular symptoms (Fig. 23-6).[24,25]

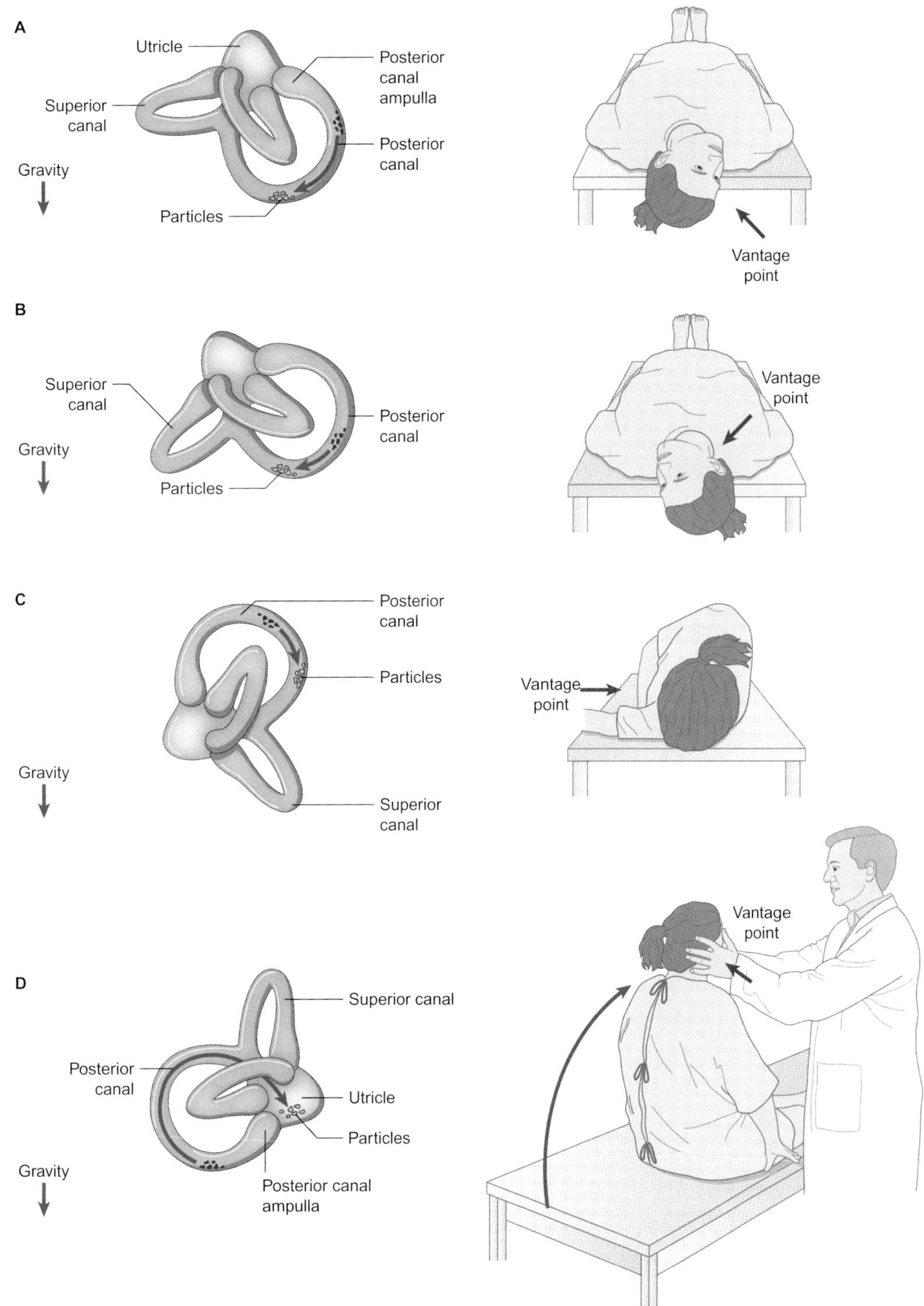

FIGURE 23-4 ■ Particle repositioning maneuver for the bedside treatment of a patient with benign paroxysmal positional vertigo affecting the right ear. The presumed position of the debris within the labyrinth during the maneuver is shown in each panel. The maneuver is a three-step procedure. First, a Dix–Hallpike test is performed with the patient's head rotated 45 degrees toward the right ear and the neck slightly extended with the chin pointed slightly upward. This position results in the patient's head hanging to the right (**A**). Once the vertigo and nystagmus provoked by the Dix–Hallpike test cease, the patient's head is rotated about the rostral-caudal body axis until the left ear is down (**B**). Then the head and body are further rotated until the head is face down (**C**). The vertex of the head is kept tilted downward throughout the rotation. The maneuver usually provokes brief vertigo. The patient should be kept in the final, face-down position for about 10 to 15 seconds. With the head kept turned toward the left shoulder, the patient is brought into the seated position (**D**). Once the patient is upright, the head is tilted so that the chin is pointed slightly downward. (From Furman JM, Cass SPC: Benign paroxysmal positional vertigo. N Engl J Med 341:1590, 1999, with permission.)

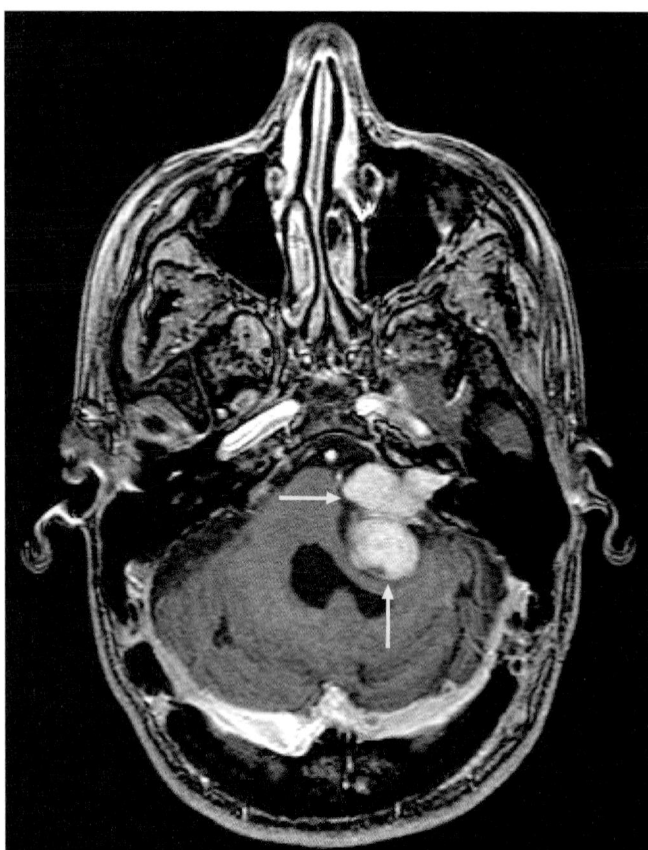

FIGURE 23-5 ■ Magnetic resonance imaging (MRI) of a large acoustic neuroma with brainstem compression. Axial contrast-enhanced T1-weighted MRI reveals a large, lobulated, enhancing mass (*arrows*) filling the left cerebellopontine angle, with compression of the pons and thinning of the brachium pontis. The patient was known to have neurofibromatosis type 2, and this lesion is most likely a schwannoma of the eighth cranial nerve. (Courtesy of Barton F. Branstetter, MD, University of Pittsburgh.)

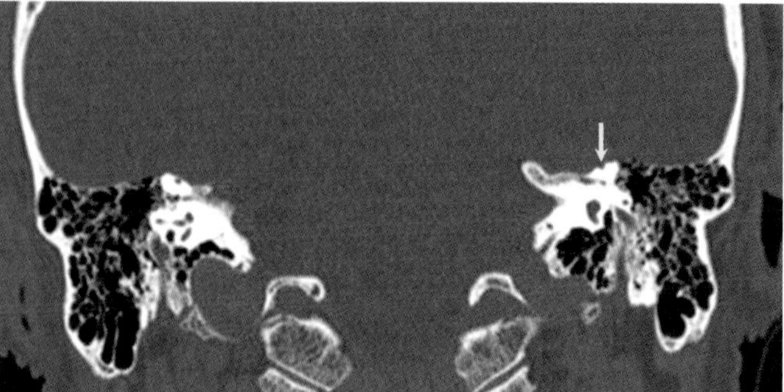

FIGURE 23-6 ■ Coronal CT scan through the level of the temporal bone demonstrating superior canal dehiscence. Arrow points to the left superior semicircular canal dehiscence. The membranous superior semicircular canal (seen in cross section) is in contact with the overlying contents of the middle cranial fossa. Compare this with the right side, where a very thin plate of bone is separating the superior semicircular canal from the middle cranial fossa. (Courtesy of Andrew A. McCall, MD, University of Pittsburgh.)

Central Vestibular Disorders

The most common central vestibular disorders include migraine-related dizziness, vascular disease affecting the brainstem and cerebellar vestibular pathways, cerebellar degeneration, and Chiari malformation. Migraine-related dizziness, which can be considered a migraine variant, affects women more often than men, particularly women in their child-bearing years. As with migraine headache, it is a diagnosis of exclusion, since there are no pathognomonic tests for this condition. Diagnostic criteria consist of a combination of the International Headache Society criteria for migraine headache and criteria developed specifically for migraine-related dizziness.[26] Establishing a diagnosis of migraine-related dizziness requires a temporal association between dizziness and either migraine headache or typical migrainous symptoms and the absence of another diagnosis that can account for the dizziness. The pathophysiology is uncertain but is likely to be related to serotonin effects on central vestibular structures. Treatment is similar to the treatment for migraine headache and includes both decreasing triggers for migraine and use of pharmacotherapy. For patients with frequent (greater than 1 per week) episodes of migraine-related dizziness, prophylactic medications are indicated to reduce the frequency and severity of attacks and include antidepressants, beta-blockers, anticonvulsants, and calcium-channel blockers. Some patients may benefit from triptans for acute attacks.

Central vestibular structures in the brainstem and cerebellum are supplied by the posterior inferior cerebellar artery and the anterior inferior cerebellar artery. Infarction of the lateral medulla in the territory of the posterior inferior cerebellar artery leads to a Wallenberg syndrome, wherein one of two vestibular nuclear complexes is damaged, leading to central vestibular imbalance. Accompanying symptoms are caused by involvement of the ascending spinothalamic tract and descending sympathetic tracts. Patients with Wallenberg syndrome may experience lateropulsion (i.e., a sense of being pushed or pulled to one side). Infarction in the territory of the anterior inferior cerebellar artery leads to a similar syndrome but may also include the presence of unilateral hearing loss resulting from cochlear ischemia because the internal auditory artery arises from the anterior inferior cerebellar artery.

Another condition to be considered in patients with acute vertigo and accompanying neurologic disturbances referable to the brainstem and cerebellum is that of cerebellar hemorrhage or infarction with concomitant brainstem compression, or even of brainstem stroke alone. This condition represents a neurosurgical emergency. Brain imaging provides definitive diagnostic information.

Vertebrobasilar insufficiency may present with various neurologic symptoms including vertigo and changes in hearing as well as symptoms referable to parenchymal posterior fossa structures, such as changes in vision, sensation, strength, or level of consciousness. Symptoms typically last for minutes. Isolated vertigo is rarely a result of vertebrobasilar insufficiency.[27,28] Diagnostic imaging such as MR or CT angiography is helpful in establishing a diagnosis of vertebrobasilar insufficiency in the context of appropriate symptoms. Treatment with antiplatelet agents and management of risk factors for cardiovascular disease are warranted for most cases; endovascular treatment with angioplasty, stenting, or both, is rarely employed.

Cerebellar degeneration can be associated with dizziness and dysequilibrium. Some types of cerebellar degeneration (particularly spinocerebellar ataxia, type 6) can also be associated with episodic features including episodic vertigo and dysequilibrium. In association with such symptoms, patients with cerebellar degeneration often demonstrate limb ataxia and sometimes long-tract signs. Chiari malformations sometimes present with "dizziness" and dysequilibrium. Physical examination may disclose down-beating nystagmus (i.e., vertical nystagmus with a downward fast component), which may reflect a central vestibular imbalance. Additionally, patients with a Chiari malformation often have nonvestibular symptoms such as dysphagia and long-tract signs. A diagnosis of a Chiari malformation can be confirmed by sagittal MRI (Fig. 23-7). Treatment is surgical and involves suboccipital craniotomy.

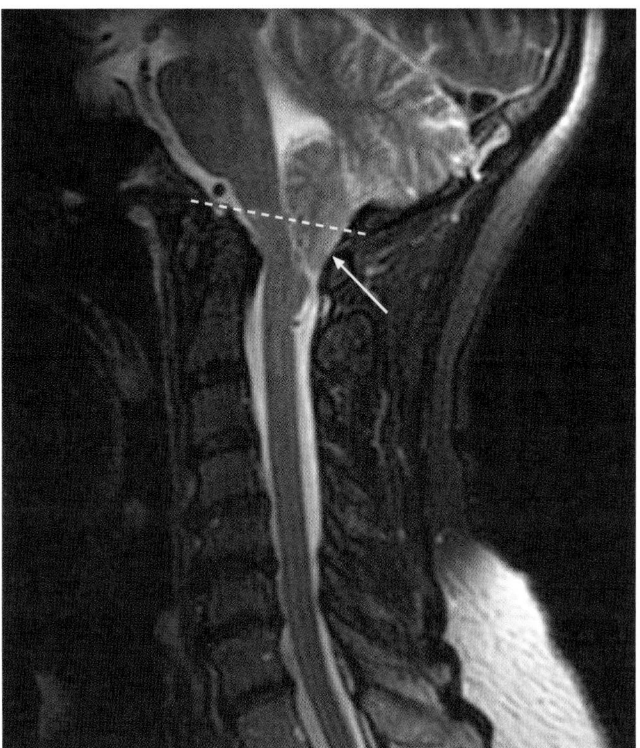

FIGURE 23-7 ■ Chiari malformation. Sagittal T2-weighted MRI through the cranio-cervical junction shows the cerebellar tonsils (*solid arrow*) extending far below the foramen magnum (*dashed line*). The medulla is compressed. (Courtesy of Barton F. Branstetter, MD, University of Pittsburgh.)

Central Auditory Processing Disorder

Central auditory processing disorder, as its name implies, is characterized by defects in higher-level processing of auditory information in the setting of normal hearing as measured by conventional audiometry. This disorder leads to difficulty in understanding oral communication, particularly when there is background noise, and can be associated with attention deficit–hyperactivity disorder, learning disabilities, head trauma, and other neurologic disorders.[29–31] Psychoacoustic testing often identifies specific deficits that correlate with patients' symptoms.[32] Treatment consists of improving the signal-to-noise ratio with amplification or reduction of background noise, as well as auditory training.[31]

OTONEUROLOGIC MANIFESTATIONS OF SYSTEMIC DISEASE

Infection

Many infections can cause otoneurologic symptoms and signs. Viral infection, in particular herpes simplex virus, has been implicated in Bell palsy.[33,34] Figure 23-8 shows herpes simplex virus type 1

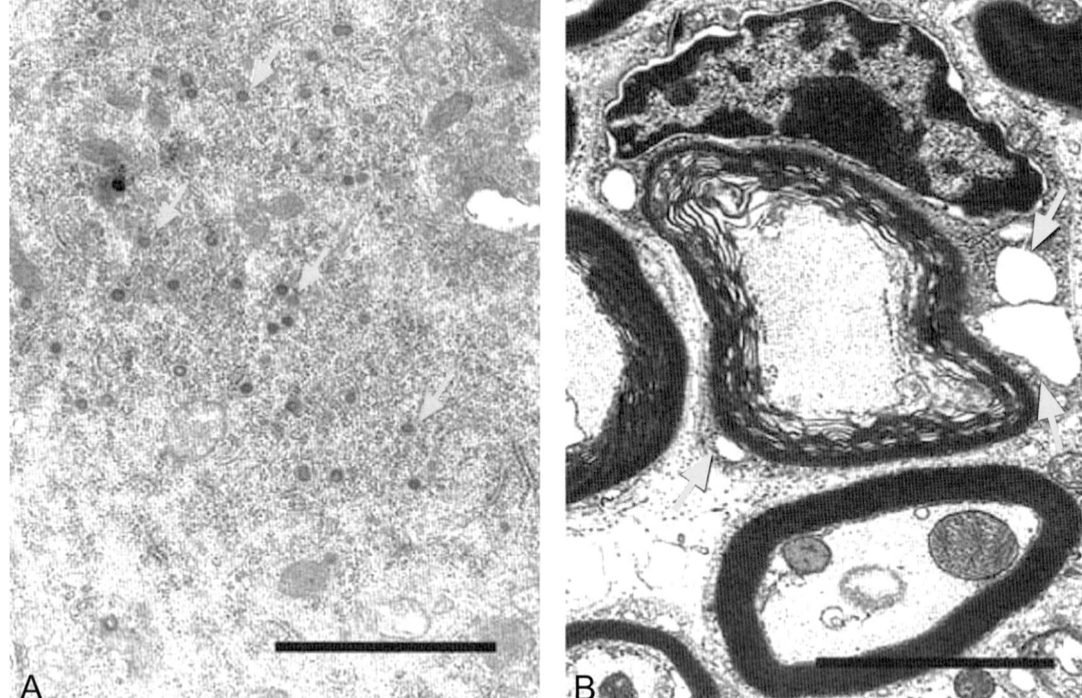

FIGURE 23-8 ▪ Herpes simplex virus (HSV) in a mouse model of Bell palsy. **A**, The intratemporal portion of the facial nerve from the paralyzed side showing a neuron in the geniculate ganglion. Replicating HSV-1 viruses in the rough endoplasmic reticulum of a neuron in the geniculate ganglion are indicated by the arrows. **B**, The geniculate portion of the facial motor nerve. Arrows indicate vacuolar changes in the cytoplasm of a Schwann cell which resulted in demyelination. Scale bars: A, 1 µm; B, 5 µm. (From Takahashi H, Hitsumoto Y, Honda N, et al: Mouse model of Bell's palsy induced by reactivation of herpes simplex virus type 1. J Neuropathol Exp Neurol 60:621, 2001, with permission.)

particles seen by electron microscopy in the geniculate ganglion of mice with experimentally induced Bell palsy. Corticosteroids are used for treatment. Viral infection is also thought to play a role in idiopathic sudden sensorineural hearing loss[35] and vestibular neuronitis.[36] Mumps, measles, and congenital rubella infection may cause significant hearing loss.[37]

Another member of the herpes virus family, varicella-zoster virus, causes herpes zoster oticus, often referred to as Ramsay Hunt syndrome. This syndrome, from reactivation of varicella-zoster virus in the geniculate ganglion, is characterized by facial weakness associated with vesicular lesions in the external auditory canal and auricle.[38] The symptoms are typically preceded by otalgia.[38] Sensorineural hearing loss and vertigo are sometimes present. Investigators have postulated that the reactivation of varicella-zoster virus may occur in the vestibular and spiral ganglia as well.[39] Ramsay Hunt syndrome may involve other cranial nerves; polymerase chain reaction has localized viral material to the CSF in some cases. MRI typically reveals enhancement of the geniculate ganglion on the affected side. Treatment is with antiviral agents and corticosteroids. The facial palsy associated with Ramsay Hunt syndrome has a poorer prognosis than that of Bell palsy.[40]

Otosyphilis was first described in 1887 by Politzer.[41] Following the introduction of penicillin, it became rare. However, with the emergence of human immunodeficiency virus (HIV) infection, syphilis has experienced a resurgence in the United States and Western Europe.[42,43] Otoneurologic manifestations may occur in secondary, tertiary, or congenital syphilis. Sensorineural hearing loss and hydropic symptoms of episodic tinnitus and vertigo may occur. Treatment is with penicillin G and corticosteroids.

Lyme disease may cause sudden sensorineural hearing loss or facial palsy.[44] Vertigo is uncommon but has been reported.[45] The mainstay of treatment is intravenous ceftriaxone; corticosteroids may be added for treatment of hearing loss.

Tuberculosis may affect the ear. As with syphilis, tuberculosis has become increasingly common in patients with HIV infection.[46] Tuberculous otitis media remains rare.[46] The classic description of mycobacterial otitis media is of chronic otorrhea and multiple perforations of the tympanic membrane.[47] Polyps and granulation tissue may also be seen. Treatment is primarily medical, with surgery reserved for complications.[46]

HIV infection and immunodeficiency may cause otologic symptoms. Otitis externa may be caused by common pathogens such as *P. aeruginosa*; however, opportunistic infections such as *Pneumocystis* species may also be responsible in these populations.[48] There are also reports of malignant otitis externa (i.e., skull base osteomyelitis secondary to otitis externa) in individuals with HIV infection,[49] although some authors note that the incidence of malignant otitis externa is not increased in the HIV-infected population as a whole.[50] Children with HIV infection often suffer from chronic otitis media. Serous otitis media may result from eustachian tube obstruction secondary to adenoid hypertrophy. Sensorineural hearing loss occurs in 21 to 49 percent of HIV-positive patients and is thought to be multifactorial.[51] Possible causes include secondary infection, central nervous system (CNS) involvement, and ototoxicity.[48] Finally, facial palsy is more common in HIV-positive patients.[52]

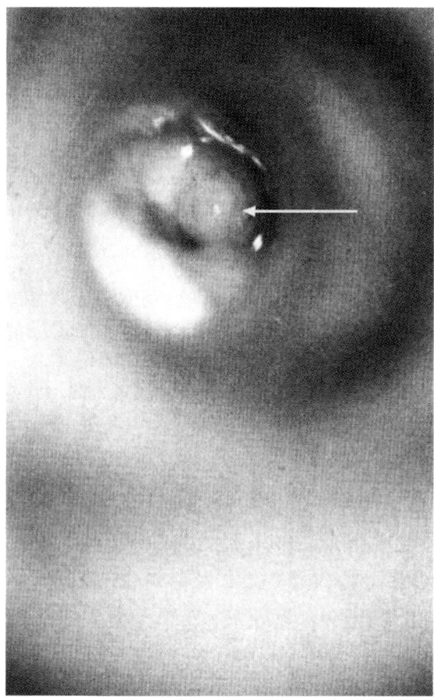

FIGURE 23-9 ▪ Chronic otitis media in Wegener granulomatosis. Granulomatous swelling of the posterior part of the left eardrum viewed through an otomicroscope (*arrow*). The large white area inferior and to the left of the eardrum is the anterior wall of the external ear canal. (From Rasmussen N: Management of the ear, nose, and throat manifestations of Wegener granulomatosis: an otorhinolaryngologist's perspective. Curr Opin Rheumatol 13:3, 2001, with permission.)

Immune-Mediated and Connective Tissue Disease

There are a number of autoimmune and connective tissue disorders that cause otoneurologic symptoms, ranging from otitis media to hearing loss or vertigo.

Wegener granulomatosis is characterized by vasculitis of medium and small vessels, as well as by necrotizing granulomas of the upper and lower respiratory tract. Up to 70 percent of patients with this disorder experience otologic symptoms.[53–55] The most common otoneurologic manifestation of Wegener granulomatosis is serous otitis media.[56] The middle ear space can be affected by granulomas, leading to a clinical picture resembling chronic suppurative otitis media (Fig. 23-9). Facial palsy may also result, from either vasculitis or direct involvement of the facial nerve by the granulomatous process.[53,55,56] Sensorineural hearing loss occurs in 8 percent of patients and is sometimes rapidly progressive.[54] Vertigo is uncommon. Wegener granulomatosis is diagnosed by the presence of cytoplasmic antineutrophil cytoplasmic antibodies (c-ANCA) and by the combination of necrotizing granulomas and vasculitis seen on histopathology. Treatment is with high-dose corticosteroids and immunosuppressive agents.[53,54]

Sarcoidosis is an immune-mediated disease of unknown etiology characterized by hilar adenopathy, pulmonary infiltrates, peripheral lymphadenopathy, and cutaneous and splenic involvement that can involve the CNS. The characteristic histopathologic finding is of noncaseating granulomas, although they are nonspecific. The most common otoneurologic manifestation of sarcoidosis is facial palsy, which may be unilateral or bilateral and can be associated with parotiditis, fever, and uveitis (uveoparotid fever or Heerfordt disease). Multiple cranial nerve palsies are common in neurosarcoidosis, occurring in approximately 5 percent of patients with sarcoidosis due to involvement of the meninges of the skull base.[57,58] Hearing loss and vertigo are less common symptoms. The presentation of hearing loss is variable, ranging from mild to severe, and may be unilateral or bilateral.[57,59] Vestibular testing may be abnormal.[59] Auditory and vestibular symptoms are thought to reflect involvement of the eighth cranial nerve by neurosarcoidosis rather than a direct effect on the inner ear end organs.[59] Contrast-enhanced MRI may show enhancement of the basal leptomeninges; intracranial mass lesions can also be seen.[58]

Systemic lupus erythematosus may cause sensorineural hearing loss that is unilateral or bilateral in 8 to 31 percent of patients and can be rapidly progressive.[60–62] The hearing loss appears to be associated with elevated anticardiolipin antibodies but not with ANA titer and frequently improves with treatment.[61,62] Vestibular symptoms are less common.[62]

Hearing loss is also commonly seen in rheumatoid arthritis, manifesting in 29 to 48 percent of patients.[60,63] It may be sensorineural, conductive, or mixed in type, and its severity is correlated with disease activity.[63] Conductive hearing loss is thought to be secondary to involvement of the ossicular chain by rheumatoid arthritis, whereas sensorineural hearing loss may be due to immunocomplex deposition, antibodies against inner ear antigens, or cell-mediated immune processes.[63] Investigations into the vestibular function of patients with rheumatoid arthritis have revealed no significant differences from controls.[64]

Other immune-mediated diseases causing otologic symptoms include polyarteritis nodosa, Cogan syndrome, Behçet syndrome, relapsing polychondritis, Sjögren syndrome, and Churg–Strauss syndrome. Polyarteritis nodosa, a small-vessel vasculitis, may cause sudden sensorineural hearing loss.[60] Cogan syndrome is characterized by sudden or rapidly progressive sensorineural hearing loss, vestibular dysfunction, and interstitial keratitis, mimicking syphilis or Meniere disease. Symptoms often respond to treatment with corticosteroids.[60] Behçet syndrome may cause hearing loss, tinnitus, and vertigo.[60] Relapsing polychondritis typically involves the cartilage of the external ear and nose; however, as the disease progresses, hearing loss and vertigo sometimes develop. The disorder is discussed further in Chapter 22.[60] High-frequency hearing loss may also be seen in 25 percent of patients with Sjögren syndrome.[60,65] Churg–Strauss syndrome causes hearing loss in rare instances.[61]

Autoimmune hearing loss also may occur in the absence of systemic illness. It is characterized by fluctuating or rapidly progressive bilateral sensorineural hearing loss that is responsive to immunosuppressive therapy.[60]

Neurocutaneous Syndromes

The most common neurocutaneous syndrome causing otoneurologic symptoms is neurofibromatosis type 2, which is discussed in detail in Chapter 21. This disease is characterized by bilateral vestibular schwannomas, eventually causing bilateral deafness and vestibular dysfunction. Other features of neurofibromatosis type 2 can include meningiomas, ependymomas, gliomas, and juvenile posterior subcapsular lens opacities.[66] Otologic manifestations consist of progressive hearing loss that may be unilateral or bilateral, tinnitus, vestibular dysfunction, and facial weakness. Genetic testing is available to detect mutations in the neurofibromin 2 (*merlin*) tumor suppressor gene.[66] Auditory rehabilitation of affected patients is complex owing to the presence of bilateral acoustic neuroma; auditory brainstem implants have been used in this population with fair results.[67]

Metabolic and Endocrine Disorders

Certain metabolic or endocrine disorders are known to contribute to hearing loss. Diabetes mellitus has been linked to hearing loss,[68,69] perhaps secondary to microangiopathy and neuropathy.[70,71] A small subset of diabetic patients have been found to have a mitochondrial mutation causing both hearing loss and diabetes, termed *maternally inherited diabetes and deafness*.[72] Diabetic patients frequently suffer from "dizziness" and imbalance, and peripheral neuropathy, autonomic dysfunction, and peripheral vestibular deficits all probably play a role in etiology.[73]

Renal failure in the absence of diabetes is also associated with high-frequency hearing loss.[74] Alport syndrome is characterized by congenital hearing loss and renal failure. Neonatal jaundice may cause sensorineural hearing loss.[37] Hyperlipidemia has also been associated with fluctuating hearing loss and vestibular dysfunction.[37]

An association between thyroid disease and otologic symptoms exists. Vertigo and hearing loss have been described in the setting of hypothyroidism.[75] Pendred syndrome is characterized by congenital

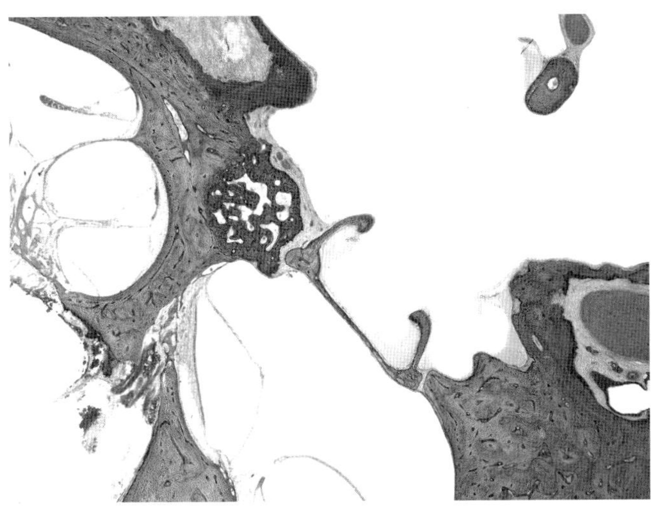

FIGURE 23-10 ■ Osteogenesis imperfecta of the temporal bone. Histologic section of the right temporal bone from a patient with osteogenesis imperfecta, showing an otosclerotic lesion anterior to the oval window. (From Santos F, McCall A, Chein W, et al: Otopathology in osteogenesis imperfecta. Otol Neurotol 33:1562, 2012, with permission.)

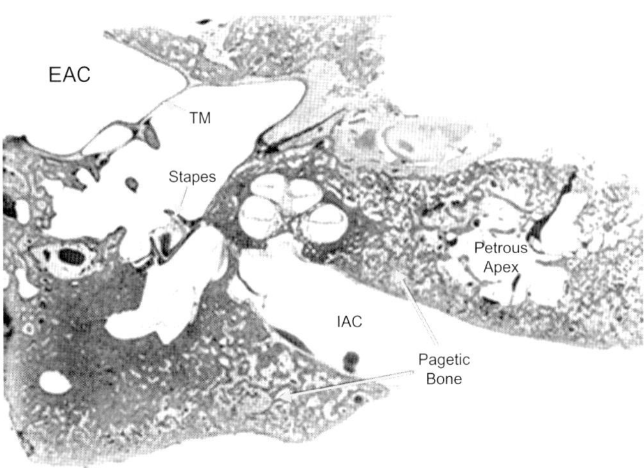

FIGURE 23-11 ■ Paget disease of the temporal bone. Histologic section through the left temporal bone showing pagetic bone surrounding the internal auditory canal. (From Bahmad F Jr, Merchant SN: Paget disease of the temporal bone. Otol Neurotol 28:1157, 2007, with permission.)

hearing loss, reduced vestibular responses, and goiter. In a study of 42 kindreds, resistance to thyroid hormone was found to be associated with hearing loss in 21 percent of individuals.[76]

Certain mucopolysaccharidoses are associated with hearing loss, and many forms predispose to otitis media. The Hurler and Hunter forms (MPS I and II) cause sensorineural hearing loss. The mechanism of loss is unclear and may involve deposition of glycosaminoglycans in the cochlea.[77]

Diseases of Bone

Several disorders of bone, discussed in Chapter 22, lead to otoneurologic manifestations, most notably hearing loss. These include osteogenesis imperfecta, Paget disease, fibrous dysplasia, and osteopetrosis.

Osteogenesis imperfecta is usually an autosomal-dominant disease caused mainly by mutations in the *COL1A1* or *COL1A2* genes, which code for type 1 collagen. The disorder is characterized by fragility of bones, hearing loss, and blue sclera. Eight major types are currently described; hearing loss is most common in types IA and IB. Hearing loss occurs in 23 to 58 percent of patients with osteogenesis imperfecta and typically presents in the second or third decade.[78] Histologic examination of temporal bones from individuals with type I osteogenesis imperfecta demonstrates otosclerosis-like lesions (Fig. 23-10). The hearing loss typically begins as a conductive loss and progresses to become mixed or largely sensorineural in nature; both ears are eventually affected. Hearing loss may be treated with amplification or stapedectomy. Tinnitus and vertigo are also common in osteogenesis imperfecta, particularly in those patients with sensorineural hearing loss. Vertigo is typically mild, triggered by head movements or position change, and brief in duration.[79] Abnormalities are frequently seen on electronystagmography but do not necessarily correlate with subjective vertigo.[79]

Paget disease is caused by increased bone absorption and repair, leading to an overall increase in the amount of bone. There are monostotic and polyostotic forms. Hearing loss is common in Paget disease and is usually mixed conductive and sensorineural. Conductive hearing loss may be caused by ossicular fixation or obliteration of the oval or round window. Bony changes in the cochlea may also contribute.[80] Involvement of the petrous portion of the temporal bone may alter the shape of the internal auditory canal, potentially impairing the function of the eighth cranial nerve. Histologically, Paget disease is characterized by disordered lamellar bone (Fig. 23-11). CT may reveal demineralization of the temporal bone. Treatment is with bisphosphonates and calcitonin, which may prevent further hearing loss.

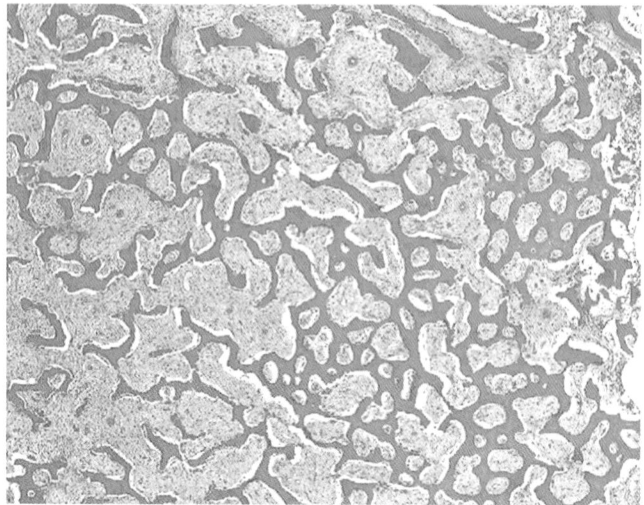

FIGURE 23-12 ■ Histology of fibrous dysplasia. Note the irregular shapes of woven bone. (From Speight PM, Carlos R: Maxillofacial fibro-osseous lesions. Curr Diagn Pathol 12:1, 2006, with permission.)

Fibrous dysplasia, like Paget disease, also has monostotic and polyostotic forms. It is nonfamilial but usually caused by mutations in the *GNAS1* gene, which codes for a second messenger G protein. The disease is characterized by expansile bony lesions (Fig. 23-12). Involvement of the temporal bone can cause narrowing of the external auditory canal, resulting in conductive hearing loss. A lesser percentage of patients will manifest sensorineural hearing loss, labyrinthitis, or facial weakness.[80] Treatment is with bisphosphonates or surgical resection. Irradiation increases the risk of malignant transformation and is not indicated.

Osteopetrosis is characterized by decreased osteoclastic activity, leading to constriction of various skull base foramina. Hearing loss, vertigo, and facial palsy or spasm may develop secondary to compression. Eustachian tube dysfunction and middle ear effusions may be seen.[81] Treatment is with vitamin D (calcitriol), prednisone, and interferon-gamma.[82]

Drug-Induced Disorders

There are numerous medications that exert ototoxic effects on the cochlea and labyrinth. The most commonly encountered ototoxic medications are chemotherapeutic agents, antibiotics, and loop diuretics. Cochlear ototoxicity is typically heralded by tinnitus or a sense of fullness in the ear; however, high-frequency hearing loss may also occur without the patient's knowledge. Hearing loss due to certain drugs, most notably salicylates and furosemide, can be reversible, whereas toxicity secondary to cisplatin and aminoglycosides is most often permanent. Vertigo and disequilibrium may result from vestibular toxicity; bobbing oscillopsia is a common symptom.[83] Conditions contributing to a higher risk for ototoxicity include renal insufficiency, hepatic insufficiency, elevated serum levels of medication, preexisting hearing loss or vestibular dysfunction, use of multiple ototoxic medications or a previous history of ototoxic medication use, treatment for more than 14 days, prior exposure to noise, hypovolemia, bacteremia, fever, and age over 65 years.[83,84]

Ototoxicity leads to distinct histologic changes within the cochlea and labyrinth, and the histologic manifestations are typically either hair cell loss (Fig. 23-13) or changes in the stria vascularis.

Aminoglycoside antibiotics have been known to be ototoxic since the parenteral use of streptomycin for tuberculosis in the early twentieth century. Symptomatic hearing loss occurs in 2 to 14 percent of patients treated with aminoglycosides[85]; however, high-frequency (10 to 20 kHz) audiometry reveals the incidence of hearing loss to be as high as 62 percent.[86] Certain aminoglycosides, such as streptomycin and gentamicin, preferentially lead to vestibular toxicity but also cause cochlear toxicity. It is unclear whether elevated serum levels of antibiotic correlate with increased risk of toxicity. The pathogenesis is thought to involve generation of free radicals leading to apoptosis of hair cells.[87] There is evidence that certain mitochondrial mutations cause increased susceptibility to the ototoxic effects of aminoglycosides.[88] Animal studies are ongoing to evaluate potential protective agents such as antioxidants or iron chelators that may be administered concomitantly.[84,87] Other anti-infective agents reported to cause ototoxicity less frequently include vancomycin, macrolides, fluoroquinolones, tetracycline, antivirals, amphotericin, flucytosine, and antimalarials.

Cisplatin is the chemotherapy agent most frequently associated with ototoxicity, with an incidence of 20 to 65 percent.[89–91] Hearing loss initially manifests in the high frequencies and progressively worsens with continued administration. Tinnitus is a common presenting complaint. Ototoxicity appears related to the cumulative dose. Histologic findings in cisplatin ototoxicity include damage to the stria vascularis and hair cell loss.[83] Ongoing studies are

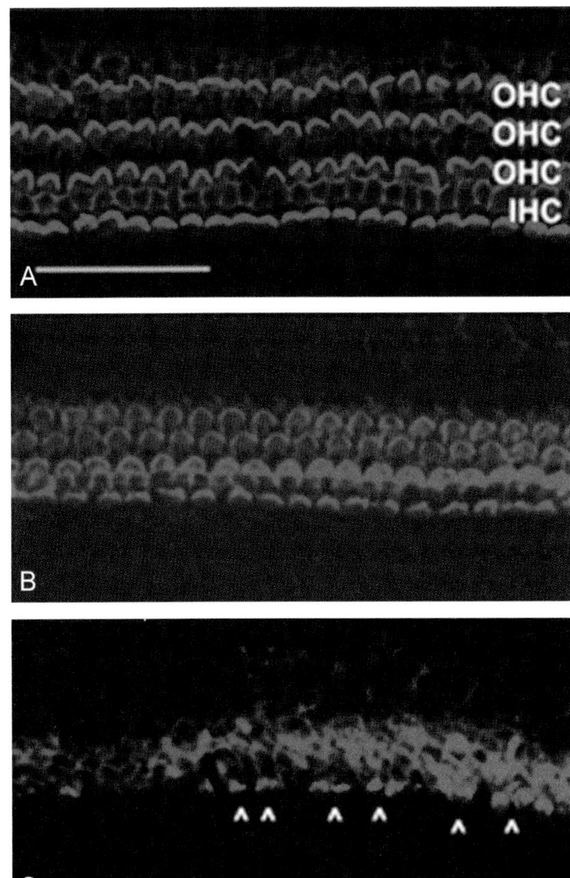

FIGURE 23-13 ■ Hair cell loss from gentamicin ototoxicity. **A** and **B** demonstrate a normal complement of inner (IHC) and outer hair cells (OHC) of the cochlea. **C** shows severe loss of outer hair cells and many inner hair cells after exposure to gentamicin (mouse cochlea). (From Matt T, Ng CL, Lang K, et al: Dissociation of antibacterial activity and aminoglycoside ototoxicity in the 4-monosubstituted 2-deoxystreptamine apramycin. Proc Natl Acad Sci USA 109:10988, 2012, with permission.)

evaluating agents that may protect against cisplatin-induced ototoxicity. Owing to the high incidence of ototoxicity with aminoglycosides and cisplatin, patient monitoring with high-frequency audiometry and careful attention to symptoms is recommended for early diagnosis and management. Other ototoxic chemotherapeutic agents include carboplatin, oxiliplatin, vinca alkaloids, bexarotene, and taxanes.

Loop diuretics can cause hearing loss, tinnitus, and occasionally vertigo, perhaps because disturbances in the sodium and potassium concentrations in endolymph cause edema of the stria vascularis. Hearing loss is typically reversible and is usually seen with parenteral rather than oral administration of the offending medication.[83] Bumetanide may be less ototoxic than furosemide or ethacrynic acid.

Salicylates can cause tinnitus and reversible hearing loss, although some cases of permanent hearing impairment have been reported following overdoses.

Environmental Disorders

Numerous types of environmental injury can result in otoneurologic symptoms. Noise exposure is well known to cause hearing loss. The typical audiometric configuration is a sensorineural hearing loss with a notched pattern around 4000 Hz. Both occupational and recreational exposure can cause significant loss. Some individuals appear more likely than others to sustain noise-induced loss.[70] The best treatment of noise-induced hearing loss is prevention. Hearing protection with earplugs or earmuffs can decrease exposure to sound. Maximum allowable amount and duration of noise exposure are available through the Occupational Health and Safety Administration (OSHA). The National Institute of Occupational Safety and Health (NIOSH) also has guidelines on the amount and duration of exposure that is safe, but the levels differ between the two agencies.[92]

Barotrauma may cause otologic injury through multiple mechanisms. The most common injury is perforation of the tympanic membrane. Barotrauma may also lead to conductive hearing loss from fracture or dislocation of the ossicles. Rarely, facial nerve paresis can result.[93] Inner ear barotrauma can manifest as a perilymphatic fistula, manifest by hearing loss, vertigo, nausea, and vomiting following exposure to increased atmospheric pressure. Inner ear decompression sickness causes similar symptoms, usually manifesting itself after surfacing from a dive.[94] The prognosis for recovery is good for inner ear barotrauma, but progressive damage to the cochlear and vestibular organs often occurs following inner ear decompression sickness.[95]

Lightning strikes (discussed in Chapter 36) have also been documented to have otoneurologic sequelae. Lightning may produce injury either through a direct strike or over telephone lines.[96,97] Hearing loss, tinnitus, tympanic membrane perforation, facial palsy, and vertigo have been reported.[98] Hearing loss is nonprogressive and may have a mixed conductive and sensorineural pattern.[99]

Blast injuries to the ear may lead to tympanic membrane rupture and resulting conductive hearing

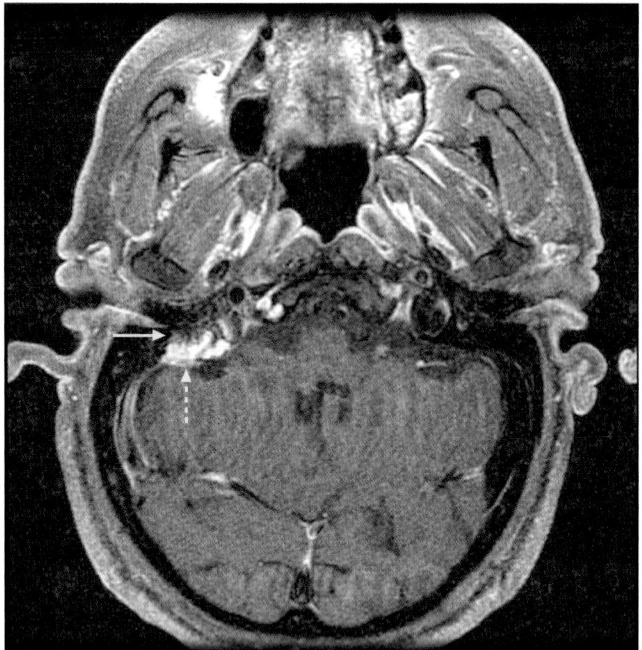

FIGURE 23-14 ▪ MRI of endolymphatic sac tumor. Axial contrast-enhanced T1-weighted MRI demonstrates an irregular, enhancing mass along the posterior border of the petrous apex, at the expected location of the endolymphatic sac (*dashed arrow*). The mass erodes into the underlying temporal bone (*solid arrow*). (Courtesy of Barton F. Branstetter, MD, University of Pittsburgh.)

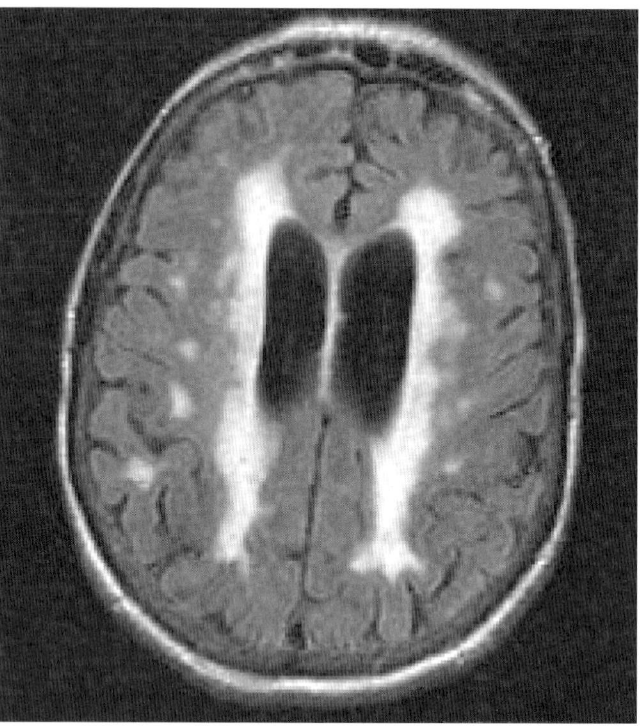

FIGURE 23-15 ▪ MRI of a patient with microvascular disease seen in disequilibrium of aging. Axial fluid-attenuated inversion recovery (FLAIR) sequence through the bodies of the lateral ventricles shows extensive, confluent areas of abnormal signal in a periventricular and subcortical distribution, consistent with white matter microvascular disease. The ventricles are slightly enlarged from associated central volume loss. (Courtesy of Barton F. Branstetter, MD, University of Pittsburgh.)

loss. Sensorineural hearing loss is also common and appears to occur via a different mechanism from noise-induced hearing loss, as the audiometric pattern lacks a notch at 4000 Hz.[100] Tinnitus can result from blast injury and may be particularly noticeable in that disorder because of its sudden onset.[101] Balance disorders can also manifest following blast and mild traumatic brain injury.[102]

Severe thermal injury to the ear may result from slag burns from welding. Often non-healing perforations of the tympanic membrane are seen. Facial paralysis, sensorineural hearing loss, and vertigo have also been reported.[103]

Nutritional Disease

Wernicke encephalopathy, which results from hypovitaminosis B_1 (thiamine), manifests with ataxia, abnormal eye movements, and mental status change. Vestibular laboratory testing of patients with Wernicke encephalopathy typically indicates bilaterally reduced vestibular responses and abnormal central vestibular processing.[104] Treatment is by replacement of thiamine, which usually corrects the abnormal eye movements and ataxia. Vestibular function remains abnormal.

Neoplastic Disease

The temporal bone is affected by primary malignancies as well as metastatic disease. Primary tumors may originate in the external ear, middle ear and mastoid, or inner ear structures. Squamous cell carcinoma and basal cell carcinoma can arise from the auricle and external auditory canal or they may spread from adjacent sites. Pain is a common complaint, although hearing loss and facial weakness may also occur.[105] Rhabdomyosarcoma may originate in the temporal bone in children. Endolymphatic sac tumors occur both sporadically and associated with von Hippel–Lindau disease[106] (Fig. 23-14). Symptoms arise from local extension of the tumor and may include pain,

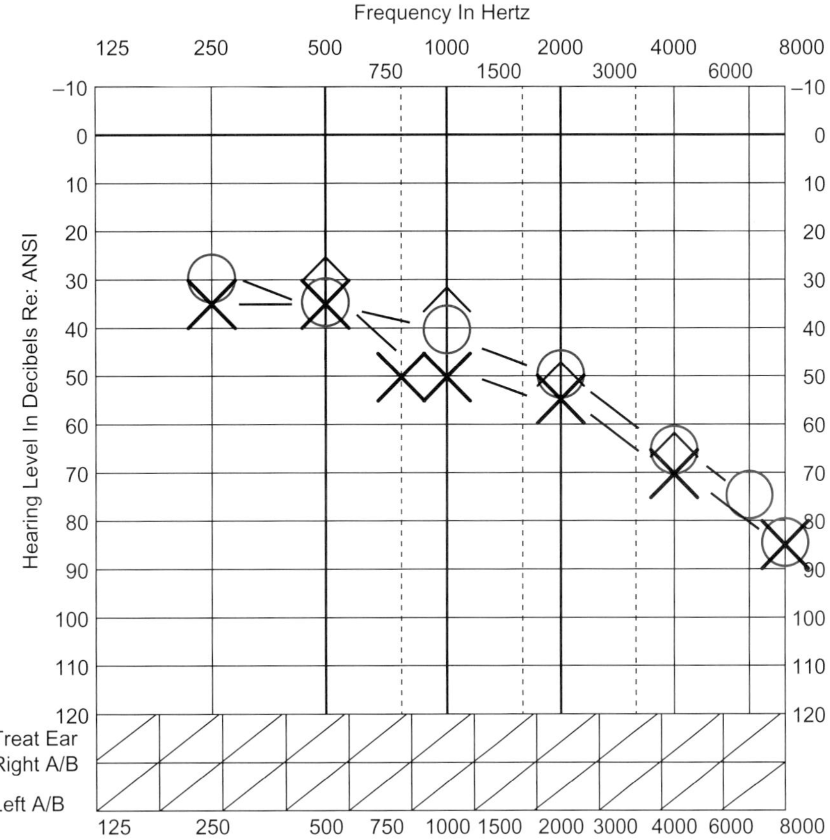

FIGURE 23-16 ■ Audiogram of presbycusis. This audiogram shows sensorineural hearing loss in a downsloping pattern, typical of presbycusis.

hearing loss, and, less commonly, vertigo.[106] Cancers of the breast, kidney, lung, stomach, thyroid gland, and prostate all may metastasize to the temporal bone.[105]

NEURO-OTOLOGIC MANIFESTATIONS OF AGING

Dysequilibrium of Aging

Dysequilibrium of aging refers to a loss of balance in association with advanced age in individuals who have no other known etiology for their balance disturbance. Patients with dysequilibrium of aging are generally in their seventies and demonstrate white matter disease on MRI including periventricular and subcortical white matter disease (Fig. 23-15) that may relate to microvascular ischemic changes.[107] Treatment consists of managing risk factors for cerebrovascular disease and balance therapy. Vestibular-suppressant medications should be discontinued.

Presbycusis

Sensorineural hearing loss related to aging is termed presbycusis. Approximately one-third of persons between the ages of 60 and 70, and up to half of those between 70 and 80, have hearing loss.[70] Four subtypes of presbycusis have been described, relating to different audiometric patterns.[108] The most common type is called sensory presbycusis, manifesting as a symmetric high-frequency sensorineural hearing loss that progressively worsens with age (Fig. 23-16). Both genetic and environmental factors play a role in etiology.[70] Patients typically complain of difficulty in understanding speech, especially when there is background noise, and they may also suffer from tinnitus.[109]

REFERENCES

1. Habib RG, Girgis NI, Abu el Ella AH, et al: The treatment and outcome of intracranial infections of otogenic origin. J Trop Med Hyg 91:83, 1988.

2. Neely JG: Intratemporal and intracranial complications of otitis media. In Bailey BJ (ed): Head and Neck Surgery—Otolaryngology. JB Lippincott, Philadelphia, 1993.
3. Brydoy B, Ellekjaer EF: Otogenic meningitis: a five-year study. J Laryngol Otol 86:871, 1972.
4. Singh B, Maharaj TJ: Radical mastoidectomy: its place in otitic intracranial complications. J Laryngol Otol 107:1113, 1993.
5. Wolfowitz BL: Otogenic intracranial complications. Arch Otolaryngol 96:220, 1972.
6. Barry B, Delattre J, Vie F, et al: Otogenic intracranial infections in adults. Laryngoscope 109:483, 1999.
7. Levine S, deSouza C: Intracranial complications of otitis media. In: Glasscock ME, Gulya AJ (eds): Surgery of the Ear. BC Decker, Ontario, 2003.
8. Winkler J, Bogdahn U, Becker G, et al: Surgical intervention and heparin-anticoagulation improve prognosis of rhinogenic/otogenic and posttraumatic meningitis. Acta Neurol Scand 89:293, 1994.
9. Samuel J, Fernandes CM, Steinberg JL: Intracranial otogenic complications: a persisting problem. Laryngoscope 96:272, 1986.
10. Hilsinger Jr RL, Caparosa RJ: Otogenic brain abscess. Laryngoscope 80:697, 1970.
11. McIntyre PB, Berkey CS, King SM, et al: Dexamethasone as adjunctive therapy in bacterial meningitis. A meta-analysis of randomized clinical trials since 1988. JAMA 278:925, 1997.
12. Paparella MM: The cause (multifactorial inheritance) and pathogenesis (endolymphatic malabsorption) of Meniere's disease and its symptoms (mechanical and chemical). Acta Otolaryngol 99:445, 1985.
13. Boleas-Aguirre MS, Lin FR, Della Santina CC, et al: Longitudinal results with intratympanic dexamethasone in the treatment of Meniere's disease. Otol Neurotol 29:33, 2008.
14. Pullens B, van Benthem PP: Intratympanic gentamicin for Meniere's disease or syndrome. Cochrane Database Syst Rev:CD008234, 2011.
15. Furman JM, Cass SP: Benign paroxysmal positional vertigo. N Engl J Med 341:1590, 1999.
16. Starr A, Picton TW, Sininger Y, et al: Auditory neuropathy. Brain 119:741, 1996.
17. Starr A, Isaacson B, Michalewski HJ, et al: A dominantly inherited progressive deafness affecting distal auditory nerve and hair cells. J Assoc Res Otolaryngol 5:411, 2004.
18. Giraudet F, Avan P: Auditory neuropathies: understanding their pathogenesis to illuminate intervention strategies. Curr Opin Neurol 25:50, 2012.
19. Madden C, Rutter M, Hilbert L, et al: Clinical and audiological features in auditory neuropathy. Arch Otolaryngol Head Neck Surg 128:1026, 2002.
20. Rance G, Beer DE, Cone-Wesson B, et al: Clinical findings for a group of infants and young children with auditory neuropathy. Ear Hear 20:238, 1999.
21. Nadol Jr JB: Vestibular neuritis. Otolaryngol Head Neck Surg 112:162, 1995.
22. Minor LB, Solomon D, Zinreich JS, et al: Sound- and/or pressure-induced vertigo due to bone dehiscence of the superior semicircular canal. Arch Otolaryngol Head Neck Surg 124:249, 1998.
23. Merchant SN, Rosowski JJ: Conductive hearing loss caused by third-window lesions of the inner ear. Otol Neurotol 29:282, 2008.
24. Mikulec AA, Poe DS, McKenna MJ: Operative management of superior semicircular canal dehiscence. Laryngoscope 115:501, 2005.
25. McCall AA, McKenna MJ, Merchant SN, et al: Superior canal dehiscence syndrome associated with the superior petrosal sinus in pediatric and adult patients. Otol Neurotol 32:1312, 2011.
26. Neuhauser H, Lempert T: Vertigo and dizziness related to migraine: a diagnostic challenge. Cephalalgia 24:83, 2004.
27. Fisher CM: Vertigo in cerebrovascular disease. Arch Otolaryngol 85:529, 1967.
28. Grad A, Baloh RW: Vertigo of vascular origin. Clinical and Electronystagmographic Features in 84 Cases. Arch Neurol 46:281, 1989.
29. Gomez R, Condon M: Central auditory processing ability in children with ADHD with and without learning disabilities. J Learn Disabil 32:150, 1999.
30. Bergemalm PO, Lyxell B: Appearances are deceptive? Long-term cognitive and central auditory sequelae from closed head injury. Int J Audiol 44:39, 2005.
31. Bamiou DE, Musiek FE, Luxon LM: Aetiology and clinical presentations of auditory processing disorders—a review. Arch Dis Child 85:361, 2001.
32. Griffiths TD: Central auditory processing disorders. Curr Opin Neurol 15:31, 2002.
33. Murakami S, Mizobuchi M, Nakashiro Y, et al: Bell palsy and herpes simplex virus: identification of viral DNA in endoneurial fluid and muscle. Ann Intern Med 124:27, 1996.
34. Furuta Y, Fukuda S, Chida E, et al: Reactivation of herpes simplex virus type 1 in patients with Bell's palsy. J Med Virol 54:162, 1998.
35. Hughes GB, Freedman MA, Haberkamp TJ, et al: Sudden sensorineural hearing loss. Otolaryngol Clin North Am 29:393, 1996.
36. Strupp M, Zingler VC, Arbusow V, et al: Methylprednisolone, valacyclovir, or the combination for vestibular neuritis. N Engl J Med 351:354, 2004.
37. Sataloff RT: Hearing loss associated with non-hereditary systemic disease. Ear Nose Throat J 62:621, 1983.
38. Hunt JR: On herpetic inflammations of the geniculate ganglion. A new syndrome and its complications. J Nerv Ment Dis 34:73, 1907.
39. Kuhweide R, Van de Steene V, Vlaminck S, et al: Ramsay Hunt syndrome: pathophysiology of cochleovestibular symptoms. J Laryngol Otol 116:844, 2002.

40. May M, Podvinec M, Ulrich J, et al: Idiopathic (Bell's) palsy, herpes zoster cephalicus and other facial nerve disorders of viral origin. In May M (ed): The Facial Nerve. Thieme, New York, 1986.
41. Politzer A: Lehrbuch der Ohrenheilkunde fur praktische Arzte und Studierende. Verlag von Ferdinand Enke (Ferdinand Enke), Stuttgart, 1887.
42. Pletcher SD, Cheung SW: Syphilis and otolaryngology. Otolaryngol Clin North Am 36:595, 2003.
43. Klemm E, Wollina U: Otosyphilis: report on six cases. J Eur Acad Dermatol Venereol 18:429, 2004.
44. Belman AL, Iyer M, Coyle PK, et al: Neurologic manifestations in children with North American Lyme disease. Neurology 43:2609, 1993.
45. Peltomaa M, Pyykko I, Seppala I, et al: Lyme borreliosis—an unusual cause of vertigo. Auris Nasus Larynx 25:233, 1998.
46. Munck K, Mandpe AH: Mycobacterial infections of the head and neck. Otolaryngol Clin North Am 36:569, 2003.
47. Greenfield BJ, Selesnick SH, Fisher L, et al: Aural tuberculosis. Am J Otol 16:175, 1995.
48. Gurney TA, Murr AH: Otolaryngologic manifestations of human immunodeficiency virus infection. Otolaryngol Clin North Am 36:607, 2003.
49. Hern JD, Almeyda J, Thomas DM, et al: Malignant otitis externa in HIV and AIDS. J Laryngol Otol 110:770, 1996.
50. Truitt TO, Tami TA: Otolaryngologic manifestations of human immunodeficiency virus infection. Med Clin North Am 83:303, 1999.
51. Lalwani AK, Sooy CD: Otologic and neurotologic manifestations of acquired immunodeficiency syndrome. Otolaryngol Clin N Am 25:1183, 1992.
52. Belec L, Georges AJ, Bouree P, et al: Peripheral facial nerve palsy related to HIV infection: relationship with the immunological status and the HIV staging in Central Africa. Cent Afr J Med 37:88, 1991.
53. Takagi D, Nakamaru Y, Maguchi S, et al: Otologic manifestations of Wegener's granulomatosis. Laryngoscope 112:1684, 2002.
54. Gubbels SP, Barkhuizen A, Hwang PH: Head and neck manifestations of Wegener's granulomatosis. Otolaryngol Clin North Am 36:685, 2003.
55. Hartl DM, Aidan P, Brugiere O, et al: Wegener's granulomatosis presenting as a recurrence of chronic otitis media. Am J Otolaryngol 19:54, 1998.
56. Rasmussen N: Management of the ear, nose, and throat manifestations of Wegener granulomatosis: an otorhinolaryngologist's perspective. Curr Opin Rheumatol 13:3, 2001.
57. Schwartzbauer HR, Tami TA: Ear, nose, and throat manifestations of sarcoidosis. Otolaryngol Clin North Am 36:673, 2003.
58. Nowak DA, Widenka DC: Neurosarcoidosis: a review of its intracranial manifestation. J Neurol 248:363, 2001.
59. Colvin IB: Audiovestibular manifestations of sarcoidosis: a review of the literature. Laryngoscope 116:75, 2006.
60. Barna BP, Hughes GB: Autoimmunity and otologic disease: clinical and experimental aspects. Clin Lab Med 8:385, 1988.
61. Papadimitraki ED, Kyrmizakis DE, Kritikos I, et al: Ear-nose-throat manifestations of autoimmune rheumatic diseases. Clin Exp Rheumatol 22:485, 2004.
62. Sperling NM, Tehrani K, Liebling A, et al: Aural symptoms and hearing loss in patients with lupus. Otolaryngol Head Neck Surg 118:762, 1998.
63. Salvinelli F, Cancilleri F, Casale M, et al: Hearing thresholds in patients affected by rheumatoid arthritis. Clin Otolaryngol Allied Sci 29:75, 2004.
64. King J, Young C, Highton J, et al: Vestibulo-ocular, optokinetic and postural function in humans with rheumatoid arthritis. Neurosci Lett 328:77, 2002.
65. Mahoney EJ, Spiegel JH: Sjogren's disease. Otolaryngol Clin North Am 36:733, 2003.
66. Neff BA, Welling DB: Current concepts in the evaluation and treatment of neurofibromatosis type II. Otolaryngol Clin North Am 38:671, 2005.
67. Toh EH, Luxford WM: Cochlear and brainstem implantation. Otolaryngol Clin North Am 35:325, 2002.
68. Kurien M, Thomas K, Bhanu TS: Hearing threshold in patients with diabetes mellitus. J Laryngol Otol 103:164, 1989.
69. Kakarlapudi V, Sawyer R, Staecker H: The effect of diabetes on sensorineural hearing loss. Otol Neurotol 24:382, 2003.
70. Fransen E, Lemkens N, Van Laer L, et al: Age-related hearing impairment (ARHI): environmental risk factors and genetic prospects. Exp Gerontol 38:353, 2003.
71. Maia CA, Campos CA: Diabetes mellitus as etiological factor of hearing loss. Rev Bras Otorrinolaringol (Engl Ed) 71:208, 2005.
72. Guillausseau PJ, Massin P, Dubois-LaForgue D, et al: Maternally inherited diabetes and deafness: a multicenter study. Ann Intern Med 134:721, 2001.
73. Lucente FE: Endocrine problems in otolaryngology. Ann Otol Rhinol Laryngol 82:131, 1973.
74. Antonelli AR, Bonfioli F, Garrubba V, et al: Audiological findings in elderly patients with chronic renal failure. Acta Otolaryngol Suppl 476:54, 1990.
75. Moehlig RC: Vertigo and deafness associated with hypothyroidism. Endocrinology 11:229, 1927.
76. Brucker-Davis F, Skarulis MC, Grace MB, et al: Genetic and clinical features of 42 kindreds with resistance to thyroid hormone. The National Institutes of Health Prospective Study. Ann Intern Med 123:572, 1995.
77. Simmons MA, Bruce IA, Penney S, et al: Otorhinolaryngological manifestations of the mucopolysaccharidoses. Int J Pediatr Otorhinolaryngol 69:589, 2005.

78. Kuurila K, Kaitila I, Johansson R, et al: Hearing loss in Finnish adults with osteogenesis imperfecta: a nationwide survey. Ann Otol Rhinol Laryngol 111:939, 2002.
79. Kuurila K, Kentala E, Karjalainen S, et al: Vestibular dysfunction in adult patients with osteogenesis imperfecta. Am J Med Genet A 120:350, 2003.
80. Hullar TE, Lustig LR: Paget's disease and fibrous dysplasia. Otolaryngol Clin North Am 36:707, 2003.
81. Steward CG: Neurological aspects of osteopetrosis. Neuropathol Appl Neurobiol 29:87, 2003.
82. Dozier TS, Duncan IM, Klein AJ, et al: Otologic manifestations of malignant osteopetrosis. Otol Neurotol 26:762, 2005.
83. Tange RA: Ototoxicity. Adverse Drug React Toxicol Rev 17:75, 1998.
84. Bates DE: Aminoglycoside ototoxicity. Drugs Today (Barc) 39:277, 2003.
85. Kahlmeter G, Dahlager JI: Aminoglycoside toxicity—a review of clinical studies published between 1975 and 1982. J Antimicrob Chemother 13(suppl A):9, 1984.
86. Fausti SA, Henry JA, Schaffer HI, et al: High-frequency audiometric monitoring for early detection of aminoglycoside ototoxicity. J Infect Dis 165:1026, 1992.
87. Rybak LP, Whitworth CA: Ototoxicity: therapeutic opportunities. Drug Discov Today 10:1313, 2005.
88. Usami S, Abe S, Kasai M, et al: Genetic and clinical features of sensorineural hearing loss associated with the 1555 mitochondrial mutation. Laryngoscope 107:483, 1997.
89. Vermorken JB, Kapteijn TS, Hart AA, et al: Ototoxicity of *cis*-diamminedichloroplatinum (II): influence of dose, schedule and mode of administration. Eur J Cancer Clin Oncol 19:53, 1983.
90. Bokemeyer C, Berger CC, Hartmann JT, et al: Analysis of risk factors for cisplatin-induced ototoxicity in patients with testicular cancer. Br J Cancer 77:1355, 1998.
91. van Zeijl LG, Conijn EA, Rodenburg M, et al: Analysis of hearing loss due to *cis*-diamminedichloroplatinum-II. Arch Otorhinolaryngol 239:255, 1984.
92. Sriwattanatamma P, Breysse P: Comparison of NIOSH noise criteria and OSHA hearing conservation criteria. Am J Ind Med 37:334, 2000.
93. Hamilton-Farrell M, Bhattacharyya A: Barotrauma. Injury 35:359, 2004.
94. Newton HB: Neurologic complications of scuba diving. Am Fam Physician 63:2211, 2001.
95. Shupak A, Gil A, Nachum Z, et al: Inner ear decompression sickness and inner ear barotrauma in recreational divers: a long-term follow-up. Laryngoscope 113:2141, 2003.
96. Weiss KS: Otologic lightning bolts. Am J Otolaryngol 1:334, 1980.
97. Poulsen P, Knudstrup P: Lightning causing inner ear damage and intracranial haematoma. J Laryngol Otol 100:1067, 1986.
98. Bergstrom L, Neblett LW, Sando I, et al: The lightning-damaged ear. Arch Otolaryngol 100:117, 1974.
99. Gluncic I, Roje Z, Gluncic V, et al: Ear injuries caused by lightning: report of 18 cases. J Laryngol Otol 115:4, 2001.
100. Kerr AG: Trauma and the temporal bone. The effects of blast on the ear. J Laryngol Otol 94:107, 1980.
101. Fausti SA, Wilmington DJ, Gallun FJ, et al: Auditory and vestibular dysfunction associated with blast-related traumatic brain injury. J Rehabil Res Dev 46:797, 2009.
102. Akin FW, Murnane OD: Head injury and blast exposure: vestibular consequences. Otolaryngol Clin North Am 44:323, 2011.
103. Panosian MS, Wayman JW, Dutcher Jr PO: Facial nerve paralysis from slag injury to the ear. Arch Otolaryngol Head Neck Surg 119:548, 1993.
104. Furman JM, Becker JT: Vestibular responses in Wernicke's encephalopathy. Ann Neurol 26:667, 1989.
105. Leonetti JP, Marzo SJ: Malignancy of the temporal bone. Otolaryngol Clin North Am 35:405, 2002.
106. Devaney KO, Ferlito A, Rinaldo A: Endolymphatic sac tumor (low-grade papillary adenocarcinoma) of the temporal bone. Acta Otolaryngol 123:1022, 2003.
107. Briley DP, Wasay M, Sergent S, et al: Cerebral white matter changes (leukoaraiosis), stroke, and gait disturbance. J Am Geriatr Soc 45:1434, 1997.
108. Schuknecht HF, Gacek MR: Cochlear pathology in presbycusis. Ann Otol Rhinol Laryngol 102:1, 1993.
109. Sahoo GC: Gerontology in ENT (geriatric otolaryngology)—an overview. J Indian Med Assoc 96:145, 1998.

CHAPTER

24

Neuro-ophthalmology in Medicine

E.R. EGGENBERGER ■ J.H. PULA

Although rarely a comforting topic for the general neurologist, neuro-ophthalmologic disorders are best diagnosed using a systematic approach that emphasizes the patient's history followed by confirmation of the localization with specific examination maneuvers. The neurologist needs be familiar with a few specialized techniques concerning ocular misalignment, fundus examination, and pupillary assessment in order to examine patients properly and guide their evaluation.[1]

AFFERENT VISUAL DISTURBANCES

Afferent neuro-ophthalmologic disorders may be limited to the eye (e.g., optic neuropathy), may be secondary to a primary neurologic disorder (e.g., papilledema from an intracranial tumor), or may be related to a systemic medical disorder (e.g., giant cell arteritis). The neuro-ophthalmologic examination provides a window to the diagnosis and natural history of the variety of medical conditions that present with afferent disturbances (Table 24-1).

Optic Neuropathy

The optic nerve is approximately 50 mm in length and is anatomically separated into intraocular, intraorbital, intracanalicular, and intracranial regions. Damage to the optic nerve can occur anywhere along its course, and optic neuropathy may result from ischemic, demyelinating, compressive, genetic, infiltrative, nutritional, traumatic, or toxic causes (Table 24-2).

Although the term "optic neuritis" is often used to describe any type of optic neuropathy, it is most appropriately used only to denote the inflammatory,

Aminoff's Neurology and General Medicine, Fifth Edition.

TABLE 24-1 ■ Selected Manifestations of Neuro-Ophthalmologic Disease Across the Spectrum of Organ Systems

Organ System	Disease State	Example of Neuro-Ophthalmologic Manifestation
Psychiatry	Conversion disorder	Functional blindness
Hematology	Sickle cell disease	Retrobulbar ischemic optic neuropathy
Cardiovascular	Endocarditis	Embolic retinal artery occlusion
Pulmonary	Pulmonary hypertension	Papilledema
Renal	Chronic renal failure	Intracranial hypertension
Gastrointestinal	Pancreatitis	Purtscher syndrome
Genitourinary	Ovarian cancer	Paraneoplastic syndromes with cerebellar degeneration (e.g., with anti-Yo antibodies)
Endocrine	Graves disease	Compressive optic neuropathy due to increased orbital fat content and enlarged extraocular muscles
Obstetric	Eclampsia	Cerebral blindness from posterior reversible encephalopathy syndrome (PRES)

TABLE 24-2 ■ Classification of Optic Neuropathy

Category	Prototypic Examples	Comment
Inflammatory/demyelinating	Optic neuritis	Usually associated with multiple sclerosis or neuromyelitis optica
Paraneoplastic	CRMP5, an autoantibody directed against collapsin response-mediator family	Reported with small cell lung cancer, lymphoma, nasopharyngeal carcinoma, and neuroblastoma
Infectious	Tuberculosis, cryptococcosis, human herpesvirus 6 infection, *Bartonella* infection	These infections causing optic neuropathy should prompt evaluation for infection with human immunodeficiency virus
Ischemic	Ischemic optic neuropathy (arteritic and nonarteritic), retinal artery occlusion (central or branch)	Funduscopy may show occlusive material (Hollenhorst plaque) in retinal artery occlusions
Compressive	Optic nerve sheath meningioma, Graves ophthalmopathy	Proptosis often present. Exophthalmos is synonymous with proptosis but is specifically used in reference to Graves disease
Infiltrative	Sarcoidosis, metastasis, lymphoma	Orbit MRI often shows persistent enhancement of the optic nerve
Traumatic	Direct (penetrating) trauma, indirect trauma (often frontal or midfacial), or chiasmal	Injury due to compression, avulsion, or shear injury. No evidence-based guidelines regarding optimal treatment
Nutritional	Deficiency of vitamin B_1, B_2, B_{12}, or folate	Slowly progressive, symmetric optic neuropathy. Does not present acutely
Toxic	Ethambutol, carbon monoxide, methanol, tobacco-alcohol amblyopia, amiodarone	Typically bilateral and symmetric. May improve with removal of offending agent
Hereditary	Leber, Kjer (dominant optic atrophy) optic neuropathies	Leber optic neuropathy is transmitted via maternally inherited mitochondrial mutation

demyelinating optic neuropathy that is either idiopathic or related to demyelinating disease such as multiple sclerosis (MS) or neuromyelitis optica (NMO). Inflammatory or infectious optic neuropathies from other known etiologies are best described in specific terms (e.g., sarcoid or syphilitic optic neuropathy).[2,3]

Optic neuropathy may be classified anatomically as retrobulbar (i.e., posterior to the globe without disc swelling), or bulbar/anterior (usually associated with acute disc edema) (Fig. 24-1). Optic neuropathy from any cause that results in retinal nerve fiber loss will eventually produce optic atrophy, appearing on funduscopic examination as visible

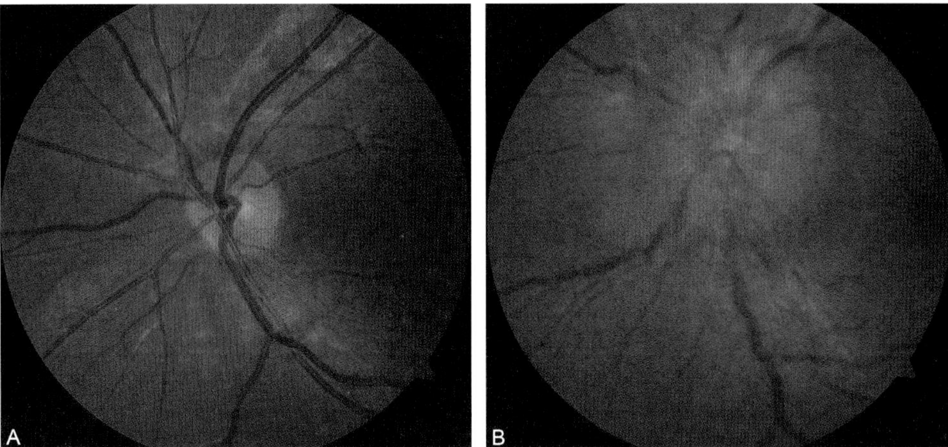

FIGURE 24-1 ▪ **A**, Normal optic nerve. Note clearly visible vessels coursing over the disc edge, small central disc depression of the physiologic cup, and visible nerve fiber layer, especially in the superior and inferior arcades. **B**, Disc edema. Note obscurations of vessels coursing over the disc and swollen peripapillary nerve fiber layer causing disc elevation.

nerve fiber layer loss and disc pallor, although disc coloration may be influenced by genetic, media, and retinal factors (Fig. 24-2). Decreased visual function, as measured by visual acuity, perimetry, and color vision, may result from several causes, including etiologies that are not neuro-ophthalmic; however, the presence of a relative afferent pupillary defect strongly suggests the presence of optic nerve dysfunction, although occasionally a mild relative afferent pupillary defect may be present with widespread retinal dysfunction. Bilateral symmetric optic nerve dysfunction does not produce a relative afferent pupillary defect as there is no interside difference in light transmission in the optic nerve, although both pupils will react sluggishly.

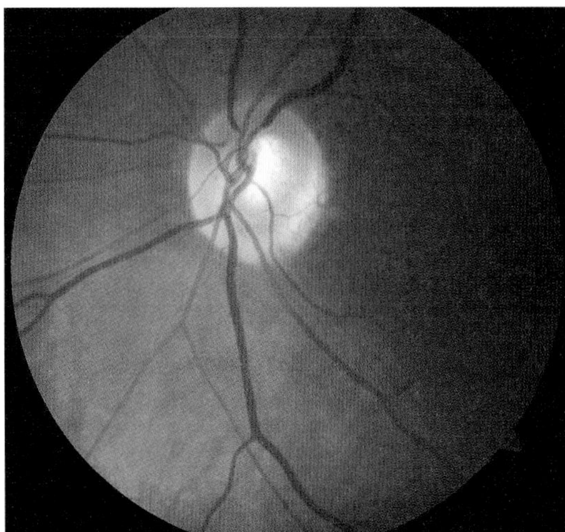

FIGURE 24-2 ▪ Optic atrophy. Note disc pallor and lack of visible nerve fiber layer striations.

Inflammatory Demyelinating Optic Neuritis

Optic neuritis may be idiopathic or associated with demyelinating disease, most commonly MS. The clinical course is characterized by a relatively sudden onset of typically unilateral visual loss. The condition worsens to a nadir over several days, and then recovery begins, typically within several weeks, independent of corticosteroid treatment (although intravenous corticosteroids given in a 3-day course followed by a 2-week oral prednisone course and taper is a frequently used therapy for optic neuritis).

Visual acuity at nadir ranges from 20/20 to no light perception. Pain occurs in more than 90 percent of cases, and often worsens with eye movement. Although centrocecal scotomas are classically associated with demyelinating optic neuritis, other types of field defects (e.g., central, altitudinal, diffuse, paracentral, and arcuate) frequently occur.

Demyelinating optic neuritis is retrobulbar in two-thirds of instances; the remainder of cases display disc edema acutely ("papillitis"). When disc swelling does occur, it is usually mild and diffuse. Magnetic resonance imaging (MRI) demonstrates contrast enhancement of the optic nerve in approximately 90 percent of cases of demyelinating optic neuritis within the first several weeks (Fig. 24-3).[4] Between 3 and 6 months after optic neuritis, optic atrophy becomes visible if there is nerve fiber loss, and visual evoked potentials may document delayed latencies. Not all cases of optic neuritis result in such optic atrophy.

The Optic Neuritis Treatment Trial followed patients with optic neuritis longitudinally and found that 72 percent of subjects had recovered

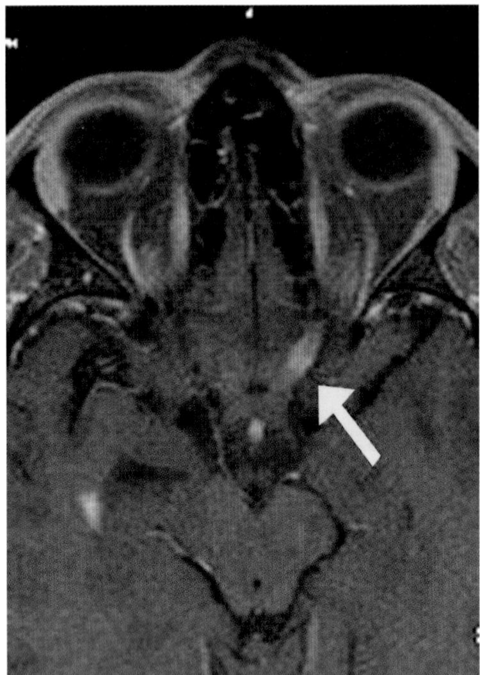

FIGURE 24-3 ■ Axial T1-weighted magnetic resonance imaging (MRI) demonstrating gadolinium enhancement of the left retrobulbar portion of the optic nerve (*arrow*).

visual acuity to at least 20/20, and 85 percent had acuity of at least 20/25 at 15 years after onset.[5] If the initial visual acuity was limited to counting fingers or worse, there was a decreased chance of 20/20 (49%) or 20/25 (63%) visual recovery at 15 years. There was only a weak correlation between the severity of visual loss at baseline and recovery of vision in patients with an initial visual acuity between 20/20 and 20/200.

The baseline brain MRI predicts the risk of developing MS in the decades following optic neuritis, and accordingly is an important test following a first attack of optic neuritis.[5] The number of T2-weighted hyperintensities at least 3 mm in size on baseline MRI reflects the likelihood that a patient with optic neuritis will develop MS. A normal baseline MRI is associated with a 25 percent chance of developing MS in 15 years. The presence of just one lesion increases the 15-year cumulative probability of MS to 60 percent, while three or more lesions on the baseline brain MRI increase the likelihood to approximately 80 percent. Optic nerve enhancement itself is not counted as a lesion. The majority of patients developing MS do so within the first 5 years. The overall risk of developing MS within 15 years after optic neuritis is 50 percent, independent of MRI findings, a figure that can be used to counsel those patients who cannot obtain an MRI.

MRI characteristics also predict future disability in patients with optic neuritis. Spinal cord and infratentorial lesions as well as enhancing lesions are associated with a higher future disability. In patients with optic neuritis who go on to develop MS, lesions in the spinal cord have the highest correlation with disability.[6]

Neuromyelitis Optica

Optic neuritis from neuromyelitis optica (NMO) is more likely to be bilateral, involve the chiasm, and result in more severe vision loss (Fig. 24-4). Optical coherence tomography is a noninvasive means of quantifying retinal nerve fiber layer atrophy or

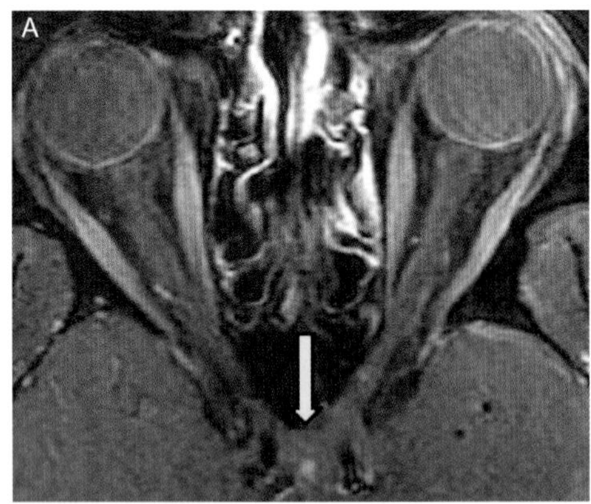

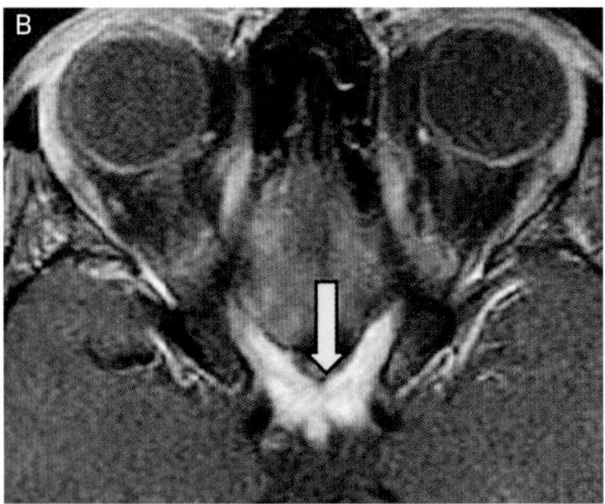

FIGURE 24-4 ■ Axial T1-weighted gadolinium-enhanced brain MRI at the level of the optic chiasm. **A**, Normal optic chiasm (*arrow*) does not enhance. **B**, An acute attack of neuromyelitis optica (NMO) resulting in abnormal enhancement of the optic chiasm (*arrow*).

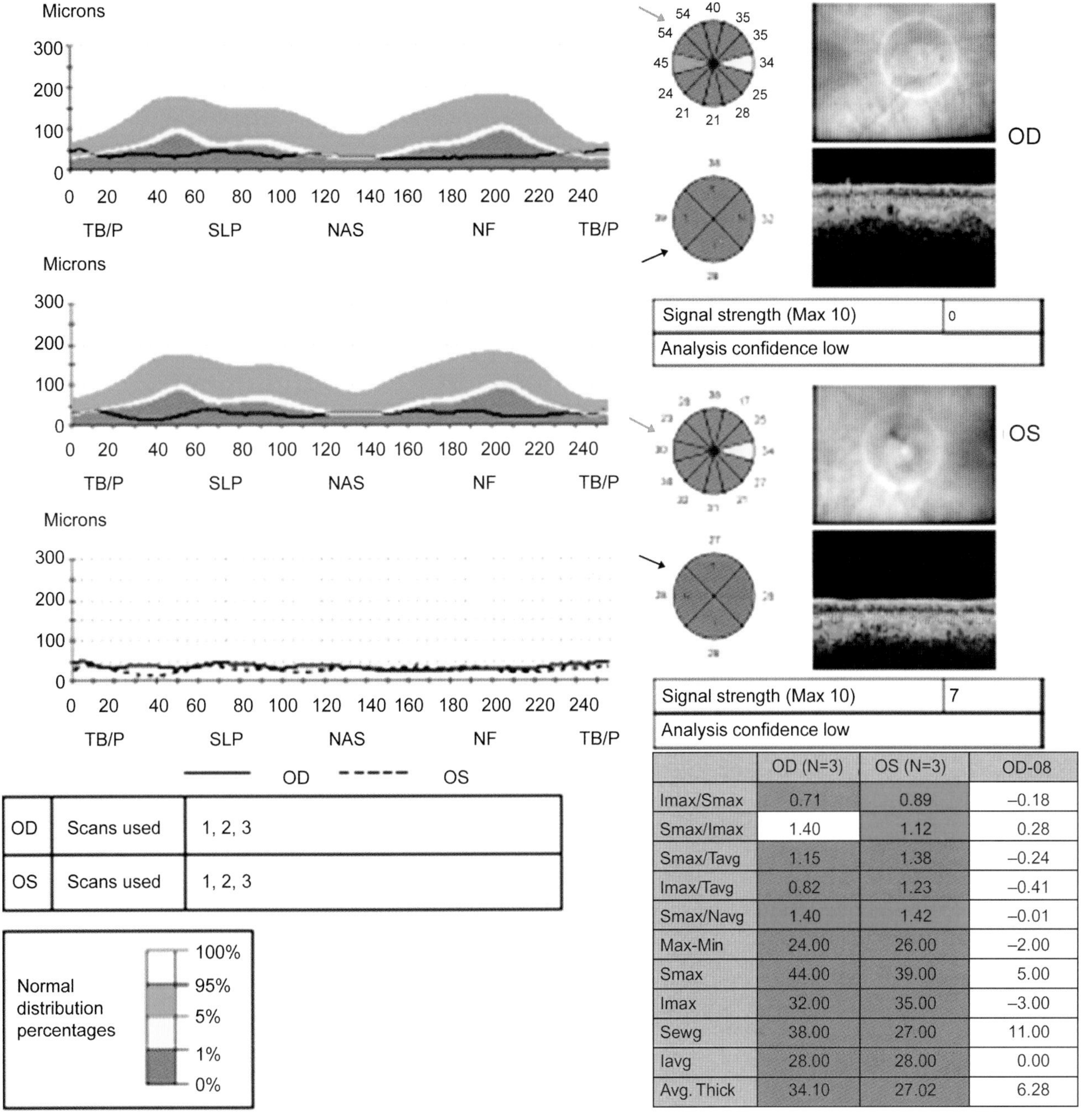

	OD (N=3)	OS (N=3)	OD-08
Imax/Smax	0.71	0.89	–0.18
Smax/Imax	1.40	1.12	0.28
Smax/Tavg	1.15	1.38	–0.24
Imax/Tavg	0.82	1.23	–0.41
Smax/Navg	1.40	1.42	–0.01
Max-Min	24.00	26.00	–2.00
Smax	44.00	39.00	5.00
Imax	32.00	35.00	–3.00
Sewg	38.00	27.00	11.00
lavg	28.00	28.00	0.00
Avg. Thick	34.10	27.02	6.28

FIGURE 24-5 ■ Optical coherence tomography demonstrating severe optic atrophy. Note sector (green arrow) and quadrant (black arrow) maps depicting dramatic nerve fiber layer (RNFL) loss in all quadrants. The average RNFL values of 34.1 (OD) and 27.02 (OS) microns indicate extreme optic atrophy (normal average RNFL ~104).

elevation. These axons comprise the optic nerve, and axonal thickness correlates with visual function. NMO-related optic neuritis is associated with greater retinal nerve fiber layer loss than MS, corresponding to the more severe vision loss in these patients (Fig. 24-5).[7]

Early treatment of NMO-associated optic neuritis with high-dose corticosteroids is associated with preservation of retinal nerve fiber layer.[8] In contrast to typical MS-related optic neuritis in which the final visual acuity is not influenced by corticosteroid treatment, visual outcomes in NMO patients may be improved with early corticosteroid therapy. Consequently, it is imperative to attempt to distinguish MS from NMO in the acute stage; bilaterality, severe visual acuity loss at onset, and

TABLE 24-3 ■ Neuro-Ophthalmologic Disorders Due to Ischemic Disease

Category	Funduscopic Features	Systemic Associations
Nonarteritic anterior ischemic optic neuropathy (NAION)	Generalized or sectoral disc edema, flame-shaped peripapillary hemorrhages, disc-at-risk in opposite eye	Diabetes, nocturnal hypotension, antihypertensive medications, sleep apnea
Nonarteritic posterior ischemic optic neuropathy	Normal in acute stage. May result in disc atrophy chronically	Severe systemic hypotension or anemia, sepsis
Arteritic ischemic optic neuropathy	Pallidedema, evidence of choroidal ischemia, infarction in distribution of cilio-retinal artery, if present	Giant-cell arteritis, polymyalgia rheumatica, thrombocytosis, inflammatory aortitis
Diabetic papillopathy	Similar in appearance to NAION, but severity of fundus appearance may be out of proportion to relative sparing of visual function	Diabetes mellitus, diabetic retinopathy
Central retinal artery occlusion	Normal optic disc, but with generalized retinal edema with cherry-red macular spot	Carotid atherosclerosis, hypertension, tobacco use, hyperhomocysteinemia
Branch retinal artery occlusion	Normal optic disc with focal area of retinal edema, at times associated with a visible occlusive plaque	Carotid atherosclerosis, hypertension, tobacco use

recurrent visual decline following corticosteroid treatment are factors suggestive of NMO. In cases where corticosteroids are ineffective or only transiently helpful, plasma exchange can be utilized; the effectiveness may depend on how early treatment is initiated.[9]

Ischemic Optic Neuropathy

Several different ischemic conditions may cause visual loss (Table 24-3). Ischemic optic neuropathy is the most common cause of acute visual loss in older patients, and may be divided into arteritic (e.g., giant cell arteritis) and nonateritic varieties. Nonarteritic anterior ischemic optic neuropathy (NAION) is always associated with disc edema acutely; the pathophysiologic mechanism of cell death is presumed to be mainly ischemic, but cellular infiltration with polymorphonuclear cells and macrophages also occurs as a response to the initial insult.[10]

NAION typically presents with sudden, painless, unilateral vision loss, often with an altitudinal visual field defect (Fig. 24-6). Acutely disc edema may be focal or diffuse. The optic disc has a characteristic "disc-at-risk" appearance, defined by a small cup-to-disc ratio that is best observed in the opposite eye in the acute phase. Treatment for NAION is limited—systemic high-dose corticosteroids, intravitreal bevacizumab, and optic nerve decompression surgery are not effective.[11–14] The risk to the opposite eye is approximately 15 percent over the next several years, and efforts should be made to address vascular risk factors such as hypertension, hyperlipidemia, and tobacco abuse.

Giant-cell arteritis (arteritic anterior ischemic optic neuropathy) is a neuro-ophthalmic emergency, which may cause ischemia to the optic or oculomotor nerve, retina, orbit, or extraocular muscles, leading to permanent visual loss, diplopia, or both. Arteritic anterior ischemic optic neuropathy occurs in elderly patients with systemic symptoms such as tongue or jaw claudication, headache, scalp tenderness, fever, anorexia, weight loss, or polymyalgia rheumatica. Laboratory abnormalities include

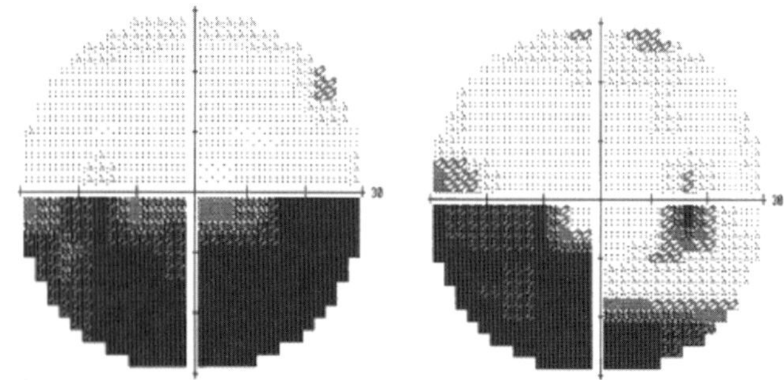

FIGURE 24-6 ■ Bilateral visual field defects in sequential nonarteritic anterior ischemic optic neuropathy. The right eye demonstrates an inferior arcuate defect with "nasal step" while the left eye reveals denser inferior field defect.

TABLE 24-4 ■ Compressive Optic Neuropathy Locations and Etiology

Orbit	Sellar Region
Optic nerve sheath meningioma	Pituitary adenoma
Orbital metastases	Craniopharyngioma
Graves ophthalmopathy	Meningioma
Idiopathic orbital inflammatory pseudotumor	Internal carotid aneurysm
Primary bone lesions (fibrous dysplasia, Paget disease)	Histiocytosis
Orbital fracture or hemorrhage	

elevation of the erythrocyte sedimentation rate (ESR) and C-reactive protein (CRP), and thrombocytosis; a normal ESR may be present in up to one-third of patients, so CRP and ESR should be ordered together and have a combined sensitivity of 99 percent. The diagnosis is made clinically; temporal artery biopsy often demonstrates characteristic giant cells, noninfectious granulomas, inflammatory infiltrates, and interruption of the internal elastic lamina. Immediate treatment with corticosteroids is indicated when giant cell arteritis is suspected and should be initiated even before biopsy, as histopathologic findings will persist for some time following corticosteroid exposure.

Posterior ischemic optic neuropathy is extremely rare, and usually follows profound hypotension as a complication of surgery (especially prolonged spinal surgeries in the prone position), with severe anemia, or as a result of giant cell arteritis. Because the responsible lesion occurs distal to the lamina cribosa of the optic nerve, the disc is not swollen (thus "posterior").

Compressive Optic Neuropathy

Compression of the optic nerve can occur anywhere along its pathway, with distinct pathophysiologies corresponding to various locations (Table 24-4). Clinical characteristics of compressive optic neuropathies are dependent on the nature of the particular lesion. In general, these lesions are usually painless (unless other cranial nerves are affected) and subacutely progressive. Associated features of an orbital process may include proptosis and diplopia, the latter related to restricted extraocular muscles or ocular motor nerve involvement. MRI including fat-saturated post-gadolinium images is often the diagnostic tool of choice.

Genetic Optic Neuropathy

Several inherited optic neuropathies have been characterized, including Leber hereditary optic neuropathy (LHON), a maternally inherited mitochondrial optic neuropathy most common in younger males. Leber hereditary optic neuropathy typically produces bilateral, sequential, painless optic neuropathy with central scotomas. Acutely, the disc may appear erythematous with telangectactic vessels, but no true disc edema is present. Genetic testing for the major mutations is commercially available. There is currently no proven therapy, although idebenone has shown some promise.[12]

Papilledema

Papilledema is defined as optic disc edema caused by elevated intracranial pressure (ICP) and should be distinguished from papillitis. Papilledema is nearly always bilateral, is accompanied by loss of venous pulsations, and varies in appearance from mild to severe (Fig. 24-7). This range of appearances can be described by using the Frisén scale (Table 24-5). The clinical features of papilledema often reflect those of elevated ICP and may include headache, diplopia related to abducens neuropathy, and transient visual obscurations; advanced papilledema produces visual field loss, often starting with an enlarging blind spot and progressing to arcuate nerve fiber layer defects, which may advance toward central visual loss if unchecked. Treatment is directed at the underlying pathology; optic nerve

TABLE 24-5 ■ Frisén Scale for Rating Papilledema

Frisen Grade	Funduscopic Features
0	Normal except for mild blurring of the nasal and temporal disc
1	C-shaped peripapillary gray halo sparing temporal quadrant
2	360-degree gray peripapillary halo, nasal elevation
3	Obscuration of ≥ 1 major vessel segment at disc border, 360-degree elevation
4	Total obscuration of a major vessel on the disc
5	Partial obscuration of all vessels on the disc

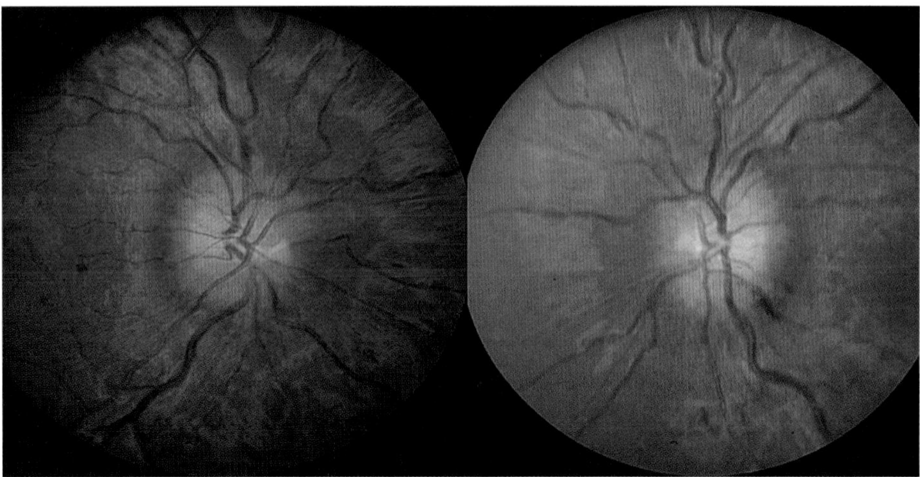

FIGURE 24-7 ■ Fundus photos showing papilledema. Both eyes are affected, as is typical. Features demonstrated include elevation of the retinal nerve layers, resulting in the appearance of a "doughnut"-shaped opacity around the optic disc. Peripapillary flame-shaped hemorrhages are visible, as well as engorgement of the retinal veins. Obscuration of the peripapillary blood vessels as they pass across the disc can be appreciated. The physiologic cups have disappeared.

sheath fenestration is sometimes performed to help preserve vision by relieving direct optic nerve pressure. The most common causes of papilledema are listed in Table 24-6.

Idiopathic Intracranial Hypertension

Idiopathic intracranial hypertension (IIH), or pseudotumor cerebri, is most characteristically a syndrome of obese females of childbearing age. Pediatric IIH is distinct in that the predisposition for obesity and female gender does not apply. The clinical characteristics of IIH include headache, pulsatile tinnitus, transient visual obscurations, and diplopia related to abducens nerve palsy.[13] Patients with IIH may have variable Frisén grades of optic disc edema. Spontaneous venous pulsations are absent on funduscopic examination in patients with increased ICP, and lack of these may precede papilledema. The pathophysiology of IIH is not fully understood, but vitamin A metabolism, endocrine-secreting adipose tissue, and cerebral venous dysregulation are all proposed possibilities.[14]

The diagnostic workup of IIH requires brain imaging to exclude other etiologies of papilledema including venous sinus thrombosis and mass lesions; this is best accomplished with MRI. Radiologic features of IIH that are supportive of the diagnosis include an enlarged optic nerve sheath, optic nerve tortuosity, protrusion of the optic nerve head, an empty sella, and concavity or flattening of the

TABLE 24-6 ■ Causes of Increased Intracranial Pressure Resulting in Papilledema

Etiology	Concomitant Features
Space-occupying brain lesion	Subacutely worsening headache. Various neurologic defects depending on location
Meningoencephalitis	Meningismus, abnormal cerebrospinal fluid chemistries
Subarachnoid hemorrhage	Terson syndrome (intravitreal hemorrhage)
Cerebral edema	Vasogenic (due to loss of intracranial capillary integrity), cytotoxic (due to cell death, often as a result of ischemic stroke), or interstitial edema
Venous sinus thrombosis	Triad of seizure, encephalopathy, and headache is classic acute presentation
Cerebral aqueductal stenosis	May be asymptomatic until critical stenosis causes drowsiness and stupor
Superior vena cava syndrome	Dyspnea, face and arm swelling, Pemberton sign
Right heart failure	Peripheral edema, ascites, hepatomegaly
Sleep apnea	Hypertension, frequent napping, crowded oropharynx
Pulmonary hypertension	Parasternal heave, jugular venous distention, clubbing
Idiopathic intracranial hypertension	Obesity, female gender, childbearing age

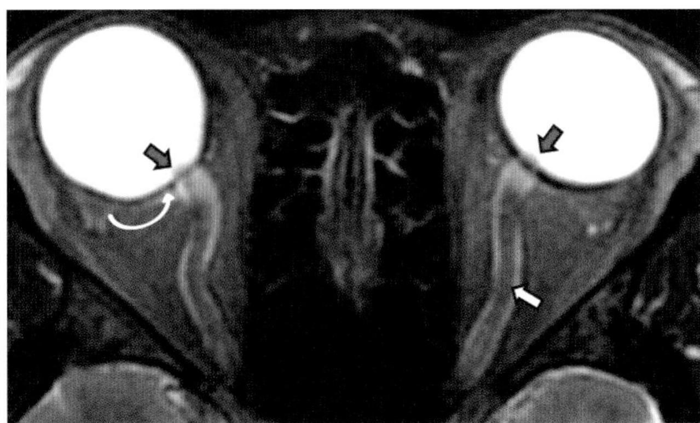

FIGURE 24-8 ■ Axial T2-weighted orbital MRI from a patient with idiopathic intracranial hypertension showing bulging of the papilla (*red arrows*), flattening of the posterior globe (*curved arrow*), and intraorbital nerve tortuosity (*white arrow*).

posterior globes (Fig. 24-8).[15] Conversely, the commonly described "slit-like ventricles" are not helpful in diagnosing IIH, and may reflect a normal imaging feature in young patients without brain atrophy.

Initial treatment for IIH may include weight loss, low-salt diet, and pharmacotherapy with acetazolamide.[16] In some cases, the cause is not idiopathic, and predisposing factors may include obstructive sleep apnea, vitamin A supplementation, tetracycline, or chronic anemia. When visual loss is severe and progressive despite medical management, or when headaches are intractable, surgical options include optic nerve sheath fenestration or lumboperitoneal or ventriculoperitoneal shunting.

Retrochiasmal Vision Loss

Lesions affecting postchiasmal afferent nerve pathways generally produce homonymous visual field loss, which may be a hemianopia or quadrantanopia depending on the location of the lesion. Unless there is concomitant involvement of the optic nerve or the field loss is bilateral, visual acuity is typically spared. The most common causes of homonymous visual field loss are stroke (69%), trauma (13%), tumor (11%), brain surgery (2%), and demyelinating lesions.[17]

In addition to primary visual loss, compromise of visuospatial function, recognition of objects and faces (prosopagnosia), and motion perception can occur with damage to visual association areas. Current theory hypothesizes a ventral visual stream involving the temporal lobe (the "what" pathway) that is concerned with object recognition, and a dorsal stream connected to the parietal lobe (the "how" pathway) involved with object spatial location and motion. Ventral pathway dysfunction may produce difficulty with object recognition, whereas dorsal pathway lesions are associated with difficulty orienting to a location, which requires spatial attention. Spatial attention is also important for searching through a cluttered visual scene; as distracters are added to the environment, patients may demonstrate more difficulty in quickly identifying a target.

Early involvement with predominant visual deficits in neurodegenerative disorders occurs in Lewy body dementia and some forms of Alzheimer disease that involve the occipital and parietal lobes early in the course. Posterior cortical atrophy has been regarded by some as a variant of Alzheimer disease because of histologic similarities.[18] The Heidenhain variant of Creutzfeldt–Jakob disease affects the occipital regions first.

EFFERENT VISUAL DISTURBANCES

Clinical Assessment

The history in patients with diplopia should concentrate on whether the disorder is binocular or monocular, the orientation of the images, and symptom modifiers. Diplopia is always sudden in onset. Monocular diplopia—diplopia that remains when one eye is closed—is generally related to ocular causes (e.g., corneal or lens opacity, refractive error), and is not neurologic in origin.[19] It typically resolves with the pinhole test and should prompt ophthalmology referral. Binocular diplopia—related to misalignment of the eyes—resolves with closure of either eye, and is typically neurogenic in origin. The direction of misalignment and presence or change with position of gaze provide clues to the diagnosis. Other factors such as age, associated features (e.g., ptosis, pain), modifiers, and diurnal variation (e.g., fluctuations) guide the localization and differential diagnosis as discussed below.

Ocular misalignment refers to any deviation of the visual axis of one eye compared to the other. Ocular alignment can be measured on examination in several ways. The least precise method involves estimation of misalignment by displacement of the corneal light reflex (Hirschberg method). Light reflects from the same position on both corneas if the eyes are orthophoric, whereas the light is displaced from the center in one eye when misalignment exists; each millimeter of light reflex displacement equals approximately 7 to 10 deg or 15 to 20 prism diopters.

The red Maddox rod is a simple method to quantify even very small amounts of ocular misalignment. The Maddox rod is composed of a series of parallel cylindrical grooves in a piece of red glass, mounted in a circular rim. (The original consisted of a single cylindrical rod, hence the name.) The device converts a light source into a red line perpendicular to the axis of the rod. The patient views a white light source with the left eye, while the Maddox rod is placed over the right eye. The position of the red line relative to the light source (seen by the left eye) indicates the presence and amount of misalignment. The red line can be made to appear vertically (to measure horizontal deviation from the light) or horizontally (to measure vertical deviation from the light), and prisms can be placed over the Maddox rod until the line dissects the light. If the red line appears to the left of the light, then an exotropia exists. If the line appears to the right of the light, an esotropia is present. If the line appears below the light, then a right hypertropia is present, and red line above the light indicates a left hypertropia. Vertical misalignment is by convention always quantified by the hypertropic eye.

The alternate cover test is more difficult to perform, but is reliable and the most widely used method. The patient fixates on a specific letter of the Snellen chart at distance or near, while the examiner alternately covers one eye and then the other, thus forcing the patient to fixate with the uncovered eye. If the eyes are orthophoric, then no corrective eye movement will be required to fixate on the target when the occluded eye is switched. If the right eye moves down to fix the target immediately after it is uncovered and the left eye is occluded, then a hypertropia exists, while an eye that has to move in toward the nose to fixate the target represents an exotropia, and eye movement out to fixate a target indicates an esotropia. A prism can be placed over one eye to neutralize this shift and quantify the misalignment. These alignment tests are repeated in the nine cardinal positions of gaze to discern the pattern of involvement.

The motility examination also includes assessment of pursuit, saccades, ductions, and versions. Pursuit is tested with the patient following a target (a large letter on the near card) moving slowly (less than 20 deg/sec) in the horizontal and vertical gaze. Saccades are rapid eye movements that "jump" fixation from one target to another. Saccadic assessment highlights certain abnormalities, such as a subtle internuclear ophthalmoparesis (see later) with adduction lag; some diseases preferentially affect saccades, producing slowing or inaccuracies. Binocular movements in various directions are known as versions (e.g., leftward version, rightward version), while ductions refer to monocular eye movements (e.g., supraduction in the right eye, indicating elevation of that eye). Ductions can be semiquantified in millimeters of "scleral show" in a position of gaze.

Patients with diplopia may adopt a head posture to avoid the position of diplopia; patients with impaired abduction of one eye may turn the head toward the side of the palsy, thus placing the eyes in contraversion. Patients with trochlear nerve palsy may present with a contralateral head tilt and chin-down position to avoid gaze into the diplopic field. Ptosis should be quantified through measurement of the height of the palpebral fissure in millimeters. Pupil size should be measured in light, in dark, and with reactivity. Proptosis can be measured in millimeters of anterior displacement of each eye from the lateral canthus.

Anatomic location is always the first task for a neurologist, and the site of lesions causing binocular diplopia may be supranuclear (e.g., skew deviation or vergence dysfunction) or involve the ocular motor nerve nuclei (cranial nerves nuclei III, IV, and VI), infranuclear segment (cranial nerves III, IV, and VI), internuclear segment (i.e., medial longitudinal fasciculus [internuclear ophthalmoplegia]), neuromuscular junction (e.g., myasthenia gravis), or muscle (e.g., trauma, thyroid eye disease, neoplasm).

A first step in localization is to consider the most specific patterns of ocular misalignment related to the ocular motor nerves or their nuclei as well as supranuclear and internuclear lesions. Even if the pattern fits that of an ocular motor nerve, nucleus, or internuclear ophthalmoplegia, mimics such as myasthenia gravis, which can masquerade as any pupil-sparing, painless, nonproptotic cause of diplopia, must also be considered. If the misalignment pattern does not conform to these specific patterns, attention should be directed toward neuromuscular junction disease, myopathy, or multiple cranial nerve palsies (e.g., Miller Fisher syndrome,

Wernicke encephalopathy). In such cases, it may be helpful to consider each eye separately to arrive at a differential diagnosis.

Supranuclear Causes of Ocular Dysmotility

The supranuclear ocular motor system is principally concerned with bilateral eye movements, and when injured, produces gaze preferences or palsies. Supranuclear causes of dysmotility may also produce binocular diplopia. The supranuclear ocular motor system includes premotor afferent connections from the cerebral hemispheres, cerebellum, and brainstem projecting to the ocular motor nuclei, which govern distinct classes of eye movements including saccades, pursuit, the vestibular ocular reflex, gaze-holding, fixation, optokinetic nystagmus, and vergence.[20]

Burst neurons facilitating vertical saccades reside within the rostral interstitial medial longitudinal fasciculus, which is situated rostral to the oculomotor nucleus[21]; dysfunction of the rostral portion of this fasciculus produces slow or absent vertical saccades, and may result from infarct, demyelination, neoplasm, or neurodegenerative processes.[22] Given that the deficit is supranuclear, intact vertical eye movements may be possible when bypassing volitional pathways (such as with the oculocephalic reflex—eye movements in response to head movement while foveating).

The cerebellum performs critical coordination and calibration functions for the ocular motor system, particularly the vestibulocerebellum (i.e., flocculus, paraflocculus, nodulus, and uvula), vermis, and fastigial nuclei. The flocculus and paraflocculus are involved in smooth pursuit, gaze holding, and calibration of the vestibular ocular reflex. The vermis and fastigial nuclei are involved in saccadic and pursuit control. The nodulus and uvula participate in modulation of the vestibular system.

Parinaud dorsal midbrain syndrome is one of the most common and distinct supranuclear causes of ocular motor dysfunction.[23] Lesions within the dorsal midbrain, typically affecting the posterior commissure and neighboring structures (often infarcts, neoplasms of pineal origin, hydrocephalus, or demyelinated plaques) produce combinations of vertical gaze palsy, vergence dysfunction, light-near dissociation of the pupils, lid retraction, square-wave jerks, convergence retraction nystagmus, and skew deviation.

Skew deviation is among the most common supranuclear causes of diplopia and produces a vertical misalignment of the eyes (hypertropia).[24] As a supranuclear problem, all ductions in the eyes are full in contrast to a cranial nerve palsy, for example, which as an infranuclear process produces limitations of ductions in one eye. The vertical misalignment with skew may be comitant (the same in all positions of gaze) or incomitant; uncrossed hypertropia is a relatively common pattern (right hypertropia in right gaze with left hypertropia in left gaze).[25] The vertical misalignment tends to be similar in up- or downgaze for any given horizontal eye position.

Skew deviation may be difficult to localize precisely within the posterior fossa, but connections from the vestibular nuclei, the medial longitudinal fasciculus, or connecting pathways involving the cerebellum are often implicated. With lesions above the level of the pontine vestibular decussation, the ipsilesional eye is often hypertropic, while lesions below this decussation more often produce a contralesional hypertropia. The ocular tilt reaction is a special circumstance of skew deviation with the additional features of head tilt and torsion of both eyes.[26]

Supranuclear networks control vergence eye movements, and with dysfunction of this circuitry, binocular horizontal diplopia results. Both divergence and convergence dysfunction produce differing horizontal misalignment at distance compared to near viewing. In addition, supranuclear circuitry is responsible for fusion of any phorias; most normal patients have small horizontal phorias that are asymptomatic due to proper functioning of the vergence networks, which serve to fuse small amounts of misalignment. Occasionally dysfunction of these pathways (from medications, structural disease, fatigue, or idiopathic causes) produces intermittent binocular horizontal diplopia.[27] Convergence insufficiency is perhaps the most common of these vergence dysfunction patterns, producing a larger exophoria (with diplopia) at near than far distance.[28]

Supranuclear lesions may also produce limitations of horizontal gaze. Within the pons, the paramedian pontine reticular formation (PPRF) just rostral to the abducens (VI) nucleus houses horizontal burst neurons. Lesions in this region produce slow or absent ipsilesional saccades. The frontal eye fields of the cerebral hemispheres generate volitional contralateral saccades, and cerebral hemispheric lesions affecting these regions produce a supranuclear gaze preference. In this situation, horizontal eye

TABLE 24-7 ■ Limitation of Upgaze

Entity	Motility	Globe Position	Eyelid	Pupil
Thyroid eye disease	Gaze in all directions may be limited	Proptosis, retropulsion*	Eyelid retraction with lagophthalmos	Usually normal; RAPD if ON present
Orbital myositis	Gaze in all directions may be limited	Proptosis, retropulsion*	None	Usually normal
Blow-out fracture with muscle entrapment	Isolated limitation of upgaze	Enophthalmos	Normal	Normal
Myasthenia gravis	Gaze in all directions may be limited; intrasaccadic slowing characteristic	Normal	Ptosis may be present	Normal
Parinaud syndrome	Skew deviation may be present	Normal	Eyelid retraction without lagophthalmos	Normal
Progressive supranuclear palsy	Symmetric limitation of vertical movement	Normal	Normal	Normal
Chronic progressive external ophthalmoplegia	Eventually gaze in all directions is limited	Normal	Normal	Normal
Superior division cranial nerve III	Isolated limitation of upgaze	Normal	Ptosis	Normal

From Cockerham KP, Olmos A: Orbital and ocular manifestations of neurological disease. p. 483. In Aminoff MJ (ed): Neurology and General Medicine. 4th Ed. Elsevier Churchill Livingstone, Philadelphia, 2008, with permission.
ON, optic neuropathy; RAPD, relative afferent pupillary defect.
*Retropulsion indicates increased resistance to retropulsion.

movements can typically be bypassed by employing the vestibular ocular reflex, which serves to maintain foveation during angular head acceleration.

Ocular Motor Nuclei and Nerves

Dysfunction of the oculomotor (III), trochlear (IV), or abducens (VI) nerves is the most common cause of diplopia.[29] Etiologies are varied and include compression, infection, inflammation, and ischemia.

Oculomotor Nerve (III) Palsy

The third cranial nerve innervates the superior, inferior, and medial recti, inferior oblique, levator palpebrae, iris sphincter, and ciliary muscles, thus controlling adduction, extorsion, supraduction, most of infraduction, lid opening, and pupil miosis. The collection of nuclei lie in the midline of the dorsal midbrain and are composed of a complex arrangement of subnuclei. The oculomotor nerve fascicles travel ventrally, traversing the red nucleus, substantia nigra, and cerebral peduncle before entering the subarachnoid space within the interpeduncular fossa. Within the subarachnoid space, the nerve projects between the superior cerebellar and posterior cerebral arteries, adjacent to the posterior communicating artery. It has an important anatomic relationship to the uncus, rendering the nerve vulnerable to compression with uncal herniation. Within the cavernous sinus, the nerve resides within the superior wall and divides into a superior division (innervating the levator palpebrae and superior rectus) and inferior division (innervating all its other muscles) prior to passing through the superior orbital fissure.

The oculomotor nerve has unique features of clinical importance including the potential for aberrant regeneration. Lesions of the oculomotor nucleus are uncommon, and have patterns dictated by the anatomy including bilateral involvement or sparing of the pupils and levator palpebrae.[30] Complete unilateral oculomotor nerve palsy produces complete ptosis, a mid-position light-fixed pupil, and an inability to adduct, supraduct, or infraduct the eye. The eye may appear depressed and abducted (e.g., "down and out"), and patients report binocular oblique diplopia when the lid is elevated. Partial oculomotor palsies may spare some aspects of this

TABLE 24-8 ■ Limitation of Medial Ocular Movement

Disorder	Motility	Globe Position	Eyelid	Pupil
Thyroid eye disease	Gaze in all directions may be limited	Proptosis, retropulsion*	Retraction/ lagophthalmos	Usually normal; RAPD should be sought
Orbital myositis	Any or all muscles may be affected	Proptosis, retropulsion*	Usually normal	Usually normal
Myasthenia gravis	Gaze in all or any direction may be limited. Fatigue is common	Normal	Ptosis especially with fatigue or sustained upgaze	Usually normal
Internuclear ophthalmoplegia	Limitation of medial gaze, abducting nystagmus	Normal	Normal	Normal
Partial CN III palsy	Limitation of medial gaze is usually associated with limitation of upgaze and ptosis; in a complete third nerve palsy, the eye is exotropic	Normal	Ptosis is present if the superior division of CN III is affected	Pupillary fibers travel with the inferior division of CN III; if affected, the pupil will be dilated and have a decreased reaction to light

From Cockerham KP, Olmos A: Orbital and ocular manifestations of neurological disease. p. 483. In Aminoff MJ (ed): Neurology and General Medicine. 4th Ed. Elsevier Churchill Livingstone, Philadelphia, 2008, with permission.
CN, cranial nerve; RAPD, relative afferent pupillary defect.
*Retropulsion indicates increased resistance to retropulsion.

function.[31] Any abnormality of extraocular movement must be distinguished from other possible causes (Tables 24-7 and 24-8).

Oculomotor nerve axons can be affected anywhere along their course. Lesions of the midbrain, often related to ischemia, are usually accompanied by hemiataxia, tremor, or hemiparesis.[32] Lesions within the subarachnoid space are typically unilateral and isolated without other neurologic features. Aneurysmal compression is often the primary consideration, most commonly related to the posterior communicating artery; rupture or enlargement of such aneurysms typically produces an acute, painful, pupil-involved ipsilateral oculomotor nerve palsy. Prompt diagnosis is critical in facilitating treatment and reducing mortality.[33] In contrast to potentially life-threatening aneurysmal oculomotor nerve palsies, ischemic (i.e., microvascular, "diabetic") palsies are much more common and nearly always improve. Ischemic injury often presents with pain, which may be indistinguishable from aneurysmal pain. The features are of a complete oculomotor palsy although the pupil is typically spared. Most patients with ischemic oculomotor nerve palsies are older, with some combination of vascular risk factors such as diabetes, hypertension, hyperlipidemia, and tobacco abuse.

The "rule of the pupil" is helpful in the evaluation, but must be applied correctly: in the face of a complete motor paresis, a normal pupil effectively eliminates compressive pathophysiologies such as aneurysm.[34] Because the pupillomotor fibers reside on the dorsomedial oculomotor nerve, and microvascular ischemic palsies tend to infarct the center part of the nerve, sparing the pupil occurs in approximately 70 percent of ischemic palsies, whereas the pupil is involved in over 90 percent of aneurysmal palsies. Although up to 30 percent of patients with ischemic palsies demonstrate some degree of anisocoria, the pupillary inequality is typically less than 1 mm. Ischemic oculomotor palsies nearly always improve, never demonstrate aberrant regeneration, and usually resolve, typically within approximately 3 months. Treatment of ischemic palsies is focused on symptomatic relief, exclusion of other causes, and ischemic risk-factor modification. The rule of the pupil cannot be applied to rule out compression for incomplete motor palsies.[35]

Oculomotor palsy from uncal herniation is related to ICP gradients, and is always attended, in short order, by other features such as hemiparesis, diminished consciousness, or visual field defects. This neurologic emergency requires prompt therapy directed at the underlying cause as well as the intracranial hypertension itself in order to avoid morbidity and mortality.

Many other pathophysiologies can cause oculomotor nerve palsy including pituitary apoplexy, giant cell arteritis, trauma, infection, and tumor.

Because the oculomotor nerve innervates several muscles, palsies can heal with aberrant regeneration (synkinesis). The presence of such regeneration implies disruption of the perineural sheath from compression or trauma, and never follows microvascular palsies. Common aberrancy patterns include lid elevation with eye adduction or depression, eye adduction with vertical movements, and pupillary constriction with eye movements.

Trochlear Nerve (IV) Palsy

The nucleus of the trochlear nerve resides in the dorsal periaqueductal gray of the caudal midbrain ventral to the aqueduct and dorsal to the medial longitudinal fasciculus. The fascicles of the trochlear nerve cross and exit the brainstem dorsally, tracing a long subarachnoid course around the midbrain and then through the cavernous sinus in its lateral wall. The nerve then passes through the superior orbital fissure to innervate the superior oblique muscle, which primarily intorts the eye (depression of the adducted eye is a secondary action).

Trochlear nerve palsies produce ipsilateral hypertropia and excyclotorsion, resulting in binocular oblique diplopia in contralateral and downgaze. The patient usually adopts a chin-down and contralateral head-tilt posture to diminish object separation. Examination of ductions, pursuits, and saccades is typically normal. A hypertropia is typically seen that is worse on contralateral gaze with an ipsilateral head tilt. The presence of ocular torsion can be demonstrated when viewing a straight horizontal line in a position of diplopia; the two horizontal lines will appear to converge toward the ipsilateral side with a trochlear nerve palsy.

Trauma is the most common cause of CN IV palsy, probably related to the long subarachnoid course of the nerve around the midbrain. Most patients with traumatic or ischemic (microvascular) trochlear nerve palsies improve with time; vertical prism may be useful if improvement is incomplete.

Abducens Nerve (VI) Palsy

The nucleus of the sixth cranial nerve resides in the dorsal pons, ventral to the facial nerve colliculus, and adjacent to the medial longitudinal fasciculus. The nucleus contains abducens neurons innervating the lateral rectus, and also internuclear neurons destined for the medial longitudinal fasciculus mediating ipsilateral gaze. The fascicles of the abducens nerve emanate ventrally to emerge at the pontomedullary junction before ascending the clivus to enter the cavernous sinus and the superior orbital fissure.

Abducens nuclear lesions cause an ipsilateral gaze palsy, while abducens nerve lesions cause binocular horizontal diplopia with an esotropia in ipsilateral gaze. In partial abducens nerve palsies, abduction may be only minimally impaired; alternate cover or red Maddox rod testing will demonstrate the incomitant esotropia. The causes of limited lateral ocular movement are indicated in Table 24-9.

Neoplasm and ischemia are important causes of abducens nerve palsy.[36] Neoplasms such as gliomas can directly affect the pontine portion of the nerve or the nucleus, but can also infiltrate the subarachnoid or cavernous sinus segments of the nerve or indirectly cause injury to the nerve through elevated ICP. Other important causes include intracranial hypotension (e.g., after lumbar puncture), Wernicke encephalopathy, and demyelination.

The majority of abducens palsies improve, although the best prognosis is for microvascular or traumatic etiologies.[37] Occlusion initially will resolve diplopia, while prism or strabismus surgery may help those with persistent dysfunction.

Duane type I retraction syndrome is relatively common, and may be mistaken for an abducens palsy.[38] This congenital dysinnervation syndrome results from hypoplasia of the abducens nucleus, producing decreased abduction; however, in contrast to abducens palsies, patients with Duane type 1 retraction syndrome demonstrate near orthophoria (i.e., normal balance of the eye muscles for near sight) in primary position and palpebral fissure narrowing (globe retraction) with adduction.

Multiple Ocular Motor Nerve Palsies

Multiple ocular motor palsies should be localized either anatomically (e.g., all related to cavernous sinus disease), via "common denominators" (e.g., all lesions share meningeal or bone passage) or through pattern recognition (e.g., ophthalmoplegia, ataxia, and confusion related to Wernicke encephalopathy). Cavernous sinus lesions commonly produce multiple cranial neuropathies, and may be related to neoplasms (e.g., meningioma, metastasis), vascular causes (e.g., aneurysm, thrombosis or carotid-cavernous fistulas), or of inflammatory origin (e.g., Tolosa–Hunt syndrome).

TABLE 24-9 ■ Limitation of Lateral Ocular Movement

Disorder	Motility	Globe Position	Eyelid	Pupil
Thyroid eye disease	Gaze in all directions may be limited	Proptosis, retropulsion*	Retraction/lagophthalmos	Usually normal; RAPD should be sought
Orbital myositis	Any or all muscles may be affected	Proptosis, retropulsion*	Usually normal	Usually normal
Medial wall fracture with entrapment	Isolated limitation of lateral gaze	Normal or enophthalmos	Acute, edema and ecchymosis; chronic, normal	Usually normal
Myasthenia gravis	Gaze in all or any direction may be limited; fatigue is common; intrasaccadic delay is characteristic†	Normal	Ptosis especially with fatigue or sustained upgaze	Usually normal
Cancer (paraneoplastic)	Gaze in all directions may be limited	Normal	Usually normal; may resemble myasthenia gravis	Normal
Sixth nerve palsy	Slowed saccades; esotropia in primary gaze	Normal	Normal	Normal

From Cockerham KP, Olmos A: Orbital and ocular manifestations of neurological disease. p. 483. In Aminoff MJ (ed): Neurology and General Medicine. 4th Ed. Elsevier Churchill Livingstone, Philadelphia, 2008, with permission.
RAPD, relative afferent pupillary defect.
*Retropulsion indicates increased resistance to retropulsion.
†Intrasaccadic delay refers to a saccade that is initially of normal or brisk velocity but slows as the eye moves laterally due to the decreased number and efficacy of the acetylcholine receptors.

Miller Fisher Syndrome

Miller Fisher syndrome is an inflammatory polyneuropathy producing the classic triad of ophthalmoplegia, areflexia, and ataxia. It shares some features with acute inflammatory demyelinating polyradiculoneuropathy (AIDP) including antecedent infection in some, areflexia, and increased cerebrospinal fluid (CSF) protein concentration without pleocytosis.[39] Anti-GQ1b antibodies are present in the serum of most patients with Miller Fisher syndrome.[40] Symptoms typically spontaneously remit in 2 to 3 months, with perhaps faster rates of improvement following intravenous immunoglobulin or plasma exchange therapy.[41]

Internuclear Ophthalmoplegia

Internuclear ophthalmoplegia is related to dysfunction of the medial longitudinal fasciculus, serving to connect the abducens nucleus to the contralateral oculomotor nucleus, coordinating binocular horizontal eye movements.[42] Lesions may be unilateral or bilateral, and commonly result from demyelination (the prototypic cause of diplopia in MS) or ischemia from basilar perforators.

Patients may report frank binocular horizontal (or oblique if associated skew deviation exists) diplopia, but otherwise may note "dizziness" or visual blurring, or are asymptomatic. Slow adduction of the ipsilateral eye is the essential element; incomplete adduction is only present in a minority of cases, emphasizing the need to examine horizontal saccades to make the diagnosis. Abducting and vertical gaze-evoked nystagmus are common accompaniments. Most improve spontaneously, whether due to demyelination or ischemia; the prognosis is less favorable with larger lesions accompanied by other signs of brainstem dysfunction.

Neuromuscular Junction Dysfunction

Myasthenia gravis (MG) is the prototypic neuromuscular junction disease, and is important to recognize not only because of diplopic-related morbidity but as it has the potential to produce life-threatening generalized weakness.[43]

The estimated prevalence of myasthenia gravis is around 15 to 20 per 100,000 population in the United States. The most common age at onset is the third decade for women and the seventh decade for men. MG presents with ocular signs and symptoms in up to 70 percent of cases; ocular forms of MG may precede the development of generalized MG.[44] Although the rate of generalized MG conversion from pure ocular disease is usually said to approximate 50 percent, in the authors' clinic the rate of generalization more closely approximates 30 percent.

Antibodies against the nicotinic postsynaptic acetylcholine receptor lead to increased degradation of the receptor; if the number of functioning receptors is sufficiently reduced, weakness may result. Antibodies against the receptor are present in the serum of approximately 90 percent of patients with generalized MG but only about 50 percent of those with purely ocular MG. Some patients without these antibodies harbor antibodies to other neuromuscular junction components, such as muscle-specific kinase (MuSK).

Classically, MG causes ptosis of one or both eyelids and diplopia, but there are numerous variations.[45] Ptosis or diplopia may be absent or intermittent, especially early in the course of the disease. Diplopia may be vertical, horizontal, oblique, or torsional, depending on the extraocular muscle involvement. The orientation of degree of diplopic object separation often varies over time. This variability is diagnostically important. Associated clinical features of generalized MG other than limb weakness may include dysarthria, dysphagia, or facial and orbicularis oculi weakness.

MG can cause weakness in any pattern of extraocular muscles; weakness of the medial rectus muscle is relatively common, mimicking the pattern seen with an internuclear ophthalmoplegia including slowed adduction saccades, abducting nystagmus, and an exotropia increasing with side gaze. This can be distinguished from a true medial longitudinal fasciculus lesion by response to therapy, variability, associated features, and lack of vertical gaze-evoked nystagmus. Saccadic and gaze-related extraocular movement dysfunction may be present in the form of gaze fatigue (gradual onset of extraocular weakness while attempting to hold eccentric gaze), gradually increasing gaze-evoked nystagmus during maintenance of eccentric gaze, and abnormal saccadic speed or amplitude. Lid findings can be particularly helpful, such as the Cogan lid twitch; this sign is elicited by having the patient look at a target in downgaze for a few seconds, then saccade back to the primary position. A Cogan eyelid twitch appears as a 1- to 2-mm drop of eyelid elevation immediately after return to the primary position, and is a sensitive sign of MG with ocular involvement although it may be seen in several other conditions involving the eyelids. Variable palpebral fissure height over the course of minutes and fatigable ptosis with sustained upgaze are also diagnostically helpful.

The ice and rest tests may be useful in the evaluation of suspected MG.[46] The ice test is performed by placing an ice pack over a ptotic eyelid for 1 to 2 minutes and noting whether this reduces ptosis; it is likely that at least part of the ice test effect involves rest, as it is common for ptosis of both eyelids to improve somewhat after application of ice to one eyelid. Rest or sleep for 10 minutes may produce dramatic improvement in ptosis, and this is highly suggestive of a neuromuscular junction disorder.

Other than antibody testing, edrophonium (Tensilon), a short-acting acetylcholinesterase inhibitor, can be used to demonstrate transient improvement in ocular signs related to neuromuscular junction defects. Dramatic improvement in ptosis is diagnostically useful, but has a limited duration of effect, false-positive and false-negative results, and potentially dangerous side effects including bradycardia. Due to these limitations, Tensilon testing is rarely performed.

Nerve conduction studies and electromyography provide the most sensitive method of quantifying neuromuscular defects. A decremental response to repetitive stimulation of a motor nerve is seen with postsynaptic neuromuscular junction disorders such as MG but is rarely seen in the pure ocular form of the disease. Single-fiber electromyography demonstrates increased jitter in over 90 percent of MG cases, but is a time-consuming technique that requires especial expertise to perform.

Approximately 15 percent of patients with MG also have thyroid alteration; some of these patients may have ocular dysmotility related to coexistent thyroid eye disease.

Thymoma is present in approximately 10 percent of patients with MG (thymic hyperplasia is present in approximately 70%). Thymectomy is routinely considered in thymoma cases or in young patients with generalized MG; the decision to perform thymectomy in patients with purely ocular MG is made on an individual basis depending on the medication requirements for adequate symptom control, general medical health of the patient, and patient input.

Cholinesterase inhibitors such as pyridostigmine started at 30 to 60 mg three times daily are usually the first-line therapy in patients with ocular MG because of their relatively rapid onset of action and tolerable side-effect profile; however, most patients will also require immunomodulatory medications such as prednisone. Prednisone can be started in low-dose alternate-day regimens, escalating as required; a corticosteroid-sparing medication such as mycophenolate mofetil can be started if long-term corticosteroid therapy is required.

Mechanical Causes of Diplopia

The most common acquired adult causes of extraocular muscle dysfunction are thyroid eye disease, orbital trauma, and neoplasm.

Thyroid eye disease may occur with hyper-, hypo-, or euthyroid states and usually runs a course independent of the underlying thyroid disease (see Chapter 18).[47] Thyroid eye disease typically produces painless proptosis, restriction of extraocular muscles with diplopia, eyelid retraction, and variable orbital inflammatory features.[48] Lid retraction commonly leads to dry eye and corneal irritation, prompting treatment with corneal lubrication.

The medial and inferior recti are the most commonly involved muscles (typically with sparing of the tendinous insertions), producing esotropia and hypertropia. In approximately 10 percent of cases, extraocular muscle enlargement may produce an orbital apex syndrome resulting in compressive optic neuropathy. The diagnosis of thyroid eye disease is clinical, with imaging confirmation. Treatment begins with correction of any thyroid derangements. Diplopia may be addressed with prisms or strabismus surgery once stability has been established; compressive optic neuropathy is typically treated with orbital decompression.

Orbital trauma not infrequently causes diplopia, often in the form of extraocular muscle entrapment. Blow-out fractures of the orbital floor may produce inferior rectus entrapment; diplopia in such patients may resolve spontaneously, although surgical decompression may be required in some.

Orbital neoplasms (e.g., lymphoma, metastasis) or sinus-related processes (e.g., infection, nasopharyngeal carcinoma, mucoceles) may also produce mechanical dysfunction of the extraocular muscles and diplopia.

Excellent orbital imaging is achievable with computerized tomography or MRI, and the choice depends on the individual case and institution. The advantages of computerized tomography include speed, multiplanar capability with newer scanners, and excellent bone detail, while disadvantages include radiation exposure and lack of soft tissue detail. MRI advantages include superior soft tissue resolution, multiplanar capability, and the lack of ionizing radiation. However, MRI scanner time is lengthy, prohibiting patient movement; pacemakers and other metal implants or shrapnel may be contraindications.

Nystagmus and other Abnormal Eye Movements

Several networks within the brain contribute to normal eye movements and suppression of abnormal spontaneous eye movements; dysfunction of these networks produces nystagmus or saccadic intrusions.[49] Nystagmus by definition must include a slow phase. Jerk nystagmus has a slow phase followed by a fast phase, while pendular nystagmus has back-to-back slow phases, and any fast phases are due to saccadic intrusions. Although nystagmus by convention is named for the direction of the fast phase, it is the slow phase that informs the clinician more about the pathophysiology.

The history of patients with nystagmus is not infrequently dominated by related symptoms from other aspects of the causative lesion, such as vertigo or diplopia. The primary symptom of nystagmus is oscillopsia, defined as the illusion of environmental movement, although patients with infantile-onset nystagmus are often asymptomatic.

Examination should emphasize looking for stability of the eyes in the primary position with and without ocular fixation, in addition to observing lateral or other positions of gaze and posture as well as vestibular ocular reflex integrity and suppression. Any abnormal involuntary eye movements should be evaluated for the presence of slow and fast phases, directionality, and presence in one or both eyes, and whether it is influenced by position of gaze, posture, or time. Peripheral vestibular nystagmus is best observed without patient fixation, which can suppress the abnormality. Frenzel lenses provide a highly magnified view of the eyes and prohibit patient viewing, but this can also be accomplished by ophthalmoscopy while occluding the opposite eye. Video-oculographic recordings provide objective and quantifiable assessment of ocular oscillations, but are rarely required in general practice. The widespread availability of video recording often captures abnormalities and facilitates documentation. The key patterns of commonly encountered nystagmus include gaze-evoked, peripheral vestibular, central vestibular, see-saw, and congenital patterns.

Gaze-Evoked Nystagmus

Eccentric gaze-holding is accomplished by a neural network that matches innervation against the elastic forces of the orbit pulling the eyes back toward midline. With dysfunction of this network, known as the neural integrator, the eyes develop slow phases back toward the primary position and require a fast corrective phase to return to eccentric gaze; the slow phase is always toward primary position. The neural integrator includes the flocculus and nodulus of the cerebellum, the nucleus prepositus hypoglossi, and the medial vestibular nuclei for horizontal movements, and the interstitial nucleus of Cajal for vertical gaze-holding. Many normal patients will demonstrate a few beats of symmetric jerk nystagmus at the extremes of horizontal gaze without other features. Pathologic gaze-evoked nystagmus is characterized by sustained nystagmus, asymmetry (e.g., present in right but not left gaze), and sometimes other features such as rebound nystagmus. Rebound nystagmus is demonstrable by holding lateral gaze for several seconds during which sustained gaze-evoked nystagmus occurs, then observing the eyes after a return to primary position; while gaze-evoked nystagmus produces a slow phase toward the primary position, rebound causes a reversal of this direction upon return to the primary position (e.g., gaze-evoked nystagmus in right gaze with slow phases leftward back to the midline is followed by a few slow phases rightward after return to the primary position). Pathologic gaze-evoked nystagmus typically localizes to the ipsilateral cerebellum or connections. Medications including anticonvulsants and sedatives may produce symmetric sustained gaze-evoked nystagmus.

Peripheral Vestibular Nystagmus

Peripheral vestibular nystagmus typically contains torsional and either horizontal or vertical waveforms, and can be partially suppressed with visual fixation. It most commonly appears in two recognizable patterns. The first is associated with an acute vestibular syndrome, and results from dysfunction of all three semicircular canals or the entire vestibular nerve.[50] This form produces a slow phase with horizontal and torsional components "rolling" toward the paretic vestibular side (e.g., section of the right vestibular nerve produces rightward and clockwise slow phases, followed by left and counterclockwise corrective fast phases). This acute vestibular syndrome may result from several etiologies including vestibular neuritis or Ménière disease. The second common pattern is that associated with benign paroxysmal positional vertigo (BPPV). Because BPPV usually results from involvement of the posterior semicircular canal (with afferent connections to the ipsilateral superior oblique and contralateral inferior rectus), testing of the right ear with the Dix–Hallpike maneuver, for example, will produce slow phases that are downbeating and counterclockwise.

Peripheral vestibular nystagmus generally obeys Alexander law: nystagmus is more pronounced in gaze in the direction of the fast phase. Depending on lesion severity, nystagmus may only appear in gaze toward the fast phase. Large cerebellopontine angle tumors may produce Bruns nystagmus, which is the combination of ipsilesional gaze-evoked nystagmus and contralesional peripheral vestibular nystagmus.

Central Vestibular Nystagmus

Central vestibular nystagmus is not influenced by visual fixation, and includes the common patterns of downbeat and pendular nystagmus, typically resulting from lesions of the vestibulocerebellum (i.e., flocculus, nodulus, and vermis) or associated connections within the brainstem. Downbeat is the most common direction of central vestibular nystagmus; it is accentuated by, or may only be present in, down and lateral gaze. Etiologies include brainstem and cerebellar processes such as infarcts, demyelination, neurodegenerative disorders, toxins, neoplasms, or Chiari malformations.[51] Upbeating mystagmus is much less common than downbeat nystagmus, and is usually associated with lesions in the medulla or cerebellum, often related to demyelination, ischemia, or nutritional deficiency (e.g., Wernicke encephalopathy). Some patients with central vestibular nystagmus may respond partially to medications such as clonazepam, baclofen, gabapentin, memantine, or 4-diaminopyridine.[52]

Periodic alternating nystagmus is horizontal jerk nystagmus that rhythmically oscillates in direction, amplitude, and frequency; for example, nystagmus with slow phases leftward that increase in amplitude and frequency over 45 to 90 seconds, then wane and are followed by the development of nystagmus with slow phases to the right with predictable periodicity. Periodic alternating nystagmus may be congenital or acquired, localizes to the cerebellar nodulus, and often is related to multiple sclerosis, cerebellar degeneration, Chiari malformation, infarct, or bilateral visual loss. It is important to recognize due to its localizing value and may respond to baclofen.

Pendular nystagmus is characterized by sequential slow phases in the horizontal, vertical, or torsional planes, often combined into elliptical waveforms. Acquired pendular nystagmus is most commonly related to multiple sclerosis. Oculopalatal myoclonus or tremor is a special circumstance of pendular nystagmus with palatal myoclonus synchronous with nystagmus that persists even during sleep. This syndrome develops months to years after a lesion within the Mollaret triangle (i.e., cerebellar dentate nuclei, red nucleus, through the central tegmental tract to the inferior olivary nucleus in the medulla). Oculopalatal myoclonus may be characterized by the MRI appearance of hyperintensities on T2-weighted sequences within one or both inferior olivary nuclei.

See-saw Nystagmus

See-saw nystagmus involves dysconjugate oscillations with one eye elevating and intorting, while the contralateral eye depresses and extorts. See-saw nystagmus is often pendular, but may be jerk, and is more commonly acquired than congenital. It is typically associated with parasellar lesions (e.g., craniopharyngioma) often accompanied by bitemporal hemianopia.

Congenital Nystagmus

Congenital nystagmus, or infantile nystagmus syndrome, typically appears in the first few months of life as conjugate horizontal nystagmus that remains horizontal even in vertical gaze. It may have a complex waveform with both slow phase velocity-increasing jerk nystagmus as well as pendular movements in varying positions of gaze. Patients with congenital nystagmus often turn the head to place the eyes in a direction of gaze with the least nystagmus (i.e., the null position), and do not typically report oscillopsia. Decreased visual acuity may result from congenital nystagmus itself or from associated afferent conditions such as optic nerve hypoplasia or ocular albinism.

Latent nystagmus, or fusional maldevelopment nystagmus syndrome, involves horizontal jerk nystagmus that appears under monocular viewing conditions with the slow phase toward the nose; the slow phase reverses direction when occlusion is switched from one eye to the other. Latent nystagmus is always accompanied by esotropia.

Monocular "shimmering" nystagmus in childhood is unilateral, with very-low-amplitude vertical or elliptical movements that raise concern for anterior visual pathway glioma, thus requiring neuroimaging.

Saccadic Intrusions

Saccadic intrusions are composed entirely of fast phases, in contrast to nystagmus. They can be divided into forms with a normal intersaccadic interval of around 200 msec, and those with back-to-back saccades without such an interval. Square-wave jerks are horizontal small-amplitude (<5 deg) saccades separated by a normal intersaccadic interval. Square-wave jerks are very common, and normal elderly patients may exhibit a few per minute; however, they indicate underlying pathology when they are continuous or accompanied by other features such as extrapyramidal signs.[53] Ocular flutter is a horizontal saccadic intrusion without an intersaccadic interval, and opsoclonus consists of multiplanar saccadic intrusions without an intersaccadic interval. These disorders typically result from paraneoplastic conditions, multiple sclerosis, brainstem encephalitis, toxins, or severe metabolic derangements (e.g., hyperosmolar coma). Voluntary "nystagmus," which has no slow phase and accordingly is not truly nystagmus, resembles flutter, with rapidly oscillating horizontal conjugate back-to-back saccades without an intersaccadic interval. Most patients are unable to sustain voluntary nystagmus for more than a few seconds, and often converge when inducing this movement.

Other Ocular Movements

Superior oblique myokymia consists of paroxysmal, monocular, very low-amplitude, high-frequency torsional oscillations. Episodes typically last only seconds, but may recur numerous times throughout the day. These movements are usually only detectable with magnification, such as during slit-lamp biomicroscopy. The condition is benign and often responds to carbamazepine, baclofen, gabapentin, or topical β-blockers.

Oculomasticatory myorhythmia is a pendular, vergence oscillation that occurs in synchrony with contractions of the masticatory muscles; it is pathognomonic of Whipple disease, a rare infection caused by *Tropheryma whipplei*, which may also produce fever, diarrhea, cognitive dysfunction, and arthralgias (see Chapter 13).

Coma is caused by lesions involving either the brainstem or cerebral hemispheres bilaterally, and the eye examination can assist in this differentiation. Slow conjugate roving horizontal eye movements generally indicate a structurally intact brainstem. In contrast, rare "ping-pong" gaze, consisting of rapidly alternating conjugate horizontal gaze every few seconds, indicates destructive lesions of both cerebral hemispheres.

Ocular bobbing is a rare but ominous sign consisting of rapid conjugate downward eye movements followed by a slow return to primary position, usually accompanied by bilateral horizontal gaze palsies. Ocular bobbing indicates a destructive pontine lesion and very poor prognosis for neurologic recovery. Ocular bobbing should not be confused with ocular dipping (slow downward movement followed by rapid return), reverse bobbing (fast upward, then rapid return to primary), or other variants which do not have localizing or prognostic value.

THE PUPIL

Examination of the pupils provides objective, and occasionally critical, visual or cerebral information. In contrast to other examinations of visual function such as of acuity, color discrimination, and visual fields, pupil testing is objective and requires minimal patient cooperation.

Anatomy

The iris sphincter and dilator muscles control pupil size, with parasympathetic sphincter muscle innervation originating in the Edinger–Westphal subnucleus of the third cranial nerve in the midbrain. Light stimulation of retinal ganglion cells travels through the optic nerve and then through the optic chiasm, where just over 50 percent of the fibers decussate to the contralateral optic tract. Within the optic tract, some axons bypass the lateral geniculate body to enter the brachium of the superior colliculus and synapse in the pretectal nucleus, which also receives light input from the opposite side. The pretectal nuclei efferents project to the Edinger–Westphal nuclei, which innervate the iris sphincter via the oculomotor nerve. Pupil dilatation involves the sympathetic pathways, which begin with first-order cell bodies in the hypothalamus. Axons from these neurons traverse the brainstem to the thoracic cord level, where the second-order cell bodies reside. Axons from these neurons enter the paravertebral sympathetic chain, before coursing over the lung apex to the superior cervical ganglion, where the final third-order cell body originates. These third-order sympathetic axons ascend as a plexus surrounding the internal carotid artery to enter the cavernous sinus before passing through the superior orbital fissure into the orbit to innervate the iris dilator muscles.

Because the midbrain receives a composite of retinal input, the pupils remain isocoric in the face of afferent visual dysfunction. For example, unilateral optic nerve section does not produce anisocoria; the pupil will not exhibit a direct light reaction, but will react consensually to light stimulation of the opposite eye.

A relative afferent pupillary defect results from asymmetric light input and is elicited by the swinging flashlight test. With the patient viewing a distance object, the examiner shines a bright light alternately in each eye for 1 to 2 seconds. Normally, each pupil constricts in response to the light—a relative afferent pupillary defect exists if, instead, the pupil dilates to the light. This phenomenon occurs because the brain perceives less light when stimulating the diseased optic nerve compared to the amount of light perceived with stimulation of the normal optic nerve, and appropriately enlarges the pupil for this relatively darker condition. A relative afferent pupillary defect is a sensitive and objective indication of asymmetric optic nerve dysfunction and does not occur with functional visual loss, refractive error, media opacity, or mild retinopathies. The swinging flashlight test requires two eyes, but just one working pupil (the pupils are isocoric with afferent lesions, so viewing either pupil provides the same information).

The near response consists of convergence, pupillary miosis, and accommodation. If the examiner encounters a pupil with an impaired light reaction, the next step should be to assess the pupillary response to a near target. Several conditions are characterized by light-near dissociation, most notably Argyll Robertson pupils, Parinaud dorsal midbrain syndrome, Adie tonic pupil (see later), and severe afferent visual loss. Argyll Robertson pupils are bilaterally small, irregular pupils with limited light response compared to a brisk near response and prompt dilatation to distance viewing. This pupil abnormality is most associated with neurosyphilis. Parinaud syndrome was discussed earlier and the Adie tonic pupil is considered in the next section. Oculomotor nerve aberrancy with a pupil that constricts in attempted adduction also produces light-near dissociation, as can a widespread neuropathy with autonomic involvement (e.g., severe diabetic neuropathy). Severe afferent visual loss from pregeniculate causes such as optic neuropathy or widespread retinopathy will also produce light-near dissociation, but the clinical picture is dominated by the visual loss in this setting.

Anisocoria

Anisocoria may have many causes ranging from benign to life-threatening.[54] Physiologic anisocoria is characterized by briskly reactive pupils that differ in size by less than 1 mm. Patients are asymptomatic, and, accordingly, old photographs may assist in dating the onset of the asymmetry. An approach emphasizing the pupil reaction to light and dark, and the pupil size in light in dark will help categorize possible causes.[55]

Transient Anisocoria

Transient anisocoria is usually related to benign etiologies such as migraine[56]; ominous potential causes include aneurysm or uncal herniation, but are unlikely in the asymptomatic patient with a normal examination.

Anisocoria Greater in Dark with Normally Reactive Pupils to Light

This common condition generally indicates either Horner syndrome or physiologic anisocoria. Rarely, pharmacologic instillation with miotics such as pilocarpine will result in changes of similar type. Physiologic anisocoria is present in 20 percent of the population and typically produces anisocoria that is equal in light and darkness or slightly greater in the dark with normally reactive pupils to light, darkness, and accommodation.

Horner Syndrome

Horner syndrome is related to sympathetic paresis of the eye. It produces miosis, ptosis and anhidrosis, although the full triad is rarely present. Responsible lesions that can affect the sympathetic pathway include lateral medullary syndromes in the brainstem, apical lung lesions, and internal carotid artery dissections.

Sympathetic fibers from the hypothalamus descend through the brainstem, where they may be affected by Wallenberg lateral medullary syndrome, into the spinal cord to the level of C8–T1, where the second-order fibers begin. Radiculopathy may affect this segment of the nerve before it ascends the lung apex to reach the carotid artery, moving toward the superior cervical ganglia, the site of the third-order neuron. The third-order fibers ascend on the carotid artery (pupillomotor fibers via internal carotid, and vasomotor plus sudomotor fibers via external carotid arteries) into the cavernous sinus, and then traverse the superior orbital fissure with V1 of the trigeminal nerve into the orbit to innervate Müller muscle and the pupil dilators.

Horner miosis is related to impaired dilatation, and accordingly the anisocoria is greatest in the dark. Slowed dilatation to dark is quite specific for sympathetic paresis. The ptosis of Horner syndrome relates to impairment of Müller muscle, a small ancillary muscle that assists in lid opening. Upper-lid ptosis in Horner is always less than 1 to 2 mm, and lower-lid or "upside down" ptosis is also present. The anhidrosis in Horner syndrome varies with the site of the sympathetic lesion, ranging from hemibody with lesions of the first-order neurons to a small patch above the brow in distal lesions of the third-order neurons; the symptom is rarely noted by patients. Many Horner syndromes are incomplete; the miosis is the most recognizable and reliable feature to guide diagnosis.

Pharmacologic studies may aid in the diagnosis. Cocaine instilled into the eye blocks norepinephrine reuptake, thus increasing norepinephrine's action at the synapse and producing pupil dilatation if the sympathetic chain is intact. In addition to mydriasis, cocaine causes lid retraction and blanching of the conjunctiva. Postcocaine anisocoria of greater than 0.8 mm increases the likelihood of a Horner syndrome; 1 mm anisocoria is often used as a convenient diagnostic cut-off.[57] Apraclonidine is an α_2-adrenergic agonist, but also has weak α_1 agonist properties. This α_1 activation is too weak to affect a normal pupil, but will dilate denervated, supersensitive iris dilators, thus producing a reversal of the preexisting anisocoria.[58] Differentiating Horner syndromes due to involvement of third-order neurons from preganglionic (first- or second-order neurons) syndromes involves the instillation of hydroxyamphetamine drops. This agent releases acetylcholine from intact third-order neurons; an increase in preinstillation to postinstillation anisocoria of 1 mm generally indicates a Horner syndrome due to a lesion of third-order neurons.

Localization of the lesion causing Horner syndrome greatly assists in the evaluation. Lesions of first-order neurons are always associated with other central nervous system features. Lesions of second-order neurons may be caused by lung lesions (Pancoast tumor) or tumors within the neck or mediastinum. Postganglionic (third-order) Horner syndromes when isolated without other features are likely to be benign, and are often associated with a primary headache history; approximately 25 percent of cluster headaches are associated with Horner syndrome. Pain or cephalgia with a third-order Horner syndrome raises concern for carotid dissection, or skull-base neoplasm.

Anisocoria Greater in Light with Abnormal Pupillary Light Reaction

Mechanical disruption of the iris may produce a pupil that reacts poorly to light (and often dark). Surgery is the most common mechanism that mechanically impairs the iris, but infection or inflammation with synechiae tethering the iris to the lens, trauma, and angle-closure glaucoma may also be responsible. Distorted pupil shape, a history of intraocular surgery, and poor reaction to mydriatic drops are all clues of a mechanical origin.

Angle-closure glaucoma is an important condition to recognize as it may lead to irreversible visual loss. In its most severe form, the pupil is mid-position and light fixed, with a "steamy"-appearing edematous cornea, conjunctival injection, and pain, which is often supraorbital. Precipitating factors include darkness or mydriatic drops. The diagnosis is made clinically including documentation of elevated intraocular pressure, and treatment involves an urgent reduction in pressure by pharmacologic and then surgical means.

The parasympathetic fibers innervating the pupil sphincter travel with the oculomotor nerve; however, palsies of the third cranial nerve never cause isolated mydriasis as a general rule, even if the only other finding is subtle ocular misalignment in extremes of gaze.

Several pharmacologic agents may produce mydriasis if instilled in the eye, either intentionally or by accident. Both anticholinergics and sympathomimetics will produce mydriasis. Commonly encountered anticholinergic agents include atropine and other "red top" drops, scopolamine patches, inhalers, insecticides, and many plant sources (e.g., belladonna). These agents typically produce light- and near-fixed maximal mydriasis (around 9 mm) with no response to 1 percent pilocarpine drops. Sympathomimetics such as epinephrine, phenylephrine, hydroxyamphetamine, cocaine, decongestants, and adrenergic inhalers produce mydriasis with a dampened light response in addition to conjunctival blanching and lid retraction. These pupils retain reaction to 1 percent pilocarpine drops.

Adie Tonic Pupil

Adie tonic pupil results from an idiopathic parasympathetic lesion involving the ciliary ganglion or postganglionic short ciliary nerves within the orbit. Acutely, the pupil is dilated with partial paresis of accommodation and light reaction. This partial paresis produces sector palsy of the iris, with limited sections partially reacting; this phenomenon is best observed with the slit lamp. Patients may report photophobia, complain of blurring of vision when reading or looking at near objects, or are asymptomatic. The muscle stretch reflexes in the legs may be depressed and some patients develop segmental anhidrosis (Ross syndrome). With time (at least 1 week), supersensitivity develops, and even dilute pilocarpine (0.1%) may produce pupillary miosis (a normal pupil has no response to this dilute preparation of pilocarpine).[59] The short ciliary nerves regenerate as accommodative fibers to the ciliary muscle along with aberrant innervation of the iris sphincter subserving the near response, thus creating light-near dissociation. Dilatation occurs only very slowly on release of accommodation following convergence. Over years, the Adie pupil tends to become the smaller pupil, but retains the light-near dissociation and tonic response to accommodation.

REFERENCES

1. Miller NR, Biousse V, Kerrison JB, et al: Walsh & Hoyt's Clinical Neuro-Ophthalmology. 6th Ed. Lippincott Williams & Wilkins, Baltimore, 2004.
2. Pau D, Al Zubidi N, Yalamanchili S, et al: Optic neuritis. Eye 25:833, 2011.
3. Koczman JJ, Rouleau J, Gaunt M, et al: Neuro-ophthalmic sarcoidiosis, the University of Iowa experience. Semin Ophthalmol 23:157, 2008.
4. Beck RW, Gal RL, Bhatti MT, et al: Visual function more than 10 years after optic neuritis: experience of the optic neuritis treatment trial. Am J Ophthalmol 137:77, 2004.
5. Biousse V, Calvetti O, Drews-Botsch C, et al: Management of optic neuritis and impact of clinical trials: an international survey. J Neurol Sci 276:69, 2009.
6. Swanton J, Fernando K, Dalton C, et al: Early MRI in optic neuritis. Neurology 72:542, 2009.
7. Naismith RT, Tutlam NT, Xu J, et al: Optical coherence tomography differs in neuromyelitis optica compared with multiple sclerosis. Neurology 72:1077, 2009.
8. Nakamura M, Nakazawa T, Doi H, et al: Early high-dose intravenous methylprednisolone is effective in preserving retinal nerve fiber layer thickness in patients with neuromyelitis optica. Graefes Arch Clin Exp Ophthalmol 248:1777, 2010.
9. Keegan M, Pineda AA, McClelland RL, et al: Plasma exchange for severe attacks of CNS demyelination: predictors of response. Neurology 58:143, 2002.
10. Salgado C, Vilson F, Miller NR, et al: Cellular inflammation in nonarteritic anterior ischemic optic neuropathy and its primate model. Arch Ophthalmol 129:1583, 2011.
11. Dickersin K, Manheimer E, Li T: Surgery for nonarteritis anterior ischemic optic neuropathy. Cochrane Database Syst Rev 1:CD001538, 2012.
12. Klopstock T, Yu-Wai-Man P, Dimitriadis K, et al: A randomized placebo-controlled trial of idebenone in Leber's hereditary optic neuropathy. Brain 134:2677, 2011.
13. Round R, Keane J: The minor symptoms of increased intracranial pressure: 101 patients with benign intracranial hypertension. Neurology 38:1461, 1988.
14. Biousse V, Bruce BB, Newman NJ: Update on the pathophysiology and management of ideopathic intracranial hypertension. J Neurol Neurosurg Psychiatry 83:488, 2012.
15. Degnan AJ, Levy LM: Pseudotumor cerebri: brief review of clinical syndrome and imaging findings. AJNR Am J Neuroradiol 32:1986, 2011.
16. Thurtell MJ, Wall M: Idiopathic intracranial hypertension (pseudotumor cerebri): recognition, treatment, and ongoing management. Curr Treat Options Neurol 15:1, 2013.
17. Zhang X, Kedar S, Lynn MJ, et al: Homonymous hemianopias: clinical antatomic correlations in 904 cases. Neurology 66:906, 2006.
18. Lee A, Martin C: Neuro-ophthalmic findings in the visual variant of Alzheimer's disease. Ophthalmology 111:376, 2004.
19. Barton JJ: "Retinal diplopia" associated with macular wrinkling. Neurology 63:925, 2004.
20. Leigh RJ, Zee DS: The Neurology of Eye Movements. 4th Ed. Oxford University Press, New York, 2006.
21. Scudder CA, Kaneko CS, Fuchs AF: The brainstem burst generator for saccadic eye movements: a modern synthesis. Exp Brain Res 142:439, 2002.
22. Pierrot-Deseilligny CH, Ploner CJ, Muri RM, et al: Effects of cerebral lesions on saccadic eye movements in humans. Ann NY Acad Sci 956:216, 2002.
23. Keane JR: The pretectal syndrome: 206 patients. Neurology 40:684, 1990.
24. Brodsky MC, Donahue SP, Vaphiades M, et al: Skew deviation revisited. Surv Ophthalmol 51:105, 2006.
25. Parulekar MV, Dai S, Buncic JR, et al: Head position-dependent changes in ocular torsion and vertical misalignment in skew deviation. Arch Ophthalmol 126:899, 2008.
26. Brandt T, Strupp M: General vestibular testing. Clin Neurophysiol 116:406, 2005.
27. Pullicino P, Lincoff N, Truax BT: Abnormal vergence with upper brainstem infarcts. Pseudoabducens palsy. Neurology 55:352, 2000.
28. Lavrich JB: Convergence insufficiency and its current treatment. Curr Opin Ophthalmol 21:356, 2010.
29. Richards B, Jones F, Younge B: Causes and prognosis in 4,278 cases of paralysis of the oculomotor, trochlear, and abducens cranial nerves. Am J Ophthalmol 113:489, 1992.
30. Jacobson DM: Pupil involvement in patients with diabetes-associated oculomotor nerve palsy. Arch Ophthalmol 116:723, 1998.
31. Rabadi MH, Beltmann MA: Midbrain infarction presenting isolated medial rectus nuclear palsy. Am J Med 118:836, 2005.
32. Sitthinamsuwan B, Nunta-aree S, Sitthinamsuwan P, et al: Two patients with rare cases of Weber's syndrome. J Clin Neurosci 18:578, 2011.
33. Kupersmith MJ, Heller G, Cox TA: Magnetic resonance angiography and clinical evaluation of third nerve palsies and posterior communicating artery aneurysms. J Neurosurg 105:228, 2006.

34. Jacobson D: Relative pupil-sparing third nerve palsy: etiology and clinical variables predictive of a mass. Neurology 56:797, 2001.
35. Lee A, Hayman L, Brazis P: The evaluation of isolated third nerve palsy revisited: an update on the evolving role of magnetic resonance, computed tomography, and catheter angiography. Surv Ophthalmol 47:137, 2002.
36. Peters GB, Bakri SJ, Krohel GB: Cause and prognosis of nontraumatic sixth nerve palsies in young adults. Ophthalmology 109:1925, 2002.
37. Holmes JM, Beck RW, Kip KE, et al: Predictors of nonrecovery in acute traumatic sixth nerve palsy and paresis. Ophthalmology 108:1457, 2001.
38. DeRespinis P, Caputo A, Wagner R, et al: Duane's retraction syndrome. Surv Ophthalmol 38:257, 1993.
39. Mori M, Kuwabara S, Fukutake T, et al: Clinical features and prognosis of Miller Fisher syndrome. Neurology 56:1104, 2001.
40. Chiba A, Kusunoki S, Obata H, et al: Serum anti-GQ1b IgG antibody is associated with ophthalmoplegia in Miller Fisher syndrome and Guillain-Barré syndrome. Neurology 43:1911, 1993.
41. Mori M, Kuwabara S, Fukutake T, et al: Intravenous immunoglobulin therapy for Miller Fisher syndrome. Neurology 68:1144, 2007.
42. Kim JS: Internuclear ophthalmoplegia as an isolated or predominant symptom of brainstem infarction. Neurology 62:1491, 2004.
43. Drachman DB: Myasthenia gravis. N Engl J Med 330:1797, 1994.
44. Kaminski HJ, Ruff RL: Ocular involvement by myasthenia gravis. Ann Neurol 41:419, 1997.
45. Scherer K, Bedlack RS, Simel DL: Does this patient have myasthenia gravis? JAMA 293:1906, 2005.
46. Golnik KC, Pena R, Lee AG, et al: An ice test for the diagnosis of myasthenia gravis. Ophthalmology 106:1282, 1999.
47. Char DH: Thyroid eye disease. Br J Ophthalmol 80:922, 1996.
48. Bartley GB, Fatourechi V, Kadrmas EF, et al: Clinical features of Graves ophthalmopathy in an incident cohort. Am J Ophthalmol 121:4284, 1996.
49. Eggenberger ER: Nystagmus. p. 85. In: Levin LA, Arnold AC (eds): Neuro-Ophthalmology: The Practical Guide. Thieme Medical Publishers, New York, 2005.
50. Baloh RW: Vestibular neuritis. N Engl J Med 348:1027, 2003.
51. Pelak VS, Hall DA: Neuro-ophthalmic manifestations of neurodegenerative disease. Ophthalmol Clin North Am 17:311, 2004.
52. Straube A, Leigh RJ, Bronstein A, et al: EFNS task force—therapy of nystagmus and oscillopsia. Eur J Neurol 11:83, 2004.
53. Altiparmak U, Eggenberger E, Coleman A, et al: The ratio of square wave jerk rates to blink rates distinguishes progressive supranuclear palsy from Parkinson disease. J Neuroophthalmol 26:257, 2006.
54. Jacobson DM: Benign episodic unilateral mydriasis: clinical characteristics. Ophthalmology 102:1623, 1995.
55. Weinstein JM: The pupil. p. 51. In: Slamovitis TL, Burde R (eds): Neuroophthalmology. (Podos and Yanoff's Textbook of Ophthalmology, Vol VI). Mosby Year Book, St Louis, 1994.
56. DeMarinis M, Assenza S, Carletto F: Oculosympathetic alterations in migraine patients. Cephalgia 18:77, 1998.
57. Kardon RH, Denison CE, Brown CK, et al: Critical evaluation of the cocaine test in the diagnosis of Horner's syndrome. Arch Ophthalmol 108:387, 1990.
58. Brown SM, Aouchiche R, Freedman KA: The utility of 0.5% apraclonidine in the diagnosis of Horner syndrome. Arch Ophthalmol 121:1201, 2003.
59. Jacobson DM, Vierkant RA: Comparison of cholinergic supersensitivity in third nerve palsy and Adie's syndrome. J Neuroophthalmol 18:171, 1998.

SECTION

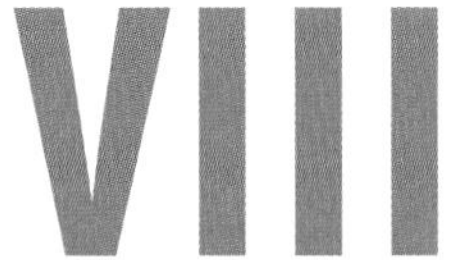

Hematologic and Neoplastic Disease

CHAPTER

25

Neurologic Manifestations of Hematologic Disorders

J.D. SUSSMAN ■ G.A.B. DAVIES-JONES

Aminoff's Neurology and General Medicine, Fifth Edition.

ANEMIA

Iron-Deficiency Anemia

Nonspecific neurologic symptoms of tiredness, fatigue, weakness, poor concentration, irritability, faintness, dizziness, tinnitus, and headache are commonly associated with anemia. Occasionally, more concrete neurologic syndromes arise, such as the association of both pseudotumor cerebri and cerebral venous sinus thrombosis with iron-deficiency anemia.[1] The pseudotumor cerebri may resolve and recur with resolution and recurrence of the iron-deficiency anemia. In some patients with iron-deficiency anemia, thrombocytosis may be so high that it suggests a myeloproliferative disorder. The increased platelet mass may result in transient ischemic attacks (TIAs) or cerebral infarction. Profound anemia, particularly when associated with thrombocytopenia, may produce a retinopathy with papilledema, cotton-wool exudates, flame-shaped hemorrhages, retinal edema, and even retinal detachment. Blindness is a rare but well-recognized complication of massive hemorrhage; swelling of the optic discs is followed within a few weeks by optic atrophy.

Focal neurologic signs may arise from severe anemia in conjunction with severe cerebral atherosclerosis; symptoms may resolve completely over hours as the hemoglobin is increased. Severe anemia may also produce signs and symptoms that mimic Guillain–Barré syndrome.[2]

Transient erythroblastopenia of childhood may present with papilledema and transient hemiparesis. Restless legs syndrome may also be associated with various forms of iron-deficiency anemia including frequent blood donation. Iron deficiency and a strong family history (present in 72%) are characteristic of childhood-onset restless legs syndrome.[3]

Vitamin B_{12} Deficiency

Caution must be exercised when interpreting serum vitamin B_{12} values as there are no well-defined cut-offs for deficiency—likely deficiency has been defined as a value of less than 148 pmol/L and possible deficiency as a value between 148 and 258 pmol/L. Falsely low levels have been associated with multiple myeloma, oral contraceptive use, folate deficiency, and pregnancy. Elevated total serum homocysteine is a sensitive marker of vitamin deficiency but may also be related to familial hyperhomocysteinemia, levodopa therapy, renal insufficiency, and folate deficiency. Methylmalonic acid levels increase in the presence of vitamin B_{12} deficiency, often preceding reduced cobalamin levels. A low vitamin B_{12} level alone does not automatically define a deficiency. Among elderly individuals with low vitamin B_{12} levels, 20 to 40 percent have normal homocysteine and methylmalonic acid blood levels and therefore should not be considered deficient in vitamin B_{12}. Holotranscobalamin may be the most sensitive measure of erythrocyte cobalamin deficiency but is rarely used in clinical practice.[4]

Vitamin B_{12} deficiency may be caused by Addisonian pernicious anemia, vitamin B_{12} malabsorption syndromes (including gastric and ileal resections, terminal ileal removal for lower urinary tract reconstruction, blind loops, and infestation with fish tapeworm), and dietary deficiency particularly in vegans. The neurologic complications of vitamin B_{12} deficiency may occur without appreciable alteration in the peripheral blood; erythropoiesis may even be normoblastic, particularly when vitamin B_{12} deficiency coincides with iron-deficiency anemia. Elevated serum methylmalonic acid and total homocysteine are useful in the diagnosis of vitamin B_{12} deficiency. Failure of intracellular transport of vitamin B_{12} by transcobalamin 2 can lead to functional deficiency, but with normal serum vitamin B_{12}; it is suggested by the presence of elevated serum methylmalonic acid or homocysteine, with low levels of transcobalamin 2. Such patients may respond to high-dose injections of vitamin B_{12}.[5]

PERIPHERAL NEUROPATHY

Sensory symptoms of peripheral neuropathy may be identical to those of vitamin B_{12} myelopathy. Somatosensory evoked potentials become abnormal before changes develop in peripheral nerves. Electrophysiologic studies indicate that the length-dependent neuropathy is secondary to a dying-back type of axonal degeneration, and neuropathologic studies have demonstrated loss of large myelinated fibers in distal sensory nerves as well as axonal degeneration in teased-fiber preparations.

MYELOPATHY

Demyelination followed by axonal degeneration affects the most heavily myelinated fibers first, which may explain why lesions appear primarily in the posterior columns and then later in the lateral columns. Progression may be subacute or rapid.

Suspicion that a sensory neuropathy may be related to vitamin B_{12} deficiency should be raised by upper-limb onset or an associated Lhermitte phenomenon. Myelopathy is accompanied by early and severe impairment of proprioception and vibration sense, sometimes accompanied by motor signs of the neuropathy. A severe sensory ataxic spastic paraparesis may be the sole manifestation of the myelopathy. Bladder symptoms may occur later. Pseudoathetosis is rare but may be prominent. Magnetic resonance imaging (MRI) may reveal hyperintense T2 signal in the dorsal cervical cord. Similar changes may occur with copper deficiency that may also arise from malabsorption following upper gastrointestinal surgery.

Encephalopathy

Multiple foci or diffuse areas of demyelination occur with little evidence of glial cell proliferation or axonal degeneration. Symptoms include disorders of mood, mental slowing, poor memory, confusion, agitation, delusions, visual and auditory hallucinations, aggression, dysphasia, and incontinence.

Neuropsychiatric assessment in patients presenting to general physicians with vitamin B_{12} or folic acid deficiency identifies organic mental change of unspecified nature in around 25 percent of patients, and affective disorders in around 20 percent of patients.

Optic Neuropathy

Optic neuropathy is rare and may be the presenting feature. Optic atrophy may ensue.

Disordered Eye Movements

Downbeat nystagmus, paralysis of upward gaze, and internuclear ophthalmoplegia have all been attributed to vitamin B_{12} deficiency and have responded to therapy.[6]

Infantile Vitamin B_{12} Deficiency

Infantile vitamin B_{12} deficiency may result from maternal vitamin B_{12} deficiency causing encephalopathy, epilepsy, and microcephaly.[7] Long-term cognitive impairment and developmental delay may ensue.

Imerslund–Graesbeck Syndrome

This is an autosomal recessive condition caused by a defect in the receptor of the vitamin B_{12}–intrinsic factor complex of the ileal enterocyte and resulting in megaloblastic anemia, proteinuria, and multiple neurologic abnormalities.

Folate Deficiency

Cerebral folate deficiency typically presents in early infancy with seizures, delayed motor and cognitive development, cerebellar ataxia, spasticity, and visual and hearing impairment. Juvenile and adult-onset cases also occur. Peripheral neuropathy has been described in a few patients. Subacute combined degeneration of the cord accompanying diet-induced folic acid deficiency may occur and improves after treatment with folic acid.[8] A variety of folate transport and metabolic disorders have been described, and blocking antibodies against folate receptors have been found in the serum in 25 of 28 children with cerebral folate deficiency and in none of matched controls.[9] There is evidence from studies in animals that abnormal cerebrospinal fluid (CSF) circulation may result in impaired cortical development along with hydrocephalus and neural tube defects as a result of disturbed folate metabolite delivery.[10]

Sickle Cell Disease

Most of the complications of sickle cell anemia (Hb SS) or of sickle C disease (Hb SC) relate to the formation of sickle cells, which occurs because of the insolubility of deoxygenated hemoglobin S polymers. These sickle cells adhere to various receptors on the vascular endothelium, producing aggregates and vessel occlusion.[11] Children with sickle cell disease have reduced levels of the majority of endothelial coagulation inhibitors, further enhancing the adhesive interactions between sickle cells with injured cell membranes and endothelial cells.[12]

Sickling occurs when PO_2 is low. In the presence of circulatory stasis or reduced cardiac output, oxygen extraction is increased such that sickling is more likely to occur. In sickle cell trait, the severity of sickling depends on the amount of Hb S; the percentage of Hb S in sickle cell trait can vary from 25 to 45 percent. In circumstances of severe hypoxemia, even patients with sickle cell trait (Hb SA) may develop symptoms.

One-quarter of patients with sickle cell disease have neurologic manifestations, with cerebral infarction being most common. Cerebral infarction on brain MRI in the absence of a history or physical findings of stroke occurs in 27 percent of patients before their 6th birthday, and 37 percent by their 14th birthday. Intracranial hemorrhage is much rarer; subarachnoid hemorrhage is the most common form and is usually aneurysmal in etiology. In children, hemorrhage tends to be primary and possibly related to vasculopathy leading to stenosis of large extracranial or intracranial vessels from fibrous proliferation of the intima. Moyamoya syndrome has been described in sickle cell disease and trait.

Less common neurologic features include cranial neuropathies, radiculopathy, ischemic mononeuropathy, radiculomyelopathy from vertebral collapse as a result of bone infarction, spinal cord infarction, hypopituitarism, ischemic optic neuropathy, TIAs, and seizures. Subcortical cerebral infarction and venous sinus thrombosis have also been described in sickle cell trait.[13] Measurement of IQ in children with hemoglobin SS demonstrates modest reductions, suggesting diffuse brain injury.

Cerebrovascular complications are relatively uncommon in Hb SC disease but a proliferative retinopathy is described. Recurrent transient impairment of vision due to occlusion of major retinal vessels is an unusual manifestation of Hb SS disease.

Thalassemia

Chronic anemias are associated with extramedullary hematopoiesis. There have been a few reports of spinal cord compression, most commonly in the middle to lower thoracic region. Surgical decompression plus radiotherapy is curative. Treatment with corticosteroids, blood transfusions, and local radiotherapy has also been successful. Transfusion to maintain the hemoglobin level above 12.5 g/dl may resolve minor compression of the spinal cord, with near-complete resolution of the extradural hematopoietic mass.[14] Visual failure secondary to suprasellar extramedullary hematopoiesis in β-thalassemia has been described.

Severe forms of β-thalassemia, particularly following splenectomy, can be associated with hypercoagulability, with an increased risk of cerebral venous thrombosis.[15] There is a reported association with moyamoya syndrome. Axonal sensorimotor neuropathy may also be a feature of β-thalassemia.

Hereditary Spherocytosis

Hereditary spherocytosis has few neurologic sequelae. It is associated with a state of chronic anemia which results in a reduced cholesterol level and therefore a reduced rate of carotid occlusion and stroke.[16] There have been reports of moyamoya syndrome in children with hereditary spherocytosis.

Paroxysmal Nocturnal Hemoglobinuria

Paroxysmal nocturnal hemoglobinuria is a rare acquired hematopoietic stem-cell disorder arising from a range of mutations in the phosphatidylinositol glycan class A (*PIGA*) gene, resulting in a deficiency of a glycosyl phosphatidylinositol–anchored protein. It may occur de novo or in association with marrow hypoplasia, ranging from pancytopenia to aplastic anemia. It results in deficiency in the binding of several protective red cell membrane proteins and leads to hypersensitivity to complement. The disorder is characterized by intravascular hemolysis and manifested by episodes of hemoglobinuria and venous thrombosis. Hemolysis occurs throughout the day and is not paroxysmal, but hemoglobinuria is seen when the first concentrated urine is passed in the morning. The commonest manifestation is large-vessel venous thrombosis particularly in the brain and portal system. The spinal cord is not affected. An occasional patient suffers TIAs that have been attributed to the hypercoagulable state induced when excess thromboplastin is released from lysing red blood cells. Increased sensitivity of the red cells to lysis by complement stimulates platelet aggregation and leads to the hypercoagulability. The hemoglobin released by hemolysis binds with circulating nitric oxide and inhibits the relaxation of smooth muscle, which results in abnormal tone of vascular smooth muscle, vasculopathy, and endothelial dysfunction. A neurologic cause of death was found in 10 percent of patients, including cerebral venous thrombosis, subarachnoid hemorrhage, and intracerebral hemorrhage.[17] Eculizumab is an effective treatment.

Cold Agglutinin Disease

Cold agglutinin disease is a form of autoimmune hemolytic anemia usually associated with IgM antibodies (rarely IgG and IgA cold-reactive autoantibodies) directed against erythrocytes with binding activity that increases as the temperature approaches 0°C. Cold-associated circulatory symptoms are very common. It is associated with a low-grade lymphoproliferative B-cell disorder in 90 percent of cases, but with a very low rate of developing overt lymphoma. Cold-induced circulatory symptoms with characteristic seasonal variations in anemia occur. The anemia is variable and usually not severe, though approximately 50 percent of patients are transfusion dependent at some time during the disease. Cold agglutinin–associated asymmetric sensory-motor neuropathy has been described as a feature of transformation to Waldenström macroglobulinemia.

Cryoglobulinemia

Cryoglobulins are serum proteins or protein complexes that undergo reversible precipitation at low temperatures. Three main types are recognized. Type I, most commonly monoclonal IgM or IgG, is seen in association with multiple myeloma, Waldenström macroglobulinemia, and other lymphoproliferative disorders. Type II consists of mixed immunoglobulin complexes in which the monoclonal antibody has specificity for polyclonal IgG and occurs in association with lymphoproliferative diseases, autoimmune disorders, and hepatitis. Type III cryoglobulin is composed of polyclonal immunoglobulin and is found in infections and autoimmune disorders. Neurologic complications are common in types II and III, with mononeuritis multiplex, peripheral symmetric sensorimotor axonal or demyelinating polyneuropathy, and small-fiber sensory neuropathy being the most common findings. More rarely, cerebral ischemia or vasculitis may occur.

Kernicterus

Kernicterus may be produced by any hemolytic process of sufficient severity in neonates, particularly in premature infants with physiologic jaundice. Whenever the serum unconjugated bilirubin level exceeds 20 mg/dl during the first few weeks of life, kernicterus may occur, though there is a poor correlation between bilirubin levels and disease severity. Unconjugated bilirubin is highly lipid soluble; it enters the brain and binds to neurons, resulting in neuronal loss, demyelination, and gliosis particularly in the basal ganglia and cerebellum. The neurologic features range from decreased alertness, hypotonia, and poor feeding to retrocollis, opisthotonus, and long-term sequelae. Chronic changes may evolve over a number of years, including the development of eye movement abnormalities, hearing loss, and extrapyramidal disorders (particularly athetosis and, less commonly, chorea). Cognitive function is relatively well preserved.

RARE NEUROLOGIC SYNDROMES AND RED CELL ABNORMALITIES

The term *neuroacanthocytosis* describes a number of conditions associated with abnormal erythrocyte membrane constituents, resulting in the formation of spiculated cells.

Pantothenate kinase–associated neurodegeneration, or neurodegeneration with brain iron accumulation type I (NBIA-1), is an autosomal recessive disorder in which classic forms are associated with *PANK2* mutations in chromosome 20. Patients are normal at birth but then develop acanthocytosis, dystonia, dysarthria, rigidity, occasional spasticity, cognitive impairment and dementia, pigmentary retinal degeneration, optic atrophy, and iron accumulation in the brain, particularly in the globus pallidus. MRI shows the “eye-of-the-tiger sign”—hyperintensity within the hypointense medial globus pallidus—but this sign may not be present in early cases. The classic form presents in the first decade, with progression and loss of independent ambulation within 15 years. Atypical forms develop in the second decade and progress slowly, with retained independent ambulation up to 40 years later. Intermediate forms are described. Early onset is associated with pigmentary retinopathy, whereas a later onset is associated with speech disorders and psychiatric features. Pantothenate kinase catalyzes the first committed step in the universal biosynthetic pathway leading to CoA, and is located in the mitochondrial intermembrane space.[18,19] Mutations in *PANK2* are also found in HARP syndrome (hypoprebetalipoproteinemia, acanthocytosis, retinitis pigmentosa, and pallidal degeneration)

Bassen–Kornzweig disease (neuroacanthocytosis with abetalipoproteinemia) is a recessively inherited syndrome characterized by acanthocytosis, retinitis pigmentosa, increasing cerebellar ataxia, peripheral neuropathy, steatorrhea, and complete or almost complete lack of serum β-lipoproteins, with onset during childhood. The microsomal triglyceride transfer protein (*MTTP*) gene is essential for synthesizing β-lipoproteins for the absorption and transport of fats and cholesterol. Mutations in the gene result in deficiency of fat-soluble vitamins, A, D, E, and K, though deficiency of vitamin E is the primary cause of the degeneration in spinocerebellar and dorsal columns of the spinal cord. Treatment with vitamins A and E as early as possible is helpful.

Chorea-acanthocytosis is an autosomal recessive disorder linked to the *VPS13A* gene on chromosome 9 which encodes chorein. The neurologic features commence between 25 and 45 years with behavioral change and obsessive compulsive disorder, followed later by the development of progressive choreiform movements of the limbs, face, mouth, lips, and throat—lip and tongue biting is characteristic. Myopathy and neuropathy may occur. In addition, motor or vocal tics, dystonia, parkinsonism, progressive supranuclear palsy, and apraxia of eyelid opening have been described. Serum creatine kinase levels are elevated; serum lipoproteins are normal.

McLeod neuroacanthosis is an X-linked syndrome with absent expression of Kx erythrocyte antigens, weak expression of Kell glycoprotein antigens, and increased serum creatinine kinase levels. A range of other features may include hemolytic anemia, myopathy, limb chorea, facial tics, lip and tongue biting, neuropathy, dystonia, seizures, psychiatric changes, cognitive impairment, and dilated cardiomyopathy.

Huntington disease–like syndrome (HDL2) is an autosomal dominant disorder found almost exclusively in people of African ancestry. It is characterized by a trinucleotide repeat in the junctophilin-3 gene. Acanthocytosis is a variable feature. There is striatal and cortical atrophy, as well as intranuclear protein aggregates. HDL2 is clinically and radiologically indistinguishable from Huntington disease, with typical juvenile and late-onset forms.

A progressive spinocerebellar syndrome and sideroblastic anemia occur together in an X-linked recessive mutation in the *ABCB7* gene that encodes the ATP-binding cassette subfamily B member 7, mitochondrial. It is a mitochondrial disorder caused by a mutation in the nuclear genome. Cerebellar ataxia and dysarthria develop by 1 year of age, with accompanying long-tract signs. The neurologic signs tend to be stable until the fifth decade, when slow progression may occur. Neuropathy and myopathy have been described in association with sideroblastic anemia.

Triosephosphate isomerase deficiency is characterized by chronic hemolytic anemia, progressive neurologic dysfunction, and an increased susceptibility to infection. The neurologic features consist of a dystonic-dyskinetic syndrome with gross intention tremor and amyotrophy and hypotonia of the trunk and limbs, sometimes with corticospinal signs. There is electromyographic evidence of denervation with normal nerve conduction velocities, suggestive of anterior horn cell impairment. It has been suggested that low triosephosphate isomerase activity leads to a metabolic block in the glycolytic pathway and hence to an impairment of the cellular energy supply.

PROLIFERATIVE DISORDERS

Leukemia

Involvement of the CNS is primarily due to infiltration with leukemic cells, but may occur as the result of hemorrhage, infection, drug- and radiation-induced neurotoxicity, electrolyte disturbance, and impairment of cerebral circulation from leukostasis.

Meningeal Leukemia

The most common presenting symptoms are headaches, nausea, and vomiting, sometimes associated with lethargy and irritability, neck stiffness, drowsiness, coma, and convulsions. Diffuse meningeal infiltration impairs the circulation of CSF and can result in communicating hydrocephalus. Papilledema is the commonest sign. The leukemic deposits may compress or infiltrate the cranial nerves or spinal nerve roots and spread between the nerve fibers.

The diagnosis of meningeal leukemia is confirmed on CSF examination in approximately 90 percent of

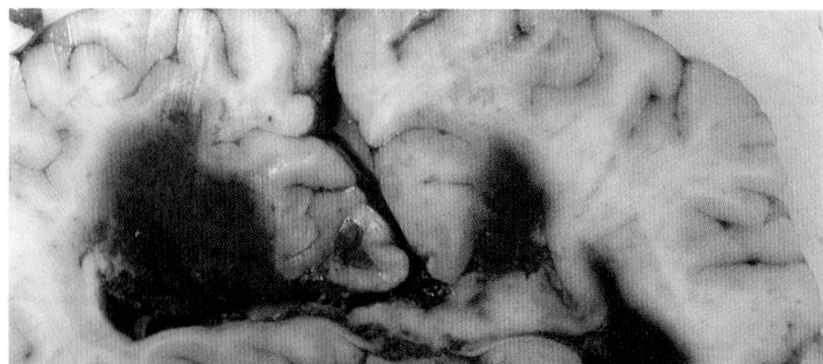

FIGURE 25-1 ■ Young male with relapse of acute B lymphoblastic leukemia complicated by multicentric intracerebral leukemic infiltrates with secondary intratumoral hemorrhage.

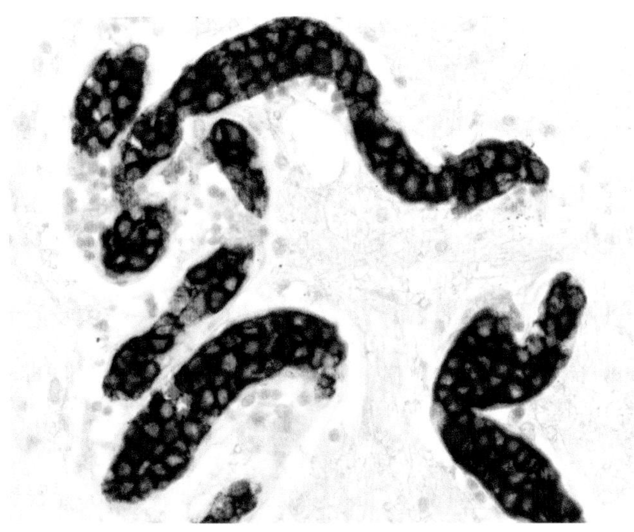

FIGURE 25-2 ▪ Magnified image from Figure 25-1 showing B-cell leukemic cells. Hematoxylin and eosin. Original magnification × 200

cases. Flow cytometric analysis of CSF has the highest diagnostic yield. The CSF pressure is usually elevated and reduced glucose concentration may be found. In 10 percent of cases the CSF is normal.

Acute myelomonocytic leukemia accompanied by pericentric inversion of chromosome 16 is a unique subtype associated with a high incidence of CNS involvement in the form of leptomeningeal deposits and granulocytic sarcoma (chloroma).

Localized Leukemic Deposits

Leukemic deposits may involve any part of the CNS (Figs. 25-1 and 25-2). The symptoms and signs are therefore numerous, varied, and depend on the extent and site of infiltration. Blindness may occur from infiltration of the optic nerve head or chiasm, and visual impairment from retinal infiltration.[20] Bilateral serous macular detachment with visual blurring may be the presenting symptom of acute lymphoblastic leukemia. Mental nerve involvement that produces sensory impairment of the lower lip and painless traumatic ulceration of the buccal mucosa along with "numb chin syndrome" has been reported.[21]

Hypothalamic and pituitary dysfunction is well recognized and may be associated with hydrocephalus.

Clinically significant spinal cord involvement is unusual in leukemia; it is encountered most commonly with acute myeloid leukemia. Spinal cord syndromes arise from compression by extradural deposits; direct infiltration of the spinal cord and nerve roots; vascular occlusion by thrombus, leukemic cells, or some combination of these; or hemorrhage. Exceptionally, an acute paraneoplastic necrotizing myelopathy occurs, often with retinal changes.

Peripheral neuropathy caused directly by leukemia is rare.

Chloromas (Granulocytic Sarcoma or Extramedullary Myeloblastoma)

Chloromas are solid tumors of nonlymphatic leukemia that are more common in children than adults. Granulocytic sarcoma develops in approximately 2.5 percent of cases of acute myeloid leukemia, and it may occur in myelofibrosis or myelodysplastic syndromes as part of transformation to acute leukemia. The majority of chloromas have a distinctive green color that fades on exposure to light. Most occur subperiosteally, usually in the cranial and facial bones, especially the paranasal sinuses, mastoid air cells, or orbits; they are usually attached to the dura mater and rarely invade cerebral tissue. Chloromas are radiosensitive.

Intracranial Hemorrhage and Thrombosis

The overall incidence of intracranial hemorrhage (ICH) is around 3 percent among adult patients with hematologic malignancies. The incidence is greatest in patients with acute myeloid leukemia. Patients with intracranial lymphoma are more prone to ICH than those with acute leukemia. Chemotherapy-related endothelial injury and reduction of coagulation factors may each play a role in the pathogenesis.

Thrombocytopenia is a frequent feature of ICH and may in some cases be the result of disseminated intravascular coagulation (DIC) or leukemic infiltration of the bone marrow. Platelet production may also be impaired as a result of the myelotoxic effects of chemotherapy. Bleeding in the CNS is usually multifocal and may be confluent. DIC is a prominent feature of promyelocytic leukemia but, in other forms of leukemia, DIC is particularly marked in those with high peripheral white cell counts. It appears soon after the beginning of chemotherapy, presumably because tissue thromboplastins are released from destroyed leukocytes.

Both acute and chronic subdural hematoma may occur. Cisternal, cervical, or lumbar puncture in a thrombocytopenic patient with acute leukemia may cause a spinal subdural hematoma with resulting compression of the spinal cord or cauda equina. Cranial irradiation causes intracranial vessel narrowing and thrombotic occlusion in later life. Weakening of the vessel wall can also result in arterial dilatation and tortuosity. The sequelae of these changes are vascular malformation, aneurysmal dilatation, and arterial thrombosis.

CELLULAR HYPERVISCOSITY

Marked elevation of the white cell count may produce a significant increase in whole-blood viscosity. The signs and symptoms include headache, somnolence, and impairment of consciousness. All types of leukemia may produce this syndrome, but neurologic symptoms may occur more readily in myelogenous leukemias at lower leukocyte counts, reflecting the larger cell size.

Treatment with leukapheresis may abolish the symptoms. Blood transfusions may be hazardous because they may further elevate viscosity.

INFECTIONS

In all leukemias, but particularly in the lymphoblastic leukemia of childhood, viruses (especially mumps, measles, and varicella) are the most common infective organisms of the CNS. Bacterial and fungal infections, especially aspergillosis, also occur. The increased incidence of involvement of the CNS with rare organisms or organisms that are normally nonpathogenic is contributed to by the widespread use of corticosteroids, chemotherapy, and broad-spectrum antibiotics.

LEUKOENCEPHALOPATHY AND OTHER ENCEPHALOPATHIES

A variety of encephalopathic complications of chemotherapy, radiotherapy, and opportunistic infection are discussed in detail in Chapters 28 and 45.

Myelomatosis

Myelomatosis is the best-recognized expression of the plasma cell dyscrasias, which include Waldenström macroglobulinemia, monoclonal gammopathy of unknown significance (MGUS), paraproteinemias, plasmacytoma, plasma cell leukemia, primary amyloidosis, and the heavy-chain diseases. The major neurologic complications are: (1) compression of the spinal cord, cauda equina, or solitary nerve roots; (2) cranial nerve involvement; (3) intracranial myeloma; and (4) peripheral neuropathy. Pure meningeal myeloma is rare and presents with confusion, altered consciousness, and cranial nerve palsies. In 20 percent of cases, it is associated with plasma cell leukemia.[22] Multiple myeloma with hyperviscosity may result in cerebral infarction.

SPINAL MYELOMA

The vertebrae are commonly infiltrated by myeloma cells, which may extend into the extradural space. Vertebral body collapse may produce neurologic deficits. Acute paraplegia sometimes occurs due to spontaneous epidural hematoma.

Extradural myeloma tumor may occur without local bone involvement, and intradural deposits may arise by spread along nerve roots via intervertebral foramina, causing radicular symptoms and signs. Spinal cord compression is sometimes caused by amyloid deposits. Infiltration of the spinal cord by myeloma cells and paraneoplastic myelopathy are rare. The lower thoracic area of the spinal cord is the most commonly affected. Patients with IgA myeloma seem to be at greater risk of spinal cord compression.

Neurologic symptoms usually develop comparatively slowly but may do so over one or two weeks. Back pain for several weeks or months commonly precedes evidence of spinal cord compression.

CRANIAL MYELOMA

Cranial myeloma is rare. The predominant sites of occurrence are the region of the sella and cavernous sinus, the body of the sphenoid, and the apex of the petrous bones. Orbital myeloma is well recognized and may present as an orbital mass with proptosis and ophthalmoplegia. Infiltration of the optic nerve may occur with features of optic neuritis. Ophthalmoplegia results from amyloid infiltration of the extraocular muscles. Primary plasmacytomas may originate in the cranial vault or the dura. Direct infiltration of the brain by myeloma cells is exceptionally rare, as is diffuse meningeal involvement.

Symptoms and signs of elevated intracranial pressure are often the earliest indications of intracranial myeloma. Other manifestations depend on the site of the lesion. Concomitant renal failure, anemia, hypercalcemia, and hyperviscosity contribute to symptoms.

PERIPHERAL NEUROPATHY

Five types of neuropathy have been described in association with myelomatosis:

1. Paraneoplastic neuropathy producing demyelination and axis cylinder degeneration
2. Ischemic neuropathy due to amyloid deposition in the vasa nervorum
3. Amyloid infiltration of the peripheral nerves
4. Infiltration of the peripheral nerves by myeloma tissue
5. Drug-induced neuropathy

Neuropathy occurring in myelomatosis is heterogeneous, arising from perineural or perivascular immunoglobulin deposition, with or without amyloid infiltration. It is particularly associated with IgG and IgM myeloma. The neuropathy is a typically mild, progressive, length-dependent, symmetric, sensory-motor neuropathy, with sensory involvement being predominant. Amyloid deposition leads to a painful small fiber neuropathy. Direct infiltration by myeloma or amyloid tissue may produce an asymmetric or mononeuritic picture.

Although it is a complication of the established disease in diffuse myelomatosis, a paraneoplastic neuropathy is usually the presenting feature of a solitary, commonly sclerotic, plasmacytoma. This combination has a distinct male predominance. The neuropathy is usually sensory-motor, with the motor component predominating. Localized radiotherapy to the bone lesion effectively arrests and usually alleviates the neuropathy with good long-term survival.

The POEMS syndrome (polyneuropathy, organomegally, endocrinopathy, monoclonal gammopathy, and skin changes) is a type of plasma cell dyscrasia associated with osteosclerotic myeloma. The major criteria for the diagnosis are the presence of polyneuropathy, with a clonal plasma cell disorder, sclerotic bone lesions, elevated vascular endothelial growth factor, and the presence of Castleman disease (lymphoid hyperplasia with marked follicular capillary proliferation and endothelial hyperplasia, which may be restricted to a single lymph node or may be a more generalized lymphadenopathy).

The bone marrow contains less than 5 percent plasma cells (in multiple myeloma, the bone marrow contains more than 10% plasma cells), but demonstrates megakaryocyte hyperplasia and clustering reminiscent of a myeloproliferative disorder (significantly, the *JAK2* V617F mutation is absent). Patients with osteosclerotic myeloma usually have multiorgan involvement including skin change, lymphadenopathy, papilledema, peripheral edema, hepatomegaly, splenomegaly, and ascites. Dispenzieri has proposed new criteria for POEMS syndrome.[23–25]

The neuropathy is of a symmetric sensory-motor demyelinating type, with clinical similarities to chronic inflammatory demyelinating polyneuropathy, including an elevated CSF protein.[26] Possibly as a result of thrombocytosis, there is a 13 percent risk of stroke over 5 years.[27]

A particularly localized form of neuropathy due to infiltration of the carpal tunnel by amyloid deposits is well recognized. Concurrent neuropathy and myositis due to sarcolemmal deposits of IgD in IgD myeloma has been described.

Neuropathy may also be a consequence of drug treatments for myeloma. Thalidomide induces a length-dependent sensory-motor neuropathy with autonomic involvement in 70 percent of patients treated for 12 months.[28] Bortezomib and vincristine may also result in neuropathy, although there appears to be an interaction between myeloma-related factors and the patient's genetic background in the development of treatment-induced peripheral neuropathy.[29]

NEUROLOGIC EFFECTS OF METABOLIC COMPLICATIONS

Neurologic complications may result from hypercalcemia, uremia, and hyperviscosity. Symptomatic hyperviscosity is much more common in Waldenström macroglobulinemia (10 to 30%) than it is in myeloma (2 to 6%). Symptoms of hyperviscosity usually appear when the normal serum viscosity of 1.4 to 1.8 centipoise (cP) reaches 4 to 5 cP, corresponding to a serum IgM level of at least 3 g/dl, an IgG level of 4 g/dl, and an IgA level of 6 g/dl.[30]

Hypercalcemia and uremia cause increasing headaches, confusion, disorientation, somnolence, stupor, coma, uremic convulsions, and myoclonic twitching.

NEUROLOGIC COMPLICATIONS OF IMMUNODEFICIENCY

Immunodeficiency is a common feature of myelomatosis. In the CNS, this is reflected by the development of meningitis (bacterial, viral, fungal) and cerebral abscess. Pneumococcal infection is particularly implicated, as is herpes zoster virus and, more rarely, cryptococcosis and toxoplasmosis. Profound septicemia may be complicated by cerebral DIC. Progressive multifocal leukoencephalopathy may also occur.

Macroglobulinemia (Waldenström Disease)

Neurologic symptoms occur in 25 percent of patients with macroglobulinemia. An antibody-related neuropathy is found in 5 to 10 percent of cases and is associated with IgM kappa, some of which has specificity for myelin-associated glycoprotein. Other mechanisms such as lymphocytic infiltration of the peripheral nerves, amyloidosis, and a bleeding tendency have also been suggested as an explanation for the neuropathy. Patients have been reported with lymphoplasmacytic cells infiltrating meninges and nerve roots, producing progressive leg weakness from lumbar radiculopathy. Chemotherapy and irradiation of the involved nerve roots may lead to significant improvement.

Complete unilateral ophthalmoplegia has been described, as has an isolated lesion of the fourth cranial nerve.

Other neurologic complications relate to hyperviscosity and bleeding tendency. Exceptionally, Waldenström disease is complicated by primary intracerebral lymphoma, progressive multifocal leukoencephalopathy, or a humorally mediated immune myopathy from IgM-kappa antibodies directed against muscle surface protein.[31,32]

Light/Heavy Chain Deposition Disease

A variety of lymphoplasmacytic processes may produce abnormal light or heavy chains such as chronic lymphocytic leukemia or lymphoma and nodal marginal cell lymphoma. These may be the result of the emergence of a mutated clone of plasma cells that occurs after the use of certain chemotherapeutic agents such as melphalan. Light/heavy chain deposition disease may occur in the absence of detectable underlying systemic neoplastic lymphoproliferative processes, even after prolonged follow-up for more than 10 years. Light chain deposition disease may be associated with a local clone of plasma cells (extramedullary plasmacytomas). They are most common in the sixth decade.

Peripheral neuropathy is found in approximately 20 percent of cases. Light chain deposits may be seen in the endoneurium. In cases of light chain deposition disease, peripheral nerve involvement has been reported occasionally.

Paraproteinemias

Monoclonal gammopathy of unknown significance (MGUS) is characterized by low-titer (<3 g/dl) bands of IgM, IgG, or IgA. They are found in 1 percent of healthy individuals over the age of 25 years, increasing to 3 percent in those over 70 years. The majority are IgG, and less than 15 percent are IgM. The prevalence of MGUS in those with idiopathic neuropathy is 10 percent, of which IgM accounts for 50 percent of cases, especially those with demyelinating neuropathies. Immunoelectrophoresis or immunofixation may be required to detect smaller bands. Urine light chains are rare. In MGUS, the marrow contains less than 5 percent plasma cells; blood counts are normal, and lymphadenopathy, organomegaly, and skeletal lesions do not occur. Investigation may identify primary systemic amyloidosis, myeloma, macroglobulinemia, cryoglobulinemia, lymphoma, or lymphoproliferative disorder. Approximately one-third of patients with MGUS will develop myeloma, macroglobulinemia, amyloidosis, or a lymphoproliferative disorder over 20 years; this is sometimes heralded by an unusually rapid, progressive course of the neuropathy. The risk of progression of MGUS to multiple myeloma or related disorders is about 1 percent per year.[33]

Approximately 5 percent of patients with MGUS will develop a polyneuropathy, associated in the majority with an IgM band. The median age of onset is in the sixth decade with a slowly progressive, distal, symmetric sensory-motor polyneuropathy or, less commonly, a predominantly sensory neuropathy. A presentation resembling chronic inflammatory demyelinating polyneuropathy is well recognized, although this condition differs from the typical form due to more dominant sensory symptoms, an older age at onset, and a slower, more progressive course.[34] Neurophysiologic studies commonly demonstrate a mixed axonal and demyelinating picture. Predominant axonal degeneration is uncommon; pure demyelination is particularly associated with IgM MGUS. CSF protein levels may be markedly elevated.

Antibody to myelin-associated glycoprotein may be identified in paraproteinemic neuropathy and in as many as half of the cases of IgM MGUS. It has a particular phenotype of a distal acquired demyelinating symmetric sensory and motor neuropathy. It is slowly progressive with prominent sensory ataxia and tremor. Histologically there is widening of the myelin lamellae. A neuropathy associated with antibody to myelin-associated glycoprotein may also occur with concurrent Waldenström macroglobulinemia or B-cell lymphoma.

The clinical pattern of antisulfatide antibody neuropathy is a sensory-predominant, distal, symmetric polyneuropathy, which may be axonal or demyelinating in type. Antisulfatide antibody–associated neuropathy accounts for about 5 percent of the cases of IgM gammopathy. The clinical pattern is similar to that of the neuropathy associated with anti–myelin-associated glycoprotein, but pain and small-fiber symptoms are more common.

Other binding specificities are described, including GM1 ganglioside and disialosyl gangliosides, but the pathogenic role of these antibodies is unclear. IgG and IgA MGUS are less likely than IgM MGUS to be associated with identifiable antineuronal antibodies and are comparatively less common than IgM neuropathies, less likely to be demyelinating or sensory, and more likely to respond to plasmapheresis.

Chronic ataxic neuropathy with ophthalmoplegia, M-protein, cold agglutinins, and disialsyl antibodies (CANOMAD) is an IgM MGUS with a characteristic phenotype. Pathologically, anti-ganglioside antibodies, anti-GD1b and anti-GQ1b, produce both demyelinating and axonal features. Weakness affects oculomotor and bulbar muscles with similarities to Miller Fisher syndrome and may either be fixed or follow a relapsing-remitting course.[35]

A condition of gait ataxia and late-onset polyneuropathy (GALOP syndrome) is also seen in the presence of serum IgM gammopathy. The features include prominent falls in patients aged 60 to 85 years with a gradually progressive, distal, symmetric sensory-predominant polyneuropathy with demyelinating features on nerve conduction studies.[36]

Lymphoma

The nervous system is involved through direct spread from primary nodal and extranodal sites. Occasionally, primary Hodgkin disease and primary non-Hodgkin lymphoma (including microglioma, reticulum cell sarcoma, and histiocytic lymphoma) of the CNS are seen.[37] Neurologic complications result from direct invasion and compression of the nervous system or from secondary paraneoplastic syndromes. CNS involvement occurs most commonly with lymphoblastic lymphoma, large B-cell lymphoma, diffuse undifferentiated lymphoma, and diffuse histiocytic lymphoma.

Spinal Cord and Meningeal Involvement

Spinal cord and meningeal involvement is relatively common. Extradural deposits arise as the result of direct spread from the retroperitoneal or postmediastinal spaces via the intervertebral foramina from tumor growth along nerve roots, or by direct invasion from an affected vertebral body. Intramedullary metastases of lymphoblastic lymphoma are a rare but recognized complication. The segmental arterial supply may also become compressed, resulting in ischemic myelopathy. Rarely, an acute necrotizing myelopathy appears as a remote paraneoplastic effect of a lymphoma. Subacute paraneoplastic myelopathy may occur in Hodgkin disease.[38]

Spinal cord segments C5 to T8 are most commonly involved, although compression may occur at any level, including the cauda equina. Nerve roots may be invaded and enlarged by the lymphoma, causing pain and sensorimotor segmental syndromes.

Intracranial Involvement

Intracranial involvement usually arises from infiltration via the skull base by direct extension from involved cervical lymph nodes, or by lymphatic spread. On rare occasions, lymphoma of the skull bones spreads to form an intracranial mass. Tumor is usually found extradurally but may present as a subdural mass that sometimes invades the underlying brain, or it may be purely intracerebral. Almost all cases of lymphomatous meningitis are found in patients with diffuse non-Hodgkin lymphoma.

Meningeal lymphoma may have a protracted course with spontaneous remission. Intracranial deposits seem to be associated more often with histiocytic lymphoma, and orbital deposits more commonly with lymphocytic lymphoma. Intracranial deposits are rarely seen in lymphocytic lymphoma unless leukemia has supervened.

Paraneoplastic Syndromes and other Neurologic Complications

A range of paraneoplastic syndromes and treatment-associated complications associated with the lymphomas are discussed in Chapters 27 and 28.

Burkitt Lymphoma

Burkitt lymphoma is an aggressive peripheral B-cell lymphoma. It is endemic in equatorial Africa where it is frequently found in children with reduced immunity to Epstein–Barr virus (EBV), often affecting the mandible. It is found internationally in a sporadic form in adolescents and young adults, but is also common in individuals infected with human immunodeficiency virus (HIV); 90 percent of the endemic form, 20 percent of sporadic cases, and 40 percent of HIV-related cases are associated with EBV infection, which causes an upregulation of *c-myc*, a gene controlling transcription regulation.

Burkitt lymphoma is frequently complicated by nervous system involvement, most commonly paraplegia, cranial neuropathies, and CSF pleocytosis. Tumor spreads through the bones of the face, skull, and orbit and along cranial nerves. Spinal cord compression from direct extension from the vertebral bodies or via the intervertebral foramina is well recognized, and ischemic myelopathy may result from compression of radicular arteries. Patients with facial tumors are likely to develop orbital involvement and ophthalmoplegia. Infiltration of the skull base may produce other cranial nerve palsies and an inflammatory CSF.

Primary CNS Lymphoma

Primary CNS lymphoma (PCNSL) is rare, accounting for about 2.5 percent of primary brain tumors. Recently reported incidence rates in the United States population increased from 0.02/100,000 persons in the first two decades of life, to 0.3/100,000 in patients aged 35 to 44 years, and up to 2.13/100,000 in patients 75 to 84 years old.

Although all cytologic types are observed, 90 percent belong to the high-grade category of non-Hodgkin lymphoma, the majority being clonal and of B-cell origin, as evidenced by their monoclonal expression of either kappa or lambda light-chain immunoglobulin. Less common histologic types include low-grade lymphomas, Burkitt lymphomas, and T-cell lymphomas. Non-Hodgkin PCNSL has an extremely poor prognosis. Tumor masses are usually multicentric and ill-defined. Immunocompromised individuals are at greatest risk. The incidence of these tumors is increasing, and their association with HIV only partly accounts for this rise. Primary CNS lymphoma in immunodeficient patients is often associated with EBV, which is detected frequently in the CSF.[39]

Imaging displays discrete, often large, enhancing tumors with bilateral hemispheric involvement spreading through the corpus callosum. Despite the fact that these tumors are highly radiosensitive, the prognosis for PCNSL is worse than for other extranodal lymphomas, and late morbidity and mortality may occur from radiation necrosis. Treatment with chemotherapy and radiation usually leads to remission but with a significant recurrence rate.

Primary lymphoma of the spinal cord is exceptionally rare, as is primary lymphoma of the nerve roots, including the cauda equina.

Peripheral neuropathy of the paraneoplastic type may occur in association with PCNSL.

Intravascular Lymphoma

Intravascular lymphoma is a rarely diagnosed subtype of generalized lymphoma, usually of large B-cell origin, producing vascular occlusion of arterioles, capillaries, and venules (Figs. 25-3 and 25-4). More

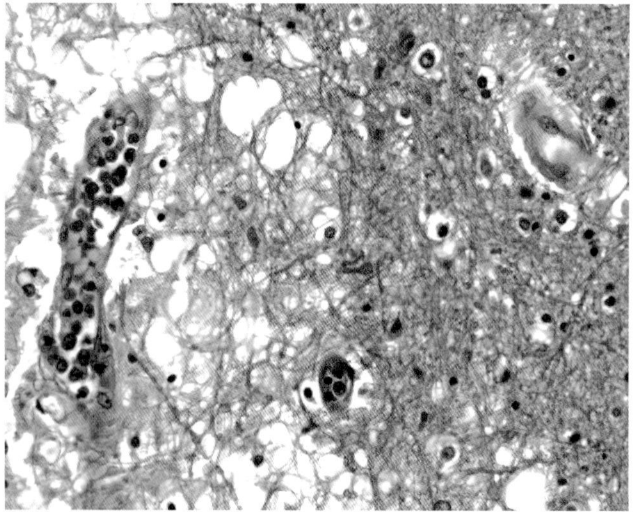

FIGURE 25-3 ■ Intravascular lymphoma. Section showing focus of cerebral ischemia with blood vessels plugged by large atypical lymphocytes (on left). Vessels in adjacent brain (right) not affected. (Hematoxylin and eosin. Original magnification × 400.)

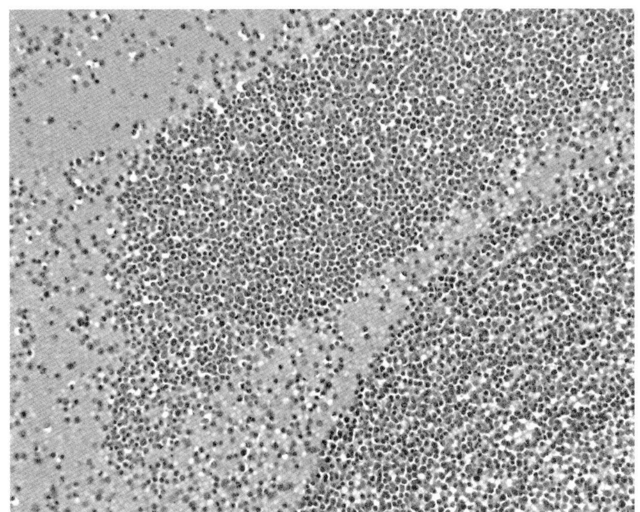

FIGURE 25-4 ■ Immunostained brain section showing distension and plugging of intracerebral vessels by CD20 stained malignant B-lymphocytes confirming intravascular lymphoma. (Original magnification × 400.)

than 25 to 50 percent of cases present with neurologic symptoms, and two-thirds develop neurologic symptoms during the course of the disease. The presentation may be diffuse or focal, and suggestive of vascular disease. Dementia, stroke-like episodes, myelopathy, cranial neuropathy, peripheral neuropathy, and brainstem syndromes predominate. The diagnosis is often difficult because of marked variability in clinical presentation and nonspecific laboratory and radiologic findings, especially when CNS symptoms are the only manifestation. Imaging demonstrates multifocal lesions in the brain suggestive of microvascular or demyelinating disease. Angiography may show a beaded appearance reminiscent of vasculitis. The CSF findings are nonspecific, and cerebral biopsy should be undertaken in suspected cases.[40]

Lymphomatoid Granulomatosis

Lymphomatoid granulomatosis is a rare, aggressive extranodal EBV-positive B-cell lymphoproliferative disease involving predominantly the lung. The nervous system is involved in one-third of patients. It may occur in patients with Sjögren syndrome, chronic viral hepatitis, rheumatoid arthritis, renal transplantation, and HIV infection. The usual presenting symptoms are fever, weight loss, malaise, cough, dyspnea, and neurologic symptoms, which can include encephalopathy, seizures, hemiparesis, cranial neuropathy, optic neuropathy, peripheral neuropathy, and mononeuritis multiplex. Pathologically, there is a nodular polymorphous mononuclear cell infiltrate with prominent vascular infiltration and often necrosis. Varying numbers of large, often atypical, CD20-positive B-lymphocytes are present within a background containing numerous polyclonal reactive CD3-positive small T-lymphocytes and scattered admixed plasma cells. There is extensive infiltration of T-lymphocytes and histiocytes in the meninges and cerebral blood vessel walls within the brain parenchyma and along nerve roots and peripheral nerves that mimics vasculitis and can result in vascular occlusion. Morphologically, there is an overlap in higher-grade forms (grades 2 and 3) with variants of large B-cell lymphoma, and multiple lesions in a single patient may show wide variation in histologic grade. Treatment depends on grade, with grade 3 being managed as diffuse large B-cell lymphoma.[41]

Polycythemia

A group of conditions previously thought to be distinct entities have been shown to have a common genetic etiology in exon 14 V617F mutations of the *JAK2* (Janus kinase 2) gene, including essential polycythemia, essential thrombocythemia, and myelofibrosis—the classic *bcr/abl*-negative myeloproliferative disorders. Each disease represents a stem cell–derived clonal myeloproliferation. The presence of this *JAK2* mutation may be used as a diagnostic test.[42]

There are many causes of polycythemia, including erythropoietin-producing neoplasms and nonmalignant renal cysts and inappropriately elevated erythropoiesis induced by hypoxemia such as from right-to-left cardiac or pulmonary shunts. The term idiopathic erythrocytosis has been used to describe patients with primary polycythemia who do not fulfill the criteria for polycythemia vera, including testing negative for the *JAK2* exon 14 V617F mutation; however, some patients considered to have idiopathic erythrocytosis on clinical grounds have been found to have *JAK2* mutations within exon 12.

An increased incidence of thrombotic and hemorrhagic complications is a well-recognized phenomenon in polycythemia, in part arising from accelerated atherosclerosis. There is growing evidence that the increased risk of thrombosis is not caused by erythrocytosis or thrombosis but by interactions amongst white cells, red cells, platelets, and endothelium. The high incidence of thrombosis is attributed to an increased blood viscosity, reduced perfusion, vascular engorgement, atheromatous degeneration of vessel walls, and possibly to chronic DIC. Patients with polycythemia whose hematocrit is below 45 percent have a significantly lower rate of cardiovascular death and major thrombosis than those with a hematocrit of 45 to 50 percent. Approximately 15 percent of patients with polycythemia die of cerebral thrombosis, 87 percent of them after repeated episodes. Thromboembolism often continues to be a major clinical problem even after hematologic control has been achieved. Hemorrhage may be related to imperfect clot retraction, abnormal thromboplastin generation, and abnormalities of platelet count and function. CNS hemorrhage may be cerebral, epidural, subdural, or subarachnoid.

The clinical course of polycythemia vera is often complicated by the transition to myeloid metaplasia with myelofibrosis or acute myeloid leukemia.

Nonspecific symptoms of fullness in the head, vertigo, tinnitus, and lack of concentration are common. More specific signs such as hemiparesis, hemianesthesia, hemianopia, and aphasia depend on the site of infarction or hemorrhage. Brainstem vascular syndromes occur, as do bulbar and pseudobulbar palsy, convulsions, and coma. Amaurosis fugax, blindness, scotomas, and cerebral or brainstem transient ischemic attacks are features as well. More rarely, signs and symptoms of a progressive cerebral lesion arise because of a subdural hematoma, an expanding intracerebral blood clot, or cerebral infarction accompanied by edema. Distention and congestion of the retinal veins, central retinal venous or arterial occlusion, and papilledema may be present. Pseudotumor cerebri has been reported. Aseptic cavernous sinus thrombosis associated with internal carotid artery occlusion may occur; treatment with repeated phlebotomies and heparin may result in resolution of proptosis, pain, periorbital edema, lacrimation, venous congestion, ptosis, and ophthalmoplegia, and may restore sight. The one-and-a-half syndrome may occur and has been ascribed to brainstem ischemia.

Transient spinal cord ischemia may be the presenting feature of polycythemia vera, but spinal cord infarction is an exceptionally rare complication. Spinal cord compression due to spontaneous subdural hematoma and extramedullary hematopoiesis in the proliferative phase of polycythemia is uncommon.

Chorea, dystonia, and hyperkinetic movement disorders are also uncommon complications of polycythemia. Chorea may be of sudden onset and tends to occur in women older than 50 years. It may resolve before any significant reduction of the red cell count, but more often it resolves with correction of the polycythemia. The chorea is generalized, with predominant involvement of the face, mouth, tongue, and arms. It is not apparently related to the rare finding of a small infarct in the caudate nucleus.

Although paresthesias are not uncommon symptoms in the extremities, peripheral neuropathy due to polycythemia was previously thought to be rare. However, a prospective clinical and electrophysiologic study of 28 patients with polycythemia identified 46 percent with clinical features of neuropathy and 71 percent with neurophysiologic evidence of sensory axonal polyneuropathy, probably arising from endoneurial ischemia.[43] Oculomotor nerve paresis as a presenting sign of acute myeloblastic leukemia complicating polycythemia has been reported.

Mutations in the *SLC30A10* gene, which is highly expressed in the liver and brain and encodes a protein belonging to a large family of membrane transporters, may result in polycythemia with parkinsonism and dystonia.[44]

Cerebellar Hemangioblastoma

Cerebellar hemangioblastoma may be associated with polycythemia, and 34 percent of these patients have von Hippell–Lindau disease, which is caused by mutations in the *VHL* gene. The VHL protein is involved in the inhibition of hypoxia inducible factor 1 α, which accumulates, causing the production of vascular endothelial growth factor, platelet derived growth factor B, erythropoietin, and transforming growth factor α. VHL is subdivided according to clinical manifestations, which largely correlate with the types of mutations present. Type 1 mostly have hemangioblastoma, and renal carcinoma and pheochromocytoma are rare. Patients with type 2A are at risk of both hemangioblastoma and pheochromocytoma, but not renal carcinoma. Those with type 2B are at risk of all three tumors, with a higher risk of clear-cell renal carcinoma; persons with type 2C are only at risk of pheochromocytoma. Type 3 disease has a risk of Chuvash polycythemia.

The symptoms of cerebellar hemangioblastoma are those of increased intracranial pressure and "dizziness," with either truncal and gait ataxia or hemiataxia with accompanying nystagmus. Neck stiffness and rarely cerebellar "fits" may occur. On examination, the symmetric or lateralized cerebellar ataxia is associated with papilledema, hemiparesis, bilateral pyramidal signs, or any combination of deficits from cranial nerve V, VI, VII, or VIII involvement. Recurrence many years after surgical treatment is typical of hemangioblastoma.

Pseudopolycythemia

Pseudopolycythemia is a condition in which an increased hematocrit is associated with normal red cell mass; plasma volume may be reduced in the absence of apparent fluid loss, related to aberrations in catecholamine metabolism. It is associated with hypertension, obesity, and stress, especially in middle-aged men who are smokers. In this condition, as in polycythemia, there is an increased risk of thromboembolism because the increased packed cell volume is associated with an increase in whole blood viscosity and reduced cerebral blood flow, predisposing to vascular occlusive episodes. In patients with a packed cell volume exceeding 54 percent, regular venipuncture with withdrawal of 100 to 250 ml blood is recommended to reduce the packed cell volume to around 46 percent.

Essential Thrombocythemia

Essential thrombocythemia is a clonal stem cell disorder, and the *JAK2* V617F mutation has been identified in approximately 50 percent of patients. Mutations in *MPL* (thrombopoietic receptor) have been reported in approximately 4 percent of patients, and mutations in *TET2* have been observed in a variety of myeloid malignancies, including *JAK2* V617F–positive and –negative essential thrombocythemia.

Essential thrombocythemia is characterized more frequently by thrombotic than hemorrhagic complications. The condition is diagnosed on the basis of a persistently elevated platelet count without evidence of trauma, inflammation, hemorrhage, hyposplenism, or any other condition known to be associated with thrombocytosis.

Amaurosis fugax, transient hemiparesis or hemianesthesia, recurrent vertigo, and confusion are the characteristic symptoms. Most patients have circulating platelet aggregates or spontaneous platelet aggregation, and reduced platelet survival. Considerable clinical improvement can be achieved with antiplatelet drugs and, where appropriate, by reduction of platelet count. Evolution to myelofibrosis occurs in 3 to 10 percent of patients in the first decade after diagnosis, and in 6 to 30 percent in the second decade. Progression to acute myeloid leukemia occurs in 1 to 2.5 percent in the first decade after diagnosis, 5 to 8 percent in the second decade, and continues to increase subsequently, though this may be a consequence of treatment rather than due to the underlying disorder.

Myelofibrosis

Myelofibrosis is an uncommon myeloproliferative disorder arising predominantly in patients older than 50 years and characterized by replacement of the bone marrow by fibrous tissue associated with extramedullary hematopoiesis and marked hepatosplenomegaly. Patients are anemic, may be slightly jaundiced, and have a leukoerythroblastic blood picture. Neurologic complications are rare. A number of reports describe meningeal hematopoietic masses. Spinal cord compression from extramedullary hematopoiesis due to myelofibrosis is recognized but uncommon.

The *JAK2* V617F mutation is found in about half of cases. Other mutations in the *JAK2* and *MPL* genes have been identified, also resulting in exaggerated JAK2 signaling.

Eosinophilic Syndromes

Eosinophilia is defined as an increase in peripheral blood eosinophil count to greater than 450 cells/µl, with accompanying eosinophilic infiltration of muscle, nerve, or CSF. Eosinophilia may be observed in a wide range of conditions (Table 25-1).

Eosinophilic infiltration into skeletal muscle is rare. It has been described in parasitic infection as focal eosinophilic myositis, in systemic hypereosinophilic conditions such as the eosinophilia-myalgia syndrome, and in idiopathic hypereosinophilic syndrome. Diffuse fasciitis or Shulman syndrome can be limited to the fascia or associated with perimyositis. Eosinophilic myositis corresponds to focal muscle involvement, and it is associated with skin lesions in approximately 40 percent of cases, including deep subcutaneous induration, erythema, angioedema,

TABLE 25-1 ■ Nervous System Involvement with Eosinophilic Syndromes

Trichinosis
Eosinophilic meningitis or meningoencephalitis (angiostrongyliasis, gnathostomiasis, visceral larva migrans)
Connective tissue diseases
Churg–Strauss vasculitis
Eosinophilic fasciitis
Polyarteritis nodosa
Eosinophilia-myalgia syndrome (due to tryptophan in the United States in 1989)
Toxic-oil syndrome (due to contaminated rapeseed oil in Spain in 1981)
Coccidioidomycosis
Helminth infections
Ascariasis
Schistosomiasis
Trichinosis
Visceral larva migrans
Gnathostomiasis
Strongyloidiasis
Fascioliasis
Paragonimiasis
Neoplasia
Lymphoma (e.g., Hodgkin lymphoma, non-Hodgkin lymphoma)
Human T-cell lymphotropic virus I (HTLV-I)
Adult T-cell leukemia/lymphoma (ATLL)
Eosinophilic leukemia
Gastric or lung carcinoma (i.e., paraneoplastic eosinophilia)
Allergic/atopic diseases
Adrenal insufficiency in ill patients

urticaria, and papular lesions. The overall prognosis of eosinophilic myositis is good, particularly when muscle lesions are focal and the principal histopathologic finding is perimysial infiltrates.[45]

Compound heterozygous or homozygous *CAPN3* mutations have been found in a subgroup of children in the first decade of life with autosomal recessive inheritance, variable peripheral eosinophilia, and elevated serum creatine kinase levels, but with little or no weakness. The *CAPN3* gene encodes calpain-3, a muscle-specific intracellular nonlysosomal protease. Mutations in this gene are responsible for the commonest autosomal recessive limb-girdle muscular dystrophy, calpainopathy (LGMD2A). Very rare cases of adult-onset eosinophilic polymyositis have now been described with mutations in the calpain-3 gene.[46] Whether this represents the well-known inflammatory feature of muscular dystrophy or is a true eosinophilic myositis is uncertain.

When it is a manifestation of the hypereosinophilic syndrome, eosinophilic myositis may be life-threatening. Hypereosinophilic syndrome is a heterogeneous group of rare disorders defined by persistent blood eosinophilia of at least 1500 eosinophils/μl without a cause, along with evidence of eosinophil-associated organ damage. There are a number of subtypes which may overlap with chronic eosinophilic leukemia. These subtypes are associated with dramatic differences in clinical presentation, prognosis, and responses to therapy. Abnormal or clonal T-cell populations are present in 17 percent of cases. There is pathologic evidence of multiorgan infiltration by eosinophils. Cardiac disease is common with valvular disease resulting in embolization. Systemic manifestations other than eosinophilia include anemia, hypergammaglobulinemia, vascular involvement (subungual petechiae, livedo reticularis, diffuse microangiopathy, Raynaud phenomenon), skin rash and subcutaneous edema, pulmonary infiltrates and pleuritis, cardiac involvement (congestive heart failure, arrhythmias, heart block, pericarditis, myocardial and endocardial fibrosis), and peripheral neuropathy. One-third of the patients have neurologic symptoms such as encephalopathy, multiple cerebral infarcts (possibly embolic in origin), peripheral neuropathy, and mononeuropathy multiplex. Patients may respond well to corticosteroids, and newer agents such as anti–IL-5 therapy and imatinib show promise, though specific therapeutic agents appear to have efficacy for particular genetic subgroups.[47]

HEMORRHAGIC DISORDERS

Hemophilia A

The severity of bleeding in hemophilic patients correlates with the factor VIII level. Severely affected hemophiliacs with levels of less than 1 percent commonly have spontaneous bleeding into muscles and joints. With factor VIII levels of 1 to 5 percent, spontaneous bleeding is much less frequent. Patients with factor VIII levels greater than 10 percent can lead normal lives, as excessive blood loss occurs only after more severe trauma and surgery. Hypertension is an important additional factor in older patients. Lyonization (X-inactivation) may result in severe factor VIII deficiency in some females.

Intracranial bleeding is the leading cause of death. The incidence of intracranial hemorrhage ranges approximately from 2 to 14 percent. Bleeding tends to occur predominantly in young hemophiliacs, and may occur into the subdural, epidural, or subarachnoid spaces or into the cerebral hemispheres, cerebellar hemispheres, and brainstem. The symptoms and signs depend on the site of the hemorrhage and its extent. Prognosis in intracranial hemorrhage has been considerably improved by the early use of factor VIII concentrates, and there is now no contraindication to surgical intervention, provided that adequate control of coagulation factors is maintained. Seizures occur in 25 percent of survivors of intracranial hemorrhage.

Bleeding into the spinal canal is rare. Patients with small epidural hemorrhages and only minimal nonprogressive signs of spinal cord dysfunction may recover completely with intensive factor VIII replacement therapy alone.

Peripheral nerve lesions are the most frequent neurologic complication of hemophilia. In most instances, nerve involvement is a complication of intramuscular hemorrhage, most commonly into the iliac muscle leading to femoral neuropathy. Median, ulnar, and radial neuropathies result from hemorrhage into the arm or forearm muscles. Nerve compression by pseudotumors (subperiosteal hemorrhages producing expanding lesions) also occurs. Severe hemophilic arthropathy of the elbow may result in ulnar nerve palsy. Intraneural hemorrhage as a cause of peripheral nerve palsy is exceptional but may, for example, affect the ulnar nerve in the cubital tunnel. On exploration of the ulnar nerve, free blood may be seen when the epineurium is divided; recovery is rapid and complete.

During the early to the mid-1980s, many patients with severe hemophilia became infected with HIV through contaminated plasma-derived clotting factors. From 1979 to 1998, 47 percent of people with hemophilia A died of HIV-related disease.

Von Willebrand Disease

Von Willebrand disease consists of a family of related disorders characterized by deficiency or malfunction of von Willebrand factor, a protein that mediates platelet adhesion to the endothelium and protects factor VIII from degradation. Most cases are inherited in an autosomal dominant fashion. Rarer acquired forms are associated with hematologic malignancies, systemic lupus erythematosus (SLE) and other autoimmune disorders, and with the use of valproic acid, griseofulvin, and ciprofloxacin. The bleeding complications of von Willebrand disease are relatively mild, and spontaneous hemorrhage into joints and muscles does not occur. Acute onset of neurologic dysfunction is not a feature of this disease. Nevertheless, serious hemorrhage may result from trauma, and patients who sustain head injuries should receive immediate factor VIII replacement therapy. The rare types 2N and 3 are inherited as autosomal recessive traits and result in more significant hemorrhage.

Hemophilia B: Factor IX deficiency

Hemophilia B (Christmas disease) is an X-linked recessive disorder, but approximately one-third of patients have no family history and have novel mutations. The neurologic complications are identical to those of hemophilia A. Thus, peripheral nerve compression occurs as a consequence of spontaneous intramuscular hemorrhage, and intracranial hemorrhage, an important cause of death in both disorders, may occur spontaneously in severely affected patients or following trauma in less severely affected individuals. Clotting factor IX is the deficient factor requiring replacement.

Other Clotting Factor Deficiencies

Spontaneous and post-traumatic hemorrhages are features of disorders resulting from deficiencies of other clotting factors. Surgical evacuation of any intracranial hemorrhage, when indicated, must be done in the setting of adequate replacement therapy with the relevant deficient factor or with fresh frozen plasma or cryoprecipitate if the specific factor is not available. Replacement therapy should probably be given routinely following head injuries in these patients.

Acquired Hemophilia A

Acquired hemophilia is a rare condition resulting from the production of autoantibodies against factor VIII. The mean age at diagnosis is 74 and both sexes are affected. Cutaneous purpura and internal hemorrhage are common, whereas extensive bleeding into the joints is not a prominent feature. The condition is associated with systemic autoimmune disorders; malignancies such as lymphoma, acute or chronic lymphocytic leukemias, and solid tumors; and pregnancy. Drugs such as the penicillins, phenytoin, phenylbutazones, or chloramphenicol have also been implicated. No cause can be found in half of patients. Neurologic involvement is rare, but cases of life-threatening intracranial hemorrhage and recurrent spontaneous subdural hematoma have been reported.[48]

The diagnosis is based on unexpected prolongation of the activated partial thromboplastin time (aPTT) and the identification of a low factor VIII level associated with the presence of a time-dependent inhibitor in the plasma. Treatment of bleeding episodes requires the use of an activated prothrombin complex concentrate or recombinant activated factor VIII. Immunoglobulin administration does not improve outcome. Immunosuppression with corticosteroids, cyclophosphamide, or rituximab achieves a 73 percent complete remission, and is usually effective at reducing inhibitor production and bringing about a sustained rise in the factor VIII level.[49]

Hemorrhagic Disease of the Newborn

Hemorrhagic disease of the newborn is a coagulation disorder that occurs as a result of vitamin K deficiency resulting in a deficiency of factors II, VII, IX, X, along with protein C and protein S. Intracranial hemorrhage represents the most serious complication and occurs from the second day to the end of the first week of life, particularly after breech deliveries. Bleeding appears to occur from capillary lesions rather than major vessels. Subdural and subarachnoid hemorrhages are the most frequent forms of intracranial bleeding, and intracerebral hemorrhage is rare. Intracranial bleeding occurs earlier and with greater frequency in infants born to mothers receiving anticonvulsant therapy because of interference of anticonvulsant medication with vitamin K–dependent clotting factors.

Late-onset vitamin K deficiency usually occurs 2 to 12 weeks after birth but may occur up to 6 months of age. It is associated with failure to receive vitamin K prophylaxis at birth but also occurs in exclusively breast-fed babies. The majority present with acute intracerebral bleeding.[50]

Thrombocytopenia

If platelet function is normal, satisfactory hemostasis may be achieved with a platelet count as low as $80 \times 10^9/L$. Clinically significant spontaneous hemorrhage does not usually occur if the platelet count exceeds $25 \times 10^9/L$, but below $20 \times 10^9/L$ spontaneous hemorrhage is not uncommon. Intracerebral, subarachnoid, and subdural hemorrhages are the most serious complications; the risk of spontaneous intracranial hemorrhage appears to be greatest during the first 2 weeks after onset of the disorder. An uncommon complication of recurrent bleeding is superficial siderosis.

Drug-induced immune thrombocytopenias arise when a drug functions as a hapten, binding to platelets and resulting in complement fixation and intravascular lysis. The platelet count typically falls within 7 or more days after initiation of the responsible drug.

Heparin-induced thrombocytopenia is the commonest disorder of this type. It is defined as a platelet count that drops below 100 to $150 \times 10^9/L$ for no apparent reason other than heparin administration. Type I heparin-induced thrombocytopenia is characterized by a moderate reduction in platelet counts, usually within the first 7 to 12 days of the initiation of heparin therapy. The platelet count rarely drops below $100 \times 10^9/L$ and normalizes in spite of continued heparin therapy. Type II heparin-induced thrombocytopenia is immunologically mediated and paradoxically is often associated with thrombosis. Most patients produce IgG antibodies against complexes of platelet factor 4 and heparin.

Delayed-onset thrombocytopenia a mean of 14 days after initiation of therapy is increasingly being recognized, and is usually associated with heparin-induced antibodies. It may begin rapidly in patients who have received heparin any time within the previous 100 days. Heparin-dependent antibodies do not invariably reappear with subsequent heparin use. Up to 60 percent or more develop serious thrombotic complications, including ischemic damage to limbs, CNS, myocardium, and lungs.[51] A study of 120 cases of immune-mediated heparin-induced thrombocytopenia showed that 9 percent developed neurologic complications, including ischemic cerebrovascular events (6%), cerebral venous sinus thrombosis (2.5%), and a transient confusional state in one case. Primary intracerebral hemorrhage was not observed. Importantly in three cases, neurologic complications preceded the onset of thrombocytopenia.[52]

In severe thrombocytopenia, massive intracranial hemorrhage may be instantaneous and treatment of no avail. The onset of intracranial bleeding is often heralded by headaches of varying severity. In these circumstances, platelet transfusion should be instituted without delay, as it should after head injury in patients who have significantly reduced platelet counts.

Disorders of Platelet Function

Regardless of the platelet count, abnormal bleeding states may result from abnormalities of platelet function, that is, disorders of platelet adhesion, aggregation, secretion, and procoagulant activity, or a combination of abnormalities of number and function. Bleeding due to these disorders is treated primarily with platelet transfusions.

Bernard–Soulier syndrome is an inherited, usually autosomal recessive disorder of platelet adhesion caused by deficiency of the component subunits of the glycoprotein 1b-IX-V complex. As a result, platelets fail to stick and clump together at the site of the injury.

Glanzmann thrombasthenia is caused by the absence of platelet aggregation due to deficiencies of αIIbβ3 integrin, an aggregation receptor on platelets. This absence prevents fibrinogen bridging from occurring and thus prevents clot retraction and significantly prolongs bleeding time. It has been associated with fatal cerebral hemorrhage. Platelet count, volume, and morphology are normal in classic Glanzmann thrombasthenia, though some reports have suggested a role for αIIbβ3 in megakaryocytopoiesis, and point mutations have been described that lead to platelet anisotropy and thrombocytopenia.

The gray platelet syndrome, a rare inherited disorder of the megakaryocyte lineage, is characterized by thrombocytopenia and enlarged platelets with absence of α-granules and their contents. Storage pool deficiency and abnormalities of the granule secretion mechanism all result in malfunction of platelet secretion of substances required for platelet adhesion and aggregation.

Scott syndrome is characterized by the absence of calcium-stimulated exposure of phosphatidylserine from the inner leaflet of the plasma membrane bilayer to the cell surface, which is required to provide an appropriate surface for the assembly of the complexes of the coagulation network, resulting in moderately severe bleeding.

A variety of hereditary disorders may be associated with low platelet counts or platelets of abnormal size, including Wiskott–Aldrich syndrome.

The commonest acquired disorders of platelet function arise from drugs such as aspirin, nonsteroidal anti-inflammatory drugs, and ticlopidine. A wide range of other drugs may affect platelet function, including antihistamines, some antibiotics, antidepressants, and anesthetics. Platelet function may also be affected by chronic renal failure, the use of blood-bank platelets, leukemia, and cardiopulmonary bypass. In myelomatosis or macroglobulinemia, abnormal platelet function results from interference by circulating paraproteins, and bleeding may be readily controlled by plasmapheresis.

Disseminated Intravascular Coagulation

DIC should be considered as indicative of the presence of an underlying disorder. At the most basic level, DIC is the clinical manifestation of inappropriate thrombin activation. The coagulation system is activated by the rapid release of thromboplastic substances into the circulation to form either soluble or insoluble fibrin. Clotting factors and platelets are consumed, and there is defective and activated fibrinolysis and impairment of the coagulation inhibition system. The clinical syndromes result from vascular obstruction from fibrin-rich thrombi. Globules of fibrin are occasionally seen free in the circulating blood, red blood cells are forced through fine networks of fibrin resulting in fragmentation, and a microangiopathic hemolytic anemia is present. The overwhelming consumption of α_2-antiplasmin and platelets together with the anticoagulant properties of fibrin degradation products may also result in a bleeding tendency that can vary in severity from slight oozing at venipuncture sites with purpura and spontaneous bruising to massive uncontrollable hemorrhage (Fig. 25-5). Simultaneous hemorrhage and thrombosis may occur. Primary brain damage releases powerful thromboplastins into the circulation that may precipitate DIC, and all patients with evidence of brain

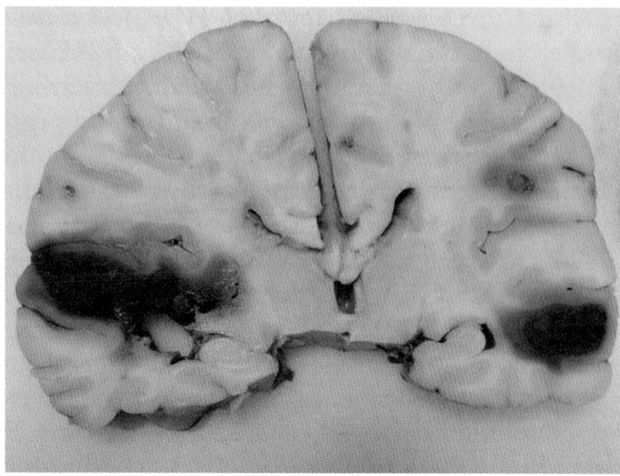

FIGURE 25-5 ▪ Young male with promyelocytic acute myeloid leukemia complicated by DIC resulting in intracerebral and intraventricular hemorrhage.

injury are at risk for its development. DIC has been described in association with status epilepticus, possibly related to widespread endothelial injury secondary to seizure-induced hyperpyrexia.[53]

The hemorrhagic complication may be so marked that massive cerebral, intraventricular, or subarachnoid hemorrhage may occur. When DIC affects the nervous system, the symptoms and signs are related to the thrombotic and hemorrhagic complications as well as to the primary disorder triggering the DIC (Table 25-2). Any part of the brain may be affected, producing focal or generalized encephalopathic manifestations. Symptoms and signs may fluctuate markedly with time, presumably because of the continuing deposition and lysis of fibrin, which results in intermittent obstruction of vessels and blood flow. Patients may remain in a coma for several days, but may make a good recovery if the circulation is reestablished.

In DIC secondary to carcinoma, microvascular obstruction of the brain may produce signs indistinguishable from those of metastatic deposits. Such signs may be found before clinical recognition of the underlying malignancy. Ischemic myelopathy due to DIC is rare.

No single test is available that is sufficiently sensitive or specific to permit a diagnosis of DIC. The presence of soluble fibrin in plasma has high sensitivity but low specificity for the diagnosis. The protamine sulfate test detects circulating fibrin monomers and is specific but not sensitive. The diagnosis frequently may be made using a combination of platelet count, measurement of global clotting times, measurement of one or two clotting factors and inhibitors (e.g., antithrombin), and a test for fibrin degradation products. Serial coagulation tests are often helpful and a reduced platelet count or a clear downward trend is a sensitive if not specific sign of DIC.

It is important to recognize coagulation syndromes that resemble DIC, especially thrombocytopenic purpura and fulminant antiphospholipid antibody syndrome. At the onset of the neurologic disorder in DIC, the coagulation profile may be normal. During pregnancy, postoperatively, following trauma, and in association with malignancy, plasma fibrinogen, an acute-phase reactant, is invariably elevated so that increased fibrinogen consumption serves only to reduce plasma fibrinogen to normal. For this reason, the only laboratory evidence of DIC in this situation may be thrombocytopenia and an elevated level of fibrin degradation products. The International Society on Thrombosis and Haemostasis has proposed a useful algorithm for the diagnosis of DIC.[54]

Thrombotic Thrombocytopenic Purpura

Thrombotic thrombocytopenic purpura (TTP) is a severe form of thrombotic microangiopathy resulting in organ failure of variable severity. The only consistent abnormalities are red cell fragmentation and thrombocytopenia, which are also found in other conditions. The condition results from excessive systemic platelet aggregation caused by the accumulation of unfolded high-molecular-weight von Willebrand factor multimers in plasma. The failure to degrade the multimers into less adhesive forms is related to a severe deficiency in a von Willebrand factor cleaving protease, ADAMTS13 (a disintegrin and metalloproteinase with a thrombospondin type 1 motif, member 13). There are three types: (1) hereditary TTP, caused by mutations in *ADAMTS13* gene; (2) acquired idiopathic TTP, caused mainly by polyclonal IgG that inhibits plasma ADAMTS13 activity; and (3) acquired nonidiopathic TTP, which is associated with pregnancy, hematopoietic progenitor cell transplantation, infection, disseminated malignancy, and certain drugs such as ticlopidine and clopidogrel.[55]

Severe deficiency of plasma ADAMTS13 activity or the presence of anti-ADAMTS13 autoantibodies

TABLE 25-2 ■ Clinical Conditions Complicated by Disseminated Intravascular Coagulation

Mechanism	Clinical Condition
Tissue damage	Trauma (including neurotrauma), fat embolism
	Surgery
	Heat stroke
	Burns
	Dissecting aneurysm
	Neuroleptic malignant syndrome
	Pancreatitis
	Status epilepticus
Infection	Bacterial
	Viral
	Protozoal
	Rickettsial
Immunologic disturbance	Immune complex disorders
	Allograft rejection
	Incompatible blood transfusion
Obstetric complications	Abruptio placentae
	Amniotic fluid embolism
	Retained fetal products
	Eclampsia
Metabolic disorder	Diabetic ketoacidosis
Neoplasms	Myeloproliferative and lymphoproliferative disorders
	Mucin-secreting adenocarcinoma
Miscellaneous	Cyanotic congenital heart disease
	Hepatic failure
	Cavernous hemangioma
	Shock
	Snake venoms

is highly specific for the diagnosis. Treatments that eliminate anti-ADAMTS13 autoantibodies such as cyclosporine, cyclophosphamide, and rituximab are effective in treating acquired TTP.

TTP presents most commonly between the ages of 20 and 50, and affects women more commonly than men. Neurologic deficits may not be present, and the current diagnostic criteria no longer require the presence of renal and neurologic abnormalities or fever.[56] Plasma exchange may therefore be introduced earlier, with a corresponding decline in the mortality rate.[57] There may be complete recovery, but a chronic relapsing form has been described.

With use of less restrictive diagnostic criteria, care must be taken to exclude conditions that may mimic TTP such as DIC, disseminated malignancy, Evans syndrome (simultaneous or sequential development of autoimmune hemolytic anemia and immune thrombocytopenia with or without immune neutropenia), sepsis, accelerated hypertension, eclampsia, the catastrophic form of the antiphospholipid antibody syndrome, and HELLP syndrome (hemolysis, elevated liver function tests, low platelets), which is found in 10 percent of cases of eclampsia and preeclampsia. Unlike TTP, fetal involvement is present in the HELLP syndrome, with fetal thrombocytopenia reported in 30 percent of cases.

Pathologically, TTP is characterized by hyperplasia of endothelial and adventitial cells in arterioles, capillaries, and venules associated with platelet-rich and hyaline thrombi in these vessels, in which microaneurysms may also form.

Neurologic features are the most frequent presenting manifestations of TTP, occurring in 60 percent of cases. As the result of involvement of any part of the CNS, there is an endless variety of neurologic manifestations. Symptoms are typically transient and fluctuating and sometimes may resemble TIAs. Permanent neurologic complications may occur, and therefore neurologic symptoms should be treated vigorously with daily repeated plasma exchange, antiplatelet drugs, corticosteroids, and possibly chemotherapeutic agents such as vincristine.

The neurologic abnormalities in TTP may precede the full syndrome by months or even years. In a typical case, there may be a variety of nonspecific prodromal symptoms. At the time of presentation, the patient is usually pale, icteric, and febrile; has petechial hemorrhages in the skin; exhibits mental changes and neurologic abnormalities; and has splenomegaly, hepatomegaly, lymphadenopathy, arthropathy, and some degree of hypertension and renal insufficiency.

Posterior reversible encephalopathy syndrome is the most common brain imaging abnormality in severe TTP. The main laboratory abnormalities are microangiopathic hemolytic anemia, thrombocytopenia, hyperbilirubinemia, uremia, and erythroid and myeloid hyperplasia of the bone marrow with increased megakaryocytic activity. Although laboratory evidence of DIC may be present, it occurs in only a few patients. Demonstration of low levels (≤5%) of normal ADAMTS13 is indicative of the diagnosis.

Hemolytic-Uremic Syndrome

The hemolytic-uremic syndrome (HUS) is characterized by renal impairment, thrombocytopenia, and microangiopathic hemolytic anemia, typically preceded by abdominal pain and diarrhea. Involvement of the nervous system is common. As with TTP, the diagnosis may be made on the basis of microangiopathic hemolytic anemia and thrombocytopenia, but there are important differences between the two entities. Deficiency of von Willebrand factor–cleaving protease has not been shown in HUS.[58] Unlike TTP, 91 percent of children with HUS survive with only supportive care, and plasma exchange treatment is not indicated.[59] Most cases arise as a complication of gastroenterologic infections by organisms producing Shiga toxins such as *Escherichia coli* O157:H7 or *Shigella*. Sporadic cases result from familial or autoimmune diseases, a variety of drugs (cyclosporine, mitomycin, and other forms of chemotherapy), tumors, bone marrow transplant, HIV infection, or are idiopathic.

Familial HUS constitutes 5 to 10 percent of cases. Several members of the alternative complement pathway are mutated in these patients resulting in overactivation of the alternative pathway, either by losing regulatory functions or by gaining persistent or enhanced activation. Mutations in thrombomodulin, which regulates complement and the coagulation cascade, have also been described. There is thought to be a role for complement in diarrhea-associated HUS; Shiga toxin circulates bound to blood cells but not attached to Gb3 receptors. Instead, it binds to an as-yet undetermined receptor for which it has less affinity. Therefore, when the Shiga toxin finds its way to an organ which expresses Gb3, it preferentially detaches from circulating blood cells and binds to these receptors.[60,61]

The most common neurologic manifestations are seizures, but behavioral changes and cerebral, cerebellar, and brainstem syndromes may occur. Axonal neuropathy has been described in a patient with *E. coli* serotype O157:H7–associated HUS.[62] Striatal involvement due to small areas of infarction, with resulting involuntary movements, may occur. MRI of the brain may show features of infarction or hemorrhage, and changes characteristic of posterior reversible encephalopathy syndrome are sometimes found.[63] Patients in coma or with pyramidal signs may have normal imaging.[64] In the German Shiga toxin–producing *E. coli* 0104:H4 outbreak, cognitive impairment, aphasia, and seizures were common but the outcome was good. There were no signs of microbleeds, thrombotic occlusions, or infarction. MR imaging and neuropathology seemed to indicate mixed toxic and inflammatory mechanisms.[65] There is a risk of residual hypertension and chronic renal failure, which is greatest in those children with neurologic complications. Seizures, alone or as part of an encephalopathic illness, are associated with mortality or long-term neurologic sequelae.[66] There is anecdotal experience of the use of plasma exchange, immunabsorption, and eculizumab in the management of severe diarrhea-associated HUS.[61]

Gaucher Disease

Gaucher disease is the commonest lipid storage disorder. An autosomal recessive condition, it is characterized by a deficiency of glucocerebrosidase and an accumulation of glucocerebroside in lipid-laden macrophages (Gaucher cells) in various organs.

Type 1 is the non-neuronopathic type. It results from accumulation in bones, liver, spleen, and lungs and is characterized by hepatosplenomegaly, bone pain and fractures, thrombocytopenia, and bleeding diathesis. It may develop at any time in childhood. It occurs worldwide in all populations, but 60 percent of cases are found in Ashkenazi Jews. The prevalence and incidence of polyneuropathy is increased in type 1 Gaucher disease.

Type 2, the acute neuronopathic form, shows no ethnic predilection, Hepatosplenomegaly arises in the first few months of life. Characteristic brainstem abnormalities then develop with strabismus, horizontal supranuclear palsy, opisthotonic posturing, and trismus arising in response to noxious stimuli. There is diffuse spasticity and developmental regression, and the disease is usually fatal during the first 3 years of life.

Type 3 Gaucher disease, the chronic neuronopathic form, is also without ethnic predilection and is estimated to occur in 1 in 50,000 live births. The neurologic symptoms are slowly progressive and appear later in childhood than the symptoms of type 2 disease. The disease has a more chronic course, with variable hepatosplenomegaly and the progressive development of incoordination, myoclonic seizures, impairment of olfaction, parkinsonian motor signs, pyramidal signs, cerebellar ataxia, and cranial nerve palsies.[67] The cognitive disturbance ranges from a mild memory disorder to severe dementia, which is most frequent. Seizures may be tonic-clonic, focal with dyscognitive features, or myoclonic with prominent jerking of the face, limbs, or palate. Oculomotor apraxia has been described as the presenting feature. In addition, thrombocytopenia and prolonged prothrombin and partial thromboplastin times may cause bleeding. The patient may be anemic, and Gaucher cells may be found on bone marrow examination. Symptoms vary between individuals, so that some children have cirrhosis with portal hypertension, varices, pulmonary interstitial involvement, and heart disease. Type 3 Gaucher disease has been classified further as types 3a and 3b based on the extent of neurologic involvement and the presence of progressive myotonia and dementia (type 3a) or isolated supranuclear gaze palsy (type 3b).

Norbottnian Gaucher disease, a genetic form identified in Sweden, has features of types 2 and 3. The slowly progressive neurologic symptoms may not occur until early adulthood.

Enzyme replacement therapy with recombinant forms of macrophage-targeted acid β-glucosidase is beneficial for types 1 and 3 Gaucher disease, reducing liver and spleen size, improving blood counts, and reducing skeletal anomalies. It does not cross the blood–brain barrier and is therefore not effective in the management of neurologic symptoms. Substrate reduction therapy with *N*-butyl-deoxynojirimycin is available for patients unable to take enzyme replacement therapy. This compound inhibits the enzyme glucosylceramide synthase, a glucosyl transferase responsible for the first step in the synthesis of glycosphingolipids. Unlike enzyme replacement therapy, this drug does cross the blood–brain barrier, but no data are yet available on whether it has a role in neuronopathic Gaucher disease.

Bleeding and the New Anticoagulants

Several new oral anticoagulant drugs have been introduced in recent years which act by direct thrombin or factor Xa inhibition and are considered to have the advantage of providing a stable level of anticoagulation on a regular dose, and to not require monitoring and dose adjustment as with warfarin.

Dabigatran is used for the prevention of stroke in patients with non-valvular atrial fibrillation. When compared to people treated with warfarin, patients taking dabigatran have fewer life-threatening bleeds and fewer minor and major bleeds, including intracranial bleeds, but the rate of gastroenterologic bleeding is higher, mostly in patients over 75 years old. The most common side effect of dabigatran, seen in more than 10 percent of patients, is bleeding. No specific method exists to reverse the anticoagulant effect of dabigatran in the event of major bleeding. Supportive care and discontinuation of anticoagulant is recommended together with activated charcoal if ingestion was in the previous few hours. Hemodialysis has also been recommended.

The lack of a reliable blood test to monitor dabigatran makes it difficult to determine if a patient is experiencing a drug interaction. The aPTT is typically elevated, so a normal level within 2 hours of ingestion might exclude overanticoagulation. An elevated level cannot be used to quantify anticoagulation accurately. The ecarin clotting time can monitor direct thrombin inhibitors but is not widely available.

Drugs such as rivaroxaban and apixaban work by inhibiting factor Xa directly. They have been trialed successfully for postoperative thromboembolic prophylaxis and for the prevention of stroke associated with atrial fibrillation. The effects of rivaroxaban may be reversed by prothrombin complex concentrate.

COAGULATION DISORDERS

Thrombosis may arise from abnormalities of the blood-vessel wall, alterations in blood composition, and abnormalities in the dynamics of blood flow—the triad of Virchow. The intact vessel wall modulates thrombin activity, platelet reactivity, and the release of vasodilators, and it promotes local fibrinolytic activity. Injury of a vessel wall may therefore lead to the exposure of the prothrombotic subendothelium as well as interfere with its antithrombotic properties.

A number of blood components exhibit prothrombotic and antithrombotic effects, so that under normal circumstances platelet degranulation and aggregation as well as thrombin generation occur only at sites of tissue injury. Thrombin production is the major step in thrombosis that results in fibrin deposition. The fibrinolytic system prevents the deposition of excess fibrin, a negative-feedback process that is catalyzed by fibrin through plasmin production and also breaks down platelet-adhesive glycoproteins, further reducing platelet recruitment. The balance between prothrombotic and antithrombotic activity determines the degree of thrombus progression.

There are a number of well-recognized circumstances under which this balance may be altered. Tissue injury may lead to increased synthesis of plasminogen activator inhibitor type 1, with an increased risk of thrombosis. Congenital deficiencies of anticoagulant proteins are well recognized. Antiphospholipid antibodies are associated with venous and arterial thrombosis. Pregnancy is associated with a variety of changes in hemostatic components, giving rise to thrombosis or hemorrhage; increased fibrinogen production and placental production of a plasminogen activator inhibitor type 2 contributes to the increased risk of thrombosis in the later stages of pregnancy. Cigarette smoking, estrogen use, tissue injury, infection, and inflammation each result in increased production of components of the cascade, particularly fibrinogen.

Diminished blood flow may lead to the local accumulation of platelets and thrombin, and, if the stasis is sufficient, endothelial hypoxia may result in impairment of the antithrombotic properties of the endothelium. Blood viscosity is a significant determinant of blood flow. Under low-flow conditions, platelets have only a minor role in the generation of thrombosis; stasis is the dominant factor in the pathogenesis of venous thrombosis in which activated clotting factors circulate to areas of venous stasis, where fibrin is generated. This process is exacerbated by defects in innate anticoagulant mechanisms. In the arterial system, thrombosis usually arises from endothelial damage, commonly in association with atherosclerosis. Procoagulant mechanisms may be involved in the initiation and progression of atherosclerosis, but local platelet degranulation results in plaque growth. Plaque rupture or ulceration is often the final event that exposes procoagulant material with rapid formation of platelet thrombus, which may break up and embolize or become consolidated and enlarged by fibrin deposition.

It follows from the physiology of thrombosis that differing risk factors are responsible for the generation of venous and arterial thrombosis. Furthermore, the multifactorial nature of thrombophilia is becoming increasingly apparent, and individuals with more than one inherited thrombophilia risk factor or those with an inherited and an acquired risk factor are particularly prone to thrombosis.

Routine evaluation for hypercoagulability, such as assays for deficiencies of coagulation inhibitors or genetic analysis for the factor V Leiden or prothrombin 20210 mutation, is not helpful in identifying risk factors for adult patients with stroke, other than in the context of an associated systemic venous clot that may travel through a right-to-left shunt, such as a patent foramen ovale (PFO).

Antiphospholipid Antibodies

The lupus anticoagulant and anticardiolipin are members of a group of antiphospholipid antibodies which are associated with venous and to a lesser degree arterial thrombosis. A diagnosis of antiphospholipid syndrome requires the combination of at least one clinical and one laboratory criterion which is persistent over time. Anticardiolipin and anti–β_2-glycoprotein I antibodies, detected by the use of enzyme-linked immunosorbent assay, and the lupus anticoagulant, detected by clotting assays, are the recommended tests for the syndrome. Antiphospholipid antibodies comprise a family of antibodies that react with serum phospholipid-binding plasma proteins, among which β_2-glycoprotein I is the most important. Antibodies to protein S, protein C, prothrombin, annexin V, and annexin II have also been described. Affinity for coagulation-active negatively charged lipids is the basis for phospholipid-dependent coagulation assays for lupus anticoagulant.

In SLE, predisposition to thrombosis is associated with the presence of antinuclear antibodies and antiphospholipid antibodies. The primary antiphospholipid syndrome is the association between arterial and venous thrombosis with the lupus anticoagulant, anticardiolipin, or other phospholipid antibodies, along with a history of recurrent early miscarriage and sometimes thrombocytopenia, in the absence of SLE or other connective tissue disorders. In a cohort of 1,000 patients with the antiphospholipid syndrome, 82 percent were female, primary antiphospholipid syndrome was present in 53 percent, and SLE was associated in 36 percent. Antiphospholipid antibodies may arise de novo or may be associated with a variety of underlying disorders, as discussed in Chapters 11 and 50. The risk of thrombosis is variable; antiphospholipid antibodies associated with infections and a variety of drugs are associated with a smaller risk of thrombosis than those of primary or secondary antiphospholipid syndromes. The presence of more than one class of antiphospholipid antibody increases thrombotic risk. Patients with triple positivity (anticardiolipin, the lupus anticoagulant, and anti–β_2-glycoprotein I) have a 30 percent chance of thrombosis even when anticoagulated.[68]

Since patients with clinical manifestations may have multiple antiphospholipid antibodies, testing must include at least two sensitive coagulation assays, usually the kaolin-cephalin clotting time (KCCT) and the dilute Russell viper venom time (DRVVT) with a platelet neutralization step, as well as the solid-phase assays for IgG and IgM anticardiolipin antibody. Long kaolin-cephalin clotting times may arise from coagulation factor deficiency, and false-negative antiphospholipid antibody testing may occur from binding of the antibodies to platelets in samples not processed rapidly and appropriately. Low-titer antibodies and IgM antibodies are most likely to be nonpathogenic. Transient positive antibodies, particularly IgM, may follow a variety of infections, so positive tests should be repeated after at least 12 weeks as in the current Sapporo classification criteria.[69]

The precise significance of anti–β_2-glycoprotein I antibodies remains to be fully elucidated. They have not been associated with thrombosis in systematic reviews. However, they were found to double the risk of stroke in a case-controlled study and there is an increased risk of thrombosis in patients with concomitant lupus anticoagulant.[70]

Antiprothrombin antibodies are found in a higher percentage (50 to 60%) of patients with SLE than are anticardiolipin antibodies and anti–β_2-glycoprotein I antibodies, and they also constitute an independent risk factor for venous thrombosis.[71–73] The simultaneous presence of antiprothrombin antibodies is also associated with a higher risk of thrombotic events in patients with primary antiphospholipid syndrome.[74]

Annexin V is a natural anticoagulant with a high calcium-dependent binding affinity for negatively charged phospholipids that acts competitively with coagulation factors to inhibit the prothrombin complex. High levels of anti–annexin V antibodies have been found in 20 to 30 percent of patients with SLE.[75,76] There is growing evidence that the antiphospholipid antibody–mediated disruption of the annexin V anticoagulant crystal shield is a mechanism for pregnancy losses and thrombosis in patients with antiphospholipid syndrome.[77]

Depression, cognitive dysfunction, psychosis, seizures, chorea, and transverse myelitis have been associated with the presence of antiphospholipid antibodies, although there is evidence that not all arise from ischemia.[78] Neuropsychiatric lupus seems to be associated with the presence of antiphospholipid antibodies and presence of anti-Ro antibodies. An interaction between these antibodies and CNS cellular elements may account for some of these manifestations. Sneddon syndrome of cerebral thrombosis in association with livedo reticularis is strongly associated with the presence of antiphospholipid antibodies.

Epilepsy occurs in 8.6 percent of patients with the antiphospholipid syndrome. Multivariate logistic regression analysis identified CNS thromboembolic events as the most significant risk factor for epilepsy in these patients, with an odds ratio (OR) of 4.1, followed by SLE (OR 1.4) and valvular vegetations (OR 2.9).[79]

The clinical features have been described in 1,000 patients with antiphospholipid syndrome.[80] Neurologic manifestations include migraine (20.2%), stroke (19.8%), TIA (11.1%), epilepsy (7.0%), amaurosis fugax (5.4%), vascular dementia (2.5%), retinal artery thrombosis (1.5%), chorea (1.3%), acute encephalopathy (1.1%), optic neuropathy (1.0%), retinal vein thrombosis (0.9%), transient amnesia (0.7%), cerebral venous sinus thrombosis (0.7%), cerebellar ataxia (0.7%), transverse myelopathy (0.4%), and hemiballismus (0.3%).

Many studies have examined the association between antiphospholipid antibodies and stroke. A study of unselected adults presenting with stroke suggested that the presence of anticardiolipin antibodies is an independent risk factor for stroke but does not predispose to subsequent thrombotic events.[81,82] Another study showed that presence of an antiphospholipid antibody (either the lupus anticoagulant or anticardiolipin) among patients with ischemic stroke did not predict either increased risk of subsequent vascular occlusive events over 2 years or a differential response to aspirin or warfarin therapy. Routine screening for antiphospholipid antibodies in unselected adults with ischemic stroke is therefore not recommended.[83] With the introduction of assays for antibodies directed specifically against β_2-glycoprotein I, however, a relative risk of stroke of 2 to 3 has been suggested.[84] Studies of a wider range of antiphospholipid antibodies in the pathogenesis of cerebral ischemia suggest a relevant role for a combination of antiphosphatidylserine IgG and anti–β_2-glycoprotein-I IgA in stroke etiology.[85] A consensus is forming that one or a number of the antiphospholipid antibodies have an association with stroke in adults; whether this is a risk factor for recurrent vascular events is uncertain.

Among younger patients, the association appears stronger, with antiphospholipid antibodies present in 46 percent of patients younger than 50 years who present with stroke or TIA compared with 8 percent of matched control subjects with nonthrombotic neurologic disease. In young adults, the presence of antiphospholipid antibodies, particularly the lupus anticoagulant, has been identified as an independent risk factor for first and possibly also for recurrent ischemic stroke,[86] although a prospective study of young patients with recent TIA or ischemic stroke failed to show that antiphospholipid antibodies are a strong risk factor for recurrent stroke or TIA.[87] Some type of prothrombotic abnormality has been identified in 20 to 50 percent of children presenting with acute ischemic stroke, suggesting that screening for antiphospholipid antibodies in this population may be of value.[88]

Hereditary Thrombophilia

The inherited thrombophilias are a group of disorders in which a defect or deficiency in the natural anticoagulant mechanisms predisposes to the development of venous thrombosis. Genetic or acquired predisposing factors can now be identified in as many as 80 percent of patients who develop cerebral venous sinus thrombosis. A genetic risk factor is identifiable in up to 50 percent of unselected patients with venous thromboembolism.[89] Investigation into potentially inherited disorders must include assessment of family members.

Within the cerebral venous sinuses, the superior sagittal and transverse sinuses are frequently involved, whereas cavernous sinus thrombosis is much less common. Antithrombin III, protein C, and protein S deficiencies, factor V Leiden mutations, the prothrombin G20210A gene mutation, and MTHFR C677T mutations (resulting in hyperhomocysteinemia) all predispose to thrombosis. Other inherited disorders, such as deficiency of heparin cofactor 2, plasminogen, tissue plasminogen activator, factor XII, or prekallikrein may result in a modestly increased risk of thrombosis.

The genetic risk factors for venous thrombosis can be subdivided based on their level of increased risk. Strong risk factors including deficiencies of antithrombin III, protein C, and protein S, which collectively affect less than 1 percent of the population. Because these deficiencies are rare, most reports on risk come from family studies, which suggest that these deficiencies can lead to highly penetrant phenotypes with a 10-fold risk for heterozygote carriers. Studies from unselected consecutive patients, however, indicate that the risks are much less, raising the possibility that these families may carry other unrecognized defects.[90] Moderately strong risk factors for thrombosis are the factor V Leiden mutation, prothrombin 20210A mutations, non-O blood group mutations, and the fibrinogen 10034T mutation. There are many weak genetic risk factors identified, including fibrinogen, factor XIII, and factor XI variants. Even for moderately strong risk factors (relative risks 2 to5), the majority of carriers will never develop thrombosis.[90]

A large genome-wide association study suggested that common variants could explain about 35 percent of venous thrombosis susceptibility, of which 3 percent only could be attributable to the main identified genes. The relevance of the findings to cerebral venous thrombosis remains unclear [91]

Antithrombin III Deficiency

Antithrombin is a plasma glycoprotein that inhibits thrombin and other activated serine proteases, including factors IXa, Xa, XIa, XIIa, and kallikrein. Heterozygous antithrombin III deficiency affects 1 in 2,000 to 5,000 of the population and may arise as a new mutation. Deficiency is associated with sagittal sinus and other cerebral venous sinus thromboses. A rarer disorder is recognized in which a nonsense mutation results in a dysfunctional variant of antithrombin causing recurrent venous thrombosis.[92] Acquired antithrombin III deficiency associated with cerebral venous sinus thrombosis may also arise from reduced antithrombin synthesis due to liver disease or increased loss in nephrotic syndrome, oral contraceptive use, DIC, protein malnutrition, and heparin therapy.[93] A retrospective cohort family study that assessed the risk of venous thromboembolism in individuals with thrombophilia suggested that antithrombin III deficiency may be associated with a higher risk of thrombosis than the other genetic defects.[94]

Protein C Deficiency

Cerebral venous sinus thrombosis is associated with deficiency of protein C, which is a vitamin K–dependent protein that binds to thrombomodulin, an endothelial cell surface protein, and is converted to an active protease by the action of thrombin. In conjunction with protein S, protein C proteolyses factors Va and VIIIa, thereby reducing thrombin formation and promoting fibrinolysis. Inheritance of protein C deficiency is usually autosomal dominant, although in some families heterozygotes with plasma concentrations of less than 50 percent of normal remain asymptomatic, giving an autosomal recessive–like pattern of inheritance. Dysfunctional molecules that are present in normal levels are described.

Population studies suggest that 1 in 200 to 300 subjects have levels of protein C consistent with congenital deficiency, although the incidence of protein C deficiency and venous thromboembolism suggests a prevalence of 1 in 30,000. This represents 4 percent of subjects with venous thromboembolism presenting before the age of 45 and demonstrates that other inherited and acquired risk factors are frequently required for thrombosis to occur.

Thrombomodulin is a cell surface endothelial glycoprotein with anticoagulant properties that activates protein C. Antibodies to thrombomudulin have been identified in patients with cerebral venous sinus thrombosis.[95]

Protein S Deficiency

Sagittal sinus and other cerebral venous sinus thromboses are reported in association with deficiency of protein S, which is a vitamin K–dependent glycoprotein that acts as a cofactor for activated protein C. Approximately 60 percent of protein S is protein bound, so that total and free levels must be measured. Only the unbound protein is biologically active, and since its level may fall in acute disease, repeat measurement and the demonstration of a persistently reduced level is required to prove association. Acquired protein S deficiency has been identified in hepatic disease, vitamin K deficiency, pregnancy, and hormonal contraceptive use. In the presence of the factor V Leiden mutation, functional assays of protein S may give a falsely low reading.

Factor V Leiden (RQ506Q)

The factor V Leiden mutation is a common gain-of-function mutation in factor V at Arg 506. Protein C cleaves and inactivates the Va procoagulant, resulting in factor V Leiden becoming resistant to inactivation by activated protein C. Factor V Leiden is the most commonly inherited prothrombotic state, accounting for at least 90 percent of the cases of resistance to activated protein C. The mutation is inherited as an autosomal dominant trait and has a prevalence of approximately 5 percent in the Caucasian population. It is found in 20 percent of patients with venous thrombosis and approximately 50 percent with familial thrombophilia.[90] A number of clinical studies, using different inclusion criteria, show a prevalence of activated protein C resistance ranging from 20 to 60 percent among patients with venous thromboembolism at any site, and 20 to 25 percent in cerebral venous sinus thrombosis. The actual thrombotic risk is moderate, but its high prevalence makes it by far the most important inherited risk factor.

Aquired activated protein C resistance, not due to the factor V Leiden mutation, is also a risk factor for venous thrombosis. Thrombotic events often occur in the presence of noninherited risk factors (e.g., oral contraceptive intake, pregnancy, puerperium, trauma, or prolonged immobilization) which are also present in many cases of cerebral venous sinus thrombosis with the factor V Leiden mutation.

Prothrombin G:A 20210 Mutation

Prothrombin is a precursor of the serine protease thrombin, a key enzyme in the production of fibrin from fibrinogen. A single nucleotide substitution (G to A) at position 20210 is associated with an increased risk of deep venous thrombosis and cerebral venous sinus thrombosis.[96] Carriers have a two- to threefold increased risk of venous thrombosis at any site, and the variant is found in approximately 6 percent of patients with venous thrombosis. The mutation is found in 18 percent of selected patients with a family history of venous thrombosis, and 1 to 2 percent of control subjects, making it the second most common cause of hereditary thrombophilia after the factor V Leiden mutation.[96] The prevalence of the prothrombin gene mutation is 20 percent in patients with cerebral venous sinus thrombosis in comparison with 3 percent of healthy control subjects.[97]

Fibrinogen Gamma 10034 T

Genetic variation in the fibrinogen gamma gene increases thrombotic risk approximately twofold. Around 6 percent of healthy individuals carry this variant, which is associated with an increased risk of venous thrombosis.[98] The relevance of this variant to cerebral venous sinus thrombosis remains unclear.

Hyperhomocysteinemia

Hyperhomocysteinemia is a risk factor for arterial and venous thrombosis. A C-to-T mutation at position 677 in the methylene tetrahydrofolate reductase gene (*MTHFR*) gives rise to a thermolabile variant with reduced activity accompanied by elevated plasma homocysteine. Homozygosity for the thermolabile form is found in 5 to 15 percent of the general population who have significantly elevated plasma homocysteine levels.[99,100]

Moderate hyperhomocysteinemia is now recognized as a risk factor for arterial disease, including carotid artery stenosis[101] and stroke.[102] It has also been suggested that hyperhomocysteinemia plays a role in the development of small vessel ischemia. Further discussion of hyperhomocysteinemia is provided in Chapter 11.

Factor VIII

Levels of the procoagulant factor VIII are associated with an increased risk of arterial and venous thrombosis. High factor VIII levels appear particularly to be a risk factor for thrombosis in children.[103,104]

Interactions Between Inherited Thrombophilias

The multifactorial nature of thrombophilia is well-recognized. Among 162 patients and 336 control subjects, two or more polymorphisms were detected in 16.7 percent of patients and 0.9 percent of controls. The odds ratios for venous thrombosis with the joint occurrence of the factor V Leiden and prothrombin G20210A mutations was 58.6; for the factor V Leiden mutation and MTHFR polymorphisms was 35.0; and for the prothrombin G20210A mutation and MTHFR polymorphisms was 7.7.[100] Coexistence of additional antithrombin III, protein C, or protein S deficiency has been reported in 14.5 percent of patients with the factor V Leiden mutation.[105] As factor V Leiden and prothrombin 20210A mutations are both common, compound heterozygotes are not particularly rare and have a 20-fold increased risk of thrombosis;[90] this combination of thrombophilias is associated with an increase in the prevalence of more unusual sites of venous thrombosis, such as the cerebral venous sinuses.[106]

Thrombophilic Disorders and Arterial Thrombosis

Although there are numerous reports of cerebral arterial thrombosis and infarction occurring in antithrombin III, protein C, and protein S deficiencies, as well as with factor V Leiden mutations,[107] the risk is extremely small compared with the risk of venous thrombosis. A stroke in the presence of a strong risk factor for venous thrombosis should therefore always raise the suspicion of paradoxical venous embolism.

Only rarely has familial thrombophilia been diagnosed conclusively following arterial thrombosis, by demonstrating that the deficiency persists after the acute event is over. This is particularly important in the case of protein S, since it binds to an acute-phase reactant (C4bBP), resulting in an acquired reduction in free or functional protein S. Low protein S levels are also found in acute nonvascular illness and during pregnancy, and protein C levels may fall in liver disease, postoperatively, and in association with DIC. Serial protein C measurements demonstrate that it may take 3 months for levels to return to normal following a stroke.[108] Case-control studies have failed to identify an association between factor V Leiden and arterial stroke.[109,110]

A number of reports suggest that hereditary thrombophilia may be associated with stroke in childhood, but reference ranges are lower than for adults, so the association may be erroneous.[111] Ethnic differences have also been noted in the levels of markers of thrombophilia in stroke, emphasizing the need for care in interpreting these tests.[112]

Interactions between genetic and noninherited risk factors, particularly oral contraceptives, should be considered, although progesterone-only contraceptives do not add to risks of thrombosis.[113] Any association between the inherited thrombophilias and arterial stroke is therefore weak and is likely to be enhanced by other prothrombotic risk factors.

Patent Foramen Ovale

In patients 55 years or younger with cryptogenic (presumed embolic) stroke, patent foramen ovale has been shown to be a more common finding (56%) than in controls (18%) and in those patients with stroke of undetermined cause (17%).[114,115] An association has been shown between the presence of coagulation abnormalities, especially the factor V Leiden and prothrombin G20210A mutations, and a history of Valsalva maneuver–like activity at stroke onset. Such activity was more common at stroke onset in patients with, rather than without, patent foramen ovale, suggesting paradoxical embolism as a mechanism. Coagulation abnormalities have been found in 30 percent of patients with cryptogenic infarction who also had patent foramen ovale[116]; however, the combined presence of patent foramen ovale and antiphospholipid syndrome does not increase the risk of subsequent cerebrovascular events.[117] Interestingly, the prevalence of prothrombin mutations is higher in patients with a patent foramen ovale as compared to stroke patients without a patent foramen ovale, raising the possibility that there may be an association between the coagulopathy and the formation of intracardiac shunts.[118] No significant association was found between the *MTHFR* genotype and strokes related to patent foramen ovale.[119]

REFERENCES

1. Benedict SL, Bonkowski JL, Thompson JA, et al: Cerebral sinovenous thrombosis in children: another reason to treat iron deficiency anaemia. J Child Neurol 19:526, 2004.
2. Leis AA, Stokie DS, Shepherd JM: Depression of spinal motoneurons may underlie weakness associated with severe anemia. Muscle Nerve 27:108, 2003.
3. Kotagal S, Silber MH: Childhood onset restless legs syndrome. Ann Neurol 58:341, 2005.
4. Valente E, Scott JM, Ueland PM, et al: Diagnostic accuracy of holotranscobalamin, methylmalonic acid, serum cobalamin, and other indicators of tissue vitamin B_{12} status in the elderly. Clin Chem 57:6856, 2011.
5. Turner MR, Talbot K: Functional vitamin B_{12} deficiency. Pract Neurol 9:37, 2009.
6. Akdal G, Yener GG, Ada E, Halmagyi GM: Eye movement disorders in vitamin B_{12} deficiency: two new cases and a review of the literature. Eur J Neurol 14:1170, 2007.
7. Korenke GC, Hunneman DH, Eber S, et al: Severe encephalopathy with epilepsy in an infant caused by subclinical maternal pernicious anaemia: case report and review of the literature. Eur J Pediatr 163:196, 2004.
8. Donnelly S, Callaghan N: Subacute combined degeneration of the spinal cord due to folate deficiency in association with a psychotic illness. Ir Med J 83:73, 1990.
9. Ramaekers VT, Rothenberg SP, Sequeira JM, et al: Autoantibodies to folate receptors in the cerebral folate deficiency syndrome. N Engl J Med 352:1985, 2005.
10. Cains S, Shepherd A, Nabiuni M, et al: Addressing a folate imbalance in fetal cerebrospinal fluid can decrease the incidence of congenital hydrocephalus. J Neuropathol Exp Neurol 68:404, 2009.
11. Prengler M, et al: Sickle cell disease: the neurological complications. Ann Neurol 51:543, 2002.
12. Liesner R, Mackie J, Cookson J, et al: Prothrombotic changes in children with sickle cell disease: relationship to cerebrovascular disease and transfusion. Br J Haematol 103:1037, 1998.
13. van Mierlo TD, Van den Berg HM, Nievelstein RAJ, et al: An unconscious girl with sickle cell disease. Lancet 361:136, 2003.
14. Lee AC, Chiu M, Wong V, et al: Hypertransfusion for spinal cord compression secondary to extramedullary haematopoiesis. Pediatr Hematol Oncol 13:89, 1996.
15. Eldor A, Rachmilewitz EA: The hypercoagulable state in thalassemia. Blood 99:36, 2002.
16. Schilling RF, Gangnon RE, Traver M: Arteriosclerotic events are less frequent in persons with chronic anemia: evidence from families with hereditary spherocytosis. Am J Hematol 81:315, 2006.
17. Hillmen P, Lewis SM, Bessler M: Natural history of paroxysmal nocturnal haemoglobinuria. N Engl J Med 333:1253, 1995.
18. Rampoldi L, Danek A, Monaco AP: Clinical features and molecular bases of neuroacanthocytosis. J Mol Med 80:475, 2002.
19. Bindu PS, Desai S, Shehanaz KE, et al: Clinical heterogeneity in Hallervorden-Spatz syndrome: a clinicoradiological study in 13 patients from South India. Brain Dev 28:343, 2006.
20. Rudolph G, Haritoglou C, Schmid I, et al: Visual loss as a first sign of adult-type chronic myeloid leukemia in a child. Am J Ophthalmol 140:750, 2005.
21. Hiraki A, Nakamura S, Abe K, et al: Numb chin syndrome as an initial symptom of acute lymphocytic

leukaemia: report of three cases. Oral Surg Oral Med Oral Pathol Oral Radiol Endod 83:555, 1997.
22. Pizzuti P, Pertuiset E, Chaumonnot F, et al: Neuromeningeal sites of multiple myeloma. Rev Med Interne 18:646, 1997.
23. Dispenzieri A: POEMS syndrome: 2011 update on diagnosis, risk-stratification, and management. Am J Hematol 86:592, 2011.
24. Li J, Zhou DB: New advances in the diagnosis and treatment of POEMS syndrome. Br J Hematol 161:303, 2013.
25. Levinson SS: POEMS syndrome: importance of the clinical laboratory practitioner's role. Clin Chim Acta 413:1800, 2012.
26. Scarlato M, Previtali SC: POEMS syndrome: the matter-of-fact approach. Curr Opin Neurol 24:491, 2011.
27. Dupont SA, Dispenzieri A, Mauermann ML, et al: Cerebral infarction in POEMS syndrome. Incidence, risk factors and imaging characteristics. Neurology 73:1308, 2009.
28. Palumbo A, Facon T, Sonneveld P, et al: Thalidomide for treatment of multiple myeloma: 10 years later. Blood 111:3968, 2008.
29. Broyl A, Corthals SL, Jongen JL, et al: Mechanisms of peripheral neuropathy associated with bortezomib and vincristine in patients with newly diagnosed multiple myeloma: a prospective analysis of data from the HOVON-65/GMMG-HD4 trial. Lancet Oncol 11:1057, 2010.
30. Mehta J, Singhal S: Hyperviscosity syndrome in plasma cell dyscrasias. Semin Thromb Hemost 29:467, 2003.
31. Ng C, Slavin MA, Seymour JF: Progressive multifocal leukoencephalopathy complicating Waldenström's macroglobulinaemia. Leuk Lymphoma 44:1819, 2003.
32. Al-Lozi MT, Pestronk A, Yee WC, et al: Myopathy and paraproteinemia with serum IgM binding to a high-molecular-weight muscle fiber surface protein. Ann Neurol 37:41, 1995.
33. Kyle RA, Therneau TM, Rajkumar SV, et al: A long term study of monoclonal gammopathy of undetermined significance. N Engl J Med 346:564, 2002.
34. Simmons Z, Albers JW, Bromberg MB, et al: Long-term follow-up of patients with chronic inflammatory demyelinating polyradiculopathy, without and with monoclonal gammopathy. Brain 118:359, 1995.
35. Willison HJ, O'Leary CP, Veitch J: The clinical and laboratory features of chronic sensory ataxic neuropathy with anti-disialosyl IgM antibodies. Brain 124:1968, 2001.
36. Ramchandren S, Lewis RA: Monoclonal gammopathy and neuropathy. Cur Opin Neurol 22:480, 2009.
37. Nuckols JD, Liu K, Burchette JL, et al: Primary central nervous system lymphomas: a 30-year experience at a single institution. Mod Pathol 12:1167, 1999.
38. Hughes M, Ahern V, Kefford R, et al: Paraneoplastic myelopathy at diagnosis in a patient with pathologic stage 1A Hodgkin disease. Cancer 70:1598, 1992.
39. Roychowdhury S, Peng R, Baiocchi RA, et al: Experimental treatment of Epstein-Barr virus-associated primary central nervous system lymphoma. Cancer Res 63:965, 2003.
40. Heesen C, Bergmann M, Figge C, et al: Intravascular lymphomatosis of the nervous system. Fortschr Neurol Psychiatr 64:234, 1996.
41. Colby TV: Current histological diagnosis of lymphomatoid granulomatosis. Mod Pathol 25(suppl 1):S39, 2012.
42. Tefferi A, Barbui T: bcr/abl-Negative, classic myeloproliferative disorders: diagnosis and treatment. Mayo Clin Proc 80:1220, 2005.
43. Poza JJ, Cobo AM, Marti-Masso JF: Peripheral neuropathy associated with polycythemia vera. Neurologia 11:276, 1996.
44. Quadri M, Federico A, Zhao T, et al: Mutations in SLC30A10 cause parkinsonism and dystonia with hypermanganesemia, polycythemia, and chronic liver disease. Am J Hum Genet 90:467, 2012.
45. Trueb RM, Pericin M, Winzeler B, et al: Eosinophilic myopathies should be distinguished from the commoner idiopathic inflammatory myopathies such as polymyositis and dermatomyositis. J Am Acad Derm 37:385, 1997.
46. Amato AA: Adults with eosinophilic myositis and calpain-3 mutations. Neurology 70:730, 2008.
47. Ogbogu PU, Bochner BS, Butterfield JH, et al: Hypereosinophilic syndrome: a multicenter, retrospective analysis of clinical characteristics and response to therapy. J Allergy Clin Immunol 124:1319, 2009.
48. Bonnaud I, Saudeau D, de Toffol B, et al: Recurrence of spontaneous subdural haematoma revealing acquired haemophilia. Eur Neurol 49:253, 2003.
49. Knoebl P, Marco P, Baudo F, et al: Demographic and clinical data in acquired hemophilia A: results from the European Acquired Haemophilia Registry (EACH2). J Thromb Haemost 10:622, 2012.
50. Pichler E, Pichler L: The neonatal coagulation system and the vitamin K deficiency bleeding—a mini review. Wien Med Wochenschr 158:385, 2008.
51. Raible MD: Hematologic complications of heparin-induced thrombocytopenia. Semin Thromb Hemost 25(suppl 1):17, 1999.
52. Pohl C, Harbrecht U, Greinacher A, et al: Neurologic complications in immune-mediated heparin-induced thrombocytopenia. Neurology 54:1240, 2000.
53. Felcher A, Commichau C, Brown MJ, et al: Disseminated intravascular coagulation and status epilepticus. Neurology 51:629, 1998.
54. Levi M, Toh CH, Thachil J, et al: Guidelines for the diagnosis and management of disseminated intravascular coagulation. British Committee for Standards in Haematology. Br J Haematol 145:24, 2009.
55. Tsai HM: Is severe deficiency of ADAMTS-13 specific for thrombotic thrombocytopenic purpura? Yes. J Thromb Haemost 1:625, 2003.

56. Vesely SK, George JN, Lammle B, et al: ADAMTS13 activity in thrombotic thrombocytopenic purpura–hemolytic uremic syndrome: relation to presenting features and clinical outcomes in a prospective cohort of 142 patients. Blood 102:60, 2003.
57. Rock G, Shumak K, Kelton J, et al: Thrombotic thrombocytopenic purpura: outcome in 24 patients with renal impairment treated with plasma exchange. Transfusion 32:719, 1992.
58. Furlan M, Robles R, Galbusera M, et al: Von Willebrand factor-cleaving proteinase in thrombotic thrombocytopaenic purpura and the hemolytic-uremic syndrome. N Engl J Med 339:1578, 1998.
59. Garg AX, Suri RS, Barrowman N, et al: Long-term renal prognosis of diarrhea-associated hemolytic uremic syndrome: a systematic review, meta-analysis, and meta-regression. JAMA 290:1360, 2003.
60. Boyer O, Niaudet P: Hemolytic uremic syndrome: new developments in pathogenesis and treatment. Int J Nephrol 2011:908407, 2011.
61. Keir LS, Marks SD, Kim JJ: Shigatoxin-associated hemolytic uremic syndrome: current molecular mechanisms and future therapies. Drug Des Devel Ther 6:195, 2012.
62. Sakakibara R, Hattori T, Mizobuchi K, et al: Axonal polyneuropathy and encephalopathy in a patient with verotoxin producing *Escherichia coli* (VTEC) infection. J Neurol Neurosurg Psychiatry 67:254, 1999.
63. Taylor MB, Jackson A, Weller JM: Dynamic susceptibility contrast enhanced MRI in reversible posterior leukoencephalopathy syndrome associated with haemolytic uraemic syndrome. Br J Radiol 73:438, 2000.
64. Nathanson S, Kwon T, Elmaleh M, et al: Acute neurological involvement in diarrhea-associated hemolytic uremic syndrome. Clin J Am Soc Nephrol 5:1218, 2010.
65. Magnus T, Rother J, Simova O, et al: The neurological syndrome in adults during the 2011 Northern German *E coli* serotype 0104:H4 outbreak. Brain 135:1850, 2012.
66. Eriksson KJ, Boyd SG, Tasker RC: Acute neurology and neurophysiology of haemolytic-uraemic syndrome. Arch Dis Child 84:434, 2001.
67. McNeill A, Duran R, Proukakis C: Hyposmia and cognitive impairment in Gaucher's disease patients and carriers. Mov Disord 27:526, 2012.
68. Pengo V, Ruffatti A, Legnani C, et al: Clinical course of high-risk patients diagnosed with antiphospholipid syndrome. J Thromb Hemost 8:237, 2010.
69. Miyakis S, Lockshin MD, Atsuma T, et al: International consensus statement on an update of the classification criteria for definite antiphospholipid syndrome (APS). J Thromb Haemost 4:295, 2006.
70. Ruiz-Irastorza G, Crowther M, Branch W, et al: Antiphospholipid syndrome. Lancet 376:1498, 2010.
71. Von Landenberg P, Matthias T, Zaech J, et al: Antiprothrombin antibodies are associated with pregnancy loss in patients with the antiphospholipid syndrome. Am J Reprod Immunol 49:51, 2003.
72. Forastiero RR, Martinuzzo ME, Cerrato GS, et al: Relationship of anti-β_2-glycoprotein I and anti-prothrombin antibodies to thrombosis and pregnancy loss in patients with antiphospholipid antibodies. Thromb Haemost 78:967, 1997.
73. Nojima J, Kuratsune H, Suehisa E, et al: Anti-prothrombin antibodies combined with lupus anticoagulant activity is an essential risk factor for venous thromboembolism in patients with systemic lupus erythematosus. Br J Haematol 114:647, 2001.
74. Lakos G, Kiss E, Regeczy N, et al: Antiprothrombin and antiannexin V antibodies imply risk of thrombosis in patients with systemic autoimmune diseases. J Rheumatol 27:924, 2000.
75. Nojima J, Kuratsune H, Suehisa E, et al: Association between the prevalence of antibodies to β_2-glycoprotein I, prothrombin, protein C, protein S, and annexin V in patients with systemic lupus erythematosus and thrombotic and thrombocytopenic complications. Clin Chem 47:1008, 2001.
76. Ogawa H, Zhao D, Dlott JS, et al: Elevated antiannexin V antibody levels in antiphospholipid syndrome and their involvement in antiphospholipid antibody specificities. Am J Clin Pathol 114:619, 2000.
77. Rand JH, Wu XX, Quinn AS, et al: The annexin A5-mediated pathogenic mechanism in the antiphospholipid syndrome: role in pregnancy losses and thrombosis. Lupus 19:460, 2010.
78. Cavaco S, Martins da Silva A, Santos E, et al: Are cognitive and olfactory dysfunctions in neuropsychiatric lupus erythematosus dependent on anxiety or depression? J Rheumatol 39:770, 2012.
79. Shoenfeld Y, Lev S, Blatt I, et al: Features associated with epilepsy in the antiphospholipid syndrome. J Rheumatol 31:1344, 2004.
80. Cervera R, Piette J-C, Font J, et al: Antiphospholipid syndrome: clinical and immunologic manifestations and patterns of disease expression in a cohort of 1,000 patients. Arthritis Rheum 46:1019, 2002.
81. Antiphospholipid Antibodies in Stroke Study Group Clinical and laboratory findings in patients with antiphospholid antibodies and cerebral ischemia. Stroke 21:1268, 1990.
82. Antiphospholipid Antibodies Stroke Study Group (APASS) Anticardiolipin antibodies and the risk of recurrent thrombo-occlusive events and death. Neurology 44:1238, 1994.
83. Levine SR, Brey RL, Tilley BC: Antiphospholipid antibodies and subsequent thrombo-occlusive events in patients with ischemic stroke. JAMA 291:576, 2004.
84. Brey RL, Abbott RD, Curb JD, et al: β_2-Glycoprotein 1-dependent anticardiolipin antibodies and risk of ischemic stroke and myocardial infarction: The Honolulu Heart Program. Stroke 32:1701, 2001.

85. Kahles T, Humpich M, Steinmetz H, et al: Phosphatidylserine IgG and β_2-glycoprotein I IgA antibodies may be a risk factor for ischaemic stroke. Rheumatology 44:1161, 2005.
86. Brey RL: Antiphospholipid antibodies in young adults with stroke. J Thromb Thrombolysis 20:105, 2005.
87. Van Goor MP, Alblas CL, Leebeck FW, et al: Do antiphospholipid antibodies increase the long-term risk of thrombotic complications in young patients with a recent TIA or ischemic stroke? Acta Neurol Scand 109:410, 2004.
88. Barnes C, Deveber G: Prothrombotic abnormalities in childhood ischaemic stroke. Thromb Res 118:67, 2006.
89. De Brujin SFT, Stam J, Koopman MMW, et al: Case-control study of risk of cerebral sinus thrombosis in oral contraceptive users who are carriers of hereditary prothrombotic conditions. BMJ 316:589, 1998.
90. Rosendaal FR, Reitsma PH: Genetics of venous thrombosis. J Thromb Haemost 7(suppl 1):301, 2009.
91. Germain M, Saut N, Greliche N, et al: Genetics of venous thrombosis: insights from a new genome wide association study. PLoS One 6:e25581, 2011.
92. Saleun S, De Moerloose P, Bura A, et al: A novel nonsense mutation in the antithrombin III gene (Cys-4→stop) causing recurrent venous thrombosis. Blood Coagul Fibrinolysis 7:578, 1996.
93. Akatsu H, Vaysburd M, Fervenza F, et al: Cerebral venous thrombosis in nephrotic syndrome. Clin Nephrol 48:317, 1997.
94. Bucciarelli P, Rosendaal FR, Tripodi A, et al: Risk of venous thromboembolism and clinical manifestations in carriers of antithrombin, protein C, protein S deficiency, or activated protein C resistance: a multicenter collaborative family study. Arterioscler Thromb Vasc Biol 19:1026, 1999.
95. Guermanzi S, Melloulli F, Trabelsi S, et al: Antithrombomodulin antibodies and venous thrombosis. Blood Coagul Fibrinolysis 15:553, 2004.
96. Dahlback B, Hillarp A, Rosen S, et al: Resistance to activated protein C, the FV:Q506 allele, and venous thrombosis. Ann Haematol 72:166, 1996.
97. Martinelli I, Landi G, Merati G, et al: Factor V gene mutation is a risk factor for cerebral venous thrombosis. Thromb Haemost 75:393, 1996.
98. Grunbacher G, Weger W, Marx-Neuhold E, et al: The fibrinogen gamma (FGG) 10034C > T polymorphism is associated with venous thrombosis. Thromb Res 121:33, 2007.
99. Arruda VR, Von Zuben PM, Chiaparini LC, et al: The mutation Ala677→Val in the methylene tetrahydrofolate reductase gene: a risk factor for arterial disease and venous thrombosis. Thromb Haemost 77:818, 1997.
100. Salomon O, Steinberg DM, Zivelin A, et al: Single and combined prothrombotic factors in patients with idiopathic venous thromboembolism: prevalence and risk assessment. Arterioscler Thromb Vasc Biol 19:511, 1999.
101. Aronow WS, Ahn C, Schoenfeld MR: Association between plasma homocysteine and extracranial carotid arterial disease in older persons. Am J Cardiol 79:1432, 1997.
102. Perry IJ, Refsum H, Morris RW, et al: Prospective study of serum total homocysteine concentration and risk of stroke in middle-aged British men. Lancet 346:1395, 1995.
103. Jenkins PV, Rawley O, Smith OP, et al: Elevated factor VIII levels and risk of venous thrombosis. Br J Haematol 157:653, 2012.
104. Bank I, Libourel EJ, Middeldorp S, et al: Elevated levels of FVIII: C within families are associated with an increased risk for venous and arterial thrombosis. J Thromb Haemost 3:79, 2005.
105. Crisan D, Mattson JC, Ahmad E, et al: Factor V Leiden detection in patients presenting with thrombotic episodes: clinical characteristics. J Clin Ligand Assay 21:418, 1998.
106. Ehrenforth S, Von Depka Prondsinski M, Aygoren Pursun E, et al: Study of the prothrombin gene 20201GA variant in FV:Q(506) carriers in relationship to the presence or absence of juvenile venous thromboembolism. Arterioscler Thromb Vasc Biol 19:276, 1999.
107. Hamedani AG, Cole JW, Mitchell BD, et al: Meta-analysis of factor V Leiden and ischaemic stroke in young adults. Stroke 41:1599, 2010.
108. Kennedy CR, Warner G, Kai M, et al: Protein C deficiency and stroke in early life. Dev Med Child Neurol 37:723, 1995.
109. Markus HS, Zhang Y, Jeffrey S: Screening for the factor-V Arg 506 Gln mutation in patients with TIA and stroke. Cerebrovasc Dis 6:360, 1996.
110. Press RD, Liu X-Y, Breamer N, et al: Ischaemic stroke in the elderly: role of the common factor V mutation causing resistance to activated protein C. Stroke 27:44, 1996.
111. Andrew M, Vegh P, Johnston M, et al: Maturation of the hemostatic system during childhood. Blood 80:1998, 1992.
112. Jerrard-Dunne P, Evans A, McGovern R, et al: Ethnic differences in markers of thrombophilia: implications for the investigation of ischemic stroke in multiethnic populations: the South London Ethnicity and Stroke Study. Stroke 34:1821, 2003.
113. Petitti DB: Hormonal contraceptives and arterial thrombosis—not risk-free but safe enough. N Engl J Med 366:2316, 2012.
114. Overell JR, Bone I, Lees KR: Interatrial septal abnormalities and stroke: a meta-analysis of case-control studies. Neurology 55:1172, 2000.
115. Chant H, McCollum C: Stroke in young adults: the role of paradoxical embolism. Thromb Haemost 85:22, 2001.

116. Karttunen V, Hiltunen L, Rasi V, et al: Factor V Leiden and prothrombin gene mutation may predispose to paradoxical embolism in subjects with patent foramen ovale. Blood Coagul Fibrinolysis 14:261, 2003.
117. Rajamani K, Chaturvedi S, Jin Z, et al: Patent foramen ovale, cardiac valve thickening, and antiphospholipid antibodies as risk factors for subsequent vascular events: the PICSS-APASS study. Stroke 40:2337, 2009.
118. Botto N, Spadoni I, Giusti S, et al: Prothrombotic mutations as risk factors for cryptogenic ischemic cerebrovascular events in young subjects with patent foramen ovale. Stroke 38:2070, 2007.
119. Pezzini A, Del Zotto E, Magoni M, et al: Inherited thrombophilic disorders in young adults with ischemic stroke and patent foramen ovale. Stroke 34:28, 2003.

CHAPTER

26

Metastatic Disease and the Nervous System

JASMIN JO ■ DAVID SCHIFF

The entire nervous system is potentially vulnerable to metastatic disease, typically occurring in the setting of a known disseminated systemic malignancy. Approximately 45 percent of patients with systemic cancer and neurologic deficits are found to have metastatic involvement of the nervous system. The most common cancer-related neurologic diagnosis is brain metastasis (16%), followed by bone metastasis (10%) and epidural metastasis (9%).[1] The incidence of metastatic involvement of the nervous system continues to rise due to improved treatment strategies directed towards primary cancers and systemic metastases. In 2012, estimated new cancer cases in the United States totaled 1.6 million people.[2]

Metastatic involvement of the central nervous system, including its overlying structures, and the peripheral nervous system causes significant neurologic morbidity and mortality. The skeletal muscles

Aminoff's Neurology and General Medicine, Fifth Edition.

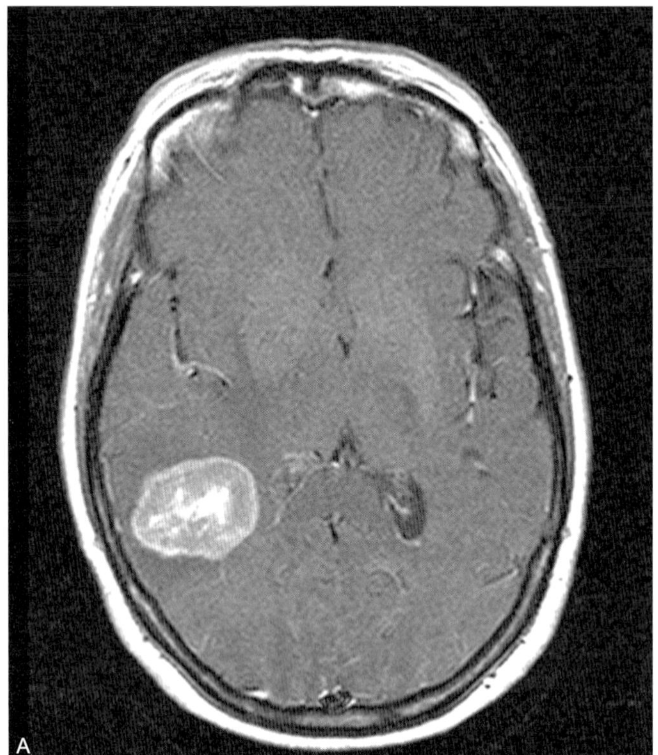

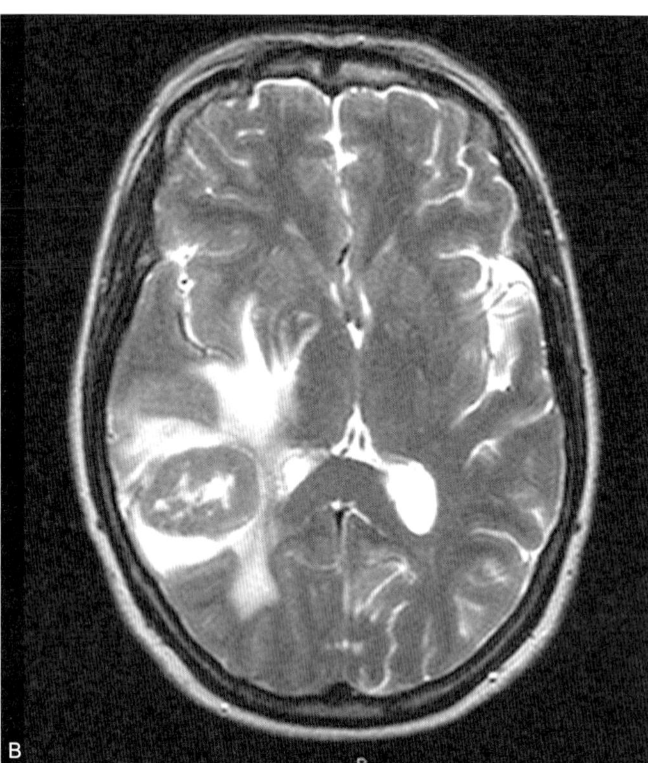

FIGURE 26-1 ■ Solitary brain metastasis in a patient with breast carcinoma. **A,** Postcontrast T1-weighted gadolinium magnetic resonance imaging (MRI) sequence demonstrating peripheral and central enhancement of a mass in the right posterior temporal lobe; **B,** T2-weighted MRI sequence demonstrates a large field of high signal with finger-like projections in the white matter extending anteriorly within the temporal lobe and posteriorly within the parietal lobe, consistent with vasogenic edema.

are affected only rarely. Early diagnosis and treatment may prevent disability in these groups of patients, who have a limited life expectancy.

METASTASES TO THE CENTRAL NERVOUS SYSTEM AND RELATED STRUCTURES

Brain

EPIDEMIOLOGY

Approximately 150,000 new cases of brain metastases occur annually in the United States, making metastases the most common intracranial tumor in adults. Brain metastases are more common in African-Americans than other ethnic groups.[3] Two population-based studies demonstrated that 8 to 10 percent of patients diagnosed with a single primary cancer develop brain metastases during their lifetime.[3,4] The incidence is highest for lung cancer (20%), followed by melanoma (7%) and then by renal (7%), breast (5%) and colorectal (2%) cancer.[3] Unknown primary sources account for up to 14 percent of cases.[5]

PATHOPHYSIOLOGY

The most common mechanism of spread to the brain is hematogenous dissemination. The "anatomic or mechanical" hypothesis states that the distribution of metastases is related to the amount of blood flow to the brain. This phenomenon explains the predilection for brain metastases to involve the cerebral hemisphere in 80 percent, cerebellum in 15 percent, and brainstem in 5 percent of cases. As cancer cells travel through the arterial circulation, they become trapped in the end arteries at the gray-white matter junction (Fig. 26-1).[6] Only about two-thirds of metastases can be explained by blood flow alone, suggesting that other factors play a role.[7] The "seed and soil" mechanism postulates that appropriate tumor cells or "seeds" grow in site-specific hosts or "soil." Brain metastases are hypothesized to result from neurotropic factors facilitating "brain-homing" and direct interaction with neural substance. The vascular basement membrane of preexisting blood vessels promotes nonsprouting angiogenesis and proliferation of metastatic tumor cells by means of tumor cell vascular endothelial growth factor (VEGF).[8–10] Contiguous brain invasion from intracranial dural and skull-base metastases is another mechanism by which brain metastases occur.[11,12]

Pathology

Grossly, metastatic tumors in the brain are well circumscribed and surrounded by edematous white matter; cystic degeneration, necrosis, and hemorrhage can be seen. Metastatic lesions from melanoma, choriocarcinoma, and renal cell carcinoma have a high tendency for intratumoral hemorrhage. Microscopically, brain metastases are usually well demarcated and generally appear histologically similar to the primary tumor. Vascular proliferation within the lesions and reactive astrocytosis in the surrounding brain parenchyma may be encountered.[13,14] Metastases from breast, kidney, and colon are usually solitary, whereas multiple metastases are common from melanoma and lung carcinoma.[15]

Clinical Features

Neurologic manifestations in patients with brain metastases may be focal, resulting from local displacement or destruction of the surrounding parenchyma by the tumor or edema, or generalized due to increased intracranial pressure (ICP) or hydrocephalus. Patients usually present with subacute or chronic progressive neurologic signs and symptoms. Headache, typically worse in the morning, is the most common presenting symptom, affecting approximately 50 percent of patients. Focal neurologic deficits are present in 30 to 40 percent of patients, and seizures are the presenting feature in 15 to 20 percent[16]; nearly 15 percent are asymptomatic.

Over 80 percent of patients diagnosed with brain metastases have a known systemic malignancy or a metachronous presentation. In 5 to 10 percent, brain metastases are diagnosed at the same time as the primary malignancy and in another 5 to 10 percent the brain metastases are the presenting manifestation. A majority of patients (more than 30%) have multiple metastases with more than four lesions, 20 to 30 percent have two to three lesions ("oligometastases"), and another 20 to 30 percent have a solitary metastasis.[11,12]

Diagnostic Studies

Magnetic resonance imaging (MRI) is the diagnostic modality of choice for the evaluation and monitoring of patients with brain metastases and is much more sensitive than computed tomography (CT) in detecting the number, size, location, and secondary effects of the lesions. Brain metastases tend to be multiple, spherical, and located at the gray-white matter junction, with surrounding vasogenic edema. These lesions appear isointense or hypointense on precontrast T1-weighted MRI sequences and enhance avidly upon contrast administration due to a disrupted blood–brain barrier. The surrounding edema is hyperintense on T2-weighted and fluid attenuated inversion recovery (FLAIR) sequences (Fig. 26-1).[17] The amount of surrounding edema is often disproportionate to the size of the lesions. Intratumoral hemorrhage within the tumor, when present, is evident on precontrast T1 and gradient recalled echo (GRE) sequencing (Fig. 26-2). CT studies are generally utilized in acute settings to determine the presence of hemorrhage, herniation, or hydrocephalus. For patients previously treated with radiation, the differentiation of tumor recurrence from radiation effects with routine MRI may be challenging. Increased glucose metabolism with [^{18}F]fluorodeoxyglucose positron emission tomography (FDG-PET) studies is characteristic for brain metastases, whereas lesions composed of radiation necrosis are frequently hypometabolic; MR perfusion imaging may also allow this distinction.

A search for primary malignancy should be performed in patients with suspected brain metastases without a known systemic cancer. CT of the chest takes precedence over abdominal and pelvic evaluation because of the high frequency of brain metastases originating from the lungs. Whole-body FDG-PET is also helpful in investigating the primary source, although it has low specificity in differentiating malignant from benign inflammatory lesions. Biopsy of tumors discovered upon systemic evaluation is often easier than biopsy or resection of the brain lesion.[13,16]

Differential Diagnosis

Several conditions mimic the radiologic findings of brain metastases including high-grade glioma,

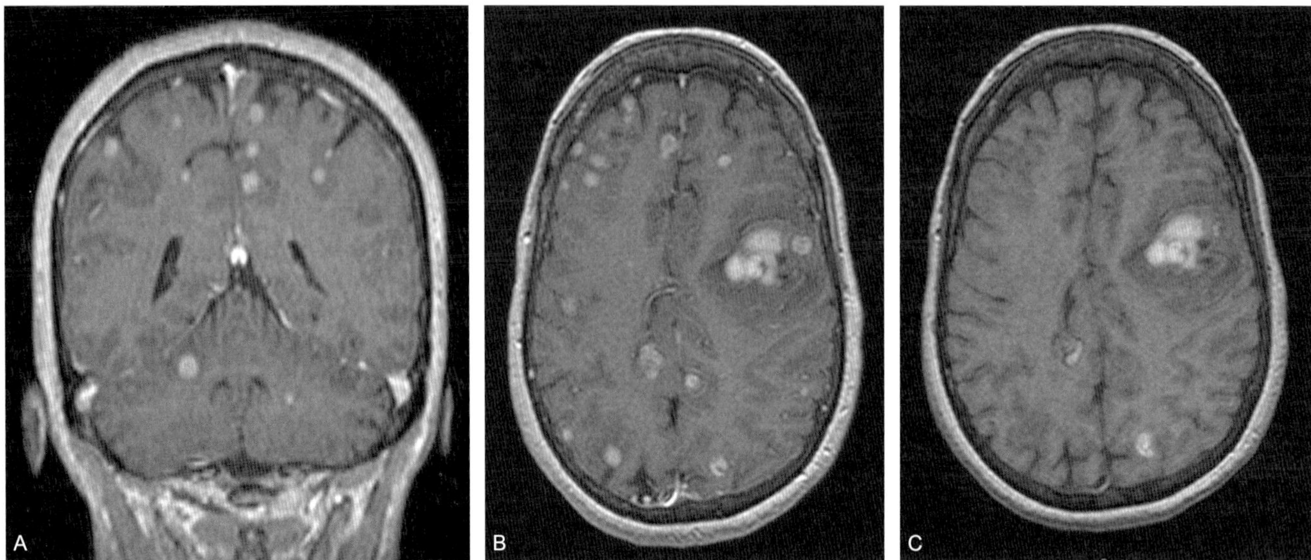

FIGURE 26-2 ■ Multiple metastases with intratumoral hemorrhage from metastatic melanoma. **A** and **B,** Numerous contrast enhancing lesions are present on T1-weighted postcontrast MR images of the supratentorial and infratentorial brain. **C,** Several lesions are present, the largest in the left frontal lobe, and show T1 shortening consistent with the presence of blood, with surrounding edema resulting in midline shift towards the contralateral side.

lymphoma, abscess, stroke, and demyelinating disorders. Different imaging techniques and special characteristics of the lesions may help distinguish between these clinical entities. An elevated cerebral blood volume in perfusion studies reflects tumor vascularity and is diminished in edema, radiation necrosis, or infarct.[18] MR spectroscopy (MRS) detects the metabolic characteristics of these lesions, differentiating spectra of metastases, gliomas, vasogenic edema, or gliosis, and other mass lesions.[17,18] Diffusion-weighted imaging (DWI) detects areas of the brain with decreased proton mobility, while the apparent diffusion coefficient (ADC) characterizes the rate of diffusional motion; unrestricted diffusion in DWI and high ADC value in the center of a ring-enhancing mass are suggestive of a necrotic mass as seen in metastasis or high-grade glioma. Restricted diffusion represents cytotoxic edema in an acute infarct, and is also seen in highly cellular lesions such as cerebral abscess, infectious encephalitis, or primary CNS lymphoma,[17,18] In many cases, brain biopsy is required for definitive diagnosis.

Prognostic Variables

Classifying patients with brain metastases based on prognosis helps clinicians maximize survival while avoiding unnecessary treatments. Important factors that predict outcomes are age, performance status, status of primary tumor, and extent of extracranial disease. The Radiation Therapy Oncology Group (RTOG) used recursive partitioning analysis (RPA) to categorize patients into three prognostic classes. Patients harboring all four favorable prognostic factors (age less than 65 years, Karnofsky performance status (KPS) of at least 70, controlled primary tumor, and no extracranial metastases) had the best prognosis, with expected median survival of 7.1 months. Patients with KPS of 70 or more but at least one other unfavorable factor have an intermediate prognosis, with expected median survival of 4.2 months. A KPS of less than 70 is a poor prognostic factor, with median survival of 2.3 months (Table 26-1).[19,20] Important prognostic factors also vary depending on tumor type. The KPS, age, presence of extracranial metastases, and number of brain metastases are prognostic factors for patients with lung cancer; KPS and number of brain metastases are prognostic factors for melanoma and renal cell carcinoma; tumor subtype, KPS, and age for breast cancer; and KPS alone for gastrointestinal cancer.[21]

Treatment

Management includes supportive care for palliation of symptoms and definitive treatment directed

TABLE 26-1 ■ Recursive Partitioning Analysis (RPA) Categorization of Patients into Three Prognostic Classes[19,20]

RPA Class	Factors	Median Survival
1	Age <65 years old KPS ≥70 Controlled primary tumor No extracranial metastases	7.1 months
2	All patients not in class 1 or 3	4.2 months
3	KPS <70	2.3 months

KPS, Karnofsky peformance status.

toward the metastases, aiming to prolong survival while preserving quality of life. Most patients die from their systemic disease rather than from their metastases.

Supportive Treatment

Dexamethasone is the corticosteroid of choice in controlling vasogenic edema, as it has a long half-life, the best CNS penetration, the fewest mineralocorticoid side effects, and is the least protein bound.[12] The recommended starting dose is 4 to 8 mg daily for symptomatic patients, and this can be increased up to 16 mg daily for patients presenting with acute signs of increased ICP. Its therapeutic effects are usually evident within 24 to 72 hours. Once clinical benefit occurs, dexamethasone should be titrated down to the lowest possible dose that provides relief of symptoms, in order to minimize adverse effects. Prophylactic treatment for peptic ulcers is generally not recommended, except for patients with a history of previous ulcer, those taking concurrent nonsteroidal anti-inflammatory drugs, or the elderly.[22,23] Among patients with brain metastases, 20 percent experience seizures, and antiepileptic drugs (AEDs) should be given when they occur. Older AEDs such as phenytoin, phenobarbital, and carbamazepine induce cytochrome P450 hepatic enzymes, which potentially can accelerate the metabolism of many chemotherapeutic agents. Because of these drug interactions, non-enzyme-inducing AEDs such as levetiracetam are preferable.[22,23] Evidence has failed to show benefit of prophylactic AEDs in decreasing the incidence of new-onset seizures, and therefore prophylaxis is not recommended.[24] The evidence of benefit for prophylactic AEDs taken only in the perioperative period is equivocal; when AEDs are utilized in this manner, they should be discontinued 1 to 2 weeks postoperatively.[23]

Surgery

Resection of brain metastases is performed to achieve local disease control, provide a histologic diagnosis, promote decompression from elevated ICP, and allow tapering of corticosteroids. Three randomized controlled trials have addressed the benefit of surgery combined with whole-brain radiation therapy (WBRT) compared to WBRT alone in patients with a solitary brain metastasis; a fourth randomized trial compared both treatments to surgery alone. These studies demonstrated significant benefits in local disease control and prolongation of functional independence from combination treatment compared to resection or radiotherapy alone, when given to patients with a single metastasis who were 60 years old or less and had controlled systemic disease and good KPS (Table 26-2).[25–28] For patients with more than one metastasis, surgery is generally limited to removal of the dominant, life-threatening lesion, and to obtain a histologic diagnosis.

Whole-Brain Radiotherapy

Treatment with WBRT targets both gross and microscopic metastases. Significant reduction of local and remote intracranial recurrence has been demonstrated in patients with solitary and oligometastases who received WBRT following surgical resection or stereotactic radiosurgery (SRS); however, overall survival and preservation of functional independence did not differ between those with or without adjuvant WBRT.[28–32] Neurocognitive complications from radiation therapy range from mild short-term memory loss to severe irreversible dementia, which may occur acutely or may be delayed for years.[33,34] Severe radiation-induced dementia is more frequent in patients who receive a short course of radiotherapy given in daily fractions, and the risk is increased for higher daily doses, particularly those exceeding 2 Gy.[34,35] Because of the lack of significant benefit in overall survival and function, it is recommended to withhold WBRT after local control with either surgery or SRS. At present, there is no recommended standard dose-fractionation

TABLE 26-2 ■ Randomized Controlled Trials of Patients with Single Brain Metastasis Treated with Surgery, Radiotherapy, or Both

	Median Survival			Duration of Functional Independence		
Population Studies	**Test Group**	**Standard**	**Result**	**Test Group**	**Standard**	**Result**
Surgery + WBRT vs WBRT $N = 48$ [Ref 25]	40 weeks	15 weeks	S	38 weeks	8 weeks	S
Surgery + WBRT vs WBRT $N = 63$ [Ref 26]	12 months	7 months	S	9 months	4 months	S
Surgery + WBRT vs WBRT $N = 84$ [Ref 27]	5.6 months	6.3 months	NS	–	–	–
Surgery + WBRT vs Surgery $N = 95$ [Ref 28]	48 weeks	43 weeks	NS	37 weeks	35 weeks	NS

WBRT, whole-brain radiotherapy; S, significant; NS, not significant.

schedule, but 30 Gy divided into 10 fractions and 20 Gy divided into 5 fractions are commonly utilized regimens. For patients with multiple metastases, WBRT is used for palliation of symptoms and is standard treatment, prolonging overall survival for up to 3 to 4 months.[36]

Stereotactic Radiosurgery

Stereotactic radiosurgery (SRS) is focused radiotherapy in which high-dose, single-fraction irradiation is directed at metastases while sparing the surrounding normal brain tissues from radiation exposure. SRS can be delivered by linear accelerator or gamma knife.[16] It is beneficial in treating lesions less than 3 cm in size that are located in the eloquent areas, in the deep structures of the brain, or both, when these are not amenable to surgery. The risk of radiation-induced neurocognitive dysfunction is markedly less than with WBRT. For patients with unresectable solitary or oligometastases with good prognostic factors (RPA class I), SRS following WBRT confers better local control of lesions and stabilization or improvement of performance status compared to WBRT alone.[37] Randomized controlled trials comparing SRS alone to SRS followed by WBRT showed improved local and remote intracranial control with combined treatment; however, overall survival and performance status were similar in both groups.[30–32]

Based on these randomized trials, close monitoring without WBRT following SRS is a reasonable option for patients with one to four brain metastases and good performance status.

Chemotherapy

Chemotherapy is recommended as first-line treatment for chemosensitive brain metastases such as germ cell tumors and non-Hodgkin lymphoma. For tumors not highly responsive to chemotherapy such as breast cancer, non–small cell lung cancer (NSCLC), and melanoma, chemotherapy is utilized as salvage therapy after radiotherapy has been exhausted.[38] Treatment response is higher for chemotherapy-naïve tumors, but as most of these patients have already failed previous chemotherapy, radiotherapy is a more effective option in the treatment of brain metastases. Agents such as capecitabine for breast cancers, temozolomide for NSCLC, and fotemustine, temozolomide, and dacarbazine for melanoma may be used.[16,38]

Targeted Therapies

Molecular targeted therapies have shown promising roles in the treatment of recurrent brain metastases, including gefitinib and erlotinib (epidermal growth factor receptor [EGFR] inhibitors) for NSCLC,[39,40] lapatinib (EGFR and HER2 inhibitors) for HER2-positive breast cancer,[41,42] sunitinib and sorafenib (VEGF receptor and platelet-derived growth factor [PDGFR] inhibitors) for renal cell carcinoma,[43,44] and dabrafenib (a B-raf inhibitor) for melanoma.[45,46]

Other Therapeutic Options

Local forms of both adjuvant chemotherapy and radiotherapy have shown some benefit in controlling local tumor recurrence. Local chemotherapy with carmustine wafers (Gliadel) placed directly in the tumor bed has shown low local recurrence rates following resection and radiotherapy. [47] Brachytherapy is a form of localized radiotherapy where a radioactive source is placed in the surgical cavity; brachytherapy using the GliaSite Radiotherapy System has demonstrated local control comparable to WBRT and SRS.[48]

Prophylactic Cranial Irradiation

In malignancies with a high predilection to metastasize to the brain such as small cell lung cancer (SCLC), prophylactic cranial radiation may be used. Patients with SCLC and limited or extensive systemic disease who respond to chemotherapy have decreased incidence of brain metastases from 40 to 14.6 percent, improvement of disease-free survival from 12 to 14.7 weeks, and overall survival improvement from 5.4 to 6.7 months with prophylactic cranial irradiation.[49,50] This prophylactic strategy did not show the same degree of benefit in NSCLC.[51] In long-term survivors of operable NSCLC treated with neoadjuvant chemoradiotherapy, neurocognitive function was not affected by whether prophylactic cranial irradiation was provided.[52]

Skull Base

Definition and Epidemiology

The base of the skull forms the floor of the cranial cavity and is composed of the ethmoid, sphenoid, occipital, paired frontal, and paired parietal bones. Metastases to the skull base may involve the cranial nerves and blood vessels that pass through foramina in these bones.[53] Skull-base metastases occur in 4 percent of cancer patients, frequently late in the course of the disease. The most common responsible primary malignancies are prostate (38.5%), breast (20.5%), lymphoma (8%), and lung (6%).[54]

Pathophysiology

The skull base may become involved directly from hematogenous spread of malignant cells or by retrograde seeding through the Batson plexus, a common route in prostate carcinoma.[54] Osseous metastases may entrap and compress the nearby cranial nerves and vessels, producing neurologic signs and symptoms. Direct extension from head and neck malignancies may also involve the skull base.[55]

Clinical Features

Skull-base metastases produce symptoms when they enlarge and compress surrounding structures, causing pain and neurologic deficits. The development of cranial neuropathies or craniofacial pain in patients with malignancy should raise the suspicion of skull-base metastases.[55] Cranial neuropathies are the presenting symptom in 28 percent of patients with such metastases.[54] The anatomic location involved can lead to specific clinical syndromes, including parasellar and sellar syndromes in 29 percent, middle fossa syndromes in 6 percent, and jugular foramen syndromes in 3.5 percent of patients (Table 26-3).[54]

Diagnostic Studies

Advances in MRI techniques have greatly improved the identification and evaluation of the extent of skull-base metastases, including bone marrow invasion, perineural spread, and cranial nerve, leptomeningeal, and brain parenchymal involvement (Fig 26-3).[56] Radionuclide bone scanning can detect skull-base metastases in 30 to 50 percent of these patients, but it has a relatively poor sensitivity in detecting purely lytic lesions.[57] CT using bone windowing is the best means of detecting lytic bone destruction.[54] Dual-isotope single-photon emission computed tomography (SPECT) may show increased uptake in the skull base. CSF examination and biopsy are sometimes indicated to establish the diagnosis of skull-base metastases.[53,54]

Differential Diagnosis

Primary skull tumors, such as osteoma and chondrosarcoma, and benign tumor-like lesions including fibrous dysplasia may appear radiographically similar to skull-base metastases. Patients with metastases

TABLE 26-3 ■ Skull-Base Syndromes, Associated Cranial Neuropathies, Accompanying Findings, and Most Common Primary Malignancies[53,54]

Skull-Base Syndromes	Cranial Neuropathies	Associated Findings	Common Primary Malignancies
Orbital syndrome	CN II, III, IV, VI and V-1	Supraorbital frontal headache, pain, diplopia, proptosis, periorbital swelling, decreased vision	Prostate cancer Lymphoma Breast cancer
Parasellar/Cavernous sinus syndrome	CN III, IV, VI and V-1 and V-2	Supraorbital frontal headache, no proptosis, vision may be affected late in the course	Lymphoma
Middle fossa/Gasserian ganglion syndrome	CN V-2 and V-3 sensory and motor roots; CN III, IV, VI and VII (less common)	Lightning-like facial pain, sparing the forehead; headache is uncommon	Breast cancer Lung cancer
Jugular foramen syndrome	CN IX, X and XI (Vernet syndrome) plus CN XII (Collet–Sicard syndrome)	Unilateral occipital and postauricular pain; Horner syndrome (Villaret syndrome)	Breast cancer Melanoma Ewing sarcoma Prostate cancer
Occipital condyle	CN XII	Occipital pain, stiff neck	Breast cancer Prostate cancer
Numb chin syndrome	Mental nerve	Unilateral anesthesia of chin and lower lip	Breast cancer Lymphoma Melanoma Lung cancer Prostate

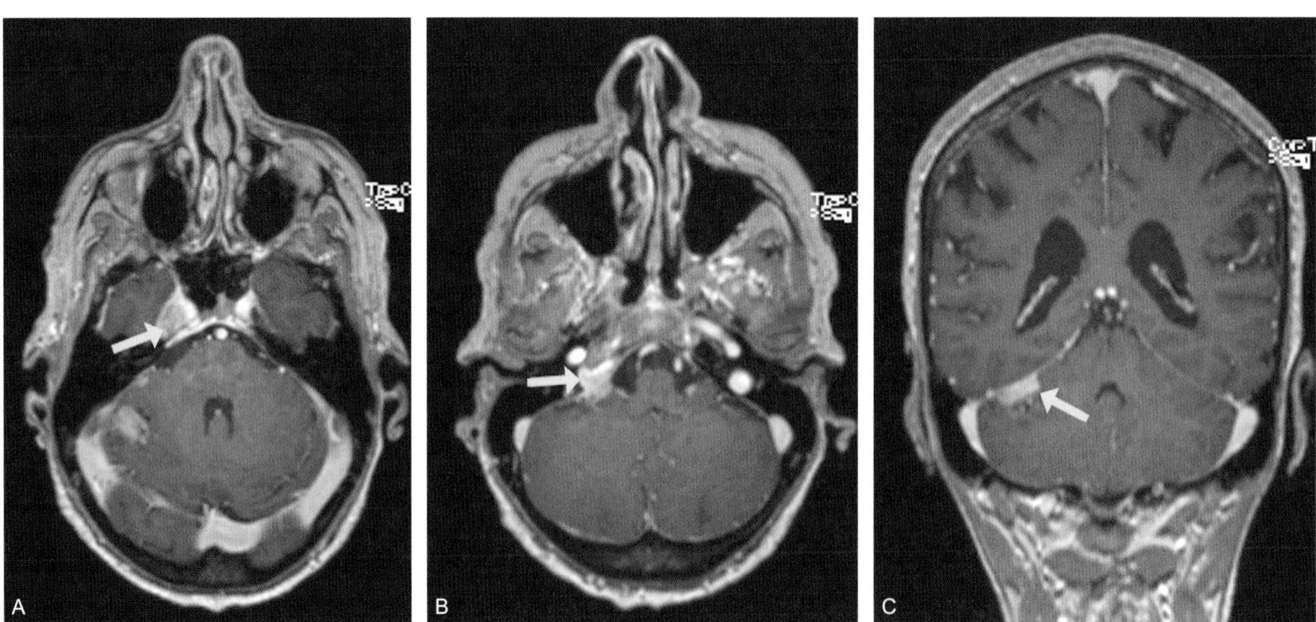

FIGURE 26-3 ■ Skull-base metastases. A 73-year-old patient with history of non–small cell lung carcinoma presented with right cavernous sinus syndrome. MRI demonstrates multiple avidly enhancing lesions within (**A**) the right Meckel cave and (**B**) the right jugular foramen. Dural-based metastases also are seen (**C**) along the inferior surface of the right tentorium.

are generally older, with a median age of 70 years, have shorter duration of symptoms (median of 2 months), and present less frequently with neurologic deficits than patients with these other lesions.[58]

Treatment

Radiation therapy is the standard treatment, providing pain relief and improvement of cranial nerve dysfunction.[54] The beneficial effects parallel the timing of irradiation—87 percent of patients who receive radiation within 1 month of symptom onset show clinical improvement compared with 25 percent of patients treated after 3 months.[59] Stereotactic radiosurgery provides clinical improvement in 62 percent and tumor control in 67 percent of patients, and can be used as an initial treatment, especially for lesions near neural structures and for previously irradiated tumors.[54] For chemosensitive tumors such as breast and prostate carcinomas, chemotherapy and hormonal therapy in combination with radiation therapy offer survival benefits.[54,60] Surgery may be considered for radioresistant tumors such as melanoma, renal cell carcinomas, and sarcomas, as well as in patients with rapid neurologic decline, such as visual loss, with the goal of preserving neurologic status and symptom relief.[55,60]

Prognosis

Skull-base metastases are typically seen in disseminated malignancies, and the overall median survival is 31 months. Patients with metastases from breast carcinoma have the best survival (60 months); prostate carcinoma and lymphoma, intermediate survival; and lung and colon carcinomas the worst survival (2.5 and 2.1 months, respectively).[54]

Intracranial Dura

Definition and Epidemiology

Carcinomatous infiltration of the dura and epidural space is found at autopsy in 9 percent of patients with primary malignancies.[61] Common primary tumors include breast, prostate, and lung carcinomas. They are more common in women; the mean age at diagnosis is 59 years.[62,63]

Pathophysiology

A majority of patients develop intracranial dural metastases by direct extension from skull metastases, whereas hematogenous spread accounts for 33 to 43 percent.[62,63] Nontraumatic subdural hematoma occurs in 15 to 40 percent of patients, presumably due to rupture of fragile tumor vessels and to mechanical obstruction of external dural vessels leading to dilation and rupture of dural capillaries.[62] Chronic subdural hematoma alters the barrier properties of the dura, promoting tumor infiltration.[64]

Clinical Features

Dural metastases produce symptoms through traction of the dura, invasion of venous sinuses, elevation of ICP, and compression of the underlying brain parenchyma, cavernous sinus, and surrounding neural structures. Common presentations include headache, cranial neuropathies, visual changes, altered mentation, and seizures.[63] The presence of new or localized headache in these patients is suggestive of subdural hematoma and should prompt imaging.[62] Between 11 and 20 percent of patients are asymptomatic, diagnosed incidentally on imaging or at autopsy.[62,63]

Diagnostic Studies and Differential Diagnosis

Gadolinium-enhanced MRI is the imaging study of choice for identification of dural metastases. These lesions typically enhance homogeneously and may be single or multiple. They may appear as localized or diffuse thickening or nodular enhancement of the dura (Fig. 26-4). CT scan can detect bony involvement.[53,62,63] The main differential diagnosis is meningioma, which also presents as an extraaxial, well-circumscribed, hyperdense, contrast-enhancing lesion with a dural tail and hyperostosis of overlying bone. High lipid signal in MR spectroscopy, a low relative cerebral blood volume in dynamic contrast (perfusion) MRI, increased FDG-PET uptake, and accumulation of tracer in octreotide brain scintigraphy all favor metastasis over meningioma.[65–67] Pachymeningeal metastases demonstrate dural enhancement localized under the inner table of the skull and do not follow the contour of the gyri in contrast to leptomeningeal involvement.[62]

Treatment

Surgical resection improves overall survival and should be considered as initial treatment for patients

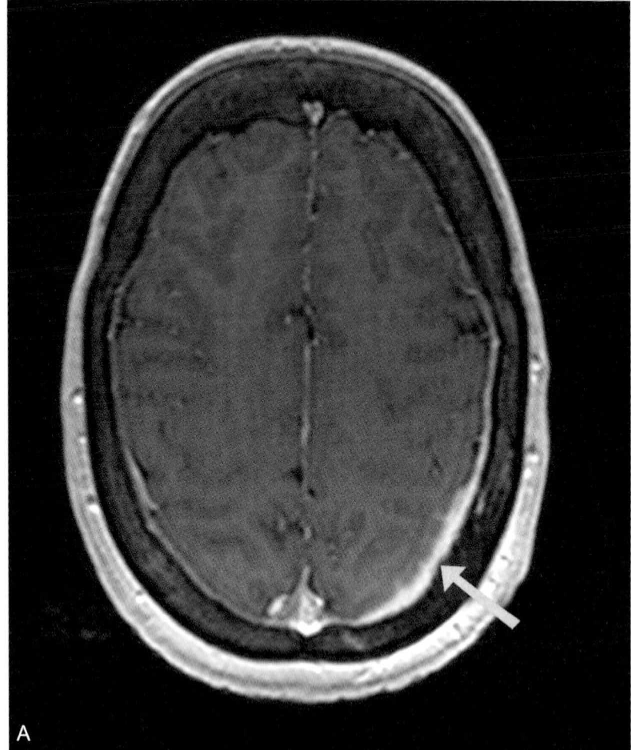

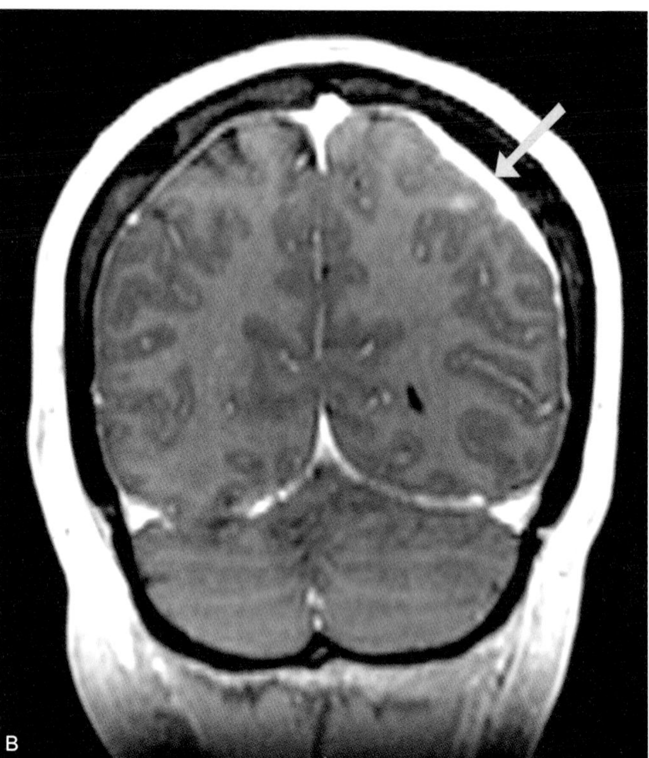

FIGURE 26-4 ■ Dural metastasis from breast cancer. Axial (**A**) and coronal (**B**) T1-weighted, contrast-enhanced brain MR images demonstrating dural thickening along the left parietal convexity.

with controlled systemic disease and a single, symptomatic, resectable intracranial dural metastasis.[63] Systemic chemotherapy also prolongs progression-free survival perhaps due to breakdown of the blood–brain barrier in dural metastases.[63] For patients who are not candidates for surgery, have poor performance status, and short life expectancy, focal or whole-brain radiation is considered.[53,62,63]

Prognosis

The overall median survival is 6 to 9.5 months and progression-free survival is 3.7 months with dural metastases.[62,63] Patients with primary hematologic malignancies or breast and prostate carcinomas have relatively favorable courses compared to those with other primary cancers.[62] Poor performance status and lung carcinoma are adverse prognostic factors, while treatment with resection and chemotherapy is associated with improved overall and progression-free survival.[63]

Spine and Spinal Cord

Epidemiology

Bone is the most common site of metastases, and the axial skeleton is the most frequent site affected. Autopsy series reveal spinal metastasis in more than 70 percent of patients with disseminated cancer. The incidence is greatest for breast (73%) and prostate (68%) cancers, followed by thyroid (42%), kidney (35%), and lung (36%) cancers.[68] Spinal metastases are 20 times more common than primary spinal tumors.[69]

Classification by Anatomic Location

Spinal tumors are classified according to anatomic location (Table 26-4).[70] Extradural metastases account for more than 94 percent of secondary spinal tumors. Most arise from the vertebral bodies and extend to the spinal canal, eventually compressing the spinal cord or cauda equina. Intradural

TABLE 26-4 ■ Anatomic Categories of Spinal Cord Tumors

Anatomic Locations	Tumors
Extradural	Metastases Chordomas Sarcomas Lymphomas Plasmacytomas and multiple myeloma
Intradural, extramedullary	Meningioma Nerve sheath tumors
Intramedullary	Ependymomas Astrocytomas Metastases

extramedullary metastases are rare and usually represent tertiary spread via CSF from cerebral metastases to the cauda equina, termed "drop metastasis." Intramedullary metastases account for about 3.5 percent of spinal metastases and are increasing in frequency, likely due to improvement in detection.[69]

Epidural Spinal Cord Compression

Epidemiology

The annual incidence of hospitalization related to epidural spinal cord compression among patients with cancer is 3.4 percent. The most common primary sources are lung and prostate cancer, and multiple myeloma.[71] The thoracic spine is most commonly involved (70%), followed by the lumbar (20%) and cervical (10%) spine; this distribution reflects the number and volume of vertebral bodies in each spinal segment. Multiple noncontiguous lesions are common, occurring in 10 to 40 percent of cases.[72,73]

Pathophysiology

Epidural spinal cord compression results from several mechanisms. Hematogenous spread is the most common route, occurring in 85 percent of cases. The Batson venous plexus drains the vertebrae and skull and forms anastomoses with veins draining the thoracic, abdominal, and pelvic organs and breast. This valveless venous system serves as a pathway to transmit metastatic cells to the spinal column. Tumor cells may also seed via the arterial circulation to the vertebral bodies, which have a relatively large blood flow. Metastatic cells cause vertebral bone destruction, mass expansion within the vertebral body, and eventual outgrowth into the epidural space. Less commonly, tumor cells from the paraspinal region reach the epidural space directly through the intervertebral foramen, particularly in patients with lymphoma and neuroblastoma. Direct hematogenous metastasis to the epidural space is rare.[69,74–76]

Direct mechanical injury to the axons and myelin, along with secondary vascular compromise of the epidural venous plexus and spinal arteries, results in spinal cord edema, infarction, and subsequent dysfunction. Tumor production of VEGF is also associated with spinal cord hypoxia.[74–76] In addition, tumor invasion of the bony spine can harm the spinal cord by destabilization of the spinal column.[76]

Clinical Features

Back pain is the most common presenting symptom, affecting more than 95 percent of patients with epidural spinal cord compression. The pain is initially localized over the involved vertebral bodies and is attributable to stretching of the periosteum and other adjacent pain-sensitive structures. It is typically chronic, with a median duration of 2 months, and increases in severity over time. It is frequently worse with the Valsalva maneuver and recumbency as a result of distention of the venous plexus. When nerve roots are involved, patients may complain of radicular pain or a tight band around the chest and abdomen. Acute pain raises the suspicion of pathologic compression fracture.[74–76] Motor deficits are the second most common symptom (60 to 85%) followed by sensory symptoms (60%). The weakness may be upper motor neuron in type from compression of the spinal cord when the lesion is above the L1-2 vertebral bodies, or lower motor neuron in type from compression of the cauda equina when the lesion is below this level. More than half of patients with epidural spinal cord compression are nonambulatory upon diagnosis.[74,75] Spinal cord compression produces a sensory level at or above the level of epidural involvement, and nerve root compression results in a dermatomal pattern of sensory deficits. Patients with compression of the posterior columns in the cervical and upper thoracic segments of the spinal cord may experience Lhermitte phenomenon. Autonomic symptoms, including bowel and

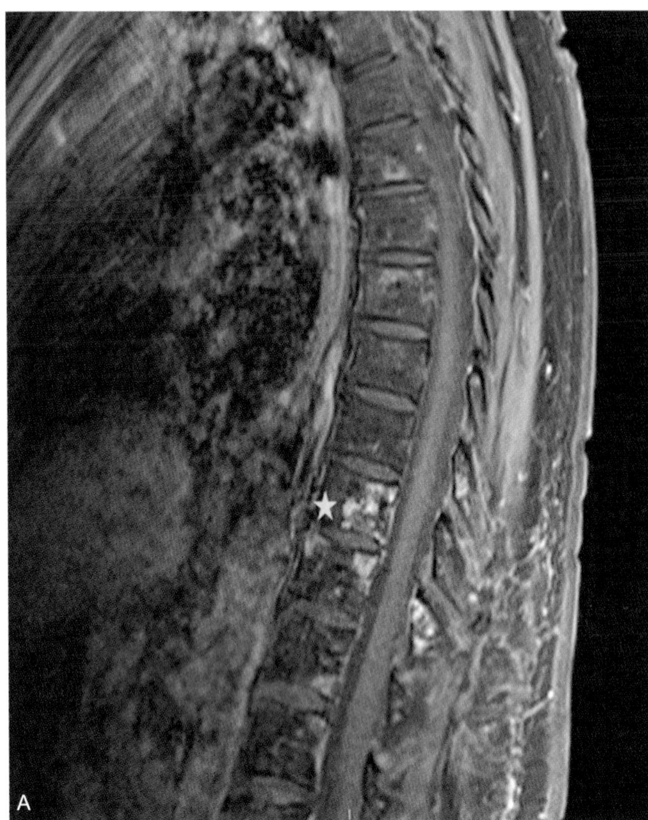

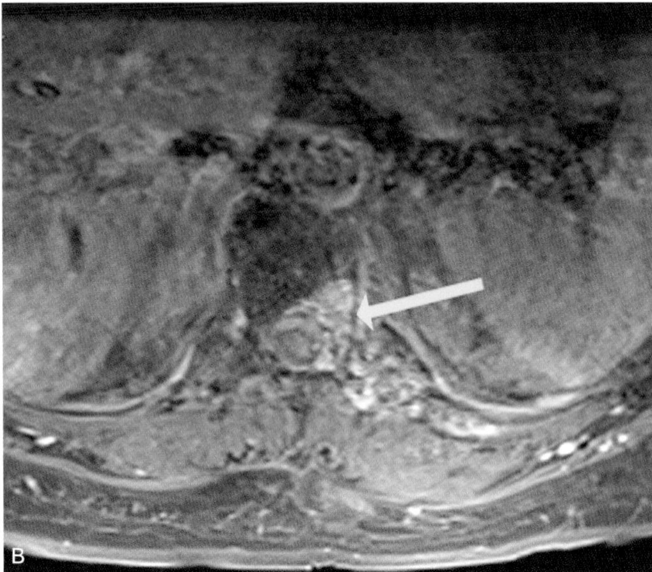

FIGURE 26-5 ■ Epidural spinal cord compression secondary to metastatic breast cancer. Postcontrast MRI demonstrates (**A**) numerous metastatic lesions involving nearly all the thoracic vertebral bodies, with greatest involvement at the T9 vertebral body (*star*). There is mild neuroforaminal encroachment by the tumor at the left T9-10 level (**B**).

bladder dysfunction, sexual disturbance, and orthostatic hypotension, tend to occur late in the course of epidural spinal cord compression.[74,75]

Diagnostic Studies

Epidural spinal cord compression is a neuro-oncologic emergency as neurologic deficits may progress rapidly. MRI is optimal for detecting the lesion, with an overall accuracy of at least 95 percent.[77] Because multiple lesions are common, the entire spine should be imaged.[78] Vertebral metastases appear hypointense on T1-weighted MRI sequences, hyperintense on T2-weighted sequences, and show postgadolinium enhancement (Fig. 26-5). Increased T2 signal within the spinal cord represents venous congestion or ischemia.[75] For patients in whom MRI is contraindicated, CT myelography is an acceptable alternative.[73] Plain radiography, bone scans, and spinal CT do not adequately depict the tumor, spinal cord, and paraspinal region.[74,75] Around 80 percent of patients with epidural spinal cord compression have a known systemic malignancy, and immediate treatment should be initiated once the diagnosis is made.[75] For patients without prior history of cancer, biopsy of the paraspinal or vertebral lesion to make a tissue diagnosis is warranted.

Treatment

The goals of treatment are pain relief and preservation or recovery of neurologic function. Corticosteroids, typically dexamethasone, are recommended for patients with neurologic deficits.[79] They may temporarily stabilize neurologic dysfunction by reducing tumor and spinal cord edema, alleviate pain through antiprostaglandin effects, and have a direct cytotoxic effect on certain malignancies such as lymphoma and multiple myeloma.[75,76] Patients with minimal or nonprogressive weakness may receive moderate dexamethasone doses (e.g., 8 to 10 mg loading dose, followed by 16 mg/d in divided doses). Some treat patients with rapidly progressive motor symptoms with higher doses, such as with a 100 mg loading dose followed by up to 96 mg/d.[76,80] When these high doses are used, rapid taper is important to minimize the risk of complications such as steroid myopathies and peptic ulcers.

Prompt surgical consultation following radiographic diagnosis is recommended. The objectives of surgery include obtaining a histologic diagnosis, local tumor control, pain relief, spinal cord decompression, restoration of neurologic status, reestablishment of spine stability, and correction of deformity.[80] Compared to patients treated with radiotherapy alone, patients undergoing timely surgery followed by radiation are more likely to recover or maintain ambulation, achieve better pain control, have preservation of continence, and experience longer median survival.[81] Patients with a good prognosis, who are medically and surgically operable, benefit from surgery, but those patients with life expectancy of less than 3 to 6 months are poor surgical candidates.[79,80]

All patients who are not candidates for surgery should be treated with radiotherapy, which improves back pain (in 60% of patients), ambulation (70%), and continence (90%).[82] Important predictors of response to radiotherapy include performance status at the start of treatment, tumor radiosensitivity, and rapidity of onset of neurologic deficits.[74,75] Radiosensitive tumors such as myeloma, lymphoma, seminoma, and prostate and breast carcinomas respond better than generally radioresistant metastases such as melanoma, osteosarcoma, and renal cell carcinoma.[74,75] For patients with a poor prognosis, two fractions of 8 Gy given 1 week apart are recommended, while those with a good prognosis are given higher total doses with more fractions.[79] The most common dose and fractionation schedule being utilized in the United States is 30 Gy divided into 10 fractions.[75]

The effectiveness of conventional radiotherapy to spinal metastases is limited due to poor radiation tolerance of the spinal cord. For this reason, the role of SRS in the treatment of spinal metastases is under investigation, allowing safe delivery of high-dose radiation to metastases within or adjacent to the vertebral bodies and spinal cord, while minimizing toxicity to the surrounding structures.[80,83,84] SRS is highly effective in reducing pain, with an overall improvement rate of approximately 85 to 100 percent, leading to long-term radiographic tumor control in 88 to 90 percent of patients.[83,85] SRS can be used both in previously irradiated patients and with relatively radioresistant tumors.[80] Because SRS has a steep fall-off gradient of target dose with negligible skin effects, it can be given soon after surgery without concern for wound complications. Complications of SRS are generally mild and self-limited.[83] However, despite promising preliminary results, high-quality data on SRS for spine metastases are still lacking.

Chemotherapy has a limited role in patients with epidural spinal cord compression because of the need to decompress the spinal cord urgently in order to preserve neurologic functions. In patients with chemosensitive tumors such as lymphoma and seminoma who have minimal or no neurologic deficits, chemotherapy may be considered.[75]

Prognosis

The median survival following diagnosis of metastatic epidural spinal cord compression is 3 to 6 months. The strongest factors affecting survival include the degree of neurologic deficit at the time of diagnosis and the primary tumor type. Patients with breast cancer have the longest survival, while those with carcinoma of the lung have the shortest. Nonambulatory patients do poorly, and those with bladder and bowel dysfunction have the worst prognosis.[73]

Intramedullary Spinal Cord Metastases

Epidemiology and Pathophysiology

Intramedullary spinal cord metastases are rare, usually encountered in the setting of extensive metastatic disease. These metastases are typically solitary and can occur in any segment of spinal cord.[86] The majority of patients have concomitant brain metastases and around 25 percent have leptomeningeal carcinomatosis. Almost half of intramedullary spinal cord metastases originate from lung cancer, particularly small cell lung cancer; less common primary neoplasms are melanoma, lymphoma, and breast, colorectal, and renal cell cancer.[74,75,87] Tumor cells reach the parenchyma of the spinal cord by hematogenous dissemination, direct extension from leptomeninges, along nerve roots, or through Virchow–Robin spaces.[75]

Clinical Features

Weakness is present in 90 percent of patients at the time of diagnosis. Other common presentations are

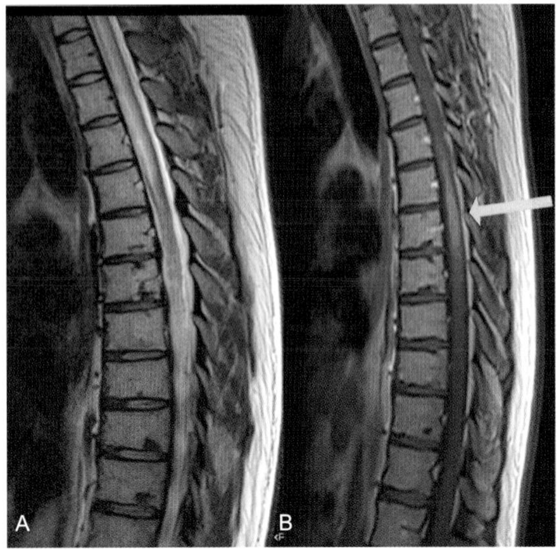

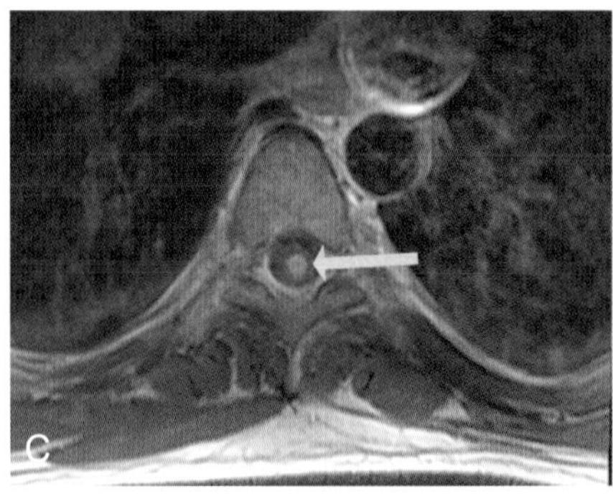

FIGURE 26-6 ■ Intramedullary spinal cord metastases from parotid salivary ductal carcinoma. **A,** Diffuse expansile hyperintense T2 signal within the thoracic cord. **B** and **C,** Enhancing intramedullary lesion, centered at the level of T6.

sensory loss, sphincter dysfunction, back pain, and radicular pain.[88] Neurologic deficits develop much earlier, usually soon after the onset of spinal or radicular pain, than in patients with epidural spinal cord compression. The presence of a Brown-Séquard syndrome or asymmetric myelopathy strongly suggests intramedullary rather than epidural metastases.[87] Intramedullary metastases may be mistaken for radiation myelopathy, but can be differentiated by the slow and relatively painless presentation of the latter.[75]

Diagnostic Studies

MRI with gadolinium enhancement reliably identifies intramedullary metastases, which appear as well-defined lesions with avid contrast enhancement that are hypointense on T1- and hyperintense on T2-weighted sequences; prominent surrounding edema is common (Fig. 26-6). Spinal MRI may also detect concomitant leptomeningeal involvement.[74] Brain MRI should be performed even in the absence of cerebral symptoms, as concurrent brain metastases are common.[75]

Treatment and Prognosis

Fractionated radiotherapy is the main treatment modality for intramedullary metastases. The goals of radiotherapy are to control tumor growth, palliate symptoms, and improve neurologic deficits.[74,75] With the development of new techniques including MR or CT navigation, cavitron ultrasonic surgical aspiration, and intraoperative electrophysiologic monitoring, surgical excision has been used increasingly in patients with limited systemic disease and radioresistant tumors.[75,88] In general, patients with intramedullary spinal cord metastases have a limited response to treatment and a very poor prognosis, with a median survival of 4 months.[86]

Leptomeninges

DEFINITION

Leptomeningeal metastasis or neoplastic meningitis refers to the dissemination of cancer cells to the CSF, pia, and arachnoid mater.[89] Depending on the underlying malignancy, this condition may be termed leptomeningeal carcinomatosis, lymphomatous meningitis, or leukemic meningitis.[90]

EPIDEMIOLOGY

Leptomeningeal carcinomatosis is diagnosed in 1 to 5 percent of patients with solid cancers and 5 to 15 percent of those with hematologic malignancies. It also occurs in 1 to 2 percent of patients with primary brain tumors.[91] The most common solid tumor sources are breast (43%) and lung (31%) carcinomas, while the most common hematologic tumor sources are lymphoma (57%) and leukemia

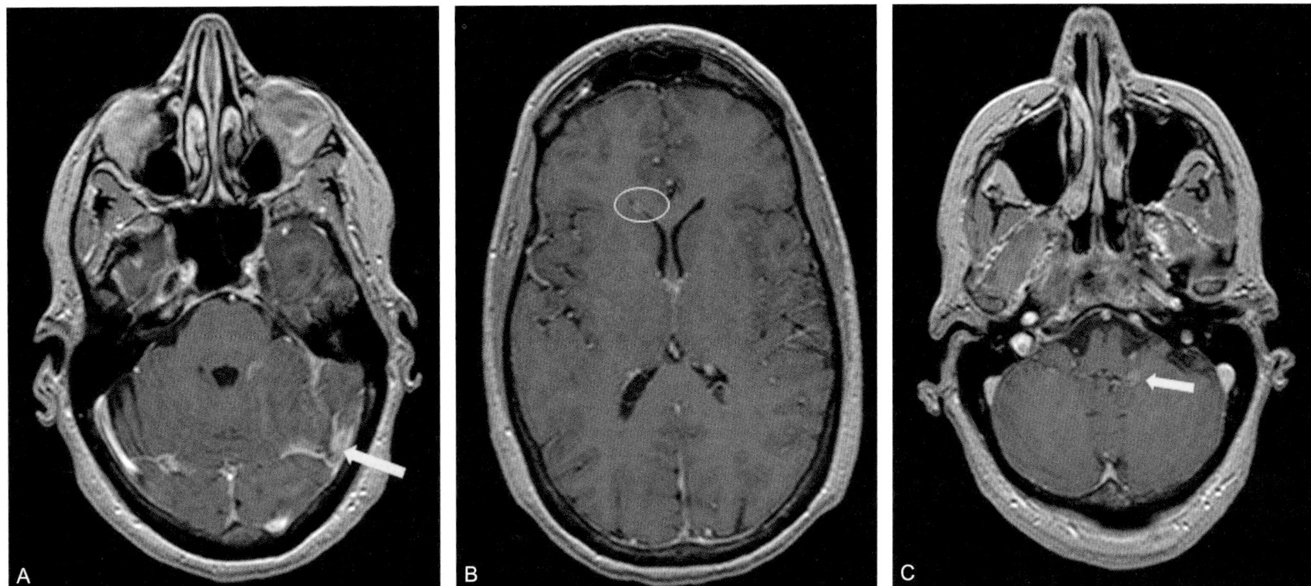

FIGURE 26-7 ■ Leptomeningeal metastasis from breast carcinoma. Postcontrast MRI demonstrates leptomeningeal enhancement along the left superior cerebellar surface (**A**), the margin of the frontal horn of the right lateral ventricle (**B**), and the left foramen of Luschka (**C**).

(41%). The median age of diagnosis is 56 years and median KPS is 70.[92] Approximately 19 percent of cancer patients with neurologic signs and symptoms have evidence of leptomeningeal metastases on autopsy studies.[93]

Pathophysiology

Leptomeningeal seeding occurs through several mechanisms, including hematogenous spread via Batson plexus or arterial dissemination, direct extension from adjacent structures, and migration from systemic tumors along perineural or perivascular spaces. Once tumor cells reach the leptomeninges, they can spread throughout the CNS via the CSF, resulting in multifocal neuraxis seeding. Tumor infiltration is most prominent in the skull base, the posterior surface of the spinal cord, and cauda equina, producing cranial nerve palsies and radiculopathies. Tumor deposits may result in obstruction of CSF flow, leading to hydrocephalus and sometimes to increased ICP. Blood vessels crossing the subarachnoid space may become occluded, leading to cerebral or spinal infarction.[89–91]

Clinical Features

Clinical manifestations of leptomeningeal metastases can be classified into three categories: cerebral involvement resulting in headache, altered mental status, nausea, vomiting, gait disturbance, and cerebellar signs; cranial nerve involvement presenting with diplopia, visual loss, hearing changes, and facial weakness; and spinal symptoms including weakness, paresthesias, radicular neck or back pain, and bowel or bladder dysfunction.[89,90] The majority of patients present with multifocal symptoms.[90]

Diagnostic Studies

Gadolinium-enhanced MRI of the entire neuraxis is warranted to evaluate the extent of CNS disease and plan treatment. Neuroimaging should precede lumbar puncture as intracranial hypotension from lumbar puncture may produce pachymeningeal enhancement that mimics leptomeningeal metastases.[90]

MRI findings that are highly suggestive of leptomeningeal metastases include linear or nodular enhancement of leptomeninges, which is often visible in the cerebral sulci, cerebellar folia, basal cisterns, and cauda equina; enhancement of the subependyma, and cranial or spinal nerves; and hydrocephalus (Fig. 26-7).[89,90] A high clinical suspicion of leptomeningeal metastases coupled with consistent MRI findings is sufficient to establish the diagnosis, even in the absence of a positive CSF cytology.

While identifying malignant cells in the CSF is the gold standard for diagnosis, its sensitivity is low. To minimize false-negative studies, the following measures are recommended: withdrawal of at least 10.5 ml of CSF for analysis; immediate processing of the sample; obtaining CSF from a site adjacent to the affected CNS region; and repeated CSF sampling and analysis.[94] The sensitivity of CSF cytology is 71 percent for the first sample, 86 percent after two samples, 90 percent following three samples, and up to 93 percent after more than three samples.[94] Flow cytometry analysis improves this sensitivity for patients with hematologic malignancies.[89] Other CSF parameters suggestive of leptomeningeal metastases are elevated opening pressure, elevated leukocyte count, increased protein content, and decreased glucose level.[92] CSF flow block develops at various levels in 30 to70 percent of patients with leptomeningeal metastases and can be seen with radionuclide studies.[91]

Treatment

Goals of treatment are to improve or stabilize neurologic function, maintain quality of life, and prolong survival.[91] Treatment optimally should be directed towards the entire neuraxis, as tumor cells are disseminated widely throughout the CSF. Radiotherapy provides palliation of symptoms, treatment of bulky disease, and restoration of CSF flow. Patients with breast cancer, leukemia, and lymphoma have a higher likelihood than those with other malignancies of responding to radiotherapy.[89] However, craniospinal radiotherapy is rarely employed because of its significant adverse effects such as gastrointestinal toxicity, mucositis, and bone marrow suppression, and the lack of significant improvement in survival compared to chemotherapy.[90,91]

Chemotherapy can be given systemically or by the intrathecal route. For systemic chemotherapy, penetration of the blood–brain barrier is an important goal. Certain chemotherapeutic drugs achieve a therapeutic level of CSF penetration when given in high doses, including methotrexate (3 to 8 g/m^2) or cytarabine (3 g/m^2). Other drugs that can cross the blood–brain barrier are capecitabine, thiotepa, and temozolomide. Tumor histology and response to prior drug exposure guide the choice of chemotherapeutic agent.[90,91]

Intrathecal delivery has several advantages over systemic chemotherapy, including circumvention of the blood–brain barrier and reduction of systemic adverse effects because the drug is delivered directly into the subarachnoid space, and reduced overall dosage.[95] Agents primarily given by the intrathecal route are methotrexate, cytarabine (Ara-C), and the longer-acting liposomal cytarabine (Depocyt). Randomized trials demonstrated no difference in survival using single-agent methotrexate or thiotepa compared to a combination of methotrexate, thiotepa, and cytarabine.[91,96] Intrathecal administration of rituximab, an anti-CD20 monoclonal antibody, and trastuzumab, an anti–human epidermal growth factor receptor (HER-2) monoclonal antibody, has been investigated for lymphomatous meningitis and HER-2–positive breast leptomeningeal metastases, respectively.[97–99]

Intrathecal agents can be delivered via lumbar puncture or intraventricular (Ommaya) reservoir. Repeated lumbar punctures are inconvenient for patients, may result in inadvertent delivery of drugs outside the thecal sac, and produce a more variable drug concentration than intraventricular administration. Although ventricular reservoirs are usually well tolerated, complications such as misplacement, catheter tip occlusion, and infection may occur.[89]

Aggressive supportive treatment should be given to all patients with leptomeningeal metastases including corticosteroids for vasogenic edema and increased ICP, AEDs for seizures, opioid drugs for adequate analgesia, and antidepressants and anxiolytics as needed.[89,91]

Prognosis

The median survival for untreated leptomeningeal metastases is 4 to 6 weeks, and death often results from progressive neurologic dysfunction. With treatment, median survival is increased to 4 to 8 months.[89,91] Patients with hematologic tumors have improved survival (median of 4.7 months) compared with solid tumors (median of 2.3 months).[92] The National Comprehensive Cancer Network suggests stratifying patients into either good- or poor-risk groups to guide decision-making regarding treatment. Patients with poor risk are those with low KPS, multiple, serious, or major neurologic deficits, extensive systemic disease with few treatment options, bulky CNS disease, leptomeningeal disease–related encephalopathy, and the presence of CSF block. The goal of treatment for these poor-risk patients is palliation of symptoms. For patients with better risk factors, a more aggressive treatment approach is recommended.[89,91]

METASTASES TO THE PERIPHERAL NERVOUS SYSTEM

Plexuses

Definition and Epidemiology

Metastatic plexopathy affects 1 percent of cancer patients and may involve the cervical, brachial, or lumbosacral plexus.[100]

Pathophysiology

Involvement of the plexus can occur by direct extension from contiguous tumors, from metastases to adjacent soft tissue, bony structures, or lymph nodes, or rarely by direct metastases to the nerves within the plexuses.[100,101]

Anatomic Considerations and Clinical Features

Neurologic manifestations depend on the involved plexus. Patients typically present with new localized pain that is burning and aching in quality, progressive in nature, and increases in severity and frequency over days to weeks. Focal deficits, such as weakness, numbness, and areflexia, develop over weeks or months.[101,102]

Cervical Plexus

The cervical plexus, composed of the anterior rami of C1 to C4 cervical roots, innervates most neck muscles and provides sensory innervation to anterior and lateral neck. Cervical plexopathy commonly occurs as a result of direct invasion from contiguous neck soft tissue tumors or indirectly from regional lymph node metastases from head and neck squamous cell carcinomas, lymphoma, or lung and breast adenocarcinomas.[100,101] Involvement of the cervical plexus is less common than the brachial or lumbosacral plexus.[101]

Patients with metastases of the cervical plexus typically complain of pain within the submandibular and subglottic area, posterior or lateral neck, or around the shoulder. Coughing, neck movement, or assuming a recumbent position exacerbates the pain. Sensory loss commonly develops along the C2, C3, and C4 dermatomal distribution. This is in contrast to sensory loss from surgical neck dissection, which occurs in the distribution of the superficial branches of the greater auricular nerve or transverse cervical branches. Involvement of the distal spinal accessory nerve produces partial trapezius and sternocleidomastoid weakness. Paralysis of the hemidiaphragm, causing dyspnea when supine or upon exertion, results from phrenic nerve involvement.[100,101]

Brachial Plexus

The anterior rami of the lower four cervical and first thoracic nerve roots form the brachial plexus, providing motor and sensory innervation to most of the upper limb except the trapezius muscle and area of skin near the axilla. The lower trunk (C8 and T1) is closely related to the axillary lymph nodes and is most often involved in metastatic cancer. The upper trunk is free of lymph nodes and is less frequently affected.[100] However, primary head and neck squamous cell carcinoma can invade the brachial plexus from above, affecting the upper plexus preferentially. Brachial plexopathy occurs in 0.43 percent of cancer patients, with breast and lung carcinomas being the most common associated malignancies.[103]

Pain is the most common presenting symptom of metastatic brachial plexopathy, and is moderate-to-severe in intensity, beginning in the shoulder girdle and radiating to the elbow, medial side of the forearm, and the fourth and fifth fingers, often exacerbated by shoulder movement. Focal weakness, atrophy, or sensory changes in the distribution of the C7 to T1 dermatomes are common.[103] Involvement of the inferior trunk and medial cord of the brachial plexus from a carcinoma of the lung apex results in the superior sulcus or Pancoast syndrome; patients present with pain and numbness along the ulnar border of the hand and forearm, intrinsic hand muscle weakness, and a palpable mass in the supraclavicular area or axilla. Tumors located near the T1 nerve root involving the stellate ganglion may result in ipsilateral Horner syndrome, which occurs in 25 percent of patients with Pancoast syndrome. Lymphedema secondary to lymphatic obstruction is present in 17 percent.[100,101]

Lumbosacral Plexus

The lumbar plexus is formed from the anterior rami of the T12 to L4 nerves, while nerve roots from L4 to S3 merge to form the sacral plexus. These plexuses supply motor and sensory innervation to the lower extremities and parts of the pelvis. Metastatic involvement of the lumbosacral plexus occurs in

0.71 percent of cancer patients.[104] Tumors within the abdomen and pelvis may directly infiltrate the lumbosacral plexus, and the most common responsible tumors are cervical, uterine, colorectal, bladder, and prostate carcinomas, retroperitoneal sarcomas, and lymphomas.[100,101]

More than 90 percent of patients with lumbosacral plexopathy present with pain. Lumbar plexus involvement results in pain in the costovertebral angle, whereas involvement of the lower sacral plexus causes pain in the hip and buttock, or radiating pain in the ipsilateral lower extremity. Pain is worsened by Valsalva maneuver, prolonged weight bearing, ambulation, sitting, or supine positioning.[100,101] Motor and sensory loss develops in 60 percent of patients. The most common clinical signs are leg weakness (86% of these patients), sensory loss (73%), areflexia (64%), and leg edema (47%). Up to 25 percent of patients suffer from incontinence or impotence, which usually signifies bilateral involvement.[101]

Diagnostic Studies

MRI is the neuroimaging study of choice for neoplastic plexopathy, typically showing a mass adjacent to the plexus or evidence of metastatic infiltration with hypointensity on T1-weighted imaging, hyperintensity on T2-weighted imaging, and gadolinium enhancement.[102] These MRI findings are nonspecific and may occur in both metastatic and radiation plexopathy; the finding of linear or nodular enhancement along the nerves favors plexus metastases.[101] Electrophysiologic studies can demonstrate the degree, type, and distribution of plexus involvement.[105] Electromyography is helpful in delineating metastatic from radiation plexopathy, as myokymic discharges are common in the latter.[100,101,105] Nerve conduction studies reveal variable axonal loss in both types of plexopathy, but patients with radiation plexopathy may also show signs of focal conduction block.[105] FDG-PET studies aid in distinguishing neoplastic disease from radiation plexopathy—in metastatic disease there is increased uptake in the involved region whereas radiation plexopathy is typically hypometabolic. Nevertheless, normal neuroimaging and electrophysiologic studies do not always exclude a metastatic plexopathy.[101]

Differential Diagnosis

Radiation plexopathy is the main differential diagnosis to consider in patients with suspected metastatic plexopathy. The incidence of radiation-induced brachial plexopathy in women with breast carcinoma is 1.8 to 9 percent, with 5 percent having disabling symptoms.[106,107] Typically, radiation plexopathy develops from 0.5 to 20 years after treatment when the brachial plexus is affected, and 1 to 5 years after treatment with lumbosacral involvement.[101] The risk of radiation plexopathy increases with radiation dose; the tolerance dose for brachial plexus (5 percent risk at 5 years) is 60 Gy for conventional fractionation regimens.[108] Mechanisms of radiation injury include direct toxic effects on axons and indirect damage from fibrosis or fibrinoid necrosis within the vasa nervorum, resulting in microinfarctions.[101] Usual presentations of radiation plexopathy include paresthesias and hypesthesia, followed by weakness and amyotrophy. In contrast to metastatic plexopathy, pain is usually mild and follows the sensory symptoms; the lower trunk is less likely to be involved as it is protected by the clavicle during radiation therapy. Horner syndrome is similarly uncommon, whereas lymphedema is more common than in metastatic plexopathy. MRI generally reveals hypointensity on T1- and T2-weighted sequences, reflecting fibrosis without nerve enhancement; however, fibrotic changes with substantial inflammation can demonstrate both hyperintensity on T2-weighted images and contrast enhancement.[109,110]

Other differential diagnoses include plexopathy from intra-arterial chemotherapy, diabetes, infection, and hemorrhage, as well as infectious and paraneoplastic syndromes.[101]

Treatment and Prognosis

The prognosis for most patients with metastatic plexopathy is generally poor because of the presence of advanced disease, and the primary therapeutic goal is palliation of symptoms. Aggressive pain management and prevention of complications of immobility are the focus of treatment. Radiation therapy can control local tumor growth, providing pain relief in 46 percent of patients with neoplastic brachial plexopathy and 85 percent of those with lumbosacral plexopathy.[100,103,111] Intra-arterial chemotherapy has limited use in the treatment of intractable pain due to plexopathy, and paradoxically can also cause plexopathy.[110] A multimodal approach in treating cancer pain should utilize opiate analgesics, infusion pumps, local and regional blocks, sympathetic ganglionic blocks, and epidural anesthetics.[100] Dysesthesias and paresthesias can be managed with transcutaneous nerve stimulation, tricyclic antidepressants, gabapentin, lamotrigine, topiramate, carbamazepine, phenytoin, and valproic acid.[100,101] Rhizotomy and neurotractomy may be used in selected cases of chronic pain. Physical and occupational therapy and decreasing lymphedema by using compressive devices and diuretics can also be beneficial.[101]

Radiation-induced malignancies (e.g., sarcomas) and atypical peripheral nerve sheath tumors develop rarely in patients with metastatic plexopathy treated with radiation. These neoplasms may appear from 4 to 41 years after radiation treatment, presenting as painful masses and leading to progressive neurologic deficits.[112] Genetic conditions such as neurofibromatosis type 1 or ataxia-telangiectasia may predispose to these tumors.[113] Patients with radiation-induced sarcomas warrant surgical excision with adjuvant chemoradiotherapy, whereas surgical resection is the main treatment for radiation-induced peripheral nerve sheath tumors.[114]

Peripheral Nerves

Definition and Epidemiology

Metastases to the peripheral and cranial nerves are relatively rare. Peripheral nerve dysfunction in cancer patients is commonly due to effects of chemotherapy, as is discussed in Chapter 28.

Mechanisms, Clinical Features, and Diagnosis

Peripheral nerves may be involved through extension or compression from adjacent bony or soft tissue structures such as the skull base, vertebrae, pelvis, lymph nodes, muscles, connective tissue, or nearby organs. Ulnar nerves may be affected by tumors at the elbow or axilla, radial nerves from the humerus, intercostal nerves by rib metastases, sciatic nerves from the bony pelvis, and fibular (peroneal) nerves behind the fibular head. Tumor invasion or metastasis to the mediastinal lymph nodes can cause hoarseness and vocal cord paralysis from involvement of the recurrent laryngeal nerve. Breast, prostate, lung, kidney, and thyroid cancers are the most common cause of peripheral nerve involvement.[100,101] The recurrent laryngeal nerve, phrenic nerve, and cervical sympathetic nerves may be affected in lung cancers. Patients commonly present with severe, lancinating pain. Focal weakness, numbness, fasciculations, cramping, muscle atrophy, and reflex loss can help localize the involved peripheral nerve.[101] Tinel sign and local tenderness can be elicited at the site of metastasis.[100]

Metastases from solid tumors within the peripheral nerves themselves are exceedingly rare. Intraneural metastases resembling multiple neuropathies were reported in a patient with carcinoid tumor.[115] Increasing pain, numbness, and weakness relating to the involved nerves are the usual presenting symptoms. Hematogenous spread to the posterior root ganglia has been reported in patients with colon and lung carcinoma.[116]

Occlusion of nerve vessels from ischemia is another mechanism for nerve injury from tumors such as intravascular lymphoma, a rare, high-grade, extranodal non-Hodgkin lymphoma with a tropism for the endothelium, commonly affecting the CNS and skin.[117,118] Infiltration of lymphoma cells into the peripheral nervous system is referred to as neurolymphomatosis and signifies local invasion occurring outside the arachnoid investment of the nerves. This mechanism is distinct from infiltration associated with subarachnoid seeding from perineural tumors seen in epidural lymphoma.[119] The malignant lymphocytes in neurolymphomatosis are clustered in perivascular sites, in contrast to meningeal lymphoma where the lymphocytes are in the epineurium. Large B-cell lymphoma is the most common cause; less frequent are T-cell, natural killer cell, and Hodgkin lymphomas.[100,102] Four patterns of presentations have been identified in patients with neurolymphomatosis: painful involvement of nerves or roots, cranial neuropathy with or without pain, painless involvement of peripheral nerves, and painful or painless involvement of a single peripheral nerve. Neurologic dysfunction usually antedates discovery of systemic lymphoma and is responsive to corticosteroids.[119] Clinical findings suggesting neurolymphomatosis rather than paraneoplastic or inflammatory processes include severe pain, asymmetric distribution, and rapid evolution.[119] MRI reveals enhancement or T2-weighted hyperintensity within the peripheral nerves. PET-CT is helpful in visualizing the involved nerve, which demonstrates hypermetabolism when the lesion is sufficiently large.[120] Electrophysiologic studies reveal an axonal neuropathy. CSF examination may be normal or may show increased protein concentration or a pleocytosis; these findings may be confused with acute or chronic inflammatory demyelinating polyneuropathy. Biopsy of a clinically affected nerve is strongly recommended to enable a definite diagnosis to be made.[121] Histopathologic findings show tumor cell infiltration of the endoneurium and perineurium, displaying B-cell–associated surface antigens (CD19 and CD20) with high proliferation index.[122] Although biopsy is sensitive, it still may be falsely negative despite widespread lymphomatous involvement of peripheral nerves.[121] In these cases, integration of clinical information, imaging findings, morphologic data from neural and non-neural tissues, and CSF studies may be helpful in establishing the clinical diagnosis. The response to empiric treatment may also lead to the correct diagnosis.[119]

Treatment and Prognosis

Systemic chemotherapy addressing multiple sites of involvement together with focal radiotherapy may offer relief of symptoms.[101] For neurolymphomatosis, treatment principles are similar to primary CNS lymphoma.[122] Methotrexate treatment in patients with neurolymphomatosis may provide clinical improvement and at least partial radiographic improvement. Radiotherapy is indicated for drug-refractory localized lymphomatous aggregates.[122] When treated promptly and properly, neurolymphomatosis carries a similar prognosis to primary CNS lymphoma.[119]

METASTASES TO MUSCLES

Epidemiology and Pathophysiology

Skeletal muscle metastases are a rare occurrence in patients with malignancy, despite the fact that skeletal muscle comprises 50 percent of total body mass. The prevalence of metastases to muscles in autopsy studies ranges from 0.03 to 17.5 percent, and a retrospective study demonstrated that 1.2 percent of oncologic patients had muscle metastases based on CT studies.[123] The rarity of these metastases is due to a number of factors, including blood flow variability between resting and exercise states causing a reduction of tumor cell adherence to underlying tissues,[124] skeletal muscles producing anticancer factors such as leukemia inhibitory factor and interleukin-6,[125] skeletal muscle microvasculature having the biochemical ability to destroy the cancer cells,[126] and the skeletal muscles removing lactic acid, which plays a role in neovascularization.[127]

The hypothesized mechanisms of metastases include hematogenous dissemination by arterial emboli or venous spread (especially through the Batson plexus), extension from intramuscular lymph nodes, or perineural spread.[123] The most frequent primary tumors are lung, gastrointestinal, breast and genitourinary cancers, lymphoma, and melanoma.[124] Metastases are most commonly located in paravertebral, iliopsoas, and gluteal muscles.[123]

Clinical Features

Most patients with skeletal muscle metastases are asymptomatic, and these metastases are found incidentally during staging. Local pain and swelling occurs in 14 percent, usually in patients with large lesions with massive infiltration or destruction. Painless palpable masses arise in 10 percent of patients.[123]

Diagnostic Studies

The advent of CT, MRI, and FDG PET has facilitated detection of skeletal muscle metastases. Different types of CT findings have been recognized, including focal intramuscular masses with homogeneous contrast enhancement, abscess-like intramuscular lesions, diffuse metastatic muscle infiltration, multifocal intramuscular calcification, and intramuscular bleeding.[123] MRI with gadolinium is superior to CT both in diagnosis and in planning treatment. The majority of patients with skeletal muscle metastases demonstrate extensive peritumoral enhancement associated with central necrosis.[128] The increasing use of FDG PET/CT for staging and follow-up has resulted in the detection of many unsuspected cases of skeletal muscle metastases, which show high tumor-to-background contrast resolution.[124] Needle biopsy establishes the diagnosis definitively.[128]

Differential Diagnosis

Conditions that may mimic skeletal muscle metastases are muscle hemangioma, intramuscular ganglion, myxoma, ischiorectal bursitis, benign muscle calcifications such as myositis ossificans, calcific tendinitis, angiomatosis, systemic sclerosis, and calcific myonecrosis.[123]

Treatment and Prognosis

As most patients have widespread systemic disease, the prognosis is generally poor. The main goal of treatment is therefore palliation, and therapeutic options include radiotherapy or chemotherapy. Surgical excision is considered for lesions larger than 4 cm and recommended for rapidly expanding lesions or those producing neurologic deficits.[129] Reports have shown effective control of local tumor recurrence after wide excision that includes the infiltrative borders of the tumor.[128]

CONCLUDING COMMENTS

Cancer can involve any part of the nervous system and lead to significant neurologic morbidity, at times representing a catastrophic event for patients with cancer. Knowledge of both common and rare manifestations of nervous system metastases aids clinicians in early recognition and proper localization. Distinguishing metastatic from nonmetastatic diseases such as those with infectious, inflammatory, and vascular etiologies or from complications of cancer therapy is imperative. The appropriate use of neurodiagnostic modalities such as MRI frequently assists in reaching a correct diagnosis. Clinicians should establish realistic therapeutic goals, including symptomatic treatment to maintain quality of life of these patients. A multidisciplinary approach involving neurologists, neurooncologists, medical oncologists, radiation oncologists, neurosurgeons, specialists in palliative care, and rehabilitation experts is necessary.

REFERENCES

1. Clouston PD, DeAngelis LM, Posner JB: The spectrum of neurological disease in patients with systemic cancer. Ann Neurol 31:268, 1992.
2. American Cancer Society Cancer Facts & Figures 2012. American Cancer Society, Atlanta, 2012.
3. Barnholtz-Sloan JS, Sloan AE, Davis FG, et al: Incidence proportions of brain metastases in patients diagnosed (1973 to 2001) in the Metropolitan Detroit Cancer Surveillance System. J Clin Oncol 22:2865, 2004.
4. Schouten LJ, Rutten J, Huveneers HA, et al: Incidence of brain metastases in a cohort of patients with carcinoma of the breast, colon, kidney, and lung and melanoma. Cancer 94:2698, 2002.
5. Nayak L, Lee EQ, Wen PY: Epidemiology of brain metastases. Curr Oncol Rep 14:48, 2012.
6. Delattre JY, Krol G, Thaler HT, et al: Distribution of brain metastases. Arch Neurol 45:741, 1988.
7. Gavrilovic IT, Posner JB: Brain metastases: epidemiology and pathophysiology. J Neurooncol 75:5, 2005.
8. Zhang C, Yu D: Microenvironment determinants of brain metastasis. Cell Biosci 1:8, 2011.
9. Fidler IJ: The role of the organ microenvironment in brain metastasis. Semin Cancer Biol 21:107, 2011.
10. Carbonell W, Ansorge O, Sibson N, et al: The vascular basement membrane as "soil" in brain metastasis. PLoS One 4:e5857, 2009.
11. Dorai Z, Sawaya R, Yung WKA: Brain metastasis. p. 345. In: Tonn JC, Westphal M, Rutka JT (eds): Oncology of CNS Tumors, Part 1. Springer, Berlin, 2010.
12. Chamberlain MC: Brain metastases: a medical neuro-oncology perspective. Expert Rev Neurother 10:563, 2010.
13. American College of Surgical Oncology CNS Working Group The management of brain metastases. p. 553. In: Schiff D, O'Neill BP (eds): Principles of Neuro-Oncology. McGraw-Hill, New York, 2005.
14. Burger PC, Scheithauer B: Metastatic and secondary neoplasms. p. 553. In: Burger PC, Scheithauer BW (eds): Tumors of the Central Nervous System. Part 7 of AFIP Atlas of Tumor Pathology, Series 4. American Registry of Pathology Press, Washington DC, 2007.
15. Shaffrey ME, Mut M, Asher AL, et al: Brain metastases. Curr Probl Surg 41:665, 2004.
16. Soffietti R, Cornu P, Delattre JY, et al: Brain metastases. p. 437. In: Gilhus NE, Barnes MP, Brainin M (eds): European Handbook of Neurological Management. 2nd Ed. Blackwell-Wiley, Oxford, 2011.
17. Cha S: Neuroimaging in neuro-oncology. Neurotherapeutics 6:465, 2009.
18. Walker MT, Kapoor V: Neuroimaging of parenchymal brain metastases. Cancer Treat Res 136:31, 2007.
19. Gaspar L, Scott C, Rotman M, et al: Recursive partitioning analysis (RPA) of prognostic factors in three Radiation Therapy Oncology Group (RTOG) brain metastases trials. Int J Radiat Oncol Biol Phys 37:745, 1997.
20. Gaspar LE, Scott C, Murray K, et al: Validation of the RTOG recursive partitioning analysis (RPA) classification for brain metastases. Int J Radiat Oncol Biol Phys 47:1001, 2000.
21. Sperduto PW, Kased N, Roberge D, et al: Summary report on the graded prognostic assessment: an accurate and facile diagnosis-specific tool to estimate survival for patients with brain metastases. J Clin Oncol 30:419, 2012.
22. Wen PY, Schiff D, Kesari S, et al: Medical mangement of patients with brain tumors. J Neurooncol 80:313, 2006.
23. Kamar FG, Posner JB: Brain metastases. Semin Neurol 30:217, 2010.
24. Glantz MJ, Cole BF, Forsyth PA, et al: Practice parameter: anticonvulsant prophylaxis in patients with newly diagnosed brain tumors. Report of the Quality Standards Subcommittee of the American Academy of Neurology. Neurology 54:1886, 2000.
25. Patchell RA, Tibbs PA, Walsh JW, et al: A randomized trial of surgery in the treatment of single metastases to the brain. N Engl J Med 322:494, 1990.

26. Vecht CJ, Haaxma-Reiche H, Noordijk EM, et al: Treatment of single brain metastasis: radiotherapy alone or combined with neurosurgery? Ann Neurol 33:583, 1993.
27. Mintz AH, Kestle J, Rathbone MP, et al: A randomized trial to assess the efficacy of surgery in addition to radiotherapy in patients with a single cerebral metastasis. Cancer 78:1470, 1996.
28. Patchell RA, Tibbs PA, Regine WF, et al: Postoperative radiotherapy in the treatment of single metastases to the brain: a randomized trial. JAMA 280:1485, 1998.
29. Aoyama H, Shirato H, Tago M, et al: Stereotactic radiosurgery plus whole-brain radiation therapy vs stereotactic radiosurgery alone for treatment of brain metastases: a randomized controlled trial. JAMA 295:2483, 2006.
30. Aoyama H, Tago M, Kato N, et al: Neurocognitive function of patients with brain metastasis who received either whole brain radiotherapy plus stereotactic radiosurgery or radiosurgery alone. Int J Radiat Oncol Biol Phys 68:1388, 2007.
31. Chang EL, Wefel JS, Hess KR, et al: Neurocognition in patients with brain metastases treated with radiosurgery or radiosurgery plus whole-brain irradiation: a randomised controlled trial. Lancet Oncol 10:1037, 2009.
32. Kocher M, Soffietti R, Abacioglu U, et al: Adjuvant whole-brain radiotherapy versus observation after radiosurgery or surgical resection of one to three cerebral metastases: results of the EORTC 22952-26001 study. J Clin Oncol 29:134, 2011.
33. Abe E, Aoyama H: The role of whole brain radiation therapy for the management of brain metastases in the era of stereotactic radiosurgery. Curr Oncol Rep 14:79, 2012.
34. Ricard D, Psimaras D, Soussain C, et al: Central nervous system complications of radiation therapy. p. 301. In: Wen PY, Schiff D, Quant Lee E (eds): Neurologic Complications of Cancer Therapy. Demos, New York, 2012.
35. DeAngelis LM, Mandell LR, Thaler HT, et al: The role of postoperative radiotherapy after resection of single brain metastases. Neurosurgery 24:798, 1989.
36. Goetz P, Ebinu JO, Roberge D, et al: Current standards in the management of cerebral metastases. Int J Surg Oncol 2012:493426, 2012.
37. Andrews DW, Scott C, Sperduto P, et al: Whole brain radiation therapy with or without stereotactic radiosurgery boost for patients with one to three brain metastases: phase III results of the RTOG 9508 randomised trial. Lancet 363:1665, 2004.
38. Cavaliere R, Schiff D: Chemotherapy and cerebral metastases: misperception or reality? Neurosurg Focus 22:E6, 2007.
39. Inoue A, Suzuki T, Fukuhara T, et al: Prospective phase II study of gefitinib for chemotherapy-naive patients with advanced non-small-cell lung cancer with epidermal growth factor receptor gene mutations. J Clin Oncol 24:3340, 2006.
40. Paz-Ares L, Sanchez JM, Garcia-Velasco A: A prospective phase II trial of erlotinib in advanced nonsmall-cell lung cancer (NSCLC) patients (p) with mutations in the tyrosine kinase (TK) domain of the epidermal growth factor receptor (EGFR). J Clin Oncol 24:369s, 2006.
41. Lin NU, Dieras V, Paul D, et al: Multicenter phase II study of lapatinib in patients with brain metastases from HER2-positive breast cancer. Clin Cancer Res 15:1452, 2009.
42. Lin NU, Eierman W, Greil R, et al: Randomized phase II study of lapatinib plus capecitabine or lapatinib plus topotecan for patients with HER2-positive breast cancer brain metastases. J Neurooncol 105:613, 2011.
43. Gore ME, Hariharan S, Porta C, et al: Sunitinib in metastatic renal cell carcinoma patients with brain metastases. Cancer 117:501, 2011.
44. Stadler WM, Figlin RA, McDermott DF, et al: Safety and efficacy results of the advanced renal cell carcinoma sorafenib expanded access program in North America. Cancer 116:1272, 2010.
45. Long GV, Kefford RF, Carr P, et al: Phase 1/2 study of GSK2118436, a selective inhibitor of V600 mutant (Mut) BRAF kinase: evidence of activity in melanoma brain metastases (Mets). Ann Oncol 21:12, 2010.
46. Falchook GS, Long GV, Kurzrock R, et al: Dabrafenib in patients with melanoma, untreated brain metastases, and other solid tumours: a phase 1 dose-escalation trial. Lancet 379:1893, 2012.
47. Ewend MG, Brem S, Gilbert M, et al: Treatment of single brain metastases with resection, intracavitary carmustine polymer wafers, and radiation therapy is safe and provides excellent local control. Clin Cancer Res 13:3637, 2007.
48. Rogers LR, Rock JP, Sills AK, et al: Results of a phase II trial of the GliaSite radiation therapy system for the treatment of newly diagnosed, resected single brain metastases. J Neurosurg 105:375, 2006.
49. Auperin A, Arriagada R, Pignon JP: Prophylactic cranial irradiation for patients with small-cell lung cancer in complete remission: Prophylactic Cranial Irradiation Overview Collaborative Group. N Engl J Med 341:476, 1999.
50. Slotman B, Faivre-Finn C, Kramer G: Prophylactic cranial irradiation in extensive small cell lung cancer. N Engl J Med 357:664, 2007.
51. Gore EM, Bae K, Wong S: A phase III comparison of prophylactic cranial irradiation versus observation in patients with locally advanced non-small cell lung cancer: primary analysis of radiation therapy oncology group RTOG 0214. J Clin Oncol 29:272, 2009.
52. Pottgen C, Eberhardt W, Grannass A, et al: Prophylactic cranial irradiation in operable stage IIIA non small-cell lung cancer treated with neoadjuvant chemoradiotherapy: results from a German multicenter randomized trial. J Clin Oncol 25:4987, 2007.

53. Da Silva AN, Schiff D: Dural and skull base metastases. Cancer Treat Res 136:117, 2007.
54. Laigle-Donadey F, Taillibert S, Martin-Duverneuil N, et al: Skull-base metastases. J Neurooncol 75:63, 2005.
55. Chamoun RB, Suki D, DeMonte F: Surgical management of cranial base metastases. Neurosurgery 70:802, 2012.
56. Glenn LW: Innovations in neuroimaging of skull base pathology. Otolaryngol Clin North Am 38:613, 2005.
57. Mitsuya K, Nakasu Y, Horiguchi S, et al: Metastatic skull tumors: MRI features and a new conventional classification. J Neurooncol 104:239, 2011.
58. Stark AM, Eichmann T, Mehdorn HM: Skull metastases: clinical features, differential diagnosis, and review of the literature. Surg Neurol 60:219, 2003.
59. Vikram B, Chu FC: Radiation therapy for metastases to the base of the skull. Radiology 130:465, 1979.
60. Chamoun RB, DeMonte F: Management of skull base metastases. Neurosurg Clin N Am 22:61, 2011.
61. Posner JB, Chernik NL: Intracranial metastases from systemic cancer. Adv Neurol 19:579, 1978.
62. Laigle-Donadey F, Taillibert S, Mokhtari K, et al: Dural metastases. J Neurooncol 75:57, 2005.
63. Nayak L, Abrey LE, Iwamoto FM: Intracranial dural metastases. Cancer 115:1947, 2009.
64. Cheng CL, Greenberg J: Prostatic adenocarcinoma metastatic to chronic subdural hematoma membranes. Case repot. J Neurosurg 68:642, 1988.
65. Bendzus M, Warmuth-Metz M, Burger R: Diagnosing dural metastases: the value of ^{1}H magnetic resonance spectroscopy. Neuroradiology 43:285, 2001.
66. Kremer S, Grand S, Remy C, et al: Contribution of dynamic contrast MR imaging to the differentiation between dural metastasis and meningioma. Neuroradiology 46:642, 2004.
67. Nathoo N, Ugokwe K, Chang AS: The role of ^{111}indium-octreotide brain scintigraphy in the diagnosis of cranial, dural-based meningiomas. J Neurooncol 81:167, 2006.
68. Coleman RE: Clinical features of metastatic bone disease and risk of skeletal morbidity. Clin Cancer Res 12:6243s, 2006.
69. Perrin RG, Laxton AW: Metastatic spine disease: epidemiology, pathophysiology, and evaluation of patients. Neurosurg Clin N Am 15:365, 2004.
70. Welch WC, Schiff D, Gerszten PC: Spinal cord tumors. www.Uptodate.com, 2013.
71. Mak KS, Lee LK, Mak RH, et al: Incidence and treatment patterns in hospitalizations for malignant spinal cord compression in the United States, 1998-2006. Int J Radiat Oncol Biol Phys 80:824, 2011.
72. Klimo Jr P, Schmidt MH: Surgical management of spinal metastases. Oncologist 9:188, 2004.
73. Spinazze S, Caraceni A, Schrijvers D: Epidural spinal cord compression. Crit Rev Oncol Hematol 56:397, 2005.
74. Schiff D: Spinal cord compression. Neurol Clin 21:67, 2003.
75. Hammack JE: Spinal cord disease in patients with cancer. Continuum (Minneap Minn) 18:312, 2012.
76. Sun H, Nemecek AN: Optimal management of malignant epidural spinal cord compression. Hematol Oncol Clin North Am 24:537, 2010.
77. Li KC, Poon PY: Sensitivity and specificity of MRI in detecting malignant spinal cord compression and in distinguishing malignant from benign compression fractures of vertebrae. Magn Reson Imaging 6:547, 1988.
78. Schiff D, O'Neill BP, Wang CH, et al: Neuroimaging and treatment implications of patients with multiple epidural spinal metastases. Cancer 83:1593, 1998.
79. Loblaw A, Mitera G, Ford M, et al: A 2011 updated systemic review and clinical practice guideline for the management of malignant extradural spinal cord compression. Int J Radiat Oncol Biol Phys 84:312, 2012.
80. Ribas ES, Schiff D: Spinal cord compression. Curr Treat Options Neurol 14:391, 2012.
81. Patchell RA, Tibbs PA, Regine WF, et al: Direct decompressive surgical resection in the treatment of spinal cord compression caused by metastatic cancer: a randomised trial. Lancet 366:643, 2005.
82. Maranzano E, Bellavita R, Rossi R, et al: Short-course versus split-course radiotherapy in metastatic spinal cord compression: results of a phase III, randomized, multicenter trial. J Clin Oncol 23:3358, 2005.
83. Sohn S, Chung CK: The role of stereotactic radiosurgery in metastasis to the spine. J Korean Neurosurg Soc 51:1, 2012.
84. Sheehan JP, Shaffrey CI, Schlesinger D, et al: Radiosurgery in the treatment of spinal metastases: tumor control, survival, and quality of life after helical tomotherapy. Neurosurgery 65:1052, 2009.
85. Gerszten PC, Burton SA, Ozhasoglu C, et al: Radiosurgery for spinal metastases: clinical experience in 500 cases from a single institution. Spine 32:193, 2007.
86. Sung WS, Sung MJ, Chan JH, et al: Intramedullary spinal cord metastases: a 20-year institutional experience with a comprehensive literature review. World Neurosurg 79:576, 2013.
87. Schiff D, O'Neill BP: Intramedullary spinal cord metastases: clinical features and treatment outcome. Neurology 47:906, 1996.
88. Kalita O: Current insights into surgery for intramedullary spinal cord metastases: a literature review. Int J Surg Oncol 2011:989506, 2011.
89. Groves MD: Leptomeningeal disease. Neurosurg Clin N Am 22:67, 2011.
90. Clarke JI: Leptomeningeal metastasis from systemic cancer. Continuum (Minneap Minn) 18:328, 2012.
91. Chamberlain MC: Leptomeningeal metastasis. Curr Opin Oncol 22:627, 2010.

92. Clarke JL, Perez HR, Jacks LM, et al: Leptomeningeal metastases in the MRI era. Neurology 74:1449, 2010.
93. Glass JP, Melamed M, Chernik NL, et al: Malignant cells in cerebrospinal fluid (CSF): the meaning of a positive CSF cytology. Neurology 29:1369, 1979.
94. Glantz MJ, Cole BF, Glantz LK: Cerebrospinal fluid cytology in patients with cancer: minimizing false-negative results. Cancer 82:733, 1988.
95. Grewal J, Saria MG, Kesari S: Novel approaches to treating leptomeningeal metastases. J Neurooncol 106:225, 2012.
96. Jaeckle KA: Neoplastic meningitis from systemic malignancies: diagnosis, prognosis and treatment. Semin Oncol 33:312, 2006.
97. Perissinotti AJ, Reeves DJ: Role of intrathecal rituximab and trastuzumab in the management of leptomeningeal carcinomatosis. Ann Pharmacother 44:1633, 2010.
98. Chamberlain MC, Johnston SK, Van Horn A, et al: Recurrent lymphomatous meningitis treated with intra-CSF rituximab and liposomal ara-C. J Neurooncol 91:271, 2009.
99. Mir O, Ropert S, Alexandre J, et al: High-dose intrathecal trastuzumab for leptomeningeal metastases secondary to HER-2 overexpressing breast cancer. Ann Oncol 19:1978, 2008.
100. Ramchandren S, Dalmau J: Metastases to the peripheral nervous system. J Neurooncol 75:101, 2005.
101. Jaeckle KA: Metastases involving spinal cord, roots, and plexus. Continuum (Minneap Minn) 17:855, 2011.
102. Antoine JC, Camdessanche JP: Peripheral nervous system involvement in patients with cancer. Lancet Neurol 6:75, 2007.
103. Kori SH, Foley KM, Posner JB: Brachial plexus lesions in patients with cancer: 100 cases. Neurology 31:45, 1981.
104. Jaeckle KA, Young DF, Foley KM: The natural history of lumbosacral plexopathy in cancer. Neurology 35:8, 1985.
105. Krarup C, Crone C: Neurophysiological studies in malignant disease with particular reference to involvement of peripheral nerves. J Neurol 249:651, 2002.
106. Pierce SM, Recht A, Lingos TI, et al: Long-term radiation complications following conservative surgery (CS) and radiation therapy (RT) in patients with early stage breast cancer. Int J Radiat Oncol Biol Phys 23:915, 1992.
107. Olsen NK, Pfeiffer P, Johannsen L, et al: Radiation-induced brachial plexopathy: neurological follow-up in 161 recurrence-free breast cancer patients. Int J Radiat Oncol Biol Phys 26:43, 1993.
108. Emami B, Lyman J, Brown A, et al: Tolerance of normal tissue to therapeutic irradiation. Int J Radiat Oncol Biol Phys 21:109, 1991.
109. Qayyum A, MacVicar AD, Padhani AR, et al: Symptomatic brachial plexopathy following treatment for breast cancer: utility of MR imaging with surface-coil techniques. Radiology 214:837, 2000.
110. Jaeckle KA: Neurologic manifestations of neoplastic and radiation-induced plexopathies. Semin Neurol 30:254, 2010.
111. Pettigrew LC, Glass JP, Maor M, et al: Diagnosis and treatment of lumbosacral plexopathies in patients with cancer. Arch Neurol 41:1282, 1984.
112. Foley KM, Woodruff JM, Ellis FT, et al: Radiation-induced malignant and atypical peripheral nerve sheath tumors. Ann Neurol 7:311, 1980.
113. Cross NE, Glantz MJ: Neurologic complications of radiation therapy. Neurol Clin 21:249, 2003.
114. Somerset HL, Kleinschmidt-DeMasters BK, Lillehei KO: Radiation-induced tumors. p. 315. In: Wen PY, Schiff D, Quant Lee E (eds): Neurologic Complications of Cancer Therapy. Demos, New York, 2012.
115. Grisold W, Piza-Katzer H, Jahn R, et al: Intraneural nerve metastasis with multiple mononeuropathies. J Peripher Nerv Syst 5:163, 2000.
116. Johnson PC: Hematogenous metastases of carcinoma to dorsal root ganglia. Acta Neuropathol 38:171, 1977.
117. Baumann TP, Hurwitz N, Karamitopolou-Diamantis E, et al: Diagnosis and treatment of intravascular lymphomatosis. Arch Neurol 57:374, 2000.
118. Levin KH, Lutz G: Angiotropic large-cell lymphoma with peripheral nerve and skeletal muscle involvement: early diagnosis and treatment. Neurology 47:1009, 1996.
119. Baehring JM, Damek D, Martin EC, et al: Neurolymphomatosis. Neuro-Oncology 5:104, 2003.
120. Trojan A, Jermann M, Taverna C, et al: Fusion PET-CT imaging of neurolymphomatosis. Ann Oncol 13:802, 2002.
121. van den Bent MJ, de Bruin HG, Bos GM, et al: Negative sural nerve biopsy in neurolymphomatosis. J Neurol 246:1159, 1999.
122. Baehring JM, Batchelor TT: Diagnosis and management of neurolymphomatosis. Cancer J 18:463, 2012.
123. Surov A, Hainz M, Holzhausen HJ, et al: Skeletal muscle metastases: primary tumours, prevalence, and radiological features. Eur Radiol 20:649, 2010.
124. Khandelwal AR, Takalkar AM, Lilien DL, et al: Skeletal muscle metastases on FDG PET/CT imaging. Clin Nucl Med 37:575, 2012.
125. Kurek JB, Nouri S, Kannourakis G, et al: Leukemia inhibitory factor and interleukin-6 are produced by diseased and regenerating skeletal muscle. Muscle Nerve 19:1291, 1996.
126. Weiss L: Biomechanical destruction of cancer cells in skeletal muscles: a rate-regulator for hematogenous metastasis. Clin Exp Metastasis 5:483, 1989.
127. Seely S: Possible reasons for the high resistance of muscle to cancer. Med Hypotheses 6:133, 1980.
128. Tuoheti Y, Okada K, Osanai T, et al: Skeletal muscle metastases of carcinoma: a clinicopathological study of 21 cases. Jpn J Clin Oncol 4:210, 2004.
129. LaBan MM, Nagarajan R, Riutta JC: Paucity of muscle metastasis in otherwise widely disseminated cancer: a conundrum. Am J Phys Med Rehabil 89:931, 2010.

CHAPTER

27

Paraneoplastic Syndromes Involving the Nervous System

JEROME B. POSNER

The term *paraneoplastic syndrome* refers to symptoms or signs resulting from dysfunction of organs or tissues caused by a cancer, but which are not a direct effect of invasion by the neoplasm or its metastases. Paraneoplastic syndromes may affect virtually any organ or tissue (Table 27-1), including the nervous system. Table 27-2 provides a classification of the wide variety of paraneoplastic disorders that affect the nervous system (a comprehensive review is provided elsewhere[1]). Although all of the disorders in Table 27-2 are paraneoplastic in nature, some neurologists use the term paraneoplastic syndrome in a more restricted sense to refer to neurologic disorders that occur with increased frequency in patients with cancer and are not caused by infection, systemic metabolic disorders, vascular disease, or side effects of cancer therapy. These disorders, also termed *remote effects of cancer on the nervous system*, detailed in Table 27-3, encompass a much less common and a clinically and pathologically more restricted group of disorders than the other nonmetastatic effects of cancer.[2] These latter disorders are the focus of this chapter.

GENERAL CONSIDERATIONS

Incidence

Several studies have addressed the frequency of paraneoplastic syndromes. Wide-ranging estimates from these studies are due to: (1) varied definitions; (2) the rigor used to exclude other causes of neurologic dysfunction; (3) the care with which the neurologic evaluation was performed; and (4) biases introduced by referral patterns. For example, the Lambert–Eaton myasthenic syndrome (LEMS) occurs in 3 percent or less of patients with small cell lung cancer (SCLC), but about 50 percent of SCLC patients have either subjective or objective muscle weakness.[3] While in one study only 7 percent of

Aminoff's Neurology and General Medicine, Fifth Edition.

TABLE 27-1 ■ Selected Non-Neurologic Paraneoplastic Syndromes

General Physiologic (Host-Reactive) Syndromes
Fever
Anorexia and cachexia
Fatigue and "weakness"
Dysgeusia
Hematologic and Vascular Syndromes
Anemia
Leukemoid reaction
Eosinophilia, basophilia
Thrombocytoses
Thrombocytopenia
Hypercoagulability (Trousseau syndrome)
Erythrocytosis
Hyperviscosity
Skin and Connective Tissue Syndromes
Acanthosis nigricans
Tripe palms
Erythemas
Pruritus
Vasculitis
Flushing
Sweet syndrome
Ichthyosis
Hypertrichosis
Pachydermoperiostosis
Melanosis, vitiligo
Endocrine-Metabolic Syndromes
Cushing syndrome
Hypoglycemia and hyperglycemia
Syndrome of inappropriate secretion of antidiuretic hormone (SIADH)
Carcinoid syndrome
Hypercalcemia and hypocalcemia
Systemic nodular panniculitis
Acromegaly
Gynecomastia
Hypernatremia
Gastrointestinal Syndromes
Protein-losing enteropathy
Malabsorption
Exudative enteropathy
Zollinger–Ellison syndrome
Collagen-Vascular Syndromes
Arthritides
Scleroderma
Lupus erythematosus
Amyloidosis
Palmar fasciitis
Renal Syndromes
Glomerulonephritis
Nephrotic syndrome
Renal failure
Hypokalemia
Bone Syndromes
Hypophosphatemic osteomalacia
Pulmonary Osteoarthropathy
Clubbing
Synovitis

1,476 cancer patients had a "neuromyopathy" on physical examination,[4] in another, abnormalities of peripheral nerve function were found by quantitative sensory testing in 44 percent.[5] Myopathic changes are found on muscle biopsy in 33 percent of patients with lung cancer.[6] These neurologic symptoms can predate the detection of cancer; in one study of 51 patients with peripheral sensory neuropathy of unknown cause, 18 patients (35%) were found who developed cancer within 6 years.[7]

True incidence figures for paraneoplastic syndromes are rare. Population-based data are available for myasthenia gravis, LEMS, and dermatomyositis. A study from the Netherlands identified the age-corrected point prevalence of myasthenia gravis as 106.1 per million persons, with an annual incidence of 6.48 per million.[8] A total of 5 percent of these patients had a paraneoplastic form of myasthenia gravis. In another study, the annual incidence of LEMS was 0.4 per million persons, equally divided between those with SCLC and those with non–small cell lung cancer (NSCLC) with a prevalence of 2.5 per million persons.[9]

For dermatomyositis, a population-based study from Olmsted County, Minnesota, identified the overall age- and sex-adjusted incidence as 9.63 per million persons; 20 percent had cancer.[10] The overall prevalence was 21.42 per 100,000 persons, and 21 percent suffered from the amyopathic subtype (rash but no muscle weakness).

Other studies have addressed the percentage of patients with a given tumor likely to have a paraneoplastic syndrome. Myasthenia gravis occurs in 10 to 15 percent of patients with thymoma.[11] LEMS has been found in about 3 percent of patients with lung cancer.[12] Paraneoplastic peripheral neuropathy occurs in 10 percent of malignant monoclonal gammopathies, and in 50 percent of patients with osteosclerotic myeloma.[13,14] Most known paraneoplastic syndromes are so uncommon that exact incidence

TABLE 27-2 ■ Nonmetastatic Complications of Cancer on the Nervous System

Disorder	Example(s)
Vascular disorders	Hemorrhage/infarction
Infections	Meningitis/abscess
Nutritional disorders	Wernicke encephalopathy
Metabolic disorders	Hypocalcemia
Side effects of therapy	
Surgery and other diagnostic or therapeutic procedures	Meningitis/CSF leak
Radiation therapy	Brain/spinal cord necrosis
Chemotherapy/small molecules	Peripheral neuropathy
Biologic therapy	PML
"Remote" or paraneoplastic syndromes	(see Table 27-3)

CSF, cerebrospinal fluid; PML, progressive multifocal leukoencephalopathy.

TABLE 27-3 ■ Neurologic Paraneoplastic Syndromes

Brain

- Limbic encephalitis*
- Encephalomyelitis*
  - Hypothalamic encephalitis
  - Brainstem/basal ganglia encephalitis
- Cerebellar degeneration*
- Opsoclonus myoclonus*
- Visual loss
  - Carcinoma/melanoma retinopathy*
  - Optic neuropathy

Spinal Cord

- Myelitis/Myelopathy
  - Demyelinating myelopathy
    - Neuromyelitis optica
  - Necrotizing myelopathy
- Motor neuron syndromes
  - Subacute motor neuronopathy
  - Amyotrophic lateral sclerosis (ALS)
- Stiff-person syndrome

Peripheral Nerve/Dorsal Root Ganglia

- Subacute sensory neuronopathy*
- Chronic/subacute sensory or sensorimotor neuropathy
- Autonomic neuropathy*
- Acute sensorimotor neuropathy (Guillain–Barré syndrome)
- Plexitis (e.g., brachial neuritis)
- Vasculitic neuropathy
- Association with plasma cell dyscrasias

Neuromuscular Junction

- Lambert–Eaton myasthenic syndrome*
- Myasthenia gravis*
- Neuromyotonia

Muscle

- Dermatomyositis*
- Polymyositis
- Inclusion-body myositis
- Necrotizing myopathy
- Cachectic myopathy
- Myotonia

*Indicates "classic" paraneoplastic syndrome.

figures cannot be established, but they probably occur in less than 0.01 percent of cancer patients.

A higher yield is found when patients whose symptoms suggest the possibility of a paraneoplastic syndrome have serum sent for examination for paraneoplastic antibodies. Dalmau and Rosenfeld found that 163 of 649 (25%) consecutive patients examined over 23 months had well-defined antineuronal autoantibodies.[15]

Pathogenesis

Although the exact pathogenesis of most paraneoplastic syndromes has not been established, the consensus is that most, or perhaps all, neurologic paraneoplastic syndromes are immune-mediated. Evidence for this hypothesis includes the presence of antibodies that recognize antigens present in both the cancer and the normal nervous system. Some of these so-called paraneoplastic or onconeural antigens are also expressed in normal testes, an organ that, like the brain, is an immunologically privileged site.[16] If the antigen cannot be identified in a cancer with a known serum paraneoplastic antibody, it must be suspected that either the patient does not have a paraneoplastic syndrome or that some other cancer is present and caused the disorder. Examination of the cerebrospinal fluid (CSF) of patients with paraneoplastic syndromes involving the central nervous system (e.g., limbic encephalitis) usually reveals a pleocytosis, at least early in the course of the disease, with a persistently slightly elevated protein level, an increased IgG Index, and oligoclonal bands. Some of these oligoclonal bands in the CSF have been identified as paraneoplastic antibodies.[17,18] The relative specific activity of the paraneoplastic antibody in CSF (expressed as a concentration of antibody against total IgG) is substantially higher than that in the serum, indicating that the antibody was synthesized within the central nervous system (CNS) rather than simply diffusing across the blood–brain barrier.[17–20] Serial plasma exchanges, although effective in substantially lowering antibody titer in the serum, have no effect on CSF antibody titers.[17] The tumors of patients with paraneoplastic syndromes, although identical in histologic type to tumors of patients without paraneoplastic syndromes, are more likely to be heavily infiltrated with inflammatory cells including T cells, B cells, and plasma cells. The nervous system is usually also infiltrated by inflammatory cells, and some paraneoplastic syndromes respond to treatment with immunosuppression.[21,22]

The current concept of the pathogenesis of paraneoplastic syndromes is that the tumor ectopically expresses an antigen that normally is expressed exclusively in the nervous system.[21] Onconeural antigens are present in the tumors of all patients with antibody-positive paraneoplastic syndromes. In some tumors, such as SCLC, onconeural antigens are present in all tumors, even in those patients who do not develop paraneoplastic antibodies or a paraneoplastic syndrome. The onconeural antigen in the tumor cell is probably recognized by the immune system when tumor cells spontaneously undergo apoptosis and the apoptotic bodies containing the antigen are phagocytized by dendritic cells.[22] Current evidence suggests that the antigens in the tumor are identical in structure to normal neural antigens but, nevertheless, are seen by the immune system as foreign, leading to development of paraneoplastic antibodies.[23,24] Others have found that some paraneoplastic antigens are mutated cancers such as SCLC.[25] The body's immune system attacks structures expressing the paraneoplastic antigen, resulting in two effects. First, the immune attack may control the growth of the tumor and in rare instances obliterate it.[26,27] Second, the immune response also attacks the nervous system itself; both B and T cells can be found in the CNS of patients with CNS paraneoplastic syndromes. The B cells generally reside in the perivascular spaces and the T cells in both perivascular spaces and in the brain parenchyma.[28,29] The T cells found in the nervous system are either mono- or oligoclonal and respond only to a specific antigen.[30]

Paraneoplastic antibodies have also been identified within neurons of some patients who died of paraneoplastic encephalomyelitis.[28] This finding is complemented by the finding of antibodies inside neurons of patients with cancer-associated retinopathy and stiff-person syndrome. Furthermore, experimental evidence indicates that infusion of paraneoplastic IgG antibodies into animals can reproduce the neurologic signs of stiff-person syndrome.[31,32]

Two paraneoplastic syndromes, LEMS and myasthenia gravis, meet formal criteria for an antibody-mediated autoimmune disease.[33] Other paraneoplastic syndromes in which antibodies appear to play a causal a role include stiff-person syndrome, autonomic neuropathy with antibodies to the ganglionic acetylcholine receptor, NMDA receptor antibody–associated limbic encephalopathy, and carcinoma-associated retinopathy.[31–36] Increasing evidence, particularly concerning paraneoplastic syndromes of the CNS, suggests a major T cell component in addition to the B cell–driven antibody response.[37–39] Tumors express paraneoplastic antigens relatively commonly, raising the question of why more cancer patients do not develop immune responses to their tumors. Activation of the $CD8^+$ T cells in lymph nodes relies on the presence of $CD4^+$ helper cells and the absence of inhibitory factors. Imbalance in these regulatory pathways might underlie the presence or absence of paraneoplastic syndrome antigen–specific $CD8^+$ T cells in individual cancer patients.

Diagnosis

Recommended criteria for the diagnosis of a neurologic paraneoplastic syndrome are listed in Table 27-4. Alternative causes that might explain the clinical symptoms must be excluded. "Classic" refers to those neurologic disorders characteristic of a paraneoplastic syndrome as indicated in Table 27-5. "Onconeural" refers to antibodies that recognize antigens that are restricted to the nervous system (or testes) and to some cancers. Originally, when the antigens were unknown, two separate nomenclatures were devised to designate these antibodies. The nomenclature applied at Memorial Sloan-Kettering Cancer Center (e.g., anti-Yo, anti-Hu) refers to the first two letters of the last name of the index patient while the Mayo Clinic terminology (e.g., anti-PCA-1, anti-ANNA-1) refers to the staining pattern by immunohistochemistry. In Table 27-5 the latter system is identified in parentheses. Once these antigens have been identified, the antigen's name is used to designate the antibody in question

TABLE 27-4 ■ Diagnostic Criteria for Paraneoplastic Neurologic Syndromes (PNS)

Definite PNS

1. A classic syndrome and cancer that develops within 5 years of the diagnosis of the neurological disorder.
2. A non-classic syndrome that resolves or significantly improves after cancer treatment without concomitant immunotherapy provided that the syndrome is not susceptible to spontaneous remission.
3. A non-classic syndrome with onconeural antibodies (well-characterized or not) and cancer that develops within 5 years of the diagnosis of the neurologic disorder.
4. A neurologic syndrome (classic or not) with well-characterized onconeural antibodies (e.g., anti-Hu, Yo, CV2, Ri, Ma-2, or amphiphysin), and no cancer.

Possible PNS

1. A classic syndrome, no onconeural antibodies, no cancer but at high risk to have an underlying tumor.
2. A neurologic syndrome (classic or not) with partially characterized onconeural antibodies and no cancer.
3. A non-classic syndrome, no onconeural antibodies, and cancer present within two years of diagnosis.

From Graus F, Delattre JY, Antoine JC, et al: Recommended diagnostic criteria for paraneoplastic neurological syndromes. J Neurol Neurosurg Psychiatry 75:1135, 2004, with permission.

(e.g., anti-VGCC, an antibody against voltage-gated calcium channels). The term "well-characterized" refers to an antibody whose antigen has been identified and whose gene has been cloned and sequenced.

The 5-year period identified in the criteria for the development of cancer is reasonable but problematic. Although in most patients with a paraneoplastic syndrome the cancer is identified within a year or so, in an occasional patient, even when the neurologic syndrome and the antibody clearly have been recognized, more than 5 years may elapse before the cancer is found. The inability to find a cancer, even after 5 years, does not mean that the patient does not have a paraneoplastic syndrome; there are rare, but well-documented, cases of a paraneoplastic syndrome being associated with spontaneous remission of a cancer.[26,27,40] There are occasional patients with high-titer, well-characterized paraneoplastic antibodies who almost certainly never have had or will develop a cancer.

The only unequivocal method of determining whether a given patient has a paraneoplastic syndrome is by identifying an antibody in the serum that reacts with the portion of the nervous system suffering damage and subsequently finding a neoplasm whose cells express the antigen. If the antigen is not found in the neoplasm, the patient either does not have a paraneoplastic syndrome or has another cancer—as yet unfound—that expresses the antigen, and a new search should be considered. One possible exception has been the failure to identify the antigen in many patients with anti-Tr antibodies and paraneoplastic cerebellar degeneration associated with Hodgkin lymphoma.[41]

Although the clinical presentation varies, several clinical features can assist in the diagnosis. Most paraneoplastic syndromes develop rapidly, progress over weeks to months, and then stabilize; syndromes that begin insidiously or are characterized by exacerbations and remissions are less likely to be paraneoplastic. Most paraneoplastic syndromes result in serious neurologic disability. Paraneoplastic syndromes affecting the CNS are often associated with an inflammatory CSF, including pleocytosis, elevated levels of protein, and oligoclonal bands; one of these features is present in nearly every patient with a CNS paraneoplastic syndrome. MRI may be normal or have abnormalities consistent with the clinical findings (e.g., medial temporal lobe T2-weighted hyperintensity in patients with limbic encephalitis or cerebellar atrophy in patients with paraneoplastic cerebellar degeneration). When the MRI is normal, fluorodeoxyglucose positron emission tomography (PET) scans may reveal hypometabolism in the brain that is either diffuse or focal, although these findings are nonspecific.[42] Several of the paraneoplastic syndromes (e.g., LEMS) are so stereotypic that the correct diagnosis can be strongly suspected even before additional diagnostic testing has excluded alternative diagnoses.

ANTIBODIES

Many paraneoplastic syndromes are characterized by serum and CSF autoantibodies which react with both the areas of the nervous system involved and the underlying cancer. Some autoantibodies (e.g., acetylcholine receptor antibodies), however, are found in patients both with and without cancer. Others (e.g., anti-Hu, anti-Ri, and anti-Yo antibodies) are highly specific for the presence of an underlying cancer and strongly suggest a specific cancer that can guide workup. For example, the anti-Yo antibody is strongly associated with breast and gynecologic tumors and requires careful mammography as well as pelvic imaging. However, because

TABLE 27-5 ■ Antibody-Associated Neurologic Paraneoplastic Disorders

Antibody	Location	Antigen/Gene(s)	Usual Tumor or Site of Origin	Neurologic Disorder
Antibody Markers of Neurologic Paraneoplastic Syndromes and Tumor, Requiring a Search for Cancer				
Anti-Hu (ANNA-1)	Nucleus > cytoplasm (all neurons)	HuD (Elavl4); Elavl2, 3	SCLC, neuroblastoma, prostate	PEM, PSN, autonomic dysfunction
Anti-Yo (PCA-1)	Cytoplasm, Purkinje cells	CDR2, Cdr2L	Ovary, breast, lung	PCD
Anti-Ri (ANNA-2)	Nucleus > cytoplasm (CNS neurons)	Nova 1,2	Breast, gynecologic, lung, bladder	Ataxia/opsoclonus; brainstem encephalitis
Anti-CRMP5 (anti-CV2)	Cytoplasm, oligodendrocytes, neurons	CRMP5	SCLC, thymoma	PEM, PCD, chorea, optic, sensory neuropathy
Anti-Ma2 (ANNA-3)	Neurons (nucleolus)	Ma2	Testis	Limbic, brainstem (diencephalic) encephalitis
Anti-amphiphysin	Presynaptic	Amphiphysin	Breast, SCLC	SPS
Anti-Sox (AGNA-1)	Nucleus of Bergman glia, other neurons	SOX1	SCLC	LEMS
Anti-Tr (PCA-Tr)	Cytoplasm, dendrites of Purkinje cells	DNER	Hodgkin	PCD
Anti-recoverin	Photoreceptor, ganglion cells	Recoverin	SCLC	CAR
Anti-bipolar	Bipolar retinal cells	??	Melanoma	MAR
Anti-Titin	Skeletal muscle	Titin	Thymoma	MG
Anti-AChR	Postsynaptic NMJ (electron immunohistochemistry)	AChR	Thymoma	MG
Anti-Ryanodine receptor	Skeletal muscle	Ryanodine receptor	Thymoma	MG (severe form)
Antibody Markers of Autoimmune Neurologic Dysfunction that Do Not Always Require a Search for Cancer				
Anti-VGCC	Presynaptic NMJ	P/Q VGCC	SCLC	LEMS
Anti-NMDAR	Neuronal cell surface, hippocampus, other brain regions	NR1/NR2	Ovarian teratoma	PEM
Anti-AMPAR	Neuronal cell surface	GluR1,2 AMPA receptor	Thymoma, breast, lung	LE
Anti-AChR	Postsynaptic NMJ	AChR	Thymoma	MG
Anti-nAChR	Postsynaptic ganglia	α3 subunit nAChR	SCLC, thymoma	Autonomic neuropathy
Anti-VGKC -anti-LGI1	Neuropile	Antibody binds to potassium channels	Thymoma	LE
Anti-VGKC- anti-CASPR2	Neuropile	Antibody binds to potassium channels		Peripheral nerve hyperexcitability, Morvan Syndrome
Anti-GAD	Purkinje cell cytoplasm, nerve terminals, other neurons	Glutamic acid decarboxylase	Several (renal, Hodgkin, SCLC)	SPS, cerebellar ataxia
Anti-glycine receptor	Brainstem, spinal cord neurons	Glycine receptor	Lung	PERM

(Continued)

TABLE 27-5 ■ (Continued)

Antibody	Location	Antigen/Gene(s)	Usual Tumor or Site of Origin	Neurologic Disorder
Anti-GABA-AR	Neuronal surface	GABA-A receptor associated protein	?	SPS
Anti-GABA-BR	Neuronal surface	GABA-B receptor	SCLC	LE
Anti-MuSK	Muscle	MuSK	Thymoma	MG
Anti-α-enolase	Multiple retinal cells	α-Enolase	SCLC	CAR
Uncommon Antibody Markers of Neurologic Disorders. Some Are Paraneoplastic Single Case Reports or Very Small Series				
Anti-PCA-2	Purkinje cytoplasm and other neurons		SCLC	PCD
Anti-Ma	Neurons (subnucleus)	Ma1 and Ma2	Lung, others	PEM, brainstem
ANNA 3	Nuclei, Purkinje cells	?	Lung	Sensory neuronopathy, PEM
Anti-mGluR1, mGluR5	Purkinje cells, olfactory neurons, hippocampus	Metabotropic glutamate receptor	Hodgkin	PCD
Anti-Zic4	Nuclei of cerebellar	Zic4	SCLC	PCD
Anti-PKC-gamma	Purkinje cells	PKCγ	NSCLC	PCD
Anti-gephyrin	Postsynaptic membranes	Gephyrin	Unknown primary	SPS
Anti-synaptotagmin	Presynaptic junction	Vesicle protein	?	LEMS
Anti-synaptophysin	Presynaptic junction	Vesicle protein	SCLC	Neuropathy
Anti-BRKSK2	Neuronal cytoplasm	BRSK2	SCLC	LE
Anti-adenylate kinase	Neuronal cytoplasm	Adenylate kinase 5	No identified cancer	LE
Anti-CARP VIII	Purkinje cells	CARP VIII	Melanoma	PCD
Anti-Homer 3	Neuropile cerebellum	Homer 3	None known	PCD
Anti-Aquaporin4	Glia			Neuromyelitis optica
Anti-GABA-AR	Neuronal surface	GABA-A receptor associated protein	?	SPS

many paraneoplastic syndromes can be caused by many tumors, a more widespread search including total body CT or PET scan is frequently necessary.[43] Table 27-5 lists many of the antibodies that can be found in the serum of patients with paraneoplastic syndromes. It is usually not necessary to measure antibodies in the CSF of patients in whom serum antibodies are negative. However, in a few instances, the CSF may be positive when there is a very low or undetectable level in the serum. Such instances have been reported in patients with paraneoplastic cerebellar degeneration associated with Hodgkin disease and the anti-Tr antibody and in patients with paraneoplastic limbic encephalopathy associated with ovarian teratomas and anti-NMDA receptor antibodies.[43,44] In patients with CNS paraneoplastic syndromes, the relative activity of the antibody is higher in spinal fluid than in serum, indicating intrathecal synthesis of the antibody.[17,45] One study suggests that CSF titers of anti-Hu antibody are higher in patients with encephalomyelitis than in those with sensory neuronopathy, despite similar serum titers.[46]

Most paraneoplastic antibodies are usually associated with specific paraneoplastic syndromes and a limited number of implicated cancers (Table 27-5). For example, the anti-Hu antibody is more likely to cause encephalomyelitis and is usually associated with SCLC. Honnorat and colleagues compared 37 patients with the anti-CRMP5 antibody and 324 patients with the anti-Hu antibody.[47] The anti-CRMP5 antibody was more likely to be associated with cerebellar ataxia, chorea, optic neuritis, uveitis, and LEMS, whereas the anti-Hu antibody was associated with dysautonomia, brainstem encephalitis, and peripheral neuropathy. Both of these antibodies were associated with SCLC, but only the anti-CRMP5 antibody was associated with thymoma. Regardless of the tumor type, patients with the anti-CRMP5 antibody survived significantly longer, a finding that did not appear to be related to a less severe neurologic disorder than those patients with the anti-Hu antibody.

Antigens can be divided into two large groups: group 1 consists of intracellular antigens, either cytoplasmic or nuclear, and group 2 consists of antigens on the surface of neurons or at synapses.[48,49] This division identifies paraneoplastic disorders that usually respond to treatment and in which antibodies are probably causal (group 2), and those that usually do not respond to treatment and where the pathogenesis is T-cell mediated (group 1).

Group 1 antigens that usually are paraneoplastic, including anti-Hu, anti-Yo and several others, may occur occasionally in patients without cancer.[49] In one series of 68 anti-Hu antibody–positive patients, 3 percent with clinical follow-up of more than 3 years did not develop an identifiable cancer, and there was no difference between those patients who did and did not develop cancer.[50] One possible explanation is that a cancer was present but spontaneously regressed. Both spontaneous regression of the cancer and anti-neuronal antibodies are common in infants with neuroblastoma.[51,52]

Group 1 also consists of intracellular antigens that are cancer-specific but not helpful in diagnosis, including Sox 1 and Zic. Others of these intracellular antigens are associated with autoimmune disorders of the nervous system that are only sometimes paraneoplastic, including anti–glutamic acid decarboxylase (anti-GAD).

Group 2 antigens can be divided into those surface antigens associated with autoimmune CNS syndromes that are only sometimes paraneoplastic, including voltage-gated potassium-related proteins (LGI1, CASPR2), and those surface antigens usually associated with paraneoplastic disorders.

Others authors have divided the antibodies into three groups. Group 1 consists of antibodies that recognize intracellular antigens, either nucleolar or cytoplasmic; group 2 antibodies recognize cell surface synaptic antigens; and group 3 antibodies recognize intracellular synaptic antigens.[53]

Treatment

There are two general approaches to the treatment of paraneoplastic neurologic disorders.[54] The most effective therapy is typically treatment of the underlying tumor, which often prevents progression of the disease and, in some instances, leads to substantial improvement or complete amelioration of the neurologic symptoms.[55,56] Effective treatment of the tumor should remove the inciting antigen and thus temper the immune response causing the neurologic damage.

Because paraneoplastic syndromes are believed to be immune mediated, the second approach to treatment is to suppress the immune response. This immunosuppression does not appear to worsen the outcome of the tumor.[55] Several different forms of immunosuppression, including corticosteroids, plasma exchange, intravenous immunoglobulin, cyclophosphamide, and cyclosporine or tacrolimus, have been used to treat the paraneoplastic syndromes (Table 27-6).[53]

The earlier in the course of the neurologic syndrome that immunosuppressive treatment or treatment of the cancer is begun, the more likely the patient is to stabilize or improve.[57] Cell surface antibodies (e.g., anti-NMDA receptor, anti-VGCC) are highly likely to respond to immunotherapy; many such patients do not have cancer. Antigens located within the cell body, often the nucleus (e.g., anti-Yo and anti-Hu antibodies), are found in patients who are highly likely to have cancer and generally respond poorly to immunosuppression. A third group consists of antibodies that lie intracellularly within synapses (e.g., anti-GAD and anti-amphiphysin antibodies); these patients may or may not have cancer and may not respond well to immunosuppression. Two recent reviews summarize the approach to treatment[58] and the effects of treatment in patients with specific antibodies.[53,58]

SPECIFIC SYNDROMES

Paraneoplastic syndromes that affect the nervous system are classified in Table 27-5. Only some of the more common syndromes are considered in this chapter, and more extensive reviews are available elsewhere.[59]

Limbic Encephalitis

Limbic encephalitis is characterized by the acute-to-subacute onset of short-term memory loss, seizures,

TABLE 27-6 ■ Treatment of Neurologic Paraneoplastic Syndromes

Syndrome	Treatment
*Syndromes That Usually Respond to Treatment**	
Lambert–Eaton myasthenic syndrome	IV immunoglobulin, plasma exchange, 2,3 diaminopyridine, immunosuppression†
Myasthenia gravis	IV immunoglobulin, plasma exchange, immunosuppression, anticholinesterases
Dermatomyositis	IV immunoglobulin, immunosuppression
Opsoclonus-myoclonus (pediatric)	IV immunoglobulin, corticosteroids, ACTH, rituximab
Neuropathy associated with osteosclerotic myeloma	Radiation, chemotherapy
Anti-NMDAR	First line: corticosteroids, IV immunoglobulin, plasma exchange Second line: cyclophosphamide, rituximab
Anti-LGI1	Corticosteroids, IV immunoglobulin, plasma exchange
Anti-cell surface antigens other than NMDAR and LGI1 (AMPA receptor, GABA(B) receptor, CASPR2)	Corticosteroids, IVIg, plasma exchange, cyclophosphamide
*Syndromes That May Respond to Treatment**	
Stiff-person syndrome	IV immunoglobulin, corticosteroids, diazepam, baclofen
Neuromyotonia	IV immunoglobulin, plasma exchange, phenytoin, carbamazepine
Guillain–Barré (Hodgkin lymphoma)	IV immunoglobulin, plasma exchange
Vasculitis of nerve and muscle	Corticosteroids, cyclophosphamide
Limbic encephalitis	IV immunoglobulin, corticosteroids
Opsoclonus-myoclonus (adults)	Corticosteroids, cyclophosphamide, protein A column, clonazepam, thiamine
Anti–MAG-associated peripheral neuropathy (Waldenström macroglobulinemia)	IV immunoglobulin, plasma exchange, chlorambucil, cyclophosphamide, fludarabine, rituximab
Acute necrotizing myopathy	Immunosuppression

In all cases, initial treatment should focus on identifying and treating the tumor.
*Syndromes that usually do not respond to treatment include encephalomyelitis, sensory neuronopathy, autonomic dysfunction, cerebellar degeneration, and cancer- and melanoma-associated retinopathy.
†Immunosuppression includes corticosteroids or azothioprine.

and behavioral abnormalities.[60,61] The disorder has been reported in association with a variety of tumors including SCLC and ovarian teratoma. A clinically identical autoimmune disorder occurs in patients without cancer. Both paraneoplastic and nonparaneoplastic limbic encephalitis can be associated with a variety of different antibodies.[60]

Paraneoplastic limbic encephalitis usually begins with changes in mood and personality that worsen over days to weeks.[62,63] Accompanying the mood changes is severe impairment of recent memory with relatively preserved remote memory. Patients are often agitated and confused, with hallucinations and generalized or complex partial seizures. Symptoms can begin quite abruptly or the onset may be more gradual, occurring over several weeks to even a few months. When behavioral changes dominate the symptomatology, particularly when the disorder affects young women, a diagnosis of psychiatric disease may occur before a correct diagnosis is made.

Loss of short-term memory with preservation of other cognitive function (the "Ophelia syndrome") is a hallmark of the syndrome.[64,65] Behavioral changes, ranging from depression through agitation to a florid delirium, are often present. Alterations of consciousness may progress to stupor or coma. Coma (often reversible) is particularly characteristic of the ovarian teratoma syndrome associated with anti-NMDA receptor antibodies.[35]

LABORATORY FINDINGS

The CSF is typically inflammatory, at least early in the course of the disease. The MRI may be normal although abnormalities, particularly hyperintensity on the T2-weighted or fluid-attenuated inversion recovery (FLAIR) sequences (Fig. 27-1), sometimes with contrast enhancement, are common.[62,66] At times, the medial temporal lobe changes are more subtle. Electroencephalographic (EEG) findings include focal or generalized slowing and occasional epileptiform activity, particularly in the temporal areas. Measurement of brain metabolism with PET or SPECT scanning shows abnormalities in the medial temporal lobes. The areas may be either hypermetabolic due to seizure activity or inflammation or may be hypometabolic late in the course, related to neuronal degeneration.[67]

The most important diagnostic test is measurement of paraneoplastic antibodies.[60,68] The most

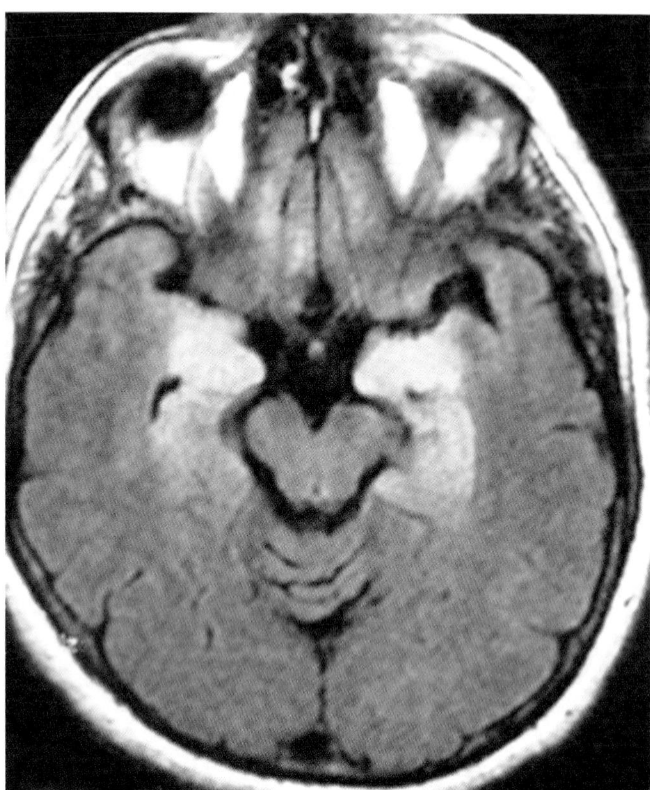

FIGURE 27-1 ▪ Axial fluid-attenuated inversion recovery (FLAIR) magnetic resonance imaging (MRI) of a patient with paraneoplastic limbic encephalopathy. There is marked hyperintensity in the medial temporal lobes bilaterally. In addition, there is slight dilatation of the temporal horns, suggesting atrophy.

common antibodies found in paraneoplastic limbic encephalitis are anti-Hu (SCLC), anti-Ma2 (testicular cancer), anti-CRMP5/CV2 (SCLC-thymoma), anti-NMDA receptor (ovarian teratoma) and anti-$GABA_B$ (SCLC).[35,69] Antibodies found in patients who frequently do not have cancer include antibodies against LGI1 and CASPR2 (these antibodies were previously referred to as voltage-gated potassium channel antibodies). LGI1 is associated with typical limbic encephalitis, whereas CASPR2 generally is associated with peripheral nerve hyperexcitability. CASPR2 antibodies may occasionally be associated with thymic tumors.

Pathology

Typical paraneoplastic limbic encephalopathy is characterized by the destruction of hippocampal neurons along with inflammatory infiltrates both in the perivascular spaces and in the brain parenchyma. Parenchymal infiltrates consist largely of T cells, and those in the perivascular spaces feature a combination of B cells and T cells. In some patients, particularly those who die many years after the disorder begins, findings are consistent with sclerosis of the hippocampus, without inflammatory infiltrates, particularly in patients with Hodgkin disease. Whether inflammation was present at onset and disappeared over time is unclear. One report describes hypometabolism in the medial temporal lobe and evidence of hippocampal sclerosis within 6 months of the onset of clinical symptoms, suggesting this may be an earlier change than previously suspected.[70]

Diagnosis

Depending on the clinical presentation, the two most important alternate diagnoses to consider are herpes simplex encephalitis and acute psychosis.[35,61] Other diagnostic considerations include temporal lobe tumors, systemic lupus erythematosus, Hashimoto encephalopathy, human herpes virus type 6 (especially after bone marrow transplantation), and a variety of metabolic abnormalities causing delirium.

The other important diagnostic consideration is to differentiate paraneoplastic limbic encephalitis from nonparaneoplastic autoimmune limbic encephalitis.[71] These two disorders are clinically indistinguishable.[71] All patients require at least an initial search for an underlying neoplasm.

Treatment

Aside from treatment of the tumor, immunosuppression is the mainstay of therapy, which is similar to that for other paraneoplastic and autoimmune disorders.[68] The earlier treatment has started, the more likely the illness will either stabilize or improve. In some of these disorders, particularly those associated with cell surface antibodies (e.g., NMDA receptor antibodies), even late treatment of comatose patients may lead to resolution of the neurologic symptoms.[35]

Encephalomyelitis

Paraneoplastic limbic encephalopathy may also occur as part of a more widespread disorder (encephalomyelitis) that is associated with carcinoma.[72] The clinical presentation often includes subacute sensory neuronopathy, cerebellar degeneration, myelopathy, and sometimes peripheral neuropathy or myopathy; these disorders are discussed in other sections of this chapter.

Hypothalamic Dysfunction

Isolated paraneoplastic hypothalamic dysfunction is rare. The disorder usually occurs in conjunction with a more widespread encephalomyelitis. Hypothalamic dysfunction characteristically occurs in patients with anti-Ma2 (anti-Ta) antibodies and testicular cancer, anti-CRMP5 (CV2) encephalomyelitis associated with thymoma, and anti-NMDA receptor encephalitis associated with ovarian teratoma.[35,73–75] The disorder, which is sometime responsive to immunoglobulin therapy, also occurs in children with neuroblastoma and sometimes in children without known cancer.[76–78] Symptoms of hypothalamic dysfunction include somnolence, temperature dysregulation with hyperhidrosis, endocrinopathies including diabetes insipidus and hypothyroidism, narcolepsy or somnolence, weight gain, and loss of libido.[63,79,80]

Brain MRI may reveal evidence of inflammation in the hypothalamus including contrast enhancement. Treatment consists of discovery and treatment of the underlying tumor as well as immunosuppression. Patients with testicular cancer and anti-Ma2 antibodies sometimes stabilize and even improve, at least partially, but patients harboring other antibodies, such as anti-Hu, do less well.[81]

Brainstem or Basal Ganglia Encephalitis

Paraneoplastic brainstem encephalitis, characterized by the subacute development of bulbar, midbrain, or basal ganglia signs, usually occurs as part of the more diffuse syndrome of encephalomyelitis, although it sometimes presents as a dominant or isolated clinical finding.[82,83] The syndrome usually affects the lower brainstem preferentially, causing diplopia, vertigo, oscillopsia, dysarthria, dysphagia, hypoventilation, hearing loss, facial weakness, myokymia, facial numbness, or opsoclonus in various combinations.[83] When the upper brainstem or basal ganglia are affected, movement disorders including chorea, dystonia, bradykinesia, myoclonus, and parkinsonism may occur along with daytime sleepiness.[84,85] The disorder has been associated with a number of antibodies including anti-Hu (usually with more widespread encephalomyelitis symptoms), anti-Ri (typically with opsoclonus), anti-Ma2 (featuring prominent midbrain and diencephalic dysfunction), and anti-NMDA (with central respiratory failure and coma). In one report of 36 patients with adult-onset autoimmune chorea, the disorder was paraneoplastic in 14; CV2/CRMP5 and anti-Hu were the major associated antibodies.[84]

Cerebellum

Of the paraneoplastic disorders affecting the brain, paraneoplastic cerebellar degeneration is perhaps the most easily recognized and best characterized. It is characterized pathologically by loss of cerebellar Purkinje cells and is associated with several different cancers.

Clinical Findings

Paraneoplastic cerebellar degeneration was first described in 1919, but the association between it and cancer was not recognized until 1938.[86,87] Paraneoplastic cerebellar degeneration can be associated with any malignancy, but the most common culprits include lung cancer, particularly SCLC, ovarian or uterine cancer, and lymphoma, particularly Hodgkin disease.[88,89] In most patients, neurologic symptoms prompt medical attention before the cancer itself has been identified. The cancer is usually then found within months to a year after the onset of neurologic symptoms; however, occasionally it may elude detection for several years and in some instances is found only at autopsy.

Typically, the disorder begins with dizziness or vertigo, nausea, and vomiting followed rapidly by gait ataxia evolving rapidly over days to a few months to include incoordination in the arms, legs, and trunk; dysarthria is also often present, as is nystagmus associated with oscillopsia. Within a few months, the illness usually reaches its peak and then stabilizes. By this time, most patients cannot walk and many cannot sit unsupported. Handwriting is impossible, independent eating is difficult, and speech may be difficult to understand. Oscillopsia may prevent reading or even watching television. The neurologic signs are always bilateral and usually symmetric, although at times one side may be more affected than the other. In occasional patients, this asymmetry is quite prominent. Diplopia is an early symptom in many patients, although abnormalities of ocular muscles are often not detected by the examiner. Exceptions include those with abrupt onset and patients with a more mild course so that the patient can walk, write, and be understood, albeit with some difficulty.[90]

The signs and symptoms are frequently limited to those of cerebellar or cerebellar pathway dysfunction but, in as many as 50 percent of patients, other neurologic abnormalities, usually mild, may be found on careful examination, including sensorineural hearing loss, dysphagia, hyperreflexia with or without extensor plantar responses, extrapyramidal signs, peripheral neuropathy, and cognitive abnormalities including dementia.[91–93] One study using formal neuropsychologic testing challenged the notion of cognitive dysfunction, finding that dementia was not common when testing was controlled for impaired motor and speech production.[94]

Laboratory Evaluation

Early in the course of the disease, the brain MRI is usually normal (Fig. 27-2A). However, a study described a reduced NAA/Cr ratio on MR spectroscopy of the cerebellar vermis in two patients with paraneoplastic cerebellar degeneration in whom routine MRI was normal.[95] If patients are followed for months to a few years, diffuse cerebellar atrophy appears (Fig. 27-2B). Occasional patients have been reported in whom hyperintensity is found in the cerebral and cerebellar white matter on T2-weighted images. Rarely, transient contrast enhancement of the cerebellar folia may suggest leptomeningeal tumor along with associated edema, which may cause hydrocephalus.

In most patients who are studied early in the course of the disease, the CSF contains an increased number of lymphocytes, slightly elevated protein level and increased IgG index along with oligoclonal bands. The pleocytosis usually resolves with time. Some, but not all, patients with paraneoplastic cerebellar degeneration have autoantibodies in serum and CSF that react with Purkinje cells of the cerebellum and the causal tumor.

The antibody most frequently associated with pure cerebellar degeneration is anti-Yo, so named based on the first two letters of the last name of the index patient (Table 27-5).[88–91] This antibody recognizes a major protein antigen termed CDR2, an approximately 62-kDa protein expressed in Purkinje cells of the cerebellum. All patients with anti-Yo paraneoplastic cerebellar degeneration who have ovarian or breast cancer express the Purkinje cell antigens in the tumor cells. About 60 percent of patients with ovarian cancer who do not have paraneoplastic cerebellar degeneration also express CDR2 in their tumors.[96] The antibody is found at higher titer in the spinal fluid than in the serum, suggesting intrathecal synthesis from B cells that have crossed into the brain.[17] In addition to the antibody response, cytotoxic T cells against CDR2 have also been described, although some question their specificity.[97] Patients with breast cancer and anti-Yo cerebellar degeneration also usually overexpress HER2.[98]

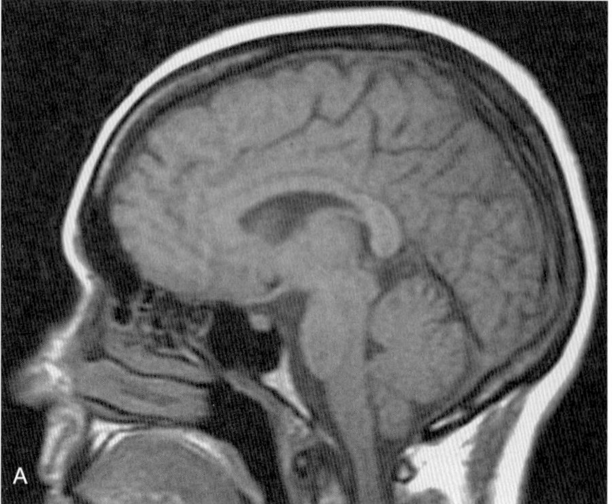

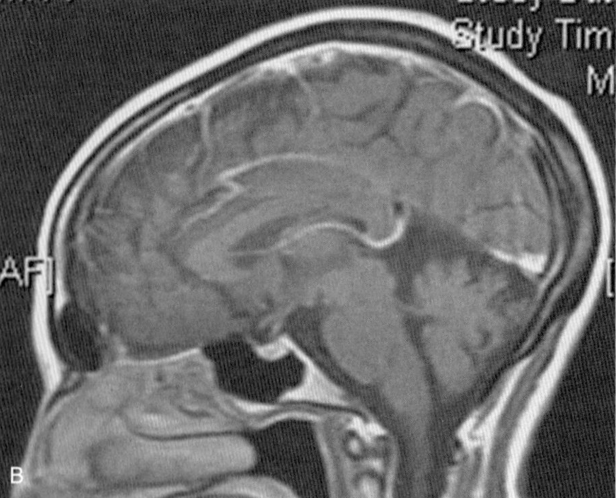

FIGURE 27-2 ■ **A**, Normal sagittal MRI of the brain. **B**, T1 contrast-enhanced sagittal MRI of the brain in a patient with paraneoplastic cerebellar degeneration. The cerebellum is atrophic, but the rest of the brain is normal.

A second antibody commonly found in patients with paraneoplastic cerebellar degeneration is the anti-Tr antibody that occurs in patients with paraneoplastic cerebellar degeneration related to Hodgkin disease.[99,100] The disorder often begins after the diagnosis of Hodgkin disease and sometimes when patients are in remission.[89] The clinical presentation is generally less severe than in patients with the anti-Yo antibody. The prognosis for successful treatment of the underlying tumor is good. One report identified the responsible antigen as delta/notch-like epidermal growth factor–related receptor.[101]

Anti-Hu antibodies usually cause cerebellar degeneration as a part of a more widespread encephalomyelitis syndrome. In some patients, cerebellar symptoms outweigh other symptoms; in other patients, sensory neuronopathy is prominent so that it is difficult to discern whether the ataxia is due to sensory loss or cerebellar dysfunction.[102] As with the anti-Yo antibody syndrome, symptoms may be sudden in onset and pathologic examination reveals substantial loss of Purkinje cells. Inflammatory infiltrates in Purkinje cells or the cerebellar dentate nucleus are often found in patients with the anti-Hu antibody, perhaps because patients only survive for a short period of time, although one report seems to suggest otherwise.[88,103]

Other less common antibodies include anti-Ma, an antibody that recognizes both Ma1 and Ma2, antigens restricted to brain and testis.[16] The paraneoplastic disorder usually is associated with encephalomyelitis, particularly brainstem and hypothalamic dysfunction, and is associated with a variety of tumors including those of breast and colon. The anti-Ri antibody (discussed later in the section on opsoclonus) is also associated with paraneoplastic cerebellar degeneration, usually as part of the opsoclonus-myoclonus syndrome. Anti-CRMP5 (anti-CV2) antibodies are directed against an antigen in some glial cells and against peripheral nerve antigens; the disorder has been associated with a number of neurologic problems including optic neuritis and paraneoplastic cerebellar degeneration.[104,105] The most common tumor is thymoma, although some patients have SCLC and gynecologic malignancies. Anti-P/Q VGCC antibodies associated with LEMS and SCLC are also occasionally associated with paraneoplastic cerebellar degeneration.[106] Anti-mGluR1 antibodies have been reported in patients with Hodgkin disease and paraneoplastic cerebellar degeneration.[107,108] Anti-Zic4 antibodies have also been associated with cerebellar degeneration as well as encephalomyelitis in patients with SCLC, as have anti-PCA2 and anti-ANNA-3 antibodies.[109–111] Other rarer antibodies include anti-CARP VIII antibodies (usually with melanoma), anti-proteasome in association with anti-Yo antibodies (ovary and breast cancers), anti-PKC gamma (NSCLC), anti-Ca (no cancer yet identified), and an unnamed antibody associated with prostate cancer.[112–116]

Pathology

The CNS may appear grossly normal when examined at autopsy, but usually the cerebellum is atrophic, with abnormally widened sulci and small gyri. Microscopically, the hallmark of paraneoplastic cerebellar degeneration is severe, often complete, loss of the Purkinje cells of the cerebellar cortex (Fig. 27-3).[117] Degenerating Purkinje cells may have swellings, called torpedoes, along the course of their axons. Other pathologic features may include thinning of the molecular and granular layers of the cerebellar cortex, often without marked cell loss, and proliferation of astrocytes. The deep cerebellar nuclei are usually well preserved, although rarefied white matter may surround the nuclei, caused by the loss of Purkinje cell axons. Basket cells and tangential fibers are usually intact. Lymphocytic infiltrates, if present, are usually found in the leptomeninges around the cerebellum, in the dentate nucleus, and throughout the surrounding white matter; they are rare in the Purkinje cell layer.

In many patients, the disorder is noninflammatory, with all pathologic changes restricted to the Purkinje cell layer of the cerebellum. However, pathologic changes outside the cerebellum do occur in some patients, including degeneration of the dorsal columns and pyramidal tracts of the spinal cord, degeneration of the basal ganglia (specifically the pallidum), loss of peripheral nerve fibers, and inflammatory infiltrates in the brainstem, spinal cord, and cerebral cortex.

The tumors associated with paraneoplastic cerebellar degeneration do not differ histologically from similar tumors unassociated with paraneoplastic symptoms except that the tumors are usually found to be infiltrated with lymphocytes and plasma cells.[20] In many patients, the tumor, when identified, is still localized. Metastases, if present, are usually found only in regional lymph nodes.

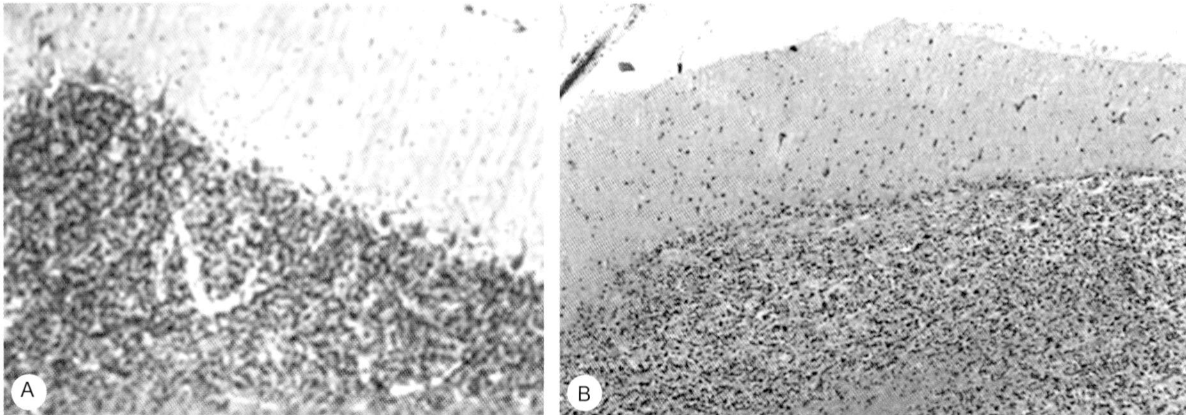

FIGURE 27-3 ■ Paraneoplastic cerebellar degeneration. **A**, Section of cerebellum of a patient who died of cancer without cerebellar symptoms. Multiple Purkinje cells are identified between the molecular (top) and granule cell (bottom) layers, both of which are normal. (Hematoxylin–eosin × 25.) **B**, Section of cerebellum from a patient with autoantibody-positive paraneoplastic cerebellar degeneration. The molecular and granular cell layers are relatively normal, but Purkinje cells are absent, and there is a slight increase in Bergmann astroglia along with some inflammatory cells in the leptomeninges. (Hematoxylin–eosin × 25.)

Diagnosis

The diagnosis depends on recognizing the characteristic clinical syndrome and excluding other cancer-associated causes of late-onset cerebellar dysfunction, such as parenchymal or leptomeningeal metastases, infections, and toxicity of therapies such as cytarabine (see Chapter 28). Causes unrelated to cancer, such as viral brainstem encephalitis or cerebellitis, demyelinating disease, Creutzfeldt–Jakob disease, infarction, hypothyroidism, and alcoholic and hereditary cerebellar degeneration, must also be excluded.

A disorder clinically identical to paraneoplastic cerebellar degeneration may occur without a cancer being identified. How often subacute cerebellar degeneration is nonparaneoplastic is uncertain, but it may be 50 percent or higher.[118,119] In patients with rapidly developing cerebellar syndromes, the physician should suspect a paraneoplastic disorder, particularly when the CSF contains a lymphocytic pleocytosis. The detection of autoantibodies will identify the neurologic disorder as being paraneoplastic and suggest the likely location of the tumor, although these tumors may be very small and difficult to identify. If evaluation including total-body PET scanning fails to identify a tumor, repeated searches may be necessary.[120] Exploratory laparotomy with salpingo-oophorectomy has been recommended in postmenopausal women who are anti-Yo positive and whose evaluation, including pelvic scans and mammograms, is negative.[121] The author has used this approach in several patients, and in all except one (in whom breast cancer was identified 4 months later) a tumor of the gynecologic tract was found; the tumor is sometimes apparent only microscopically.

Treatment

Reviews addressing the treatment of paraneoplastic cerebellar degeneration are available elsewhere.[122] Treatment is commonly unsuccessful, perhaps in part due to death of Purkinje cells. The general treatment approach requires identifying and treating the causal tumor and then attempting immunosuppression. Immunosuppressive treatments have included corticosteroids, usually at a dose of 1000 mg of methylprednisolone daily followed by oral prednisone in a tapering dose. If the treatment is partially successful, consideration can be given to repeated courses of intravenous immunoglobulin (IVIg) at a dose of 2 g/kg administered over either 2 or 5 days and repeated every 3 to 4 weeks.[123] Cyclophosphamide, tacrolimus (0.15 to 0.3 mg/kg daily), rituximab (usually 375 mg/m^2 weekly for 4 weeks), mycophenolate (1 to 1.5 g twice daily), and plasma exchange are additional treatments that have been used.[108,122,124–127]

Individual case reports indicate that treatment of the tumor and immunosuppression either stabilize or improve paraneoplastic cerebellar degeneration.[88,128,129] In general, however, the anti-Hu and anti-Yo antibody patients rarely improve, whereas anti-Tr or anti-CRMP5 antibody disorders may have a better prognosis. Symptomatic improvement in the ataxia occurs in a few patients using clonazepam in daily doses varying from 0.5 to 1.5 mg. Buspirone may also give modest relief.[130]

Opsoclonus-Myoclonus

Opsoclonus consists of involuntary, arrhythmic, multidirectional, high-amplitude conjugate saccades. Opsoclonus is often associated with diffuse or focal myoclonus as well as truncal titubation, with or without other cerebellar signs. Opsoclonus-myoclonus occurs primarily in children as a self-limited illness, probably the result of a viral infection affecting the brainstem. The disorder is paraneoplastic in about 40 percent of children.[131,132] Although neuroblastoma is the common associated tumor, less than 2 percent of children with neuroblastoma have opsoclonus.[52,133] However, given the known tendency of neuroblastoma to resolve spontaneously, some patients with opsoclonus-myoclonus without tumor may, in fact, have had a paraneoplastic form. These children are more likely to suffer from intrathoracic tumors with a benign pathology.[134] Neuroblastoma prognosis is better in patients who have a paraneoplastic syndrome.[135]

The age at peak incidence is 18 months, with more girls than boys affected. Neurologic signs precede identification of the tumor at least 50 percent of the time, making recognition of the neurologic syndrome an important clue to the presence of neuroblastoma. Ataxia, irritability, vomiting, and dementia may accompany opsoclonus-myoclonus.

A number of autoantibodies have been described in neuroblastoma-related opsoclonus.[52,136,137] Affected children have a high incidence of antibodies that react with CNS antigens, but no particular antibody is pathognomonic for the syndrome. An autoantibody that binds the surface of cerebellar granule cells and is cytotoxic to neuroblastoma cell lines has been identified in pediatric patients with opsoclonus-myoclonus, with or without neuroblastoma.[137] Some of the children had other antibodies that also reacted with cerebellar structures, including the anti-Hu antibody.[52] Another report has identified elevated serum concentration of Th2-attracting chemokines in this disorder.[138]

Opsoclonus may respond to treatment with corticotropin (ACTH), plasma exchange, intravenous immunoglobulin, or rituximab and may improve after chemotherapy for the tumor. Multimodal therapy is better than corticotrophin alone.[139] Unfortunately, many patients develop relapses and are left with significant cognitive deficits.[137]

The disorder is less common in adults and is paraneoplastic in 15 to 20 percent of adults.[140] Lung cancer is the most common cause, followed by ovarian teratoma. Neurologic symptoms usually precede the diagnosis of tumor and progress over several weeks, although more rapid or slower progression is observed in some instances. Opsoclonus is often associated with truncal ataxia, dysarthria, myoclonus, vertigo, and encephalopathy; some patients appear to have paraneoplastic cerebellar degeneration as well, and ophthalmoplegia has been reported.[141] A mild CSF pleocytosis and a slightly elevated protein level are present in most patients. The results of neuroimaging are usually normal; in a few patients, an abnormality in the brainstem or cerebellum is detected by MRI. The anti-Ri antibody is the most common culprit, occurring in women with breast cancer and other gynecologic tumors most commonly.[140,142–144] This antibody identifies a protein called Nova, an RNA-binding protein that regulates encoding synaptic proteins, including the glycine and $GABA_A$ receptors in the brainstem.[145,146] Identifiable antibodies are usually not found in patients with opsoclonus and SCLC or ovarian teratomas.

Nonparaneoplastic causes of opsoclonus-myoclonus include viral infections, parainfectious syndromes, infection with human immunodeficiency virus (HIV), and toxic or metabolic encephalopathies. In many instances the cause is unknown.[140] Immunosuppressive agents sometimes appear to be effective, although spontaneous remissions have also been described, making it difficult to interpret positive results.[147] In the paraneoplastic form, the syndrome responds less well to immunotherapy unless the tumor is also treated.[148]

Visual Loss

Paraneoplastic syndromes can cause visual loss by affecting either the retina or the optic nerve.[149–152] They can affect photoreceptors (either rods, cones, or both) or can cause a retinal vasculitis. A paraneoplastic visual disorder can occur either as an isolated phenomenon or as part of a more widespread encephalomyelopathy.

Retinopathy

Although all paraneoplastic visual disorders are rare, paraneoplastic retinal degeneration, also called cancer-associated retinopathy, is the most common. The two most common disorders are cancer-associated retinopathy (CAR) and melanoma-associated retinopathy (MAR). The former disorder usually occurs in association with SCLC and gynecologic tumors. Typically, the visual symptoms, which include episodic visual obscurations, night blindness, light-induced glare, photosensitivity, and impaired color vision, precede the diagnosis of cancer.[149] The symptoms progress to painless visual loss and may begin unilaterally before usually becoming bilateral. Visual testing demonstrates peripheral and ring scotomas along with loss of acuity. Funduscopic examination may reveal arteriolar narrowing and abnormal mottling of the retinal pigment epithelium; the electroretinogram is abnormal. The CSF is typically normal, although elevated immunoglobulin levels have been reported. Inflammatory cells are sometimes seen in the vitreous using slit-lamp examination. Pathologically, a loss of photoreceptors and ganglion cells with inflammatory infiltrates and macrophages is usually found. Other parts of the optic pathway are preserved, although a loss of myelin and lymphocytic infiltration of the optic nerve may occur. The melanoma-associated form is usually less severe, and generally occurs in patients already known to have melanoma; symptoms include night blindness, photopsias, and visual glare.[153]

Several autoantibodies have been identified in patients with cancer-associated retinopathy, the most common of which is recoverin.[149,154] Recoverin is a 23-kDa protein that modulates dark and light adaptation through calcium-dependent regulation of rhodopsin phosphorylation in photoreceptor cells. Recoverin antibodies can cross the blood–brain barrier, gaining access to photoreceptor cells within the aqueous humor.[155] Several other autoantibodies may also occur in patients with paraneoplastic visual loss. Treatment of cancer-associated retinopathy is usually unsuccessful, despite immunosuppression and treatment of the cancer.[149] A number of different antibodies have been detected in the serum of patients with melanoma-associated retinopathy and, like cancer-associated retinopathy, treatment is usually not effective.[153,156]

Optic Neuropathy

Paraneoplastic optic neuropathy occurring in the absence of other neurologic symptoms is extremely uncommon.[157] Cross and colleagues described 16 patients with optic neuritis (5 of whom also had retinitis) who harbored antibodies to collapsin response-mediator protein (CRMP5).[105] These patients had subacute visual loss; optic discs were swollen and visual field defects were present. All of the patients had a variety of other neurologic symptoms including cognitive changes, ataxia, sensory neuropathy, and myelopathy. In some patients the disorder resembled neuromyelitis optica.[158,159] The most common associated cancer is SCLC.

Spinal Cord Syndromes

Paraneoplastic disorders may affect the spinal cord, either in isolation or as part of a more widespread encephalomyelitis.[160–162]

Myelitis

Paraneoplastic non-necrotizing myelitis occurs rarely as an isolated syndrome and more commonly as a part of diffuse encephalomyelitis. Patients present with progressive weakness, sometimes with lower motor neuron signs including fasciculations, in association with sensory loss and autonomic dysfunction (e.g., incontinence and postural hypotension). The disorder may rarely be episodic or primarily involve posterior column function. Early in its evolution, the disorder may clinically resemble motor neuron disease. Upper extremity findings often predominate owing to cervical cord involvement, and respiratory failure may occur. The differential diagnosis includes compressive or intrinsic spinal cord masses, other inflammatory or infectious myelopathies, and radiation injury. The CSF is typically inflammatory. Neuroimaging usually shows a normal spinal cord but, occasionally, expansion or hyperintensity of the spinal cord can be identified on T2-weighted MRI; rarely, contrast enhancement is present. No treatment is effective.

Pathologically, an intense inflammatory reaction with neuronal loss in the anterior and posterior horns is seen, with secondary nerve root degeneration and neurogenic muscle atrophy. Inflammation and degeneration of white matter tracts also can occur. A number of antibodies have been reported, including anti-CV2/CRMP5, anti-amphiphysin, anti-Hu, and anti-Ri.[160]

Subacute necrotizing myelopathy is a rare syndrome that occurs with lymphoma, leukemia, or lung cancers most commonly.[163] The onset of the paraneoplastic disorder may precede or follow the diagnosis of cancer. Patients typically present with rapidly ascending flaccid paraplegia; back pain or radicular pain may herald the onset of neurologic dysfunction. The disease may ascend in the spinal cord, leading to respiratory failure. Inflammatory cells are usually present in the CSF. The MRI may be normal or show spinal cord swelling or contrast enhancement.[163] The absence of an epidural mass or discrete intramedullary enhancement rules out metastatic myelopathy, which is much more common. Treatment is usually unsuccessful, although some patients respond to immunosuppression including corticosteroids.[160,163] Pathologically, there is widespread necrosis involving all components of the spinal cord, but with some white matter predominance.[163] Inflammatory infiltrates are not typical.

Motor neuron disease may occasionally occur as a paraneoplastic syndrome.[164,165] Paraneoplastic motor neuron disease can resemble amyotrophic lateral sclerosis with both upper and lower motor neuron dysfunction or it may present as progressive muscular atrophy, a pure lower motor neuron syndrome that is sometimes reversible and is associated with lymphoproliferative disorders. Subacute, nonreversible lower motor neuron syndromes have been reported in patients with anti-Hu antibodies and SCLC.[166] Primary lateral sclerosis, a pure upper motor neuron syndrome, is associated with solid tumors as well as with lymphoproliferative disorders.[164] The clinical and pathologic characteristics differ little from nonparaneoplastic motor neuron disease except that the paraneoplastic disorders are often more rapid in onset and evolution, sometimes reverse spontaneously, and, at autopsy, may have more inflammatory cells than the nonparaneoplastic forms.

Neuromyelitis optica is usually nonparaneoplastic and associated with antibodies against aquaporin-4; however, the disorder is occasionally paraneoplastic.[159,167,168]

Stiff-Person Syndrome

Originally called the stiff-man syndrome, although it affects more women than men, this disorder is characterized by muscle stiffness and rigidity that are usually painful.[169,170] The muscles involved almost always include the paraspinal and abdominal muscles and usually those of the lower extremities. In some instances, the illness is restricted to a single extremity. Sustained muscle contraction results in abnormal postures, such as an exaggerated lumbar lordosis. In addition to the chronic contractions, severe episodic muscle spasms may be precipitated by voluntary movements, unexpected environmental stimuli, and emotional upset. The arms are less commonly involved, and although stiffness of the neck and face can occur, it is rarely severe. On examination, the muscles feel hard and may be difficult to move passively. An unexpected external stimulus or a voluntary movement may precipitate an observable spasm. The electromyogram (EMG) is characterized by sustained continuous motor-unit activity that disappears during sleep and general anesthesia.

The nonparaneoplastic form of the disorder is associated with diabetes and antibodies to GAD.[171] The paraneoplastic disorder is associated with antibodies against amphiphysin, GAD, anti-Ri, gephyrin, and the glycine receptor α-1 subunit antibody.[172,173] The common associated tumors include breast cancer, SCLC, Hodgkin disease, and colon cancer.

Although the pathogenesis of the disorder is not fully understood, the disorder may be antibody mediated.[170] Injection of either anti-Gad65 or anti-amphiphysin antibodies into animals reproduces the syndrome.[32,174]

Benzodiazepines and baclofen may relieve symptoms. Treatment of the tumor and immunosuppression with corticosteroids, intravenous immunoglobulin, or repeated plasmapheresis are sometimes effective.[175]

Peripheral Nerve and Dorsal Root Ganglion Syndromes

Virtually any of the abnormalities that can affect the peripheral nervous system of patients without cancer can also occur as a paraneoplastic syndrome, including subacute sensory neuronopathy (dorsal root ganglionitis), sensory peripheral neuropathy, sensorimotor peripheral neuropathy (either axonal or demyelinating), autonomic neuropathy, paraproteinemic neuropathy, vasculitic neuropathy (presenting as mononeuritis multiplex), and a pure motor neuropathy or neuronopathy.[176,177] Motor neuronopathy was discussed earlier with the spinal cord syndromes. The exact incidence of these disorders is not established. In a review of 979 patients referred to the paraneoplastic Euronetwork database, the most common syndrome was sensory neuronopathy, occurring in 238 patients.[176] All other causes of neuropathy were found in a total of only 86 patients. In another series of 422 consecutive patients with peripheral neuropathy referred to a tertiary center, 26 were believed to have a paraneoplastic peripheral neuropathy and 7 had onconeuronal antibodies.[178] The overall incidence of presumed paraneoplastic peripheral neuropathy in this study was 6 to 8 percent, varying with the type of neuropathy.

Subacute sensory neuronopathy is the most common type of paraneoplastic peripheral neuropathy and is usually associated with SCLC. Symptoms typically begin before the cancer is identified with dysesthetic pain and numbness in the distal extremities or occasionally in the face or trunk. The symptoms may be asymmetric at onset, but progress over days to several weeks to involve all limbs, causing a severe sensory ataxia. All sensory modalities are affected, distinguishing this disorder from cisplatin neuropathy, in which pinprick and temperature sensation are typically spared. Pain is occasionally a prominent symptom.[179] Muscle stretch reflexes are usually lost, but motor function is preserved. The CSF typically contains a mild lymphocytic pleocytosis, particularly when the sensory changes are associated with encephalomyelitis. On nerve conduction studies, sensory nerve action potentials are diminished or absent, and compound muscle action potentials are normal; EMG evidence of denervation is absent.

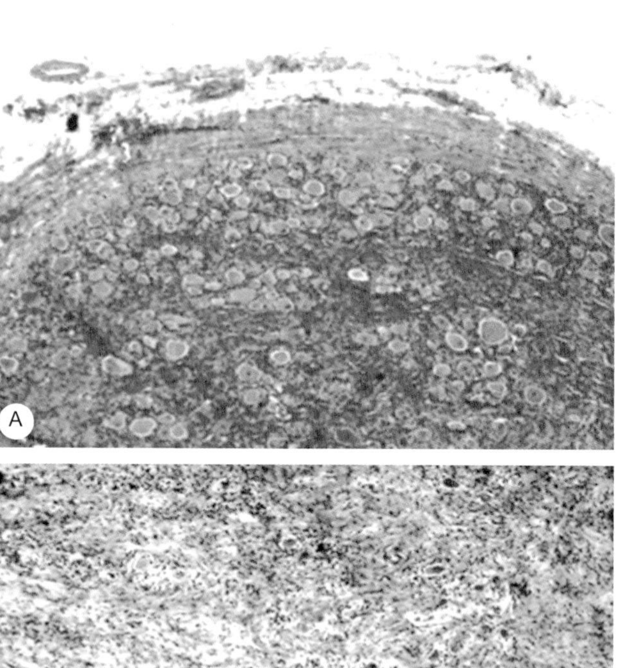

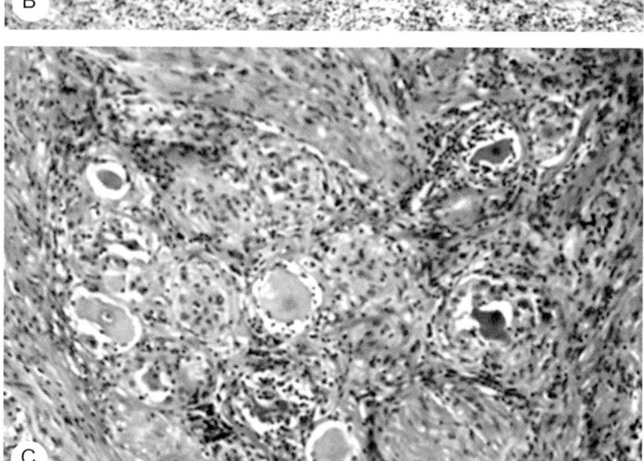

FIGURE 27-4 ■ Paraneoplastic sensory neuronopathy. **A**, Dorsal root ganglion obtained at autopsy from a patient without neurologic disease. **B**, Dorsal root ganglion obtained from a patient with paraneoplastic sensory neuronopathy and anti-Hu antibodies. Note that there are virtually no normal dorsal root ganglion neurons in the entire section. A few scattered inflammatory infiltrates are present. (Hematoxylin–eosin × 40.) **C**, The dorsal root ganglion of another patient with anti-Hu-related subacute sensory neuronopathy. Degenerating neurons can be seen surrounded by inflammatory cells. (Hematoxylin–eosin × 40.)

Pathologic changes may be limited to the dorsal root ganglia, with neuronal loss and lymphocytic inflammatory infiltrates (Fig. 27-4). Secondary changes seen on sural nerve biopsy are usually characterized by a substantial reduction in myelinated fiber density with a lesser reduction in small fibers; however, in those patients with severe painful neuropathy, small fibers are reduced more than myelinated fibers.[179] In about 50 percent of patients, clinically inapparent pathologic changes are found in other regions of the nervous system. Treatment of the underlying tumor and removal of the autoantibody by plasmapheresis or immunosuppressive therapy may stabilize or sometimes improve symptoms, particularly when given early.[58,180] Occasional patients have a mild and indolent sensory neuropathy.[181]

Sensory neuronopathy can occur in previously healthy individuals or in those with a variety of underlying autoimmune conditions, including Sjögren syndrome. It can also be caused by heavy metal intoxication, including the platinum analogue chemotherapeutic agents. The disorder is paraneoplastic in only a minority of patients.[182] At least two-thirds of patients with paraneoplastic sensory neuronopathy have SCLC as the cause. Criteria for distinguishing subacute sensory neuronopathy from other sensory neuropathies include the early development of sensory ataxia, an asymmetric distribution of sensory loss, sensory loss occurring in a non–length-dependent manner beyond the distal lower extremities, and relatively normal motor but abnormal sensory conduction studies.[183] Criteria for separating paraneoplastic subacute sensory neuropathy from other causes include an acute or subacute onset in four limbs, early pain, and its occurrence in men more than 60 years old.[184] The presence of anti-Hu antibodies is useful to confirm the paraneoplastic etiology, having a specificity of 99 percent and sensitivity of 82 percent. [185]

Subacute sensorimotor neuropathy is predominantly a distal symmetric polyneuropathy that is more marked in the lower than upper extremities and is characterized by weakness, stocking-and-glove sensory impairment to all modalities, and a loss of muscle stretch reflexes. Bulbar involvement is uncommon. Patients with mild sensory or sensorimotor neuropathy that evolves slowly over many months to years are unlikely to have carcinoma as the underlying cause. Patients with subacutely developing severe peripheral neuropathy leading to substantial paralysis and sensory loss are much more likely to have a paraneoplastic syndrome. A few patients with paraneoplastic sensorimotor neuropathy follow the remitting and relapsing course typical of chronic inflammatory demyelinating polyneuropathy; these patients may respond to corticosteroid therapy. Guillain–Barré syndrome, acute brachial neuritis, cauda equina syndrome, and dysfunction of individual nerves are occasionally paraneoplastic.[186–189]

In most paraneoplastic sensorimotor neuropathies, the CSF is typically acellular with a normal or slightly elevated protein concentration. Nerve conduction studies are consistent with an axonal neuropathy, with low-amplitude or absent sensory nerve action potentials and normal or decreased motor nerve conduction velocities. A few patients have marked slowing of motor conduction velocities consistent with a demyelinating process. Pathologically, there is usually axonal degeneration; in a few patients, demyelination is prominent.

A relatively pure *paraneoplastic sensory neuropathy* (not neuronopathy) occurs with a variety of malignancies, but cannot be distinguished from other causes of sensory neuropathy. When no cause of a sensory neuropathy is identified, cancer is subsequently found as the etiology in approximately one-third of patients. The mean time to cancer diagnosis following the neurologic disorder is more than 2 years.[14]

Peripheral neuropathy due to microvasculitis is rare as a paraneoplastic syndrome and is found without obvious antibody involvement in patients with a variety of cancers. Vasculitic neuropathy can present either as a diffuse polyneuropathy or as mononeuritis multiplex. It can involve both peripheral and cranial nerves. The importance of making a diagnosis, which may require nerve biopsy, is that the condition may respond to corticosteroid treatment.

Peripheral neuropathy may be associated with multiple myeloma and Waldenström macroglobulinemia.[190] With the rare osteosclerotic form of myeloma, peripheral neuropathy is present in about 50 percent of patients. Successful treatment of the myeloma often leads to amelioration of the neurologic symptoms. Amyloidosis associated with myeloma can also cause a peripheral neuropathy that responds poorly to treatment. Options for therapy include both tumor treatment and immunosuppression.[58] Rituximab is effective in treating some neuropathies associated with IgM antibodies.[190,191] A Cochrane review found no controlled trials addressing the effectiveness of treatment, only case series and expert opinions.[180]

AUTONOMIC NEUROPATHY

Paraneoplastic autonomic neuropathy is a rare syndrome that occurs alone or along with a sensory neuronopathy.[192,193] Usually associated with SCLC, it may occur with other cancers and may present before or after the cancer is diagnosed. Patients present with the subacute onset of postural hypotension, pupillary abnormalities, a neurogenic bladder, or some combination of these signs. Severe constipation may be the only symptom of this paraneoplastic disorder. The syndrome is generally progressive but may stabilize or improve with treatment of the underlying tumor. When autonomic neuropathy occurs with lung cancer, it is usually part of the anti-Hu syndrome. Autonomic neuropathy also occurs with an antibody against the ganglionic acetylcholine receptor (anti-nAChR). Immunization with the protein produces an autonomic neuropathy, as does passive transfer of antibodies, indicating a B cell–mediated disease.[194] Immunosuppression with a combination of rituximab and cyclophosphamide has proved effective in one instance.[195]

Neuromuscular Junction Syndromes

Paraneoplastic disorders of the neuromuscular junction include LEMS and myasthenia gravis.[196] These disorders have a common pathogenetic mechanism in that they are caused by antibodies against ion channels and, whether paraneoplastic or not, they often respond to immunologic treatment.

LEMS is characterized by progressive proximal weakness and fatigability, but, unlike myasthenia gravis, cranial nerve symptoms are usually not severe.[197] Respiratory weakness may occur. Power initially increases with effort, so that reported weakness may seem out of proportion to the examiner's findings; however, with continued effort, weakness returns. Muscle stretch reflexes, especially those in the legs, are diminished or absent but may reappear after exercise. Cholinergic dysautonomia occurs in more than 50 percent of patients, causing dry mouth and impotence. Characteristic abnormalities are found on electrophysiologic testing, including very small compound muscle action potentials that may increase to normal after brief exercise. Repetitive stimulation causes a decrement of the compound muscle action potentials at low rates of stimulation and an increment at high rates of stimulation. About 60 percent of patients with LEMS have SCLC; a few have other cancers. Some of the 40 percent who do not have cancer may have evidence of other autoimmune diseases.

The disorder results from reduced release of acetylcholine at presynaptic nerve terminals. Antibodies that react with the P/Q-type VGCC are found in patients with or without paraneoplastic syndromes.[147] The same P/Q-type VGCC antibodies are found in SCLC; the richest source of these channels is the cerebellum, perhaps explaining the occasional relationship of paraneoplastic cerebellar degeneration and LEMS.

LEMS is a classic autoimmune disease in that binding of circulating IgG antibodies to the VGCC reproduces the electrophysiologic abnormalities in animals; removal of IgG antibodies from humans with the disorder improves neurologic function. Accordingly, LEMS can be treated either by immunosuppression or by treatment of the underlying cancer when present.[198] 3,4-Diaminopyridine (3,4-DAP) may improve the muscle weakness but can be difficult to obtain.[198] Patients with SCLC-associated LEMS have a better prognosis than patients with SCLC who do not develop a paraneoplastic disorder.[199] SOX1 antibodies are reported in 64 percent of patients with paraneoplastic LEMS but are not found in nonparaneoplastic LEMS.[200]

Myasthenia gravis usually affects ocular, bulbar, and respiratory muscles, often sparing the extremities. In contrast to LEMS, patients grow weaker with exercise and improve with rest; repetitive stimulation decreases the compound muscle action potentials on EMG. Myasthenia gravis is usually not associated with cancer, but about 15 percent of patients have thymoma, and a rare patient develops the syndrome when Hodgkin disease directly affects the thymus. The disorder is caused by antibodies against the acetylcholine receptor at the postsynaptic myoneural junction. Patients with thymoma-associated myasthenia are more likely to also have other antibodies against muscle proteins such as ryanodine receptors. Myasthenia gravis usually responds to immunosuppression, acetylcholinesterase inhibitors, and thymectomy. Thymectomy is more effective for the treatment of myasthenia gravis in patients without thymomas than with thymomas.

Peripheral Nerve Hyperexcitability (Neuromyotonia)

Several disorders characterized by hyperexcitability of terminal arborizations of peripheral nerves occur in patients with paraneoplastic syndromes, including neuromyotonia, the cramp-fasciculation syndrome, and Morvan syndrome.[201,202]

Neuromyotonia occurs when single motor unit potentials fire spontaneously at 150 to 300 Hz, leading to chronic contraction of muscles that can be either focal or generalized; the disorder is sometimes associated with neuropathic pain and autonomic dysfunction, especially hyperhidrosis. There are several underlying causes, including nerve damage associated with radiation therapy, snake bites, ion channel mutations, and inherited neuropathies. The disorder is often autoimmune and related to antibodies against CASPR2, a part of the voltage-gated potassium channel complex.[203] When the disorder is paraneoplastic, antibodies against amphiphysin may also be found.[172] In its mildest form it is called myokymia (repetitive and recurrent firing of a motor unit potential at 2 to 60 Hz), clinically visible as undulating muscle twitching. Patients may also demonstrate pseudomyotonia (failure of muscles to relax after contraction), and intestinal pseudo-obstruction. Some patients develop CNS symptoms of memory loss, hallucinations, insomnia, and changes in mood (Morvan syndrome).[204]

The serum creatine kinase level is elevated in about one-half of patients. The diagnosis can be made electrophysiologically when needle EMG reveals spontaneous firing of single or multiple motor units at a rate of 150 to 300 Hz. These units fire at irregular intervals and may persist during sleep, general anesthesia, and even when peripheral nerves are blocked at proximal sites. Symptoms are relieved by blocking the neuromuscular junction, indicating that the action potentials arise from terminal arborizations of the motor nerve. When these disorders are paraneoplastic, thymoma is the most common cause, but SCLC and Hodgkin disease have also been reported.

The pathophysiology of the central and peripheral nervous system signs and symptoms is unknown. The fact that symptoms are relieved by plasma exchange suggests that the disorder, or at least the major part of it, is antibody mediated. These antibodies have been shown to bind to neurons in areas of brain likely to cause the CNS symptoms.[180] Some patients respond well to anticonvulsants, such as phenytoin or carbamazepine, or to muscle relaxants such as diazepam. However, the treatment of choice is immunosuppression with plasma exchange or intravenous immunoglobulin; one report suggests that plasma exchange is superior.[205,206]

Muscle Syndromes

Polymyositis and dermatomyositis are common inflammatory autoimmune muscle diseases.[207–209] Only a minority of patients suffering from these disorders have an underlying malignancy as the cause, particularly in older patients. Dermatomyositis with typical cutaneous changes is more likely than polymyositis to be paraneoplastic. Females and males are affected in approximately equal numbers. Symptoms of muscle weakness generally precede identification of the cancer, which may be at any site; breast, lung, ovarian, and gastric malignancies are the most common. Hodgkin disease and prostate and colon cancer have also been reported.

The clinical and laboratory findings in dermatomyositis and polymyositis associated with malignancy resemble those in the idiopathic disease, although cancer patients often have more striking abnormalities on muscle biopsy specimens. Patients characteristically present with proximal muscle weakness, elevated levels of serum creatine kinase, and EMG evidence suggesting a myopathic process. A muscle biopsy specimen showing an inflammatory myopathy confirms the diagnosis. Although laboratory findings do not distinguish paraneoplastic from nonparaneoplastic forms, the presence of the anti-p155 antibody is more common in patients with cancer, whereas anti-synthetase antibodies suggest an etiology not related to cancer.[208] Normal serum creatine kinase levels are occasionally found even in patients with profound muscle weakness, with or without malignancy; abnormal levels indicate a poor prognosis for the muscle disease. Weakness of respiratory and pharyngeal muscles may be life-threatening. The prognosis is not as good for the paraneoplastic disorder as it is for nonparaneoplastic forms. Corticosteroids, cyclosporine, and other immune suppressants have been used successfully. High-dose intravenous immunoglobulin therapy is sometimes helpful in patients unresponsive to other forms of immunosuppression.

A necrotizing myopathy, with or without marked inflammation, has also been reported in patients with cancer, as has inclusion-body myositis.[210–212] The necrotizing myopathy has been reported to respond to intravenous immunoglobulin, sometimes in spite of tumor progression.[213] Corticosteroids, cyclosporine, and other immunosuppressants have also been used successfully.

REFERENCES

1. DeAngelis LM, Posner JB: Neurologic Complications of Cancer. 2nd Ed. Oxford University Press, New York, 2009.

2. Brain WR: Norris FHE. The Remote Effects of Cancer on the Nervous System. Grune & Stratton, New York, 1965.
3. Erlington GM, Murray NM, Spiro SG, et al: Neurological paraneoplastic syndromes in patients with small cell lung cancer. A prospective survey of 150 patients. J Neurol Neurosurg Psychiatry 54:764, 1991.
4. Croft PB, Wilkinson M: The incidence of carcinomatous neuromyopathy in patients with various types of carcinomas. Brain 88:427, 1965.
5. Lipton RB, Galer BS, Dutcher JP, et al: Quantitative sensory testing demonstrates that subclinical sensory neuropathy is prevalent in patients with cancer. Arch Neurol 44:944, 1997.
6. Gomm SA, Thatcher N, Barber PV, et al: A clinicopathological study of the paraneoplastic neuromuscular syndromes associated with lung cancer. QJM 278:577, 1990.
7. Camerlingo M, Nemni R, Ferraro B, et al: Malignancy and sensory neuropathy of unexplained cause. Arch Neurol 55:981, 1998.
8. Wirtz PW, Nijnuis MG, Sotodeh M, et al: The epidemiology of myasthenia gravis, Lambert-Eaton myasthenic syndrome and their associated tumours in the northern part of the province of South Holland. J Neurol 250:698, 2003.
9. Wirtz PW, Van Dijk JG, Van Doorn PA, et al: The epidemiology of the Lambert-Eaton myasthenic syndrome in the Netherlands. Neurology 63:397, 2004.
10. Bendewald MJ, Wetter DA, Li X, et al: Incidence of dermatomyositis and clinically amyopathic dermatomyositis: a population-based study in Olmsted County, Minnesota. Arch Dermatol 146:26, 2010.
11. Marx A, Muller-Hermelink HK, Strobel P: The role of thymomas in the development of myasthenia gravis. Ann NY Acad Sci 998:223, 2003.
12. Seute T, Leffers P, Ten Velde GP, et al: Neurologic disorders in 432 consecutive patients with small cell lung carcinoma. Cancer 100:801, 2004.
13. Drappatz J, Batchelor T: Neurologic complications of plasma cell disorders. Clin Lymphoma 5:163, 2004.
14. Kelly Jr JJ, Kyle RA, Miles JM, et al: Osteosclerotic myeloma and peripheral neuropathy. Neurology 33: 202, 1983.
15. Dalmau J, Rosenfeld MR: Paraneoplastic syndromes of the CNS. Lancet Neurol 7:327, 2008.
16. Dalmau J, Gultekin SH, Voltz R, et al: Ma1, a novel neuronal and testis specific protein, is recognized by the serum of patients with paraneoplastic neurologic disorders. Brain 122:27, 1999.
17. Furneaux HM, Reich L, Posner JB: Autoantibody synthesis in the central nervous system of patients with paraneoplastic syndromes. Neurology 40:1085, 1990.
18. Jarius S, Stich O, Rasiah C, et al: Qualitative evidence of Ri specific IgG-synthesis in the cerebrospinal fluid from patients with paraneoplastic neurological syndromes. J Neurol Sci 268:65, 2008.
19. Stich O, Rauer S: Antigen-specific oligoclonal bands in cerebrospinal fluid and serum from patients with anti-amphiphysin- and anti-CV2/CRMP5 associated paraneoplastic neurological syndromes. Eur J Neurol 14:650, 2007.
20. Hetzel DJ, Stanhope CR, O'Neil BP, et al: Gynecologic cancer in patients with subacute cerebellar degeneration predicted by anti-Purkinje cell antibodies and limited in metastatic volume. Mayo Clin Proc 65:1558, 1990.
21. Darnell RB, Posner JB: Paraneoplastic syndromes affecting the nervous system. Semin Oncol 33:270, 2006.
22. Albert ML, Darnell RB: Paraneoplastic neurological degenerations: keys to tumour immunity. Nat Rev Cancer 4:36, 2004.
23. Schreiber H, Rowley DA: Cancer. Quo vadis, specificity? Science 319:164, 2008.
24. Carpentier AF, Voltz R, Dechamps T, et al: Absence of HuD gene mutations in paraneoplastic small cell lung cancer tissue. Neurology 50:1919, 1998.
25. D'Alessandro V, Muscarella LA, la Torre A, et al: Molecular analysis of the HuD gene in neuroendocrine lung cancers. Lung Cancer 67:69, 2009.
26. Byrne T, Mason WP, Posner JB, et al: Spontaneous neurological improvement in anti-Hu associated encephalomyelitis. J Neurol Neurosurg Psychiatry 62:276, 1997.
27. Darnell RB, DeAngelis LM: Regression of small-cell lung carcinoma in patients with paraneoplastic neuronal antibodies. Lancet 341:21, 1993.
28. Dalmau J, Furneaux HM, Rosenblum MK, et al: Detection of the anti-Hu antibody in specific regions of the nervous system and tumor from patients with paraneoplastic encephalomyelitis/sensory neuronopathy. Neurology 41:1757, 1991.
29. Hormigo A, Dalmau J, Rosenblum MK, et al: Immunological and pathological study of anti-Ri-associated encephalopathy. Ann Neurol 36:896, 1994.
30. Voltz R, Dalmau J, Posner JB, et al: T-cell receptor analysis in anti-Hu associated paraneoplastic encephalomyelitis. Neurology 51:1146, 1998.
31. Geis C, Weishaupt A, Hallermann S, et al: Stiff person syndrome–associated autoantibodies to amphiphysin mediate reduced GABAergic inhibition. Brain 133:3166, 2010.
32. Hansen N, Grunewald B, Weishaupt A, et al: Human stiff person syndrome IgG-containing high-titer anti-GAD65 autoantibodies induce motor dysfunction in rats. Exp Neurol 239:202, 2013.
33. Drachman DB: How to recognize an antibody-mediated autoimmune disease: criteria. Res Publ Assoc Res Nerv Ment Dis 68:183, 1990.
34. Vernino S, Low PA, Fealey RD, et al: Autoantibodies to ganglionic acetylcholine receptors in autoimmune autonomic neuropathies. N Engl J Med 343:847, 2000.
35. Dalmau J, Lancaster E, Martinez-Hernandez E, et al: Clinical experience and laboratory investigations in patients with anti-NMDAR encephalitis. Lancet Neurol 10:63, 2011.

36. Magrys A, Anekonda T, Ren G, et al: The role of anti-alpha-enolase autoantibodies in pathogenicity of autoimmune-mediated retinopathy. J Clin Immunol 27:181, 2007.
37. Roberts WK, Posner JB, Darnell RB: Patients with lung cancer and the paraneoplastic Hu syndrome harbor HuD-specific Type 2 CD8+ T cells. J Clin Invest 119:2042, 2009.
38. Santomasso BD, Roberts WK, Thomas A, et al: A T-cell receptor associated with naturally occurring human tumor immunity. Proc Natl Acad Sci USA 104:19073, 2007.
39. Rousseau A, Benyahia B, Dalmau J, et al: T cell response to Hu-D peptides in patients with anti-Hu syndrome. J Neurooncol 71:231, 2005.
40. Graus F, Delattre JY, Antoine JC, et al: Recommended diagnostic criteria for paraneoplastic neurological syndromes. J Neurol Neurosurg Psychiatry 75:1135, 2004.
41. Bernal F, Shams'ili S, Rojas I, et al: Anti-Tr antibodies as markers of paraneoplastic cerebellar degeneration and Hodgkin's disease. Neurology 60:230, 2003.
42. Clapp AJ, Hunt CH, Johnson GB, et al: Semiquantitative analysis of brain metabolism in patients with paraneoplastic neurologic syndromes. Clin Nucl Med 38:241, 2013.
43. Titulaer MJ, Soffietti R, Dalmau J, et al: Screening for tumours in paraneoplastic syndromes: report of an EFNS Task Force. Eur J Neurol 18:19, 2010.
44. Dalmau J, Gleichman AJ, Hughes EG, et al: Anti-NMDA-receptor encephalitis: case series and analysis of the effects of antibodies. Lancet Neurol 7:1091, 2008.
45. Stich O, Graus F, Rasiah C, et al: Qualitative evidence of anti-Yo-specific intrathecal antibody synthesis in patients with paraneoplastic cerebellar degeneration. J Neuroimmunol 141:165, 2003.
46. Vega F, Graus F, Chen QM, et al: Intrathecal synthesis of the anti-Hu antibody in patients with paraneoplastic encephalomyelitis or sensory neuronopathy: clinical-immunologic correlation. Neurology 44:2145, 1994.
47. Honnorat J, Cartalat-Carel S, Ricard D, et al: Onco-neural antibodies and tumor type determine survival and neurological symptoms in paraneoplastic neurological syndromes with Hu or CV2/CRMP5 antibodies. J Neurol Neurosurg Psychiatry 80:412, 2009.
48. Hoftberger R, Dalmau J, Graus F: Clinical neuropathology practice guide 5-2012: updated guideline for the diagnosis of antineuronal antibodies. Clin Neuropathol 31:337, 2012.
49. Graus F, Saiz A, Dalmau J: Antibodies and neuronal autoimmune disorders of the CNS. J Neurol 257:509, 2009.
50. Llado A, Carpentier AF, Honnorat J, et al: Hu-antibody-positive patients with or without cancer have similar clinical profiles. J Neurol Neurosurg Psychiatry 77:996, 2006.
51. Hero B, Simon T, Spitz R, et al: Localized infant neuroblastomas often show spontaneous regression: results of the prospective trials NB95-S and NB97. J Clin Oncol 26:1504, 2008.
52. Antunes NL, Khakoo Y, Matthay KK, et al: Antineuronal antibodies in patients with neuroblastoma and paraneoplastic opsoclonus-myoclonus. J Pediatr Hematol Oncol 22:315, 2000.
53. Viaccoz A, Honnorat J: Paraneoplastic neurological syndromes: general treatment overview. Curr Treat Options Neurol 15:150, 2013.
54. Vedeler CA: Management of paraneoplastic neurological syndromes: report of an EFNS Task Force. Eur J Neurol 13:682, 2006.
55. Keime-Guibert F, Graus F, Broet P, et al: Clinical outcome of patients with anti-Hu-associated encephalomyelitis after treatment of the tumor. Neurology 53:1719, 1999.
56. Douglas CA, Ellershaw J: Anti-Hu antibodies may indicate a positive response to chemotherapy in paraneoplastic syndrome secondary to small cell lung cancer. Palliat Med 17:638, 2003.
57. Sillevis SP, Grefkens J, De Leeuw B, et al: Survival and outcome in 73 anti-Hu positive patients with paraneoplastic encephalomyelitis/sensory neuronopathy. J Neurol 249:745, 2002.
58. Antoine JC, Camdessanche JP: Treatment options in paraneoplastic disorders of the peripheral nervous system. Curr Treat Options Neurol 15:210, 2013.
59. Darnell RB, Posner JB: Paraneoplastic Syndromes. Oxford University Press, New York, 2011.
60. Rubio-Agusti I, Salavert M, Bataller L: Limbic encephalitis and related cortical syndromes. Curr Treat Options Neurol 15:169, 2013.
61. Rosenfeld MR, Dalmau JO: Paraneoplastic disorders of the CNS and autoimmune synaptic encephalitis. Continuum (Minneap Minn) 18:366, 2012.
62. Tuzun E, Dalmau J: Limbic encephalitis and variants: classification, diagnosis and treatment. Neurologist 13:261, 2007.
63. Gultekin SH, Rosenfeld MR, Voltz R, et al: Paraneoplastic limbic encephalitis: neurological symptoms, immunological findings and tumour association in 50 patients. Brain 123:1481, 2000.
64. Carr I: The Ophelia syndrome: memory loss in Hodgkin's disease. Lancet 1:844, 1982.
65. Lancaster E, Martinez-Hernandez E, Titulaer MJ, et al: Antibodies to metabotropic glutamate receptor 5 in the Ophelia syndrome. Neurology 77:1698, 2011.
66. Sureka J, Jakkani RK: Clinico-radiological spectrum of bilateral temporal lobe hyperintensity: a retrospective review. Br J Radiol 85:e782, 2012.
67. Basu S, Alavi A: Role of FDG-PET in the clinical management of paraneoplastic neurological syndrome: detection of the underlying malignancy and the brain PET-MRI correlates. Mol Imaging Biol 10:131, 2008.
68. Grisold W, Giometto B, Vitaliani R, et al: Current approaches to the treatment of paraneoplastic encephalitis. Ther Adv Neurol Disord 4:237, 2011.

69. Jarius S, Steinmeyer F, Knobel A, et al: GABAB receptor antibodies in paraneoplastic cerebellar ataxia. J Neuroimmunol 256:94, 2013.
70. Scheid R, Lincke T, Voltz R, et al: Serial ^{18}F-fluoro-2-deoxy-D-glucose positron emission tomography and magnetic resonance imaging of paraneoplastic limbic encephalitis. Arch Neurol 61:1785, 2004.
71. Irani SR, Vincent A: Autoimmune encephalitis —new awareness, challenging questions. Discov Med 11:449, 2011.
72. Henson RA, Hoffman HL, Urich H: Encephalomyelitis with carcinoma. Brain 88:449, 1965.
73. Dalmau J, Graus F, Villarejo A, et al: Clinical analysis of anti-Ma2-associated encephalitis. Brain 127:1831, 2004.
74. Voltz R, Gultekin SH, Rosenfeld MR, et al: A serologic marker of paraneoplastic limbic and brain-stem encephalitis in patients with testicular cancer. N Engl J Med 340:1788, 1999.
75. Vernino S, Lennon VA: Autoantibody profiles and neurological correlations of thymoma. Clin Cancer Res 10:7270, 2004.
76. Sirvent N, Berard E, Chastagner P, et al: Hypothalamic dysfunction associated with neuroblastoma: evidence for a new paraneoplastic syndrome? Med Pediatr Oncol 40:326, 2003.
77. Nunn K, Ouvrier R, Sprague T, et al: Idiopathic hypothalamic dysfunction: a paraneoplastic syndrome? J Child Neurol 12:276, 1997.
78. Huppke P, Heise A, Rostasy K, et al: Immunoglobulin therapy in idiopathic hypothalamic dysfunction. Pediatr Neurol 41:232, 2009.
79. Landolfi JC: Paraneoplastic limbic encephalitis and possible narcolepsy in a patient with testicular cancer: case study. Neuro-Oncology 5:214, 2003.
80. Ahern GL, O'Connor M, Dalmau J, et al: Paraneoplastic temporal lobe epilepsy with testicular neoplasm and atypical amnesia. Neurology 44:1270, 1994.
81. Buckley C, Vincent A: Autoimmune channelopathies. Nature Clin Prac Neurol 1:22, 2005.
82. Blaes F: Paraneoplastic brain stem encephalitis. Curr Treat Options Neurol 15:201, 2013.
83. Jubelt B, Mihai C, Li TM, Veerapaneni P: Rhombencephalitis / brainstem encephalitis. Curr Neurol Neurosci Rep 11:543, 2011.
84. O'Toole O, Lennon VA, Ahlskog JE, et al: Autoimmune chorea in adults. Neurology 80:1133, 2013.
85. Golbe LI, Miller DC, Duvoisin RC: Paraneoplastic degeneration of the substantia nigra with dystonia and parkinsonism. Mov Dis 4:147, 1989.
86. Brouwer B: Beitrag zur Kenntnis der chronischen diffusen Kleinhirnerkrankungen. Neurol Zentralbl 38:674, 1919.
87. Brouwer B, Biemond A: Les affections parenchymateuses du cervelet et leur signification du point de vue de l'anatomie et la physiologie de cet organe. J Belg Neurol Psychiatrie 38:691, 1938.
88. Shams'ili S, Grefkens J, de Leeuw B, et al: Paraneoplastic cerebellar degeneration associated with antineuronal antibodies: analysis of 50 patients. Brain 126:1409, 2003.
89. Hammack J, Kotanides H, Rosenblum MK, et al: Paraneoplastic cerebellar degeneration: II. Clinical and immunologic findings in 21 patients with Hodgkin's disease. Neurology 42:1938, 1992.
90. Bonakis A: Acute onset paraneoplastic cerebellar degeneration. J Neurooncol 84:329, 2007.
91. Peterson K, Rosenblum MK, Kotanides H, et al: Paraneoplastic cerebellar degeneration. I. A clinical analysis of 55 anti-Yo antibody positive patients. Neurology 42:1931, 1992.
92. Collinson SL, Anthonisz B, Courtenay D, et al: Frontal executive impairment associated with paraneoplastic cerebellar degeneration: a case study. Neurocase 12:350, 2006.
93. Schmahmann JD, Sherman JC: The cerebellar cognitive affective syndrome. Brain 121:561, 1998.
94. Anderson NE, Posner JB, Sidtis JJ, et al: The metabolic anatomy of paraneoplastic cerebellar degeneration. Ann Neurol 23:533, 1998.
95. Hadjivassiliou M, Currie S, Hoggard N: MR spectroscopy in paraneoplastic cerebellar degeneration. J Neuroradiol 40:310, 2013.
96. Darnell JC, Albert ML, Darnell RB: Cdr2, a target antigen of naturally occuring human tumor immunity, is widely expressed in gynecological tumors. Cancer Res 60:2136, 2000.
97. Carpenter EL, Vance BA, Klein RS, et al: Functional analysis of $CD8^+$ T cell responses to the onconeural self protein cdr2 in patients with paraneoplastic cerebellar degeneration. J Neuroimmunol 193:173, 2008.
98. Rojas-Marcos I, Picard G, Chinchon D, et al: Human epidermal growth factor receptor 2 overexpression in breast cancer of patients with anti-Yo-associated paraneoplastic cerebellar degeneration. Neuro Oncol 14:506, 2012.
99. Trotter JL, Hendin BA, Osterland K: Cerebellar degeneration with Hodgkin's disease. An immunological study. Arch Neurol 33:660, 1976.
100. Briani C, Vitaliani R, Grisold W, et al: Spectrum of paraneoplastic disease associated with lymphoma. Neurology 76:705, 2011.
101. deGraaf E, Maat P, Hulsenboom E, et al: Identification of delta/notch-like epidermal growth factor-related receptor as the Tr antigen in paraneoplastic cerebellar degeneration. Ann Neurol 71:815, 2012.
102. Graus F, Keime-Guibert F, Reñe R, et al: Anti-Hu-associated paraneoplastic encephalomyelitis: analysis of 200 patients. Brain 124:1138, 2001.
103. Aye MM, Kasai T, Tashiro Y, et al: CD8 positive T-cell infiltration in the dentate nucleus of paraneoplastic cerebellar degeneration. J Neuroimmunol 208:136, 2009.

104. Saloustros E, Zaganas I, Mavridis M, et al: Anti-CV2 associated cerebellar degeneration after complete response to chemoradiation of head and neck carcinoma. J Neurooncol 97:291, 2009.
105. Cross SA, Salomao DR, Parisi JE, et al: Paraneoplastic autoimmune optic neuritis with retinitis defined by CRMP-5-IgG. Ann Neurol 54:38, 2003.
106. Clouston PD, Saper CB, Arbizu T, et al: Paraneoplastic cerebellar degeneration. III. Cerebellar degeneration, cancer and the Lambert-Eaton myasthenic syndrome. Neurology 42:1944, 1992.
107. Sillevis-Smitt P, Kinoshita A, De Leeuw B, et al: Paraneoplastic cerebellar ataxia due to autoantibodies against a glutamate receptor. N Engl J Med 342:21, 2000.
108. Marignier R, Chenevier F, Rogemond V, et al: Metabotropic glutamate receptor type 1 autoantibody-associated cerebellitis: a primary autoimmune disease? Arch Neurol 67:627, 2010.
109. Bataller L, Wade DF, Graus F, et al: Antibodies to Zic4 in paraneoplastic neurologic disorders and small-cell lung cancer. Neurology 62:778, 2004.
110. Vernino S, Lennon VA: New Purkinje cell antibody (PCA-2): marker of lung cancer-related neurological autoimmunity. Ann Neurol 47:297, 2000.
111. Chan KH, Vernino S, Lennon VA: ANNA-3 anti-neuronal nuclear antibody: marker of lung cancer-related autoimmunity. Ann Neurol 50:301, 2001.
112. Bataller L, Sabater L, Saiz A, et al: Carbonic anhydrase-related protein VIII: autoantigen in paraneoplastic cerebellar degeneration. Ann Neurol 56:575, 2004.
113. Storstein A, Knudsen A, Vedeler CA: Proteasome antibodies in paraneoplastic cerebellar degeneration. J Neuroimmunol 165:172, 2005.
114. Sabater L, Bataller L, Carpentier A, et al: Protein kinase Cγ autoimmunity in paraneoplastic cerebellar degeneration and non-small-cell lung cancer. J Neurol Neurosurg Psychiatry 77:1359, 2006.
115. Jarius S, Wandinger KP, Horn S, et al: A new Purkinje cell antibody (anti-Ca) associated with subacute cerebellar ataxia: immunological characterization. J Neuroinflammation 7:21, 2010.
116. Greenlee JE, Clawson SA, Hill KE, et al: Antineuronal autoantibodies in paraneoplastic cerebellar degeneration associated with adenocarcinoma of the prostate. J Neurol Sci 291:74, 2010.
117. Verschuuren J, Chuang L, Rosenblum MK, et al: Inflammatory infiltrates and complete absence of Purkinje cells in anti-Yo associated paraneoplastic cerebellar degeneration. Acta Neuropathol 91:519, 1996.
118. Henson RA, Urich H: Cancer and the Nervous System: The Neurological Manifestations of Systemic Malignant Disease. Blackwell Scientific, London, 1982.
119. Ropper AH: Seronegative, non-neoplastic acute cerebellar degeneration. Neurology 43:1602, 1993.
120. Rees JH, Hain SF, Johnson MR, et al: The role of [^{18}F] fluoro-2-deoxyglucose-PET scanning in the diagnosis of paraneoplastic neurological disorders. Brain 24:2223, 2001.
121. Hammack JE, Kimmel DW, O'Neill BP, et al: Paraneoplastic cerebellar degeneration: a clinical comparison of patients with and without Purkinje cell cytoplasmic antibodies. Mayo Clinic Proc 65:1423, 1990.
122. Greenlee JE: Treatment of paraneoplastic cerebellar degeneration. Curr Treat Options Neurol 15:185, 2013.
123. Schessl J, Schuberth M, Reilich P, et al: Long-term efficiency of intravenously administered immunoglobulin in anti-Yo syndrome with paraneoplastic cerebellar degeneration. J Neurol 258:946, 2011.
124. Pelosof LC, Gerber DE: Paraneoplastic syndromes: an approach to diagnosis and treatment. Mayo Clin Proc 85:838, 2010.
125. Orange D, Frank M, Tian S, et al: Cellular immune suppression in paraneoplastic neurologic syndromes targeting intracellular antigens. Arch Neurol 69:1132, 2012.
126. Yeo KK, Walter AW, Miller RE, et al: Rituximab as potential therapy for paraneoplastic cerebellar degeneration in pediatric Hodgkin disease. Pediatr Blood Cancer 58:986, 2012.
127. Esposito M, Penza P, Orefice G, et al: Successful treatment of paraneoplastic cerebellar degeneration with Rituximab. J Neurooncol 86:363, 2008.
128. Keime-Guibert F, Graus F, Fleury A, et al: Treatment of paraneoplastic neurological syndromes with antineuronal antibodies (anti-Hu, anti-Yo) with a combination of immunoglobulins, cyclophosphamide, and methylprednisolone. J Neurol Neurosurg Psychiatry 68:479, 2000.
129. Widdess-Walsh P, Tavee JO, Schuele S, et al: Response to intravenous immunoglobulin in anti-Yo associated paraneoplastic cerebellar degeneration: case report and review of the literature. J Neurooncol 63:187, 2003.
130. Trouillas P, Xie J, Adeleine P, et al: Buspirone, a 5-hydroxytryptamine$_{1A}$ agonist, is active in cerebellar ataxia - Results of a double-blind drug placebo study in patients with cerebellar cortical atrophy. Arch Neurol 54:749, 1997.
131. Tate ED, Allison TJ, Pranzatelli MR, et al: Neuroepidemiologic trends in 105 US cases of pediatric opsoclonus-myoclonus syndrome. J Pediatr Oncol Nurs 22:8, 2005.
132. Singhi P, Sahu JK, Sarkar J, et al: Clinical profile and outcome of children with opsoclonus-myoclonus syndrome. J Child Neurol in press, 2013.
133. Rudnick E, Khakoo Y, Antunes NL, et al: Opsoclonus-myoclonus-ataxia syndrome in neuroblastoma: clinical outcome and antineuronal antibodies—a report from the Children's Cancer Group Study. Med Pediatr Oncol 36:612, 2001.

134. Stefanowicz J, Izycka-Swieszewska E, Drozynska E, et al: Neuroblastoma and opsoclonus-myoclonus-ataxia syndrome—clinical and pathological characteristics. Folia Neuropathol 46:176, 2008.
135. Krug P, Schleiermacher G, Michon J, et al: Opsoclonus-myoclonus in children associated or not with neuroblastoma. Eur J Paediatr Neurol 14:400, 2010.
136. Connolly AM, Pestronk A, Mehta S, et al: Serum autoantibodies in childhood opsoclonus-myoclonus syndrome: an analysis of antigenic targets in neural tissues. J Pediatr 130:878, 1997.
137. Gorman MP: Update on diagnosis, treatment, and prognosis in opsoclonus-myoclonus-ataxia syndrome. Curr Opin Pediatr 22:745, 2010.
138. Pranzatelli MR, Tate ED, McGee NR, et al: CCR4 agonists CCL22 and CCL17 are elevated in pediatric OMS sera: rapid and selective down-regulation of CCL22 by ACTH or corticosteroids. J Clin Immunol 33:817, 2013.
139. Tate ED, Pranzatelli MR, Verhulst SJ, et al: Active comparator-controlled, rater-blinded study of corticotropin-based immunotherapies for opsoclonus-myoclonus syndrome. J Child Neurol 27:875, 2012.
140. Klaas JP, Ahlskog JE, Pittock SJ, et al: Adult-onset opsoclonus-myoclonus syndrome. Arch Neurol 69: 1598, 2012.
141. Ohmer R, Golnik KC, Richards AI, et al: Ophthalmoplegia associated with the anti-Ri antibody. J Neuroophthalmol 19:246, 1999.
142. Mancuso M, Orsucci D, Bacci A, et al: Anti-Ri-associated paraneoplastic cerebellar degeneration. Report of a case and revision of the literature. Arch Ital Biol 149:318, 2011.
143. Luque FA, Furneaux HM, Ferziger R, et al: Anti-Ri: an antibody associated with paraneoplastic opsoclonus and breast cancer. Ann Neurol 29:241, 1991.
144. Pittock SJ, Lucchinetti CF, Lennon VA: Anti-neuronal nuclear autoantibody type 2: paraneoplastic accompaniments. Ann Neurol 53:580, 2003.
145. Allen SE, Darnell RB, Lipscombe D: The neuronal splicing factor Nova controls alternative splicing in N-type and P-type CaV2 calcium channels. Channels (Austin) 4:483, 2010.
146. Ule J, Ule A, Spencer J, et al: Nova regulates brain-specific splicing to shape the synapse. Nat Genet 37:844, 2005.
147. Cher LM, Hochberg FH, Teruya J, et al: Therapy for paraneoplastic neurologic syndromes in six patients with protein A column immunoadsorption. Cancer 75:1678, 1995.
148. Bataller L, Graus F, Saiz A, et al: Clinical outcome in adult onset idiopathic or paraneoplastic opsoclonus-myoclonus. Brain 124:437, 2001.
149. Shildkrot Y, Sobrin L, Gragoudas ES: Cancer-associated retinopathy: update on pathogenesis and therapy. Semin Ophthalmol 26:321, 2011.
150. Braithwaite T, Vugler A, Tufail A: Autoimmune retinopathy. Ophthalmologica 228:131, 2012.
151. Cornblath WT: Paraneoplastic disorders of ophthalmic interest. Ophthalmol Clin North Am 17:447, 2004.
152. Thirkill CE: Cancer-induced, immune-mediated ocular degenerations. Ocul Immunol Inflamm 13:119, 2005.
153. Dhingra A, Fina ME, Neinstein A, et al: Autoantibodies in melanoma-associated retinopathy target TRPM1 cation channels of retinal ON bipolar cells. J Neurosci 31:3962, 2011.
154. Faez S, Loewenstein J, Sobrin L: Concordance of antiretinal antibody testing results between laboratories in autoimmune retinopathy. JAMA Ophthalmol 131:113, 2013.
155. Ohguro H, Maruyama I, Nakazawa M, et al: Antirecoverin antibody in the aqueous humor of a patient with cancer-associated retinopathy. Am J Ophthalmol 134:605, 2002.
156. Lu Y, Jia L, He S, et al: Melanoma-associated retinopathy: a paraneoplastic autoimmune complication. Arch Ophthalmol 127:1572, 2009.
157. Ko MW, Dalmau J, Galetta SL: Neuro-ophthalmologic manifestations of paraneoplastic syndromes. J Neuro-ophthalmol 28:58, 2008.
158. Jarius S, Wandinger KP, Borowski K, et al: Antibodies to CV2/CRMP5 in neuromyelitis optica-like disease: case report and review of the literature. Clin Neurol Neurosurg 114:331, 2012.
159. Cree B: Neuromyelitis optica: diagnosis, pathogenesis, and treatment. Curr Neurol Neurosci Rep 8:427, 2008.
160. Flanagan EP, McKeon A, Lennon VA, et al: Paraneoplastic isolated myelopathy: clinical course and neuroimaging clues. Neurology 76:2089, 2011.
161. Sa MJ: Acute transverse myelitis: a practical reappraisal. Autoimmun Rev 9:128, 2009.
162. Flanagan EP, Keegan BM: Paraneoplastic myelopathy. Neurol Clin 31:307, 2013.
163. Urai Y, Matsumoto K, Shimamura M, et al: Paraneoplastic necrotizing myelopathy in a patient with advanced esophageal cancer: an autopsied case report. J Neurol Sci 280:113, 2009.
164. Flanagan EP, Sandroni P, Pittock SJ, et al: Paraneoplastic lower motor neuronopathy associated with Hodgkin lymphoma. Muscle Nerve 46:823, 2012.
165. Rosenfeld MR, Posner JB: Paraneoplastic motor neuron disease. p. 445. In Rowland LP (ed): Advances in Neurology, Vol 56: Amyotrophic Lateral Sclerosis and Other Motor Neuron Diseases. Raven Press, New York, 1991.
166. Forsyth PA, Dalmau J, Graus F, et al: Motor neuron syndromes in cancer patients. Ann Neurol 41:722, 1997.
167. Jarius S, Ruprecht K, Wildemann B, et al: Contrasting disease patterns in seropositive and seronegative

neuromyelitis optica: a multicentre study of 175 patients. J Neuroinflammation 9:14, 2012.
168. Pittock SJ, Lennon VA: Aquaporin-4 autoantibodies in a paraneoplastic context. Arch Neurol 65:629, 2008.
169. Ciccoto G, Blaya M, Kelley RE: Stiff person syndrome. Neurol Clin 31:319, 2013.
170. Rakocevic G, Floeter MK: Autoimmune stiff person syndrome and related myelopathies: understanding of electrophysiological and immunological processes. Muscle Nerve 45:623, 2012.
171. Pittock SJ, Yoshikawa H, Ahlskog JE, et al: Glutamic acid decarboxylase autoimmunity with brainstem, extrapyramidal, and spinal cord dysfunction. Mayo Clin Proc 81:1207, 2006.
172. Pittock SJ, Lucchinetti CF, Parisi JE, et al: Amphiphysin autoimmunity: paraneoplastic accompaniments. Ann Neurol 58:96, 2005.
173. McKeon A, Martinez-Hernandez E, Lancaster E, et al: Glycine receptor autoimmune spectrum with stiff-man syndrome phenotype. JAMA Neurol 70:44, 2013.
174. Geis C, Beck M, Jablonka S, et al: Stiff person syndrome associated anti-amphiphysin antibodies reduce GABA associated $[Ca^{2+}]i$ rise in embryonic motoneurons. Neurobiol Dis 36:191, 2009.
175. Casa-Fages B, Anaya F, Gabriel-Ortemberg M, et al: Treatment of stiff-person syndrome with chronic plasmapheresis. Mov Disord 28:396, 2013.
176. Giometto B, Grisold W, Vitaliani R, et al: Paraneoplastic neurologic syndrome in the PNS Euronetwork Database: a European study from 20 centers. Arch Neurol 67:330, 2010.
177. Koike H, Tanaka F, Sobue G: Paraneoplastic neuropathy: wide-ranging clinicopathological manifestations. Curr Opin Neurol 24:504, 2011.
178. Antoine JC, Mosnier JF, Absi L, et al: Carcinoma associated paraneoplastic peripheral neuropathies in patients with and without anti-onconeural antibodies. J Neurol Neurosurg Psychiatry 67:7, 1999.
179. Oki Y: Ataxic vs painful form of paraneoplastic neuropathy. Neurology 69:564, 2007.
180. Giometto B, Vitaliani R, Lindeck-Pozza E, et al: Treatment for paraneoplastic neuropathies. Cochrane Database Syst Rev:CD007625, 2012.
181. Graus F, Bonaventura I, Uchuya M, et al: Indolent anti-Hu-associated paraneoplastic sensory neuropathy. Neurology 44:2258, 1994.
182. Kuntzer T, Antoine JC, Steck AJ: Clinical features and pathophysiological basis of sensory neuronopathies (ganglionopathies). Muscle Nerve 30:255, 2004.
183. Camdessanche JP, Jousserand G, Ferraud K, et al: The pattern and diagnostic criteria of sensory neuronopathy: a case-control study. Brain 132:1723, 2009.
184. Camdessanche JP, Jousserand G, Franques J, et al: A clinical pattern-based etiological diagnostic strategy for sensory neuronopathies: a French collaborative study. J Peripher Nerv Syst 17:331, 2012.
185. Molinuevo JL, Graus F, Serrano C, et al: Utility of anti-Hu antibodies in the diagnosis of paraneoplastic sensory neuropathy. Ann Neurol 44:976, 1998.
186. Vigliani MC, Magistrello M, Polo P, et al: Risk of cancer in patients with Guillain-Barré syndrome (GBS). A population-based study. J Neurol 251:321, 2004.
187. Martinelli P, Macri S, Scaglione C, et al: Acute brachial plexus neuropathy as a presenting sign of peripheral nervous system involvement in paraproteinaemia. Acta Neurol Scand 95:319, 1997.
188. Kumar N: Hypertrophy of the nerve roots of the cauda equina as a paraneoplastic manifestation of lymphoma. Arch Neurol 62:1776, 2005.
189. Otrock ZK, Barada WM, Sawaya RA, et al: Bilateral phrenic nerve paralysis as a manifestation of paraneoplastic syndrome. Acta Oncol 49:264, 2010.
190. Hadden RD, Nobile-Orazio E, Sommer C, et al: European Federation of Neurological Societies/Peripheral Nerve Society guideline on management of paraproteinaemic demyelinating neuropathies: report of a joint task force of the European Federation of Neurological Societies and the Peripheral Nerve Society. Eur J Neurol 13:809, 2006.
191. Goldfarb AR, Weimer LH, Brannagan TH: Rituximab treatment of an IgM monoclonal autonomic and sensory neuropathy. Muscle Nerve 31:510, 2005.
192. Koike H, Watanabe H, Sobue G: The spectrum of immune-mediated autonomic neuropathies: insights from the clinicopathological features. J Neurol Neurosurg Psychiatry 84:98, 2013.
193. Vernino S, Adamski J, Kryzer TJ, et al: Neuronal nicotinic ACh receptor antibody in subacute autonomic neuropathy and cancer-related syndromes. Neurology 50:1806, 1998.
194. Lennon VA, Ermilov LG, Szurszewski JH, et al: Immunization with neuronal nicotinic acetylcholine receptor induces neurological autoimmune disease. J Clin Invest 111:907, 2003.
195. Badari A, Farolino D, Nasser E, et al: A novel approach to paraneoplastic intestinal pseudo-obstruction. Support Care Cancer 20:425, 2012.
196. van Sonderen SA, Wirtz PW, Verschuuren JJ, et al: Paraneoplastic syndromes of the neuromuscular junction: therapeutic options in myasthenia gravis, Lambert-Eaton myasthenic syndrome, and neuromyotonia. Curr Treat Options Neurol 15:224, 2013.
197. Titulaer MJ, Lang B, Verschuuren JJ: Lambert-Eaton myasthenic syndrome: from clinical characteristics to therapeutic strategies. Lancet Neurol 10:1098, 2011.
198. Maddison P: Treatment in Lambert-Eaton myasthenic syndrome. Ann NY Acad Sci 1275:78, 2012.
199. Maddison P, Newsom-Davis J, Mills KR, et al: Favourable prognosis in Lambert-Eaton myasthenic syndrome and small-cell lung carcinoma. Lancet 353:117, 1999.
200. Sabater L, Titulaer M, Saiz A, et al: SOX1 antibodies are markers of paraneoplastic Lambert-Eaton myasthenic syndrome. Neurology 70:924, 2008.

201. Rubio-Agusti I, Perez-Miralles F, Sevilla T, et al: Peripheral nerve hyperexcitability: a clinical and immunologic study of 38 patients. Neurology 76:172, 2011.
202. Irani SR, Pettingill P, Kleopa KA, et al: Morvan syndrome: clinical and serological observations in 29 cases. Ann Neurol 72:241, 2012.
203. Klein CJ, Lennon VA, Aston PA, et al: Insights From LGI1 and CASPR2 potassium channel complex autoantibody subtyping. JAMA Neurol 70:229, 2013.
204. Abou-Zeid E, Boursoulian LJ, Metzer WS, et al: Morvan syndrome: a case report and review of the literature. J Clin Neuromuscul Dis 13:214, 2012.
205. Rana SS, Ramanathan RS, Small G, et al: Paraneoplastic Isaacs' syndrome: a case series and review of the literature. J Clin Neuromuscul Dis 13:228, 2012.
206. van den Berg JS, van Engelen BG, Boerman RH, et al: Acquired neuromyotonia: superiority of plasma exchange over high-dose intravenous human immunoglobulin. J Neurol 246:623, 1999.
207. Danko K, Ponyi A, Molnar AP, et al: Paraneoplastic myopathy. Curr Opin Rheumatol 21:594, 2009.
208. Aggarwal R, Oddis CV: Paraneoplastic myalgias and myositis. Rheum Dis Clin North Am 37:607, 2011.
209. Zahr ZA, Baer AN: Malignancy in myositis. Curr Rheumatol Rep 13:208, 2011.
210. Samuels N, Applbaum YH, Esayag Y: Paraneoplastic necrotizing myopathy and dermatomyositis in a patient with rectosigmoid carcinoma. Rheumatol Int 33:1619, 2013.
211. Wegener S, Bremer J, Komminoth P, et al: Paraneoplastic necrotizing myopathy with a mild inflammatory component: a case report and review of the literature. Case Rep Oncol 3:88, 2012.
212. Buchbinder R, Forbes A, Hall S, et al: Incidence of malignant disease in biopsy-proven inflammatory myopathy. A population-based cohort study. Ann Intern Med 134:1087, 2001.
213. Sampson JB: Paraneoplastic myopathy: response to intravenous immunoglobulin. Neuromuscul Disord 17:404, 2007.

CHAPTER

28

Neurologic Complications of Chemotherapy and Radiation Therapy

MARIEL B. DEUTSCH ■ LISA M. DEANGELIS

Chemotherapy and radiation therapy (RT) are two of the major modalities used to treat cancer. Their goal is to kill or inactivate enough cancer cells so that the body's own defenses can control the disease without unacceptable damage to normal tissue. Unfortunately, both RT and chemotherapy are relatively nonspecific and depend on their ability to damage rapidly dividing cells. The therapeutic/toxic ratio is often low; even in highly sensitive tumors such as acute lymphoblastic leukemia, Hodgkin disease, and germ cell tumors, for which the cure rate is high, many patients suffer serious side effects of therapy, either immediately or months to years later.

The nervous system may be expected to be relatively insensitive to the side effects of cancer therapy. It is protected from exposure to many chemotherapeutic agents by the blood–brain, blood–cerebrospinal fluid (CSF), and blood–nerve barriers. Furthermore, most neurons do not reproduce, and glial cells reproduce only slowly, thus affording protection against agents directed against dividing cells. Nevertheless, nervous system toxicity is common, second only to myelosuppression as a reason for limiting the dose of chemotherapy, and often is also dose limiting for RT. This chapter describes the side effects of these therapeutic modalities on both the central and peripheral nervous systems. Chemotherapeutic agents and radiotherapeutic approaches that are used widely in clinical practice are emphasized, with particular attention to newer agents.

CHEMOTHERAPY

Table 28-1 classifies the major chemotherapeutic agents that have been reported to cause central nervous system (CNS) or peripheral nervous system (PNS) toxicity. Table 28-2 lists the neurotoxic signs caused by agents commonly used in cancer patients; details can be found elsewhere.[1–9]

TABLE 28-1 ■ Neurotoxicity of Chemotherapeutic Agents in Humans

		Neurotoxicity					Neurotoxicity		
Agents	**Drug**	**PNS**	**CNS†**	**Muscle**	**Agents**	**Drug**	**PNS**	**CNS†**	**Muscle**
Antimetabolites	5-Azacitidine	+	+	?+	Podophyllotoxins	Etoposide (VP-16)	?+	?+	–
	5-Fluorouracil	–	++	–		Teniposide (VM-26)	?+	?+	–
	Capecitabine	?+	+	–	Monoclonal antibodies	Bevacizumab	–	+	–
	Cladribine	–	+	–		Ipilimumab	+	+	–
	Cytarabine	+	+	–		Rituximab	–	+	–
	Fludarabine	–	++	–	Small molecule inhibitors	Bortezomib	++	–	–
	Gemcitabine	?+	?+	+		Carfilzomib	+	+	–
	Methotrexate	–	++	–		Gefitinib	–	+	–
	Nelarabine	++	+	–		Imatinib	–	+	–
	Pemetrexed	+	–	–		Selumetinib	–	+	+
	Pentostatin	+	+	–		Sorafenib	++	+	–
Alkylating agents	Carmustine (BCNU)	–	+	–		Sunitinib	–	++	–
	Chlorambucil	–	?+	–		Tipifarnib	++	+	–
	Cyclophosphamide	–	?+	–		Vemurafenib	–	+	–
	Ifosfamide	–	++	–	Other Biologics	Cyclosporine	+	+	+
	Lomustine (CCNU)	–	+	–		Interferons	+	++	–
	Temozolomide	–	+	–		Interleukins	–	++	–
	Thiotepa	–	+	–		Lenalidomide	+	–	–
Platinums	Carboplatin	+	–	–		Mycophenolate mofetil	+	+	–
	Cisplatin	++	++	–		Tacrolimus	–	+	–
	Oxaliplatin	++	–	–		Thalidomide	++	–	–
Taxanes	Cabazitaxel	++	–	+	Miscellaneous	Dexamethasone	–	++	++
	Docetaxel	+	–	+		DTIC (Dacarbazine)	–	?+	–
	Nab-paclitaxel	++	–	+		Hexamethylmelamine	+	+	–
	Paclitaxel	++	–	+		Ixabepilone	++	–	–
Vinca alkaloids	Vinblastine	+	–	–		L-Asparaginase	–	+	–
	Vincristine	++	+	?+		Procarbazine	+	+	–
	Vinorelbine	+	–	–		Retinoids	+	++	–
						Suramin	++	+	–
						Tamoxifen	–	+	–

?+, questionable; +, rare; ++, common; –, none; CNS, central nervous system; PNS, peripheral nervous system.
†CNS and cranial nerves.

Antimetabolites

FLUDARABINE

Fludarabine (2-fluoroadenosine arabinoside) is active against a variety of lymphoproliferative neoplasms. It is highly immunosuppressive and has been associated with the development of progressive multifocal leukoencephalopathy (PML) in some patients.[10] In addition, fludarabine can cause delayed neurotoxicity leading to a severe

TABLE 28-2 ■ Neurotoxic Signs Caused by Agents Commonly Used in Cancer Patients

Acute Encephalopathy (Delirium)
5-Azacytidine, 5-fluorouracil, asparaginase, bevacizumab, capecitabine, carmustine, cisplatin, cladribine, corticosteroids, cyclophosphamide, cyclosporin A, cytarabine, dacarbazine, docetaxel, etoposide (HD), fludarabine, gemcitabine, hydroxyurea, ifosfamide, imatinib, interferons, interleukins 1 and 2, methotrexate (HD, IV, IT), nelarabine, nitrosoureas (HD or arterial), paclitaxel, pentostatin, procarbazine, tacrolimus, tamoxifen, thalidomide, thiotepa (HD), tipifarnib, vincristine
Seizures
5-Fluorouracil, amifostine, asparaginase, bevacizumab, busulfan (HD), carmustine, cisplatin, corticosteroids, cyclophosphamide (HD), cyclosporin A, cytarabine, dacarbazine, docetaxel, erythropoietin, etanercept, etoposide (HD), fludarabine (HD), gemcitabine, hydroxyurea, ifosfamide, interferon, interleukin-2, letrozole, leuprolide, methotrexate, nelarabine, octreotide, paclitaxel, pentostatin (HD), temozolomide, teniposide, thalidomide, topotecan (IT), vincristine
Headaches Without Meningitis
5-Fluorouracil, anastrozole, asparaginase, carmustine, capecitabine, cetuximab, cisplatin, cladribine, corticosteroids, cytarabine, erlotinib, estramustine, etoposide, fludarabine, gefitinib, gemtuzamab, hydroxyurea, ibritumomab, imatinib, interferons, interleukins, isotretinoin, ixabepilone, letrozole, leuprolide, methotrexate, nelarabine, panitumumab, procarbazine, retinoic acid, rituximab (IV & IT), sorafenib, sunitinib, tamoxifen, temozolomide, thalidomide, thiotepa, topotecan, traztusumab, vemurafenib, vincristine
Visual Loss
5-Fluorouracil, bevacizumab, carboplatin, carmustine, cisplatin, cytarabine, etanercept, etoposide, fludarabine, interferon, interleukin, ipilimumab, isotretinoin, methotrexate, nitrosoureas (IA), oxaliplatin, paclitaxel, pentostatin, tamoxifen, vincristine
Chronic Encephalopathy (Dementia)
5-Fluorouracil, carmofur, carmustine, cisplatin, cytarabine, dacarbazine, fludarabine, ifosfamide, interferon-alpha, methotrexate, rituximab (IT), topotecan (IT)
Peripheral Neuropathy
5-Azacitidine, 5-fluorouracil, bortezomib, cabazitaxel, capecitabine, carboplatin, carfilzomib, cisplatin, cladribine, cytarabine, docetaxel, etoposide, fludarabine, gemcitabine, ifosfamide, interferon, ipilimumab, ixabepilone, lenalidomide, nab-paclitaxel, nelarabine, oxaliplatin, paclitaxel, pemetrexed, pentostatin, procarbazine, sorafenib, sunitinib, teniposide, thalidomide, tipifarnib, vinca alkaloids
Cerebellar Dysfunction (Ataxia)
5-Fluorouracil, cyclosporin A, cytarabine, nelarabine, procarbazine, vinblastine, vincristine
Myelopathy (Intrathecal Drugs)
Cytarabine, methotrexate, thiotepa
Aseptic Meningitis
Cytarabine (IT), IVIg, methotrexate (IT), monoclonal antibodies, rituximab (IT), thiotepa (IT), topotecan (IT)

HD, high dose; IT, intrathecal; IV, intravenous; IVIg, intravenous γ-globulin factor.

encephalopathy and occasionally cortical blindness.[11] Older patients and those receiving higher doses of the drug are at greatest risk.

METHOTREXATE

Methotrexate causes both acute and delayed neurotoxicity.[6,12] The side effects associated with intrathecal administration are discussed on page 599, where the various neurologic side effects of methotrexate are also tabulated.

A stroke-like syndrome affecting adults or children occasionally follows systemic high-dose methotrexate infusion. The disorder usually follows the second or third treatment by 5 or 6 days and is characterized by alternating hemiparesis associated with aphasia and sometimes encephalopathy or coma. Seizure activity is rare, and the electroencephalogram (EEG) is typically slow. Magnetic resonance imaging (MRI) shows foci of hyperintensity on fluid-attenuated inversion recovery (FLAIR) sequences, and diffusion-weighted imaging (DWI) sequences display well-delineated hyperintense areas affecting the deep white matter that do not conform to a single vascular territory. Apparent diffusion coefficient maps demonstrate decreased signal intensity in a corresponding distribution, suggesting restricted diffusion, similar to an acute vascular event.[13] Patients generally recover spontaneously in 48 to 72 hours with complete or partial resolution of the imaging abnormalities. Recurrences are rare with subsequent treatments. The pathogenesis is unknown, but it may be related to brain glucose metabolism, which decreases following intravenous infusion of high-dose methotrexate in rats.[14]

Leukoencephalopathy may appear months to years following therapy, beginning either insidiously or abruptly. The disorder generally follows repeated doses of intravenous high-dose methotrexate or intrathecal methotrexate, but it may occur after standard doses as well.[4] Although the syndrome can be caused by methotrexate alone, it is enhanced by brain RT and the combination of systemic and intrathecal drug. The sequence of administration is probably also important; when methotrexate is administered concurrently with or follows cranial RT, the synergy is particularly toxic. Patients may recover slowly over weeks or months, their symptoms may stabilize with a mild-to-moderate cognitive deficit, or there may be relentless progression with spastic hemiparesis or quadriparesis, severe dementia, and coma, ending in death. Seizures can occur, usually late in the course. The MRI reveals cerebral atrophy, bilateral and diffuse periventricular white matter hyperintensities on T2-weighted or FLAIR sequences, ventricular dilatation, and, sometimes, cortical calcifications (Fig. 28-1). Neurologic signs are usually preceded by radiographic white matter changes, and identical radiographic findings may be seen in patients years after prophylactic treatment with intrathecal or intravenous methotrexate, even in the absence of RT. Similar findings may occasionally be seen in asymptomatic patients who have received methotrexate.[15] Focal gadolinium enhancement may be present in the early stages, but it typically does not persist. No effective treatment exists.

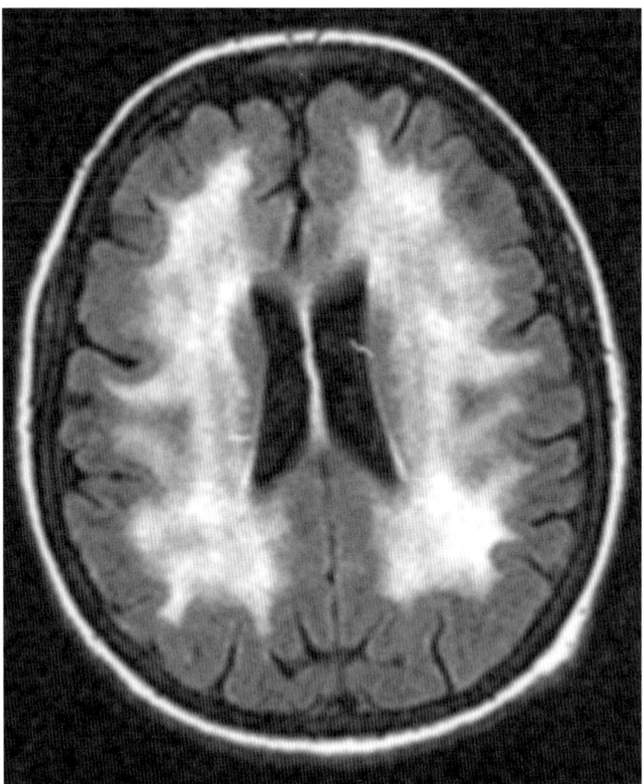

FIGURE 28-1 ■ Treatment-induced leukoencephalopathy. Fluid-attenuated inversion recovery MRI of the brain demonstrating diffuse periventricular white matter hyperintensity following treatment with methotrexate and whole-brain radiotherapy.

Cytarabine (Cytosine Arabinoside)

Intravenous high-dose cytarabine (ara-C) may cause central or peripheral neurologic disorders.[6] Cerebellar dysfunction occurs most frequently in older patients and in those with preexisting renal dysfunction, usually at a cumulative dose $\geq 36\,g/m^2$; however, it has been reported after a single dose of $3\,g/m^2$. Patients develop dysarthria, nystagmus, and appendicular and gait ataxia. Confusion, lethargy, and somnolence may also occur. With cessation of the drug, complete resolution of symptoms and signs generally occurs within 2 weeks, but some have persistent deficits.

Peripheral neuropathy, which may be axonal or demyelinating, is a rare complication of ara-C. Other reported toxicities include seizures, intracranial hypertension, reversible ocular toxicity (blurred vision, photophobia, burning eye pain, and blindness), pseudobulbar palsy, Horner syndrome, the "painful legs, moving toes" syndrome, brachial plexopathy, bilateral lateral rectus palsies, and acute aseptic meningitis following intravenous injection. There is no treatment for any of the neurotoxic effects of ara-C, but many patients recover spontaneously.

Nelarabine

Nelarabine is a purine analog that is used in the treatment of T-cell acute lymphoblastic leukemia. Motor or sensory neuropathy, or both, occurs in approximately 20 percent of patients. Central neurotoxicity most frequently involves somnolence and fatigue that begins approximately 1 week after drug administration. Other symptoms may include headache, seizures, ataxia, tremor, amnesia, and paraplegia.[16,17] The deficits may not be reversible, and drug discontinuation is recommended.

GEMCITABINE

Gemcitabine is a deoxycytidine analogue. Sensory neuropathy occurs in approximately 10 percent of patients, and an autonomic neuropathy has been reported.[18] Gemcitabine may also cause an acute myositis. Patients present with painful symmetric weakness of the proximal muscles, with elevation of serum creatine kinase levels. Symptoms resolve rapidly with discontinuation of the drug and may respond to corticosteroids. Patients often do not have symptoms following additional doses of the drug.[19] Gemcitabine may also cause a focal myositis hours to days after administration, in a muscle group within a field previously irradiated months or years earlier, a phenomenon referred to as "radiation recall."[20] Many other agents have also been associated with radiation recall, including capecitabine and docetaxel.[20]

Microtubule Agents

IXABEPILONE

Ixabepilone is an epothilone that stabilizes microtubules and induces apoptosis.[5,21,22] A predominantly sensory neuropathy is the most common neurotoxicity, occurring in more than 60 percent of patients.[22–24] The neuropathy is generally mild-to-moderate and improves with drug discontinuation, typically within 1 to 2 months. Alternatively, the dose can be reduced if the severity is no worse than grade 2 by National Cancer Institute common toxicity criteria, being discontinued if the severity reaches grade 3. Less common neurologic side effects include headache and dizziness.

TAXANES

Paclitaxel and Docetaxel

Approximately 60 percent of patients receiving paclitaxel (Taxol) at $\leq 250\,mg/m^2$ per dose develop paresthesias of the hands and feet that do not usually progress and may resolve even with continued therapy.[25] The neuropathy is predominantly sensory, affecting all modalities. Paclitaxel causes axonal damage with secondary demyelination, probably reflecting cell body damage. A few patients also develop proximal muscle weakness that resolves; it is usually associated with the peripheral neuropathy.[26] Acute arthralgias and myalgias of the legs that curtail activity may occur 2 to 3 days after a course of paclitaxel and can last for 2 to 4 days.[27] Rarely, encephalopathy and seizures occur. Docetaxel causes the same type of sensory neuropathy as paclitaxel but in general has less neurotoxicity. Paclitaxel or docetaxel neuropathy is enhanced by prior or subsequent neurotoxic chemotherapy, particularly with cisplatin or vinorelbine.[28] Data from animal models suggest that lithium, ibudilast, and cannabinoid receptor agonists may be neuroprotective against paclitaxel-induced peripheral neuropathy, but to date there are insufficient human data to support any neuroprotective agents against taxane-induced (or any chemotherapy-induced) peripheral neuropathy.[29–34]

Nab-paclitaxel

Nab-paclitaxel, an albumin-bound formulation of paclitaxel, has a higher incidence of grade 3 sensory neuropathy compared to standard paclitaxel.[35] Patients may improve with discontinuation, and the drug may be rechallenged at a reduced dose.[5,8]

Cabazitaxel

Cabazitaxel is a semisynthetic taxane that can be effective in docetaxel- and paclitaxel-resistant tumors.[36,37] Peripheral neuropathy can occur but is rarely severe.[37]

VINCRISTINE

Vincristine affects primarily the peripheral nerves but can also be toxic to the CNS, cranial nerves, and autonomic nervous system (Table 28-3). Vinorelbine and vinblastine are much less neurotoxic. A dose-limiting sensorimotor neuropathy appears in virtually all patients.[2] The earliest complaint is of tingling and paresthesias of the fingertips and later of the toes. Fine movements of the fingers and toes are often eventually impaired. Objective sensory loss is uncommon, but weakness, especially of the extensors of the feet and hands, is frequent. Foot drop

TABLE 28-3 ■ The Spectrum of Vincristine Neurotoxicity

Toxic Effect	Subacute (1 Day to 2 Weeks)	Intermediate (1 to 4 Weeks)	Chronic (>3 Weeks)
Peripheral neuropathy	Depressed Achilles reflex (universal)	Other tendon reflexes depressed, paresthesias	Sensory loss, weakness, "foot drop" gait
Myopathy?	Muscle pain, tenderness (especially quadriceps); jaw pain	–	–
Autonomic neuropathy	Ileus with cramping abdominal pain	Constipation, urinary hesitancy, impotence, orthostatic hypotension	–
Cranial neuropathy (uncommon)	–	–	Optic atrophy; ptosis; sixth, seventh, and eighth cranial nerve dysfunction; hoarseness; dysphagia
"Central" toxicity	–	Seizure, SIADH	–

Modified from DeAngelis LM, Posner JB. Neurologic Complications of Cancer. 2nd Ed. Oxford University Press, Oxford, 2009.
SIADH, syndrome of inappropriate antidiuretic hormone secretion.

is either unilateral or bilateral; unilateral foot drop is more common in patients who have lost weight and habitually sit with crossed legs, causing fibular (peroneal) nerve compression. The weakness is usually tolerable, but rarely patients may become bedbound or quadriparetic, particularly if there is a preexisting neuropathy. The sensory symptoms, weakness, and loss of muscle-stretch reflexes are reversible, but may require months to improve after the medication is stopped. Neurophysiologic studies show an axonal neuropathy.

Muscle cramps, usually diurnal, affecting the arms and legs, may also be an early symptom of neurotoxicity. These cramps are also particularly common in the jaw and tend to occur within 1 day to 2 weeks of drug administration.

Vincristine occasionally causes focal neuropathies of cranial (as well as peripheral) nerves.[4] The most common is oculomotor nerve involvement, characterized by isolated ptosis. Less frequently, ophthalmoplegia with diplopia occurs. The recurrent laryngeal nerve, facial nerve, vestibulocochlear nerve, and optic nerve are also affected occasionally. These cranial neuropathies may be bilateral or unilateral. Night blindness due to retinal damage has also been reported.

Autonomic neuropathy, characterized by colicky abdominal pain and constipation, occurs in almost all patients. Rarely, paralytic ileus develops and may be fatal. Prevention of constipation is essential, and all patients should receive a prophylactic bowel regimen. Other manifestations of autonomic dysfunction include bladder atony, impotence, and postural hypotension.

CNS toxicity may result from hyponatremia due to inappropriate secretion of antidiuretic hormone (SIADH). Encephalopathy and focal or generalized seizures not associated with SIADH have also been reported. Cortical blindness and other CNS signs, including athetosis, ataxia, and parkinsonian-like symptoms, usually reverse after treatment is discontinued.

DNA-Damaging Drugs

Alkylating Agents

Ifosfamide

High-dose ifosfamide has been associated with a reversible encephalopathy of varying severity, which is dose limiting.[38] The most common manifestations include confusion, stupor, and mutism, rarely evolving into coma; less common features include seizures, hallucinations, personality changes, blurred vision, extrapyramidal signs, cerebellar symptoms, and urinary incontinence. EEG abnormalities are found in 65 percent of patients, and nonconvulsive status epilepticus has been reported.[39] Although death or permanent disability can occur, the encephalopathy is usually reversible and can be treated with methylene blue.[12]

TABLE 28-4 ■ Neurotoxicity of Cisplatin

Common
Peripheral neuropathy (large fiber, sensory)
Lhermitte sign
Hearing loss (high frequency)
Tinnitus
Uncommon
Encephalopathy
Visual loss (retinal, optic nerve, cortical)
Seizures
Herniation (hydration-related)
Electrolyte imbalance (Ca^{2+}, Mg^{2+}, Na^{+}, SIADH)
Vestibular toxicity
Autonomic neuropathy

SIADH, syndrome of inappropriate antidiuretic hormone secretion.

Temozolomide

Temozolomide is standard chemotherapy for high-grade gliomas, and common side effects include nausea, fatigue, myelosuppression, and constipation. It rarely produces significant neurologic toxicity, although headaches may occur in up to 40 percent of patients.[40,41]

PLATINUMS

The platinums (cisplatin, oxaliplatin, carboplatin) contain a heavy-metal moiety, and therefore may cause a peripheral neuropathy in addition to other CNS and peripheral nervous system manifestations (Table 28-4).

Cisplatin

The peripheral neuropathy associated with cisplatin is dose dependent and usually follows cumulative doses exceeding 400 mg/m^2. It is characterized by numbness and tingling in the extremities, which are occasionally painful. The first symptoms usually appear during treatment and typically progress for several months after therapy is completed. The disorder affects predominantly the large sensory fibers; the muscle stretch reflexes disappear and proprioception is lost, often resulting in a sensory ataxia. Pain and temperature sensation are spared, and power may be normal. The disorder may be confused with paraneoplastic sensory neuronopathy, which usually affects all sensory modalities equally. Nerve conduction studies reveal a sensory axonopathy. With discontinuation of the drug, the neuropathy may improve and the patient's condition may return to normal after many months; however, many are left with permanent disability. Because maximal injury is not observed until months after discontinuation of the drug, dose adjustment is not possible to accommodate ongoing neural damage. There is no known treatment and there are insufficient data to support preventive pretreatment with acetylcysteine, acetyl-L-carnitine, amifostine, calcium and magnesium, growth factors, glutathione, Org 2766, oxcarbazepine, or vitamin E.[31,42,43]

Lhermitte sign appearing during or shortly after treatment with cisplatin suggests a demyelinating lesion in the posterior columns of the spinal cord. In some instances, patients may experience paresthesias down the arms when the upper limbs are abducted, suggesting that the brachial plexus may be affected as well. Lhermitte sign resolves completely and is not associated with any permanent damage.

Muscle cramps not related to electrolyte imbalance (see later) are also common but usually resolve spontaneously.

Ototoxicity is caused by cisplatin. Hearing loss results from hair cell damage.[44] The hearing loss is often subclinical and affects primarily the high-frequency ranges (>4,000 Hz). Tinnitus may precede hearing loss; rarely, high-dose cisplatin causes sudden deafness. Animal studies suggest that prophylactic vitamin E or sodium thiosulfate may reduce this toxicity.[45,46] Human data on amifostine are insufficient to support its use as an otoprotective agent.[31,47] Radiotherapy that encompasses the VIII nerve complex and hearing apparatus can enhance the ototoxicity of cisplatin regardless of the sequence of the two modalities. Vestibular toxicity is much less common than hearing loss.

Encephalopathy is rare following intravenous infusion and is characterized by seizures and focal brain dysfunction, particularly cortical blindness. The symptoms are usually reversible. Encephalopathy due to the drug must be differentiated from the electrolyte disorders that result from its administration. Vigorous hydration precedes cisplatin use and can therefore lead to dilutional hyponatremia and cerebral herniation. SIADH with hyponatremia and seizures may also occur.

Cisplatin has been implicated in late vascular toxicity, such as Raynaud phenomenon and the cardiac and cerebral infarction that sometimes follows multiagent chemotherapy. Vascular toxicity can also be subacute and occur within days to weeks of cisplatin administration. Other rare complications of cisplatin include irreversible myelopathy, taste disturbances, and a myasthenic syndrome.

Oxaliplatin

Oxaliplatin produces two types of peripheral neuropathy.[48] The first occurs during or shortly after infusion and consists of paresthesias and dysesthesias of the hands, feet, and perioral region with jaw tightness. These symptoms are usually transient, may be triggered by cold, and may increase in both duration and severity with repeated drug administration. A pharyngolaryngeal dysesthesia syndrome accompanied by a sensation of shortness of breath without any objective evidence of respiratory distress has also been described. Second, oxaliplatin can induce a peripheral sensory neuropathy similar to that seen with cisplatin. This neurotoxicity generally follows a cumulative dose greater than 540 mg/m^2 and is characterized by sensory ataxia, jaw pain, eye pain, ptosis, leg cramps, visual changes, and voice changes. Although reversible, these clinical findings may persist for months and require discontinuation of treatment. Less common neurologic complications include Lhermitte phenomenon and urinary retention.[49] Ototoxicity is rare.

Carboplatin

Carboplatin is less neurotoxic than cisplatin or oxaliplatin. Rare cases of peripheral neuropathy have been reported after high doses of carboplatin in patients treated with combinations of other cytotoxic agents.[50]

Monoclonal Antibodies

Bevacizumab

Bevacizumab is a monoclonal antibody that binds to and inhibits soluble vascular endothelial growth factor (VEGF), a mediator of tumor angiogenesis.[51] Patients treated with bevacizumab have an increased incidence of systemic hemorrhage as well as thromboembolism, including stroke, and transient ischemic attack.[52] The risk of CNS hemorrhage in patients with glioblastoma is under 4 percent,[53] and comparable to the risk associated with the disease itself. Bevacizumab's most common side effect is hypertension, which may lead to the posterior reversible encephalopathy syndrome (PRES) in some patients. Symptoms include headache, lethargy, visual disturbances including blindness, and seizures.[54–57] Symptoms usually resolve with discontinuation of the drug and blood pressure control, although permanent deficits can occur.[58] Rarely, bevacizumab may cause visual loss due to optic neuropathy.[59]

Ipilimumab

Ipilimumab is a monoclonal antibody directed against a cytotoxic T-cell receptor (CTLA-4) that is effective against melanoma.[60] Neurologic toxicity results from activation of the immune system and includes motor and sensory neuropathy, Guillain–Barré syndrome, giant cell arteritis, hypophysitis, and myasthenia gravis.[61,62] Depending on the severity of the side effects, ipilimumab should be withheld or discontinued. Corticosteroids are suggested for giant cell arteritis, hypophysitis, and severe neuropathy.[62]

Rituximab

Rituximab is a monoclonal antibody directed against the CD20 antigen found on the surface of malignant and normal B lymphocytes. It is used to treat non-Hodgkin lymphoma as well as other disorders in which B lymphocytes are implicated in disease pathogenesis. Neurologic side effects are uncommon but can include myalgias, dizziness, and headache.[63] Rituximab has also been associated rarely with PML.[40,64]

Small Molecule Inhibitors

Bortezomib and Carfilzomib

Bortezomib is a proteosome inhibitor that is primarily effective against multiple myeloma. Bortezomib causes a cumulative dose-dependent painful peripheral neuropathy that is predominantly sensory,[65] but is also associated with enhanced vulnerability to pressure-point neuropathies such as fibular (peroneal) nerve compression. Symptoms usually improve even without stopping treatment, but some patients are left with fixed deficits. Carfilzomib is a second-generation proteasome inhibitor; it causes a peripheral neuropathy that tends to be less severe than bortezomib.[66]

SELUMETINIB

Selumetinib is a small molecule inhibitor of MEK, a mitogen-activated protein kinase, used in clinical trials against solid tumors and melanoma. It can cause dropped head syndrome: a focal noninflammatory myopathy characterized by neck pain, neck extensor weakness, and elevated serum creatine kinase levels. ^{18}F-fluorodeoxyglucose positron emission tomography (FDG-PET) scan may show abnormal uptake in the affected muscles. Corticosteroids do not improve the condition, but discontinuation of the drug leads to recovery.[67]

Retinoids

The retinoids are a group of compounds consisting of vitamin A and related derivatives. They are used to treat acute promyelocytic leukemia (APL) as well as other malignancies.[68] Pediatric patients with a variety of cancers in a phase I trial of all-*trans* retinoic acid (ATRA) reported headache unassociated with pseudotumor cerebri in 7 of 17 patients (41%), and associated with it in 4 of 17 patients (24%).[69] In another ATRA trial in children with APL, severe headache occurred in 13 percent of patients and pseudotumor cerebri in 10 percent.[70] Adults have a lower incidence of intracranial hypertension.[71] Several reports also suggest an increased risk of suicide and depression in patients treated with 13-*cis* retinoic acid.[72]

Intrathecal Chemotherapy

Chemotherapy is sometimes given directly into the subarachnoid space as part of treatment for or prophylaxis against leptomeningeal metastases. It can either be injected into the lumbar thecal sac via lumbar puncture or into the lateral ventricle through an Ommaya reservoir. Intrathecal chemotherapy is contraindicated in patients who have elevated intracranial pressure (ICP). Increased ICP may cause plateau waves, which consist of waves of elevated ICP associated with transient neurologic symptoms such as visual changes, leg buckling, vertigo, or loss of consciousness in the setting of positional change or Valsalva maneuver. In patients with elevated ICP, intrathecally administered chemotherapy will not circulate properly through the CSF and may accumulate in the ventricle, causing toxicity when administered through an Ommaya reservoir.

TABLE 28-5 ■ Methotrexate Toxicity*

Route of Administration	Dose	Toxic Effect
Oral or intravenous	Standard	Leukoencephalopathy
Intravenous	High	Acute transient encephalopathy
		Chronic leukoencephalopathy
Intra-arterial	Standard	Hemorrhagic cerebral infarction
Intrathecal	Standard	Acute aseptic meningitis, paraplegia, seizures
		Chronic leukoencephalopathy, cerebral atrophy, and calcification

*Toxicity may be enhanced by cranial irradiation and/or other systemic chemotherapeutic agents.

Intrathecal methotrexate causes an aseptic meningitis in 10 to 50 percent of patients, primarily after administration by lumbar puncture rather than via ventricular cannula (Table 28-5).[6] Patients complain of headache, nausea, vomiting, and neck stiffness, and may become febrile and lethargic. Symptoms usually begin 2 to 4 hours after drug administration and may last up to a few days. A CSF pleocytosis is often present and can mimic acute bacterial meningitis, except that it occurs too soon after injection to be caused by bacterial growth. The symptoms are self-limited, and there is no specific treatment, although corticosteroids may reduce the inflammation and have been used as therapy.[73] The drug may be readministered without recurrent aseptic meningitis, but prophylactic oral corticosteroids may help. Transverse myelopathy is a less common complication of intrathecal methotrexate.[6] The symptoms include back pain followed by weakness, sensory changes, and sphincter dysfunction; they usually start between 30 minutes and 2 days after drug administration, but can be delayed by up to 2 weeks.[4] Concurrent radiotherapy may be a risk factor. Recovery may be incomplete and further intrathecal chemotherapy is contraindicated.[6] Acute encephalopathy is rare, but can occur if the intraventricular catheter is misplaced into the brain parenchyma rather than in the ventricle. Other complications include seizures, cranial neuropathies, the posterior reversible encephalopathy syndrome (PRES), lumbosacral polyradiculopathy, and sudden death.[6]

Intrathecal cytarabine causes aseptic meningitis in approximately 10 percent of patients, but it occurs in 40 percent when the cytarabine is given as the liposomal preparation DepoCyt. Dexamethasone should be taken prophylactically at a dose of 4 mg twice daily for 5 days, starting the day prior to administration, in order to decrease the risk of aseptic meningitis and arachnoiditis.[73] Transverse myelopathy can develop a few days to months following treatment. Other complications include seizures, headaches, and encephalopathy.[6]

Intrathecal thiotepa may cause aseptic meningitis and rarely a myelopathy. Topotecan intrathecally may also cause an aseptic meningitis[74] and less commonly seizure; leukoencephalopathy occurred in 36 percent of patients in one study.[75]

Rituximab is given intrathecally to treat leptomeningeal lymphoma. Headache, cramps, and reversible back pain associated with paraparesis have been reported,[76,77] as well as neuropathic pain,[78] leukoencephalopathy, transient diplopia, nausea and vomiting, and paresthesias.[79] Intrathecal traztuzumab has been used for leptomeningeal metastases from HER2-positive breast cancer. Aseptic meningitis has not been reported with intrathecal rituximab or intrathecal traztuzumab,[80] but use of those drugs via the intrathecal route is relatively recent.

RADIATION THERAPY

Therapeutic ionizing irradiation may damage neural structures when they are included in the radiation portal, whether the cancer undergoing RT is within or outside the nervous system. Nervous system injury can also occur secondarily when irradiation damages blood vessels supplying the brain or the endocrine organs necessary for normal nervous system function, or when the irradiation leads to tumors that compress or destroy nervous system structures. Nervous system dysfunction caused by RT can occur acutely or may be delayed by weeks, months, or even years following the successful completion of treatment. The likelihood that RT will damage the nervous system depends on the total dose delivered to the nervous system, the dose per fraction, the total volume of nervous system irradiated, the time after completion of RT, the presence of other systemic diseases that enhance the side effects of irradiation (e.g., diabetes, hypertension), and other unidentifiable host factors. Detailed reviews of RT-induced neurotoxicity can be found elsewhere.[4,81]

Primary Neurologic Damage

Brain

Encephalopathy caused by RT occurs in three forms: acute, early delayed (weeks to months), and late delayed (months to years) (Table 28-6).

Acute Encephalopathy

Acute encephalopathy usually follows large RT fractions given to patients with increased ICP from primary or metastatic brain tumor, particularly in the absence of corticosteroids.[4] Immediately following treatment, susceptible patients develop headache, nausea, vomiting, somnolence, fever, and worsening of neurologic symptoms, rarely severe enough to cause cerebral herniation. Acute encephalopathy usually follows the first radiation fraction and becomes progressively less severe with each ensuing fraction. Usually the disorder is mild, with the patient developing only headache and nausea in the evening following irradiation.

The pathogenesis of the disorder is uncertain. There are variable data to suggest it is secondary to a rise in ICP, with cerebral edema following breakdown of the blood–brain barrier by ionizing irradiation, particularly with fractions of 300 cGy or more. Therefore, patients harboring large brain tumors, particularly with signs of increased ICP, should be treated with doses of 200 cGy or less per fraction. All patients undergoing brain irradiation should be protected with corticosteroids (8 to 16 mg of dexamethasone daily) preferably for at least 24 hours before the start of RT. Both clinical and experimental evidence indicates that corticosteroids ameliorate the acute complications of irradiation.

Early Delayed Encephalopathy

Early delayed encephalopathy, which is thought to be due to demyelination, usually begins in the second or third month after irradiation but can begin anywhere from 2 weeks to 4 months after treatment.

TABLE 28-6 ■ Radiation-Induced Injury: Direct Damage to the Central Nervous System

Time After Radiation	Clinical Findings	Possible Mechanisms
Brain		
Acute (minutes to days)	Increased intracranial pressure	Acute vasogenic edema
Early delayed (weeks)	Pseudoprogression Brainstem encephalopathy Somnolence syndrome	Demyelination
Delayed (months to years)		
Necrosis	Diffuse: dementia (rare) Focal: simulates recurrent tumor	Glial and vascular destruction
Leukoencephalopathy	Asymptomatic or dementia	Unknown (Atrophy) (Spongiosis of white matter) (Normal-pressure hydrocephalus)
Spinal Cord		
Early delayed (weeks)	Lhermitte sign	Demyelination
Delayed (months to years)		
Spinal cord necrosis	Transverse myelopathy	Glial and vascular destruction
Motor neuron disease	Flaccid paraparesis, amyotrophy	Unknown
Arachnoiditis	Often asymptomatic	Radiation-induced damage to the leptomeninges
Hemorrhage	Acute myelopathy	Vascular lesions

If the patient has a glioblastoma, the symptoms of early delayed encephalopathy often simulate tumor progression ("pseudoprogression").[4,82] The risk of pseudoprogression is increased in those patients whose tumor contains a methylated promoter of the O^6-methylguanine-DNA methyltransferase (*MGMT*) gene, a DNA repair enzyme. Changes on neuroimaging may include an increase in the size of the lesion or the new appearance of contrast enhancement. These changes resolve spontaneously if the disorder is due to radiation encephalopathy rather than tumor recurrence, and resolution can be hastened by corticosteroids. The patient and the scan remain improved after corticosteroids are discontinued, indicating that the disorder was indeed not recurrence of tumor.

A rare and serious early delayed neurologic syndrome is brainstem encephalopathy, following irradiation of posterior fossa tumors or when the brainstem has been included in the irradiated field for head and neck cancer. The most frequent symptoms are ataxia, diplopia, dysarthria, and nystagmus. Most patients recover spontaneously within 6 to 8 weeks. Rarely, the symptoms progress to stupor, coma, and death.

Late Delayed Radiation Injury

Radiation Necrosis

Late delayed radiation necrosis usually begins 1 to 2 years after the completion of RT. In patients who are treated for primary or metastatic brain tumors, symptoms generally recapitulate those of the brain tumor itself, leading the physician to suspect tumor recurrence. A second clinical picture occurs when the patient's brain was included in the radiation portal but there was no underlying brain tumor. Examples include irradiation of head and neck tumors, including pituitary tumors, as well as prophylactic cranial irradiation.[4] Because only a portion of the brain has usually been irradiated and there was no previous brain damage, new focal neurologic signs are the rule. For example, bilateral medial temporal destruction sometimes follows irradiation for nasopharyngeal or pituitary tumors, and frontal or temporal lobe destruction follows

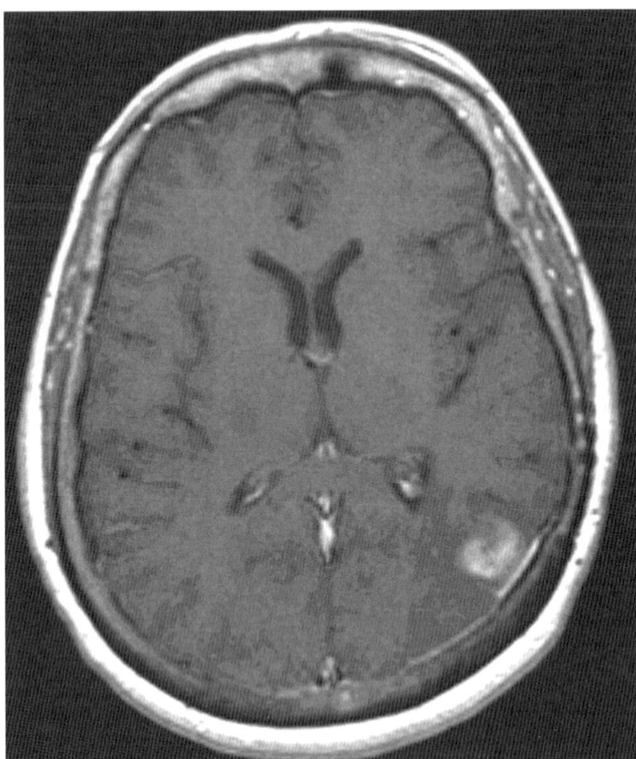

FIGURE 28-2 ■ Radiation necrosis. T1-weighted, post-contrast MRI 9 months after stereotactic radiosurgery for a left parietal, solitary dural-based metastasis. The lesion was hypointense on pre-contrast T1-weighted sequences.

treatment for ocular or maxillary sinus tumors.[83] The clinical features are similar to those of a brain tumor, with focal signs depending on the site of brain damage, and increased ICP if the lesion is sufficiently large. The MRI usually reveals a mass, often with contrast enhancement (Fig. 28-2). Elevated cerebral blood volume on MR perfusion sequences, restricted diffusion on MRI, and hypermetabolism on FDG-PET all favor recurrent tumor rather than radiation necrosis, but a definitive diagnosis can be made only pathologically.[84–86]

Radiation necrosis is often treated initially with corticosteroids; however, patients may respond only transiently. Bevacizumab has also shown clinical and radiographic benefit in the treatment of radiation necrosis and can allow corticosteroid dosage to be decreased.[82,87] When patients are symptomatic despite medical therapy or they develop morbidity from treatment, radiation necrosis may be treated with resection. Other suggested treatments, such as vitamin E, pentoxifylline, hyperbaric oxygen, antiplatelet agents, and anticoagulation, are based on the rationale that the disorder is characterized by fibrinoid necrosis of vessels, but they have not proved useful in most patients.[82]

SMART Syndrome

Stroke-like migraine attacks after RT, or SMART syndrome, is a rare complication of cranial irradiation that may occur 1 to 10 years after treatment. The syndrome is characterized by migraine-like headaches associated with transient neurologic signs that may be accompanied by seizures. MRI may show focal contrast enhancement that resolves over time without intervention.[88] The mechanism is thought to be due to neuronal dysfunction and not cerebral vascular activity.[89]

Cerebral Atrophy

Cerebral atrophy often follows whole-brain irradiation, and may be accompanied by periventricular leukoencephalopathy. The atrophy may occur in patients irradiated prophylactically or in those with a brain tumor that was eradicated by radiotherapy. It usually begins 6 to 12 months after RT. The patient may be asymptomatic or suffer memory loss, which may be severe. Some patients have gait abnormalities and urgency incontinence, suggesting communicating hydrocephalus, and they may respond to ventriculoperitoneal shunting. Symptomatic patients generally have greater degrees of atrophy and ventricular dilatation than asymptomatic patients. Cerebral atrophy also occurs in children receiving prophylactic brain irradiation for acute leukemia and is associated with a learning disability.[90]

SPINAL CORD

There are no acute effects of radiation on the spinal cord.

Early Delayed Radiation Myelopathy

Early delayed radiation myelopathy is common following irradiation of the neck (Table 28-6). Several weeks after irradiation, the patient develops Lhermitte sign that persists for weeks or months and then disappears spontaneously. Some but not all investigators have reported delayed somatosensory evoked potentials.[91,92] Symptoms are thought to be due to demyelination of the posterior columns of the spinal cord. They do not predict the development of late delayed radiation spinal cord injury.

Late Delayed Radiation Myelopathy

Late delayed radiation myelopathy appears in two forms. The first and most common is characterized by progressive myelopathy, often beginning as a Brown-Séquard syndrome and progressing over weeks or months to cause paraparesis or quadriparesis.[93] Usually the symptoms progress subacutely, but in some instances they progress over several years and, at times, may stabilize, leaving the patient with only mild or moderate paraparesis. MRI is usually nonspecific but helps to exclude metastatic spinal cord compression or intramedullary metastasis. Hyperintense changes of the irradiated vertebral bodies due to fat replacement of bone marrow may outline the radiation field even if the details of the RT port are unknown. In the acute stages, the spinal cord is swollen, and the damaged area may enhance with contrast material; spinal cord atrophy develops later.[94] There is no good treatment, although corticosteroids sometimes delay progression. Other potential therapies include hyperbaric oxygen and anticoagulation but they do not give benefit reliably.[95,96]

A second form of late delayed radiation myelopathy is a rare motor neuron syndrome that characteristically follows pelvic irradiation for testicular tumors or craniospinal irradiation for medulloblastoma.[97] This disorder occurs 3 months to 23 years following irradiation and is characterized by the subacute onset of flaccid leg weakness affecting both distal and proximal muscles accompanied by atrophy, fasciculations, and areflexia.[98] It is usually bilateral and symmetric but may be asymmetric or restricted to one leg. Sensory, sphincter, and sexual functions are all normal. The CSF may contain an increased protein concentration. Imaging is typically normal. Although electromyography reveals varying degrees of denervation, sensory and motor nerve conduction velocities are normal. It is difficult to differentiate the disorder from a pure motor polyneuropathy, isolated motor neuron loss, or the paraneoplastic syndrome of subacute motor neuronopathy. The deficit usually stabilizes after several months to a few years; often patients are still able to walk, but some may become paraplegic.

Another lower motor neuron syndrome caused by irradiation is the dropped-head syndrome, which can occur after mantle field radiation in the treatment of Hodgkin lymphoma. Amyotrophy of the neck and shoulder muscles is associated with reduced cervical range of motion, weakness in the neck flexors and extensors, neck pain, and a posture in which the head is dropped forward and resting on the chest.[99]

Cranial Nerves

The clinical features of radiation injury to the cranial and peripheral nerves and the special senses are shown in Table 28-7. Anosmia may follow irradiation. Taste is affected in almost every patient who undergoes cranial radiotherapy and is the main clinical complaint of those affected by anosmia. Visual loss may follow irradiation of the eye or brain. It can be caused by radiation-induced "dry eye syndrome," glaucoma, or cataract; more commonly, it results from retinopathy or optic neuropathy. The optic neuropathy following irradiation begins 7 to 26 months after RT and is characterized by progressive painless monocular or bilateral blindness. Papilledema and retinal hemorrhages may be present on fundoscopy. Hearing loss may also follow RT to the brain or ear. Radiation-induced otitis media appears during or shortly following cranial RT and causes a conductive hearing loss that may require myringotomy for relief. It is distinct from the sensorineural hearing loss that is a late delayed RT effect and has been attributed to an endarteritis producing vascular damage to the cochlear or eighth

TABLE 28-7 ■ Radiation-Induced Injury: Damage to the Cranial and Peripheral Nerves and Organs of Special Sense

Cranial Nerves
Visual system
Retinopathy
Optic neuropathy
Central retinal artery occlusion
Taste and smell
Acute, transient loss of taste and smell during radiation therapy
Chronic loss of smell (rare)
Involvement of the lower cranial nerves
Twelfth nerve most frequently affected
Brachial Plexopathies
Acute?
Early delayed (rare)
Delayed
Delayed Lumbosacral Plexopathy

cranial nerve.[4] The lower cranial nerves, particularly the hypoglossal nerve, are often involved as a late delayed effect of RT delivered to the neck. Lower cranial neuropathy can be delayed over 10 years.[100] Electrophysiologic studies commonly show myokymia and myokymic discharges in the tongue.[101] Recurrent laryngeal, vagal, and sympathetic fibers (Horner syndrome) may be involved as well.

Peripheral Nerves

There are no acute changes in peripheral nerve function following RT. Early delayed brachial plexus dysfunction is characterized by paresthesias in the hand and forearm, sometimes associated with pain and accompanied by weakness and atrophy in a C6 to T1 distribution.[4] Nerve conduction studies reveal segmental slowing, and the course is characterized by recovery over a few weeks or months. This disorder is particularly common in patients with breast cancer because the brachial plexus is frequently included in the radiotherapy port.

Late delayed radiation plexopathy has been reported after irradiation of either the brachial or lumbosacral plexus, although the former is more common.[4] The disorder usually occurs a year or more after RT doses of or exceeding 5,000 cGy. Late delayed brachial plexopathy is characterized by paresthesias and weakness of the hand or arm. Sensory loss, particularly in the fingers and hand, is seen early but the numbness and weakness often progress to a complete plexopathy affecting the entire arm. This disorder is frequently accompanied by lymphedema and palpable induration in the supraclavicular fossa. Radiation-induced plexopathy is usually painless, which distinguishes it from tumor plexopathy, which is typically painful. Myokymia on needle electromyography in the territory of affected nerves is characteristic of radiation damage as opposed to tumor infiltration of the plexus. CT scan or MRI usually reveals a diffuse loss of tissue planes without a mass. Occasionally, radiation damage can produce a marked fibrotic reaction causing a mass of fibrosis that can be distinguished from tumor with FDG-PET. There is no treatment for radiation plexopathy,[102] although painful paresthesias may be relieved by amitriptyline or gabapentin.

Lumbosacral plexopathy causes painless weakness of one or both legs. The disorder often affects the foot, and sensory impairment as well as weakness is present in most cases. Electromyography frequently reveals myokymic discharges, which differentiate the process from tumor recurrence. Radiation-induced lumbosacral plexopathy is often slowly progressive over many years. The pathogenesis is thought to be related to fibrosis causing damage to Schwann cells, rather than stemming from direct damage to the nerves themselves.

Secondary Neurologic Involvement

Radiogenic Tumors

The manner in which the nervous system may be affected secondarily after RT is summarized in Table 28-8.

Radiation-induced tumors, including meningiomas,[103,104] sarcomas,[105,106] and, less frequently, gliomas[107–109] and malignant schwannomas,[110,111] may appear years to decades after irradiation of nervous system tissue; secondary tumors may develop even after low doses of RT.[112] Children who received low-dose scalp RT for tinea capitis had a 9.5-fold increase in the incidence of meningiomas[113] and higher rates of multiple meningiomas and recurrence compared

TABLE 28-8 ■ Secondary Involvement of the Nervous System Following Radiation Therapy

Radiation-Induced Tumors
Meningiomas (atypical, malignant)
Sarcomas (malignant)
Gliomas (malignant)
Schwannomas (malignant)
Vascular Lesions
Stenosis/occlusion of the supraclinoid internal carotid
Moyamoya syndrome
Extracranial stenosis/occlusion
Carotid rupture (rare)
Endocrinopathy
Primary hypothyroidism
Hyperparathyroidism
Hypothalamic pituitary dysfunction
Growth hormone deficiency (most frequent)
Hyperprolactinemia
Cortisol deficiency (rare)
Gonadotropin deficiency (rare)

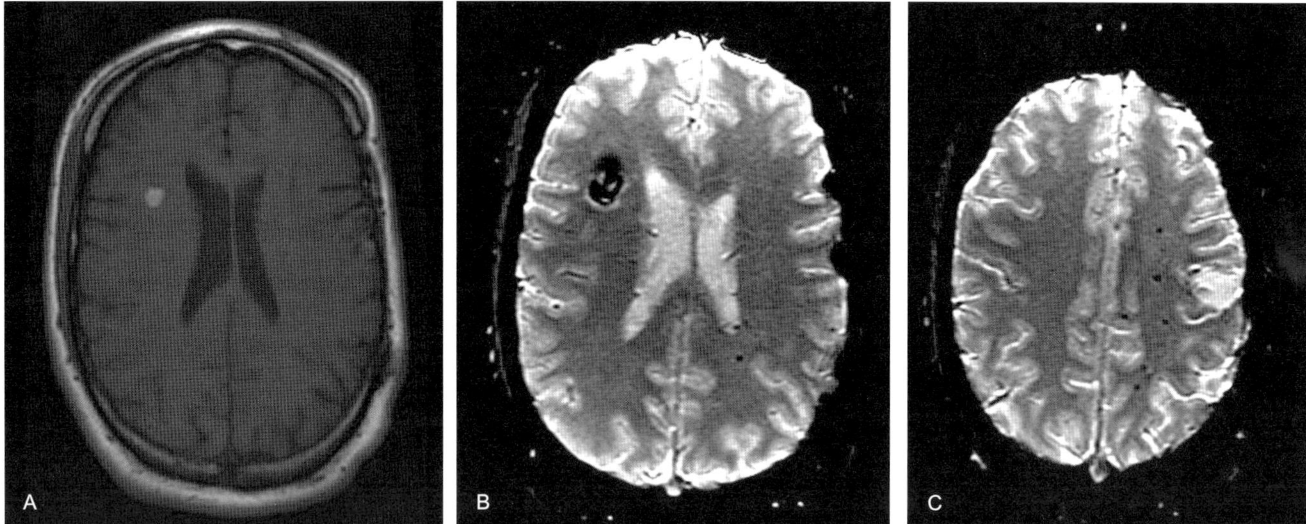

FIGURE 28-3 ■ Radiation-induced cavernomas (images **A-C** are different sequences from the same MRI). **A**, T1-weighted, precontrast MRI 6 years after focal radiation for a left frontal grade 2 astrocytoma showing hemorrhage. **B**, Susceptibility-weighted imaging (SWI) demonstrating a hemorrhagic cavernoma in the right frontal lobe. **C**, SWI demonstrating multiple microbleeds in the left hemisphere.

to non-irradiated control patients.[114] Malignant or atypical nerve sheath tumors may follow irradiation of the brachial, cervical, or lumbar plexuses. Signs and symptoms of radiogenic tumors are no different from tumors that arise without prior radiation therapy, and their surgical treatment is similar. Some patients may be able to tolerate additional RT or chemotherapy if the tumor is malignant and cannot be excised totally.

Vascular Abnormalities

Narrowing of large intracranial or extracranial blood vessels may follow RT by months to years. Patients may develop transient ischemic attacks or cerebral infarcts. Arteriography reveals stenosis or occlusion of the artery within the radiation portal. A particularly vulnerable area is the supraclinoid portion of the internal carotid artery in children who received brain irradiation; this occlusion is sometimes associated with moyamoya syndrome. The pathology of radiation-induced vascular occlusion is similar to severe atherosclerosis,[115] although there may be marked periarterial fibrosis as well. This condition is characterized by arteriopathy restricted to the vessel segment within the RT field without evidence of widespread involvement elsewhere, by the younger age of the affected patients, and by the atypical location of the stenotic carotid segments.[115] If appropriate, carotid stenting can be performed successfully on patients with extracranial vascular disease.

Cavernomas may also develop as a complication of cranial or spinal RT, occurring 1 to 26 years after treatment.[116–118] These lesions may be at higher risk of bleeding compared to cavernomas unassociated with prior radiation therapy (Fig. 28-3).

A few patients have been described with hemorrhage in the spinal cord developing many years after irradiation. Characteristically, 8 to 30 years after RT to the spine, a patient without prior neurologic symptoms suddenly develops back pain and leg weakness. MRI suggests acute or subacute hemorrhage, but no other lesions are found. The patient typically improves, and the symptoms may resolve entirely. A few patients have had recurrent episodes of spinal cord hemorrhage. The pathogenesis is probably related to telangiectatic vascular changes caused by the RT,[119] but anecdotally hemorrhages are often preceded by heavy use of nonsteroidal anti-inflammatory drugs.

REFERENCES

1. Plotkin SR, Wen PY: Neurologic complications of cancer therapy. Neurol Clin 21:279, 2003.
2. Sul JK, Deangelis LM: Neurologic complications of cancer chemotherapy. Semin Oncol 33:324, 2006.
3. Hildebrand J: Neurological complications of cancer chemotherapy. Curr Opin Oncol 18:321, 2006.

4. DeAngelis LM, Posner JB: Neurologic Complications of Cancer. 2nd ed. Oxford University Press, New York, 2009.
5. Schiff D: Neurological side-effects caused by recently approved chemotherapy drugs. Cancer World 13, 2010.
6. Quant EC, Fisher DC, Wen PY: Neurological complications of chemotherapy in lymphoma and leukemia patients. In: Batchelor T, DeAngelis LM (eds): Lymphoma and Leukemia of the Nervous System. Springer, New York, 2012.
7. Lee EQ, Arrillaga-Romany IC, Wen PY: Neurologic complications of cancer drug therapies. Continuum (Minneap Minn) 18:355, 2012.
8. Kannarkat G, Lasher EE, Schiff D: Neurologic complications of chemotherapy agents. Curr Opin Neurol 20:719, 2007.
9. Giglio P, Gilbert MR: Neurologic complications of cancer and its treatment. Curr Oncol Rep 12:50, 2010.
10. Vidarsson B, Mosher DF, Salamat MS, et al: Progressive multifocal leukoencephalopathy after fludarabine therapy for low-grade lymphoproliferative disease. Am J Hematol 70:51, 2002.
11. Shvidel L, Shtalrid M, Bairey O, et al: Conventional dose fludarabine-based regimens are effective but have excessive toxicity in elderly patients with refractory chronic lymphocytic leukemia. Leuk Lymphoma 44:1947, 2003.
12. Khasraw M, Posner JB: Neurological complications of systemic cancer. Lancet Neurol 9:1214, 2010.
13. Haykin ME, Gorman M, van Hoff J, et al: Diffusion-weighted MRI correlates of subacute methotrexate-related neurotoxicity. J Neurooncol 76:153, 2006.
14. Phillips PC, Dhawan V, Strother SC, et al: Reduced cerebral glucose metabolism and increased brain capillary permeability following high-dose methotrexate chemotherapy: a positron emission tomographic study. Ann Neurol 21:59, 1987.
15. Laitt RD, Chambers EJ, Goddard PR, et al: Magnetic resonance imaging and magnetic resonance angiography in long term survivors of acute lymphoblastic leukemia treated with cranial irradiation. Cancer 76:1846, 1995.
16. Cohen MH, Johnson JR, Massie T, et al: Approval summary: nelarabine for the treatment of T-cell lymphoblastic leukemia/lymphoma. Clin Cancer Res 12:5329, 2006.
17. Roecker AM, Stockert A, Kisor DF: Nelarabine in the treatment of refractory T-cell malignancies. Clin Med Insights Oncol 4:133, 2010.
18. Dormann AJ, Grunewald T, Wigginghaus B, et al: Gemcitabine-associated autonomic neuropathy. Lancet 351:644, 1998.
19. Pentsova E, Liu A, Rosenblum M, et al: Gemcitabine induced myositis in patients with pancreatic cancer: case reports and topic review. J Neurooncol 106:15, 2012.
20. Burris 3rd HA, Hurtig J: Radiation recall with anticancer agents. Oncologist 15:1227, 2010.
21. Schiff D, Wen PY, van den Bent MJ: Neurological adverse effects caused by cytotoxic and targeted therapies. Nat Rev Clin Oncol 6:596, 2009.
22. Roche H, Yelle L, Cognetti F, et al: Phase II clinical trial of ixabepilone (BMS-247550), an epothilone B analog, as first-line therapy in patients with metastatic breast cancer previously treated with anthracycline chemotherapy. J Clin Oncol 25:3415, 2007.
23. Perez EA, Lerzo G, Pivot X, et al: Efficacy and safety of ixabepilone (BMS-247550) in a phase II study of patients with advanced breast cancer resistant to an anthracycline, a taxane, and capecitabine. J Clin Oncol 25:3407, 2007.
24. Galsky MD, Small EJ, Oh WK, et al: Multi-institutional randomized phase II trial of the epothilone B analog ixabepilone (BMS-247550) with or without estramustine phosphate in patients with progressive castrate metastatic prostate cancer. J Clin Oncol 23:1439, 2005.
25. Gelmon K, Eisenhauer E, Bryce C, et al: Randomized phase II study of high-dose paclitaxel with or without amifostine in patients with metastatic breast cancer. J Clin Oncol 17:3038, 1999.
26. Freilich RJ, Balmaceda C, Seidman AD, et al: Motor neuropathy due to docetaxel and paclitaxel. Neurology 47:115, 1996.
27. Loprinzi CL, Reeves BN, Dakhil SR, et al: Natural history of paclitaxel-associated acute pain syndrome: prospective cohort study NCCTG N08C1. J Clin Oncol 29:1472, 2011.
28. Lee JJ, Swain SM: Peripheral neuropathy induced by microtubule-stabilizing agents. J Clin Oncol 24:1633, 2006.
29. Mo M, Erdelyi I, Szigeti-Buck K, et al: Prevention of paclitaxel-induced peripheral neuropathy by lithium pretreatment. FASEB J 26:4696, 2012.
30. Naguib M, Xu JJ, Diaz P, et al: Prevention of paclitaxel-induced neuropathy through activation of the central cannabinoid type 2 receptor system. Anesth Analg 114:1104, 2012.
31. Hensley ML, Hagerty KL, Kewalramani T, et al: American Society of Clinical Oncology 2008 clinical practice guideline update: use of chemotherapy and radiation therapy protectants. J Clin Oncol 27:127, 2009.
32. Kaley TJ, Deangelis LM: Therapy of chemotherapy-induced peripheral neuropathy. Br J Haematol 145:3, 2009.
33. Kottschade LA, Sloan JA, Mazurczak MA, et al: The use of vitamin E for the prevention of chemotherapy-induced peripheral neuropathy: results of a randomized phase III clinical trial. Support Care Cancer 19:1769, 2011.
34. Kottschade L, Sloan J, Loprinzi C: Second response to the letter to the editor referencing the manuscript the "Use of vitamin E for the prevention of

chemotherapy-induced peripheral neuropathy: results of a randomized phase III clinical trial". Support Care Cancer 21:3, 2013.
35. Gradishar WJ, Tjulandin S, Davidson N, et al: Phase III trial of nanoparticle albumin-bound paclitaxel compared with polyethylated castor oil-based paclitaxel in women with breast cancer. J Clin Oncol 23:7794, 2005.
36. Bilusic M, Dahut WL: Cabazitaxel: a new drug for metastatic prostate cancer. Asian J Androl 13:185, 2011.
37. de Bono JS, Oudard S, Ozguroglu M, et al: Prednisone plus cabazitaxel or mitoxantrone for metastatic castration-resistant prostate cancer progressing after docetaxel treatment: a randomised open-label trial. Lancet 376:1147, 2010.
38. Nicolao P, Giometto B: Neurological toxicity of ifosfamide. Oncology 65(suppl 2):11, 2003.
39. Kilickap S, Cakar M, Onal IK, et al: Nonconvulsive status epilepticus due to ifosfamide. Ann Pharmacother 40:332, 2006.
40. Dietrich J, Wen PY: Neurologic complications of chemotherapy. In: Schiff D, Kesari S, Wen PY (eds): Cancer Neurology in Clinical Practice. Humana Press, Totowa, NJ, 2008.
41. Yung WK, Prados MD, Yaya-Tur R, et al: Multicenter phase II trial of temozolomide in patients with anaplastic astrocytoma or anaplastic oligoastrocytoma at first relapse. Temodal Brain Tumor Group. J Clin Oncol 17:2762, 1999.
42. Albers JW, Chaudhry V, Cavaletti G, et al: Interventions for preventing neuropathy caused by cisplatin and related compounds. Cochrane Database Syst Rev:CD005228, 2011.
43. Wolf S, Barton D, Kottschade L, et al: Chemotherapy-induced peripheral neuropathy: prevention and treatment strategies. Eur J Cancer 44:1507, 2008.
44. Rybak LP: Mechanisms of cisplatin ototoxicity and progress in otoprotection. Curr Opin Otolaryngol Head Neck Surg 15:364, 2007.
45. Kalkanis JG, Whitworth C, Rybak LP: Vitamin E reduces cisplatin ototoxicity. Laryngoscope 114:538, 2004.
46. Dickey DT, Wu YJ, Muldoon LL, et al: Protection against cisplatin-induced toxicities by *N*-acetylcysteine and sodium thiosulfate as assessed at the molecular, cellular, and in vivo levels. J Pharmacol Exp Ther 314:1052, 2005.
47. van As JW, van den Berg H, van Dalen EC: Medical interventions for the prevention of platinum-induced hearing loss in children with cancer. Cochrane Database Syst Rev 5:CD009219, 2012.
48. Pasetto LM, D'Andrea MR, Rossi E, et al: Oxaliplatin-related neurotoxicity: how and why? Crit Rev Oncol Hematol 59:159, 2006.
49. Taieb S, Trillet-Lenoir V, Rambaud L, et al: Lhermitte sign and urinary retention: atypical presentation of oxaliplatin neurotoxicity in four patients. Cancer 94:2434, 2002.
50. Heinzlef O, Lotz JP, Roullet E: Severe neuropathy after high dose carboplatin in three patients receiving multidrug chemotherapy. J Neurol Neurosurg Psychiatry 64:667, 1998.
51. Verhoef C, de Wilt JH, Verheul HM: Angiogenesis inhibitors: perspectives for medical, surgical and radiation oncology. Curr Pharm Des 12:2623, 2006.
52. Kreisl TN, Kim L, Moore K, et al: Phase II trial of single-agent bevacizumab followed by bevacizumab plus irinotecan at tumor progression in recurrent glioblastoma. J Clin Oncol 27:740, 2009.
53. Friedman HS, Prados MD, Wen PY, et al: Bevacizumab alone and in combination with irinotecan in recurrent glioblastoma. J Clin Oncol 27:4733, 2009.
54. Glusker P, Recht L, Lane B: Reversible posterior leukoencephalopathy syndrome and bevacizumab. N Engl J Med 354:980, 2006.
55. Ozcan C, Wong SJ, Hari P: Reversible posterior leukoencephalopathy syndrome and bevacizumab. N Engl J Med 354:981, 2006.
56. Allen JA, Adlakha A, Bergethon PR: Reversible posterior leukoencephalopathy syndrome after bevacizumab/FOLFIRI regimen for metastatic colon cancer. Arch Neurol 63:1475, 2006.
57. Seet RC, Rabinstein AA: Clinical features and outcomes of posterior reversible encephalopathy syndrome following bevacizumab treatment. QJM 105:69, 2012.
58. Lazarus M, Amundson S, Belani R: An Association between bevacizumab and recurrent posterior reversible encephalopathy syndrome in a patient presenting with deep vein thrombosis: a case report and review of the literature. Case Rep Oncol Med 2012:819546, 2012.
59. Sherman JH, Aregawi DG, Lai A, et al: Optic neuropathy in patients with glioblastoma receiving bevacizumab. Neurology 73:1924, 2009.
60. Hersh EM, O'Day SJ, Powderly J, et al: A phase II multicenter study of ipilimumab with or without dacarbazine in chemotherapy-naive patients with advanced melanoma. Invest New Drugs 29:489, 2011.
61. Andrews S, Holden R: Characteristics and management of immune related adverse effects associated with ipilimumab, a new immunotherapy for metastatic melanoma. Cancer Manag Res 4:299, 2012.
62. Fellner C: Ipilimumab (Yervoy) prolongs survival in advanced melanoma: serious side effects and a hefty price tag may limit its use. P&T 37:503, 2012.
63. Maloney DG, Grillo-Lopez AJ, White CA, et al: IDEC-C2B8 (rituximab) anti-CD20 monoclonal antibody therapy in patients with relapsed low-grade non-Hodgkin's lymphoma. Blood 90:2188, 1997.
64. Carson KR, Evens AM, Richey EA, et al: Progressive multifocal leukoencephalopathy after rituximab therapy in HIV-negative patients: a report of 57 cases from the Research on Adverse Drug Events and Reports project. Blood 113:4834, 2009.

65. Richardson PG, Briemberg H, Jagannath S, et al: Frequency, characteristics, and reversibility of peripheral neuropathy during treatment of advanced multiple myeloma with bortezomib. J Clin Oncol 24:3113, 2006.
66. Siegel DS, Martin T, Wang M, et al: A phase 2 study of single-agent carfilzomib (PX-171-003-A1) in patients with relapsed and refractory multiple myeloma. Blood 120:2817, 2012.
67. Chen X, Schwartz GK, DeAngelis LM, et al: Dropped head syndrome: report of three cases during treatment with a MEK inhibitor. Neurology 79:1929, 2012.
68. Freemantle SJ, Spinella MJ, Dmitrovsky E: Retinoids in cancer therapy and chemoprevention: promise meets resistance. Oncogene 22:7305, 2003.
69. Smith MA, Adamson PC, Balis FM, et al: Phase I and pharmacokinetic evaluation of all-*trans*-retinoic acid in pediatric patients with cancer. J Clin Oncol 10:1666, 1992.
70. Testi AM, Biondi A, Lo Coco F, et al: GIMEMA-AIEOPAIDA protocol for the treatment of newly diagnosed acute promyelocytic leukemia (APL) in children. Blood 106:447, 2005.
71. Labrador J, Puig N, Ortin A, et al: Multiple cranial neuropathy and intracranial hypertension associated with all–*trans* retinoic acid treatment in a young adult patient with acute promyelocytic leukemia. Int J Hematol 96:383, 2012.
72. Hull PR, D'Arcy C: Acne, depression, and suicide. Dermatol Clin 23:665, 2005.
73. Glantz MJ, Jaeckle KA, Chamberlain MC, et al: A randomized controlled trial comparing intrathecal sustained-release cytarabine (DepoCyt) to intrathecal methotrexate in patients with neoplastic meningitis from solid tumors. Clin Cancer Res 5:3394, 1999.
74. Gammon DC, Bhatt MS, Tran L, et al: Intrathecal topotecan in adult patients with neoplastic meningitis. Am J Health Syst Pharm 63:2083, 2006.
75. Groves MD, Glantz MJ, Chamberlain MC, et al: A multicenter phase II trial of intrathecal topotecan in patients with meningeal malignancies. Neuro Oncol 10:208, 2008.
76. Antonini G, Cox MC, Montefusco E, et al: Intrathecal anti-CD20 antibody: an effective and safe treatment for leptomeningeal lymphoma. J Neurooncol 81:197, 2007.
77. Schulz H, Pels H, Schmidt-Wolf I, et al: Intraventricular treatment of relapsed central nervous system lymphoma with the anti-CD20 antibody rituximab. Haematologica 89:753, 2004.
78. Villela L, Garcia M, Caballero R, et al: Rapid complete response using intrathecal rituximab in a patient with leptomeningeal lymphomatosis due to mantle cell lymphoma. Anticancer Drugs 19:917, 2008.
79. Rubenstein JL, Fridlyand J, Abrey L, et al: Phase I study of intraventricular administration of rituximab in patients with recurrent CNS and intraocular lymphoma. J Clin Oncol 25:1350, 2007.
80. Chamberlain MC, Johnston SK, Van Horn A, et al: Recurrent lymphomatous meningitis treated with intra-CSF rituximab and liposomal ara-C. J Neurooncol 91:271, 2009.
81. Rogers LR: Neurologic complications of radiation. Continuum (Minneap Minn) 18:343, 2012.
82. Fink J, Born D, Chamberlain MC: Radiation necrosis: relevance with respect to treatment of primary and secondary brain tumors. Curr Neurol Neurosci Rep 12:276, 2012.
83. Lam TC, Wong FC, Leung TW, et al: Clinical outcomes of 174 nasopharyngeal carcinoma patients with radiation-induced temporal lobe necrosis. Int J Radiat Oncol Biol Phys 82:e57, 2012.
84. Shah R, Vattoth S, Jacob R, et al: Radiation necrosis in the brain: imaging features and differentiation from tumor recurrence. Radiographics 32:1343, 2012.
85. Larsen VA, Simonsen HJ, Law I, et al: Evaluation of dynamic contrast-enhanced T1-weighted perfusion MRI in the differentiation of tumor recurrence from radiation necrosis. Neuroradiology 55:361, 2013.
86. Hollingworth W, Medina LS, Lenkinski RE, et al: A systematic literature review of magnetic resonance spectroscopy for the characterization of brain tumors. AJNR Am J Neuroradiol 27:1404, 2006.
87. Wang Y, Pan L, Sheng X, et al: Reversal of cerebral radiation necrosis with bevacizumab treatment in 17 Chinese patients. Eur J Med Res 17:25, 2012.
88. Kerklaan JP, Lycklama á Nijeholt GJ, Wiggenraad RG, et al: SMART syndrome: a late reversible complication after radiation therapy for brain tumours. J Neurol 258:1098, 2011.
89. Farid K, Meissner WG, Samier-Foubert A, et al: Normal cerebrovascular reactivity in stroke-like migraine attacks after radiation therapy syndrome. Clin Nucl Med 35:583, 2010.
90. Pavlovsky S, Fisman N, Arizaga R, et al: Neuropsychological study in patients with ALL. Two different CNS prevention therapies–cranial irradiation plus IT methotrexate vs. IT methotrexate alone. Am J Pediatr Hematol Oncol 5:79, 1983.
91. Dorfman LJ, Donaldson SS, Gupta PR, et al: Electrophysiologic evidence of subclinical injury to the posterior columns of the human spinal cord after therapeutic radiation. Cancer 50:2815, 1982.
92. Lecky BR, Murray NM, Berry RJ: Transient radiation myelopathy: spinal somatosensory evoked responses following incidental cord exposure during radiotherapy. J Neurol Neurosurg Psychiatry 43:747, 1980.
93. Behin A, Delattre JY: Complications of radiation therapy on the brain and spinal cord. Semin Neurol 24:405, 2004.
94. Mahta A, Borys E, Kanakamedala MR, et al: Radiation induced myelopathy in a patient with tongue cancer: a case report. Acta Oncol 51:409, 2012.
95. Glantz MJ, Burger PC, Friedman AH, et al: Treatment of radiation-induced nervous system injury with heparin and warfarin. Neurology 44:2020, 1994.

96. Feldmeier JJ, Hampson NB: A systematic review of the literature reporting the application of hyperbaric oxygen prevention and treatment of delayed radiation injuries: an evidence based approach. Undersea Hyperb Med 29:4, 2002.
97. Grunewald RA, Chroni E, Panayiotopoulos CP, et al: Late onset radiation-induced motor neuron syndrome. J Neurol Neurosurg Psychiatry 55:741, 1992.
98. Tallaksen CM, Jetne V, Fossa S: Postradiation lower motor neuron syndrome–a case report and brief literature review. Acta Oncol 36:345, 1997.
99. Rowin J, Cheng G, Lewis SL, et al: Late appearance of dropped head syndrome after radiotherapy for Hodgkin's disease. Muscle Nerve 34:666, 2006.
100. Rong X, Tang Y, Chen M, et al: Radiation-induced cranial neuropathy in patients with nasopharyngeal carcinoma. A follow-up study. Strahlenther Onkol 188:282, 2012.
101. Shin HY, Park HJ, Choi YC, et al: Clinical and electromyographic features of radiation-induced lower cranial neuropathy. Clin Neurophysiol 124:598, 2013.
102. Delanian S, Lefaix JL, Pradat PF: Radiation-induced neuropathy in cancer survivors. Radiother Oncol 105:273, 2012.
103. Harrison MJ, Wolfe DE, Lau TS, et al: Radiation-induced meningiomas: experience at the Mount Sinai Hospital and review of the literature. J Neurosurg 75:564, 1991.
104. Oikonomou A, Birbilis T, Daskalogiannakis G, et al: Meningioma of the conus medullaris mimicking neurofibroma–possibly radiation induced. Spine J 11:e11, 2011.
105. Sanno N, Hayashi S, Shimura T, et al: Intracranial osteosarcoma after radiosurgery–case report. Neurol Med Chir (Tokyo) 44:29, 2004.
106. Carlson ML, Babovic-Vuksanovic D, Messiaen L, et al: Radiation-induced rhabdomyosarcoma of the brainstem in a patient with neurofibromatosis type 2. J Neurosurg 112:81, 2010.
107. Salvati M, Frati A, Russo N, et al: Radiation-induced gliomas: report of 10 cases and review of the literature. Surg Neurol 60:60, 2003.
108. Balasubramaniam A, Shannon P, Hodaie M, et al: Glioblastoma multiforme after stereotactic radiotherapy for acoustic neuroma: case report and review of the literature. Neuro Oncol 9:447, 2007.
109. Abedalthagafi M, Bakhshwin A: Radiation-induced glioma following CyberKnife® treatment of metastatic renal cell carcinoma: a case report. J Med Case Rep 6:271, 2012.
110. Baser ME, Evans DG, Jackler RK, et al: Neurofibromatosis 2, radiosurgery and malignant nervous system tumours. Br J Cancer 82:998, 2000.
111. Shin M, Ueki K, Kurita H, et al: Malignant transformation of a vestibular schwannoma after gamma knife radiosurgery. Lancet 360:309, 2002.
112. Loeffler JS, Niemierko A, Chapman PH: Second tumors after radiosurgery: tip of the iceberg or a bump in the road? Neurosurgery 52:1436, 2003.
113. Ron E, Modan B, Boice Jr JD, et al: Tumors of the brain and nervous system after radiotherapy in childhood. N Engl J Med 319:1033, 1988.
114. Sadetzki S, Flint-Richter P, Ben-Tal T, et al: Radiation-induced meningioma: a descriptive study of 253 cases. J Neurosurg 97:1078, 2002.
115. O'Connor MM, Mayberg MR: Effects of radiation on cerebral vasculature: a review. Neurosurgery 46:138, 2000.
116. Jain R, Robertson PL, Gandhi D, et al: Radiation-induced cavernomas of the brain. AJNR Am J Neuroradiol 26:1158, 2005.
117. Kamide T, Nakada M, Hayashi Y, et al: Radiation-induced cerebellar high-grade glioma accompanied by meningioma and cavernoma 29 years after the treatment of medulloblastoma: a case report. J Neurooncol 100:299, 2010.
118. Paramanathan N, Ooi KG, Reeves D, et al: Synchronous radiation-induced orbital meningioma and multiple cavernomas. Clin Experiment Ophthalmol 38:414, 2010.
119. Allen JC, Miller DC, Budzilovich GN, et al: Brain and spinal cord hemorrhage in long-term survivors of malignant pediatric brain tumors: a possible late effect of therapy. Neurology 41:148, 1991.

SECTION

IX

Genitourinary System and Pregnancy

CHAPTER

29

Lower Urinary Tract Dysfunction and the Nervous System

AMIT BATLA ■ JALESH N. PANICKER

Lower urinary tract dysfunction is common in patients with neurologic disease. The neurogenic bladder can result from lesions affecting any part of the nervous system. Symptoms are often bothersome and may have a significant impact on quality of life. Some patients may also be at risk of developing changes in the upper urinary tract and even renal impairment.

NEUROLOGIC CONTROL OF THE BLADDER

The essential function of the lower urinary tract (bladder and urethra) is storage of urine and its elimination at appropriate times. This ultimately depends on a local spinal reflex arc which is regulated by supraspinal input to preserve continence until appropriate.

Neurologic control of the key bladder functions of storage and voiding is accomplished by a neural network involving regions of the cortex, brainstem, and spinal cord. The peripheral innervation of the detrusor and sphincter is vital in the execution of this central control. Understanding of the neurologic control of the bladder was derived initially from animal studies, and then refined using

Aminoff's Neurology and General Medicine, Fifth Edition.

functional imaging studies. Experiments on decerebrate cats in the 1920s led to the understanding that the mid-pons played an integral role in micturition.[1] The same region was later stimulated electrically in cats to produce detrusor contractions.[2–4] Subsequent work demonstrated that stimulation of the medial region of the dorsomedial pontine tegmentum led to relaxation of urethral pressure, silence of the pelvic floor electromyogram, and an increase of detrusor pressures, so that this area became known as the pontine micturition center.[5–8] Later studies established functional continuity of the intermediolateral cell column in the sacral spinal cord to this region.

Brain Centers

The development of functional imaging modalities such as positron emission tomography (PET) and functional magnetic resonance imaging (MRI) has allowed further understanding of the central control of micturition.[9,10] Activation occurs in the region of the medioposterior pons during voiding, and in the region of the ventrolateral pontine tegmentum in subjects unable to void in the scanner.[9,10] In the cortex, PET studies have suggested that the right inferior frontal gyrus and the right anterior cingulate gyrus are activated during voiding along with several other regions including the cerebellum, hypothalamus, thalamus, subthalamic nucleus, and the periaqueductal gray.[11,12]

Innervation of the Lower Urinary Tract

The bladder is one of the few visceral organs with voluntary control; it has innervation from both the autonomic and somatic systems (Fig. 29-1). Parasympathetic fibers arise from neurons in the S2 to S4 segments, activating muscarinic receptors of the detrusor muscle. Sympathetic fibers from the thoracolumbar segments (T11 to L1) pass through the hypogastric nerve and pelvic plexus and activate the β3 receptors of the detrusor muscle and α-adrenergic receptors of the internal urethral sphincter and bladder neck. Somatic fibers pass through the pudendal nerve and activate nicotinic receptors of the external urethral (and anal) sphincter. Sensations of bladder fullness are conveyed to the spinal cord through all these sets of nerves.

Storage Phase

The bladder is in the storage phase for 98 percent of the time. During this phase, passive distension of the bladder results in low-level afferent firing. This firing leads to reflex inhibition of parasympathetic efferents, and activation of the sympathetic outflow innervating the internal urethral sphincter and pudendal outflow innervating the external urethral sphincter; these responses promote continence. Ascending afferent signals relay at the periaqueductal gray before reaching cortical centers. Signals from the pontine micturition center are essentially inhibitory and promote storage.

Voiding Phase

When the bladder is perceived to be full and it is a socially appropriate time and place to void, facilitatory signals from the pontine micturition center result in parasympathetically mediated contractions of the detrusor muscle and inhibition of the sympathetic and pudendal outflow (leading to sphincter relaxation).

Central Mediation of Voiding

The decision to void is based on a combination of factors, including emotional state, an appreciation of the social environment, and sensory signals arising from the bladder. Knowledge of the extent to which one's bladder content is comfortable and "safe" is central in this process. Thus, voluntary control of the bladder and the urethra has two important aspects: registration of bladder filling sensations and manipulation of the firing of the voiding reflex, both of which are dependent on the periaqueductal gray.[13]

Neurochemistry of Urothelium and Bladder Pharmacology

The urothelium (the bladder epithelium) has specialized sensory and signaling properties that allow the bladder to respond to chemical and mechanical stimuli and to engage in reciprocal chemical communication with nerves in the bladder wall.[14] The urothelium expresses nicotinic, muscarinic, tachykinin, adrenergic, bradykinin, and transient-receptor-potential vanilloid receptors.[15] It has the ability to release chemical mediators such as adenosine triphosphate (ATP), acetylcholine, and nitric

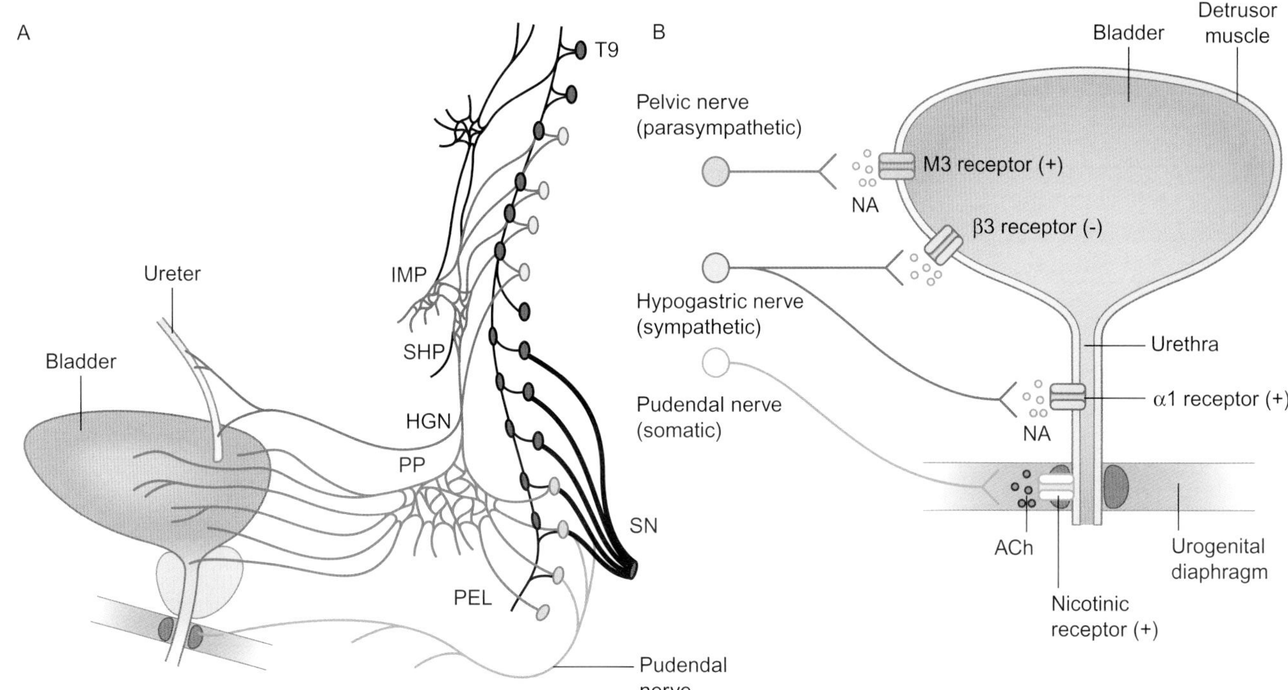

FIGURE 29-1 ■ Innervation of the lower urinary tract **A**, Sympathetic fibers (shown in blue) originate in the T11–L2 segments in the spinal cord and run through the inferior mesenteric ganglia (inferior mesenteric plexus, IMP) and the hypogastric nerve (HGN) or through the paravertebral chain to enter the pelvic nerves at the base of the bladder and the urethra. Parasympathetic preganglionic fibers (shown in green) arise from the S2–S4 spinal segments and travel in sacral roots and pelvic nerves (PEL) to ganglia in the pelvic plexus (PP) and in the bladder wall, which then supply parasympathetic innervation to the bladder. Somatic motor nerves (shown in yellow) that supply the striated muscles of the external urethral sphincter arise from S2–S4 motor neurons and pass through the pudendal nerves. SHP, superior hypogastric plexus; SN, sciatic nerve; T9, ninth thoracic root **B**, Efferent pathways and neurotransmitter mechanisms that regulate the lower urinary tract. Parasympathetic postganglionic axons in the pelvic nerve release acetylcholine (ACh), which produces a bladder contraction by stimulating M3 muscarinic receptors in the bladder smooth muscle. Sympathetic postganglionic neurons release norepinephrine (NA), which activates β3 adrenergic receptors to relax bladder smooth muscle and activates β1 adrenergic receptors to contract urethral smooth muscle. Somatic axons in the pudendal nerve also release ACh, which produces a contraction of the external sphincter striated muscle by activating nicotinic cholinergic receptors. (From Fowler CJ, Griffiths D, de Groat WC: The neural control of micturition. Nat Rev Neurosci 9:453, 2008, with permission.)

oxide, which can regulate the activity of adjacent nerves and trigger local vascular changes or reflex bladder contractions.

The presence of muscarinic and nicotinic receptors in the urothelium has focused attention on the role of acetylcholine as a chemical mediator of neural–urothelial interactions.[16] Acetylcholine is released from the urothelium in response to chemical or mechanical stimuli. Thus, the clinical effect of antimuscarinic agents in overactive bladder conditions might not only lead to a motor response, but also influence the afferent pathway.

Various neurotransmitters have been implicated in the central control of the lower urinary tract. Putative excitatory transmitters include glutamate, tachykinins, pituitary-adenylate-cyclase-activating polypeptide, nitric oxide, and ATP.[17] Glutamate seems to be the essential transmitter in spinal and supraspinal reflex pathways that control the bladder and the external urethral sphincter.[18] Inhibitory amino acids (γ-aminobutyric acid and glycine) and opioid peptides (enkephalins) exert a tonic inhibitory control in the pontine micturition center and regulate bladder capacity.[19] These substances also have inhibitory actions in the spinal cord. Drugs used in management of the bladder symptoms have mainly developed in accordance with this neurochemistry. Although antimuscarinics are the mainstay of therapy, other agents have been developed that influence the vanilloid, cannabinoid, and β3 receptors, which are discussed further in the section on treatment.

NEUROGENIC BLADDER DYSFUNCTION

Lower urinary tract symptoms usually consist of problems with storage or problems with voiding (Table 29-1). The pattern of bladder dysfunction following neurologic disease depends to a large extent upon the level of the lesion.[20] The storage function of the bladder is affected following suprapontine or lesions below the pons but above the sacral spinal cord (Table 29-2) resulting in involuntary, spontaneous, or induced contractions of the detrusor muscle (detrusor overactivity), which can be identified during the filling phase of urodynamic testing. The voiding function can be affected by infrapontine lesions. Following spinal cord damage interrupting the connections between sacral and pontine centres, detrusor-sphincter dyssynergia may also occur and results in incomplete bladder emptying and abnormally high bladder pressures. With lesions of the conus medullaris, cauda equina, or peripheral nerves, voiding dysfunction predominates and results in poor detrusor contraction and nonrelaxing urethral sphincters.

TABLE 29-1 ■ Storage and Voiding Symptoms

Storage symptoms	Voiding symptoms
Urgency	Hesitancy
Daytime frequency	Poor flow
Nocturia	Intermittent flow
	Straining
	Incomplete voiding

Cerebral Lesions

Disorders affecting the cortex or subcortical white matter often result in lower urinary tract symptoms. This is most commonly seen with lesions of the anteromedial frontal lobe including the anterior part of the cingulate gyrus.[21] The clinical picture is one of severe urgency and frequency of micturition with urge incontinence; the patient is usually socially aware and embarrassed by the incontinence. Urinary retention also has been described but is less common; a small number of patients have been described with urinary retention that resolved with treatment of the frontal lobe disorder.[8]

Urinary incontinence may follow stroke, often with more anteriorly placed infarcts.[22] It has not been possible to demonstrate a correlation between any specific lesion site and the urodynamic findings. The most common cystometric finding is that of detrusor overactivity, and voiding is usually coordinated. Patients with hemorrhagic stroke are more likely to have detrusor underactivity.[23] Urinary incontinence at 7 days after stroke is predictive of poor survival, disability, and institutionalization independent of the patient's level of consciousness.

Small-vessel disease of the white matter (leukoaraiosis) has been associated with urgency incontinence as well as falls and cognitive disturbance, especially when it involves the frontal lobes. This may be an important cause of incontinence in functionally independent elderly persons.[24]

TABLE 29-2 ■ Results of the Diagnostic Evaluation for Patients with Suspected Neurogenic Bladder Dysfunction

	Suprapontine lesion e.g., stroke, Parkinson disease	Infrapontine-suprasacral lesion e.g., spinal cord injury, multiple sclerosis	Infrasacral lesion e.g., conus medullaris tumor, cauda equina syndrome, peripheral neuropathy
History/bladder diary	Urgency, frequency, urgency incontinence	Urgency, frequency, urgency incontinence, hesitancy, interrupted stream	Hesitancy, interrupted stream
Postvoid residual urine	PVR <100 ml	±Elevated PVR	PVR >100 ml
Uroflowmetry	Normal flow	Interrupted flow	Poor/absent flow
Urodynamics	Detrusor overactivity	Detrusor overactivity Detrusor-sphincter dyssynergia	Detrusor underactivity, sphincter insufficiency

PVR, postvoid residual urine. (From Panicker JN, Fowler CJ: The bare essentials: uro-neurology. Pract Neurol 10:178, 2010 with permission.)

A much less common cause of frontal involvement with urinary incontinence is normal pressure hydrocephalus, where incontinence is a cardinal feature. Improvement in urodynamic function has been demonstrated within hours of lumbar puncture or shunting procedures.

The cause of urinary incontinence in patients with dementia is probably multifactorial, but frontal lobe degeneration probably plays a role. In a study of patients with progressive cognitive decline, incontinence was observed to not occur until more advanced stages of Alzheimer disease but occurred earlier in the course of dementia with Lewy bodies.[25]

Basal Ganglia Lesions

Parkinson Disease

Lower urinary tract symptoms are reported in 38 to 71 percent of patients with Parkinson disease (PD).[26,27] Storage symptoms are the most common problem, seen in more than 60 percent of these patients, with considerable impact on their quality of life.[28–30] Nocturia is the most common symptom followed by urinary urgency; these are among the most common nonmotor symptoms of PD. Urodynamic studies typically show detrusor overactivity probably due to neuronal loss in the substantia nigra disinhibiting the normal effect of the basal ganglia on the micturition reflex.[31] Dopamine receptor stimulation through D1 receptors provides the main inhibitory influence on the micturition reflex normally, although dopaminergic stimulation in PD has little apparent impact.[32]

Overactive bladder is common in patients with PD, and many patients have nocturnal polyuria. Patients may also report voiding difficulties and bradykinesia of the pelvic floor muscles resulting in pseudo-dyssynergia. Lower urinary tract symptoms may be multifactorial and other non-neurogenic factors such as prostatic enlargement may contribute. Other medical comorbidities such as diabetes mellitus, congestive cardiac failure, medications such as diuretics, cerebrovascular disease, and cervical spondylosis may also play a role.[33] Sleep disturbances and disturbed circadian rhythm, which are common in PD, may be closely associated with nocturia.[34–36]

Multiple System Atrophy

Patients with parkinsonism and early and prominent urogenital complaints may have multiple system atrophy. Around 40 percent of these patients first present with lower urinary tract symptoms and 97 percent will experience these symptoms during the disease course.[37–40] Presentations include daytime frequency (about 45%), nocturnal frequency (nearly 70%), urinary urgency (60%), and urge incontinence (66 to 75%).[41]

Bladder symptoms occur much earlier and are more disabling in multiple system atrophy than PD. Although urgency and frequency occur in both conditions, patients with multiple system atrophy are more likely than those with PD to have a high (>100 ml) postvoid residual volume, detrusor-sphincter dyssynergia, an open bladder neck at the start of bladder filling on videocystometrogram, and evidence of neurogenic changes in the electromyography of the anal sphincter.[42–47]

Brainstem Lesions

Although the pontine micturition center is essential for micturition, the rarity of brainstem lesions in clinical practice makes it less common to encounter bladder dysfunction secondary to brainstem lesions. In cases with brainstem tumors or other mass lesions, the clinical picture is usually dominated by other long-tract and ocular features. Due to the proximity of the pontine micturition center to the medial longitudinal fasciculus, internuclear ophthalmoplegia is a common accompanying finding. Voiding difficulty is a rare but well-recognized symptom of a posterior fossa tumor.[48] In an analysis of urinary symptoms in 39 patients with brainstem stroke, lesions that resulted in micturition disturbance usually were situated dorsally.[49] Brainstem involvement in multiple sclerosis is discussed separately.

Spinal Cord Lesions

The spinobulbar reflex arc is crucial in the control of bladder function in health. Following spinal cord lesions, interruption of this reflex, along with loss of supraspinal control, results in a local spinal reflex that drives bladder contractions. The localization of lesions can be guided by the type of bladder dysfunction observed.

The hyperreflexic neurogenic (spastic) bladder occurs following lesions that interrupt the connections between the pontine micturition center and sacral cord micturition centers. Commonly these myelopathic conditions cause quadriplegia or paraplegia. Clinically, patients present with detrusor contraction during bladder filling leading to detrusor overactivity, characterized by urinary frequency, urgency, urge incontinence, and inability to initiate micturition voluntarily. Bladder capacity is reduced, although residual urine may be increased. On examination, the bulbocavernosus and anal reflexes are preserved.

Autonomous neurogenic bladder (detrusor areflexia) may occur with complete lesions below the T12 segment that involve the conus medullaris and cauda equina. Common pathologies include sacral myelomeningoceles and tumors of the conus medullaris and cauda equina. This type of neurogenic bladder also occurs during the initial shock phase following spinal cord injury; gradually over the course of weeks new reflexes emerge to drive bladder emptying and cause detrusor contractions in response to low filling volumes. Clinically there is urinary retention since the tone of the detrusor muscle is abolished and there is no awareness of fullness. Overflow incontinence and increased residual urine develop later. On examination, associated saddle anesthesia with absence of the bulbocavernosus and superficial anal reflexes are common. Anal sphincter control is often affected similarly.

Motor paralytic bladder results from lesions involving the efferent motor fibers to the detrusor or the detrusor motor neurons in the sacral spinal cord. Common pathologies include lumbar spinal stenosis, lumbosacral meningomyelocele, or following abdominoperineal resection or radical hysterectomy. Clinically painful urinary retention or impaired bladder emptying is the presenting feature, and residual urine is markedly increased. The bulbocavernosus and superficial anal reflexes are usually absent, but sacral and bladder sensation are preserved.

Sensory paralytic bladder is caused by impairment of the afferent pathways innervating the bladder or by dysfunction of the posterior columns or lateral spinothalamic tract in the spinal cord. Classically, this condition has been described in tabes dorsalis, syringomyelia, and diabetes mellitus. Voluntary initiation of micturition may be retained. On examination, the bulbocavernosus and superficial anal reflexes are variably absent, decreased, or present.

This classification system does not often reflect clinical practice and deviations from these descriptions often exist. Spinal shock is quite variable in presentation, and the neurophysiology of recovery from spinal shock has been characterized mainly in cats where, following injury, C fibers emerge as the major afferents, forming a spinal segmental reflex that results in automatic voiding. The abnormally overactive, small-capacity bladder that characterizes spinal cord disease causes patients to experience urinary urgency and frequency; however, patients with complete transection of the cord may not complain of urgency. If detrusor overactivity is severe, incontinence is highly likely.

Bladder Dysfunction in Multiple Sclerosis

Lower urinary tract dysfunction can be one of the main features of multiple sclerosis.[50] Urinary incontinence impacts quality of life for patients and is associated with considerable costs.[50,51] Up to 75 percent of patients with multiple sclerosis have lower urinary tract symptoms, and overactive bladder and dyssynergia are the commonest presentations.[52] Urinary tract infections are common; infection is found in 30 percent of those reporting urinary symptoms.[53] The incidence of lower urinary tract symptoms increases with lower extremity weakness from corticospinal tract dysfunction (usually from spinal cord involvement) and longer disease duration.[54] As the neurologic condition progresses, lower urinary tract dysfunction may become more difficult to treat.[55]

The most common urinary symptom in these patients is urgency, and detrusor overactivity is often seen on urodynamic testing. Patients sometimes initially report hesitancy, but those with more severe symptoms may be unable to initiate micturition voluntarily, emptying their bladders only through involuntary overactive contractions followed by interrupted urinary flow. Evidence of incomplete emptying may come from the need to pass urine again within 5 to 10 minutes (double voiding).

Multiple sclerosis is a dynamic disease, and symptoms may appear or worsen during a relapse and then remit or improve with neurologic remissions. Neurologic symptoms may deteriorate acutely when the patient has an infection, including that of the urinary tract. As the disease progresses, recurrent infections may result in the accumulation of deficits.[56]

Disturbances of Peripheral Innervation

Peripheral neuropathies may result in autonomic symptoms including bladder dysfunction.

Diabetic Neuropathy

Lower urinary tract symptoms are common, although often asymptomatic, in patients with diabetes. Bladder dysfunction is generally accompanied by other symptoms and signs of generalized neuropathy. The onset of the bladder dysfunction is insidious, with progressive loss of bladder sensation and impairment of bladder emptying over years, finally leading to chronic low-pressure urinary retention.[57] Urodynamic studies demonstrate impaired detrusor contractility, reduced urine flow, increased postmicturition residual volume, and reduced bladder sensation. It seems likely that both afferent and efferent fibers of the local spinal reflex arc are involved, causing reduced awareness of bladder filling and decreased contractility.

Amyloid Neuropathy

Lower urinary tract symptoms generally appear early in the course of amyloid neuropathy and are present in 50 percent of patients within the first 3 years of the disease. Patients most often complain of difficulty in bladder emptying and incontinence, although bladder dysfunction may be asymptomatic.[58] Urodynamic studies have demonstrated reduced bladder sensations, underactive detrusor, poor urinary flow, and inappropriate opening of the bladder neck. Bladder wall thickening may be seen on ultrasound. Up to 10 percent of patients with familial amyloid neuropathy type I may proceed to end-stage renal disease, often reporting polyuria as an early symptom.[59] These patients may be treated with liver transplantation, and the presence of postoperative urinary incontinence is associated with a higher post-transplant mortality.[60]

Immune-Mediated Neuropathies

Traditionally immune-mediated neuropathies have not been associated with bladder dysfunction. However, many patients with Guillain–Barré syndrome (as high as 25 percent) report bladder symptoms; these are more common with more severe neuropathies, appearing after limb weakness is established. Both detrusor areflexia and bladder overactivity have been described. Long-term complications are unusual and recovery of lower urinary tract symptoms follows the course of the neuropathy.

Autoimmune Autonomic Ganglionopathy

Bladder dysfunction is well-recognized in patients with autoimmune autonomic ganglionopathy. The usual presentation is that of the rapid onset of severe autonomic failure, with orthostatic hypotension, gastrointestinal dysmotility, anhidrosis, erectile dysfunction, and sicca symptoms, often with ganglionic acetylcholine receptor (AChR) antibodies. Bladder dysfunction generally manifests as voiding difficulty and incomplete emptying. The severity and distribution of autonomic dysfunction appear to depend upon the level of antibody titers.[61]

Pure Autonomic Failure

Pure autonomic failure is a synucleinopathy affecting the postganglionic fibers and may mimic multiple system atrophy. Lewy body deposition is confined primarily to the autonomic ganglia. Nocturia and voiding dysfunction are common, and bladder emptying is often affected.

Myotonic Dystrophy

Although myotonic activity has not been found in either the sphincter or pelvic floor of patients with myotonic dystrophy, bladder symptoms may be prominent and difficult to treat, presumably because bladder smooth muscle is affected. With advancing disease, megacolon and fecal incontinence also may become intractable problems.

Urinary Retention

Urinary retention occurring in isolation is most often due to a urologic cause. However, in some cases a neurologic cause is responsible. The differential diagnosis that should be considered once a structural urologic lesion is excluded is found in Table 29-3.

Fowler Syndrome

Urinary retention or symptoms of obstructed voiding in young women in the absence of overt neurologic disease have long puzzled urologists and neurologists alike; in the absence of any convincing organic cause, the condition was thought be hysterical. A primary disorder of urethral sphincter relaxation (Fowler syndrome) is typically seen in young women postmenarche who present with retention and bladder capacities often exceeding a liter

TABLE 29-3 ■ Differential Diagnosis in a Patient Presenting with Urinary Retention

Lesions of the conus medullaris or cauda equina
Compressive lesions
Trauma
Intervertebral disc prolapse
Tumor
Granuloma
Abscess
Non-compressive lesions
Vascular: infarction, ischemia (arteriovenous malformation)
Inflammation: myelitis, meningitis retention syndrome
Infection: herpes simplex, varicella zoster, cytomegalovirus,
Other neurologic conditions
Spina bifida
Multiple system atrophy
Conditions associated with dysautonomia (e.g,, pure autonomic failure, autonomic neuropathies)
Miscellaneous causes
Medications (e.g.,opiates, anticholinergics, retigabine)
Fowler syndrome
Radical pelvic surgery
Chronic intestinal pseudo-obstruction
Primary detrusor muscle failure
Idiopathic

Modified from Smith MD, Seth JH, Fowler CJ, et al: Urinary retention for the neurologist. Pract Neurol 13:288, 2013.

without experiencing expected urgency. Polycystic ovaries are often associated. Electromyography of striated muscle of the urethral sphincter reveals complex repetitive discharges and myotonia-like activity, called decelerating bursts. The urethral pressure profile and urethral sphincter volume are elevated. Urinary retention is often successfully managed by sacral neuromodulation.

DIAGNOSTIC EVALUATION

History

The history of patients with suspected lower urinary tract dysfunction should address both storage and voiding. Patients with storage dysfunction complain of frequency of micturition, nocturia, urgency, and urge incontinence. Urgency, frequency, and nocturia, with or without incontinence, is called the "overactive bladder syndrome," "urge syndrome," or "urgency-frequency syndrome."[62] Patients experiencing voiding dysfunction report hesitancy for micturition, a slow and interrupted urinary stream, the need to strain to pass urine, and double voiding. The history of voiding dysfunction is often unreliable as patients may be unaware of incomplete bladder emptying; therefore, the history should be supplemented by a bladder scan, as discussed later. Occasionally, these patients with voiding dysfunction may experience complete urinary retention.

The pattern of lower urinary tract dysfunction is influenced by the site of the neurologic lesion (Table 29-2), and variation from this expected pattern warrants a search for additional problems such as urologic disease.

Bladder Diary

A bladder diary provides a real-time assessment of bladder symptoms and is considered an extension of the history. It provides an opportunity to record the frequency of micturition, volumes voided, episodes of incontinence, and fluid intake over the course of a few days and should be a part of the evaluation of suspected lower urinary tract dysfunction (Fig. 29-2).

Physical Examination

In patients without an established diagnosis, the neurologic examination helps guide whether urologic complaints are neurologic in origin. Bradykinesia or rigidity can point to basal ganglia disorders. Cerebellar ataxia, parkinsonism, and symptomatic postural hypotension should raise the suspicion of multiple system atrophy. Other autonomic features such as erectile dysfunction, orthostatic hypotension, and constipation may suggest autonomic failure. The findings of saddle anaesthesia and absent sacral reflexes (anal or bulbocavernous) point to a lesion of the conus medullaris or cauda equina. The lumbosacral spine should be examined for dimples, tufts of hair, nevi, or sinus, which can be signs of occult spina bifida.

If the neurologic examination is normal in a patient reporting only bladder dysfunction, more

		Time / Volume (mL)					Total Fluid intake	Episodes of leakage
Day 1	Time	6 AM	10 AM	12 30 PM	3 30 PM	5 PM		
26/4/2009	Volume	160	120	130	190	140		
	Time	7 PM	8 45 PM	2 30 AM	4 AM		1700	4
Time out of bed (am) - 6 AM	Volume	150	170	200	180			
Time to bed (pm)-	Time							
9 PM	Volume							

FIGURE 29-2 ■ Bladder diary recorded over 24 hours demonstrating increased daytime and nocturnal urinary frequency, low voided volumes, and incontinence. These findings are seen in patients with detrusor overactivity. (From Panicker JN, Kalsi V, de Seze M: Approach and evaluation of neurogenic bladder dysfunction. p. 61. In Fowler CJ, Panicker JN, Emmanuel A (eds): Pelvic Organ Dysfunction in Neurological Disease: Clinical Management and Rehabilitation. Cambridge University Press, Cambridge, 2010, with permission).

detailed investigations such as neuroimaging or physiologic testing are unlikely to reveal an underlying neurologic cause.

In the general physical examination, palpating the abdomen for an enlarged bladder may suggest upper urinary tract damage including stones; tenderness over the loins may occur as well. Digital rectal examination helps to evaluate for prostate enlargement.

INVESTIGATIONS

Bladder Scan

Estimating the postvoid residual of urine is an essential step in the investigation of a neurogenic bladder. This assessment is most commonly carried out with a portable bladder scanner or by "in-out" catheterization, especially in patients who perform intermittent self-catheterization. A single measurement of a postvoid residual may not be reliable, and therefore a series of measurements should be made over the course of 1 or 2 weeks.

Screening for Urinary Tract Infections

All patients with lower urinary tract symptoms should be screened for urinary tract infection. Combined rapid tests of urine using reagent strips ("dipstick" tests) have a negative predictive value of 98 percent. However, since the positive predictive value is only 50 percent, a positive test should be followed by a urine culture to confirm infection.[63]

Ultrasound Scan

In patients known to be at risk of upper urinary tract disease, surveillance ultrasonography should be performed periodically to evaluate for upper urinary tract dilatation or renal scarring. Ultrasound may also detect complications of neurogenic bladder dysfunction such as bladder stones.

Urodynamic Studies

Urodynamic studies include measurements of urine flow rate and residual volume, cystometry during both filling and voiding, videocystometry, and urethral pressure profilometry. The term *urodynamics* is often used incorrectly as a synonym for cystometry. From the patient's point of view, urodynamic studies can be divided into noninvasive tests and those tests requiring urethral catheterization.

NONINVASIVE BLADDER INVESTIGATIONS

Uroflowmetry is a valuable test that assesses voiding function. The urinary flow is calculated through a flow meter, usually fitted in a commode or urinal, based upon the power necessary to maintain a rotation speed. A graphic printout of the urinary flow is obtained and time taken to reach maximum flow, maximum and average flow rates, and the voided volume are analyzed (Fig. 29-3). It is important that the patient performs the test with a comfortably full bladder, preferably voiding volumes of at least 150 ml; privacy is essential and a spurious result may

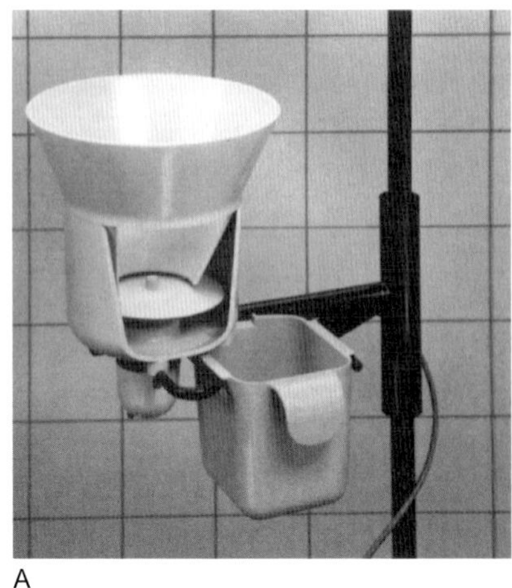

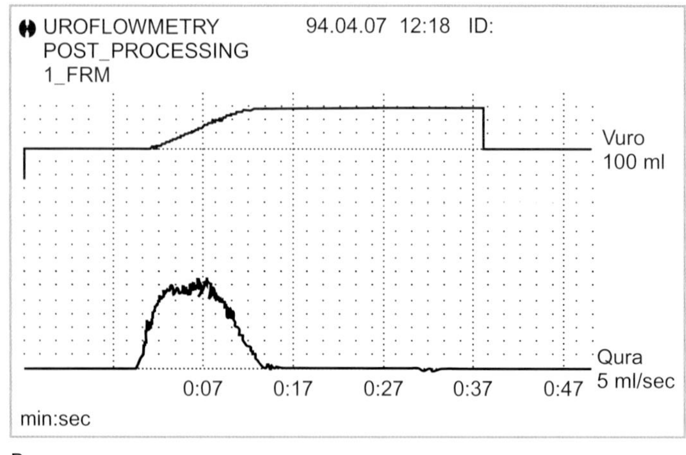

A B

FIGURE 29-3 ■ **A**, Urinary flow meter. The side of the uroflow transducer has been cut away to show the disc at the base of the funnel, which rotates as urine passes into the collecting vessel. **B**, A normal printout from the uroflowmeter. A total of 290 ml was voided *(upper trace)*, with a maximum flow rate of 30 ml per second *(lower trace)*. (From Dantec Medical A/S, Copenhagen, with permission.)

be obtained if the patient is not fully relaxed. The test usually complements a bladder scan, and significant outflow obstruction is unlikely if uroflowmetry demonstrates a normal urine flow rate with no significant postvoid residual in the bladder scan.

Investigations Requiring Catheterization

Cystometry assesses changes in the bladder during nonphysiologic filling and also the pressure–flow relationship during voiding. The detrusor pressure is derived by subtraction of the abdominal pressure (measured from a pressure transducer attached to a catheter inserted into the rectum) from the intravesical pressure (measured from a pressure transducer attached to a catheter inserted into the bladder). The rate of filling is recorded by a machine that pumps sterile water or saline through the catheter into the bladder. For speed and convenience, most laboratories use filling rates of between 50 and 100 ml per minute. This non-physiologic rapid filling means that the full bladder capacity can be reached usually within 7 or 8 minutes. First sensation of bladder filling may be reported at around 100 ml, and full capacity is reached between 400 and 600 ml. In healthy subjects with a "stable" bladder, the bladder expands to contain this amount of fluid without an increase of pressure above 15 cmH_2O. The main abnormality sought during filling cystometry in patients with a neurologic disease is the presence of detrusor overactivity (Fig. 29-4) characterized by involuntary detrusor contractions which may be spontaneous or provoked. Detrusor overactivity of neurogenic origin is indistinguishable from other causes of detrusor overactivity on urodynamic testing. When bladder filling has been completed, the patient voids into the flow meter with the bladder and rectal lines still in place as valuable information can be obtained by measuring detrusor pressure and urine flow simultaneously.

Cystometry may be valuable in demonstrating the underlying pathophysiology of the lower urinary tract and may identify concomitant urologic conditions such as bladder outflow obstruction or stress incontinence. A general criticism is that findings on cystometry contribute little to elucidating the underlying disorder. In many patients with a neurogenic bladder, the "urodynamic diagnosis" does not influence management, and the need to perform a complete urodynamic study in all patients with a suspected neurogenic bladder is therefore unclear. The decision to carry out cystometry should include consideration of the underlying neurologic diagnosis, the perceived risk of upper tract damage, and sometimes, response to initial treatment.[64] Patients with spinal cord injury, spina bifida, and possibly advanced multiple sclerosis should undergo urodynamic studies as they are at higher risk of upper tract involvement and renal impairment (although ultrasound is a less invasive method for monitoring the upper tract). In other conditions such as early multiple sclerosis, stroke, and PD, some authors

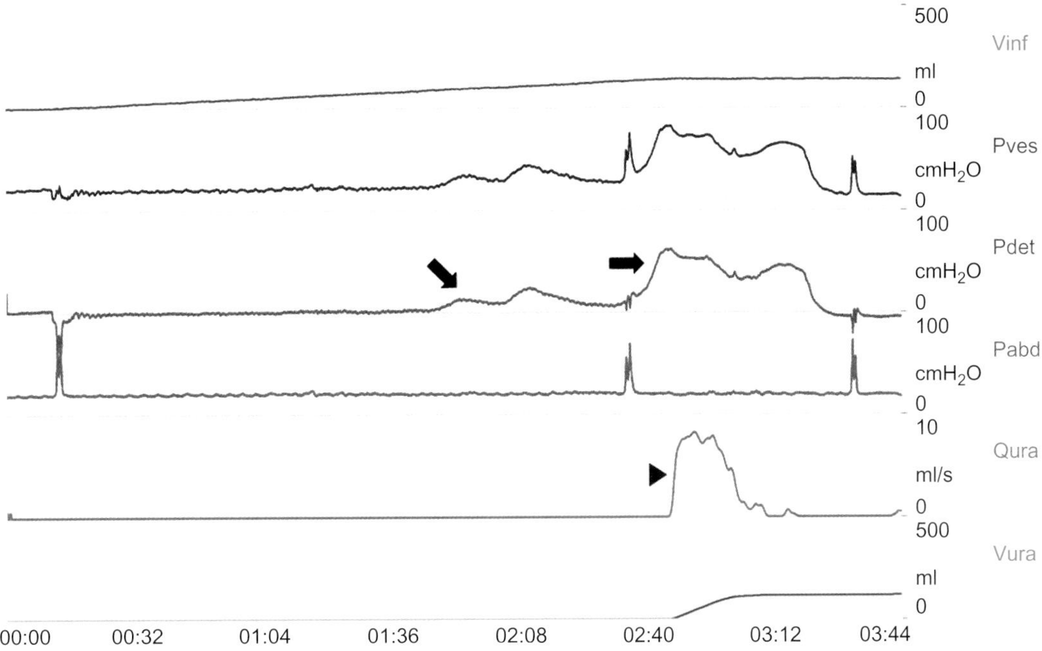

FIGURE 29-4 ■ Filling cystometry demonstrating detrusor overactivity. The dark orange line (Pabd) is the intra-abdominal pressure recorded by the rectal catheter, the dark blue line (Pves) is the intravesical pressure recorded by the bladder catheter. The pink line (Pdet) is the subtracted detrusor pressure (Pves − Pabd). Green lines represent volume infused during the test (Vinf) and volume voided (Vura) while the orange line represents urinary flow (Qura). The black arrows demonstrate detrusor overactivity and the black arrowhead indicates associated incontinence. (From Panicker JN, Fowler CJ: The bare essentials: uro-neurology. Pract Neurol 10:178, 2010, with permission.)

have recommended that the initial evaluation be restricted to noninvasive tests as the risk of upper urinary tract damage is less.[50]

Videocystometry

Videocystometry is cystometry carried out using a contrast-filling medium visualized radiographically. Urologists and urogynecologists have found videocystometry useful in detecting sphincter or bladder neck incompetence in patients with stress incontinence. The technique also gives additional information regarding morphologic changes that may occur as a consequence of neurogenic bladder dysfunction, including the presence of vesicoureteric reflux. The opportunity to inspect the outflow tract during voiding is of great value in patients with suspected obstruction.

Uro-Neurophysiology

Various neurophysiologic investigations of the pelvic floor have been developed for assessing the innervation of muscles that are difficult to test clinically. Their clinical utility has been debated, and they currently play a role only in the assessment of patients presenting in specific clinical situations.

Electromyography

Pelvic floor electromyography was first introduced with the aim of recognizing detrusor-sphincter dyssynergia, but it is currently performed only rarely. Technically the best signal is obtained using a needle electrode, but the discomfort from the needle itself can impair normal relaxation of the pelvic floor. Surface recording electrodes have been used, but they may record a considerable amount of noise artifact, which makes interpretation difficult. The value of the information provided is limited, and the demonstration of detrusor-sphincter dyssynergia is most often achieved by less invasive techniques such as videourodynamics.

Concentric needle electromyography of the pelvic floor is possible since motor units of the pelvic floor and sphincters fire tonically; they therefore may be captured conveniently using a trigger and delay line and subjected to individual motor unit analysis. Well-established normative values exist for the normal duration and amplitude of motor units recorded from these sphincter muscles.

Sphincter Electromyography for Suspected Cauda Equina Lesions

Lesions of the cauda equina are an important cause of pelvic floor dysfunction. Although electromyography may demonstrate pathologic spontaneous activity 3 weeks or more after injury, these changes of denervation often become lost in the tonically firing motor units of the sphincter. Most often with long-standing cauda equina syndrome, electromyography of the external anal sphincter demonstrates changes of chronic reinnervation, with a reduced interference pattern and enlarged motor units (>1 mV amplitude) along with polyphasic potentials.[65]

Sphincter Electromyography in Multiple System Atrophy

Postmortem studies of multiple system atrophy have demonstrated a selective loss of anterior horn cells in Onuf nuclei, which are spared in PD.[66,67] This finding may explain the early urinary symptoms and sphincter involvement in multiple system atrophy. Sacral cord involvement may precede central changes responsible for lower urinary tract symptoms in these patients. The central pathology of multiple system atrophy may explain the symptoms of overactive bladder that may occur.[68,69] The characteristic Onuf nucleus involvement may account for the abnormalities seen in the external urethral sphincter. These changes can be detected easily using electromyography (Fig. 29-5). There is debate on the role of anal sphincter electromyography in the diagnosis of multiple system atrophy.[45,46,70]

Sphincter Electromyography for Urinary Retention in Young Women

A characteristic abnormality in isolated urinary retention in young women can be found on urethral sphincter electromyography; complex repetitive discharges, akin to the sound of "helicopters" along with decelerating bursts, a signal somewhat like myotonia and akin to the sound of "underwater recording of whales," can be found. It has been proposed that this abnormal spontaneous activity results in an impairment of relaxation of the urethral sphincter, which may cause urinary retention in some women and obstructed voiding in others. This condition, known as Fowler syndrome, is also characterized by elevated urethral pressures.

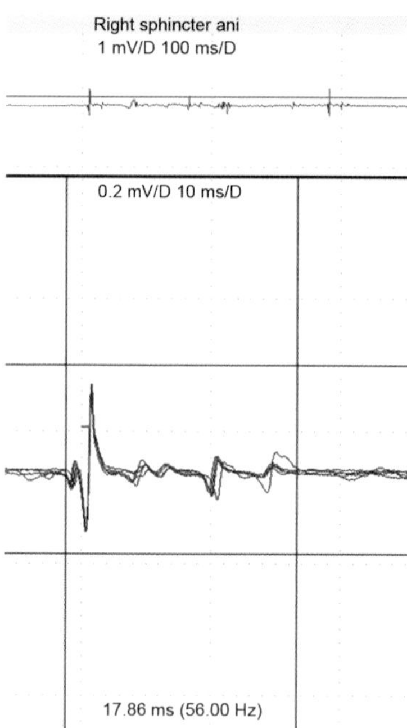

FIGURE 29-5 ■ Concentric needle electromyogram (EMG) of the external anal sphincter from a 64-year-old man presenting with parkinsonism and urinary retention. Duration of the motor unit is 17.9 msec (normal <10 msec) with a mean duration of all the motor units recorded during the study of 22.9 msec; these prolonged motor units suggest chronic reinnervation and are compatible with a diagnosis of multiple system atrophy.

Penilo-Cavernosus Reflex

The penilo-cavernosus reflex, formally known as the "bulbocavernosus" reflex, assesses the sacral root afferent and efferent pathways. The dorsal nerve of the penis (or clitoris) is electrically stimulated and recordings are made from the bulbocavernosus muscle, usually with a concentric needle. This test may be of value in patients with bladder dysfunction suspected to be secondary to cauda equina or lower motor neuron pathway damage. A normal response does not completely exclude the possibility of an axonal lesion.

Pudendal Nerve Terminal Motor Latency

The only test of motor conduction for the pelvic floor is the pudendal nerve terminal motor latency. The response is obtained by stimulating the pudendal nerve either rectally or vaginally, adjacent to the ischial spine using a finger-mounted stimulating device with a recording electrode around the base of the finger that records from the external anal sphincter. Prolongation suggests pudendal nerve damage. However, as a prolonged latency is a relatively poor marker of denervation, the test has not proved contributory in the investigation of patients with suspected pudendal neuralgia.

Pudendal Somatosensory Evoked Potentials

Pudendal somatosensory evoked potentials can be recorded from the scalp following electric stimulation of the dorsal nerve of the penis or clitoris. Although abnormal when a spinal cord lesion is the cause of sacral sensory loss or neurogenic detrusor overactivity, such pathology is usually apparent from the clinical examination. The latencies of the evoked potentials recorded are compared to those found with stimulation of the posterior tibial nerve.

COMPLICATIONS OF NEUROGENIC BLADDER DYSFUNCTION

Detrusor overactivity and reduced bladder wall compliance may lead to raised intravesical pressure, which can, in turn, lead to structural changes in the bladder wall such as trabeculations and diverticuli. The upper urinary tract (kidney and ureter) can also be affected through the vesicoureteric reflux, resulting in hydronephrosis along with renal impairment and possible failure. For reasons that are unclear, upper urinary tract damage and renal failure are less common in multiple sclerosis than in traumatic spinal cord injury or spina bifida. The risk of upper urinary tract damage is highest in patients who have raised intravesical pressure due to detrusor overactivity, low bladder compliance, and a competent bladder neck. Patients with a neurogenic bladder are prone to genitourinary tract infections such as cystitis, pyelonephritis, and epididymo-orchitis as well as bladder stones.

MANAGEMENT OF NEUROGENIC BLADDER DYSFUNCTION

The goals of managing neurogenic bladder dysfunction are to achieve urinary continence, prevent urinary tract infections, and preserve upper urinary tract function, which all may improve the quality of life of patients with neurologic disease.[71] The management of neurogenic bladder dysfunction must address both voiding and storage dysfunction (Fig. 29-6).

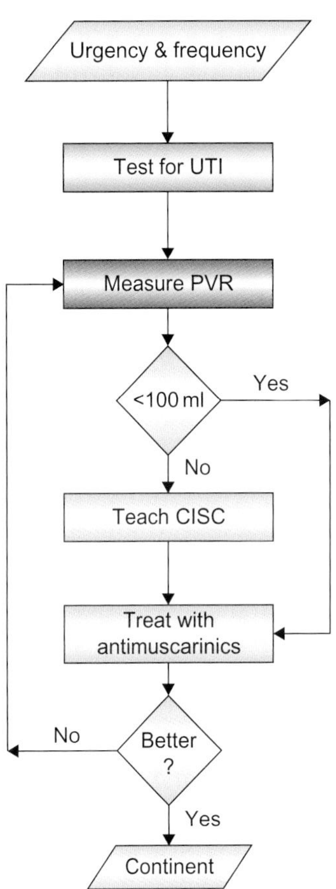

FIGURE 29-6 ■ Algorithm for the management of neurogenic lower urinary tract dysfunction. (From Fowler CJ, Panicker JN, Drake M, et al: A UK consensus on the management of the bladder in multiple sclerosis. J Neurol Neurosurg Psychiatry 80:470, 2009, with permission.)

Management of Voiding Dysfunction

A postvoid residual volume of more than 100 ml, or more than one-third of bladder capacity, is considered incomplete emptying.[50] This voiding dysfunction can exacerbate detrusor overactivity, and an overactive bladder constantly stimulated by a residual volume responds with contraction, producing symptoms of urgency and frequency, making antimuscarinic medications less effective.

The widespread use of intermittent self-catheterization has greatly improved the management of neurogenic bladder dysfunction. There is no consensus regarding the amount of residual volume at which intermittent self-catheterization should be initiated. Sterile intermittent catheterization was previously the standard, but a clean, rather than sterile, technique has been found to be adequate. Intermittent catheterization is best performed by the patient, who should be taught by an experienced provider such as a nurse continence advisor. Neurologic lesions affecting manual dexterity, visual acuity, or cognitive function may require the patient to be assisted by a partner or other provider. The incidence of symptomatic urinary tract infections is low when catheterization is performed regularly.

Alpha blockers can relax the internal urethral sphincter in men, and although they improve bladder emptying and reduce postvoid residual volumes, their use is usually not recommended unless concomitant prostatic enlargement is present.[72] Botulinum toxin injections into the external urethral sphincter may improve bladder emptying in patients with spinal cord injury and significant voiding dysfunction.[73] Suprapubic vibration using a mechanical "buzzer" is modestly effective in patients with multiple sclerosis who have incomplete bladder emptying and detrusor overactivity.[74] The Credé maneuver (pressure applied from the umbilicus towards the pubis) and reflex voiding using nonforceful trigger techniques are usually not recommended as they may result in high detrusor pressure and incomplete bladder emptying during voiding.[50]

Management of Storage Dysfunction

General Measures

Nonpharmacologic strategies are useful in the early stages of storage dysfunction when symptoms are mild. A restriction of fluid intake to around 1 to 2 liters daily is suggested, and it is often helpful to assess fluid balance by means of a bladder diary.[75] Reduction of caffeine intake may reduce urgency and frequency especially in patients who drink coffee or tea excessively. Bladder retraining, whereby patients void at regular timed intervals and then voluntarily "hold on" for increasingly longer periods of time, aims to restore the normal pattern of micturition. Pelvic floor exercises and neuromuscular stimulation may also be useful, once voiding dysfunction has been excluded, in the symptomatic treatment of an overactive bladder.

Antimuscarinic Medications

Detrusor overactivity is a major cause of incontinence in patients with neurogenic bladder disorders. The first-line treatment of detrusor overactivity is with antimuscarinic drugs, but the evidence for their efficacy is limited, with only five high-quality published studies in adults.[76–80] A systematic review found no significant difference in efficacy between the various antimuscarinic drugs in patients with neurogenic bladder.[81] Oxybutinin was one of the earlier drugs introduced, but propiverine, trospium, propantheline, and tolterodine have all been shown to produce clinical and some urodynamic improvement in detrusor overactivity. Adverse events are due to nonspecific anticholinergic actions and include dry mouth, blurred vision for near objects, tachycardia, and constipation. These drugs can also block central muscarinic receptors and cause impairment of cognition and consciousness. Medications that have low selectivity for the M1 receptor, such as darifenacin, or restricted permeability across the blood–brain barrier, such as trospium, are probably less likely to cause cognitive disturbances. The postvoid residual urine volume may increase following treatment and should be monitored by serial bladder scans. Many patients also have underlying voiding dysfunction, and it is often judicious to use antimuscarinic medications along with clean intermittent self-catheterization.[50]

Desmopressin

Desmopressin, a synthetic analogue of arginine vasopressin, reduces urine production and volume by promoting water reabsorption at the distal collecting tubules of the kidney. The evidence for its efficacy in the treatment of nocturia and daytime frequency in patients with multiple sclerosis is based on a meta-analysis that suggested it provides symptom relief for up to 6 hours.[82] Desmopressin is useful also in managing patients with orthostatic hypotension.[83] Side effects include the risk of hyponatremia, particularly in older patients, and it should be prescribed with caution in those with dependent leg edema or congestive heart failure. In patients over 65 years of age who are taking the drug, serum sodium levels should be measured at baseline and again at 3 and 7 days at the beginning of treatment or when the dose is changed.[84]

Cannabinoids

Cannabinoids have limited efficacy on urinary disturbances in patients with multiple sclerosis. In one study of orally administered Δ^9-tetrahydrocannabinol extract, frequency, nocturia, and incontinence episodes were diminished.[85] In another study, oral nabiximols showed significant reduction in the number of episodes of nocturia and of voids per day, and improvement in overall bladder control.[86]

Botulinum Toxin

Botulinum toxin was used initially on the basis that it blocks synaptic release of acetylcholine from parasympathetic nerve endings and produces paralysis of the detrusor muscle along with a demonstrable increase in bladder capacity. Accumulating evidence indicates that the mechanism of action is more complex, however, and may involve afferent bladder innervation as well. Botulinum toxin type A injections of the detrusor muscle under cystoscopic guidance are now licensed for managing refractory neurogenic detrusor overactivity in several countries, including the United States. The duration of effect is 9 to 13 months. Two pivotal phase III studies demonstrated that onabotulinumtoxinA significantly improves overactive bladder symptoms, urodynamic parameters, and quality of life, although patients often have to perform clean intermittent self-catheterization afterwards depending on the dose administered (30 to 42% in one study).[84,87–89] Evidence also supports the efficacy of detrusor injections of botulinum toxin A in the treatment of neurogenic detrusor overactivity in adults with multiple sclerosis and spinal cord injury, as well as in myelodysplasia in children.[84] Studies also suggest that patients receiving botulinum toxin injections have fewer urinary tract infections and reduced catheter bypassing (urethral leakage while using an indwelling catheter).

Vanilloids

Despite the initial enthusiasm for its use, intravesical vanilloid therapy generally has been superseded by botulinum toxin treatments. Only a few centers worldwide offer resiniferatoxin treatment.

Nerve Stimulation

Sacral Neuromodulation

An extradural sacral nerve stimulator can be useful in conditions resistant to antimuscarinic medications. The mechanism of action is likely stimulation of pelvic afferents, which are known to have an inhibitory effect on the detrusor. Implanting the stimulator requires evaluation during a test phase to determine whether the patient's symptoms are improved as judged by bladder diaries and measurement of residual volumes. If effective, the battery is implanted in a subcutaneous pocket and connected to the stimulating lead. The stimulator is continuously active, although it can be maintained at a subsensory level. There is only limited evidence supporting sacral neuromodulation in patients with progressive neurologic conditions.

Percutaneous Tibial Nerve Stimulation

Percutaneous stimulation of the posterior tibial nerve for an overactive bladder involves inserting a fine needle into the nerve, just above the ankle. A mild electric current is passed through the needle and is carried to the nerves that control bladder function. Studies of such stimulation for overactive bladder show that it reduces symptoms in the short and medium term without major safety concerns.

Nerve Root Stimulators

In patients with complete spinal cord transection, but in whom the caudal section of the cord and its roots are intact, implantation of a nerve root stimulator should be considered. Stimulating electrodes are placed around the lower sacral roots (S2 to S4) and activated by an external switching device. The stimulating electrodes are usually applied intrathecally to the anterior roots, and the posterior roots are severed at the same time. After the implant, adjustments are made to stimulation parameters so that the patient obtains maximum benefit in terms of making the bladder contract for voiding, assisting defecation, or producing penile erection. Although such devices are highly effective in selected cases, the additional neurologic deficit caused by the need for sectioning of the dorsal roots and resulting erectile dysfunction has reduced its acceptance. These stimulators are suitable only for patients with complete spinal cord lesions and are not effective in partial cord lesions or chronic neurologic disease.

Surgery

Various surgical procedures to rectify a disorder causing incontinence in otherwise fit and healthy persons are often highly successful. Even after

TABLE 29-4 ■ Situations Prompting Early Referral to a Urologist

Hematuria
Renal impairment
Frequent urinary tract infections
Suspicion of concomitant urologic pathologies such as bladder outlet obstruction due to prostate enlargement in men or stress incontinence in women
Symptoms refractory to treatment
Consideration of suprapubic catheterization
Consideration of urologic procedures such as intradetrusor injections of botulinum toxin A or surgeries such as augmentation cystoplasty or urinary diversion

spinal cord injury, a surgical option might be the best solution for long-term bladder management. These procedures are typically not effective in chronic and progressive neurologic conditions such as multiple sclerosis.

Permanent Indwelling Catheters

When incontinence is refractory to management or the patient is no longer able to perform self-catheterization, an indwelling catheter may become necessary. The long-term complications of urethral catheters are well-known and include catheter bypassing, which occurs when strong detrusor contractions produce a rapid urine flow that cannot drain sufficiently quickly. A common response to bypassing is to use a wider-caliber catheter, and consequently the bladder closure mechanism becomes progressively stretched and destroyed. Bladder stones and recurrent infections are also more likely in patients with an indwelling catheter.

A preferred alternative to an indwelling urethral catheter is a suprapubic catheter, which can be inserted by a urologist. Extreme care is required since these patients often have small, contracted bladders, contributing to the risk of bowel perforation during placement. A suprapubic catheter is a better long-term alternative to urethral catheters since it preserves urethral integrity and sexual function, while leading to fewer problems with perineal hygiene.

Stepwise Approach to Neurogenic Bladder Dysfunction

The treatment options offered to a patient with lower urinary tract dysfunction should reflect the severity of bladder problems, which generally parallel the extent of neurologic disease. There are specific situations where patients should be seen early by a urology consultant (Table 29-4).

REFERENCES

1. Barrington FJ: Affections of micturition resulting from lesions of the nervous system. Proc R Soc Med 20:722, 1927.
2. Kuru M, Yamamoto H: Fiber connections of the pontine detrusor nucleus (Barrington). J Comp Neurol 123:161, 1964.
3. De Groat WC: Nervous control of the urinary bladder of the cat. Brain Res 87:201, 1975.
4. Kuru M, Makuya A, Koyama Y: Fiber connections between the mesencephalic micturition facilitory area and the bulbar vesico-motor centers. J Comp Neurol 117:161, 1961.
5. Griffiths D, Tadic SD: Bladder control, urgency, and urge incontinence: evidence from functional brain imaging. Neurourol Urodyn 27:466, 2008.
6. Griffiths D, Derbyshire S, Stenger A, et al: Brain control of normal and overactive bladder. J Urol 174:1862, 2005.
7. Holstege G, Griffiths D, de Wall H, et al: Anatomical and physiological observations on supraspinal control of bladder and urethral sphincter muscles in the cat. J Comp Neurol 250:449, 1986.
8. Fowler CJ: Neurological disorders of micturition and their treatment. Brain 122:1213, 1999.
9. Blok BF, Willemsen AT, Holstege G: A PET study on brain control of micturition in humans. Brain 120:111, 1997.
10. Blok BF, Sturms LM, Holstege G: Brain activation during micturition in women. Brain 121:2033, 1998.
11. Nour S, Svarer C, Kristensen JK, et al: Cerebral activation during micturition in normal men. Brain 123:781, 2000.
12. Fowler CJ, Griffiths DJ: A decade of functional brain imaging applied to bladder control. Neurourol Urodyn 29:49, 2010.
13. Blok BF, De Weerd H, Holstege G: Ultrastructural evidence for a paucity of projections from the lumbosacral cord to the pontine micturition center or M-region in the cat: a new concept for the organization of the micturition reflex with the periaqueductal gray as central relay. J Comp Neurol 359:300, 1995.
14. Apodaca G: The uroepithelium: not just a passive barrier. Traffic 5:117, 2004.
15. Birder LA, Nakamura Y, Kiss S, et al: Altered urinary bladder function in mice lacking the vanilloid receptor TRPV1. Nat Neurosci 5:856, 2002.
16. Hanna-Mitchell AT, Beckel JM, Barbadora S, et al: Non-neuronal acetylcholine and urinary bladder urothelium. Life Sci 80:2298, 2007.

17. Andersson KE, Wein AJ: Pharmacology of the lower urinary tract: basis for current and future treatments of urinary incontinence. Pharmacol Rev 56:581, 2004.
18. Chang HY, Cheng CL, Chen JJ, et al: Roles of glutamatergic and serotonergic mechanisms in reflex control of the external urethral sphincter in urethane-anesthetized female rats. Am J Physiol Regul Integr Comp Physiol 291:R224, 2006.
19. Andersson KE, Pehrson R: CNS involvement in overactive bladder: pathophysiology and opportunities for pharmacological intervention. Drugs 63:2595, 2003.
20. Panicker JN, Kalsi V, de Seze M: Approach and evaluation of neurogenic bladder dysfunction. p. 61. In Fowler CJ, Panicker JN, Emmanuel A (eds): Pelvic Organ Dysfunction in Neurological Disease: Clinical Management and Rehabilitation. Cambridge University Press, Cambridge, 2010.
21. Andrew J, Nathan PW: Lesions on the anterior frontal lobes and disturbances of micturition and defaecation. Brain 87:233, 1964.
22. Sakakibara R, Hattori T, Uchiyama T, et al: Urinary function in elderly people with and without leukoaraiosis: relation to cognitive and gait function. J Neurol Neurosurg Psychiatry 67:658, 1999.
23. Han KS, Heo SH, Lee SJ, et al: Comparison of urodynamics between ischemic and hemorrhagic stroke patients; can we suggest the category of urinary dysfunction in patients with cerebrovascular accident according to type of stroke? Neurourol Urodyn 29:387, 2010.
24. Tadic SD, Griffiths D, Murrin A, et al: Brain activity during bladder filling is related to white matter structural changes in older women with urinary incontinence. Neuroimage 51:1294, 2010.
25. Ransmayr GN, Holliger S, Schletterer K, et al: Lower urinary tract symptoms in dementia with Lewy bodies, Parkinson disease, and Alzheimer disease. Neurology 70:299, 2008.
26. Andersen JT: Disturbances of bladder and urethral function in Parkinson's disease. Int Urol Nephrol 17:35, 1985.
27. Berger Y, Blaivas JG, DeLaRocha ER, et al: Urodynamic findings in Parkinson's disease. J Urol 138:836, 1987.
28. Sakakibara R, Shinotoh H, Uchiyama T, et al: Questionnaire-based assessment of pelvic organ dysfunction in Parkinson's disease. Auton Neurosci 92:76, 2001.
29. Araki I, Kitahara M, Oida T, et al: Voiding dysfunction and Parkinson's Disease: urodynamic abnormalities and urinary symptoms. J Urol 164:1640, 2000.
30. Campos-Sousa RN, Quagliato E, da Silva BB, et al: Urinary symptoms in Parkinson's disease: prevalence and associated factors. Arq Neuropsiquiatr 61:359, 2003.
31. Araki I, Kitahara M, Oida T, et al: Voiding dysfunction and Parkinson's disease: urodynamic abnormalities and urinary symptoms. J Urol 164:1640, 2000.
32. Yoshimura N, Kuno S, Chancellor MB, et al: Dopaminergic mechanisms underlying bladder hyperactivity in rats with a unilateral 6-hydroxydopamine (6-OHDA) lesion of the nigrostriatal pathway. Br J Pharmacol 139:1425, 2003.
33. Saunders JB, Schuckit MA: The development of a research agenda for substance use disorders diagnosis in the Diagnostic and Statistical Manual of Mental Disorders. 5th edition (DSM-V). Addiction 101(suppl 1):1, 2006.
34. Gomez-Esteban JC, Zarranz JJ, Lezcano E, et al: Sleep complaints and their relation with drug treatment in patients suffering from Parkinson's disease. Mov Disord 21:983, 2006.
35. Cochen De Cock V, Abouda M, Leu S, et al: Is obstructive sleep apnea a problem in Parkinson's disease? Sleep Med 11:247, 2010.
36. Menza M, Dobkin RD, Marin H, et al: Sleep disturbances in Parkinson's disease. Mov Disord 25(suppl 1):S117, 2010.
37. Sakakibara R, Kishi M, Ogawa E, et al: Bladder, bowel, and sexual dysfunction in Parkinson's disease. Parkinsons Dis 2011:924605, 2011.
38. Sakakibara R, Uchiyama T, Yamanishi T, et al: Genitourinary dysfunction in Parkinson's disease. Mov Disord 25:2, 2010.
39. Sakakibara R, Uchiyama T, Yoshiyama M, et al: Disturbance of micturition in Parkinson's disease. No To Shinkei 53:1009, 2001.
40. Sammour ZM, Gomes CM, Barbosa ER, et al: Voiding dysfunction in patients with Parkinson's disease: impact of neurological impairment and clinical parameters. Neurourol Urodyn 28:510, 2009.
41. Saunders JB: Substance dependence and non-dependence in the Diagnostic and Statistical Manual of Mental Disorders (DSM) and the International Classification of Diseases (ICD): can an identical conceptualization be achieved? Addiction 101(suppl 1):48, 2006.
42. Hahn K, Ebersbach G: Sonographic assessment of urinary retention in multiple system atrophy and idiopathic Parkinson's disease. Mov Disord 20:1499, 2005.
43. Regier D: Interview with Darrel A. Regier. The developmental process for the diagnostic and statistical manual of mental disorders, fifth edition. Interview by Norman Sussman. CNS Spectr 13:120, 2008.
44. Sakakibara R, Hattori T, Uchiyama T, et al: Videourodynamic and sphincter motor unit potential analyses in Parkinson's disease and multiple system atrophy. J Neurol Neurosurg Psychiatry 71:600, 2001.
45. Palace J, Chandiramani VA, Fowler CJ: Value of sphincter electromyography in the diagnosis of multiple system atrophy. Muscle Nerve 20:1396, 1997.
46. Tison F, Arne P, Sourgen C, et al: The value of external anal sphincter electromyography for the diagnsosi of multiple system atrophy. Mov Disord 15:1148, 2000.
47. Kirby R, Fowler C, Gosling J, et al: Urethro-vesical dysfunction in progressive autonomic failure with multiple

system atrophy. J Neurol Neurosurg Psychiatry 49:554, 1986.
48. Komiyama A: Urinary retention associated with a unilateral lesion in the dorsolateral tegmentum of the rostral pons. J Neurol Neurosurg Psychiatry 65:953, 1998.
49. Sakakibara R, Hattori T, Yasuda K, et al: Micturitional disturbance and the pontine tegmental lesion: urodynamic and MRI analyses of vascular cases. J Neurol Sci 141:105, 1996.
50. Fowler CJ, Panicker JN, Drake M, et al: A UK consensus on the management of the bladder in multiple sclerosis. J Neurol Neurosurg Psychiatry 80:470, 2009.
51. Hemmett L, Holmes J, Barnes M, et al: What drives quality of life in multiple sclerosis? QJM 97:671, 2004.
52. Marrie RA, Cutter G, Tyry T, et al: Disparities in the management of multiple sclerosis-related bladder symptoms. Neurology 68:1971, 2007.
53. Hennessey A, Robertson NP, Swingler R, et al: Urinary, faecal and sexual dysfunction in patients with multiple sclerosis. J Neurol 246:1027, 1999.
54. Giannantoni A, Scivoletto G, Di Stasi SM, et al: Urological dysfunctions and upper urinary tract involvement in multiple sclerosis patients. Neurourol Urodyn 17:89, 1998.
55. Litwiller SE, Frohman EM, Zimmern PE: Multiple sclerosis and the urologist. J Urol 161:743, 1999.
56. Buljevac D, Flach HZ, Hop WC, et al: Prospective study on the relationship between infections and multiple sclerosis exacerbations. Brain 125:952, 2002.
57. Hill SR, Fayyad AM, Jones GR: Diabetes mellitus and female lower urinary tract symptoms: a review. Neurourol Urodyn 27:362, 2008.
58. Andrade MJ: Lower urinary tract dysfunction in familial amyloidotic polyneuropathy, Portuguese type. Neurourol Urodyn 28:26, 2009.
59. Lobato L: Portuguese-type amyloidosis (transthyretin amyloidosis, ATTR V30M). J Nephrol 16:438, 2003.
60. Adams D, Samuel D, Goulon-Goeau C, et al: The course and prognostic factors of familial amyloid polyneuropathy after liver transplantation. Brain 123:1495, 2000.
61. Gibbons CH, Freeman R: Antibody titers predict clinical features of autoimmune autonomic ganglionopathy. Auton Neurosci 146:8, 2009.
62. Abrams P, Cardozo L, Fall M, et al: The standardisation of terminology of lower urinary tract function: report from the Standardisation Sub-committee of the International Continence Society. Neurourol Urodyn 21:167, 2002.
63. Fowlis GA, Waters J, Williams G: The cost effectiveness of combined rapid tests (Multistix) in screening for urinary tract infections. J R Soc Med 87:681, 1994.
64. Schafer W, Abrams P, Liao L, et al: Good urodynamic practices: uroflowmetry, filling cystometry, and pressure-flow studies. Neurourol Urodyn 21:261, 2002.
65. Podnar S, Trsinar B, Vodusek DB: Bladder dysfunction in patients with cauda equina lesions. Neurourol Urodyn 25:23, 2006.
66. Mannen T, Iwata M, Toyokura Y, et al: The Onuf's nucleus and the external anal sphincter muscle in ALS and Shy-Drager syndrome. Acta Neuropathol 58:255, 1982.
67. Sakakibara R, Uchiyama T, Yamanishi T, et al: Bladder and bowel dysfunction in Parkinson's disease. J Neural Transm 115:443, 2008.
68. Yoshida M: Multiple system atrophy: alpha-synuclein and neuronal degeneration. Neuropathology 27:484, 2007.
69. Benarroch EE, Schmeichel AM, Low PA, et al: Involvement of medullary serotonergic groups in multiple system atrophy. Ann Neurol 55:418, 2004.
70. Giladi N, Simon ES, Korczyn AD, et al: Anal sphincter EMG does not distinguish between multiple system atrophy and parkinson's disease. Muscle Nerve 23:731, 2000.
71. Stohrer M, Castro-Diaz D, Chartier-Kastler E, et al: EAU Guidelines on Neurogenic Lower Urinary Tract Dysfunction. Eur Urol 56:81, 2009.
72. O'Riordan JI, Doherty C, Javed M, et al: Do alpha-blockers have a role in lower urinary tract dysfunction in multiple sclerosis? J Urol 153:1114, 1995.
73. Naumann M, So Y, Argoff CE, et al: Assessment: botulinum neurotoxin in the treatment of autonomic disorders and pain (an evidence-based review): report of the Therapeutics and Technology Assessment Subcommittee of the American Academy of Neurology. Neurology 70:1707, 2008.
74. Prasad RS, Smith SJ, Wright H: Lower abdominal pressure versus external bladder stimulation to aid bladder emptying in multiple sclerosis: a randomized controlled study. Clin Rehabil 17:42, 2003.
75. Hashim H, Abrams P: How should patients with an overactive bladder manipulate their fluid intake? BJU Int 102:62, 2008.
76. Madersbacher H, Stohrer M, Richter R, et al: Trospium chloride versus oxybutynin: a randomized, double-blind, multicentre trial in the treatment of detrusor hyper-reflexia. Br J Urol 75:452, 1995.
77. Gajewski JB, Awad SA: Oxybutynin versus propantheline in patients with multiple sclerosis and detrusor hyperreflexia. J Urol 135:966, 1986.
78. Stohrer M, Madersbacher H, Richter R, et al: Efficacy and safety of propiverine in SCI-patients suffering from detrusor hyperreflexia—a double-blind, placebo-controlled clinical trial. Spinal Cord 37:196, 1999.
79. Fader M, Glickman S, Haggar V, et al: Intravesical atropine compared to oral oxybutynin for neurogenic detrusor overactivity: a double-blind, randomized crossover trial. J Urol 177:208, 2007.
80. Stohrer M, Murtz G, Kramer G, et al: Propiverine compared to oxybutynin in neurogenic detrusor overactivity—results of a randomized, double-blind, multicenter clinical study. Eur Urol 51:235, 2007.
81. Madhuvrata P, Singh M, Hasafa Z, et al: Anticholinergic drugs for adult neurogenic detrusor overactivity: a

systematic review and meta-analysis. Eur Urol 62:816, 2012.
82. Bosma R, Wynia K, Havlikova E, et al: Efficacy of desmopressin in patients with multiple sclerosis suffering from bladder dysfunction: a meta-analysis. Acta Neurol Scand 112:1, 2005.
83. Suchowersky O, Furtado S, Rohs G: Beneficial effect of intranasal desmopressin for nocturnal polyuria in Parkinson's disease. Mov Disord 10:337, 1995.
84. Fowler CJ: Systematic review of therapy for neurogenic detrusor overactivity. Can Urol Assoc J 5:S146, 2011.
85. Freeman RM, Adekanmi O, Waterfield MR, et al: The effect of cannabis on urge incontinence in patients with multiple sclerosis: a multicentre, randomised placebo-controlled trial (CAMS-LUTS). Int Urogynecol J Pelvic Floor Dysfunct 17:636, 2006.
86. Kavia RB, De Ridder D, Constantinescu CS, et al: Randomized controlled trial of Sativex to treat detrusor overactivity in multiple sclerosis. Mult Scler 16:1349, 2010.
87. Giannantoni A, Rossi A, Mearini E, et al: Botulinum toxin A for overactive bladder and detrusor muscle overactivity in patients with Parkinson's disease and multiple system atrophy. J Urol 182:1453, 2009.
88. Kulaksizoglu H, Parman Y: Use of botulinim toxin-A for the treatment of overactive bladder symptoms in patients with Parkinsons's disease. Parkinsonism Relat Disord 16:531, 2010.
89. Kalsi V, Gonzales G, Popat R, et al: Botulinum injections for the treatment of bladder symptoms of multiple sclerosis. Ann Neurol 62:452, 2007.

CHAPTER

30

Sexual Dysfunction in Patients with Neurologic Disorders

DAVID B. VODUŠEK ■ MICHAEL J. AMINOFF

Sexual excitement and satisfaction from adequate stimuli are a normal component of a fulfilled life. The somatic and psychosocial factors involved may be compromised by neurologic disease. Sexual dysfunction may occur as the presenting symptom of a developing neurologic disease (e.g., erectile dysfunction in multiple system atrophy) or as an isolated phenomenon after local nerve injury (e.g., painful clitoral dysesthesia after pudendal nerve lesion), or it may be due to more general effects of a neurologic disorder. It is helpful to conceptualize sexual dysfunction in neurologic disease as Foley and Iverson[1] did for multiple sclerosis: there are primary effects stemming from physiologic or pharmacologic factors; secondary problems related to sensorimotor, bladder, and bowel disturbances and higher brain dysfunction; and tertiary issues related to psychosocial and cultural changes resulting from the disease.

Sexual disorders, such as loss of sexual desire, erectile dysfunction in men, decreased lubrication in women, and disturbances of ejaculation and orgasm, are common in patients with neurologic disorders but are usually not communicated by them

Aminoff's Neurology and General Medicine, Fifth Edition.

to the neurologist. Sexual functioning needs to be addressed because it may be relevant for diagnosis, is a major determinant of quality of life, and may be responsive to treatment. The focus of this chapter is on the more classic neurologic dimension of sexuality as a physiologic function dependent on the integrity of neural control, on sexual dysfunction as a consequence of neurologic disease, and on management of neurologic patients with sexual dysfunction.

SEXUAL FUNCTION AND THE NERVOUS SYSTEM

To the neurologist, sexual behavior involves a series of neurally controlled phenomena occurring in a hormonally defined milieu. Sexuality depends also on psychosocial factors, but the neurologist's interest is necessarily focused more on physiologic aspects; nevertheless, the perspective of partnership and social issues should not be forgotten.

The normal sexual response is traditionally conceptualized as consisting of several phases, including desire, excitation, and orgasm.[2] Although the distinction of phases has been criticized and reformulated by different authors, it still serves to structure the relevant observational, neuroanatomic, physiologic and clinical issues for both genders. Differences in sexual behavior between men and women exist and are determined also by biologic factors. Neural control areas in the central nervous system are dimorphic. This has been studied mostly in rodents; major issues in humans remain to be resolved.[3]

Any lesion involving neural tissue relevant for sexual responses may cause dysfunction, as also may lesions of other neural structures more generally involved in control of sensation, motor function, cognition, and behavior (Fig. 30-1). Thus, all primary sensory areas plus the parietal and inferior temporal lobes process sexual stimuli, the forebrain regulates the initiation and the execution of sexual behavior, the medial preoptic area integrates sensory and hormonal signals, and the amygdala plays a role in the reward aspects of sexual function. Neurons from the paraventricular nucleus project to the thoracic and lumbosacral nuclei concerned with the sexual response, the hypothalamospinal projections being situated in the posterolateral funiculus of the spinal cord. Finally, the sympathetic, parasympathetic, and somatic efferents affect the sexual response, with genital afferents playing a part in the initiation of the cycle and in reinforcing the response.[4] Furthermore, the hypothalamus controls the gonadotropic functions of the pituitary gland and thus prenatal development of genital organs, pubertal development, and the menstrual cycle; hormones finally influence the development of the nervous system.

Fertility and procreation are importantly linked to sexuality, but will not be discussed in depth here.

Desire

Desire or sexual interest (libido) refers to the extent that an individual responds to or seeks out erotic stimuli. This varies with time and circumstances, and its measurement depends on self-ratings of such items as the frequency of spontaneous sexual thoughts, the excitement provoked by them, and the resulting behavioral response. Desire is enhanced by sexual activity itself, exciting circumstances, new sexual partners, hypomania, and certain focal brain lesions (particularly of the frontal and temporal lobes). Depressed patients may develop more than their premorbid levels of sexual desire in response to antidepressant medication and patients with Parkinson disease in response to dopaminergic therapy. Sexual interest may be lowered by lack of opportunity, age, malnutrition, certain addictive or sedative drugs, debilitating illness, depression, epilepsy, and certain focal brain lesions.

Animal experiments have revealed dopaminergic-stimulating and serotonergic-inhibiting mechanisms controlling sexual interest. Androgens are necessary for normal libido, although there are some uncertainties related to this issue. In women, sexual desire is also associated with levels of free testosterone.[5]

The rhinencephalon, including the limbic cortex, is important for sexual desire and behavior. The basal hypothalamus is particularly relevant; it is affected by tissue levels of the sex steroid hormones, and lesions involving it may lead to loss of desire. The medial preoptic area is involved in regulating sexual motivation and performance, and dopamine may regulate penile erection at this level.[6] A functional magnetic resonance imaging (fMRI) study of sexual interest in men (by comparing erotic to sport clips) showed activation in the right parietooccipital sulcus, the left superior occipital gyrus, and the precentral gyri.[7] Functional imaging studies have demonstrated that the ovulatory cycle influences sexual interest[8] and that activations in relevant brain areas are relatively greater in premenopausal than menopausal women.[9]

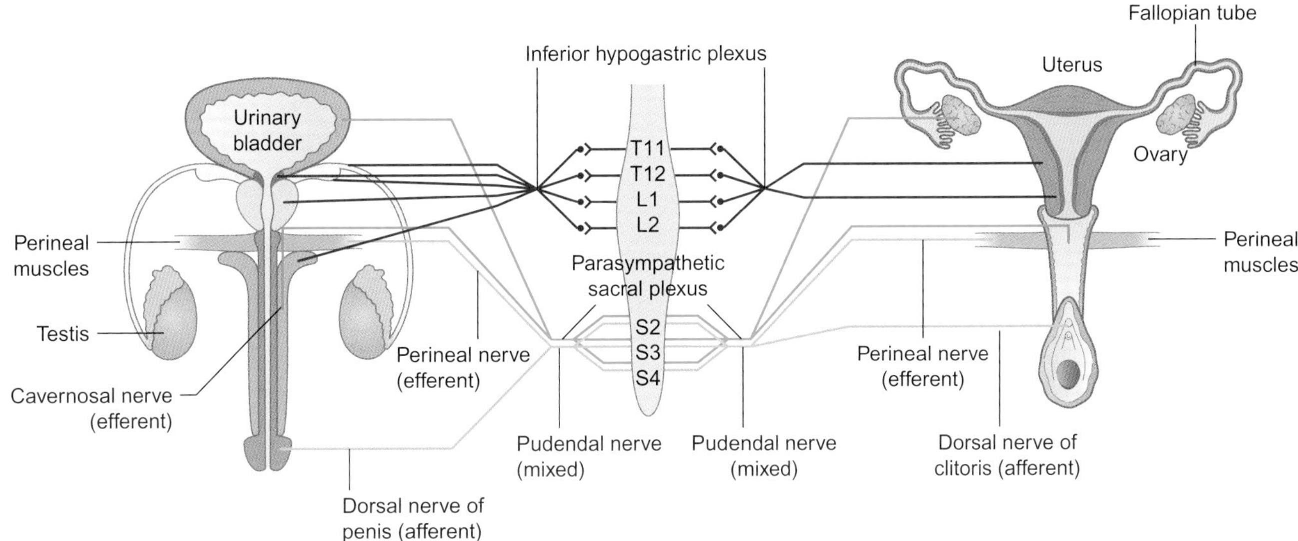

FIGURE 30-1 ■ Schematic representation of the autonomic and somatic innervation of the male (left) and female (right) sexual organs.

Arousal

Sexual excitement results from genital stimulation, other sensory stimuli, or sexual ideation. The glans in both genders has a high receptor density: up to 80 to 90 percent of the nerve endings are free in the most superficial layer of mucosa. There are also corpuscular-type endings beneath the mucosal layer. The receptors are of two types: slowly adapting distally and rapidly adapting proximally, with afferent C and A delta fibers. Surrounding the cavernous bodies are large nerve endings that resemble onions, with thick lamellae and a central nerve fiber connected to thick, myelinated nerve fibers. These nerve endings respond to deep pressure and vigorous movement. Receptors close to the cavernous bodies are influenced by the amount of engorgement of cavernous tissues so that touch may be experienced simply as touch or as a sexual stimulus depending on the degree of engorgement.

Sensory information from the glans and skin of the penis and clitoris is conveyed through bilateral branches of the pudendal nerve (the dorsal nerves of penis/clitoris), as shown schematically in Figure 30-1. The afferents from the root of the penis (and from the anterior part of the scrotum) join the ilioinguinal nerve. Genital afferents synapse in the spinal cord via interneurons with both somatic and autonomic motor neurons; those afferents destined for supraspinal structures travel in the anterolateral funiculus. "Erotically colored" sensations from the genital region are conveyed by the spinothalamic pathways, and patients with selective damage to these tracts may complain of anorgasmia and ejaculatory failure. Orgasmic sensation is blocked by bilateral anterolateral section of the spinal cord (cordotomy).[10]

Somatic sensory afferents deliver information on tactile sexual stimuli that, after synapsing in the sacral spinal cord, induce local sexual responses (i.e., erectile and glandular responses). Sensory information also passes to suprasacral regions and is operative in other reflex activity, leading to awareness of sexual excitation. Both thalamic and cortical areas receive sensory input from the genitals, and sexual feelings may be elicited when such areas are stimulated. In the primary sensory cortex the genitals are traditionally thought to be represented in the parasagittal area; localization on the medial edge of the hemispheric convexity is claimed by a recent functional imaging study.[11]

Somatosensory input from other body parts ("erogenic zones") may—subject to somatic and individual psychologic factors and dependent on context—also lead to sexual excitement. Adequate sexual excitation can be achieved by stimuli delivered through cranial nerves. Although such "extrinsic" excitation—similarly to that achieved by stimulation of sexual organs—should also be called reflex (because there may be little "intrinsic" contribution to the excitatory response), it has traditionally been called "psychogenic." Cortical and subcortical structures related to the limbic system elicit erection when stimulated. (Mental imagery is the "real" psychogenic activator.)

In men during visually evoked sexual arousal, regional cerebral blood-flow measurements by positron emission tomography have demonstrated activation of the inferior temporal cortex (a visual association region) bilaterally, of the right insula and inferior frontal cortex (regions processing sensory information and motivational state), and the left anterior cingulate cortex (involved in neuroendocrine function).[12] Sexual arousal correlated with the magnitude of hypothalamic activation but was more pronounced in men than women. The occipitotemporal region was more activated in men, and the parietal lobe in women.[13]

Sexual excitement leads to a complex response of the autonomic nervous system, and also to typical posturing in different species; in humans this behavior has been studied little but is understood to be influenced by psychosocial and cultural factors.

Parasympathetic efferents from the S2 to S4 spinal segments, traveling through the sacral plexus and cavernosal nerves, initiate erection (Fig. 30-1). (The male erection has to be firm enough for vaginal penetration, and maintained throughout intercourse to bring about ejaculation, which in turn should deliver sperm to the uterine cervix.)

Blood flow in the penile artery, or the corresponding artery in the clitoris, increases. The smooth muscle of the cavernosal sinuses in the penile corpora relax, and the helicine arterioles branching from cavernosal arteries, selectively shunt blood flow to the lacunar spaces of the cavernosal bodies, filling them with blood. Subtunical venules are compressed so that corporeal venous return is restricted, resulting in increasing intracorporeal pressure. The pressure stabilizes at approximately systolic blood pressure, resulting in penile (and clitoral) tumescence and rigidity. Continued sacral parasympathetic activity maintains this erection.

The nerves of the corpora cavernosa have anatomic characteristics different from other nerves. The intracavernous nerves are located in fibrous tunnels, into which numerous fibrous bundles are attached. Contraction of striated pelvic floor muscles, the ischiocavernous muscles in particular, brought about through pudendal nerve activity, increases the rigidity of erection.

In women, parasympathetic activity causes clitoral erection, engorgement of the labia, and vaginal lubrication. The lubrication during sexual arousal is due to transudation through the vaginal wall. Another source is secretion from paraurethral glands (emptying into the urethra). Increased vaginal blood-flow, lubrication, and erection of cavernous tissue in the clitoris and around the outer part of the vagina are the female homologues of the male erectile response; indeed, lubrication occurs during rapid-eye-movement sleep in women. The response is dependent on innervation and a normal estrogen level.[14]

In the periphery, the main proerectile transmitter is nitric oxide, which is co-localized with vasoactive intestinal peptide and acetylcholine; the main antierectile neurotransmitter is norepinephrine.[4] The same mechanisms are responsible for clitoral erection.

Erections can still occur in men and animals after lesions of the sacral cord and pelvic nerves. This is due to the "alternative" proerectile pathway mediated through the hypogastric nerve. This explains the so-called psychogenic erections of paraplegics with conus or cauda equina lesions but preserved thoracolumbar segments.[15] Similarly, women with injury to the sacral spinal cord and an ability to perceive pinprick in the T12 to L2 segments may retain the capacity for psychogenic genital vasocongestion.[16] In women with complete spinal cord injuries and preserved sacral segments, such a response is as a rule obtained only by manual genital stimulation. Thus, the reflex–"psychogenic" dichotomy of the genital sexual response can be seen in both genders.

Inhibitory influences on the sexual response also exist. In nucleus paragigantocellularis a majority of the serotonergic neurons project to the spinal cord (traveling in the lateral funiculus) and provide tonic inhibition of sexual reflexes in the rat.[17]

Orgasm

Seminal emission begins during arousal and, with continued sensory stimulation, orgasm is triggered, with ejaculation of the urethral contents resulting from the rhythmic phasic contractions of perineal and pelvic floor muscles. Ejaculation is effected by integrated sympathetic outflow from T11 to L2 segments traveling through the sympathetic chain and hypogastric plexus and along the pelvic and pudendal nerves, and by somatic efferents traveling through the pudendal nerves. Although the predominant neural control of the male accessory sexual organs is sympathetic (adrenergic and purinergic), the secretion of seminal fluid is under parasympathetic control. Sympathetic activity causes smooth muscle contraction in the seminal vesicles, vas deferens, and prostate to deliver seminal fluid to the posterior urethra; in the bladder neck to prevent retrograde ejaculation; and in the corpora cavernosa to cause detumescence. The latter "antierectile" activity is inhibited during erection through spinal coordination of reflex action.

The female orgasmic response consists of rhythmic contractions of pelvic floor muscles, the uterus, fallopian tubes, and paraurethral glands; expulsions from the paraurethral glands through the urethra may occur (so-called female ejaculation).[18] Women may achieve orgasms by stimulation outside the genital region and probably do so more easily than men, but the most notable difference from men is that women may achieve multiple consecutive orgasms.

Motor innervation of the pelvic floor muscles as well as the ischiocavernosus and bulbocavernosus muscles is conveyed through pudendal nerve branches from below. However, the most relevant motor innervation of the levator ani ("pelvic floor") muscle is directly from the sacral plexus via the levator ani nerve. Electromyographic recording of the pelvic floor muscles in women during vibratory clitoral stimulation shows intermittent activity associated with contractions on a background of continuous activity.[19] During ejaculation in males, repeated bursts of electromyographic activity have been recorded that preceded and followed expulsion of semen. The sensation of orgasm, however, is not dependent on pelvic muscle contractions. Men reported that orgasmic sensation began before, and lasted longer than, bursts of electromyographic activity in the perineal muscles.[20]

Orgasm can be separated conceptually (but not easily physiologically) from emission and ejaculation. Positron emission tomography (PET) imaging during orgasm has shown deactivation of frontal regions and the left temporal lobe; cerebellum and pons were activated (Fig. 30-2). There were only minor differences between genders.[13]

After orgasm (during the "resolution" or "refractory" phase), fMRI revealed activation of amygdala and the temporal lobes, and—for a short period—of the septal area.[21]

Anorgasmia is very rare in neurologically normal men, but 13 percent of women between the ages of 18 and 26 years have never achieved orgasm, with the incidence declining to a minimum of 3 percent in women between the ages of 51 and 64 years.[22]

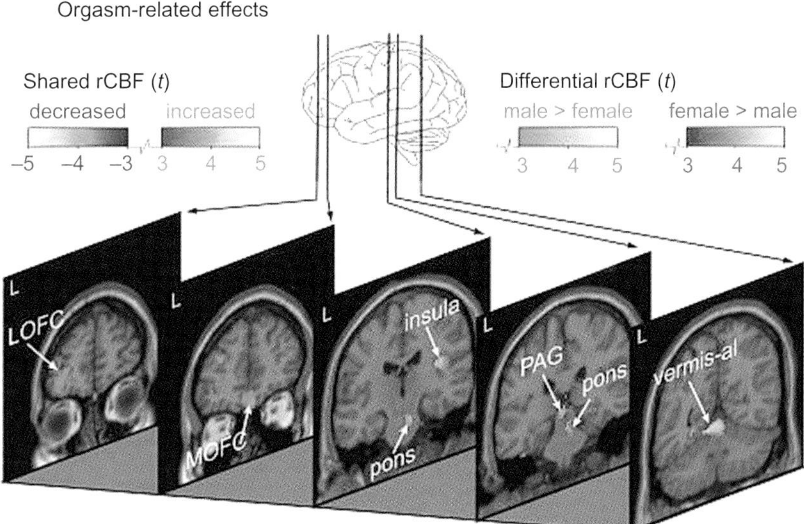

FIGURE 30-2 ■ Functional neuroimaging during male and female orgasm. Orgasm-related effects were evaluated by comparing scans of orgasm with scans of sexual tactile genital stimulation. Activated (orange) and inactivated (blue) areas are the same in men and women. However, certain parts of the brain are more active only in men (green) or in women (red). LOFC, lateral orbitofrontal cortex; MOFC, medial orbitofrontal cortex: PAG, periaqueductal gray: rCBF, regional cerebral blood flow. (From Georgiadis JR, Reinders AA, Paans AM, et al: Men versus women on sexual brain function: prominent differences during tactile genital stimulation, but not during orgasm. Hum Brain Mapp 30:3089, 2009, with permission.)

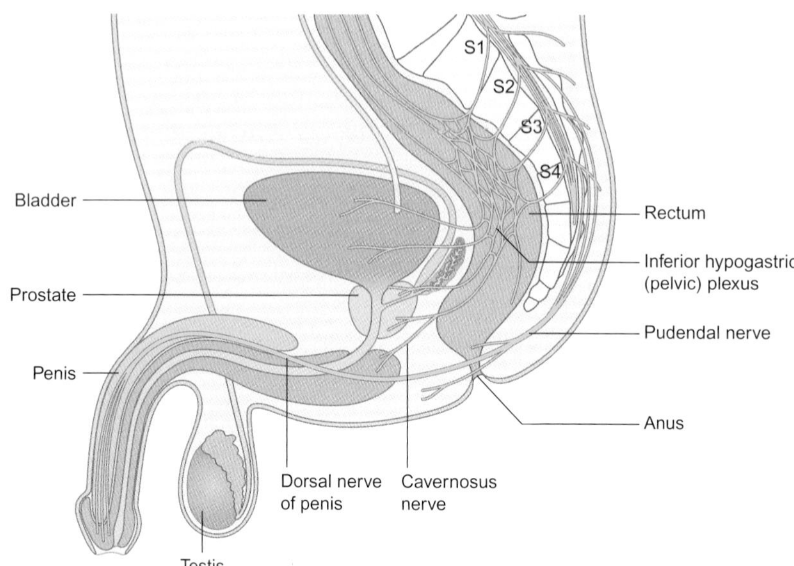

FIGURE 30-3 ■ Anatomy in males of the pudendal nerve (indicating its vulnerability to compression during cycling), and of the pelvic plexus and cavernous nerves (indicating their vulnerability during perineal or pelvic surgery).

Ejaculation can be absent with an intact orgasm in lesions of the hypogastric plexus and under the influence of some drugs.

Topographic Anatomy of Nerves in the Pelvis

The topographic anatomy is important as preservation of the peripheral nerves related to sexual (and bladder and bowel) function during abdominal and pelvic surgery is necessary for good postoperative results. In the pelvis and abdomen, autonomic structures related to genital innervation are situated in the retroperitoneal space. The superior hypogastric plexus is located anterior to the aortic bifurcation at the level of the fifth lumbar vertebral body and sacral promontory between the common iliac arteries. It divides caudally into the right and left hypogastric nerves. Within the pelvis, these nerves become the inferior hypogastric (pelvic) plexus, which is joined on each side by the pelvic nerves. In males, the inferior hypogastric plexus is lateral to the rectum, seminal vesicle, prostate, and the posterior part of the urinary bladder (Fig. 30-3). The lesser and greater cavernosal nerves originate from the anterior part, are joined by fibers from the pudendal nerves, and pass below the pubic arch. In females, the inferior hypogastric (pelvic) plexus gives off uterine nerves, branches for the vagina and cervix, and connections with the paracervical plexus.

Awareness of the anatomy, careful surgical technique and specific intraoperative "mapping" and "monitoring" procedures have been suggested to preserve neural structures relevant for sexual function.[23]

Change in Sexual Function with Aging

There is great variability of sexual functioning in the elderly. The frequency of intercourse as a rule decreases; nevertheless, 26 percent of those aged 75 to 85 years report sexual activity during the past 12 months.[24] Males need more time and stimuli to achieve erection and orgasm. They have a decreased sensation of impending ejaculation and decreased ejaculatory volume. Their refractory period after detumescence is prolonged.[25]

Hormonal changes in menopause lead to decreased libido and thinning of the vaginal wall with decreased elasticity and lubrication. Decreased sexual thoughts and frequency of intercourse after menopause are more closely correlated with testosterone than estrogen levels, but so far most studies have failed to demonstrate a clear relationship between low sexual desire and serum testosterone.[26]

EVALUATION OF PATIENTS WITH SEXUAL DYSFUNCTION AND NEUROLOGIC DISORDERS

The breadth of the history and clinical examination will be tailored by the individual physician's interests and practice habits, but inquiry about sexual function should not be reserved for male patients. With the advent of effective treatment for erectile dysfunction, many physicians take a pragmatic approach to treatment and inquire about little more than whether erectile dysfunction is present. However, there is more to sexual dysfunction than erectile dysfunction, and more to treating any dysfunction than simply prescribing a pill. Dysfunction in an individual patient—even in the presence of neurologic disease—may be due entirely or in part to psychosocial, vascular, endocrine, or other causes.

History

The history should include details of neurologic disease as well as any past history of urologic/gynecologic, cardiovascular, endocrine, psychologic, and psychiatric disturbances. History of disorders of the sex organs, trauma and surgical procedures, the use of prescription drugs, smoking and alcohol habits, and possible drug abuse should also be elicited. The patient's sexual expectations, needs, and behavior should be defined as well as any misconceptions. Before diagnosing dysfunction of sexual organs, the level of actual desire should be established. The term *hypoactive sexual desire disorder* (HSDD) is used to define a persistent or recurrent reduction in desire for sexual activity, alone or with a partner, with inability to respond to sexual cues that would be expected to trigger a sexual response; symptoms need to be associated with personal distress. If present in men, it may be associated with impotence; in women it often occurs with the female sexual arousal disorder (FSAD), which is a persistent or recurrent inability to attain or maintain sufficient sexual excitement that causes personal distress.[14]

Men should be asked about erectile function (the occurrence of nocturnal erections, morning erections, and erections evoked by genital, visual, auditory, or psychogenic stimuli) and women about vaginal lubrication. The nature of ejaculation should be determined, and in particular whether it is premature, retarded, absent, or dribbling (i.e., emissions occur through the urethra without the activity of pelvic floor muscles). Retrograde ejaculation, described as "dry ejaculation," means that ejaculum has entered the bladder. Finally it should be clarified whether the patient can achieve orgasm, and the quality of orgasmic sensations and experiences should be noted. In some circumstances it may be helpful to interview the patient's partner.

Formal questionnaires can be used to obtain standardized information on male sexual function.[27,28] These questionnaires mostly focus on erectile dysfunction (the persistent inability to develop and maintain an erection sufficient for satisfactory sexual activity). The impact on quality of life is covered by another inventory.[29] Questionnaires have also been formulated to assess sexual function in women, for instance the female sexual function index.[30] Formal questionnaires are particularly relevant in research.

Clinical Examination

Sexual development, body length and weight, changes in pigmentation and body hair, and the presence of galactorrhea should be noted. The external genitalia should be examined. Palpation of peripheral pulses (arms, legs, penis), auscultation of the heart, and blood pressure measurement are recommended.

A standard neurologic examination, with inspection of the lower back (for nevus, hypertrichosis, or sinus), the feet (for deformity or muscle atrophy), and the anogenital area may reveal signs of underlying neurologic disease. Examination of the anogenital region involves palpation of the bulbocavernosus muscles in the male, testing for voluntary contraction ("move the penis") and reflex contraction. The anal sphincter (also levator ani) is palpated for tone, voluntary contraction, and reflex contraction in both sexes by rectal examination. The cremasteric reflex (the L1 segment) and the bulbocavernosus and anal reflexes (S2 to S4/5 segments) should be tested.

Investigation of Genital Reaction and Arousal

In men, spontaneous and physiologically induced erection can be studied with a variety of techniques. Spontaneous nocturnal penile tumescence and rigidity can be measured in the sleep laboratory using mercury strain gauges (measuring penile expansion), visual inspection, measurement of buckling force (for assessment of rigidity), and polygraphic confirmation of sleep phases. Continuous monitoring of nocturnal penile tumescence and rigidity can be obtained by a rigidometer during normal sleeping conditions at home and also during daytime napping or in the awake, sexually stimulated state. Various low-cost screening tests for nocturnal penile expansion have been proposed, but their validity is questionable. Testing for nocturnal erections, however, does not reliably distinguish psychologic from central nervous system (CNS) causes of erectile dysfunction, as has been suggested by studies in men with multiple sclerosis.[31] The aforementioned testing remains mainly of research interest.

An intracorporeal penile injection of a vasoactive substance, such as prostaglandin E_1, will induce an erection (in the absence of major vascular pathology), thus strengthening the suspicion of a neurogenic or psychogenic cause of erectile dysfunction. Intracorporeal injection of vasoactive agents has been proposed as an established diagnostic tool in patients undergoing assessment for possible neurogenic erectile dysfunction and is safe when performed by experienced physicians, with an acceptable complication rate.[32]

Suspected vasogenic erectile dysfunction may require the testing of penile vasculature (blood pressure and vascular competence) by a urologist. The purpose of testing should always be defined; pharmacologic testing may be sufficient for the majority of patients, and invasive tests reserved for those in whom surgery is contemplated.

In women, both direct and indirect methods are used to measure blood-flow changes in the labia and vagina. Noncontrast dynamic magnetic resonance imaging (MRI) can assess female sexual arousal quantitatively.[33] All these tests are only of research interest; it has been stressed that vaginal vasocongestion to erotic stimuli may be unaccompanied by erotic feelings, and subjective indices should therefore be obtained when physiologic measurements are made.[34]

Investigations of Neurologic Function

Functional tests are direct extensions of the clinical examination. Special devices and algorithms can be used for quantifying sensory perception on the genital organs and in the perineum. The measurement of vibratory perception (biothesiometry; measuring the vibration perception threshold) on the glans have been advocated for diagnosing sensory neuropathy in male and female patients. The vibration perception threshold on the penis (glans and shaft) in neurologically healthy men is similar to that of the feet, whereas in females this threshold (best measured on the clitoris, labia majora, and perineum[35]) is the same as in the hands. Tests evaluating small-fiber function (e.g., testing for penile thermal sensation) may be more informative about the neural control of erection.

Several neurophysiologic tests have been suggested for assessing sacral or suprasegmental lesions (Table 30-1). Tests measuring conduction through somatic nervous pathways (motor, sensory, and reflex) might be expected to be useful because most lesions should involve both somatic and autonomic neural pathways, and abnormalities obtained on testing the former could be extrapolated to the latter. Even so, these tests are sensitive only to demyelination and not to axonal lesions, which predominate in clinical practice. Electromyography may demonstrate the activation patterns of striated

TABLE 30-1 ■ Tests for Assessing Sacral or Suprasegmental Neural Lesions

Somatic Sensory
Quantitative sensory testing
Dorsal penile nerve neurography
Pudendal somatosensory evoked potentials
Visceral Sensory
Somatosensory evoked potentials to proximal urethra/bladder neck stimulation
Bladder sensitivity testing
Somatic Motor
Electromyography
Motor evoked potentials
Sacral Reflex
Bulbocavernosus reflex
Anal reflex
Sacral reflex to proximal urethra/bladder neck stimulation
Autonomic
Sympathetic skin response
Neurocardiac testing
Cystometry

muscles but is mainly used to differentiate normal from denervated (reinnervated) muscle, discussed in detail elsewhere.[36] Controversy exists about the source and nature of the signals recorded in penile and clitoral electromyography, and the findings have no diagnostic relevance. The lumbosacral sympathetic system may be tested by the sympathetic skin response from the perineum (and penis).[37]

The role in clinical practice of these and the other tests shown in Table 30-1 is limited. In terms of validity, experience, and available normative values, only electromyography (in muscles of the lower sacral myotomes) and the recording of sacral reflex responses and somatosensory evoked potentials to pudendal nerve stimulation are recommended.[38] The patients with possible or probable neurogenic sexual dysfunction in whom such testing might yield a result relevant for diagnosis and prognosis (though rarely important for decisions on therapy) are those with suspected lesions in the peripheral sacral reflex arc. In these patients, support for the presence or absence of a neurologic lesion can be obtained; this may have medicolegal implications. The relationship between a neurologic lesion (or, for that matter, any neurophysiologic test abnormality) and sexual dysfunction is complex; in women with multiple sclerosis, for instance, latency of pudendal (and tibial) somatosensory evoked potentials failed to predict the extent of sexual dysfunction.[39]

Hormone Measurement

When patients with sexual dysfunction have symptoms or signs indicating endocrine dysfunction, hormone assays—or rather, endocrinologic consultation—may be necessary. The hormones to be studied depend on the circumstances (sex, age, and onset and nature of symptoms).

SEXUAL DYSFUNCTION IN PATIENTS WITH NEUROLOGIC DISEASE

Sexual dysfunction, such as lack of libido (in both sexes), erectile dysfunction and disturbances of ejaculation (in men), and deficient lubrication, dyspareunia, and problems with orgasm (in women), is not uncommon in the general population.[40] In patient populations with disorders of the CNS, the prevalence of sexual dysfunction is reportedly higher, although few comparative studies have been done.

Insofar as many neurologic diseases affect primarily elderly patients and also carry the burdens of any chronic affection, the sexual dysfunction "specific" to the neurologic lesion(s) has to be ascertained against the background of valid control groups.

Head and Brain Injuries

Some cognitive impairment, personality change, and sensorimotor disability often remain after traumatic brain injury and may be accompanied by sexual dysfunction as a consequence of either the cerebral lesion or psychosocial factors. Among patients with closed-head injury admitted for 24 hours or more, significant sexual dysfunction was found in 50 percent over a 15-year time span.[41] Decreased or increased sexual desire, erectile failure, and retarded ejaculation may occur, at least in part as a consequence of post-traumatic pituitary dysfunction.[42] Frontal and temporal lesions seem to result more often in sexual disturbances than parieto-occipital lesions. Hypersexuality, disinhibited and inappropriate sexual behavior, sexually aggressive behavior, and changes in sexual preference sometimes follow basal frontal and limbic brain injury and may lead to sex offences. Bilateral anterior temporal lesions may result in the Klüver–Bucy syndrome with hypersexuality and pansexuality (i.e., sexual drive that is directed not only toward humans but also toward animals and inanimate objects).[43]

Cerebrovascular Disease

Decline in desire and the frequency of intercourse after stroke is not unexpected[44]; the best predictor of decreased sexuality between partners is the degree of dependence in activities of daily living. From various studies, about 75 percent of patients who were sexually active before the stroke report a subsequent decrease in coital frequency.[45] Late outcome studies are scant; poor sexual functioning may persist even with otherwise good improvement.

Many men (up to 65%) have erectile dysfunction after a stroke.[46] Erectile dysfunction has been associated with abnormal nocturnal tumescence.[47] Orgasmic and ejaculatory dysfunction after stroke is also common; nevertheless, both erections and ejaculation may return within a year after stroke. Decreased vaginal lubrication and inability to achieve orgasm occur in female patients.[45]

Sexual problems after a stroke may be complicated by other deficits, poor personal image, and lack of coping.

Patients and their partners may avoid sexual intercourse out of concern that another stroke may be precipitated. The heart rate during sexual activity may exceed 180 beats per minute in men and reach similar values in women; the workload during sexual activity is similar to that of climbing stairs or walking briskly. Although the exact risk of stroke during sexual activity is not known, it seems to be low.[48] Patients and their partners may thus be reassured that, in resuming sexual activity, the gains in most instances outweigh any slight risks. These issues should be addressed in counseling.

Hypersexuality after stroke has also been described, but seems to be rare.[49]

Epilepsy

Epilepsy is associated with sexual problems, more often in men than women. Various types of abnormal behavior, hypersexuality, and, most commonly, hyposexuality have been reported, particularly in temporal lobe epilepsy. Satisfaction with life and sexuality is better in patients who are seizure free. The extent to which social and psychologic factors bear on sexual dysfunction is not clear. It is helpful to determine whether disturbances relate to seizures or occur during the interictal period.

Seizures and Sexual Symptoms

Arousal and intercourse can provoke an epileptic attack through several pathophysiologic mechanisms; sexual phenomena may occur as part of an epileptic seizure; and sexual behavior may change in epileptic patients. Hyperventilation accompanying sexual activity can provoke generalized epileptic seizures. Sexual fantasies as well as genital stimuli (masturbation) or orgasm may trigger reflex epilepsy.[50] Sensations in the genital organs may be manifestations of a partial epileptic seizure arising from a genital sensory cortical area. Motor symptoms such as erection and ejaculation or the sensory experience of an orgasm may also occur, the latter particularly from right mesiotemporal foci.[51]

Such events may be experienced by patients as sexual or nonsexual. Pelvic sexual movements, as a part of epileptic automatisms, or compulsive masturbation in front of others may occur during or after a seizure. Complex sexual experiences may occur during an epileptic seizure in patients with complex partial epilepsy, most often in patients with temporal lobe lesions. Sexual automatisms may also occur with frontal lobe lesions.

Deviant sexual behaviors (e.g., exhibitionism, fetishism, or violent sexual behavior) have been related to epilepsy and interpreted as ictal phenomena. Only a few cases have been reported, but the episodic nature of the behavior and its occasional disappearance after treatment favors a causal connection between the behavior and the epilepsy. Complex partial seizures usually occurred, and lesions were present in one or both temporal lobes. Deviant behavior sometimes correlates with the presence of continuous seizure discharges in the electroencephalogram (psychomotor status).[50]

Interictal Phenomena

Patients with epilepsy, regardless of gender, often report a loss of sexual desire, reduced sexual activity, or inhibited sexual arousal; the prevalence of these complaints varies in different studies. Sexual interest is more reduced in patients with left temporal lobe lesions.[52] Paranoid delusions of a sexual nature (such as of being violated) occur in some epileptic patients.[50]

In men with temporal lobe damage and epilepsy, however, desire is sometimes preserved but erectile function is impaired and ejaculatory dysfunction may occur. Nocturnal tumescence may be lost.[53]

Antiepileptic drugs, especially the older agents (phenytoin, phenobarbital, primidone, carbamazepine, and valproate), may lead to hormonal changes (particularly increased estradiol and decreased free testosterone levels in men), as well as decreased sexual desire and performance in both sexes. Menstrual irregularities are common among women with epilepsy. Antiepileptic drugs may influence morphology and motility of spermatozoa.[54] The effect of the newer anticonvulsant drugs on sexual function is claimed to be less (for instance, for oxcarbazepine and lamotrigine).[55] Sexual function is occasionally restored by surgery for epilepsy, but this has been little studied.

Parkinson Disease

Bladder and bowel dysfunction in Parkinson disease are related to specific autonomic nervous system involvement, and the same is probably true for some of the abnormalities in sexuality. The dopaminergic system is intimately involved in neural circuits controlling desire and arousal. In comparison to controls, parkinsonian patients of both genders show a decrease in libido, frequency of intercourse, and ability to reach orgasm; in men, erection and ejaculation are disproportionately affected.[56] Depression is common in parkinsonian patients and may affect sexual activity; its treatment may further compromise sexual function.

Sexual dysfunction is common even in young male parkinsonian patients. In comparison with age-matched controls, in whom the prevalence of impotence was 37.5 percent, the corresponding number in patients with Parkinson disease was 60 percent.[57] An inability to maintain erections occurs in approximately half of parkinsonian men[58]; nocturnal and morning erections may be absent. Many men cannot ejaculate or reach orgasm. As for women with parkinsonism, vaginal tightness, involuntary urination, anxiety, and inhibition are more prevalent than in matched controls.[59]

Tremor may be enhanced during sexual arousal, thereby limiting the patient. Muscle rigidity and bradykinesia may also make sexual activities more difficult and may be worse in the late evenings if dose scheduling is aimed at favoring daytime activities.

Dopaminergic treatment may result in an apparent increase, or normalization, of libido without corresponding improvement in parkinsonism. A true increase in desire and hypersexuality may occur as an adverse reaction to treatment with levodopa[60] and, particularly, with dopamine agonists.[61] On the order of 3 percent of treated patients demonstrate hypersexuality and probably even more do so among those treated with dopamine agonists[62]; this has been attributed to D3 receptor hyperactivation.[63] Spontaneous erections have been reported in patients receiving levodopa. Apomorphine treatment may result in erections and benefits sexual function, as does cabergoline.[64]

Deep brain stimulation of the subthalamic nucleus may have a positive influence on sexual well-being in Parkinson disease, in that male (but not female) patients are reportedly more satisfied with their sexual life.[65] Hypersexuality has been reported as a side effect.[66]

Multiple System Atrophy

Erectile dysfunction is an early sign of multiple system atrophy (MSA) and precedes bladder dysfunction and orthostatic hypotension.[67] In a retrospective study of 46 men, 96 percent had erectile dysfunction at the time of diagnosis; it occurred alone as the first symptom in 37 percent and was part of the presenting symptom-complex in 59 percent.[68] Erectile dysfunction usually began several years before the onset of other neurologic symptoms, often in patients in their early 50s or late 40s. By the time of diagnosis, 30 percent of male patients were also unable to ejaculate. In women, reduced genital sensitivity (as compared to parkinsonian patients and controls) has been reported.[69]

MSA patients have a decrease in desire, the ability to reach orgasm, and the frequency of intercourse.[70] They may, however, develop hypersexuality with dopaminergic treatment.[61]

Other Extrapyramidal Disorders

In families with Huntington disease, members who ultimately develop the disease tend to have more children than those who are spared. Approximately 10 percent of patients with Huntington disease have increased sexual activity, sometimes associated with mania or hypomania. Habitual promiscuity and marital infidelity may be early or initial symptoms of the disease. However, patients may have difficulty in becoming sexually aroused. Paraphilias such as sexual aggression, exhibitionism, and pedophilia may occur.[71]

Disinhibited sexual behavior is common in patients with Gilles de la Tourette syndrome,[72] and increased sexual activity has been reported in patients with Wilson disease.[73]

Hypothalamopituitary Disorders

Hypothalamopituitary dysfunction is usually caused by a pituitary adenoma; less common types of tumors in this region include craniopharyngiomas, meningiomas, optic gliomas, hypothalamic hamartomas, and metastases. Three-fourths of patients with hypothalamopituitary tumors have decreased or absent libido at the time of diagnosis. The figures are higher for large tumors that extend into the suprasellar region than for intrasellar tumors. Decreased libido (related to low serum testosterone levels) is also the first symptom in most men with small pituitary tumors and hyperprolactinemia, but is not a symptom for which patients commonly seek medical advice. Hence, the diagnosis is usually postponed until other symptoms appear, and it may be as long as a decade after the onset of changes in sexual behavior before the pituitary tumor becomes apparent.[74] Erectile dysfunction is also common[50] but, because of reduced sexual interest, is less distressing.

Most women with hypothalamopituitary disorders have amenorrhea. Women with hypoprolactinemia reportedly complain more commonly of loss of sexual desire than those with normal serum prolactin levels.[75]

A low serum testosterone level in patients with erectile dysfunction does not necessarily signify a space-occupying lesion in the hypothalamopituitary region: a neuroimaging study of 164 impotent men with repeatedly low serum testosterone levels detected potentially serious lesions (pituitary lesions greater than 5 mm or any hypothalamic lesion) in 11, including 5 pituitary microadenomas (5 mm or more), 4 pituitary macroadenomas, and 2 hypothalamic lesions.[76]

Multiple Sclerosis

Disturbances of sexual function are common in patients with multiple sclerosis, regardless of gender,[77] and affect eventually the majority of patients.[78] Sexual dysfunction is proven to decrease the quality of life in patients.[79] Most such disturbances relate to spinal cord involvement and are generally, but not always, associated with urinary symptoms and lower limb involvement. Sexual dysfunction has also been correlated with destructive lesions in the pons, as detected by magnetic resonance imaging, in patients with relapsing-remitting multiple sclerosis.[80]

Erectile dysfunction is rare initially, but becomes more common with evolution of multiple sclerosis.[78] Interest in resuming sexual activity persists in 75 percent of patients.[81] Spontaneous improvement in erectile function sometimes occurs. Problems with ejaculation are frequent and are often coupled to the erectile dysfunction. Anorgasmia has been correlated with evidence on magnetic resonance imaging of brainstem and corticospinal abnormalities as well as with total area of lesions.[82]

Decreased vaginal lubrication and sensory disturbances involving the genital region (hypoesthesia, hyperesthesia, and different types of pain) are common and may be apparent already in the early stages of multiple sclerosis.[83] Sacral-segment dysesthesias may be so severe that patients are unable to bear direct genital or nongenital contact. Electrodiagnostic data—cortical evoked potentials of the dorsal nerve of the clitoris[84]—suggest that pudendal somatosensory input is necessary for female orgasmic function, and that this may be disturbed even in early MS.

Some patients experience decreased libido; emotional and cognitive disturbances may be contributory. Increased sexual desire occasionally constitutes a problem. Other symptoms related to multiple sclerosis, such as fatigue, depression, cognitive dysfunction, spasticity in the lower limbs, urinary and bowel disturbances, and the use of aids to manage incontinence, can inhibit sexuality, as can paroxysmal motor and sensory disturbances triggered by sexual intercourse.

Lesions of the Spinal Cord

A spinal cord injury (SCI) or lesion may lead to major neurologic deficits that in men initially often overshadow sexual disturbances such as a loss of normal erectile and ejaculatory function and of the ability to procreate naturally. For women, the resulting sexual dysfunction is often regarded as less limiting but is definitely important. The effects on erection, ejaculation, vaginal lubrication, and orgasm relate to the level and completeness of the lesion.

After complete cord transection, reflex function in all segments of the isolated spinal cord is completely lost (spinal shock) for a variable period lasting from a few hours to several weeks. Incomplete or slowly developing lesions may be associated with little or no spinal shock. The male genital reflexes (reflex penile erection and the bulbocavernosus and cremaster reflexes) are abolished or profoundly depressed during the period of spinal shock, and erectile and ejaculatory functions are abolished. Because of the occurrence of spinal shock, it is usually impossible to predict the extent or severity of sexual dysfunction, including whether erectile and ejaculatory functions will recover, in men within the first weeks after injury. With complete lesions of the spinal cord, the penis may become enlarged and semierect from passive engorgement of the corpora cavernosa due to paralytic vasodilation after the interruption of vasoconstrictor fibers in the anterolateral tracts of the spinal cord. As spinal shock subsides, reflex activity and spasticity may develop in the lower extremities and reflex functioning is regained of the bladder and bowels. In patients with upper motor neuron lesions, the erection reflex becomes part of the autonomic function of the isolated cord and may appear with tactile stimuli of various types and intensity, including stimuli to the penis, independent of cerebral participation and before the reflex responses of skeletal muscles are fully developed.

With complete destruction of the lower sacral spinal cord segments (the conus medullaris), reflex erection and lubrication are usually lost and the striated ejaculatory muscles are paralyzed. With spinal cord lesion between the level of the lower thoracic segments and the conus, both cerebral and reflex erection and lubrication may be possible, even though the patient cannot feel the sexual organs. Loss of sacral sensation does not necessarily imply anorgasmia. Although ejaculatory contractions cannot be felt when a complete lesion of the spinal cord exists above the conus, autonomic components of the orgasm can be experienced. Hyperesthesia often occurs just above or at the level of the spinal cord lesion, and may be useful as an erogenous zone. Although bladder, bowel, and sexual dysfunction often coexist, this is not necessarily the case; sexual function may be preserved in spite of severe neurogenic bladder dysfunction, presumably owing to preservation of the thoracic sympathetic outflow.

A meta-analysis of 24 studies of more than 2,500 men with spinal cord injuries showed that a median of 80 percent (range, 54 to 95%) reported spontaneous erections.[85] The percentage of men reporting ejaculation without therapeutic assistance was much lower (median, 15%; range, 0 to 52%). Fewer (26%) of the patients with complete lower sacral lesions had erectile capacity than those with complete upper cord lesions or incomplete lesions at any level (90 to 99%). However, there is much individual variation, and an accurate prognosis for future sexual function may not be possible in individual cases.

Patients with incomplete spinal cord injury retain the ability for psychogenic genital vasocongestion if pinprick sensation is preserved in the T11 to T12 segments; only reflexogenic responses are obtained in those with complete spinal cord injury.[15,16] After spinal cord injury, women menstruate and are able to conceive and give birth, although those with a paralyzed pelvic floor are at risk of overstretching and perineal tears. Autonomic hyperreflexia (Chapter 8) may occur in those with a lesion above T6–7.

Preoccupation with future sexual performance occurs early after injury, and it may be easier for men to accept motor deficits than sexual problems. Sexual readjustment depends on the individual, on previous sexual habits, and on the cooperation of partners. In one study, sexual readjustment was closely and positively correlated with a young age at injury, frequency of sexual intercourse, and willingness to experiment with alternative sexual expressions. Physical and social independence and a high mood level were further positive determinants of sexual adaptation after injury.[86]

The semen of men with spinal cord injury is characterized by small volume, low sperm count, and low sperm mobility. Reduced fertility cannot therefore be attributed completely to ejaculatory dysfunction.[87] Collection of semen very early after the injury makes it possible to store semen of good quality for future insemination.

The ability to ejaculate by masturbation or sexual intercourse is impaired in most men with severe injury of the spinal cord; consequently, pregnancies caused by such men are rare without medical intervention. Ejaculation can be provoked in many paraplegic men through vibratory stimulation or electrostimulation (with careful blood pressure monitoring because of the risk of autonomic dysreflexia). Repeated vibration-induced ejaculations result in increased volume of semen, a larger number of motile sperms, and improved sperm penetration capacity. Insemination with autologous semen obtained in such a way has resulted in pregnancies.

Orgasms may occur in men with spinal cord injury but may differ from those that occurred before the injury.[88] Women with such injuries may also achieve orgasm; indeed, some women with apparently complete lesions can do so, perhaps because of afferents from the cervix traveling with the vagus nerve.[89] Latency to orgasm is greater in women with spinal cord injury than in normal subjects, but the descriptions of orgasm are indistinguishable.[90]

Cauda Equina Lesions and Lumbar Stenosis

Although complete lesions of the cauda equina damage the parasympathetic erectile pathways to the penis, a number of men (approximately one-fourth) are still able to achieve an erection psychogenically, mediated probably by the sympathetic erectile pathway involving the hypogastric plexus. There are also ejaculatory disturbances (delayed or absent, but occasionally premature ejaculation), penile sensory loss, paresthesias, dysesthesias, and even pain syndromes. In a group of men with cauda equina lesions of differing causes and variable severity, only 15 percent reported normal sexual function.[91] Women report loss of erotic sensation, dyspareunia, loss of lubrication, loss of feeling during vaginal intercourse, difficulties in achieving orgasm, and changes in the feeling of orgasm.[92]

Involvement of lower sacral nerve roots by any process can lead to "positive" as well as "negative" functional symptoms. Sensory symptoms and deficits involving the genitals are not necessarily accompanied by impotence. Spontaneous erections on walking are occasionally reported in patients with symptomatic lumbar stenosis.

Spinal Malformations

Any type of dysraphism may be associated with neurologic symptoms that may include sexual disturbances, but data from large patient populations are lacking. Meningomyelocele as a rule gives rise, among other disturbances, to sexual dysfunction, depending on the severity of the malformation. Some boys have no genital sensations at all, with loss of erection and orgasm; some have isolated erections without emission.[93] Loss of genital sensations is the major complaint in girls.[94]

Erectile dysfunction may occur in patients with Arnold–Chiari malformations; the onset of sexual symptoms is generally after the development of other neurologic disturbances.

Localized Nerve Lesions

Trauma may cause pudendal nerve injury, leading to loss of penile sensation, dysesthesias, pain syndromes, and dribbling ejaculation because of perineal muscle denervation. Among long-distance cyclists, it was found in one study that 22 percent had penile sensory symptoms and 13 percent had erectile dysfunction; symptoms were transient but persisted for up to 8 months.[95]

Erectile dysfunction may follow pelvic fracture, especially when urethral injury has occurred, owing to involvement of the neurovascular bundles. The peripheral autonomic nerves to the genitalia may be injured also by surgical procedures, leading to erectile and ejaculatory dysfunction in men and loss of lubrication in women. The sympathetic thoracolumbar fibers may be injured by retroperitoneal lymph node dissections. Pelvic plexus and cavernosal nerves may be injured by such operations as abdominoperineal resection for carcinoma, hysterectomy, radical prostatectomy, or sphincterotomy, thus significantly impairing the quality of life in patients after otherwise successful surgery (cf. Fig. 30-3). Surgeons are increasingly aware of the need to preserve relevant neural tissue even during radical surgery and have developed "nerve-sparing" operations.[96]

Erectile dysfunction has also been reported after injection of sclerosing agents to treat hemorrhoids and hypersensitive bladder.[97]

Diabetic Polyneuropathy

Diabetes is the most common cause of polyneuropathy in developed countries, and the most frequent type of neuropathy is the distal symmetric sensorimotor variety, in which small nerve fibers may be involved earlier than large fibers. This polyneuropathy is frequently accompanied by autonomic involvement, and dysautonomia is occasionally the predominant clinical presentation, with bladder, bowel, and sexual dysfunction. Hyperglycemia and some glycosylation products promote inactivation of nitric oxide and there seems to be a selective nitrergic neurodegeneration in diabetes.[98] Further discussion of diabetic neuropathy is provided in Chapter 19.

Sexual dysfunction, especially erectile dysfunction, is common in diabetic men. Erectile dysfunction has been reported in 9 percent of diabetic men aged 20 to 29 years, rising to 95 percent of diabetics by age 70. Overall the incidence in a population of 9,500 diabetic men (20 to 70 years old) was 38 percent. Patients had the onset of impotence within the first 10 years of their disease in 50 percent of cases.[99] Men with diabetic polyneuropathy have fewer sleep-related erections, shorter tumescence time, diminished penile circumference increase, and weaker penile rigidity than do nondiabetic men. Erectile dysfunction is usually considered neurogenic when there are other signs of neuropathy, although alternative etiologic possibilities cannot be excluded. There is little correlation with neurophysiologic abnormalities in peripheral nerve function.[100] Although the bulbocavernosus reflex latencies and penile (pudendal) evoked potentials are more often abnormal in impotent than potent diabetic men, neurophysiologic testing of pudendal nerve function is less sensitive in diagnosing neuropathy in impotent diabetics than limb nerve conduction studies.[101]

In patients with cystopathy, retrograde ejaculation is sometimes an additional problem; failure of normal closure of the bladder neck by sympathetic activation during ejaculation leads to semen passing retrogradely into the bladder.

Among women, those with more diabetic complications have greater sexual dysfunction. A correlation in diabetic women of sexual dysfunction with the presence of neuropathy has not been found in all studies. Reduced sexual desire, decreased vaginal lubrication, and decreased capacity to achieve orgasm compared with age-matched controls have been reported.[102]

Chronic Renal Failure

Male patients on hemodialysis have a similar prevalence of erectile dysfunction (71%) to patients on peritoneal dialysis (80%).[103] Neuropathy is not the only possible cause; primary hypogonadism has been reported, and involvement of the testes also leads to low sperm counts and azoospermia. However, even in nondiabetic men with erectile dysfunction who were undergoing hemodialysis, the etiology was usually neuropathic rather than endocrinologic or vascular.[104] On the whole, there is a tendency for preexistent erectile dysfunction to improve after transplantation.[105]

Among women with uremia, one-half have decreased desire, and one-third have decreased lubrication; dysfunction improves after transplantation.[105]

Other Acquired Polyneuropathies

Autonomic dysfunction, including erectile dysfunction, occurs in other peripheral neuropathies, including those due to infectious agents, chemical toxins, secondary amyloidosis, prescription or street drugs, and vitamin B_1 or vitamin B_{12} deficiency, or those that are parainfectious or paraneoplastic. Autonomic involvement may lead to erectile dysfunction in the Guillain–Barré syndrome and may also occur in patients with chronic inflammatory demyelinating polyneuropathy. Reversal of erectile dysfunction and penile sensory loss may follow effective treatment.

In persons infected with the human immunodeficiency virus (HIV), peripheral nerve disorders occur commonly and may be accompanied by a dysautonomia. Slowed sural and dorsal penile sensory conduction velocities suggest that neuropathy is important in the genesis of erectile dysfunction in HIV-positive men.[106] Counseling and treatment may be especially important in AIDS patients with sexual dysfunction, since the use of condoms often precipitates the problem, and men are therefore unwilling to use protection.

Hereditary Polyneuropathies

Erectile dysfunction and ejaculatory problems may occur in patients with hereditary sensory neuropathy and Charcot–Marie–Tooth syndrome.[107] Erectile dysfunction also occurs in primary amyloidotic polyneuropathy[108] and adrenoleukodystrophies. Men with hereditary motor and sensory neuropathy and electrophysiologically proven involvement of the pudendal nerves may nevertheless have normal sexual function.[109]

Amyotrophic Lateral Sclerosis

Sexual function is normal in men with amyotrophic lateral sclerosis. Even when severe weakness makes intercourse impractical, erection and ejaculation are possible through partner masturbation, and the sensation of orgasm may be experienced as normal. These factors are highly relevant with regard to the patient's quality of life and may be important in counseling patients and their partners.

Hereditary Neuromuscular Diseases

The early onset and progressive course of certain hereditary neuromuscular diseases may restrict psychosocial and psychosexual development and limit sexual activity. Nevertheless, the capacity for sexual satisfaction remains unaffected in many patients who survive to adulthood and consequently has led to more awareness of the need for appropriate counseling.

In Kennedy syndrome (X-linked bulbospinal muscular atrophy), gynecomastia is common and testicular atrophy, decreased libido, and erectile dysfunction may occur. Hypogonadism, diminished libido, erectile dysfunction, and amenorrhea occur in certain muscular dystrophies (myotonic dystrophy[110] but also others) and in mitochondrial encephalomyopathies.[111]

Adverse Sexual Reactions to Medications

Many medications used in patients with neurologic disorders have adverse effects on sexuality (Table 30-2). At least until recently, however, the occurrence of sexual dysfunction was rarely monitored in clinical drug trials, and our data are collated from postregistration use, mostly uncontrolled studies and case reports. Further discussion of this aspect is beyond the scope of this chapter.

TABLE 30-2 ■ The Effects on Sexual Function of Some Common Medications Used for Neurologic or Related Purposes

Drug	Effects on Sexual Function
Anticholinergics (e.g., for movement disorders, depression, overactive bladder)	Vaginal dryness
Antihypertensives	Erectile dysfunction
Antipsychotics	Erectile dysfunction Reduced libido
Antidepressants	
Selective/nonselective serotonin reuptake inhibitors	Reduced libido Anorgasmia Delayed ejaculation Erectile dysfunction
Duloxetine	Reduced libido Anorgasmia Delayed ejaculation Erectile dysfunction
Trazodone	Priapism
Tricyclic agents (e.g., for depression, pain)	Erectile dysfunction Reduced libido Anorgasmia Delayed ejaculation
Antiparkinsonian agents	
Levodopa, dopamine agonists	Hypersexuality
Amantadine	Reduced libido
Antispasticity agents	
Baclofen	Erectile dysfunction Delayed ejaculation
Dantrolene	Erectile dysfunction Reduced libido
Antiepileptic drugs	
Enzyme-inducing antiepileptic drugs (e.g., phenytoin, carbamazepine, barbiturates)	Erectile dysfunction Reduced libido
Valproate	Erectile dysfunction Reduced libido Anorgasmia
Topiramate	Erectile dysfunction Anorgasmia
Pregabalin	Erectile dysfunction Delayed ejaculation
Oxcarbazepine	Anorgasmia
Levetiracetam	Reduced libido
Lamotrigine	Hypersexuality*

*Improved sexual function has been reported when patients are switched to lamotrigine.

THERAPY

Sexual dysfunction associated with neurologic disease often increases patients' distress. Discussion with patients and partners about their sexual life should be part of any rehabilitation strategy. In all instances, drug regimens should be reviewed for possible effects on sexual function. Sexual education, counseling, and specific suggestions about therapeutic methods are important, and should be provided by the treating physician. In a limited number of patients, referral to a sexual therapist may be indicated. Methods for sexual rehabilitation in the context of neurologic disorders have been described.[112]

Treatment of Neurogenic Erectile Dysfunction

The development of drug treatments by the oral and intracavernous routes has revolutionized the outlook for men with erectile failure. In neurogenic erectile dysfunction, part of the problem may be penile sensory loss. Additional vibratory stimulation may help in producing a rigid erection sufficient for vaginal penetration. As a last resort, surgical treatment is also possible.

Oral Agents

Specific phosphodiesterase-5 inhibitors continue to be developed to treat erectile dysfunction; the first was sildenafil. These drugs have already been used by several million men. The selective inhibitors of type 5 cyclic guanosine monophosphate phosphodiesterase augment the nitric oxide–mediated relaxation pathway in penile tissues by increasing available cyclic guanosine monophosphate in the corpus cavernosum. These medications therefore do not cause erection but enhance the response to sexual arousal. Sildenafil taken at bedtime also significantly increases nocturnal erections.[113]

Sildenafil is an effective treatment for erectile dysfunction in men with diabetes,[114] patients on dialysis and after renal transplantation,[115] multiple sclerosis,[81] Parkinson disease,[116] spinal cord injury,[117] spina bifida,[118] and familial amyloidotic polyneuropathy.[119] In men with erectile dysfunction after radical prostatectomy, sildenafil is ineffective when a nerve-sparing procedure was not performed on at least one side, but it is effective if the cavernous nerves were spared, although it may take up to 18 months to obtain the best response.[120] Overall, its efficacy in patients with an organic etiology of erectile dysfunction was reported to be 68 percent, being lower in diabetics (59%) and in nonselected post-prostatectomy patients (43%).[121]

Sildenafil (25, 50, or 100 mg) can be taken orally 1 hour before intended sexual activity. (Significant effects have been reported between 30 minutes and 4 to 6 hours after taking the medication.) It should be noted that a meal delays absorption of the drug, and so does slowed gastric emptying such as seen in Parkinson disease and autonomic neuropathy. Treatment should be begun with 25 mg or 50 mg, and the same dose taken several times before it is increased. Dose-finding studies have demonstrated a dose-response curve. Sildenafil can be used repeatedly, and if used once or twice per week there should be no fear of tachyphylaxis.

In men with diabetes mellitus or spinal cord injury, vardenafil (5 to 20 mg)[122] and tadalafil (2.5 to 20 mg) have been used with similar efficacy.[123] Tadalafil has a longer half-life and is thus longer acting.[123]

Phosphodiesterase-5 inhibitors are contraindicated in combination with vasodilator drugs of the nitro type and nitric oxide donors, but a cardiologist can change such drug regimens in suitable patients with erectile difficulties requiring treatment. Phosphodiesterase-5 inhibitors should not be used in patients with retinitis pigmentosa. They are contraindicated in men with hypotension (blood pressure below 90/50 mmHg). Care should be taken to identify men with multiple system atrophy who may have erectile dysfunction, atypical parkinsonism, and asymptomatic postural hypotension. In our experience, an intelligent patient can use sildenafil after clear explanation, with careful planning of activity during the several hours after drug intake and performing sexual activity in the recumbent position.

No evidence was found of sildenafil effects on the myocardium or the conduction system. However, evaluation of functional capacity is necessary in patients with coronary artery disease, who need to know the risks of physical (and sexual) activity. Patients who can exercise to 4.5 metabolic equivalents without angina or hypotension can probably use sildenafil safely. Recommendations for the use of sildenafil in patients with cardiovascular disease have been published.[123] In controlled and open-label studies, no increased risk of cerebrovascular events has been reported, although one patient has shown a temporal association of sildenafil use with a transient ischemic attack and then a stroke.[124]

The most common adverse events of sildenafil are headache, flushing, and dyspepsia. Temporary visual symptoms (mainly color-vision disturbances) may occur with higher doses (100 mg), and nonvasculitic anterior optic neuropathy has been described in rare instances. Adverse effects are mostly transitory and of minor intensity.

Treatment with apomorphine sublingually has been introduced as another therapeutic option for men with erectile dysfunction, but due to its relatively weaker effect and obnoxious side effect (nausea) it is less effective than phosphodiesterase-5 inhibitors.

Yohimbine is an ancient aphrodisiac that is produced from the yohimbine tree (*Pausinystalia yohimbine* of the Rubiaceae family), which grows in West Africa. It has little to offer in the presence of modern drugs.

INTRACAVERNOUS INJECTION THERAPY

Intrapenile injections of papaverine have been used extensively in the treatment of erectile dysfunction in men with spinal cord injury, multiple sclerosis, and other neurogenic conditions. Doses did not relate statistically to the level or extent of spinal injury.[125] Prostaglandin E_1, papaverine, and a papaverine-phentolamine mixture all showed an efficacy rate of more than 70 percent. Acute complications such as priapism were, however, lower with prostaglandin (25%) than papaverine (65%) or a papaverine-phentolamine mixture (63%); the risk of local long-term complications was also lower with prostaglandin (8%) than with papaverine (57%) or a papaverine-phentolamine mixture (12.4%).[126]

Prostaglandin E_1 (alprostadil) is now the preferred drug for self-injection therapy in erectile dysfunction. Intracavernous injection should be taught under medical supervision before self-administration is attempted by the patient or his partner. The effect is very rapid and may last for 2 to 4 hours. Its efficacy in diabetic patients with impotence has been confirmed.[127] Local bleeding, pain, and fibrosis may develop in the corpora cavernosa, leading to loss of effectiveness. This treatment is contraindicated in patients taking anticoagulants or with hematologic malignancies.

Long-lasting erections—priapism—as an adverse drug reaction usually have a good prognosis with conservative treatment. Painless priapism of less than 6 hours' duration should be treated at first by cooling. If present for more than 6 but less than 24 hours, intracavernous injection of an alpha-adrenergic agonist such as metaraminol is recommended. In painful priapism or with failure of conservative methods, penile puncture should be performed, at which time a cavernosal blood sample should be obtained to assess cavernosal hypoxia.[128]

Intraurethral Therapy

Intraurethral therapy with alprostadil (prostaglandin E_1) has been introduced as a less invasive alternative; in a study of patients with spinal cord injury, it was found to be of variable effectiveness and less satisfactory than intracavernosal injection therapy.[129]

Vacuum Devices

Rigidity adequate for penetration occurs in 90 percent of patients with neurogenic erectile dysfunction when a vacuum device is used. Satisfaction of partners was initially reported as high (70%), but after months of treatment, and despite an increase in sexual activity, only 41 percent of patients were satisfied.[130] Premature loss of rigidity and difficulty in placing and removing the constriction bands are common complaints. The most common complications are bruises, petechiae, and skin edema. The constriction band should not stay in place for longer than 30 minutes; major complications such as penile gangrene, severe erosion, and cellulitis have been associated with prolonged wearing of the band.

The use of a constriction band (on its own) may help patients who can obtain an erection, albeit not a durable one; the same restrictions concerning the duration of application should be observed.

Surgical Treatment

Penile prostheses (implanted semi-firm or inflatable rods) were introduced in the 1970s, but, with the advent of pharmacologic treatment options, have limited utility in neurologic patients. They may still be useful as a last resort, but are not considered further here. Surgical arterial revascularization and procedures to treat cavernous insufficiency (i.e., venous leakage) are not indicated in patients with neurologic disorders.

Ejaculatory Dysfunction in Men with Neurologic Disorders

In cases of anejaculation/anorgasmia, vibratory stimulation may be helpful. The presence of functional penile nerves is necessary for orgasm achieved by penile vibratory stimulation. (Interestingly, penile vibration has a significant antispastic effect.)

Diabetes mellitus, retroperineal lymph node resection, and certain pharmacologic agents may render the patient effectively sympathectomized, leading to failure of seminal emission or to retrograde ejaculation. Patients may respond to a variable extent to sympathomimetic pharmacologic agents such as imipramine, phenylpropanolamine, or ephedrine. If retrograde ejaculation persists, sperm retrieval from the bladder is usually all that is required when insemination is contemplated. If unsuccessful, procedures such as surgical sperm retrieval from the testis, epididymis, or vas deferens may be necessary. Such patients are usually poor candidates for the assisted ejaculation procedure of penile vibratory stimulation because the sympathetic innervation necessary for seminal emission is not intact.

Treatment options for insemination in other neuropathic conditions include assisted ejaculation or surgical sperm retrieval. The choice of treatment depends on the patient's ability to respond to methods of assisted ejaculation and on the quantity and quality of sperm in the ejaculate. With surgical methods, the assisted reproductive technology of intracytoplasmic sperm injection will probably be required owing to the low numbers of sperm obtained with these methods. Assisted ejaculation methods generally result in higher numbers of sperm, thus allowing for more assisted reproductive technology options.[131]

Premature (or rapid) ejaculation has been associated with myelopathy and neuropathy, but is nowadays usually considered to be constitutional, with psychogenic contributory mechanisms. Counseling on the use of particular techniques may lead to improvement. Pharmacotherapeutic options include topical anesthetics, antidepressants (selective serotonin reuptake inhibitors such as paroxetine), and phosphodiesterase-5 inhibitors, all used off-label.[132]

Treatment of Abnormalities of Libido

Hormone insufficiency, testosterone in men and estrogens in women, should be corrected. Hyperprolactinaemia should be treated.

For abnormally increased libido, pharmacologic treatment should be checked. Androgen antagonists (cyproterone acetate, medroxyprogesterone acetate) may be effective. In resistant cases, neuroleptics are usually helpful.

Treatment in Women with Sexual Dysfunction

Vibratory stimulation and dildos may be helpful and are routinely advised in patients with genital sensory disturbances and in those with weakness or motor disorders.

Sildenafil has been well tolerated in women with neurologic disorders causing lack of sexual arousal, such as multiple sclerosis[39] and spinal cord injury,[133] with few benefits or side effects. In multiple sclerosis, there was an effect on lubrication, but quality of life did not improve significantly although some women opted to continue on the drug after conclusion of the study.[39] Clearly sildenafil does not produce the same spectacular results in women as it does in men with disturbed sexual responses related to underlying neurologic disorders.

In women with dysesthetic or painful sensations in the genitalia that are not alleviated by improving lubrication, antiepileptic drugs such as gabapentin, pregabalin, and carbamazepine may help. Women showing signs of estrogen insufficiency should be referred to a gynecologist for hormone replacement therapy.

NEUROLOGIC PROBLEMS ASSOCIATED WITH SEXUAL ACTIVITY

Headache

Headaches related to sexual activity must be treated as potentially serious because subarachnoid hemorrhage may occur during exertion and headaches of other cause may also be exacerbated in the sexual context. Vascular mechanisms are the probable cause of headaches that occur during sexual arousal in patients with unruptured aneurysms, cerebral tumors, and subdural hematomas. Pain due to angina pectoris or myocardial infarction may be referred to the head. Low-pressure postcoital headache, analogous to that following lumbar puncture, may also occur; symptoms are relieved by recumbency.

Regardless of cause, a headache developing for the first time during sexual activity, particularly if it is of sudden onset and occurs at orgasm, is usually alarming; many patients are convinced that they have had a cerebral hemorrhage. Luckily, most sexual headaches are benign and self-limiting.

The designation *benign coital cephalalgia* refers to a severe, usually sudden, occipital headache that occurs at orgasm. The pain, which is pulsatile, may not end with the cessation of sexual activity; its mean duration is 30 minutes (10 to 180 minutes).[134] Headache may also begin during sexual activity but before orgasm (typically 2 to 3 minutes before; so-called *preorgasmic headache*) and generally worsens as orgasm approaches; it may last from 10 minutes to several hours. The headache is usually occipital in location but may spread diffusely. It may be pulsatile but is more often felt as pressure on the head.[134] A dull, long-lasting, tension-type discomfort can outlast the headache. The headache may be accompanied by nausea, vertigo, and other symptoms, but often stops after cessation of sexual activity. These types of headache are rare; orgasmic headache is about four times more frequent than preorgasmic headache. Men are afflicted more often than women (3–4:1); the first peak of occurrence is early in the third decade, with the second late in the fourth decade. Comorbidity with migraine, tension-type headache, and exertional headache is common. The headaches may be recurrent, but spontaneous remission is the rule. There have been no controlled studies of treatment; short-term prophylaxis with indomethacin has been recommended.

Postcoital migraine is well documented and may occur in patients with benign coital cephalalgia. Its character is identical to the patient's usual pattern of migraine, and the onset is postorgasmic, beginning minutes or hours after the event. On occasion, particularly in women, sexual arousal forms part of the aura of migraine.

Ampoules of amyl nitrite, crushed and inhaled immediately before the event, are sometimes used in an attempt to enhance orgasm. A potent vasodilator, this drug may produce severe vascular headache. More often "sexual activity–associated" headache is nowadays a side effect of the use of phosphodiesterase inhibitors taken for treatment (or sport).

Transient Global Amnesia

Transient global amnesia is sometimes associated with a precipitating event. "Emotional" events predominate in women, "physical" events in men. Sexual intercourse may qualify for both categories and has been regularly reported among provoking events in both genders.[135]

CONCLUDING COMMENTS

Many questions regarding the neuroanatomy and neurophysiology of sexual function remain to be answered. The fine neural control of human sexual behavior by the cerebral hemispheres, brainstem, and spinal cord is far from elucidated. Tools to define the role of psychosocial and biologic factors (such as endocrine, neurologic, vascular, endothelial, and other factors) in the individual with sexual dysfunction are still crude. The options to help patients have nevertheless improved significantly in the last decades. Patients need the interest and support of their physicians in the realm of sexuality; they deserve no less.

ACKNOWLEDGMENT

D. B. Vodušek acknowledges previous collaborations with C. J. Fowler and P. O. Lundberg on texts related to sexual dysfunction in neurologic patients. Some of the material in this chapter appeared in an earlier edition of this book in a chapter co-authored by C. J. Fowler. We thank Ms. Vanja Škedelj for help with manuscript preparation.

REFERENCES

1. Foley FW, Iverson J: Sexuality and MS. p. 63. In: Kalb RC, Scheinberg LC (eds): Multiple Sclerosis and the Family. Demos, New York, 1992.
2. Lue TF, Basson R, Rosen R, et al (eds): Sexual Medicine. Editions 21, Paris, 2004.
3. Sakamoto H: Brain–spinal cord neural circuits controlling male sexual function and behavior. Neurosci Res 72:103, 2012.
4. Giuliano FA, Rampin O, Benoit G, et al: Neural control of penile erection. Urol Clin North Am 22:747, 1995.
5. Meston CM, Frohlich PF: Update on female sexual function. Curr Opin Urol 11:603, 2001.
6. McKenna KE: Neural circuitry involved in sexual function. J Spinal Cord Med 24:148, 2001.
7. Mouras H, Stoleru S, Bittoun J, et al: Brain processing of visual sexual stimuli in healthy men: a functional magnetic resonance imaging study. Neuroimage 20: 855, 2003.
8. Zhu X, Wang X, Parkinson C, et al: Brain activation evoked by erotic films varies with different menstrual phases: an fMRI study. Behav Brain Res 206:279, 2010.
9. Jeong GW, Park K, Youn G, et al: Assessment of cerebrocortical regions associated with sexual arousal in premenopausal and menopausal women by using BOLD-based functional MRI. J Sex Med 2:645, 2005.
10. Beric A, Light JK: Anorgasmia in anterior spinal cord syndrome. J Neurol Neurosurg Psychiatry 56:548, 1993.
11. Kell CA, von Kriegstein K, Rosler A, et al: The sensory cortical representation of the human penis: revisiting somatotopy in the male homunculus. J Neurosci 25:5984, 2005.
12. Stoléru S, Grégoire M-C, Gérard D, et al: Neuroanatomical correlates of visually evoked sexual arousal in human males. Arch Sex Behav 28:1, 1999.
13. Georgiadis JR, Reinders AA, Paans AM, et al: Men versus women on sexual brain function: prominent differences during tactile genital stimulation, but not during orgasm. Hum Brain Mapp 30:3089, 2009.
14. Basson R, Weijmar Shultz WCM, Binik YM, et al: Women's sexual desire and arousal disorders and sexual pain. p. 851. In Lue TF, Basson R, Rosen R, et al (eds): Sexual Medicine. Editions 21, Paris, 2004.
15. Benevento BT, Sipski ML: Neurogenic bladder, neurogenic bowel, and sexual dysfunction in people with spinal cord injury. Phys Ther 82:601, 2002.
16. Sipski ML, Alexander CJ, Rosen RC: Physiologic parameters associated with sexual arousal in women with incomplete spinal cord injuries. Arch Phys Med Rehabil 78:305, 1997.
17. McKenna KE, Chung SK, McVary KT: A model for the study of sexual function in anesthetized male and female rats. Am J Physiol 261:R1276, 1991.

18. Whipple B: Beyond the G spot: new research on human female sexual anatomy and physiology. Scand J Sexol 3:35, 2000.
19. Gillan P, Brindley GS: Vaginal and pelvic floor responses to sexual stimulation. Psychophysiology 16:471, 1979.
20. Gerstenberg TC, Levin RJ, Wagner G: Erection and ejaculation in man: assessment of the electromyographic activity of the bulbocavernosus and ischiocavernosus muscles. Br J Urol 65:395, 1990.
21. Mallick HN, Tandon S, Jagannathan NR, et al: Brain areas activated after ejaculation in healthy young human subjects. Indian J Physiol Pharmacol 51:81, 2007.
22. Janus SS, Janus CL: The Janus Report on Sexual Behavior. John Wiley & Sons, New York, 1993.
23. Rodi Z, Vodušek DB: Monitoring of neural structures involved in micturition and sexual function. p. 739. In Nuwer MR ed: Intraoperative Monitoring of Neural Function. Handbook of Clinical Neurophysiology Vol 8. Elsevier, Amsterdam, 2008.
24. Lindau St, Schumm LP, Laumann EO, et al: A study of sexuality and health among older adults in the United States. N Engl J Med 357:762, 2007.
25. Rowland DL, Greenleaf WJ, Dorfman LJ, et al: Aging and sexual function in men. Arch Sex Behav 22:545, 1993.
26. Gracia CR, Freeman EW, Sammel MD, et al: Hormones and sexuality during transition to menopause. Obstet Gynecol 109:831, 2007.
27. O'Leary MP, Fowler FJ, Lenderking WR, et al: A brief male sexual function inventory for urology. Urology 46:697, 1995.
28. Rosen RC, Riley A, Wagner G, et al: An international index of erectile function (IIEF): a multidimensional scale for assessment of erectile dysfunction. Urology 49:822, 1997.
29. Wagner TH, Patrick DL, McKenna SP, et al: Cross-cultural development of a quality of life measure for men with erection difficulties. Qual Life Res 5:443, 1996.
30. Rosen R, Brown C, Heiman J, et al: The Female Sexual Function Index (FSFI): a multidimensional self-report instrument for the assessment of female sexual function. J Sex Marital Ther 26:191, 2000.
31. Ghezzi A, Zaffaroni M, Baldini S, et al: Sexual dysfunction in male multiple sclerosis patients in relation to clinical findings. Eur J Neurol 3:462, 1996.
32. Therapeutics and Technology Assessment Subcommittee American Academy of Neurology Assessment: neurological evaluation of male sexual dysfunction. Neurology 45:2287, 1995.
33. Maravilla KR, Cao Y, Hewman JR, et al: Noncontrast dynamic magnetic resonance imaging for quantitative assessment of female sexual arousal. J Urol 173:162, 2005.
34. Laan E, Everaerd W: Physiological measures of vaginal vasocongestion. Int J Impot Res 10(suppl 2):S107, 1998.
35. Hulter BM, Lundberg PO: Genital vibratory perception threshold (VPT) measurements in women with sexual dysfunction and/or sexual pain disorders. Eur J Sexual Health 15(suppl):S33, 2006.
36. Vodušek DB, Fowler CJ: Pelvic floor clinical neurophysiology. p. 281. In: Binnie C, Cooper R, Mauguière F (eds): Clinical Neurophysiology. Vol 1. EMG, Nerve Conduction and Evoked Potentials. Elsevier, Amsterdam, 2004.
37. Vodušek DB: Pelvic floor conduction studies. p. 295. In Kimura J ed: Peripheral Nerve Diseases. Handbook of Clinical Neurophysiology Vol 7. Elsevier, Edinburgh, 2006.
38. Vodušek DB, Amarenco G, Podnar S: Clinical neurophysiological tests. p. 523. In Abrams P, Cardozo L, Khoury S, et al (eds): Incontinence. 4th International Consultation on Incontinence, Paris, July 5–8, 2008. Health Publication, Paris, 2009.
39. Dasgupta R, Wiseman OJ, Kanabar G, et al: Efficacy of sildenafil in the treatment of female sexual dysfunction due to multiple sclerosis. J Urol 171:1189, 2004.
40. Addis IB, Van Den Eeden SK, Wassel-Fyr CL, et al: Sexual activity and function in middle aged and older women. Obstet Gynecol 107:755, 2006.
41. O'Carroll R, Woodrow J, Maroun F: Psychosexual and psychosocial sequelae of closed head injury. Brain Inj 5:303, 1991.
42. Agha A, Rogers B, Sherlock M, et al: Anterior pituitary dysfunction in survivors of traumatic brain injury. J Clin Endocrinol Metab 89:4929, 2004.
43. Hayman LA, Rexer JL, Pavol MA, et al: Klüver-Bucy syndrome after bilateral selective damage of amygdala and its cortical connections. J Neuropsych Clin Neurosci 10:354, 1998.
44. Giaquinto S, Buzzelli S, Di Francesco L, et al: Evaluation of sexual changes after stroke. J Clin Psychiatry 64:302, 2003.
45. Korpelainen JT, Kaulhanen M-L, Kemola H, et al: Sexual dysfunction in stroke patients. Acta Neurol Scand 98:400, 1998.
46. Aloni R, Schwartz J, Ring H: Sexual function in male patients after stroke—a follow up study. Sex Disabil 11:121, 1993.
47. Nakayama H, Jorgensen HS, Pedersen PM, et al: Prevalence and risk factors of incontinence after stroke. The Copenhagen Stroke Study. Stroke 28:58, 1997.
48. Monga TN, Ostermann HJ: Sexuality and sexual adjustment in stroke patients. Phys Med Rehabil State of Art Rev 9:345, 1995.
49. Mutarelli EG, Omuro AM, Adoni T: Hypersexuality following bilateral thalamic infarction: case report. Arq Neuropsiquiatr 64:146, 2006.

50. Lundberg PO: Sexual dysfunction in patients with neurological disorders. Annu Rev Sex Res 23:121, 1992.
51. Janszky J, Szucs A, Halasz P, et al: Orgasmic aura originates from the right hemisphere. Neurology 58:302, 2002.
52. Braun CM, Dumont M, Duval J, et al: Opposed left and right brain hemisphere contributions to sexual drive: a multiple lesion case analysis. Behav Neurol 14:55, 2003.
53. Goldner GT, Morrell MJ: Nocturnal penile tumescence and rigidity evaluation in men with epilepsy. Epilepsia 37:1211, 1996.
54. Isojärvi JI, Lofgren E, Juntunen KS, et al: Effect of epilepsy and antiepileptic drugs on male reproductive health. Neurology 62:247, 2004.
55. Sachdeo R, Sathyan RR: Amelioration of erectile dysfunction following a switch from carbamazepine to oxcarbazepine: recent clinical experience. Curr Med Res Opin 21:1065, 2005.
56. Sakakibara R, Shinotoh H, Uchiyama T, et al: Questionnaire-based assessment of pelvic organ dysfunction in Parkinson's disease. Auton Neurosci 92:76, 2001.
57. Singer C, Weiner WJ, Sanchez-Ramos IR, et al: Sexual function in patients with Parkinson's disease. J Neurol Neurosurg Psychiatry 54:942, 1991.
58. Wermuth L, Stenager E: Sexual problems in young patients with Parkinson's disease. Acta Neurol Scand 91:453, 1995.
59. Welsh M, Hung L, Waters CH: Sexuality in women with Parkinson's disease. Mov Disord 12:923, 1997.
60. Uitii R, Tanner C, Rajput A, et al: Hypersexuality with antiparkinsonism therapy. Clin Neuropharmacol 5:375, 1989.
61. Klos KJ, Bower JH, Josephs KA, et al: Pathological hypersexuality predominantly linked to adjuvant dopamine agonist therapy in Parkinson's disease and multiple system atrophy. Parkinsonism Relat Disord 11:381, 2005.
62. Voon V, Hassan K, Zurowski M, et al: Prevalence of repetitive and reward-seeking behaviors in Parkinson disease. Neurology 67:1254, 2006.
63. Fenu S, Wardas J, Morelli M: Impulse control disorders and dopamine dysregulation syndrome associated with dopamine agonist therapy in Parkinson's disease. Behav Pharmacol 20:363, 2009.
64. Safarinejad MR: Salvage of sildenafil failures with cabergoline: a randomized, double-blind, placebo-controlled study. Int J Impot Res 18:550, 2006.
65. Castelli L, Perozzo P, Genesia ML, et al: Sexual well being in parkinsonian patients after deep brain stimulation of the subthalamic nucleus. J Neurol Neurosurg Psychiatry 75:1260, 2004.
66. Romito LM, Raja M, Daniele A, et al: Transient mania with hypersexuality after surgery for high frequency stimulation of the subthalamic nucleus in Parkinson's disease. Mov Disord 17:1371, 2002.
67. Kirchhof K, Apostolidis AN, Mathias CJ, et al: Erectile and urinary dysfunction may be the presenting features in patients with multiple system atrophy: a retrospective study. Int J Impot Res 15:293, 2003.
68. Beck RO, Betts CD, Fowler CJ: Genitourinary dysfunction in multiple system atrophy: clinical features and treatment in 62 cases. J Urol 151:1336, 1994.
69. Oertel WJ, Wachter T, Quinn NP, et al: Reduced genital sensitivity in female patients with multiple system atrophy of parkinsonian type. Mov Disord 18:430, 2003.
70. Yamamoto T, Sakakibara R, Uchiyama T, et al: Questionnaire-based assessment of pelvic organ dysfunction in multiple system atrophy. Mov Disord 24:972, 2009.
71. Morris M: Dementia and cognitive changes in Huntington's disease. Adv Neurol 65:187, 1995.
72. Lombroso PJ, Scahill LD, Chappell PB, et al: Tourette's syndrome: a multigenerational, neuropsychiatric disorder. Adv Neurol 65:305, 1995.
73. Akil M, Brewer GJ: Psychiatric and behavioral abnormalities in Wilson's disease. Adv Neurol 65:171, 1995.
74. Lundberg P, Hulter B: Sexual dysfunction in patients with hypothalamo-pituitary disorders. Exp Clin Endocrinol 98:81, 1991.
75. Hulter BM, Lundberg PO: Sexual function in women with hypothalamo-pituitary disorders. Arch Sex Behav 23:171, 1994.
76. Citron JT, Ettinger B, Rubinoff H, et al: Prevalence of hypothalamic-pituitary imaging abnormalities in impotent men with secondary hypogonadism. J Urol 155:529, 1996.
77. McCabe MP: Exacerbation of symptoms among people with multiple sclerosis: impact of sexuality. Arch Sex Behav 33:593, 2004.
78. Zorzon M, Zivadinov R, Monti Bragadin L, et al: Sexual dysfunction in multiple sclerosis: a 2-year follow-up study. J Neurol Sci 187:1, 2001.
79. Nortvedt MW, Riise T, Myhr KM, et al: Reduced quality of life among multiple sclerosis patients with sexual disturbance and bladder dysfunction. Mult Scler 7:231, 2001.
80. Zivadinov R, Zorzon M, Locatelli L, et al: Sexual function in multiple sclerosis: a MRI, neurophysiological and urodynamic study. J Neurol Sci 210:73, 2003.
81. Fowler CJ, Miller JR, Sharief MK, et al: A double blind, randomised study of sildenafil citrate for erectile dysfunction in men with multiple sclerosis. J Neurol Neurosurg Psychiatry 76:700, 2005.
82. Barak Y, Achiron A, Elizur A, et al: Sexual dysfunction in relapsing-remitting multiple sclerosis: magnetic resonance imaging, clinical, and psychological correlates. J Psychiatry Neurosci 21:255, 1996.
83. Tzortzis V, Skriapas K, Hadjigeorgiou G, et al: Sexual dysfunction in newly diagnosed multiple sclerosis women. Mult Scler 14:561, 2008.

84. Yang CC, Bowen JR, Kraft GH, et al: Cortical evoked potentials of the dorsal nerve of the clitoris and female sexual dysfunction in multiple sclerosis. J Urol 164:2010, 2000.
85. Lundberg PO, Brackett LB, Denys P, et al: Neurological disorders: erectile and ejaculatory dysfunction. p. 591. In Jardin A, Wagner G, Khoury S, et al (eds): Erectile Dysfunction. Plymbridge, Plymouth, UK, 2000.
86. Siösteen A, Lundqvist C, Blomstrand C, et al: Sexual ability, activity, attitudes and satisfaction as part of adjustment in spinal cord-injured subjects. Paraplegia 28:285, 1990.
87. Brackett NL, Bloch WE, Lynne CM: Predictors of necrospermia in men with spinal cord injury. J Urol 159:844, 1998.
88. Alexander CJ, Sipski ML, Findley TW: Sexual activities, desire and satisfaction in males pre- and post-spinal cord injury. Arch Sex Behav 22:217, 1993.
89. Whipple B, Komisaruk BR: Sexuality and women with complete spinal cord injury. Spinal Cord 35:136, 1997.
90. Sipski ML, Alexander CJ, Rosen RC: Sexual arousal and orgasm in women: effects of spinal cord injury. Ann Neurol 49:35, 2001.
91. Podnar S, Oblak C, Vodušek DB: Sexual function in men with cauda equina lesions: a clinical and electromyographic study. J Neurol Neurosurg Psychiatry 73:715, 2002.
92. Sipski ML, Alexander CJ, Rosen R: Sexual arousal and orgasm in women: effects of spinal cord injury. Ann Neurol 49:35, 2001.
93. Joyner BD, McLorie GA, Khoury AE: Sexuality and reproductive issues in children with myelomeningocele. Eur J Pediatr Surg 8:29, 1998.
94. Sawyer SM, Roberts KV: Sexual and reproductive health in young people with spina bifida. Dev Med Child Neurol 41:671, 1999.
95. Andersen KV, Bovim G: Impotence and nerve entrapment in long distance amateur cyclists. Acta Neurol Scand 95:233, 1997.
96. Klotz L: Cavernosal nerve mapping: current data and applications. BJU Int 93:9, 2004.
97. Bullock N: Impotence after sclerotherapy of haemorrhoids: case report. BMJ 314:419, 1997.
98. Cellek S, Rodrigo J, Lobos E, et al: Selective nitrergic neurodegeneration in diabetes mellitus—a nitric oxide–dependent phenomenon. Br J Pharmacol 128: 1804, 1999.
99. Fedele D, Bortolotti A, Coscelli C, et al: Erectile dysfunction in type 1 and type 2 diabetics in Italy. On behalf of Gruppo Italiano Studio Deficit Erettile nei Diabetici. Int J Epidemiol 29:524, 2000.
100. Žgur T, Vodušek DB, Krzan M, et al: Autonomic system dysfunction in moderate diabetic polyneuropathy assessed by sympathetic skin response and Valsalva index. Electromyogr Clin Neurophysiol 33:433, 1993.
101. Vodušek DB, Ravnik-Oblak M, Oblak C: Pudendal versus limb nerves electrophysiologic abnormalities in diabetics with erectile dysfunction. Int J Impot Res 2:37, 1993.
102. Enzlin P, Mathieu C, Van Den Bruel A, et al: Sexual dysfunction in women with type 1 diabetes: a controlled study. Diabetes Care 25:672, 2002.
103. Turk S, Karalezli G, Tomnbul HZ, et al: Erectile dysfunction and the effects of sildenafil treatment in patients on haemodialysis and continuous ambulatory peritoneal dialysis. Nephrol Dial Transplant 16:1818, 2001.
104. Suzuki N, Kumamoto Y: Study of sexual function in male hemodialysis patients—analysis of the cause of erectile dysfunction. Jpn J Urol 86:1098, 1995.
105. Shamsa A, Motavalli SM, Aghdam B: Erectile function in end-stage renal disease before and after renal transplantation. Transplant Proc 37:3087, 2005.
106. Ali ST, Shaikh RN, Siddiqi A: HIV-1 associated neuropathies in males: impotence and penile electrodiagnosis. Acta Neurol Belg 94:194, 1994.
107. Bird TD, Lipe HP, Crabtree LD: Impotence associated with Charcot–Marie–Tooth syndrome. Eur Neurol 34:155, 1994.
108. Alves M, Conceição I, Sales Luis ML: Neurophysiological evaluation of sexual dysfunction in familial amyloidotic polyneuropathy—Portuguese type. Acta Neurol Scand 96:163, 1997.
109. Vodušek DB, Zidar J: Pudendal nerve involvement in patients with hereditary motor and sensory neuropathy. Acta Neurol Scand 76:457, 1987.
110. Olsson T, Olofsson B-O, Hägg E, et al: Adrenocortical and gonadal abnormalities in dystrophiamyotonica—a common enzyme defect? Eur J Intern Med 7:29, 1996.
111. Chen CM, Huang CC: Gonadal dysfunction in mitochondrial encephalomyopathies. Eur Neurol 35:281, 1995.
112. Bronner G, Vodušek DB: Management of sexual dysfunction in Parkinson's disease. Ther Adv Neurol Disord 4:375, 2011.
113. Montorsi F, Maga T, Strambi LF, et al: Sildenafil taken at bedtime significantly increases nocturnal erection: results of a placebo-controlled study. Urology 56:906, 2000.
114. Ng KK, Lim HCP, Ng FC, et al: The use of sildenafil in patients with erectile dysfunction in relation to diabetes mellitus—a study of 1,511 patients. Singapore Med J 43:387, 2002.
115. Sharma RK, Prasad N, Gupta A, et al: Treatment of erectile dysfunction with sildenafil citrate in renal allograft recipients: a randomized, double-blind, placebo-controlled, crossover trial. Am J Kidney Dis 48:128, 2006.
116. Hussain IF, Brady CM, Swinn MJ, et al: Treatment of erectile dysfunction with sildenafil citrate (Viagra) in parkinsonism due to Parkinson's disease or multiple

system atrophy with observation on orthostatic hypotension. J Neurol Neurosurg Psychiatry 71:371, 2001.

117. Sanchez Ramos A, Vidal J, Jáuregui ML, et al: Efficacy, safety and predictive factors of therapeutic success with sildenafil for erectile dysfunction in patients with different spinal cord injuries. Spinal Cord 39:637, 2001.
118. Palmer JS, Kaplan WE, Firlit CF: Erectile dysfunction in spina bifida is treatable. Lancet 354:125, 1999.
119. Obayashi K, Ando Y, Terazaki H, et al: Effect of sildenafil citrate (Viagra) on erectile dysfunction in a patient with familial amyloidotic polyneuropathy ATTR Val30Met. J Auton Nerv Syst 80:89, 2000.
120. Lowentritt B, Scardino P, Miles B, et al: Sildenafil citrate after radical retropubic prostatectomy. J Urol 162:1614, 1999.
121. Salonia A, Rigatti P, Montorsi F: Sildenafil in erectile dysfunction: a critical review. Curr Med Res Opin 19:241, 2003.
122. Goldstein I, Young JM, Fischer J, et al: Vardenafil, a new phosphodiesterase type 5 inhibitor, in the treatment of erectile dysfunction in men with diabetes: a multicenter double-blind placebo-controlled fixed-dose study. Diabetes Care 26:77, 2003.
123. Saenz de Tejada I, Anglin G, Knight JR, et al: Effects of tadalafil on erectile dysfunction in men with diabetes. Diabetes Care 25:2159, 2002.
124. Zusman RM, Morales A, Glasser DB, et al: Overall cardiovascular profile of sildenafil citrate. Am J Cardiol 83:35C, 1999.
125. Yarkony G, Chen D, Palmer J, et al: Management of impotence due to spinal cord injury using low dose papaverine. Paraplegia 33:77, 1995.
126. Porst H: The rationale for prostaglandin E_1 in erectile failure: a survey of worldwide experience. J Urol 155:802, 1996.
127. Heaton JP, Lording D, Liu SN, et al: Intracavernosal alprostadil is effective for the treatment of erectile dysfunction in diabetic men. Int J Impot Res 13:317, 2001.
128. Lundberg PO: Priapism: review. Scand J Sexol 3:13, 2000.
129. Bodner DR, Haas CA, Krueger B, et al: Intraurethral alprostadil for treatment of erectile dysfunction in patients with spinal cord injury. Urology 53:199, 1999.
130. Denil J, Ohl D, Smythe C: Vacuum erection device in spinal cord injured men: patient and partner satisfaction. Arch Phys Med Rehabil 77:750, 1996.
131. Fodde M, Krogh-Jespersen S, Brackett NL, et al: Male sexual dysfunction and infertility associated with neurological disorders. Asian J Androl 14:61, 2012.
132. Perelman MA: A new combination treatment for premature ejaculation: a sex therapist's perspective. J Sex Med 3:1004, 2006.
133. Sipski ML, Rosen RC, Alexander CJ, et al: Sildenafil effects on sexual and cardiovascular responses in women with spinal cord injury. Urology 55:812, 2000.
134. Frese A, Eikermann A, Frese K, et al: Headache associated with sexual activity: demography, clinical features, and comorbidity. Neurology 61:796, 2003.
135. Gallagher J, Murphy MS, Carroll J: Transient global amnesia after sexual intercourse. Ir J Med Sci 174:86, 2005.
136. Morgan JC, Alhatou M, Oberlies J, et al: Transient ischemic attack and stroke associated with sildenafil (Viagra) use. Neurology 57:1730, 2001.

CHAPTER

31

Pregnancy and Disorders of the Nervous System

MICHAEL J. AMINOFF

Neurologic disorders may first present during pregnancy, and their investigation and treatment may be complicated by concerns for the safety of the developing fetus. Furthermore, the natural history of certain preexisting diseases may be affected by pregnancy, and obstetric management may be influenced by the neurologic disturbance. These aspects are considered in this chapter.

EPILEPSY

Many of the pregnancies that occur in the United States are unplanned, so that regular counseling of women with epilepsy during the reproductive years is important.[1] Pregnancy may affect the natural history and management of patients with epilepsy in several ways. In addition, antiepileptic management may affect the developing fetus and obstetric management.

Effect of Pregnancy on Maternal Seizures

In recent series, an increase in seizures occurred during pregnancy in 23 to 75 percent of cases[2]; between 53 and 67 percent had unchanged seizure control.[3] It is not possible to predict in advance whether or how seizure frequency will be altered during pregnancy, but certain general points can be made. Seizure frequency is more likely to increase in poorly controlled epileptic patients than in those with infrequent seizures, and in those with focal seizures[4]; any increase is most likely to occur during the first trimester. Any change in seizure frequency usually reverses after the birth of the

Aminoff's Neurology and General Medicine, Fifth Edition.

infant, although occasional patients whose seizures increase during pregnancy remain more difficult to control thereafter. For patients without seizures for at least 9 months prior to conception, the likelihood of remaining seizure-free during pregnancy ranges between 84 and 92 percent in different series.[5] The influence of a particular pregnancy cannot be predicted by the outcome of previous pregnancies, any relationship between seizures and the menstrual cycle, or maternal age. Seizures may occur for the first time during or immediately after pregnancy and in some instances occur only in relation to pregnancy. Even in patients with such true gestational epilepsy, however, it is not possible to predict the course of subsequent pregnancies from the occurrence of seizures during one pregnancy.

Status epilepticus may complicate pregnancy and sometimes occurs before there is any other evidence that seizures have become more difficult to control. It may take the form of tonic-clonic (major motor) or nonconvulsive status. The former is easy to recognize, but a transient alteration in mental status and level of arousal may not be attributed to nonconvulsive status epilepticus unless an electroencephalogram is performed. As in the nonparous woman, it is important to obtain control of the seizures rapidly, but therapeutic termination of pregnancy is usually unnecessary. There is no evidence that anticonvulsant drugs administered intravenously to treat status epilepticus affect the fetus adversely.

The reason that seizure frequency sometimes increases during pregnancy is not clear, but a change in drug requirements during the gestational period may sometimes be responsible. Pregnancy probably causes an increase in the clearance and a decrease in the blood concentrations of lamotrigine, phenytoin, and, to a lesser extent, carbamazepine, and possibly decreases the blood level of levetiracetam and the active oxcarbazepine metabolite, the monohydroxy derivative (MHD).[6] Evidence of a change in clearance or blood level of phenobarbital, valproate, primidone, and ethosuximide is inadequate to permit a definite conclusion to be reached.[6] Other possible reasons for the increased dose requirements of anticonvulsants during pregnancy include poor compliance with the drug regimen, changes in drug absorption and excretion, and the dilutional effects of increasing plasma volume and extracellular fluid volume. Changes in drug absorption may relate to nausea, vomiting, or reduced gastric motility. Antacids are frequently prescribed during pregnancy and are known to adsorb to medications, preventing absorption. An increased metabolic capacity of maternal liver and metabolism of part of the anticonvulsant dose by the fetus, placenta, or both may also be important. Folic acid therapy (which may reduce the risk of major congenital malformations when taken preconceptionally[6]), prescribed routinely by many obstetricians, sometimes lowers the plasma phenytoin level. The effects of pregnancy on the pharmacokinetics of other antiseizure agents, such as felbamate, gabapentin, pregabalin, zonisamide, topiramate, and lacosamide, have not been defined.

Whether hormonal factors contribute to an increase in seizure frequency during pregnancy is unclear, but estrogens are epileptogenic in animals, and progesterone is said to have both convulsant and anticonvulsant properties. Finally, fatigue and sleep deprivation may influence seizure frequency during pregnancy.

The reason that seizure frequency decreases in some epileptic patients is also unclear, but improved compliance with the anticonvulsant drug regimen may be responsible.

Effects of Maternal Epilepsy on the Fetus

Seizures

A major concern in the management of epileptic women during pregnancy is the possible effect of the seizure disorder and of anticonvulsant drugs on the developing fetus. It is difficult to determine the precise risk that a seizure disorder will also develop in the offspring of epileptic parents. The risk depends in part on whether the parental epilepsy is idiopathic (constitutional) or acquired; such risk appears to be increased among the offspring of epileptic mothers but not when only the father is epileptic. The reason for the increased risk is unclear, but genetic factors may be important, as may the consequences of maternal seizures or anticonvulsant drugs taken during pregnancy.

Fetal Malformations

For many years, concern has existed that anticonvulsant drugs are teratogenic. Epidemiologic studies are difficult to interpret because epilepsy occurs for many reasons, varies in severity between patients and in the same patient at different times, may itself increase the risk of fetal malformation, and is treated by many drugs in different doses and combinations; environmental factors also bear on the development of fetal malformations and are difficult to control. Nevertheless, numerous reports suggest that certain anticonvulsant drugs are indeed teratogenic in humans, and the risk of malformation among the offspring of epileptic women is approximately double that for nonepileptic women.[7] In a prospective study involving the UK Epilepsy and Pregnancy Register, however, the rate of major congenital malformation was 3.5 percent for women with epilepsy who had not taken antiseizure medication during pregnancy compared with 4.2 percent among those who had (3.7% with monotherapy and 6% for those on polytherapy).[8] The failure of this study to show an increased risk of major malformations among women on antiseizure medication may have been because the study was not sufficiently sensitive.[9] It seems that a greater teratogenic risk exists when polypharmacy is used,[7,9] and the combination of lamotrigine and valproate is particularly teratogenic.[10] Cognitive and behavioral development may also be affected,[11] and the evidence is most suggestive for valproate, phenytoin, and phenobarbital.[9]

The older antiepileptic drugs taken during the first trimester of pregnancy are probably all teratogenic to some extent, especially when taken in combination.[8,9] However, it cannot be determined whether the increased risk relates to all or to only some antiseizure medications. Trimethadione, which is now rarely used and should be avoided during pregnancy, is particularly dangerous and causes fetal malformations and mental retardation in more than 50 percent of exposed infants. The absolute risk of major congenital malformations is also especially marked for valproate,[8,9,12,13] which is associated with a high (1%) rate of neural tube defects and may also cause cleft lip or palate, polydactyly, hypospadias, craniosynostosis, atrial septal defect, developmental delay, and other disorders.[8,14] It is not clear whether the rates and types of major congenital malformations differ in epileptic women taking specific antiseizure drugs (other than valproate). Existing data suggest that phenytoin and carbamazepine are associated with cleft palate, and phenobarbital may be associated with cardiac malformations; a relationship probably exists between the risk of developing major congenital malformations and the dose of valproate or lamotrigine.[9] The data concerning the teratogenic risks of monotherapy with the newer anticonvulsant drugs such as levetiracetam, topiramate, and oxcarbazepine are still unclear and incomplete.

A specific syndrome has been described among some of the offspring born to mothers taking phenytoin, phenobarbital, or carbamazepine during pregnancy and bears some resemblance to the fetal alcohol syndrome. It is characterized by prenatal and postnatal growth deficiency, microcephaly, a dysmorphic appearance, hypoplasia of the distal phalanges, and mental deficiency. A characteristic facial phenotype in children exposed to valproic acid or sodium valproate in utero has also been described.[15] Some of these children may have educational difficulties.

The mechanisms involved in teratogenesis of anticonvulsant drugs are not known but may include folate deficiency (Fig. 31-1) or antagonism[16] and production of toxic intermediary metabolites during biotransformation of the parent compound.[17] Specific oxidative intermediates such as epoxide, for example, have been suggested as the ultimate teratogen in patients receiving phenytoin.[17]

Bleeding Disorders

A clinical or subclinical bleeding disorder may occur in neonates exposed to anticonvulsant drugs in utero, without evidence of coagulopathy in the mothers. Although a number of anecdotal cases have been reported, the evidence is insufficient to determine whether the risk is, in fact, substantially increased in the newborns of women with epilepsy.[6] Factors II, VII, IX, and X are decreased, whereas factors V and VIII and fibrinogen are normal. Bleeding usually occurred within 24 hours of birth, sometimes in unusual sites (e.g., the pleural or abdominal cavities). Bleeding has also been reported to occur in utero, leading to stillbirth. It has been suggested that the bleeding disorder may be prevented by the maternal ingestion of vitamin K_1 during the last month of pregnancy. The recommended dose of vitamin K is 10 mg daily for 30 days before delivery. However, other studies suggest that this hemorrhagic disorder is rare and that routine prophylaxis by maternal treatment with vitamin K_1 is unjustified.[18,19] Indeed, it has even been questioned whether maternal use of antiseizure medication leads to a coagulopathy at all, and certainly the evidence is insufficient to support or refute this association.[6] In any event, the routine

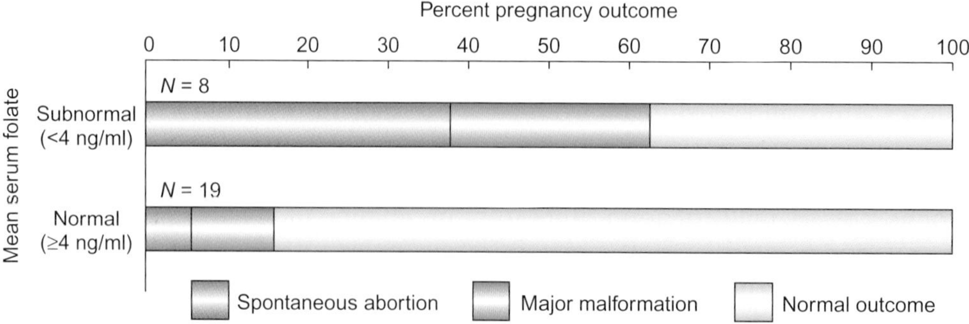

FIGURE 31-1 ▪ Percentages of pregnancy outcome in relationship to mean serum folate levels in the first trimester dichotomized as less than 4 (subnormal) or at least 4 ng/ml. N = number of pregnancies with subnormal or normal serum folate levels. A significantly higher number of pregnancies with subnormal levels resulted in an abnormal outcome than did pregnancies with normal levels. Using Fisher's exact test, $P = 0.05$ for spontaneous abortion and $P = 0.03$ for total abnormal outcomes. (From Dansky LV, Andermann E, Rosenblatt D, et al: Anticonvulsants, folate levels, and pregnancy outcome: a prospective study. Ann Neurol 21:176, 1987, with permission.)

administration of vitamin K_1 (1 mg/kg intramuscularly) to newborns of women receiving anticonvulsant drugs during pregnancy is sufficient to prevent such a coagulopathy.

Withdrawal Symptoms

Maternal use of barbiturates may be associated with barbiturate withdrawal symptoms in the neonate, with restlessness, irritability, tremulousness, difficulty in sleeping, and vasomotor instability, usually beginning a week after birth.

Breast-Feeding

Although certain anticonvulsant drugs (primidone, ethosuximide, gabapentin, lamotrigine, levetiracetam, and topiramate) taken by the mother may be present in breast milk, there is no evidence that these have symptomatic effects on the newborn.[6] Breast-feeding therefore need not be discouraged on this account; however, when obvious sedation develops in an infant that could relate to anticonvulsants in the maternal milk, breast-feeding should be discontinued and the child observed for signs of drug withdrawal. A literature review found evidence that phenobarbital, phenytoin, valproate, and carbamazepine do not penetrate the breast milk in a clinically important amount.[6]

Management of Epilepsy

Little or no information is available in the published literature to guide decision making with regard to certain management issues in women with epilepsy.[20] Epilepsy must be managed during pregnancy, as at other times, by prophylactic anticonvulsant drugs. Management should be by monotherapy whenever possible, with selection of the anticonvulsant that is most appropriate for seizure type. As indicated earlier, trimethadione and valproic acid are best avoided, but available data concerning relative safety and therapeutic utility of the various anticonvulsant drugs during pregnancy are insufficient to provide any more detailed guidelines at this time for the management of epileptic patients or of women wishing to become pregnant. Moreover, there is little point in substituting one anticonvulsant drug for another after the first 2 to 3 months of pregnancy because major fetal malformations will probably have occurred already if they are going to occur at all. Folate supplementation (4 mg daily) may help, however, to reduce the risk of teratogenicity,[16] although the optimal dose is unclear.

Anticonvulsant drug treatment should be monitored during pregnancy by serial measurement of plasma drug levels, depending on the drug that is being taken, as discussed earlier. Patients should be seen monthly, and as the pregnancy continues the dose of medication may need to be increased to maintain plasma concentrations at previously effective levels. If increases are made during pregnancy, dose reductions will be necessary at some point (usually within 8 weeks) after delivery to prevent toxicity, but at a time that must be determined individually based on clinical evaluation and plasma drug levels.

If patients inquire, it is appropriate to indicate that there is a slightly increased risk of fetal malformation due either to the seizure disorder itself or to the drugs used in its treatment. Nevertheless, there is still a very good chance (90 to 95%) that offspring will be normal. It must also be emphasized that the risks to both mother and fetus of noncompliance with anticonvulsant drug regimen are considerable, in that an increased seizure frequency or even status epilepticus may occur, with its associated morbidity and mortality.

Obstetric Management

Increased incidences of vaginal hemorrhage and toxemia, and an increased stillbirth rate are reported in epileptic women by some authors but not others. For women with epilepsy taking antiepileptic medication, there is probably no substantially increased risk (greater than two times expected) of cesarian delivery or late-pregnancy bleeding, and no moderately increased risk (greater than 1.5 times expected) of premature contractions or premature labor and delivery.[5] Any increase in cesarian deliveries has been attributed to uncertainty in guiding the delivery of epileptic women and the misperception of an increased risk of complications.[20] An increased incidence of neonatal death has sometimes been reported, perhaps owing to an increased incidence of congenital malformations, iatrogenic neonatal hemorrhage, the metabolic or toxic effects of seizures or anticonvulsant drugs, or socioeconomic factors.

Targeted ultrasonography can be used to diagnose most neural tube defects at 12 to 22 weeks of pregnancy as well as other major structural abnormalities.

Interactions Between Oral Contraceptives and Anticonvulsant Agents

Certain anticonvulsants (including phenytoin, carbamazepine, felbamate, topiramate, oxcarbazepine, phenobarbital, and primidone) may alter the effectiveness of oral contraceptives, leading to unwanted pregnancy.[21] Thus, the risk of contraceptive failure in patients taking these anticonvulsants should be discussed in advance and documented in the patient's records; in some instances, use of an additional backup contraceptive method should be considered. The incidence of breakthrough bleeding is also increased in women taking these anticonvulsants and concurrent oral contraceptives, and such bleeding may point to the possibility of contraceptive failure.[21] Valproic acid and the newer anticonvulsants, zonisamide, vigabatrin, gabapentin, lamotrigine, levetiracetam, pregabalin, and tiagabine (at low doses), have not been reported to cause contraceptive failure.[1,5,21] When oral contraception is to be used in a woman taking enzyme-inducing anticonvulsants, a formulation that includes at least 50 μg ethinyl estradiol or mestranol should be used. Oral contraceptives may also affect seizure frequency or blood levels of anticonvulsant medication, but this is less clear.

MIGRAINE

Migraine is often influenced by pregnancy. Most commonly, symptoms improve after the first trimester, but occasionally they worsen or occur for the first time during pregnancy. The influence of pregnancy on migraine does not depend on any relationship of migraine to the menstrual cycle. Similarly, it does not relate to the sex of the fetus or to differences in plasma progesterone levels, although there may be some relationship to changes in the pattern of circulating estrogens. Treatment of migraine during pregnancy is similar to that at other times, with emphasis on the avoidance of precipitating factors together with the use of simple analgesics as necessary. However, acetaminophen should be used in preference to aspirin because there is some evidence that aspirin use in large dosages in the later stages of pregnancy may prolong labor, increase the incidence of stillbirth, impair neonatal hemostasis, and cause premature closure of the ductus arteriosus. Nonsteroidal anti-inflammatory drugs are best avoided for similar reasons,[22] except in severe cases. If acetaminophen is insufficient, partial opioid agonists may be used on a limited basis. Ergot-containing preparations should be avoided when possible because of possible teratogenicity[23] and the effect this drug may have on the gravid uterus. Propranolol should similarly be avoided during pregnancy when possible because animal studies have shown that it may impair fetal growth and that β-adrenergic blockade may inhibit the normal responsiveness of the fetus to asphyxia or other stresses. Other reported complications in neonates include prematurity, respiratory depression, hypoglycemia, and hyperbilirubinemia.[24] Triptans are also best avoided because they have been associated with premature labor.[25]

Many women, often with a past or family history of migraine, experience mild bifrontal headaches in the week after delivery. These headaches usually respond to simple analgesics and settle spontaneously.

The association between migraine and oral contraceptive preparations is discussed in Chapter 20.

TUMORS

Although any type of intracranial tumor occasionally presents during pregnancy, pituitary adenomas, meningiomas, neurofibromas, hemangioblastomas, and certain vascular malformations sometimes exhibit relapses during pregnancy, with partial or complete remission occurring after delivery. The basis of this relationship is unclear, but it seems likely that pregnancy produces a slight increase in tumor size. The enlargement of certain pituitary adenomas during pregnancy may be due to the trophic effects of increased circulating estradiol. Similarly, an increase in size of meningiomas may relate to a direct trophic effect of gonadal hormones on tumor cells; sex steroid–binding sites have been found in human meningiomas, but there are marked differences in their reported prevalence and concentration.[26] Tumors with symptoms that show a consistent temporal relationship to pregnancy are usually so situated that significant neurologic involvement, with the development of new symptoms or signs, occurs with only slight expansion of the underlying lesion. Thus, spinal meningiomas are more likely than convexity meningiomas to show a relationship of symptoms to pregnancy. Visual field defects are unlikely to develop during pregnancy in patients with pituitary microadenomas, but may certainly occur with larger tumors.[27]

Patients with suspected intracranial neoplasms should be managed during pregnancy as at other times. Magnetic resonance imaging (MRI) is generally the best noninvasive means of establishing the diagnosis and does not involve exposing the fetus to irradiation. Essential operative treatment should not be delayed. However, surgery for pituitary adenomas or other benign tumors diagnosed toward the end of pregnancy can often be delayed until after delivery, provided that the patient is followed closely. Radiation therapy or chemotherapy may be required during pregnancy. Radiation therapy is associated with a risk of fetal loss or teratogenicity depending on the level of fetal exposure, especially if administered during the first trimester; in later pregnancy it carries an increased risk of childhood cancer or leukemia.[28] However, tumors of the brain or head and neck can usually be irradiated satisfactorily without dangerous fetal exposure.[28] Therapeutic abortion may need to be considered in some patients with malignant brain tumors, depending on the therapy required and especially when it cannot be delayed to the latter half of pregnancy or postponed until after delivery, or when significant symptoms, such as uncontrollable seizures, complicate the pregnancy.

The pregnancy itself can usually be managed normally in patients with intracranial tumors. Concerns that vaginal delivery may exacerbate any existing increase in intracranial pressure due to the tumor are usually misplaced, especially if adequate regional anesthesia is employed and low forceps are used, if necessary, to shorten the second stage of labor.

The long survival associated with low-grade gliomas suggests that some women with such tumors may wish to become pregnant after the diagnosis has been established. Such decisions need to be made on an individual basis, but patients with these lesions may certainly go through pregnancy without further complications.

Choriocarcinoma may develop after a normal pregnancy or follow a molar, ectopic, or terminated pregnancy. Intracranial metastases are common, and hemorrhage may occur into the cerebral lesions. Early diagnosis and treatment are important for survival.

PSEUDOTUMOR CEREBRI

Idiopathic intracranial hypertension, also known as pseudotumor cerebri, has a clear association with pregnancy and is especially likely to occur during the first trimester or postpartum. It therefore seems sensible that women with this disorder should defer pregnancy until their disease is controlled and important that all pregnant patients with new-onset headaches be examined funduscopically to exclude the diagnosis. Headache and visual disturbances due to papilledema may be accompanied by diplopia from sixth nerve palsy. Investigations reveal no space-occupying lesion, but the cerebrospinal fluid (CSF) pressure is increased. The disorder is self-limiting, but it may not remit for weeks after delivery, and there may be recurrences during subsequent pregnancies.[29] Treatment, as in the nonpregnant woman, consists of measures to lower the intracranial pressure to prevent secondary optic atrophy. It may require the use of acetazolamide, furosemide, corticosteroids, repeated lumbar punctures, or a surgical shunting procedure. Optic nerve decompression and early delivery of the fetus may have to be considered if the intracranial pressure remains high despite these measures. There are no specific obstetric complications, and a normal birth can be expected.

Intracranial venous sinus thrombosis may simulate pseudotumor cerebri and is discussed later.

CEREBROVASCULAR DISEASE

A significant number of pregnancy-related maternal deaths result from stroke. An increased incidence of stroke has been associated particularly with the puerperium.[30] Pregnancy itself appears to be associated with an increased risk of stroke,[30,31] and this probably relates at least in part to various hormonal changes.

Sex steroids can affect several physiologic and metabolic factors that predispose to cerebral thromboembolic or venous infarction, as discussed in Chapter 20. The association of stroke with oral contraceptives is well recognized. Estrogens increase blood coagulability and platelet aggregation.[32] Sex hormones may also predispose to aneurysm formation or rupture, as suggested by observations that early menarche or oral contraceptive use is associated with an increased risk of subarachnoid hemorrhage,[33] that the risk of hemorrhage is greatest in the perimenstrual period,[34] and that premenopausal women are at reduced risk of subarachnoid hemorrhage.[34] Whether pregnancy influences intracranial arteriovenous malformations (AVMs) is unclear, but it may certainly aggravate spinal arteriovenous fistulas (p. 667). Eclampsia or pre-eclampsia is the most common cause of stroke during pregnancy, and the microangiopathic syndromes of pre-eclampsia, thrombotic thrombocytopenic purpura, and hemolytic-uremic syndrome are considered on p. 677.

Occlusive Arterial Disease

Most cases of nonhemorrhagic hemiplegia developing during pregnancy or the postpartum period are due to arterial occlusion.[35] As in nonpregnant patients, this may relate to thrombus formation on an atheromatous plaque; inflammatory disorders such as arteritis or meningovascular syphilis; hematologic disorders such as polycythemia and sickle cell disease; and cardiac disorders such as a cardiomyopathy, rheumatic or ischemic heart disease, intracardiac shunts, cardiac dysrhythmias, subacute bacterial endocarditis, use of prosthetic heart valves, and cardiac myxoma. It may be associated with diabetes, cigarette smoking, and migrainous headaches. During pregnancy, in addition, stroke may be predisposed to by anemia, hormonal factors, changes in blood coagulation factors (see Chapter 25), increased platelet aggregation, hypertension, and puerperal septicemia.

The blood is in a hypercoagulable state during pregnancy; there is a rise in all procoagulant factors except XI and XIII, and increased thrombin activity. Circulating inhibitors of coagulation, such as protein C and protein S, are reduced during normal pregnancy, and antithrombin III may be reduced, as is discussed in Chapter 25. The activity of the fibrinolytic system is also reduced during pregnancy. These various changes predispose pregnant women to stroke. Hemoglobinopathies may also lead to significant maternal morbidity during pregnancy. Thus, women with sickle cell disease are especially likely to experience crises, usually vaso-occlusive, during pregnancy.[36] Sickle cell disease is also associated with an increased incidence of obstetric complication—including abortion, growth retardation, preterm birth, and stillbirth—although fetal wastage has been reduced considerably by improved prenatal care.[36]

The presence of circulating antiphospholipid autoantibodies (discussed in Chapters 11 and 25) is similarly associated with a high rate of maternal arterial and venous thrombotic events and transient ischemic attacks, as well as with obstetric complications such as an increased rate of spontaneous abortion and of early-onset, atypical pre-eclampsia.[37] Pregnancy may represent an especially high risk of thromboembolic disease in patients with these antibodies.[37] Treatment recommendations are limited by a lack of clinical evidence but may involve low-dose aspirin, unfractionated heparin, or low-molecular-weight heparin.[38]

A peripartum cardiomyopathy may occur during the last trimester of pregnancy or the puerperium, especially in the presence of twinning, toxemia, or postpartum hypertension; it sometimes presents with embolic phenomena necessitating anticoagulation. Its precise cause is unclear, but nutritional, hormonal, viral, and immunologic mechanisms have been suggested.[39] Subsequent pregnancies are associated with a significant reduction in left ventricular function and may lead to clinical deterioration and death.[40]

A postpartum cerebral angiopathy may occur during an otherwise normal pregnancy or the postpartum period and lead to a fatal outcome.[41] It has been associated with hypertension and use of vasoconstrictive drugs and may be mistaken for cerebral vasculitis.[42,43] Presentation is commonly with thunderclap headache; focal deficits and seizures may also occur. Cerebral infarction, intracranial bleeding, or vasogenic edema may be associated. The disorder follows a self-limiting course. Treatment is with calcium-channel blockers, but benefit is uncertain. The outcome is variable; full recovery occurs in many patients, but in others the disorder has a fulminant course and may have a fatal outcome or lead to residual deficits.[41]

A reversible intimal hyperplasia of the cerebral vasculature during pregnancy has been described as a rare cause of stroke or transient ischemic attack during the gestational period, but such cases are poorly documented and hard to interpret. There are rare reports of arterial occlusion by paradoxical embolization from a pelvic vein through a patent foramen ovale. Fat, air, or amniotic fluid embolism may also occur during childbirth but usually presents with dyspnea, shock, and acute encephalopathy. Amniotic fluid embolism is an important cause of stroke and maternal death. In the United Kingdom and France, it is the fifth and third highest direct cause of maternal death, respectively, and in Singapore an autopsy study revealed that it was responsible for more than 30 percent of direct maternal deaths.[44] Hemodynamic collapse and disseminated intravascular coagulopathy may lead to focal neurologic signs from cerebral hypoperfusion or hemorrhage. Plasma exchange may be helpful after initial resuscitation.

The role of thrombolytic agents (e.g., tissue plasminogen activator) for treating acute ischemic stroke in pregnant women or nursing mothers is unclear. Hemorrhagic complications are more likely, especially in the first few days after delivery; any effects on the fetus and the extent to which these agents are excreted in breast milk are uncertain. Nevertheless, tissue plasminogen activator has been used safely and effectively during pregnancy although it may increase the risk of miscarriage.[45]

As in nonpregnant women, transient cerebral ischemic attacks may precede occlusion of one of the major intracranial arteries. Neurologic investigation and management should not be influenced by the pregnancy, but special shielding during radiologic studies may help to protect the developing fetus. Angiographic delineation of degenerative atherosclerotic disease in a localized arterial segment that is surgically accessible may permit disobliterative surgery, especially when stenosis is severe (70 to 99% in the internal carotid artery). If surgery is decided against or there is more widespread atherosclerotic disease, treatment is with low-dose aspirin. A cardiac source of emboli usually necessitates treatment with warfarin (as also do certain hypercoagulable states or venous occlusive disease). This drug is associated with risks of teratogenicity and fetal wastage when used during the first trimester, and it crosses the placenta, thereby increasing the risk of hemorrhagic complications. Accordingly, patients requiring anticoagulation during pregnancy are best maintained on subcutaneous heparin, which is discontinued with the onset of labor and restarted approximately 12 hours after vaginal delivery (or 24 hours after cesarean section).

The optimal management of labor and delivery in patients who have had a stroke during pregnancy is unclear. In most cases, vaginal delivery assisted by forceps is probably satisfactory. The blood pressure needs to be monitored closely, however, to avoid excessively high or low levels.

Occlusive Venous Disease

Aseptic intracranial venous thrombosis may occur during pregnancy, during the puerperium, or with the use of oral contraceptives for reasons that are unclear.[46] It has been attributed to coagulation abnormalities, changes in the constituents of peripheral blood, and intimal damage to dural sinuses (see Chapter 25). The extent to which it relates to hormonal changes is unknown, but such changes probably have an important etiologic role, as discussed in Chapters 11 and 20. In many instances there is no evidence of thrombosis in the

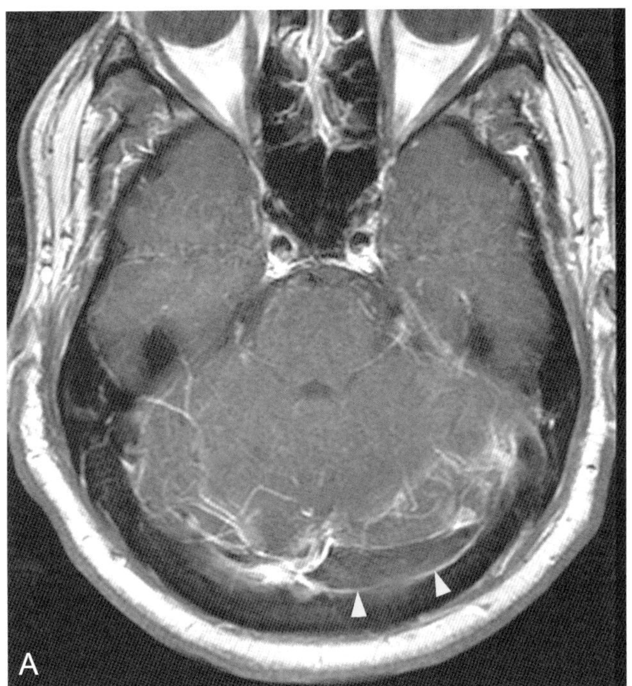

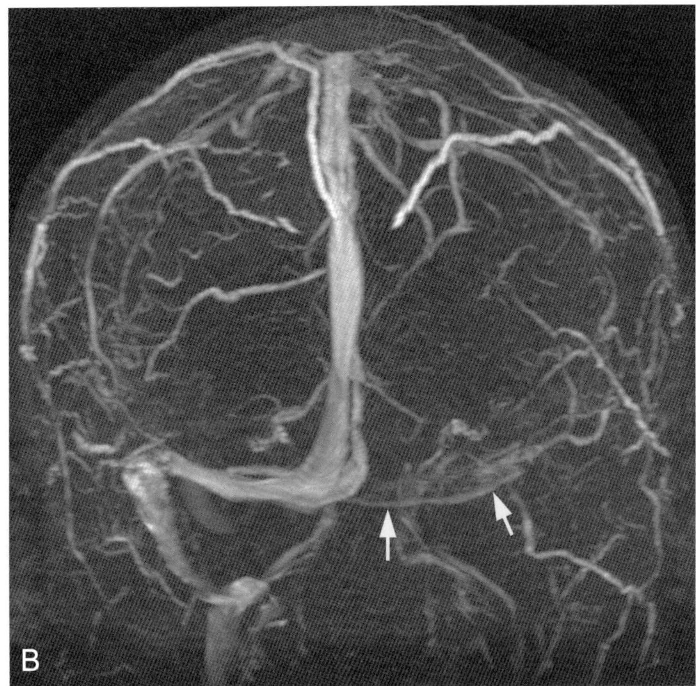

FIGURE 31-2 ■ Thrombosis of the left transverse sinus. **A**, Axial postcontrast T1-weighted MR image shows a filling defect within the left transverse sinus consistent with thrombosis (arrowheads). **B**, Coronal MR venogram confirms thrombosis of the left transverse sinus (arrows). (Courtesy of William P. Dillon, MD, University of California, San Francisco.)

pelvic or leg veins. Inherited prothrombotic states associated with intracranial venous thrombosis include protein C, protein S, antithrombin III, and factor V Leiden deficiency, and hyperhomocyteinemia (see Chapter 25); the antiphospholipid antibody syndrome and systemic malignancy may also be associated, and thus require exclusion.[47]

Intracranial venous thrombosis (Fig. 31-2) occurs most commonly during the third trimester of pregnancy or the postpartum period, sometimes in relation to pre-eclampsia. Although it may, in fact, occur at any time during a normal pregnancy, when it develops during the first trimester it usually is in relation to some complication such as spontaneous or therapeutic abortion. It is characterized clinically by headache, seizures, obtundation, confusion, and sometimes focal neurologic disturbances.[46] Examination commonly reveals papilledema, and there may be signs of meningeal irritation from subarachnoid bleeding secondary to cortical infarction. Cerebrospinal fluid pressure is often increased, and its protein or cell content may be increased. Radiologic imaging procedures (computed tomography [CT] scan, MRI, and arteriography) confirm the diagnosis and help to exclude arterial disease.

Treatment of intracranial venous thrombosis is controversial.[46] Anticonvulsant drugs and antiedema agents may be helpful. Anticoagulation with dose-adjusted intravenous heparin may also be worthwhile despite the risk of provoking hemorrhagic complications.[48,49] The role of thrombolytic therapy to prevent extension of the thrombus in pregnant or postpartum women is not clear. Different mortality rates have been reported in various series, but a rate of 15 percent is based on the pooled outcomes in a number of studies.[47] Survivors may experience recurrence of thrombosis later in the same pregnancy or in subsequent ones. The outcome is better, however, than when intracranial venous thrombosis is a sequel to inherited thrombophilia or systemic disease.[49]

Cesarean section may be necessary if venous thrombosis has occurred before or during labor. If it occurs early in the pregnancy, labor can generally be allowed to commence spontaneously, with forceps-assisted delivery if necessary.

Pituitary Infarction or Hemorrhage

Acute infarction or hemorrhage of the pituitary gland, especially around the time of delivery, is a well-recognized complication that leads to hypopituitarism if the patient survives the acute event. The disorder may occur in patients with preexisting diabetes or in those who experience such obstetric complications as postpartum hemorrhage with vascular collapse. It may also occur in patients with coagulopathies or a pituitary adenoma. The extent of pituitary damage governs the severity of pituitary hypofunction. The initial symptom may be failure of lactation. Emergency treatment with corticosteroids and trans-sphenoidal decompression of the intrasellar content may need to be considered to preserve life and vision. Management otherwise is with hormone replacement therapy.

Disseminated Intravascular Coagulation

Disseminated intravascular coagulation may occur in patients with a variety of obstetric complications. It is discussed in detail in Chapter 25 and further consideration here is unnecessary.

Subarachnoid Hemorrhage from Intracranial Vascular Anomalies

Subarachnoid hemorrhage may occur during pregnancy from an aneurysm or cerebral AVM (Fig. 31-3). The morbidity and mortality rates are greater with the former. It is unclear whether intracranial AVMs are more likely to bleed during pregnancy, but recent data do not support this belief.[50,51]

Symptoms and signs of subarachnoid hemorrhage are as in nonpregnant patients. The hemorrhage may be the first indication of the underlying lesion. An AVM is somewhat more likely than an aneurysm to be responsible if subarachnoid hemorrhage is accompanied by a major focal neurologic deficit (suggesting an intracerebral hematoma). CT scan of the head detects recent subarachnoid or intracerebral bleeding and may permit the causal lesion to be identified and localized. Arteriography confirms the identity of the lesion and provides information about its anatomic characteristics that is especially important in planning operative treatment. All of the major intracranial vessels should be opacified because feeders to AVMs sometimes arise from the contralateral side and aneurysms may be multiple. Special shielding during radiologic studies is necessary for pregnant women to protect the developing fetus.

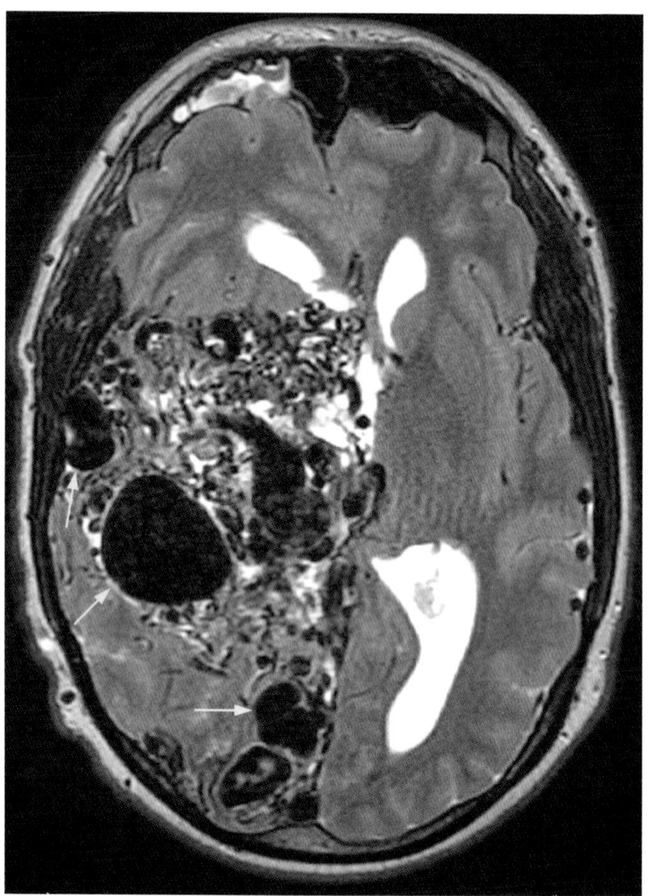

FIGURE 31-3 ■ Axial T2-weighted MR scan showing a large mass of flow voids involving the thalamus, typical of an arteriovenous malformation. The large flow voids (arrows) are venous varices, indicating possible outflow obstruction and increased risk of hemorrhage. Midline shift of the lateral ventricle is evident. (Courtesy of William P. Dillon, MD, University of California, San Francisco.)

The management of subarachnoid hemorrhage is as for nonpregnant women. Because of the high risk of rebleeding in survivors of a ruptured aneurysm, operative or endovascular treatment should not be delayed because of pregnancy if the clinical and arteriographic findings indicate its feasibility. Although ruptured AVMs may also bleed again, this may not be for months or years after the initial hemorrhage, and neurosurgical treatment can often be postponed until the pregnancy is over.

The obstetric management of survivors of a subarachnoid hemorrhage is controversial. In patients with aneurysms that have been successfully treated by surgery or in whom rupture occurred before the last trimester, pregnancy and delivery can generally be permitted to continue normally. In patients with unoperated or incompletely obliterated aneurysms that ruptured during the last trimester of pregnancy, cesarean section at 38 weeks' gestation is probably appropriate. Some have also suggested delivery by cesarean section at 38 weeks for women with AVMs, but this measure seems more difficult to justify.

Intracranial hemorrhage during pregnancy or the postpartum period may also occur in association with hypertension, vasculitis, various hematologic disorders, mycotic aneurysms, cocaine abuse,[52] and moyamoya disease[53] and as a manifestation of choriocarcinoma.[54] Treatment is of the underlying cause.

The relationship of oral contraceptive use to intracranial hemorrhage is considered in Chapter 20.

Intracranial Dural Arteriovenous Fistulas

Dural arteriovenous fistulas may present during pregnancy, after abortion, or during the postpartum period. Some are developmental anomalies, but others are acquired in adult life, occasionally following trauma. The anomalous arteriovenous shunt may involve either the anterior-inferior group of dural sinuses (cavernous, intercavernous, sphenoparietal, superior and inferior petrosal, and basilar plexus) or the superior-posterior group (superior and inferior sagittal, straight, transverse, sigmoid, and occipital). Anomalies involving the former group lead typically to unilateral orbital or head pain, diplopia, a proptosed or red eye, tinnitus, or some combination of these symptoms. Malformations involving the superior-posterior dural sinuses may lead to subarachnoid hemorrhage, increased intracranial pressure, tinnitus, seizures, or focal neurologic deficits due to cerebral ischemia. In either case, there may be papilledema, and a bruit is often present either over the eye (with involvement of the anterior-inferior sinuses) or about the mastoid region or ear (superior-posterior sinuses involved).

Arteriography is necessary to localize the shunt with certainty and determine its anatomic features. With shunts to the anterior-inferior dural sinuses, embolization of feeding vessels may help preserve vision or relieve intolerable symptoms. Ligation or embolization of feeding vessels is often helpful in relieving symptoms from shunts to the superior-posterior dural sinuses, and a direct surgical approach is also sometimes feasible.

Spinal Arteriovenous Fistulas and Malformations

Spinal fistulas and AVMs are usually either dural or intradural in location. They may lead to spinal subarachnoid hemorrhage or to a myeloradiculopathy that can either present acutely or develop insidiously. Symptoms usually are progressive. At least one-half of the survivors of subarachnoid hemorrhage from these spinal lesions have further episodes of bleeding, and one-half of the subsequent survivors bleed again unless the underlying lesion is treated.[55] Similarly, once there is any functional impairment in the legs due to the myeloradiculopathy, disability is likely to worsen, so that 50 percent of patients become unable to walk at all or require two sticks or crutches to do so, within 3 years.[55] Spinal cord or root symptoms may show a characteristic relationship to exercise or posture and occasionally to pregnancy or the menstrual cycle.

Typically, examination reveals a mixed upper and lower motor neuron deficit in the legs, often with an associated sensory disturbance that occasionally has a radicular distribution. There may be a coexisting cutaneous malformation that sometimes relates segmentally to the spinal lesion. A spinal bruit may be present.

Unruptured dural arteriovenous fistulas and spinal AVMs probably produce symptoms by causing venous hypertension. Although they are usually extramedullary, their draining veins connect with veins draining the spinal cord. The increased venous pressure leads to a reduction in the arteriovenous pressure gradient across the cord and thus to a reduction in spinal blood-flow.[55] Pressure on pelvic or abdominal veins by the gravid uterus could aggravate symptoms of caudally situated dural arteriovenous fistulas and AVMs by obstructing venous return to the heart, thereby reducing still more the arteriovenous pressure gradient across the cord. Whether anemia and hemodilution are also partly responsible for exacerbations of symptoms during pregnancy is unclear, and it is not known whether sex hormones exert direct trophic influences on these lesions.

Advances in imaging procedures have revealed that the nidus of many spinal vascular lesions is situated durally. Spinal MRI is an excellent screening procedure (Fig. 31-4); if the findings suggest an arteriovenous fistula, spinal angiography is performed to determine its anatomy, the anatomy of the spinal circulation, and the precise level of the

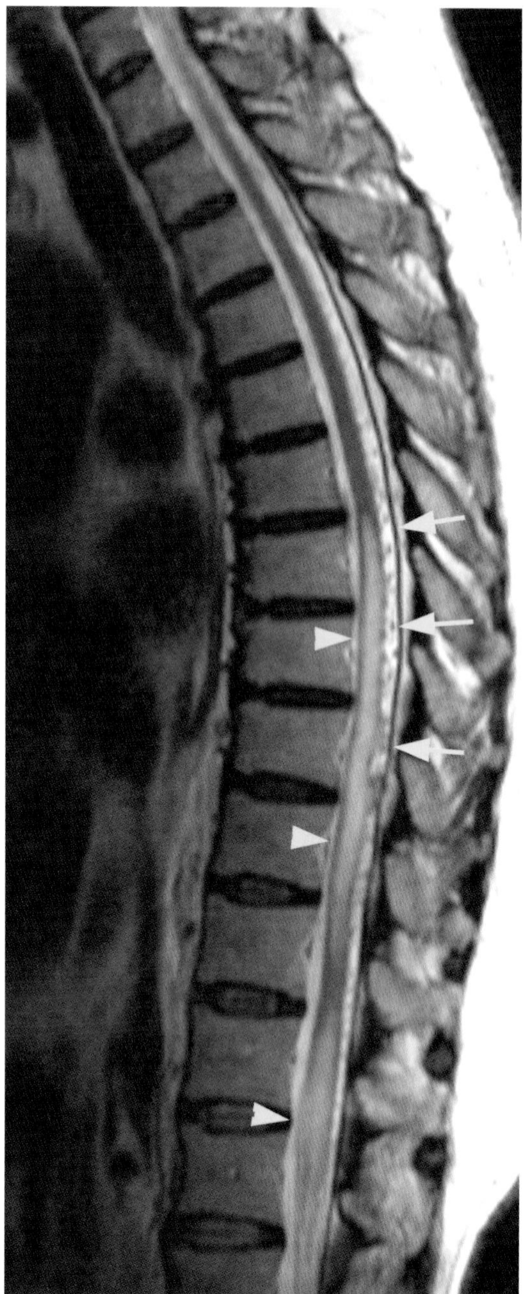

FIGURE 31-4 ■ Sagittal T2-weighted MR scan of the thoracic spine illustrates edema of the central spinal cord (arrowheads) and enlarged flow voids posteriorly (arrows). The findings are typical of a spinal dural arteriovenous fistula. (Courtesy of William P. Dillon, MD, University of California, San Francisco.)

abnormal fistula. Treatment of dural lesions is indicated in patients with progressive symptoms, functional incapacity, or a history of hemorrhage, and consists of embolization, surgical excision, or both. Treatment is clearly more difficult for vascular anomalies located anteriorly or within the spinal cord, but in some of these, also, the actual nidus of the lesion is dural and thus operable.

INFECTIONS

A variety of organisms may infect the nervous system, as discussed in Chapters 39 to 47. Pregnancy may interfere with resistance to specific infectious agents, thereby endangering maternal health. Treatment of various infections may also be complicated during pregnancy because of the need to avoid certain antimicrobial agents if possible. When infection occurs during pregnancy, it may pose risks to the developing fetus from the infective organism and the drugs used in its treatment. Thus, obstetric management may be complicated.

Pregnancy increases the susceptibility of women to clinical *poliomyelitis,* but it is not clear whether this is because pregnant women are more susceptible to the initial viral infection or to invasion of the nervous system. Weakness tends to be more severe and widespread when poliomyelitis develops during the late stages of pregnancy. Poliomyelitis affects the course of pregnancy. During the first trimester, spontaneous abortion may occur with apparently mild nonparalytic attacks of the disease or in conjunction with a febrile reaction in its acute phase. Abortion or fetal loss may also occur during later stages of pregnancy, but usually in conjunction with severe poliomyelitis. Successful pregnancy may occur, however, even in patients who are dependent on continuous noninvasive positive pressure ventilation.[56] The uterine muscle is not paralyzed in women with poliomyelitis, and labor can usually be managed as in normal women unless there are specific obstetric indications for cesarean section or induction of labor. Normal offspring can be anticipated, although neonatal poliomyelitis may occur. Neonatal involvement within the first 5 days of life is generally assumed to follow transplacental transmission of the virus and is associated with a 50 percent or greater mortality rate.

Tetanus is an important complication of abortion or delivery, especially in developing countries, and is associated with a high mortality rate. In addition to treating the tetanus, any retained products must be evacuated from the uterus, and hysterectomy is sometimes necessary. Neonatal tetanus results from contamination of the umbilical cord, and in some areas the mortality rate is a high (but uncertain and geographically variable) proportion of all births.[57] Infants are usually diagnosed within 10 days; the history is typically that of increased irritability for up to 48 hours, followed by cessation of sucking and crying, accompanied by convulsions and often by fever. Improved maternity facilities and the active immunization of women who are pregnant or of childbearing age are important public health measures to counter this disorder.[58]

Maternal infection with *Listeria monocytogenes* may lead to abortion or stillbirth as well as to a number of other manifestations including meningitis; in neonates it leads to either an early-onset, predominantly septicemic infection or a late-onset, predominantly meningitic or meningoencephalitic infection. The bacteriologic and serologic findings suggest the diagnosis, and treatment is with appropriate antibiotics.

Maternal *rubella*, especially during the first trimester, may lead to congenital fetal malformations. Ocular abnormalities, seizures, mental retardation, deafness, focal neurologic deficits, and other abnormalities, including cardiac anomalies, occur in a variety of combinations. Much more rarely, a panencephalitic illness has been reported during the second decade of life in patients with congenital rubella and leads to pyramidal and extrapyramidal signs, seizures, and dementia. High antibody titers to rubella virus occur in the blood and CSF, and the virus may be isolated from the brain. The topic is reviewed in detail elsewhere.[59]

Congenital *toxoplasmosis* causes meningoencephalitis, chorioretinitis, obstructive hydrocephalus, and cerebral calcification. Pregnant women should therefore be advised to keep away from cat feces and to avoid ingestion of raw or undercooked meat or eggs.

Fetal infection with *cytomegalovirus* may lead to a variety of somatic manifestations. Neurologic involvement may be manifested by cerebral malformation, microcephaly, mental retardation, seizures, obstructive hydrocephalus, cerebral calcification, deafness, chorioretinitis, or some combination of these disorders.

Neonatal infection with *herpes simplex virus* leads primarily to visceral involvement. When there is neurologic involvement, manifestations may include seizures, irritability, increased intracranial pressure, depressed level of consciousness, and motor deficits.

Maternal *syphilis* is an important disorder to recognize and treat. It is associated with an increased rate of spontaneous abortion and increased perinatal mortality. Offspring of affected mothers may have symptomatic congenital syphilis. Infection may also occur at birth if infants come into contact with an infective lesion. The clinical features of congenital neurosyphilis are similar to those of neurosyphilis in adults. They may become apparent at any time after the first few weeks of life, or they can be delayed for several years. Treatment is of the underlying infection, penicillin being the drug of choice. Fetal infection usually occurs in the second half of pregnancy. Thus, treatment at an early stage of pregnancy generally prevents fetal involvement, emphasizing the importance of serologic testing during antenatal care. Details of treatment are provided in Chapter 40.

Tuberculous meningitis may occur during pregnancy and is then associated with higher mortality and neurologic morbidity rates than otherwise. Its treatment is discussed in Chapter 41.

Children born to women with *acquired immunodeficiency syndrome* (AIDS) are at risk of development of the disease after an interval that varies from several months to several years. Children infected transplacentally may be born with congenital AIDS. Infection may occur not during fetal development but at birth or from breast milk. Neurologic manifestations of the disorder are particularly frequent in such children and are due to a progressive encephalopathy that leads to developmental delay or regression, with evidence of cortical atrophy on neuroimaging studies. Calcification of the basal ganglia also occurs. Other manifestations of the disease include failure to thrive, interstitial pneumonitis, hepatosplenomegaly, and increased susceptibility to bacterial infections. Secondary opportunistic infections of the immunocompromised mother are potentially a risk to the fetus or child. The availability of effective antiretroviral agents and access to infant formula (to prevent postnatal transmission through breast milk) have reduced the incidence of perinatal infections with human immunodeficiency virus in developed countries. Combination antiretroviral therapy of infected pregnant women and nevirapine therapy with or without zidovudine for 6 or 14 weeks to neonates are helpful in preventing mother-to-child transmission without an increase in fetal adverse events.[60,61] Compared with no antiretroviral treatment or monotherapy, combination therapy does not seem to be associated with increased risks of prematurity or other adverse outcomes of pregnancy.[62]

Because some of the antiviral agents used for AIDS may be teratogenic (in many instances no pharmacokinetic or safety data related to pregnancy are available),[63,64] infants born of mothers treated with them during pregnancy may have nervous system malformations from the virus itself, from the medications used in its treatment, or both. The virus invades endothelial cells, causes a vasculitis, and leads to microinfarcts in the fetal brain; its teratogenic effects depend upon the developmental stage of the fetus when it is exposed to the virus, but even late gestational exposures may affect brain development.

Children of women infected with human T-cell leukemia virus, type I (HTLV-I) may acquire the infection through breast-feeding and develop a resulting myelopathy in adult life. This is considered further in Chapter 44.

METABOLIC AND TOXIC DISORDERS

In parts of the world where malnutrition is common, many pregnant women have a deficient intake of diverse nutrients including proteins, vitamins, and minerals. The incidence of malformed fetuses is high in this circumstance, but it is generally not possible to recognize the specific deficiency that is responsible. Fetuses exhibit intrauterine growth retardation, and organ development, including that of the brain, is sometimes affected.

Clinical presentation of the neurologic manifestations of *vitamin B_{12} deficiency* (myelopathy, polyneuropathy, mental changes, optic neuropathy) do not differ during pregnancy, but any accompanying megaloblastic anemia may be obscured by folic acid supplements. As in the nonpregnant patient, treatment is with parenteral vitamin B_{12} to arrest progression and correct reversible neurologic deficits. Maternal vitamin B_{12} deficiency during pregnancy may lead to similar deficiency in neonates, exacerbated in breast-fed infants by the reduced content of vitamin B_{12} in maternal milk. Clinically, such infants exhibit apathy, developmental delay or regression, involuntary movements, cutaneous pigmentation, and megaloblastic anemia. Treatment is with vitamin supplementation.

Phenylketonuria, with its autosomal-recessive inheritance, is an important cause of mental retardation. Neonatal screening programs can identify affected infants so they can be treated before intellectual function deteriorates. Affected women have a high rate of spontaneous abortion. Offspring of untreated women have a high incidence of facial dysmorphism, developmental delay, microcephaly, and congenital heart disease. Family planning and preconception counseling are important, as dietary treatment before conception or as soon as possible thereafter may prevent or lessen some of these features.[65–68] To ensure that the diagnosis is not missed, antenatal screening for maternal phenylketonuria or testing at the first antenatal visit of women with a positive family history, low intelligence of uncertain cause, or a history of microcephalic offspring is justifiable. The homozygous offspring of an affected mother requires a diet low in phenylalanine, but the most appropriate nutritional management of heterozygotes is less certain. In any event, the affected mother should avoid breast-feeding because of the high concentration of phenylalanine in her milk.

Many *toxins* and *drugs* are teratogenic and may affect the developing nervous system. The teratogenic effects of antiepileptic drugs taken during pregnancy were considered earlier. Excessive maternal alcohol intake may lead to the fetal alcohol syndrome, in which intrauterine growth retardation and dysmorphic facies are common, but cerebral abnormalities (cortical changes, hypoplasia or agenesis of the corpus callosum, and microcephaly) may lead to seizures, mental deficiency, and motor deficits.[69] Excessive vitamin A intake early in gestation may be teratogenic (cleft palate, spina bifida).[70] Many other agents that are seemingly innocuous to the mother may affect the fetus,[64] and the topic is too extensive to be reviewed here. Most drugs are not labeled for use in pregnancy, and there are few or no data on human fetal effects at the time of marketing. The use of medication or recreational agents during pregnancy should therefore be as limited as possible.

MOVEMENT DISORDERS

Movement disorders of any type may occur during pregnancy, as at other times. Comment here is restricted to those related more specifically to pregnancy or posing obstetric problems.

Chorea gravidarum occurs most often in primigravidas, frequently without evidence of preceding streptococcal infection, as a variant of Sydenham chorea. Approximately two-thirds of patients have a history of chorea or rheumatic fever, and most of the others have signs of rheumatic heart disease. Symptoms usually begin early in pregnancy; they remit after delivery but may recur during subsequent pregnancies. Altered patterns of circulating sex hormones during pregnancy may account for the chorea by their effects on previously damaged basal ganglia (Chapter 20). The chorea improves after delivery or abortion, as sex hormone levels return to prepregnancy values. The prognosis relates to cardiac complications. The neurologic disorder generally benefits from bed rest and sedation. It is not an indication for termination of pregnancy, and there are no specific obstetric complications.

Chorea developing for the first time during pregnancy does not necessarily represent a variant of Sydenham chorea. Huntington chorea may occasionally present during pregnancy, and chorea may also develop at this time as a result of systemic lupus erythematosus, polycythemia vera rubra, thyrotoxicosis, hypocalcemia, encephalitis, cerebrovascular disease, or Wilson disease, or as a drug-induced reaction. Further discussion is provided in Chapter 58.

Chorea may be induced by oral contraceptives, sometimes in women with preexisting abnormalities of the basal ganglia. It usually begins approximately 3 months after contraceptives are started, tends to evolve subacutely, may be asymmetric or unilateral, and settles with discontinuation of the causal agent. Its pathophysiologic basis is unknown, but vascular mechanisms, immunologic mechanisms, and a hormone-dependent alteration in central dopaminergic activity have been proposed.

A number of pregnant women have the *restless legs syndrome*, usually during the latter part of pregnancy, for uncertain reasons. Among pregnant Japanese women, almost 20 percent reportedly have symptoms of restless legs syndrome[71]; the corresponding number in pregnant women in northern Italy was 27 percent.[72] Unpleasant creeping sensations occur in the legs and occasionally the arms, usually at night or during relaxation, leading to a compelling need to move about. The cause is unknown. Neurologic examination reveals no abnormalities. Treatment of coexisting anemia or iron deficiency may improve symptoms, and treatment with clonazepam is sometimes worthwhile. Other drugs that may be helpful include carbidopa-levodopa (Sinemet), pramipexole, ropinirole, gabapentin, carbamazepine, propranolol, and opiates, but these drugs are usually best avoided during pregnancy. Symptoms generally resolve spontaneously in the first few weeks postpartum.

Untreated *Wilson disease*, an autosomal-recessive disorder, is associated with a high miscarriage rate, but pregnancy poses no special problems in patients receiving adequate chelation treatment. Penicillamine therapy may be associated with mesenchymal birth defects, but a number of reports document an uneventful pregnancy with birth of a normal infant in patients treated with penicillamine or zinc sulfate.[73–75] When acute *dystonia* develops during pregnancy, the most probable cause is use of a dopamine antagonist antiemetic or neuroleptic, such as metoclopramide. In patients with long-standing dystonia of either the idiopathic or secondary variety, there is no evidence that pregnancy affects the neurologic outcome adversely. Pregnant patients with dystonia should be offered genetic counseling if the disorder has a hereditary basis; the conduct of labor depends on the severity and nature of the abnormal posturing.

Parkinson disease may develop in women who are still young enough to bear children, and concerns are sometimes expressed about the possible effects of pregnancy on the neurologic disorder. There is no consistent effect on overall parkinsonian disability, although some patients may show a worsening of their neurologic symptoms; the incidence of obstetric complications or fetal defects is not increased.

MULTIPLE SCLEROSIS

The classic, unpredictable relapses and remissions that occur in multiple sclerosis make it difficult to determine whether pregnancy influences the disorder. However, several epidemiologic studies have suggested that the relapse rate is reduced during pregnancy but increased during the 3 to 6 months immediately after childbirth.[76–80] The postpartum increase in relapse rate may relate to fatigue, stress, or a reduction in antenatal immunosuppression. Neither pregnancy itself nor the number of pregnancies affects the degree of subsequent neurologic disability.[77,81] In some studies multiple sclerosis did not seem to influence the course of pregnancy or childbirth, but in others it was associated with smaller babies for age and more frequent deliveries involving the use of forceps, vacuum extractors, or cesarian section than in controls.[82–84] Patients receiving beta-interferon therapy when they became pregnant had a higher rate of fetal wastage (miscarriages or stillbirths) and of low-birth-weight babies.[85] If possible, patients should stop beta-interferon therapy before becoming pregnant; failure to do so, however, does not necessarily imply a bad outcome, and most patients will produce a healthy infant.[86] Other disease-modifying therapies such as glatiramer acetate, natalizumab, fingolimod, and mitoxantrone are also best avoided by women who are pregnant or planning to become pregnant because limited evidence is available concerning their safety during pregnancy; they can be started or restarted in the immediate postpartum period. Intravenous corticosteroids are used to treat acute relapses during pregnancy.

Pregnant women with multiple sclerosis are often concerned about development of the disease in their offspring. Although multiple sclerosis may indeed show a familial incidence, this association is uncommon and tends to involve siblings rather than different generations, so that firm reassurance can generally be given. Pregnancy and parenthood should not be discouraged unless the patient is incapable of coping with the demands involved. Neurologic management during pregnancy is as at other times, but patients with sphincter disturbances or a paraparesis may pose particular problems. The method of delivery should be guided by obstetric factors alone.

OPTIC NEURITIS

Optic neuritis of any type may occur fortuitously during pregnancy. Optic nerve involvement is a rare complication of hyperemesis gravidarum, and uncontrollable vomiting may necessitate termination of pregnancy. Optic nerve involvement may occur during pregnancy or the postpartum period in patients with multiple sclerosis or tumors that enlarge slightly during the gestational period. Genetic counseling is important if there is a history of hereditary optic atrophy.

TRAUMATIC PARAPLEGIA

When spinal injury occurs during pregnancy, the patient must be investigated and managed with her own best interests in mind. Despite concerns that radiologic studies might affect the developing fetus, such studies should not be postponed if indicated neurologically.

Patients with established paraplegia should be educated about (1) the importance of avoiding urinary infection by ensuring a minimal amount of residual urine after micturition, and (2) the best means of avoiding pressure sores. Unless a paraplegic woman has a gross impairment of renal function, however, she need not be discouraged from pregnancy if she wishes to have a family. Care should be taken to prevent anemia during pregnancy.

The conduct of labor is complicated in paraplegic women. With complete cord lesions above T10, onset of labor is unrecognized and labor is painless. For this reason, the cervix is usually examined at each antenatal visit after approximately the 26th week of pregnancy; patients are hospitalized if the cervix is dilated, or routinely after about 32 weeks of pregnancy. With cord lesions below T10, uterine contractions are accompanied by normal pain sensations.

Complete cord lesions above T5 or T6 may be associated with *autonomic hyperreflexia.* Headache, sweating, nasal congestion, hypertension, reflex bradycardia, and cutaneous vasodilation and piloerection above the level of the lesion are often conspicuous during the uterine contractions of labor, becoming especially marked just before delivery. If unrecognized, the disorder is sometimes mistaken for pre-eclampsia. Symptoms have been attributed to release of catecholamines. Treatment in the past has included reserpine (to deplete catecholamines from sympathetic nerve terminals), atropine, clonidine, glyceryl trinitrate, or hexamethonium. Continuous lumbar epidural anesthesia can block or prevent autonomic hyperreflexia.

Cesarean section is not necessarily indicated by the paraplegia itself but may be required if there is bony deformity of the spine or pelvis. Forceps delivery may be necessary to compensate for paralysis of muscle involved in the expulsive efforts of the second stage or to shorten delivery time because of severe hypertension. Paraplegic and even quadriplegic patients have a normal milk ejection reflex during suckling and can breast-feed their infants.

ROOT AND PLEXUS LESIONS

Low back pain is common during pregnancy. There is usually no serious underlying neurologic cause, so that management is generally conservative.

Acute prolapse of a lumbar intervertebral disc, for example, is rare during pregnancy. Management of the acute prolapse is as in nonpregnant women, but it is important to distinguish the disorder from conditions simulating it. This may require imaging. MRI during pregnancy is without known adverse effects on the fetus, but the use of contrast agents is best avoided if possible.[87] Compressive injuries of the lumbosacral plexus may occur during labor and can be difficult to distinguish from an acutely prolapsed lumbar intervertebral disc. However, the latter is associated with tenderness and rigidity of the lumbar spine, sciatica, and signs of root tension. Electrophysiologic studies may also clarify the diagnosis, depending on whether there is evidence of involvement of the paraspinal muscles (which are supplied proximally from the nerve roots).

Lumbosacral plexus lesions result from compression by the fetal head or obstetric forceps of the roots of the sciatic nerve. This injury is especially likely when there is minor disproportion or when midforceps are used during delivery because of malpresentation. Anatomic features of the pelvis that predispose to this complication include a straight sacrum; a flat, wide posterior pelvis; posterior displacement of the transverse diameter of the inlet; wide sacroiliac notches; and prominent ischial spines. Symptoms are usually unilateral and develop immediately after delivery. There is often predominant involvement of fibular (peroneal) fibers, as reflected by the distribution of motor and sensory findings. With mild injuries, the prognosis for recovery is excellent, but recovery may be prolonged and incomplete if axonal degeneration has occurred. Electrophysiologic studies therefore assist in determining prognosis. Treatment of severe cases with calipers and a night cast prevents contractures.

Despite an obstetric lumbosacral plexus palsy, delivery in subsequent pregnancies need not be by cesarean section. However, cesarean section is appropriate if the infant is large or there are premonitory symptoms suggesting nerve compression with attempted engagement of the fetal head during the last 4 weeks of pregnancy.

Brachial plexopathy may occur on a familial basis, and in some of the reported cases there has been a clear association of attacks with pregnancy or the puerperium; inflammation, probably immune-based, appears pathogenic at least in some instances.[88]

PERIPHERAL NERVE DISORDERS

Entrapment Neuropathies

Two entrapment neuropathies are especially likely to occur during pregnancy.[89] *Carpal tunnel syndrome* occurs often, possibly because of fluid retention. Nocturnal pain and paresthesias in the hand disturb sleep. Weakness of the thenar muscles occurs in more advanced cases. The clinical and electrophysiologic features of the disorder do not require description here. When the syndrome develops during pregnancy, it most often does so in the third trimester (although it may present earlier), and typically settles within approximately 3 months of delivery, often within 2 weeks[90]; however, symptoms with onset in early pregnancy are less likely to improve after delivery.[91] Treatment should be conservative. The use of a nocturnal wrist splint is often helpful for alleviating symptoms; the splint is placed on the dorsal surface with the aim of maintaining the wrist in a neutral or slightly flexed position. [92] Salt restriction, local injection of corticosteroids into the carpal tunnel, or treatment with diuretics sometimes helps. The patient should be reassured about the benign nature of her symptoms. Surgical division of the anterior carpal ligament is usually unnecessary unless symptoms become intolerable or continue to progress in the weeks after delivery. In some instances, carpal tunnel syndrome develops in the puerperium; it may then relate to the position of the hand and wrist during breast-feeding. Treatment is conservative, but the wearing of wrist splints at such a time may be difficult.

Entrapment of the lateral femoral cutaneous nerve is also common during pregnancy, especially in its later stages, and leads to the syndrome of *meralgia paresthetica*.[93] Pain, paresthesias, and numbness occur about the outer aspect of the thigh, usually unilaterally, and are sometimes relieved by sitting. Clinical examination reveals no abnormality except in advanced cases, when cutaneous sensation may be disturbed in the affected area. Symptoms generally settle spontaneously within a few weeks of delivery, and the patient can therefore be reassured. In rare instances, however, the pain has reportedly been so severe that labor has been induced early. Local injection of hydrocortisone about the region where the nerve lies medial to the anterior superior iliac spine may provide temporary benefit. Symptomatic relief may also follow treatment with low-dose tricyclic antidepressants; anticonvulsant drugs such as carbamazepine should be avoided during pregnancy.

Traumatic Mononeuropathies

A number of isolated nerve lesions may occur as a complication of various obstetric maneuvers. Lower-limb nerve injury has been associated with nulliparity and a prolonged second stage of labor.[94] The *obturator nerve* may be injured when the patient is in the lithotomy position because of angulation as the nerve leaves the obturator foramen. It may also be compressed between the fetal head and the bony pelvic wall.[95] Similarly, an isolated *femoral neuropathy* may occur by angulation and pressure from the inguinal ligament when the thighs are markedly flexed and abducted, as when anesthetized patients are placed in the lithotomy position; stretch of the nerve by excessive hip abduction and external rotation may also occur. The *saphenous nerve* is sometimes injured by pressure from leg braces when the patient is improperly suspended in the lithotomy position. The most common cause of *sciatic nerve* palsy is a misplaced deep intramuscular injection, but this nerve can also be injured by stretch when a patient is placed in stirrups on the obstetric table. To avoid such injury, the knee and hip joints should be well flexed and extreme external rotation of the hip avoided. The *common fibular (peroneal) nerve* may be injured in the region of the head of the fibula by pressure from the leg braces of the obstetric table, especially in anesthetized women.[96] The clinical features of all these neuropathies are well known and are not recapitulated here.

Damage during labor and delivery to the innervation of the sphincter muscles in the pelvic floor may be responsible for stress incontinence of urine or feces, as discussed in Chapter 29.

Bell Palsy

Idiopathic lower motor neuron facial palsy is common and shows a definite association with pregnancy, speculatively attributed by some to fluid retention, a viral inflammatory reaction, or pregnancy-related immunosuppression.[97] Approximately 85 percent of cases occurred during the third trimester of pregnancy or the puerperium. The onset of Bell palsy during pregnancy has been related to hypertensive disorders, implying that patients who develop Bell palsy during pregnancy should be monitored closely for hypertension or pre-eclampsia.[98] Diabetes should be excluded. Although most patients with Bell palsy recover completely without treatment, such recovery may be less likely for women with a complete palsy developing during pregnancy than for the general population.[99] Despite questions concerning its efficacy, treatment with corticosteroids is generally prescribed for Bell palsy, especially if a poor prognosis is anticipated because of severe pain or a clinically complete palsy and if patients are seen within the first week of the disorder. Antiviral therapies are probably not effective.[100] In patients with a complete facial palsy, protection of the cornea should be ensured. Electrodiagnostic evaluation after the first week provides a guide to prognosis.

Polyneuropathies

There is no specific polyneuropathy of pregnancy, but any type may occur during the gestational period. *Nutritional deficiency* is probably the most likely cause in patients from one of the developing nations or in those with hyperemesis. There may be evidence of peripheral nerve involvement in patients with hyperemesis gravidarum complicated by Wernicke encephalopathy and sometimes by Korsakoff syndrome. Diagnosis is confirmed by finding a marked reduction in blood transketolase activity and a marked thiamine pyrophosphate effect. As in nonpregnant women, treatment is with thiamine, 100 mg being given once intravenously and then intramuscularly for several days until a satisfactory diet is ensured. Vitamin B_{12} deficiency was discussed earlier (see p. 670).

Guillain–Barré syndrome may occur during any stage of pregnancy. A Scandinavian epidemiologic study has suggested that the disorder has a lower incidence during pregnancy but an increased incidence in the first month of the postpartum period.[101] It may be associated with antecedent infections such as with *Campylobacter jejuni* or cytomegalovirus.[102,103] Its course is not influenced by pregnancy. Approximately 3 percent of patients have one or more relapses, sometimes several years after the initial illness, and they occasionally occur in relation to pregnancy. There has been a case reported of a mother with cytomegalovirus-related acute inflammatory neuropathy that developed approximately 10 weeks before delivery of a healthy infant who, in turn, developed a neonatal inflammatory neuropathy after several days.[104]

Serial ultrasonographic fetal monitoring has sometimes been performed but usually reveals normal fetal movement, even when paralysis is severe in the mother. Early ventilatory support may be helpful in preventing fetal hypoxia.[105] Hypotensive episodes due to autonomic involvement may necessitate volume expansion to ensure adequate placental perfusion. The maternal outcome appears unaffected by early delivery. The Guillain–Barré syndrome is treated as in nonpregnant women; experience with plasmapheresis or intravenous immunoglobulin therapy is more limited in this circumstance but both have been used safely during pregnancy. Delivery may require forceps or assisted extraction devices because of weakness of the abdominal muscles, which may reduce the ability to increase the intra-abdominal pressure voluntarily; uterine contractions are normal.

When relapse of *chronic inflammatory demyelinating polyneuropathy occurs* during pregnancy, it is usually late in pregnancy or in the puerperium. There are no specific fetal complications. Treatment is as in nonpregnant women, but concerns regarding plasmapheresis and intravenous immunoglobulin merit reiteration; there is further concern about the use of azathioprine, cyclosporine, and cyclophosphamide, which may retard fetal growth and have other adverse effects, including potential teratogenicity. *Multifocal motor neuropathy* with conduction block may be exacerbated during pregnancy but responds to intravenous immunoglobulin therapy; after pregnancy, power reverted to its previous level.[106]

Pregnancy may lead to acute exacerbations in the hepatic type of *porphyria*. The usual neurologic manifestation is a polyneuropathy that is predominantly motor but sometimes has pronounced autonomic accompaniments. Cerebral manifestations may also occur. In many patients with hepatic porphyria, however, pregnancy is well tolerated. Relapses may occur at any time, but are most likely during early pregnancy and may then lead to spontaneous abortion. Patients with this disorder who are contemplating pregnancy must therefore understand the implications and uncertain outcome, and they must be monitored closely during the gestational period. Caution must also be exercised in the medications used during and after labor because they may provoke exacerbations.

MYASTHENIA GRAVIS

Myasthenia gravis, an autoimmune disorder of neuromuscular transmission, is associated most commonly with antibodies against muscle nicotinic acetylcholine receptors; in seronegative cases, antibodies against muscle-specific kinase (MuSK) are often present. Exacerbations of myasthenia gravis may occur in relation to the menstrual period. The disorder may be influenced in an unpredictable manner by pregnancy, and the effect of pregnancy may vary in the same patient on different occasions. Pregnancy does not worsen the long-term outlook.[107] The severity of the myasthenia at the time of the pregnancy does not predict the occurrence of exacerbation or remission. Remission occurs during pregnancy in approximately one-third of cases, relapse in another one-third,[108] and no change in the remainder. A significant additional number of relapses occur in the postpartum period, when they tend to be particularly severe[109]; these may relate in part to postpartum infection. Relapses may occur at any time during the pregnancy. Severe relapse of the disorder may suggest the need for termination of pregnancy, but termination does not necessarily lead to clinical benefit. The myasthenia must be treated effectively but, as indicated earlier, the safety (to mother or fetus) of cholinesterase inhibitors, immunosuppressive agents, plasmapheresis, and intravenous immunoglobulins during pregnancy is not completely clear; the potential risks of such treatment, however, must be balanced against the risks to both mother and fetus of myasthenic crisis.[110] Plasmapheresis or intravenous immunoglobulin therapy has been used safely and effectively in myasthenic patients during pregnancy.[108]

Myasthenia gravis has little effect on pregnancy itself, unless it leads to maternal respiratory inadequacy; weakness of the respiratory muscles may be exacerbated by a restriction of diaphragmatic excursions by the growing fetus. There is sometimes a marked contrast between the strength of uterine contractions during the second stage of labor and the severity of skeletal muscle weakness. Enemas should not be given because they may precipitate a myasthenic crisis. Cesarean section is best reserved for patients in whom it is indicated for obstetric reasons.[111] Regional anesthesia rather than general anesthesia is desirable, and the use of muscle relaxant drugs should be avoided if possible. Magnesium sulfate should not be used in myasthenic patients with toxemia because of its effects on neuromuscular transmission. In a population-based cohort study, no significant differences were found in perinatal mortality, mean gestational age, or birth weight between the offspring of myasthenic and nonmyasthenic women.[112] Breast-feeding is not contraindicated.

Neonatal myasthenia, a transient disorder that may relate to placental transfer of maternal antibodies against acetylcholine receptors, occurs in approximately 10 to 15 percent of the newborn infants of myasthenic women, regardless of the duration or severity of the maternal illness or anti–acetylcholine receptor antibody titer.[107] Infants of myasthenic mothers should therefore be watched carefully for clinical signs of the disorder: a poor cry, respiratory difficulties, weakness in sucking, feeble limb movements, and a weak Moro reflex. Symptoms generally become apparent within the first 3 days of birth but are not usually evident immediately after birth. The neonatal disorder can be treated with anticholinesterase drugs if necessary, and it usually subsides within 6 weeks of delivery. Its occurrence in one child does not imply that subsequent children born to the same mother will have the disorder.

The transient neonatal form of myasthenia is distinct from congenital myasthenia, which is rare, occurs in children born to healthy mothers, and is a life-long disorder that varies in type with age of onset, severity, and pathogenesis.

MYOTONIC DYSTROPHY

The weakness and myotonia of myotonic dystrophy type 1 may worsen during pregnancy, and the course of the disorder sometimes appears to accelerate during the gestational period. Women with early-onset myotonic dystrophy are more likely to experience a complicated pregnancy than those with later onset.[113] A number of obstetric complications have been reported, including threatened, spontaneous, and habitual abortion; ectopic pregnancy; and placenta praevia. Perinatal loss (stillbirths or neonatal deaths) is increased and has been related to congenitally affected fetuses and associated complications of the pregnancy.[113] Hydramnios has been attributed to diminished fetal swallowing. Premature onset of labor in patients with myotonic dystrophy has sometimes been attributed to abnormalities of uterine muscle. The uterus may fail to contract normally during labor, so that the first stage is prolonged, and retention of the placenta and postpartum hemorrhage may occur. Skeletal muscle weakness may also lead to difficulties during the second stage of labor. If anesthesia is required for obstetric reasons, depolarizing muscle relaxant drugs should be avoided because they may cause myotonic spasm, and nondepolarizing drugs are given in reduced dosage to patients who are taking quinine for their myotonia. Electrocardiographic monitoring facilitates the early recognition of cardiac arrhythmias, to which patients with myotonic dystrophy are prone, and which may require a pacemaker. General anesthetics may lead to marked respiratory depression, and regional analgesia is the preferred method of management.

Type 2 myotonic dystrophy (CCTG expansion in intron 1 of the *ZNF9* gene on chromosome 3q 21.3) may first become manifest during pregnancy, with worsening occurring in subsequent pregnancies, for uncertain reasons. When initial symptoms occur before or during pregnancy, marked improvement often follows delivery, with a recurrence of symptoms in subsequent pregnancies.[114,115] In one series, preterm labor occurred in 50 percent of pregnancies and was more likely in women who developed the first symptoms or a deterioration of the myotonic dystrophy during pregnancy compared with those in whom an influence of gestation on the disease course was inapparent. No increased obstetric risk was found, and early pregnancy loss rate was normal.[114]

Myotonic dystrophy type 1 may occur congenitally among the offspring of mothers with the disease. Magee and colleagues calculated that the risk of a child having congenital myotonic dystrophy is 59 to 100 percent if the maternal CTG expansion is greater than 1 to 4 kb, as opposed to 17 percent if the expansion is less than 1 kb.[116] An affected mother is more likely to have a child with congenital myotonic dystrophy in a first pregnancy if she has multisystem disease when pregnant, age at onset is less than 30 years, her father is the affected parent, and CTG expansion is more than 1 kb; however, even subclinically affected women with low repeat sizes can have congenitally affected offspring.[116] Recurrence risk to further children is high if an affected woman has given birth to one child with congenital myotonic dystrophy and has been estimated as nearly 100 percent.[116] There may be a history of hydramnios or reduced fetal activity during late pregnancy. Affected infants may die within hours or a few days of birth. Clinical features of the disorder in such infants include facial diplegia, hypotonia, respiratory distress, feeding difficulties, delayed motor development, and mental retardation. Talipes is also common. Myotonia is absent clinically in neonates with the congenital form of myotonic dystrophy but is uniformly present in children 10 years or older. Myotonic dystrophy type 2 has not been reported in congenital form.[114,117]

In congenital myotonic dystrophy, transmission is generally via the mother. The data suggest that the disorder results from the combination of the gene responsible for the disorder in adults, with some additional maternally transmitted factor.

The gene causing myotonic dystrophy type 1 is on chromosome 19q13.2-q13.3 and has variable penetrance; increasing numbers of triplet repeat expansions govern development of clinical disease. Genetic counseling is an important consideration for women with myotonic dystrophy who are contemplating pregnancy. Counseling and planning of pregnancy may be difficult in patients with mild cognitive impairment or behavioral disturbances. Prenatal detection of the disorder provides the opportunity for abortion of an affected fetus.

ECLAMPSIA AND PRE-ECLAMPSIA

Reference has not been made in this chapter to eclampsia (defined as the occurrence of seizures or coma in a patient with pre-eclampsia, i.e., the onset of hypertension and proteinuria during the second half of pregnancy), which is usually treated by obstetricians rather than neurologists. The neurologic manifestations of pre-eclampsia or eclampsia include headache, tinnitus, diplopia, visual blurring, scotomas, and transient blindness that may arise cortically. The pathophysiologic basis of the seizures or coma that occur in patients with eclampsia is unclear, but the cerebral dysfunction has been attributed to a number of factors, including intensive vasoconstriction, endothelial damage, cerebral edema, and disseminated intravascular coagulation in the cerebral microcirculation. The relationship between hypertension, seizures, and cerebral dysfunction is unclear and unpredictable, but a further increment in the previously elevated blood pressure or an exacerbation of headache may be noted. Imaging (CT scans or MRI) may reveal cerebral edema, ischemia, infarction, or hemorrhage, and angiographic evidence of vasospasm is sometimes found; the radiologic findings resemble those in hypertensive encephalopathy. Treatment generally consists of controlling hypertension, preventing convulsions, and reducing cerebral edema. In extreme cases, termination of pregnancy may be necessary. In general, seizures can be controlled with intravenous diazepam, with the addition of phenytoin if necessary. Many obstetricians prefer to use magnesium sulfate to control eclamptic seizures, and some justification exists for this approach, which may be superior in this context to phenytoin[118,119] or diazepam.[120] A common regimen is to administer 10g intramuscularly followed by 5g intramuscularly every 4 hours, depending on renal output. The aim is to achieve a serum magnesium level of 5 to 8mEq/L. Other therapeutic approaches reflect obstetric management and include prompt delivery, and need not be recapitulated here.

Pre-eclampsia (hypertension, proteinuria, and edema, occurring between the 20th week of gestation and 48 hours postpartum) may present with a variety of manifestations due to involvement of such different organs as the kidney, liver, heart, central nervous system (CNS), or blood-clotting system. It may be clinically impossible to distinguish between pre-eclampsia and either thrombotic thrombocytopenic purpura or the hemolytic-uremic syndrome. Hematologically, however, pre-eclampsia is characterized by disseminated intravascular coagulation and reduction of plasma antithrombin III activity, in contrast to thrombotic thrombocytopenic purpura and hemolytic-uremic syndrome. The so-called HELLP syndrome (hemolysis, elevated liver enzymes, and low platelet count), probably a variant of pre-eclampsia, frequently has major neurologic consequences such as intracerebral hemorrhage.

The posterior reversible leukoencephalopathy syndrome (PRES) is sometimes considered to be indicative of eclampsia, even when there are no other features of eclampsia (proteinuria, hypertension).[121] It is characterized by the gradual onset of headache, confusion or an impairment of consciousness, visual changes, and seizures, associated with edema of the posterior cerebral (parieto-occipital) white matter on imaging studies. The MRI findings consist most often of punctate or confluent areas of increased signal on proton density and T2-weighted images (Fig. 31-5).[122] Treatment is as for pre-eclampsia or eclampsia.

Thrombotic thrombocytopenic purpura is characterized by fever, Coombs-negative hemolytic anemia, thrombocytopenic purpura, fluctuating neurologic

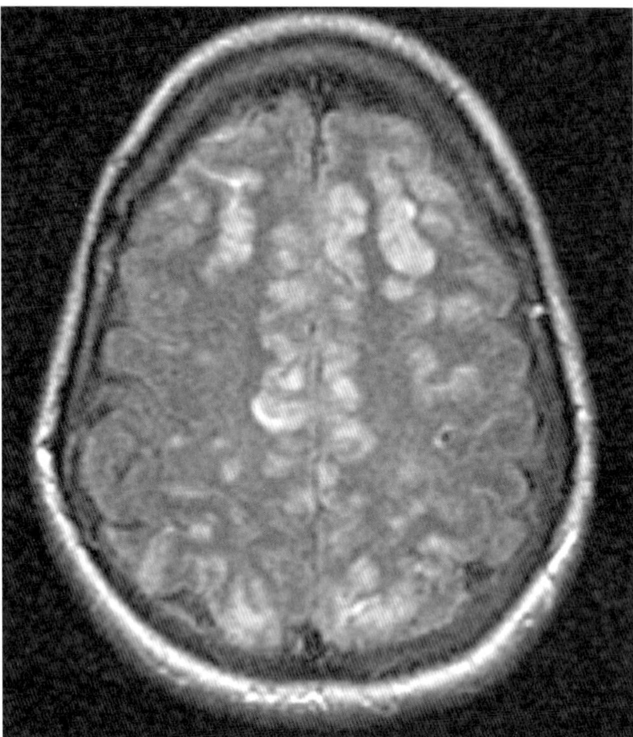

FIGURE 31-5 ■ Posterior reversible leukoencephalopathy syndrome (PRES) in a patient with eclampsia, following a seizure. Axial T2-weighted FLAIR MR image demonstrates symmetric high signal intensity, in this instance involving also the cortex of the frontal and parietal lobes bilaterally. (Courtesy of William P. Dillon, MD, University of California, San Francisco.)

involvement, and renal disease, and it may simulate pre-eclampsia. Its neurologic features are discussed in Chapter 25. Thrombotic thrombocytopenic purpura may develop during the antepartum period, often before approximately 24 weeks of gestation, and may result in infant death, although successful treatment may permit prolongation of the pregnancy. Treatment is by plasma exchange or infusion. Platelet transfusions should be avoided because they may trigger an exacerbation. Antiplatelet agents (such as aspirin or dipyridamole) usually are not effective, but treatment with corticosteroids may be helpful. Postpartum *hemolytic-uremic syndrome* is similar to thrombotic thrombocytopenic purpura, and many consider it within the same spectrum.

REFERENCES

1. Quality Standards Subcommittee, American Academy of Neurology: Practice parameter: management issues for women with epilepsy (summary statement). Neurology 51:944, 1998.
2. Yerby MS: Pregnancy and epilepsy. Epilepsia 32(suppl 6): S51, 1991.
3. EURAP Study Group: Seizure control and treatment in pregnancy: observations from the EURAP Epilepsy Pregnancy Registry. Neurology 66:354, 2006.
4. Tanganelli P, Regesta G: Epilepsy, pregnancy, and major birth anomalies: an Italian prospective, controlled study. Neurology 42:89, 1992.
5. Harden CL, Hopp J, Ting TY, et al: Practice parameter update: management issues for women with epilepsy—focus on pregnancy (an evidence-based review): obstetrical complications and change in seizure frequency: report of the Quality Standards Subcommittee and Therapeutics and Technology Assessment Subcommittee of the American Academy of Neurology and American Epilepsy Society. Neurology 73:126, 2009.
6. Harden CL, Pennell PB, Koppel BS, et al: Practice parameter update: management issues for women with epilepsy—focus on pregnancy (an evidence-based review): vitamin K, folic acid, blood levels, and breastfeeding: report of the Quality Standards Subcommittee and Therapeutics and Technology Assessment Subcommittee of the American Academy of Neurology and American Epilepsy Society. Neurology 73:142, 2009.
7. Perucca E: Birth defects after prenatal exposure to antiepileptic drugs. Lancet Neurol 4:781, 2005.
8. Morrow J, Russell A, Guthrie E, et al: Malformation risks of antiepileptic drugs in pregnancy: a prospective study from the UK Epilepsy and Pregnancy Register. J Neurol Neurosurg Psychiatry 77:193, 2006.
9. Harden CL, Meador KJ, Pennell PB, et al: Practice parameter update: management issues for women with epilepsy—focus on pregnancy (an evidence-based review): teratogenesis and perinatal outcomes: report of the Quality Standards Subcommittee and Therapeutics and Technology Assessment Subcommittee of the American Academy of Neurology and American Epilepsy Society. Neurology 73:133, 2009.
10. Crawford P: Best practice guidelines for the management of women with epilepsy. Epilepsia 46(suppl 9): 117, 2005.
11. Hunt SJ, Morrow JI: Safety of antiepileptic drugs during pregnancy. Expert Opin Drug Saf 4:869, 2005.
12. Alsdorf R, Wyszynski DF: Teratogenicity of sodium valproate. Expert Opin Drug Saf 4:345, 2005.
13. Wyszynski DF, Nambisan M, Surve T, et al: Increased rate of major malformations in offspring exposed to valproate during pregnancy. Neurology 64:961, 2005.
14. Jentink J, Loane MA, Dolk H, et al: Valproic acid monotherapy in pregnancy and major congenital malformations. N Engl J Med 362:2185, 2010.
15. Kini U, Adab N, Vinten J, et al: Dysmorphic features: an important clue to the diagnosis and severity of fetal anticonvulsant syndromes. Arch Dis Child Fetal Neonatal Ed 91:F90, 2006.

16. Dansky LV, Rosenblatt DS, Andermann E: Mechanisms of teratogenesis: folic acid and antiepileptic therapy. Neurology 42(suppl 5):32, 1992.
17. Finnell RH, Buehler BA, Kerr BM, et al: Clinical and experimental studies linking oxidative metabolism to phenytoin-induced teratogenesis. Neurology 42(suppl 5):25, 1992.
18. Hey E: Effect of maternal anticonvulsant treatment on neonatal blood coagulation. Arch Dis Child Fetal Neonatal Ed 81:F208, 1999.
19. Choulika S, Grabowski E, Holmes LB: Is antenatal vitamin K prophylaxis needed for pregnant women taking anticonvulsants? Am J Obstet Gynecol 190:882, 2004.
20. Katz O, Levy A, Wiznitzer A, et al: Pregnancy and perinatal outcome in epileptic women: a population-based study. J Matern Fetal Neonatal Med 19:21, 2006.
21. Zupanc ML: Antiepileptic drugs and hormonal contraceptives in adolescent women with epilepsy. Neurology 66(suppl 3):S37, 2006.
22. Silberstein SD: Headaches and women: treatment of the pregnant and lactating migraineur. Headache 33:533, 1993.
23. Fox AW, Diamond ML, Spierings EL: Migraine during pregnancy: options for therapy. CNS Drugs 19:465, 2005.
24. Contag SA, Bushnell C: Contemporary management of migrainous disorders in pregnancy. Curr Opin Obstet Gynecol 22:437, 2010.
25. Soldin OP, Dahlin J, O'Mara DM: Triptans in pregnancy. Ther Drug Monit 30:5, 2008.
26. Hsu DW, Efird JT, Hedley-Whyte ET: Progesterone and estrogen receptors in meningiomas: prognostic considerations. J Neurosurg 86:113, 1997.
27. Kupersmith MJ, Rosenberg C, Kleinberg D: Visual loss in pregnant women with pituitary adenomas. Ann Intern Med 121:473, 1994.
28. Kal HB, Struikmans H: Radiotherapy during pregnancy: fact and fiction. Lancet Oncol 6:328, 2005.
29. Gumma AD: Recurrent benign intracranial hypertension in pregnancy. Eur J Obstet Gynecol Reprod Biol 115:244, 2004.
30. Kittner SJ, Stern BJ, Feeser BR, et al: Pregnancy and the risk of stroke. N Engl J Med 335:768, 1996.
31. Grosset DG, Ebrahim S, Bone I, et al: Stroke in pregnancy and the puerperium: what magnitude of risk? J Neurol Neurosurg Psychiatry 58:129, 1995.
32. Schipper HM: Sex hormones and the nervous system. p. 409. In Aminoff MJ (ed): Neurology and General Medicine. 4th Ed. Churchill Livingstone Elsevier, Philadelphia, 2008.
33. Okamoto K, Horisawa R, Kawamura T, et al: Menstrual and reproductive factors for subarachnoid hemorrhage risk in women: a case-control study in Nagoya, Japan. Stroke 32:2841, 2001.
34. Longstreth WT, Nelson LM, Koepsell TD, et al: Subarachnoid hemorrhage and hormonal factors in women: a population-based case-control study. Ann Intern Med 121:168, 1994.
35. Jaigobin C, Silver FL: Stroke and pregnancy. Stroke 31:2948, 2000.
36. Perry KG, Morrison JC: The diagnosis and management of hemoglobinopathies during pregnancy. Semin Perinatol 14:90, 1990.
37. Branch DW: Antiphospholipid antibodies and pregnancy: maternal implications. Semin Perinatol 14:139, 1990.
38. Ziakas PD, Pavlou M, Voulgarelis M: Heparin treatment in antiphospholipid syndrome with recurrent pregnancy loss: a systematic review and meta-analysis. Obstet Gynecol 115:1256, 2010.
39. Ro A, Frishman WH: Peripartum cardiomyopathy. Cardiol Rev 14:35, 2006.
40. Elkayam U, Tummala PP, Rao K, et al: Maternal and fetal outcomes of subsequent pregnancies in women with peripartum cardiomyopathy. N Engl J Med 344:1567, 2001.
41. Fugate JE, Ameriso SF, Ortiz G, et al: Variable presentations of postpartum angiopathy. Stroke 43:670, 2012.
42. Ducros A, Boukobza M, Porcher R, et al: The clinical and radiological spectrum of reversible cerebral vasoconstriction syndrome. A prospective series of 67 patients. Brain 130:3091, 2007.
43. Singhal AB, Hajj-Ali RA, Topcuoglu MA, et al: Reversible cerebral vasoconstriction syndromes: analysis of 139 cases. Arch Neurol 68:100, 2011.
44. Tuffnell DJ: Amniotic fluid embolism. Curr Opin Obstet Gynecol 15:119, 2003.
45. Leonhardt G, Gaul C, Nietsch HH, et al: Thrombolytic therapy in pregnancy. J Thromb Thrombolysis 21:271, 2006.
46. Ehtisham A, Stern BJ: Cerebral venous thrombosis: a review. Neurologist 12:32–, 2006.38.
47. Saposnik G, Barinagarrementeria F, Brown Jr RD, et al: Diagnosis and management of cerebral venous thrombosis: a statement for healthcare professionals from the American Heart Association/American Stroke Association. Stroke 42:1158, 2011.
48. Einhaupl KM, Villringer A, Meister W, et al: Heparin treatment in sinus venous thrombosis. Lancet 338:597, 1991.
49. Appenzeller S, Zeller CB, Annichino-Bizzachi JM, et al: Cerebral venous thrombosis: influence of risk factors and imaging findings on prognosis. Clin Neurol Neurosurg 107:371, 2005.
50. Horton JC, Chambers WA, Lyons SL, et al: Pregnancy and the risk of hemorrhage from cerebral arteriovenous malformations. Neurosurgery 27:867, 1990.
51. Friedlander RM: Arteriovenous malformations of the brain. N Engl J Med 356:2704, 2007.
52. Witlin AG, Mattar F, Sibai BM: Postpartum stroke: a twenty-year experience. Am J Obstet Gynecol 183:83, 2000.
53. Komiyama M, Yasui T, Kitano S, et al: Moyamoya disease and pregnancy: case report and review of the literature. Neurosurgery 43:360, 1998.

54. Fadli M, Lmejjati M, Amarti A, et al: Metastatic and hemorrhagic brain arteriovenous fistulae due to a choriocarcinoma: case report. Neurochirurgie 48:39, 2002.
55. Aminoff MJ: Spinal vascular disease. p. 423. In: Critchley EMR, Eisen A (eds): Diseases of the Spinal Cord. 2nd Ed.. Springer, London, 1997.
56. Bach JR: Successful pregnancies for ventilator users. Am J Phys Med Rehabil 82:226, 2003.
57. Lawn JE, Wilczynska-Ketende K, Cousens SN: Estimating the causes of 4 million neonatal deaths in the year 2000. Int J Epidemiol 35:706, 2006.
58. Demicheli V, Barale A, Rivetti A: Vaccines for women to prevent neonatal tetanus. Cochrane Database Syst Rev:CD002959, 2005.
59. Frey TK: Neurological aspects of rubella virus infection. Intervirology 40:167, 1997.
60. Sturt AS, Dokubo EK, Sint TT: Antiretroviral therapy (ART) for treating HIV infection in ART-eligible pregnant women. Cochrane Database Syst Rev:CD008440, 2010.
61. Horvath T, Madi BC, Iuppa IM, et al: Interventions for preventing late postnatal mother-to-child transmission of HIV. Cochrane Database Syst Rev:CD006734, 2009.
62. Tuomala RE, Shapiro DE, Mofenson LM, et al: Antiretroviral therapy during pregnancy and the risk of an adverse outcome. N Engl J Med 346:1863, 2002.
63. Capparelli E, Rakhmanina N, Mirochnick M: Pharmacotherapy of perinatal HIV. Semin Fetal Neonatal Med 10:161, 2005.
64. Jacqz-Aigrain E, Koren G: Effects of drugs on the fetus. Semin Fetal Neonatal Med 10:139, 2005.
65. Waisbren SE, Azen C: Cognitive and behavioral development in maternal phenylketonuria offspring. Pediatrics 112:1544, 2003.
66. Clarke JT: The Maternal Phenylketonuria Project: a summary of progress and challenges for the future. Pediatrics 112:1584, 2003.
67. Feillet F, Abadie V, Berthelot J, et al: Maternal phenylketonuria: the French survey. Eur J Pediatr 163:540, 2004.
68. Lee PJ, Ridout D, Walter JH, et al: Maternal phenylketonuria: report from the United Kingdom Registry 1978–97. Arch Dis Child 90:143, 2005.
69. Chen WJ, Maier SE, Parnell SE, et al: Alcohol and the developing brain: neuroanatomical studies. Alcohol Res Health 27:174, 2003.
70. Ackermans MM, Zhou H, Carels CE, et al: Vitamin A and clefting: putative biological mechanisms. Nutr Rev 69:613, 2011.
71. Suzuki K, Ohida T, Sone T, et al: The prevalence of restless legs syndrome among pregnant women in Japan and the relationship between restless legs syndrome and sleep problems. Sleep 26:673, 2003.
72. Manconi M, Govoni V, De Vito A, et al: Restless legs syndrome and pregnancy. Neurology 63:1065, 2004.
73. Furman B, Bashiri A, Wiznitzer A, et al: Wilson's disease in pregnancy: five successful consecutive pregnancies of the same woman. Eur J Obstet Gynecol Reprod Biol 96:232, 2001.
74. Pellecchia MT, Criscuolo C, Longo K, et al: Clinical presentation and treatment of Wilson's disease: a single-centre experience. Eur Neurol 50:48, 2003.
75. Sinha S, Taly AB, Prashanth LK, et al: Successful pregnancies and abortions in symptomatic and asymptomatic Wilson's disease. J Neurol Sci 217:37, 2004.
76. Birk K, Ford C, Smeltzer S, et al: The clinical course of multiple sclerosis during pregnancy and the puerperium. Arch Neurol 47:738, 1990.
77. Roullet E, Verdier-Taillefer M-H, Amarenco P, et al: Pregnancy and multiple sclerosis: a longitudinal study of 125 remittent patients. J Neurol Neurosurg Psychiatry 56:1062, 1993.
78. Finkelsztejn A, Brooks JB, Paschoal Jr FM, et al: What can we really tell women with multiple sclerosis regarding pregnancy? A systematic review and meta-analysis of the literature. BJOG 118:790, 2011.
79. Confavreux C, Hutchinson M, Hours MM, et al: Rate of pregnancy-related relapse in multiple sclerosis. Pregnancy in Multiple Sclerosis Group. N Engl J Med 339:285, 1998.
80. Vukusic S, Hutchinson M, Hours M, et al: Pregnancy and multiple sclerosis (the PRIMS study): clinical predictors of post-partum relapse. Brain 127:1353, 2004.
81. Stenager E, Stenager EN, Jensen K: Effect of pregnancy on the prognosis for multiple sclerosis. A 5-year follow up investigation. Acta Neurol Scand 90:305, 1994.
82. Dahl J, Myhr KM, Daltveit AK, et al: Pregnancy, delivery, and birth outcome in women with multiple sclerosis. Neurology 65:1961, 2005.
83. Kelly VM, Nelson LM, Chakravarty EF: Obstetric outcomes in women with multiple sclerosis and epilepsy. Neurology 73:1831, 2009.
84. Dahl J, Myhr KM, Daltveit AK, et al: Pregnancy, delivery, and birth outcome in women with multiple sclerosis. Neurology 65:1961, 2005.
85. Boskovic R, Wide R, Wolpin J, et al: The reproductive effects of beta interferon therapy in pregnancy: a longitudinal cohort. Neurology 65:807, 2005.
86. Sandberg-Wollheim M, Frank D, Goodwin TM, et al: Pregnancy outcomes during treatment with interferon beta-1a in patients with multiple sclerosis. Neurology 65:802, 2005.
87. ACOG Committee on Obstetric Practice: ACOG Committee Opinion. No. 299, September 2004 (replaces No. 158, September 1995). Guidelines for diagnostic imaging during pregnancy. Obstet Gynecol 104:647, 2004.
88. Klein CJ, Dyck PJ, Friedenberg SM, et al: Inflammation and neuropathic attacks in hereditary brachial plexus neuropathy. J Neurol Neurosurg Psychiatry 73:45, 2002.

89. Sax TW, Rosenbaum RB: Neuromuscular disorders in pregnancy. Muscle Nerve 34:559, 2006.
90. Finsen V, Zeitlmann H: Carpal tunnel syndrome during pregnancy. Scand J Plast Reconstr Surg Hand Surg 40:41, 2006.
91. Padua L, Aprile I, Caliandro P, et al: Carpal tunnel syndrome in pregnancy: multiperspective follow-up of untreated cases. Neurology 59:1643, 2002.
92. Weimer LH, Yin J, Lovelace RE, et al: Serial studies of carpal tunnel syndrome during and after pregnancy. Muscle Nerve 25:914, 2002.
93. van Slobbe AM, Bohnen AM, Bernsen RM, et al: Incidence rates and determinants in meralgia paresthetica in general practice. J Neurol 251:294, 2004.
94. Wong CA, Scavone BM, Dugan S, et al: Incidence of postpartum lumbosacral spine and lower extremity nerve injuries. Obstet Gynecol 101:279, 2003.
95. Nogajski JH, Shnier RC, Zagami AS: Postpartum obturator neuropathy. Neurology 63:2450, 2004.
96. Mabie WC: Peripheral neuropathies during pregnancy. Clin Obstet Gynecol 48:57, 2005.
97. Cohen Y, Lavie O, Granovsky-Grisaru S, et al: Bell palsy complicating pregnancy: a review. Obstet Gynecol Surv 55:184, 2000.
98. Shmorgun D, Chan WS, Ray JG: Association between Bell's palsy in pregnancy and pre-eclampsia. QJM 95:359, 2002.
99. Gillman GS, Schaitkin BM, May M, et al: Bell's palsy in pregnancy: a study of recovery outcomes. Otolaryngol Head Neck Surg 126:26, 2002.
100. Lockhart P, Daly F, Pitkethly M, et al: Antiviral treatment for Bell's palsy (idiopathic facial paralysis). Cochrane Database Syst Rev:CD001869, 2009.
101. Jiang GX, De Pedro-Cuesta J, Strigard K, et al: Pregnancy and Guillain–Barré syndrome: a nationwide register cohort study. Neuroepidemiology 15:192, 1996.
102. Hurley TJ, Brunson AD, Archer RL, et al: Landry Guillain–Barré Strohl syndrome in pregnancy: report of three cases treated with plasmapheresis. Obstet Gynecol 78:482, 1991.
103. Mendizabal JE, Bassam BA: Guillain–Barré syndrome and cytomegalovirus infection during pregnancy. South Med J 90:63, 1997.
104. Luijckx GJ, Vles J, de Baets M, et al: Guillain–Barré syndrome in mother and newborn child. Lancet 349:27, 1997.
105. Gauthier PE, Hantson P, Vekemans MC, et al: Intensive care management of Guillain–Barré syndrome during pregnancy. Intensive Care Med 16:460, 1990.
106. Chaudhry V, Escolar DM, Cornblath DR: Worsening of multifocal motor neuropathy during pregnancy. Neurology 59:139, 2002.
107. Batocchi AP, Majolini L, Evoli A, et al: Course and treatment of myasthenia gravis during pregnancy. Neurology 52:447, 1999.
108. Ferrero S, Pretta S, Nicoletti A, et al: Myasthenia gravis: management issues during pregnancy. Eur J Obstet Gynecol Reprod Biol 121:129, 2005.
109. Plauché WC: Myasthenia gravis in mothers and their newborns. Clin Obstet Gynecol 34:82, 1991.
110. Ciafaloni E, Massey JM: The management of myasthenia gravis in pregnancy. Semin Neurol 24:95, 2004.
111. Ferrero S, Esposito F, Biamonti M, et al: Myasthenia gravis during pregnancy. Expert Rev Neurother 8:979, 2008.
112. Hoff JM, Daltveit AK, Gilhus NE: Myasthenia gravis: consequences for pregnancy, delivery, and the newborn. Neurology 61:1362, 2003.
113. Rudnik-Schoneborn S, Zerres K: Outcome in pregnancies complicated by myotonic dystrophy: a study of 31 patients and review of the literature. Eur J Obstet Gynecol Reprod Biol 114:44, 2004.
114. Rudnik-Schoneborn S, Schneider-Gold C, Raabe U, et al: Outcome and effect of pregnancy in myotonic dystrophy type 2. Neurology 66:579, 2006.
115. Newman B, Meola G, O'Donovan DG, et al: Proximal myotonic myopathy (PROMM) presenting as myotonia during pregnancy. Neuromuscul Disord 9:144, 1999.
116. Magee AC, Hughes AE, Kidd A, et al: Reproductive counselling for women with myotonic dystrophy. J Med Genet 39:E15, 2002.
117. Day JW, Ricker K, Jacobsen JF, et al: Myotonic dystrophy type 2: molecular, diagnostic and clinical spectrum. Neurology 60:657, 2003.
118. Lucas MJ, Leveno KJ, Cunningham FG: A comparison of magnesium sulfate with phenytoin for the prevention of eclampsia. N Engl J Med 333:201, 1995.
119. Duley L, Henderson-Smart D: Magnesium sulphate versus phenytoin for eclampsia. Cochrane Database Syst Rev:CD000128, 2003.
120. Duley L, Henderson-Smart D: Magnesium sulphate versus diazepam for eclampsia. Cochrane Database Syst Rev:CD000127, 2003.
121. Raps EC, Galetta SL, Broderick M, et al: Delayed peripartum vasculopathy: cerebral eclampsia revisited. Ann Neurol 33:222, 1993.
122. Lamy C, Oppenheim C, Meder JF, et al: Neuroimaging in posterior reversible encephalopathy syndrome. J Neuroimaging 14:89, 2004.

SECTION

X

Toxic, Environmental, and Traumatic Disorders

CHAPTER

32

Drug-Induced Disorders of the Nervous System

KEVIN D.J. O'CONNOR ■ FRANK L. MASTAGLIA

Adverse drug reactions are a frequent cause of morbidity and hospital admission and are a major burden on the health care system.[1] Drug reactions commonly involve the nervous system, causing a variety of disorders that may be serious and even life-threatening, and may mimic other neurologic disorders. Most drug-induced disorders are potentially reversible if the offending agent is identified early and withdrawn. The possibility of an iatrogenic condition should be considered, therefore, in any patient with neurologic symptoms, and a full drug history should always be obtained. The spectrum

Aminoff's Neurology and General Medicine, Fifth Edition.

of drug-induced disorders is wide, as is discussed in this chapter. Only relatively recent references are cited; references to the earlier literature can be found in previous editions of this book.

HEADACHE

Drugs may cause headache by inducing vasodilation, raised intracranial pressure, or aseptic meningitis, and may exacerbate a preexisting headache disorder such as migraine.[2] In addition, medication-induced headache accounts for up to 5 to 10 percent of patients with headache[3] and is often unrecognized.[4,5]

Vascular Headaches

Many drugs cause headaches by inducing cerebral vasodilation or vasoconstriction. These include antihistamines, sympathomimetics, amyl nitrate, nitroglycerin, nicotinic acid, hydralazine, prazosin, pentoxifylline, cyclandelate, nifedipine, perhexiline, theophylline, aminophylline, terbutaline, and dipyridamole.[6]

Headache may also occur during treatment with cyclosporine,[7] bromocriptine, dopamine, and some nonsteroidal anti-inflammatory drugs such as naproxen, ketoprofen, diclofenac, alclofenac, and ibuprofen. Severe and persistent headache may also occur in some patients treated with H_2-receptor antagonists (e.g., cimetidine and ranitidine) and proton pump inhibitors (e.g., omeprazole and lansoprazole).

Headache is a common transient reaction with intravenous immunoglobulin therapy, particularly in migraine patients, perhaps due to reversible cerebral vasoconstriction syndrome.[8] This syndrome has also been reported with illicit drugs such as cannabis, cocaine, amphetamines, and lysergic acid diethylamide (LSD). Selective serotonin reuptake inhibitors (SSRIs), serotonin-noradrenaline reuptake inhibitors (SNRIs), α-sympathomimetics, nasal decongestants, triptans, ergot alkaloid derivatives, nicotine patches, and herbal medications such as ginseng have also been implicated.[9]

Medication Overuse Headache

Medication overuse headache is now recognized as the third most frequent form of headache encountered in clinical practice[10,11] and one of the most costly neurologic disorders[12,13]; it is often unrecognized and is a significant contributor to health care costs. A paradoxical increase in headache frequency commonly occurs in migraine or cluster headache patients taking excessive ergotamine-containing preparations or triptans on a regular basis.[14–17] Treatment involves gradual withdrawal of the offending medications and commencement of another prophylactic medication.[13,18] Chronic analgesic dependency may have a similar effect in patients with primary headache disorders, leading to rebound headaches and chronic daily headache.[17,19]

Idiopathic Intracranial Hypertension (Pseudotumor Cerebri)

A number of drugs may cause idiopathic intracranial hypertension (pseudotumor cerebri), characterized by headache, papilledema, diplopia, and visual impairment. These include oral contraceptives, estrogens and progestational agents, growth hormone, anabolic steroids, antibiotics (tetracyclines, minocycline,[20,21] ampicillin, nalidixic acid, nitrofurantoin), nonsteroidal anti-inflammatory drugs (naproxen, ibuprofen, indomethacin), vitamin A, retinoids (isotretinoin, etretinate), danazol, amiodarone, perhexiline, thyroxine, ketamine, nitrous oxide, corticosteroids (or corticosteroid withdrawal),[22,23] and intrathecal liposomal cytarabine.[24]

Aseptic Meningitis

Drug-induced aseptic meningitis may occur with the use of nonsteroidal anti-inflammatory drugs or cotrimoxazole,[25–28] particularly in patients with systemic connective tissue diseases, and occasionally with other antimicrobials, such as sulfasalazine, penicillin, amoxicillin,[29] ciprofloxacin, and cephalosporins, and with carbamazepine and pentoxifylline.[30–32] Aseptic meningitis may also develop after intravenous immunoglobulin therapy, and treatment with other immunomodulatory agents such as infliximab, leflunomide, azathioprine, and muromonab-CD3.[8,28] Intrathecal anesthetics, contrast media, methylprednisolone, methotrexate, and cytarabine may also cause aseptic meningitis.[28,31]

STROKE

Women taking oral contraceptives have an increased risk of both cerebral venous sinus thrombosis[33] and ischemic stroke, although the absolute risk is small.

The risk of stroke was previously greater with the higher-dose estrogen preparations but is not significantly increased in women taking current low-dose oral contraceptives, although there is an increased risk in women who are older and smoke cigarettes.[34,35] Oral contraceptives have also been implicated in subarachnoid hemorrhage, particularly in smokers. The risk of ischemic stroke is increased by tamoxifen treatment for breast cancer.[36]

Excessive use of antihypertensive drugs leading to hypotension is an important cause of iatrogenic stroke, particularly in the elderly and in patients with cerebrovascular disease. Patients taking anticoagulant drugs have an increased risk of intracerebral and other forms of intracranial hemorrhage, particularly with poorly controlled or long-term therapy. In addition, patients with heparin-induced thrombocytopenia have an increased risk of both ischemic stroke and hemorrhage.[37] The use of aspirin for primary or secondary prevention of ischemic stroke may be a possible risk factor for intracerebral hemorrhage, although a meta-analysis did not show a significant increase.[38]

Intracerebral or subarachnoid hemorrhage may occur after intravenous, oral, or intranasal use of amphetamines and related compounds such as cocaine that can cause acute blood pressure elevation.[39–42] Intracranial hemorrhage has also been reported in patients taking diet pills, decongestants, stimulants containing phenylpropanolamine,[42] and pseudoephedrine. Intracerebral hemorrhage or ischemic stroke may occur in individuals taking high doses of ephedrine-containing preparations including those that were previously available without prescription as decongestants.[43–45] These drugs, as well as phenylpropanolamine, pseudoephedrine, oxymetazoline, allopurinol, penicillin, and ergot alkaloids, have also been associated with cerebral vasculopathy.[31] Cerebral and myocardial ischemia may also occur in patients given cisplatin-based combination chemotherapy.[46]

TABLE 32-1 ■ Drugs that May Cause Seizures

Antidepressants	Tricyclics, mianserin, monoamine oxidase inhibitors, SSRIs
Antipsychotics	Phenothiazines, butyrophenones, lithium, clozapine, olanzapine
Analgesics	Fentanyl, alfentanil, morphine, meperidine, pentazocine, propoxyphene, mefenamic acid
Local Anesthetics	Lidocaine, mepivacaine, procaine, bupivacaine, etidocaine
General Anesthetics	Ketamine, halothane, althesin, enflurane, propanidid, methohexital, propofol, isoflurane
Antimicrobials	Penicillins, ampicillin, cephalosporins, imipenem, metronidazole, nalidixic acid, isoniazid, cycloserine, pyrimethamine, acyclovir, ganciclovir, foscarnet
Antineoplastics	Chlorambucil, vincristine, methotrexate, cytarabine, misonidazole, carmustine (BCNU), *N*-phosphonacetyl-L-aspartic acid (PALA)
Bronchodilators	Aminophylline, theophylline
Sympathomimetics	Ephedrine, terbutaline, phenylpropanolamine
Other Drugs	Insulin, antihistamines, anticholinergics, anticonvulsants, chloroquine, baclofen, cyclosporine, azathioprine, β-adrenergic blockers, flumazenil, disopyramide, digoxin, methyldopa, levodopa, bromocriptine, domperidone, phencyclidine, amphetamines, methylphenidate, famotidine, isotretinoin, ondansetron, allopurinol, doxapram, camphor, oxytocin, erythropoietin

SEIZURES

Many drugs may induce seizures in healthy individuals (Table 32-1).[31,47,48] One study showed that 6.1 percent of new-onset seizures were drug related,[49] and a prospective study of status epilepticus demonstrated an association with ethanol and drug overdose in 18 percent of cases.[50] Another study found that 9 percent of cases of status epilepticus presenting to an emergency department resulted from drug toxicity.[51] Some drugs are more likely than others to cause seizures, particularly those administered in high doses by the intrathecal or intravenous routes and those that cross the blood–brain barrier. The following drugs or classes of drugs have been reported repeatedly to induce seizures, in decreasing order of frequency: antidepressants, stimulants, anticholinergics, antiepileptics, diphenhydramine, antipyschotics, naproxen, ditropan, meperidine, isoniazid, ethylene glycol, lindane, baclofen, propoxyphene, methylphenidate, lithium, lidocaine, cyproheptadine, bupivicaine, acetylsalicylic acid, and glipizide.[51,52] With a number of the drugs listed in Table 32-1, seizures have been reported only rarely and the association remains circumstantial.

A number of factors may predispose to drug-induced seizures. Patients often have a family history of epilepsy and a genetically determined low seizure threshold. Penicillin-induced seizures usually develop with high-dose intravenous or intrathecal administration and in patients with renal failure who develop high blood levels. Other drugs that may accumulate as a result of reduced renal excretion and cause seizures with high serum levels include meperidine, imipenem, nalidixic acid, cephalosporins, cimetidine, lithium, and erythropoietin.[53] Seizures have been reported to occur in 1.5 to 6 percent of patients treated with cyclosporine, especially in renal or liver transplant patients with high blood levels.[7]

A number of therapeutic agents such as oxytocin, carbamazepine, and SSRIs can induce seizures by causing hyponatremia.[6,54] Withdrawal of benzodiazepines, barbiturates, tricyclic antidepressants, alcohol, or baclofen is an important cause of seizures, particularly if these drugs are discontinued too abruptly. Withdrawal of anticonvulsant drugs in epileptic patients can lead to seizures or status epilepticus and should always be gradual.

Conversely, excessively high doses and serum concentrations of phenytoin, carbamazepine, and other anticonvulsants may aggravate epilepsy or induce new seizure types or status epilepticus.[55–58] Carbamazepine may aggravate primary generalized seizure disorders including those presenting with absence, myoclonic, or atonic seizures. Benzodiazepines may induce tonic seizures and status epilepticus in patients with Lennox–Gastaut syndrome. Valproic acid and vigabatrin may also occasionally induce status epilepticus.[31] Gabapentin may have an adverse effect on myoclonic epilepsy, as may topiramate on focal epilepsy, and tiagabine may induce nonconvulsive status epilepticus.[58]

The proconvulsant effects of isoniazid, aminophylline, local anesthetics, phencyclidine, and meperidine are dose related,[51,52] but other drugs may cause seizures even with normal therapeutic doses and blood levels. These include theophylline,[59] tricyclic antidepressants,[60] and phenothiazines, the latter of which induces seizures in 1 to 2 percent of patients.[61] The aliphatic phenothiazines chlorpromazine, promazine, and prochlorperazine are more likely to induce seizures than the piperazine group, such as fluphenazine and trifluoperazine.[61] Seizures have also been reported with the atypical neuroleptics clozapine, olanzapine, risperidone, and sertindole.[47] Of the antidepressants, bupropion, tricyclic antidepressants and venlafaxine induce seizures more frequently than pure SSRI medications.[52] Lithium-induced seizures are well known, and generally occur with plasma levels exceeding 3.0 mEq/L.[61]

COMA

Drugs are a common and important cause of coma, which may result from accidental or self-administered overdosage. These drugs can be classified into those that have a direct effect on the brain such as hypnotics, sedatives, antidepressants, analgesics, or various drug combinations, and those that cause coma through more indirect effects, such as insulin, antihypertensives, and antiarrhythmics.[62] Other drugs that may cause depression of consciousness include phenothiazines, salicylates, acetaminophen (which produces severe hepatic damage), paraldehyde, acyclovir, and valproic acid.[6,62]

Certain neurologic findings are characteristic of drug-induced coma. The pupils are typically small and reactive, but may be dilated and fixed in severe barbiturate intoxication or pinpoint in opiate poisoning. The corneal reflexes are preserved but may be lost in profound drug-induced coma. Ocular movements are depressed early, particularly with barbiturate, tricyclic, and phenytoin intoxication, the eyes being fixed and divergent, without spontaneous roving eye movements, and with impaired or absent oculocephalic and oculovestibular reflexes. Muscle tone is usually reduced, and the muscle stretch reflexes are depressed, with flexor plantar responses, although in some cases there may be hypertonia, hyperreflexia, decerebrate posturing, and extensor plantar responses, particularly if there has been superimposed hypoxia. Muscle twitching, choreoathetosis, myoclonus, and seizures may occur in coma caused by tricyclic agents or lithium toxicity.[62]

The electroencephalogram (EEG) usually shows diffuse slowing or, with barbiturate or benzodiazepine intoxication, prominent beta activity. Alpha-pattern coma, or mixed alpha and beta rhythms, may occur in benzodiazepine or chlormethiazole intoxication.[63]

ENCEPHALOPATHY

Certain drugs such as lithium and acyclovir may lead to a diffuse disturbance of cerebral function leading to tremor, asterixis, myoclonus, seizures, ataxia, confusion, and obtundation, at times progressing to coma. Such a syndrome may be caused by lithium toxicity and may occur even when blood levels are within the recommended therapeutic range.[64]

A myoclonic encephalopathy may occur in patients with prolonged exposure to bismuth-containing preparations, or with aluminum toxicity in patients with renal failure undergoing hemodialysis (although current dialysate preparations have reduced this risk),[31] and with carisoprodol overdosage.[65]

Penicillin and cephalosporins may cause encephalopathy in high doses,[60] particularly in patients with renal failure, as well as lidocaine, tocainide, benzodiazepines, vigabatrin, valproic acid, phenytoin, carbamazepine, baclofen, isoniazid, levodopa, mefloquine, sulfonamides, podophyllin, L-asparaginase, thymidine, 5-fluorouracil, carmustine (BCNU), mechlorethamine, *N*-phosphonacetyl-L-aspartic acid (PALA), cytarabine, fludarabine, doxorubicin, and intrathecal metrizamide and iohexol.[31] Cephalosporins, and particularly cefepime, have been reported to cause a severe but reversible encephalopathy, with global aphasia or myoclonus.[66,67]

A severe progressive leukoencephalopathy characterized by dementia, dysarthria, ataxia, and paralysis, at times followed by seizures, coma, and death, may occur in patients treated with high-dose intrathecal, intraventricular, or intravenous methotrexate, particularly after cranial or craniospinal radiotherapy. A posterior reversible encephalopathy syndrome presenting with headache, seizures, cortical blindness, and white matter lesions has been increasingly recognized in patients treated with cyclosporine (Fig. 32-1).[7] The condition is often associated with hypertension and high serum drug levels and is usually reversible. A similar condition may also occur with bevacizumab,[68] cisplatin, cytarabine, 5-fluorouracil, fludarabine, ifosfamide, amphotericin B, interferons, interleukin-2, levamisole, tacrolimus, and melarsoprol.[31]

NEUROPSYCHIATRIC DISORDERS

Psychiatric adverse drug reactions are common in clinical practice and may take various forms.[6,69]

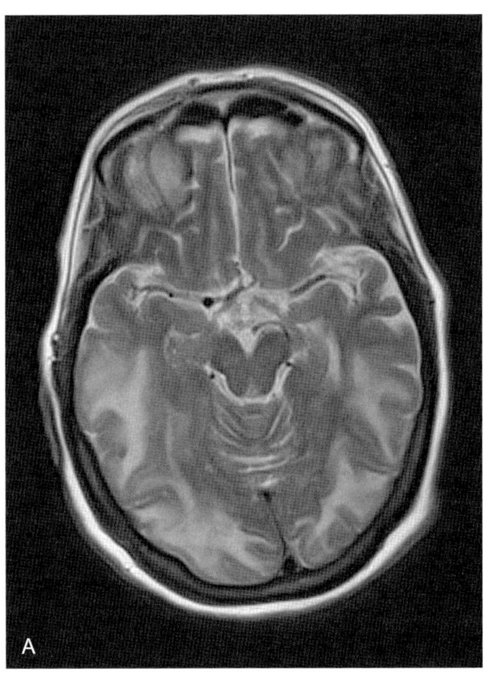

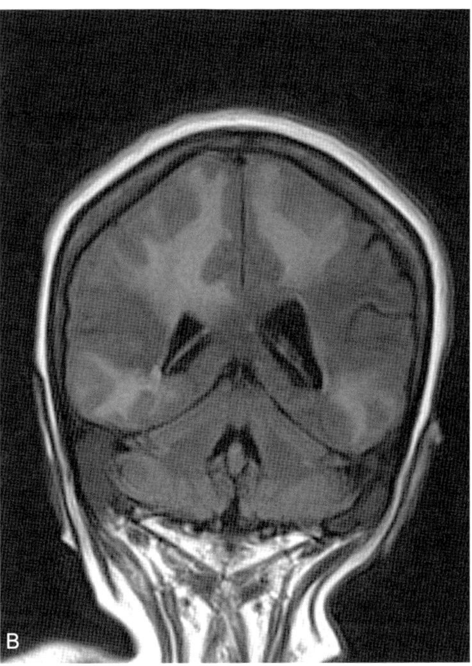

FIGURE 32-1 ■ Axial (**A**) and coronal (**B**) T2-weighted MRI of the brain showing findings of posterior reversible encephalopathy syndrome in a patient with mixed connective tissue disease receiving cyclosporine.

Behavioral Toxicity

Nonspecific symptoms such as drowsiness, insomnia, irritability, restlessness, anxiety, mood changes, vivid dreams and nightmares, and increased sensitivity to light and sound may occur with a wide range of medications. These symptoms may be the prelude to a more florid delirious state, and usually subside with dose reduction. They are encountered most frequently with tricyclic antidepressants, lithium, amphetamines, phenothiazines, barbiturates, glucocorticoids, cholinergic drugs, levodopa, anticonvulsants, some antihistamines, and acetylcholinesterase inhibitors.[6] Similar symptoms may occur after withdrawal of drugs such as benzodiazepines and SSRIs.

Delirium and Confusional States

Drugs are an important cause of delirium and confusional states, particularly in the elderly. Although various drugs may cause such reactions, the sedatives and hypnotics are the most common. Other important causative agents include benzodiazepines, antiparkinsonian drugs, and antidepressants, including the SSRIs.[31] SSRIs also can lead to the serotonin syndrome, which usually results from an interaction between serotonergic drugs and monoamine oxidase inhibitors or tricyclic agents and is characterized by an altered mental state with fever, confusion, agitation, tremor, myoclonus, shivering, hyperreflexia, and incoordination.[70–72] Abrupt withdrawal of SSRI drugs may also result in a confusional or delirious state with twitching, hypertonia, and sensory symptoms. With the recent influenza epidemics and increased use of oseltamivir, delirious states with increased motor activity have been frequently reported.[73]

Affective Disorders

Drug-induced depressive reactions are common and represent approximately 1 percent of reported adverse drug reactions.[6] Reserpine and α-methyldopa were among the first drugs recognized to cause depression, but the newer antihypertensive agents do not commonly depress mood. Depression may occur in patients on corticosteroids, and is the most common psychiatric symptom in patients receiving levodopa. Oral contraceptives, anabolic steroids, digoxin, indomethacin and naproxen, sulfonamides, retinoids, disulfiram, cycloserine, antineoplastic and antiepileptic drugs, baclofen, barbiturates, benzodiazepines, phenothiazines, butyrophenones, interferons[31] as well as withdrawal from benzodiazepines, amphetamines, and fenfluramines may also cause depression. A review of depression as an adverse drug reaction found that the best evidence supporting this association related to corticosteroids, contraceptive implants (progestin-releasing), gonadotropin-releasing hormone agonists, interferon-α, interleukin-2, mefloquine, and to a lesser extent propranolol.[74]

Although euphoria is common in patients on various drugs, manic or hypomanic reactions are uncommon.[6] Such reactions may occur with glucocorticoids or corticotropin, anabolic steroids, thyroid hormone, captopril, chloroquine, isoniazid, ranitidine and cimetidine, dopaminergic agents, baclofen, opiates, pentazocine, monoamine oxidase inhibitors, tricyclic antidepressants, iproniazid, cyclosporine, sympathomimetic amines, amphetamines, benzodiazepines, procyclidine, phenylpropanolamine, and hallucinogens.[31,75] A mood disturbance with manic features is the commonest psychiatric condition caused by corticosteroids, considered responsible for 54 percent of cases of organic mania in one study.[76] In another study it was found that 13 of 50 individuals receiving between 50 and 150mg of methylprednisolone or fluocortolone developed manic-like episodes.[76]

Antidepressants may induce mania in those who have bipolar affective disorder. An increased risk of a manic episode has been reported with the introduction of tricyclic antidepressants or monoamine oxidase inhibitors, but not with standard-dose SSRIs.[77] Agitation and hypomania may also occur in the serotonin syndrome.[70]

Psychoses

Various drugs have been reported to cause paranoid and schizophreniform psychotic reactions characterized by delusions, hallucinations, and emotional and thought disorder, particularly in the elderly.[6,69] Although these drug-induced disorders closely resemble the naturally occurring psychoses, such individuals do not appear predisposed to develop a chronic psychotic condition.

Hallucinatory States

Various drugs may cause hallucinations without other features of delirium or psychosis. The hallucinations are usually visual, extremely vivid and colored, and often of animals, sometimes having microptic or lilliputian dimensions. The most common drugs are tricyclic antidepressants, benzodiazepines, vigabatrin, bromides, methylphenidate, atropine and other anticholinergic drugs after parenteral (or even topical) administration, ephedrine, amantadine, bromocriptine, pergolide, levodopa, digoxin, diltiazem, β-adrenergic blockers, prazosin, captopril, disopyramide, pentazocine, buprenorphine, indomethacin, salicylates, cimetidine, aminophylline, acyclovir, and cyproheptadine, as well as cannabis and LSD. Hallucinations, usually auditory and less often visual, are also a feature of withdrawal from alcohol, barbiturates, benzodiazepines, and baclofen.

Cognitive Impairment

A number of drugs may cause transient memory impairment, including clioquinol, isoniazid, baclofen, benzhexol, and antidepressant drugs that have a central anticholinergic action. More severe, but reversible, cognitive impairment that may mimic dementia sometimes develops with chronic use of benzodiazepines, barbiturates, bromides, and chlorpromazine, and with glucocorticoid[78] and interleukin administration. A number of antiepileptic drugs may adversely affect cognitive functions. Early studies suggested that such effects were less frequent with carbamazepine or sodium valproate than with phenytoin or phenobarbital. However, more recent studies have shown that, at therapeutic serum concentrations, the adverse effects are comparable for these four drugs.[79] The newer antiepileptics gabapentin, lamotrigine, vigabatrin, tiagabine, remacemide, topiramate, and levetiracetam likely have fewer cognitive effects.[79,80] In a review of cognitive toxicity of agents used to treat social anxiety disorder, impairment was least with fluvoxamine, paroxetine, and escitalopram, moderate with propranolol, sertraline, and dothiepin, and more severe with pregabalin, amitriptyline, lorazepam, and mianserin.[81]

MOVEMENT DISORDERS

Several groups of drugs may induce involuntary movements or abnormalities of movement, posture, or muscle tone that resemble primary extrapyramidal disorders.[82–85] All of the typical neuroleptic drugs (phenothiazines, reserpine, benzoquinolizines, thioxanthenes, and butyrophenones) and some of the atypical neuroleptics such as risperidone,[86] clozapine,[87] and olanzapine,[88] as well as tricyclic antidepressants, SSRIs,[89] and antiparkinsonian medications can induce such syndromes, which may take a number of different forms (Table 32-2).[90,91] These drugs may also aggravate preexisting extrapyramidal disorders such as Parkinson disease and should be avoided or used with caution in such patients.

TABLE 32-2 ■ Drug-Induced Movement Disorders

Acute dystonic-dyskinetic reactions
Akathisia
Tardive dyskinesia
Tardive dystonia
Chorea and choreoathetosis
Drug-induced parkinsonism
Neuroleptic malignant syndrome
Tremor
Tics
Myoclonus

The reported incidence of drug-induced extrapyramidal disorders varies considerably according to the diagnostic criteria used and patient group studied. It is now well recognized that there is a marked individual variability in the susceptibility to these reactions; some patients develop side effects even after small doses of a drug, whereas others on much higher doses are unaffected. Age, gender, and genetic factors probably contribute to determining individual susceptibility.

Dystonic-Dyskinetic Reactions

Acute dystonic reactions are well recognized with neuroleptic drugs such as the phenothiazines and butyrophenones, metoclopamide, tricyclic antidepressants, and, less frequently, phenytoin, carbamazepine, propranolol, ondansetron, fluoxetine, flunarizine, and cinnarizine.[6,92] The onset is usually within the first few days of starting treatment and may be abrupt. The dystonia may be confined to the head and neck, causing facial grimacing, trismus, abnormal tongue movements, oculogyric crises, orofacial dyskinesias, torticollis, and retrocollis, but may also be more generalized, with slow writhing movements of the limbs and more prolonged tonic contractions of the axial and limb muscles leading to opisthotonos, lordosis, tortipelvis, and bizarre gait. The character of the movements may lead to a mistaken diagnosis of hysteria, tetanus, tetany, or epilepsy. Such reactions occur in around 6 percent of patients exposed to typical neuroleptics and 1 to 2 percent of those taking atypical neuroleptics.[92] Despite their dramatic and at times alarming nature, the acute dystonias are usually self-limited and remit once the drug is discontinued; severe reactions may be terminated by the intravenous administration of benztropine or diazepam.

Dyskinetic reactions involving the lips, face, and tongue, and at times the limbs and trunk, are common in parkinsonian patients treated with levodopa. These dyskinesias may develop early during the course of treatment with levodopa (or with various dopamine agonists) and respond to a reduction in dose. With prolonged treatment, dyskinesias become an increasing problem, tending to occur at times of maximal response to levodopa and alternating with periods of akinesia and severe rigidity (the "on-off" phenomenon). The administration of smaller, more frequent doses of levodopa, or a reduction in overall dose and the introduction of a dopamine agonist, is sometimes helpful in alleviating this common complication of chronic levodopa therapy. More severe cases may require alternative approaches including deep brain stimulation.[92]

Akathisia

Akathisia is a state of motor restlessness characterized by an uncontrollable urge to move about, pace, or even run incessantly.[64] The condition is typically seen in patients taking dopamine-blocking agents such as phenothiazine derivatives and less frequently with the butyrophenones, benzodiazepines, tricyclic antidepressants, SSRIs, levodopa, lithium, monoamine oxidase inhibitors, and vigabatrin. The reported incidence of akathisia with antipsychotic drugs has ranged from 20 to 75 percent and is less frequent with the atypical neuroleptics.[6,64] It usually remits within days or weeks of withdrawal of the drug, but it may persist for several months and is occasionally permanent.

The most effective treatment for akathisia is to withdraw the offending drug or lower the dose. Benztropine or diphenhydramine is usually effective in controlling akathisia when given by the intramuscular or intravenous route. Propranolol, clonazepam, mirtazapine, amantadine, and mianserin may also be beneficial.[64]

Tardive Dyskinesia and Other Disorders

Tardive dyskinesia is an involuntary movement disorder that occurs most frequently after prolonged treatment with dopamine antagonists, particularly antipsychotic drugs, but also with metoclopramide, promethazine, prochlorperazine, amoxapine, perphenazine, flunarizine, cinnarizine, and tricyclic antidepressants.[84] Early studies found tardive dyskinesia in up to 50 percent of patients treated with antipsychotic drugs, but this frequency appears to be declining since the introduction of the atypical antipsychotic agents.[93] Tardive dyskinesia usually develops after more than 12 months of continuous therapy, although it has been reported with periods as short as 3 months. The condition is more common and more severe in the elderly, in whom it is less likely to remit.

The condition typically takes the form of orobuccal dyskinesias with lip smacking and pursing; sucking; jaw opening and closing; protruding, side-to-side, or writhing movements of the tongue; and facial grimacing. The movements tend to be stereotyped and, when severe, may interfere with speech or swallowing. In some cases, more generalized choreoathetotic movements of the limbs and trunk and repetitive foot tapping are present, at times resembling Huntington chorea. Less frequently, dystonic posturing of the neck and myoclonic jerking of the distal extremities are present as well. Concomitant akathisia or parkinsonism may also occur. Dystonia or dyskinesia may also occur occasionally with abrupt withdrawal of clozapine and other neuroleptic agents.[94]

The pathophysiologic basis for tardive dyskinesia has not been clearly established. The most widely held theory is that, as a result of prolonged dopamine receptor blockade in the corpus striatum, a state of hypersensitivity to endogenous dopamine develops owing to changes in receptor properties or numbers.[84,95]

The severity of tardive dyskinesia is variable, and the condition is not often disabling. It may remit in up to 40 percent of cases, even on continued therapy, but in some cases the condition persists. Occasionally, remission may occur even several years after withdrawal of antipsychotic drugs. Interruption of therapy when dyskinesia first develops may be beneficial, but there is some evidence that repeated interruptions paradoxically may increase the risk of dyskinesia and its persistence.[83,84]

The risks of developing tardive dyskinesia should be reduced by using the lowest effective dose of a neuroleptic for the shortest amount of time that is necessary. If tardive dyskinesia is diagnosed, the causative drug should be discontinued when possible. Many drugs have been used to treat established tardive dykinesia, including dopaminergic agents, such as tetrabenazine, bromocriptine, and levodopa, along with drugs with a cholinergic action such as choline, deanol, and lecithin. None has been consistently effective. Other drugs reported to be beneficial in individual cases include baclofen, propranolol, diazepam, tocopherol, levetiracetam, melatonin, and the calcium-channel blockers.[64]

Tardive dystonia may be focal or more generalized and may involve the neck, jaw, limbs, or trunk. It is distinguished from the more frequent orobuccal dyskinesia by the dystonic nature of the disorder. It is often more disabling than tardive dyskinesia. Other tardive syndromes include akathisia, chorea, myoclonus, tremor, tics, or oculogyric crises.[83]

Choreoathetosis

A number of drugs may cause chorea, which is characterized by multifocal, nonstereotyped, "fidgety" or jerky movements[92] and may be associated with the slower movements of athetosis or with dystonia. Chorea has been reported with anticonvulsants (phenytoin overdose, ethosuximide, valproic acid, carbamazepine, phenobarbital), clonazepam withdrawal, anticholinergic drugs (e.g., high doses of benzhexol), tricyclic antidepressants, fluoxetine, amphetamines, methylphenidate, amoxapine, pemoline, cimetidine, theophylline, aminophylline, lithium, methadone, antihistamines, cyclosporine, oxymetholone, intrathecal baclofen, and oral contraceptives.[31] Chorea has also been well described with cocaine use ("crack dancing").[92]

Parkinsonism

Drug-induced parkinsonism can occur at any age, but it is more common in the elderly and is probably the most common drug-induced movement disorder. It closely resembles idiopathic Parkinson disease. Bradykinesia is usually the most prominent feature, and may be accompanied by facial masking, rigidity, tremor, and gait disturbance. The incidence of tremor is lower than in idiopathic Parkinson disease but has been as high as 50 percent in some series.[91] The drugs most frequently implicated are the phenothiazines, most frequently prochlorperazine, but not clozapine[91]; haloperidol; the tricyclic andtidepressants; metoclopramide; lithium; and the calcium-channel blockers cinnarizine, flunarizine, and verapamil.[96,97] The condition is usually reversible after drug withdrawal or dose reduction. In a study of 36 cases of parkinsonism induced by calcium-channel blockers, most patients were found to improve after drug discontinuation, but tremor usually persisted.[96]

In patients who need to continue on neuroleptic therapy, administration of anticholinergic agents such as benzhexol or benztropine may alleviate some of their parkinsonian symptoms; levodopa may aggravate the underlying psychotic disorder and is best avoided or used with caution. Consideration should be given to switching to a drug with fewer parkinsonian risks, such as clozapine.[64]

In some cases, spontaneous improvement occurs even if the causative agent is continued. Prophylactic treatment with anticholinergic agents is not advocated, since it may predispose to the development of an irreversible form of tardive dyskinesia.[64]

Neuroleptic Malignant Syndrome

The neuroleptic malignant syndrome is a serious and potentially lethal complication of treatment with antipsychotic drugs. It is characterized by hyperpyrexia, severe muscular rigidity, and elevated serum creatine kinase (CK) levels (which are considered major diagnostic criteria). Tachycardia, abnormal blood pressure, tachypnea, altered consciousness, diaphoresis, and leukocytosis also occur (and are minor diagnostic criteria). Three major criteria or two major and four minor criteria are considered very suggestive of the diagnosis in the correct clinical context. Other movement disorders associated with the neuroleptic malignant syndrome include tremor, myoclonus, and dystonia.[92]

The drugs most frequently implicated are haloperidol, fluphenazine and other phenothiazines, thioxanthenes, olanzapine, clozapine, and combinations of these drugs either with each other or with lithium, metoclopramide, loxapine, or tricyclic antidepressants.[98,99] The condition may occur with both high and low doses of either high- or low-potency neuroleptic drugs and may develop after neuroleptic therapy is begun, after an increase in dose, or after the introduction of a second more potent drug. A similar syndrome has been reported after abrupt levodopa withdrawal in patients with Parkinson disease.[100]

In mild cases, complete recovery may occur within days or weeks of stopping the causative drug, but in severe cases metabolic acidosis, myoglobinuria, renal failure, coagulation defects, respiratory failure, shock, seizures, and coma can develop, leading to a mortality rate of up to 20 percent, with persistent neurologic sequelae in 10 percent of survivors.[92]

The underlying pathophysiologic mechanism is uncertain, but the current view is that the condition relates to profound dopamine receptor blockade in the striatum and in the thermoregulatory and vasomotor centers of the hypothalamus.

Treatment involves discontinuation of the causative drug together with vigorous cooling, restoration of fluid and electrolyte balance, and management of any other complications. Specific medications that may be beneficial in reversing the rigidity and akinesia include levodopa, pancuronium, bromocriptine, dantrolene, or a combination of these drugs.[64,92]

Tremor

Various drugs may cause or aggravate tremor.[101] These include β-adrenergic agonists (e.g., salbutamol, salmeterol), sympathomimetic drugs (e.g., ephedrine, pseudoephedrine, phenylpropanolamine), antiepileptic agents (e.g., sodium valproate), antidepressants and mood stabilizers (e.g., tricyclic antidepressants, SSRIs, lithium), neuroleptic agents (e.g., phenothiazines, butyrophenones), antiarrhythmics (e.g., amiodarone, procainamide, mexiletine), chemotherapeutic agents (e.g., doxorubicin, cytarabine, thalidomide), and immunosuppressants (e.g., cyclosporine, tacrolimus), as well as thyroxine, glucocorticoids, oral hypoglycemic drugs, levodopa, amphetamines, theophylline, and aminophylline.

A postural tremor of the hands, head, and trunk resembling essential tremor is not uncommon in patients treated with sodium valproate.[102] The tremor develops over a period of several months and usually remits when the drug is stopped or the dose is reduced. Treatment with propranolol or amantadine may alleviate the tremor.

Postural or action tremor is an early manifestation of lithium intoxication and is common even at therapeutic doses.[64] A postural tremor has been reported in up to 40 percent of patients on cyclosporine.[7] A flapping tremor (asterixis) may occur in patients treated with phenytoin, phenobarbital, carbamazepine, sodium valproate, methyldopa, ceftazidime, lithium, or tocainide.[31]

Tics

A syndrome resembling Gilles de la Tourette syndrome has been reported after the administration of dextroamphetamine, methylphenidate, pemoline, or haloperidol in children.[103] Other antipsychotic drugs as well as opiates, clonazepam, carbamazepine, phenobarbital, and fluoxetine have also been reported to cause tics.[84]

Myoclonus

Drug-induced myoclonus may occur in patients treated with antipsychotic and tricyclic antidepressant drugs or lithium. Myoclonus has been reported in patients treated with clozapine,[104,105] propofol, vigabatrin,[106] fluvoxamine,[107] chlorambucil,[108] opioids,[109] antibiotics (e.g., penicillin, ticarcillin, carbenicillin, imipenem, cephalosporins), and calcium-channel blockers.[110] A clinical picture resembling that of Creutzfeldt–Jakob disease with myoclonus, tremor, cerebellar and extrapyramidal manifestations, cognitive impairment, and periodic sharp-wave complexes on EEG has been reported in patients with lithium toxicity.[111] Posturally induced myoclonic jerks in the upper limbs have been described in patients on phenytoin,[112] and with long-term antipsychotic drug therapy; the myoclonus may also be associated with tardive dyskinesia.

CEREBELLAR SYNDROMES

Various drugs may cause ataxia, incoordination, and other manifestations of cerebellar dysfunction. Sedatives (e.g., chloral hydrate, barbiturates, benzodiazepines, and paraldehyde) and anticonvulsants (e.g., phenytoin, carbamazepine, primidone) are most often responsible, their effects being dependent on dose. Individual tolerance to these drugs varies considerably, but in general symptoms are more likely to develop when high doses are administered too quickly; however, with newer anticonvulsants such as pregabalin or gabapentin, relatively low doses may cause these symptoms, especially if titration is too rapid. Ataxia may occur with high doses of most tranquilizers, including diazepam, chlordiazepoxide, and meprobamate; signs of cerebellar dysfunction may be caused more rarely by phenothiazines, monoamine oxidase inhibitors, reserpine, thioxanthenes, and lithium. Lithium may cause an isolated cerebellar ataxia or a more diffuse encephalopathy, even with blood levels within the therapeutic range. A cerebellar syndrome has also been reported in bone marrow and liver transplant recipients treated with cyclosporine,[7] in patients with leukemia or lymphoma on high doses of cytarabine,[114] in cancer patients treated with high- or low-dose fluorouracil,[113] and in patients with impaired renal function taking nitrofurantoin or perhexiline.

All of these disorders are usually reversible when the causative agent is withdrawn or the dose adjusted, but there are occasional reports of permanent cerebellar atrophy or dysfunction in patients treated with lithium or phenytoin.[113,114] A preexisting cerebellar disorder may also be unmasked by use of these drugs.

OTOTOXICITY

Over 100 drugs are known to have ototoxic effects, causing cochlear or vestibular damage to the inner ear.[115] Tinnitus is often the first symptom of cochleotoxicity and, when persistent, is suggestive of impending hearing loss. Vestibulotoxicity results in vertigo, oscillopsia, and balance impairment that is particularly prominent in dark environments.

The most important ototoxic drugs are the aminoglycoside antibiotics, which may cause irreversible inner ear damage after parenteral, oral, or even topical administration. Since these agents are excreted through the kidneys, ototoxicity is more likely to develop in those with renal insufficiency.[116] All of the aminoglycosides can cause cochlear or vestibular toxicity; some are more cochleotoxic (e.g., neomycin, kanamycin, amikacin, and vancomycin), whereas others are preferentially vestibulotoxic (e.g. gentamicin, streptomycin); tobramycin is equally vestibulotoxic and cochleotoxic.

Vertical oscillation of the surroundings on movement ("bobbing oscillopsia") is highly characteristic of the vestibulopathy caused by the aminoglycoside antibiotics. Hearing loss affects the high frequencies initially and is usually irreversible. It may develop within a few days of beginning treatment, but is more often delayed, and may even develop after the drug is stopped. The aminoglycosides as a class cause degeneration of the sensory hair cells of the cochlea, the outer hair cells being most severely affected, accounting for the preferential loss of high frequencies; gentamycin is unique in its selective destruction of the vestibular hair cells.[116,117] It is important to have a high level of awareness of this serious complication, to monitor blood levels of the drug, to avoid prolonged courses of gentamycin, and to discontinue the drug if any symptoms of vestibulotoxicity develop. However, some patients may develop irreversible vestibulotoxicity even when blood levels of gentamycin are maintained within the recommended range, and the onset of symptoms may be delayed even after discontinuation.[116,118]

Other ototoxic antibiotics include minocycline (which is almost exclusively vestibulotoxic), colistin, polymyxin B, erythromycin (which may cause reversible deafness after oral or intravenous administration), metronidazole, vancomycin, and rarely, procaine penicillin, cephalexin, and chloramphenicol.

The loop diuretics furosemide, ethacrynic acid, and bumetanide may also be ototoxic, especially in patients with renal or hepatic impairment or those taking concurrent aminoglycoside antibiotics. Salicylates, in particular aspirin, may cause tinnitus, deafness, and vertigo when the serum concentration approaches 300 mg/L. Quinine may cause tinnitus and reversible low-tone hearing loss in a small proportion of patients taking the drug; an idiosyncratic mechanism seems to be involved. Prolonged high-dose administration of chloroquine may cause irreversible tinnitus and deafness. A number of cytotoxic drugs including cisplatin, vincristine, misonidazole, bleomycin, and mustine hydrochloride may cause hearing loss. Cisplatin causes a high incidence of tinnitus and high-tone hearing loss; recording of brainstem auditory evoked potentials is helpful in detecting early involvement of the auditory pathway.[117]

Other ototoxic drugs include quinidine, deferoxamine, sildenafil,[119] and the β-adrenergic blocker practolol, which caused combined sensorineural deafness and conductive hearing loss due to serous otitis media when it was in use. There are also rare reports of hearing loss or vestibular dysfunction in patients taking propoxyphene, naproxen, indomethacin, sulindac, metoprolol, nortriptyline, propylthiouracil, flecainide, and interferon-α.[120]

VISUAL DISORDERS

Drug-induced visual disorders may result from effects on the pupil, lens, retina, optic nerve, and central visual pathways.

Pupillary Changes

Parasympathomimetic drugs such as carbachol and neostigmine cause miosis, as can morphine, chloral hydrate, and phenothiazines.[121] Mydriasis is more often drug-induced and potentially more serious as it may precipitate acute angle-closure glaucoma in susceptible individuals. Drugs that may cause mydriasis and cycloplegia with blurring of near vision include anticholinergics, antihistamines, monoamine oxidase inhibitors, tricyclic antidepressants, chlorpropamide, indomethacin, hexamethonium, fenfluramine, oral contraceptives, amphetamines, and LSD.

Refractive Changes

In addition to the drugs mentioned that may cause cycloplegia and induce hypermetropia, certain drugs cause a transient myopia as a result of fluid shifts between the lens and the aqueous humor. These include oral diuretics (chlorothiazide, hydrochlorothiazide, chlorthalidone, and acetazolamide), tetracyclines, sulfonamides, corticosteroids and corticotropin, stilbestrol, phenytoin, thiamine, bromocriptine, and arsenicals, as well as insulin and oral hypoglycemic agents.

Retinopathy

Chloroquine, hydroxychloroquine, mepacrine, and amodiaquine may cause a pigmentary maculopathy and retinopathy with central and peripheral field defects and impairment of central vision after prolonged administration. Patients taking these drugs should have regular neuro-ophthalmic examinations, electroretinography, and electro-oculography to detect early signs of retinopathy. Phenothiazines in high doses may produce a progressive choroidoretinopathy; cardiac glycosides, methylphenidate, and cephaloridine have also been reported to cause pigmentary retinopathy. Macular edema may be caused by fingolimod, a novel oral therapeutic agent for multiple sclerosis, with an incidence of around 0.5 percent; the edema normally resolves on cessation of treatment.[122] Macular edema may also be caused by contraceptives and, rarely, by chlorothiazide and acetazolamide. Other drugs that may interfere with vision through retinal effects include indomethacin, quinine, tamoxifen, ethambutol, diethylcarbamazine, and vigabatrin, the latter of which has been found to cause symptomatic—or more commonly asymptomatic—visual field constriction.[123]

Optic Neuropathy

Optic atrophy occurred as part of the subacute myelo-opticoneuropathy syndrome associated with clioquinol when it was in use for the treatment of enteric infections. A number of other antimicrobial agents including linezolid, chloramphenicol, isoniazid, paraminosalicylate, streptomycin, ethambutol, sulfonamides, griseofulvin, dapsone, and chlorpropamide may also cause optic neuropathy.[124] In the case of chloramphenicol, this may be prevented by the prophylactic administration of vitamin B_{12}.

There have been case reports of tumor necrosis factor alpha (TNF-α) inhibitors infliximab, adalimumab, and entancercept causing optic neuritis with enhancement of the optic nerve on MRI in some cases; some patients have associated cerebral demyelinating lesions.[125]

Other drugs implicated in causing optic neuropathy include amiodarone, chlorambucil, cisplatin, 5-fluorouracil, vincristine, penicillamine, disulfiram, phenylbutazone, indomethacin, ibuprofen, naproxen, benoxaprofen, morphine, monoamine oxidase inhibitors, retinoids, organic arsenicals, cardiac glycosides, ergotamine, dideoxyinosine, omeprazole, and interferon-α.[31,124,126]

Disorders of Color Vision

Disturbances of color vision may result from the effects of various drugs on retinal cone receptors or from direct injury to the optic nerve. Xanthopsia (yellow vision) may be caused by sulfonamides, streptomycin, methaqualone, barbiturates, digitalis derivatives, thiazide diuretics, and the anthelmintic agent santonin.[127] Other drugs that may cause altered color vision include nalidixic acid, oral contraceptives, cannabis, LSD, and the older anticonvulsants troxidone and paramethadione.

Cortical Blindness

Cortical blindness may rarely occur after episodes of severe hypotension during anesthesia or after aggressive treatment of hypertension. It has also been reported as a complication of chemotherapy during childhood; with excessive doses of salicylates or barbiturates; and in those treated with drugs such as cyclosporine causing a posterior reversible encephalopathy syndrome (Fig. 32-1).[7]

Diplopia

Certain drugs commonly cause diplopia through breakdown of a latent squint. These include benzodiazepines, indomethacin, chlorpropamide, quinine, methaqualone, fenfluramine, tricyclic antidepressants, and anticonvulsants.

Nystagmus

Drug-induced nystagmus is common in hospital practice. Horizontal vestibular nystagmus occurs in patients on high doses of barbiturates, benzodiazepines, anticonvulsants, and other sedative and hypnotic drugs. It is a useful sign of toxicity in patients on anticonvulsant therapy and may occur even with therapeutic serum levels. Other drugs reported to cause nystagmus include monoamine oxidase inhibitors, salicylates, gold, neostigmine, chlordiazepoxide, fenfluramine, and amitriptyline, as well as the ototoxic antibiotics.[31] Lithium and various other drugs may cause downbeat nystagmus.

DISORDERS OF TASTE AND SMELL

Drug-induced disorders of taste are common. Many drugs cause metallic, bitter, salty, or other distortions of taste (phantogeusia). These include biguanides, ethambutol, vitamin D, gold, allopurinol, penicillin, metronidazole, tinidazole, lincomycin, clindamycin, terbinafine, aspirin, and phenindione. A number of other drugs may cause a reduction or loss in taste, the perception of sweet being most often affected. These include D-penicillamine (which causes marked hypogeusia in up to 30 percent of patients that can be corrected by the administration of copper), levodopa, captopril, enalapril, etidronate, oxyfedrine, methimazole, carbimazole, thiouracil, phenylbutazone, amphotericin B, griseofulvin, terbinafine, azathioprine, salazosulfapyridine, chlormezanone, carbamazepine, and baclofen.[128]

Distortion of the sense of smell or complete anosmia, which may be irreversible, has been associated with a number of drugs including amoxicillin/clavulanate potassium, intranasal beclomethasone, captopril, doxycycline, and erythromycin. A more complete list of drugs affecting smell and taste is provided elsewhere.[128]

SPINAL DISORDERS

Intrathecal injections may be complicated by infective or aseptic meningitis, adhesive arachnoiditis, or toxic myeloradiculopathy. Injection of methylprednisolone can cause an acute meningeal reaction thought to be due to the polyethylene glycol detergent in the preparation; patients may present with back and limb pain and paresthesias, bladder disturbances, and an acute spinal cord syndrome. Other drugs that may be toxic when given intrathecally include baclofen, lidocaine, morphine, chymopapain, methotrexate, cytarabine, and radiologic contrast materials.[31]

Epidural injections are not associated with such reactions unless there is inadvertent dural penetration. Spinal anesthesia is associated with a low incidence of lower-limb numbness, paresthesias, or weakness attributable to toxic effects of the anesthetic agent or accidental injury to the nerve roots.

A syndrome of myeloneuropathy with sensory dysesthesia, Lhermitte sign, leg weakness and spasticity, ataxia, and sphincter dysfunction has been described after prolonged exposure to nitrous oxide, often as a recreational drug. The condition is thought to be due to the inhibitory effects of nitrous oxide on vitamin B_{12} utilization. Recovery may occur after exposure is stopped.[129]

Spinal cord compression due to increased extradural adipose tissue may occur in rare patients after prolonged corticosteroid therapy. Cord compression may also occur as a result of hemorrhage into the extradural space in patients taking anticoagulants. Acute ischemic myelopathy may occur in heroin addicts due to vasculopathy. Spinal cord infarction has also been reported as a result of accidental injection of penicillin into the superior gluteal artery during intramuscular injection.[130]

AUTONOMIC DISORDERS

Postural Hypotension

Many drugs may cause postural hypotension, resulting in dizziness, falls, or syncope; focal cerebral ischemic events sometimes occur in patients with preexisting narrow intracranial or cervical vessels. The drugs most frequently implicated are antihypertensives, vasodilators, diuretics, tricyclic antidepressants, and levodopa.

Bladder Dysfunction

Anticholinergic drugs may cause urinary retention by inhibiting parasympathetic postganglionic cholinergic neurons, particularly if there is bladder outflow obstruction due to prostatic hypertrophy. These agents commonly include atropine, hyoscine, propantheline, benzhexol, benztropine, methixene, orphenadrine, dicyclomine, and belladonna derivatives. Tricyclic antidepressants and phenothiazines may also precipitate acute urinary retention due to their anticholinergic effects. Other drugs that may cause urinary retention include monoamine oxidase inhibitors, disopyramide, ephedrine, salbutamol, terbutaline, and theophylline.[131]

A number of other drugs may also interfere with control of micturition, causing urinary incontinence, including prazosin, metoprolol, benoxaprofen, depot phenothiazines, clonazepam, phenoxybenzamine, and methyldopa.[132]

Sexual Dysfunction

Many drugs interfere with normal sexual function, causing loss of libido, impotence, impaired ejaculation, or orgasmic dysfunction. Those most commonly implicated include antihypertensives, tricyclic antidepressants, monoamine oxidase inhibitors, SSRIs, tranquilizers, antihistamines, anticholinergics, baclofen, cimetidine, clofibrate, disopyramide, dopamine agonists, and levodopa.[6]

NEUROMUSCULAR DISORDERS

Peripheral Neuropathies

Various drugs may interfere with peripheral nerve function, causing an axonal, or less often a demyelinating, neuropathy.[133] The risk of drug-induced neuropathy is greater in patients with preexisting neuropathy, including diabetics and alcoholics, and with combinations of more than one potentially neurotoxic drug. Some drugs principally affect sensory nerve function, causing peripheral paresthesias and possibly other signs of a sensory neuropathy. Conversely, drugs such as dapsone and gold cause a predominantly motor neuropathy with absent or inconspicuous sensory findings. Most drugs, however, produce a mixed sensory and motor neuropathy presenting initially with sensory symptoms, followed by progressive motor symptoms later if the drug is not stopped. Muscle pain and cramps are prominent early symptoms in some cases. Tendon reflexes may be preserved in the early stages but are usually depressed or lost later, even when motor involvement is absent or inconspicuous.

Antineoplastic Drugs

The vinca alkaloids, platinum compounds, taxanes, and suramin have the greatest potential to cause neuropathy.[134] Vincristine and other vinca alkaloids that interfere with intracellular microtubules are particularly neurotoxic. Most patients treated with these drugs will develop a sensorimotor polyneuropathy with early loss of tendon reflexes and possibly associated autonomic symptoms.[135] Muscle cramps may be prominent in the early stages, and some patients also develop a painful proximal myopathy. Recovery may occur if the drug is stopped or reduced, but mild sensory symptoms and areflexia usually persist. In some patients treated with these drugs, symptoms of neuropathy may not develop until after the treatment is completed, or may progress despite cessation of treatment, a phenomenon referred to as "coasting."[134]

The platinum compounds are all potentially neurotoxic and can cause a painful sensory neuropathy with impairment of proprioception accompanied by a sensory ataxia. Cisplatin and carboplatin cause a dorsal root ganglion neuronopathy rather than an axonopathy. Oxaliplatin, which interferes with axonal ionic conductance, causes transient sensory symptoms after intravenous administration, but persistent symptoms of neuropathy may develop after repeated infusions.[134,136]

The taxanes paclitaxel and docetaxel, which act by causing aggregation of microtubules, can cause a predominantly sensory or sensorimotor axonal neuropathy affecting large-diameter myelinated sensory and motor fibers.[137] Coadministration of other neurotoxic drugs such as cisplatin increases this risk.[138] The recently introduced epothilone group of drugs, which also act on microtubules, may also cause a neuropathy.[139]

The proteasome inhibitor bortezomib, an agent used to treat multiple myeloma, commonly presents with a length-dependent sensory neuropathy, with an incidence of 30 percent; motor involvement is rare.[140] Small sensory fibers are usually affected, and therefore a painful neuropathy is common. Autonomic neuropathy has been reported with an incidence of 10 to 15 percent, and the neuropathic effects may be reversed with dose reduction or withdrawal of the drug. The mechanism of injury involves bortezomib causing intracytoplasmic vacuolization of satellite cells in the dorsal root ganglion.[135,140]

Misonidazole and other compounds related to metronidazole are used as radiosensitizing agents in cancer therapy, and may also cause a sensory neuropathy. Suramin produces a dose-related axonal sensorimotor neuropathy with lamellar inclusions in dorsal root ganglia and Schwann cells, mimicking Guillain–Barré syndrome.[133,135] Podophyllin derivatives, which have been used to treat disseminated malignancy and also are constituents of certain laxative preparations and topical agents, may cause a peripheral neuropathy that is sometimes associated with signs of myelopathy. A severe demyelinating peripheral neuropathy has been reported after high-dose cytarabine therapy in leukemia patients.[141] Additional discussion of these drugs can be found in Chapter 28.

Unfortunately no agent has been shown to be neuroprotective to date; erythropoietin shows some promise, but further study is required.[142,143]

ANTIMICROBIAL AGENTS

A number of antimicrobials may cause neuropathy. The best-known example is the mixed sensorimotor neuropathy caused by isoniazid, which is due to the effect of the drug on pyridoxine metabolism and can be prevented with vitamin B_6 supplementation. Ethambutol may cause a sensory or sensorimotor neuropathy or lead to an optic neuropathy. Ethionamide and streptomycin may rarely also cause a peripheral neuropathy, but the ototoxic effects of streptomycin are usually the most prominent feature. Sensorimotor, or occasionally motor, peripheral neuropathy is a well-documented complication of nitrofurantoin, especially in patients with renal insufficiency. Chloramphenicol rarely causes a mild sensory neuropathy.[133]

The triazole antifungals voriconazole and itraconazole have been reported to cause a sensorimotor neuropathy in conjunction with neurotoxic chemotherapy or in the treatment of invasive aspergillosis and fluconazole-resistant candida infections.[140]

Although peripheral neuropathy was a recognized complication of sulfonamide treatment in the past, none of the drugs in current use has this effect. Prolonged metronidazole therapy can lead to a reversible sensory neuropathy.[133] A peripheral neuropathy has also been reported in patients treated with fluoroquinolones[140] and sodium stibogluconate.[144]

ANTIRHEUMATIC DRUGS

Peripheral neuropathy is a well-recognized complication of gold treatment in rheumatoid arthritis, occurring in 0.5 to 1 percent of patients. Motor involvement is usually prominent and sensory symptoms inconspicuous. The onset may be abrupt and the progression rapid, and in some cases may mimic Guillain–Barré syndrome, particularly in patients who develop facial diplegia and have elevated cerebrospinal fluid protein levels. A sensory or mixed neuropathy has also been reported in patients treated with leflunomide for rheumatoid arthritis.[145]

Chloroquine may cause a mild sensorimotor neuropathy, with a severe proximal myopathy in some cases. A neuropathy occurs rarely in patients treated with D-penicillamine.[6] A mixed sensorimotor neuropathy usually associated with a proximal myopathy may develop in patients treated with colchicine for long periods.[6]

Several types of neuropathy have been described with the TNF-α inhibitors etanercept and infliximab, including Guillain–Barré syndrome, the Miller Fisher syndrome, chronic inflammatory demyelinating neuropathy, multifocal motor neuropathy, mononeuritis multiplex, and axonal sensory or sensorimotor polyneuropathy.[146] These neuropathies usually resolve only incompletely on cessation of therapy.[147] The pathogenesis is thought to involve a T-cell and humoral immune attack against peripheral nerve myelin, inhibition of axonal signaling functions, and vasculitis-induced ischemia.[146,147] Adalimumab is less clearly associated with a peripheral neuropathy, but cases of multifocal motor neuropathy, Guillain–Barré syndrome, and acute bilateral phrenic neuropathy have been reported.[147–149]

Cardiovascular Drugs

A demyelinating sensorimotor polyneuropathy occurred in about 0.1 percent of patients treated with the coronary vasodilator perhexiline, which is no longer widely used, and is also well documented in patients treated with the antiarrhythmic agent amiodarone. Streptokinase has been associated with the development of Guillain–Barré syndrome.[150] Peripheral neuropathy occurs rarely in patients treated with disopyramide, hydralazine, flecainide, enalapril, and captopril.[151,152]

Lipid-Lowering Agents

A number of reports have documented the development of neuropathy in patients treated with various statin drugs.[153–155] This has usually been an axonal sensorimotor polyneuropathy, but there have also been case reports of a neuropathy resembling Guillain–Barré syndrome[156] and of a reversible small-fiber neuropathy.[157] In Australia, the National Adverse Drug Reactions Advisory Committee has received reports of 281 patients with peripheral neuropathy attributed to statins since 1993.[158] Most cases were associated with simvastatin or atorvastatin and, less frequently, pravastatin and fluvastatin. Recovery occurred in about 50 percent of cases after stopping the drug but symptoms may persist for months or even years in some cases.[155] Population-based studies in the United Kingdom and Denmark have shown an increased incidence of idiopathic peripheral neuropathy in patients taking statins.[159,160] A mild reversible sensory neuropathy has also been reported with bezafibrate treatment, and a motor neuropathy with clofibrate.[161] However, the confounding effects of glucose intolerance and hyperlipidemia could not be excluded in many of these studies, and the Fremantle Diabetes Study, including nearly 1,300 patients, showed a decreased risk of neuropathy in patients treated with statins and fibrates.[147]

Hypnotic and Psychotropic Drugs

There have been occasional reports of neuropathy developing in patients taking phenelzine,[162] methaqualone, glutethimide, imipramine, amitriptyline, lithium carbonate, and perazine.

Other Drugs

Various other drugs have been found occasionally to cause neuropathy. A mild peripheral neuropathy can occur in patients on chronic treatment with phenytoin, but it is only rarely symptomatic. Disulfiram, used in the treatment of alcoholism, may cause an axonal sensorimotor polyneuropathy as well as an optic neuropathy. Dapsone may cause a predominantly motor neuropathy after prolonged high-dose therapy for leprosy, certain dermatologic conditions, or for prophylaxis of *Pneumocystis carinii* pneumonia. A sensory or mixed axonal neuropathy is well documented in patients treated with thalidomide.[163–165]

Chronic administration of high doses of pyridoxine may cause a severe sensory polyneuropathy of insidious onset, and paresthesias may develop even in some patients taking conventional doses.[6]

There have been a number of reports of an axonal polyneuropathy developing in patients with hepatitis C treated with interferon-α, and more recently cases of Guillain–Barré syndrome have been reported with polyethylene glycol interferon-α, which is now more commonly used.[146] A reversible sensorimotor neuropathy has also been reported with high doses of deferoxamine.[166]

A number of drugs including gangliosides,[167] streptokinase,[150] zimeldine, D-penicillamine, interferon-α, captopril, and danazol have been associated with the development of Guillain–Barré syndrome.[168,169] A demyelinating neuropathy resembling chronic inflammatory demyelinating polyneuropathy has been reported in patients treated with tacrolimus,[135,170,171] and in a patient treated with interferon-α.[172]

Trigeminal neuropathy has occurred in a patient with hepatitis C treated with interferon-α.[173] Peripheral neuropathy has also been reported in a number of patients with multiple sclerosis treated with interferon-β.[174] Dichloroacetate may lead to or worsen peripheral neuropathy in patients with the syndrome of mitochondrial myopathy, lactic acidosis, and stroke-like episodes (MELAS).[175]

Neuromuscular Transmission Disorders

Various drugs may interfere with neuromuscular transmission by causing a postsynaptic blockade or through a presynaptic effect on neurotransmitter release, as occurs with botulinum toxin (Table 32-3).[176] The most common clinical manifestation is postoperative ventilatory depression in patients treated with aminoglycoside antibiotics or drugs that potentiate the muscle relaxants used during anesthesia. Many of the drugs shown in Table 32-3 may also unmask or aggravate preexisting myasthenia gravis by further reducing the safety factor for neuromuscular transmission and should be avoided or used with caution in such patients. In particular, the choice of antibiotics for use in myasthenic patients is important; aminoglycosides, tetracyclines, sulfonamides, and polypeptide antibiotics should be avoided, whereas cephalosporins, macrolides, and penicillins (with the exception of ampicillin) are generally considered to be safe. The antifungal agent voriconazole has been reported to transiently exacerbate ocular myasthenia through direct blocking of acetylcholine receptors.[177] Deterioration of myasthenia gravis and even myasthenic crisis may occur after botulinum toxin injections.[178,179]

TABLE 32-3 ■ Drugs that May Interfere with Neuromuscular Transmission

Antibiotics	*Anesthetic Agents*
Aminoglycosides	Muscle relaxants
Colistin	Diazepam
Ciprofloxacin	Ketamine
Ampicillin	Propanidid
Clarithromycin	Lidocaine
Erythromycin	Procaine
Clindamycin	*Other Drugs*
Lincomycin	Glucocorticoids
Sulfonamides	Corticotropin
Antirheumatic Drugs	Oral contraceptives
D-Penicillamine	Thyroxine
Chloroquine	Quinine
Cardiovascular Drugs	Diuretics
β-Adrenergic blockers	Magnesium salts
Procainamide	Cholinesterase inhibitors
Quinidine	Anticholinergics
Verapamil	Oxytocin
Statins	Carnitine
Anticonvulsants	Interferon-α
Phenytoin	Deferoxamine
Trimethadione	Ritonavir
Antipsychotics	Botulinum toxin
Lithium	
Phenothiazines	

A syndrome indistinguishable from myasthenia gravis sometimes develop in patients receiving long-term D-penicillamine treatment.[180] These patients have acetylcholine receptor antibodies in the serum, and rarely muscle-specific kinase antibodies, suggesting that the drug initiates a humoral autoimmune response.[180] Other drugs reported to induce myasthenia include interferon-α, captopril, and thiopronine.[181–183] An association between commencement of statin treatment and the development of autoimmune myasthenia gravis (and its exacerbation) is described.[184]

Muscle Disorders

A variety of drugs may cause muscular symptoms through a direct toxic effect on skeletal muscle (Table 32-4).[185] Other drugs that are not intrinsically myotoxic may cause myopathy through a variety of mechanisms including immunologic processes, severe hypokalemia, ischemia, muscle compression (crush syndrome) from prolonged periods of immobility after drug overdosage, and excessive neural driving.[186]

Lipid-Lowering Agents

Myopathy is an important side effect of treatment with statins and fibrate drugs used in the treatment of hyperlipidemia.[185,187] The risk of developing myopathy was shown to be increased 8-fold in patients on statins and 42-fold in patients taking fibrates in a case-control study in the United Kingdom.[188] Myopathy may also develop with high doses of nicotinic acid, and in some patients treated with ezetimibe.[189]

Statins may cause asymptomatic elevated serum CK levels or a more severe necrotizing myopathy with myalgias and proximal muscle weakness (Fig. 32-2). Symptoms usually resolve over a period of 2 to 3 months once the drug is discontinued but may persist chronically in some patients.[190] The risk of myopathy is greater with the lipophilic statins such as simvastatin, atorvastatin, and lovastatin than with hydrophilic compounds such as pravastatin. Acute rhabdomyolysis is the most severe form of statin myopathy and was associated particularly with cerivastatin, which was withdrawn from the market in 2001 after the occurrence of over 100 fatal cases. Rhabdomyolysis occurs rarely with the other statins, with an estimated mortality rate of 0.15 per 1 million prescriptions.[191] Risk factors for statin myopathy include older age, high drug doses, diabetes, hypothyroidism, renal failure, and hepatobiliary disease. Other risk factors include coadministration of statins with fibrate drugs or drugs that compete with or inhibit the CYP3A4 enzyme system[185,192] including cyclosporine, macrolide antibiotics, azole antifungal agents, calcium-channel blockers, SSRIs, and grapefruit juice,[185,193] which should be avoided or restricted during statin therapy. Genetic factors may also predispose to susceptibility.[185,194,195]

In patients whose symptoms fail to improve following withdrawal of the statin, further investigations including a muscle biopsy should be performed since statins may rarely induce or unmask a previously asymptomatic mitochondrial or other metabolic myopathy,[196] or an immune-mediated inflammatory myopathy,[190] such as necrotizing autoimmune myopathy.[185,195,197,198] Detection of an antibody against HMGCR protein is sensitive and specific for necrotizing autoimmune myopathy, with the muscle biopsy showing muscle fiber necrosis with regenerating fibers and upregulation of MCH-1 even in non-necrotic fibers[190] with little or no accompanying inflammatory infiltrate.[185,195,197] Autoantibodies against HMGCR protein are not found in the majority of patients who have been exposed to statins and are without an autoimmune myopathy, but have been found rarely without statin exposure in patients with connective tissue diseases; in spite of this, the condition responds to immunosuppression, with a corresponding decrease in serum CK levels even though the titers of HMGCR autoantibodies remain high.[195] Patients may need multiple agents to control necrotizing autoimmune myopathy, and commonly relapse on withdrawal or weaning of immunotherapy.[198]

There has also been a report of rippling muscle disease brought on by simvastatin.[199]

TABLE 32-4 ■ Therapeutic Agents that May Cause Myopathy

Lipid-Lowering Agents	*Cardiovascular Drugs*
Statins	Amiodarone
Fibrates	Perhexiline
Nicotinic acid	*Other Drugs*
Ezetimibe	Emetine
Antirheumatic Drugs	ε-Aminocaproic acid
Colchicine	Etretinate
Chloroquine	Zidovudine
Hydroxychloroquine	Interferon-α
Glucocorticoids	D-Penicillamine
Prednisone and prednisolone	Streptokinase
Methylprednisolone	
Dexamethasone	
Inhaled steroids	

Acute Rhabdomyolysis

Rhabdomyolysis is the most serious form of drug-induced myopathy, and it has been associated with statin treatment and a number of other drugs. Acute rhabdomyolysis may also occur following self-administration of heroin, cocaine, and other narcotic drugs, alcohol intoxication, and with drug-induced coma, seizures, dyskinesias, or the neuroleptic malignant syndrome. Severe muscle pain, tenderness, and weakness develop over a period of 24 to 48 hours, often with marked limb swelling and the development of a secondary compartment syndrome. The serum CK level is markedly elevated, and myoglobinuria is an early feature, possibly leading to acute oliguric renal failure. Muscle biopsy shows widespread muscle fiber necrosis. The prognosis for recovery is generally good, but some patients die as a result of multiple organ failure. The management of patients with acute rhabdomyolysis is primarily supportive, with careful monitoring of renal function and fluid and electrolyte balance, urinary alkalization, and early treatment of any metabolic derangements. Monitoring of intracompartment pressures is important in patients with muscle swelling as some patients require fasciotomy and muscle decompression.

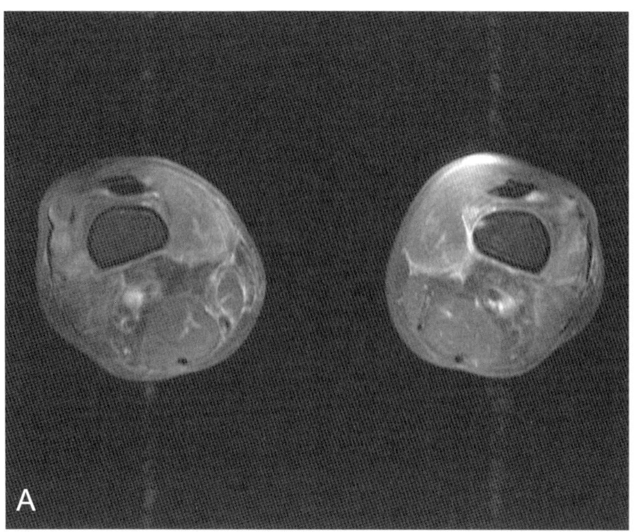

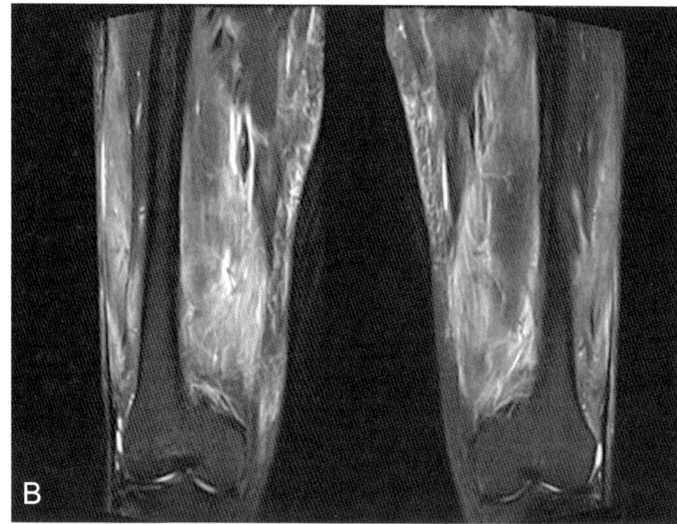

FIGURE 32-2 ■ Axial (**A**) and coronal (**B**) MRI of the proximal lower extremities showing extensive signal change in the quadriceps muscles in a 54-year-old man with a necrotizing myopathy that developed after he started atorvastatin.

Mitochondrial Myopathies

A myopathy with ragged-red fibers and paracrystalline mitochondrial inclusions along with mtDNA depletion may occur in patients infected with human immunodeficiency virus (HIV) on long-term treatment with zidovudine (AZT).[190,203] It is characterized by myalgia, fatigue, proximal or generalized muscle weakness, and elevated serum CK levels, and usually improves when the drug is withdrawn. Other forms of antiretroviral therapy, including the nucleoside analogues didanosine and stavudine, may also cause a mitochondrial myopathy with a clinical phenotype resembling chronic progressive external ophthalmoplegia.[185]

A slowly progressive proximal myopathy has been reported in Korean patients treated with the pyrimidine nucleoside analogue clevudine for chronic hepatitis B infection, with marked serum CK elevation and muscle biopsy changes consistent with a mitochondrial myopathy.[185]

A mitochondrial myopathy with normal CK levels has occurred in some patients taking statins[200] or germanium, which is a constituent of a number of dietary supplements and elixirs.[201,202]

Dyskalemic Myopathies

Severe weakness with depressed tendon reflexes and marked serum CK elevation may develop in patients who become hypokalemic as a result of treatment with diuretics, nasal sprays containing fluoroprednisolone, or as a result of purgative abuse or consumption of large quantities of licorice or licorice extracts (which are ingredients of some traditional Chinese drugs and which contain the potent mineralocorticoid analogue glycyrrhizinic acid).[186] Hypokalemia and myopathy may also complicate treatment with amphotericin B due to renal tubular acidosis.[203] Profound muscle weakness due to hyperkalemia may occur in patients taking potassium-retaining diuretics.

Inflammatory Myopathies

Some drugs may initiate an immune-mediated inflammatory myopathy. The best known are D-penicillamine and interferon-α, both of which may cause polymyositis or dermatomyositis.[204] More recently the main drugs implicated are the TNF-α inhibitors, particularly etanercept and adalimumab, and statins.[205] In the case of statins, apart from necrotizing autoimmune myopathy, dermatomyositis and polymyositis have been described.[185,195,205] An immune-mediated inflammatory myopathy has also been reported as a complication of treatment with streptokinase.[206]

A condition referred to as macrophagic myofasciitis was first recognized in the 1990s in France, where over 130 cases were documented.[207] It is characterized by diffuse myalgia, arthralgia, and fatigue, with a good response to corticosteroid therapy, and is now thought to have been caused by intramuscularly injected vaccines containing aluminum hydroxide.[207]

An interstitial form of myositis characterized by muscle pain, stiffness, and mild weakness has been reported rarely in patients treated with procainamide, hydralazine, phenytoin, levodopa, cimetidine, leuprolide, or propylthiouracil.[203]

Eosinophilic myositis and fasciitis characterized by severe myalgia, edema, and induration of the skin (the eosinophilia-myalgia syndrome) was reported in the early 1990s in patients taking a contaminated preparation of L-tryptophan as a hypnotic, which is no longer in use.

GLUCOCORTICOID MYOPATHY

Glucocorticoid myopathy is common with prolonged treatment and is probably the most common drug-induced myopathy in clinical practice. A symptomatic myopathy is most likely to develop with the 9α-fluorinated corticosteroids triamcinolone, betamethasone, and dexamethasone, but may also occur with prolonged administration of prednisolone (over 10 mg per day). Those taking daily doses of 40 mg or more of prednisolone are at particular risk, whereas patients on an alternate-day regimen are not usually affected.[208,209] The muscles of the pelvic girdle and thighs are most severely affected; myalgia may occur but is not usually a feature. Muscles innervated by the cranial nerves are spared, but involvement of the laryngeal muscles leading to dysphonia can occur in patients using inhaled corticosteroids such as beclomethasone. Diaphragmatic weakness may develop in asthmatic patients taking corticosteroids,[210] and weakness of the respiratory muscles has been reported with corticosteroids in patients with chronic obstructive pulmonary disease and in cancer patients.[211,212] Serum CK levels are usually normal in corticosteroid-induced myopathy and elevated levels should suggest the possibility of another type of myopathy. Muscle biopsy shows selective atrophy of type II muscle fibers.

Glucocorticoid myopathy is usually reversible if the drug is stopped or the dose reduced, and may be attenuated if an alternate-day regimen is implemented. Glucocorticoid-induced muscle atrophy and weakness can be prevented at least in part or reversed by a regular program of physical exercise.[213] Growth hormone and insulin-like growth factor–1 may also be protective.[209,214]

ACUTE QUADRIPLEGIC MYOPATHY

Acute quadriplegic myopathy, also referred to as "acute steroid myopathy" or "critical-illness myopathy," occurs particularly in patients with severe sepsis treated with high intravenous doses of glucocorticoids usually in combination with nondepolarizing neuromuscular blocking agents in the setting of an intensive care unit.[215] There is profound muscle weakness, hypotonia, and depressed tendon reflexes along with respiratory muscle weakness that often leads to difficulties in weaning from the ventilator. The serum CK level is usually normal but may be moderately elevated. Muscle biopsy shows myofiber atrophy, necrosis, and loss of ATPase activity with a selective pattern of myosin filament loss on electron microscopy. Its electrophysiologic hallmark is a markedly reduced excitability of muscles with direct electric stimulation. Nerve conduction studies show only reduced amplitude of the compound muscle action potentials, but can be performed to exclude superimposed critical illness neuropathy, Guillain–Barré syndrome, or a myasthenic disorder. Gradual recovery usually occurs over a period of several months with the help of an intensive program of physiotherapy.

AUTOPHAGIC MYOPATHIES

A number of amphiphilic cationic drugs may cause autophagic degeneration and accumulation of phospholipids in muscle and other tissues. These include chloroquine and hydroxychloroquine, which can cause a painless proximal myopathy or neuromyopathy after prolonged periods of administration, and perhexiline and amiodarone,[185] which lead to the development of a demyelinating sensorimotor peripheral neuropathy at times associated with a proximal myopathy. Immunohistochemistry for microtubule-associated protein light chain 3 and p62 can facilitate tissue-based diagnosis of drug-induced autophagic vacuolar myopathies without the need for electron microscopy, making the diagnosis potentially more accurate and efficient.[216]

MALIGNANT HYPERTHERMIA

Malignant hyperthermia is a condition in which susceptible individuals may develop a potentially fatal state of severe generalized muscular rigidity, hyperpyrexia, metabolic acidosis, and myoglobinuria when exposed to certain anesthetic agents or other drugs.[217] Susceptibility is usually transmitted as an autosomal dominant trait and may be associated with a myopathy that may be subclinical. Mutations in the ryanodine receptor gene (*RYR1*) on chromosome 19q account for over 70 percent of susceptible individuals.[218,219] A number of other susceptibility loci have been reported, and mutations have also been found in the *CACNA1S* gene that encodes the α_1-subunit of the voltage-gated dihydropyridine receptor.[218,219] The most reliable method of identifying individuals at risk is still through demonstration of abnormal sensitivity of muscle tissue to halothane and caffeine (in vitro contracture test). A similar susceptibility to anesthetic reactions may rarely occur in patients with Duchenne or Becker muscular dystrophy, myotonia congenita, myotonic dystrophy, central core disease, and hypokalemic periodic paralysis.

The malignant hyperthermia crisis is thought to be caused by an intrinsic abnormality of the excitation–contraction coupling mechanism in skeletal muscle, as a result of which exposure to anesthetic agents leads to the excessive release of calcium ions from the sarcoplasmic reticulum, causing sustained myofibrillar contraction. Management involves the urgent administration of dantrolene, cooling, correction of fluid and electrolyte balance, and prompt treatment of complications.[218]

Myalgia and Cramps

Many drugs have been reported to cause muscle pain, stiffness, and cramping that are reversible when the drug is withdrawn (Table 32-5). In some cases, serum CK levels may be elevated transiently. Similar symptoms may occur in patients with drug-induced myotonia and may herald a more severe necrotizing myopathy. Muscle pain and fasciculations are commonly induced during anesthesia by succinylcholine. Fasciculations and myokymia have also been reported in patients treated with gold or D-penicillamine.

Drug-Induced Myotonia

A number of drugs may induce myotonia either in humans or experimentally in animals. These include the lipid-lowering agents 20,25-diazacholesterol, clofibrate, triparanol, and zuclomiphene. In addition, some drugs may exacerbate a preexisting myotonic disorder or unmask previously undetected myotonia including the depolarizing muscle relaxants such as succinylcholine, the β-adrenergic blockers (e.g., propranolol and pindolol), and β_2-agonists (e.g., fenoterol and ritodrine). A number of diuretics including furosemide, ethacrynic acid, mersalyl, and acetazolamide can induce myotonia in animals and should be used with caution in patients with genetic forms of myotonia.

TABLE 32-5 ■ Miscellaneous Drugs that May Cause Myalgia or Muscle Cramps

Suxamethonium	Rifampicin
Danazol	Cyclosporine
Clofibrate	Labetalol
Gemfibrozil	Procainamide
Statins	Clonidine
Salbutamol	Pindolol
Lithium	Cimetidine
Captopril	D-Penicillamine
Enalapril	Gold
Bumetanide	Nifedipine
Cytotoxics	Ethchlorvynol
Colchicine	L-Tryptophan
Zidovudine	

Other Drugs

Myopathy is an uncommon complication of treatment with the antifibrinolytic agent ε-aminocaproic acid.[220] Muscle weakness is a common side effect of treatment with emetine in patients with amebiasis, and a severe myopathy has been reported in individuals using ipecac syrup as an emetic agent.[221,222] A proximal myopathy with myalgia and myasthenic features along with a marked elevation of the serum CK level has been reported with the consumption of large quantities of the cough-suppressant codeine linctus, one of the components of which is squill, which contains the cardiac glycosides scillarin A and B that inhibit the cell membrane sodium-potassium pump.

Other drugs rarely implicated in causing myopathy include rifampicin, cimetidine, tetracycline, griseofulvin, sulfasalazine,[223] mercaptopropionyl glycine, vidarabine, ethchlorvynol, finasteride,[224] etretinate, and isotretinoin. Selumetinib, a mitogen-activated protein kinase inhibitor, has caused a focal myopathy of the neck extensors resulting in head drop, with mild elevation in serum CK levels, resolving on cessation of the medication.[225] The recombinant DNA–origin human parathyroid hormone teriparatide, used to treat osteoporosis in postmenopausal women, has been reported to cause muscle cramping and a mild proximal lower-limb myopathy involving the gluteal muscles, which resolves after discontinuation of its use.[226] Severe muscle fibrosis and contracture may develop after repeated intramuscular injections in illicit drug abusers or after prolonged courses of antibiotic injections.

REFERENCES

1. Pirmohamed M, James S, Meakin S, et al: Adverse drug reactions as cause of admission to hospital: prospective analysis of 18 820 patients. BMJ 329:15, 2004.
2. Silberstein SD: Drug-induced headache. Neurol Clin 16:107, 1998.
3. Evers S, Suhr B, Bauer B, et al: A retrospective long-term analysis of the epidemiology and features of drug-induced headache. J Neurol 246:802, 1999.
4. Zed PJ, Loewen PS, Robinson G: Medication-induced headache: overview and systematic review of therapeutic approaches. Ann Pharmacother 33:61, 1999.
5. Allena M, Katsarava Z, Nappi G: From drug-induced headache to medication overuse headache. A short epidemiological review, with a focus on Latin American countries. J Headache Pain 10:71, 2009.
6. Needleman F, Grosset D: Neurological disorders. p. 399. In Lee A (ed): Adverse Drug Reactions. 2nd Ed. Pharmaceutical Press, London, 2006.
7. Gijtenbeek JM, van den Bent MJ, Vecht CJ: Cyclosporine neurotoxicity: a review. J Neurol 246:339, 1999.
8. Bertorini TE, Nance AM, Horner LH, et al: Complications of intravenous gammaglobulin in neuromuscular and other diseases. Muscle Nerve 19:388, 1996.
9. Ducros A: Reversible cerebral vasoconstriction syndrome. Lancet Neurol 11:906, 2012.
10. Diener HC, Limmroth V: Medication-overuse headache: a worldwide problem. Lancet Neurol 3:475, 2004.
11. Limmroth V, Katsarava Z: Medication overuse headache. Curr Opin Neurol 17:301, 2004.
12. Andlin-Sobocki P, Jonsson B, Wittchen HU, et al: Cost of disorders of the brain in Europe. Eur J Neurol 12(suppl 1):1, 2005.
13. Russell MB, Lundqvist C: Prevention and management of medication overuse headache. Curr Opin Neurol 25:290, 2012.
14. Goadsby PJ: Is medication-overuse headache a distinct biological entity? Nat Clin Pract Neurol 2:401, 2006.
15. Limmroth V, Katsarava Z, Fritsche G, et al: Features of medication overuse headache following overuse of different acute headache drugs. Neurology 59:1011, 2002.
16. Paemeleire K, Bahra A, Evers S, et al: Medication-overuse headache in patients with cluster headache. Neurology 67:109, 2006.
17. Evers S, Marziniak M: Clinical features, pathophysiology, and treatment of medication-overuse headache. Lancet Neurol 9:391, 2010.
18. Silberstein SD, Welch KM: Painkiller headache. Neurology 59:972, 2002.
19. Dowson AJ, Dodick DW, Limmroth V: Medication overuse headache in patients with primary headache disorders: epidemiology, management and pathogenesis. CNS Drugs 19:483, 2005.
20. Bandini F: Minocycline in neurological diseases. Lancet Neurol 4:138, 2005.
21. Fraser CL, Biousse V, Newman NJ: Minocycline-induced fulminant intracranial hypertension. Arch Neurol 69:1067, 2012.
22. Spennato P, Ruggiero C, Parlato RS, et al: Pseudotumor cerebri. Childs Nerv Syst 27:215, 2011.
23. Ball AK, Clarke CE: Idiopathic intracranial hypertension. Lancet Neurol 5:433, 2006.
24. Gallego Perez-Larraya J, Palma JA, Carmona-Iragui M, et al: Neurologic complications of intrathecal liposomal cytarabine administered prophylactically to patients with non-Hodgkin lymphoma. J Neurooncol 103:603, 2011.
25. Chazan B, Weiss A, Weiner Z, et al: Drug induced aseptic meningitis due to diclofenac. J Neurol 250:1503, 2003.
26. Gordon MF, Allon M, Coyle PK: Drug-induced meningitis. Neurology 40:163, 1990.
27. Kepa L, Oczko-Grzesik B, Stolarz W, et al: Drug-induced aseptic meningitis in suspected central nervous system infections. J Clin Neurosci 12:562, 2005.
28. Hopkins S, Jolles S: Drug-induced aseptic meningitis. Exp Opin Drug Saf 4:285, 2005.
29. Wittmann A, Wooten GF: Amoxicillin-induced aseptic meningitis. Neurology 57:1734, 2001.
30. Creel GB, Hurtt M: Cephalosporin-induced recurrent aseptic meningitis. Ann Neurol 37:815, 1995.
31. Jain KK: Drug-Induced Neurological Disorders. Hogrefe & Huber, Seattle, 1996.
32. Mathian A, Amoura Z, Piette JC: Pentoxifylline-induced aseptic meningitis in a patient with mixed connective tissue disease. Neurology 59:1468, 2002.
33. de Bruijn SF, Stam J, Koopman MM, et al: Case-control study of risk of cerebral sinus thrombosis in oral contraceptive users and in [correction of who are] carriers of hereditary prothrombotic conditions.

The Cerebral Venous Sinus Thrombosis Study Group. BMJ 316:589, 1998.

34. Petitti DB, Sidney S, Bernstein A, et al: Stroke in users of low-dose oral contraceptives. N Engl J Med 335:8, 1996.
35. Zeitoun K, Carr BR: Is there an increased risk of stroke associated with oral contraceptives? Drug Saf 20:467, 1999.
36. Bushnell CD, Goldstein LB: Risk of ischemic stroke with tamoxifen treatment for breast cancer: a meta-analysis. Neurology 63:1230, 2004.
37. LaMonte MP, Brown PM, Hursting MJ: Stroke in patients with heparin-induced thrombocytopenia and the effect of argatroban therapy. Crit Care Med 32:976, 2004.
38. Baigent C, Blackwell L, Collins R, et al: Aspirin in the primary and secondary prevention of vascular disease: collaborative meta-analysis of individual participant data from randomised trials. Lancet 373:1849, 2009.
39. Pozzi M, Roccatagliata D, Sterzi R: Drug abuse and intracranial hemorrhage. Neurol Sci 29(suppl 2): S269, 2008.
40. Geibprasert S, Gallucci M, Krings T: Addictive illegal drugs: structural neuroimaging. AJNR Am J Neuroradiol 31:803, 2010.
41. McEvoy AW, Kitchen ND, Thomas DG: Lesson of the week: intracerebral haemorrhage in young adults: the emerging importance of drug misuse. BMJ 320:1322, 2000.
42. Bruno A: Cerebrovascular complications of alcohol and sympathomimetic drug abuse. Curr Neurol Neurosci 3:40, 2003.
43. Kase CS, Foster TE, Reed JE, et al: Intracerebral hemorrhage and phenylpropanolamine use. Neurology 37:399, 1987.
44. Bruno A, Nolte KB, Chapin J: Stroke associated with ephedrine use. Neurology 43:1313, 1993.
45. Morgenstern LB, Viscoli CM, Kernan WN, et al: Use of Ephedra-containing products and risk for hemorrhagic stroke. Neurology 60:132, 2003.
46. Li SH, Chen WH, Tang Y, et al: Incidence of ischemic stroke post-chemotherapy: a retrospective review of 10,963 patients. Clin Neurol Neurosurg 108:150, 2006.
47. Murphy K, Delanty N: Drug-induced seizures: general principles in assessment, management and prevention. CNS Drugs 14:135, 2000.
48. Zaccara G, Muscas GC, Messori A: Clinical features, pathogenesis and management of drug-induced seizures. Drug Saf 5:109, 1990.
49. Pesola GR, Avasarala J: Bupropion seizure proportion among new-onset generalized seizures and drug related seizures presenting to an emergency department. J Emerg Med 22:235, 2002.
50. DeLorenzo RJ, Hauser WA, Towne AR, et al: A prospective, population-based epidemiologic study of status epilepticus in Richmond, Virginia. Neurology 46:1029, 1996.
51. Thundiyil JG, Rowley F, Papa L, et al: Risk factors for complications of drug-induced seizures. J Med Toxicol 7:16, 2011.
52. Thundiyil JG, Kearney TE, Olson KR: Evolving epidemiology of drug-induced seizures reported to a Poison Control Center System. J Med Toxicol 3:15, 2007.
53. Jackson GD, Berkovic SF: Ceftazidime encephalopathy: absence status and toxic hallucinations. J Neurol Neurosurg Psychiatry 55:333, 1992.
54. Degner D, Grohmann R, Kropp S, et al: Severe adverse drug reactions of antidepressants: results of the German multicenter drug surveillance program AMSP. Pharmacopsychiatry 37(suppl 1):S39, 2004.
55. Chaves J, Sander JW: Seizure aggravation in idiopathic generalized epilepsies. Epilepsia 46(suppl 9): 133, 2005.
56. Perucca E, Gram L, Avanzini G, et al: Antiepileptic drugs as a cause of worsening seizures. Epilepsia 39:5, 1998.
57. Sazgar M, Bourgeois BF: Aggravation of epilepsy by antiepileptic drugs. Pediatr Neurol 33:227, 2005.
58. Ettinger AB, Bernal OG, Andriola MR, et al: Two cases of nonconvulsive status epilepticus in association with tiagabine therapy. Epilepsia 40:1159, 1999.
59. Bahls FH, Ma KK, Bird TD: Theophylline-associated seizures with "therapeutic" or low toxic serum concentrations: risk factors for serious outcome in adults. Neurology 41:1309, 1991.
60. Dailey JW, Naritoku DK: Antidepressants and seizures: clinical anecdotes overshadow neuroscience. Biochem Pharmacol 52:1323, 1996.
61. Lee KC, Finley PR, Alldredge BK: Risk of seizures associated with psychotropic medications: emphasis on new drugs and new findings. Expert Opin Drug Saf 2:233, 2003.
62. De Paepe P, Calle PA, Buylaert WA: Coma induced by intoxication. Handb Clin Neurol 90:175, 2008.
63. Husain AM: Electroencephalographic assessment of coma. J Clin Neurophysiol 23:208, 2006.
64. Taylor D, Paton C, Kapur S: The Maudsley Prescribing Guidelines in Psychiatry. 11th Ed. Wiley-Blackwell, Chichester, 2012.
65. Roth BA, Vinson DR, Kim S: Carisoprodol-induced myoclonic encephalopathy. J Toxicol Clin Toxicol 36:609, 1998.
66. Grill MF, Maganti R: Cephalosporin-induced neurotoxicity: clinical manifestations, potential pathogenic mechanisms, and the role of electroencephalographic monitoring. Ann Pharmacother 42:1843, 2008.
67. Lam S, Gomolin IH: Cefepime neurotoxicity: case report, pharmacokinetic considerations, and literature review. Pharmacotherapy 26:1169, 2006.
68. Tlemsani C, Mir O, Boudou-Rouquette P, et al: Posterior reversible encephalopathy syndrome

induced by anti-VEGF agents. Target Oncol 6:253, 2011.
69. Poole R, Brabbins C: Drug induced psychosis. Br J Psychiatry 168:135, 1996.
70. Sternbach H: The serotonin syndrome. Am J Psychiatry 148:705, 1991.
71. Brown TM, Skop BP, Mareth TR: Pathophysiology and management of the serotonin syndrome. Ann Pharmacother 30:527, 1996.
72. Gillman PK: The serotonin syndrome and its treatment. J Psychopharmacol 13:100, 1999.
73. Toovey S, Rayner C, Prinssen E, et al: Assessment of neuropsychiatric adverse events in influenza patients treated with oseltamivir: a comprehensive review. Drug Saf 31:1097, 2008.
74. Patten SB, Barbui C: Drug-induced depression: a systematic review to inform clinical practice. Psychother Psychosom 73:207, 2004.
75. Peet M, Peters S: Drug-induced mania. Drug Saf 12:146, 1995.
76. Patten SB, Neutel CI: Corticosteroid-induced adverse psychiatric effects: incidence, diagnosis and management. Drug Saf 22:111, 2000.
77. Parker G, Parker K: Which antidepressants flick the switch? Aust NZ J Psychiatry 37:464, 2003.
78. Sacks O, Shulman M: Steroid dementia: an overlooked diagnosis? Neurology 64:707, 2005.
79. Kälviäinen R, Äikiä M, Riekkinen Sr P: Cognitive adverse effects of antiepileptic drugs. CNS Drugs 5:358, 1996.
80. Aarsen FK, van den Akker EL, Drop SL, et al: Effect of topiramate on cognition in obese children. Neurology 67:1307, 2006.
81. Hindmarch I: Cognitive toxicity of pharmacotherapeutic agents used in social anxiety disorder. Int J Clin Pract 63:1085, 2009.
82. Factor S, Lang A, Weiner W: Drug Induced Movement Disorders. Blackwell, Oxford, 2005.
83. Jankovic J: Tardive syndromes and other drug-induced movement disorders. Clin Neuropharmacol 18:197, 1995.
84. Jimenez-Jimenez FJ, Garcia-Ruiz PJ, Molina JA: Drug-induced movement disorders. Drug Saf 16:180, 1997.
85. Sethi KD (ed): Drug-Induced Movement Disorders. Marcel Dekker, New York, 2004.
86. Rosebush PI, Mazurek MF: Neurologic side effects in neuroleptic-naive patients treated with haloperidol or risperidone. Neurology 52:782, 1999.
87. Miller CH, Mohr F, Umbricht D, et al: The prevalence of acute extrapyramidal signs and symptoms in patients treated with clozapine, risperidone, and conventional antipsychotics. J Clin Psychiatry 59:69, 1998.
88. Molho ES, Factor SA: Worsening of motor features of parkinsonism with olanzapine. Mov Disord 14:1014, 1999.
89. Gerber PE, Lynd LD: Selective serotonin-reuptake inhibitor-induced movement disorders. Ann Pharmacother 32:692, 1998.
90. Blanchet PJ: Antipsychotic drug-induced movement disorders. Can J Neurol Sci 30(suppl 1):S101, 2003.
91. Rodnitzky RL: Drug-induced movement disorders. Clin Neuropharmacol 25:142, 2002.
92. Robottom BJ, Shulman LM, Weiner WJ: Drug-induced movement disorders: emergencies and management. Neurol Clin 30:309, 2012.
93. Tarsy D, Baldessarini RJ: Epidemiology of tardive dyskinesia: is risk declining with modern antipsychotics? Mov Dis 21:589, 2006.
94. Ahmed S, Chengappa KN, Naidu VR, et al: Clozapine withdrawal-emergent dystonias and dyskinesias: a case series. J Clin Psychiatry 59:472, 1998.
95. Teo JT, Edwards MJ, Bhatia K: Tardive dyskinesia is caused by maladaptive synaptic plasticity: a hypothesis. Mov Dis 27:1205, 2012.
96. Garcia-Ruiz PJ, Jimenez-Jimenez FJ, Garcia de Yebenes J: Calcium channel blocker-induced parkinsonism: clinical features and comparisons with Parkinson's disease. Parkinsonism Relat Disord 4:211, 1998.
97. Negrotti A, Calzetti S, Sasso E: Calcium-entry blockers-induced parkinsonism: possible role of inherited susceptibility. Neurotoxicology 13:261, 1992.
98. Johnson V, Bruxner G: Neuroleptic malignant syndrome associated with olanzapine. Aus NZ J Psychiatry 32:884, 1998.
99. Karagianis JL, Phillips LC, Hogan KP, et al: Clozapine-associated neuroleptic malignant syndrome: two new cases and a review of the literature. Ann Pharmacother 33:623, 1999.
100. Reutens DC, Harrison WB, Goldswain PR: Neuroleptic malignant syndrome complicating levodopa withdrawal. Med J Aust 155:53, 1991.
101. Morgan JC, Sethi KD: Drug-induced tremors. Lancet Neurol 4:866, 2005.
102. Alty JE, Kempster PA: A practical guide to the differential diagnosis of tremor. Postgrad Med J 87:623, 2011.
103. Gilbert DL: Drug-induced movement disorders in children. Ann NY Acad Sci 1142:72, 2008.
104. Bak TH, Bauer M, Schaub RT, et al: Myoclonus in patients treated with clozapine: a case series. J Clin Psychiatry 56:418, 1995.
105. Barak Y, Levine J, Weisz R: Clozapine-induced myoclonus: two case reports. J Clin Psychopharmacol 16:339, 1996.
106. Neufeld MY, Vishnevska S: Vigabatrin and multifocal myoclonus in adults with partial seizures. Clin Neuropharmacol 18:280, 1995.
107. Bauer M: Severe myoclonus produced by fluvoxamine. J Clin Psychiatry 56:589, 1995.
108. Wyllie AR, Bayliff CD, Kovacs MJ: Myoclonus due to chlorambucil in two adults with lymphoma. Ann Pharmacother 31:171, 1997.

109. Mercadante S: Pathophysiology and treatment of opioid-related myoclonus in cancer patients. Pain 74:5, 1998.
110. Vadlamudi L, Wijdicks EF: Multifocal myoclonus due to verapamil overdose. Neurology 58:984, 2002.
111. Fear CF: Drug-induced Creutzfeldt-Jakob like syndrome: a review. Hum Psychopharmacol Clin Exp 7:89, 1992.
112. Duarte J, Sempere AP, Cabezas MC, et al: Postural myoclonus induced by phenytoin. Clin Neuropharmacol 19:536, 1996.
113. Manto M: Toxic agents causing cerebellar ataxias. Handb Clin Neurol 103:201, 2012.
114. Niethammer M, Ford B: Permanent lithium-induced cerebellar toxicity: three cases and review of literature. Mov Disord 22:570, 2007.
115. Seligmann H, Podoshin L, Ben-David J, et al: Drug-induced tinnitus and other hearing disorders. Drug Saf 14:198, 1996.
116. Halmagyi GM, Fattore CM, Curthoys IS, et al: Gentamicin vestibulotoxicity. Otolaryngol Head Neck Surg 111:571, 1994.
117. Yorgason JG, Fayad JN, Kalinec F: Understanding drug ototoxicity: molecular insights for prevention and clinical management. Expert Opin Drug Saf 5:383, 2006.
118. Black FO, Pesznecker S, Stallings V: Permanent gentamicin vestibulotoxicity. Otol Neurotol 25:559, 2004.
119. McGwin Jr G: Phosphodiesterase type 5 inhibitor use and hearing impairment. Arch Otolaryngol Head Neck Surg 136:488, 2010.
120. Kanda Y, Shigeno K, Kinoshita N, et al: Sudden hearing loss associated with interferon. Lancet 343:1134, 1994.
121. Li J, Tripathi RC, Tripathi BJ: Drug-induced ocular disorders. Drug Saf 31:127, 2008.
122. Jain N, Bhatti MT: Fingolimod-associated macular edema: incidence, detection, and management. Neurology 78:672, 2012.
123. Fecarotta C, Sergott RC: Vigabatrin-associated visual field loss. Int Ophthalmol Clin 52:87, 2012.
124. Kerrison JB: Optic neuropathies caused by toxins and adverse drug reactions. Ophthalmol Clin North Am 17:481, 2004.
125. Li SY, Birnbaum AD, Goldstein DA: Optic neuritis associated with adalimumab in the treatment of uveitis. Ocular Immunol Inflamm 18:475, 2010.
126. Lafeuillade A, Aubert L, Chaffanjon P, et al: Optic neuritis associated with dideoxyinosine. Lancet 337:615, 1991.
127. [No authors listed]: Drug-induced colour vision disorders. Prescrire Int 21:126, 2012.
128. Naik BS, Shetty N, Maben EV: Drug-induced taste disorders. Eur J Intern Med 21:240, 2010.
129. Sotirchos ES, Saidha S, Becker D: Neurological picture. Nitrous oxide-induced myelopathy with inverted V-sign on spinal MRI. J Neurol Neurosurg Psychiatry 83:915, 2012.
130. Tesio L, Bassi L, Strada L: Spinal cord lesion after penicillin gluteal injection. Paraplegia 30:442, 1992.
131. Verhamme KM, Sturkenboom MC, Stricker BH, et al: Drug-induced urinary retention: incidence, management and prevention. Drug Saf 31:373, 2008.
132. Tsakiris P, Oelke M, Michel MC: Drug-induced urinary incontinence. Drugs Aging 25:541, 2008.
133. Windebank AJ: Drug-induced neuropathies. Baillieres Clin Neurol 4:529, 1995.
134. Quasthoff S, Hartung HP: Chemotherapy-induced peripheral neuropathy. J Neurol 249:9, 2002.
135. Postma TJ, Heimans JJ: Neurological complications of chemotherapy to the peripheral nervous system. Handb Clin Neurol 105:917, 2012.
136. Krishnan AV, Goldstein D, Friedlander M, et al: Oxaliplatin-induced neurotoxicity and the development of neuropathy. Muscle Nerve 32:51, 2005.
137. Freilich RJ, Balmaceda C, Seidman AD, et al: Motor neuropathy due to docetaxel and paclitaxel. Neurology 47:115, 1996.
138. Argyriou AA, Polychronopoulos P, Iconomou G, et al: Paclitaxel plus carboplatin-induced peripheral neuropathy. A prospective clinical and electrophysiological study in patients suffering from solid malignancies. J Neurol 252:1459, 2005.
139. Zhuang SH, Agrawal M, Edgerly M, et al: A Phase I clinical trial of ixabepilone (BMS-247550), an epothilone B analog, administered intravenously on a daily schedule for 3 days. Cancer 103:1932, 2005.
140. Manji H: Toxic neuropathy. Curr Opin Neurol 24:484, 2011.
141. Openshaw H, Slatkin NE, Stein AS, et al: Acute polyneuropathy after high dose cytosine arabinoside in patients with leukemia. Cancer 78:1899, 1996.
142. Albers JW, Chaudhry V, Cavaletti G, et al: Interventions for preventing neuropathy caused by cisplatin and related compounds. Cochrane Database Syst Rev:CD005228, 2011.
143. Beijers AJ, Jongen JL, Vreugdenhil G: Chemotherapy-induced neurotoxicity: the value of neuroprotective strategies. Neth J Med 70:18, 2012.
144. Brummitt CF, Porter JA, Herwaldt BL: Reversible peripheral neuropathy associated with sodium stibogluconate therapy for American cutaneous leishmaniasis. Clin Infect Dis 22:878, 1996.
145. Martin K, Bentaberry F, Dumoulin C, et al: Neuropathy associated with leflunomide: a case series. Ann Rheum Dis 64:649, 2005.
146. Toyooka K, Fujimura H: Iatrogenic neuropathies. Curr Opin Neurol 22:475, 2009.
147. Weimer LH, Sachdev N: Update on medication-induced peripheral neuropathy. Curr Neurol Neurosci Rep 9:69, 2009.
148. Alentorn A, Alberti MA, Montero J, et al: Monofocal motor neuropathy with conduction block associated with adalimumab in rheumatoid arthritis. Joint Bone Spine 78:536, 2011.

149. Alexopoulou A, Koskinas J, Soultati A, et al: Acute bilateral phrenic neuropathy following treatment with adalimumab. Clin Rheumatol 28:1337, 2009.
150. Taylor BV, Mastaglia FL, Stell R: Guillain-Barré syndrome complicating treatment with streptokinase. Med J Aust 162:214, 1995.
151. Hormigo A, Alves M: Peripheral neuropathy in a patient receiving enalapril. BMJ 305:1332, 1992.
152. Palace J, Shah R, Clough C: Flecainide induced peripheral neuropathy. BMJ 305:810, 1992.
153. Umapathi T, Chaudhry V: Toxic neuropathy. Curr Opin Neurol 18:574, 2005.
154. Jeppesen U, Gaist D, Smith T, et al: Statins and peripheral neuropathy. Eur J Clin Pharmacol 54:835, 1999.
155. Phan T, McLeod JG, Pollard JD, et al: Peripheral neuropathy associated with simvastatin. J Neurol Neurosurg Psychiatry 58:625, 1995.
156. Rajabally YA, Varakantam V, Abbott RJ: Disorder resembling Guillain-Barré syndrome on initiation of statin therapy. Muscle Nerve 30:663, 2004.
157. Lo YL, Leoh TH, Loh LM, et al: Statin therapy and small fibre neuropathy: a serial electrophysiological study. J Neurol Sci 208:105, 2003.
158. Australian Adverse Drug Reactions Advisory Committee Statins and peripheral neuropathy. Aust Adv Drug Reactions Bull 24:6, 2005.
159. Gaist D, Jeppesen U, Andersen M, et al: Statins and risk of polyneuropathy: a case-control study. Neurology 58:1333, 2002.
160. Gaist D, Rodriguez LA, Huerta C, et al: Lipid-lowering drugs and risk of myopathy: a population-based follow-up study. Epidemiology 12:565, 2001.
161. Ellis CJ, Wallis WE, Caruana M: Peripheral neuropathy with bezafibrate. BMJ 309:929, 1994.
162. Goodheart RS, Dunne JW, Edis RH: Phenelzine associated peripheral neuropathy–clinical and electrophysiologic findings. Aust NZ J Med 21:339, 1991.
163. Briani C, Zara G, Rondinone R, et al: Thalidomide neurotoxicity: prospective study in patients with lupus erythematosus. Neurology 62:2288, 2004.
164. Chaudhry V, Cornblath DR, Corse A, et al: Thalidomide-induced neuropathy. Neurology 59:1872, 2002.
165. Ochonisky S, Verroust J, Bastuji-Garin S, et al: Thalidomide neuropathy incidence and clinico-electrophysiologic findings in 42 patients. Arch Dermatol 130:66, 1994.
166. Levine JE, Cohen A, MacQueen M, et al: Sensorimotor neurotoxicity associated with high-dose deferoxamine treatment. J Ped Hematol Oncol 19:139, 1997.
167. Illa I, Ortiz N, Gallard E, et al: Acute axonal Guillain-Barré syndrome with IgG antibodies against motor axons following parenteral gangliosides. Ann Neurol 38:218, 1995.
168. Awong IE, Dandurand KR, Keeys CA, et al: Drug-associated Guillain-Barré syndrome: a literature review. Ann Pharmacother 30:173, 1996.
169. Boz C, Ozmenoglu M, Aktoz G, et al: Guillain-Barré syndrome during treatment with interferon alpha for hepatitis B. J Clin Neurosci 11:523, 2004.
170. Bronster DJ, Yonover P, Stein J, et al: Demyelinating sensorimotor polyneuropathy after administration of FK506. Transplantation 59:1066, 1995.
171. Wilson JR, Conwit RA, Eidelman BH, et al: Sensorimotor neuropathy resembling CIDP in patients receiving FK506. Muscle Nerve 17:528, 1994.
172. Marzo ME, Tintore M, Fabregues O, et al: Chronic inflammatory demyelinating polyneuropathy during treatment with interferon-alpha. J Neurol Neurosurg Psychiatry 65:604, 1998.
173. Marey-Lopez J, Sousa CP: Trigeminal sensory neuropathy related to interferon-alpha treatment. Muscle Nerve 33:581, 2006.
174. Ekstein D, Linetsky E, Abramsky O, et al: Polyneuropathy associated with interferon beta treatment in patients with multiple sclerosis. Neurology 65:456, 2005.
175. Kaufmann P, Engelstad K, Wei Y, et al: Dichloroacetate causes toxic neuropathy in MELAS: a randomized, controlled clinical trial. Neurology 66:324, 2006.
176. Wittbrodt ET: Drugs and myasthenia gravis. An update. Arch Intern Med 157:399, 1997.
177. Azzam R, Shaikh AG, Serra A, et al: Exacerbation of myasthenia gravis with voriconazole. Muscle Nerve 47:928, 2013.
178. Bhatia KP, Munchau A, Thompson PD, et al: Generalised muscular weakness after botulinum toxin injections for dystonia: a report of three cases. J Neurol Neurosurg Psychiatry 67:90, 1999.
179. Borodic G: Myasthenic crisis after botulinum toxin. Lancet 352:1832, 1998.
180. Poulas K, Koutsouraki E, Kordas G, et al: Anti-MuSK- and anti-AChR-positive myasthenia gravis induced by D-penicillamine. J Neuroimmunol 250:94, 2012.
181. Penn AS, Low BW, Jaffe IA, et al: Drug-induced autoimmune myasthenia gravis. Ann NY Acad Sci 841:433, 1998.
182. Batocchi AP, Evoli A, Servidei S, et al: Myasthenia gravis during interferon alfa therapy. Neurology 45:382, 1995.
183. Bora I, Karli N, Bakar M, et al: Myasthenia gravis following IFN-alpha-2a treatment. Eur Neurol 38:68, 1997.
184. de Sousa E, Howard J: More evidence for the association between statins and myasthenia gravis. Muscle Nerve 38:1085, 2008.
185. Mastaglia FL, Needham M: Update on toxic myopathies. Curr Neurol Neurosci Rep 12:54, 2012.
186. Mastaglia FL: Toxic myopathies. Handb Clin Neurol 62:595, 1992.
187. Mastaglia FL: Drug-induced myopathies. Pract Neurol 6:4, 2006.
188. Gaist D, Garcia Rodriguez LA, Huerta C, et al: Are users of lipid-lowering drugs at increased risk of

peripheral neuropathy? Eur J Clin Pharmacol 56:931, 2001.
189. Fux R, Morike K, Gundel UF, et al: Ezetimibe and statin-associated myopathy. Ann Intern Med 140:671, 2004.
190. Needham M, Fabian V, Knezevic W, et al: Progressive myopathy with up-regulation of MHC-I associated with statin therapy. Neuromuscul Disord 17:194, 2007.
191. Staffa JA, Chang J, Green L: Cerivastatin and reports of fatal rhabdomyolysis. N Engl J Med 346:539, 2002.
192. Worz CR, Bottorff M: The role of cytochrome P450-mediated drug-drug interactions in determining the safety of statins. Expert Opin Pharmacother 2:1119, 2001.
193. Lilja JJ, Neuvonen M, Neuvonen PJ: Effects of regular consumption of grapefruit juice on the pharmacokinetics of simvastatin. Br J Clin Pharmacol 58:56, 2004.
194. Vladutiu GD, Simmons Z, Isackson PJ, et al: Genetic risk factors associated with lipid-lowering drug-induced myopathies. Muscle Nerve 34:153, 2006.
195. Mohassel P, Mammen AL: Statin-associated autoimmune myopathy and anti-HMGCR autoantibodies: a review. Muscle Nerve 48:477, 2013.
196. Tsivgoulis G, Spengos K, Karandreas N, et al: Presymptomatic neuromuscular disorders disclosed following statin treatment. Arch Intern Med 166:1519, 2006.
197. Sathasivam S: Statin induced myotoxicity. Eur J Intern Med 23:317, 2012.
198. Grable-Esposito P, Katzberg HD, Greenberg SA, et al: Immune-mediated necrotizing myopathy associated with statins. Muscle Nerve 41:185, 2010.
199. Baker SK, Tarnopolsky MA: Sporadic rippling muscle disease unmasked by simvastatin. Muscle Nerve 34:478, 2006.
200. Phillips PS, Haas RH, Bannykh S, et al: Statin-associated myopathy with normal creatine kinase levels. Ann Intern Med 137:581, 2002.
201. Higuchi I, Takahashi K, Nakahara K, et al: Experimental germanium myopathy. Acta Neuropathol 82:55, 1991.
202. Wu CM, Matsuoka T, Takemitsu M, et al: An experimental model of mitochondrial myopathy: germanium-induced myopathy and coenzyme Q10 administration. Muscle Nerve 15:1258, 1992.
203. George KK, Pourmand R: Toxic myopathies. Neurol Clin 15:711, 1997.
204. Hengstman GJ, Vogels OJ, ter Laak HJ, et al: Myositis during long-term interferon-alpha treatment. Neurology 54:2186, 2000.
205. Bukhari M: Drug-induced rheumatic diseases: a review of published case reports from the last two years. Curr Opin Rheumatol 24:182, 2012.
206. Di Muzio A, Di Guglielmo G, Feliciani C, et al: Inflammatory myopathy after intravenous streptokinase. Muscle Nerve 20:619, 1997.
207. Gherardi RK, Coquet M, Cherin P, et al: Macrophagic myofasciitis lesions assess long-term persistence of vaccine-derived aluminium hydroxide in muscle. Brain 124:1821, 2001.
208. Minetto MA, Lanfranco F, Motta G, et al: Steroid myopathy: some unresolved issues. J Endocrinol Invest 34:370, 2011.
209. Pereira RM, Freire de Carvalho J: Glucocorticoid-induced myopathy. Joint Bone Spine 78:41, 2011.
210. Dekhuijzen PN, Decramer M: Steroid-induced myopathy and its significance to respiratory disease: a known disease rediscovered. Eur Resp J 5:997, 1992.
211. Batchelor TT, Taylor LP, Thaler HT, et al: Steroid myopathy in cancer patients. Neurology 48:1234, 1997.
212. van Balkom RH, van der Heijden HF, van Herwaarden CL, et al: Corticosteroid-induced myopathy of the respiratory muscles. Neth J Med 45:114, 1994.
213. LaPier TK: Glucocorticoid-induced muscle atrophy. The role of exercise in treatment and prevention. J Cardiopulm Rehab 17:76, 1997.
214. Kanda F, Takatani K, Okuda S, et al: Preventive effects of insulinlike growth factor-I on steroid-induced muscle atrophy. Muscle Nerve 22:213, 1999.
215. Latronico N, Tomelleri G, Filosto M: Critical illness myopathy. Curr Opin Rheumatol 24:616, 2012.
216. Lee HS, Daniels BH, Salas E, et al: Clinical utility of LC3 and p62 immunohistochemistry in diagnosis of drug-induced autophagic vacuolar myopathies: a case-control study. PLoS One 7:e36221, 2012.
217. Bandschapp O, Girard T: Malignant hyperthermia. Swiss Med Wkly 142:w13652, 2012.
218. Halsall PJ, Robinson RL: Malignant hyperthermia and associated conditions. Handb Clin Neurol 85:107, 2007.
219. Hogan K: The anesthetic myopathies and malignant hyperthermias. Curr Opin Neurol 11:469, 1998.
220. Seymour BD, Rubinger M: Rhabdomyolysis induced by epsilon-aminocaproic acid. Ann Pharmacother 31:56, 1997.
221. Dresser LP, Massey EW, Johnson EE, et al: Ipecac myopathy and cardiomyopathy. J Neurol Neurosurg Psychiatry 56:560, 1993.
222. Lacomis D: Case of the month. June 1996—anorexia nervosa. Brain Pathol 6:535, 1996.
223. Norden DK, Lichtenstein GR, Williams WV: Sulfasalazine-induced myopathy. Am J Gastroenterol 89:801, 1994.
224. Haan J, Hollander JM, van Duinen SG, et al: Reversible severe myopathy during treatment with finasteride. Muscle Nerve 20:502, 1997.
225. Chen X, Schwartz GK, DeAngelis LM, et al: Dropped head syndrome: report of three cases during treatment with a MEK inhibitor. Neurology 79:1929, 2012.
226. Luigetti M, Capone F, Monforte M, et al: Muscle cramps and weakness after teriparatide therapy: A new drug-induced myopathy? Muscle Nerve 47:615, 2013.

CHAPTER

33

Alcohol and the Nervous System

ROBERT O. MESSING

Who could have foretold, from the structure of the brain, that wine could derange its functions?

Hippocrates

Alcohol is the most commonly used recreational psychoactive substance worldwide. While moderate drinking can be beneficial to health, excessive use can result in serious medical disorders. Excessive alcohol consumption has been implicated in diseases affecting virtually every level of the neuraxis (Fig. 33-1). Despite its protean nature, alcoholic neurologic disease often involves select anatomic structures or cell populations, suggesting that multiple, discrete pathophysiologic processes are involved.

ALCOHOL INTOXICATION AND WITHDRAWAL

Intoxication

In nonalcoholics, early signs of intoxication occur at blood alcohol concentrations less than 50 mg/dl (11 mmol/L) and include relaxation, loss of social inhibitions, increased talking, and impairment in some skilled tasks.[1] Ataxia, nystagmus, slurred speech, impaired judgment, and changes in mood and behavior generally occur at blood alcohol levels above 100 mg/dl (22 mmol/L) and are followed by findings of central nervous system depression as blood levels increase. Blood levels above 300 mg/dl (65 mmol/L) can lead to coma, hyporeflexia, respiratory compromise, and hypotension. Although the behavioral effects of alcohol generally correlate with blood concentrations, tolerance may occur rapidly and greatly modify the clinical response to a specific blood level. Acute tolerance develops even during a single bout of drinking, and can cause the drinker to become sober at blood alcohol concentrations higher than those at which intoxication previously developed.[2] In chronic alcoholics, the degree of tolerance can be extensive, permitting sobriety at blood concentrations above 120 mg/dl and survival above 700 mg/dl.[3]

Minor Withdrawal Syndrome

Characteristic symptoms of alcohol withdrawal follow abrupt cessation of drinking.[4] Tremulousness

Aminoff's Neurology and General Medicine, Fifth Edition.

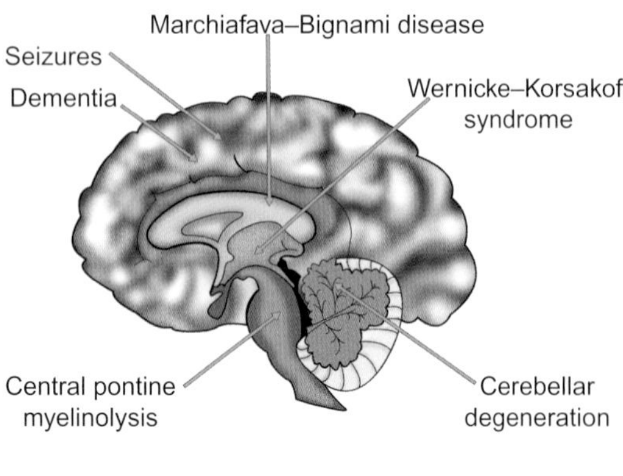

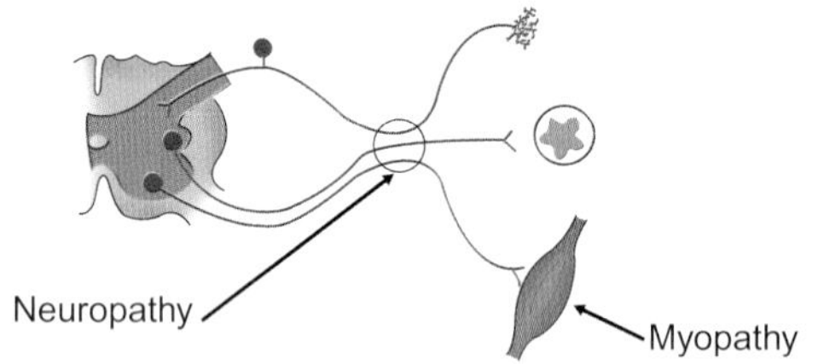

FIGURE 33-1 ■ Alcohol-related disorders affecting different levels of the neuraxis.

is the most common early symptom, becoming most marked 24 to 36 hours after the last drink. The tremor is generalized, resembles an accentuated physiologic tremor, and is accompanied by signs of autonomic hyperactivity such as increased arousal, tachycardia, flushing, and hyperreflexia. These signs are associated with elevated blood and urinary catecholamine levels and increased levels of catecholamine metabolites in the cerebrospinal fluid (CSF).[5,6]

Withdrawal Seizures

Seizures may occur shortly after chronic ethanol intake is discontinued.[7] Alcohol withdrawal seizures are usually associated with a history of daily alcohol consumption, but briefer drinking sprees may also culminate in seizures following cessation. Generalized tonic-clonic seizures are most common; focal seizures suggest an etiology other than alcohol withdrawal, although alcohol can lower the seizure threshold in a patient otherwise predisposed to focal seizures. The majority of seizures occur 6 to 48 hours after cessation of drinking. Approximately 60 percent of patients have more than one seizure, but usually less than four, over a period of less than 12 hours.[3] Among patients undergoing withdrawal, status epilepticus is unusual, but among patients with status epilepticus, alcohol withdrawal is responsible in approximately 9 to 25 percent.[7]

In patients with repeated seizures, benzodiazepines (e.g., diazepam, chlordiazepoxide, and lorazepam) prevent seizure recurrence, but the evidence is not adequate to support the use of non-benzodiazepine anticonvulsants.[8–11] Status epilepticus that is suspected to be due to alcohol withdrawal is a medical emergency and should be treated with anticonvulsants in the same fashion as status epilepticus due to any other etiology, beginning with doses of benzodiazepines. It is important to recognize that alcoholics are at risk of a variety of other treatable conditions that may cause status epilepticus, including occult head trauma, meningitis, hypoglycemia, hyponatremia, and other drug ingestions.

Delirium Tremens

Approximately 20 percent of patients become delirious 2 to 5 days after ethanol withdrawal, and in up to one-half of these patients the syndrome of delirium tremens may develop, with marked confusion, hallucinations, tremor, hyperpyrexia, and sympathetic hyperactivity.[12] The risk of development of delirium tremens is higher in alcoholics with heavy daily alcohol intake, prior alcohol withdrawal seizures or delirium, decreased serum chloride and potassium concentrations, elevated serum levels of alanine aminotransferase and γ-glutamyltransferase, and findings of tachycardia (≥100 bpm), ataxia, and polyneuropathy on admission.[12–14] The major threat to life is from associated illnesses or injuries, hyperthermia, dehydration, and hypotension. Although initial studies reported mortality rates as high as 15 percent, rates with current treatment have declined to 1 percent or less.[12] A variety of sedatives, anticonvulsants, sympatholytics, and neuroleptics have been administered to patients with alcohol-withdrawal delirium, usually in uncontrolled trials.[8,12] Several double-blind studies have suggested that benzodiazepines are effective in controlling the symptoms of alcohol withdrawal.[10,13,14] Benzodiazepines and barbiturates are better than neuroleptics in reducing mortality from the delirium associated with alcohol withdrawal and should be used preferentially.[12]

The dose of medication required to control alcohol-withdrawal symptoms can vary greatly among different patients and over time in the same patient.

A typical regimen is to administer 5 to 10 mg of diazepam intravenously every 5 to 10 minutes until the patient is lightly somnolent, followed by 5 to 20 mg every few hours as needed to control delirium and agitation.[12] Shorter-acting benzodiazepines such as oxazepam or lorazepam may be safer in patients with liver disease.[15] Patients refractory to benzodiazepines may respond to addition of a different class of sedative-hypnotic (e.g., barbituates or propofol). Neuroleptics, such as haloperidol, are reserved for severe agitation as adjunctive therapy. Fluid and electrolyte abnormalities can be severe and require prompt therapy. Dehydration accompanying delirium tremens may require replacement of up to 4 to 10 liters of fluid during the first 24 hours. Hypomagnesemia is common and should be treated with magnesium sulfate (e.g., 1 g intravenously every 6 hours during the first day in patients with adequate renal function). Potassium should be included in intravenous solutions because hypokalemia may be exacerbated by glucose administration, leading to cardiac arrhythmias.

DISORDERS OF COGNITION

More than 10 percent of patients with alcohol use disorders develop cognitive dysfunction.[16] The pathogenic mechanisms are often multiple and include the neurotoxic effects of ethanol, nutritional deficiencies, and electrolyte disturbances. Several alcohol-related clinical syndromes with cognitive dysfunction as the predominant feature are described in this section.

Alcoholic Dementia

Alcohol-induced dementia is a recognized form of substance-induced dementia.[17] It presents in the context of chronic, excessive alcohol use and is characterized by progressive memory impairment along with aphasia, agnosia, apraxia, or impaired executive function that persists beyond periods of intoxication or withdrawal and cannot be attributed to other causes. Heavy alcohol use can result in brain atrophy with neuronal loss in the frontal cortex, hypothalamus, and cerebellum; a reduction in the size of cell bodies and dendritic arbors in layer III pyramidal neurons of the superior frontal gyrus and motor cortices; and white matter loss, particularly in the hippocampus, corpus callosum, and cerebellum.[16,18] With several years of abstinence, cognitive function can improve.

Brain imaging studies have shown widespread volume loss affecting cortical gray and white matter.[19–23] In addition, magnetic resonance imaging (MRI) studies show signal abnormalities in several subcortical structures, including the corpus callosum, pons, cerebellar hemispheres, and vermis.[21] These regions are less affected in patients with uncomplicated alcoholism free of alcohol-associated electrolyte and nutritional disturbances.[21] White matter abnormalities may be observed with greater sensitivity and detail using diffusion tensor imaging.[19] These imaging and neuropsychiatric abnormalities are partly reversible during abstinence.[21] Volume loss and recovery during abstinence may reflect changes in brain water, but longitudinal studies using MR spectroscopy have shown increases in *N*-acetyl aspartate and phospholipids in certain brain regions, suggesting actual recovery of neurons and white matter during abstinence.[24,25]

Pellagra

Endemic pellagra, which results from deficiency of nicotinic acid (niacin) or its amino acid precursor tryptophan, is uncommon in developed countries because of fortification of processed foods with niacin (vitamin B_3). However, alcoholic pellagra is an underappreciated cause of confusion and delirium in malnourished alcoholics.[26,27] Neuropathologic changes are most prominent in neurons of the pons and deep cerebellar nuclei, though neurons elsewhere are also involved. Affected neurons show chromatolysis, appearing swollen and rounded, with eccentric nuclei and loss of Nissl substance. Systemic manifestations of pellagra include diarrhea, glossitis, anemia, and erythematous cutaneous lesions that appear in sun-exposed areas. Although pellagra was named for the characteristic skin lesions, they are not always present. Early mental symptoms of irritability, depression, fatigue, insomnia, and inability to concentrate are nonspecific and suggest a psychiatric disorder. However, the later development of confusion, hallucinosis, or paranoid ideation confirms the presence of an encephalopathy, and is usually accompanied by spastic weakness and extensor plantar responses. Tremor, rigidity, polyneuropathy, optic neuritis, and deafness may also be present. Pellagra responds readily to administration of niacin, although cerebral symptoms may not be completely reversible. Further details are given in Chapter 15.

Marchiafava–Bignami Disease

Marchiafava–Bignami disease is a rare disorder characterized by destruction of myelin mainly in the corpus callosum and anterior commissure.[28,29] Exceptionally, lesions extend laterally to involve the centrum semiovale, and in some instances the middle cerebellar peduncles are demyelinated. Neurons in layer III of the cerebral cortex may be replaced by gliosis, possibly owing to disruption of involved callosal fibers. The disease is usually diagnosed postmortem because the clinical signs are nonspecific, although MRI has made diagnosis more feasible during life. Most patients are alcoholics of long standing and many have associated malnutrition or liver disease, although the disease has appeared in a few nondrinkers. The etiology is not known.

Patients may present acutely with seizures and coma often accompanied by signs of upper motor neuron dysfunction, or alternatively they may follow a subacute course with gait disturbance, dysarthria, hyperreflexia, cognitive impairment, neuropsychiatric symptoms, and signs of interhemispheric disconnection. Brain MRI demonstrates T2-hyperintense swelling of the corpus callosum, followed later in the course by callosal atrophy along with cortical and subcortical atrophy. T1-weighted images may show hypointense necrotic lesions of the corpus callosum. Motor deficits, such as pyramidal tract signs and gait disturbances, tend to recover with abstinence from alcohol and improved nutrition, but many patients show residual cognitive impairment and a disconnection syndrome. Patients who develop coma carry the greatest risk of serious disability or death, whereas those with little impairment in consciousness may recover with only mild disability.

Hepatocerebral Disorders

Severe alcoholism can cause hepatic cirrhosis with portocaval shunting and hepatic insufficiency, leading to serious secondary neurologic disorders. In its mildest, covert form, hepatic encephalopathy presents with a normal neurologic examination and deficits apparent only on psychometric testing, termed "minimal hepatic encephalopathy."[30] Overt hepatic encephalopathy presents as a confusional state with deficits in awareness, attention, and calculation ability or, in severe cases, somnolence, stupor, and coma. The pathogenesis and treatment of hepatic encephalopathy are discussed in Chapter 12.

Acquired (non-Wilsonian) hepatocerebral degeneration is a less common disorder that can accompany advanced liver disease and is characterized by parkinsonism, ataxia and, in some patients, dystonia, chorea, and orobuccolingual dyskinesia.[31] Cognitive dysfunction is common but is not always present. Occasional patients show signs of a myelopathy with corticospinal tract signs. Acquired hepatocerebral degeneration begins insidiously after many weeks or years of hepatic dysfunction and is usually progressive, with episodes of stability or spontaneous remissions and relapses. It is characterized by neuropathologic lesions that resemble those found in Wilson disease with diffuse, patchy necrosis and microcavitation at the junction of cerebral gray and white matter, and a loss of neurons and myelinated fibers in the basal ganglia and cerebellum. Protoplasmic type II (Alzheimer) astrocytes are increased in number, and Opalski cells may be present.

Acquired hepatocerebral degeneration is thought to result from central nervous system exposure to neurotoxic substances present in the portal circulation, such as ammonia, aromatic amino acids, and metals.[31,32] A role for manganese in particular is supported by elevated serum and CSF manganese levels and by pallidal hyperintensities on T1-weighted MRI images of patients with severe liver disease, reminiscent of findings in occupational manganese toxicity. Dopaminergic drugs may reduce parkinsonian symptoms, although less effectively than in patients with Parkinson disease. Death usually occurs as a complication of advanced liver disease or intercurrent infection.

WERNICKE ENCEPHALOPATHY

Wernicke encephalopathy is an acute disorder manifested by nystagmus, ophthalmoplegia, gait ataxia, and an acute confusional state.[33] Neuropathologic findings include neuronal loss, demyelination, glial and vascular proliferation, hemorrhage, and necrosis, particularly affecting the anterior and mediodorsal thalamus, mammillary bodies, basal forebrain, raphe nuclei, and cerebellar vermis.[34] An underlying disorder that predisposes to malnutrition appears to be common to all cases. Alcoholism is the most frequent predisposing factor, but persistent vomiting due to a variety of causes, starvation, and malignancy or other chronic systemic diseases, and other causes of malabsorption have also been implicated. A detailed account of its clinical features is provided in Chapter 13.

The link between malnutrition and Wernicke encephalopathy is a deficiency of vitamin B_1 (thiamine). With chronic alcoholism, decreased dietary intake of thiamine may be compounded by alcohol-induced defects in intestinal absorption, metabolism, and hepatic storage of thiamine. However, the manner in which thiamine depletion produces neurologic dysfunction is unknown. Thiamine pyrophosphate is a required cofactor for at least four enzymes involved in intermediary metabolism: pyruvate dehydrogenase, α-ketoglutarate dehydrogenase, transketolase, and branched-chain α-ketoacid dehydrogenase. Variant forms of transketolase and thiamine transport genes could provide a basis for the preferential vulnerability of certain alcoholic patients to develop Wernicke encephalopathy.[35–37]

The diagnosis of Wernicke encephalopathy has historically been made by the presence of the clinical triad of ophthalmoplegia, ataxia, and confusion. In patients who present with this triad, the differential diagnosis includes sedative drug intoxication and structural lesions of the posterior fossa. In the absence of overt ocular signs in patients with confusion or ataxia, the differential diagnosis includes ethanol intoxication and encephalopathy due to other causes such as hepatic insufficiency or infection.

Over the past 20 years, careful neuropathologic studies have raised concern that reliance on this classic clinical triad has led to underdiagnosis, resulting in establishment of modified diagnostic criteria that have been validated at autopsy.[38] These criteria require two of the following four signs to be present for diagnosis: dietary deficiency, oculomotor abnormalities, cerebellar dysfunction, and either an altered mental state or memory impairment. Application of these criteria leads to nearly 100 percent diagnostic specificity, while greatly improving sensitivity to 85 percent from only 22 percent using the classic clinical triad.[38]

In addition to modified clinical criteria, the advent of MRI and sensitive measures for serum thiamine have also served to improve diagnostic accuracy.[39] The most characteristic MRI findings are of cytotoxic and vasogenic edema involving the thalamus, hypothalamus, and brainstem, appearing as symmetric signal intensities on T2-weighted images of medial thalamic nuclei, periventricular gray matter, midbrain tectum, and the mammillary bodies.[40,41] Less common are symmetric alterations in the cerebellum, dentate nuclei, cranial nerve nuclei, caudate, splenium of the corpus callosum, and cerebral cortex.

Treatment of Wernicke encephalopathy is by repletion of thiamine. Patients should be hospitalized and receive 200 mg of thiamine intravenously three times daily for several days until there is no further improvement in signs and symptoms.[42] It is important that thiamine replacement is started prior to administering glucose, to avoid worsening the encephalopathy. Improvement with therapy is considered evidence of correct diagnosis. Acute, reversible MRI abnormalities have also been described, and may be helpful in confirming the diagnosis in mild cases or those with atypical clinical features.[43,44] Detection of a low blood thiamine level may also be useful; current guidelines recommend that total blood thiamine levels be sent at first diagnosis, immediately before beginning thiamine replacement.[42]

The prognosis of Wernicke encephalopathy depends on the prompt institution of appropriate treatment. The overall mortality rate is 10 to 20 percent. After the institution of treatment, ocular and gaze palsies begin to improve within hours to days, and nystagmus, gait ataxia, and confusion within days to weeks. Long-term sequelae include residual nystagmus or gait ataxia in approximately 60 percent of patients and a chronic memory disorder (Korsakoff amnestic syndrome) in more than 80 percent.

KORSAKOFF SYNDROME

Korsakoff syndrome is a selective disorder of memory that typically arises in chronic alcoholics in the wake of one or more episodes of Wernicke encephalopathy. The distribution of histopathologic lesions is identical to that seen in Wernicke encephalopathy.[34] The main additional behavioral deficits in Korsakoff syndrome are impairment of anterograde episodic memory, with semantic and retrograde memory affected to a lesser extent; in many patients there is also evidence of frontal lobe dysfunction.[45] Both encoding and retrieval of memories are affected. Episodic memory processing requires a network of limbic structures, many of which are damaged in Korsakoff syndrome. Biochemical studies have provided evidence of oxidative stress, glutamate-mediated excitotoxicity, and inflammation in vulnerable brain regions as major mechanisms for brain damage due to thiamine deficiency.[46]

Although a causal relationship between (acute) Wernicke encephalopathy due to thiamine deficiency and (chronic) Korsakoff syndrome is generally assumed, this issue is not completely resolved.[47] Korsakoff syndrome was rarely a consequence of Wernicke encephalopathy in malnourished prisoners of war in the Pacific theater during World War II. A review of cases of nonalcoholic Wernicke encephalopathy found that patients who developed subsequent amnestic syndromes showed a substantial improvement in memory over time compared to alcoholics with Wernicke encephalopathy.[47] This difference in recovery may be due to the duration of malnutrition being briefer in nonalcoholics than is usually the case in chronic alcoholics or alternatively because alcohol itself contributes to development of the syndrome. The latter possibility is supported by the finding that alcoholics who develop Wernicke encephalopathy after a period of vomiting perform better on tests of memory than those without vomiting, possibly because emesis helps to clear alcohol from the body.[48]

The disability afflicting patients with Korsakoff syndrome is one of the most striking in clinical neurology. There is an inability to incorporate new memories (anterograde amnesia) and impaired retrieval of previously established, especially recent, memories (retrograde amnesia). Immediate recall is intact. Patients are typically disoriented to time and place, and hospitalized patients are characteristically unaware of their room numbers or hospital floor, how long they have been in the hospital, what they had for their last meal, or who visited them. At the same time, very distant memories may be preserved in detail; some patients appear to be stuck in time, insisting that the year is one from decades past. Patients with Korsakoff syndrome appear to be unaware of their deficit and commonly attempt to reassure the examiner that nothing is seriously wrong. Confabulation, the invention of material to fill in gaps in memory, is often but not invariably seen. Other aspects of cognitive function may exhibit subtle impairment, but alertness and language are intact.

Patients with Korsakoff syndrome may show evidence of other alcohol-related neurologic disorders. Nystagmus and gait ataxia related to past bouts of Wernicke disease are common, as are signs of a peripheral neuropathy.

Korsakoff syndrome is a clinical diagnosis. This relatively selective memory disorder must be distinguished from the more global cognitive impairment that occurs in dementia due to a variety of causes including alcoholism. The differential diagnosis of a chronic amnestic syndrome resembling Korsakoff syndrome includes pancerebral hypoxia or ischemia, bilateral posterior cerebral artery strokes, herpes simplex virus encephalitis, paraneoplastic limbic encephalitis, and brain tumors in the vicinity of the third ventricle.

Although acute Wernicke encephalopathy should always be treated with thiamine, the effectiveness of thiamine in preventing the subsequent development of the chronic amnestic syndrome is uncertain.[49] Similarly, thiamine has not been shown to be effective for the treatment of established Korsakoff syndrome, although patients with this disorder may improve spontaneously and likely warrant a trial of this treatment, which has few side effects.[47]

ALCOHOLIC CEREBELLAR DEGENERATION

In some alcoholic patients, a chronic cerebellar syndrome develops, sometimes as a long-term sequela of Wernicke encephalopathy. The neuropathologic features of alcoholic cerebellar degeneration include loss of cerebellar cortical neurons, especially Purkinje cells, with a particular predilection for the anterior and superior vermis; the anterior and superior cerebellar hemispheres are affected less often.[50] The distribution of this cerebellar pathologic process is strikingly similar to that seen in Wernicke encephalopathy, suggesting that the two disorders are linked pathophysiologically. Alcoholic cerebellar degeneration may also result from a direct toxic effect of alcohol on the cerebellum, or from a combination of thiamine deficiency and alcohol neurotoxicity.[51,52]

The natural history of alcoholic cerebellar degeneration is variable. The syndrome usually occurs in the setting of chronic alcoholism of 10 years' or more duration. The most frequent mode of onset is with ataxia that progresses steadily for weeks to months. A more gradually progressive disorder that evolves over years is also common. Less often, a mild and stable chronic deficit may suddenly worsen.

Although gait ataxia is the most prominent manifestation of both alcoholic cerebellar degeneration and Wernicke encephalopathy, the pattern of involvement in the two disorders may differ.[3,53] Limb ataxia, which is absent in most patients with Wernicke encephalopathy, is usually detectable in alcoholic cerebellar degeneration. Examination of such patients typically discloses severe ataxia of the legs, with milder involvement of the arms. Dysarthria, which is usually mild, is also more frequent in alcoholic cerebellar degeneration than Wernicke encephalopathy. In contrast, nystagmus is present less often than in Wernicke encephalopathy.

Patients with alcoholic cerebellar degeneration may also exhibit signs of a polyneuropathy (see later). Uncommon manifestations of alcoholic cerebellar degeneration include hypotonia, ocular dysmetria, and postural tremor.

Alcoholic cerebellar degeneration is a clinical diagnosis. Neuroimaging may show cerebellar cortical atrophy, but laboratory findings usually are helpful only for excluding other causes of ataxia. Other conditions that must be considered in the differential diagnosis of subacute or chronic cerebellar ataxia in middle life include multiple sclerosis, hypothyroidism, paraneoplastic cerebellar degeneration, idiopathic cerebellar or olivopontocerebellar degeneration, Creutzfeldt–Jakob disease, and posterior fossa tumors. Like alcoholic cerebellar degeneration, many of these disorders can produce ataxia that preferentially affects gait.

Ataxia due to alcoholic cerebellar degeneration often stabilizes or improves with cessation of drinking and improved nutritional status,[3] although the relative importance of each of these two factors is uncertain. Patients should receive parenteral thiamine, although it is not yet known whether thiamine improves outcome, as it clearly does in Wernicke encephalopathy.[51]

CENTRAL PONTINE MYELINOLYSIS

Central pontine myelinolysis is manifested by rapidly evolving paraparesis or quadriparesis, pseudobulbar palsy, and impaired consciousness and is further discussed in Chapter 17. A history of alcoholism is common and found in 39 percent of affected patients.[54] Recent liver transplantation accounts for 17 percent of cases and as many as 7 percent of patients with burns may develop the disorder. Less often, it develops after prolonged use of diuretics, psychogenic polydipsia, or pituitary or urologic surgery.[55]

Central pontine myelinolysis is mainly an iatrogenic disorder, and its appearance coincided with the widespread use of intravenous therapy for correction of fluid and electrolyte disorders.[54–56] Hyponatremia frequently precedes central pontine myelinolysis, and aggressive correction of hyponatremia appears to be the precipitating factor in most cases.[54,55,57] However, there are reports of central pontine myelinolysis in patients with hypernatremia or normal serum sodium levels, although a rise in serum osmolality may have been an important factor in such cases.[54,58,59]

The characteristic pathologic lesion in central pontine myelinolysis is bilaterally symmetric, focal destruction of myelin in the ventral pons.[54,55] Histologically, there is severe loss of myelin, and oligodendroglia are reduced in number. Neurons and axons are relatively spared, although axonal swelling and neuronal shrinkage may occur, particularly in the center of lesions. There is no inflammation, and blood vessels appear normal.

In approximately 50 percent of cases, characteristic lesions are present outside the basis pontis, and in half of these cases with extrapontine lesions, no pontine lesions are present. Extrapontine myelinolysis has been observed in the cerebellum, thalamus (especially the lateral geniculate body), external and extreme capsules, basal ganglia, deep layers of cerebral cortex and adjacent white matter, and rarely in the fornix, anterior commissure, subthalamic nucleus, amygdala, optic tract, and spinal cord.[54]

Coexistent illnesses often influence the clinical manifestations of central pontine myelinolysis, making it difficult to diagnose in some cases. Although some small lesions detected postmortem can be asymptomatic, certain clinical features are typical.[57] Central pontine myelinolysis often evolves over several days to weeks in a severely ill patient, and mental confusion is a prominent feature in almost all cases. Demyelination of pontine corticobulbar fibers leads to early dysarthria or mutism. Spastic quadriparesis and pseudobulbar palsy are common, occurring in more than 90 percent of patients. When lesions extend into the midbrain, medulla, or pontine tegmentum, there may be pupillary and oculomotor signs, depressed consciousness or coma, and dysfunction of cranial nerves. Progressive demyelination of corticospinal and corticobulbar tracts in the basis pontis may produce a locked-in syndrome. Extrapontine lesions may cause ataxia, parkinsonism, choreoathetosis, and dystonia.[55,57] Cognitive and behavioral symptoms include restlessness, emotional lability, apathy, agitation, insomnia, paranoia, delusions, rage, and disinhibition.[54]

The CSF is normal in up to 72 percent of patients.[56] Elevated CSF pressure, increased protein concentration, and a mononuclear pleocytosis occur in a few. Because MRI is more sensitive and allows better visualization of the brainstem, it is preferable to CT for detecting the characteristic lesions.[55] MRI scans may be normal during the first 2 weeks of illness, but eventually affected regions appear hyperintense on T2-weighted sequences and hypointense on corresponding T1-weighted sequences; they usually do not enhance with gadolinium.[57,60] Diffusion-weighted MRI may be more sensitive and show lesions within the first few days after onset of symptoms, prior to abnormalities developing on T2-weighted sequences.

Although the disorder has historically been considered to carry a poor prognosis, as many as 50 percent of patients show improvement after several weeks.[61,62] In general, outcome does not correlate with the severity of neurologic deficits during the acute phase of illness or with the degree of hyponatremia. Therefore, all patients with suspected central pontine myelinolysis should be supported aggressively, especially since substantial improvement may occur after several weeks to months.

Over the past 20 years there has developed a consensus on the treatment of hyponatremia to minimize the risk of myelinolysis. Severe hyponatremia (≤120 mEq/L), if it develops rapidly, can cause life-threatening symptoms such as coma and seizures, and demands prompt treatment. If hyponatremia occurs slowly, however, symptoms are generally less severe and include malaise, nausea, headache, lethargy, and confusion. In rats, the brain adapts to hyponatremia over the course of several days by losing electrolytes and other osmolytes, including phosphocreatinine, *myo*-inositol, and several amino acids, so that brain volumes return to normal within 2 to 3 weeks.[58,63] Once the brain adapts, it is vulnerable to osmotic stress that occurs with rapid correction of the hyponatremia.[64] The general consensus is to increase the serum sodium level by no more than 12 meq/L in 24 hours in patients with chronic hyponatremia.[65]

ALCOHOLIC NEUROPATHY

Neuropathy is the most frequently encountered chronic neurologic disorder related to alcohol abuse. Both nutritional deficiency and a direct, toxic, dose-dependent effect of alcohol have been invoked as etiologies.[66,67] Support for a toxic effect of ethanol comes from studies in rats demonstrating hyperalgesia following several weeks of ethanol ingestion.[68,69] Axonal degeneration appears to be the principal pathogenic process. Segmental demyelination also occurs and may be secondary to the primary axonal disorder or a consequence of concomitant nutritional deficiency.

Alcoholic neuropathy usually presents after several years of alcohol abuse as a distal, symmetric, sensorimotor polyneuropathy that is gradual in onset. Symptoms include weakness, pain, paresthesias, muscle cramps, numbness, gait ataxia, and burning dysesthesias. Neurologic examination may reveal any combination of reflex, sensory, and motor abnormalities, with predominant involvement of the legs. Absent or decreased muscle stretch reflexes and impaired vibration sense in the lower extremities are virtually universal findings. Defective appreciation of light touch and weakness are also seen in most patients. Pain and temperature sensation are affected less often, and symptomatic autonomic dysfunction and cranial nerve involvement are comparatively rare. In addition to the neurologic abnormalities, affected limbs may exhibit edema, hyperpigmentation or ulceration of the skin, along with bony deformities.

Nerve conduction studies are useful for documenting the presence of neuropathy and for demonstrating the predominantly axonal pathologic process. Laboratory studies on blood and CSF can exclude other causes of polyneuropathy including diabetes, chronic inflammatory demyelinating polyneuropathy, uremia, dysproteinemia, and vasculitis.

Vitamin supplementation (especially thiamine) and abstinence from alcohol can often arrest the progression of alcoholic polyneuropathy and in some cases lead to clinical improvement. Neuropathic pain may respond to anticonvulsants or tricyclic antidepressants.

Rarely, alcoholic neuropathy develops acutely over several days with severe weakness, absent tendon reflexes, and multimodal sensory loss in the limbs.[70] This condition can be distinguished from acute inflammatory demyelinating neuropathy

(Guillain–Barré syndrome) by the absence of bulbar and respiratory muscle weakness, normal or only mild elevations in CSF concentration, and electrophysiologic and pathologic findings of primarily axonal damage. With abstinence from alcohol, most patients regain their ability to walk after several months.

ALCOHOLIC MYOPATHY

Chronic alcoholism has adverse effects on both skeletal and cardiac muscle.[71–73] Both acute and chronic clinical presentations of alcoholic myopathy are recognized.

Acute Necrotizing Myopathy

An acute, necrotizing myopathy may develop over the course of 1 to 2 days in the setting of heavy binge drinking, and affects up to 2 percent of heavy drinkers. Symptoms include muscle pain and weakness, which, although classically symmetric and proximal in distribution, may be asymmetric or focal in nature. Neurologic examination shows tender, swollen muscles in the affected areas. Weakness is a prominent finding and may be associated with dysphagia. Signs of congestive heart failure are sometimes present.

Laboratory abnormalities include moderate to severe elevation of serum creatine kinase levels and in some cases myoglobinuria. The electrocardiogram may reveal arrhythmias or conduction defects. Electromyography discloses myopathic changes in configuration and recruitment of motor unit potentials, as well as fibrillation potentials. The muscle biopsy shows necrosis of muscle fibers.

Acute alcoholic myopathy must be distinguished from other causes of acute weakness in alcoholic patients, such as hypokalemia and hypophosphatemia. In hypokalemia, weakness is not accompanied by muscle pain, and myoglobinuria does not occur. Hypophosphatemia closely reproduces the clinical features of acute alcoholic myopathy and may also contribute to its pathogenesis.[74] Consequently, serum potassium and phosphorus concentrations should always be measured in acutely weak alcoholic patients.

Complications of acute alcoholic myopathy, such as cardiac disturbances and renal compromise due to myoglobinuria, should be treated urgently. Electrolyte abnormalities should be monitored carefully and corrected if necessary. Muscle pain and tenderness may improve with analgesics. With abstinence, recovery within weeks to months is the rule, but some patients exhibit residual weakness and long-standing cardiac conduction abnormalities.

Chronic Myopathy

The much more common form of alcoholic myopathy is a chronic condition which develops insidiously over weeks to months, and is seen in 40 to 60 percent of patients, typically those with a history of more than 10 years of heavy alcohol use.[72,73] In animal and cell-culture studies, alcohol reversibly inhibits initiation of translation and protein synthesis in skeletal muscle.[71] In addition, disruption of carbohydrate and energy metabolism, oxidative stress, and apoptosis appear to contribute to myopathy.[73] Chronic alcoholic myopathy is characterized by proximal weakness involving pelvic and shoulder girdles, with relative preservation of muscle stretch reflexes. In contrast to acute necrotizing alcoholic myopathy, muscle pain is uncommon or mild. Patients often show signs of other ethanol-induced end-organ damage such as cirrhosis or cardiomyopathy. Serum creatine kinase levels are elevated three- to sixfold in 40 percent of patients. When the clinical diagnosis is uncertain, chronic alcoholic myopathy can be distinguished from polyneuropathy by electrodiagnostic studies or by muscle biopsy, which shows atrophy mainly of type II muscle fibers and myocyte necrosis without inflammation.[73] The chronic form of myopathy is related to lifetime alcohol dose and may improve with abstinence or decreased drinking.[73]

ALCOHOL AND STROKE

Epidemiologic studies suggest that alcohol consumption influences the risk of stroke.[75,76] For intracerebral and subarachnoid hemorrhage, the risk increases linearly with increasing daily alcohol intake. Possible explanations for this association include alcohol-induced disorders of coagulation or fibrinolysis, thrombocytopenia or impaired platelet function, and acute or chronic hypertension.

In contrast, the relationship between daily alcohol intake and ischemic stroke is J-shaped. Thus, moderate drinking—two or fewer drinks per day—appears to reduce ischemic stroke risk compared with that observed in nondrinkers, whereas less temperate drinking patterns predispose to ischemic stroke. The protective effect of small amounts of alcohol has been attributed to elevated levels of prostacyclin, decreased platelet activation, enhanced fibrinolysis, increased levels of high-density lipoprotein cholesterol, and activation of signaling mechanisms involved in ischemic preconditioning.[77] In some studies, the protective effect is more significant for red wine, possibly due to phenolic components of wine that promote vasodilation, impair plaque formation, and have antioxidant activity; other studies have suggested the effect is independent of the type of alcohol consumed.[78] Mechanisms that could be responsible for an increased risk of ischemic stroke in heavy drinkers include alcohol-related cardiomyopathy or arrhythmias, alcohol-induced hypertension, the increased incidence of cigarette smoking in heavy drinkers, rebound thrombocytosis occurring with alcohol withdrawal, and hypercoagulable states.[75,76]

ACKNOWLEDGMENTS

The author's work is supported by grants AA013588, AA017072, and AA018316 from the US Public Health Service.

REFERENCES

1. Vonghia L, Leggio L, Ferrulli A, et al: Acute alcohol intoxication. Eur J Intern Med 19:561, 2008.
2. Kalant H: Current state of knowledge about the mechanisms of alcohol tolerance. Addict Biol 1:133, 1996.
3. Messing RO: Alcohol and the nervous system. p. 721. In Aminoff MJ (ed): Neurology and General Medicine. 4th Ed. Churchill Livingstone Elsevier, Philadelphia, 2008.
4. Hall W, Zador D: The alcohol withdrawal syndrome. Lancet 349:1897, 1997.
5. Hawley RJ, Nemeroff CB, Bissette G, et al: Neurochemical correlates of sympathetic activation during severe alcohol withdrawal. Alcohol Clin Exp Res 18:1312, 1994.
6. Patkar AA, Gopalakrishnan R, Naik PC, et al: Changes in plasma noradrenaline and serotonin levels and craving during alcohol withdrawal. Alcohol Alcohol 38:224, 2003.
7. Hillbom M, Pieninkeroinen I, Leone M: Seizures in alcohol-dependent patients: epidemiology, pathophysiology and management. CNS Drugs 17:1013, 2003.
8. Mayo-Smith MF: Pharmacological management of alcohol withdrawal. A meta-analysis and evidence-based practice guideline. American Society of Addiction Medicine Working Group on Pharmacological Management of Alcohol Withdrawal. JAMA 278:144, 1997.
9. Amato L, Minozzi S, Davoli M: Efficacy and safety of pharmacological interventions for the treatment of the Alcohol Withdrawal Syndrome. Cochrane Database Syst Rev CD008537, 2011.
10. Muzyk AJ, Leung JG, Nelson S, et al: The role of diazepam loading for the treatment of alcohol withdrawal syndrome in hospitalized patients. Am J Addict 22:113, 2013.
11. Rathlev NK, Ulrich A, Shieh TC, et al: Etiology and weekly occurrence of alcohol-related seizures. Acad Emerg Med 9:824, 2002.
12. Mayo-Smith MF, Beecher LH, Fischer TL, et al: Management of alcohol withdrawal delirium. An evidence-based practice guideline. Arch Intern Med 164:1405, 2004.
13. Wetterling T, Kanitz RD, Veltrup C, et al: Clinical predictors of alcohol withdrawal delirium. Alcohol Clin Exp Res 18:1100, 1994.
14. Lee JH, Jang MK, Lee JY, et al: Clinical predictors for delirium tremens in alcohol dependence. J Gastroenterol Hepatol 20:1833, 2005.
15. Peppers MP: Benzodiazepines for alcohol withdrawal in the elderly and in patients with liver disease. Pharmacotherapy 16:49, 1996.
16. Vetreno RP, Hall JM, Savage LM: Alcohol-related amnesia and dementia: animal models have revealed the contributions of different etiological factors on neuropathology, neurochemical dysfunction and cognitive impairment. Neurobiol Learn Mem 96:596, 2011.
17. American Psychiatric Association Diagnostic and Statistical Manual of Mental Disorders. Version IV-TR. American Psychiatric Association, Washington DC, 2000.
18. Harper CG, Kril JJ: Neuropathology of alcoholism. Alcohol Alcohol 25:207, 1990.
19. Pfefferbaum A, Adalsteinsson E, Sullivan EV: Supratentorial profile of white matter microstructural integrity in recovering alcoholic men and women. Biol Psychiatry 59:364, 2006.
20. Pfefferbaum A, Lim KO, Zipursky RB, et al: Brain gray and white matter volume loss accelerates with aging in chronic alcoholics: a quantitative MRI study. Alcohol Clin Exp Res 16:1078, 1992.
21. Sullivan EV, Pfefferbaum A: Neurocircuitry in alcoholism: a substrate of disruption and repair. Psychopharmacology (Berl) 180:583, 2005.
22. Jernigan TL, Butters N, DiTraglia G, et al: Reduced cerebral grey matter observed in alcoholics using magnetic resonance imaging. Alcohol Clin Exp Res 15:418, 1991.
23. Fein G, Di Sclafani V, Cardenas VA, et al: Cortical gray matter loss in treatment-naive alcohol dependent individuals. Alcohol Clin Exp Res 26:558, 2002.

24. Estilaei MR, Matson GB, Payne GS, et al: Effects of abstinence from alcohol on the broad phospholipid signal in human brain: an in vivo ^{31}P magnetic resonance spectroscopy study. Alcohol Clin Exp Res 25:1213, 2001.
25. Parks MH, Dawant BM, Riddle WR, et al: Longitudinal brain metabolic characterization of chronic alcoholics with proton magnetic resonance spectroscopy. Alcohol Clin Exp Res 26:1368, 2002.
26. Oldham MA, Ivkovic A: Pellagrous encephalopathy presenting as alcohol withdrawal delirium: a case series and literature review. Addict Sci Clin Pract 7:12, 2012.
27. Cook CC, Hallwood PM, Thomson AD: B vitamin deficiency and neuropsychiatric syndromes in alcohol misuse. Alcohol Alcohol 33:317, 1998.
28. Kohler CG, Ances BM, Coleman AR, et al: Marchiafava-Bignami disease: literature review and case report. Neuropsychiatry Neuropsych Behav Neurol 13:67, 2000.
29. Heinrich A, Runge U, Khaw AV: Clinicoradiologic subtypes of Marchiafava-Bignami disease. J Neurol 251:1050, 2004.
30. Atluri DK, Prakash R, Mullen KD: Pathogenesis, diagnosis, and treatment of hepatic encephalopathy. J Clin Exp Hepatol 1:77, 2011.
31. Ferrara J, Jankovic J: Acquired hepatocerebral degeneration. J Neurol 256:320, 2009.
32. Butterworth RF: Metal toxicity, liver disease and neurodegeneration. Neurotox Res 18:100, 2010.
33. Thomson AD, Marshall EJ: The natural history and pathophysiology of Wernicke's encephalopathy and Korsakoff's psychosis. Alcohol Alcohol 41:151, 2006.
34. Harper C: The neuropathology of alcohol-specific brain damage, or does alcohol damage the brain? J Neuropathol Exp Neurol 57:101, 1998.
35. Heap LC, Pratt OE, Ward RJ, et al: Individual susceptibility to Wernicke-Korsakoff syndrome and alcoholism-induced cognitive deficit: impaired thiamine utilization found in alcoholics and alcohol abusers. Psychiatr Genet 12:217, 2002.
36. Martin PR, McCool BA, Singleton CK: Molecular genetics of transketolase in the pathogenesis of the Wernicke-Korsakoff syndrome. Metab Brain Dis 10:45, 1995.
37. Guerrini I, Thomson AD, Gurling HM: Molecular genetics of alcohol-related brain damage. Alcohol Alcohol 44:166, 2009.
38. Caine D, Halliday GM, Kril JJ, et al: Operational criteria for the classification of chronic alcoholics: identification of Wernicke's encephalopathy. J Neurol Neurosurg Psychiatry 62:51, 1997.
39. Lough ME: Wernicke's encephalopathy: expanding the diagnostic toolbox. Neuropsychol Rev 22:181, 2012.
40. Zuccoli G, Pipitone N: Neuroimaging findings in acute Wernicke's encephalopathy: review of the literature. AJR Am J Roentgenol 192:501, 2009.
41. Jung YC, Chanraud S, Sullivan EV: Neuroimaging of Wernicke's encephalopathy and Korsakoff's syndrome. Neuropsychol Rev 22:170, 2012.
42. Galvin R, Brathen G, Ivashynka A, et al: EFNS guidelines for diagnosis, therapy and prevention of Wernicke encephalopathy. Eur J Neurol 17:1408, 2010.
43. Gallucci M, Bozzao A, Splendiani A, et al: Wernicke encephalopathy: MR findings in five patients. AJNR Am J Neuroradiol 11:887, 1990.
44. Donnal JF, Heinz ER, Burger PC: MR of reversible thalamic lesions in Wernicke syndrome. AJNR Am J Neuroradiol 11:893, 1990.
45. Fama R, Pitel AL, Sullivan EV: Anterograde episodic memory in Korsakoff syndrome. Neuropsychol Rev 22:93, 2012.
46. Hazell AS, Butterworth RF: Update of cell damage mechanisms in thiamine deficiency: focus on oxidative stress, excitotoxicity and inflammation. Alcohol Alcohol 44:141, 2009.
47. Homewood J, Bond NW: Thiamin deficiency and Korsakoff's syndrome: failure to find memory impairments following nonalcoholic Wernicke's encephalopathy. Alcohol 19:75, 1999.
48. Price J, Hicks M, Williams G: A feature of alcoholic Wernicke's encephalopathy favourable to the maintenance of memory function: vomiting. Alcohol Alcohol 28:339, 1993.
49. Day E, Bentham P, Callaghan R, et al: Thiamine for Wernicke-Korsakoff syndrome in people at risk from alcohol abuse. Cochrane Database Syst Rev CD004033, 2004.
50. Kril JJ: Neuropathology of thiamine deficiency disorders. Metab Brain Dis 11:9, 1996.
51. Jaatinen P, Rintala J: Mechanisms of ethanol-induced degeneration in the developing, mature, and aging cerebellum. Cerebellum 7:332, 2008.
52. Mulholland PJ, Self RL, Stepanyan TD, et al: Thiamine deficiency in the pathogenesis of chronic ethanol-associated cerebellar damage in vitro. Neuroscience 135:1129, 2005.
53. Fitzpatrick LE, Jackson M, Crowe SF: Characterization of cerebellar ataxia in chronic alcoholics using the International Cooperative Ataxia Rating Scale (ICARS). Alcohol Clin Exp Res 36:1942, 2012.
54. Kleinschmidt-Demasters BK, Rojiani AM, Filley CM: Central and extrapontine myelinolysis: then...and now. J Neuropathol Exp Neurol 65:1, 2006.
55. Martin RJ: Central pontine and extrapontine myelinolysis: the osmotic demyelination syndromes. J Neurol Neurosurg Psychiatry 75(suppl 3):iii22, 2004.
56. Fishman RA: Cerebrospinal Fluid in Diseases of the Nervous System. WB Saunders, Philadelphia, 1992.
57. Laureno R, Karp BI: Myelinolysis after correction of hyponatremia. Ann Intern Med 126:57, 1997.
58. Norenberg MD: Central pontine myelinolysis: historical and mechanistic considerations. Metab Brain Dis 25:97, 2010.

59. Levin J, Hogen T, Patzig M, et al: Pontine and extrapontine myolinolysis associated with hypernatraemia. Clin Neurol Neurosurg 114:1290, 2012.
60. Hurley RA, Filley CM, Taber KH: Central pontine myelinolysis: a metabolic disorder of myelin. J Neuropsychiatry Clin Neurosci 23:369, 2011.
61. Menger H, Jörg J: Outcome of central pontine and extrapontine myelinolysis (n = 44). J Neurol 246:700, 1999.
62. Louis G, Megarbane B, Lavoue S, et al: Long-term outcome of patients hospitalized in intensive care units with central or extrapontine myelinolysis. Crit Care Med 40:970, 2012.
63. Sterns RH, Baer J, Ebersol S, et al: Organic osmolytes in acute hyponatremia. Am J Physiol 264:F833, 1993.
64. Verbalis JG, Martinez AJ: Neurological and neuropathological sequelae of correction of chronic hyponatremia. Kidney Int 39:1274, 1991.
65. Lien YH, Shapiro JI: Hyponatremia: clinical diagnosis and management. Am J Med 120:653, 2007.
66. Koike H, Sobue G: Alcoholic neuropathy. Curr Opin Neurol 19:481, 2006.
67. Mellion M, Gilchrist JM, de la Monte S: Alcohol-related peripheral neuropathy: nutritional, toxic, or both? Muscle Nerve 43:309, 2011.
68. Dina OA, Barletta J, Chen X, et al: Key role for the epsilon isoform of protein kinase C in painful alcoholic neuropathy in the rat. J Neurosci 20:8614, 2000.
69. Dina OA, Khasar SG, Alessandri-Haber N, et al: Alcohol-induced stress in painful alcoholic neuropathy. Eur J Neurosci 27:83, 2008.
70. Wohrle JC, Spengos K, Steinke W, et al: Alcohol-related acute axonal polyneuropathy: a differential diagnosis of Guillain-Barre syndrome. Arch Neurol 55:1329, 1998.
71. Lang CH, Frost RA, Summer AD, et al: Molecular mechanisms responsible for alcohol-induced myopathy in skeletal muscle and heart. Int J Biochem Cell Biol 37:2180, 2005.
72. Preedy VR, Ohlendieck K, Adachi J, et al: The importance of alcohol-induced muscle disease. J Muscle Res Cell Motil 24:55, 2003.
73. Urbano-Marquez A, Fernandez-Sola J: Effects of alcohol on skeletal and cardiac muscle. Muscle Nerve 30:689, 2004.
74. Felsenfeld AJ, Levine BS: Approach to treatment of hypophosphatemia. Am J Kidney Dis 60:655, 2012.
75. Reynolds K, Lewis B, Nolen JD, et al: Alcohol consumption and risk of stroke: a meta-analysis. JAMA 289:579, 2003.
76. Patra J, Taylor B, Irving H, et al: Alcohol consumption and the risk of morbidity and mortality for different stroke types–a systematic review and meta-analysis. BMC Public Health 10:258, 2010.
77. Krenz M, Korthuis RJ: Moderate ethanol ingestion and cardiovascular protection: from epidemiologic associations to cellular mechanisms. J Mol Cell Cardiol 52:93, 2012.
78. Szmitko PE, Verma S: Antiatherogenic potential of red wine: clinician update. Am J Physiol Heart Circ Physiol 288:H2023, 2005.

CHAPTER

34

Neurologic Complications of Recreational Drugs

S. ANDREW JOSEPHSON

Recreational drug use can lead to neurologic problems stemming from both acute intoxication and chronic use, and physicians must be aware of these complications when faced with any patient having a neurologic disorder. In the past decade, the landscape of drug use has shifted from primarily illicit substances manufactured with the sole purpose of recreational drug use, to an ever-increasingly common realization that many drugs of abuse are medications prescribed for a variety of medical conditions. No longer do abusers need to obtain drugs exclusively on the street; physician offices, pharmacies, and medicine cabinets now have become common sources of these substances. Practitioners need to be aware not only of the potential for abuse by patients when prescribing these substances but also of the potential for these drugs to fall into the hands of other users, including family members and acquaintances of patients. This shift to abuse of prescription drugs has also likely changed the demographics of those at risk of drug abuse; young and old alike, spanning the full array of socioeconomic backgrounds, are at risk of abuse in the setting of relatively easy accessibility to these substances.

Standard urinary drug screens are inexpensive and utilized in most emergency departments when concern exists for acute intoxication. These screens also are employed in drug treatment programs and employee screens in order to monitor compliance with abstinence. They test for commonly used recreational drugs or their metabolites including alcohol, amphetamines, barbiturates, benzodiazepines, cannabis, and cocaine. Although this list captures many drugs of abuse, other agents discussed here are not included in typical urinary screens and either cannot be tested for easily or are only detected using serum screens that tend to be expensive and time-consuming. These serum screens remain the gold standard for testing, especially outside the emergency setting. Other options for testing are employed much less commonly and include saliva and hair analysis, the latter having the advantage of detecting drugs of abuse weeks to even months after ingestion.

COCAINE

Cocaine is a widely used, highly addictive stimulant that increases monoamine neurotransmitters through inhibition of reuptake. It is taken in a variety of different ways including by snorting, smoking (often as "crack" cocaine), and intravenous injection. Acute intoxication effects and risk depend on the method of ingestion and dose but, in general, as with other stimulants, a variety of neuropsychiatric

Aminoff's Neurology and General Medicine, Fifth Edition.

effects—including psychosis and paranoia—can occur in addition to the expected euphoria and increased energy.

Adverse neurologic effects may include tremor and a number of other movement disorders including acute dystonia, tics, and dyskinesias, the latter of which can be long-lasting in some patients.[1] As with other stimulant drugs, seizures can occur with acute intoxication and are difficult to predict by dose or route of drug administration; generalized tonic-clonic seizures are most common, but cocaine lowers the seizure threshold and can lead to focal-onset seizures in patients with an underlying brain lesion. Thus, any focality to seizures occurring in the setting of cocaine use should lead to urgent neuroimaging to exclude an underlying structural cause.

The most recognizable of the acute neurologic complications associated with cocaine are cerebrovascular in nature.[2] Dramatic rises in blood pressure shortly after use can lead to intracerebral hemorrhage as a result of exceeding the upper limits of the cerebral autoregulatory curve.[3] In addition, patients with intracranial aneurysms may be at risk of rupture with the hypertension that accompanies intoxication. Ischemic stroke can also occur shortly after use due to the promotion of thrombosis via platelet activation and other downstream mechanisms; indeed this hypercoagulability was first described in myocardial infarction but likely applies similarly to ischemic stroke.

In contrast to the acute effects, chronic cocaine use can lead to ischemic stroke and cerebral transient ischemic attacks through a variety of mechanisms, many of which remain incompletely understood. Some cocaine abusers appear to develop a non-inflammatory vasculopathy similar to accelerated atherosclerosis in both large and small vessels of the intracranial circulation, predisposing them to stroke at a young age.[4] It has been suggested that part of the rise in stroke incidence in younger populations is accounted for by the increased use of recreational stimulants such as cocaine.[5,6] Other purported mechanisms of cocaine-induced stroke have included vasospasm of small arteries and an increased incidence of cervical artery dissection—these appear to be less common than atherosclerotic-like changes but should be considered in cocaine-related stroke and transient ischemic attacks.

In addition to direct effects on the cerebral circulation, a variety of ischemic cocaine-related complications stem from the varied effects of the drug on the heart. Cocaine-induced arrhythmias, both atrial and ventricular, can predispose to cardioembolic events with either acute or chronic use of the drug.[7] The cardiomyopathy that accompanies cocaine-related myocarditis can also lead to cardioembolic disease when the ejection fraction is moderately-to-severely depressed. Myocardial infarction in the setting of acute use is one of the more common causes of concern when a cocaine user presents to the emergency department with chest pain.[8] Stroke can occur when wall motion abnormalities of the heart or an apical aneurysm set the stage for stasis and intracardiac clot formation that can subsequently embolize to the cerebral circulation. Finally, acute aortic dissection, which is well described in cocaine users due to effects on the aortic endothelium and to acute hypertension, can lead to cerebrovascular events when the dissection involves the origins of the great vessels, leading to either hypoperfusion or a proximal embolic source.[9]

METHAMPHETAMINES

The numerous methamphetamine-containing compounds that are available to recreational users all work through a common mechanism of increased norepinephrine, epinephrine, and serotonin transmission at the synapse while also activating dopamine receptors. The stimulant effects of acute intoxication are therefore similar in many respects to those occurring with cocaine, with euphoria and increased energy predominating along with the risk of occasional paradoxical reactions including agitation and paranoia. As the effects of the drug wear off, dysphoria and increased sleep commonly occur, mimicking some of the effects of sedatives.

Other neurologic effects of acute intoxication involve intracerebral hemorrhage due presumably in part to severe hypertension, even in patients without a history of chronic use; subcortical locations of hemorrhage are most common. As with other stimulants, tremor and tonic-clonic seizures can occur with acute intoxication. Any focal features of the seizure or in the postictal period should trigger a neuroimaging search for an underlying lesion.

A number of neuropsychatric complications are well described in chronic users of methamphetamines. Psychosis, attention-deficit hyperactivity disorder, and chronic memory and executive function deficits may occur, with resultant poor psychosocial and behavioral outcomes.[10] Individuals who chronically abuse methamphetamines typically require psychologic assistance in addition to substance abuse counseling. The chronic neurotoxicity that leads to these complications is thought to involve both dopaminergic and serotonergic fronto-striatal-thalamocortical networks. Compulsive performance of repetitive, mechanical tasks such as assembling or disassembling an object, termed "punding," is likely the result of this dopaminergic overactivity and is well-described in chronic users of methamphetamines (termed "tweaking" by some users).[11] Although studies have been mixed, users of methamphetamines may have an increased risk of developing parkinsonism later in life due to involvement of striatal dopamine pathways; ongoing longitudinal investigations are addressing this possibility.[12]

Cerebrovascular complications of chronic methamphetamine use include the development of an often dramatic cerebral vasculopathy with fusiform enlargement of the large vessels of the brain with a tendency toward aneurysm formation (Fig. 34-1). These aneurysms can be large enough to contain clot, which serves as an embolic source for ischemic stroke. Other patients with vasculopathy in the setting of methamphetamine use demonstrate narrowing of some distal branches of the cerebral vessels, leading to ischemia.[13] It is likely that this vasculopathy is a result, at least in part, of direct toxicity of the drug or adulterants rather than simply the consequence of hypertension. Some have suggested an inflammatory process (e.g., cerebral vasculitis) within the vessel wall, although studies supporting this have been mixed, and typical findings in the cerebrospinal fluid and on histologic and gross pathologic examination are non-inflammatory.

In addition to an increased risk of ischemic stroke, methamphetamine abusers have an increased risk of subarachnoid hemorrhage relating to their tendency to aneurysm formation. In patients with methamphetamine-related subarachnoid hemorrhage, the complications of vasospasm and delayed cerebral ischemia are particularly common and severe, even when adjusted for severity of bleed. These effects are apparently more long-lasting than in most patients with aneurysmal subarachnoid hemorrhage and require vigilance for 3 to 4 weeks following initial bleed. As a result, subarachnoid hemorrhage has a worse prognosis when related to methamphetamine use than otherwise, when adjusted for Hunt and Hess grade.[14] Similar to cocaine, methamphetamines can also importantly lead to a cardiomyopathy, myocardial ischemia, or aortic dissection, all of which predispose patients to stroke via the mechanisms discussed earlier.

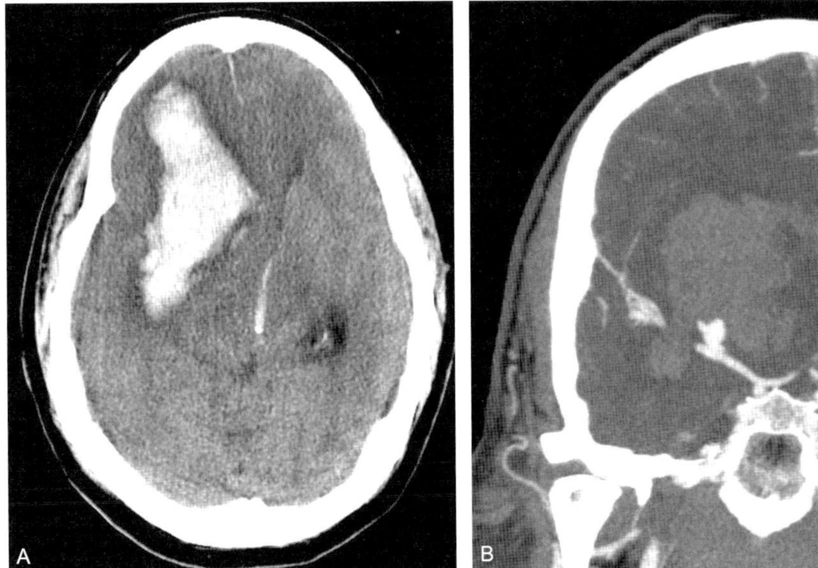

FIGURE 34-1 ■ Noncontrast CT (**A**) and CT angiogram (**B**) of the brain in a 41-year-old man with a history of chronic methamphetamine abuse who presented with confusion and left hemiparesis. A large right-hemispheric intracerebral hemorrhage is demonstrated, resulting from a bilobed 8 × 8 × 6-mm aneurysm in the region of the right middle cerebral artery bifurcation.

BATH SALTS

A recent increase of the use of so-called "bath salts" has been observed particularly in the United States. These compounds, which contain various synthetic cathinones and have no relationship with actual substances used in bathing, are usually swallowed or snorted with effects similar to other stimulants, leading to the moniker "fake cocaine" due in part to their addictive properties.[15,16] The mechanism of action involves interactions with plasma membrane transporters for dopamine, norepinephrine, and serotonin; the duration of action is typically 3 to 4 hours.[17] Low doses often produce euphoria and increased alertness, but neurologic side effects include tremors and seizures as well as hallucinations, agitation, and dysphoria among some users.[18] An agitated delirium can result that is often accompanied by tachycardia and hyperthermia; this constellation of findings should alert health care workers to possible ingestion of these substances, which are not detected by typical drug screens.[19,20] These compounds until recently have been widely available in over-the-counter form. Although various governments have recently made these compounds illegal, new cathinones have been introduced, staying one step ahead of regulatory bodies.

MDMA (ECSTASY)

The synthetic compound 3,4 methylenedioxymethamphetamine (MDMA, ecstasy) is a serotonergic amphetamine that became popular at dance parties ("raves") and can be taken in combination with other psychotropic drugs. As with other stimulants, the desired effects among users are euphoria and a sense of well-being. Ecstasy is also known for leading to disinhibition and sexual arousal. In some patients, agitation and anxiety can paradoxically occur at the time of intoxication or once the acute effects of the drug have worn off.

The association between severe hyponatremia and MDMA ingestion is important and can lead to serious neurologic complications. Users of the drug develop both a primary polydipsia and a drug-induced increase in antidiuretic hormone secretion, limiting the ability of the kidneys to secrete water and leading to, at times, a precipitous decline in the serum sodium level.[21] The polydipsia may be in part due to an attempt among users to avoid hyperthermia in crowded dance arenas. The resultant hyponatremia may lead to seizures as well as potentially fatal cerebral edema; therefore, serum sodium measurement is important in any patient presenting with altered mental status or seizures following MDMA use.[22] Careful correction is important to avoid osmotic demyelination, as discussed in Chapters 13, 15, and 17, although in the setting of life-threatening neurologic complications, more rapid correction may be necessary. As is the case with most stimulants, seizures can also occur with MDMA ingestion independent of the serum sodium level.

Use of MDMA can also lead to a serotonin syndrome characterized by altered mental status, fever, and other neurologic abnormalities such as clonus, myoclonus, and tremor. There is likely a spectrum of this disorder ranging from mild confusion to life-threatening circulatory collapse when autonomic instability occurs. The risk of serotonin syndrome increases when MDMA is combined with other serotonergic drugs such as selective serotonin reuptake inhibitors.[23] Treatment options include supportive care in a cool environment for milder cases to treatment with cyproheptadine in more severe instances.

Individuals with a history of heavy use of MDMA appear to demonstrate cognitive problems in memory and attentional domains that may be long-lasting.[24] Some studies, however, have suggested that these cognitive deficits may relate, at least in part, to underlying comorbidities, including the behavioral and psychologic disturbances that led originally to use of recreational drugs. These chronic cognitive effects seem to be mainly observed in those with a history of heavy use rather than in those with more infrequent use of the drug.[25]

GAMMA HYDROXYBUTYRATE (GHB)

Gamma hydroxybutyrate (GHB) leads to both euphoria and stimulant effects with purported sexual enhancement and disinhibition. The drug is the precursor to γ-aminobutyric acid (GABA), one of the most common inhibitory neurotransmitters in the central nervous system. Previously marketed for bodybuilding, it is now used recreationally, often simultaneously with other "club drugs" including MDMA.[26] The drug is ingested orally, usually in liquid form. GHB has a narrow window of safety and therefore overdosing and emergency department visits are common.[27] Interestingly, the drug has found a therapeutic purpose and is marketed in the

United States and Europe for treatment of narcolepsy with cataplexy or excessive daytime sleepiness.

The most commonly cited neurologic effect of GHB intoxication is coma, which may occur rapidly after ingestion and necessitate intubation and admission to the hospital in order to protect the airway and avoid fatal ventilatory failure. Since GHB is not detected in most routine urine toxicology screens, neurologists are often consulted for an otherwise unexplained coma in a young person. An impressively sudden reversal of coma is sometimes observed, which is strongly suggestive of GHB intoxication. Other neurologic complications of acute use include ataxia and nystagmus; the effects on consciousness may preclude safe driving.[28]

When GHB wears off, an agitated delirium with self-injurious behavior may be observed, and some patients will alternate quickly between agitated and sedated states. Patients with GHB intoxication are at risk of seizures, and myoclonus is typically seen especially when patients are in the agitated phase.[29] Patients using GHB are usually quite amnestic to events, even when they are conscious, leading to its use in sexual assault as a "date rape" drug.[30]

SEDATIVE-HYPNOTICS

The sedative-hypnotic class of drugs is mainly used for medical purposes including induction of sleep and relief of anxiety. However, these compounds have developed into common drugs of abuse with a potential for dependence as prescription drug abuse has increased. Historically, barbiturates were replaced by the benzodiazepine class of drugs in part due to an increased safety profile in overdose; however, both classes of drug have a similar potential for abuse.[31] The sedative and anxiolytic properties of all of these medications resemble those of alcohol since both act in part at the level of the GABA system in the brain, and alcohol withdrawal syndromes are treated with long-acting forms of these drugs.

The sedation that accompanies acute intoxication represents an important neurologic manifestation of these compounds that is typically easy to recognize. Reversal of acute intoxication with benzodiazepines by flumazenil, a benzodiazepine receptor antagonist, for purely diagnostic purposes is generally discouraged, and its use is limited to life-threatening situations, given its tendency to produce seizures and rapidly induce withdrawal.

The most important neurologic effects of sedative medications involve withdrawal, which can lead to tachycardia, agitation, tremor, and hallucinations that may develop into frank psychosis. Seizures are an important concern, and abrupt withdrawal of these medications can lead to ictal events even in those without an underlying epileptic disorder. Treatment for these seizures usually involves administration of benzodiazepines, often in intravenous form, followed by a slow taper which may need to last for days or weeks depending on the duration and dose of use prior to withdrawal. As a general rule, traditional antiepileptic medications that are not of the benzodiazepine or barbiturate class are ineffective.

Recently, a number of benzodiazepine-related substances including zolpidem, zaleplon, and eszopiclone have emerged with a safety profile that is so favorable that they are available in many countries without a prescription for use as a short-term sleeping aid. With this greater availability has emerged a potential for abuse as well as symptoms of withdrawal with prolonged exposure.[32] Zolpidem in particular has been widely used by teenagers in the United States to produce a high rather than induction of sleep. Neurologic symptoms that have been described include depression, behavioral changes including irritability, unusual complex behaviors similar to sleepwalking, and severe amnesia for events, leading it to be used by sexual predators.[33]

OPIATES

Abuse of opiates remains an extremely important public health concern. In the last decade, the emphasis has shifted from abuse of intravenous heroin and similar substances to recreational use of opiates prescribed for pain relief. Physicians need to be particularly aware of this possibility when prescribing these medications—many of these drugs end up either for sale on the street or abused by persons other than the individual for whom the prescription was intended.

The neurologic effects of opiate intoxication are well known and include miosis and an altered mental status that can progress to coma with high doses, especially in those without previous exposure to this class of medications. Some specific opiates can lead to seizures, including fentanyl, meperidine (particularly in the setting of renal insufficiency), tramadol, and pentazocine.[34,35] Individuals taking opiates reliably demonstrate diffuse myoclonus, which can be mistaken for seizures, often leading to neurologic consultation; this condition is generally self-limited and of no consequence, reversing with discontinuation of the drug. Patients in whom opiate intoxication has led to profound respiratory depression are at risk of hypoxic-ischemic injury to the brain and may present with persistent coma even after withdrawal or reversal of opiates. Changes on neuroimaging may be nonexistent or subtle in cases of hypoxic-ischemic injury, and therefore the condition is a diagnosis of exclusion.

There are a number of neuromuscular complications of which opiate abusers are at risk. Myalgias can represent direct muscle involvement from opiate intoxication; frank rhabdomyolysis remains a rare but important complication that needs to be treated aggressively in order to prevent acute kidney injury.[36] Repeated intramuscular injections of opiates may lead to a fibrotic myopathy due to a local direct toxic effect, and therefore users who inject opiates should be asked regarding site of injection.[37]

Beginning in the mid-1990s, an epidemic of wound botulism was described, mainly in California, in users of so-called "black tar heroin" when the drug was administered via skin popping.[38] This important public health concern can present with "outbreaks" of multiple cases of botulism in a single community when a batch of the substance becomes contaminated with *C. botulinum*.[39] Patients present with weakness and depressed muscle stretch reflexes, often along with bulbar signs that include difficulty swallowing, double vision, and slurred speech from facial weakness. The pupils may be dilated and poorly reactive to light, but this varies with the serotype of the offending organism and therefore should not be used to make or exclude the diagnosis. If botulism is recognized at an early stage, antitoxin administration is important to avoid ventilatory failure from neuromuscular weakness, which in many cases may be prolonged and necessitate tracheostomy.

Withdrawal from opiate medications reliably leads to dysphoria and akathisia. Muscle pain, nausea, vomiting, yawning, and rhinorrhea are a few of the non-neurologic symptoms of withdrawal that are well-recognized. Treatment of life-threatening acute intoxication involves administration of opiate antagonists such as naloxone; complications from withdrawal symptoms should be anticipated when these antagonists are given, especially in patients who are chronic users or in whom use involves longer-acting opiate preparations.

When an opiate, often heroin, is inhaled by the user after vaporization on a piece of aluminum foil ("chasing the dragon"), a toxic leukoencephalopathy may result and is characterized on magnetic resonance imaging (MRI) by diffuse and symmetric T2 hyperintensities in the white matter (Fig. 34-2).[40,41] Symptoms range from mild abulia and parkinsonism to akinetic mutism or coma. Onset of the disorder may be delayed by days to weeks following opiate exposure, and clinical and neuroimaging features may progress before reaching a plateau after a few weeks. There is no effective treatment. Postmortem examination reveals a spongiform-like degeneration in the white matter that spares the U-fibers.

An important, mainly historical, opiate compound is 1-methyl-4-phenyl-1,2,3,6-tetrahydropyridine, which in the early 1980s was found to cause a parkinsonian syndrome when the drug was inadvertently created in an attempt to create a synthetic form of meperidine.[42] 1-Methyl-4-phenyl-1,2,3,6-tetrahydropyridine leads to neuronal death over a fairly short period of time in neurons in the substantia nigra pars compacta and has led to the development of an important animal model of Parkinson disease.[43]

HALLUCINOGENS

The intent of use of hallucinogens is to alter neurologic perception and mood, often leading to vivid visual illusions which may be colorful and well-formed. A distortion of sensory input and synesthesia occurs with the prototypic drug, lysergic acid diethylamide (LSD). At times, LSD ingestion can be characterized paradoxically by agitation, panic, or dysphoria in what is termed a "bad trip" by users. Rare adverse effects that may be due to LSD or its adulterants include more permanent visual disturbances and vasospasm leading to cerebral ischemia.[44,45] Due to its effects on the serotonin receptors in the brain, serotonin syndrome can result, especially when LSD is combined with other serotonergic drugs including prescription antidepressants.

Long-term effects of LSD use may include "flashbacks," where a hallucination that accompanied intoxication is experienced again months to years later and is usually not distressing. Exposure to serotonergic drugs may be the trigger for such flashbacks in some patients.[46] In contrast, hallucinogen

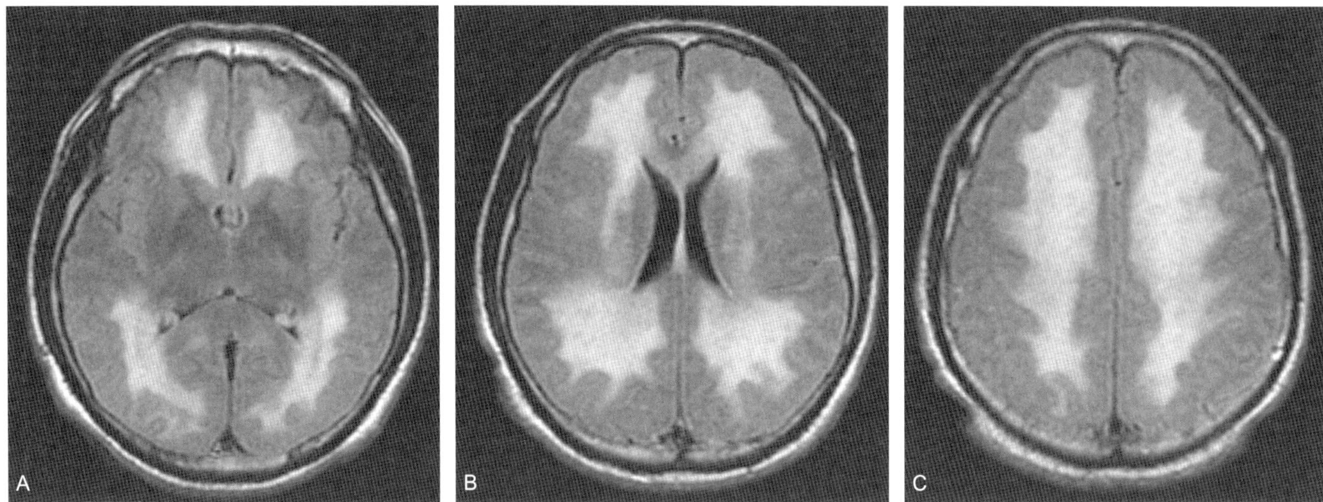

FIGURE 34-2 ▪ Axial FLAIR MRI images of the brain from a 39-year-old man presenting with progressive altered mental status and parkinsonism 7 days after inhalation of vaporized heroin ("chasing the dragon"). Extensive white matter hyperintensities spare the subcortical U-fibers. No enhancement occurred on postcontrast images (not shown).

persisting perception disorder is a long-term and potentially disabling recurrent condition in which hallucinations are experienced again; the disorder is unpleasant, disruptive, and difficult to treat.[47]

Other important drugs of abuse with properties similar to LSD include mescaline, which is found in the peyote cactus in the southwestern United States. Ingestion leads to tachycardia, agitation, and mydriasis along with hallucinations and altered perceptions.[48] Mushroom intoxication recreationally involves those that contain psilocybin and are consumed often in dried form; headache often accompanies intoxication with these so-called "magic mushrooms."[49,50]

N-METHYL-D-ASPARTATE ANTAGONISTS

Phencyclidine (PCP, "Angel dust") was first developed as a surgical anesthetic but some patients developed a long-lasting psychotic syndrome following its administration.[51] The drug subsequently emerged as a recreational drug of abuse due to its dissociative effects. One important site of action for PCP is antagonism of *N*-methyl-D-aspartate (NMDA) glutamate receptors, which are widely distributed in the brain, especially in the medial temporal lobes and throughout the limbic system.

Manifestations of PCP intoxication in the emergency setting include tachycardia, hypertension, violent outbursts, and nystagmus, which classically can be vertical in direction.[51] Higher doses of PCP may induce an acute psychosis with hallucinations and agitation, whereas a striking akinetic mutism with unresponsiveness and preserved eye opening may accompany overdose. PCP's stimulant effects can lead to hyperreflexia as well as dystonia and occasionally seizures.[52] The agitation that results may itself cause rhabdomyolysis, which has otherwise been attributed to a direct toxic effect of the drug. Long-term use of PCP can lead to a condition resembling chronic schizophrenia, and the drug has been used to create animal models of schizophrenia for research purposes.[53]

The anesthetic ketamine has also emerged as a recreational drug of abuse, sometimes in those prescribed the medication for chronic pain. The main mechanism of action involves NMDA antagonism similar to PCP. One of the advantages of its use in anesthetic settings is its relatively favorable safety profile in high doses and, similarly, respiratory depression is an extremely rare occurrence in abusers. Intoxication is characterized by acute CNS depressant effects of slurred speech and impaired consciousness and can lead to injury.[54] Long-term effects of use may not only partially mimic schizophrenia as is the case with PCP, but may also lead to a more subtle permanent cognitive disorder with deficits of memory and mood.[55]

DEXTROMETHORPHAN

Dextromethorphan has been used for decades as a cough suppressant but has emerged more recently as a recreational drug of abuse, especially among teenagers due to its stimulant and dissociative properties.[56] At high doses, dextromethorphan can present with PCP-like effects on NMDA receptors.[57] Patients may present with hallucinations, agitation, and ataxia; although in its extreme form coma can result.[58,59] Elevated blood pressure and heart rate are common along with stimulant and perceptual effects similar to psilocybin. Serotonin syndrome can result from overdose, especially when combined with other serotonergic agents.[60] Widespread abuse of the drug has led to regulatory controls in many states of over-the-counter sale of dextromethorphan-containing compounds.

NITROUS OXIDE

Nitrous oxide is often used recreationally by inhaling the gas from a balloon ("whippet") or other canisters such as those that deliver whipped cream, where the gas is used as a propellant. Although commonly used by young people recreationally, abuse among health care providers with access to nitrous oxide, such as among those in the dental field, is also well documented.[61] The neurologic manifestations result from effects on vitamin B_{12} pathways. Under normal conditions, nitrous oxide converts vitamin B_{12} to an inactive form that inhibits a key enzyme used in DNA and RNA synthesis, methionine synthase. Patients present with similar symptoms and signs to those occurring with vitamin B_{12} deficiency, although the serum B_{12} level may be normal. Some patients who are exposed to nitrous oxide anesthesia may develop a similar syndrome if they have preexisting vitamin B_{12} deficiency from, for example, pernicious anemia.[62]

Central nervous system manifestations include psychosis and cognitive decline, but far more common is a myeloneuropathy with prominent posterior column signs.[63] MR imaging may demonstrate increased T2 signal in the posterior columns, often with a predilection for the cervical spinal cord (Fig. 34-3).[64] Patients present with a sensory ataxia, decreased vibratory and proprioceptive thresholds, and a spastic gait with or without weakness of the limbs. Some of these abnormalities can be reversed with vitamin B_{12} supplementation and abstinence from nitrous oxide use, but chronic users may not seek medical attention until the condition is irreversible.

MARIJUANA AND RELATED COMPOUNDS

Tetrahydrocannabinol (THC) is the principal active component of marijuana, which is typically smoked recreationally but can also be consumed orally, where its effects are more delayed. Marijuana use typically leads to euphoria as well as a decrease in anxiety and perceptual changes that can involve slowing of time and vivid colors. There may be relatively mild psychedelic effects in comparison with the hallucinogen class of drugs. Intoxicated patients

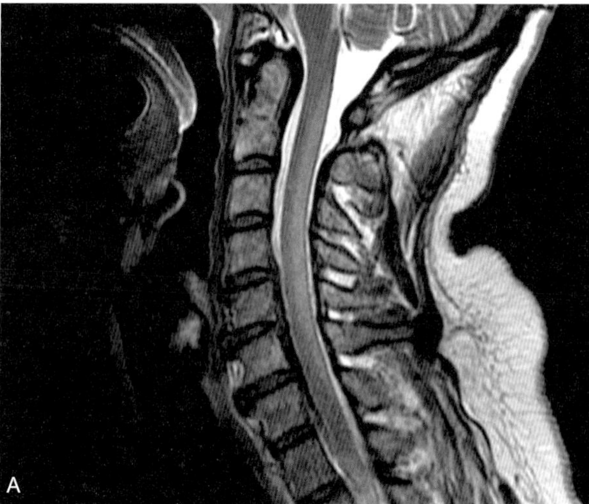

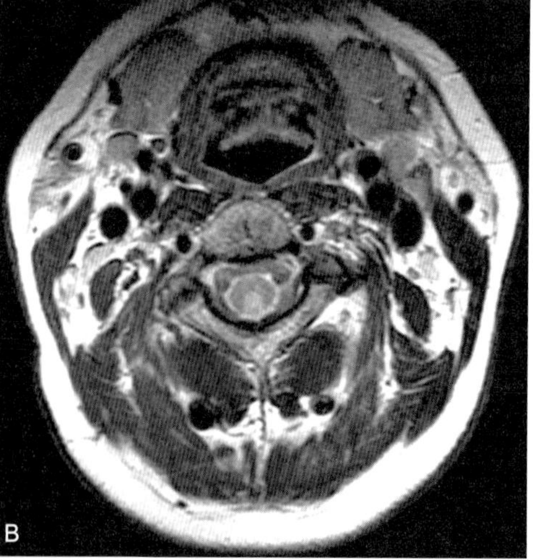

FIGURE 34-3 ▪ Sagittal (**A**) and axial (**B**) T2-weighted MR images of the cervical spine in a 51-year-old woman presenting with gait difficulties and ataxia following a 6-month history of recreational nitrous oxide abuse. Hyperintensity is demonstrated in the posterior portion of the cord, corresponding to the location of the dorsal column pathways.

demonstrate decreased coordination and gait along with psychomotor slowing that can impair safe driving.[65] Some reports have rarely associated marijuana use with stroke, presumably on the basis of vasoconstriction as the likely mechanism.[66] Some chronic heavy users may develop a withdrawal syndrome of irritability, fatigue, anxiety, and difficulty sleeping.[67]

Chronic users of the drug may exhibit an amotivational syndrome characterized by apathy and lack of ambition and drive. It is unclear from the literature whether heavy users of marijuana can develop more permanent cognitive sequelae including deficits of executive function, memory, and attention.[68–70] Marijuana users appear to be at increased risk of developing psychotic disorders or affective symptoms, but these studies may be confounded by any underlying psychiatric disorder (or tendency) leading to marijuana or other drug use.[71]

The terms "Spice" or "K2" are brand names used to describe a variety of herbal medicines that are widely available and mimic the effects of marijuana.[72] These compounds may be labeled as "incense" or "herbal smoking products" and have only recently been banned from over-the-counter sale in the United States. Although these drugs include synthetic compounds that resemble cannabanoids, they are not detectable in the usual screens for THC in the urine; emergency medical personal should be aware of these drugs in patients presenting with symptoms and signs of marijuana intoxication with negative drug screens.

INFECTIOUS COMPLICATIONS OF INJECTION DRUG USE

Many of the recreational drugs discussed earlier are administered intravenously, and the risk of infectious complications is substantial. This risk is due not only to sharing of needles with associated bacterial and viral contaminants, but also to a lack of sterile technique that can introduce skin flora and other nearby bacteria into the blood stream.

Endocarditis remains an important cause of stroke and cerebral abscess among those with intravenous drug abuse. Staphylococcus and streptococcus species are particularly common culprits. Embolic ischemic strokes from endocarditis have a propensity for hemorrhagic transformation, and septic emboli should be considered in patients presenting with multiple hemorrhagic strokes. Subarachnoid hemorrhage may result from ruptured mycotic aneurysms. Those that are ruptured should be secured, usually via surgical clipping; unruptured mycotic aneurysms that are stable are usually treated with antibiotics alone despite the lack of good data supporting this practice. Intracerebral abscess is a dreaded complication that usually begins as a less walled-off cerebritis, occasionally in the setting of endocarditis; early surgical management is typically recommended along with administration of broad-spectrum intravenously administered antibiotics with good penetration across the blood–brain barrier.

Bacteremia can also lead to seeding of the spinal column and thus to discitis, osteomyelitis, and epidural abscess, important considerations when patients with a history of intravenous drug use present with new back pain, with or without fever. MR imaging is the modality of choice for the spinal cord, and surgery with intravenous administration of antibiotics is the preferred treatment when clinical signs of spinal cord compression are present.

Sharing of needles can also lead to infections such as with human immunodeficiency virus, human T-lymphotropic virus types 1 and 2, and hepatitis virus. Their neurologic presentations are discussed in Chapter 44. Clinicians need to be aware of these infections and their neurologic complications in patients with a history of intravenous drug use.

CONCLUDING COMMENTS

Neurologic complications of drug abuse continue to be common, and knowledge of these substances and their effects, both during intoxication and with chronic use, is essential for evaluation of patients presenting with neurologic disorders. Because new substances and methods of ingestion are continually emerging, all physicians should remain familiar with current recognition and management decisions in this rapidly changing field.

REFERENCES

1. Brust JC: Substance abuse and movement disorders. Mov Disord 25:2010, 2010.
2. Toossi S, Hess CP, Hills NK, et al: Neurovascular complications of cocaine use at a tertiary stroke center. J Stroke Cerebrovasc Dis 19:273, 2010.
3. Martin-Schild S, Albright KC, Hallevi H, et al: Intracerebral hemorrhage in cocaine users. Stroke 41:680, 2010.
4. De Giorgi A, Fabbian F, Pala M, et al: Cocaine and acute vascular diseases. Curr Drug Abuse Rev 5:129, 2012.

5. Kaku DA, Lowenstein DH: Emergence of recreational drug abuse as a major risk factor for stroke in young adults. Ann Intern Med 113:821, 1990.
6. de Los Rios F, Kleindorfer DO, Khoury J, et al: Trends in substance abuse preceding stroke among young adults: a population-based study. Stroke 43:3179, 2012.
7. Kloner RA, Hale S, Alker K, et al: The effects of acute and chronic cocaine use on the heart. Circulation 85:407, 1992.
8. Finkel JB, Marhefka GD: Rethinking cocaine-associated chest pain and acute coronary syndromes. Mayo Clin Proc 86:1198, 2011.
9. Singh A, Khaja A, Alpert MA: Cocaine and aortic dissection. Vasc Med 15:127, 2010.
10. Scott JC, Woods SP, Matt GE, et al: Neurocognitive effects of methamphetamine: a critical review and meta-analysis. Neuropsychol Rev 17:275, 2007.
11. Rusyniak DE: Neurologic manifestations of chronic methamphetamine abuse. Neurol Clin 29:641, 2011.
12. Callaghan RC, Cunningham JK, Sykes J, et al: Increased risk of Parkinson's disease in individuals hospitalized with conditions related to the use of methamphetamine or other amphetamine-type drugs. Drug Alcohol Depend 120:35, 2012.
13. Ho EL, Josephson SA, Lee HS, et al: Cerebrovascular complications of methamphetamine abuse. Neurocrit Care 10:295, 2009.
14. Beadell NC, Thompson EM, Delashaw JB, et al: The deleterious effects of methamphetamine use on initial presentation and clinical outcomes in aneurysmal subarachnoid hemorrhage. J Neurosurg 117:781, 2012.
15. Penders TM: How to recognize a patient who's high on "bath salts". J Fam Pract 61:210, 2012.
16. Prosser JM, Nelson LS: The toxicology of bath salts: a review of synthetic cathinones. J Med Toxicol 8:33, 2012.
17. Gershman JA, Fass AD: Synthetic cathinones ('bath salts'): legal and health care challenges. P T 37:571, 2012.
18. Antoniou T, Juurlink DN: Five things to know about..."bath salts". CMAJ 184:1713, 2012.
19. Baumann MH, Partilla JS, Lehner KR: Psychoactive "bath salts": not so soothing. Eur J Pharmacol 698:1, 2013.
20. Jerry J, Collins G, Streem D: Synthetic legal intoxicating drugs: the emerging 'incense' and 'bath salt' phenomenon. Cleve Clin J Med 79:258, 2012.
21. Campbell GA, Rosner MH: The agony of ecstasy: MDMA (3,4-methylenedioxymethamphetamine) and the kidney. Clin J Am Soc Nephrol 3:1852, 2008.
22. Rosenson J, Smollin C, Sporer KA, et al: Patterns of ecstasy-associated hyponatremia in California. Ann Emerg Med 49:164, 2007.
23. Silins E, Copeland J, Dillon P: Qualitative review of serotonin syndrome, ecstasy (MDMA) and the use of other serotonergic substances: hierarchy of risk. Aust NZ J Psychiatry 41:649, 2007.
24. Cuyas E, Verdejo-Garcia A, Fagundo AB, et al: The influence of genetic and environmental factors among MDMA users in cognitive performance. PLoS One 6:e27206, 2011.
25. Hanson KL, Luciana M: Neurocognitive impairments in MDMA and other drug users: MDMA alone may not be a cognitive risk factor. J Clin Exp Neuropsychol 32:337, 2010.
26. Galicia M, Nogue S, Miro O: Liquid ecstasy intoxication: clinical features of 505 consecutive emergency department patients. Emerg Med J 28:462, 2011.
27. Munir VL, Hutton JE, Harney JP, et al: Gamma-hydroxybutyrate: a 30 month emergency department review. Emerg Med Australas 20:521, 2008.
28. Couper FJ, Logan BK: GHB and driving impairment. J Forensic Sci 46:919, 2001.
29. Cagnin A, Pompanin S, Manfioli V, et al: Gamma-hydroxybutyric acid-induced psychosis and seizures. Epilepsy Behav 21:203, 2011.
30. Nemeth Z, Kun B, Demetrovics Z: The involvement of gamma-hydroxybutyrate in reported sexual assaults: a systematic review. J Psychopharmacol 24:1281, 2010.
31. Lader M: Benzodiazepines revisited–will we ever learn? Addiction 106:2086, 2011.
32. Hajak G, Muller WE, Wittchen HU, et al: Abuse and dependence potential for the non-benzodiazepine hypnotics zolpidem and zopiclone: a review of case reports and epidemiological data. Addiction 98:1371, 2003.
33. Ben-Hamou M, Marshall NS, Grunstein RR, et al: Spontaneous adverse event reports associated with zolpidem in Australia 2001-2008. J Sleep Res 20:559, 2011.
34. Hagmeyer KO, Mauro LS, Mauro VF: Meperidine-related seizures associated with patient-controlled analgesia pumps. Ann Pharmacother 27:29, 1993.
35. Talaie H, Panahandeh R, Fayaznouri M, et al: Dose-independent occurrence of seizure with tramadol. J Med Toxicol 5:63, 2009.
36. O'Connor G, McMahon G: Complications of heroin abuse. Eur J Emerg Med 15:104, 2008.
37. Weber M, Diener HC, Voit T, et al: Focal myopathy induced by chronic heroin injection is reversible. Muscle Nerve 23:274, 2000.
38. Werner SB, Passaro D, McGee J, et al: Wound botulism in California, 1951-1998: recent epidemic in heroin injectors. Clin Infect Dis 31:1018, 2000.
39. Yuan J, Inami G, Mohle-Boetani J, et al: Recurrent wound botulism among injection drug users in California. Clin Infect Dis 52:862, 2011.
40. Kriegstein AR, Armitage BA, Kim PY: Heroin inhalation and progressive spongiform leukoencephalopathy. N Engl J Med 336:589, 1997.
41. Keogh CF, Andrews GT, Spacey SD, et al: Neuroimaging features of heroin inhalation toxicity: "chasing the dragon". AJR Am J Roentgenol 180:847, 2003.

42. Langston JW, Ballard P, Tetrud JW, et al: Chronic parkinsonism in humans due to a product of meperidine-analog synthesis. Science 219:979, 1983.
43. Blesa J, Phani S, Jackson-Lewis V, et al: Classic and new animal models of Parkinson's disease. J Biomed Biotechnol 2012:845618, 2012.
44. Kawasaki A, Purvin V: Persistent palinopsia following ingestion of lysergic acid diethylamide (LSD). Arch Ophthalmol 114:47, 1996.
45. Lieberman AN, Bloom W, Kishore PS, et al: Carotid artery occlusion following ingestion of LSD. Stroke 5:213, 1974.
46. Goldman S, Galarneau D, Friedman R: New onset LSD flashback syndrome triggered by the initiation of SSRIs. Ochsner J 7:37, 2007.
47. Lerner AG, Gelkopf M, Skladman I, et al: Flashback and hallucinogen persisting perception disorder: clinical aspects and pharmacological treatment approach. Isr J Psychiatry Relat Sci 39:92, 2002.
48. Carstairs SD, Cantrell FL: Peyote and mescaline exposures: a 12-year review of a statewide poison center database. Clin Toxicol (Phila) 48:350, 2010.
49. Griffiths RR, Johnson MW, Richards WA, et al: Psilocybin occasioned mystical-type experiences: immediate and persisting dose-related effects. Psychopharmacology (Berl) 218:649, 2011.
50. Johnson MW, Sewell RA, Griffiths RR: Psilocybin dose-dependently causes delayed, transient headaches in healthy volunteers. Drug Alcohol Depend 123:132, 2012.
51. Bey T, Patel A: Phencyclidine intoxication and adverse effects: a clinical and pharmacological review of an illicit drug. Cal J Emerg Med 8:9, 2007.
52. McCarron MM, Schulze BW, Thompson GA, et al: Acute phencyclidine intoxication: incidence of clinical findings in 1,000 cases. Ann Emerg Med 10:237, 1981.
53. Mouri A, Noda Y, Enomoto T, et al: Phencyclidine animal models of schizophrenia: approaches from abnormality of glutamatergic neurotransmission and neurodevelopment. Neurochem Int 51:173, 2007.
54. Ng SH, Tse ML, Ng HW, et al: Emergency department presentation of ketamine abusers in Hong Kong: a review of 233 cases. Hong Kong Med J 16:6, 2010.
55. Morgan CJ, Muetzelfeldt L, Curran HV: Consequences of chronic ketamine self-administration upon neurocognitive function and psychological wellbeing: a 1-year longitudinal study. Addiction 105:121, 2010.
56. Wilson MD, Ferguson RW, Mazer ME, et al: Monitoring trends in dextromethorphan abuse using the national poison data system: 2000-2010. Clin Toxicol (Phila) 49:409, 2011.
57. Pungente MD, Jubeli E, Opstad CL, et al: Synthesis and preliminary investigations of the siRNA delivery potential of novel, single-chain rigid cationic carotenoid lipids. Molecules 17:3484, 2012.
58. Reissig CJ, Carter LP, Johnson MW, et al: High doses of dextromethorphan, an NMDA antagonist, produce effects similar to classic hallucinogens. Psychopharmacology (Berl) 223:1, 2012.
59. Romanelli F, Smith KM: Dextromethorphan abuse: clinical effects and management. J Am Pharm Assoc (2003) 49:e20, 2009.
60. Monte AA, Chuang R, Bodmer M: Dextromethorphan, chlorphenamine and serotonin toxicity: case report and systematic literature review. Br J Clin Pharmacol 70:794, 2010.
61. Layzer RB, Fishman RA, Schafer JA: Neuropathy following abuse of nitrous oxide. Neurology 28:504, 1978.
62. Singer MA, Lazaridis C: Nations SP, et al: Reversible nitrous oxide-induced myeloneuropathy with pernicious anemia: case report and literature review. Muscle Nerve 37:125, 2008.
63. Sethi NK, Mullin P, Torgovnick J, et al: Nitrous oxide "whippit" abuse presenting with cobalamin responsive psychosis. J Med Toxicol 2:71, 2006.
64. Hsu CK, Chen YQ, Lung VZ, et al: Myelopathy and polyneuropathy caused by nitrous oxide toxicity: a case report. Am J Emerg Med 30:1016.e3, 2012.
65. Asbridge M, Hayden JA, Cartwright JL: Acute cannabis consumption and motor vehicle collision risk: systematic review of observational studies and meta-analysis. BMJ 344:e536, 2012.
66. Thanvi BR, Treadwell SD: Cannabis and stroke: is there a link? Postgrad Med J 85:80, 2009.
67. Budney AJ, Hughes JR: The cannabis withdrawal syndrome. Curr Opin Psychiatry 19:233, 2006.
68. Pope Jr HG, Gruber AJ, Yurgelun-Todd D: Residual neuropsychologic effects of cannabis. Curr Psychiatry Rep 3:507, 2001.
69. Grant I, Gonzalez R, Carey CL, et al: Non-acute (residual) neurocognitive effects of cannabis use: a meta-analytic study. J Int Neuropsychol Soc 9:679, 2003.
70. Bolla KI, Brown K, Eldreth D, et al: Dose-related neurocognitive effects of marijuana use. Neurology 59:1337, 2002.
71. Moore TH, Zammit S, Lingford-Hughes A, et al: Cannabis use and risk of psychotic or affective mental health outcomes: a systematic review. Lancet 370:319, 2007.
72. Harris CR, Brown A: Synthetic cannabinoid intoxication: a case series and review. J Emerg Med 44:360, 2013.

CHAPTER

35

Neurotoxin Exposure in the Workplace

MICHAEL J. AMINOFF

Occupationally related disorders may result from injury, which is not the focus of this chapter, or from exposure to toxins. Many of the chemical agents that are present or are being introduced into the workplace environment may produce behavioral, cognitive, motor, sensory, or autonomic disturbances resulting from disorders of the central or peripheral nervous system (CNS or PNS). In this chapter, attention is focused on some of the main neurotoxic agents to which exposure occurs in the workplace. These may affect workers using or involved in the manufacture of potentially neurotoxic substances and those subject to industrial, agricultural, horticultural, or military exposure.

In order to demonstrate that a particular chemical is neurotoxic or that a certain syndrome is due to neurotoxin exposure, it must be shown that the suspected neurotoxin causes neurologic dysfunction of a consistent nature in exposed humans. The dysfunction may vary in severity between individuals but—depending on their level of exposure—all exposed workers should have some signs of neurotoxicity. Involvement of a single worker suggests that the disorder is not due to a toxin, that toxin exposure did not occur at work, or that exposure resulted from some individual work habit, such as failure to use a protective mask. In practice, many disorders that are presumed to be occupationally related consist of nonspecific symptoms that are common and may occur for a variety of reasons. Furthermore, any publicity about the outbreak of a neurotoxic disorder may lead to identical symptoms in suggestible subjects with less or no exposure to the suspected toxin.[1]

It is often difficult to reproduce a suspected neurotoxic syndrome in animals and thereby provide support for the belief that a substance is indeed neurotoxic. Failure to reproduce in animals a suspected human neurotoxic disorder does not exclude this possibility, as differences in species susceptibility may be responsible and certain impairments, such as of cognitive function, are anyway difficult to reproduce in animals.[2] Moreover, human exposure is often to combinations of several chemicals,

Aminoff's Neurology and General Medicine, Fifth Edition.

which individually may be harmless but in combination lead to neurologic dysfunction. This is because the effects of the different chemicals may be additive or one may potentiate the neurotoxic effects of another, as is illustrated by the effect of adding the nontoxic methyl ethyl ketone to a lowered concentration of the known neurotoxin *n*-hexane, a practice that led in the past to an outbreak of toxic neuropathy.

Ideally, to establish the toxic basis of a neurologic disorder, it should be possible to identify reproducible pathologic or pathophysiologic changes in the nervous system in humans or animals, and these should account for the clinical features of the disorder. In practice, this is often not possible or feasible.

The temporal profile of the clinical disorder may suggest a neurotoxic disorder. Depending on the toxic agent, there is often little or no latent period between the time of exposure and onset of symptoms, but certain toxic neuropathies (arsenic, thallium, organophosphates) occur after a delay on the order of 2 to 3 weeks. Although cessation of exposure may lead to clinical stabilization or improvement, deterioration may continue for some days to weeks after termination of exposure to certain neurotoxins, a phenomenon termed "coasting."

Improvement of symptoms during periods away from work, such as at weekends or during vacations, may raise the possibility of a work-related exposure to a neurotoxin, but other factors may be responsible, such as anxiety or disputes with co-workers. These various points are summarized in Table 35-1.

TABLE 35-1 ■ Features Suggestive of an Occupational Neurotoxic Disorder

History of exposure to a potential neurotoxin
Pattern of neurologic dysfunction accords with previously reported cases
Exposed co-workers also affected
A temporal relation exists between toxin exposure and onset of symptoms, and between cessation of exposure and arrest of progression (sometimes after coasting)
If the pathologic and pathophysiologic basis of the disorder have been identified, they should be reproducible and account for the clinical disturbance; an animal model of the disorder may exist
Other causes of the disorder have been excluded

MANIFESTATIONS OF OCCUPATIONAL NEUROTOXIC DISORDERS

Acute Encephalopathy

An acute encephalopathy is a common but nonspecific manifestation that may consist solely of headache and malaise that settle shortly after exposure is discontinued. With more severe involvement, symptoms may come to include confusion, irritability, poor concentration, impaired judgment, drowsiness, vertigo, tinnitus, sensory complaints, ataxia, weakness or fatigue, and nausea and vomiting. Neurologic examination is usually normal. Neuropsychologic examination may be abnormal but, because recovery is rapid and complete (usually within 24 hours), is rarely performed. With continued exposure, level of consciousness becomes depressed, sometimes leading to coma; seizures may also occur. Recovery is then likely to be more protracted and may be incomplete. The cause of this acute syndrome usually is easy to determine because of the history of exposure, because many workers are affected, and because a variety of other manifestations are common, such as conjunctival, mucosal, and cutaneous irritation, and respiratory difficulties.

Chronic Encephalopathy

The occurrence of a chronic encephalopathy relating to long-term low-level neurotoxin exposure is widely reported but of uncertain validity. Its symptoms include headache, "dizziness," poor concentration, memory impairment, irritability, affective disorders, various sleep disturbances, loss of libido, numbness and paresthesias, and "weakness." Such symptoms are nonspecific in nature, usually mild in degree, but may lead to surprising disability. Examination is typically normal, but ataxia and nystagmus are sometimes found; the results of laboratory and electrophysiologic studies are generally unhelpful or of questionable significance or relevance. Neurobehavioral studies may be abnormal, but often the findings are inconsistent, difficult to interpret in the absence of premorbid baseline studies, and of uncertain relevance. At present, then, whether such an entity truly exists—and its pathophysiologic basis—remains unclear.

Peripheral Neuropathy

Peripheral neuropathy is a better understood consequence of toxin exposure in the workplace. It may occur as a delayed effect of single high-dose exposure or after short-term repeated exposure to certain organophosphates, arsenic, or thallium. Chronic exposure to these and other neurotoxins, such as acrylamide and many organic solvents, also leads to neuropathy, causing that portion of the axon farthest from the cell body to degenerate, a phenomenon described as a *distal axonal neuropathy* or *axonopathy*, or a *dying-back neuropathy*. Symptoms and signs begin distally in the legs and then progress proximally depending on the severity of exposure. Sensory axons pass both peripherally to the limbs and centrally into the spinal cord; both degenerate toward the cell body. Some of the central sensory fibers ascend in the posterior columns to the cuneate and gracile nuclei in the medulla and, because of their length, are often among the first to degenerate. As regeneration does not occur in the CNS, recovery after axonal degeneration will be incomplete despite effective regeneration of the peripheral nerves.

In subjects who are chronically exposed to other neurotoxins in the workplace but who have no clinical deficit, minor electrodiagnostic abnormalities are sometimes found. Although these will not necessarily progress to clinical neuropathy, such subjects need careful monitoring to limit exposure and minimize any risk of progression.

SCREENING AT-RISK WORKERS

Screening workers for signs of toxicity may help to identify individuals with incipient or subclinical neurologic dysfunction or exposure to low levels of a neurotoxin, and thereby limit further exposure. Screening of fellow workers may also be diagnostically helpful when a subject with a suspected, occupationally related, neurotoxic disorder is encountered, because similarly exposed workers are likely to have at least some symptoms and signs of intoxication, although to a varying degree that probably relates to differences in age, gender, ethnicity, genetic background, health status, and other factors. In general, however, screening techniques are insensitive, nonspecific, time-consuming, costly, or poorly tolerated by patients.[1]

Clinical Evaluation

An occupational history is an important part of the medical record, especially when patients with obscure neurologic disorders are encountered. Job titles may need clarification for the nature of an occupation to be appreciated. If exposure to toxins is suspected, a detailed list of chemicals used in the workplace—and at previous places of employment, if symptoms are longstanding—should be obtained. Details of the work environment are also important, such as whether it is well ventilated, the nature of any protective measures (such as a requirement to wear special clothing and gloves, and the use of other devices including masks and goggles), and the provisions made for washing after exposure and for storage of food. The most common routes of occupational exposure are inhalation and through the skin.

It may be necessary to question co-workers to determine whether they have similar symptoms to those of a subject with a suspected neurotoxic disorder, and even to examine those working in a similar environment. When asymptomatic but exposed co-workers are screened, questioning may be focused, based on the clinical features in recognized cases; self-administered, standardized symptom questionnaires may be especially helpful.[1]

Neurotoxin exposure may also relate to environmental factors (such as a subject's residence or its location close to, for example, an industrial plant) and to social and personal factors (such as hobbies, other recreational activities, or dietary peculiarities) rather than to the workplace. The history must therefore exclude these possibilities.

Routine neurologic examination is of limited utility for screening purposes, its principal role being to exclude other conditions that might underlie the patient's symptoms. Generalized rather than focal neurologic abnormalities are the expected finding in many neurotoxic disorders. In some instances, however, focal findings—such as parkinsonism from manganese exposure—may be conspicuous. Techniques have been developed for quantifying aspects of the neurologic—especially the sensory—examination for screening purposes and for following changes over time. These include quantitative tests of muscle strength, coordination, body sway, balance, vibration and discriminative tactile sensibility, cold and warm thermal thresholds, and heat pain thresholds.[1,3]

Electrodiagnostic Testing and Neuroimaging

Electroencephalography (EEG) and evoked potential studies can be used to assess CNS function. The EEG is commonly slowed diffusely—but occasionally more focally—in patients with acute toxic or metabolic encephalopathies, but may be normal in chronic encephalopathies. It is therefore of little use in screening patients for neurotoxic injury. Changes are nonspecific and do not distinguish between toxic and other encephalopathies or between different toxic disorders. Evoked potentials provide some measure of the functional integrity of certain afferent CNS pathways, but normal responses may show marked amplitude variation between subjects and on the two sides of the same subject. Because most neurotoxins produce axonal degeneration, which causes changes in amplitude rather than latency of responses, evoked potentials are of limited utility in evaluating patients with suspected neurotoxicity.

Electromyography (EMG) and nerve conduction studies evaluate the function of the PNS, neuromuscular junctions, and muscle. The findings help to identify subclinical disease, follow the progression of disorders, and characterize the pathophysiologic basis of symptoms.[4] Nerve conduction studies are useful in studying both axonal and demyelinating neuropathies. Needle EMG can indicate the cause of weakness and localize pathologic processes to different regions of the motor units (spinal cord, nerve root, plexus, peripheral nerve, neuromuscular junction, or muscle). When evaluating exposed workers, comparison with appropriate control subjects is important. For example, sedentary office workers should not be used as controls for manual workers, who frequently develop minor abnormalities of nerve conduction as a result of occupationally related, repeated minor trauma or subclinical entrapment neuropathies.[3]

Neuroimaging of the CNS, when normal, does not exclude a neurotoxic disorder. In some instances, however, the findings may show characteristic abnormalities, such as in manganese poisoning, discussed later.

Neuropsychologic Evaluation

Advances in neuropsychologic test procedures in recent years have improved their utility as a screening device.[5] Such test procedures may reveal subtle cognitive dysfunction but the findings are not diagnostic of toxic encephalopathy. Moreover, testing is time-consuming even when self-administered questionnaires and computerized test procedures are used, and thus costly and impractical for screening large numbers of subjects. Careful matching for age, gender, ethnicity, and social, cultural, and educational background is necessary when making comparisons between groups.

Other Laboratory Testing

With the exception of screening for heavy metal excretion in the urine or their presence in other tissues, laboratory studies are generally unhelpful in screening for neurotoxic disorders.

SELECTED NEUROTOXIC DISORDERS

Only a limited number of neurotoxins and the disorders that they produce can be discussed in the space available here, and readers seeking more specialized information should consult standard textbooks or compendia on neurotoxicology.

Organic Solvents

Organic solvents, either individually or in combinations, are widely used in the workplace, for example, as cleaners, degreasers, and thinners, and in manufacturing other chemicals. Most are highly volatile liquids. Accordingly, exposure occurs primarily by inhalation, so the risk of toxicity is greatest in poorly ventilated areas. Some absorption also takes place through the skin, especially of those solvents that are both lipid and water soluble and are somewhat less volatile.

Ridgway and co-workers assessed the published evidence that industrial organic solvents as a generic group can induce long-term neurologic damage detectable by brain imaging, neurophysiologic testing, or postmortem studies of exposed workers.[6] Some of the studies provided evidence for marginal atrophic abnormalities in the brain or deficits in nerve conduction velocity in solvent-exposed workers. However, methodologic limitations, absence of a consistently strong association between exposure and effect, lack of a dose–response relationship, the nonspecific nature of the reported changes, and the lack of coherence between the human and experimental animal data were problematic. Overall they were unable to draw reliable conclusions with respect to the presence or absence of nervous system damage related to the common properties of organic solvents.

Central Effects

Most organic solvents have high lipid solubility, so that they rapidly enter the brain and act as nonspecific depressants of the CNS. Acute exposure can cause the syndrome of acute encephalopathy described earlier. The exposed individual must be removed from exposure; recovery after mild exposure occurs rapidly (minutes to hours), usually without sequelae, although headache may continue for longer. When exposure has led to coma, however, recovery may be incomplete, perhaps because of hypoxic brain damage.

Several epidemiologic studies have suggested that neuropsychologic dysfunction has an increased prevalence in spray painters, who are chronically exposed to solvents used as thinners. Both level and duration of exposure may be important in its development. Using sophisticated imaging techniques, pronounced disturbances within the frontostriatothalamic circuitry were found in subjects with *painters' encephalopathy* and in asymptomatic but exposed house painters, and related to the clinical findings and to exposure severity to solvents.[7] However, it is unclear whether the entity of painters' encephalopathy truly exists, because it is based on studies, mainly from the 1970s, which are so methodologically flawed that they are invalid.[8–11] These studies were primarily epidemiologic in nature. Objections to them include concerns about the manner in which neuropsychologic tests were conducted and that other factors (such as alcohol, medications, or the residual effect of acute solvent exposure) may have caused the encephalopathic features ascribed to chronic exposure. Details concerning work conditions and extent of solvent exposure were often not provided or based on subjective recall. Some studies failed to allow for the influence of various confounding factors on neuropsychologic test results. In others, inappropriate controls may have confounded any comparisons that were made. This is well exemplified by the study of Gade and co-workers, in which 20 solvent-exposed workers, mostly painters, were re-examined 2 years after the diagnosis of chronic toxic encephalopathy was made.[12] Neuropsychologic test results were unchanged, but the earlier impression of significant cognitive decline was not confirmed when comparison was now made to a non-exposed control group and allowance was made for age, educational background, and level of intelligence.

Nevertheless, the concept of painters' encephalopathy has come to be accepted by many authorities even though no scientific consensus has been reached to establish it as a diagnosable disorder.[13] It appears to be nonprogressive, with no deterioration of functioning—or, in some cases, improvement—occurring after diagnosis, presumably because of cessation of exposure.[14] If such a syndrome of chronic painters' encephalopathy exists, it may have been caused by toluene, as most subjects were exposed to solvent mixtures, often of unknown composition, and toluene is a common constituent of such mixtures.

Chronic abuse of toluene in large doses taken for recreational purposes may cause dementia, ataxia, dysarthria, nystagmus, tremor, and spasticity.[15] Magnetic resonance imaging (MRI) shows diffuse cerebral and cerebellar atrophy and widespread periventricular white matter lesions. Brainstem auditory evoked potentials (BAEPs) may be abnormal, even in the absence of clinical or neuroimaging abnormalities, suggesting that the BAEP may be useful for screening at-risk workers.[15] A similar syndrome has not been seen with occupational exposure, perhaps because of the prolonged exposure to very large doses during abuse, but contamination of the solvents with other toxins or the concomitant use of other chemicals and drugs may also be relevant.

A more persuasive example of toxic encephalopathy with chronic exposure to organic solvents is the chronic encephalopathy that follows long-term exposure to carbon disulfide, used to manufacture cellophane and rayon.[16]

Peripheral Neuropathy

Relatively few organic solvents or solvent mixtures used industrially are known to be toxic to peripheral nerves. Discussion here focuses on *n*-hexane and methyl *n*-butyl ketone (MnBK) because the use of these hexacarbons has led to several outbreaks of neuropathy. Their metabolite, 2,5-hexanedione, is primarily responsible for the distal axonopathy that occurs with repeated and prolonged exposure to *n*-hexane. Methyl ethyl ketone, a common constituent of organic solvent mixtures, potentiates the neurotoxic properties of *n*-hexane and MnBK.

Onset is typically insidious and progression occurs slowly. Numbness begins distally in the feet, spreading proximally with continuing exposure and then coming to involve the hands. Motor disturbances are less conspicuous but, in severe cases, mild footdrop and weakness of the intrinsic hand muscles develop. With recreational exposure, which is typically heavier than occupational exposure, more rapid progression occurs and symptoms may be more extensive and severe. Examination shows significant cutaneous sensory deficits, and loss or attenuation of muscle stretch reflexes, especially distally. Gradual improvement (by axonal regeneration) eventually follows cessation of exposure, but coasting may occur for a period of several weeks.

Electrodiagnostic screening is useful in the detection of subclinical hexacarbon neuropathy. In a major outbreak of MnBK neuropathy in Ohio, 43 percent of cases had characteristic electrophysiologic abnormalities in the absence of symptoms and signs of neuropathy.[17] Needle electromyography usually showed signs of active denervation in distal leg muscles, and motor conduction velocity was slowed. Pathologically, the neuropathy is characterized by defective axonal transport, axonal degeneration, and secondary demyelination. Such changes may be seen on sural nerve biopsy and are also present at autopsy in the distal (i.e., most rostral) portion of the sensory axons in the posterior columns of the spinal cord.

A distal axonopathy can also result from exposure to trichloroethylene, which has been used as a degreaser. It is confined to the cranial nerves, initially the trigeminal nerve, with early onset of facial numbness, analgesia, or dysesthesias and later weakness of the masticatory muscles. The lower cranial nerves are involved in some patients; optic neuropathy (with an enlarged blind spot, paracentral scotoma, or constricted fields) has also been described. Recovery occurs with time after discontinuation of exposure, but patchy facial sensory loss may persist indefinitely. The neuropathy has been attributed to dichloroacetylene, which is formed by decomposition when trichloroethylene is exposed to alkalis.

Heavy Metals

Heavy metals accumulate, especially in bone, during lengthy periods of low-level exposure, as in the workplace, and it may take years to eliminate them from the body. Heavy metals are neurotoxic but also have other effects, particularly on the hematopoietic and gastrointestinal systems. The present discussion focuses on lead and arsenic, as exposure to these is most likely to occur, on mercury because of the large outbreaks that have occurred in the past (to environmental rather than occupational exposure), and on manganese because of suggestions that it may be a cause of classic Parkinson disease.

Lead

Industrial exposure is mainly to inorganic lead and occurs by inhalation of fine particulate matter; lead may also be absorbed after ingestion, as occurs in children. Occupational exposure occurs in the construction industry as well as in various other industrial settings (such as lead production or smelting; scrap metal handling; battery manufacturing; lead and other metal foundries; lead soldering; metal radiator repair; firing ranges; and ceramics or plastics manufacturing). Lead is taken up into bone and then slowly released into the blood over many years and excreted primarily through the urine, with smaller amounts in feces, hair, nails, and sweat. There is increasing concern about the health effects of lead at blood levels once thought to be harmless.[18] For example, a causal relationship of lead exposure to hypertension has been suggested, with implications for stroke prevention,[19] as has an association of blood lead levels with declining cognitive function.[20] Recent studies have led to a reappraisal of the levels of lead exposure that may be safely tolerated in the workplace.[18] It is important that workers are in well-ventilated premises; wear appropriate personal protective equipment such as goggles, boots, special clothing, and proper respiratory protection; shower after work; and undergo routine determination of blood lead level.

Lead Encephalopathy

Acute occupational exposure to lead results mainly in systemic effects involving the hematopoietic, gastrointestinal, and renal systems, rather than the nervous system. An acute lead encephalopathy, resulting from increasing cerebral edema, tends to occur in children rather than exposed workers and is therefore not considered further here. A chronic encephalopathy may follow long-term exposure to low levels of lead,[21] and progressive cerebral atrophy can occur long after further exposure is prevented.[22–24] Symptoms may include apathy, fatigue, insomnia, reduced libido, headache, irritability, memory loss, and difficulty in concentration; testing reveals neuropsychologic and neurophysiologic abnormalities.

Lead Neuropathy

Chronic exposure (i.e., for several years) to lead causes neuropathy. In one study, the average duration of exposure in subjects with lead neuropathy was almost 22 years.[25,26] Nerve conduction slowing may occur earlier, increasing with duration of exposure and blood lead levels, but whether these neurophysiologic changes progress to overt neuropathy is unclear.

Lead neuropathy, when it develops subacutely, is unusual in that it is predominantly motor, often asymmetric, and affects the arms more than the legs, and the wrist and finger extensors more than other muscles. Wrist drop is characteristic. This form of neuropathy typically develops after a relatively short period of intense exposure.[25,26] A more typical toxic neuropathy, with distal sensory impairment and weakness, may also occur, however, especially after prolonged exposure.[25,26] Individuals with lead neuropathy generally have a microcytic, hypochromic anemia; basophilic stippling of red blood cells is not always present and is not specific for lead poisoning. In patients with continuing exposure to lead, neuropathy is unlikely if the urinary δ-aminolevulinic acid (δALA) is normal. Lead interferes with hemoglobin synthesis by inhibiting the enzyme δALA dehydrase, and the enzyme substrate begins to appear in the urine when the blood lead level reaches 40 to 50 μg/dl, which is less than the level at which neuropathy usually results. An increased blood lead level or increased 24-hour urinary excretion should also be present in patients with suspected lead neuropathy, provided that exposure to lead is ongoing. A 24-hour urinary excretion of lead exceeding 2 mg after an intravenous dose of the chelator ethylenediamine tetra-acetic acid (EDTA) helps to confirm the diagnosis and distinguish it from porphyria. Past excessive exposure to lead can be measured through its accumulation in teeth or bones, but this is seldom practical.

The pathophysiologic basis of lead neuropathy in humans is unknown. There are species differences in the effects of lead on the nervous system. The early development of slowed conduction velocity suggests that the primary pathologic process is demyelination, but in established neuropathy the predominant abnormality is axonal degeneration.[26]

Management involves removal of the individual from the toxic environment to prevent further exposure. Workers exposed to lead occupationally should undergo regular determination of the blood lead level, and exposure terminated in those with an increased level before neuropathy develops. The blood lead level reflects the amount of lead in the blood and soft tissues but does not indicate either previous or current exposure, or total body burden.[27] National and state guidelines indicate surveillance requirements (including blood level monitoring requirements) for at-risk workers, such as those of the California Department of Public Health Occupational Lead Poisoning Prevention Program.[28] Based on a literature review and their own experience in evaluating lead-exposed adults, Kosnett and colleagues recommended in 2007 that subjects should be removed from occupational lead exposure if a single blood lead level exceeds 30 μg/dl or two successive blood lead levels measured over a 4-week interval exceed 19 μg/dl.[18] Removal of individuals from lead exposure should be considered to avoid long-term risk to health if exposure control measures over an extended period do not decrease blood lead concentrations to less than 10 μg/dl or if selected medical conditions exist that would increase the risk of continued exposure. They recommended that medical surveillance for all lead-exposed workers should include quarterly blood lead measurements for individuals with blood lead concentrations between 10 and 19 μg/dl and semi-annual blood lead measurements when sustained blood lead concentrations are less than 10 μg/dl.

It is unclear whether chelation therapy, which accelerates removal of lead from the blood and soft tissues (but less so from bone), benefits the clinical neuropathy.[26,29] Clinical trials are lacking. Guidelines are controversial and liable to change. One therapeutic approach has been with EDTA (with or without dimercaprol) followed by oral penicillamine; another oral agent, 2,3-dimercaptosuccinic acid (DMSA; succimer), seems equally effective and can be used alone or after EDTA.[30,31] Regardless of the treatment chosen, it should be continued until a steady-state level of lead excretion has been achieved. In patients with large lead stores in bone, chelation may be followed by movement of lead from bone back into the blood and soft tissues, leading to a rebound increase in blood lead level after an initial drop. Chelation therapy is not appropriate for workers with continuing lead exposure as prophylaxis against rising blood lead levels.[32]

ARSENIC

Arsenic intoxication may occur occupationally but more commonly by ingestion of contaminated food or water. It may relate to attempted homicide. Occupational exposures may occur in the manufacture of paints, fungicides, wood preservatives, and semiconductors; in certain mining and smelting operations; from combustion of arsenic-containing coal or incineration of certain preserved wood products; and in pesticide spraying. A hemorrhagic encephalopathy and various systemic effects (including QTc prolongation on the electrocardiogram and subsequent ventricular tachycardias) occur with acute intoxication; the role of arsenic in the development of a chronic encephalopathy is controversial. Arsenic leads to a peripheral neuropathy that is a predominantly sensory, distal axonopathy and occurs after exposure to high levels of arsenic, usually by ingestion with suicidal or homicidal intent, or after long-duration low-level exposure.[33] Chronic exposure is associated also with an increased risk of skin and various other cancers. Acute intoxication leads to prominent gastrointestinal symptoms followed, after 1 to 3 weeks, by the onset of neuropathy. Numbness, burning, and paresthesias begin in the feet and spread to the legs, hands, and arms. Pain is sometimes prominent. Sensory ataxia occurs in severe cases. Weakness is usually mild and overshadowed by the sensory disturbances, but marked weakness and respiratory insufficiency may occur with severe intoxication. Autonomic instability is usually a minor feature. Examination confirms that there is symmetrical, distally conspicuous sensory loss and weakness.

Other toxic effects of arsenic accompany the neuropathy and include hyperkeratosis and desquamation of the skin, particularly in the palms (Fig. 35-1) and soles; redness and swelling of the hands and feet; patchy areas of skin discoloration with chronic intoxication; and, particularly with acute poisoning, transverse gray lines in the nails (Mees lines; Fig. 35-2). Kidney failure may occur. Anemia is common, and red blood cells may show basophilic stippling.

An acutely evolving neuropathy may be misdiagnosed as Guillain–Barré syndrome, especially if the initial gastrointestinal symptoms are mistaken for a prodromal illness and the cerebrospinal fluid shows an albuminocytologic dissociation, as sometimes occurs in early arsenic neuropathy.[34] The electrodiagnostic findings may also resemble those of Guillain–Barré syndrome because the underlying axonal degeneration is accompanied by proximal demyelination. The diagnosis requires the demonstration of arsenic in blood, urine, or tissues. Measurement of blood levels is usually diagnostically unhelpful because arsenic is cleared very rapidly, but urinary excretion is increased for weeks. The most reliable means of monitoring exposure in at-risk occupations is by determining the 24-hour urinary arsenic level, which should be determined after subjects have abstained from eating fish, seaweed, or shellfish for 48 to 72 hours. Arsenic is cleared from blood into tissues; for example, it comes to be bound to keratin of growing hair or

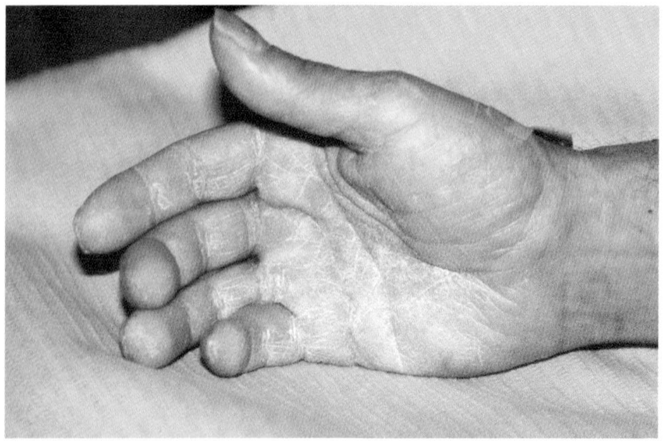

FIGURE 35-1 ■ Hyperkeratosis and desquamation of the skin of the palms of the hands from arsenic toxicity. (Courtesy of J. Richard Baringer, MD, University of Utah.)

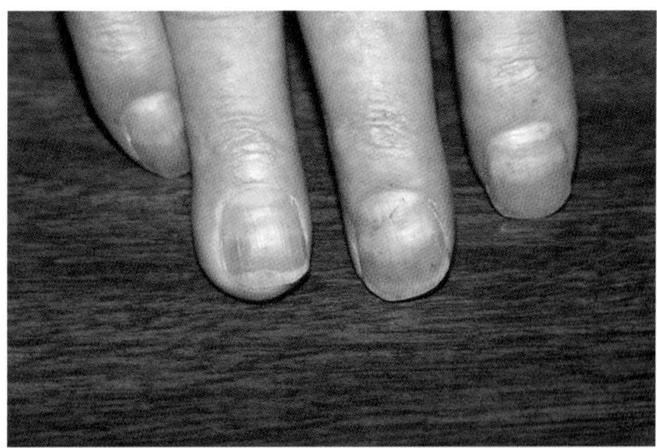

FIGURE 35-2 ■ Transverse gray lines in the nails (Mees lines) related to arsenic toxicity. (Courtesy of J. Richard Baringer, MD, University of Utah.)

nails and may be found in slow-growing hair, such as pubic or axillary hair, for months or even years after exposure. This is important when exposure is not suspected until long after the event. The results of such analyses when performed in commercial laboratories, however, are often quite inaccurate.[35]

Treatment consists of removing the subject from further exposure. Removal of clothing and cleaning the skin and hair to prevent further contamination is particularly important in those exposed to pesticides. Chelation therapy hastens the excretion of arsenic,[36] but there is no evidence that it increases the rate of recovery from neuropathy, which takes months to years. There is little evidence to recommend a specific chelating regimen.[36] Patients with mild neuropathy may recover completely, but those with a severe neuropathy are likely to have a residual deficit.

MERCURY

Both organic and inorganic mercury may cause toxicity. Ingestion of methyl mercury in contaminated food such as fish leads to optic neuropathy, hearing loss, cerebellar deficits, and cognitive or behavioral changes. There are also prominent sensory abnormalities that are probably also central in origin.

Inorganic mercury is mainly absorbed by inhalation during smelting, which is the major means of occupational exposure. Occupational exposure also occurs in chloralkali plants, during mining operations,[37] during the manufacture of medical appliances, glassware and jewelry, and in dental offices during the preparation of fillings. Neurotoxicity is common in the workplace with exposure to mercury vapour levels exceeding 50 µg Hg/m^3.[3,38,39] It can manifest as a toxic encephalopathy. The past use of mercury in felt hat production led to many symptoms of high-level mercury neurotoxicity, and thus to the popular phrase "mad as a hatter." Signs include irritability, anxiety, agitation, social withdrawal, and insomnia; continuing exposure leads to development of a fine tremor of the hands ("hatter's shakes") and then of the facial muscles and tongue. Clinical and quantitative methods have been used to assess the tremor.[40] In mild cases, encephalopathy and tremor improve gradually over several years once exposure is discontinued. Peripheral neuropathy resembling an inflammatory polyneuropathy has also been attributed to exposure to both forms of mercury, but with only limited supportive evidence. The neuropathy may still be detected many years after the end of exposure, depending on its severity.[41]

MANGANESE

Inhalation of dust or vapor during the mining or smelting of manganese may lead to intoxication. Occupational exposure also occurs in manganese alloy producers, cell-battery factory workers, and farmers using manganese-containing fungicides.[42] As much of the dietary intake of manganese is cleared by the liver, liver failure[43] or even asymptomatic hepatitis may precipitate manganese neurotoxicity in exposed workers.[44] The earliest manifestation is a toxic psychosis, with behavioral and cognitive abnormalities; headache, dysarthria, tremor, and incoordination may develop later. Extrapyramidal changes, with dystonia (such as involuntary plantar flexion of the feet) or parkinsonism (abnormalities of gait and balance, bradykinesia, rigidity, rest and action tremor, hypomimia) may eventually develop. After exposure is terminated, early behavioral changes may stabilize and reverse, but extrapyramidal deficits may continue to progress for several years before reaching a plateau.[45]

MRI, positron emission tomography (PET) and single-photon emission computed tomography (SPECT) have been used to study manganese-induced parkinsonism.[46] T1-weighted MRI (Fig. 35-3) shows increased signal intensity in the globus pallidus and midbrain bilaterally in exposed workers who are either asymptomatic or have signs of manganese intoxication. [^{18}F]dopa PET and

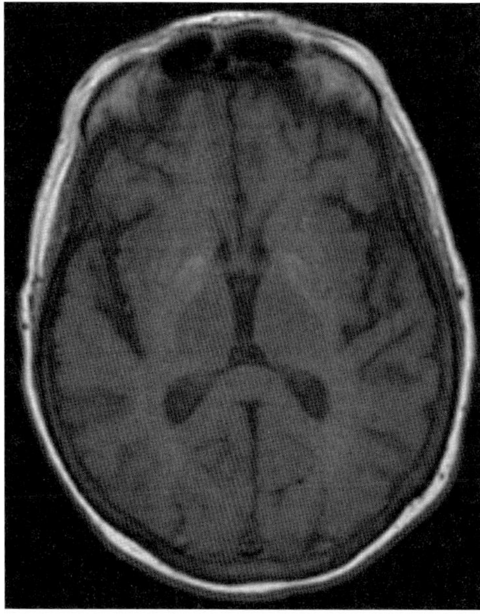

FIGURE 35-3 ■ Bilateral globus pallidus hyperintensity in T1-weighted axial MRI suggestive of manganese accumulation. (Courtesy of William P. Dillon, MD, University of California, San Francisco.)

SPECT are normal, indicating the integrity of the nigrostriatal dopaminergic system.[47] Thus, the damage in manganese toxicity is presumably downstream of the nigrostriatal system, and this would account for the poor response to levodopa in such patients.[48]

Manganese-induced parkinsonism is distinguished from classic Parkinson disease by the history of manganese exposure, usually symmetric clinical features, neuroimaging findings (abnormal T1-weighted MRI and normal fluorodopa PET and SPECT scans), and poor response to levodopa.[49,50] There are also pathologic differences at autopsy.[49] Exposure to manganese in low dose, as in welders,[51] has been incriminated as a risk factor for the early onset of Parkinson disease,[52] but no relationship between welding and Parkinson disease could be identified in other studies.[53,54]

Organophosphate and Carbamate Pesticides

Organophosphates and carbamates are used as pesticides or herbicides, and some organophosphates have also been used for terrorism or as warfare agents. Inhibition of acetylcholinesterase (AChE) accounts for their early acute toxicity, and inhibition of neuropathy target esterase (NTE) relates to the delayed neuropathy that occurs after exposure to some of them. Although inhibition of NTE is necessary for the development of peripheral neurotoxicity, not all organophosphates that inhibit NTE cause neuropathy; other factors are also involved. Different organophosphates have differing potencies against these enzymes, although almost all have some anticholinesterase effects. Most organophosphates and carbamates are readily absorbed transdermally during and after spraying, as well as by inhalation and ingestion.

Early (Type I) Syndrome

The earliest manifestations represent inhibition of AChE at CNS cholinergic and postganglionic parasympathetic receptors (Table 35-2).[55] The CNS effects are characterized by behavioral changes, mainly agitation, and may progress to convulsions, obtundation, and even coma, which sometimes has a delayed onset. Life-threatening peripheral muscarinic effects include bradycardia and hypotension, or even complete cardiovascular collapse. Bronchospasm, increased secretions, and pulmonary edema can occur. Less threatening peripheral muscarinic effects include meiosis, diarrhea, urinary urgency or incontinence, and increased salivation, lacrimation, and sweating. Muscle fasciculations and weakness reflect nicotinic (neuromuscular junction) effects. In severe intoxication, death occurs from respiratory failure or cardiac arrhythmias. The cholinergic effects of organophosphate poisoning usually begin within hours of exposure. AChE inhibition by carbamates is reversible, and symptoms and signs of carbamate toxicity are generally less severe and of shorter duration than with organophosphate poisoning.

Diagnosis is clinical and is suggested by signs of cholinergic overactivity. Electrodiagnostic studies

TABLE 35-2 ■ Effects of Organophosphate Poisoning

Muscarinic Effects
Respiratory
Smooth muscle (contraction): bronchoconstriction; dyspnea
Glandular secretions (increased): bronchorrhea; pulmonary edema
Multifactorial: cough; dyspnea
Cardiac
Conducting system: bradycardia; arrhythmias; heart block
Gastrointestinal
Smooth muscle (contraction): nausea; vomiting; abdominal cramps; diarrhea
Secretions (increased): nausea; vomiting; diarrhea
Sphincter (relaxation): fecal incontinence
Urinary bladder
Contraction: frequency; urgency
Sphincter (relaxation): urgency; incontinence
Eye
Contraction of iris and ciliary muscle: meiosis; blurred vision
Other
Secretions (increased): sweating; salivation; lacrimation
Nicotinic Effects
Skeletal muscle
Excitation: fasciculations; cramps; followed by weakness, paralysis; areflexia
CNS Effects
Excitation: agitation; headache; ataxia; confusion; delirium; behavioral abnormalities; convulsions
Depression: obtundation; coma; respiratory depression

initially reveal repetitive firing of the compound muscle action potential after a single stimulus to the motor nerve, and later a decremental muscle response to repetitive nerve stimulation.[56] Measurement of AChE activity in plasma or red blood cells to confirm suspected intoxication or to monitor exposed subjects is of dubious value.[57]

Prompt treatment is essential. Atropine blocks the binding of acetylcholine to muscarinic receptors; a test dose of 0.5 mg intravenously causes tachycardia and mydriasis in normal subjects but has little effect in organophosphate-intoxicated subjects. After this, 1 mg is administered intravenously and repeated every 10 to 20 minutes until clinical evidence of atropinization is achieved, and then maintained for 24 to 48 hours. In severe cases, continuous intravenous infusion of atropine is required. Patients should be managed in the intensive care unit because atropine can precipitate cardiac arrhythmias, especially in the setting of hypoxemia. Atropine has no effect on nicotinic neuromuscular receptors and thus fails to help any weakness or respiratory impairment, and similarly does not influence the CNS effects (agitation and convulsions).

Reactivators of phosphorylated AChE, such as pralidoxime, are also utilized in organophosphate poisoning, but are of uncertain benefit. Effectiveness is independent of receptor type. The complex that forms between the organophosphate and cholinesterase is initially reversible, but subsequently configurational changes occur, and pralidoxime is then ineffective.[58] Treatment is started early with pralidoxime (1 g) intravenously; in the absence of improvement, the dose is repeated after 30 minutes or continuous infusion is commenced at 0.5 g/hour. Treatment with oxime is not necessary for carbamate poisoning, because spontaneous reactivation of AChE occurs rapidly. Diazepam and supportive therapy (such as with anticonvulsants and artificial ventilation) are important.

Prognosis depends on the severity of poisoning and on how it is managed. Neurobehavioral sequelae unrelated to structural brain damage have been noted after recovery from acute poisoning.[59,60] It is unclear whether long-term low-level exposures to anticholinesterases have neurologic or behavioral consequences.[61–63]

Intermediate (Type II) Syndrome

This occurs a few days after exposure in up to 50 percent of cases of severe organophosphate poisoning. Its pathogenesis is unknown, but does not relate directly to AChE inhibition and it does not respond to atropine or pralidoxime. Presentation is with acute respiratory failure, weakness of neck flexors and proximal limb muscles, and cranial neuropathies. An acute, reversible extrapyramidal disorder has also been attributed to organophosphate poisoning following massive exposure.[64] Treatment is supportive. Recovery may take several weeks.

Delayed Syndrome: Polyneuropathy

Certain organophosphates cause a distal, predominantly motor, subacute axonal neuropathy that manifests about 1 to 3 weeks after exposure. With those insecticides currently in use, the neuropathy follows an episode of severe cholinergic toxicity.[65,66] It is unclear whether neuropathy also follows severe carbamate intoxication.[67] The neuropathy relates to inhibition of NTE, followed by "aging" of the phosphoryl–NTE complex, but how this leads to development of the neuropathy is unknown.

The usual initial symptoms are of cramping muscle pain in the calves, followed by distal paresthesias in the feet. Lower-extremity weakness and areflexia then occur, beginning distally and speading proximally. The upper limbs are involved in severe cases, but the cranial nerves are not affected. Progression occurs over 2 or 3 weeks, followed by gradual improvement. CNS involvement is common after severe exposure but is obscured initially by the peripheral neuropathy; spasticity and ataxia become apparent as the neuropathy improves. Organophosphate toxicity should be considered in any subacute, progressive distal axonopathy even in the absence of a history of exposure. The electrodiagnostic findings are abnormal but nonspecific. There is no specific treatment.

There is no evidence that long-term low-level exposure to organophosphates causes this or any other type of neuropathy.[62]

Organochlorine and Pyrethroid Insecticides

Dichlorodiphenyltrichlorethane (DDT) and various organochlorines, such as aldrin, dieldrin, and lindane, were previously used widely as insecticides. Because of their slow degradation, they persist for long periods in animals and the environment. Their use is now banned. Decline in neurobehavioral functioning and increase of neuropsychologic and psychiatric symptoms have been reported in retired DDT workers.[68] Cognitive performance deteriorated with increasing duration of exposure to DDT. Although such data suggest that exposure to DDT may be associated with permanent decline in neurobehavioral functioning, the limited number of studies and uncertainties about exposure levels prevent a firm conclusion from being drawn.[69] Because organochlorine pesticides are potent tremor-producing agents, exposure to DDT, dieldrin, and certain other chlorinated hydrocarbons was examined as a possible etiologic factor for the development of essential tremor, but no association was found.[70] Similarly, studies in animals have failed to show any effect of DDT or dieldrin on the nigrostriatal system, making unlikely a relationship between exposure to these insecticide and development of Parkinson disease.[71]

Chlordecone, another persistent chlorinated hydrocarbon, was involved in a major industrial exposure and environmental contamination in the 1970s from a manufacturing plant in Hopewell, Virginia. Some workers developed a neurologic illness from dust inhalation, characterized by opsoclonus, postural and intention tremor, clumsiness, and mild gait ataxia. Benign intracranial hypertension occurred in a few cases. Recovery occurred slowly over several years and was sometimes incomplete.[72] Use of chlordecone is now banned.

Pyrethrins are now preferred over organophosphates or organochlorines as pesticides because of their biodegradability. They occur in the seed cases of the perennial plant pyrethrum, and have been synthesized to produce the pyrethroid insecticides. DDT, the pyrethrins, and the synthetic pyrethroids (which account for about 20 percent of the world insecticide market) act on the voltage-gated sodium channel proteins of insect neuronal membranes. Transmission of nerve impulses is disrupted by binding of the insecticides, leading to paralysis and eventual death.

Occupational exposure to pyrethroids occurs primarily through the skin but sometimes by inhalation, in professional sprayers for agricultural purposes or to control vector-borne diseases. Reports of human poisoning are relatively few.[73] Pyrethroid toxicity in humans causes paresthesias affecting the face and hands. This has been attributed to an effect on voltage-dependent sodium channels, resulting in prolonged inward sodium currents leading to repetitive firing and subsequently to membrane depolarization.[74] There is no correlation between the occurrence of paresthesias and urinary excretion of pyrethroids or their metabolites. Paresthesias generally disappear within 24 hours and there is no specific treatment. Other common symptoms are "dizziness," headache, and fatigue; palpitations, chest tightness and blurred vision are less frequent.[73] Coma and convulsions occur in rare instances and may then be life-threatening.

A slowly progressive motor neuron disease simulating amyotrophic lateral sclerosis has been reported after heavy and prolonged exposure to various pyrethroids,[75] but further studies of this association are required before any conclusions can be reached about its significance.

Pesticides, Herbicides, and Parkinsonism

The pathogenesis of Parkinson disease probably involves both genetic and environmental factors. Case-control studies in humans have related parkinsonism to farming, rural living and well-water consumption.[76] Pesticide exposure is one risk factor for developing the disease, but it is difficult to expand on this effect. Exposures typically occur many years before the development of clinical parkinsonism, probably involve several pesticides that may have had additive effects, and often are of unknown duration and severity.[77] Genetic factors may affect the response to environmental factors.[78] Furthermore, toxin-mediated effects may remain clinically silent until normal age-related dopaminergic cell loss reaches a certain critical level, accounting for the delay between exposure and clinical disease.

Parkinsonism has developed in humans who took methylphenyl tetrahydropyridine (MPTP) for recreational purposes. MPTP is converted in the body to methylphenyl pyridinium (MPP), which causes selective degeneration of the dopaminergic nigrostriatal system involved in the genesis of the motor deficits of parkinsonism. MPP structurally resembles paraquat, a herbicide. New models of selective nigrostriatal damage, such as neurotoxicity induced by the pesticides rotenone and paraquat, indicate that these environmental agents may indeed contribute to the neurodegenerative process in parkinsonism.[77] Mitochondrial complex I activity is reduced in Parkinson disease; MPP inhibits mitochondrial complex I, as does rotenone. Epidemiologic studies have found an association of Parkinson disease with pesticide exposure, depending on duration of exposure.[79–81] Petrovitch and colleagues undertook a prospective cohort study with 30-year follow up of Hawaiian plantation workers, and found a relative risk of Parkinson disease of 1.0, 1.7 and 1.9 for those who had worked on the plantation for 1 to 10, 11 to 20, and more than 20 years, respectively, compared to those who had never done plantation work.[81] Participants were exposed to pesticides but also to many other substances, and the findings from this study cannot determine which exposures influenced the development of parkinsonism. In Taiwan, a history of rural living, farming, use of herbicides/pesticides, and use of paraquat were associated with an increased risk of parkinsonism in a dose–response manner. After adjustment for multiple risk factors, the relationship between Parkinson disease and previous use of herbicides/pesticides and paraquat remained significant, the risk being greater among subjects who had used paraquat plus other herbicides/pesticides rather than in those who had not used paraquat.[79] The risk of developing Parkinson disease was increased more than six times in those exposed for more than 20 years to paraquat.[79]

At the present time, then, it seems that exposure to certain pesticides increases the risk of developing Parkinson disease, but the precise mechanisms and pesticides involved are not known and probably vary depending on genetic and other factors. By assessing lifetime use of pesticides selected by mechanism in a case-control study, however, Parkinson disease was associated with use of pesticides that inhibit mitochondrial complex I, including rotenone, and with use of pesticides causing oxidative stress, including paraquat.[82]

CONCLUDING COMMENTS

Most physicians have only limited experience of occupationally related neurotoxic disorders, even though the majority of patients with such disorders come under the care of neurologists, primary care physicians, or internists, at least at some point during the course of their disorder. It is therefore important that physicians become and remain sensitive to the possibility that their patients may have diseases induced by toxic exposures occurring at work. Unfortunately, there remains a shortage of physicians with expertise in occupational medicine who can act as clinical or educational resources, and this shortage has proved difficult to remedy. The emphasis has moved to the prevention of occupationally related disorders. In the United States, federal and state legislation regulates and enforces comprehensive safety and health programs in the workplace and also provides for various informational and educational services to improve occupational safety. Nevertheless, physicians must be aware of the basic principles of occupational medicine and understand how to screen for possible neurotoxic disorders, as well as the limitations of the screening process. They must also know the implications of making such diagnoses, understand their responsibilities within the framework of any local or national workers' compensation system, and be aware of any requirements to alert health or regulatory agencies to suspected occupationally related neurotoxic disorders.

REFERENCES

1. Parry GJ: Neurological complications of toxin exposure in the workplace. p. 749. In Aminoff MJ (ed): Neurology and General Medicine. 4th Ed. Elsevier, Philadelphia, 2008.
2. Becker CE, Lash A: Detecting subtle human CNS dysfunction: challenge for toxicologists in the 1990's. J Toxicol Clin Toxicol 28:7, 1990.
3. Aminoff MJ, Lotti M: Neurotoxic effects of workplace exposures. p. 1151. In: Baxter PJ, Aw T-C, Cockcroft A (eds): Hunter's Diseases of Occupations. 10th Ed. Hodder Arnold, London, 2010.
4. Aminoff MJ, Albers JW: Electrophysiologic techniques in the evaluation of patients with suspected neurotoxic disorders. p. 813. In Aminoff MJ (ed): Aminoff's Electrodiagnosis in Clinical Neurology. 6th Ed. Elsevier, London, 2012.
5. Singer R: Neuropsychological assessment of toxic exposures. p. 357. In Horton Jr AM, Wedding D, Webster J (eds): The Neuropsychology Handbook Vol 2. 2nd Ed. Springer, New York, 1997.
6. Ridgway P, Nixon TE, Leach JP: Occupational exposure to organic solvents and long-term nervous system damage detectable by brain imaging, neurophysiology or histopathology. Food Chem Toxicol 41:153, 2003.
7. Visser I, Lavini C, Booij J, et al: Cerebral impairment in chronic solvent-induced encephalopathy. Ann Neurol 63:572, 2008.
8. Van Hout MS, Schmand B, Wekking EM, et al: Suboptimal performance on neuropsychological testing in patients with suspected chronic toxic encephalopathy. Neurotoxicology 24:547, 2003.
9. Van Hout MS, Schmand B, Wekking EM, et al: Cognitive functioning in patients with suspected chronic toxic encephalopathy: evidence for neuropsychological

disturbances after controlling for insufficient effort. J Neurol Neurosurg Psychiatry 77:296, 2006.

10. Errebo-Knudsen EO, Olsen F: Organic solvents and presenile dementia (the painters' syndrome). A critical review of the Danish literature. Sci Total Environ 48:45, 1986.
11. Lees-Haley PR, Williams CW: Neurotoxicity of chronic low-dose exposure to organic solvents: a skeptical review. J Clin Psychol 53:699, 1997.
12. Gade A, Mortensen EL, Bruhn P: 'Chronic painter's syndrome'. A reanalysis of psychological test data in a group of diagnosed cases, based on comparisons with matched controls. Acta Neurol Scand 77:293, 1988.
13. Albers JW, Berent S: Controversies in neurotoxicology: current status. Neurol Clin 18:741, 2000.
14. van Valen E, Wekking E, van der Laan G, et al: The course of chronic solvent induced encephalopathy: a systematic review. Neurotoxicology 30:1172, 2009.
15. Filley CM, Halliday W, Kleinschmidt-DeMasters BK: The effects of toluene on the central nervous system. J Neuropathol Exp Neurol 63:1, 2004.
16. Aaserud O, Hommeren OJ, Tvedt B, et al: Carbon disulfide exposure and neurotoxic sequelae among viscose rayon workers. Am J Ind Med 18:25, 1990.
17. Allen N, Mendell JR, Billmaier DJ, et al: Toxic polyneuropathy due to methyl n-butyl ketone: an industrial outbreak. Arch Neurol 32:209, 1975.
18. Kosnett MJ, Wedeen RP, Rothenberg SJ, et al: Recommendations for medical management of adult lead exposure. Environ Health Perspect 115:463, 2007.
19. Navas-Acien A, Guallar E, Silbergeld EK, et al: Lead exposure and cardiovascular disease–a systematic review. Environ Health Perspect 115:472, 2007.
20. Shih RA, Hu H, Weisskopf MG, et al: Cumulative lead dose and cognitive function in adults: a review of studies that measured both blood lead and bone lead. Environ Health Perspect 115:483, 2007.
21. Pasternak G, Becker CE, Lash A, et al: Cross-sectional neurotoxicology study of lead-exposed cohort. J Toxicol Clin Toxicol 27:37, 1989.
22. Schwartz BS, Stewart WF, Bolla KI, et al: Past adult lead exposure is associated with longitudinal decline in cognitive dysfunction. Neurology 55:1144, 2000.
23. Links JM, Schwartz BS, Simon D, et al: Characterization of toxicokinetics and toxicodynamics with linear systems theory: application to lead-associated cognitive decline. Environ Health Perspect 109:361, 2001.
24. Stewart WF, Schwartz BS, Davatzikos C, et al: Past adult lead exposure is linked to neurodegeneration measured by brain MRI. Neurology 66:1476, 2006.
25. Rubens O, Logina I, Kravale I, et al: Peripheral neuropathy in chronic occupational inorganic lead exposure: a clinical and electrophysiological study. J Neurol Neurosurg Psychiatry 71:200, 2001.
26. Thompson RM, Parry GJ: Neuropathies associated with excessive exposure to lead. Muscle Nerve 33:732, 2006.
27. Hu H, Shih R, Rothenberg S, et al: The epidemiology of lead toxicity in adults: measuring dose and consideration of other methodologic issues. Environ Health Perspect 115:455, 2007.
28. California Department of Public Health, Occupational lead Poisoning Prevention Program: Medical Guidelines for the Lead-Exposed Worker. California Department of Public Health, Richmond, CA, 2009.
29. Windebank AJ: Metal neuropathy. p. 1549. In: Dyck PJ, Thomas PK, Griffin JW (eds): Peripheral Neuropathy. 3rd Ed. WB Saunders, Philadelphia, 1993.
30. Porru S, Alessio L: The use of chelating agents in occupational lead poisoning. Occup Med 46:41, 1996.
31. Bradberry S, Sheehan T, Vale A: Use of oral dimercaptosuccinic acid (succimer) in adult patients with inorganic lead poisoning. QJM 102:721, 2009.
32. Royce S, Rosenberg J: Chelation therapy in workers with lead exposure. West J Med 158:372, 1993.
33. Lagerkvist BJ, Zetterlund B: Assessment of exposure to arsenic among smelter workers: a five-year follow-up. Am J Ind Med 25:477, 1994.
34. Windebank AJ: Arsenic. p. 203. In: Spencer PS, Schaumburg HH (eds): Experimental and Clinical Neurotoxicology. 2nd Ed. Oxford University Press, New York, 2000.
35. Seidel S, Kreutzer R, Smith D, et al: Assessment of commercial laboratories performing hair mineral analysis. JAMA 285:67, 2001.
36. Kalia K, Flora SJ: Strategies for safe and effective therapeutic measures for chronic arsenic and lead poisoning. J Occup Health 47:1, 2005.
37. Drake PL, Rojas M, Reh CM, et al: Occupational exposure to airborne mercury during gold mining operations near El Callao, Venezuela. Int Arch Occup Environ Health 74:206, 2001.
38. Magos L, Clarkson TW: Overview of the clinical toxicity of mercury. Ann Clin Biochem 43:257, 2006.
39. Clarkson TW, Magos L, Myers GJ: The toxicology of mercury—current exposures and clinical manifestations. N Engl J Med 349:1731, 2003.
40. Wastensson G, Lamoureux D, Sällsten G, et al: Quantitative tremor assessment in workers with current low exposure to mercury vapor. Neurotoxicol Teratol 28:681, 2006.
41. Albers JW, Kallenbach LR, Fine LJ, et al: Neurological abnormalities associated with remote occupational elemental mercury exposure. Ann Neurol 24:651, 1988.
42. Levy BS, Nassetta WJ: Neurologic effects of manganese in humans: a review. Int J Occup Environ Health 9:153, 2003.
43. Hauser RA, Zesiewicz TA, Rosemurgy AS, et al: Manganese intoxication and chronic liver failure. Ann Neurol 36:871, 1994.
44. Schaumburg HH, Herskovitz S, Cassano VA: Occupational manganese neurotoxicity provoked by hepatitis C. Neurology 67:322, 2006.

45. Huang CC, Chu NS, Lu CS, et al: The natural history of neurological manganism over 18 years. Parkinsonism Relat Disord 13:143, 2007.
46. Kim Y: Neuroimaging in manganism. Neurotoxicology 27:369, 2006.
47. Shinotoh H, Snow BJ, Chu NS, et al: Presynaptic and postsynaptic striatal dopaminergic function in patients with manganese intoxication: a positron emission tomography study. Neurology 48:1053, 1997.
48. Lu C, Huang C, Chu N, et al: Levodopa failure in chronic manganism. Neurology 44:1600, 1994.
49. Olanow CW: Manganese-induced parkinsonism and Parkinson's disease. Ann NY Acad Sci 1012:209, 2004.
50. Cersosimo MG, Koller WC: The diagnosis of manganese-induced parkinsonism. Neurotoxicology 27:340, 2006.
51. Racette BA, McGee-Minnich L, Moerlein SM, et al: Welding-related parkinsonism: clinical features, treatment, and pathophysiology. Neurology 56:8, 2001.
52. Racette BA, Tabbal SD, Jennings D, et al: Prevalence of parkinsonism and relationship to exposure in a large sample of Alabama welders. Neurology 64:230, 2005.
53. Fored CM, Fryzek JP, Brandt L, et al: Parkinson's disease and other basal ganglia or movement disorders in a large nationwide cohort of Swedish welders. Occup Environ Med 63:135, 2006.
54. Jankovic J: Searching for a relationship between manganese and welding and Parkinson's disease. Neurology 64:2021, 2005.
55. Costa LG: Current issues in organophosphate toxicology. Clin Chim Acta 366:1, 2006.
56. Besser R, Gutmann L, Dillmann U, et al: End-plate dysfunction in acute organophosphate intoxication. Neurology 39:561, 1989.
57. Lotti M: Cholinesterase inhibition: complexities in interpretation. Clin Chem 41:1814, 1995.
58. Lotti M: Organophosphorus compounds. p. 897. In: Spencer PS, Schaumburg HH (eds): Experimental and Clinical Neurotoxicology. 2nd Ed. Oxford University Press, New York, 2000.
59. Rosenstock L, Keifer M, Daniell WE, et al: Chronic central nervous system effects of acute organophosphate pesticide intoxication. The Pesticide Health Effects Study Group. Lancet 338:223, 1991.
60. Roldán-Tapia L, Leyva A, Laynez F, et al: Chronic neuropsychological sequelae of cholinesterase inhibitors in the absence of structural brain damage: two cases of acute poisoning. Environ Health Perspect 113:762, 2005.
61. Jamal GA, Hansen S, Julu PO: Low level exposures to organophosphorus esters may cause neurotoxicity. Toxicology 181:23, 2002.
62. Lotti M: Low-level exposures to organophosphorus esters and peripheral nerve function. Muscle Nerve 25:492, 2002.
63. Solomon C, Poole J, Palmer KT, et al: Neuropsychiatric symptoms in past users of sheep dip and other pesticides. Occup Environ Med 64:259, 2007.
64. Bhatt MH, Elias MA, Mankodi AK: Acute and reversible parkinsonism due to organophosphate intoxication: five cases. Neurology 52:1467, 1999.
65. Lotti M: Clinical toxicology of anticholinesterase agents in humans. p. 1043. In: Krieger RI, Doull J (eds): Handbook of Pesticide Toxicology. Academic Press, San Diego, 2001.
66. Lotti M, Moretto A: Organophosphate-induced delayed polyneuropathy. Toxicol Rev 24:37, 2005.
67. Lotti M, Moretto A: Do carbamates cause polyneuropathy? Muscle Nerve 34:499, 2006.
68. van Wendel de Joode B, Wesseling C, Kromhout H, et al: Chronic nervous-system effects of long-term occupational exposure to DDT. Lancet 357:1014, 2001.
69. Colosio C, Tiramani M, Maroni M: Neurobehavioral effects of pesticides: state of the art. Neurotoxicology 24:577, 2003.
70. Louis ED, Factor-Litvak P, Parides M, et al: Organochlorine pesticide exposure in essential tremor: a case-control study using biological and occupational exposure assessments. Neurotoxicology 27:579, 2006.
71. Hatcher JM, Delea KC, Richardson JR, et al: Disruption of dopamine transport by DDT and its metabolites. Neurotoxicology 29:682, 2008.
72. Taylor JR: Neurological manifestations in humans exposed to chlordecone: follow-up results. Neurotoxicology 6:231, 1985.
73. Bradberry SM, Cage SA, Proudfoot AT, et al: Poisoning due to pyrethroids. Toxicol Rev 24:93, 2005.
74. Ray DE, Fry JR: A reassessment of the neurotoxicity of pyrethroid insecticides. Pharmacol Ther 111:174, 2006.
75. Doi H, Kikuchi H, Murai H, et al: Motor neuron disorder simulating ALS induced by chronic inhalation of pyrethroid insecticides. Neurology 67:1894, 2006.
76. Priyadarshi A, Khuder SA, Schaub EA, et al: Environmental risk factors and Parkinson's disease: a metaanalysis. Environ Res 86:122, 2001.
77. DiMonte DA: The environment and Parkinson's disease: is the nigrostriatal system preferentially targeted by neurotoxins? Lancet Neurol 2:531, 2003.
78. Goldman SM, Kamel F, Ross GW, et al: Genetic modification of the association of paraquat and Parkinson's disease. Mov Disord 27:1652, 2012.
79. Liou HH, Tsai MC, Chen CJ, et al: Environmental risk factors and Parkinson's disease: a case–control study in Taiwan. Neurology 48:1583, 1997.
80. Gorell JM, Johnson CC, Rybicki BA, et al: The risk of Parkinson's disease with exposure to pesticides, farming, well water, and rural living. Neurology 50:1346, 1998.
81. Petrovitch H, Ross W, Abbott RD, et al: Plantation work and risk of Parkinson disease in a population-based longitudinal study. Arch Neurol 59:1787, 2002.
82. Tanner CM, Kamel F, Ross GW, et al: Rotenone, paraquat, and Parkinson's disease. Environ Health Perspect 119:866, 2011.

CHAPTER

36

Neurologic Complications of Thermal and Electric Burns

MARC D. WINKELMAN

Fires and burns are the fifth leading cause of accidental death in the United States. Each year 1.2 million people seek medical attention for a burn, 50,000 are hospitalized, and 3,900 die.[1] Serious neurologic complications can follow a severe burn. The complications of thermal burns differ considerably from those of electric burns and therefore are considered separately. Electricity is encountered in two forms: lightning and man-made current. Their neurologic effects are much the same and they are considered together. Versions of the chapter in previous editions of this book contain references to earlier literature to which some readers may want to refer because they are rich in clinical detail.

THERMAL BURNS

The term *thermal burn* refers to a burn caused by contact with flames, hot metal, hot water, or by the flash of radiant heat from an explosion. The extent of a burn is expressed as the percentage of the total body surface area involved. The depth is gauged as *full thickness* when the dermal appendages are destroyed and *partial thickness* when they are spared. Patients with extensive, full-thickness burns are more likely to sustain neurologic complications than those with less severe burns.

Neurologic diagnosis is difficult because extensively burned patients are difficult to examine. Their burned eyelids are swollen shut, and their faces are swollen and move poorly. It is hard for the patient to move swollen and bandaged limbs and for the clinician to assess tone and reflexes. Under these circumstances a full neurologic examination cannot be performed; hence, focal signs may escape detection. Peripheral neuropathies may go unnoticed, and symptoms of focal, structural cerebral lesions may be attributed to metabolic or toxic encephalopathies. The neurologist must appreciate the limitations of the neurologic examination and resort to imaging, examination of the cerebrospinal fluid (CSF), and nerve conduction studies more often than for other types of patients.

Central Nervous System Complications

Because the brain and spinal cord lie deep in the body, they are not injured by the heat of flash or flame. Most victims are neurologically normal immediately after their burn. Those who are not

Aminoff's Neurology and General Medicine, Fifth Edition.

have usually sustained head trauma or anoxic encephalopathy caused by carbon monoxide poisoning or cardiopulmonary arrest due to smoke inhalation.[2,3] Most disorders of the central nervous system (CNS) arise later, during hospitalization, not as a direct consequence of the burn but as a result of some other complication: a systemic infection, disseminated intravascular coagulation (DIC), hypotension, or metabolic abnormalities.[3] Most of them bear a characteristic temporal relationship to the burn, which may provide a valuable clue in diagnosis.

The overall frequency of CNS complications was 14 percent in a large clinical series of patients with burns.[4] Metabolic encephalopathies, cerebrovascular lesions, and CNS infections are the major types of complications and occur in that order of frequency.[3,4] Adults and children are equally affected.[3] Many patients have more than one CNS complication, for several reasons. First, a systemic infection can affect the brain by direct invasion, by an intermediary mechanism of disease, such as DIC and septic shock, or by leading to systemic metabolic abnormalities. A patient may be affected in more than one way. Second, patients may have several independent CNS complications (e.g., infectious and noninfectious, metabolic and structural). Third, elderly patients may have coexisting cerebral diseases in addition to complications of their burn. Often a single diagnosis is an adequate but incomplete explanation for a cerebral symptom. For example, a patient with an atherosclerotic cerebral infarct or a metabolic encephalopathy may also have a CNS infection. Therefore, diagnostic evaluations must be extensive, and the response to treatment may be difficult to interpret.

Metabolic and Other Encephalopathies

Anoxic Encephalopathy

A severe burn is attended by the rapid and massive accumulation of edema in the burned and unburned skin (burn edema).[1] Intravascular volume depletion and hypotension follow and lead to ischemic tissue damage. This state is called burn shock. Anoxic encephalopathy is the most common neurologic complication of a burn, and burn shock is its most common cause in the first few days after a burn.[3,4] After the first week, septic shock becomes the major cause.[3]

Other Encephalopathies

Burned patients are liable to a variety of metabolic derangements, many of which cause encephalopathy. Fluid resuscitation for burn shock can result in dilutional hyponatremia, the most common cause of early confusion and seizures in burned patients, especially children.[4] Later in the hospital course, hyponatremia is most often associated with systemic infection.[3] Uremic encephalopathy is most often due to acute renal failure, which is common in the burn unit. In patients with chronic liver disease, hepatic encephalopathy can develop during convalescence from a burn.[3] Precipitating causes include a systemic infection, narcotic analgesics, hypovolemia, and gastrointestinal bleeding. Hypernatremia, caused by insensible water loss through the burn wound, is the most common electrolyte abnormality. A burn causes a marked increase in metabolic rate. There is increased production of glucose, and this may lead to hyperglycemia. Insulin resistance and intravenous hyperalimentation are other causes of hyperglycemia in burned patients. Hypoglycemia is usually associated with overwhelming systemic infection. Sequestration of calcium in burned skin may cause hypocalcemia, which can lead to seizures and confusion. Hypomagnesemia, with muscle cramps or hallucinations, occurs occasionally. Septic encephalopathy, caused by systemic infection, and toxic encephalopathy, caused by sedating and analgesic medicines, are common problems in the burn unit.

Central Pontine Myelinolysis

Burned patients, like people with alcoholism, are especially susceptible to central pontine myelinolysis (CPM; see Chapter 17). In a retrospective autopsy study, this disorder was found 25 times more often in burned patients than in the general autopsy population.[5] It was associated with a prolonged period (>3 days) of extreme serum hyperosmolality (>360 mOsm/kg). Infection was a major factor in the genesis of the hypernatremia, azotemia, and hyperglycemia that contributed to hyperosmolality. CPM was a late complication; it began after the second hospital week in most cases and never in the first week. A case of CPM occurring early was caused by rapid correction of hyponatremia, in turn caused by fluid resuscitation of burn shock.[6]

The diagnosis of CPM is difficult in burned patients. Metabolic coma may hide the motor signs of CPM, or they may be missed because of the difficulties of neurologic examination described earlier. Late development of quadriplegia, pseudobulbar palsy, the locked-in syndrome, or coma suggests the diagnosis. Magnetic resonance imaging (MRI) can confirm it.

CENTRAL NERVOUS SYSTEM INFECTIONS

Infection is the most common cause of morbidity and mortality in burned patients, because they are immunocompromised in several ways. The burn destroys the skin barrier to microorganisms, and the devitalized eschar of the burn wound is a good culture medium for them. Inhalation of smoke injures the local defense mechanisms of the tracheobronchial tree. Intravenous and urethral catheters and endotracheal tubes promote intraluminal ingress of microorganisms. In addition, both the cellular and the humoral immune systems sustain complex impairments.[7]

CNS infection is the result of hematogenous spread of microorganisms from a source outside the nervous system.[3] Burn wound infection, pneumonia, suppurative thrombophlebitis, and infective endocarditis are the most common sources. *Candida* species, *Pseudomonas aeruginosa*, and *Staphylococcus aureus* are the most common pathogens.[3] Most CNS infections arise in the second and third weeks after the burn; they occur only rarely in the first week and never in the first few days.[3,4] This delay occurs because the CNS is a secondary rather than a primary target of invading microorganisms. Serious infections, including those of the CNS, do not follow minor burns but follow extensive, deep ones (i.e., full-thickness burns that involve at least 30 percent of total body surface area).[7]

These facts may help in neurologic diagnosis. A week or more after a severe burn, a patient with a systemic infection is at high risk of developing a CNS infection. In contrast, patients without a known site of infection, positive blood cultures, or systemic signs of infection and those in the first week after their burn are unlikely to have an infection of the CNS.[3] Similarly, a patient with a burn involving less than 30 percent of total body surface is unlikely to have a CNS infection, even if there is a systemic source.[3] Such patients have less suppression of systemic immune function than those with a major burn and are better able to contain a local infection.[7]

Pseudomonas aeruginosa

Bacterial meningitis develops in 0.1 to 4 percent of extensively burned patients.[3,8] *P. aeruginosa* is the most common etiology.[3,4] Moreover, in one autopsy series, meningitis developed in 15 percent of burned patients who had a systemic *Pseudomonas* infection.[3] A burn wound infection was the most common source, and blood cultures were positive. This is the only CNS infection that has been reported in the first week after a burn.[3,4] Other gram-negative enteric organisms, such as *Escherichia coli* and *Acinetobacter baumannii*, and *Staphylococcus aureus*, but not fungi, have been reported to cause meningitis in burned patients.[3,8] Gram-negative rods have not been reported to cause other types of intracranial infection, such as brain abscess.

The diagnosis of meningitis may be difficult because the burn surgeon will probably have started to treat the primary (source) infection by the time of neurologic consultation. This may eliminate the headache and stiff neck of meningitis without eradicating the infection. In some patients, only confusion, stupor, or coma is found. Hence, a metabolic or septic encephalopathy may be diagnosed. However, a gram-negative infection outside the CNS, especially one due to *P. aeruginosa*, occurring in a patient with an extensive burn that is more than 1 week old, should prompt lumbar puncture. Evidence of meningitis, perhaps partially treated, may be found. If cultures and smears of CSF are negative, antibiotics effective against *P. aeruginosa* meningitis should be prescribed because that is the likeliest pathogen. Many burned patients have more than one systemic infection.[3] Adequate coverage should also be provided for meningitis due to all other microorganisms grown in systemic culture.

If the skin of the back is burned, it may be impossible to do a lumbar or cervical puncture. This is the case in the most extensively burned patients, and they are the ones most likely to develop meningitis. If such a patient has a systemic infection due to a gram-negative rod, particularly *P. aeruginosa*, an antibiotic with good CSF penetration should be prescribed so that meningitis, although impossible to document, should not go untreated.

Candida Species

The frequency of *Candida* infections is increasing among burned patients, because of the use of broad-spectrum antibiotics for bacterial infections, longer survival of older and more extensively burned patients, and the use of central intravenous catheters and intravenous hyperalimentation.[3,7] Half of the patients with invasive candidiasis have cerebral involvement at autopsy.[3] This most often takes the form of disseminated microabscesses; large abscesses, meningitis and mycotic aneurysms are much less common.[3] Patients infected with *Candida* have almost always had at least one previously treated bacterial infection.[3] This is reflected in the relatively late onset of cerebral candidiasis—usually late in the second hospital week and never in the first week.[3]

The antemortem diagnosis of disseminated cerebral microabscesses is difficult.[9] They typically produce drowsiness, confusion, stupor, or coma. Fixed, focal cerebral signs and seizures are unusual. The CSF remains normal. Often less than 3 mm in diameter, the abscesses are too small to be detected by computed tomography (CT), but MRI shows larger ones as small ring-enhancing lesions.[10] Thus, it may require MRI to distinguish multiple cerebral microabscesses from a metabolic or septic encephalopathy.

The diagnosis of cerebral candidiasis may be difficult because the CSF is usually normal, and the diagnosis therefore requires the demonstration of infection outside the CNS. The primary site of infection may not be apparent, and metastatic foci of infection may be hidden as microabscesses in the myocardium or kidney. Pneumonia, evidence of which can be seen on a chest radiograph, is not common. Positive urine, sputum, fecal, and wound cultures can mean colonization rather than infection. Blood cultures are often negative. Without candidemia, the diagnosis is usually made only after death.[3] There is currently no single test that identifies every case of invasive candidiasis. The diagnosis begins with a high index of suspicion in patients with unexplained systemic signs of infection, deep extensive burns, and a prior bacterial infection. Blood cultures, serologic tests, and repeated clinical evaluation for involvement of the skin and eye may help in diagnosis. In an autopsy study, almost half of burned patients with candidemia had cerebral involvement.[3] Therefore, a positive blood culture should prompt systemic antifungal therapy.

Staphylococcus aureus

S. aureus spreads to the brain by way of endocarditis in burned patients.[3] Intracranial spread from other sites has been reported but rarely.[8,11] The sequence of events is burn wound infection, bacteremia, infection of a heart valve, and embolism of infected material to the brain, with infarction or microabscess formation. Other cerebral complications of endocarditis, such as meningitis and mycotic aneurysm, probably occur in burned patients but have not been reported. Intracranial staphylococcal infections begin relatively late—in most cases more than 10 days after the burn—because the brain is infected after the burn wound and endocardium. The frequency of CNS infection with this organism has declined since the mid-1970s because better antibiotic treatment of burn wound infection prevents the development of endocarditis. The diagnosis of staphylococcal cerebral microabscesses is as hard as that of microabscesses due to *Candida*, but the identification of *S. aureus* as the cause is easier because blood cultures are positive. The diagnosis of a staphylococcal CNS infection should prompt a search for endocarditis.

STROKE

Cerebrovascular lesions typically present as a stroke (i.e., the sudden onset of a focal neurologic deficit), but in burned patients this often is not the case, for three reasons. First, there is the difficulty of neurologic examination, described earlier. Second, multiple cerebral complications, the general debility of patients, and the use of narcotic analgesics may obscure the acute onset of a stroke. And third, cerebral infarcts and hemorrhages are often multiple and bilateral in patients with burns,[3] and that may convert an asymmetric neurologic picture into one of relative symmetry. Thus, an infarct or hemorrhage may present not as a stroke but in the guise of a metabolic encephalopathy. Therefore, any unexplained cerebral symptom or sign should lead to brain imaging.

Septic Infarction

Cerebral infarction is due more often to complications of the burn than atherosclerosis, atrial fibrillation, and other premorbid conditions unrelated to the burn.[3,12] Each infection discussed earlier can cause septic occlusion of cerebral blood vessels, with infarction of brain. Meningeal infection can extend into the walls of arteries and veins that run through the subarachnoid space, and that may lead to inflammation and occlusion of affected vessels. This is a common complication of *P. aeruginosa* meningitis and can occur in the first week of disease.[3] Embolism of infected material with occlusion of cerebral arteries is a classic complication of infective endocarditis. Invasive cerebral candidiasis causes mainly microabscesses; infarcts are fewer.[3] Only one burned patient with cerebral aspergillosis has been reported, and it took the form of septic infarction, but *Aspergillus* is a common cause of systemic infection in patients with burns.

Radiologic features do not distinguish septic infarcts from those caused by premorbid vascular disease, but certain clinical points are helpful.[3] Septic infarction may affect patients of any age and does not occur during the first week after a burn. Patients have extensive burns and systemic signs of sepsis. Focal neurologic deficits do not improve. In contrast, infarction caused by premorbid conditions may occur at any time during the hospital course and regardless of the severity of the burn or of the presence of systemic infection. Patients are usually elderly, have conventional risk factors for cerebral infarction, and may have had previous cerebral infarcts or coronary or peripheral vascular disease.

When a burned patient has a cerebral infarct and a septic cause seems likely, it is important to determine the mechanism involved—meningitis, endocarditis, or fungal invasion of a vessel—and the responsible microorganism. If the patient was neurologically normal before cerebral infarction, meningitis is unlikely. Physical signs of meningitis, infective endocarditis, or disseminated candidiasis may be found. The mechanism and etiology of septic infarcts correlate with one another. Cerebral infarction in a patient with *S. aureus* bacteremia suggests the presence of endocarditis. A systemic *P. aeruginosa* infection suggests that meningitis due to that organism underlies the infarct. If meningitis is found, it is the likely mechanism of infarction, and *P. aeruginosa* is the probable cause. Thus, examination of the CSF should always be considered in a burned patient who has had a cerebral infarct. If neither meningitis nor endocarditis is found, fungal invasion of cerebral blood vessels should be suspected. Cerebral infarction in a patient with invasive candidiasis or aspergillosis suggests that the infection has spread to the brain. A cerebral infarct in a patient with systemic signs of sepsis but negative cultures suggests the possibility of infection with *Candida* or *Aspergillus*.

Disseminated Intravascular Coagulation and other Causes of Cerebral Infarction

DIC is a well-known complication of deep, extensive burns.[13] Fibrin thrombi occlude capillaries and small arteries and veins throughout the body. In the brain, disseminated hemorrhagic infarcts and microinfarcts are the result.[3,12] They may or may not produce focal cerebral signs.[14] DIC, like disseminated microabscesses, may simulate a metabolic or toxic encephalopathy. CT detects the larger infarcts, and micro-infarcts may appear on MRI. DIC is unlikely to be the cause of early neurologic symptoms; it usually begins later than the first week after a burn, and never before the fourth day.[3] Heparin has not proved helpful in treating DIC in patients with burns. Treatment of the infection and hypotension causing DIC and replacement of depleted platelets and clotting factors are the recommended approaches.[15]

Cerebral infarction in the arterial borderzone may occur early in the hospital course as a complication of burn shock and, later, with septic shock.[3] The location of the infarct on brain imaging and the clinical setting suggest the diagnosis. Cerebral infarction caused by occlusion of dural sinuses and large and small cerebral veins has been reported in burned patients.[16] Meningitis is not associated. DIC or intravascular volume depletion may be responsible. Magnetic resonance venography or routine MRI can detect occlusion of large venous channels. Nonbacterial thrombotic endocarditis and deep venous thrombosis with paradoxical cerebral embolism are possible, but unreported, causes of cerebral infarction in burned patients.

Intracranial Hemorrhage

Intracranial hemorrhage occurs much less often than cerebral infarction in burned patients.[3] Lobar hemorrhage, subarachnoid hemorrhage, and widespread parenchymal petechiae (brain purpura) have been reported.[3] A bleeding diathesis related to DIC or thrombocytopenia is the cause.[3] Cerebral hematomas and infarcts may both be present in patients with DIC.[3]

BLINDNESS

Several burn patients with blindness not caused by a lesion of the eye have been reported.[17–24] The cases are heterogeneous and no syndrome of blindness emerges that is specifically related to thermal-burn injury. Cortical blindness appeared suddenly and resolved substantially in three patients during their convalescence from a burn.[18,20,21] Bilateral occipital lobe infarction or posterior reversible encephalopathy syndrome was the likely cause. Various optic neuropathies caused blindness in the other patients. The underlying causes included nutritional deficiency,[19] bacterial meningitis,[18] dural venous sinus thrombosis,[18] hypotension,[17,23,24] and neuromyelitis optica.[18] In some patients, blindness and signs of optic neuropathy were part of an acute, widespread cerebral disease that probably caused increased intracranial pressure but went undiagnosed.[17,18] Unsold and colleagues, reporting two cases of burn-associated optic neuropathy and reviewing the literature, speculated that demyelination caused by a circulating toxin released from burned skin could be the cause.[22]

Peripheral Nervous System Complications

Mononeuropathy

In a retrospective study, 10 percent of patients hospitalized with burns developed a mononeuropathy.[25] There are many different causes. Heat may cause coagulation necrosis of nerve trunks involved in a thermal burn.[26] Superficial nerves, such as the ulnar nerve at the elbow and the sensory branch of the radial nerve in the hand, are more liable than deep nerves to thermal damage. Such injuries cannot be treated surgically. Many limbs burned deeply enough to involve nerves require amputation. Blunt trauma from a fall is another cause of nerve injury that presents at the time of a burn; it may affect nerves in unburned and burned limbs.

Reference was made earlier to burn edema, the massive swelling that follows a serious burn. In the wrist it may cause acute carpal tunnel syndrome.[27] There is another mechanism of nerve compression that presents in the first day or two after a burn. When the indistensible eschar of a burn surrounds a limb, the hydrostatic pressure within may be sufficient to shut off the flow of blood. Thus, in a circumferential burn, a tourniquet effect may lead to ischemic necrosis of distal muscle and nerve.[26]

Nerve injury may also occur as a complication of treatment.[26,28] Nerves can be lacerated during escharotomy. The ulnar nerve at the elbow, the fibular (peroneal) nerve as it winds around the head of the fibula, and the sensory branch of the radial nerve are especially vulnerable because they are superficial. The same nerves are liable to compression by tight dressings or malpositioning.

Heterotopic bone formation can cause a mononeuropathy late in the hospital course.[26] The ossification is usually periarticular. The elbow is the joint affected most often, and the ulnar nerve may be compressed. Treatment consists of decompression and transposition of the nerve. The cause of heterotopic bone formation is unknown and recurrence is common. Another cause of late-onset entrapment neuropathy is compression by post-burn scar.[29]

Burned patients with multiple mononeuropathies, in burned and unburned limbs, which could not be attributed to the mechanisms of injury discussed previously, have been described.[30,31] Possible causes include thrombosis of vasa nervorum, a circulating neurotoxin derived from burned tissue, and an autoimmune mechanism, as in post-surgical inflammatory neuropathy.[30,32]

Polyneuropathy

In two prospective studies, polyneuropathy developed in 37 and 41 percent of patients with severe burns.[33,34] These figures may be unreliable because the studies included only 74 patients. The cause of burn-associated polyneuropathy is unknown. Critical illness polyneuropathy (discussed in Chapters 56 and 59) has been reported in burned patients.[30,35] Perhaps burn-associated polyneuropathy represents critical illness polyneuropathy that develops in the burn unit. The two are similar in several respects: weakness in the distal muscles of the limbs is the major sign; sensation is relatively spared; and most patients recover after their burns have healed.[28,36] Also, the occurrence of polyneuropathy in burned patients correlates with measures of severity of illness, such as multiple-organ failure, sepsis, depth and extent of burn, and length of stay in the intensive care unit.[25,37,38] Margherita and associates suggested that burn-associated polyneuropathy is a direct specific result of thermal injury, but they did not offer a precise idea of pathogenesis.[33]

ELECTRICITY AND LIGHTNING

Serious electric injuries are much less common than serious thermal burns. They account for only 3 to 7 percent of admissions to burn units.[1,39] Electricity causes three types of burns. High-voltage current often jumps a gap between its source and a victim. This arc can attain a temperature of 4,000 °C and cause a severe burn, identical to a flash burn. Ignition of a victim's clothing may cause a flame burn. These thermal burns make the victim of electric trauma liable to the neurologic complications discussed earlier. The third type of burn is produced only when the victim becomes part of an electric circuit, and current flows through the body on its way to ground. Burns mark the points of entry and exit. These *contact burns* are much deeper than flash and flame burns and often involve nerves. Structures between the entry and the exit wounds, including nerves, spinal cord, and brain, conduct the current and sustain its direct effects. Also of importance are two indirect mechanisms of neurologic damage: cardiac arrest and trauma. Passage of an electric current through the heart causes asystole or ventricular fibrillation, with resulting syncope or anoxic encephalopathy. An electric shock often causes the victim to fall, and this may result in head injury. A lightning bolt has the force of an explosion, which may cause trauma directly or by throwing the victim to the ground.

General Effect on the Nervous System

Man-made electricity and lightning can injure any structure in the peripheral or central nervous system through which it passes. The degree of damage is directly related to the amount of current.[40] A small current produces only a derangement of function, and clinical manifestations are transient. Larger currents cause structural damage that may be reversible or irreversible; neurologic deficits may be permanent or may resolve with time.

The quantity of current varies directly with its voltage and the duration of its passage and inversely with the resistance of the skin, which it must breach before it reaches neural structures.[40] An arbitrary division is made at 1,000V between high-tension and low-tension electric current. Household current is 110 or 220V; high-tension wires carry current of several thousand volts. Alternating current causes muscle tetany, which may prolong an electrical shock by causing the victim's hand to grip the contact. Thus, alternating current is more dangerous than direct current. A high-tension circuit is often completed by arcing before contact is made. A massive contraction of axial and limb musculature ensues, and this can throw the victim to safety. Thus, low-tension alternating current may cause more damage to the nervous system than high-tension current.

Electricity takes the shortest pathway through the body to ground.[41] Identifying the entry and exit wounds is important, because the current injures only structures between them. When current travels from hand to hand, the nerves and muscles in the arms, the brachial plexus, and the cervical spinal cord lie in its pathway, but the brain does not. A current pathway from head to feet includes the brain, the entire spinal cord, and the nerves and muscles in the legs.

A bolt of lightning can exceed 200 million volts, which is far larger than the voltage of the highest-tension electric wire. A direct strike need not, however, be fatal, for two reasons. First, the duration of the electric discharge is short, approximately 1 millisecond.[42] Second, most of the current flows over the surface of the body, not through it. Lightning, considerably attenuated after striking a tree, can "splash" or "spray" onto a nearby person. Moreover, once lightning has struck the ground, the weakened current can run up one leg and down the other leg of a bystander (stride potential). In addition to entrance and exit burns, lightning figures may be present on the skin. They are arborescent red lines that indicate the path of lightning over the surface of the body.[43] As they fade, they may leave pigmentary changes in their place. Their presence on a victim's back may help account for myelopathy after a stroke of lightning.

As current flows through the resistance of tissue, electric energy is turned into heat (Joule effect). This is the cause of many electric lesions of the nervous system, but some may be due to nonthermal effects. Lee has suggested electric breakdown of cell membranes—electroporation—as a nonthermal mechanism of tissue injury.[44]

Specific Effects

Transient Loss of Consciousness

Lightning or man-made electric current passing through the head causes immediate loss of consciousness. Patients awaken in minutes to hours. Agitation, confusion, retrograde amnesia, headache, and even a convulsive seizure often follow, but complete recovery is to be expected.[39,41] Some patients may have sustained cerebral concussion caused by a fall or the force of a lightning bolt, but electrically induced seizure activity or inhibition of cerebral function is the likely pathophysiologic mechanism in most cases. Brief loss of consciousness often follows passage of lightning or high-tension current outside the head. Transient cardiac asystole, ventilatory failure caused by tetanic contraction or paralysis of the thoracic musculature, and acute intracranial hypertension are possible mechanisms. Loss of consciousness is sometimes delayed rather than immediate, or it may occur immediately and then again somewhat later.[45] A similar phenomenon can follow mild head trauma and probably represents vasodepressor syncope. Patients who lose consciousness for more than a few hours or have focal cerebral signs do not fall into this category; anoxic encephalopathy or a serious head injury should be suspected.

Transient Paralysis

Immediate and transitory sensorimotor paralysis is the neurologic syndrome that typically results from lightning strike. Charcot coined the term *keraunoparalysis* (lightning paralysis). Symptoms and signs correspond to the sites in the peripheral nervous system, spinal cord, and occasionally the brain through which lightning has passed. Paraplegia is most common, but quadriplegia, monoplegia, bibrachial paralysis, hemiplegia, ventilatory paralysis, cranial neuropathies, and aphasia have been reported.[42] Signs of involvement of the autonomic nervous system are common and include pupillary abnormalities and loss of peripheral pulses, as well as coldness and pallor or cyanosis of the weak limbs.[46] Prolonged ventilatory paralysis and binocular mydriasis can simulate death. Lightning paralysis lasts minutes to hours and seldom more than a day, although minor paresthesias may linger for weeks.[42] High-tension electric current can occasionally produce the same syndrome, and one case following a low-voltage shock has been reported.[39,47] The pathophysiologic basis of the syndrome is unknown.

Injury of Peripheral and Cranial Nerves

High-Tension Current

A focal peripheral or cranial neuropathy is the most common serious neurologic complication of a high-tension electric burn. In a large series of patients the frequency was 22 percent.[39] The lesion is usually located in the midst of a contact burn but may be elsewhere in the pathway of the current.[48] It consists of coagulation necrosis and is caused by heat.[49] Its severity parallels that of thermal damage to surrounding muscle, blood vessels, and tendons.[40] Symptoms begin immediately. If the nerve sheath and vasculature are intact, some function may return.[39] Permanent damage to peripheral nerves does not extend beyond the area of local tissue damage.

High-tension electric current, including lightning, causes coagulation necrosis of muscle in its pathway.[1] Swelling begins within hours. Massively swollen muscles, encased in compartments of fascia and bone, may compress adjacent blood vessels. The result is ischemic necrosis of tissue, including muscle and nerve. The diagnosis of this compartment syndrome can be difficult. Unburned skin may cover a vast extent of burned muscle ("hidden muscle damage"). The swollen muscle is confined by fascia, over which the skin may be loose, not taut. Distal pulses may be present. Myoglobinuria and acute renal failure are clues to the diagnosis. More than one peripheral nerve may be affected (e.g., the median, musculocutaneous, and radial nerves in the anterior arm and the median and ulnar nerves in the anterior forearm). Wick catheters (to measure the pressure inside a muscle compartment) and nerve conduction studies may help in diagnosis, but most surgeons perform emergency fasciotomy on clinical indication.

Swelling of burned tissue can cause acute entrapment of nerves that pass through tight anatomic canals. The median nerve may be affected in the carpal tunnel or between the heads of the pronator teres muscle (pronator syndrome), the ulnar nerve in the Guyon canal or the cubital tunnel, and the posterior interosseous nerve in the arcade of Frohse. The most common clinical problem is a deep burn of the anterior wrist associated with a median or ulnar neuropathy. Many surgeons routinely open the carpal tunnel and Guyon canal in such circumstances.[50] Patients who respond presumably have a compressive neuropathy; those who do not may have a primary electric neuropathy.

Scar tissue in healing electric burns may grow around or within a peripheral nerve and impede regeneration or cause a new mononeuropathy late in the hospital course. This happens most often with deep burns of the wrist.[40] The responsible scar is usually apparent on the surface of the body.

Low-Tension Current

Peripheral nerve injury by low-tension current is uncommon but can happen when the resistance of the skin is lowered by water or when contact is prolonged.[40] Electric burns, if present, are minor, and the neural lesion lies far from where current entered the body. For example, current flow from hand to hand may cause a brachial plexopathy or an axillary or radial neuropathy; from hand to foot, an ipsilateral long thoracic neuropathy; and from finger to face, a lesion of the facial nerve.[40,51,52] Usually only one nerve is involved. Pain in the limb begins with the shock, and muscle weakness appears instantly or after a delay of hours to days. Symptoms may worsen over several hours. Full or almost full spontaneous recovery is the rule, although reflex sympathetic dystrophy may ensue as a complication.[53] Focal neuropathies long delayed in onset or progressive in course may be due to heat-induced perineural fibrosis, damage to vasa nervorum, or demyelination.[54,55]

Lightning

Limb neuropathies have been reported more often than cranial neuropathies with man-made electricity, but with lightning the reverse is true. This is probably because lightning often involves the head. These cranial neuropathies resemble low-tension rather than high-tension electric neuropathies in two respects. First, they are usually reversible, probably because most of the current flows over the victim, and burns tend to be superficial. Second, their onset may be delayed for a few days. Optic neuropathy, ocular palsies, Horner syndrome, ophthalmoplegia, and lesions of the facial, vagus and glossopharyngeal nerves have been recorded.[56,57] Deafness is especially common.[58] In one case, autopsy showed loss of hair cells from the organ of Corti,[59] but most victims have conductive deafness caused by thermal injury or rupture of the tympanic membrane or middle ear.[58] Like man-made current, lightning can also cause focal neuropathy of delayed onset.[60] Three cases of acute paraplegia or tetraplegia after a lightning strike or electric shock were attributed to polyneuropathy, but the evidence was unconvincing.[40,61–63]

SPINAL CORD INJURY

Delayed Electric Myelopathy

This is the most characteristic neurologic effect of electric injury. Estimates of its frequency range from 2 to 5 percent of victims.[64] The following analysis is based on a review of 25 patients.[59,64–71] High-tension current (usually >5,000 V) or lightning, a current pathway crossing or running the length of the spinal cord, and at least some deep electric burns are typical. If the victim's skin is wet, enough household current can flow to damage the spinal cord.[71] Neurologic symptoms may appear immediately but a delay of 1 day to 6 weeks—1 week on average—is typical. Neurologic signs worsen for 2 to 14 days, usually for approximately 5 days. One-third of patients recover fully, one-third make a partial recovery, and one-third do not recover at all. Those with signs of a complete spinal cord lesion or with prolonged progression of signs do not recover completely. Almost all patients have pyramidal signs, i.e., paraparesis or quadriparesis with spasticity, hyperreflexia, and Babinski signs. Some show atrophy of muscles innervated by segments of the spinal cord through which the current flowed. Sensory signs are less prominent than motor signs and may be transitory. Joint position sense and vibratory sense are affected more than pain and temperature. Sphincter paralysis is uncommon. T2-weighted MRI shows hyperintense signal, without contrast enhancement, in a long span of the spinal cord.[72,73]

Five patients had postmortem examinations.[59,67,69,70,74] The abnormal portion of the spinal cord corresponded to the pathway of the current. The white matter was more affected than the gray matter, and the lateral and posterior columns were affected most, showing demyelination with relative preservation of axons. Central chromatolysis, necrosis, and mild loss of anterior horn cells were also found. In three patients, some segments of the cord were necrotic. There were no vascular changes. The preponderance of long-tract signs over muscle atrophy correlates with that of damage to white matter over gray matter.

Spinal cord compression due to intervertebral disc herniation or fracture of the spine—usually the thoracic spine—is the major consideration in the differential diagnosis.[75] It can result from a fall or tetanic contraction of the paraspinal muscles during electric shock. The absence of pain in electric myelopathy is a useful point in differential diagnosis.

Spinal Atrophic Paralysis

Panse coined the term *spinal atrophic paralysis* for a syndrome of focal muscular atrophy occurring after a shock from man-made electricity.[45] No figure of its frequency is available, but it must be rare, since no new case has been published since Panse's original review in 1955. Low-tension current, a pathway from hand to hand (across the cervical spinal cord), and either minor or no burns are the usual circumstances of the accident, but the syndrome may also follow lightning strike. Pain or paresthesia in the arm through which current entered begins at once but disappears within days or weeks. Weakness begins immediately or after a few days' or weeks' delay. Muscle wasting becomes evident weeks to months later. The muscles of the shoulder girdle or the hand are affected. Involvement is usually unilateral. Some but not all patients have weakness and spasticity in the legs. Sensory signs may be present in the arms or legs. Horner syndrome, cyanosis and coolness in the hand, and trophic changes in the fingernails are occasionally present, as is sphincter incontinence. The weakness and muscle atrophy worsen for a few months, then stabilize or improve. If the current flows from hand to foot or from foot to foot, the muscles of the leg may be affected.

There are no postmortem studies of the disorder, but Seo and colleagues found experimentally that the anterior horn cells of the spinal cord are especially vulnerable to low-voltage electric current, and that can explain why muscle weakness and atrophy are the major features.[76]

Amyotrophic Lateral Sclerosis

Delayed electric myelopathy and spinal atrophic paralysis resemble amyotrophic lateral sclerosis (ALS) in some respects: there are upper and lower motor neuron signs, and sensory and sphincter functions are often spared. Case reports of progressive rather than self-limited disease have advanced the idea of an association between electric shock and ALS.[77] In these patients, signs develop pointing to parts of the brain and spinal cord outside the pathway of electric current. Hence, a direct effect of current could not have caused them. Epidemiologic studies have found electric shock and lightning strike, like other types of trauma, to be more frequent in ALS than in control subjects.[78] The meaning of this finding is unclear because all these retrospective analyses depend on adequate memory of events by subjects and on valid selection of the control population. A systematic review of the literature found no convincing evidence that electric shock could cause ALS.[79] In conclusion, it seems unlikely that electric shock can cause ALS.

Brain Injury

Electric Burns of the Skull

The skull's resistance to electric current protects the brain from electric injury. Only high-voltage current passes through the skull. This happens when the head accidentally makes contact with high-voltage electric wires. The heat generated by this passage causes coagulation necrosis of the underlying brain.[80] It may also cause coagulation of the blood in a dural sinus and, as a result, infarction of the brain that the sinus drains.[81]

Lightning Strike to the Head

This is fatal in most victims. Most survivors sustain no cerebral damage but several cases of cerebellar ataxia, parkinsonism, and hemiplegia have been reported.[82,83] No pathologic data are available. Some of the patients may have had late sequelae of anoxic encephalopathy rather than electrical damage of the brain.

Stroke

A small number of cases of hemorrhage in the thalamus or basal ganglia after electric shock or lightning strike have been reported.[84,85] Possible causes include acute hypertension induced by electricity,[53] damage of intracerebral arteries due to electric current,[86] and head trauma associated with the accident. High-voltage electric shock to the head can cause occlusion of cerebral-cortical veins with subsequent lobar hemorrhage or hemorrhagic infarction of the cerebral cortex.[81,87] Bland cerebral infarction after lightning or electric shock may be ascribed to injury of arteries by current,[86] hypotension caused by cardiac arrest, and cervicocerebral arterial dissection due to trauma.[88,89]

Dystonia

Several patients with dystonia after electric shock have been reported.[90–95] Low-tension current and lightning (one patient) were involved and caused minor burns, if any. In most patients, a fixed dystonic posture developed in the upper limb through which current had entered; two patients had cervical dystonia, and two had dystonia of the tongue. The onset of dystonia was delayed by a few days to weeks in all but two patients. Reflex sympathetic dystrophy developed in the same limb in one patient.[91] No other neurologic signs, electrophysiologic evidence of peripheral nerve injury, or brain imaging abnormality was present in any of the patients. Several patients were treated with botulinum toxin and a few responded; one patient improved spontaneously. Dystonia has been reported after other types of limb trauma.[96] It is psychogenic in some patients but not in others.[97]

REFERENCES

1. Jeschke M, Williams FN, Gauglitz GG: Burns. p. 521. In: Townsend CM, Beauchamp RD, Evers MB (eds): Sabiston Textbook of Surgery. 19th Ed. Elsevier, Philadelphia, 2012.
2. Hawtof DB: Intracranial hemorrhage in burned patients: report of four cases. J Trauma 6:503, 1996.
3. Winkelman MD, Galloway PG: Central nervous system complications of thermal burns: a postmortem study of 139 patients. Medicine (Baltimore) 71:271, 1992.
4. Antoon AY, Volpe JJ, Crawford JD: Burn encephalopathy in children. Pediatrics 50:609, 1972.
5. McKee AC, Winkelman MD, Banker BQ: Central pontine myelinolysis in severely burned patients: relationship to serum hyperosmolality. Neurology 38:1211, 1988.
6. Cohen BJ, Jordan MH, Chapin SD, et al: Pontine myelinolysis after correction of hyponatremia during burn resuscitation. J Burn Care Rehabil 12:153, 1991.
7. Barillo DJ, McManus AT: Infection in burn patients. p. 903. In: Cohen J, Powderly WG, Berkley SF (eds): Infectious Diseases. 2nd Ed. Mosby, New York, 2004.
8. Calvano TP, Hospenthal DR, Renz EM, et al: Central nervous system infections in patients with severe burns. Burns 36:688, 2010.
9. Pendlebury WW, Perl DP, Munoz DG: Multiple microabscesses in the central nervous system: a clinicopathologic study. J Neuropathol Exp Neurol 48:290, 1989.
10. Lai PH, Lin SM, Pan HB, et al: Disseminated miliary cerebral abscesses. AJNR 18:1303, 1997.
11. Suzuki T, Ueki I, Isago T, et al: Multiple brain abscesses complicating treatment of a severe burn injury: an unusual case report. J Burn Care Rehabil 13:446, 1992.
12. Cho SJ, Minn YK, Kwon KH: Stroke after burn. Cerebrovasc Dis 24:261, 2007.
13. Lippi G, Ippolito L, Cervellin G: Disseminated intravascular coagulation in burn injury. Semin Thromb Hemost 36:429, 2010.
14. Schwartzman RJ, Hill JB: Neurologic complications of disseminated intravascular coagulation. Neurology 32:791, 1982.
15. Liebman HA, Weitz C: Disseminated intravascular coagulation. p. 2169. In: Hoffman R, Benz EJ, Shattil SJ (eds): Hematology: Basic Principles and Practice. Elsevier, Philadelphia, 2005.
16. Sevitt S: The nervous system. In Burns: Pathology and Therapeutic Applications. Butterworths, London, 1957.
17. Resch CS, Sullivan WG: Unexplained blindness after a major burn. Burns 14:225, 1988.
18. Salz JJ, Donin JF: Blindness after burns. Can J Ophthalmol 7:243, 1972.
19. Williams IS: Neuro-ophthalmic deterioration after burns. Proc Aust Assoc Neurol 11:49, 1974.
20. Balzar E, Reisner T, Wolf A: Acute cortical blindness: a reversible complication of acute kidney failure in a child with burns. Padiatr Padol 18:21, 1983.
21. Jie X, Hui X, Yin KF: Bilateral visual loss after severe burns in a child. Burns 17:423, 1991.
22. Unsold AS, Rizzo JF, Lessell S: Optic neuropathy after burns. Arch Ophthalmol 118:1696, 2000.
23. Pirson J, Zizi M, Jacob E, et al: Acute ischemic optic neuropathy associated with an abdominal compartment syndrome in a burn patient. Burns 30:491, 2004.
24. Vallejo A, Lorente JA, Bas ML, et al: Blindness due to anterior ischemic optic neuropathy in a burn patient. J Trauma 53:139, 2002.
25. Kowalske K, Holavanahalli R, Helm P: Neuropathy after burn injury. J Burn Care Rehabil 22:353, 2001.
26. Salisbury RE, Dingeldein GP: Peripheral nerve complications following burn injury. Clin Orthop 163:92, 1982.
27. Emecheta IE, Azzawi K, Kettle R, et al: Bilateral carpal tunnel syndrome in wrist burn: a case report. Burns 31:388, 2005.
28. Helm PA, Pandian G, Heck E: Neuromuscular problems in the burn patient: cause and prevention. Arch Phys Med Rehabil 66:451, 1985.
29. Ferguson JS, Franco J, Pollack J: Compression neuropathy: a late finding in the postburn population: a four-year institutional review. J Burn Care Res 31:458, 2010.
30. Marquez S, Turley JJE, Peters WJ: Neuropathy in burn patients. Brain 116:471, 1993.
31. Dagum AB, Peters WJ, Neligan PC, et al: Severe multiple mononeuropathy in patients with major thermal burns. J Burn Care Rehabil 14:440, 1993.
32. Staff NP, Engelstad J, Klein CJ, et al: Post-surgical inflammatory neuropathy. Brain 133:2866, 2010.
33. Margherita AJ, Robinson LR, Heimbach DM, et al: Burn-associated peripheral polyneuropathy: a search for causative factors. Am J Phys Rehabil 74:28, 1995.
34. Khedr EM, Khedr T, El-Oteify MA, et al: Peripheral neuropathy in burn patients. Burns 23:579, 1997.
35. De Saint-Victor JF, Durand G, Le Gulluche Y, et al: Neuropathies of septic syndrome with multiple organ failure in burn patients: 2 cases with review of the literature. Rev Neurol (Paris) 150:149, 1994.

36. Gabriel V, Kowalske KJ, Holavanahalli RK: Assessment of recovery from burn-related neuropathy by electrodiagnostic testing. J Burn Care Res 30:668, 2009.
37. Lee MY, Liu G, Kowlowitz V, et al: Causative factors affecting peripheral neuropathy in burn patients. Burns 35:412, 2009.
38. Chan Q, Ng K, Vandervord J: Critical illness polyneuropathy in patients with major burn injuries. Eplasty 10:e68, 2010.
39. Grube BJ, Heimbach DM, Engrav LH, et al: Neurologic consequences of electrical burns. J Trauma 30:254, 1990.
40. Wilbourn AJ: Peripheral nerve disorders in electrical and lightning injuries. Semin Neurol 15:241, 1995.
41. Cherington M: Central nervous system complications of lightning and electrical injuries. Semin Neurol 15:233, 1995.
42. Cherington M: Neurologic manifestations of lightning strikes. Neurology 60:182, 2003.
43. Domart Y, Garet E: Lichtenberg figures due to a lightning strike. N Engl J Med 343:1536, 2000.
44. Lee RC: Injury by electrical forces: pathophysiology, manifestations and therapy. Curr Probl Surg 34:679, 1997.
45. Panse F: Electrical lesions of the nervous system. In Vinken PJ Bruyn GW (eds): Handbook of Clinical Neurology Vol 7. North-Holland, Amsterdam, 1970.
46. Jost WH, Schonrock LM, Cherington M: Autonomic nervous system dysfunction in lightning and electrical injuries. Neurorehabilitation 20:19, 2005.
47. Kumar A, Sadiq SA: Transient quadriparesis after electric shock. J Accid Emerg Med 16:376, 1999.
48. Vasquez JC, Shusterman EM, Hansbrough JF: Bilateral facial nerve paralysis after high voltage electrical injury. J Burn Care Rehabil 20:307, 1999.
49. Koshima I, Moriguchi T, Soeda S, et al: High-voltage electrical injury: electron microscopic findings of injured vessel, nerve, and muscle. Ann Plast Surg 26:587, 1991.
50. Engrav LH, Gottlieb JR, Walkinshaw MD, et al: Outcome and treatment of electrical injury with immediate median and ulnar palsy at the wrist: a retrospective review and a survey of members of the American Burn Association. Ann Plast Surg 25:166, 1990.
51. Still JM, Law EJ, Duncan JW, et al: Long thoracic nerve injury due to an electric burn. J Burn Care Rehabil 17:562, 1996.
52. Ahmed I, Farhan W, Durham L: Unilateral facial nerve paralysis after electrocution injury. J Laryngol Otol 121:494, 2007.
53. Cohen JA: Autonomic nervous system disorders and reflex sympathetic dystrophy in lightning and electrical injuries. Semin Neurol 15:387, 1995.
54. Parano E, Uncini A, Incorpora G, et al: Delayed bilateral median nerve injury due to low-tension electric current. Neuropediatrics 27:105, 1996.
55. Smith MA, Muehlberger T, Dellon AL: Peripheral nerve compression associated with low-voltage electrical injury without associated significant cutaneous burn. Plast Reconstr Surg 109:137, 2002.
56. Grover S, Goodwin J: Lightning and electrical injuries: neuro-ophthalmologic aspects. Semin Neurol 15:335, 1995.
57. Saddler MC, Thomas JE: Temporary bulbar palsy following lightning strike. Cent Afr J Med 36:161, 1990.
58. Ogren FP, Edmunds AL: Neuro-otologic findings in the lightning-injured patient. Semin Neurol 15:256, 1995.
59. Davidson GS, Deck JH: Delayed myelopathy following lightning strike: a demyelinating process. Acta Neuropathol (Berl) 77:104, 1988.
60. Guiraud V, Touzé E, Cabane JP, et al: Bilateral plexopathy following lightning injury. Rev Neurol (Paris) 160:1078, 2004.
61. Baqain E, Haertsch P, Kennedy P: Complete recovery following a high voltage electrical injury associated with delayed onset of quadriplegia and multiple cranial nerves dysfunction. Burns 30:603, 2004.
62. Thaventhiran J, O'Leary MJ, Coakley JH, et al: Pathogenesis and recovery of tetraplegia after electrical injury. J Neurol Neurosurg Psychiatry 71:535, 2001.
63. Hawkes CH, Thorpe JW: Acute polyneuropathy due to lightning injury. J Neurol Neurosurg Psychiatry 55:388, 1992.
64. Arevalo JM, Lorente JA, Balseiro-Gomez J: Spinal cord injury after electrical trauma treated in a burn unit. Burns 25:449, 1999.
65. Koller J, Orsagh J: Delayed neurological sequelae of high-tension electrical burns. Burns 15:175, 1989.
66. Varghese G, Mani MM, Redford JB: Spinal cord injuries following electrical accidents. Paraplegia 24:159, 1986.
67. Levine NS, Atkins A, McKeel DW, et al: Spinal cord injury following electrical accidents: case reports. J Trauma 15:459, 1975.
68. Ko SH, Chun W, Kim HC: Delayed spinal cord injury following electrical burns: a 7-year experience. Burns 30:691, 2004.
69. Jackson FE, Martin R, Davis R: Delayed quadriplegia following electrical burn. Milit Med 130:60, 1965.
70. Gerhard L, Spancken E: Chronische Ruckenmarksschadigung nach Starkstrom-unfall. Acta Neuropathol (Berl) 20:357, 1972.
71. So SC, Lee MLK: Spastic quadriplegia due to electric shock. BMJ 2:590, 1973.
72. Freeman CB, Goyal M, Bourque PR: MR image findings in delayed reversible myelopathy from lightning strike. Am J Neuroradiol 25:851, 2004.
73. Lakshminarayanan S, Chokroverty S, Eshkar N, et al: The spinal cord in lightning injury: a report of two cases. J Neurol Sci 276:199, 2009.

74. Komar J, Komar G: Paralysie spinale atrophiante due au traumatisme electrique du chat. Schweiz Arch Tierheilkd 108:325, 1966.
75. Vazquez D, Solano I, Pages E, et al: Thoracic disc herniation, cord compression, and paraplegia caused by electrical injury: case report and review of the literature. J Trauma 37:328, 1994.
76. Seo CH, Jeong JH, Lee DH, et al: Radiological and pathological evaluation of the spinal cord in a rat model of electrical injury-induced myelopathy. Burns 38:1066, 2012.
77. Jafari H, Couratier P, Camu W: Motor neuron disease after electrical injury. J Neurol Neurosurg Psychiatry 71:265, 2001.
78. Das K, Nag C, Ghosh M: Familial, environmental, and occupational risk factors in development of amyotrophic lateral sclerosis. N Am J Med Sci 4:350, 2012.
79. Abhinav K, Al-Chalabi A, Hortobagyi T, et al: Electrical injury and amyotrophic lateral sclerosis: a systematic review of the literature. J Neurol Neurosurg Psychiatry 78:450, 2007.
80. Scholz T, Rippmann V, Wojtecki L, et al: Severe brain damage by current flow after electrical burn injury. J Burn Care Res 27:917, 2006.
81. Singh G, Kaif M, Deep A, et al: high-voltage electrical burn of the skull causing thrombosis of the superior sagittal sinus. J Clin Neurosci 18:1552, 2011.
82. Cherington M, Yarnell P: Hallmark D: MRI in lightning encephalopathy. Neurology 43:1437, 1993.
83. Yarnell PR, Cherington M: Lightning strikes to the head. Ann Neurol 38:347, 1995.
84. Ozgun B, Castillo M: Basal ganglia hemorrhage related to lightning strike. AJNR Am J Neuroradiol 16:1370, 1995.
85. Caksen H, Yuca SA, Demirtas I, et al: Right thalamic hemorrhage from high-voltage electrical injury: a case report. Brain Dev 26:134, 2004.
86. Toy J, Ball BJ, Tredget EE: Carotid rupture following electrical injury: a report of two cases. J Burn Care Res 33:e160, 2012.
87. Sure U, Kleihues P: Intracerebral venous thrombosis and hematoma secondary to high-voltage brain injury. J Trauma 42:1161, 1997.
88. Cherington M, Yarnell P, Lammereste D: Lightning strikes: nature of neurological damage in patients evaluated in hospital emergency departments. Ann Emerg Med 21:575, 1992.
89. Aslan S, Yilmaz S, Karcioglu O: Lightning: an unusual cause of cerebellar infarction. Emerg Med J 21:750, 2004.
90. Ondo W: Lingual dystonia following electrical injury. Mov Disord 12:253, 1997.
91. Tarsy D, Sudarsky L, Charness M: Limb dystonia following electrical injury. Mov Disord 9:230, 1994.
92. O'Brien C: Involuntary movement disorders following lightning and electrical injuries. Semin Neurol 15:263, 1995.
93. Adler CH, Caviness JN: Dystonia secondary to electrical injury: surface electromyographic evaluation and implications for the organicity of the condition. J Neurol Sci 148:187, 1997.
94. Broonkongchuen P, Lees A: Case of torticollis following electrical injury. Mov Disord 11:109, 1996.
95. Baskerville JR, McAninch SA: Focal lingual dystonia, urinary incontinence, and sensory deficits secondary to low voltage electrocution: case report and literature review. Emerg Med J 19:368, 2002.
96. van Rooijen DE, Geraedts EJ, Marinus J, et al: Peripheral trauma and movement disorders: a systematic review of reported cases. J Neurol Neurosurg Psychiatry 82:892, 2011.
97. Hawley JS, Weiner WJ: Psychogenic dystonia and peripheral trauma. Neurology 77:496, 2011.

CHAPTER

37

Abnormalities of Thermal Regulation and the Nervous System

DOUGLAS J. GELB

THERMOREGULATORY SYSTEM

Thermoregulatory regions in the preoptic, anterior, and dorsomedial hypothalamus integrate thermal inputs to produce an output that adjusts body temperature to match a set point.[1–8] Thermoregulatory disorders may be produced either by malfunction of this system or by conditions that overwhelm its capacity.

Thermoregulatory disorders should be distinguished from other causes of abnormal body temperature, in which the thermoregulatory system functions properly but the set point is shifted. The most common condition of this type is fever, which is produced by an abnormal upward shift of the set point.[1,9,10] Shifts in the set point may also be responsible for variations of body temperature with the menstrual cycle and for diurnal temperature fluctuations.[7]

The afferent limb of the thermoregulatory system includes skin thermosensors, visceral thermosensors, vascular thermosensors, and neurons within the hypothalamic regulatory areas that are sensitive to the temperature in the hypothalamus itself. Thermosensitive neurons are also present in the brainstem and spinal cord and, possibly, in the abdominal viscera. The molecular mechanisms mediating temperature sensitivity are not known, but the transient receptor potential family of cation channels appear to play a role, at least in the skin thermosensors.[3,6,7,11]

The efferent limb of the system generates or dissipates heat, as necessary. Basal metabolic activity produces heat, and within a narrow range of ambient temperatures called the thermoneutral zone, the core temperature can be maintained by adjusting metabolic rate. Outside this range, heat generation is achieved primarily by shivering.[12] Newborn infants do not shiver, and shivering is probably not fully effective until several years of age; before then, nonshivering thermogenesis occurs in brown adipose tissue. The mitochondria of brown adipose tissue contain an uncoupling protein that, when induced, diverts the energy generated by oxidative phosphorylation into heat production rather than ATP synthesis, so that heat becomes the primary product of metabolism rather than a byproduct as in other tissues.[13] Nonshivering thermogenesis may possibly also occur in older children and adults.[8] Heat dissipation is achieved by evaporation (sweating) and by

Aminoff's Neurology and General Medicine, Fifth Edition.

nonevaporative heat loss (conduction, convection, and radiation).[4,5,7] Evaporative heat loss is the most important of these mechanisms in most clinical situations. Nonevaporative heat loss can occur only when the ambient temperature is lower than the skin temperature. The amount of heat dissipated is then a function of vasomotor activity; increased skin blood flow promotes heat dissipation, and reduced skin blood flow minimizes it.[14–16] These thermoregulatory vasomotor effects are controlled by both the hypothalamus and local reflexes, and can be modified by exercise, reproductive hormones, aging, and disease. The local vasomotor reflexes can override the hypothalamic regulation under extreme local temperature conditions.

NEUROLOGIC CAUSES OF ABNORMAL THERMOREGULATION

The main neurologic causes of abnormal thermoregulation are diseases of the hypothalamus or its autonomic outflow. In addition, a few neurologic disorders result in excessive heat production that overwhelms the thermoregulatory system. Tables 37-1 and 37-2 summarize the main causes of hyperthermia and hypothermia.

Hypothalamic Lesions

Hypothalamic lesions may produce either hyperthermia or hypothermia, although hypothermia is more common.[17–20] Hyperthermia has been described with tumors, stroke, encephalitis, trauma, and surgery. Hypothermia has been reported with tumors, stroke, subarachnoid hemorrhage, sarcoidosis, multiple sclerosis, neuromyelitis optica, limbic encephalitis, Parkinson disease, and idiopathic gliosis. Hypothermia is common in Wernicke encephalopathy and may be the presenting feature. In contrast, although fever occurs in about 12 percent of patients with Wernicke encephalopathy, a superimposed infection is almost always responsible. Prominent abnormalities of sweating (anhidrosis or hypohidrosis) have been described in primary autonomic failure, multiple system atrophy, and as an isolated condition, and hyperthermia may develop when these patients are exposed to hot climates without air conditioning.[21]

TABLE 37-1 ■ Causes of Hyperthermia
Malfunction of Thermoregulatory System
Hypothalamic disorders
Tumor
Stroke
Encephalitis
Head trauma
Surgery
Other lesions
Hydrocephalus
Posterior fossa surgery
Interruption of Effector Pathways
Spinal cord lesions
Autonomic neuropathies
Overwhelming Heat Production or Exposure
Neurologic conditions
Status epilepticus
Delirium tremens
Tetanus
Malignant hyperthermia
Neuroleptic malignant syndrome
Serotonin syndrome
Non-neurologic conditions
Heat stress disorders (exertional or nonexertional)
Heat shock
Heat exhaustion
Endocrine disorders
Thyrotoxicosis
Pheochromocytoma
Drugs
Inadequate Heat Dissipation
Dehydration
Skin disorders
Occlusive dressings
Drugs

TABLE 37-2 ■ Causes of Hypothermia

Malfunction of Thermoregulatory System
Hypothalamic disorders
Tumor
Stroke
Subarachnoid hemorrhage
Sarcoidosis
Wernicke encephalopathy
Parkinson disease
Primary autonomic failure
Multiple system atrophy
Multiple sclerosis
Agenesis of the corpus callosum (Shapiro syndrome)
Disease at the mesencephalic-diencephalic junction
Interruption of Effector Pathways
Spinal cord lesions
Autonomic neuropathies
Neuromuscular causes of weakness
Inadequate Heat Production
Accidental hypothermia (exposure)
Endocrine disorders
Hypothyroidism
Hypoadrenalism
Hypopituitarism
Derangements of glucose regulation
Hypoglycemia
Diabetic ketoacidosis
Hyperosmolar coma
Malnutrition
Drugs
Excessive Heat Dissipation
Severe burns
Skin disorders (exfoliative dermatitis, psoriasis, ichthyosis, erythroderma)

Lesions of Effector Pathways

Interruption of the autonomic outflow from the hypothalamus may produce either hyperthermia or hypothermia by impairing the effector mechanisms necessary for heat dissipation or production, respectively.[1,21,22] Lesions of the spinal cord above the thoracic level may interrupt descending input to the thoracic intermediolateral cell column, producing both vasomotor abnormalities and disorders of sweating, or to anterior horn cells, impairing or eliminating shivering below the level of the lesion.

Any neuromuscular disease that is severe enough to cause profound weakness can impede shivering. Polyneuropathies that involve autonomic fibers can produce abnormalities of vasomotor activity and sweating, and either hypothermia or hyperthermia may result.[23] For example, hypothermia is common in patients with diabetes, probably because of impaired vasomotor reflexes. In contrast, some diabetics manifest a syndrome of heat intolerance that is attributed to anhidrosis. Because the autonomic nerve involvement in diabetes is usually predominantly distal, these patients sometimes exhibit profuse sweating over the head and upper trunk ("compensatory hyperhidrosis").

Miscellaneous Lesions

Disorders that produce widespread damage to the CNS can impair thermoregulation, but the precise mechanism is often difficult to establish.[24–33] Degenerative diseases including multiple sclerosis can be associated with hypothermia, and hyperthermia has been reported in patients with acute hydrocephalus, posterior fossa surgery, ischemic strokes, and intracranial hemorrhage. As a general rule, however, hyperthermia should not be attributed to "neurogenic factors" even when a patient has CNS disease, unless there is clear involvement of the hypothalamus or its effector pathways and other causes of fever have been excluded.

Agenesis or dysplasia of the corpus callosum may be associated with episodic hyperhidrosis and hypothermia (Shapiro syndrome).[34] There may also be associated structural abnormalities in the septal region, cingulate gyrus, and posterior hypothalamus. The periods of sweating may last from minutes to hours, and the hypothermia may last from 30 minutes up to several weeks. Episodes may be separated by intervals of months to years. There is often ataxia and impaired cognition during the hypothermic episodes. A similar syndrome has occasionally been seen without any associated abnormality of the corpus callosum, and neurotransmitter abnormalities have been identified in some cases.[34–36] Episodic hypothermia without hyperhidrosis has also been described. Recurrent hypothermia has also been attributed to "diencephalic epilepsy," but electrographic seizures have not been demonstrated consistently.

Cases of periodic hyperthermia associated with agenesis of the corpus callosum ("reverse Shapiro syndrome") have been reported.[1] Episodic hyperthermia (or hypothermia) associated with other manifestations of autonomic dysfunction has also been described after head trauma and many other neurologic disorders.[37–40]

Thermoregulatory System Overload

Several neurologic diseases produce thermoregulatory disorders by creating conditions that overwhelm the capacity of the thermoregulatory system. Just as paralysis may eliminate effective shivering and result in hypothermia, muscle hyperactivity may result in hyperthermia. Elevated body temperatures are common after generalized seizures, tetanus, and delirium tremens for example. Three important examples of hyperthermia associated with increased muscle activity are malignant hyperthermia, neuroleptic malignant syndrome, and serotonin syndrome.

Malignant Hyperthermia

Malignant hyperthermia is characterized by vigorous muscle contractions and an abrupt increase in temperature on exposure to certain drugs, most commonly inhalational anesthetics and succinylcholine.[41,42] It can occur at any time during anesthesia administration or shortly thereafter. The hyperthermia is probably a direct result of the heat produced by sustained muscle activity resulting from defective regulation of intracellular free calcium. Malignant hyperthermia is inherited as an autosomal dominant trait with variable penetrance, and a predominance of expression in young males.[43] More than 50 percent of patients have mutations in the gene for the ryanodine receptor, the primary channel for release of calcium stored in the sarcoplasmic reticulum; other cases are due to mutations in the gene encoding the main subunit of the dihydropyridine receptor, a voltage sensor that interacts closely with the ryanodine receptor, or in the gene coding for calsequestrin, a calcium-binding protein that modulates ryanodine receptor function.[44–49] Mutations in the gene for the ryanodine receptor also cause central core disease, a congenital myopathy; some, but not all, patients with central core disease are also at risk of malignant hyperthermia.[45,46,48–50] Nemaline rod myopathy and multiminicore disease are myopathies that are also caused by mutations in the ryanodine receptor, but these conditions do not appear to be associated with an increased risk of malignant hyperthermia.[50] Although patients with other myopathies, muscular dystrophies, and myotonia may have adverse effects from anesthesia (e.g., contractures after administration of succinylcholine, increased susceptibility to respiratory depression after receiving barbiturates or opiates, disease-related cardiac complications, or rhabdomyolysis), they do not appear to have an increased risk of malignant hyperthermia.[51–54]

Neuroleptic Malignant Syndrome and Serotonin Syndrome

Both neuroleptic malignant syndrome and serotonin syndrome are characterized by hyperthermia, diaphoresis, rigidity, mental status changes, tachypnea, tachycardia, and hypertension or labile blood pressure. Patients with neuroleptic malignant syndrome typically have hyporeflexia, normal pupillary responses, and normal or decreased bowel sounds, whereas serotonin syndrome is associated with hyperreflexia, dilated pupils, and hyperactive bowel sounds.[55–62] Patients with neuroleptic malignant syndrome often have laboratory abnormalities that are not present in serotonin syndrome including peripheral leukocytosis, elevated serum creatine kinase, increased liver enzymes, and low serum iron, magnesium, and calcium levels. The pathophysiology of these two syndromes is poorly understood. The elevated body temperatures are at least partly due to increased muscle activity, but there may also be an elevation of the hypothalamic temperature set point. Neuroleptic malignant syndrome is typically triggered by exposure to neuroleptic agents, including atypical antipsychotic agents, but it has also been described in patients being treated for presumed Parkinson disease after sudden withdrawal of dopaminergic agents or changes in their medication regimen.[63,64] When associated with neuroleptics, the condition typically arises within

2 weeks of starting therapy or increasing the dose, but at times it may begin within hours or after a delay of months. Serotonin syndrome can occur with any serotonergic drugs—notably tricyclic antidepressants, monoamine oxidase inhibitors, selective serotonin reuptake inhibitors, serotonin-norepinephrine reuptake inhibitors, and meperidine—especially when used in combination.

NEUROLOGIC CONSEQUENCES OF ABNORMAL THERMOREGULATION

Most cases of abnormal thermoregulation occur in individuals without a primary neurologic disease and are caused by external temperature conditions (or, less commonly, internal metabolic derangements) that overwhelm the thermoregulatory system. Regardless of the underlying cause, neurologic manifestations are often prominent.

Neuronal function is significantly affected by even moderate changes in temperature. Basic electrical parameters (such as membrane capacitance, axoplasmic resistance, maximal sodium and potassium conductances, and ion channel rate constants) vary systematically with temperature. Consequently, temperature affects the action potential amplitude, duration, maximal rate of rise, net ionic movements, and conduction velocity, and therefore changes the likelihood of signal propagation or conduction block.[65] Clinical electrophysiologic tests reflect these effects; for example, the maximal motor conduction velocity of the ulnar nerve falls by 2.4 m/sec for every 1°C decline in temperature. As the temperature drops, compound action potential amplitudes increase, the duration of motor unit action potentials increases, mean amplitude declines, and polyphasic potentials become more frequent. Hypothermia also prolongs the latencies of visual, somatosensory, and brainstem auditory evoked potentials.

Although these alterations in function can have clinical consequences, actual nervous system injury does not occur until extreme temperatures are reached. Direct thermal injury to the brain and spinal cord results in the production of a variety of cytokines and altered expression of heat-shock proteins, leading to endothelial cell injury and diffuse microvascular thrombosis, ultimately causing cell death, edema, and hemorrhage.[1,66–71]

Cerebral metabolic rate and oxygen metabolism increase with rising temperatures between 38°C and 42°C, but decline as temperatures rise further. Hypothermia leads to slowing of the rate of chemical reactions, decrease in the metabolic requirement for oxygen, and reduction of cerebral blood flow by 4.4 to 6.0 percent for every 1°C decline in temperature.[67,72–75] This reduction in metabolic rate is protective, but neural damage still occurs. It is difficult to know to what extent the neuronal damage is a direct effect of low temperatures rather than a consequence of secondary injury from the systemic effects of hypothermia (including cardiovascular collapse).

HYPERTHERMIA

The neurologic causes of hyperthermia were considered earlier.

Non-Neurologic Causes

Conditions in which the thermoregulatory system is overwhelmed by extremely high external temperatures are called *heat stress disorders*.[70,71,73,76–80] The most severe form is heat stroke, defined as a core body temperature exceeding 40°C (or 41°C according to older sources) associated with CNS dysfunction such as delirium, seizures, or coma. Heat stroke is characterized by hot, dry skin, but this is not used as a diagnostic criterion. Heat exhaustion is a milder form, characterized by progressive lethargy, headache, vomiting, tachycardia, and hypotension, with less severe neurologic impairment than occurs in heat stroke. These two conditions form a continuum: if untreated, heat exhaustion may progress to heat stroke.

Classic heat stroke results from prolonged exposure to high environmental temperatures while the individual undertakes normal activities; exertional heat stroke occurs in situations of physical exertion, typically in healthy young individuals, often athletes or military personnel. Inadequate cardiovascular conditioning, poor acclimatization, dehydration, heavy clothing, low work efficiency, and reduced ratio of skin area to body mass all are risk factors. Congenital or acquired abnormalities of sweat gland function may contribute. Classic heat stroke is typically seen in the elderly, especially in those with chronic diseases (e.g., alcoholism, malnutrition, diabetes, cardiovascular dysfunction, obesity). Some medications predispose to the condition, including anticholinergics, β-blockers, diuretics, antihistamines, antidepressants, and amphetamines. People in lower socioeconomic groups are at particular risk, especially those living in urban areas, because they may be exposed to a greater thermal load and live in apartments with inadequate ventilation.

The most common cause of hyperthermia is simple dehydration because it results in vasoconstriction and decreased sweating, interfering with heat dissipation. Heat dissipation may also be impaired in advanced scleroderma or in miliaria, or by extensive use of occlusive dressings. Both thyrotoxicosis (mainly during thyroid storm) and pheochromocytoma may cause hyperthermia on the basis of hypermetabolism. Drug exposure can also produce hyperthermia in several ways, including increased metabolic rate, hyperactivity, and impaired heat dissipation (Table 37-3).[71,73,80–82]

Neurologic Manifestations

The earliest neurologic manifestations of hyperthermia include thirst, weakness, and fatigue. Skeletal muscle cramps may occur in the exertional heat stress disorders and are probably related to hyponatremia and increased intracellular calcium release. Patients with heat exhaustion are frequently agitated and may develop delirium and incoordination. Tetany or paresthesias sometimes will occur secondary to hyperventilation.

Heat stroke may present with the sudden onset of stupor or coma, or patients may pass through a prodromal period that can include progressive headache, drowsiness, confusion, agitation, and delirium. Seizures occur in 60 to 70 percent of patients. Pupils are usually small and often pinpoint, and oculovestibular ("cold caloric") responses are intact except terminally. Diffuse hypertonia is common, but flaccidity has also been described. Hemiplegia, cerebellar deficits, and papilledema may also occur. Cerebrospinal fluid (CSF) from patients with heat stroke is usually normal but may show an increased protein concentration, xanthochromia, or mild lymphocytic pleocytosis. Slowing of the electroencephalogram (EEG) occurs at temperatures above 42°C.

Most patients who recover from heat stroke have no permanent neurologic sequelae, but some may have persistent ataxia and dysarthria; a few cases of hemiparesis, myelopathy, or quadriparesis have been reported. There are also reports of persistent polyneuropathy after patients have been treated with experimental whole-body hyperthermia for cancer, and localized neuropathies following hyperthermic isolated limb perfusion. Survivors of severe heat stroke may also develop premature cataracts, attributed to dehydration.

Systemic Manifestations

Heat stroke is associated with diffuse systemic derangements.[1,71,76,80,83,84] The mildest are dependent edema and syncope. Respiratory alkalosis is almost always present, and tetany may occur. Hypoxia, metabolic acidosis, hypokalemia, hyperkalemia, hypernatremia, hypophosphatemia, hypomagnesemia, and hypoglycemia have each been described. Peripheral leukocytosis in the range of 20,000 to 30,000 cells/mm^3 is common.

Cardiovascular manifestations include low cardiac output and low diastolic pressure. Subendocardial hemorrhages may occur. Minor electrocardiographic changes are sometimes found and include transient conduction abnormalities and inverted or flattened T waves. Apart from the respiratory alkalosis, pulmonary manifestations may include pulmonary edema and acute lung injury in the presence of disseminated intravascular coagulation.

Rhabdomyolysis is almost universal in exertional heat stroke but is uncommon in classic heat stroke. Elevated serum creatine kinase levels occur in both conditions, often followed by elevated levels of lactate dehydrogenase. Acute renal failure occurs in about 25 percent of patients with exertional heat stroke but is uncommon in classic heat stroke. Diarrhea and vomiting are common; melena and hematemesis may occur in severe cases. Elevated serum amylase and liver enzymes are common; liver injury is usually asymptomatic, but acute liver failure occurs in 5 percent of patients with exertional heat stroke. Clinically significant coagulopathies are common and, in severe heat shock, disseminated intravascular coagulation is almost always present.

Patient Management

There are three components to the management of the hyperthermic patient: treatment of the underlying cause (when possible), cooling, and treatment or prevention of common complications.[71,73,76,79,80,85–87]

TABLE 37-3 ■ Pharmacologic Agents that Promote Hyperthermia

Agent	Excess Heat Production		Impaired Heat Dissipation		Other Mechanisms
	Occurrence	Cause or Comment	Occurrence	Cause	
Anticholinergic agents			+		
Vasoconstricting agents			+		
β-Blockers			+		
Diuretics			+		
Antihistamines			+		
Barbiturates			+		
Alcohol			+		
Topiramate			+	Hypohidrosis	
Zonisamide			+	Hypohidrosis	
Tricyclic antidepressants	+	Increased motor activity	+	Anticholinergic effects	
Cocaine	+				
Amphetamines	+				
Opiates	+				
Lysergic acid diethylamide (LSD)	+				
Cannabinoids	+				
Phenothiazines	+	Neuroleptic malignant syndrome	+	Anticholinergic effects	Possible effect on hypothalamus
Butyrophenones	+	Neuroleptic malignant syndrome			Failure to recognize thirst, possible effect on hypothalamus
Atypical antipsychotics	+	Neuroleptic malignant syndrome			
Salicylate overdose	+				
Anticholinesterase agents					Cause unknown
Methyldopa					Idiosyncratic
Propylthiouracil					Idiosyncratic
Inhalational anesthetics	+	Malignant hyperthermia			
Monoamine oxidase inhibitors (overdose in conjunction with meperidine or biogenic amine precursors)	+	Serotonin syndrome			
Serotonin reuptake inhibitors	+	Serotonin syndrome			
Triptans (in conjunction with SSRIs or SNRIs)	+	Serotonin syndrome			

SNRI, serotonin-norepinephrine reuptake inhibitor; SSRI, selective serotonin reuptake inhibitor.

Most of the hypothalamic causes of hyperthermia are not amenable to acute treatment, although corticosteroid administration is appropriate when there is vasogenic edema. Compressive spinal cord lesions associated with hyperthermia (e.g., epidural hematoma or abscess) may require immediate treatment, but no acute treatment is possible for most other lesions. Hyperthermia caused by excessive muscle activity (including status epilepticus) is treated by reducing or eliminating the muscle activity.

Patients with malignant hyperthermia are treated by stopping the responsible anesthesia, instituting hyperoxygenation, and intravenously administering dantrolene, a skeletal muscle relaxant that uncouples excitation and contraction by preventing the release of calcium from the sarcoplasmic reticulum.[41,58] Although dantrolene has been used successfully to treat neuroleptic malignant syndrome, bromocriptine and amantadine have also been tried in some cases, probably because of the apparent role of dopaminergic systems in neuroleptic malignant syndrome. Electroconvulsive therapy may be useful in severe, refractory cases. Cyproheptadine is the most commonly recommended medication for serotonin syndrome, but it has not been studied rigorously.

Non neurologic causes of hyperthermia may also be amenable to specific treatment. Thyrotoxic storm or crisis is treated with β-adrenergic antagonists, glucocorticoids (because of increased requirement and reduced adrenal reserve), and administration of an antithyroid agent, as discussed in Chapter 18. Patients with pheochromocytoma are treated with α-adrenergic antagonists. Dehydrated patients are rehydrated as necessary. For hyperthermic patients in whom a precipitating drug can be identified, treatment is directed at minimizing the drug's toxicity. Patients with alcohol withdrawal and delirium tremens require large doses of benzodiazepines. For the hyperthermia of heat stress disorders, treatment of the underlying cause simply consists of removing the patient from the hot environment and cooling the patient.

Cooling may be achieved by either evaporative or direct external methods.[71,73,80,86,87] Centrally acting antipyretic medications exert their effect by lowering the temperature set point, so they are appropriate for use in fever, where the set point is abnormally high, but not in thermoregulatory disorders. Evaporative cooling methods involve wetting the skin with tepid water and directing bedside fans at the patient. Direct external cooling involves immersion of the patient in ice water, use of a hypothermic mattress, or packing the patient in ice. These direct external cooling techniques produce vasoconstriction, which impedes removal of heat from the core; therefore, in order to counteract this response, these cooling methods are applied (either simultaneously or in alternation) with vigorous skin massage, tepid (40°C) water spray, or exposure to hot moving air (45°C). Cooling is more rapid and more effective with direct external methods than with evaporative methods, but evaporative techniques are often adequate and permit easier patient management and monitoring. In rare instances where neither method is sufficient, more aggressive options include peritoneal lavage with iced saline, gastric lavage or enemas with ice water, and hemodialysis or cardiopulmonary bypass with external cooling of blood.

Regardless of the cooling method used, shivering often occurs as the body temperature falls and hampers cooling. In the case of cold water immersion, the rate of heat transfer is high enough that the heat produced by shivering is generally not a concern. If necessary, shivering can be treated with phenothiazines, benzodiazepines, meperidine, or nondepolarizing muscle relaxants; serotonin uptake inhibitors, α_2 agonists, and NMDA antagonists have also been proposed.[88,89] As the patient's core temperature reaches 38°C or 39°C, cooling should be stopped to avoid overshoot hypothermia.

The most important complication of hyperthermia is hypotension, which should be treated with fluid administration. Vasopressors may be used if necessary, but those that produce vasoconstriction should be avoided. Patients should receive 100 percent oxygen until adequate oxygenation is documented. Serum electrolyte and glucose concentrations should be assessed frequently and treated as necessary. To promote urine output, patients are often given an initial dose of mannitol or furosemide and subsequent doses of diuretics as necessary. Disseminated intravascular coagulation and seizures should be treated if they occur. Appropriate treatment of heat stroke results in a 90 to 95 percent survival rate. Poor prognosis is associated with a peak temperature higher than 41°C, prolonged symptoms before initiation of treatment, acute renal failure, elevated serum liver enzymes, red blood cell apoptosis on early peripheral blood smears, and persistence of coma after restoration of normothermia.

HYPOTHERMIA

Neurologic causes of hypothermia were discussed earlier.

Non-Neurologic Causes

As with hyperthermia, hypothermia is usually due to conditions that overwhelm the thermoregulatory system, rather than a consequence of primary malfunction in the system.[1,72–75,90–94] Accidental hypothermia is defined as an unintentional decline in the core temperature below 35°C. It is most common in neonates, the elderly, and those who are unconscious or immobile, especially from drug exposure. Alcohol, in particular, is a vasodilator, a CNS depressant, an anesthetic, and a risk factor for trauma and environmental exposure, all of which increase the risk of hypothermia. Other drugs predispose to hypothermia through a variety of mechanisms including depression of the hypothalamic center, inhibition of shivering by neuromuscular blockade, and vasodilation (Table 37-4).[72,75,90,93,95]

Patients with severe burns, exfoliative dermatitis, or other dermatologic conditions may develop hypothermia because of increased evaporative and nonevaporative heat loss and the inability to regulate these processes through vasoconstriction. Hypothermia may also occur in the setting of several endocrine disorders that impair metabolism including hypothyroidism, hypoadrenalism, and hypopituitarism. Hypoglycemia, diabetic ketoacidosis, and hyperosmolar coma are also associated with hypothermia, but it is not clear whether this is because of a hypometabolic state or a direct effect on the hypothalamus.

TABLE 37-4 ■ Pharmacologic Agents that Promote Hypothermia

Agent	Impaired Heat Production	Excessive Heat Loss	Other Mechanisms
Alcohol	+	+	Possible effect on hypothalamus
Barbiturates	+		
General anesthetics	+		
Phenothiazines	+	+	
Benzodiazepines	+		
Tricyclic antidepressants		+*	
Vasodilating agents		+	
Bromocriptine			Possible effect on hypothalamus
Reserpine			Possible effect on hypothalamus
Acetaminophen			Possible effect on hypothalamus
Lithium			Possible effect on hypothalamus
Valproic acid			Mechanism unknown
Penicillin			Mechanism unknown
Erythromycin			Mechanism unknown

*Hyperhidrosis in some subjects.

Neurologic Manifestations

The neurologic manifestations of hypothermia progress in a relatively predictable manner. Thought processes may be normal with rectal temperatures as low as 34°C, but below this temperature most patients exhibit psychomotor slowing, speech perseveration, lethargy, or confusion. A few patients have been described as alert with rectal temperatures as low as 31°C, but this is uncommon. Dysarthria develops at temperatures below 33.5°C, and below 28°C most patients only grunt in response to questions, although some patients remain verbally responsive at temperatures as low as 23.5°C. Most patients still make purposeful responses to noxious stimuli even with temperatures approaching 20°C.

Pupillary reaction to light becomes progressively more sluggish as temperatures decline below about 32°C, but pupillary size and eye movements do not correlate reliably with temperature. Deep tendon reflexes are typically normal or even increased at temperatures as low as 29.5°C, but they become progressively diminished at lower temperatures. Extensor plantar responses are rare at any level of hypothermia. Increased muscle tone is frequent even in mild hypothermia, and it is universal at temperatures below 29.5°C. Myotonia is a common finding. Focal dystonias and dyskinesias are rare, but patients may exhibit a characteristic posture consisting of flexion in all four limbs.

No specific CSF abnormalities have been described in hypothermia. The EEG frequency spectrum changes, with increased beta and theta activity and reduced alpha activity. At temperatures below 28°C, there is progressive slowing. As the temperature declines further, a burst-suppression pattern appears, with the EEG becoming isoelectric below 10°C to 20°C. Brainstem auditory evoked potentials show increasing latencies of waves I, III, and V as temperature decreases. Visual evoked potential latencies also increase progressively as temperature declines. The changes that occur in electromyographic and nerve conduction studies were discussed earlier.

Patients who recover from hypothermia usually have no long-term neurologic problems.

Systemic Manifestations

During the shivering phase (typically between 35°C and 30°C), there is an initial rise in metabolic rate and oxygen consumption, with corresponding increases in respiratory rate, heart rate, and blood pressure, but at temperatures below about 30°C shivering ceases and there is a rapid decline in metabolic rate and oxygen consumption—respiration slows and becomes shallow, the heart rate decreases, and cardiac output declines. Clinically significant hypotension typically does not occur until temperatures of 25°C and below are reached. The principal cardiac concern with hypothermia is arrhythmia. Arrhythmia is preceded by the characteristic J-point elevation (or "Osborn wave") that appears at about 33°C and becomes increasingly prominent as the temperature falls. Atrial fibrillation is common below 33°C, but all types of atrial and ventricular arrhythmias can occur.

Mild hypothermia induces diuresis because peripheral vasoconstriction redistributes blood to internal organs including the kidneys, and also because of inhibition of antidiuretic hormone release and decreased renal tubular function. As hypothermia progresses and cardiac output diminishes, renal blood flow and glomerular filtration rate decline, ultimately resulting in acute renal failure. Hemoconcentration increases the hematocrit by 2 percent for every 1°C drop in core temperature. With falling temperatures, the platelet count progressively declines due to bone marrow suppression and splenic or hepatic sequestration. Platelet function is also impaired. Cold suppresses the enzymatic function of activated clotting factors, leading to coagulopathies that may not be detected on standard laboratory tests which are performed at 37°C. Hypercoagulability can also develop due to thromboplastin release from cold tissue, catecholamine and steroid release, and circulatory collapse. Granulocytopenia may occur with temperatures below 28°C.

Hypothermia has no consistent effect on potassium, calcium, magnesium, or other electrolytes, but moderate hypoglycemia is common. Endocrine functions generally remain normal. Ileus is frequent, and ischemic pancreatitis can also occur; serum amylase levels appear to correlate with the severity of hypothermia. Depressed airway reflexes result in a high incidence of pneumonia.

Patient Management

The management of hypothermia is analogous to the management of hyperthermia. The three principal components are treatment of the underlying cause (when possible), rewarming, and treatment or prevention of common complications.

Treatment of hypothalamic and spinal cord pathology causing hypothermia is similar to that discussed for hyperthermia. In addition, thiamine should be given routinely to hypothermic patients unless Wernicke encephalopathy has been excluded. Spells of episodic hyperhidrosis and hypothermia have responded to cyproheptadine, clonidine, β-blockers, anticonvulsants, dopamine agonists, or peripheral muscarinic blockade with oxybutynin or glycopyrrolate.

Any metabolic derangement predisposing to hypothermia should be corrected. For example, exogenous thyroxine is usually required to treat myxedema coma. Patients should be evaluated for trauma and drug or toxin ingestion. For patients with dermatologic conditions and those without any predisposition to hypothermia other than environmental exposure, treatment of the underlying cause consists of drying the patient and removal from the cold environment.

There are three rewarming methods: passive external rewarming, active external rewarming, and active core rewarming.[72,74,75,90–92,94,96–104] Passive external rewarming is the slowest and least invasive of these techniques: patients are placed in a warm environment and covered with blankets or aluminized body covers, and intravenous fluids are warmed to a temperature of 36°C to 39°C. This technique is usually adequate for patients with a core temperature of 32°C or above as long as the external hypothermic stresses are removed; patients who must avoid the cardiovascular stress of shivering may require active rewarming unless the shivering can be suppressed with benzodiazepines or meperidine or eliminated through neuromuscular blockade (in patients who are already sedated and receiving mechanical ventilation).

Active external rewarming consists of heating the skin with heating pads, heated blankets, hot water bottles, or a forced air heating system; radiant heat from a light source; or immersion in warm water. Concern has been raised regarding the risk of burn injuries to the vasoconstricted skin and because warming the skin prior to the core may result in peripheral vasodilatation and abrupt return of cold, acidic blood to the core from relatively hypoperfused regions, resulting in hypotension ("core temperature after-drop").

Active core rewarming techniques include the administration of heated oxygen by face mask or endotracheal tube, warm gastric or bladder irrigation, warm lavage (peritoneal, thoracic, mediastinal, or colonic), and hemodialysis or cardiopulmonary bypass with extracorporeal blood rewarming. The relative efficacy of these methods has not been established. Extracorporeal rewarming is preferred in patients with circulatory arrest.

All hypothermic patients with a severely depressed level of consciousness should be intubated to prevent aspiration. Patients should receive 100 percent oxygen until adequate oxygenation has been documented. Blood gas interpretation is complicated in the setting of hypothermia, and the optimal strategy for managing acid-base status remains controversial.

Hypotension in hypothermic patients is generally due to dehydration resulting from increased urine output, and fluid resuscitation is usually adequate. The role of inotropic agents is debated, because they have reduced efficacy at temperatures below 30°C and may be arrhythmogenic. Similarly at temperatures below 30°C, cardiac arrhythmias are resistant to many pharmacologic agents, pacing efforts, and defibrillation. Fortunately, many atrial arrhythmias and transient ventricular arrhythmias convert spontaneously during rewarming. For persistent ventricular arrhythmias, no anti-arrhythmic agent has been shown to be safe and effective.[72–75,90,91,94,100,101,105]

Treatment of hypothermia can lead to changes in serum electrolyte levels, requiring frequent monitoring. Hyperkalemia or hypophosphatemia may be particularly severe. Patients should be assessed for coagulopathy, including disseminated intravascular coagulation. A nasogastric tube should be inserted and serum amylase level checked because of the risk of ileus and pancreatitis.

The prognosis in hypothermia is influenced more by the patient's age and underlying disease than by the magnitude of the temperature decline. Some patients have been successfully resuscitated after 2 hours of apparent arrest, and others have survived temperatures below 20°C. This has prompted some to advocate warming all patients to normal temperatures before concluding that resuscitation is futile ("patients are not dead unless they are warm and dead").

Therapeutic Hypothermia

A 12 to 24 hour period of therapeutic hypothermia to a target of 32°C to 34°C is recommended for unconscious adults who have achieved return of spontaneous circulation after out-of-hospital cardiac arrest when the initial rhythm was ventricular fibrillation or pulseless ventricular tachycardia, based on studies showing reduced mortality and improved neurologic outcome.[106–109] Further investigation is required to determine the optimal duration of treatment, target temperature, and cooling method, as well as the efficacy of hypothermia when cardiac arrest occurs in the hospital or after other rhythms.[109–111] Therapeutic hypothermia has not been demonstrated to improve outcomes after head trauma or other neurologic injury, or during neurosurgical procedures.[112–117] Clinicians assessing prognosis in patients who are comatose following cardiac arrest need to recognize that predictive clinical findings and laboratory tests may be less reliable following therapeutic hypothermia.[118–126] Even the criteria for brain death in this setting may need to be revisited.[127]

REFERENCES

1. Gelb DJ: Abnormalities of thermal regulation and the nervous system. p. 1045. In Aminoff MJ (ed): Neurology and General Medicine. 4th Ed. Churchill Livingstone Elsevier, Philadelphia, 2008.
2. DiMicco JA, Zaretsky DV: The dorsomedial hypothalamus: a new player in thermoregulation. Am J Physiol Regul Integr Comp Physiol 292:R47, 2007.

3. Benarroch EE: Thermoregulation: recent concepts and remaining questions. Neurology 69:1293, 2007.
4. Kurz A: Physiology of thermoregulation. Best Pract Res Clin Anaesthesiol 22:627, 2008.
5. Bach V, Telliez F, Chardon K, et al: Thermoregulation in wakefulness and sleep in humans. Handb Clin Neurol 98:215, 2011.
6. Nakamura K: Central circuitries for body temperature regulation and fever. Am J Physiol Regul Integr Comp Physiol 301:R1207, 2011.
7. Cranshaw LI, Nagashima K, Yoda T, et al: Thermoregulation. p. 104. In Auerbach PS (ed): Wilderness Medicine. 6th Ed. Mosby, Philadelphia, 2012.
8. Clapham JC: Central control of thermogenesis. Neuropharmacology 63:111, 2012.
9. Mackowiak PA: Concepts of fever. Arch Intern Med 158:1870, 1998.
10. Avner JR: Acute fever. Pediatr Rev 30:5, 2009.
11. Pitoni S, Sinclair HL, Andrews PJD: Aspects of thermoregulation physiology. Curr Opin Crit Care 17:115, 2011.
12. Nakamura K, Morrison SF: Central efferent pathways for cold-defensive and febrile shivering. J Physiol 589:3641, 2011.
13. Silva JE: Physiological importance and control of non-shivering facultative thermogenesis. Front Biosci (Schol Ed) 3:352, 2011.
14. Charkoudian N: Mechanisms and modifiers of reflex induced cutaneous vasodilation and vasoconstriction in humans. J Appl Physiol 109:1221, 2010.
15. Johnson JM, Kellogg DL: Local thermal control of the human cutaneous circulation. J Appl Physiol 109:1229, 2010.
16. Holowatz LA, Kenney WL: Peripheral mechanisms of thermoregulatory control of skin blood flow in aged humans. J Appl Physiol 109:1538, 2010.
17. Jacob S, Irani SR, Rajabally YA, et al: Hypothermia in VGKC antibody-associated limbic encephalitis. J Neurol Neurosurg Psychiatry 79:202, 2008.
18. Tanev KS, Roether M, Yang C: Alcohol dementia and thermal dysregulation: a case report and review of the literature. Am J Alzheimers Dis Other Demen 2:563, 2009.
19. Davis SL, Wilson TE, White AT, et al: Thermoregulation in multiple sclerosis. J Appl Physiol 109:1531, 2010.
20. Suzuki K, Nakamura T, Hashimoto K, et al: Hypothermia, hypotension, hypersomnia, and obesity associated with hypothalamic lesions in a patient positive for the anti-aquaporin 4 antibody. Arch Neurol 69:1355, 2012.
21. Palm F, Löser C, Gronau W, et al: Successful treatment of acquired idiopathic generalized anhydrosis. Neurology 68:532, 2007.
22. Di Leo R, Nolano M, Boman H, et al: Central and peripheral autonomic failure in cold-induced sweating syndrome type 1. Neurology 75:1567, 2010.
23. Figueroa JJ, Dyck PJB, Laughlin RS, et al: Autonomic dysfunction in chronic inflammatory demyelinating polyradiculoneuropathy. Neurology 78:702, 2012.
24. Thompson HJ, Pinto-Martin J, Bullock MR: Neurogenic fever after traumatic brain injury: an epidemiological study. J Neurol Neurosurg Psychiatry 74:614, 2003.
25. Dietrich WD, Bramlett HM: Hyperthermia and central nervous system injury. Prog Brain Res 162:201, 2007.
26. Fernandez A, Schmidt JM, Claassen J, et al: Fever after subarachnoid hemorrhage: risk factors and impact on outcome. Neurology 68:1013, 2007.
27. Rabinstein AA, Sandhu K: Non-infectious fever in the neurological intensive care unit: incidence, causes and predictors. J Neurol Neurosurg Psychiatry 78:1278, 2007.
28. Sreedharan J, Shaw CE, Jarosz J, et al: Alexander disease with hypothermia, microcoria, and psychiatric and endocrine disturbances. Neurology 68:1322, 2007.
29. Axelrod YK, Diringer MN: Temperature management in acute neurologic disorders. Neurol Clin 26:585, 2008.
30. Sung CY, Lee TH, Chu NS: Central hyperthermia in acute stroke. Eur Neurol 62:86, 2009.
31. Konaka K, Miyashita K, Ishibashi-Ueda H, et al: Severe hyperthermia caused by four-vessel occlusion of main cerebral arteries. Intern Med 48:2137, 2009.
32. Li G, Xu X-Y, Wang Y, et al: Mild-to-moderate neurogenic pyrexia in acute cerebral infarction. Eur Neurol 65:94, 2011.
33. Darlix A, Mathey G, Sauvée M, et al: Paroxysmal hypothermia in two patients with multiple sclerosis. Eur Neurol 67:268, 2012.
34. Belcastro V, Striano P, Pierguidi L, et al: Recurrent hypothermia with hyperhidrosis in two siblings: familial Shapiro syndrome variant. J Neurol 259:756, 2012.
35. Duman O, Durmaz E, Akcurin S, et al: Spontaneous endogenous hypermelatoninemia: a new disease? Horm Res Paediatr 74:444, 2010.
36. Rodrigues Masruha M, Lin J, Harumi Arita J, et al: Spontaneous periodic hypothermia and hyperhidrosis: a possibly novel cerebral neurotransmitter disorder. Dev Med Child Neurol 53:378, 2011.
37. Alty JE, Ford HL: Multi-system complications of hypothermia: a case of recurrent episodic hypothermia with a review of the pathophysiology of hypothermia. Postgrad Med J 84:282, 2008.
38. Weiss N, Hasboun D, Demeret S, et al: Paroxysmal hypothermia as a clinical feature of multiple sclerosis. Neurology 72:193, 2009.
39. Perkes I, Baguley IJ, Nott MT, et al: A review of paroxysmal sympathetic hyperactivity after acquired brain injury. Ann Neurol 68:126, 2010.
40. Gómez-Choco MJ, Valls-Solé J, Grau JM, et al: Episodic hyperhidrosis as the only clinical manifestation of neuromyotonia. Neurology 65:1331, 2005.
41. Rosenberg H, Davis M, James D, et al: Malignant hyperthermia. Orphanet J Rare Dis 2:21, 2007.

42. Stowell KM: Malignant hyperthermia: a pharmacogenetic disorder. Pharmacogenomics 9:1657, 2008.
43. Green Larach M, Gronert GA, Allen GC, et al: Clinical presentation, treatment, and complications of malignant hyperthermia in North America from 1987 to 2006. Anesth Analg 110:498, 2010.
44. Protasi F, Paolini C, Dainese M: Calsequestrin-1: a new candidate gene for malignant hyperthermia and exertional/environmental heat stroke. J Physiol 587:3095, 2009.
45. Betzenhauser MJ, Marks AR: Ryanodine receptor channelopathies. Eur J Physiol 460:467, 2010.
46. Hirshey Dirksen SJ, Green Larach M, Rosenberg H, et al: Future directions in malignant hyperthermia research and patient care. Anesth Analg 113:1108, 2011.
47. Rosenberg H: Continued progress in understanding the molecular genetics of malignant hyperthermia. Can J Anaesth 58:489, 2011.
48. Lanner JT: Ryanodine receptor physiology and its role in disease. Adv Exp Med Biol 740:217, 2012.
49. Van Petegem F: Ryanodine receptors: structure and function. J Biol Chem 287:31624, 2012.
50. Klingler W, Rueffert H, Lehmann-Horn F, et al: Core myopathies and risk of malignant hyperthermia. Anesth Analg 109:1167, 2009.
51. Klingler W, Lehmann-Horn F, Jurkat-Rott K: Complications of anaesthesia in neuromuscular disorders. Neuromuscul Disord 15:195, 2005.
52. Gurnaney H, Brown A, Litman RS: Malignant hyperthermia and muscular dystrophies. Anesth Analg 109:1043, 2009.
53. Parness J, Bandschapp O, Girard T: The myotonias and susceptibility to malignant hyperthermia. Anesth Analg 109:1054, 2009.
54. Benca J, Hogan K: Malignant hyperthermia, coexisting disorders, and enzymopathies: risks and management options. Anesth Analg 109:1049, 2009.
55. Eyer F, Zilker T: Bench-to-bedside review: mechanisms and management of hyperthermia due to toxicity. Crit Care 11:236, 2007.
56. Gillman PK: Neuroleptic malignant syndrome: mechanisms, interactions, and causality. Mov Disord 25:1780, 2010.
57. Margetić B, Aukst-Margetić B: Neuroleptic malignant syndrome and its controversies. Pharmacoepidemiol Drug Saf 19:429, 2010.
58. McAllen KJ, Schwartz DR: Adverse drug reactions resulting in hyperthermia in the intensive care unit. Crit Care Med 38(suppl):S244, 2010.
59. Ables AZ, Nagubilli R: Prevention, diagnosis, and management of serotonin syndrome. Am Fam Physician 81:1139, 2010.
60. Levine M, Brooks DE, Truitt CA, et al: Toxicology in the ICU part 1: general overview and approach to treatment. Chest 140:795, 2011.
61. Perry PJ, Wilborn CA: Serotonin syndrome vs neuroleptic malignant syndrome: a contrast of causes, diagnoses, and management. Ann Clin Psychiatry 24:155, 2012.
62. Bienvenu OJ, Neufeld KJ, Needham DM: Treatment of four psychiatric emergencies in the intensive care unit. Crit Care Med 40:2662, 2012.
63. Trollor JN, Chen X, Sachdev PS: Neuroleptic malignant syndrome associated with atypical antipsychotic drugs. CNS Drugs 23:477, 2009.
64. Newman EJ, Grosset DG, Kenney PGE: The parkinsonism-hyperpyrexia syndrome. Neurocrit Care 10:136, 2009.
65. Racinais S, Oksa J: Temperature and neuromuscular function. Scand J Med Sci Sports 20(suppl 3):1, 2010.
66. Haveman J, Sminia P, Wondergem J, et al: Effects of hyperthermia on the central nervous system: what was learnt from animal studies? Int J Hyperthermia 21:473, 2005.
67. Cremer OL, Kalkman CJ: Cerebral pathophysiology and clinical neurology of hyperthermia in humans. Prog Brain Res 162:153, 2007.
68. White MG, Luca LE, Nonner D, et al: Cellular mechanisms of neuronal damage from hyperthermia. Prog Brain Res 162:347, 2007.
69. Hashim IA: Clinical biochemistry of hyperthermia. Ann Clin Biochem 47:516, 2010.
70. Epstein Y, Roberts WO: The pathophysiology of heat stroke: an integrative view of the final common pathway. Scand J Med Sci Sports 21:742, 2011.
71. Leon LR, Kenefick RW: Pathophysiology of heat-related illnesses. p. 215. In Auerbach PS (ed): Wilderness Medicine. 6th Ed. Mosby, Philadelphia, 2012.
72. Leikin SM, Korley FK, Wang EE, et al: The spectrum of hypothermia: from environmental exposure to therapeutic uses and medical simulation. Dis Mon 58:6, 2012.
73. Dhillon S: Environmental hazards, hot, cold, altitude, and sun. Infect Dis Clin North Am 26:707, 2012.
74. Corneli HM: Accidental hypothermia. Pediatr Emerg Care 28:475, 2012.
75. Danzl DF: Accidental hypothermia. p. 116. In Auerbach PS (ed): Wilderness Medicine. 6th Ed. Mosby, Philadelphia, 2012.
76. Jardine DS: Heat illness and heat stroke. Pediatr Rev 28:249, 2007.
77. Rowland T: Thermoregulation during exercise in the heat in children: old concepts revisited. J Appl Physiol 105:718, 2008.
78. Leon LR, Helwig BG: Heat stroke: role of the systemic inflammatory response. J Appl Physiol 109:1980, 2010.
79. Cancio LC, Lundy JB, Sheridan RL: Evolving changes in the management of burns and environmental injuries. Surg Clin North Am 92:959, 2012.
80. O'Brien KK, Leon LR, Kenefick RW: Clinical management of heat-related illnesses. p. 232. In Auerbach PS (ed): Wilderness Medicine. 6th Ed. Mosby, Philadelphia, 2012.

81. Galicia SC, Lewis SL, Metman LV: Severe topiramate-associated hyperthermia resulting in persistent neurologic dysfunction. Clin Neuropharmacol 28:94, 2005.
82. Markowitz SY, Robbins MS, Cascella C, et al: Reversible hypohidrosis with topiramate therapy for chronic migraine. Headache 50:672, 2010.
83. Crandall CG, González-Alonso J: Cardiovascular function in the heat-stressed human. Acta Physiol 199:407, 2010.
84. Wilson TE, Crandall CG: Effect of thermal stress on cardiac function. Exerc Sport Sci Rev 39:12, 2011.
85. Hadad E, Cohen-Sivan Y, Heled Y, et al: Clinical review: treatment of heat stroke: should dantrolene be considered? Crit Care 9:86, 2005.
86. Bouchama A, Dehbi M, Chaves-Carballo E: Cooling and hemodynamic management in heatstroke: practical recommendations. Crit Care 11:R54, 2007.
87. Casa DJ, McDermott BP, Lee EC, et al: Cold water immersion: the gold standard for exertional heatstroke treatment. Exerc Sport Sci Rev 35:141, 2007.
88. Mahmood MA, Zweifler RM: Progress in shivering control. J Neurol Sci 261:47, 2007.
89. Weant KA, Martin JE, Humphries RL, et al: Pharmacologic options for reducing the shivering response to therapeutic hypothermia. Pharmacotherapy 30:830, 2010.
90. Epstein E, Anna K: Accidental hypothermia. BMJ 332:706, 2006.
91. Aslam AF, Aslam AK, Vasavada BC, et al: Hypothermia: evaluation, electrocardiographic manifestations, and management. Am J Med 119:297, 2006.
92. Jurkovich GJ: Environmental cold-induced injury. Surg Clin North Am 87:247, 2007.
93. Turk EE: Hypothermia. Forensic Sci Med Pathol 6:106, 2010.
94. Brown DJA, Brugger H, Boyd J, et al: Accidental hypothermia. N Engl J Med 367:1930, 2012.
95. Kreuzer P, Landgrebe M, Wittmann M, et al: Hypothermia associated with antipsychotic drug use: a clinical case series and review of current literature. J Clin Pharmacol 52:1090, 2012.
96. Plaisier BR: Thoracic lavage in accidental hypothermia with cardiac arrest – report of a case and review of the literature. Resuscitation 66:99, 2005.
97. Kjærgaard B, Bach P: Warming of patients with accidental hypothermia using warm water pleural lavage. Resuscitation 68:203, 2006.
98. Ruttmann E, Weissenbacher A, Ulmer H, et al: Prolonged extracorporeal membrane oxygenation-assisted support provides improved survival in hypothermic patients with cardiocirculatory arrest. J Thorac Cardiovasc Surg 134:594, 2007.
99. Seiji M, Sadaki I, Shigeaki I, et al: The efficacy of rewarming with a portable and percutaneous cardiopulmonary bypass system in accidental deep hypothermia patients with hemodynamic instability. J Trauma 65:1391, 2008.
100. Vanden Hoek TL, Morrison LJ, Shuster M, et al: Part 12: cardiac arrest in special situations: 2010 American Heart Association guidelines for cardiopulmonary resuscitation and emergency cardiovascular care. Circulation 122(suppl 3):S829, 2010.
101. Soar J, Perkins GD, Abbas G, et al: European Resucitation Council guidelines for resuscitation 2010 section 8. Cardiac arrest in special circumstances: electrolyte abnormalities, poisoning, drowning, accidental hypothermia, hyperthermia, asthma, anaphylaxis, cardiac surgery, trauma, pregnancy, electrocution. Resuscitation 81:1400, 2010.
102. van der Ploeg G-J, Goslings JC, Walpoth BH, et al: Accidental hypothermia: rewarming treatments, complications and outcomes from one university medical centre. Resuscitation 81:1550, 2010.
103. Maria Galvão C, Liang Y, Clark AM: Effectiveness of cutaneous warming systems on temperature control: meta-analysis. J Adv Nurs 66:1365, 2010.
104. Brodmann Maeder M, Dünser M, Eberle B, et al: The Bernese hypothermia algorithm: a consensus paper on in-hospital decision-making and treatment of patients in hypothermic cardiac arrest at an alpine level 1 trauma centre. Injury 42:539, 2011.
105. Wira CR, Becker JU, Martin G, et al: Anti-arrhythmic and vasopressor medications for the treatment of ventricular fibrillation in severe hypothermia: a systematic review of the literature. Resuscitation 78:21, 2008.
106. Varon J, Acosta P: Therapeutic hypothermia: past, present, and future. Chest 133:1267, 2008.
107. Janata A, Holzer M: Hypothermia after cardiac arrest. Prog Cardiovasc Dis 52:168, 2009.
108. Holzer M: Targeted temperature management for comatose survivors of cardiac arrest. N Engl J Med 363:1256, 2010.
109. Walters JH, Morley PT, Nolan JP: The role of hypothermia in post-cardiac arrest patients with return of spontaneous circulation: a systematic review. Resuscitation 82:508, 2011.
110. Lopez-de-Sa E, Rey JR, Armada E, et al: Hypothermia in comatose survivors from out-of-hospital cardiac arrest: pilot trial comparing 2 levels of target temperature. Circulation 126:2826, 2012.
111. Shinozaki K, Oda S, Sadahiro T, et al: Duration of well-controlled core temperature correlates with neurological outcome in patients with post-cardiac arrest syndrome. Am J Emerg Med 30:1838, 2012.
112. Liu-DeRyke X, Saely S, Rhoney DH: Temperature management in acute neurologic injury: to cool or not to cool. J Pharm Pract 23:483, 2010.
113. Nunnally ME, Jaeschke R, Bellingan GJ, et al: Targeted temperature management in critical care: a report and recommendations from five professional societies. Crit Care Med 39:1113, 2011.
114. Rossetti AO: What is the value of hypothermia in acute neurologic diseases and status epilepticus? Epilepsia 52(suppl 8):64, 2011.

115. Moore EM, Nichol AD, Bernard SA, et al: Therapeutic hypothermia: benefits, mechanisms, and potential clinical applications in neurological, cardiac and kidney injury. Injury 42:843, 2011.
116. El Beheiry H: Protecting the brain during neurosurgical procedures: strategies that can work. Curr Opin Anaesthesiol 25:548, 2012.
117. Georgiou AP, Manara AR: Role of therapeutic hypothermia in improving outcome after traumatic brain injury: a systematic review. Br J Anaesth 110:357, 2013.
118. Al Thenayan E, Savard M, Sharpe M, et al: Predictors of poor neurologic outcome after induced mild hypothermia following cardiac arrest. Neurology 71:1535, 2008.
119. Rossetti AO, Oddo M, Liaudet L, et al: Predictors of awakening from postanoxic status epilepticus after therapeutic hypothermia. Neurology 72:744, 2009.
120. Rossetti AO, Oddo M, Logroscino G, et al: Prognostication after cardiac arrest and hypothermia: a prospective study. Ann Neurol 67:301, 2010.
121. Leithner C, Ploner CJ, Hasper D, et al: Does hypothermia influence the predictive value of bilateral absent N20 after cardiac arrest? Neurology 74:965, 2010.
122. Cronberg T, Rundgren M, Westhall E, et al: Neuron-specific enolase correlates with other prognostic markers after cardiac arrest. Neurology 77:623, 2011.
123. Fugate JE, Wijdicks EFM, White RD, et al: Does therapeutic hypothermia affect time to awakening in cardiac arrest survivors? Neurology 77:1346, 2011.
124. Rossetti AO, Carrera E, Oddo M: Early EEG correlates of neuronal injury after brain anoxia. Neurology 78:796, 2012.
125. Bouwes A, Binnekade JM, Kuiper MA, et al: Prognosis of coma after therapeutic hypothermia: a prospective cohort study. Ann Neurol 71:206, 2012.
126. Crepeau AZ, Rabinstein AA, Fugate JE, et al: Continuous EEG in therapeutic hypothermia after cardiac arrest: prognostic and clinical value. Neurology 80:339, 2013.
127. Webb AC, Samuels OB: Reversible brain death after cardiopulmonary arrest and induced hypothermia. Crit Care Med 39:1538, 2011.

CHAPTER

38

Postconcussion Syndrome

JEFFREY S. KUTCHER

Postconcussion syndrome (PCS) is a common condition that includes physical, cognitive, and affective symptoms. PCS has a long history of controversy, is diagnostically complex, and lacks a widely accepted approach to management.[1,2] Writings on the subject appear in the medical literature as far back as the late nineteenth century, when Jean-Martin Charcot described twenty cases of "traumatic hysteria."[3] John Hughlings Jackson and Joseph Babinski followed with seminal works that further elucidated how the interactions between psychologic factors and organic pathologies work to produce self-propagating symptom complexes.[4,5] These works helped frame the early thinking of this condition, which became known as "shell shock" in relation to World War I soldiers who developed a predictable pattern of chronic symptoms after being in the proximity of an explosion while suffering no observable head wound.[1] The evolution in terminology continued in the mid-twentieth century when the term *postconcussion syndrome* was popularized, indicating a more complex pathophysiologic process that included, but was not limited to, psychologic mediators.[1] Although the accepted terminology for the condition has evolved over nearly a century, a clear understanding of the etiologies of PCS remains elusive and no single definition of PCS is accepted by the medical community.[6,7]

Scientific and clinical interest has focused on the consequences of head injuries, particularly those suffered in organized athletics and during the course of military service.[8–10] In patients suffering a mild traumatic brain injury (concussion), PCS is estimated to occur in 24 to 84 percent of cases.[11] Given that the US Centers for Disease Control and Prevention estimates that between 1.6 and 3.8 million concussions occur in the United States annually from sports and recreation activities alone, the prevalence of PCS is probably high.[12,13] Traditionally, the diagnosis of PCS has used symptom-based criteria, but the application of a more comprehensive clinical approach is now favored.[2]

TRADITIONAL DIAGNOSIS

PCS has been codified under both the International Statistical Classification of Diseases and Related Health Problems (ICD-10) and the Diagnostic and Statistical Manual of Mental Disorders (DSM-IV).[14,15] The ICD-10 criteria begin with a history of head trauma "usually sufficiently severe to result in loss of consciousness." Diagnosis then requires the presence of three or more of the following symptoms: headache, dizziness, fatigue, irritability, insomnia, concentration or memory difficulty,

Aminoff's Neurology and General Medicine, Fifth Edition.

and intolerance of stress, emotion, or alcohol.[14] The sole exclusionary criterion is the absence of an ongoing concussion. This diagnostic schema has come under criticism for three main reasons. First, observational studies have indicated that less than 10 percent of concussions involve loss of consciousness, and its presence is not a predictor of symptom duration.[8,16,17] Second, the presence of five, rather than three, of the ICD-10 symptoms has been shown to be diagnostically useful for PCS at 1 month after injury, with a sensitivity of 73 percent and specificity of 61 percent.[18] At 3 months after injury, the ICD-10 symptoms were not found to be useful for making a diagnosis of PCS.[18] The third criticism involves the absence of symptoms that pertain specifically to mood or affect, which are common in PCS.[19]

By comparison, the DSM-IV criteria do include mood- and affect-related symptoms.[20] The DSM-IV diagnostic schema begins with a history of traumatic brain injury causing "significant cerebral concussion." Cognitive deficits in attention or memory are then required, as is the presence of at least three of the following symptoms: fatigue, sleep difficulty, headache, dizziness, irritability, affective disturbance, personality change, or apathy. Symptoms must also persist for 3 months and interfere with social functioning. Dementing illnesses or other conditions that could account for symptoms need to be excluded.[6,21] As with the ICD-10 criteria, the DSM-IV criteria are notable for their lack of specific symptoms commonly seen in these patients, namely those of multi-domain cognitive dysfunction.[21] Whether the clinician opts to use the ICD-10 or DSM-IV diagnostic criteria, significant limitations exist. In one study, a consecutive series of 340 patients was evaluated with both criteria; the two criteria resulted in markedly different incidence rates without any discernible pattern to support the clinical utility of either.[21]

Several factors account for the difficulties in applying any strict diagnostic criteria to PCS. The nature of the antecedent event is usually concussion, which itself is a separate clinical entity that has diagnostic confusion and an incompletely elucidated pathophysiology.[12,20] Given that PCS is a diagnosis preceded by concussion, a certain amount of uncertainty is inherent. PCS-like symptoms may also be present in individuals who have not experienced head trauma.[20,22,23] In one healthy, noninjured population, the incidence of reporting three or more typical PCS symptoms was 80 percent.[24] Many common conditions, such as depression, attention-deficit hyperactivity disorder, migraine, and sleep disorders can easily be exacerbated by a preceding brain injury and produce symptoms similar to PCS, creating a complex differential diagnosis.[25]

CLINICAL DIAGNOSIS

Given the uncertainty produced through the application of specific, symptom-based, diagnostic schemata for PCS, an alternative approach should be taken that allows for a more open-ended interpretation of PCS symptoms and the use of basic clinical principles to dictate diagnostic accuracy. The clinician must first accurately recognize concussion and identify its resolution, before determining the presence of PCS. Symptoms of *prolonged concussion* must be distinguished from PCS.

Concussion

The American Academy of Neurology recognizes concussion as a "clinical syndrome of biomechanically induced alteration of brain function, typically affecting memory and orientation, which may involve loss of consciousness."[8] In most cases, concussion is characterized by a rapid onset of symptoms or cognitive dysfunction that resolves spontaneously.[12] Concussions typically produce no abnormalities on standard structural neuroimaging, although newer imaging technologies, such as functional magnetic resonance imaging (fMRI), do show promise as potential diagnostic tools.[9,26] The pathophysiology of concussion is not completely understood but it is assumed to have a significant metabolic component characterized by a mismatch between the amount of energy available to cortical neurons and the amount needed to perform expected neuronal functions and restore appropriate intracellular ion concentrations to their preinjury states.[27] The majority of concussions, perhaps as many as 90 percent, have complete symptom resolution in 7 days.[28] Common manifestations of concussion include physical symptoms such as headache, nausea, and photophobia; cognitive symptoms; emotional symptoms; and sleep disturbance.[28] Loss of consciousness is not required to make the diagnosis and occurs in the significant minority (less than 10 percent) of cases.[8,12]

The hallmark of concussion management in the acute phase is rest, both physical and cognitive, although there is a lack of published data that point to a particular duration or degree of rest that is beneficial.[29] There is no objective confirmatory test for concussion that is widely accepted, and the recommended clinical approach for determining the resolution of a concussion is for the patient who has recently become asymptomatic to undergo a series of increasing physical challenges, allowing enough time between each challenge (24 hours on average) for symptoms to develop.[9] If the recently concussed patient is able to tolerate significant levels of physical exertion, with heart rate elevated above 80 percent of estimated maximum heart rate for at least 30 minutes, along with complex physical tasks without the return of symptoms, it is reasonable to conclude that the concussion has resolved.[9] The approach of using stepwise physical exertion to determine a return to participation in activities is discussed below.

Prolonged Concussion

A minority of concussions will last longer than 7 days.[28] These cases can be attributed to individual variation in some combination of the degree of metabolic injury, the propensity for a particular patient to experience the symptoms of concussion, and the presence of confounding comorbidities such as migraine headache, attention deficit hyperactivity disorder, or depression.[25,30] It is assumed that continued physical exertion, and perhaps even cognitive exertion, during the acute postinjury phase (2 to 3 days) following the initial head trauma may result in deepening the causative metabolic injury and prolonging the clinical syndrome of concussion.[9] A concussed patient who experiences a second blow to the head or body resulting in an acceleration-deceleration injury of the brain may exacerbate the underlying pathophysiology.[8] In either scenario, the ensuing injury may last significantly longer than the 7-day average, producing a concussion that can persist for several weeks.[12,25]

Postconcussion Syndrome

PCS is the clinical manifestation of a pathologic process that is separate from concussion and produces a clinically distinct symptom complex. Although the nomenclature of PCS implies that it occurs following the original injury, the pathologic process actually may begin before the associated concussion has completely resolved. While the patient is still symptomatic from the initial injury, it is difficult to determine which process is contributing. PCS symptoms always eventually outlast the symptoms of concussion and become the primary clinical concern.[19]

The precise mechanism of PCS is not well understood but is thought to include both psychologic and organic factors.[31–35] Postulated organic causes include subcellular structural changes, impaired regulation of cerebral blood flow, and changes in brain network connectivity.[11,36,37] Although organic factors have been implicated more closely in the creation of PCS symptoms, psychologic factors may be responsible for their chronicity. The symptoms of PCS are widely accepted to have the potential to last for months or even years.[14,38–40]

EVALUATION

Regardless of the duration of the preceding concussion, the key to diagnosing PCS is first to determine that the concussion itself has resolved. This can be difficult given that the symptoms of concussion and PCS overlap in character and in timing. A thorough neurologic history that explicitly describes the time course of each symptom is essential. The natural history of concussion symptoms tends to be monophasic, with a gradual and progressive resolution of symptoms over time, allowing for occasional symptomatic worsening with continued exertion or subsequent injury.[9] The timing of PCS symptoms, by contrast, tends to be more variable.[7,35] PCS symptoms do not respond to continued physical or cognitive rest, whereas rest typically improves concussive symptoms.[12]

In patients with concussion whose symptoms are still present and whose history does not allow for an easy delineation between concussion and PCS, the patient can be asked to increase gradually their physical or cognitive activities while monitoring for changes in symptom duration and severity.[41,42] PCS responds favorably to a gradual introduction of physical exertion, whereas no such relationship has been described for concussion.[42] Care should be taken not to allow a symptomatic patient who may still be concussed to continue to increase their physical exertion to the point of dramatically increasing symptom severity.[12]

Currently, there are no diagnostic tests that are helpful in making a diagnosis of PCS.[8] Several technologies continue to be investigated including quantitative electroencephalography (EEG), fMRI, and magnetic resonance spectroscopy.[26,43] Neuropsychologic tests can provide important information including identifying the presence of other comorbid diagnoses but must be used as one part of a larger clinical evaluation paradigm.[6]

DIFFERENTIAL DIAGNOSIS

Given that PCS has many symptoms and features in common with other conditions, it is frequently misdiagnosed.[19,44] Some of the more common conditions that should be considered include migraine and other headache disorders, depression, attention deficit hyperactivity disorder, and sleep disorders.[25,45–49] Each of these preexisting conditions can potentially be exacerbated by a traumatic brain injury; in some instances, these conditions may only be mild, or even asymptomatic, prior to a concussion and then worsen considerably afterward, leading to diagnostic confusion with the symptoms of PCS.[25]

An alternative approach to this differential diagnosis is to use a more liberal application of the PCS diagnosis itself, allowing for these "comorbid" conditions to be considered subtypes of PCS. In this way, the diagnosis of PCS becomes more simple. The clinician need only determine that the presenting symptoms were not present, or were present to a lesser degree, prior to the inciting concussion and that the concussion itself has resolved. Using this approach, any neurologic symptom-complex that begins following a head trauma and continues beyond the course of the actual concussion may be considered to be part of PCS regardless of symptom number, type, or duration.

One additional symptom-generating mechanism that must be considered carefully is that of inappropriate rest.[50,51] Having an individual dramatically reduce their level of physical, cognitive, and social activity is a risk factor for the development of physical, cognitive, emotional, or sleep-related symptoms.[51] Identifying rest as a potential contributor to symptoms is important, given that it is also the hallmark treatment for concussion. Symptoms present due to inappropriate rest that are misinterpreted as being direct manifestations of the original brain injury will be made worse if the patient is asked to continue their period of rest. A careful history should include asking about current levels of activity and how they relate to the patient's preinjury experience.

TREATMENT AND PROGNOSIS

Once PCS has been diagnosed, the first step in developing a treatment plan involves addressing suspected symptom generators. If over-resting is suspected, the patient should be instructed to begin gradually reintroducing physical exertion, cognitive exertion, and social involvement. Ignoring this particular potential symptom generator will further propagate symptoms and potentially decrease the efficacy of other treatment modalities.[51]

Preexisting conditions should be addressed and treated symptomatically including migraine and depression. The management of PCS should then turn to addressing the specific symptoms that remain; since there are no pharmacologic therapies specifically for PCS, treatment is analogous to that of common conditions that produce the symptoms in question.[52,53] Psychologic therapy and cognitive behavioral therapy have some benefit.[54,55] Hyperbaric oxygen has been suggested as a possible treatment for PCS but its use, as yet, is not widely accepted.[56]

Despite the diagnostic complexities of PCS and a lack of specific proven therapies, prognosis is largely positive, with the majority of patients experiencing complete symptom resolution within 6 months.[7,38]

RETURN TO PARTICIPATION

One of the most critical decisions in the management of patients with PCS is deciding when to recommend a return to sports, school, or work. This decision is complex, given the multitude of variables that can effect PCS symptom development, severity, and duration.[3,35] The degree of individual variability in brain physiology, and thus response to injury, can produce different estimations of inherent risk on a case-by-case basis. Differing levels of injury risk that are associated with specific activities in question help to further define future risk of injury; players of American football are likely to be at higher risk of recurrent injury than baseball players. The amount of physical, psychologic, social, or economic benefit that may come from returning to that activity cannot be ignored as these factors define the patient's personal motivation for returning to participation.

It is essential that the clinician be confident that the patient is no longer concussed as there is clear medical consensus that individuals who are still concussed should not be exposed to additional significant risk of further head injury.[8,9,28,57] Patients who are symptomatic from a concussion should avoid the extremes of physical and cognitive exertion in an effort to minimize symptom duration and severity.[8,9,12] The decision to return to participation for a patient diagnosed with concussion involves a relatively straightforward management construct in which the resolution of the injury is determined through a series of increasing physical challenges while assessing for symptomatic worsening.[9] Unfortunately, no similarly accepted approach for returning to play with PCS exists, further highlighting the need to be certain about the diagnosis.

TABLE 38-1 ■ Suggested Return-to-Participation Protocol Following the Resolution of Concussion Symptoms

Stage	Objective	Exercise
I Stationary bike	Increase heart rate	30 minutes of sustained effort, heart rate 70–80% maximum
II Treadmill jog	Simple movement	30 minutes of sustained effort, heart rate 70–80% maximum
III Agility drills	Interval cardiovascular exertion and complex movement	30 minutes of sport-specific training drills
IV Noncontact practice	Cognitive load	Full noncontact practice
V Full game play	Return to activity	Full game play

Participation after Concussion

The majority of concussions are self-limited clinical syndromes that resolve spontaneously. It has been estimated that up to 90 percent of concussions in adults will resolve between 7 and 10 days.[12,25] The risk from returning to a contact-risk activity while still actively concussed is twofold. First, the actively concussed state appears to be a period of increased vulnerability to additional injury, and perhaps to more significant injury.[8,58] It has been suggested that during this time of physiologic vulnerability, it takes less biomechanical force to produce an additional physiologic perturbation. The diagnosis of "second-impact syndrome" has been used to refer to a potentially devastating, perhaps lethal, state of malignant cerebral edema that is induced when a patient who is actively concussed experiences another biomechanical force acting on their brain.[59] The nature of second-impact syndrome is still unclear, with some authors downplaying the importance of the second impact itself, instead postulating that the condition is a manifestation of an inherent sensitivity, perhaps at the ion-channel level, to any significant biomechanical force.[60,61] The second reason to limit contact-risk exposure while an individual is still concussed is that additional blows to the head or body that transmit biomechanical force to the brain may exacerbate the existing injury and induce greater symptom duration and severity, resulting in an overall increase in morbidity.[8,9,28]

The process for making a return-to-participation decision following concussion begins with the determination that the patient is no longer experiencing the acute symptoms of the injury. Clinicians should be careful not to insist that patients are completely asymptomatic, as the presence of some symptoms may be accounted for by other noninjury factors related to management, such as the loss of physical activity and social interaction.[12,25,51] It is more appropriate that the patient be able to tolerate a day of "regular" activities, such as going to school, without a return of bothersome symptoms and without the use of symptomatic medications or other therapies. Once this is the case, it is then best to have the patient begin a graduated set of physical challenges designed to test whether an injury might still exist that is subsymptomatic.[9,12,28]

Each stage of the return to participation protocol is designed to test a very particular demand on brain function (Table 38-1). Stage I is designed to introduce simple cardiovascular exertion that is sustained and constant. Around 30 minutes of exertion with a heart rate sustained between 70 and 80 percent of the expected maximum (which can be calculated as 220 minus the patient's age) is usually adequate. This first stage is best accomplished by the use of a stationary bike, as this minimizes other variables including movement, visual processing, and cognitive load. Stage II adds predictable, simple movement by having the patient jog on a treadmill with the same time and cardiovascular goals as stage I. Stage III adds both complex movements and interval cardiovascular exertion through the use of sport-specific agility drills; this stage can also include resistance training. As with the first two stages, at least 30 minutes of exposure is necessary. Stage IV adds the cognitive load of playing the sport in question, by having the patient participate in a typical noncontact practice that has been carefully controlled to eliminate any significant risk of head trauma. Stage IV further challenges the patient by providing a complex and dynamic visual environment. The final stage is a return to participation without restrictions.

With each stage, the patient should be asked to perform the task and note the development of any symptoms. It should be emphasized that certain symptoms, such as light-headedness or head pressure, may be the result of the exertion itself and not necessarily an indication of the presence of injury. It is perhaps more useful to ask the patient to note any symptoms that are out of proportion to what might typically be experienced with that particular challenge. Enough time should be given to allow for the development of symptoms following the challenge; typically this period involves being asymptomatic for the remainder of the day, during an evening of typical sleep, and then the following morning upon awaking. If no obvious clinical syndrome develops during this time period, the patient can than go on to the next challenge.[9,12,25,28] Once the patient is able to tolerate all stages of the protocol, it is reasonable to suggest that he or she can return to activities without restrictions.[12]

Participation after Postconcussion Syndrome

Unlike the patient who is still concussed, a patient with PCS does not have a well-described risk associated with returning to participation in contact sports or other activities with a known risk of head trauma. For patients with PCS, any additional risk of injury beyond what would be considered baseline for the particular activity is not well established, nor is the risk of more significant or permanent injury. Given the nature of PCS, however, it can be assumed that a patient with PCS who continues to participate in such activities is at an increased risk of significant symptom exacerbation if an additional head trauma is experienced.[11,20,62] However, it is also plausible that participation in sports or other activities may help to alleviate the symptoms of PCS by providing the patient with physical or psychologic benefit, or both.[2,51] The use of medications for the symptomatic management of patients with PCS is not a clear contraindication to participation in contact-risk activities, as it is in those patients with an active concussion. Given the varied pathologic mechanisms of PCS, each specific case carries its own particular risk of symptom exacerbation.

The return-to-participation process in patients with PCS, therefore, should be individualized and focused on rehabilitation efforts that allow the patient to experience gradually increasing amounts of physical and cognitive exertion without significant symptom exacerbation.[41,42] Rehabilitation plans that provide the patient with objective markers for improvement are recommended. For example, a period of exercise on a stationary bicycle, while monitoring heart rate, can be used to determine a level of exertion that does not significantly exacerbate symptoms; the patient can then use heart rate as a marker for exertion, allowing for monitoring of improvement and increase of activity tolerance.[42]

Retirement from a Contact-Risk Activity

Clinicians are frequently asked to make a recommendation as to whether a patient should retire permanently from contact-risk activities following head injury. It is often assumed that this decision is best made by determining the number of concussions the patient has experienced during their lifetime.[12] Given that concussion is a clinical diagnosis based mainly on the patient's self-reported symptoms when injured, this approach is likely an oversimplification. The number of concussions that have been experienced by a patient does not provide any clear estimate of the patient's risk of long-term consequences and, therefore, their risk of continued participation in a contact activity. At present, there are no objective tests or accepted biomarkers available to the clinician to help determine whether a patient has experienced a decrease in baseline brain function as the result of exposure to head trauma.[12,26]

The retirement decision, therefore, akin to other decisions regarding the diagnoses of concussion and PCS, is largely dependent on a comprehensive neurologic evaluation and a clinical decision-making process. Although no clear rules have been established for when to recommend retirement, there are some basic clinical principles that should be applied. If a clear pattern is established of concussions occurring with less and less biomechanical force, this may be an indication that the patient's brain has experienced some degree of altered baseline function. If a patient is clearly experiencing longer or more severe symptoms with each subsequent concussion, the clinician may reasonably conclude that additional concussions will produce a continued increase in injury-associated morbidity, making further participation in a contact-risk activity more risky. If the patient shows objective signs, or has subjective complaints, of a decrease in baseline cognitive function or a change in personality, care should be given to determine whether these changes can be attributed to other potential causes such as mood dysfunction or sleep disorders; if no other cause is found and head trauma becomes the presumed mechanism of the observed change in brain function, retirement should be recommended.

CHRONIC TRAUMATIC ENCEPHALOPATHY

PCS is not the only clinical manifestation of head trauma that can produce symptoms that last beyond the time frame of typical concussion. Recently, chronic traumatic encephalopathy (CTE) has been receiving increasing attention as a potential long-term consequence of head trauma that has some features in common with PCS.[63,64] CTE is a progressive degenerative disease of the brain that was first described in professional boxers in 1928 as a clinical syndrome that had both motor and cognitive features, including bradykinesia, gait abnormalities, changes in mood and affect, behavioral abnormalities, memory impairment, and executive dysfunction.[65–67] CTE, at the time referred to as the "punch drunk syndrome," was presumed to be caused by repetitive blows to the head. More recently, CTE has been described in a wider variety of contact-sport athletes, military personnel, and others who have experienced frequent head injuries over many years.[63,64] Despite over 80 years of clinical observation by the medical community, there is no known threshold of lifetime exposure to biomechanical force that has been shown to be associated with the development of CTE. In addition, although strongly suspected by many, the causality of CTE has not been established and the relationship between CTE and head trauma is strictly associative.[67]

Recent interest in CTE has focused on the pathologic features of the disease. Gross pathologic features of CTE include an overall decrease in brain weight, enlargement of the third and lateral ventricles, and a thinning of the corpus callosum.[64] Microscopically, CTE pathology is dominated by abnormal depositions of tau in brain structures typically deeper than those affected in Alzheimer disease. How these pathologic features relate to the clinical presentations of CTE is unclear.[67] Epidemiologic features of CTE, including its prevalence, remain unknown.[9,67]

Given that symptoms of PCS can last for many months or even years, these patients often are concerned that they are experiencing the early clinical manifestations of CTE. These two conditions offer two very different prognoses. PCS is a treatable condition with symptoms that may significantly interfere with normal function but often respond to therapy.[19] Symptoms of PCS may vary over time or even be produced largely by particular situations such as physical exertion or exposure to crowded or complex environments. CTE, in contrast, is a dementing illness with features more in common with other neurodegenerative disorders including a lack of insight, significant emotional lability, and less variability over time compared with PCS symptoms. There is no known treatment for CTE and functional morbidity tends to be progressive. While the natural history of CTE is not well understood, it is a condition that likely leads to a decreased lifespan.[67] Since there are no established diagnostic tests for either PCS or CTE, the distinction is based on a thorough clinical evaluation.

REFERENCES

1. Jones E, Fear NT, Wessely S: Shell shock and mild traumatic brain injury: a historical review. Am J Psychiatry 164:1641, 2007.
2. Silverberg ND, Iverson GL: Etiology of the post-concussion syndrome: physiogenesis and psychogenesis revisited. NeuroRehabilitation 29:317, 2011.
3. Macleod AD: Post concussion syndrome: the attraction of the psychological by the organic. Med Hypotheses 74:1033, 2010.
4. York GK, Steinberg DA: The philosophy of Hughlings Jackson. J R Soc Med 95:314, 2002.
5. Babinski J, Froment J: Hysteria of Pithiatism and Reflex Nervous Disorders in the Neurology of War. University of London Press, London, 1918.
6. Hall RC, Hall RC, Chapman MJ: Definition, diagnosis, and forensic implications of postconcussional syndrome. Psychosomatics 46:195, 2005.

7. Evans RW: The postconcussion syndrome and the sequelae of mild head injury. Neurol Clin 10:815, 1992.
8. Giza CC, Kutcher JS, Ashwal S, et al: Summary of evidence-based guideline update: evaluation and management of concussion in sports: report of the Guideline Development Subcommittee of the American Academy of Neurology. Neurology 80:2250, 2013.
9. McCrory P, Meeuwisse WH, Aubry M, et al: Consensus statement on concussion in sport: the 4th International Conference on Concussion in Sport held in Zurich, November 2012. Br J Sports Med 47:250, 2013.
10. Felber ES: Combat-related posttraumatic headache: diagnosis, mechanisms of injury, and challenges to treatment. J Am Osteopath Assoc 110:737, 2010.
11. Ryan LM, Warden DL: Post concussion syndrome. Int Rev Psychiatry 15:310, 2003.
12. Kutcher JS, Giza CC, Alessi AG: Sports concussion. Continuum 16:41, 2010.
13. Langlois JA, Rutland-Brown W, Wald MM: The epidemiology and impact of traumatic brain injury: a brief overview. J Head Trauma Rehabil 21:375, 2006.
14. Boake C, McCauley SR, Levin HS, et al: Diagnostic criteria for postconcussional syndrome after mild to moderate traumatic brain injury. J Neuropsychiatry Clin Neurosci 17:350, 2005.
15. Yeates KO, Taylor HG: Neurobehavioural outcomes of mild head injury in children and adolescents. Pediatr Rehabil 8:5, 2005.
16. Halstead ME, Walter KD: Council on Sports Medicine and Fitness: American Academy of Pediatrics. Clinical report—sport-related concussion in children and adolescents. Pediatrics 126:597, 2010.
17. Eisenberg MA, Andrea J, Meehan W, et al: Time interval between concussions and symptom duration. Pediatrics 132:8, 2013.
18. Kashluba S, Casey JE, Paniak C: Evaluating the utility of ICD-10 diagnostic criteria for postconcussion syndrome following mild traumatic brain injury. J Int Neuropsychol Soc 12:111, 2006.
19. Iverson GL, Zasler ND, Lange RT: Post-concussive disorder. p. 374. In: Zasler ND, Katz D, Zafonte RD (eds): Brain Injury Medicine: Principles and Practice. Demos Medical Publishing, New York, 2006.
20. Iverson GL: Outcome from mild traumatic brain injury. Curr Opin Psychiatry 18:301, 2005.
21. McCauley SR, Boake C, Pedroza C, et al: Postconcussional disorder: are the DSM-IV criteria an improvement over the ICD-10? J Nerv Ment Dis 193:540, 2005.
22. Edmed S, Sullivan K: Depression, anxiety, and stress as predictors of postconcussion-like symptoms in a nonclinical sample. Psychiatry Res 200:41, 2012.
23. Dean PJ, O'Neill D, Sterr A: Post-concussion syndrome: prevalence after mild traumatic brain injury in comparison with a sample without head injury. Brain Inj 26:14, 2012.
24. Anderson THM, Macleod AD: Concussion and mild head injury. Pract Neurol 6:342, 2006.
25. Kutcher JS: Management of the complicated sports concussion patient. Sports Health 2:197, 2010.
26. Kutcher JS, McCrory P, Davis G, et al: What evidence exists for new strategies or technologies in the diagnosis of sports concussion and assessment of recovery? Br J Sports Med 47:299, 2013.
27. Giza CC, Hovda DA: The neurometabolic cascade of concussion. J Athl Train 36:228, 2001.
28. Harmon KG, Drezner J: Gammons M, et al: American Medical Society for Sports Medicine position statement: concussion in sport. Clin J Sport Med 23:1, 2013.
29. Schneider KJ, Iverson GL, Emery CA, et al: The effects of rest and treatment following sport-related concussion: a systematic review of the literature. Br J Sports Med 47:304, 2013.
30. Chrisman SP, Rivara FP, Schiff MA, et al: Risk factors for concussive symptoms 1 week or longer in high school athletes. Brain Inj 27:1, 2013.
31. Datta SG, Pillai SV, Rao SL, et al: Post-concussion syndrome: correlation of neuropsychological deficits, structural lesions on magnetic resonance imaging and symptoms. Neurol India 57:594, 2009.
32. Evans RW: Persistent post-traumatic headache, postconcussion syndrome, and whiplash injuries: the evidence for a non-traumatic basis with an historical review. Headache 50:716, 2010.
33. Garden N, Sullivan KA: An examination of the base rates of post-concussion symptoms: the influence of demographics and depression. Appl Neuropsychol 17:1, 2010.
34. Garden N, Sullivan KA, Lange RT: The relationship between personality characteristics and postconcussion symptoms in a nonclinical sample. Neuropsychology 24:168, 2010.
35. Jacobson RR: The post-concussional syndrome: physiogenesis, psychogenesis and malingering. An integrative model. J Psychosom Res 39:675, 1995.
36. Messe A, Caplain S, Pelegrini-Issac M, et al: Specific and evolving resting-state network alterations in postconcussion syndrome following mild traumatic brain injury. PLoS One 8:e65470, 2013.
37. Slobounov SM, Zhang K, Pennell D, et al: Functional abnormalities in normally appearing athletes following mild traumatic brain injury: a functional MRI study. Exp Brain Res 202:341, 2010.
38. Barlow KM, Crawford S, Stevenson A, et al: Epidemiology of postconcussion syndrome in pediatric mild traumatic brain injury. Pediatrics 126:e374, 2010.
39. Dean PJ, Sterr A: Long-term effects of mild traumatic brain injury on cognitive performance. Front Hum Neurosci 7:30, 2013.

40. Falk AC, Von Wendt L, Soderkvist BK: The specificity of post-concussive symptoms in the pediatric population. J Child Health Care 13:227, 2009.
41. Leddy JJ, Kozlowski K, Donnelly JP, et al: A preliminary study of subsymptom threshold exercise training for refractory post-concussion syndrome. Clin J Sport Med 20:21, 2010.
42. Leddy JJ, Sandhu H, Sodhi V, et al: Rehabilitation of concussion and post-concussion syndrome. Sports Health 4:147, 2012.
43. Duff J: The usefulness of quantitative EEG (QEEG) and neurotherapy in the assessment and treatment of post-concussion syndrome. Clin EEG Neurosci 35:198, 2004.
44. Bryant RA: Disentangling mild traumatic brain injury and stress reactions. N Engl J Med 358:525, 2008.
45. Seifert TD: Sports concussion and associated post-traumatic headache. Headache 53:726, 2013.
46. Seifert TD, Evans RW: Posttraumatic headache: a review. Curr Pain Headache Rep 14:292, 2010.
47. Kutcher JS: Treatment of attention-deficit hyperactivity disorder in athletes. Curr Sports Med Rep 10:32, 2011.
48. Donnell AJ, Kim MS, Silva MA, et al: Incidence of post-concussion symptoms in psychiatric diagnostic groups, mild traumatic brain injury, and comorbid conditions. Clin Neuropsychol 26:1092, 2012.
49. Bryan CJ: Repetitive traumatic brain injury (or concussion) increases severity of sleep disturbance among deployed military personnel. Sleep 36:941, 2013.
50. Gibson S, Nigrovic LE, O'Brien M, et al: The effect of recommending cognitive rest on recovery from sport-related concussion. Brain Inj 27:839, 2013.
51. Silverberg ND, Iverson GL: Is rest after concussion "the best medicine?": recommendations for activity resumption following concussion in athletes, civilians, and military service members. J Head Trauma Rehabil 28:250, 2013.
52. McAllister TW, Arciniegas D: Evaluation and treatment of postconcussive symptoms. NeuroRehabilitation 17:265, 2002.
53. Watanabe TK, Bell KR, Walker WC, et al: Systematic review of interventions for post-traumatic headache. PM R 4:129, 2012.
54. Mittenberg W, Canyock EM, Condit D, et al: Treatment of post-concussion syndrome following mild head injury. J Clin Exp Neuropsychol 23:829, 2001.
55. Potter S, Brown RG: Cognitive behavioural therapy and persistent post-concussional symptoms: integrating conceptual issues and practical aspects in treatment. Neuropsychol Rehabil 22:1, 2012.
56. Harch PG, Andrews SR, Fogarty EF, et al: A phase I study of low-pressure hyperbaric oxygen therapy for blast-induced post-concussion syndrome and post-traumatic stress disorder. J Neurotrauma 29:168, 2012.
57. Schatz P, Moser RS: Current issues in pediatric sports concussion. Clin Neuropsychol 25:1042, 2011.
58. McCrea M, Guskiewicz K, Randolph C, et al: Incidence, clinical course, and predictors of prolonged recovery time following sport-related concussion in high school and college athletes. J Int Neuropsychol Soc 19:22, 2013.
59. Cantu RC: Second-impact syndrome. Clin Sports Med 17:37, 1998.
60. McCrory P: Does second impact syndrome exist? Clin J Sport Med 11:144, 2001.
61. Weinstein E, Turner M, Kuzma BB, et al: Second impact syndrome in football: new imaging and insights into a rare and devastating condition. J Neurosurg Pediatr 11:331, 2013.
62. Zemek RL, Farion KJ, Sampson M, et al: Prognosticators of persistent symptoms following pediatric concussion: a systematic review. JAMA Pediatr 167:259, 2013.
63. Saulle M, Greenwald BD: Chronic traumatic encephalopathy: a review. Rehabil Res Pract 2012:816069, 2012.
64. Yi J, Padalino DJ, Chin LS, et al: Chronic traumatic encephalopathy. Curr Sports Med Rep 12:28, 2013.
65. Courville CB: Punch drunk. Its pathogenesis and pathology on the basis of a verified case. Bull Los Angel Neuro Soc 27:160, 1962.
66. Parker HL: Traumatic encephalopathy ('punch drunk') of professional pugilists. J Neurol Psychopathol 15:20, 1934.
67. McCrory P, Meeuwisse WH, Kutcher JS, et al: What is the evidence for chronic concussion-related changes in retired athletes: behavioural, pathological and clinical outcomes? Br J Sports Med 47:327, 2013.

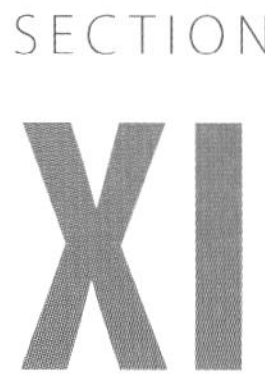

Infectious, Inflammatory, and Immunologic Disorders

CHAPTER

39

Acute Bacterial Infections of the Central Nervous System

KAREN L. ROOS

Acute bacterial infections of the central nervous system (CNS) include meningitis, brain abscess, subdural empyema, epidural abscess, and septic intracranial thrombophlebitis. The etiology, clinical presentation, diagnosis, and treatment of each of these bacterial infections are discussed in this chapter.

ACUTE BACTERIAL MENINGITIS

Bacterial meningitis is an acute purulent infection in the subarachnoid space, associated with an inflammatory reaction in the brain parenchyma and cerebral vasculature. During its treatment, not only must the meningeal pathogen be eradicated, but also the neurologic complications resulting from an often robust inflammatory reaction must be anticipated and managed. The most common causative organisms of bacterial meningitis are *Streptococcus pneumoniae, Neisseria meningitidis, Listeria monocytogenes*, group B streptococci, and gram-negative bacilli. The current epidemiology of acute bacterial meningitis, the best diagnostic tests to perform on cerebrospinal fluid (CSF), the use of dexamethasone as adjunctive therapy, and the present recommendations for the use of chemoprophylaxis and vaccination are discussed here.

Etiology

The most common etiologic organisms of acute bacterial meningitis in children and adults are *S. pneumoniae* and *N. meningitidis.*[1] Prior to the routine use of the *Haemophilus influenzae* type b conjugate vaccine, *H. influenzae* type b was the most common cause of bacterial meningitis in children

Aminoff's Neurology and General Medicine, Fifth Edition.

in the United States. This vaccine has dramatically reduced the incidence of meningitis in infants and children.[2] *H. influenzae* type b remains an important cause of bacterial meningitis in older adults, immunocompromised patients, and patients with chronic lung disease, splenectomy, leukemia, or sickle cell anemia.[2] Children too young to have completed a primary *H. influenzae* type b vaccination course are also at risk.

S. pneumoniae is the most common cause of meningitis in adults older than 18 years. A number of predisposing conditions increase the risk of pneumococcal meningitis, the most common of which is pneumonia. Acute and chronic otitis media, alcoholism, diabetes mellitus, splenectomy, hypogammaglobulinemia, and head trauma with basilar skull fracture and CSF rhinorrhea are also important risk factors. Approximately 44 percent of clinical isolates of *S. pneumoniae* in the United States have either intermediate or high levels of resistance to penicillin, and an increasing incidence of isolates are resistant to the third-generation cephalosporins, including cefotaxime and ceftriaxone.[3] It is therefore imperative that all isolates of *S. pneumoniae* be tested for penicillin and cephalosporin susceptibility and that a repeat lumbar puncture, if safe, be performed 48 hours into antimicrobial therapy in cases of penicillin-resistant pneumococcal meningitis to document microbiologic cure.[4]

N. meningitidis is the second most common cause of meningitis in adults, but has a predilection for those younger than age 60. The quadrivalent (serogroups A, C, W-135, and Y) meningococcal glycoconjugate vaccine is recommended for all 11- to 18-year olds. The vaccine does not provide immunity to *N. meningitidis* serogroup B, which is of concern as serogroups B and C cause the majority of cases of meningococcal meningitis in the United States and Europe.[5]

The Enterobacteriaceae (*Proteus* species, *Escherichia coli*, *Klebsiella* species, *Serratia* species, and *Enterobacter* species) cause meningitis in older adults; in adults with underlying diseases such as cancer, diabetes, alcoholism, congestive heart failure, chronic lung disease, and hepatic or renal dysfunction; and in neurosurgical patients.[6]

L. monocytogenes is a cause of meningitis in individuals with impaired cell-mediated immunity from older age (adults greater than 60 years), organ transplantation, pregnancy, malignancy, chronic illness, or immunosuppressive therapy. The routine use of trimethoprim-sulfamethoxazole as a prophylactic agent for the prevention of *Pneumocystis carinii* pneumonia in patients with the acquired immunodeficiency syndrome (AIDS) has the added benefit of reducing the risk of *L. monocytogenes* infection including meningitis.

Staphylococcus aureus and coagulase-negative staphylococci are the predominant organisms causing meningitis as a complication of invasive neurosurgical procedures, particularly shunting procedures for hydrocephalus and with subcutaneous Ommaya reservoirs or following lumbar puncture for the administration of intrathecal chemotherapy.

Streptococcus agalactiae, or group B streptococcus, is a leading cause of bacterial meningitis and sepsis in neonates and is increasingly recognized in two groups of adults: puerperal women and patients with serious underlying diseases.[7]

Clinical Presentation

Fever, headache, and stiff neck constitute the classic triad of symptoms and signs of bacterial meningitis. Patients are also typically lethargic or stuporous, and the level of consciousness may deteriorate rapidly. Nausea, vomiting, and photophobia are common complaints which often reflect elevated intracranial pressure (ICP). Seizure activity occurs in approximately 40 percent of patients, typically either at the onset or within the first few days of the illness.

A stiff neck, or meningismus, is the pathognomonic sign of meningeal irritation. Meningismus is present when the neck resists passive flexion. The Kernig and Brudzinski signs are classic signs of meningeal irritation, although their sensitivity is relatively low. Kernig sign is elicited with the patient in the supine position; the thigh is flexed on the abdomen, with the knee flexed. Attempts to passively extend the leg elicit pain when meningeal irritation is present. The Brudzinski sign is elicited with the patient in a supine position and is positive when passive flexion of the neck results in spontaneous flexion of the hips and knees.[8]

Increased ICP is an expected complication of bacterial meningitis and is the major cause of obtundation and coma. The most common signs of increased ICP in bacterial meningitis are an altered level of consciousness and papilledema. Cerebral arteritis and septic venous thrombosis of the cerebral dural sinuses and cortical veins are also complications of bacterial meningitis and present as focal neurologic deficits or with new-onset seizure activity.

The rash of meningococcemia begins as a diffuse erythematous maculopapular rash resembling a viral exanthem, but the lesions rapidly become petechial. This rash can be differentiated from the rash of a viremia in that petechiae are found on the trunk and lower extremities in meningococcemia. Petechiae may also be found in the mucous membranes and conjunctiva and occasionally on the palms and soles. Other infectious diseases that may manifest with a petechial, purpuric, or erythematous maculopapular rash resembling that of meningococcemia include enteroviral meningitis, Rocky Mountain spotted fever, West Nile virus encephalitis, bacterial endocarditis, echovirus type 9 viremia, and, more rarely, pneumococcal or *H. influenzae* meningitis.

Diagnosis

The diagnosis of bacterial meningitis is made by examination of the CSF. The necessity of neuroimaging prior to lumbar puncture has been debated for years. Neuroimaging prior to lumbar puncture should be performed in any patient with an altered level of consciousness, papilledema, focal neurologic deficit, an immunocompromised state, or new-onset seizure activity. When the clinical presentation is suggestive of bacterial meningitis, blood cultures should be obtained and dexamethasone and empiric antimicrobial therapy initiated immediately. If the patient is being treated with antibiotics, there is no risk in delaying lumbar puncture until after neuroimaging has been performed. Antibiotic therapy for several hours prior to lumbar puncture does not alter the CSF white blood cell (WBC) count or glucose concentration enough to obscure the diagnosis of bacterial meningitis, and it is not likely to sterilize the CSF enough to prevent the isolation of a microorganism on Gram stain or in culture.

The classic CSF abnormalities in bacterial meningitis are: (1) an increased opening pressure, (2) a pleocytosis of polymorphonuclear leukocytes (10 to 10,000 WBCs/mm^3), (3) a decreased glucose concentration (<45 mg/dl or CSF/serum glucose ratio of <0.31), and (4) an increased protein concentration. A CSF sample should be analyzed, using Gram stain and bacterial culture. The Gram stain is positive in 70 to 90 percent of untreated cases. Cerebrospinal fluid PCR assays have been developed to detect bacterial nucleic acid in CSF. A 16S rRNA conserved sequence broad-based bacterial PCR can detect small numbers of viable and nonviable organisms in the CSF. When the broad-range PCR is positive, a PCR that uses specific bacterial primers to detect the nucleic acid of *S. pneumoniae, N. meningitidis, E. coli, L. monocytogenes, H. influenzae,* and *S. agalactiae* can be performed to identify the responsible organism. It is anticipated that this broad-range PCR may eventually be used more commonly to exclude the diagnosis of bacterial meningitis.[9] The latex particle agglutination (LA) test for the detection of bacterial antigens of *S. pneumoniae, N. meningitidis, H. influenzae* type b, group B streptococcus, and *E. coli* K1 strains in CSF is useful for making a diagnosis of bacterial meningitis in patients who have been pretreated with oral or parenteral antibiotics and in whom Gram stain and CSF culture are negative; it is being replaced by PCR-based assays. The LA test has a specificity of 96 percent for *S. pneumoniae* and 100 percent for *N. meningitidis*. It has a sensitivity of 69 to 100 percent for the detection of *S. pneumoniae* in CSF and a sensitivity of 33 to 70 percent for the detection of bacterial antigens of *N. meningitidis* in CSF. A negative LA test for bacterial antigens does not exclude bacterial meningitis, and this test is therefore not recommended for deciding whether to continue or discontinue empiric antibiotic therapy. The *Limulus* amebocyte lysate assay is a rapid diagnostic test for the detection of gram-negative endotoxin in CSF to make a diagnosis of gram-negative bacterial meningitis. This test is reported to have a sensitivity of 99.5 percent and a specificity of 86 to 99.8 percent, but it is not routinely available.[10–12] In clinical practice, when bacterial meningitis is a possibility, most physicians treat with empiric therapy until the results of bacterial cultures are negative.

If there are petechial skin lesions, biopsies should be performed. The rash of meningococcemia results from the dermal seeding of organisms with vascular endothelial damage, and biopsy may reveal the organism on Gram stain.

Lumbar puncture should be performed with a 22- or 25-gauge needle, and a minimal amount of CSF removed for analysis. Approximately 6 ml of CSF is typically sufficient to obtain a cell count, determine glucose and protein concentrations, and analyze the sample using Gram stain, culture, and PCR or LA methods. An additional 1 ml of CSF can be sent for herpes simplex virus (HSV) DNA since HSV-1 encephalitis is the leading disease in the differential diagnosis of bacterial meningitis. The result of CSF RT-PCR for enteroviruses is often available within hours and, as enteroviruses are the most common viral cause of meningitis, a CSF RT-PCR should usually be sent in patients suspected of having meningitis.

Differential Diagnosis

HSV encephalitis is an important consideration in the differential diagnosis of bacterial meningitis, and arthropod-borne viral encephalitis should be considered during the summer and early fall months while mosquitoes are biting. Focal intracranial mass lesions and subarachnoid hemorrhage also need to be included in the differential diagnosis when approaching patients with suspected meningitis.

Herpes Simplex Virus Encephalitis

The clinical presentation of HSV encephalitis (discussed in detail in Chapter 43) often includes hemicranial headache, fever, behavioral abnormalities, focal or generalized seizure activity, and focal neurologic deficits (e.g., dysphasia, hemiparesis with greater involvement of the face and arm, and superior field defects). The symptoms of HSV encephalitis typically evolve over several days, and the presentation is often less acute than bacterial meningitis. In patients with HSV encephalitis, fluid-attenuated inversion recovery (FLAIR), T2-, and diffusion-weighted magnetic resonance imaging (MRI) sequences demonstrate lesions in the medial and inferior temporal lobe extending into the insula. The absence of an abnormality on MRI 48 hours after symptom onset should prompt consideration of another diagnosis. There is a distinctive electroencephalographic (EEG) pattern in HSV encephalitis, consisting of periodic, stereotyped complexes from one or both temporal areas that occur at regular intervals of 1 to 2 seconds and are typically observed between day 2 and day 15 of the illness. Examination of the CSF reveals an increased opening pressure, a lymphocytic pleocytosis of 5 to 500 cells/mm^3, a mild to moderate elevation in the protein concentration, and a normal or mildly decreased glucose concentration. There may be red blood cells or xanthochromia, findings that reflect the hemorrhagic nature of the encephalitis but are neither sensitive nor specific markers of the disorder. Results of CSF viral cultures for HSV-1 are almost always negative. The PCR is typically positive within 72 hours of symptom onset and then declines in sensitivity after the first week. If an initial CSF HSV PCR is negative within the first 72 hours of symptoms and HSV remains a major diagnostic consideration, the CSF should be resampled as the initial result may be a false negative.[13] Cerebrospinal fluid and serum samples can also be sent for HSV IgG antibody titers; antibodies to HSV appear in the CSF approximately 8 to 12 days after the onset of symptoms and can be detected for at least 30 days. A serum to CSF HSV-1 antibody ratio of less than 20 to 1 is considered diagnostic of intrathecal synthesis of antibodies and HSV encephalitis in the appropriate clinical context.

Arthropod-Borne Virus Encephalitis

During the summer and early fall months when mosquitoes are active, arthropod-borne viral encephalitis (see Chapter 43) should be included in the differential diagnosis of patients with meningitis. In the United States, the La Crosse virus, the St. Louis encephalitis virus, and the West Nile virus are the most common causes of arthropod-borne viral encephalitis. Eastern equine encephalitis virus causes the most severe arthropod-borne viral encephalitis, and the fatality rate is high. Japanese encephalitis virus is the most common cause of arthropod-borne human encephalitis worldwide. Venezuelan equine encephalitis virus is endemic in South America and is a rare cause of encephalitis in Central America and the southwestern United States, particularly in Texas.

The clinical presentation of arthropod-borne viral encephalitis, regardless of the specific virus, is fairly characteristic. The onset of encephalitic symptoms may be preceded by an influenza-like prodrome of fever, malaise, myalgias, nausea, and vomiting followed by headache, confusion, stupor, and occasionally convulsions. Focal neurologic deficits and focal seizure activity have been reported in cases of encephalitis caused by eastern equine encephalitis virus and La Crosse virus. Patients with West Nile virus encephalitis may have conjunctivitis or a maculopapular or roseolar rash. Patients with West Nile virus or St. Louis virus encephalitis may present with a polio-like acute asymmetric flaccid weakness or tremors, myoclonus, or parkinsonian features.

Japanese encephalitis virus tends to infect the basal ganglia and the thalamus, leading to tremors during the acute disease and a parkinsonian-like syndrome in survivors.

Either neuroimaging is normal or there are nonspecific abnormalities. Focal abnormalities in the basal ganglia and the thalamus have been reported in eastern equine, Japanese, and West Nile virus encephalitis.[14]

Examination of the CSF demonstrates a polymorphonuclear leukocytic pleocytosis or a lymphocytic pleocytosis. The CSF glucose concentration is usually normal. Based on criteria established by the US Centers for Disease Control and Prevention, a confirmed case of arboviral encephalitis is defined as a febrile illness with encephalitis during a period when arboviral transmission is likely to occur, plus at least one of the following: (1) fourfold or greater rise in serum antibody titer between the time of acute illness and 4 weeks later; (2) isolation of virus from tissue, blood, or CSF; or (3) a specific immunoglobulin M (IgM) antibody identified in the CSF. However, La Crosse virus has not been isolated from CSF and St. Louis encephalitis virus, eastern equine encephalitis virus, and western equine encephalitis virus are rarely isolated from CSF; therefore antibody titers are typically the diagnostic test of choice. A CSF PCR assay is available for the detection of West Nile virus nucleic acid; however, it has a low sensitivity so a negative test does not exclude the disorder. The detection of West Nile virus IgM in CSF is considered the most sensitive diagnostic test for West Nile virus encephalitis. West Nile virus IgM antibodies may persist in serum (not the CSF) for a year or more after exposure to the virus and therefore cannot be used for definitive diagnosis of recent infection.

Rocky Mountain Spotted Fever

Rocky Mountain spotted fever is caused by the bacterium *Rickettsia rickettsii*. The disease begins with high fever, prostration, myalgias, headache, nausea, and vomiting. The rash is characteristic and presents initially as a diffuse erythematous maculopapular rash appearing 2 to 4 days after the onset of symptoms, usually beginning at the wrist and ankles and then spreading distally, including to the palms and soles, and proximally within a matter of a few hours. Diagnosis is made by immunofluorescent staining of skin biopsy specimens or by the detection of IgM and IgG antibodies.

Focal Infectious Intracranial Mass Lesions

Focal infectious intracranial mass lesions, including brain abscess, subdural empyema, and epidural abscess, are discussed later in this chapter but should be included in the differential diagnosis of bacterial meningitis. The presence of a focal infectious intracranial mass lesion is suggested by focal or generalized seizure activity or focal neurologic deficits on examination and is ruled out by neuroimaging.

Subarachnoid Hemorrhage

The possibility of a subarachnoid hemorrhage should also be included in the differential diagnosis of acute bacterial meningitis. Clinical presentation is characterized by the explosive onset of a severe headache or a sudden transient loss of consciousness followed by a severe headache. Because of the presence of blood in the subarachnoid space, nuchal rigidity is frequently present, leading to diagnostic confusion with infectious meningitis. A dilated nonreactive pupil is suggestive of a subarachnoid hemorrhage from an aneurysm of the posterior communicating artery. Computed tomography (CT) of the brain may demonstrate blood in the basal cisterns. If the CT scan is normal, the spinal fluid should be examined for red blood cells and xanthochromia. Red blood cells are present in the CSF within minutes of the rupture of an intracranial aneurysm and usually fail to clear in successive tubes of CSF. A sample of the blood-tinged CSF should be centrifuged; a yellow or xanthochromic color in the supernatant is present 6 to 12 hours following subarachnoid hemorrhage and lasts for 2 to 3 weeks. Xanthochromic spinal fluid may also be seen when the CSF protein concentration is elevated (above 150 to 200 mg/dl), and therefore it can be seen in bacterial meningitis.

Treatment

Empiric Antimicrobial Therapy

When bacterial meningitis is suspected, antimicrobial therapy is initiated immediately after blood cultures are obtained and before the results of CSF Gram stain, culture, and antimicrobial susceptibility

TABLE 39-1 ■ Empiric Therapy for Acute Bacterial Meningitis in Children and Adults

Community-acquired (immunocompetent child or adult)	Cefotaxime or ceftriaxone or cefepime *plus* Vancomycin *plus* Acyclovir
Community-acquired (immunosuppressed individual)	Cefotaxime or ceftriaxone or cefepime *plus* Vancomycin *plus* Acyclovir *plus* Ampicillin
Iatrogenic (associated with neurosurgery, epidural anesthesia, intrathecal chemotherapy)	Vancomycin *plus* Ceftazidime or meropenem

tests are known. Empiric therapy should be based on the possibility that the patient has penicillin- and cephalosporin-resistant pneumococcal meningitis and should include a combination of a third- (ceftriaxone or cefotaxime) or fourth-generation cephalosporin (cefepime) plus vancomycin. Acyclovir is added to the empiric regimen to cover HSV (Table 39-1). Ampicillin should be added to cover *L. monocytogenes* if the patient is over the age of 60 years or is immunosuppressed. When the patient has been treated with trimethoprim-sulfamethoxazole for prophylaxis of toxoplasmosis or *P. carinii* pneumonia, it is less likely that the meningitis is due to *L. monocytogenes*. Meningitis that complicates a neurosurgical procedure, epidural anesthesia, or intrathecal chemotherapy should be treated empirically with a combination of vancomycin plus ceftazidime, cefepime, or meropenem. Vancomycin is used to cover staphylococci and ceftazidime, cefepime, or meropenem to cover gram-negative bacilli, specifically *Pseudomonas aeruginosa*. The doses of each of the antimicrobial agents are provided in Table 39-2, which shows both pediatric and adult dosing ranges.

SPECIFIC ANTIMICROBIAL THERAPY

All CSF bacterial isolates should be tested for antimicrobial susceptibility. In experimental models of bacterial meningitis, the maximal bactericidal activity occurs when the antibiotic concentration is 10 to 30 times greater than the minimal bactericidal concentration of the microorganism in vitro.[15]

TABLE 39-2 ■ Doses of Antimicrobial Agents

Antimicrobial Agent	Total Daily Pediatric Dose (Dosing Interval)	Total Daily Adult Dose (Dosing Interval)
Acyclovir	30 mg/kg daily (every 8 h)	30 mg/kg daily (every 8 h)
Ampicillin	300 mg/kg daily (every 6 h)	12 g/day (every 4 h)
Cefepime	150 mg/kg daily (every 8 h)	6 g/day (every 8 h)
Cefotaxime	225–300 mg/kg daily (every 6–8 h)	12 g/day (every 4–6 h)
Ceftazidime	150–200 mg/kg daily (every 8 h)	8 g/day (every 8 h)
Ceftriaxone	100 mg/kg daily (every 12 h)	4 g/day (every 12 h)
Meropenem	120 mg/kg daily (every 8 h)	6 g/day (every 8 h)
Metronidazole	30 mg/kg daily (every 6 h)	1.5–2 g/day (every 6 h)
Nafcillin	150–200 mg/kg daily (every 6 h)	12 g/day (every 4 h)
Penicillin G	0.3 million U/kg/d (every 4 h)	24 million U/day (every 4 h)
Vancomycin	45–60 mg/kg daily (every 6 h)	45–60 mg/kg daily (every 6 h)
Intrathecal vancomycin	10 mg/day	20 mg/day

Pneumococcal Meningitis

Antimicrobial therapy for pneumococcal meningitis is initiated with a third- or fourth-generation cephalosporin and vancomycin. Some strains of pneumococci are sensitive to penicillin. Once the results of antimicrobial susceptibility tests are known, therapy can be modified accordingly (Table 39-3). According to the guidelines of the National Committee for Laboratory Standards, an isolate of *S. pneumoniae* is considered to be highly resistant to penicillin with a minimal inhibitory concentration (MIC) of at least 2 μg/ml.[16] An isolate of *S. pneumoniae* is considered to have intermediate resistance to penicillin with an MIC of 0.1 to 1 μg/ml and to be susceptible to penicillin with an MIC of less than 0.1 μg/ml. Penicillin G can be used to treat susceptible strains of *S. pneumoniae* in various clinical situations. For *S. pneumoniae* meningitis, however, more rigid guidelines are applied. An isolate in this situation is defined as penicillin-susceptible when the MIC is 0.06 μg/ml or less, to have intermediate resistance when the MIC is 0.1 to 1.0 μg/ml, and to be highly

TABLE 39-3 ■ Specific Antimicrobial Therapy for Bacterial Infections of the Central Nervous System

Organism	Antibiotic
Streptococcus pneumoniae	
Sensitive to penicillin	Penicillin G *or* ceftriaxone *or* cefotaxime
Relatively resistant to penicillin	Ceftriaxone *or* cefotaxime
Resistant to penicillin	Vancomycin *plus*
	Cefotaxime *or* ceftriaxone +/− intraventricular vancomycin
Neisseria meningitidis	Ceftriaxone *or* penicillin G *or* ampicillin
Staphylococci	
Methicillin-sensitive	Nafcillin
Methicillin-resistant	Vancomycin
Listeria monocytogenes	Ampicillin
Enterobacteriaceae	Cefotaxime *or* ceftriaxone *or* cefepime
Pseudomonas aeruginosa	Ceftazidime *or* cefepime *or* meropenem
Haemophilus influenzae	Ceftriaxone
Streptococcus agalactiae	Ampicillin *or* penicillin G
Anaerobes	Metronidazole
Nocardia asteroides	Trimethoprim-sulfamethoxazole
Bacteroides species	Metronidazole

resistant when the MIC is greater than 1.0 μg/ml. Isolates of *S. pneumoniae* that have MICs of 0.5 μg/ml or less are defined as susceptible to the cephalosporins (cefotaxime, ceftriaxone, cefepime). Those with MICs of 1 μg/ml are considered to have intermediate resistance, and those with MICs of 2 μg/ml or more are considered resistant. For meningitis due to pneumococci, when the MICs of cefotaxime or ceftriaxone are 0.5 μg/ml or less, treatment with cefotaxime or ceftriaxone is probably adequate. If the MICs are 1 μg/ml or more, vancomycin is the antibiotic of choice. Rifampin can be added to vancomycin for its synergistic effect because it is highly active against most penicillin-resistant pneumococci, but rifampin is inadequate as monotherapy because resistance develops rapidly.

For pneumococcal meningitis, a repeat lumbar puncture should be performed 24 to 48 hours after the initiation of antimicrobial therapy to document eradication of the pathogen, if possible. Consideration should be given to using intraventricular vancomycin in patients not responding to parenteral vancomycin. The intraventricular route of administration is preferred over the intrathecal route because adequate concentrations of vancomycin in the cerebral ventricles are not always achieved with intrathecal administration. Intraventricular and intrathecal vancomycin is safe and is not associated with a risk of seizure activity.

A 2-week course of intravenous antimicrobial therapy is recommended for pneumococcal meningitis.

Meningococcal Meningitis

Penicillin G or a third-generation cephalosporin (Table 39-3) remains the antibiotic of choice for meningococcal meningitis. Isolates of *N. meningitidis* with moderate or relative resistance to penicillin (defined as a penicillin MIC of 0.1 to 1.0 μg/ml) and decreased susceptibility to ampicillin have been reported from a wide variety of geographic locations. All CSF isolates of *N. meningitidis* should be tested for penicillin and ampicillin susceptibility. If antimicrobial susceptibility testing demonstrates that the isolate is a relatively penicillin-resistant strain, or in areas with a high prevalence of meningococci with decreased susceptibility to penicillin, cefotaxime or ceftriaxone should be used. A 7-day course of intravenous antibiotic therapy is adequate for most uncomplicated cases of meningococcal meningitis. The index case and all close contacts should receive chemoprophylaxis with a 2-day regimen of rifampin (600 mg every 12 hours for 2 days in adults and 10 mg/kg every 12 hours for 2 days in children older than 2 years of age). Rifampin should not be used in pregnant women. Pregnant and lactating women and children less than 2 years of age may be given intravenous or intramuscular ceftriaxone, in a single injection of 250 mg for adults and 125 mg for children. Close contacts are defined as individuals who have had contact with nasopharyngeal secretions either through kissing or sharing toys, beverages, or cigarettes.

Staphylococcal Meningitis

Meningitis caused by *S. aureus* or coagulase-negative staphylococci is treated with nafcillin or oxacillin. Vancomycin is the drug of choice for methicillin-resistant staphylococci and for patients allergic to penicillin. The CSF should be monitored during therapy, and if the spinal fluid continues to yield viable organisms after 48 hours of intravenous therapy, intraventricular vancomycin, 10 mg once daily for children or 20 mg once daily for adults, should be added.

Listeria monocytogenes Meningitis

Meningitis due to *L. monocytogenes* is treated with ampicillin for at least 3 weeks. Gentamicin should be added to ampicillin in critically ill patients. Meningitis caused by this organism is seen less often today in immunosuppressed patients than in the past because of trimethoprim-sulfamethoxazole administration in these patients as prophylaxis against *P. carinii* pneumonia and toxoplasmosis.

Enterobacteriaceae Meningitis

Meningitis caused by the Enterobacteriaceae, including *Proteus* species, *E. coli*, *Klebsiella* species, *Serratia* species, and *Enterobacter* species, is treated with a third- or fourth-generation cephalosporin, either cefotaxime, ceftriaxone or cefepime, for 3 weeks.

Pseudomonas aeruginosa Meningitis

The third-generation cephalosporins cefotaxime, ceftriaxone, and ceftazidime are equally efficacious for the treatment of gram-negative bacillary meningitis, with the exception of meningitis caused by *P. aeruginosa*. Meningitis resulting from infection with this organism is treated with ceftazidime, cefepime, or meropenem intravenously for 3 weeks.

Newer Antimicrobial Agents

Meropenem is a carbapenem antibiotic structurally related to imipenem, but reportedly with less seizure proclivity.[17] In experimental models, meropenem has bactericidal activity similar to that of the combination of ceftriaxone and vancomycin against penicillin-resistant *S. pneumoniae*.[18] The safety and efficacy of meropenem were compared with those of cefotaxime in a prospective randomized trial of 190 children with bacterial meningitis (caused by *H. influenzae*, *S. pneumoniae*, and *E. coli*). Seizures occurred within 24 hours before antibiotic therapy in 16 of 98 patients (16%) randomized to receive meropenem, and in 6 of 92 patients (7%) randomized to receive cefotaxime. In patients without seizures before therapy, seizures occurred during treatment in 5 of 82 patients (6%) receiving meropenem and in 1 of 86 patients (1%) receiving cefotaxime.[19] Meropenem is highly active in vitro against *L. monocytogenes* as well as against multidrug-resistant gram-negative bacteria and *P. aeruginosa*.[19–21] The dose of meropenem is 2 g intravenously every 8 hours for adults; the pediatric dose is 40 mg/kg every 8 hours. The number of patients enrolled in clinical trials of meropenem for bacterial meningitis has not been sufficient to date to correctly assess its efficacy or epileptogenic potential.

Cefepime is a broad-spectrum fourth-generation cephalosporin with in vitro activity similar to that of cefotaxime or ceftriaxone against the common meningeal pathogens *H. influenzae*, *S. pneumoniae*, and *N. meningitidis*, and greater activity against *Enterobacter* species and *P. aeruginosa*.[22] The dose of cefepime is 3 g intravenously every 8 hours in adults. In clinical trials, cefepime has been demonstrated to be equivalent to cefotaxime in the treatment of pneumococcal and meningococcal meningitis, but its efficacy in bacterial meningitis caused by penicillin- and cephalosporin-resistant pneumococcal organisms has not been established.

Dexamethasone Therapy

The use of dexamethasone as adjunctive therapy in bacterial meningitis comes from present understanding of the pathophysiology of the neurologic complications of bacterial meningitis. The critical event in pathogenesis is the inflammatory reaction in the subarachnoid space to the invading meningeal pathogen. The pathogen itself is not responsible for most neurologic complications. In bacterial meningitis, damage to the CNS progresses long after the CSF has been sterilized by antibiotic therapy.[23] Lysis of bacteria and release of bacterial cell wall components in the subarachnoid space are the initial steps in the induction of the inflammatory process and formation of a purulent exudate in the subarachnoid space (Fig. 39-1). Components of bacterial cell walls, such as lipopolysaccharide molecules (endotoxin), a cell wall component of gram-negative bacteria, and teichoic acid and peptidoglycan, cell wall components of the pneumococcal species, induce meningeal inflammation by stimulating the production of inflammatory

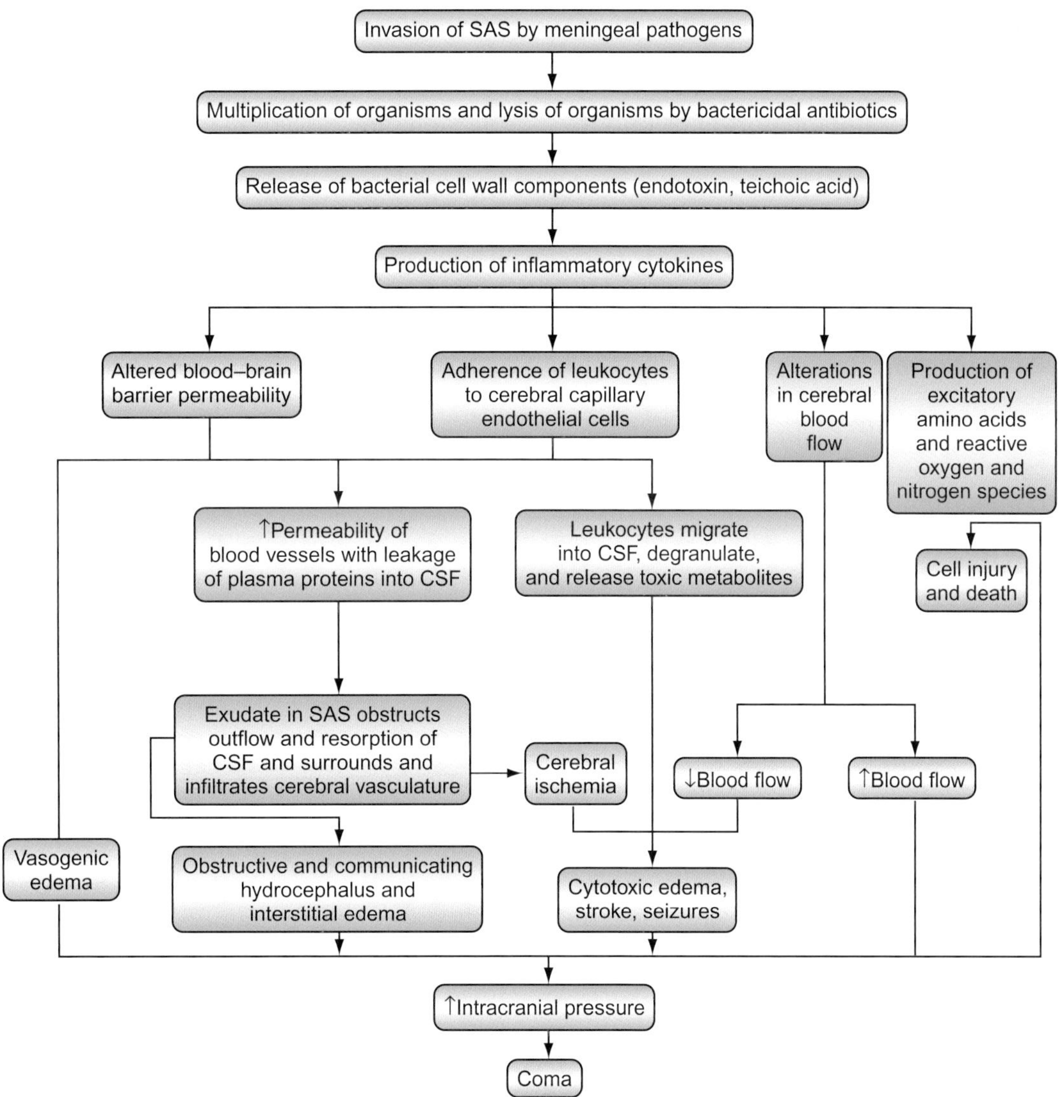

FIGURE 39-1 ■ Inflammatory cascade leading to the neurologic complications of bacterial meningitis. CSF, cerebrospinal fluid; SAS, subarachnoid space. (Reprinted by permission of Karen L. Roos, MD, Indiana University Hospital, Indianapolis.)

cytokines and chemokines by microglia (CNS macrophage-equivalent cells), astrocytes, monocytes, microvascular endothelial cells, and white blood cells in the CSF space. There are a number of consequences that result from the presence of inflammatory cytokines in CSF. Tumor necrosis factor (TNF) and interleukin-1 (IL-1) act synergistically to alter the permeability of the blood–brain barrier, allowing for the leakage of serum proteins and other molecules into the CSF and contributing to the formation of a purulent exudate. The purulent exudate may obstruct the flow of CSF through the ventricular system and diminish the resorptive capacity of the arachnoid granulations in the dural sinuses, leading to obstructive and communicating hydrocephalus and to interstitial edema. The exudate also surrounds and narrows the diameter of the lumen of the large arteries at the base of the brain with infiltration of inflammatory cells in the arterial walls (vasculitis). These inflammatory cytokines also recruit polymorphonuclear leukocytes from the bloodstream and upregulate the expression of selectins on cerebral capillary endothelial cells and leukocytes, which allow for migration of leukocytes into the CSF. Experimental models of meningitis suggest that bacterial eradication is not a leukocyte-dependent phenomenon. Neutrophils degranulate and release toxic metabolites that contribute to cytotoxic edema, cell injury, and death. The adherence of leukocytes to cerebral capillary endothelial cells increases the permeability of blood vessels, allowing for the leakage of plasma proteins into the CSF and further contributing to the inflammatory exudate in the subarachnoid space.

Dexamethasone exerts its beneficial effect by inhibiting the synthesis of IL-1 and TNF at the level of mRNA and through decreasing CSF outflow resistance and stabilizing the blood–brain barrier. The rationale for giving dexamethasone prior to antibiotic therapy is that dexamethasone inhibits the production of TNF if administered to macrophages and microglia before they are activated by endotoxin, both by diminishing the quantity of TNF mRNA in response to endotoxin and by preventing its translation. Dexamethasone is unable to regulate TNF production once induction occurs.

There have been a number of clinical trials dating back to 1950 designed to evaluate the efficacy of corticosteroids in reducing mortality and morbidity in bacterial meningitis.[24] It was the work of Tauber and co-workers in 1985 and Lebel and co-workers in 1988, however, that renewed interest in corticosteroid therapy for bacterial meningitis.[25,26] A meta-analysis of randomized, controlled trials of dexamethasone therapy in childhood bacterial meningitis published from 1988 to 1996 confirmed the benefit of dexamethasone for *H. influenzae* type b meningitis if begun with or before intravenous antibiotics and also suggested a beneficial effect for pneumococcal meningitis in children.[27] Maximal benefit from dexamethasone therapy is dependent on timing.[28]

A common early criticism of the dexamethasone trials is that in the majority of cases, the causative organism of the meningitis was *H. influenzae* type b. However, this organism no longer is one of the more common etiologic agents of bacterial meningitis because of the success of the Hib conjugate vaccine. Present understanding of the molecular basis of the neurologic complications of bacterial meningitis, however, does not suggest that the pathophysiology of the neurologic complications varies with the meningeal pathogen, with the exception of how the microorganism gains access to the CNS. In 2002, a prospective, randomized, double-blind, multicenter trial of dexamethasone in 301 patients with acute bacterial meningitis was published. *Streptococcus pneumoniae* was the causative organism in 37 percent of patients in the dexamethasone group and 44 percent of the placebo group. Among the patients with pneumococcal meningitis, 26 percent in the dexamethasone group had an unfavorable outcome, as compared with 52 percent in the placebo group.[29] After the introduction of nationwide dexamethasone therapy in adults with pneumococcal meningitis in the Netherlands, the case fatality rate declined from 30 to 20 percent; a total of 45 percent of cases of bacterial meningitis were pneumococcal.[30]

An additional concern regarding the use of dexamethasone in the treatment of bacterial meningitis is its effect on the penetration of antibiotics into the CSF. Meningeal inflammation appears to improve the penetration of vancomycin. By decreasing meningeal inflammation, dexamethasone could theoretically reduce the penetration of vancomycin into the CSF. However, in a prospective, randomized clinical trial of bactericidal activity against cephalosporin-resistant pneumococci in children with acute bacterial meningitis, vancomycin (60 mg/kg daily) reliably penetrated the CSF when the children were treated concomitantly with dexamethasone (0.6 mg/kg daily, divided into four doses for 4 days).[31] The third- and fourth-generation cephalosporins and rifampin penetrate the CSF extremely well, even in the presence of dexamethasone.

The American Academy of Pediatrics recommends the consideration of dexamethasone for bacterial meningitis in infants and children aged 2 months or older. The recommended dose is 0.6 mg/kg daily in four divided doses (0.15 mg/kg/dose) given intravenously for the first 4 days of antibiotic therapy. The first dose of dexamethasone should be administered before or at least with the first dose of antibiotics. Results of clinical trials of dexamethasone therapy in children have demonstrated its efficacy in decreasing meningeal inflammation and neurologic sequelae and in reducing the incidence of sensorineural hearing loss.

The Infectious Diseases Society of America (IDSA) practice guidelines for the management of bacterial meningitis recommend the use of dexamethasone in adults with suspected or proven pneumococcal meningitis.[32] The recommended dose is 0.6 mg/kg daily in four divided doses for the first 4 days of antimicrobial therapy, with the first dose administered 10 to 20 minutes before or at least concomitant with the first dose of antibiotic. Dexamethasone is not likely to be of much benefit if started 24 hours or more after antimicrobial therapy has been initiated. A study since publication of these guidelines also demonstrated a favorable trend toward reduced rates of death and hearing loss in patients with meningococcal meningitis treated with dexamethasone.[33]

Prevention

It is recommended that college freshmen be vaccinated against meningococcal meningitis with a quadrivalent (A, C, W135, Y) meningococcal polysaccharide vaccine. During an outbreak of meningococcal disease, individuals who have not been previously vaccinated should be treated with chemoprophylaxis. As many as 33 percent of secondary cases of meningococcal disease develop within 2 to 5 days of presentation of the index case. Vaccination is not a substitute for chemoprophylaxis to prevent secondary disease, because there is an insufficient amount of time for development of the optimum effect of vaccination, which requires approximately 1 to 2 weeks for good antibody production.[34] Adults and adolescents who have not been vaccinated but have been exposed to an individual with meningococcal disease can be treated with rifampin, 600 mg twice daily for 2 days. Children, older than age 2, can be treated with rifampin, 10 mg/kg twice daily for 2 days. Rifampin should not be used in pregnant women. Pregnant and lactating women and children under 2 years of age may be given intravenous or intramuscular ceftriaxone in a single injection of 250 mg for adults and 125 mg for children.

Vaccination against pneumococci is recommended for three at-risk populations: adults older than 65 years, adults with chronic underlying diseases (cardiopulmonary diseases, renal diseases, diabetes mellitus, splenectomy, and CSF fistula), and immunocompromised patients over 10 years of age, including those infected with the human immunodeficiency virus (HIV).[34]

BRAIN ABSCESS

A brain abscess is a focal suppurative infection in the brain parenchyma that typically begins as a localized area of cerebritis and develops into a collection of pus surrounded by a capsule.[35] It develops from a contiguous suppurative focus of infection (e.g., frontoethmoidal sinusitis, chronic otitis media, mastoiditis, or dental infections) in 25 to 50 percent of cases, hematogenous dissemination from a distant site of infection (e.g., lungs, skin, endocarditis, intra-abdominal abscess, urinary tract infection) in 15 to 30 percent of cases, and direct inoculation (head trauma or a neurosurgical procedure) in 8 to 19 percent of cases. In 20 to 30 percent of cases, no source of infection is identified.[36–38] Bacteria are not a common cause of brain abscess in immunosuppressed patients because of routine prophylaxis with antibiotics during episodes of neutropenia. The single exception to this is *Nocardia asteroides*, which is the causative organism in an increasing number of cases of brain abscess in patients with defects in cell-mediated immunity.

Etiology

The most common source of brain abscess is direct spread of infection from a contiguous suppurative focus of infection or hematogenous spread from a distant site of infection. Brain abscesses that arise from intracranial extension of paranasal sinus infections are caused usually by microaerophilic streptococci and anaerobic organisms (e.g., *Bacteroides* species, *Fusobacterium* species, and anaerobic streptococci), Enterobacteriaceae, and *Haemophilus* species.[35] Bacterial infection in the paranasal sinuses spreads intracranially to the frontal or temporal lobe either by retrograde thrombophlebitis of the diploic veins or via a contiguous area of osteomyelitis.[39] Brain abscesses associated with a dental procedure or dental abscesses are also typically due to microaerophilic streptococci and anaerobic organisms. A brain abscess may arise from direct extension of mastoid infection or via retrograde thrombophlebitis of the emissary veins within the temporal bone from mastoiditis. Middle ear infections can cause temporal lobe abscess by direct spread of infection through the tegmen antrum or petrous portion of the temporal bone.[39] Brain abscesses that arise from middle ear infections are most often due to *Streptococcus* species, Enterobacteriaceae, *Bacteroides* species (including *B. fragilis*), and *P. aeruginosa*. A brain abscess may develop from hematogenous dissemination of microorganisms from a remote site of infection such as the heart, the lungs, the abdomen, or the urinary tract. Metastatic abscesses are often multiple and tend to form primarily in areas supplied by the middle cerebral artery (i.e., posterior frontal or parietal lobes) at the interface of gray and white matter, where capillary blood flow is slowest.[39]

A common cause of brain abscess in infants and children is cyanotic congenital heart disease, with tetralogy of Fallot and transposition of the great vessels being the most frequent associated anomalies. As a general rule, a brain abscess in these patients develops only in an area of ischemic or devitalized brain tissue. The polycythemia that occurs with cyanotic congenital heart disease causes intravascular thrombosis and reduces the rate of blood flow in the microcirculation in the brain, leading to brain hypoxia or infarction. In addition, the presence of a right-to-left shunt precludes the filtering of virulent bacteria by the lungs. Bacteria in the systemic circulation are able to reach the brain and establish infection in areas of focal cerebral damage from reduced tissue oxygenation.[40,41] Anaerobic and microaerophilic streptococci are most often recovered in abscesses associated with congenital heart disease.[42] Neonatal brain abscesses occur as a complication of meningitis, a predisposing condition that is uncommon in older children and adults; the most common causative organisms of bacterial brain abscess in neonates and infants are *Proteus* species and *Citrobacter* species.[39] Brain abscess is an uncommon complication of neonatal group B streptococcal or *E. coli* meningitis.

Bacterial brain abscess is not a common intracranial infection in immunosuppressed patients because of the use of prophylactic antibiotics in patients who are neutropenic. When a bacterial brain abscess develops in the first month after organ transplantation, the source is usually infection in a surgical wound, the lungs, the urinary tract, or in intravenous lines.[43] *Nocardia asteroides* is a common etiologic organism. It is a branching, filamentous, rod-shaped aerobic, gram-positive bacterium within the order Actinomycetes, and is found in soil and decaying vegetables.[44] Infection is acquired by inhalation, and the organism spreads from the lungs to the brain.[45] Risk factors for the development of a *Nocardia* brain abscess include cytotoxic chemotherapy, pregnancy, corticosteroid therapy, organ transplantation, and lymphatic malignancy.[44] Immunosuppressed patients receiving prophylactic therapy with trimethoprim-sulfamethoxazole to prevent *P. carinii* pneumonia are less likely to have *Nocardia* as the causative organism of brain abscess, as this antimicrobial agent acts against *Nocardia*.

When a brain abscess develops as a complication of penetrating head trauma, *S. aureus* is the most common pathogen found. Such abscesses are frequently multiloculated and may contain foreign bodies.[35] A brain abscess following a neurosurgical procedure is typically due to staphylococci or gram-negative bacilli.

Clinical Presentation

Headache is the most common presenting complaint in patients with brain abscess, and fever occurs in fewer than 50 percent of patients. One-third of patients present with new-onset focal or generalized seizures. The findings on neurologic examination are related both to the site of the abscess and to the presence of increased ICP. Hemiparesis is a common localizing sign of a frontal or parietal lobe abscess. A temporal lobe abscess may be associated with dysphasia or a visual field deficit (e.g., upper homonymous quadrantanopia). A patient with a cerebellar abscess presents usually with nystagmus and ataxia. When the brain abscess is complicated by increased ICP, the clinical findings may include papilledema, deficits of the oculomotor (III) or abducens (VI) nerves, and an alteration in consciousness ranging from lethargy to irritability, confusion, or coma.

Diagnosis

Brain MRI is the best neuroimaging procedure for demonstrating a brain abscess, especially one that is in an early (i.e., cerebritis) stage. On T2-weighted images, cerebritis is evident as an area of hyperintensity. A mature brain abscess appears hypointense to CSF on T1-weighted sequences and shows ring enhancement following administration of intravenous gadolinium. On T2-weighted images, a mature brain abscess has a central area of pus that is hyperintense, is surrounded by a well-defined hypointense capsule, and has a surrounding area of hyperintense edema.[35] Diffusion-weighted MRI and magnetization transfer ratios are helpful in differentiating a brain abscess from other types of cystic lesions. Brain abscesses are hyperintense, with restricted diffusion.[46] The magnetization transfer ratio of a brain abscess is higher than that of a non-abscess cystic lesion.[47] On contrast-enhanced CT, the mature abscess has the appearance of a low-density lesion with a sharply demarcated, dense ring of contrast enhancement surrounded by a variable hypodense region of edema. In both the early (cerebritis) and mature stages, a marginal ring of density is present on contrast-enhanced images; however, in the cerebritis stage, the enhancing ring forms an inhomogeneous "halo." As the abscess matures, its margin becomes more discrete and the associated enhancement more homogeneous. There may be leakage of contrast medium into the low-density center of an abscess in the cerebritis stage.

The etiologic organism of a brain abscess is determined by stereotactic needle aspiration. This procedure not only provides diagnostic specimens for Gram stain and culture but also permits therapeutic drainage of pus. Lumbar puncture should be avoided in patients with known or suspected focal intracranial infections because of the danger of herniation and because the diagnostic yield is low. About 50 percent of patients with a brain abscess have a peripheral leukocytosis, and 60 percent have an elevated erythrocyte sedimentation rate.

Differential Diagnosis

The differential diagnosis of a brain abscess includes focal structural or space-occupying lesions such as tumor, stroke, subdural empyema, and superior sagittal sinus thrombosis.

Treatment

All abscesses that are larger than 2.5 cm in diameter or that are causing significant mass effect should be drained by stereotactic aspiration.[48] Antibiotic therapy is based on culture and sensitivity testing of the specific etiologic organism of the brain abscess. Empiric antibiotic therapy should be based on a knowledge of the organisms most frequently encountered with the suspected etiology of the brain abscess until the results of culture and sensitivity studies are available (Table 39-4).[39]

Abscesses originating from the paranasal sinuses are caused predominantly by microaerophilic streptococci, anaerobic organisms (*Bacteroides* species, *Fusobacterium* species, and anaerobic streptococci), Enterobacteriaceae, and *Haemophilus* species. A combination of penicillin G, or a third- or fourth-generation cephalosporin, along with metronidazole is recommended. The doses of these antimicrobial agents are provided in Table 39-2. A brain abscess associated with dental disease is treated with a combination of penicillin G or a third- or fourth-generation cephalosporin along with metronidazole

TABLE 39-4 ■ Etiologic Organisms of Brain Abscess and Empiric Therapy

Source	Organisms	Antibiotics
Paranasal sinuses	Microaerophilic streptococci *Bacteroides* species *Fusobacterium* species *Haemophilus* species Anaerobic streptococci *Staphylococcus aureus*	Third- or fourth-generation cephalosporin *plus* metronidazole *plus* vancomycin
Dental disease	Streptococci *Bacteroides fragilis*	Penicillin G *or* a third- or fourth-generation cephalosporin *plus* metronidazole
Otitis media or mastoiditis	*Streptococcus* species Enterobacteriaceae *Bacteroides* species (including *B. fragilis*) *Pseudomonas aeruginosa*	Penicillin G *plus* metronidazole *plus* ceftazidime *or* meropenem
Pulmonary disease	*Streptococcus* species *Actinomyces* species *Fusobacterium* species	Penicillin G *plus* metronidazole *plus* ceftazidime *or* meropenem
Endocarditis	*Staphylococcus aureus* Microaerophilic streptococci	Nafcillin *or* vancomycin *plus* Cefotaxime
Intra-abdominal site	*Streptococcus* species Enterobacteriaceae Anaerobes	Penicillin G *plus* metronidazole *plus* ceftazidime *or* meropenem
Urinary tract	*Pseudomonas* species Enterobacteriaceae	Penicillin G *plus* metronidazole *plus* ceftazidime *or* meropenem
Cyanotic congenital heart disease	Anaerobic and microaerophilic streptococci (viridans streptococci)	Penicillin G *plus* cefotaxime *plus* metronidazole
Neonatal meningitis	*Proteus* species *Citrobacter* species	Ampicillin *plus* aminoglycoside *or* cefotaxime
Immunosuppressed state	*Nocardia asteroides* *Clostridium* species *Pseudomonas aeruginosa* *Xanthomonas maltophilia* *Enterobacter cloacae* Staphylococci Gram-negative bacilli	Trimethoprim-sulfamethoxazole *plus* ceftazidime *or* meropenem *plus* vancomycin
Penetrating head injury	Staphylococci Gram-negative bacilli Anaerobes	Vancomycin *plus* ceftazidime *or* meropenem *plus* metronidazole
Neurosurgical procedure	Staphylococci Gram-negative organisms Enterobacteriaceae *Pseudomonas aeruginosa*	Vancomycin *plus* Ceftazidime *or* meropenem

to cover streptococci and *B. fragilis*. A brain abscess that complicates otitis media or mastoiditis may be caused by *Streptococcus* species, *Bacteroides* species (including *B. fragilis*), Enterobacteriaceae, or *P. aeruginosa*. A combination of penicillin G, metronidazole, and ceftazidime or meropenem is recommended. Cerebral abscesses due to bacteremia from a pyogenic lung infection, urinary sepsis, or an intra-abdominal source of infection are treated with a combination of penicillin G, metronidazole, and ceftazidime or meropenem until the results of culture and antimicrobial susceptibility tests are available. A brain abscess that develops in association with endocarditis is most often caused by *S. aureus* or microaerophilic streptococci; empiric therapy should include a combination of nafcillin or vancomycin plus a third- or fourth-generation cephalosporin (e.g., cefotaxime).

The most common organisms isolated when brain abscess complicates cyanotic congenital heart disease are viridans streptococci (microaerophilic streptococci), anaerobic streptococci, and occasionally *Haemophilus* species. A combination of penicillin G and cefotaxime plus metronidazole is recommended. Penicillin G usually adequately covers microaerophilic streptococci. Metronidazole has excellent bactericidal activity against strict anaerobes, excellent oral absorption, and good penetration into CSF and brain abscess cavities, but streptococci and aerotolerant anaerobes are resistant to metronidazole. Cefotaxime is added to cover *Haemophilus* species, and is the preferred third-generation cephalosporin because it and its lipophilic metabolite, desacetylcefotaxime, have excellent antibacterial activity and penetrate and accumulate within abscess cavities.[35]

Brain abscesses complicating neurosurgical procedures are usually due to staphylococci or gram-negative organisms. Empiric therapy should be a combination of vancomycin plus ceftazidime or meropenem. The most common pathogens recovered from brain abscesses that complicate penetrating head injuries are staphylococci and gram-negative bacteria. Anaerobes and *Nocardia* species may also be found. Empiric therapy should include a combination of vancomycin, ceftazidime, and metronidazole.

Brain abscesses are treated with a 6- to 8-week course of parenteral antimicrobial therapy, followed by an additional 2- to 3-month course of oral antimicrobial therapy. Either CT or MRI can be performed every 2 weeks and should also be undertaken at any sign of clinical deterioration.[48] A small amount of enhancement may still be seen on imaging for several months after the abscess has been treated successfully.

The majority of abscesses can be managed with stereotactic aspiration and therapeutic drainage in combination with antimicrobial therapy, with two exceptions. An abscess that is in the cerebritis stage and has not become encapsulated may respond to antimicrobial therapy alone. Brain abscesses due to *N. asteroides* usually require surgical excision and therapy with trimethoprim-sulfamethoxazole.

Corticosteroids are recommended only for those patients with significant cerebral edema and associated mass effect causing increased ICP. Corticosteroids should not be given routinely to patients with brain abscesses, as they delay the encapsulation of the abscess.

Because of the high risk of focal or generalized seizures, patients should be treated with prophylactic anticonvulsant drugs during the course of antimicrobial therapy and for at least 3 months after resolution of the abscess, at which time consideration can be given to tapering and discontinuing anticonvulsant therapy.

SUBDURAL EMPYEMA AND EPIDURAL ABSCESS

A subdural empyema is a collection of pus in the space between the dura and the arachnoid (Fig. 39-2). A cranial epidural abscess develops in the space between the dura and the inner table of the skull (Fig. 39-3). A subdural empyema is a more malignant and life-threatening infection than is an epidural abscess.

Etiology

Paranasal sinusitis, especially frontal sinusitis, is the most common predisposing condition for subdural empyema.[49] Septic thrombophlebitis of the mucosal veins of the sinuses results in retrograde extension of infection with drainage of bacteria into the dural venous sinuses and cortical veins and the formation of a subdural empyema.[50] Subdural empyema may also result from direct infection of the subdural space during a neurosurgical procedure, such as drainage of a subdural hematoma; as

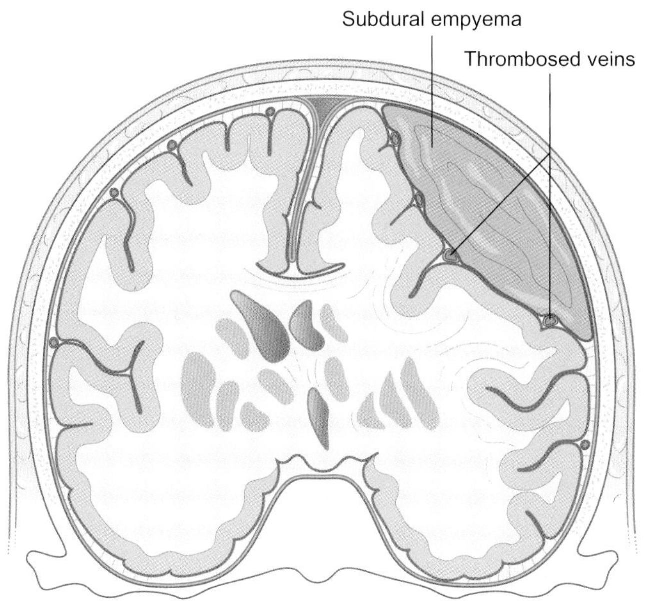

FIGURE 39-2 ▪ Schematic appearance of a subdural empyema.

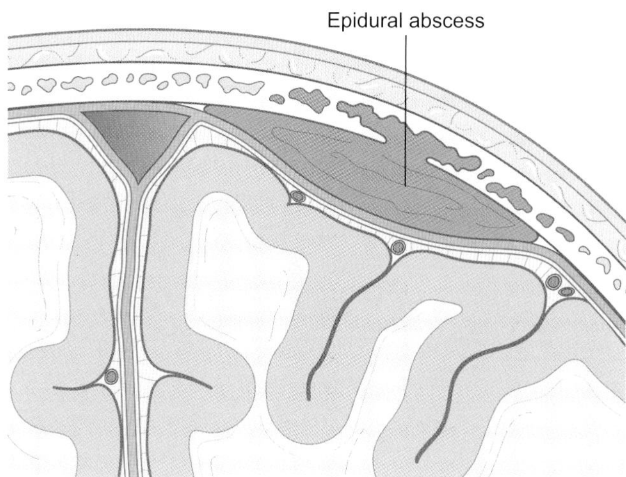

FIGURE 39-3 ▪ Cranial epidural abscess located in the space between the dura and the inner table of the skull.

a complication of head trauma; or from infection of a subdural effusion. It only rarely develops from hematogenous dissemination of bacteria from a distant focus of infection.

An epidural abscess may develop as a complication of a craniotomy or a compound skull fracture or as the result of spread of infection from the frontal sinuses, middle ear, mastoid, or orbit.[51] When an epidural abscess develops as a complication of a craniotomy, it is either from direct infection of the epidural space or as a complication of a contiguous area of osteomyelitis that develops from infection of a wound or bone flap. A cranial epidural abscess rarely results from hematogenous seeding of the epidural space from a distant site of infection.[51]

Aerobic and microaerophilic streptococci and anaerobic bacteria are the most common causative organisms of subdural empyema or epidural abscess that develops as a complication of sinusitis, middle ear infection, or mastoiditis. A subdural empyema or an epidural abscess that develops as a complication of craniotomy, compound skull fracture, or drainage of a subdural hematoma is usually caused by *S. aureus*, coagulase-negative staphylococci, or gram-negative organisms. A subdural effusion may be a complication of bacterial meningitis in infants and children. It is typically a self-limited process that resolves as the meningitis is treated. Occasionally, a subdural effusion may become infected, causing a subdural empyema—the causative organism is the organism responsible for the meningitis.

Clinical Presentation

Headache is the most common complaint with a subdural empyema and is initially localized to the side of the subdural infection. It may be accompanied by fever and symptoms of sinusitis or otitis media. The evolution of a subdural empyema tends to be remarkably rapid. There are no septations in the subdural space, and, as a result, the purulent exudate can spread quite extensively. The headache may become more severe and generalized as the infection spreads. Focal neurologic deficits or seizures may also occur. Contralateral hemiparesis or hemiplegia is the most common focal neurologic deficit. Seizures begin as focal motor type that then may become secondarily generalized. Over the course of a few days, the level of consciousness decreases from somnolence to stupor and finally to coma.[52] In a review of subdural empyema arising from sinusitis in 18 patients, headache was present in 15 patients (83%), fever in 17 patients (94%), focal neurologic signs in 17 patients (94%), nuchal rigidity in 14 patients (78%), altered level of consciousness in 10 patients (56%), seizures in 10 patients (56%), and sinus tenderness or periorbital swelling in 7 patients (39%).[52]

The clinical presentation of an epidural abscess is distinctly different from that of a subdural empyema. The patient is not as ill, and there is rarely rigidity of the neck or focal neurologic signs.[52] Presentation is typically with an unrelenting hemicranial headache accompanied by persistent fever. Focal neurologic deficits, seizures, and signs of increased ICP do not typically develop until the infection spreads into the subdural space (subdural empyema).[51]

Diagnosis

Cranial MRI is the procedure of choice for demonstrating these lesions because it is free from bony artifacts adjacent to the inner table of the skull and readily can demonstrate extracerebral fluid collections. T1-weighted postgadolinium and T2-weighted sequences are best for demonstrating subdural empyema or cranial epidural abscess. Subdural empyema is hyperintense on T1-weighted sequences. There is contrast enhancement of the rim of the empyema separating the empyema from the subjacent brain parenchyma. The empyema itself appears as a crescent-shaped lesion of hyperintensity on T2-weighted sequences.

On T1-weighted sequences, an epidural abscess has a signal intensity that is between that of normal brain parenchyma and CSF. Enhancement of the dura is seen on T1-weighted contrast-enhanced images. An epidural abscess appears as a lentiform or crescentic purulent fluid collection that is hyperintense on T2-weighted sequences.

Lumbar puncture should not be performed in patients with subdural empyema or epidural abscess. The etiologic organism is identified by Gram stain and culture of pus obtained either via burr hole or by craniotomy.

Treatment

Immediate neurosurgical drainage of a subdural empyema or a cranial epidural abscess is the definitive step in their management. At surgery, Gram stain and culture of the purulent material are performed. Empiric antimicrobial therapy pending the results of Gram stain and culture should cover aerobic and microaerophilic streptococci, anaerobic bacteria, staphylococci, and gram-negative bacilli and include a combination of a third- or fourth-generation cephalosporin (e.g., ceftriaxone, cefotaxime, or cefepime), metronidazole, and nafcillin or vancomycin. Ceftazidime or meropenem should be substituted for cefotaxime or ceftriaxone in neurosurgical patients because of better *Pseudomonas* species coverage. Antibiotics can be modified when the results of Gram stain and bacterial culture and sensitivity testing are known. A 4-week course of intravenous antibiotic therapy is recommended for subdural empyema, followed by a 2-week course of oral antibiotic therapy. A cranial epidural abscess is treated for 3 weeks with parenteral antibiotics in the absence of osteomyelitis, and for 6 to 8 weeks when it is a complication of a contiguous area of osteomyelitis.

SPINAL EPIDURAL ABSCESS

An epidural abscess may develop in the spinal epidural space (Fig. 39-4). The most common locations are either the posterior midthoracic region between the fourth and the eighth thoracic vertebrae (Fig. 39-5) or the lower lumbar epidural space. These locations are most commonly involved because the anteroposterior width of the spinal epidural space is greatest from approximately T4 to T8 and from L3 to S2.[53] Anterior abscesses occur less often than do posterior abscesses and usually occur at the cervical level.

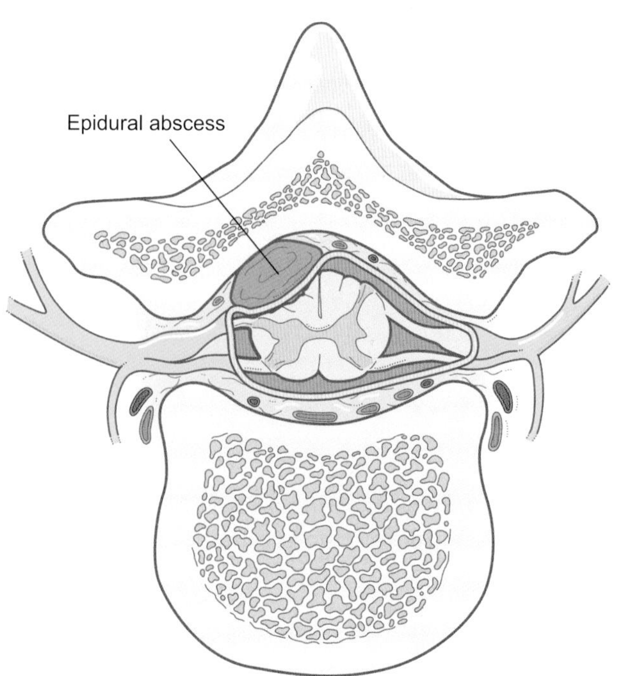

FIGURE 39-4 ■ An abscess in the epidural space posterior to the spinal cord.

Etiology

A spinal epidural abscess develops in the space outside the dura mater but within the spinal canal as the result of hematogenous spread of bacteria from a remote site of infection to the epidural space (e.g., secondary to skin infection, urinary tract infection, intra-abdominal infection, pelvic inflammatory disease, pneumonia, endocarditis, or infections from intravenous lines); by direct extension from a contiguous infection (e.g., an area of osteomyelitis in an adjacent vertebral body); by direct infection of the epidural space during spine surgery or epidural anesthesia; or by direct extension of infection from decubitus ulcers, infected abdominal wounds, retropharyngeal abscesses, or psoas muscle abscesses. Immunosuppression from chronic disease (such as diabetes or chronic renal insufficiency), HIV infection, corticosteroid therapy, and immunosuppressive therapies are increasingly reported as predisposing conditions.

The etiologic organism of the spinal epidural abscess is predictable from the predisposing condition. A spinal epidural abscess that arises from hematogenous dissemination from a skin infection or infections in intravenous lines, or as a complication of spine surgery or epidural anesthesia, is caused in the majority of cases by *S. aureus*. Infection that reaches the epidural space by hematogenous spread of bacteria from a genitourinary infection or intra-abdominal infection to the paravertebral venous plexus is usually caused by gram-negative bacilli.

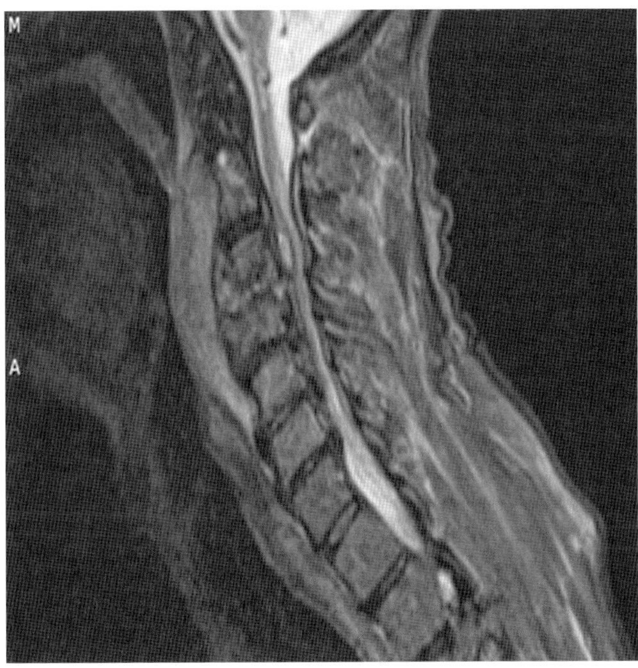

FIGURE 39-5 ▪ Sagittal T2-weighted magnetic resonance imaging (MRI) of the cervical spine demonstrating an epidural fluid collection (abscess) compressing the spinal cord.

Clinical Presentation

Patients with a bacterial spinal epidural abscess present with a classic neurologic syndrome.[54] Back pain is the initial symptom, followed within 2 to 3 days by radicular pain in the extremities or pain in an intercostal thoracic dermatomal distribution. As the disease progresses, weakness of appendicular muscles is associated with decreased sensation below the level of the lesion and loss of bowel and bladder control. Finally, there is complete paralysis of appendicular muscles and loss of all sensory modalities below the level of the lesion (i.e., a sensory level). The majority of patients also have an elevated temperature.

The possibility of a spinal epidural abscess should be considered in any patient with fever, back pain (especially focal vertebral pain and tenderness), and radicular pain in the extremities or pain in a thoracic dermatomal distribution.

Diagnosis

Gadolinium-enhanced MRI is the diagnostic procedure of choice for spinal epidural abscess. MRI of the thoracic and lumbar region should be obtained to visualize the extent of the epidural abscess, and it is reasonable to obtain images of the cervical region as well, especially if the upper extremities are involved. A lumbar puncture should not be performed at the site of a possible abscess because of the risk of spread of infection from the epidural to the subarachnoid space. The majority of patients have an elevated peripheral white blood cell count, and blood cultures may demonstrate the organism.

Treatment

A spinal epidural abscess is treated with immediate laminectomy for decompression and drainage of the epidural space. Empiric therapy depends on the predisposing condition. Because *S. aureus* is the most common etiologic agent, and given the increasing incidence of community- and hospital-acquired methicillin-resistant *S. aureus*, empiric therapy should include vancomycin. In the postneurosurgical patient, ceftazidime or meropenem should be added to the empiric regimen to cover gram-negative bacilli. When a spinal epidural abscess is the result of local extension from an adjacent infection, such as a decubitus ulcer, empiric therapy should cover *S. aureus* and gram-negative bacilli. If the source is an abdominal infection, anaerobic coverage with metronidazole should be added. Once a specific organism has been isolated, the antibiotic regimen can be modified based on the results of sensitivity studies. The duration of intravenous antibiotic therapy is usually 3 to 4 weeks in the absence of osteomyelitis, and 6 to 8 weeks when vertebral osteomyelitis is present.[55]

SEPTIC INTRACRANIAL THROMBOPHLEBITIS

Septic intracranial thrombophlebitis is a bacterial infection of the cortical veins and sinuses with resultant venous thrombosis. It is a complication of bacterial meningitis, subdural empyema, epidural abscess, or infection in the skin of the face, paranasal sinuses, middle ear, or mastoid. Textbooks tend to treat septic intracranial thrombophlebitis as a distinct entity, but in reality clinicians probably underdiagnose it as a complication of bacterial meningitis or subdural empyema. The availability of noninvasive neuroimaging procedures, such as magnetic resonance venography and CT angiography, that demonstrate dural sinus thrombosis may increase the recognition of this complication.

Etiology

The superior sagittal sinus is the largest of the venous sinuses (Fig. 39-6), and it receives blood from the frontal, parietal, and occipital superior cerebral veins and the diploic veins, which communicate with the meningeal veins. Infection can spread from the meninges to the superior sagittal sinus via the diploic veins, especially in cases with purulent exudate near the superior sagittal sinus. The cerebral veins and venous sinuses have no valves; therefore, blood within them can flow in either direction. The superior sagittal sinus drains into the transverse sinus. The transverse sinuses also receive venous drainage from small veins from both the middle ear and the mastoid cells. The transverse sinus becomes the sigmoid sinus before draining into the internal jugular vein. Septic transverse or sigmoid sinus thrombosis can be a complication of acute and chronic otitis media or mastoiditis. Infection spreads from the mastoid air cells to the transverse sinus via the emissary veins or by direct invasion.

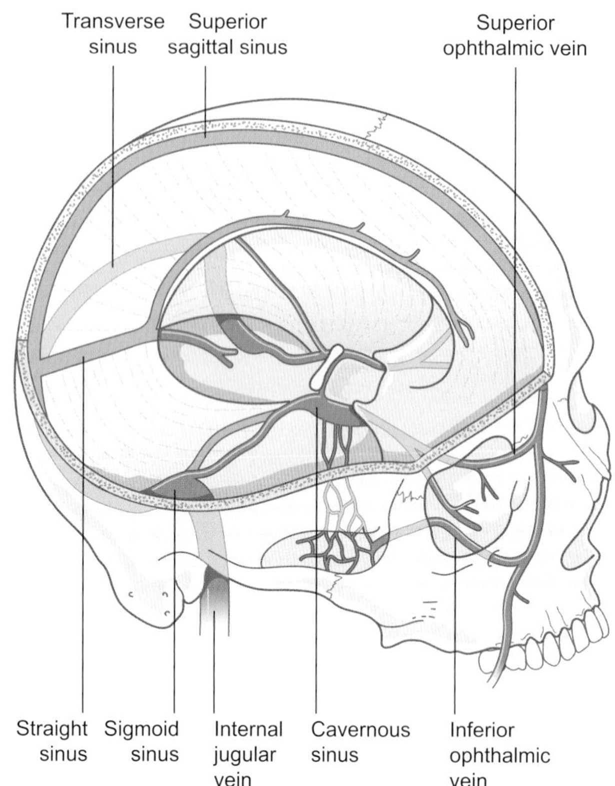

FIGURE 39-6 ■ The major cerebral venous sinuses.

The cavernous sinuses are inferior to the superior sagittal sinus at the base of the skull (Fig. 39-6). Bacteria in the sphenoid and ethmoid sinuses can spread to the cavernous sinuses via the small emissary veins, causing septic cavernous sinus thrombosis.

Dehydration from vomiting and hypercoagulable states contribute to the formation of thrombosis in the cerebral venous sinuses. Immunologic abnormalities, including the presence of circulating antiphospholipid antibodies, can also serve as risk factors. Thrombosis of a dural sinus can be associated with thrombosis of the cortical veins that drain blood into and out of the sinuses, resulting in small parenchymal hemorrhages.

Clinical Presentation

Patients with septic thrombosis of the superior sagittal sinus have headache, nausea and vomiting, weakness of the lower extremities with bilateral Babinski signs, focal or generalized seizures, and an alteration in the level of consciousness. There may be a rapid development of stupor and coma.

The signs and symptoms of septic cavernous sinus thrombosis are fever, headache, and diplopia. The oculomotor nerve (III), trochlear nerve (IV), abducens nerve (VI), and ophthalmic and maxillary branches of the trigeminal nerve (V) all pass through the cavernous sinus; therefore, the classic signs of a septic cavernous sinus thrombosis are ptosis, proptosis, and extraocular dysmotility due to deficits of cranial nerves III, IV, and VI. Hypo- or hyperesthesia of the ophthalmic and maxillary divisions of the fifth cranial nerve and a decreased corneal reflex may be detected.

Patients with septic transverse sinus thrombosis may present with Gradenigo syndrome, which is characterized by otitis media, VI nerve palsy, and retro-orbital or facial pain.

Diagnosis

The diagnosis of septic venous sinus thrombosis is suggested by an absent flow void within the sinus on MRI and is confirmed by magnetic resonance venography, CT angiography, or the venous phase of cerebral angiography.

Treatment

Septic venous sinus thrombosis has traditionally been treated with antibiotics and hydration along with removal of infected tissue and thrombus. Anticoagulation with dose-adjusted heparin is reported to be beneficial in patients with aseptic venous sinus thrombosis and is used in the treatment of septic venous sinus thrombosis when patients are worsening despite antimicrobial therapy and intravenous fluids. Occasionally good clinical results have been reported with catheter-directed urokinase therapy and intrathrombus infusion of recombinant tissue plasminogen activator for aseptic venous sinus thrombosis that clinically progresses while on anticoagulation, but there has not been enough experience with these therapies for septic venous sinus thrombosis to make recommendations regarding their use. In patients with bacterial meningitis and lower extremity weakness or a decreased level of consciousness, the use of noninvasive magnetic resonance venography and CT angiography may increase the recognition of this complication.

REFERENCES

1. van de Beek, de Gans J, Tunkel AR, et al: Community acquired bacterial meningitis in adults. N Engl J Med 354:44, 2006.
2. Bisgard KM, Kao A, Leake J, et al: *Haemophilus influenzae* invasive disease in the United States, 1994–1995: near disappearance of a vaccine-preventable childhood disease. Emerg Infect Dis 4:229, 1998.
3. Doern GV, Brueggemann AB, Blocker M, et al: Clonal relationships among high-level penicillin-resistant *Streptococcus pneumoniae* in the United States. Clin Infect Dis 27:757, 1998.
4. Leggiadro RJ: The clinical impact of resistance in the management of pneumococcal disease. Infect Dis Clin North Am 11:867, 1997.
5. Rosenstein NE, Perkins BA, Stephens DS, et al: Meningococcal disease. N Engl J Med 344:1378, 2001.
6. Harder E, Moller K, Skinhoj P: Enterobacteriaceae meningitis in adults: a review of 20 consecutive cases 1977–97. Scand J Infect Dis 31:287, 1999.
7. Domingo P, Barquet N, Alvarez M, et al: Group B streptococcal meningitis in adults: report of twelve cases and review. Clin Infect Dis 25:1180, 1997.
8. Feigin RD, McCracken GH, Klein JO: Diagnosis and management of meningitis. Pediatr Infect Dis 11:785, 1992.
9. Schuurman T, de Boer RF, Kooistra-Smid AM, et al: Prospective study of use of PCR amplification and sequencing of 16S ribosomal DNA from cerebrospinal fluid for diagnosis of bacterial meningitis in a clinical setting. J Clin Microbiol 42:734, 2004.
10. Hoban DJ, Witwicki E, Hammond GW: Bacterial antigen detection in cerebrospinal fluid of patients with meningitis. Diagn Microbiol Infect Dis 3:373, 1985.
11. Maxson S, Lewno MJ, Schutze GE: Clinical usefulness of cerebrospinal fluid bacterial antigen studies. J Pediatr 125:235, 1994.
12. Dwelle TL, Dunkle LM, Blair L: Correlation of cerebrospinal fluid endotoxin-like activity with clinical and laboratory variables in gram-negative bacterial meningitis in children. J Clin Microbiol 25:856, 1987.
13. Weil AA, Glaser CA, Amad Z, et al: Patients with suspected herpes simplex encephalitis: rethinking an initial negative polymerase chain reaction result. Clin Infect Dis 34:1154, 2002.

14. Ali M, Safriel Y, Sohi J, et al: West Nile virus infection: MR imaging findings in the nervous system. AJNR Am J Neuroradiol 26:289, 2005.
15. Hasbun R, Aronin SI, Quagliarello VJ: Treatment of bacterial meningitis. Comp Ther 25:73, 1999.
16. National Committee for Clinical Laboratory Standards: Performance Standards for Antimicrobial Susceptibility Testing. National Committee for Laboratory Standards, Villanova, PA, 1994.
17. Dupuis A, Pariat C, Courtois P, et al: Imipenem but not meropenem induces convulsions in DBA/2 mice, unrelated to cerebrospinal fluid concentrations. Fundam Clin Pharmacol 14:163, 2000.
18. Fitoussi F, Doit C, Benali K, et al: Comparative *in vitro* killing activities of meropenem, imipenem, ceftriaxone, and ceftriaxone plus vancomycin at clinically achievable cerebrospinal fluid concentrations against penicillin-resistant *Streptococcus pneumoniae* isolates from children with meningitis. Antimicrob Agents Chemother 42:942, 1998.
19. Klugman KP, Dagan R: Randomized comparison of meropenem with cefotaxime for treatment of bacterial meningitis. Meropenem Meningitis Study Group. Antimicrob Agents Chemother 39:1140, 1995.
20. Zhanel GG, Wiebe R, Dilay L, et al: Comparative review of the carbapenems. Drugs 67:1027, 2007.
21. Donnelly JP, Horrevorts AM, Sauerwein RW, et al: High dose meropenem in meningitis due to *Pseudomonas aeruginosa*. Lancet 339:1117, 1992.
22. Saez-Llorens X, Castano E, Garcia R, et al: Prospective randomized comparison of cefepime and cefotaxime for treatment of bacterial meningitis in infants and children. Antimicrob Agents Chemother 39:937, 1995.
23. Tauber MG, Moser B: Cytokines and chemokines in meningeal inflammation: biology and clinical implications. Clin Infect Dis 28:1, 1999.
24. Lepper MH, Spies HW: Treatment of pneumococcic meningitis. Arch Intern Med 104:253, 1959.
25. Tauber MG, Khayam-Bashi H, Sande M: Effects of ampicillin and corticosteroids on brain water content, cerebrospinal fluid pressure, and cerebrospinal fluid lactate levels in experimental pneumococcal meningitis. J Infect Dis 151:528, 1985.
26. Lebel MH, Freij B, Syrogiannopoulos GA, et al: Dexamethasone therapy for bacterial meningitis. N Engl J Med 319:964, 1988.
27. McIntyre PB, Berkey CS, King SM, et al: Dexamethasone as adjunctive therapy in bacterial meningitis. JAMA 278:925, 1997.
28. Odio CM, Faingezicht I, Paris M, et al: The beneficial effects of early dexamethasone administration in infants and children with bacterial meningitis. N Engl J Med 324:1525, 1991.
29. de Gans J, van de Beek D, for the European Dexamethasone in Adulthood Bacterial Meningitis Study Investigators: Dexamethasone in adults with bacterial meningitis. N Engl J Med 347:1549, 2002.
30. Brouwer MC, Heckenberg SGB, de Gans J, et al: Nationwide implementation of adjunctive dexamethasone therapy for pneumococcal meningitis. Neurology 75:1533, 2010.
31. Klugman KP, Friedland IR, Bradley JS: Bactericidal activity against cephalosporin-resistant *Streptococcus pneumoniae* in cerebrospinal fluid of children with acute bacterial meningitis. Antimicrob Agents Chemother 39:1988, 1995.
32. Tunkel AR, Hartman BJ, Kaplan BA, et al: Practice guidelines for the management of bacterial meningitis. Clin Infect Dis 39:1267, 2004.
33. Heckenberg SGB, Brouwer MC, van der Ende A, et al: Adjunctive dexamethasone in adults with meningococcal meningitis. Neurology 79:1563, 2012.
34. Peltola H: Prophylaxis of bacterial meningitis. Infect Dis Clin North Am 13:685, 1999.
35. Mathisen GE, Johnson JP: Brain abscess. Clin Infect Dis 25:763, 1997.
36. Al Masalma M, Lonjon M, Richet H, et al: Metagenomic analysis of brain abscesses identifies specific bacterial associations. Clin Infect Dis 54:202, 2012.
37. Heilpern KL, Lorber B: Focal intracranial infections. Infect Dis Clin North Am 10:876, 1996.
38. Honda H, Warren DK: Central nervous system infections: meningitis and brain abscess. Infect Dis Clin North Am 23:609, 2009.
39. Osenbach RK, Loftus CM: Diagnosis and management of brain abscess. Neurosurg Clin North Am 3:403, 1992.
40. Garvey G: Current concepts of bacterial infection of the central nervous system: bacterial meningitis and bacterial brain abscess. J Neurosurg 59:735, 1983.
41. Kagawa M, Takeshita M, Yato S: Brain abscess in congenital heart disease. J Neurosurg 58:913, 1983.
42. Brook I: Aerobic and anaerobic bacteriology of intracranial abscesses. Pediatr Neurol 8:210, 1992.
43. Fishman JA, Rubin RH: Infection in organ-transplant recipients. N Engl J Med 338:1741, 1998.
44. Braun TI, Kerson LA, Eisenberg FP: Nocardial brain abscesses in a pregnant woman. Rev Infect Dis 13:630, 1991.
45. Mamelak AN, Obana WG, Flaherty JF, et al: Nocardial brain abscess: treatment strategies and factors influencing outcome. Neurosurgery 35:622, 1994.
46. Reddy JS, Mishra AM, Behari S, et al: The role of diffusion-weighted imaging in the differential diagnosis of intracranial cystic mass lesions: a report of 147 lesions. Surg Neurol 66:246, 2006.
47. Mishra AM, Reddy SJ, Husain M, et al: Comparison of the magnetization transfer ratio and fluid-attenuated inversion recovery imaging signal intensity in differentiation of various cystic intracranial mass lesions and its correlation with biological parameters. J Magn Reson Imaging 24:52, 2006.
48. Mamelak AN, Mampalam TJ, Obana WG, et al: Improved management of multiple brain abscesses: a combined

surgical and medical approach. Neurosurgery 36:76, 1995.

49. Dill SR, Cobbs CG, McDonald CK: Subdural empyema: analysis of 32 cases and review. Clin Infect Dis 20:372, 1995.
50. Courville CB: Subdural empyema secondary to purulent frontal sinusitis: a clinicopathologic study of forty-two cases verified at autopsy. Arch Otolaryngol 39:211, 1944.
51. Silverberg AL, DiNubile MJ: Subdural empyema and cranial epidural abscess. Med Clin North Am 69:361, 1985.
52. Kubik CS, Adams RD: Subdural empyema. Brain 66:18, 1943.
53. Baker AS, Ojemann RG, Swartz MN, et al: Spinal epidural abscess. N Engl J Med 293:463, 1975.
54. Heusner AP: Nontuberculous spinal epidural infections. N Engl J Med 239:845, 1948.
55. Darouiche RO, Hamill RJ, Greensberg SB, et al: Bacterial spinal epidural abscess: review of 43 cases and literature survey. Medicine (Baltimore) 71:369, 1992.

CHAPTER

40

Spirochetal Infections of the Nervous System

JOHN J. HALPERIN

Spirochetes cause a broad range of human illnesses, including relapsing fever, yaws, pinta, leptospirosis, and periodontal disease. Although leptospirosis and relapsing fevers can cause severe headaches and myalgias in conjunction with high fever and severe systemic illness, two spirochetal infections target the nervous system specifically: syphilis and Lyme disease. Both are the subject of popular mythology and have been blamed for far more than they could possibly have done. Syphilis swept Europe at a time when medicine had yet to understand such fundamental concepts as the germ basis of infection. Even early in the twentieth century, preeminent physicians referred to syphilis as the great imitator. Notably at that time, little was understood about cerebrovascular disease or other neurologic disorders. As late as the 1950s and beyond, anecdotal reports appeared about neurosyphilis having been diagnosed on the basis of silver stains of brain tissue—a highly problematic methodology since fibrillar structures normally present in the brain stain with silver and have a corkscrew-like appearance.

Similarly, Lyme disease has been blamed for innumerable "quality-of-life" ailments. At a time when science has sequenced the human genome, can detect subtle structural abnormalities with magnetic resonance imaging (MRI), and has developed an immense and powerful pharmacopoeia, many find it difficult to accept that medicine has limitations and, in particular, cannot provide simple biologic answers to and remedies for a constellation of common and distressing symptoms, variably known over the years by terms such as *neurasthenia*, *chronic fatigue syndrome*, and *fibromyalgia*, among others. In this setting, some have chosen to extrapolate from the known phenomenology of Lyme disease, emphasizing the areas of similarity between these symptom complexes and Lyme disease and ignoring the far more glaring differences.

There are fascinating similarities between syphilis and Lyme disease that deserve emphasis, as they presumably reflect basic biologic properties of spirochetes. Both infections can be chronic, despite the presence of easily demonstrable antibodies targeted against major epitopes. Presumably, this relates to the spirochetal predisposition to present a limited range of surface antigens, and then change the expressed epitopes over time, as conditions require. Both disorders are spread almost exclusively by intimate contact with a vector, reflecting the very limited ability of spirochetes to survive in vitro. Both begin with prominent, angry-looking cutaneous abnormalities that are surprisingly painless, the lack of pain presumably reflecting the peculiarities of the limited local host immune response.

Aminoff's Neurology and General Medicine, Fifth Edition.

Both disseminate widely and rapidly, easily broaching the blood–brain barrier, probably reflecting their own inherent motility and adherence to cell-surface molecules. Both seed the nervous system frequently but cause neurologic disease only in a small subset of those seeded. Most important, both remain sensitive to fairly simple antibiotics. Although both are frequently described as presenting with protean manifestations, this reflects an approach to neurology based on phenomenology rather than pathophysiology. In fact, each infection usually causes a characteristic range of disorders. Specific manifestations in any given individual depend on the part of the nervous system involved, but the disorders are pathophysiologically related.

SYPHILIS

Background

Syphilis, caused by *Treponema pallidum*, became prominent in Europe shortly after the return of Columbus from the New World. Known at the time (in some circles) as "the French pox," the mode of transmission was recognized early on. The *Breviary of Health* of 1547 states clearly that "specially it is taken when one pocky person doth synne in lechery the one with another."[1] At that time, as with other newly introduced infectious diseases, the morbidity and mortality associated with syphilis were high. Then, presumably as the most susceptible hosts died and the bacteria self-selected for strains that could persist without killing or incapacitating their hosts, the bacteria and humankind settled into their current symbiotic relationship. Currently, there are about 14,000 cases of primary and secondary syphilis each year in the United States.[2]

Diagnosis

Diagnosis was originally clinical and rested on recognition of the characteristic chancre—a painless, ulcerated, indurated lesion at the site of primary infection that typically heals spontaneously. The lesion contains numerous spirochetes; one of the best methods of diagnosis is to scrape the lesion, place the scrapings in saline on a slide, and view the motile spirochetes with a dark-field microscope. In patients not seen at the time of the chancre, diagnosis initially rested on the recognition of one of the large number of clinical syndromes attributed to this disease.

More accurate diagnosis of later disease required advancements in laboratory techniques. Identification of the causative organism was an important first step, but growing *T. pallidum* in vitro remains essentially impossible, although inoculation into susceptible animals provides an indirect—and clinically impractical—method of propagating the organism.

The spirochete has now been very well characterized. Its length varies from 6 to 20 µm; its diameter is about 0.18 µm. It is shaped in a regular helix and exhibits corkscrew motility, propelled by its flagella.[3] Its entire genome has now been sequenced.[4] Despite this intimate knowledge of the spirochete, laboratory confirmation of infection, particularly after resolution of the chancre, remains dependent on serologic tests. All fall into one of two groups. Historically, screening has used indirect tests, measuring "reaginic" antibodies—in essence, anticardiolipin antibodies. The reason that patients with this infection have high titers of anticardiolipin antibody remains unknown, but presumably reflects an interaction of the spirochete with host lipoproteins and other lipids. Tests such as the Wasserman reaction, rapid plasma reagin (RPR), Venereal Disease Research Laboratory (VDRL), and Hinton tests all fall into this group. These tests have been thought to have very high sensitivity but, as indirect measures of infection, lack specificity. However, more recent work, using capture enzyme-linked immunosorbent assays (ELISAs) for comparison, suggest the reaginic tests are less sensitive than previously believed, leading to recommendations by some that direct tests be used for initial screening.[5–7]

Using the still recommended approach, patients with positive reaginic test results are further tested with specific antitreponemal tests, such as the FTA-Abs (fluorescent treponemal antibody, absorbed against nonpathogenic treponemata to decrease cross-reactivity) or the MHA-TP test (microhemagglutination for *T. pallidum*). Response to therapy is generally assessed by measuring titers of reaginic antibody. Typically, the serum titer in a VDRL or similar test declines steadily after successful treatment and eventually becomes negative in most cases.

When serologic testing was introduced early in the twentieth century, seroprevalence rates of 8 to 14 percent were reported in major cities.[1] It was at that time that the medical literature blossomed, attributing all manner of disease to syphilis. It may well be that at least some of this was misattribution due to coincidentally positive serologic tests, much as occurs in Lyme disease–endemic areas today (where, coincidentally, seroprevalence rates of 5 to 15% are common).

Diagnosis of nervous system disease relies heavily on examination of the cerebrospinal fluid (CSF), which is recommended in the assessment of any patient with primary or secondary syphilis and clinical suspicion of central nervous system (CNS) involvement or with tertiary syphilis.[8,9] Invasion and infection of the CNS typically result in increased protein concentration or a CSF pleocytosis, with an increased proportion of B cells.[10] Rarely there is mild hypoglycorrhachia. Active disease typically results in presence of reaginic antibodies (VDRL) in the CSF. Chronic infection and stimulation of the immune response within the CNS generally result in increased CSF IgG concentration as well as production of oligoclonal bands. Synthesis of specific anti–*T. pallidum* antibody can often be demonstrated in the CSF.[11] Successful treatment usually leads to resolution of all these abnormalities.

CSF-based diagnosis is usually straightforward but can, in some circumstances, be problematic. The CSF VDRL test is considered highly specific—a positive CSF VDRL result is regarded as diagnostic of CNS syphilis. (A CSF RPR test has far more false-positive results.) This specificity is probably related to the fact that the methodology is rather insensitive in that a fairly high concentration of antibody is needed for the test to be judged positive. Thus, the presence of a positive VDRL in the CSF is unlikely to be an artifact of contamination of CSF with peripheral blood immunoglobulin. One potential diagnostic problem arises, however, in that although the CSF VDRL typically declines after successful treatment, it may remain positive for an extended period of time. In this circumstance, the return of the CSF white blood cell count and protein concentration to normal is usually taken as evidence of adequate treatment.

With the far more technically sensitive methods used to detect actual antitreponemal antibodies (FTA-Abs, MHA-TP), contamination is a more important issue. False-positive results can occur for one of at least three reasons. Antibodies against antigenically similar organisms (e.g., *Borrelia burgdorferi*) can cross-react. More important, if the lumbar puncture is traumatic, peripheral blood can contaminate the specimen, resulting in artifactual elevations in antibody titers. Probably most important, however, is the fact that some peripheral blood immunoglobulin always filters into the CSF. In the absence of CNS inflammation, there is minimal if any intrinsic production of antibodies within the CNS. However, CSF IgG concentration is typically 2 to 3 mg/dl, approximately 0.2 percent of peripheral blood IgG concentration, representing the small amount of serum immunoglobulin that normally passes through the blood–brain barrier. Just as in testing CSF Lyme serologies, standard testing conditions (diluting CSF 1:5 for the FTA-Abs, for example) are selected to compensate for this leakage. However, artifacts may arise in two important circumstances. In patients with high serum FTA-Abs titers, CSF titers may be positive simply by virtue of the small amount of specific antibody that normally filters in. Second, in the presence either of CNS inflammation or of blood–brain barrier breakdown for other reasons, the amount of peripheral blood immunoglobulin leaking into the CNS may be greater than assumed, resulting in an apparent increase in the concentration of the tested antibody but actually simply reflecting an overall and nonspecific increase in all antibody levels. These considerations notwithstanding, the CSF FTA is a highly sensitive if not entirely specific marker of neurosyphilis.[10]

The absence of an absolute "gold standard" test for the diagnosis of neurosyphilis has resulted in controversy, differing recommendations for diagnostic strategies, and varying estimates of the sensitivity and specificity of different CSF tests. Whereas the CSF VDRL test is often said to be 100 percent specific, estimates of its sensitivity vary widely, depending on the alternative criteria used to define neurosyphilis. Screening CSF samples using the FTA-Abs and considering patients to have probable neurosyphilis if they have (1) a positive CSF FTA-Abs result, (2) a consistent clinical syndrome, and (3) elevation in either the CSF cell count, protein concentration, or both, leads to an estimated sensitivity of the CSF VDRL of 27 percent.[12] Performing a similar analysis, but using the CSF MHA-TP as the primary criterion and comparing the CSF MHA-TP, CSF FTA-Abs, and CSF VDRL,[13] suggests that the sensitivity of the CSF VDRL is about 40 percent, but that of the CSF MHA-TP is substantially greater than that of the FTA-Abs. However, there is evidence that as many as one-third of human immunodeficiency virus (HIV)–seronegative individuals with positive serum VDRL results will have inflammatory changes in the CSF,[14] but no serologic (CSF VDRL or FTA-Abs) evidence of neurosyphilis, calling into doubt the assumptions underlying the first two conclusions.

Theoretically, a more definitive approach would be to determine whether antibodies targeted against *T. pallidum* are actually being produced within the CNS. Although a variety of techniques can be used, conceptually this is accomplished by measuring the antibody concentration in CSF and serum, normalizing for the relative total immunoglobulin concentrations in both, and determining whether specific antibody is disproportionately represented in the CSF. This approach, used in many other infections,[15] should have very high specificity, although, again, sensitivity is difficult to define.[11,16–18] Despite the intuitive appeal of this approach, sensitivity estimates have varied widely, depending on underlying assumptions, making its applicability uncertain at this time.

Clinical Features

After initial inoculation of spirochetes, the organism disseminates rapidly. Within weeks of infection the chancre develops at the site of infection. Chancres contain large numbers of spirochetes and are highly infectious. Untreated, they typically subside spontaneously over weeks. This early, localized disease constitutes primary syphilis. Over the ensuing few months, spirochetes disseminate, setting the stage for secondary syphilis. In this phase, there is a high antigen load, often with a significant spirochetemia. Spirochetes can invade any organ of the body but have a particular predilection for the skin (with secondary lesions, particularly involving the palms and soles), lymph nodes (particularly the epitrochlear nodes), kidney (with an immune complex–mediated glomerulonephritis), and CNS (seeded in between 25 and 40% of infected individuals). As many as 40 percent of untreated patients develop a lymphocytic meningitis. As in other basilar meningitides, the cranial nerves, particularly II to VIII, can be compromised. Intracranial pressure may be increased.

The disease then typically enters a latent phase, during which infection—and the immune response to it—persist. In the majority, the host immune response clears the infection.[17] In a subset, late or tertiary complications develop. In some, this consists of disseminated granulomata, known as gummas, that can occur anywhere in the body, causing focal symptoms depending on location. Patients may develop gummas in the brain, causing local structural damage and symptoms. Gummas tend to be relatively benign but can be confused with neoplasms or other processes. Some patients develop an endarteritis obliterans affecting the vasa vasorum of the ascending aorta, causing characteristic aneurysmal dilatation.

Although neurologic involvement is generally divided into early or late (secondary or tertiary) manifestations, there is some variability in how different pathophysiologic entities are grouped. The acute meningitis, with or without cranial nerve involvement, typically occurs during acute spirochetal dissemination and is considered part of secondary (acute disseminated) disease. All other manifestations occur later in the disease, in what might be termed *late disseminated infection* ("tertiary syphilis"), although some tend to occur earlier in this "late" phase, others later.

Symptomatic nervous system involvement ultimately occurs in 4 to 6 percent of untreated patients[19,20] and tends to take one of several forms. One of the earlier occurring late manifestations is meningovascular syphilis, in which the characteristic obliterative endarteritis involves the intracranial vasculature, causing strokes. Although the resultant clinical phenomena are described as protean, they are no more protean than in other cerebrovascular disease—differences reflect the site of damage, not the mechanism.

Several other characteristic abnormalities may occur. Those not due to vasculitis are collectively referred to as parenchymal neurosyphilis. Involvement of the upper brainstem and surrounding basilar cisterns may lead to Argyll Robertson pupils, small irregular pupils that do not react to light but do to accommodation. Optic atrophy may develop slowly, presumably owing to both increased intracranial pressure caused by the meningitis and local infiltration of the optic nerves. *Tabes dorsalis*, consisting of damage to the dorsal roots, the dorsal root ganglia, and the posterior columns, results in marked loss of proprioception, as well as "lightning-like" shooting radicular pain. Gait is typical of that in individuals with proprioceptive loss—slapping, with poor awareness of the location of the feet in space. Loss of the dorsal root ganglion neurons and dorsal roots leads to loss of reflexes and diminished pain awareness, potentially leading to repeated injuries to lower extremity joints with severe cumulative damage (Charcot joints).

One of the most fascinating disorders associated with late neurosyphilis is the late dementia, referred to as *general paresis of the insane*, or GPI. Initial symptoms are described as personality changes with delusions and hallucinations; seizures and myoclonus may occur. Involvement tends to be frontotemporoparietal, with a slowly progressive dementia. Considered a consequence of long-standing meningitis, the pathology is rather subtle. Inflammatory changes are seen in the ventricular walls (granular ependymitis). There is brain atrophy, ventricular enlargement, and neuronal loss, with some reactive gliosis. Parenchymal inflammation is usually rather limited, without evidence of multiple infarcts—in brief, the degree of CNS dysfunction seems out of proportion to the evidence of disease activity. MRI studies have demonstrated fairly widespread abnormalities.[21]

Since the early 1980s, the HIV epidemic has led to a resurgence of neurosyphilis, raising new concerns about both the biology of the infection and its treatment. In HIV-infected individuals, early disease and asymptomatic disease each account for about one-third of the cases of coexisting neurosyphilis.[22] Of patients with early disease, one-half have meningitis and one-fourth have meningovascular syphilis. Of those with late-stage disease, the majority have general paresis, and a small subset have tabes.

Finally, congenital infection still occurs. This happens most commonly during early stages of maternal infection,[1] when spirochete dissemination is still actively occurring. Treatment during the first 4 months of gestation usually protects the fetus; after that, death of the fetus or newborn, or congenital infection, can result. The common manifestations of newborn infections include "snuffles" (rhinitis due to mucocutaneous involvement) and a diffuse rash that is unusual in that it involves the palms and soles as well as skin at mucoepithelial junctions. Involvement of the liver is common, as are osteochondritis and perichondritis, most typically manifested as a "saddle nose" and "saber shins." Unusual, centrally notched, peg-shaped upper teeth ("Hutchinson's incisors") occur, as does frontal bossing. IgM assays can be useful for diagnosis.[23,24]

Treatment

Treatment of early syphilis remains remarkably effective with simple regimens.[8,25] Primary, secondary, and latent syphilis (without CNS involvement and of less than 1-year duration) are generally treated with a single dose of intramuscular benzathine penicillin (2.4 million units). Treatment for 2 weeks with oral doxycycline (100 mg twice daily) has been recommended for patients allergic to penicillin, although few studies have evaluated this approach; recommendations are usually for desensitization to penicillin if at all possible.[8] When the nervous system is involved, high doses of intravenous penicillin are generally required (10 to 14 days, 3 to 4 million units every 4 hours). Curiously, for many years, weekly intramuscular injections of benzathine penicillin were used. This is still one of the recommended alternative regimens for neurosyphilis, even though the demonstrable levels in the CNS are subtherapeutic for *T. pallidum*, presumably reflecting the efficacy of this regimen outside the blood–brain barrier and the rather low incidence of late neurosyphilis in untreated individuals. An acceptable alternative is procaine penicillin 2.4 million units intramuscularly daily, with probenecid 500 mg orally four times daily for 10 to 14 days.[9] Ceftriaxone has been suggested as an alternative in patients allergic to penicillin and may be useful, although few studies have demonstrated its efficacy.[26–28]

Treatment has been particularly challenging in patients coinfected with HIV. Not only may syphilis cause considerably more serious symptoms, it may be much more difficult to eradicate.[29,30] Patients who have received full courses of usually curative doses of intravenous penicillin have developed clear-cut relapses, even when initial treatment was at a time when the patient was not severely immunocompromised.[29] This suggests that treatment may not eliminate these spirochetes entirely, but reduces the bacterial burden to a number that normally can be controlled by the patient's immune system.

LYME DISEASE

Background

The term *Lyme disease* was coined in the mid-1970s to describe a disorder affecting children living near Lyme, Connecticut, who developed what appeared

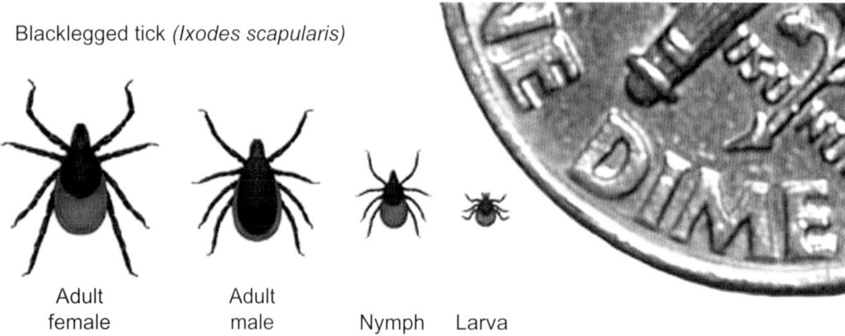

FIGURE 40-1 ▪ Ixodes ticks. (Reproduced courtesy of Centers for Disease Control and Prevention: http://www.cdc.gov/lyme/transmission/; accessed 26 February, 2013.)

to be juvenile rheumatoid arthritis. Careful epidemiologic studies demonstrated that this disorder developed following bites by hard-shelled *Ixodes* ticks (Fig. 40-1), particularly when the bites were followed by a slowly enlarging erythroderm (Fig. 40-2). It was soon recognized that this rash was identical to the one described early in the twentieth century in the European literature, known as erythema chronicum migrans (ECM or, more recently, EM), also known to develop following bites of *Ixodes* ticks. Similarly, by the late 1970s it became apparent that affected individuals frequently developed all or part of a neurologic triad of lymphocytic meningitis, cranial neuritis, and painful radiculoneuritis, virtually identical to the disorder described in the 1920s by two French physicians[31] and now known as Garin–Bujadoux–Bannwarth syndrome. A German report in 1941 even associated the disorder with "rheumatism." Although American patients appear to have more prominent rheumatologic symptoms and European patients more striking nervous system abnormalities, the European and American disorders are qualitatively similar.

In 1982, Willy Burgdorfer isolated a novel spirochete from *Ixodes* ticks collected on Shelter Island, New York (directly across Long Island Sound from Connecticut),[32] and the following year it was clearly established that this organism, named *B. burgdorferi*, was the agent responsible for Lyme disease.[33,34] Shortly thereafter, Eva Asbrink in Sweden identified a virtually identical organism as the agent responsible for European borreliosis.[35] Subsequent studies have permitted the subdivision of this group of *Borrelia* (referred to collectively as *B. burgdorferi sensu lato*) into at least three subspecies.[36] The strain responsible for North American disease has been termed *B. burgdorferi sensu stricto*, whereas European disease is attributed primarily to two strains, known as *Borrelia garinii*, responsible for most cases of neuroborreliosis, and *Borrelia afzelii*, responsible for several unique cutaneous abnormalities. These strain differences are believed to be responsible for the somewhat different range of presentations seen in Europe and North America.

B. burgdorferi spirochetes differ somewhat morphologically from *T. pallidum*. They range in length from 10 to 30 μm and are 0.2 to 0.5 μm in diameter.[37] Like treponemes, they are helical in shape and propel themselves through medium or tissue with flagella.

Lyme disease occurs worldwide, primarily in areas in which *Ixodes* ticks coexist with a reservoir of infected animal hosts and potential human victims. In temperate climates the tick goes through a 2-year life cycle. After hatching into a larva (Fig. 40-1),

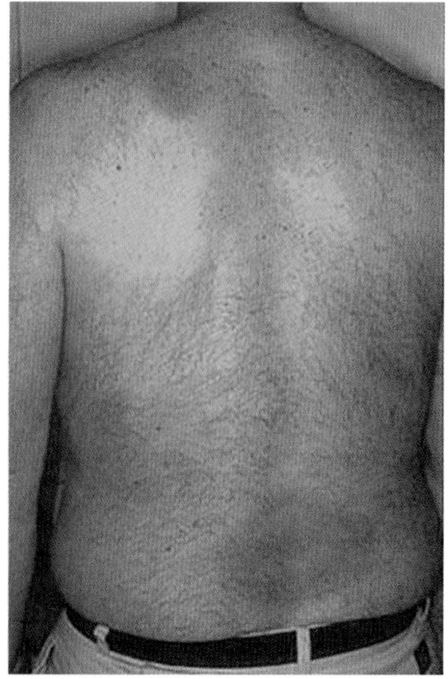

FIGURE 40-2 ▪ Multifocal erythema migrans, extending across much of the back.

it feeds once, typically on a small mammal such as a field mouse. If this host has previously been infected, the tick may ingest spirochetes and itself become infected. After feeding, the larva matures into a nymph, which will then have its next meal. As blood enters the infected tick's gut, spirochetes already present proliferate. Over a period of 24 to 48 hours, they migrate to the tick's salivary glands, from which they can be injected into the new host, again transmitting infection. Because of this process, tick attachment lasting less than 24 to 48 hours is highly unlikely to result in infection.

The tick ultimately partakes of one last meal, this time as an adult. This typically occurs on a larger mammal, such as a deer, bear, or sheep—the species of choice giving rise to the popular name given the tick. Since the tick responsible for Lyme disease in the northeastern United States (*Ixodes scapularis*) is most closely associated with deer, some control strategies have focused on reducing the deer population. Although this may be helpful in lowering tick density, host elimination must be nearly complete.[38] Similar strategies are less practical elsewhere. In much of the world, sheep provide the predominant large host. Elimination of these commercially important animals would be impractical. Other control strategies,[38] such as providing rodents—the principal reservoir host—with acaricide-containing nesting material, springtime acaricide spraying to eliminate nymphs, and creation of dry barriers between wooded and residential areas, have met with varying success. In most endemic areas, ticks feed primarily during warmer months, placing human victims at greatest risk of contracting this infection from spring through autumn. The more temperate California climate leads to less seasonal variation.

Interestingly, although Lyme arthritis was characterized only in the 1970s, identical cases of recurrent, nontraumatic knee arthritis were recognized years earlier in eastern Long Island, where this was known as Montauk knee. Some have conjectured that Lyme disease was introduced to the United States when a herd of deer was brought to Long Island, New York, from Europe early in the twentieth century, an interesting counterpoint to the theory that Columbus imported syphilis to Europe from the New World. The disease appears to have spread slowly from Long Island to Connecticut, and then to contiguous regions, and is now endemic along much of the eastern seaboard of the United States from Massachusetts to Delaware. A second endemic focus exists in the upper Midwest, and a third in northern California. These three regions account for the vast majority of cases of Lyme disease in the United States (Fig. 40-3).[39]

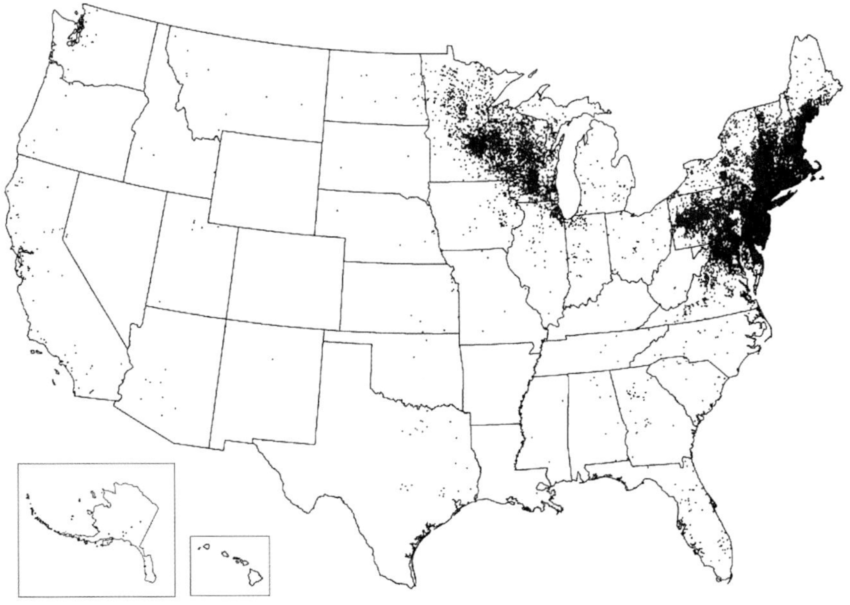

FIGURE 40-3 ▪ Reported cases of Lyme disease in the United States, 2011. One dot is placed randomly within the county of residence for each confirmed case. Though Lyme disease cases have been reported in nearly every state, cases are reported based on the county of residence, not necessarily the county of infection. (Reproduced courtesy of the Centers for Disease Control and Prevention: Reported cases of Lyme disease—2011. http://www.cdc.gov/lyme/stats/maps/map2011.html, 2012.)

Clinical Features

General

Lyme disease typically begins with a virtually pathognomonic rash, known as erythema migrans, occurring at the site of the tick bite, generally developing within 1 month of infection. Although the rash is erythematous and occasionally swollen, it typically is remarkably asymptomatic. Untreated, it expands to become many inches in diameter, potentially spanning an entire limb or occupying much of the trunk (Fig. 40-2). Between one-half and two-thirds of adults with Lyme disease recall having such a rash; in children, who are presumably under the watchful eye of a parent, the rash is seen in as many as 90 percent of infected individuals.[40] Since the rash may occur on parts of the body not readily seen and is asymptomatic, it is not surprising that a significant number of patients have no recollection of having had a rash. Like the chancre, it can resolve spontaneously without treatment, although treatment speeds resolution. Also like the chancre, the rash contains innumerable spirochetes, particularly at the leading edge. Unlike *T. pallidum*, however, it is possible to culture *B. burgdorferi* in vitro, although this requires a specialized medium that is not commonly available in most microbiology laboratories.

The spirochetes typically disseminate rapidly after inoculation. This secondary spread differentiates acute localized Lyme disease, analogous to primary syphilis, from early disseminated infection, analogous to secondary lues. Dissemination is often accompanied by fever and diffuse myalgias and arthralgias, identical to those seen in other bacteremias, often referred to as a "flu-like" syndrome. Notably, this flu-like syndrome does not include upper respiratory or gastrointestinal symptomatology. With dissemination, the rash may become multifocal (Fig. 40-2), and other organ systems may become involved.

Other cutaneous abnormalities occur infrequently in North America, but more commonly in Europe. Acrodermatitis atrophicans develops late in European borreliosis and consists of "tissue paper–like" atrophy of the skin, which becomes reddish-purple in hue. *Borrelia* lymphocytoma, a thickening of the skin due to a dense lymphocytic infiltrate, typically involving the earlobe or the areola of the breast, similarly occurs frequently in Europe but rarely in the United States.

In early series about 5 percent of patients (fewer in more recent studies[39]) developed cardiac conduction abnormalities—commonly heart block in an otherwise healthy young adult. Occasional cases of myositis have been described.[41] Mild elevations of serum creatine kinase are not uncommon, although frank muscle weakness is distinctly unusual. The myositis is typically focal, presents particularly with pain and swelling, and often occurs adjacent to areas of skin, joint, or nerve involvement.[42,43]

As in virtually every other known infection, a certain number of individuals become infected but do not become symptomatic, or develop minor symptoms that are self-limited and indistinguishable from other summertime febrile illnesses. The precise frequency with which this occurs is indeterminate, but probably is substantial.

Unlike syphilis, congenital infection does not appear to be a significant problem. Despite anecdotal reports, no characteristic "congenital Lyme disease syndrome" has been identified.[44,45] Epidemiologic studies have failed to demonstrate any increase in adverse outcomes among women with positive serologies who have not had clinical evidence of acute infection. In a few instances, infants born to women who had experienced acute infections during pregnancy have themselves been infected, so aggressive treatment in this circumstance is appropriate.

Neuroborreliosis

Among infected patients, 10 to 15 percent will develop neurologic abnormalities, most commonly a lymphocytic meningitis, cranial neuropathy, or painful radiculitis. The neurologic syndromes can be categorized (Table 40-1) as affecting primarily the peripheral nervous system or the CNS, although overlap occurs. Manifestations of each vary widely, depending on the specific site and severity of involvement. However, pathophysiologic mechanisms are limited to a small number of phenomena.

The CNS is often seeded early in infection. Precise estimates are difficult because patients do not routinely undergo CSF examination. However, it is likely that the CNS is infected in many individuals, but the infection clears spontaneously.[46–48] In many patients, acute infection is marked by an acute lymphocytic meningitis. Headache and neck stiffness are quite variable in severity and do not

TABLE 40-1 ■ Central Nervous System Manifestations of Neuroborreliosis

Infection in Subarachnoid Space (Abnormal CSF)
Meningitis
Radiculitis
Cranial neuritis
Infection in CNS Parenchyma (Abnormal Neurological Examination, MRI, CSF)
Encephalitis
Myelitis
Some cases of severe encephalopathy
Toxic or Metabolic Encephalopathy (Normal MRI, CSF)
Encephalopathy

CNS, central nervous system; CSF, cerebrospinal fluid; MRI, magnetic resonance imaging.

correlate well with the degree of CSF pleocytosis. Typically, the CSF contains 50 to several hundred lymphocytes per cubic millimeter, with mild (50 to 150 mg/dl) elevations in CSF protein concentration. CSF glucose concentration is usually normal. Although culture of *B. burgdorferi* is technically possible, generally CSF cultures are positive in less than 10 percent of patients with unequivocal Lyme meningitis,[49] probably reflecting the very low number of spirochetes free in the CSF.

Although this meningitis typically is benign and manifests primarily as a headache, in children a disorder resembling pseudotumor cerebri may occur,[50,51] with increased intracranial pressure. This generally occurs either with or following Lyme meningitis and presumably relates to impaired CSF resorption, to increased vascular permeability mediated by cytokines and therefore increased pressure, or to both. On rare occasions, this has resulted in significant visual impairment.[52]

Actual infection of the brain or spinal cord parenchyma (encephalomyelitis) is extremely rare, probably affecting fewer than 1 in 1,000 infected, untreated individuals. In these rare individuals, there is generally clear clinical and MRI evidence of focal parenchymal involvement,[54] usually affecting the white matter preferentially (perhaps reflecting preferential binding of *B. burgdorferi* to oligodendroglia).[55,56] Patients may present with focal signs that depend on the site of involvement, although a myelopathy tends to be more common. Anecdotal case reports have described a remarkable range of neurologic presentations. Establishing a causal relationship in such circumstances can be challenging. A number of case reports have suggested that, as in meningovascular syphilis, strokes may be caused by Lyme disease, but the evidence of a causal relationship is tenuous[57]; if a meningovascular form of Lyme disease exists, it must be rare. Similarly, numerous reports have suggested that optic neuritis may occur in rare instances of neuroborreliosis,[58] but this association similarly is unclear.

Despite the potential severity of CNS involvement, antimicrobial therapy is usually highly effective. As with any disorder of the nervous system, scarring may leave residual deficits, but treatment in most cases will arrest any further worsening and usually results in significant clinical improvement.

The final and most controversial CNS syndrome has been a chronic encephalopathic state, referred to as Lyme encephalopathy.[59–61] In rare, more severely affected patients, this may reflect a mild form of encephalitis. In such individuals, the CSF is virtually always abnormal and brain MRI may demonstrate focal abnormalities. In others, who have prominent non-neurologic involvement (most typically active, recurrent oligoarthritis), a mild encephalopathy occurs that is similar to that seen in patients with other chronic inflammatory disorders in whom there is a sense of chronic fatigue and malaise with blunting of intellect and memory.[62] An important corollary of this, however, is that it is difficult to attribute mental status changes to Lyme disease in the absence of either systemic inflammation or abnormal CSF.

Unfortunately, this concept has been expanded to describe a disorder referred to as "chronic Lyme disease." Such patients probably fall into one of at least three groups. Rare patients with true CNS infection will fail to respond to standard courses of antimicrobial therapy. In these, a second course may well end the symptoms.[62,63] Other individuals who clearly have Lyme disease and are microbiologically cured continue to manifest chronic and nonspecific symptoms. The etiology of these symptoms is unclear. However, these patients do not respond to additional antibiotics,[64,65] but often respond to symptomatic treatment of their symptoms with various combinations of exercise, "wellness education," and medications including anti-inflammatory and antidepressant agents. Often, a sleep disorder is a prominent part of this syndrome and correcting this can be beneficial. Finally, this group undoubtedly includes patients whose symptoms were never caused by Lyme disease in the first place. These individuals require careful evaluation to determine the original cause of their symptoms, then appropriate treatment. It needs to be emphasized in this context that no systematic study has ever indicated that Lyme disease causes psychiatric disease, beyond the usual difficulties associated with being chronically ill[66–68]; in fact, a systematic study of more than 900 psychiatric patients in a Lyme disease–endemic area suggested that no specific psychiatric disorder was associated with this infection.[69]

The cranial nerves are at particular risk in Lyme disease. As in syphilis and in basilar meningitides, cranial nerves VII and VIII are frequently affected, although cranial nerves III through VI may also be involved. The lower cranial nerves are sometimes impaired, although much less frequently. Lyme disease is one of the few disorders commonly associated with bilateral facial palsies (along with sarcoidosis and Guillain–Barré syndrome). Because these cranial neuropathies generally occur fairly early in infection and because, in the most commonly involved areas, climate dictates that ticks feed primarily from spring through autumn, patients presenting with facial palsies in summer and autumn in endemic areas should undergo serologic screening for Lyme disease. CSF examination may be helpful to address alternative diagnoses. However, numerous European studies have shown that Lyme meningitis and cranial neuritis respond well to oral doxycycline, so findings will likely not directly affect treatment.[70]

The peripheral nervous system (Table 40-2) is probably involved even more frequently than the CNS.[59,71] Most dramatic is the syndrome of Garin–Bujadoux–Bannwarth. Such patients typically have severe radicular pain that can precisely mimic the symptoms of a mechanical radiculopathy. Truncal radiculopathies occur and may lead to much diagnostic confusion. Weakness in the same nerve root distribution may be minimal or severe. A clue to this atypical etiology of a radiculopathy may be involvement of more than one dermatome. CSF is often, although not invariably, abnormal.

Patients with more longstanding infection may develop a milder more diffuse polyneuropathy.[71] This typically is not painful, but presents as a more mundane distal neuropathic sensorimotor syndrome, with both positive and negative symptoms. Some patients may develop a plexopathy or a typical mononeuropathy multiplex. Interestingly, electrophysiologic and pathologic studies indicate that all these syndromes are due to a mononeuropathy multiplex. Notably, in the rhesus macaque monkey, the only animal model of human neurologic Lyme disease, virtually all infected animals develop a mononeuropathy multiplex that subsides over time.[72]

TABLE 40-2 ■ Peripheral Nervous System Manifestations of Neuroborreliosis

Mononeuropathy Multiplex
Radiculopathy
Cranial neuropathy (particularly cranial nerves VII, VIII, III, V, VI)
Diffuse polyneuropathy (confluent mononeuropathy multiplex)
Brachial plexopathy
Lumbosacral plexopathy
Mononeuropathy multiplex
Disorder resembling Guillain–Barré syndrome
Demyelinating Polyneuropathy (Anecdotal, Rare)

Finally, occasional patients have been described with a disorder resembling Guillain–Barré syndrome.[73,74] Clinically, these individuals have had a rapidly progressive polyneuropathy, with ascending paralysis, but many have had a more prominent CSF pleocytosis than typically occurs in Guillain–Barré syndrome. Electrophysiologic changes have been varied.

Diagnosis

Accurate diagnosis requires recognition of the clinical syndrome, a reasonable epidemiologic likelihood of exposure, and laboratory confirmation.[75,76] Although much has been said in the past about the inaccuracy of testing for Lyme disease,[77] it is comparable, overall, with other serologic testing. There remain technical arguments about the best antigen to use and the best methodology to use, but it is likely that more of the difficulty arises from misinterpretation of test results than from inaccurate ones.

Laboratory diagnosis relies primarily on serologic diagnosis—the demonstration of antibody in peripheral blood that adheres to *B. burgdorferi.*

The sensitivity of microbiologic culture remains low (except in erythema migrans, where it is unnecessary) and probably reflects the small number of spirochetes present in readily accessible specimens from patients. The polymerase chain reaction (PCR) assay has remained problematic, probably for the same reason (in addition to contamination-related issues leading to false-positive results). Antigen detection methods have not been found to be reproducible. Immune complexes containing *Borrelia* antigens have been described,[78–80] but do not appear to be a reliable independent marker of infection. Hence, most laboratories rely on ELISAs to quantitate immunoreactivity.

In addition to the technical limitations listed previously, several particular problems confront serologic testing for Lyme disease. First, the disease is focally endemic. In highly endemic areas, such as areas of Long Island, 10 percent or more of the population may have been exposed. In contrast, in nearby New York City, there were about as many cases of malaria in 2010 as of confirmed Lyme disease.[2] This highly varying background prevalence has a major effect on the positive and negative predictive values of test results, which depend on the background prevalence. In areas with Lyme disease prevalence of 1 in 100,000 and a statistically defined negative cut-off of 3 standard deviations, 1 sample in 1,000 will be a false positive, but only 1 in 100,000 will be a true positive. Second, as with any antibody-based testing, it must be remembered that it takes several weeks or months to develop a detectable antibody response in blood. Thus, negative results are common at the time of the erythema migrans, but, as with the syphilitic chancre, the rash by itself is sufficiently diagnostic to mandate immediate antibiotic treatment. Third, unlike other serologic tests, most clinicians rely on a single Lyme disease ELISA value rather than comparing acute and convalescent titers. This may be reasonable in syphilis, where screening reaginic tests are typically positive only during active infection, and is understandable insofar as there is a desire to treat Lyme infection as soon as possible. However, it makes test interpretation difficult in patients who have had prior infection and have a persistently elevated titer. As in most infections, the immune system usually continues to generate detectable antibodies for an extended period after the infection has resolved, making the relevance of the infection to current symptoms difficult to judge.

TABLE 40-3 ■ Western Blot Criteria for Confirmation of Positive Serology in Lyme Disease

IgM (2 Required)	Bands (kDa)	23, 39, 41
IgG (5 Required)	Bands (kDa)	18, 23, 28, 30, 39, 41, 45, 58, 66, 93

Finally, as with most serologic tests, some cross-reactions occur. An effort to address this using a two-step test procedure,[81] comparable with that used in HIV infection, has produced even more confusion. First, the criteria for positive and negative Western blots[82] (Table 40-3) were defined in individuals with positive or borderline ELISA results; therefore, these criteria should not be applied in individuals with negative ELISA results. Second, the criteria were derived statistically. Interpretation is based not on the uniqueness of any of the bands but on the statistical probability of accurate diagnosis using the specified criteria.

As in syphilis, spinal fluid studies can be extremely useful, but they also are the source of considerable confusion. Most, if not all, patients with active CNS infection will have elevations in the CSF white blood cell count, protein concentration, or both. Chronic infection is often accompanied by increased local production of antibodies, resulting in an increased relative CSF IgG concentration and even oligoclonal bands. In most acute cases (about 90%) and in many patients with more longstanding CNS Lyme disease (at least 50% and possibly more), synthesis of specific anti–*B. burgdorferi* antibodies in the CNS can be demonstrated by appropriately comparing concentrations of specific antibody in CSF and serum.[83,84] Simple measurement of antibody concentration in the CSF alone can be very misleading in individuals with blood–brain barrier breakdown, CNS inflammation from other causes, or positive peripheral blood Lyme disease serologies, as discussed previously in considering CSF serologies in syphilis.

Treatment and Outcome

As with any infection, prevention is usually simpler than treatment. Infected ticks occur in relatively restricted locales, and avoidance is therefore a feasible strategy. Those who cannot or choose not to adopt this strategy can limit their risk by wearing light-colored clothing that covers as much of the body as possible, making it easier to spot the very small, responsible ticks. Because ticks must be attached

TABLE 40-4 ■ Treatment Regimens

Medication and Route of Administration (Duration)	Adults	Children*
Parenteral (2–4 weeks)		
Ceftriaxone†	2 g daily	50–75 mg/kg daily
Cefotaxime	2 g every 8 hours	150–200 mg/kg daily in 3–4 divided doses
Penicillin	20–24 million units daily	300,000 units/kg daily, divided every 4 hours
Oral (3, Possibly 4 Weeks)		
Doxycycline‡	100 mg twice to four times daily	4 mg/kg daily in 2 divided doses
Amoxicillin§	500 mg three times daily	50 mg/kg daily in 3 divided doses
Cefuroxime axetil§	500 mg twice daily	30 mg/kg daily in 2 divided doses

Modified from Treatment of Lyme disease. Med Lett 42:37, 2000, with permission.
*Pediatric dosage should not exceed adult recommendation.
†Ceftriaxone should not be used late in pregnancy.
‡Doxycycline should not be used in pregnant women or children younger than the age of 8 years.
§Limited data but probably effective.

and feeding for 24 to 48 hours before infection is likely, a careful tick check at the end of the day is highly effective. Attached ticks should be removed by placing a fine forceps between the tick and the skin, and gently pulling back. Efforts to suffocate ticks in petroleum products or burn them with a lit cigarette are counterproductive. Use of acaricides can help, but repeated exposures, particularly in children and with higher-concentration products, can lead to significant systemic absorption and can be neurotoxic. A vaccine was available but has been withdrawn from the market, primarily because of poor sales.

Antimicrobial therapy is highly effective, regardless of disease duration and severity. Popular mythology about the organism hibernating invisibly, only to resurface years later, is an intriguing theoretical possibility, but from a practical perspective is irrelevant.[85] Patients with the characteristic rash should be treated immediately with oral medication (Table 40-4), regardless of the results of serologic testing. Those with more disseminated disease may well respond to oral regimens,[86] and there are excellent data that Lyme arthritis and meningitis[86] will also usually respond well to oral regimens, particularly with doxycycline.[70] Although US practitioners tend to be reluctant to use oral regimens when there is evidence of CNS involvement (particularly CSF abnormalities), such patients—if there is no parenchymal CNS involvement—can be treated effectively with oral doxycycline (Table 40-4). The optimal duration of treatment remains unclear. No randomized trial has demonstrated any advantage of prolonging parenteral treatment beyond 2 weeks.[87] However, anecdotal evidence from all major centers treating patients indicates that this is occasionally insufficient. As a result, courses of 3 to 4 weeks are routinely used and, under exceptional circumstances, repeated. Despite common practice at some centers, there are no data to support longer courses or the use of more toxic antimicrobials. Several studies have now addressed the role of longer courses of antimicrobial therapy in patients with continuing but nonspecific symptoms; no sustained benefit was found over conventional treatment.[64,88]

Two studies from Lyme disease–endemic areas should be highly reassuring.[89,90] Systematic case-control studies from Connecticut and Nantucket Island, Massachusetts, both areas highly endemic for Lyme disease, provide clear evidence that long-term outlooks of treated patients are excellent. Many patients who have been diagnosed as having Lyme disease and have undergone treatment appear to develop the same transient symptoms as do normal control subjects; however, they attribute them to Lyme disease and therefore find them more distressing. By all objective measures, though, the treated patients appear indistinguishable from healthy, uninfected individuals.

REFERENCES

1. Tramont E: *Treponema pallidum* (syphilis). In: Mandell G, Bennett J, Dolin R (eds): Principles and Practice of Infectious Diseases. Churchill Livingstone, Philadelphia, 2000.
2. Centers for Disease Control and Prevention (CDC) Summary of Notifiable Diseases—United States, 2010. MMWR Morb Mortal Wkly Rep 59:25, 2012.
3. Larsen SA, Norris SJ, Pope V: *Treponema* and other host-associated spirochetes. p. 759. In: Murray PR, Baron EJ, Pfaller MA (eds): Manual of Clinical Microbiology. 7th Ed. ASM Press, Washington DC, 1999.
4. Fraser CM, Norris SJ, Weinstock GM, et al: Complete genome sequence of *Treponema pallidum*, the syphilis spirochete. Science 281:375, 1998.
5. Radolf JD, Bolan G, Park IU, et al: Discordant results from reverse sequence syphilis screening—five laboratories, United States, 2006–2010. MMWR Morb Mortal Wkly Rep 60:133, 2011.
6. Park IU, Chow JM, Bolan G, et al: Screening for syphilis with the treponemal immunoassay: analysis of discordant serology results and implications for clinical management. J Infect Dis 204:1297, 2011.
7. Knaute DF, Graf N, Lautenschlager S, et al: Serological response to treatment of syphilis according to disease stage and HIV status. Clin Infect Dis 55:1615, 2012.
8. Centers for Disease Control and Prevention, Workowski K, Berman S: Sexually transmitted diseases treatment guidelines, 2006. MMWR Morb Mortal Wkly Rep 55:1, 2006.
9. Libois A, De Wit S, Poll B, et al: HIV and syphilis: when to perform a lumbar puncture. Sex Transm Dis 34:141, 2007.
10. Marra C, Tantalo L, Maxwell C, et al: Alternative cerebrospinal fluid tests to diagnose neurosyphilis in HIV-infected individuals. Neurology 63:85, 2004.
11. Luger AF, Schmidt BL, Kaulich M: Significance of laboratory findings for the diagnosis of neurosyphilis. Int J STD AIDS 11:224, 2000.
12. Davis LE, Schmitt JW: Clinical significance of cerebrospinal fluid tests for neurosyphilis. Ann Neurol 25:50, 1989.
13. Marra CM, Critchlow CW, Hook 3rd EW, et al: Cerebrospinal fluid treponemal antibodies in untreated early syphilis. Arch Neurol 52:68, 1995.
14. Carey LA, Glesby MJ, Mundy LM, et al: Lumbar puncture for evaluation of latent syphilis in hospitalized patients. High prevalence of cerebrospinal fluid abnormalities unrelated to syphilis. Arch Intern Med 155:1657, 1995.
15. Roos KL: Pearls and pitfalls in the diagnosis and management of central nervous system infectious diseases. Semin Neurol 18:185, 1998.
16. Lowhagen GB: Syphilis: test procedures and therapeutic strategies. Semin Dermatol 9:152, 1990.
17. Marra CM, Castro CD, Kuller L, et al: Mechanisms of clearance of *Treponema pallidum* from the CSF in a nonhuman primate model. Neurology 51:957, 1998.
18. Moskophidis M, Peters S: Comparison of intrathecal synthesis of *Treponema pallidum*-specific IgG antibodies and polymerase chain reaction for the diagnosis of neurosyphilis. Zentralbl Bakteriol 283:295, 1996.
19. Rockwell DH, Yobs AR, Moore Jr MB: The Tuskegee study of untreated syphilis; the 30th year of observation. Arch Intern Med 114:792, 1964.
20. Clark E, Danbolt N: The Oslo study of the natural course of untreated syphilis. Med Clin North Am 48:613, 1964.
21. Alam F, Yasutomi H, Fukuda H, et al: Diffuse cerebral white matter T2-weighted hyperintensity: a new finding of general paresis. Acta Radiol 47:609, 2006.
22. Flood JM, Weinstock HS, Guroy ME, et al: Neurosyphilis during the AIDS epidemic, San Francisco, 1985–1992. J Infect Dis 177:931, 1998.
23. Sanchez PJ, Wendel Jr GD, Grimprel E, et al: Evaluation of molecular methodologies and rabbit infectivity testing for the diagnosis of congenital syphilis and neonatal central nervous system invasion by *Treponema pallidum*. J Infect Dis 167:148, 1993.
24. Sanchez PJ, Wendel GD, Norgard MV: IgM antibody to *Treponema pallidum* in cerebrospinal fluid of infants with congenital syphilis. Am J Dis Child 146:1171, 1992.
25. Jay CA: Treatment of neurosyphilis. Curr Treat Options Neurol 8:185, 2006.
26. Marra CM, Boutin P, McArthur JC, et al: A pilot study evaluating ceftriaxone and penicillin G as treatment agents for neurosyphilis in human immunodeficiency virus-infected individuals. Clin Infect Dis 30:540, 2000.
27. Marra CM, Slatter V, Tartaglione TA, et al: Evaluation of aqueous penicillin G and ceftriaxone for experimental neurosyphilis. J Infect Dis 165:396, 1992.
28. Shann S, Wilson J: Treatment of neurosyphilis with ceftriaxone. Sex Transm Infect 79:415, 2003.
29. Gordon S, Eaton M, George R, et al: The response of symptomatic neurosyphilis to high-dose intravenous penicillin G in patients with human immunodeficiency virus infection. N Engl J Med 331:1469, 1994.
30. Rolfs RT, Joesoef MR, Hendershot EF, et al: A randomized trial of enhanced therapy for early syphilis in patients with and without human immunodeficiency virus infection. The Syphilis and HIV Study Group. N Engl J Med 337:307, 1997.
31. Garin C, Bujadoux A: Paralysie par les tiques. J Med Lyon 71:765, 1922.
32. Burgdorfer W, Barbour AG, Hayes SF, et al: Lyme disease: a tick borne spirochetosis? Science 216:1317, 1982.
33. Benach JL, Bosler EM, Hanrahan JP, et al: Spirochetes isolated from the blood of two patients with Lyme disease. N Engl J Med 308:740, 1983.

34. Steere AC, Grodzicki RL, Kornblatt AN, et al: The spirochetal etiology of Lyme disease. N Engl J Med 308:733, 1983.
35. Asbrink E, Hederstedt B, Hovmark A: The spirochetal etiology of acrodermatitis chronica atrophicans Herxheimer. Acta Derm Venereol 64:506, 1984.
36. Baranton G, Postic D, Saint GI, et al: Delineation of *Borrelia burgdorferi* sensu stricto, *Borrelia garinii* sp. nov., and group VS461 associated with Lyme borreliosis. Int J Syst Bacteriol 42:378, 1992.
37. Rosa PA: Microbiology of *Borrelia burgdorferi*. Semin Neurol 17:5, 1997.
38. Hayes EB, Piesman J: How can we prevent Lyme disease? N Engl J Med 348:2424, 2003.
39. Bacon RM, Kugeler KJ, Mead PS: Surveillance for Lyme disease—United States, 1992–2006. MMWR Morb Mortal Wkly Rep 57:1, 2008.
40. Gerber MA, Shapiro ED, Burke GS, et al: Lyme disease in children in southeastern Connecticut. Pediatric Lyme Disease Study Group. N Engl J Med 335:1270, 1996.
41. Reimers CD, de Koning J, Neubert U, et al: *Borrelia burgdorferi* myositis: report of eight patients. J Neurol 240:278, 1993.
42. Carvounis PE, Mehta AP, Geist CE: Orbital myositis associated with *Borrelia burgdorferi* (Lyme disease) infection. Ophthalmology 111:1023, 2004.
43. Holmgren AR, Matteson EL: Lyme myositis. Arthritis Rheum 54:2697, 2006.
44. ACOG Committee Opinion: Lyme disease during pregnancy. Committee on Obstetrics Maternal and Fetal Medicine. Number 99, November 1991. Int J Gynaecol Obstet 39:59, 1992.
45. Strobino BA, Williams CL, Abid S, et al: Lyme disease and pregnancy outcome: a prospective study of two thousand prenatal patients. Am J Obstet Gynecol 169:367, 1993.
46. Luft BJ, Steinman CR, Neimark HC, et al: Invasion of the central nervous system by *Borrelia burgdorferi* in acute disseminated infection. JAMA 267:1364, 1992.
47. Keller TL, Halperin JJ, Whitman M: PCR detection of *Borrelia burgdorferi* DNA in cerebrospinal fluid of Lyme neuroborreliosis patients. Neurology 42:32, 1992.
48. Logigian EL, Steere AC: Invasion of the central nervous system by *Borrelia burgdorferi* in acute disseminated infection. JAMA 267:1364, 1992.
49. Karlsson M, Hovind HK, Svenungsson B, et al: Cultivation and characterization of spirochetes from cerebrospinal fluid of patients with Lyme borreliosis. J Clin Microbiol 28:473, 1990.
50. Kan L, Sood SK, Maytal J: Pseudotumor cerebri in Lyme disease: a case report and literature review. Pediatr Neurol 18:439, 1998.
51. Jacobson DM, Frens DB: Pseudotumor cerebri syndrome associated with Lyme disease. Am J Ophthalmol 107:81, 1989.
52. Rothermel H, Hedges 3rd TR, Steere AC: Optic neuropathy in children with Lyme disease. Pediatrics 108:477, 2001.
53. Halperin JJ, Volkman DJ, Wu P: Central nervous system abnormalities in Lyme neuroborreliosis. Neurology 41:1571, 1991.
54. Kalina P, Decker A, Kornel E, et al: Lyme disease of the brainstem. Neuroradiology 47:903, 2005.
55. Garcia-Monco JC, Fernandez-Villar B, Benach JL: Adherence of the Lyme disease spirochete to glial cells and cells of glial origin. J Infect Dis 160:497, 1989.
56. Garcia Monco JC, Fernandez VB, Rogers RC, et al: *Borrelia burgdorferi* and other related spirochetes bind to galactocerebroside. Neurology 42:1341, 1992.
57. Halperin JJ: Stroke in patients with Lyme disease. p. 59. In Caplan L (ed): Uncommon Causes of Stroke. 2nd Ed. Cambridge University Press, Cambridge, 2008.
58. Sibony P, Halperin J, Coyle P, et al: Reactive Lyme serology in patients with optic neuritis and papilledema. J Neuroophthalmol 25:71, 2005.
59. Logigian EL, Kaplan RF, Steere AC: Chronic neurologic manifestations of Lyme disease. N Engl J Med 323:1438, 1990.
60. Krupp LB, Fernquist S, Masur D, et al: Cognitive impairment in Lyme disease. Neurology 40:304, 1990.
61. Halperin JJ, Krupp LB, Golightly MG, et al: Lyme borreliosis-associated encephalopathy. Neurology 40:1340, 1990.
62. Kaplan RF, Jones-Woodward L, Workman K, et al: Neuropsychological deficits in Lyme disease patients with and without other evidence of central nervous system pathology. Appl Neuropsychol 6:3, 1999.
63. Logigian EL, Kaplan RF, Steere AC: Successful treatment of Lyme encephalopathy with intravenous ceftriaxone. J Infect Dis 180:377, 1999.
64. Krupp LB, Hyman LG, Grimson R, et al: Study and treatment of post Lyme disease (STOP-LD): a randomized double masked clinical trial. Neurology 60:1923, 2003.
65. Fallon BA, Keilp JG, Corbera KM, et al: A randomized, placebo-controlled trial of repeated IV antibiotic therapy for Lyme encephalopathy. Neurology 70:992, 2008.
66. Coyle PK, Krupp LB, Doscher C, et al: *Borrelia burgdorferi* reactivity in patients with severe persistent fatigue who are from a region in which Lyme disease is endemic. Clin Infect Dis 18:S24, 1994.
67. Elkins LE, Pollina DA, Scheffer SR, et al: Psychological states and neuropsychological performances in chronic Lyme disease. Appl Neuropsychol 6:19, 1999.
68. Gaudino EA, Coyle PK, Krupp LB: Post-Lyme syndrome and chronic fatigue syndrome. Neuropsychiatric similarities and differences. Arch Neurol 54:1372, 1997.
69. Hajek T, Libiger J, Janovska D, et al: Clinical and demographic characteristics of psychiatric patients

seropositive for *Borrelia burgdorferi*. Eur Psychiatry 21:118, 2006.
70. Halperin JJ, Shapiro ED, Logigian EL, et al: Practice parameter: treatment of nervous system Lyme disease. Neurology 69:91, 2007.
71. Halperin JJ, Luft BJ, Volkman DJ, et al: Lyme neuroborreliosis - peripheral nervous system manifestations. Brain 113:1207, 1990.
72. England JD, Bohm RP, Roberts ED, et al: Mononeuropathy multiplex in rhesus monkeys with chronic Lyme disease. Ann Neurol 41:375, 1997.
73. Shapiro EE: Guillain-Barré syndrome in a child with serologic evidence of *Borrelia*. Pediatr Infect Dis J 17:264, 1998.
74. Muley SA, Parry GJ: Antibiotic responsive demyelinating neuropathy related to Lyme disease. Neurology 72:1786, 2009.
75. Halperin J, Logigian E, Finkel M, et al: Practice parameter for the diagnosis of patients with nervous system Lyme borreliosis (Lyme disease). Neurology 46:619, 1996.
76. Golightly MG: Laboratory considerations in the diagnosis and management of Lyme borreliosis. Am J Clin Pathol 99:168, 1993.
77. Bakken LL, Case KL, Callister SM, et al: Performance of 45 laboratories participating in a proficiency testing program for Lyme disease serology. JAMA 268:891, 1992.
78. Coyle PK, Schutzer SE, Deng Z, et al: Detection of *Borrelia burgdorferi*-specific antigen in antibody-negative cerebrospinal fluid in neurologic Lyme disease. Neurology 45:2010, 1995.
79. Brunner M, Sigal LH: Immune complexes from serum of patients with Lyme disease contain *Borrelia burgdorferi* antigen and antigen-specific antibodies: potential use for improved testing. J Infect Dis 182:534, 2000.
80. Marques AR, Hornung RL, Dally L, et al: Detection of immune complexes is not independent of detection of antibodies in Lyme disease patients and does not confirm active infection with *Borrelia burgdorferi*. Clin Diagn Lab Immunol 12:1036, 2005.
81. American College of Physicians: Guidelines for laboratory evaluation in the diagnosis of Lyme disease. Ann Intern Med 127:1106, 1997.
82. Dressler F, Whalen JA, Reinhardt BN, et al: Western blotting in the serodiagnosis of Lyme disease. J Infect Dis 167:392, 1993.
83. Steere AC, Berardi VP, Weeks KE, et al: Evaluation of the intrathecal antibody response to *Borrelia burgdorferi* as a diagnostic test for Lyme neuroborreliosis. J Infect Dis 161:1203, 1990.
84. Hammers Berggren S, Hansen K, Lebech AM, et al: *Borrelia burgdorferi*-specific intrathecal antibody production in neuroborreliosis: a follow-up study. Neurology 43:169, 1993.
85. Halperin JJ, Baker P, Wormser GP: Common misconceptions about Lyme disease. Am J Med 126:264e1, 2013.
86. Wormser GP, Dattwyler RJ, Shapiro ED, et al: The clinical assessment, treatment, and prevention of Lyme disease, human granulocytic anaplasmosis, and babesiosis: clinical practice guidelines by the Infectious Diseases Society of America. Clin Infect Dis 43:1089, 2006.
87. Dattwyler RJ, Wormser GP, Rush TJ, et al: A comparison of two treatment regimens of ceftriaxone in late Lyme disease. Wien Klin Wochenschr 117:393, 2005.
88. Klempner MS, Hu LT, Evans J, et al: Two controlled trials of antibiotic treatment in patients with persistent symptoms and a history of Lyme disease. N Engl J Med 345:85, 2001.
89. Seltzer EG, Gerber MA, Cartter ML, et al: Long-term outcomes of persons with Lyme disease. JAMA 283:609, 2000.
90. Shadick NA, Phillips CB, Sangha O, et al: Musculoskeletal and neurologic outcomes in patients with previously treated Lyme disease. Ann Intern Med 131:919, 1999.

CHAPTER

41

Tuberculosis of the Central Nervous System

JOHN M. LEONARD

Tuberculosis in all its forms remains a challenging clinical problem and a public health issue of considerable magnitude.[1] Rates of new infection vary widely from country to country in relation to socioeconomic conditions. For example, the incidence is approximately 5 cases per 100,000 population in the United States, compared with rates in excess of 200 cases per 100,000 population in some developing countries of Asia and Africa.

Tuberculosis of the central nervous system (CNS) accounts for 1 to 2 percent of all cases of tuberculosis and about 8 percent of all forms of extrapulmonary infection in immunocompetent individuals. Although pulmonary tuberculosis in the United States has been on the decline, the number of reported cases of meningeal tuberculosis has changed little over the past decade. CNS tuberculosis may be considered as comprising three clinical syndromes: meningitis, intracranial tuberculoma, and spinal tuberculous arachnoiditis.[2–5] All three forms of CNS infection are encountered with about equal frequency in regions of the world where the incidence of tuberculosis is high. In areas such as Europe and North America, where the incidence is lower and extrapulmonary tuberculosis is seen primarily in adults with reactivation disease, the large majority of cases present with meningitis.

MENINGITIS

Pathogenesis

Current understanding of the pathogenesis of CNS tuberculosis is based on a series of careful clinicopathologic correlations that date to the early part of the last century.[6,7] Conceptually, there is a two-phase process, beginning with the hematogenous dissemination of *Mycobacterium tuberculosis* (bacillemia) that follows primary pulmonary infection or late reactivation elsewhere in the body. During this hematogenous phase, small numbers of bacilli are scattered throughout the substance of the brain, meninges, and adjacent tissues, leading to the formation of multiple granulomatous foci of varying size and degree of encapsulation (tubercles). In the second phase that develops over time, such lesions may coalesce to form larger caseous foci, with some lying just beneath the pia mater (the

Aminoff's Neurology and General Medicine, Fifth Edition.

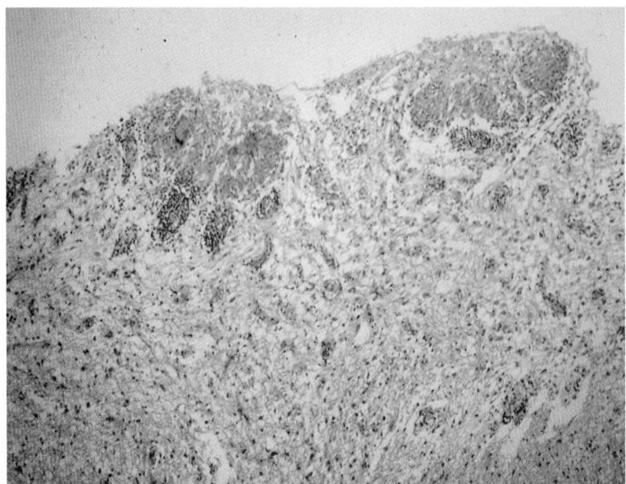

FIGURE 41-1 ■ Section from an autopsied case of tuberculous meningitis showing fresh granulomas beneath the surface of the brain, having eroded through the pia membrane into the subarachnoid space. (Hematoxylin and eosin, × 400.)

thin vascular membrane consisting of blood vessels and lymphatics that covers the entire surface of the brain) or beneath the ependyma (the thin nucleated epithelial membrane that lines the surface of the ventricles). With time and circumstance, such tuberculomas, if unstable, may erode into the subarachnoid space, producing meningitis (Fig. 41-1). It follows that the propensity for developing clinical illness is determined by the number of tubercles and their proximity to the surface of the brain, the rapidity of progression, and the rate at which encapsulation follows acquired immunity.

The widespread and dense distribution of tubercles that occurs in progressive miliary tuberculosis greatly increases the chance that a juxtapial granuloma will be established and, from this critical location, break through into the subarachnoid space.[8] This is the usual sequence in childhood tuberculous meningitis, as infants and young children are especially susceptible to progressive hematogenous dissemination after primary infection.[9] Adult cases also develop in association with clinically apparent progressive miliary disease or from other less apparent or entirely hidden foci of chronic organ tuberculosis. Reactivation of latent foci with resultant secondary hematogenous dissemination may be intermittent or chronic and progressive. In either circumstance, the spread of bacilli to distant organs produces scattered tubercles of varying size and encapsulation. Subpial tuberculous foci arising in this manner may remain quiescent for months or years, later to destabilize when local injury or a general depression in host immunity supervenes. Risk factors include advanced age, alcoholism, drug-induced immunosuppression, lymphoma, and infection with human immunodeficiency virus (HIV), all of which impair cellular immunity and, in persons with smoldering chronic organ tuberculosis, can lead to late generalized tuberculosis including meningitis.[9]

A significant proportion of adult cases of tuberculous meningitis have no demonstrable extracranial infection or apparent defect in host immune function. Occasionally, there is a history of head trauma some weeks or months prior to the onset of symptoms, suggesting that intracranial caseous foci may be destabilized by physical factors.

Pathology

The pathologic changes observed in the CNS result from an intense, cytokine-mediated hypersensitivity reaction induced by the presence of organisms and associated antigenic material in the substance of the brain and the subarachnoid space. Three features dominate the pathologic process and account for the clinical manifestations: (1) a proliferative, predominantly basilar, arachnoiditis, (2) vasculitis of the arteries and veins traversing this exudate, and (3) disturbance of cerebrospinal fluid (CSF) circulation or resorption leading to hydrocephalus.[10]

Proliferative arachnoiditis is most marked at the base of the brain and, in a matter of days, produces a thick, gelatinous exudate extending from the pons to the optic chiasm. With chronicity, the optochiasmic zone of arachnoiditis comes to resemble a fibrous mass encasing nearby cranial nerves and vessels coursing through this area.

Vasculitis with resultant thrombosis and hemorrhagic infarction may develop in vessels that traverse the basilar or spinal exudate or those that are located within the brain substance itself. The vascular inflammatory reaction is initiated by direct invasion of the adventitia by mycobacteria or by secondary extension of adjacent arachnoiditis. An early polymorphonuclear reaction followed by infiltration of lymphocytes, plasma cells, and macrophages leads to progressive destruction of the adventitia, disruption of elastic fibers, and extension of the inflammatory process to the intima. Eventually, fibrinoid degeneration in small arteries and veins produces aneurysms, multiple thrombi, and focal hemorrhage in some combination. Depending on the location and extent of the vasculitis, a variety of stroke syndromes may result.[10,11] Multiple lesions are common, and areas of ischemic injury that simulate lacunar infarctions most frequently involve the basal ganglia, cerebral cortex, pons, and cerebellum. Intracranial vasculitis and multiple infarcts are a common feature of autopsy studies, and account for many of the residual neurologic deficits in those who recover following therapy.

Extension of the inflammatory process to the basilar cisterns may also impede CSF circulation and resorption, leading to *communicating hydrocephalus* in most cases that have been symptomatic for longer than 2 to 3 weeks.[10,12] Less frequently, obstruction of the aqueduct develops from exudate surrounding the brainstem, inflammation of the ependymal lining of the ventricles, or a strategically placed tuberculoma. In far-advanced cases, increased intracranial pressure may cause brainstem compression and tentorial herniation.

Clinical Presentation

Symptoms and Signs

Typically, tuberculous meningitis begins with a prodrome of insidious onset characterized by malaise, lassitude, personality change, intermittent headache, and low-grade fever. This is followed, usually within 2 to 3 weeks, by more prominent neurologic symptoms and signs such as meningismus, protracted headache, vomiting, confusion, cranial nerve palsies, and long-tract signs. The pace of illness may accelerate rapidly at this stage; confusion gives way to stupor and coma, seizures may occur, and multiple cranial nerve palsies and hemiparesis or hemiplegia are common. In most untreated cases, death supervenes within 5 to 8 weeks of the onset of illness although in occasional patients the illness follows a more indolent, slowly progressive course over weeks or months.[13–16] In children, the condition is characterized early by irritability, loss of interest in play, restlessness, and anorexia; headache is less common and vomiting often much more prominent, especially in the very young.[15,17] Seizures are more common in children and are apt to be an early or presenting symptom. Table 41-1 lists common symptoms and signs at presentation, and the frequency range compiled from three clinical series in separate regions of the world.[13,15,16]

TABLE 41-1 ■ Presenting Symptoms and Signs of Tuberculous Meningitis

Symptoms/Signs	Frequency (%)
Fever	60–90
Headache	40–90
Vomiting	30–60
Neck stiffness	40–80
Lethargy/drowsiness	25–80
Confusion	10–30
Stupor/coma	5–30
Focal neurologic signs	15–40
Cranial nerve palsy	20–40
Hemiparesis	10–20
Seizures	
Children	40–50
Adults	5

For purposes of prognosis and therapy, it is useful to categorize patient severity on presentation based mainly on mental status and focal neurologic signs. *Stage I* comprises patients who are conscious and rational, with or without meningismus but with no focal neurologic signs or evidence of hydrocephalus; *stage II* patients exhibit lethargy and confusion and may have mild focal neurologic signs such as single cranial nerve palsies and hemiparesis; *stage III* illness includes signs of advanced disease such as stupor and coma, seizures, multiple cranial nerve palsies, dense hemiplegia, and paraplegia.[18] Some patients progress rapidly from one stage to the next within a few days. The response to treatment is influenced by the clinical stage of illness at the time therapy is initiated, with better responses obtained when it is initiated early.

Atypical Features

In some adults, the prodrome may be a slowly progressive dementia over months or even years, characterized by personality change, social withdrawal, loss of libido, and memory deficits. At the other end of the spectrum, some patients may present with an acute, rapidly progressive meningitic syndrome indistinguishable from pyogenic bacterial meningitis; at times, this accelerated form is superimposed on a chronic dementing illness. Seizures and focal neurologic disturbances such as cranial nerve palsies or hemiparesis may occur early and dominate the clinical presentation. Of the cranial nerves, the sixth is the most commonly involved, followed by the third and fourth. Occasionally the symptoms and signs of hydrocephalus with raised intracranial pressure (headache, papilledema, diplopia, and visual disturbance) precede signs of meningeal irritation. Movement disorders, including tremor, myoclonus, chorea, and ballismus, may follow basal ganglia infarction secondary to vasculitis.[19]

Tuberculous Meningitis and HIV Infection

Coinfection with HIV has been reported in 21 percent of patients with extrapulmonary tuberculosis in the United States.[20] Although CNS tuberculosis has not yet become a widespread problem in persons infected with HIV, there are reports that meningitis occurs with greater frequency in those HIV patients with active tuberculosis.[21–23] In a study of 455 HIV-positive patients with tuberculosis, 10 percent developed meningitis compared with 2 percent of HIV-negative patients; HIV-positive patients accounted for 59 percent of all cases of tuberculous meningitis seen during the study period.[21] Dube and colleagues compared the clinical features, laboratory findings, and in-hospital mortality rates in patients having tuberculous meningitis with or without HIV infection; intracerebral tuberculomas were more common in the HIV-infected group (60% compared with 14%), but otherwise, coinfection with HIV did not alter the clinical manifestations, CSF findings, or response to therapy.[22]

Diagnosis

Few problems in medicine so critically challenge the physician's diagnostic acumen and clinical judgment as a patient with CNS tuberculosis. Once the possibility of tuberculous meningitis has been considered, the central task is rapid and thorough assessment of clinical and laboratory features followed by a prompt decision regarding empiric therapy.[6,24] Clues to the diagnosis include a positive family history of tuberculosis, recent exposure to others with active tuberculosis (especially in cases involving children and immunosuppressed adults), a history of recent head trauma, and alcoholism. Evidence of active tuberculosis elsewhere in the body, observed in 20 to 70 percent of cases, provides the most reliable basis for the presumptive diagnosis in patients with CNS disease. A meticulous physical examination should include looking for lymphadenopathy, spinal and other joint lesions, splenomegaly, scrotal masses, and draining fistulas. In patients with generalized (miliary) infection, careful funduscopic examination often shows choroidal tubercles, which are multiple, ill-defined, raised yellow-white nodules (granulomas) of varying size near the optic disc.[25]

Abnormalities on chest radiography, including miliary infiltrate and, less commonly, hilar adenopathy or upper lobe nodular infiltrates, occur in most childhood cases and in approximately 50 percent of adults. Computed tomography (CT) of the chest likely has a higher yield for these findings.

Patients with tuberculous meningitis may exhibit mild anemia and leukocytosis, but often the complete blood count and even the erythrocyte sedimentation rate are entirely normal. Hyponatremia related to inappropriate secretion of antidiuretic hormone occurs commonly and is a useful, though nonspecific, clue to the diagnosis. The tuberculin skin test is of limited utility. A positive skin test is nonspecific but supports the diagnosis; however, the reaction is commonly absent in all forms of active tuberculosis.

Cerebrospinal Fluid Examination

Careful examination of the CSF is the key to diagnosis in most instances. The opening pressure is usually elevated, the fluid is clear or "ground glass" in appearance, and, on standing, a delicate, web-like clot often forms. The typical CSF formula shows elevated protein and low glucose concentrations as well as a mononuclear pleocytosis.[24]

The CSF protein concentration ranges from 100 to 500 mg/dl in most patients, is less than 100 mg/dl in 25 percent, and is more than 500 mg/dl in 10 percent. Patients with subarachnoid block may exhibit extremely high protein concentrations, in the range of 2 to 6 g/dl, associated with xanthochromia and a poor prognosis. The CSF glucose concentration is usually low, being less than 45 mg/dl in approximately 80 percent of cases. The CSF cell count is between 100 and 500/mm^3 in most patients, less than 100 cells/mm^3 in approximately 15 percent, and between 500 and 1,500 cells/mm^3 in 20 percent.

Although the characteristic cellular reaction is lymphocytic, early in the course of meningitis the findings are often atypical with only a few cells, a mixed pleocytosis, or polymorphonuclear predominance. Cases with an atypical cellular reaction at the outset evolve in the direction of more typical findings on repeat CSF examination. Misinterpretation of this sequence as improvement in response to antibacterial therapy (when an erroneous diagnosis of pyogenic meningitis is being entertained) can have serious consequences. On occasion, an initial mononuclear pleocytosis may briefly change in the direction of polymorphonuclear predominance after therapy is initiated ("therapeutic paradox"), a change that may be associated with clinical deterioration.

Bacteriology

Specific diagnosis rests on the demonstration of *Mycobacterium tuberculosis* in the CSF. Cultures are positive in approximately 75 percent of cases but often require weeks for detectable growth. Consequently, the careful examination of a stained smear for acid-fast bacilli (AFB) is the most effective means of making a prompt diagnosis. The importance of repeated, careful examination and culture of CSF specimens cannot be overemphasized; the diagnostic yield by smear and culture is enhanced when multiple CSF specimens from repeated lumbar punctures are submitted to the laboratory. In a prospective study designed specifically to evaluate the effectiveness of careful bacteriologic technique, acid-fast bacilli were seen on smear in 77 of 132 adult patients (58%) and cultured from 94 of 132 (71%); the overall sensitivity of smear and culture was 82 percent.[26] This study confirmed earlier observations regarding the importance of high CSF volume and meticulous microscopy in the bacteriologic diagnosis of tuberculous meningitis.

In suspect cases, it is recommended that at least two CSF samples from separate lumbar punctures be obtained for stain and culture. It is best to submit 5 to 10 ml of the last portion removed; the AFB stain should be examined for 30 minutes. It is not necessary to defer treatment as the yield remains high for several days after the institution of antituberculous chemotherapy.

Molecular Diagnostic Techniques

The nucleic acid–based amplification methodology, based on the polymerase chain reaction (PCR), is an effective method for the rapid detection of bacterial DNA. Although simple, rapid, and appealing in principle, the reliability of PCR for the identification of mycobacteria is not well established, in part because of variability in sensitivity and specificity across multiple laboratories.[27] In a blind comparison study of seven facilities, the rate of false-positive results ranged from 3 to 20 percent, and levels of sensitivity varied widely.[28] There are few studies comparing PCR with stains and cultures in large series of patients with suspected or confirmed infection. In one, the sensitivity of PCR testing was 60 percent in 15 patients classified as having definite or probable tuberculous meningitis.[29] In a meta-analysis of nucleic acid amplification tests used for the diagnosis of tuberculous meningitis, the pooled sensitivity was 56 percent and the specificity was 98 percent.[30] CSF should be submitted for PCR testing whenever clinical suspicion is sufficiently high to warrant empiric therapy and initial stains for acid-fast bacilli are negative, recognizing that a negative PCR test result neither excludes the diagnosis nor obviates the need for continued treatment. Work to develop more sensitive PCR-based methods is continuing.

Neuroradiologic Evaluation

CT and magnetic resonance imaging (MRI) have greatly enhanced understanding of the pathogenesis, clinical assessment, and management of all forms of CNS tuberculosis.[31–34] CT can define the presence and extent of basilar arachnoiditis, the presence of cerebral edema and infarction, and the presence and course of hydrocephalus. In a study of 289 cases (214 children and 75 adults), hydrocephalus was demonstrated in 80 percent of patients, basilar meningeal enhancement in 39 percent, cerebral infarcts in 15 percent, and tuberculomas in 5 percent.[33] Hydrocephalus was associated with a longer duration of symptoms prior to treatment and was seen more often in children than adults. The CT findings are of prognostic significance and useful to monitor the effectiveness of adjunctive therapy such as corticosteroids and neurosurgical shunting procedures. In patients presenting with tuberculous meningitis, approximately 30 percent of those with stage I and 8 percent with stage II disease have a normal CT scan. Virtually all stage III patients have abnormalities, including hydrocephalus. Hydrocephalus alone without other features is uncommon and carries a good prognosis. Any degree of basilar meningeal enhancement combined with hydrocephalus is strongly suggestive of tuberculosis, and the combination is indicative of advanced disease, correlates well with the presence of vasculitis, and portends serious risk for basal ganglia infarction.[33]

MRI is the preferred imaging modality for defining lesions of the basal ganglia, midbrain, and brainstem.[35,36] In a prospective study of 27 childhood cases, including clinical, radiographic, and pathologic findings, MRI proved superior to CT in delineating focal infarcts of the basal ganglia and diencephalon and in defining the presence and extent of associated brainstem lesions.[35] The character and severity of MRI-defined brainstem abnormalities correlates well with clinical evidence of brainstem disease.

TABLE 41-2 ■ Differential Diagnosis of Tuberculous Meningitis
Fungal meningitis (e.g., cryptococcosis, histoplasmosis, blastomycosis, coccidioidal mycosis)
Neurobrucellosis
Viral meningoencephalitis (e.g, herpes simplex virus, mumps)
Partially treated bacterial meningitis
Neurosyphilis
Focal parameningeal infection (sphenoiditis, brain abscess, endocarditis, spinal epidural abscess)
Central nervous system toxoplasmosis
Neoplastic meningitis (lymphoma, carcinoma)
Stroke
Neurosarcoidosis

DIFFERENTIAL DIAGNOSIS

A variety of inflammatory, vascular, and neoplastic conditions of the CNS may mimic tuberculosis. In most cases, the differential diagnosis involves a patient presenting with clinical features of a granulomatous meningitis syndrome: fever, headache, meningeal signs, altered mentation, and a CSF profile showing lymphocytic pleocytosis, lowered glucose concentration, and high protein content. In addition to tuberculosis, the other primary infectious considerations include fungal disease (principally cryptococcosis), brucellosis, and syphilis. On occasion subacute aseptic meningitis with these CSF findings may be encountered in patients with unrecognized parameningeal suppurative infection such as sphenoid sinusitis, brain abscess, and endocarditis. Patients with herpes simplex virus and mumps meningoencephalitis can be confusing as they may present with fever, rapid neurologic deterioration, and on occasion, mild lowering of the CSF glucose concentration (see Chapter 43). Noninfectious etiologies to be considered include neurosarcoidosis and lymphomatous or carcinomatous meningitis. A careful evaluation for tuberculosis is warranted in every patient suspected of any of the diagnoses listed in Table 41-2.

TUBERCULOMA

Tuberculomas are conglomerate caseous foci within the substance of the brain that develop from deep-seated tubercles acquired during a recent or remote period of bacillemia. Centrally located, active lesions may reach considerable size without producing signs of meningeal inflammation. Under conditions of poor host resistance, this process may result in focal areas of cerebritis or frank abscess formation, but the more usual course is coalescence of caseous foci and fibrous encapsulation (tuberculoma).[37,38] The characteristic CT finding is a nodular enhancing lesion with a central hypodense region. In the early stage, however, lesions may be isodense, often with edema out of proportion to the mass effect along with little encapsulation. Late in their development, well-encapsulated tuberculomas appear as isodense or hyperdense lesions with peripheral ring enhancement. CT is useful for assessing the presence of cerebral edema, the risk of herniation, and the response to therapy. The MRI appearance depends on the stage of tuberculoma: focal cerebritis is manifest by nonspecific edema on T2-weighted images and ill-defined enhancement, whereas a caseating lesion typically shows central hypointensity and peripheral enhancement.

Clinically silent, single or multiple, small parenchymal tuberculomas are seen commonly in cases of tuberculous meningitis and often in miliary tuberculosis without meningitis. These lesions usually disappear with medical therapy, although cases have been reported in which tuberculomas enlarged early during the course of antituberculous therapy.[39]

In contrast to lesions demonstrated by imaging studies that produce few or no symptoms, clinical tuberculomas presenting as symptomatic intracranial mass lesions are encountered frequently in areas of the world where the prevalence of tuberculosis is high. The usual patient is a child or young adult with headache, seizure, focal neurologic deficits, or signs of raised intracranial pressure. Symptoms of systemic illness and meningeal inflammation are usually lacking. The diagnosis is made with clinical, epidemiologic, and radiographic data or via needle biopsy.

Surgery for purposes other than diagnosis may be required when lesions are critically located and produce obstructive hydrocephalus or compression of the brainstem. Corticosteroids aid in selected cases in which cerebral edema disproportionate to the mass effect contributes to altered mental state or focal neurologic deficits; however, they may mask the characteristic pathology of other diagnostic mimics such as CNS lymphoma, and therefore should be reserved for patients in whom the diagnosis is secure.

SPINAL TUBERCULOUS ARACHNOIDITIS

Tuberculous arachnoiditis or tuberculoma may arise at any level of the spinal cord in association with either breakdown of a granulomatous focus in the spinal cord or nearby meninges or through extension from an adjacent area of inapparent spondylitis. The inflammatory process is usually confined locally, gradually producing partial or complete encasement of the spinal cord in a gelatinous or fibrous exudate. In other cases, tuberculomas of the extradural, intradural, or intramedullary space may produce symptoms resembling local tumor.

Patients usually present with some combination of signs of nerve root and spinal cord compression secondary to impingement by the advancing arachnoiditis. The clinical manifestations are more neurologic than infectious, protean in nature, and often take the form of an ascending or transverse radiculomyelopathy of variable pace involving single or multiple levels.[40–42] Common symptoms and signs include pain, hyperesthesia or paresthesias in the distribution of the nerve root, lower motor neuron paralysis, and urinary or fecal incontinence. On occasion, the granulomatous mass or abscess may be confined largely to the epidural space, producing symptoms of spinal cord compression with no evidence of meningeal inflammation. Localized vasculitis may lead to thrombosis of spinal arteries and infarction of the cord.

The diagnosis of spinal tuberculous arachnoiditis should be considered in the patient with any combination of the following clinical and laboratory features: subacute onset of spinal or nerve root pain; rapidly ascending transverse myelopathy or multiple-level myelopathy; increased CSF protein concentration and cell count; signs of arachnoiditis or epidural space infection by MRI; and evidence of tuberculosis elsewhere in the body. Surgical intervention and tissue biopsy are often required for diagnosis. Some patients progress from an initial spinal syndrome to tuberculous cranial meningitis; this progression carries an extremely poor prognosis.

THERAPY

Antituberculous Chemotherapy

The decision to begin antituberculous chemotherapy must be made promptly, usually based on clinical suspicion and presumptive diagnosis rather than direct evidence of mycobacterial infection. The prognosis is favorable when therapy is started before the development of focal signs and altered mentation. There are no randomized trials to establish the optimal drug combination, dosage, and duration of treatment for tuberculous meningitis; the regimens used are extrapolated from the management of pulmonary tuberculosis.[43] The use of combination drug regimens is intended to enhance the bactericidal effect, cover the possibility of drug resistance, and reduce the risk of emerging resistance while on therapy.

Isoniazid, rifampin, and pyrazinamide are each bactericidal, can be administered orally, penetrate inflamed meninges, and achieve CSF concentrations required for activity against sensitive strains.[44] These drugs, usually along with ethambutol or streptomycin, are considered first-line therapy.

Isoniazid diffuses readily into CSF and achieves concentrations many times that required for bactericidal activity. The recommended daily dose is 10 mg/kg for children and 300 mg for adults. Pyridoxine, 25 or 50 mg daily, should be given concurrently to avoid the neurologic complications of isoniazid-induced pyridoxine deficiency, including peripheral neuropathy.

Rifampin is active early against rapidly dividing organisms and achieves reliable CSF concentrations only in the presence of meningeal inflammation. Because rifampin is active against semidormant organisms, its major contribution may relate to the resolution of residual foci in the CNS and elsewhere in the body. The daily dose in children and adults is 10 mg/kg (maximum 600 mg), and an intravenous formulation is available.

Studies of pulmonary tuberculosis have demonstrated that the addition of *pyrazinamide* to regimens that include isoniazid and rifampin produces a more powerful antituberculous effect without increasing the incidence of hepatotoxicity, as long as the duration of pyrazinamide therapy is restricted to 2 months or less. CSF penetration is excellent in the presence or absence of inflammation, and the drug is highly active against intracellular mycobacteria. It is recommended that pyrazinamide be included in the treatment regimen for meningitis during the first 2 months of therapy. In children, the daily dose is 15 to 20 mg/kg (maximum 2,000 mg). In adults, the dose is based on weight: 40 to 55 kg, 1,000 mg; 56 to 75 kg, 1,500 mg; 76 to 90 kg, 2,000 mg.

Ethambutol is a weak drug that reaches the subarachnoid space in moderate concentration. Its major toxicity, optic neuropathy, occurs in as many as 3 percent of patients receiving 25 mg/kg daily but is rare at the recommended dose of 15 mg/kg. When ethambutol is used, it is advisable to check visual acuity, red-green color vision, and visual fields if possible.

Recommended Regimen

Guidelines published by American and British societies and by the Centers for Disease Control and Prevention recommend an initial intensive phase of treatment with four drugs for 2 months followed by a prolonged continuation phase with two drugs for 7 to 10 months for drug-sensitive infections.[45,46] The initial four-drug regimen includes isoniazid, rifampin, pyrazinamide, and either ethambutol or streptomycin, administered for 2 months. This is followed by isoniazid and rifampin alone if the isolate is fully susceptible, the risk of drug resistance is small, and the clinical course satisfactory. If pyrazinamide is omitted or not tolerated initially, the total course of treatment should be extended to 18 months.

The possibility of drug-resistant infection should be anticipated in high-risk individuals such as those from areas of the world where tuberculosis is endemic, the homeless, in those having received previous antituberculous drugs, and in individuals with known exposure to persons harboring resistant organisms. The impact on therapeutic outcome is variable, depending on whether the isolate is resistant to isoniazid or rifampin or both.[47] The best drug combination for resistant infection is uncertain and to some extent depends on the particular sensitivity pattern of a given isolate. The second-line drugs ethionamide and cycloserine penetrate the CSF well and may be useful. The fluoroquinolones also have good activity against mycobacteria. In addition to streptomycin, other aminoglycides such as kanamycin and amikacin are effective and have been given for resistant organisms via intrathecal injection.[48] The duration of treatment should be extended to 18 to 24 months when resistant organisms are encountered.

Adjunctive Therapy

Corticosteroids

The role of corticosteroids in the management of tuberculous meningitis has long been a matter of uncertainty. Older studies were limited by small patient numbers and failure to stratify severity of illness according to neurologic manifestations. There is, however, a growing body of clinical data demonstrating that adjunctive corticosteroid therapy is beneficial in children and adults with CNS tuberculosis.[49–52] In most major clinical centers in Europe, Asia, and Africa, corticosteroids are administered routinely to patients with clinical stage II and III disease. A meta-analysis of the various trials demonstrated a significant benefit of corticosteroids in tuberculous meningitis across a variety of patient populations.[49] In a randomized trial in 141 children, prednisone administered for the first month improved survival and intellectual outcome and enhanced resolution of basilar exudate and tuberculomas.[51] In those children with stage III disease, prednisone therapy was associated with a significant reduction in mortality (4 versus 17 percent).

Adjunctive corticosteroid therapy is recommended for all patients with convincing clinical evidence of CNS tuberculosis, the possible exception being adults with early stage I meningitis. Complications for which corticosteroids are thought to be most beneficial include increased intracranial pressure, cerebral edema, stupor, focal neurologic signs, and spinal block. Specific clinical indications based on urgent warning signs include: progression from one stage to the next at or before the start of chemotherapy, CT evidence of marked basilar enhancement, moderate or advancing hydrocephalus, spinal block, or incipient block (CSF protein ≥500 mg/dl), and intracerebral tuberculoma when edema is out of proportion to mass effect with clinical signs.

Either dexamethasone or prednisone may be used. For dexamethasone, the daily dose is 8 mg for children weighing less than 25 kg and 12 mg for adults and children weighing more than 25 kg. For prednisone, the dose is 2 to 4 mg/kg daily for children and 60 mg/day for adults. This initial dose is given for 3 weeks and then tapered gradually over the following 3 to 4 weeks.

The decision to use corticosteroids should rest on a strong presumptive or positive diagnosis. Caution is advisable in the face of diagnostic uncertainty, especially in cases in which fungal CNS infection is considered a strong possibility. The expected benefit from corticosteroids must be weighed carefully against the potential for adverse consequences, bearing in mind that initial improvement may be nonspecific for tuberculosis. In select cases, systemic antifungal therapy should be administered concurrently until a specific etiologic diagnosis has been reached.

Surgery

The management of hydrocephalus may require surgical decompression of the ventricular system in order to prevent neurologic complications of sustained raised intracranial pressure. In patients with clinical stage II disease, serial lumbar puncture combined with corticosteroids, diuretics, and osmotic agents may suffice while awaiting the early response to chemotherapy.[53] However, surgical intervention should not be delayed when these measures fail or when the clinical course while on therapy is one of progressive neurologic impairment.[34,54]

Surgical removal of intracranial tuberculoma may be necessary in the patient presenting with clinical features of a single space-occupying lesion, midline shift, raised intracranial pressure, and lack of satisfactory response to chemotherapy.

PROGNOSIS AND OUTCOME

The clinical outcome in any individual case is greatly influenced by age, duration of illness, clinical stage at the initiation of therapy, and the extent and character of optochiasmic arachnoiditis and vascular complications. In general, when antituberculous treatment is started before patients progress beyond stage I or during early stage II disease, cure rates of 85 to 90 percent may be achieved. Ages younger than 5 years and older than 50 years are associated with a poor prognosis. The observed mortality rate exceeds 50 percent in patients older than 50 years and in those with stupor and coma. The impact of stage of disease on therapeutic outcome is illustrated in a well-studied clinical series of 58 patients from Australia.[13] Of 50 patients presenting with stage I or II disease, 1 died and 5 were left with mild or moderate neurologic sequelae. Of the 8 patients with stage III disease, 3 died and 3 were left with severe neurologic impairment.[13]

The incidence of residual neurologic deficits after recovery from tuberculous meningitis varies from 10 to 30 percent in recent series. Late sequelae include cranial nerve deficits, gait disturbance, hemiplegia, blindness, deafness, learning disability, dementia, and various syndromes of hypothalamic or pituitary dysfunction.

CONCLUDING COMMENTS

Tuberculosis of the CNS, principally meningitis, remains the most devastating form of active mycobacterial infection. The natural history is that of insidious onset and subacute progression, prone to rapid deterioration once focal neurologic deficits supervene, usually resulting in stupor, coma, and death within 5 to 8 weeks of the onset of illness. Antituberculous chemotherapy is effective, but in order to achieve a favorable outcome, it is important that treatment be started promptly in the early stages of disease, before the occurrence of serious changes in mentation or progression of focal neurologic deficits. Of necessity, this requires understanding of the pathophysiology and clinical features of granulomatous meningitis. Patients with subacute meningitis syndrome and CSF findings of low glucose concentration, elevated protein level, and mononuclear pleocytosis should be treated immediately if there is evidence of tuberculosis elsewhere in the body or if prompt evaluation fails to establish an alternative diagnosis. Serial sampling of the CSF for culture and meticulous examination of stained smears remain the best means for reaching a bacteriologic diagnosis. Treatment need not be delayed as culture and stain for acid-fast bacilli remain positive for some days after antituberculous therapy has been started. In the patient with compatible clinical features, CT or MRI evidence of basilar meningeal enhancement combined with any degree of hydrocephalus is strongly suggestive of tuberculous meningitis. Serial CT or MRI is useful for following the course of therapy and for managing hydrocephalus and tuberculoma. The recommended chemotherapy regimen for presumed drug-sensitive infection is isoniazid and rifampin in all patients, together with pyrazinamide and ethambutol for the first 2 months. Adjunctive corticosteroid therapy can ameliorate complications and reduce mortality in patients with stage II and III disease. Surgical shunting should be considered early in the patient with advancing hydrocephalus and symptoms or signs attributable to raised intracranial pressure.

REFERENCES

1. Centers for Disease Control and Prevention (CDC): Trends in tuberculosis—United States, 2012. MMWR Morb Mortal Wkly Rep 62:210, 2013.
2. Bartzatt R: Tuberculosis infections of the central nervous system. Cent Nerv Syst Agents Med Chem 11:321, 2011.
3. Delance AR, Safaee M, Oh MC, et al: Tuberculoma of the central nervous system. J Clin Neurosci 20:1333, 2013.
4. Chou PS, Liu CK, Lin RT, et al: Central nervous system tuberculosis: a forgotten diagnosis. Neurologist 18:219, 2012.
5. Patkar D, Narang J, Yanamandala R, et al: Central nervous system tuberculosis: pathophysiology and imaging findings. Neuroimaging Clin N Am 22:677, 2012.
6. Thwaites GE, Schoeman JF: Update on tuberculosis of the central nervous system: pathogenesis, diagnosis, and treatment. Clin Chest Med 30:745, 2009.
7. Rock RB, Olin M, Baker CA, et al: Central nervous system tuberculosis: pathogenesis and clinical aspects. Clin Microbiol Rev 21:243, 2008.
8. Sharma SK, Mohan A, Sharma A, et al: Miliary tuberculosis: new insights into an old disease. Lancet Infect Dis 5:415, 2005.
9. Donald PR, Schaaf HS, Schoeman JF: Tuberculous meningitis and military tuberculosis: the "Rich" focus revisited. J Infect 50:193, 2005.
10. Dastur DK, Manghani DK, Udani PM: Pathology and pathogenic mechanisms in neurotuberculosis. Radiol Clin North Am 33:753, 1995.
11. Chan KH, Cheung RT, Lee R, et al: Cerebral infarcts complicating tuberculous meningitis. Cerebrovasc Dis 19:391, 2005.
12. vanWell GT, Paes BF, Terwee CB, et al: Twenty years of pediatric tuberculous meningitis: a retrospective cohort study on the western cape of South Africa. Pediatrics 123:e1, 2009.
13. Kent SJ, Crowe SM, Yung A, et al: Tuberculous meningitis: a 30-year review. Clin Infect Dis 17:987, 1993.
14. Gunawardhana SA, Somaratne SC, Fernando MA, et al: Tuberculous meningitis in adults: a prospective study at a tertiary referral centre in Sri Lanka. Ceylon Med J 58:21, 2013.
15. Farinha NJ, Razali KA, Holzel H, et al: Tuberculosis of the central nervous system in children: a 20-year survey. J Infect 41:61, 2000.
16. Verdon R, Chevert S, Laissy P, et al: Tuberculous meningitis in adults: review of 48 cases. Clin Infect Dis 22:982, 1996.
17. Yaramis A, Gurkan F, Elevli M, et al: Central nervous system tuberculosis in children: a review of 214 cases. Pediatrics 102:e49, 1998.
18. Katti MK: Pathogenesis, diagnosis, treatment, and outcome aspects of cerebral tuberculosis. Med Sci Monit 10:RA215, 2004.
19. Alacon F, Duenas G, Cevallos N, et al: Movement disorders in 30 patients with tuberculous meningitis. Mov Disord 15:561, 2000.
20. Braun MN, Byers RH, Heyward WL, et al: Acquired immunodeficiency syndrome and extrapulmonary tuberculosis in the United States. Arch Intern Med 150:1913, 1990.
21. Berenguer J, Moreno S, Laguna F, et al: Tuberculous meningitis in patients infected with the human immunodeficiency virus. N Engl J Med 326:668, 1992.
22. Dube MP, Holtom PD, Larsen RA: Tuberculous meningitis in patients with and without human immunodeficiency virus infection. Am J Med 93:520, 1992.
23. Katrak SM, Shembalkar PK, Bijwe SR, et al: The clinical, radiological, and pathological profile of tuberculous meningitis in patients with and without human immunodeficiency virus infection. J Neurol Sci 181:118, 2000.
24. Thwaites GE, Chau H, Stepnieska K, et al: Diagnosis of tuberbulous meningitis by clinical and laboratory features. Lancet 360:1287, 2002.
25. Mehta S, Gilada IS: Ocular tuberculosis in acquired immune deficiency syndrome (AIDS). Oculo Immunol Inflamm 13:87, 2005.
26. Thwaites GE, Chau TTH, Farrar JJ: Improving the bacteriologic diagnosis of tuberculous meningitis. J Clin Microbiol 42:378, 2004.
27. Mehta PK, Raj A, Singh N, et al: Diagnosis of extrapulmonary tuberculosis by PCR. FEMS Immunol Med Microbiol 66:20, 2012.

28. Noordhoek GT, Kolk AH, Bjune G, et al: Sensitivity and specificity of PCR for detection of *Mycobacterium tuberculosis:* a blind comparison study among seven laboratories. J Clin Microbiol 32:277, 1994.
29. Bonington A, Strang JI, Klapper PE, et al: Use of Roche AMPLICOR *Mycobacterium tuberculosis* PCR in early diagnosis of tuberculous meningitis. J Clin Microbiol 36:1251, 1998.
30. Pai M, Flores LL, Pai N, et al: Diagnostic accuracy of nucleic acid amplification tests for diagnosis of tuberculous meningitis: a systematic review and meta-analysis. Lancet Infect Dis 3:633, 2003.
31. Bernaerts A, Vanhoenacker FM, Parizel PM, et al: Tuberculosis of the nervous system: overview of neuroloradiological findings. Radiology 13:1876, 2003.
32. Botha A, Ackerman C, Candy S, et al: Reliability and diagnostic performance of CT imaging criteria in the diagnosis of tuberculous meningitis. PLoS One 7:e38982, 2012.
33. Ozates M, Kemaloglu S, Gurkan F, et al: CT of the brain in tuberculous meningitis. Acta Radiol 41:13, 2000.
34. Lamprecht D, Schoeman J, Donald P, et al: Ventriculoperitoneal shunting in childhood tuberculous meningitis. Br J Neurosurg 15:119, 2001.
35. Schoeman J, Hewlett R, Donald P: MR of childhood tuberculous meningitis. Neuroradiology 30:473, 1988.
36. Offenbacher H, Fazekas F, Schmidt R, et al: MRI in tuberculous meningoencephalitis: report of four cases and review of the neuroimaging literature. J Neurol 238:340, 1991.
37. Kumar R, Pandi CK, Base N, et al: Tuberculous brain abscess: clinical presentation, pathophysiology and treatment (in children). Childs Nerv Syst 18:118, 2002.
38. Wasay M, Khealani BA, Moolani MK, et al: Brain CT and MR findings in 100 consecutive patients with intracranial tuberculoma. J Neuroimaging 13:240, 2003.
39. Ravensscroft A, Schoeman JF, Donald PR: Tuberculous granulomas in childhood tuberculous meningitis: pathologic features and course. J Trop Pediatr 47:5, 2001.
40. Konar SK, Rao KN, Mahadevan A, et al: Tuberculous lumbar arachnoiditis mimicking conus cauda tumor: a case report and review of literature. J Neurosci Rural Pract 2:93, 2011.
41. Kumar A, Montanera W, Willinsky R, et al: MR features of tuberculous arachnoiditis. J Comput Assist Tomogr 17:127, 1991.
42. Wasay M, Khealani B, Ahsan H: Neuroimaging of tuberculous myelitis: analysis of ten cases and review of literature. J Neuroimaging 16:197, 2006.
43. Mitchison DA: Role of individual drugs in the chemotherapy of tuberculosis. Int J Tuberc Lung Dis 4:796, 2000.
44 Ellard GA, Humphries MJ, Allen BW: Cerebrospinal fluid drug concentrations and treatment of tuberculous meningitis. Am Rev Respir Dis 148:650, 1993.
45. Joint Tuberculosis Committee of the British Thoracic Society: Chemotherapy and management of tuberculosis in the United Kingdom: recommendations. Thorax 53:536, 1998.
46. American Thoracic Society Centers for Disease Control and Prevention, Infectious Diseases Society of America: Treatment of tuberculosis. Am J Respir Crit Care Med 167:603, 2003.
47. Thwaites GE, Lan NT, Dung NH, et al: Effect of antituberculous drug resistance on relapse to treatment and outcome in adults with tuberculous meningitis. J Infect Dis 192:79, 2005.
48. Berning SE, Cherry TA, Iseman MD: Novel treatment of meningitis caused by multi-drug resistant *Mycobacterium tuberculosis* with intrathecal levofloxacin and amikacin: case report. Clin Infect Dis 32:643, 2001.
49. Critchley JA, Young F, Orton L, et al: Corticosteroids for prevention of mortality in people with tuberculosis: a systemic review and meta-analysis. Lancet Infect Dis 13:223, 2013.
50. Girgis NI, Farid Z, Kilpatrick ME, et al: Dexamethasone adjunctive treatment for tuberculous meningitis. Pediatr Infect Dis J 10:179, 1991.
51. Schoeman JF, Van Zyl LE, Laubscher JA, et al: Effect of corticosteroids on intracranial pressure, computed tomographic findings, and clinical outcome in young children with tuberculous meningitis. Pediatrics 99:226, 1997.
52. Thwaite GE, Nguyen DB, Nguyen HD, et al: Dexamethasone for the treatment of tuberculous meningitis in adolescents and adults. N Engl J Med 351:1741, 2004.
53. Schoeman J, Donald P, van Zyl L, et al: Tuberculous hydrocephalus: comparison of different treatments with regard to ICP, ventricular size and clinical outcome. Dev Med Child Neurol 33:396, 1991.
54. Palur R, Rajshekhar V, Chandy MJ, et al: Shunt surgery for hydrocephalus in tuberculous meningitis: a log-term follow-up study. J Neurosurg 74:64, 1991.

CHAPTER

42

Neurologic Complications of Leprosy

THOMAS D. SABIN ■ THOMAS R. SWIFT

The acid-fast organism *Mycobacterium leprae*, the cause of leprosy, was the first pathogen conclusively linked to a human disease, a discovery made by Dr. G. Armauer Hansen in 1874.[1] The genome of the organism underwent dramatic "reductive evolution" with loss of the metabolic machinery that other mycobacteria retain.[2] The organism is an obligate intracellular pathogen. Single nucleotide polymorphisms indicate that leprosy originated in East Africa and passed on to Europe and Asia before explorers brought the disease to West Africa.[3] The genome has also been found in ancient remains of the Near East from biblical times.

The number of active cases in the world has fallen dramatically from 10 to 20 million in 1970 to under 200,000 in 2012 because patients are now rapidly classified as "cured" with brief courses of multidrug therapy (MDT).[4] The long-term validity of this encouraging trend, however, relies on the assumption that the relapse rate will be very low. No corresponding drop in incidence has yet occurred, but the hope of the World Health Organization program is to eliminate leprosy by effecting a critical decrease in infectious bacteria within the population.[5]

The leprosy bacillus is unique in two important ways. First, it is the only bacterial pathogen that regularly invades peripheral nerves. The molecular biology underlying this neurotropism of *M. leprae* is unique among bacteria. An α-dystroglycan in the G domain of the α_2 chain of laminin in the basal lamina of the Schwann cell–axon unit is a specific binding target for *M. leprae*.[6] After entering the Schwann cell, the organism commandeers the MEK kinase cascade, causing proliferation of more potential victim Schwann cells.[7] Macrophages are the other major target cell.

Second, *M. leprae* multiplies at temperatures that are 7° to 10°C lower than the core body temperature of 37°C.[8] These two factors account for several important clinical features of the disease. All patients with leprosy have some degree of nerve involvement, making leprous neuritis a significant cause of treatable neuropathy in the world. Visible deformities from involvement of facial structures, eyes, nerves, bones, and skin result in stigmatization and social ostracism.[9] The diagnosis of leprosy is often missed by physicians, leading to a delay in treatment during which progressive neuropathy, visual loss, and deformity may occur.

GENERAL MANIFESTATIONS

Leprosy may be spread by aerosol or rarely by skin-to-skin contact; fortunately, more than 95 percent of individuals are naturally immune.[5] Animal reservoirs have been found in chimpanzee, sooty mangaby, cynomolgus macaque, and armadillo.[10] In susceptible patients, the organisms rapidly gain access to cooler dermal tissues, primarily cutaneous and subcutaneous nerves and nerve networks, skin appendages, sweat glands, and erector pili muscles.[11]

Aminoff's Neurology and General Medicine, Fifth Edition.

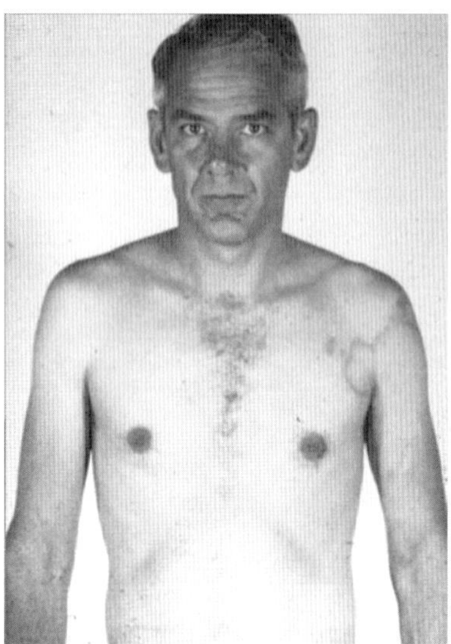

FIGURE 42-1 ■ Tuberculoid (TT) leprosy. There is complete anesthesia within this lesion, which has a raised erythematous border and a pale, dry center. (Courtesy of Gillis W. Long Hansen's Disease Center, Carville, Louisiana.)

Leprosy occurs in three major forms: tuberculoid, borderline, and lepromatous. The type of leprosy that develops depends on the degree of host resistance rather than on the bacterium. There are some genetic variations in *M. leprae*, but these do not play a role in the severity of the disease, which is the same for all three types.[12]

In patients with high resistance, the leprosy that develops is called tuberculoid (or TT) or paucibacillary. A single patch of skin is involved by a granulomatous infiltrate, often with enlargement of underlying nerve trunks, but systemic dissemination does not occur, bacterial organisms are few, and self-healing is the rule. The skin lesions have raised edges and may have one or more satellite lesions (Fig. 42-1). Within these lesions, nerves are destroyed in an epithelioid granulomatous reaction. Often, a superimposed inflammatory response, known as a reversal reaction, occurs within the lesion either spontaneously or in response to drug treatment. Such a reaction reflects altered immunologic responsiveness by the host to the organism and often results in bacteriologic clearing of the lesions.

In contrast, patients with multibacillary leprosy (called lepromatous or LL) have little or no resistance, and bacilli are disseminated throughout the body through a continuous bacteremia, multiplying to extremely high numbers. There is little histologic evidence of host resistance; histiocytes are literally packed with huge numbers of organisms that proliferate in cool areas of the body: the skin, upper respiratory tract, anterior one-third of the eye, superficial nerves, testes, and other tissues. Beading of corneal nerves may be seen. Although bacilli may be deposited passively in the deeper, and therefore warmer, vital organs, such as the lungs, heart, liver, kidneys, and brain, there is little evidence of bacterial proliferation or pathologic tissue reaction at those sites. Clinically, patients present with skin infiltration, particularly prominent in the cool areas, such as facial promontories, ears, dorsal forearms, legs, nasal mucosa, and scrotum (Fig. 42-2). Biopsy sample examination and skin scrapings of such tissues reveal innumerable acid-fast organisms. Without treatment, lepromatous leprosy continues to progress, eventually leading to severe deformities in most cases. At times spontaneously, but more often in response to antibacterial treatment, a reaction known as erythema nodosum leprosum occurs. Clinically, this is a very severe form of erythema nodosum and is a result of the deposition of antigen-antibody complexes in the walls of small arteries. Erythema nodosum leprosum occurs in areas where large amounts

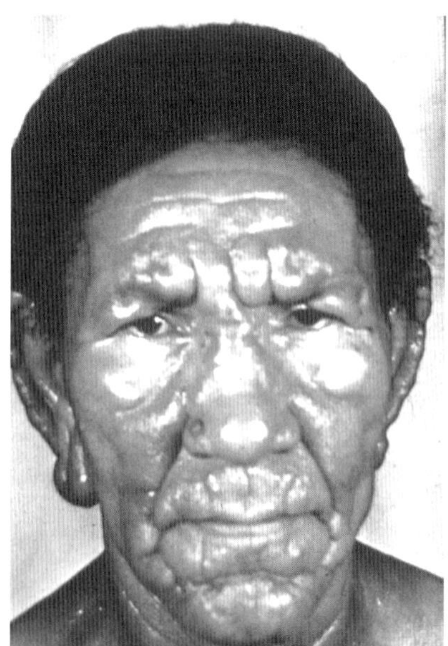

FIGURE 42-2 ■ Lepromatous (LL) leprosy. There is infiltration of the cooler facial promontories, such as the ears, upper lip, chin, and supraorbital and malar areas. (Courtesy of Gillis W. Long Hansen's Disease Center, Carville, Louisiana.)

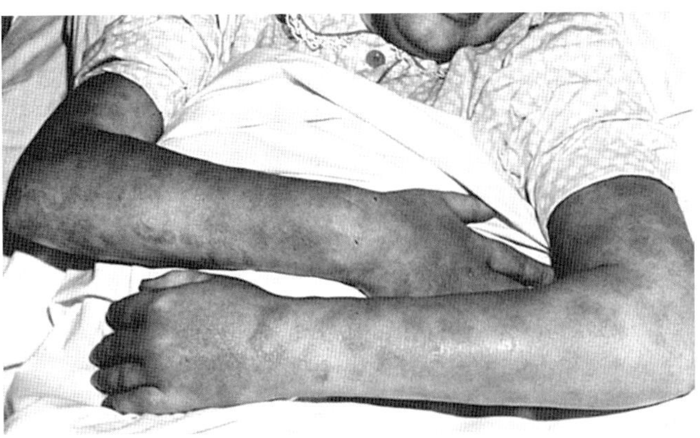

FIGURE 42-3 ▪ Erythema nodosum leprosum. Painful subcutaneous nodules cover the face and trunk (not shown) and the extremities. (Courtesy of Gillis W. Long Hansen's Disease Center, Carville, Louisiana.)

of mycobacterial antigen are present. The resulting inflammatory lesions can be devastating to the cornea and anterior eye, peripheral nerves, testes, and skin, producing multiple painful erythematous nodules (Fig. 42-3), leading to frank ulceration in some cases. During the course of erythema nodosum leprosum, iritis, neuritis, and orchitis occur and may be more damaging than the underlying leprosy itself. Erythema nodosum leprosum is a complex immunologic reaction occurring with the production of cytokines such as tumor necrosis factor α (TNF-α). It is ironic that the circulating antibodies to mycobacterial antigen, constituting the host's only immunologic responsiveness to the offending organism, appear not to benefit the host, but paradoxically to result in additional tissue damage.

In the third type of leprosy, called borderline leprosy (or BB), a variable spectrum of disease occurs, depending on the degree of host resistance. In patients having low resistance, the disease resembles lepromatous disease (BL), whereas in those with higher resistance it resembles tuberculoid disease (BT). Patients with borderline leprosy have less skin involvement than those with lepromatous disease and may have more circumscribed skin lesions, but they have more skin lesions than patients with tuberculoid disease (Fig. 42-4). A form of "pure neuritic" leprosy occurs without visible skin lesions.[13,14] Since few mycobacteria may be present, the diagnosis is confirmed by immunohistochemical techniques.[15] Increasingly in leprosy work, the terms *paucibacillary* and *multibacillary* are used in an attempt to simplify disease classifications and treatment decisions.

In the spectrum of borderline leprosy, immunity may change, with patients worsening, their disease becoming more like lepromatous (BL) disease (downgrading reaction), or evolving more toward the tuberculoid (BT) form (reversal reaction). Such shifts in the spectrum of disease may occur spontaneously or in response to drug treatment or intercurrent medical conditions, such as underlying neoplasms or secondary infections. Considering the extent of infection with human immunodeficiency virus (HIV) in leprosy-endemic areas, it is fortunate that no increase in leprosy has been associated with acquired immunodeficiency syndrome (AIDS), which may, however, precipitate reversal or downgrading reactions in leprosy patients.[16] $CD8^+$ T cells are implicated in triggering reversal reaction in HIV/ leprosy patients.[17]

NEUROPATHOLOGY

In tuberculoid leprosy, the few organisms present in peripheral nerves evoke a strong granulomatous response with early and severe nerve damage, fortunately limited to the few nerves involved. In

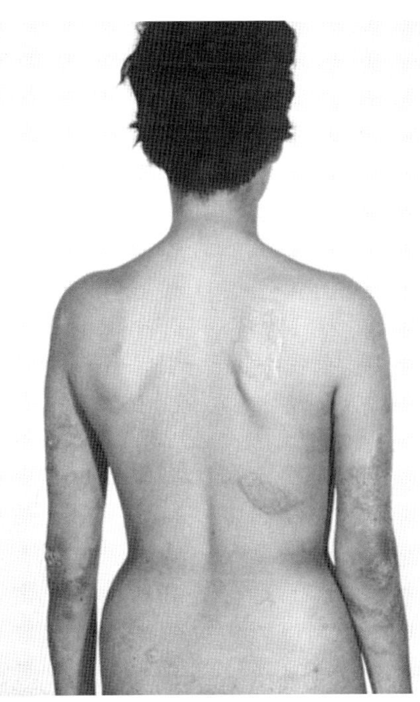

FIGURE 42-4 ▪ Borderline (BB) leprosy. The widespread symmetric skin lesions are hypesthetic. (Courtesy of Gillis W. Long Hansen's Disease Center, Carville, Louisiana.)

lepromatous leprosy, the overwhelming majority of organisms are present in Schwann cells (Fig. 42-5), but neuropathologic and electrophysiologic data indicate that there is substantial axonal destruction, and some of the demyelinating lesions themselves may be secondary to axonal changes. Complex immunologic parasite–host interactions are gradually emerging as the basis for nerve damage.[11,12]

In addition to the damage to nerves caused by the invasion of *M. leprae*, there are several types of leprosy reactions in which there is a sudden and often sustained increase in immune response to bacilli or products released by dead bacilli. Erythema nodosum leprosum occurs only in multibacillary leprosy and appears to be a clinical example of the Arthus phenomenon, with consumption of complement and an intense vasculitis.[18] The vasculitis is most severe in the regions of greatest bacterial density and therefore may result in a devastating acute neuritis. There is a high amount of TNF-α in the blood with debilitating systemic symptoms.[18] Although the nerve lesions of leprosy tend to be permanent, prompt treatment of reactions may improve neurologic deficits.[19] It is also unclear to what extent or by what mechanisms erythema nodosum leprosum produces nerve damage, but it is likely that cytokines released by immunocompetent cells are important. Exogenous interferon-γ (IFN-γ) used in an attempt to treat leprosy has caused erythema nodosum leprosum in patients, who then have increased release of TNF. Thalidomide, which controls erythema nodosum leprosum, reduces TNF secretion. Thalidomide also reduces elevated numbers of $CD4^+$ lymphocytes in the blood of patients with erythema nodosum leprosum.[20] During erythema nodosum leprosum, there is a loss of suppressor cell function and an increase in interleukin-2 (IL-2) production.[20] Cyclosporine suppresses erythema nodosum leprosum and restores suppressor cell activity, possibly by its effect on macrophages.[21,22] Infliximab, a monoclonal antibody that inhibits the production of TNF-α, has reportedly suppressed erythema nodosum leprosum in a patient in whom corticosteroid and thalidomide therapy had failed.[23]

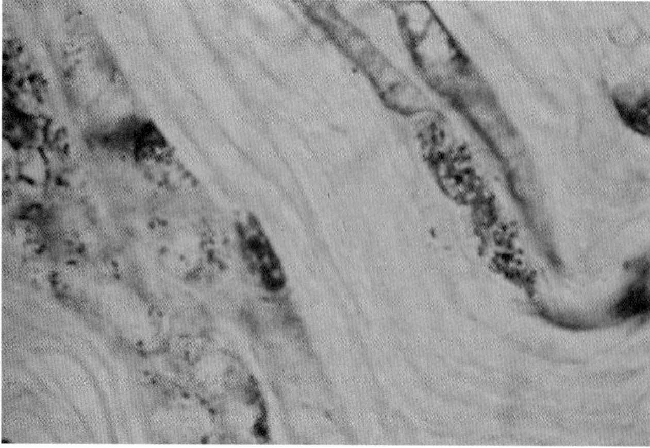

FIGURE 42-5 ■ Sural nerve biopsy, lepromatous leprosy (LL). Acid-fast stain reveals numerous organisms in endoneurial vacuoles. (Courtesy of Gillis W. Long Hansen's Disease Center, Carville, Louisiana.)

In the higher-resistance tuberculoid and borderline cases, reactions are related to increase in tissue-mediated immune factors. There is infiltration of the lesions with IFN-γ and CD4 lymphocytes producing TNF-α, which causes local redness, swelling, and rapid loss of function in any nerve coursing through the lesion.[24]

LEPROUS NEURITIS

A meticulous neurologic examination yields definitive diagnostic information of this treatable neuropathy. The diagnosis is based on the recognition of two interplaying themes that, although they produce limitless combinations in individual cases, capture the unique nature of this neuropathy once they are discerned. Both of these themes rest on the fact that *M. leprae* is the only bacterium that consistently invades peripheral nerves.

The first of the two diagnostic themes is based on the biologic feature that *M. leprae* has a highly thermosensitive growth rate that is optimal at 27° to 30°C.[8,25,26] The organism does not reproduce at all at core body temperature. This feature limits leprosy to involvement of only superficial nerves. The distinction between the "superficial" neuropathy of leprosy and a distal polyneuropathy is vital for correct diagnosis. This has been a source of confusion because long nerves tend to innervate cooler parts of the body. In leprosy, nerve damage is limited to intracutaneous nerve endings and networks and to the named nerves of gross anatomy at certain segments along their length where they course closest to the cooler surface of the body.[27] Since *M. leprae* cannot proliferate at core body temperature, peripheral nerves that are situated in deep tissues under or close to muscles, nerve roots, and the central nervous system (CNS) are not actively involved.

The second diagnostic theme relates to host factors that determine the immune resistance to the invasion and proliferation of bacilli. This host resistance has resulted in the classification of leprosy into the three subtypes mentioned earlier and is the other major determinant of the clinical features including nerve damage.

In a study of Chinese patients with leprosy, a genetic basis for vulnerability to infection by *M. leprae* was found involving 93 single-nucleotide polymorphisms in five genes (*CCDC122*, *C13orf31*, *TNFSF15*, *HLA-DR*, and *RIPK2*).[28] An additional polymorphism in the *LRRK2* gene was associated with the multibacillary form of leprosy. HLA-DR allows *M. leprae* antigen to contact and activate CD4 lymphocytes.

Leprosy bacilli are intracellular human pathogens with very limited growth in animals with the exception of the armadillo, and they do not grow in culture. Examination of the genome of *M. leprae* has shown great stability so that the large variation in clinical features of the disease must depend upon host factors. Populations vary widely in vulnerability to the infection and even in the frequency of the various subtypes, presumably because of underlying genetic differences in human hosts.

LEPROMATOUS LEPROSY

There is very little evidence of tissue-mediated immune responses to *M. leprae* in lepromatous leprosy, and lepromin skin testing is negative. The organism proliferates most rapidly in the coolest tissues, and there is a constant blood-stream dissemination of organisms. In untreated cases, this type of leprosy becomes widespread and symmetric within superficial tissues and may involve large areas of the skin, the anterior chamber of the eye, the upper respiratory tract, and the testes, as well as superficial nerves. Sensory loss is largely due to destruction of intracutaneous nerve endings and first appears in cool areas, such as the dorsal surfaces of the hands, dorsomedial surfaces of the forearms, dorsal surfaces of the feet, and ventrolateral aspects of the legs, as well as in the pinnae of the ears, especially the helices and earlobes (Fig. 42-6).[29,30] The tip of the nose, malar areas, and buttocks are often the next to show intracutaneous sensory loss (Fig. 42-7). There is a stage with sparing of the soles of the feet and palms of the hands, which may be due in part

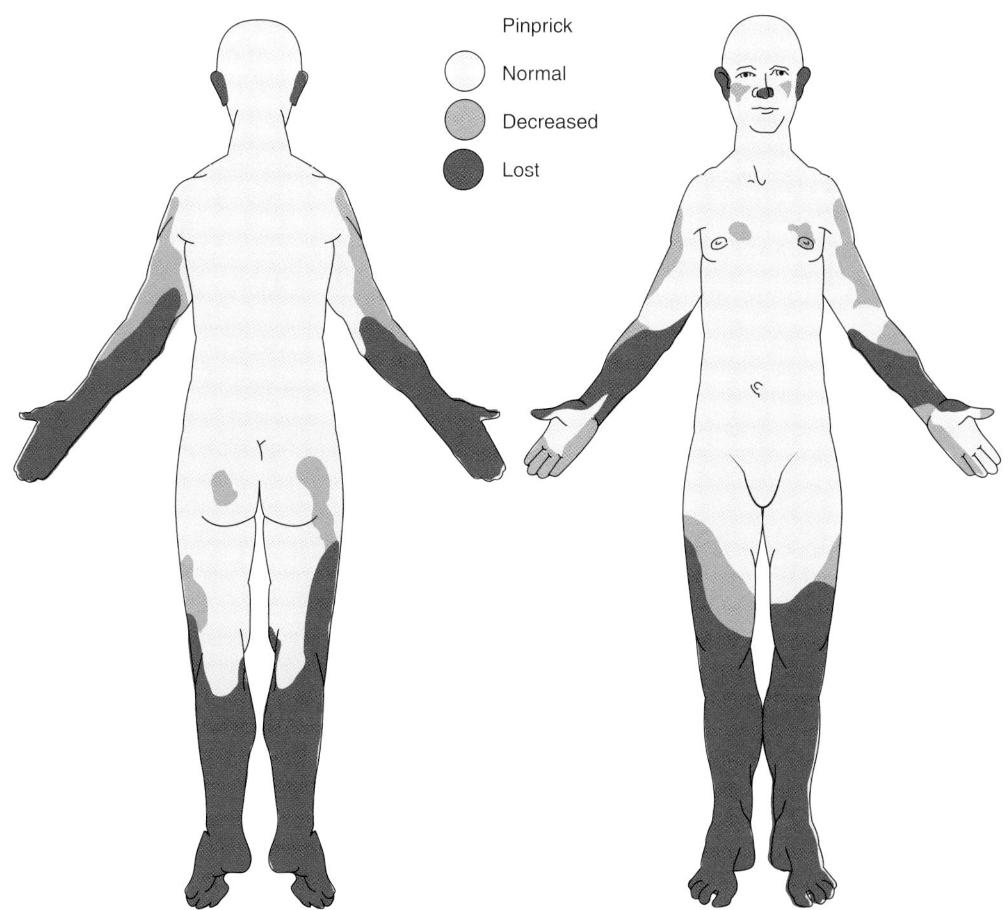

FIGURE 42-6 ■ Lepromatous leprosy (LL). Sensation is diminished in cool zones of the face, trunk, and extremities.

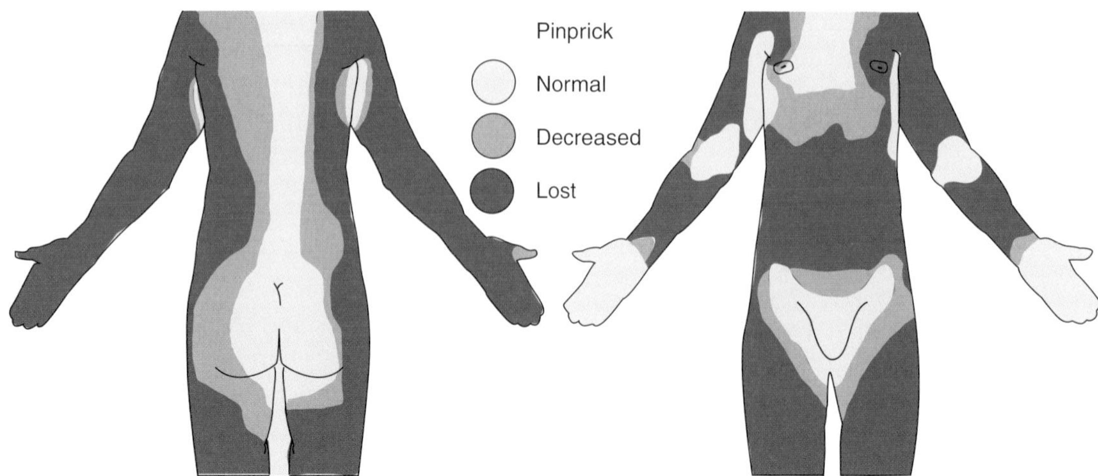

FIGURE 42-7 ▪ Lepromatous leprosy (LL). Sensation is preserved in warm areas: axillae, palms, antecubital fossae, inguinal region, gluteal cleft, and center of back and chest.

to the insulating effect of the thickened corium in these areas. If the patient is examined at the right stage, a distinct change in sensation at the cuticular border can sometimes be found in the hands or feet. When the intracutaneous pattern has evolved to this point, nerve trunk deficits supervene. Involvement of a 10- to 15-cm segment of the ulnar nerve proximal to the olecranon groove is most common, but the segment just proximal to the wrist may also be affected. Further paralysis is seen with damage to (1) the median nerve in the segment where it assumes a superficial position just proximal to the transverse carpal ligament (Fig. 42-8), (2) the fibular (peroneal) nerve where it courses around the fibular head, (3) the branch of the fibular nerve to the extensor digitorum brevis, and (4) the posterior tibial nerve at the level of the ankle.[27] There is also a unique patchy involvement of the most superficial facial nerve twigs, causing lagophthalmos and paralysis of some segments of the orbicularis oris and of the medial aspects of the corrugators of the forehead.[31]

With progression of the intracutaneous sensory loss, this pattern is more easily recognized by the areas of sparing, which include the intergluteal fold, the perineum, the anterior neck, under the scalp hair, the posterior creases at the attachment of the ears to the head, the axillae, the sternal area, and the center of the back where skin overlies the "warm" paraspinal muscles and the concavity overlying the spinous processes where cross-radiation of heat occurs. Sparing may be found in the webs of the toes or fingers and the antecubital and popliteal fossae (Fig. 42-9). A careful search may reveal unique features, such as sparing under constantly worn items of clothing (e.g., under a watchband or at a belt line) and even in small cutaneous vascular malformations.[32] A patient with chronic hemiplegia developed lepromatous leprosy with skin lesions limited to the cooler hemiplegic side.[33] Sensory examination of the distal extremities alone may result in confusion with a distal sensory polyneuropathy;

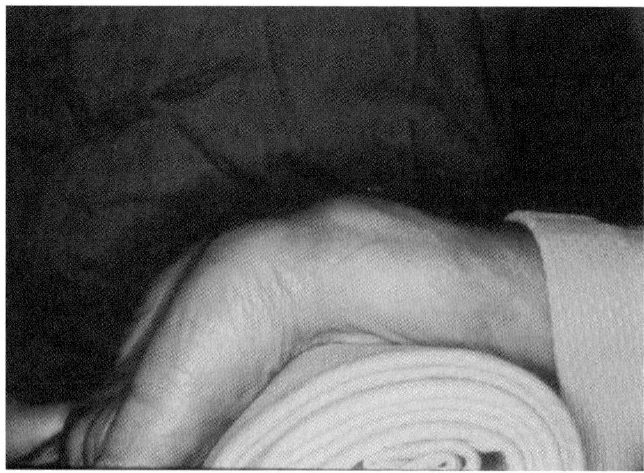

FIGURE 42-8 ▪ Lepromatous leprosy (LL). Enlargement of the median nerve proximal to the carpal tunnel is shown. (Courtesy of Dr. Paul Brand and Gillis W. Long Hansen's Disease Center, Carville, Louisiana.)

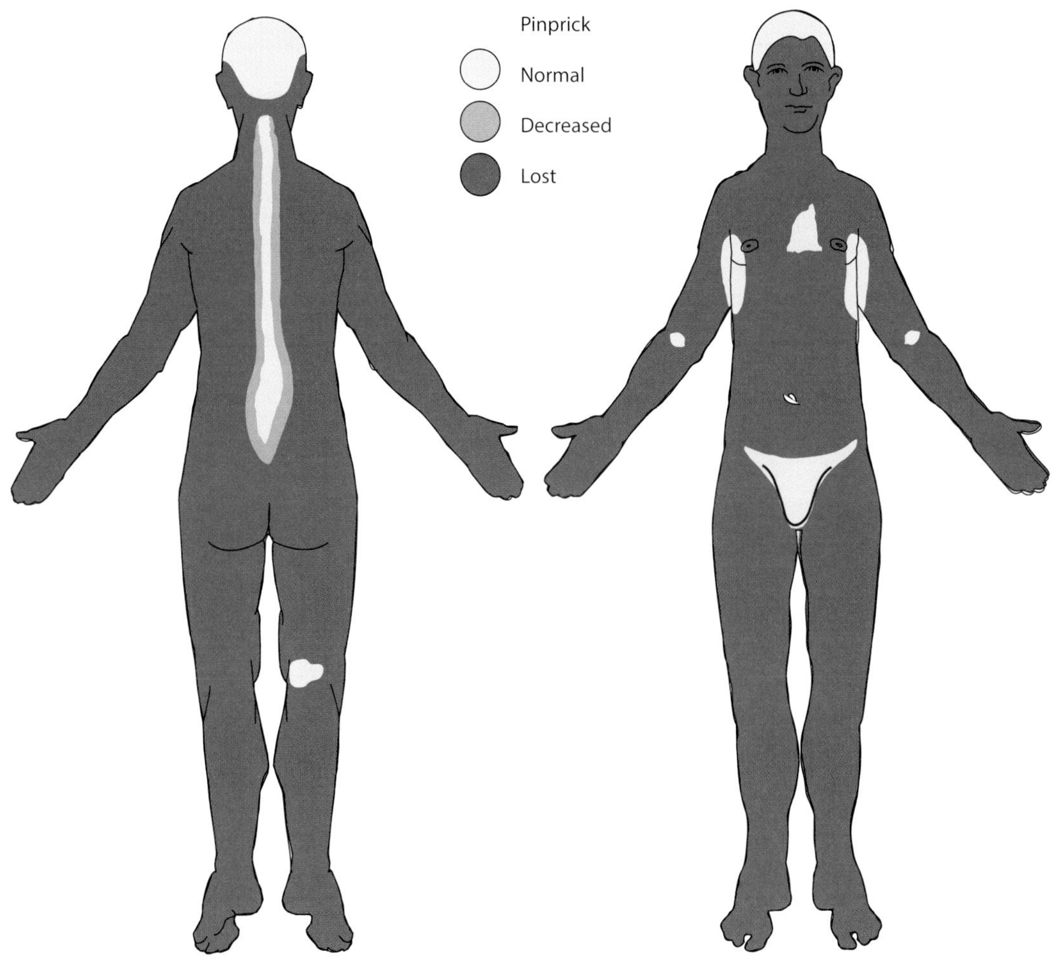

FIGURE 42-9 ■ Lepromatous leprosy (LL). There is sensory sparing of the scalp, in the axillae and the groin, in the center of the back and the chest, and in the antecubital fossae.

therefore, the search must include the ears, nose, and malar areas in order to detect the pattern of temperature-linked sensory loss. This differential diagnosis is also suggested by the preservation of muscle stretch reflexes. Even total destruction of the mixed sensorimotor nerves at the sites outlined earlier would fail to disrupt the arcs for the usually elicited stretch reflexes. Despite the appearance of an extensive sensorimotor neuropathy with clawed toes, foot drop, and clawed hands, preserved muscle stretch reflexes are the rule. Rarely, radial nerve involvement affects the segment that emerges from under the triceps, 4 to 6 cm proximal to the elbow. There is paralysis and atrophy in the wrist and finger extensors, whereas the triceps, brachioradialis, and anconeus muscles tend to be spared. The differential diagnosis of leprous neuritis is summarized in Table 42-1.

A variety of cutaneous lesions are associated with lepromatous leprosy, and they are most abundant and prominent in the areas where bacilli are most common in the cooler tissues. There is no precise linkage between those skin lesions and the intracutaneous sensory loss. Because the tissue immune response to the bacilli in lepromatous leprosy is very indolent, the neuropathy evolves over many years. Nerves that are grossly enlarged and infiltrated with abundant bacilli may still function well. These enlarged nerves are more liable to recurrent trauma, and measures must occasionally be taken to prevent the addition of mechanical damage to these already vulnerable nerves.

TABLE 42-1 ■ Differential Diagnosis of Leprous Neuritis

Neurological Disorder	Clinical Features			
	Paralysis Confined to Major Nerve Trunks	**Preserved Tendon Reflexes**	**Enlarged Nerves**	**Pattern of Sensory Loss**
Peripheral Nerve Diseases				
"Superficial" neuropathy				
Lepromatous leprosy	+	+	+	Unique: superficial loss beginning over coolest body surfaces and certain nerve trunks
Tuberculoid leprosy	+	+	+	Co-terminous with skin lesion and certain nerve trunks
Peripheral neuropathies				
Most toxic, metabolic, and nutritional neuropathies	0	0	0	"Stocking-glove"
Rare types with nerve enlargement (primary amyloidosis, Refsum, Dejerine–Sottas interstitial hypertrophic)	0	0	+	"Stocking-glove"
Mononeuropathy and mononeuropathy multiplex				
Patients with arteritis (lupus, polyarteritis), diabetes, serum neuritis, lead neuropathy, Lyme disease	+	+	0	In distribution of affected nerve trunks
Multifocal motor (and sensory) neuropathy	+	+	0	Localized, e.g., digit or single sensory nerve
Chronic pressure palsies	+	+	0	Nerve trunks
Types with nerve enlargement				
von Recklinghausen neurofibromatosis	+ (& roots)	+	+	Roots or trunks
Sarcoidosis	+ (& roots)	+	+ /0	Roots or trunks
Radiculoneuropathies				
Guillain–Barré syndrome and similar syndromes in diabetes, AIDS, porphyria, and vasculitis	0	0	0	Sensation often spared; deep sensibility loss may be present
Chronic inflammatory demyelinating polyneuropathy	0	0	+ /0	Sensory loss often involving hands, feet, mouth, genitalia
Relapsing demyelinating polyradiculoneuropathy	0	0	0	Deep sensation most affected
Diseases Confused with Leprosy Because of Painless Injuries, with Tropic Ulcers and Absorption of Digits (Not Classified Earlier)				
Syringomyelia	0	0	0	"Forequarter" or "cape" dissociated sensory loss
Universal insensitivity to pain	0	+	0	Pain loss only, whole body affected
Tabes dorsalis	0	0	0	Patchy thermoanalgesia with profound loss of deep sensation

TUBERCULOID LEPROSY

At the other end of the spectrum of host response to infection with *M. leprae* is tuberculoid leprosy. There is a vigorous tissue-mediated immune response to the invasion of bacilli that greatly limits the spread and proliferation of *M. leprae.*[5] Only rare organisms are found in the resulting epithelioid granuloma, and nerve damage occurs as the lesion develops. The lesions contain abundant activated $CD4^+$ T cells that produce IFN-γ.[34] This means that the neurologic picture is generally one of a clearly demarcated patch of sensory loss and absent sweating corresponding with a visible skin lesion that is usually hypopigmented, with an elevated border (Fig. 42-1). Bacteria have often been cleared from the center of these lesions but are still detectable in biopsy samples at the perimeter. Results of lepromin skin testing are positive in this form of the disease. Temperature has only a "permissive" role, in the sense that the lesions must occur in a region where the bacilli can reproduce; tissue temperature does not otherwise determine the precise nature of the neuropathy, as it does in lepromatous disease. Local bacillary invasion of nerves and the immediate immune tissue response are the two factors that result in focal, limited, and asymmetric disease. There is a tendency for self-healing in this type of leprosy. A mixed, motor, or sensory nerve near a solitary tuberculoid patch may also be affected.

These observations have suggested that *M. leprae* can travel from the intracutaneous endings back to the major nerve supplying the area of anesthetic skin. The major mixed nerves that are most commonly affected are the ulnar, median, fibular (peroneal), and facial. Subcutaneous sensory nerves near the tuberculoid patch are most likely to be enlarged, but one should also palpate for enlargement of distant nerves, such as the superficial cutaneous radial, digital, sural, and posterior auricular nerves. The tissue response within nerves may be so intense that there is necrosis and formation of a "cold" abscess. Intense local pain results, requiring surgical drainage of the abscess.[35] Calcification resulting in radiographically detectable linear streaks within nerves may also occur, and enlarged nerves may be demonstrable on computed tomography (CT) scans.[36] Anhidrosis is always present within tuberculoid lesions; injections or iontophoresis of cholinergic agents into the area may be helpful in establishing the diagnosis.

BORDERLINE LEPROSY

Many patients have clinical and pathologic features that fall between polar tuberculoid and lepromatous leprosy, and their conditions are thus classified as borderline leprosy.[5] Such patients demonstrate unending permutations in the roles of tissue temperatures and host resistance in the pathogenesis of their nerve dysfunction. The immunologic reactivity in these patents is unstable, and a drift toward one of the polar patterns occurs over time. The neurologist experienced in leprosy can place patients along a spectrum paralleling a pathologic classification by the pattern of cutaneous sensory loss. Cases of pure neural leprosy with no skin lesions are usually of the borderline type; they are revealed by a good neurologic examination and can be confirmed with nerve biopsy or polymerase chain reaction (PCR) testing.[24] Patients with borderline features that are nearer to tuberculoid disease have several skin lesions that tend to be larger and less distinctly demarcated than those in the pure tuberculoid cases. As one moves away from the tuberculoid end of the spectrum, there is less overlap of the sensory deficit with the visible skin lesion. In the midrange of borderline leprosy, lesions may be quite large and begin to coalesce with insensitivity covering a large area of the body, but they retain borders that do not closely reflect tissue temperature gradients beyond a general tendency to spare the warmest parts of the body (Fig. 42-10). Sensory maps in such cases may show extensive intracutaneous loss that does not conform to the disruption of named peripheral nerves, nerve roots, or any known neuropathy. Further movement toward lepromatous disease is revealed by symmetry of neural deficits and the loss of linkage between the perimeters of skin lesions and areas of sensory loss. A definite tendency toward temperature-linked patterns of sensory loss emerges, but these are not as perfectly symmetric and graduated as in pure lepromatous disease.

TREATMENT

The treatment of leprosy is threefold: (1) drug treatment aimed at the eradication of *M. leprae*, (2) drug treatment of leprosy reactions, and (3) rehabilitation, cosmetic and restorative procedures, and prevention of further deformity consequent to loss of sensation.

The drug treatment of leprosy is changing. Since 1940, sulfones have been the mainstay of treatment, replacing chaulmoogra oil, which had only limited antimycobacterial action. However, with sulfone treatment, many patients developed recurrent disease after periods during which they were apparently free from bacteria. The organisms found at recurrence were shown to be sulfone-resistant using the mouse footpad test.[37]

In addition, sulfones themselves may produce peripheral neuropathy and other idiopathic and

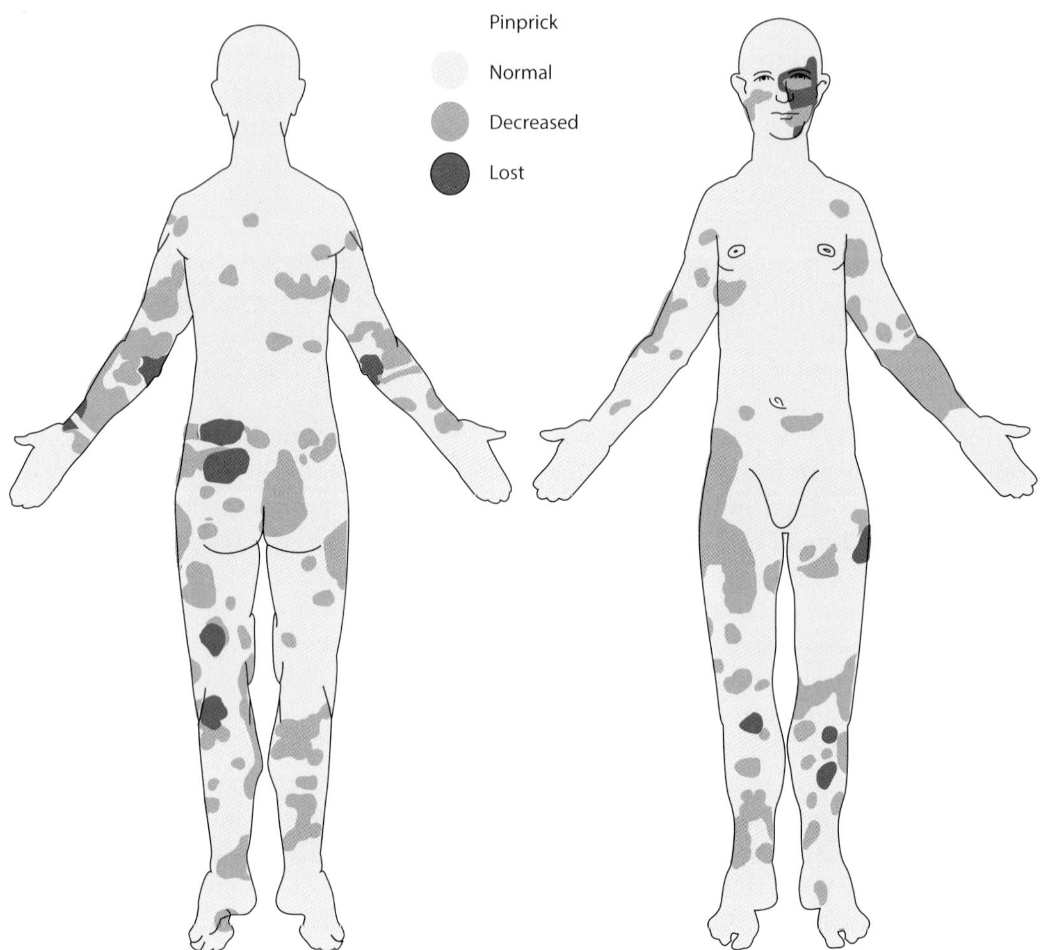

FIGURE 42-10 ▪ Borderline leprosy (BB). Sensory loss occurs in the skin lesions. Skin lesions tend to affect cooler areas.

dose-related side effects, such as hemolysis and, rarely, agranulocytosis.[38] Another useful drug is clofazimine (Lamprene, B663), a rimino phenazine dye, and this drug may be helpful in suppressing erythema nodosum leprosum.[5] However, it discolors the skin and is therefore unacceptable to many patients, and its hepatotoxicity is a major side effect.

In patients with tuberculoid or single skin lesions, current guidelines of the World Health Organization suggest a single-dose combination of rifamycin 600 mg, ofloxacin 400 mg, and minocycline 100 mg.[39] In paucibacillary intermediate disease, rifamycin 600 mg monthly and dapsone 100 mg daily are both given for 6 months. With low-resistance disease (low-resistance borderline and lepromatous leprosy), triple therapy with dapsone, rifamycin, and clofazimine is advocated. Rifamycin 600 mg monthly, clofazimine 300 mg monthly, clofazimine 50 mg daily, and dapsone 100 mg daily are given for 12 to 14 months.[39] For the most recent treatment recommendations, biopsy interpretation, patient referrals, or suggestions for management, the reader should contact the Gillis W. Long Hansen's Disease Center in Baton Rouge, Louisiana.

The treatment of leprosy reactions is important because of the threat that such reactions pose to the patient. Leprosy reactions are of three types. Erythema nodosum leprosum is treated with high-dose corticosteroids (prednisone 60 to 80 mg or more daily), particularly if accompanied by neuritis, or with thalidomide 300 to 400 mg daily. Female patients receiving thalidomide must take absolute precautions to prevent pregnancy because the drug induces phocomelia in offspring. Thalidomide reduces the secretion of TNF-α by monocytes and causes a decrease in the ratio of $CD4^+$ to $CD8^+$ lymphocytes.[20] When erythema nodosum leprosum is controlled, the dose of thalidomide is tapered to 100 mg daily. Long-term thalidomide treatment may also cause or worsen peripheral neuropathy.[40,41] The use of infliximab in resistant erythema nodosum leprosum has been described in a single patient.[23] Reversal reactions, which may be very intense, are treated with high-dose corticosteroids as necessary. Clofazimine in a dose of 200 to 300 mg daily is also of value in treating reactions, in addition to being antibacterial. After the reaction is controlled, the dose can be tapered to 100 mg daily. It is important to note that thalidomide or high doses of corticosteroids are required to treat erythema nodosum leprosum. In tuberculoid and high-resistance borderline leprosy, a reversal reaction consists of a sudden increase in tissue-mediated immunity, with flaring of the skin lesions and acute neuritis. Corticosteroids (but not thalidomide) are effective in these reactions.

Rehabilitation of leprosy patients is difficult because the associated stigma makes patients reluctant to come forward for treatment. Many such patients who have cosmetic and crippling deformities involving the face, eyes, eyelids, eyebrows, ears, nose, hands, and feet may benefit from surgical restorative procedures. The attendant peripheral neuropathy, with loss of temperature and pain sensation and of sweating but with preservation of motor function, creates the risk of progressive damage to hands and feet from painless injury followed by ulceration, infection, osteomyelitis, and eventually bone resorption. Such patients must be instructed in the care of the hands, feet, and eyes to prevent secondary disability resulting from the neuropathy, in a manner similar to patients with other neurologic conditions in which pain sensation is lost but power is retained, such as syringomyelia, hereditary sensory and autonomic neuropathies, amyloid neuropathy, certain cases of diabetic neuropathy involving small fibers, and other conditions. In fact, patients with these neurologic conditions can often be found in leprosariums, where they are mistakenly believed to have leprosy because the mutilating deformities are so similar.

REFERENCES

1. Hansen GA: Umder sogeiser angaende spedalskhedens arsager tiedels und forte sammen med forstander Hartwig. Norske Mag Laegevidensk Suppl 4:1, 1874.
2. Cole ST, Eiglmeier K, Parkhill J, et al: Massive gene decay in the leprosy bacillus. Nature 409:1007, 2001.
3. Monet M, Honore N, Garnier T, et al: On the origin of leprosy. Science 308:1040, 2005.
4. Anonymous: Global leprosy: update on the 2012 situation. WHO Weekly Epidemiol Rec 88:365, 2013.
5. Jacobson RR, Krahenbuhl JL: Leprosy. Lancet 353:655, 1999.
6. Rambukkana A, Salzer JL, Yurchenco PD, et al: Neural targeting of *Mycobacterium leprae* mediated by the G domain of the laminin-a2 chain. Cell 88:811, 1997.
7. Tapinos N, Rambukkana A: Insights into regulation of human Schwann cell proliferation by Erk1/2 via a MEK-independent and p56Lck-dependent pathway from leprosy bacilli. Proc Natl Acad Sci USA 102:9188, 2005.
8. Shepard CC: Temperature optimum of *Mycobacterium leprae* in mice. J Bacteriol 90:1271, 1965.
9. Sabin TD: Facing the human face of disease. Hosp Pract 28:86, 1993.
10. Valverde CR, Canfield O, Tarara R, et al: Spontaneous leprosy in a wild caught cynomolgus macaque. Int J Lepr Other Mycobact Dis 66:140, 1998.
11. Facer P, Mathur R, Pandya SS, et al: Correlation of quantitative tests of nerve and target organ dysfunction with skin immunohistology in leprosy. Brain 121:2239, 1998.
12. Britton WJ, Lockwood DNJ: Leprosy. Lancet 363:1209, 2004.
13. Jacob M, Mathai R: Diagnostic efficacy of cutaneous nerve biopsy in primary neuritic leprosy. Int J Lepr Other Mycobact Dis 56:56, 1988.
14. Mahajan PM, Joglekar DG, Mehta JM: A study of pure neuritic leprosy: clinical experience. Indian J Lepr 68:137, 1996.
15. Medeiros MF, Jardim MR, Vital RT, et al: An attempt to improve pure neural leprosy diagnosis using immunohistochemistry tests in peripheral nerve biopsy specimens. Appl Immunohistochem Mol Morphol in press, 2013.
16. Ustianowski AP, Lawn SD, Lockwood DN: Interactions between HIV infection and leprosy: a paradox. Lancet Infect Dis 6:350, 2006.
17 de Oliveira AL, Amadeu TP, de França Gomes AC, et al: Role of $CD8^{+}$ T cells in triggering reversal reaction in HIV/leprosy patients. Immunology 140:47, 2013.
18. Little D, Khanolkar-Young S, Coulthart A, et al: Immunohistochemical analysis of cellular infiltrate and gamma interferon, interleukin-12, and inducible nitric acid synthetase expression in leprosy type I (reversal) reactions before and during prednisolone treatment. Infect Immunol 69:3413, 2001.
19. Becx-Bleumink M, Berhe D: Occurrence of reactions, their diagnosis and management in leprosy patients treated with multidrug therapy: experience in the leprosy control program of the All Africa Leprosy and Rehabilitation Training Center (ALERT) in Ethiopia. Int J Lepr Other Mycobact Dis 60:173, 1992.
20. Shannon EJ, Ejigu M, Haile-Mariam HS, et al: Thalidomide's effectiveness in erythema nodosum leprosum is associated with a decrease in $CD4^{+}$ cells in the peripheral blood. Leprosy Rev 63:5, 1992.

21. Miller RA, Shen JY, Rea TH, et al: Treatment of chronic erythema nodosum leprosum with cyclosporine A produces clinical and immunohistologic remission. Int J Lepr Other Mycobact Dis 55:441, 1987.
22. Uyemura K, Dixon JF, Wong L, et al: Effect of cyclosporine A in erythema nodosum leprosum. J Immunol 137:3620, 1986.
23. Faber WR, Jensema AJ: Goldschmidt WFM: Treatment of recurrent erythema nodosum leprosum with infliximab. N Engl J Med 355:739, 2006.
24. Bezzera DA, Cunha FM, Werneck MC, et al: Pure neural leprosy: diagnostic value of the polymerase chain reaction. Muscle Nerve 33:409, 2006.
25. Brand PW: Temperature variation and leprosy deformity. Int J Lepr 27:1, 1959.
26. Hastings RC, Brand PW, Mansfield RE, et al: Bacterial density in the skin in lepromatous leprosy as related to temperature. Lepr Rev 39:71, 1968.
27. Sabin TD, Hackett ER, Brand PW: Temperatures along the course of certain nerves affected in leprosy. Int J Lepr Other Mycobact Dis 42:38, 1974.
28. Zhang F-R, Huang W, Chen S-M, et al: Genomewide association study of leprosy. N Engl J Med 361:2609, 2009.
29. Sabin TD: Temperature-linked sensory loss: a unique pattern in leprosy. Arch Neurol 20:257, 1969.
30. Sabin TD, Ebner JE: Patterns of sensory loss in lepromatous leprosy. Int J Lepr Other Mycobact Dis 37:239, 1969.
31. Monrad-Krohn GH: The Neurological Aspect of Leprosy. Jacob Dybward, Christiana, 1923.
32. Sabin TD: Preservation of sensation in a cutaneous vascular malformation in lepromatous leprosy. N Engl J Med 282:1084, 1970.
33. Conejo-Mir SJ, Artola-Igarzaul JL, Gareianda C, et al: Lepromatous leprosy in a patient with hemiplegia. Clin Infect Dis 1:212, 1998.
34. Yamamura M, Wang X-H, Ohman JD, et al: Cytokine patterns of immunological mediated tissue damage. J Immunol 149:1470, 1992.
35. Siddalingaswamy MK, Rao KS: Nerve abscess in leprosy: a retrospective study. Lepr Rev 64:357, 1993.
36. Barbancon O, Rath S, Alqubati Y: Hansen's disease: computed tomography findings in peripheral nerve lesions. Ann Radiol (Paris) 32:579, 1989.
37. Shepard CC: Experimental chemotherapy in leprosy, then and now. Int J Lepr Other Mycobact Dis 41:307, 1973.
38. Sirsat AM, Lalitha VS, Pandya SS: Dapsone neuropathy: report of three cases and pathologic features of a motor nerve. Int J Lepr Other Mycobact Dis 55:23, 1987.
39. WHO Expert Committee on Leprosy. World Health Organization Tech Rep Serv 874:1, 1998.
40. Awofeso N: Thalidomide peripheral neuropathy. Trop Doct 22:139, 1992.
41. Gunzler V: Thalidomide in human immunodeficiency virus (HIV) patients: a review of safety considerations. Drug Saf 7:116, 1992.

CHAPTER

43

Nervous System Complications of Systemic Viral Infections

JOHN E. GREENLEE

Invasion of the central nervous system (CNS) by viruses typically produces a meningoencephalitis in which either meningitis or encephalitis may predominate. Viruses may also infect cranial or spinal blood vessels leading to ischemic injury. Systemic or CNS infection by viruses or other infectious agents may elicit a host immune response that is cross-reactive with components of neural tissue, resulting in encephalomyelitis, transverse myelitis, injury to peripheral nerves, or optic neuritis.

PATHOGENESIS OF VIRAL CNS INFECTIONS

Before a virus can infect the CNS, it must first breach the cutaneous or mucosal barriers that protect the patient from the outside environment and then penetrate the blood–brain barrier to gain access to susceptible cells in the meninges, brain, or spinal cord. At each step, the virus must infect specific cell populations and produce progeny virus in order to continue the infection. Viruses can enter the body through ingestion, as in enterovirus infections, by the respiratory route, as in influenza or chicken pox, by inoculation across skin, as in arthropod-borne encephalitides or rabies, or across mucosal membranes, as in human immunodeficiency virus (HIV) infection. Virtually all viruses capable of infecting the CNS do so via hematogenous spread; exceptions are the rabies virus and herpes simplex viruses types 1 and 2 (HSV-1, HSV-2), all of which travel from the periphery to the CNS within peripheral nerves. Varicella zoster virus (VZV) is transported within nerves during reactivated infection.

Infection at the cellular level may occur through several mechanisms. Herpesviruses are taken into the cell following fusion of the viral envelope to the host cell.[1] The human polyomavirus, JC virus (JCV), the etiologic agent of progressive multifocal leukoencephalopathy (PML), reacts with serotonin and other receptors in this process.[2] Alphaviruses, such as St. Louis encephalitis virus, recognize cell surface laminin and heparan molecules.[3] Viral replication within the host cell may result in various outcomes including lytic infection with cell death; productive infection with budding of viruses across

Aminoff's Neurology and General Medicine, Fifth Edition.
Published by Elsevier Inc.

the cell membrane without death of the host cell; or persistent infection, with the virus remaining latent over time.[2,4] Classic examples of viruses causing latent infection include HSV-1, HSV-2, and VZV, all of which persist in sensory ganglia and may reactivate to cause several syndromes including cutaneous lesions and CNS disease.[4]

Host response to viral infections initially involves innate immune responses and natural killer cells. Resolution of infection, however, involves both production of antibody and development of specific T-cell–mediated immune responses. Antibody is required to control and clear enteroviruses, and failure of antibody response may result in progressive enteroviral encephalitis. In contrast, immune control of West Nile virus (WNV) involves both B and T cells.[5,6] Failure of host T-cell response is a major factor in the pathogenesis of PML, as is alteration in CNS T-cell immune surveillance following treatment with the immunomodulatory drug natalizumab in disorders such as multiple sclerosis.[2,7] $CD8^+$ T cells are important in maintaining HSV and VZV in their latent states and in controlling both primary and reactivated infection.[4] In general, the host immune response is protective, although the inflammatory process that results may augment cerebral edema; however, CNS or systemic infections may also elicit an immune response cross-reactive with antigens to the central or peripheral nervous system, leading to postinfectious neurologic injury.

VIRAL MENINGITIS

Acute viral meningitis is most commonly a disease of children and young adults and is the most frequent CNS complication of viral infection.[8] Viral meningitis accounts for an estimated 400,000 hospitalizations yearly in the United States. Major causative agents in Western countries are enteroviruses (accounting for up to 77% of cases), HSV-2 (10 to 20% of cases), and VZV (10 to 20% of cases) (Table 43-1).[8–12] A minority of cases are caused by WNV or other arthropod-borne agents, HIV, HSV-1, lymphocytic choriomeningitis virus (LCMV), or other agents.[13–16] In northern Europe, cases may be associated with tick-borne encephalitis virus and in southern Europe with Toscana virus.[16,17] In Asia, Japanese encephalitis virus is a common etiologic agent.[18] In 35 to 50 percent of cases, no agent is identified.[9,16]

The clinical presentation of viral meningitis in adults is similar to that of bacterial meningitis, although patients usually are less acutely ill (Table 43-2). Onset of meningeal symptoms may be preceded by fever and other symptoms of systemic illness, but viral meningitis often is of abrupt onset with severe headache and nuchal rigidity.[8] Although headache is most commonly the presenting symptom, it may be not be evident in infants and may be less prominent in young children and immunosuppressed individuals. Patients may exhibit photophobia, nausea, vomiting, and, in some cases, irritability and lethargy. Progression to obtundation or coma is rare without accompanying encephalitis. Some patients may have other evidence of systemic viral infection such as pharyngitis or rash, but abnormalities on general physical examination are often absent. Meningeal signs are typically less severe than in bacterial meningitis and may be subtle. The neurologic examination otherwise is usually unremarkable, and the presence of focal neurologic signs should raise concern that some other process is present.[8]

Enteroviruses

Enteroviruses are unenveloped single-stranded RNA viruses forming a genus in the family picornavirus. They account for 70 to 80 percent of cases of viral meningitis in which an agent is identified.[8,19] Enteroviruses survive well in water and sewage, are transmitted by fecal-oral or hand-mouth routes, and replicate initially in the gastrointestinal tract. Enteroviruses were previously subdivided into three groups: polioviruses, echoviruses, and coxsackieviruses. Newer isolated enteroviruses have been assigned numbers (e.g., enterovirus 71 or EV 71). Coxsackievirus A9 and echoviruses E7, E9, E11, E19, and E30 have accounted for 70 percent of all cultured isolates from cerebrospinal fluid (CSF) in cases of enteroviral meningitis. Polioviruses have been largely eradicated, persisting only in Nigeria, Pakistan, and Afghanistan. Other enteroviruses have a worldwide distribution, and although cases of enteroviral meningitis occur throughout the year, infection is most likely to occur during summer and early fall months when conditions of sanitation are most lax. Acute enterovirus infection is usually asymptomatic or may result in mild gastroenteritis or pharyngitis; less than 5 percent of patients will develop meningitis or encephalitis.[19]

Enteroviral CNS infection typically causes meningitis rather than encephalitis, with fever, headache, and stiff neck.[19] These symptoms commonly last for 1 to 3 weeks in older children and adults. In occasional patients, enteroviruses may cause encephalitis or rarely a paralytic disease similar to polioviruses (see below) and may cause protracted, atypical infection in immunocompromised patients.

Herpes Simplex Virus Type 2

HSV-2 is a double-stranded DNA virus that is universal in human populations. HSV-2 is usually transmitted sexually, with antiviral antibodies first appearing in adolescence or early adult life. Following acute infection, the virus persists predominantly in spinal sensory ganglia and is subject to periodic reactivation, often without cutaneous or mucosal signs of infection.[20] HSV-2 accounts for up to 10 to 20 percent of isolates in adults with viral meningitis and is roughly twice as common among women.[20,21] HSV-2 as a cause of viral meningitis should be considered particularly in young, sexually active adults.[21] Older data suggested that up to 36 percent of women and 11 percent of men had headache, fever, or nuchal rigidity at the time of their first attack of genital herpes.[21,22] Some patients with HSV-2 meningitis following genital herpes may have focal lumbosacral symptoms including urinary retention suggesting nerve root infection, and the virus may also be associated with myelitis.[20,21] HSV-2 DNA can frequently be detected in CSF by amplification using the polymerase chain reaction (PCR).[21] Approximately 20 percent of individuals with acute HSV-2 meningitis may subsequently develop recurrent episodes of meningitis (Mollaret meningitis).[21] Many individuals with recurrent meningitis have no history of genital herpes and lack genital lesions during attacks of meningitis.

Patients with HSV-2 meningitis usually recover without treatment. Although successful treatment with acyclovir has been described in individual cases, the efficacy of antiviral therapy in acute or recurrent HSV-2 meningitis is uncertain.[23,24] In a recent trial, suppressive treatment with valacyclovir did not prohibit recurrence of HSV-2 meningitis.[25]

Varicella Zoster Virus

VZV is a herpesvirus typically associated with chicken pox during acute infection and with cutaneous zoster (shingles) during reactivated infection. Like HSV-2, VZV is thought to account for 10 to 20 percent of identified cases of viral meningitis.[8–12] Meningitis may occur during either primary or reactivated infection and may do so in the absence of rash.[26–30] In contrast to many other viruses, VZV meningitis may result in significant CSF hypoglychorrachia and may be accompanied by a CSF pleocytosis characterized by atypical lymphocytes.[29,30] As with HSV-2 meningitis, most immunocompetent patients with VZV meningitis recover without treatment. VZV infection may produce a wide variety of other neurologic conditions, which are discussed in greater detail later.

Less Common Causes of Viral Meningitis

The arthropod-borne agents—WNV, St. Louis encephalitis virus, California encephalitis virus, Powassan virus, and Colorado tick fever virus—are most commonly associated with encephalitis, but may also cause meningitis. WNV, St. Louis encephalitis virus, and California encephalitis virus are transmitted by mosquitoes and tend to be more common in summer and early autumn months. The tick-borne agents Powassan virus and Colorado tick fever virus can cause a rash and most frequently occur during spring and early summer months. An important consideration in patients with suspected Colorado tick fever is the tick-borne rickettsial illness Rocky Mountain spotted fever, which also has a peak incidence in spring and summer, usually has a rash, and requires antibiotic treatment.[31]

LCMV is an arenavirus whose natural host is mice but which can cause meningitis and, less frequently, encephalitis in humans. The virus is present in mouse urine and is acquired by the respiratory route. At one time, it was thought to account for roughly 4 percent of diagnosed cases of viral meningitis, but in recent years it has become much less common, for unknown reasons.[15,32] LCMV infections are classically most common in autumn and winter. Occasional outbreaks of infection have been associated with exposure to mice in animal facilities or to pet hamsters or guinea pigs.[15] The meningitis associated with LCMV may be accompanied by low CSF glucose levels, which may persist in cases of prolonged recovery over weeks to months.[33] In neonates, LCMV may cause a fatal systemic and CNS infection.[34] Outbreaks of severe infection with high mortality have also been reported in which LCMV

TABLE 43-1 ■ Major Viral Agents Associated With Human Neurologic Disease

Viruses	Genus (Family)	Animal Reservoir	Transmission	Geographic Location	Peak Season[a]	Neurologic Syndromes	Acute Diagnosis[b,c]	Treatment
Major Viruses in North America and Europe								
Coxsackieviruses Echoviruses Enterovirus 71 and other numbered enteroviruses	Enteroviruses (Picornaviridae)	No	Fecal-oral spread	Worldwide	Summer to early autumn	Meningitis (Encephalitis)[d] (Poliomyelitis)	CSF PCR	Supportive (Pleconaril)[e]
Herpes simplex virus type 1 (HSV-1)	Herpesviruses (Herpesviridae)	No	Human contact	Worldwide	No seasonal distribution	Encephalitis	CSF PCR	Acyclovir
Herpes simplex virus type 2 (HSV-2)[f]	Herpesviruses (Herpesviridae)	No	Human contact	Worldwide	No seasonal distribution	Meningitis Recurrent meningitis Myelitis	CSF PCR	Acyclovir[g]
Varicella zoster virus	Herpesviruses (Herpesviridae)	No	Respiratory or human contact	Worldwide	No seasonal distribution	Shingles Post-herpetic neuralgia Meningitis Vasculitis involving brain, spinal cord, eye, peripheral nervous system (Encephalitis)	CSF PCR (acute infection) CSF IgM and IgG (reactivated infection)	Acyclovir Valacyclovir[g]
Cytomegalovirus[h]	Herpesviruses (Herpesviridae)	No	Human contact	Worldwide	No seasonal distribution	Encephalitis (infants or immunocompromised patients)	CSF PCR	Gancyclovir (Foscarnet)
Human herpesvirus 6[i]	Herpesviruses (Herpesviridae)	No	Human contact	Worldwide	No seasonal distribution	Meningitis Encephalitis	CSF PCR	Gancyclovir, Foscarnet
West Nile virus	Togaviruses (Flaviviridae)	Birds, esp. crows, jays, magpies	Mosquito sp. Organ transplantation	USA excepting Alaska and Hawaii[j]	Summer to early autumn	Meningitis Encephalitis Poliomyelitis	CSF IgM	Supportive
St. Louis encephalitis virus	Togaviruses (Flaviviridae)	Small mammals	Mosquito sp.	USA excepting Alaska and Hawaii	Summer to early autumn	Meningitis Encephalitis	CSF IgM	Supportive
Eastern equine encephalitis virus	Alphavirus (Togaviridae)	Salt marsh and other birds	Mosquito sp.	Atlantic seabord, Gulf coast, upper Midwest	Summer to early autumn	Meningitis Encephalitis	CSF IgM (PCR)	Supportive
California/ LaCrosse virus[i]	(Bunyaviridae)	Small mammals	Mosquito sp.	USA, esp. Midwestern and mid-Atlantic states	Summer to early autumn	Meningitis Encephalitis	CSF IgM	Supportive
Colorado tick fever	Orbivirus (Reoviridae)	Small mammals	Tick sp.	Western USA (esp. mountain states), western Canada	Spring to mid-summer	Meningitis Encephalitis	PCR CSF IgM	Supportive
Lymphocytic choriomeningitis virus (LCMV)[k]	Arenavirus (Arenaviridae)	Mice (hamsters)	Aerosol	Worldwide	Autumn to winter	Meningitis Encephalitis	PCR CSF IgM Serum and CSF IgM and IgG	Supportive

(HIV1, HIV2)	Human immunodeficiency virus (Retroviridae)	None	Intimate sexual contact; IV drug abuse	Worldwide	No seasonal distribution	Meningitis acutely	PCR Serology	Antiretroviral treatment
JC virus[h]	Polyoma virus (Polyomaviridae)	None	Unknown	Worldwide	No seasonal distribution	PML	PCR	Supportive [l]
Viruses Which Are Uncommon in North America but May Occur in Individuals Exposed in Endemic Areas								
Mumps virus[m]	Rubalavirus (Paramyxoviridae)	None	Respiratory spread	Worldwide	January to May	Meningitis Encephalitis	CSF PCR	Supportive
Toscana virus	Phlebovirus (Bunyaviridae)	Reservoir in nature unknown	Sand fly	Italy, other Mediterranean countries	May to September	Meningitis (Encephalitis)	CSF PCR	Supportive
Japanese encephalitis virus	Flavivirus (Flaviviridae)	Pigs, wild birds (herons)	Mosquito sp.	Southeast Asia and Far East	Following wet season: varies by country	Encephalitis	CSF IgM	Supportive
Nipah virus	Henipavirus (Paramyxoviridae)	Pteropid fuit bats	Consumption of food contaminated with infected bat saliva or urine Human-to-human	India, Bangladesh, Southeast Asia, Indonesia, Australia	No seasonal distribution	Encephalitis	PCR CSF IgM Serum serology	Supportive
Venezuelan equine encephalitis	Alphavirus (Togaviridae)	Birds, small mammals	Mosquito sp.	South and Central America, extreme southern USA	No seasonal distribution	Encephalitis (Meningitis)	PCR	Supportive
Tick-borne encephalitis virus	Flavivirus (Flaviviridae)	Birds, small mammals	Tick sp. Unpasteurized milk	Europe, former Soviet Union, Asia	April to November	Meningitis Encephalitis	PCR	Supportive
Rabies virus	Lissavirus (Rhabdoviridae)	Bats, skunks, foxes, raccoons Unvaccinated dogs	Animal bite Aerosol (Organ transplantation)	Worldwide	No seasonal distribution	Encephalitis ("furious" or "dumb" rabies) Ascending motor paralysis[n]	PCR (CSF) Nuchal biopsy	Supportive

[a]Sporadic cases of many agents may occur outside peak season.
[b]Retrospective diagnosis may be made by comparing antibody titers in acute and convalescent sera or by comparing serum:CSF ratios of antibody against those of other agents.
[c]Diagnostic methods for common agents such as HSV-1, HSV-2, enteroviruses, West Nile virus, and varicella zoster virus are readily available through many hospital and commercial laboratories. Advice concerning less usual infections may be obtained through the Centers for Disease Control and Prevention.
[d]Less frequent forms of illness are shown in parentheses.
[e]Not available in the United States.
[f]HSV-2 meningitis may occur as a single event but may also be recurrent and is the major cause of Mollaret meningitis.
[g]Mild cases of HSV-2 meningitis may not require treatment. Severe HSV-2 meningitis may require treatment with acyclovir. Treatment of recurrent HSV-2 meningitis may employ valacyclovir.
[h]Immunocompromised patients
[i]Predominantly an infection of children
[j]West Nile virus also present in much of Europe, Egypt, Israel, Africa, India, and western Asia.
[k]A murine virus. Infections also reported after exposure to infected pet hamsters.
[l]Treatment in AIDS involves suppression of HIV with antiretroviral therapy; treatment in patients developing PML in the setting of natalizumab therapy (and possible other monoclonal agents) has consisted of withdrawal of the monoclonal agent and plasma exchange to reduce circulating levels of the monoclonal antibody.
[m]Previously a major cause of viral meningitis in the United States. Still a major cause of meningitis in countries where vaccination is not routine. Associated with occasional outbreaks of infection in unvaccinated individuals in the United States and Europe.
[n]Incubation period may be 3 or more years. Obtaining history of exposure should take this into account.

TABLE 43-2 ■ Signs and Symptoms of Viral Meningitis

Common
Headache
Fever
Nausea, vomiting
Stiff neck (not present in all cases; may be subtle)
Less Common
Lethargy, mild confusion, irritability*
Seizures*
Systemic signs including rash, diarrhea, pharyngitis, myalgias, adenopathy (with mumps parotitis)

*Impaired consciousness, seizures, and focal neurologic signs suggest the likelihood of encephalitis or other severe infections (meningitis, parameningeal infection, brain abscess).

has been transmitted by organ transplantation.[35,36] Reliable antiviral therapy for LCMV infection is not available; one patient with transplant-acquired LCMV infection recovered after reduction of the patient's immunosuppressive regimen and treatment with ribavirin.[35]

Mumps virus, once a major cause of meningitis worldwide, is now rare in developed countries but remains a significant cause of meningitis in areas where mumps immunization is not practiced.[37] The virus has caused occasional epidemics in Western countries in unvaccinated populations exposed to individuals who have visited areas where mumps is still prevalent.[37–39]

Human Immunodeficiency Virus

CNS invasion occurs early in the course of primary HIV infection, and meningitis due directly to HIV occurs in 9 to 24 percent of patients (see Chapter 44).[40,41] The meningitis usually develops near the time of seroconversion and often occurs in the setting of an acute, mononucleosis-like retroviral syndrome characterized by fever, pharyngitis, and cervical lymphadenopathy; CNS findings of disorientation, confusion, or psychosis accompany this syndrome in some patients.[40] Primary HIV meningitis should be considered in young adults with meningitis, particularly when they have HIV risk factors or a coexistent mononucleosis-like syndrome. The symptoms of meningitis are usually not severe and resolve in most but not all cases; in some patients, HIV meningitis becomes chronic.[40] The CSF typically reveals a mild lymphocytic pleocytosis, mildly elevated protein content, and normal glucose level.[40] Standard serologic tests for HIV (as well as tests for home use) are negative in many patients with this acute syndrome; serologic tests first become positive 22 to 27 days after onset of acute infection.[41] The diagnosis of acute HIV meningitis is made by detecting viral RNA or viral p24 antigen in serum or plasma; the viral RNA usually becomes detectable 3 to 5 days prior to the detection of p24 antigen and is typically present in copy numbers greater than 50,000 copies/ml.[41] Treatment of HIV is with antiretroviral therapy, and follow-up assay for antiviral antibodies is used to confirm the diagnosis. In approaching patients with suspected HIV meningitis, it must be kept in mind that lymphocytic meningitis in patients with HIV infection may be caused by a wide variety of other agents, many of which are treatable.[40]

Approach to Patients with Viral Meningitis

Bacterial meningitis is the primary concern in any patient presenting with acute meningitis. If the patient is severely ill, bacterial meningitis should be suspected and presumptive antibiotic therapy should be initiated immediately, usually along with corticosteroids. Similarly, acyclovir should be initiated if HSV encephalitis is a significant diagnostic concern. Antibiotics and acyclovir can be discontinued once CSF studies are negative. In general, patients presenting with viral meningitis are less severely ill, and antibiotic and acyclovir treatment may often be deferred.

The diagnosis of viral meningitis is made by lumbar puncture and CSF analysis. In acute bacterial meningitis, there is often an elevated opening pressure and typically a marked neutrophilic pleocytosis, with significantly elevated protein and depressed glucose concentrations.[33] In contrast, in viral meningitis the opening pressure is usually normal or mildly elevated, and the CSF white cell count is usually in the range of 50 to 2000/ml. Although viral meningitis typically produces a lymphocytic pleocytosis, polymorphonuclear leukocytes may constitute over 50 percent of the cells during the first 24 to 36 hours of the infection and may occasionally remain the predominant cell type for longer periods of time.[33] Protein is usually elevated in the range of 50 to 100 mg/dl but is sometimes higher.[33] The CSF glucose level in viral meningitis is usually greater than 50 percent of blood glucose; the absence of CSF hypoglychorrhachia is an important consideration in differentiating viral from bacterial meningitis. Depression of glucose to levels approaching those of bacterial meningitis may occasionally occur in meningitis caused by HSV-2, VZV, mumps, and LCMV.[33] In the proper setting, lymphocytic pleocytosis with low CSF glucose may also raise concern about tuberculous or fungal meningitis.

Specific diagnosis of viral agents in CSF currently involves PCR amplification of viral RNA or DNA; at present, tissue culture isolation of virus is rarely performed for diagnostic purposes (Table 43-1).[33] PCR is rapid and has a high level of sensitivity in meningitis due to enteroviruses, HSV-2, and VZV during acute infection.[33] PCR can identify all strains of enteroviruses but does not distinguish between individual strains.[33] Enteroviral RNA can be identified in CSF in the first 1 or 2 days of meningitis, from throat for several days, and from stool for a few weeks. Because asymptomatic enterovirus infections are common in the summer months, enterovirus isolation from throat or stool does not make a definitive diagnosis of enterovirus meningitis. In one study, use of an enterovirus PCR assay in the emergency department in children with aseptic meningitis resulted in significantly less antibiotic use, shorter length of hospitalization, and lower hospital costs.[42] Although it is the diagnostic study of choice in many viral meningitides, CSF PCR may be negative early in the disease course, and diagnostic yield may be highest when CSF is obtained within 3 to 14 days of onset of meningitis.[43] In certain instances, the detection of CSF immunoglobulins may have greater diagnostic sensitivity than PCR. This is the case in WNV neuroinvasive disease and other arbovirus infections, in which detection of virus-specific immunoglobulin M (IgM) is more sensitive than PCR.[33] Similarly, detection of virus-specific IgG in CSF may prove diagnostic in infections due to protracted or reactivated VZV where PCR is negative.[44] Identification of the causative agent in viral meningitis may be made retrospectively by detecting a rise in IgG antibody titers between acute and convalescent (obtained after 3 to 6 weeks) serum or, at times, by detecting an abnormal serum:CSF ratio of antiviral antibodies.

Other laboratory studies in viral meningitis are usually unhelpful. Peripheral white blood cell count may be normal or elevated. Computed tomography (CT) scans and magnetic resonance imaging (MRI) of the brain are typically normal. The electroencephalogram (EEG) is usually normal but may occasionally show mild background slowing. Marked asymmetries or seizure foci should not be seen unless encephalitis predominates.

Viral meningitis is sometimes referred to by the older term "aseptic meningitis." This term, however, subsumes a broad range of clinical entities characterized by a meningeal reaction but distinct from purulent bacterial meningitis. It may include not only viral meningitis but also infections by bacteria that are not readily detected in routine cultures (*Leptospira icterohaemorrhagiae, Borrelia burgdorferi, Treponema pallidum, Mycoplasma pneumoniae*), meningeal involvement by *Rickettsia, Ehrlichia*, or *Anaplasma*, and infection by parasites such as *Toxoplasma gondii*. The possibility of infection by one of these agents should be kept in mind in a patient with suspected viral meningitis, since all are amenable to antibiotic treatment. In particular, *Borrelia burgdorferi* can be a major cause of lymphocytic meningitis in endemic areas (see Chapter 40).[45,46] Aseptic meningitis may also be associated with a variety of pharmacologic agents including nonsteroidal anti-inflammatory agents, trimethoprim-sulfamethoxazole, augmentin, carbamazepine, intravenous immunoglobulin G, and the murine monoclonal antibody OKT3.[47,48]

Treatment of viral meningitis is supportive in most cases. Analgesics may be required for individuals with severe headaches, and antiemetics for those with considerable nausea and vomiting. Hospitalization is seldom required except when vomiting is severe enough to cause dehydration or when bacterial meningitis cannot be excluded. Acyclovir and valacyclovir have been used to shorten the duration of illness in acute meningitis due to HSV-2 and VZV (Table 43-3).[49] However, controlled studies do not exist, and no standardized regimen has been developed.[24,50] Patients with recurrent HSV meningitis may wish to keep oral acyclovir or valacyclovir at home and take the drug at the onset of meningeal symptoms. Ongoing twice daily treatment with valacyclovir at a dose of 0.5 mg has not been shown to prevent recurrence, but higher dosages were not studied.[25] The antiviral agent pleconaril, which prevents uncoating of viral RNA, has been used in enteroviral meningitis but is not routinely available in the United States.[51,52]

As a group, patients with viral meningitis generally make a complete recovery within 1 to 2 weeks. Not all patients recover this quickly, however, and

TABLE 43-3 ■ Antiviral Agents Used for CNS Infections

Antiviral	Mechanism of Action	Indication	Regimen in Adults	Major Adverse Effects
Acyclovir	Competes with deoxyguanosine triphosphate as a substrate for DNA polymerase. Causes viral DNA chain termination. Converted to active form in infected cells	HSV encephalitis Severe HSV meningitis VZV encephalitis, CNS vasculitis or severe meningitis	10 mg/kg intravenously every 8 hours for 21 days	Nephrotoxicity: may cause renal failure if patient not adequately hydrated Psychosis Stevens–Johnson syndrome Tissue necrosis
		Recurrent HSV-2 meningitis	800 mg orally 5 times daily for 5–7 days	
		Varicella (chicken pox) or Herpes zoster (shingles)	800 mg orally 5 times daily for 5–7 days	
Valacyclovir	Same as acyclovir	HSV meningitis (esp. recurrent)	1,000 mg every 8 hours for 7 days	Similar to acyclovir
		Herpes zoster (shingles)	1,000 mg every 8 hours for 7 days	
Ganciclovir	Similar to acyclovir: inhibits viral DNA polymerization	Encephalitis due to cytomegalovirus or HHV-6	5 mg/kg every 12 hours for 14–21 days	Hematologic toxicity (anemia, leukopenia, thrombocytopenia) Nephrotoxicity: may cause renal failure if patient not adequately hydrated
Foscarnet	Selective inhibition of viral DNA polymerase	Encephalitis due to cytomegalovirus or HHV-6; acyclovir-resistant VZV	90 mg/kg intravenously every 12 hours for 14–21 days	Hematologic toxicity (anemia, leukopenia, thrombocytopenia) Nephrotoxicity: may cause renal failure if patient not adequately hydrated

HSV, herpes simplex virus; VZV, varicella zoster virus; HHV-6, human herpesvirus type 6.

symptoms such as fatigue may last for weeks or even months. CSF abnormalities may also persist for well beyond the initial period of recovery.[33] In addition, there have been occasional reports of permanent sequelae, usually but not always in small children, including cognitive impairment, deafness, and cranial nerve palsies.[53–57] Aqueductal stenosis with hydrocephalus is a rare complication of HSV-2 and mumps meningitis.[58,59]

VIRAL ENCEPHALITIS

Viral encephalitis is caused by viral infection of cells within the brain parenchyma (Table 43-4). The cell populations in which viral replication occurs differ among the various viruses and may involve neurons, glia, or, at times, vascular endothelial cells. The result of the infection may be death of specific cell populations or more widespread destruction involving multiple cell types. Viruses affecting unique populations of cells include rabies, which infects neurons exclusively; poliomyelitis, which involves spinal and other motor neurons; and JC virus, which causes lytic infection almost exclusively in oligodendrocytes. Viruses infecting multiple cell types, often with extensive parenchymal destruction, include HSV and agents of the arthropod-borne encephalitides. Parenchymal destruction in severe infections such as herpes simplex encephalitis may be accompanied by hemorrhage. Virtually all viral encephalitides are accompanied by some degree of meningeal inflammation and cerebral edema, the latter of which may be severe enough to cause death.[60,61]

Viral encephalitis occurs worldwide, with a particularly high incidence in the tropics. (Table 43-1) outlines the major viruses that cause encephalitis and lists some of their distinguishing characteristics. Each year in the United States, between 1,000 and 5,000 cases of encephalitis are reported to the Centers for Disease Control (CDC). Identification of the etiologic agent in viral encephalitis is achieved in only about 50 percent of cases.[12,62]

TABLE 43-4 ■ Signs and Symptoms of Viral Encephalitis

Common
Impairment of consciousness: confusion, lethargy, delirium, coma
Inability to recall new information/anterograde amnesia (esp. HSV-1 encephalitis)
Headache
Fever
Stiff neck (may be subtle)
Less Common
Focal or generalized seizures
Hemiparesis, spasticity, or other signs of focal CNS dysfunction including aphasia, blindness, or ataxia
Cranial nerve palsies
Tremors

HSV-1, herpes simplex virus type 1.

Herpes Simplex Virus

Herpes simplex encephalitis represents only 10 to 15 percent of cases of viral encephalitis in the United States. However, it remains the most common cause of fatal nonepidemic viral encephalitis and is the only viral encephalitis for which effective antiviral therapy has been proven in clinical trials.[20,63] HSV is ubiquitous in human populations. HSV-1 is most commonly acquired as a symptomatic or asymptomatic gingivostomatitis in early childhood.[1,4] HSV-2 is more commonly sexually transmitted and is classically acquired during adolescence or adulthood.[1,4] Both agents enter neuronal processes during primary infection and persist in neurons within sensory ganglia. HSV-1 may also persist within the CNS and is responsible for 90 percent of cases of herpes simplex encephalitis in adults; of these cases, roughly two-thirds represent reactivated infection.[64,65] HSV-2 may be associated with myelitis.[22]

The pathogenesis of herpes simplex encephalitis is not well understood. Encephalitis has been postulated to follow the spread of virus from the trigeminal ganglia through sensory fibers to the meninges overlying the temporal lobes and orbitofrontal cortex or, alternatively, to follow reactivation of virus in the olfactory bulbs prior to spread to the brain itself.[20,64] HSV infects neurons, glia, and ependyma.

Herpes simplex encephalitis occurs throughout the year without seasonal incidence, affects men and women equally, and may occur at any age.[63,66] Immunosuppression does not increase the risk of encephalitis, but the course may be atypical in these individuals.[67,68] The virus has a predilection for orbitofrontal cortex and temporal lobes, which it may involve unilaterally or bilaterally.[63] The cingulate cortex is also involved in many patients. Occasionally herpes simplex encephalitis involves the occipital cortex or brainstem, in rare cases without temporal lobe involvement.[69] Vascular congestion and petechial or larger hemorrhages may be present; progression of the infection results in extensive and frequently hemorrhagic destruction of brain.[70]

Herpes simplex encephalitis presents with an almost universal triad of headache (in over 90% of cases), fever, and alteration in mental state.[20,63] Changes in mental state at presentation may range from confusion, frank psychosis, or somnolence to stupor or coma. Temporal lobe involvement may be manifested by olfactory or gustatory hallucinations, déjà vu phenomena, and upper quadrant visual field defects.[63] Bilateral temporal involvement may result in the loss of ability to store and recall new information, and involvement of the dominant hemisphere can result in aphasia. Rare patients present with symptoms and signs referable to the occipital lobes.[71] Focal or generalized seizures may occur at any point during the acute illness or after recovery.

The CSF typically contains a lymphocytic pleocytosis of 50 or more cells/mm^3 (median, 130 cells/mm^3).[72] In occasional patients, however, the cell count is normal.[33,72] Although herpes simplex encephalitis is frequently hemorrhagic, the presence or absence of red blood cells in CSF does not differentiate HSV infection from encephalitis due to other causes.[33,72] CSF protein concentration has a median value of 80 mg/dl, but ranges from normal to over 700 mg/dl; CSF glucose is usually normal.[33,72] MRI with gadolinium enhancement is the initial diagnostic procedure of choice and will usually demonstrate hyperintense T2-weighted signal along with gadolinium enhancement within the temporal lobe; it may also show involvement of the insula, orbitofrontal cortex, and cingulate gyrus (Fig. 43-1).[63] MRI abnormalities in other regions of cortex or brainstem, without temporal lobe involvement, do not exclude the diagnosis.[73] The EEG may show temporal lobe slowing or spike-wave activity. CT with contrast and EEG are less sensitive, but used together may provide diagnostic information when MRI is not available.[74]

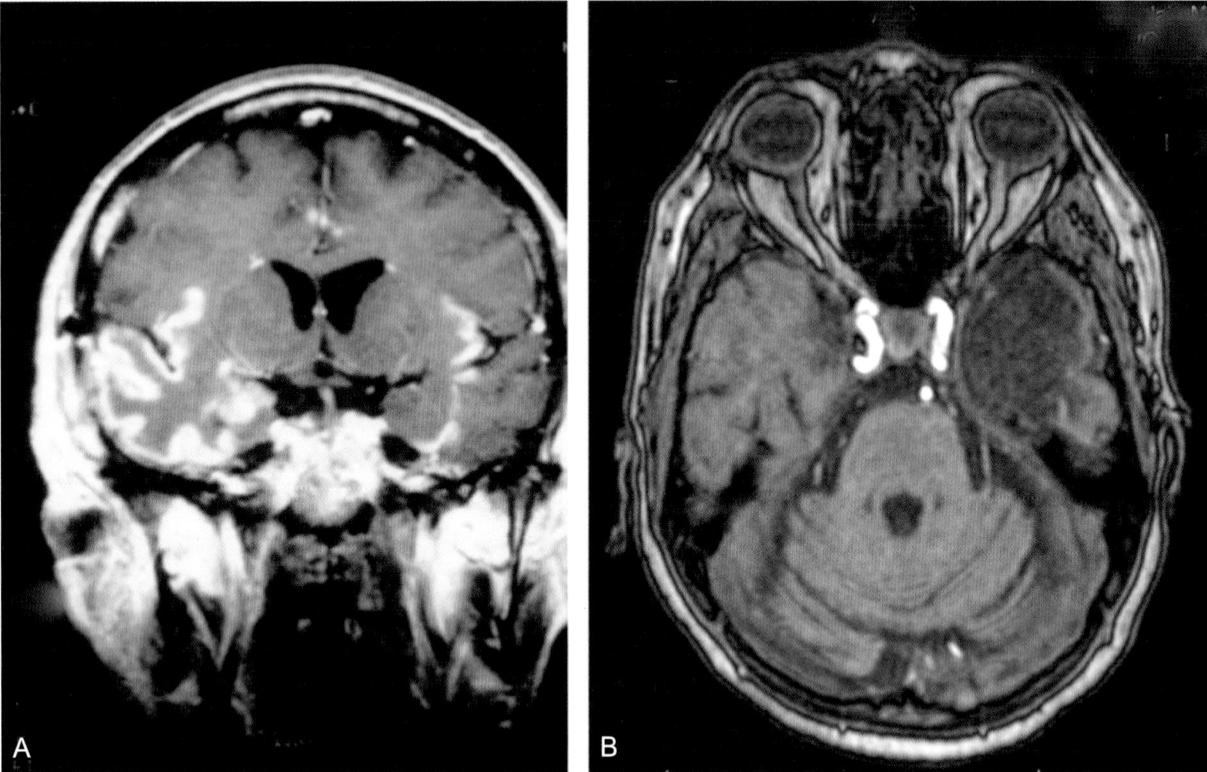

FIGURE 43-1 ■ **A**, Magnetic resonance imaging (MRI) of herpes simplex virus encephalitis. T2-weighted fluid-attenuated inversion recovery (FLAIR) sequence showing increased signal in right temporal lobe, insula, and orbitofrontal cortex. There is also involvement of the left insula. **B**, T1-weighted MRI 6 months after infection, showing massive destruction of the left temporal lobe.

A specific diagnosis of herpes simplex encephalitis is made by amplification of viral DNA from CSF using PCR. Overall diagnostic accuracy of PCR in patients with brain biopsy-proven HSV encephalitis is 98 percent.[33,75] In some patients, however, PCR may be negative at presentation due to low copy numbers of DNA in the CSF; in these cases, repeat CSF PCR after 4 to 7 days is usually positive.[76] Diagnostic yield of PCR falls to 21 percent in patients after 2 weeks of antiviral treatment.[75] Determination of acute antibody titers is not of value in the acute diagnosis of HSV encephalitis; however, comparison of acute and convalescent serum titers may be useful retrospectively and, in rare cases, provides diagnostic information when PCR was negative or when CSF was not obtained initially.[77] Retrospective serologic confirmation of herpes simplex encephalitis may also be made by determining serum:CSF ratios of HSV-specific antibodies to identify intrathecal antibody production.

Herpes simplex encephalitis is treated with intravenous acyclovir (Table 43-3), which inhibits HSV synthesis by competing with deoxyguanosine triphosphate as a substrate for DNA polymerase and causing DNA chain termination.[67] The drug is converted into its pharmacologically active monophosphate form by virally encoded thymidine kinase and thus only becomes active in infected cells.[67] Acyclovir is administered intravenously at 10 mg/kg body weight every 8 hours for 21 days. Complications of acyclovir therapy are usually mild. The major concern is nephrotoxicity due to deposition of drug crystals, which can be avoided by careful hydration. Although acyclovir resistance has been reported in other conditions, acyclovir-resistant herpes simplex encephalitis is rare.[78,79]

Prior to the introduction of acyclovir, overall mortality from herpes simplex encephalitis was over 70 percent, with mortality approaching 100 percent in patients over the age of 40 years.[80] The advent of acyclovir has reduced the overall mortality to 28 percent, and instituting antiviral therapy at presentation when the diagnosis is suspected has reduced 1-year mortality to 14 percent.[81] Patients who are alert or lethargic when treatment is initiated have an excellent likelihood of survival, but mortality in patients treated when semicomatose or comatose still approaches 25 percent.[63] The likelihood of death or serious neurologic impairment is greater when the patient is elderly, initiation of acyclovir treatment is delayed, or evidence of extensive CNS involvement is present on initial neuroimaging. Even with prompt initiation of treatment, up to two-thirds of patients are left with permanent neurologic deficits including epilepsy, impaired cognition, aphasia, anterograde amnesia, or motor deficits.[63,81,82] Neurologic improvement takes place over months, and some patients who are severely impaired immediately after treatment have a good functional recovery over time.

Varicella Zoster Virus

VZV, like HSV, is an enveloped double-stranded DNA virus that is worldwide in distribution. The virus is acquired by the respiratory route and replicates initially in tonsillar tissue to produce a viremia followed by seeding of multiple tissues including skin. Primary infection classically results in chicken pox, but individuals may also be infected acutely with little or no rash. Virus is then taken up by nerves supplying infected skin or other tissues and is transported to sensory ganglia, establishing lifelong persistence.[83] VZV thus differs from HSV in that it produces an acute viremic illness and only then persists secondarily and spreads within neurons. Viral latency in sensory ganglia is heavily controlled by T-cell–mediated immunity, and reactivation of infection may occur with waning of immune response during old age or in states of compromised host immunity.[83]

Cutaneous zoster (shingles), the most common manifestation of reactivated VZV infection, affects roughly 1 million adults in the United States annually.[83] The likelihood of developing zoster is higher in individuals who acquired chicken pox during infancy.[83] Most cases of zoster occur in patients older than 50 years. Neuropathologic correlates of cutaneous zoster include focal meningeal inflammation, necrosis of associated neurons, and degeneration of motor and sensory nerve roots in the involved area.[83] Cutaneous zoster may develop without known precipitating cause or may be triggered by systemic cancer, spinal irradiation, HIV infection or other immunosuppressed states, or spinal trauma.[83] Many patients experience a sharp, burning discomfort in a dermatomal distribution for 2 to 5 days before onset of the rash. A localized redness with red macules then develops and progresses to vesicles in the same dermatomal pattern as the pain.[83] Additional vesicles may appear over the next 2 to 7 days. The distribution of herpes zoster is usually unilateral and involves a single dermatome. The rash involves the trunk in 50 percent, the head in 20 percent, the arms in 15 percent, and the legs in 15 percent of cases. Over the next month, the dermatomal pain slowly disappears, leaving residual hypoalgesia or hyperalgesia. Occasional patients may present with dermatomal pain without rash, termed *zoster sine herpete*.[83] Treatment with oral valacyclovir (1 gram three times daily for 7 to 10 days) shortens the duration of rash and acute pain.[83,84] Recommended treatment in immunocompromised individuals is 5 to 10 mg/kg of usually intravenous acyclovir given three times daily for 5 to 7 days.[83]

Postherpetic neuralgia (PHN)—pain occurring in the distribution of the original rash and persisting for longer than 3 months—occurs in 9 to 14 percent of patients following shingles and increases with advancing age.[85] The pain may be relentless, episodic, or paroxysmal and may be elicited by cutaneous contact or stimulation. Postherpetic itch is also common. The live attenuated Oka strain VZV vaccine has been shown to reduce the incidence of cutaneous zoster in healthy individuals by 50 percent and the incidence of postherpetic neuralgia by 67 percent.[86] To what extent antiviral treatment of acute zoster lessens the likelihood of PHN has not been clearly demonstrated.[84] Symptomatic treatment of PHN is often disappointing. Tricyclic antidepressants, gabapentin, pregabalin, controlled-release morphine sulfate, oxycodone, and lidocaine patches have moderate to high efficacy, but are sometimes completely unhelpful.[87] Aspirin in cream or ointment form, topical capsaicin, and intrathecal methylprednisolone are less effective, limited by side effects, or both.[87] For most of these medications, treatment involves escalating dosages of medication until pain relief is achieved or unacceptable side effects occur.

VZV may invade the CNS during primary or reactivated infection and, in reactivated infection, may do so in the absence of cutaneous zoster.[88] Prior to the advent of PCR testing, CNS invasion by VZV was considered unusual. It is now realized, however, that CNS involvement by VZV is much more frequent; in one series VZV was found to be the most common agent identified in viral meningitis and encephalitis (29% of isolates).[88] Studies from France and England have identified the agent in 5 to 15 percent of encephalitis isolates.[89,90] The virus is now known to cause a wide range of syndromes of neurologic injury involving not only brain and spinal cord but also cranial nerves and brainstem or peripheral ganglia.[88] CNS invasion in reactivated VZV infection occurs following spread of virus from trigeminal or spinal sensory ganglia; in this process, the virus may produce ophthalmic involvement or may produce Ramsay–Hunt syndrome, in which infection of the tympanic membrane and surrounding structures is accompanied by facial nerve palsy.[88] Of greater concern and unlike HSV, VZV may infect both large and small vessels supplying the brain or spinal cord, at times followed by spread of the infection into neural parenchyma.[88,91] Involvement of vessels may produce focal or multifocal ischemic injury or may cause vessel-wall necrosis with resulting arterial dissection, aneurysm formation, or hemorrhage within the subarachnoid space or brain parenchyma.[88] The classic presentation of VZV vasculopathy is herpes zoster ophthalmicus, in which there is initial superficial zoster in the distribution of the ophthalmic branch of the trigeminal nerve followed days to weeks later by stroke in the territory of the carotid or middle cerebral artery.[88] However, VZV vasculitis may occur with or without preceding cutaneous zoster or herpes zoster ophthalmicus or oticus and may involve virtually any vascular territory within the brain or spinal cord. VZV vasculitis may be significantly more severe in HIV infection or other immunosuppressed states, and immunosuppressed patients may develop a more slowly progressive CNS vasculopathy or myelitis.[88]

CSF in acute VZV CNS infection may reveal a mononuclear pleocytosis, at times with red blood cells and sometimes hypoglychorrhachia.[33,88] VZV encephalitis in the setting of acute VZV infection may be diagnosed by PCR; however, the reaction rapidly becomes negative, so a negative PCR does not exclude the diagnosis.[88] Diagnosis of VZV vasculopathy in the setting of reactivated infection may also be made by the presence of elevated titers of anti-VZV IgG antibodies in CSF.[83,88] Oligoclonal bands are commonly present and are reactive with VZV proteins.[88]

Treatment of VZV encephalitis is with acyclovir, 10 mg/kg, usually intravenously, every 8 hours for a minimum of 14 days. Oral prednisone, 1 mg/kg, given daily for 5 days, may be used to treat the inflammatory component of the vasculitis; more prolonged treatment is avoided to prevent steroid-induced immunosuppression.[88]

West Nile Virus

WNV, a single-stranded RNA flavivirus virus, is currently the most common cause of epidemic encephalitis in the United States.[92,93] The virus infects multiple species of animals and birds, in particular crows, jays, magpies, and ravens. *Culex* species mosquitoes, predominantly *C. tarsalis* and *C. pipiens*, are the primary vectors for human infection. WNV produces infection predominantly in the summer and early autumn, when mosquitoes are most active. As of December 2012, 5,387 cases of WNV infection had been reported to the CDC for the year, with 243 deaths (Fig. 43-2). Of these cases, 2,734 (51%) represented neuroinvasive disease (Fig. 43-3). In most individuals, WNV infection is silent or produces only trivial symptoms. In 20 percent of infected patients, symptomatic West Nile fever develops, characterized by malaise, fatigue, anorexia, headache, nausea, vomiting, myalgia, fever, eye pain, and a nonspecific maculopapular rash.[92] The illness usually lasts less than 7 days, although a minority of patients may remain symptomatic for as long as 6 weeks.[92]

Less than 1 percent of infected patients develop neuroinvasive disease, which is more common in the elderly and is especially severe in immunosuppressed patients or transplant recipients.[92,94] West Nile encephalitis typically presents with fever, headache, and altered mental state, stupor, or coma. Other signs of parenchymal involvement may include cerebellar ataxia or movement disorders including tremor, myoclonus, and parkinsonian symptoms.[94,95] WNV infection may also result in a syndrome of acute flaccid paralysis similar to that seen with polio virus.[94,95] A minority of patients develop chorioretinitis or vitritis.[96] CSF in neuroinvasive WNV infection typically shows a mild elevation in opening pressure, lymphocytic pleocytosis, mild elevation of protein level, and normal glucose concentration. Cell count is usually 50 to 260 cells/mm^3 but may be as high as 2,600 and may be heavily polymorphonuclear, in particular at presentation.[33,95] In one series, cell count was normal in 20 percent of patients.[97] Occasional patients have low serum sodium levels indicative of the

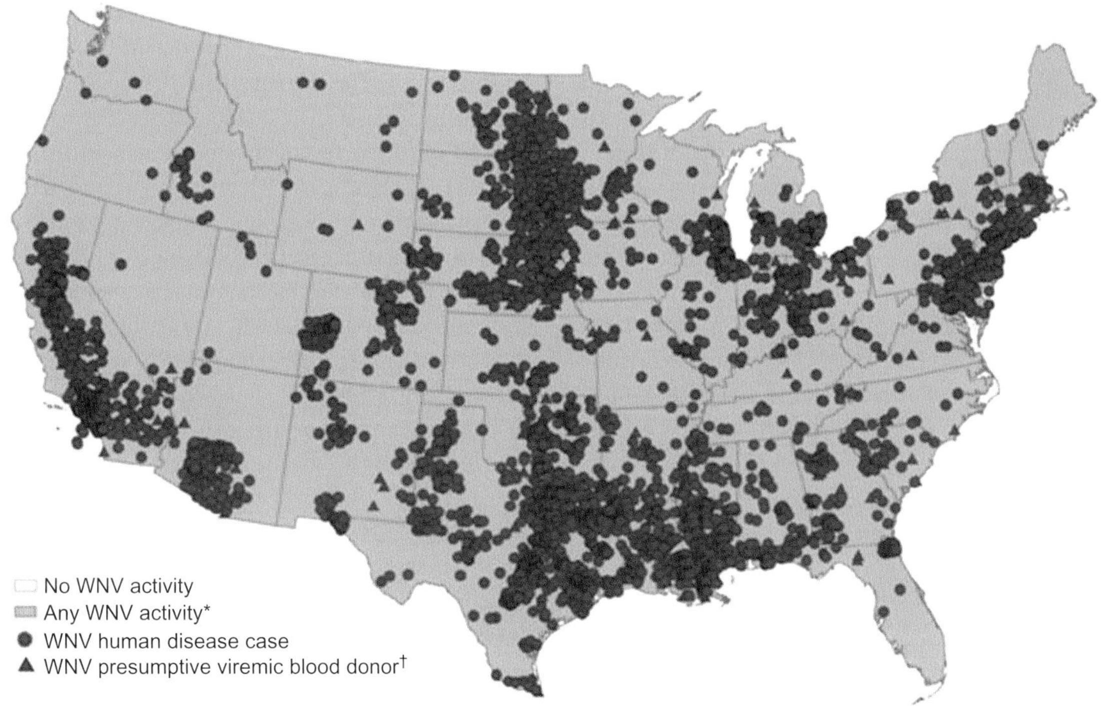

FIGURE 43-2 ▪ Distribution of West Nile virus in the United States showing cases of infection and WNV identified in blood donors, 2012. (From the US Centers for Disease Control and Prevention.)

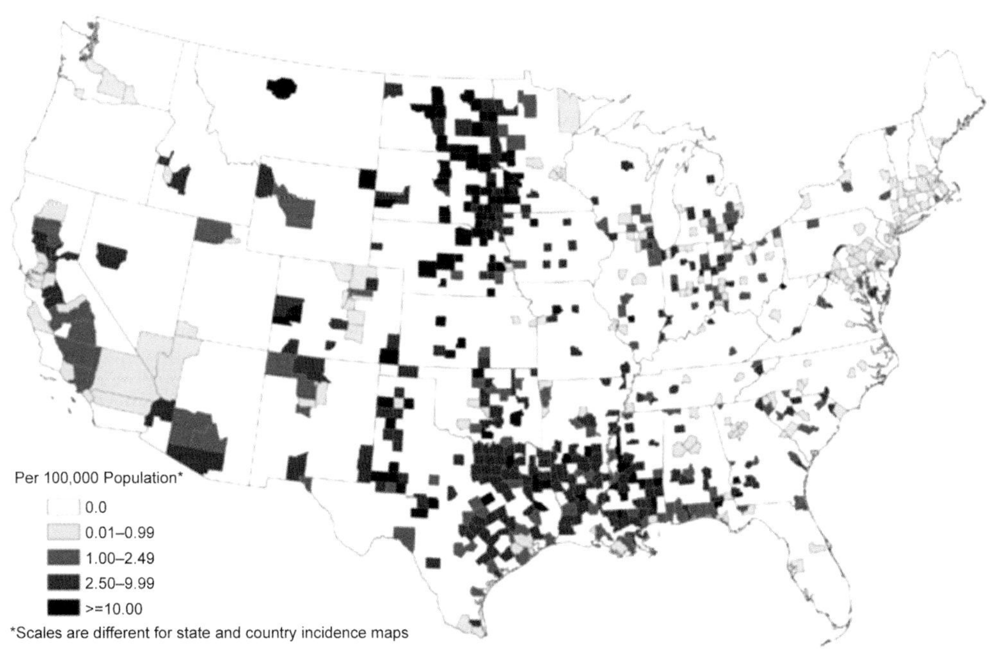

FIGURE 43-3 ▪ Distribution of cases of West Nile neuroinvasive disease in the United States, 2012. (From the US Centers for Disease Control and Prevention.)

syndrome of inappropriate antidiuretic hormone secretion (SIADH). MRI is often normal, although a minority of patients have areas of increased signal on T2-weighted and fluid-attenuated inversion recovery (FLAIR) sequences in the substantia nigra, basal ganglia, and thalamus.[98,99] Patients with WNV-induced flaccid paralysis may show increased signal in the anterior horns of the spinal cord.[99] A single, acute, cerebrospinal fluid specimen positive for WNV-specific IgM antibodies is diagnostic of WNV neuroinvasive disease.[98] PCR is less reliable. Paired sera positive for WNV-specific IgM antibodies (a fourfold or greater rise in titer from the "acute" serum, obtained 0 to 7 days after symptom onset, and the "convalescent" serum, obtained 14 to 21 days after symptom onset) also provide serologic confirmation.

Treatment of WNV encephalitis is currently supportive. Human intravenous IgG containing high titers against WNV has been used experimentally but is not available routinely.[100] Prognosis for recovery after WNV meningitis or encephalitis is good, although recovery may be extremely prolonged. The likelihood of complete recovery after West Nile flaccid paralysis is poor.[95,98]

Other Arthropod-Borne Viruses

Several arthropod-borne viruses other than WNV may infect humans and cause neurologic disease. All but two of the agents occurring in the United States and Canada are carried by mosquitoes, with rates of infection that peak in mid-summer through early autumn.[101] Colorado tick fever virus and Powassan virus are carried by ticks, and infections caused by these agents tend to occur in late spring and early summer.[31] Prior to the advent of WNV in the United States, St. Louis encephalitis was the most common arthropod-borne cause of encephalitis. Eastern equine encephalitis, although rare, remains the most deadly.[101] No human case of Western equine encephalitis virus infection has been reported since 1994.

St. Louis encephalitis virus, like WNV, is a mosquito-borne virus that is a member of the family Flaviviridae. Cases of St. Louis encephalitis have been reported from almost every area of the United States, but the majority occur in the central Midwest and Texas. The virus is usually seen with scattered rural infections but may also cause urban epidemics. St. Louis encephalitis resembles neuroinvasive West Nile disease but rarely if ever produces a flaccid, polio-like illness.[101] The two diseases are both more severe in the elderly and they have similar CSF findings. Diagnosis of St. Louis encephalitis is either by CSF IgM, by a rise in antibody titers, or both.

Eastern equine encephalitis virus is an agent of wading and migratory birds that is found predominantly along the Atlantic seaboard, the Gulf of Mexico, Indiana, Michigan, and Wisconsin.[101,102] Although the virus does not usually produce severe infection in its natural hosts, it can infect horses and may cause epizootic outbreaks of infection in flocks of turkeys or in exotic or game farm birds. Eastern equine encephalitis is rare in humans, with approximately 5 cases occurring annually.[101,102] The virus is most apt to cause encephalitis in infants and in individuals over 55 years of age. A prodromal illness which may include fever, headache, and abdominal pain frequently occurs.[103] Onset of encephalitis may be fulminant: nearly 70 percent of patients present in stupor or coma, and presentation only with meningeal symptoms is uncommon.[103] Corticospinal or extrapyramidal signs are often present, and the illness may be complicated by focal or generalized seizures. Overall mortality is around 35 percent, with one-third of survivors suffering significant neurologic impairment.[103]

Two groups of arthropod-borne infections occur outside the United States and should be considered when evaluating patients with encephalitis coming from endemic areas (Table 43-1). Tick-borne encephalitides relate to multiple viral agents existing throughout Eurasia, with greatest prevalence in northern Europe and Asia.[104] Japanese encephalitis virus, endemic in eastern and southeastern Asia, results in 15,000 deaths annually.[18] Both tick-borne encephalitis and Japanese encephalitis may present with findings similar to those produced by WNV, including flaccid paralysis.[17,18]

Rabies Virus

Rabies virus is an unenveloped single-stranded RNA virus that is a member of the Lyssavirus genus of the family Rhabdoviridae. Rabies virus exists worldwide and predominant reservoirs are bats, skunks, foxes, and raccoons in developed countries where there is mandatory rabies vaccination for dogs.[105] Most—but not all—human cases acquired in the United States have resulted from bat bites.[105] In less developed countries, dogs are the source of most human cases; other animals including infected monkeys, sometimes kept as pets, may account for a minority of cases.[105,106]

Rabies virus is typically acquired through the bite of an infected animal; rare cases have occurred following exposure to aerosolized rabies virus or after inadvertent transplantation of infected tissue.[105,107–109] The virus may remain latent at the site of an infected bite for 6 or more years before the onset of neurologic disease.[110] Unlike most other viruses causing encephalitis, rabies is specifically neurotropic: the virus enters peripheral nerve fibers at the site of inoculation, is carried proximally by reverse axoplasmic flow, and progressively infects the CNS through neuron-to-neuron spread (the centripetal phase of infection). The virus then spreads outward within nerves (the centrifugal phase of infection) to involve multiple tissues including salivary glands, corneas, and the heart. In animals, this centrifugal phase of infection, with shedding of salivary virus, may occur prior to clinical disease.[106,111,112]

Rabies classically begins with dysesthesias at the site of the bite, followed by progressive neurologic involvement with a clinical picture (termed "furious rabies") of agitated delirium, stimulus-sensitive laryngeal spasm with hydrophobia, prolonged inspiratory spasm, and progression to coma and death.[105] Rabies may also present as a more classic encephalitis with stupor and coma ("dumb rabies"), or as an ascending paralysis, similar to Guillain–Barré syndrome, followed by signs of CNS involvement.[105]

Rabies should be considered in appropriate clinical settings, in particular when there is a history of animal bite or of recent or remote travel to, or residence in, countries where rabies is a significant health problem. There may no history of bite, however; the minute punctures caused by bat bites may go unnoticed, or, alternatively, the animal bite may have occurred long enough ago to have been forgotten.[110,113] MRI may show ill-defined, mild T2-hyperintensities in the brainstem and hippocampus; early in the disease these lesions may fail to enhance with gadolinium.[114] Specific diagnosis of rabies is made by identifying rabies antigen in nuchal biopsy or by PCR from saliva or CSF.

Management of rabies consists of two strategies: prevention of clinical disease by immunotherapy and immunization at the time of the bite, and supportive treatment of clinical rabies. Preventive therapy involves washing the area of the bite thoroughly, infiltrating the area with rabies virus-specific immunoglobulin, and administration of diploid cell rabies vaccine.[105] This treatment, when administered soon after the bite, is highly effective in preventing clinical rabies.[105] Once clinical rabies develops, the patient's course may be influenced by a wide variety of CNS, autonomic, and systemic complications.[115] Rabies is almost invariably fatal; fewer than 10 patients are known to have survived, and of these, only one made a full recovery.[116] Of interest, a handful of patients known to have received infected corneal tissue or organs failed to develop clinical rabies.[107,108] One patient surviving rabies was treated with midozalam and ketamine, but the use of these agents in other cases has been unsuccessful.[117,118]

Other Viruses

Although enteroviruses are most commonly associated with viral meningitis, they may also cause encephalitis and rarely may result in paralytic disease. Enterovirus 71, a cause of hand, foot, and mouth disease and herpangina in children, may cause encephalitis with involvement of the brainstem or, less frequently, the cortex, cerebellum, or spinal ventral roots.[119] In some patients, MRI abnormalities are detected on diffusion-weighted or FLAIR sequences.[120].

The mouse arenavirus LCMV usually causes meningitis but may occasionally cause encephalitis.[121] Infection in children and adults is rarely fatal, but clinical recovery and return of CSF to normal can be prolonged. LCMV meningoencephalitis is one of the few viral CNS infections that may cause hypoglychorrhachia.[33] Parvovirus B19, the agent of the childhood condition erythema infectiosum (fifth disease), is an uncommon cause of encephalitis in both children and adults.[122] Human herpesviruses type 6 (HHV-6, associated with roseola infantum) and type 7 (HHV-7) have been associated with seizures or, rarely, encephalopathy in early childhood.[123] In one study, HHV-6 was detected in the CSF of 40 percent of patients with encephalitis of otherwise undetermined cause.[124] Important viruses to consider in patients exposed in Southeast Asia include Japanese encephalitis virus, and the bat henipavirus, Nipah virus (Thailand) (Table 43-1).[18,125]

Epstein–Barr virus (EBV), the agent of infectious mononucleosis, has been associated with a wide variety of infectious and postinfectious neurologic disorders in both immunologically normal and immunocompromised patients.[126–128] The association of EBV with specific disease presentations, however, is made difficult by two properties of the virus. First, EBV infects and can remain latent in B lymphocytes for many years. For this reason, PCR amplification of EBV DNA from CSF in patients with suspected CNS infection may simply indicate the presence of the virus in lymphocytes rather than proving it as a causative agent. Second, like HSV, EBV can reactivate under situations of physiologic stress, so that a rise in antibody titer in the setting of acute illness may or may not be indicative of disease causation.

Viral Encephalitis in Immunocompromised Patients

Impairment of host B- or T-cell response, whether because of congenital immunodeficiency, HIV infection, or iatrogenic immunosuppression, may result in infection with unusual agents or produce atypical infection by more common viruses. Because control of enteroviral infection depends heavily on antibody, enteroviruses have been associated with chronic meningitis and progressive encephalitis in children with X-linked hypogammaglobulinemia or X-linked hyper-IgM syndrome; these patients exhibit ongoing presence of enteroviral RNA in CSF and may show continued enterovirus excretion in stool.[129,130] Chronic enteroviral meningoencephalitis has also been reported in patients treated with the anti-CD20 monoclonal agent rituximab.[131,132] Impairment of T-cell immune response, as in HIV-infected or immunosuppressed patients, may lead to infection with less commonly pathogenic agents such as JC virus, cytomegalovirus, adenovirus, HHV-6, or HHV-7, or may result in prolonged or atypical presentations of infections with HSV or VZV.[68,133–140] HSV and VZV are treatable with acyclovir, as is the case in immunologically intact patients. Treatment of cytomegalovirus CNS infections has usually involved gancyclovir, foscarnet, or a combination of both agents; cidofovir has been used as a second choice (Table 43-3).[141] Cases of encephalitis associated with HHV-6 have been treated with gancyclovir, foscarnet, or a combination of the two drugs.[140,142] CNS infections in immunocompromised patients may involve common infections as well as those caused by unusual organisms. Especially in patients infected with HIV, more than one infective agent may be present.

Progressive Multifocal Leukoencephalopathy

PML is an uncommon opportunistic infection of immunocompromised patients. Its causative agent, the human polyomavirus JCV, affects over 50 percent of individuals worldwide by late adult life.[2] Acute viral infection is not known to cause symptomatic illness, but the virus establishes protracted infection of renal tubular epithelial cells and other tissues, possibly including the brain.[2,143] In PML, JCV produces lytic infection of oligodendrocytes, causing areas of demyelination; astrocytes are also infected in some cases.[2] PML was initially described as a rare disorder of patients with hematologic malignancies and in immunosuppressed patients. In untreated AIDS, however, 4 percent of patients will die of PML, which can be the presenting feature.[144] In recent years, PML has become increasingly frequent in patients treated with the more aggressive immunosuppressive regimens now used for collagen-vascular diseases and solid organ or hematopoietic stem cell transplantation.[145] PML has also become a significant—although infrequent—complication of treatment with natalizumab and other monoclonal immunosuppressive agents such as rituximab, efalizumab, alemtuzumab, and TNF-α inhibitors.[146] The course of PML is that of the progressive development of multifocal neurologic deficits that may involve motor control, sensation, speech, vision, or

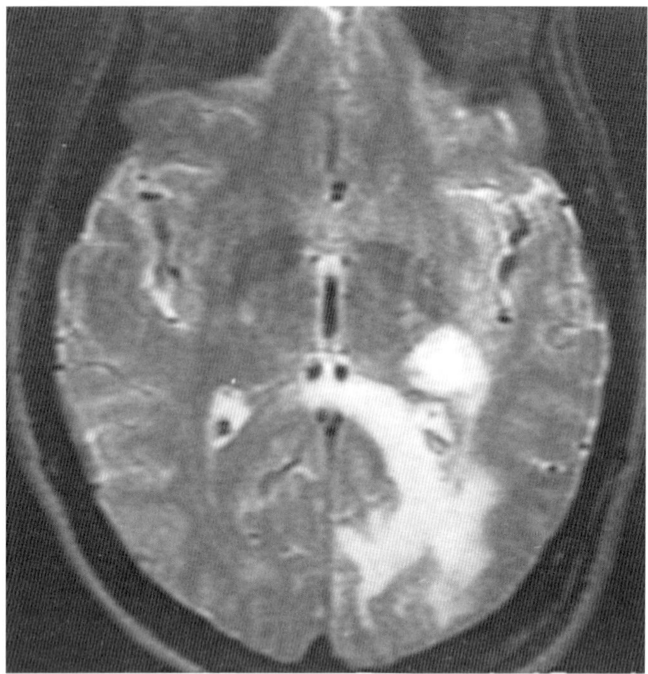

FIGURE 43-4 ■ Progressive multifocal leukoencephalopathy (PML): axial T2-weighted MRI showing multifocal involvement of cerebral white matter.

cognition. Occasional patients develop cerebellar or brainstem signs, but clinical involvement of the spinal cord is virtually never present. Rarely AIDS patients have been reported to develop JCV infection of cerebellar granule or other neurons.[147]

PML is presumptively diagnosed by MRI, which typically shows multifocal white matter lesions in the cerebrum or, less often, brainstem or cerebellum (Fig. 43-4); PML lesions are often not apparent on CT. Although PML lesions usually do not enhance, gadolinium enhancement may occur in AIDS- and natalizumab-associated PML.[2,148] A definitive diagnosis of PML is made by PCR amplification of JCV DNA from the CSF.[2,33] Sensitivity of PCR in early studies approached 80 to 90 percent.[149] However in HIV patients treated with antiretroviral therapy, PCR is positive in only 58 percent of cases[150].

There is no proven treatment for PML. Cytosine arabinoside has been reported to have limited efficacy in non-AIDS patients only.[151] Cidofovir, mefloquine, and mirtazapine have not been effective in controlled trials. Restoration of host immune function with antiretroviral therapy in AIDS patients may lead to stabilization or improvement, as may reduction of immunosuppressive therapy in transplant recipients or other patients receiving these drugs.[2] Treatment of PML in cases associated with natalizumab involves withdrawal of that agent and plasma exchange or immunoabsorption to remove natalizumab from the circulation; this approach has not been used with other monoclonal agents.[152] Improvement of immune status may cause a fulminant immune reconstitution inflammatory syndrome (IRIS) (Fig. 43-5).[153]

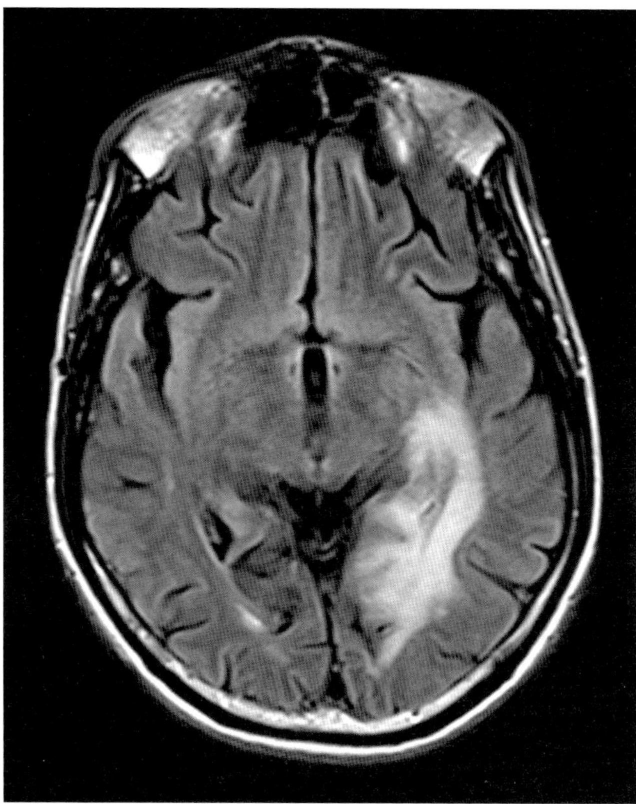

FIGURE 43-5 ▪ FLAIR MRI showing PML with immune reconstitution inflammatory syndrome (IRIS) in a patient with human immunodeficiency virus (HIV) following institution of antiretroviral therapy. There is edema in and surrounding a lesion within the left posterior cerebral white matter.

Approach to Patients with Viral Encephalitis

Viral encephalitis should be suspected in any patient presenting with signs suggesting acute involvement of the brain parenchyma, especially in individuals with fever and alteration of consciousness.[154] Meningeal signs may or may not be present. Signs indicating temporal lobe involvement suggest herpes simplex encephalitis, but other viral encephalitides may have a similar presentation as may occasional bacterial infections or autoimmune encephalitis from antineuronal antibodies. Patients often have an elevated peripheral white blood cell count, but signs of systemic infection may also be absent. Diagnosis relies heavily on clinical findings, MRI, and the results of CSF analysis. MRI in herpes simplex encephalitis characteristically shows abnormalities of one or both temporal lobes, at times with involvement of the orbitofrontal cortex, insula, or cingulate gyrus. Similar findings, however, may be seen in other potentially treatable conditions including neurosyphilis and autoimmune encephalitis.[155,156] The CSF in viral encephalitis typically shows significant pleocytosis and an elevated protein but normal glucose concentration. The pleocytosis is commonly lymphocytic, but is neutrophilic in rare cases.[33] A depressed CSF glucose level, while not typical, has been described in VZV, LCMV, mumps, and HSV-2 infections.[33] CSF should be sent for PCR for HSV, and consideration should be given to ordering PCR for other agents. Detection of virus-specific IgM in CSF is more sensitive than PCR for the diagnosis of WNV and may be useful in other arboviral infections where PCR is negative. Similarly, elevated CSF titers of IgG may be more sensitive than PCR in encephalitis due to reactivated VZV. Lumbar puncture may need to be deferred when there is evidence on examination, CT, or MRI of increased intracranial pressure or mass lesion.

Acyclovir should be initiated presumptively where viral encephalitis is strongly suspected and should be continued until PCR has been shown to be negative for HSV.[154] Because the initial PCR in herpes simplex encephalitis may rarely not be positive, acyclovir should be continued in seriously ill patients until a second CSF PCR, obtained 3 to 7 days later, is also negative.[33,76] Acyclovir should also be continued if VZV is detected by CSF PCR or serology. Gancyclovir should be instituted if CMV or HHV-6 infection is diagnosed; gancyclovir may be supplemented with foscarnet.[154] Antibacterials should be initiated if bacterial meningitis, brain abscess, or parameningeal infection is suspected.

Treatment of encephalitis is otherwise supportive.[154] Seizures may require intravenous phenytoin, levetiracetam, or other agents. Cerebral edema is a major concern in severe encephalitis; dexamethasone (10 mg orally or intravenously followed by 4 mg every 6 hours), mannitol, and hyperventilation have all been used in individual cases, but their efficacy is unproven. Decompressive craniectomy has resulted in patient survival with good initial outcome in a few cases of herpes simplex encephalitis complicated by fulminant cerebral edema.[157] Cerebral salt wasting or SIADH may require treatment with hydration and sodium supplementation, or fluid restriction, respectively. Attention must be given to preventing complications of severe illness such as pneumonia, deep venous thrombosis, and decubitus ulcers. Recovery in viral encephalitis may be extremely prolonged, with the full extent of recovery not realized for many months.

PRION DISEASES

Prion diseases represent a group of rare disorders including Creutzfeldt–Jakob disease (CJD), new variant CJD (vCJD), Gerstmann–Straussler–Schenker disease, familial fatal insomnia, kuru, and variably protease–sensitive prionopathy.[158,159] Prion diseases of animals include scrapie of sheep (the prototype for this group of conditions), bovine spongiform encephalopathy, wasting disease of deer and elk, and transmissible mink encephalopathy.[159] Prion diseases are not caused by viruses but rather by a self-replicating isoform of a normal intracellular sialoglycoprotein. The normal cellular protein is termed "PrP(c)" and the self-replicating protein causing disease is referred to as "PrP(Sc)." PrP(Sc) does not contain nucleic acid, its presence does not elicit an immune response, and it is not inactivated by many agents normally used for decontamination.[159,160] Interaction of PrP(Sc) with PrP(c) appears to be essential for disease.[159,160] Except in familial cases, PrP(Sc) is thought to arise from a spontaneous mutation in PrP(c). Several different subtypes of CJD have been associated with homozygosity or heterozygosity of methionine or valine at codon 129 of the *PrP* gene, differences in variation in glycosylation patterns of PrP(Sc), and patterns of electrophoretic mobility of PrP(Sc) after proteinase K digestion.[159,160] Prion diseases have repeatedly been shown to be transmissible through PrP(Sc)-contaminated material, including PrP(Sc)-containing human grafts of dura mater or other tissues, contaminated electrodes used for intracerebral recording, and human pituitary-derived growth hormone. In the case of vCJD, transmission has occurred predominantly through ingestion of contaminated beef, but it has also occurred through blood transfusion.[159,161]

The most common human prion disease is CJD, which occurs worldwide with 1 to 2 cases per million population per year.[159] The average age at onset is 60 years, with an equal gender distribution. Most cases are sporadic (sCJD), but 12 percent cluster in families.[159] The condition affects the CNS only, without systemic symptoms. The onset of CJD is typically with subtle changes in cognition and personality changes that may include apathy, irritability, depression, or paranoia.[159] Occasional patients present with ataxia, spasticity, or visual complaints. These initial symptoms are followed by progressive dementia, often involving parietal lobe symptoms and, at times, aphasia. As the disease progresses, over 85 percent of patients develop stimulus-sensitive myoclonic jerks that tend to disappear as the disease progresses to profound dementia and a vegetative state. CJD is untreatable, and its course is relentlessly progressive, resulting in death within 6 months to 2 years.[159]

The diagnosis of CJD is made on the basis of clinical presentation, EEG, MRI, and evaluation of CSF for the proteins 14-3-3, tau, and neuron-specific enolase. The yield of these studies, however, varies among the different subtypes of CJD.[162] CSF cell count and protein levels are usually normal, such that significant pleocytosis suggests strongly that

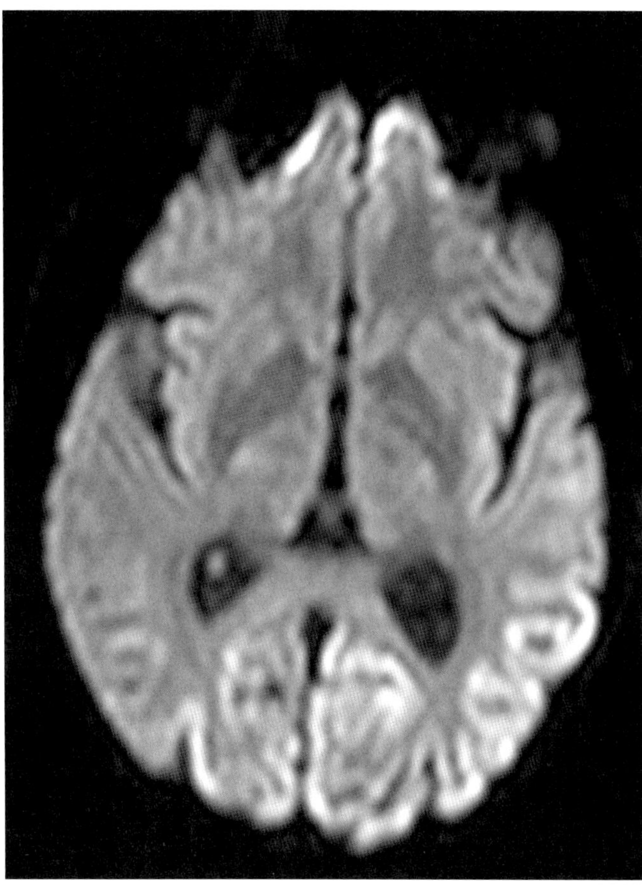

FIGURE 43-6 ▪ Creutzfeld–Jakob disease. Diffusion-weighted MRI image showing restricted diffusion within the cortical ribbon of the posterior hemispheres bilaterally.

the diagnosis is incorrect. The EEG initially may show only mild slowing but subsequently becomes strikingly abnormal, with repetitive, periodic, stereotyped, bilaterally synchronous sharp waves that usually occur at a frequency of 1 to 2 per second and are often associated with myoclonic jerks.[163,164] This periodic EEG activity may give way to generalized slowing late in the disease.[163,164] MRI has become the major diagnostic test in suspected CJD and typically shows foci of increased signal in the putamen, caudate, thalamus, and gray matter of the cerebral cortex. These findings are most prominent on diffusion-weighted sequences and, with less sensitivity, FLAIR sequences (Fig. 43-6); MRI changes are not reliably present in familial CJD.[165] Detection of 14-3-3 and tau proteins as well as neuron-specific enolase in CSF provides supportive evidence for the presence of CJD in patients with clinical, EEG, or MRI markers of the disease.[166] None of these CSF markers is specific for CJD, however, and their use in unselected patients may lead to erroneous diagnosis.[166] Postmortem diagnosis can be made by the characteristic brain histopathology and staining with specific prion antibodies or by demonstration of prions from homogenized brain using immunodiagnostic procedures.

In general, animal prion diseases such as scrapie have not been thought transmissible to humans. However, the appearance in Britain of bovine spongiform encephalopathy (BSE; mad cow disease), a prion disease, was followed by an outbreak of human cases of vCJD, which were presumably acquired by ingestion of contaminated beef.[167] Human cases peaked in 2000 after extensive culling of affected cattle.[159] Cases of vCJD have occurred primarily in younger individuals and have tended to present with psychiatric signs, with dementia and painful sensory symptoms occurring commonly. In contrast to the general population, all patients studied with vCJD have been homozygous for methionine at codon 129 of the *PrP* gene. Unlike sporadic CJD, the EEG in vCJD only rarely shows periodic activity. MRI typically shows increased signal in the pulvinar on diffusion-weighted imaging and FLAIR sequences.[168] Survival in vCJD may be more prolonged compared with sCJD.[159,160,167] Unlike sCJD, there have been cases of vCJD transmitted by blood transfusion.[159]

POSTINFECTIOUS COMPLICATIONS OF CNS VIRAL INFECTION

The interaction of an infective agent with the host immune system usually results in containment of the agent and eradication of disease. In some instances, however, systemic or CNS viral infections may induce an immune response that reacts not only with the infecting agent but also with components of nervous tissue. This interaction may result in postinfectious encephalomyelitis, acute hemorrhagic leukoencephalitis, transverse myelitis, or injury to the peripheral nervous system resulting in peripheral nerve involvement including plexopathy and the Guillain–Barré syndrome (see Chapter 59). Rarely, optic neuritis may also occur as a postinfectious condition.

Postinfectious Encephalomyelitis

Postinfectious encephalomyelitis is defined as an acute, monophasic demyelinating illness occurring

TABLE 43-5 ■ Major Viruses Associated With Postinfectious Neurologic Complications

Postinfectious Encephalomyelitis	Transverse Myelitis	Cerebellar Ataxia	Guillain–Barré Syndrome
Varicella zoster virus	Measles virus	Varicella zoster virus	Measles virus
Measles virus	Mumps virus	Measles virus	Epstein–Barr virus
Mumps virus	Varicella zoster virus	Epstein–Barr virus	Cytomegalovirus
Rubella virus	Rubella virus	Influenza virus	Influenza virus
Influenza virus	Influenza virus		Varicella zoster virus
Enteroviruses	Epstein–Barr virus		HIV
Coronaviruses	Enteroviruses		Dengue virus
HIV	HIV		
HTLV-1	HTLV-1		
Hepatitis A,B,C,E	Hepatitis A,B,C		
Herpes simplex virus	Herpes simplex virus		
Epstein–Barr virus	Human herpesvirus 6		
Cytomegalovirus	Hantavirus		
Human herpesvirus 6	Dengue virus		
Hantavirus (puumala virus)			
Dengue virus			
Smallpox (historical)			

HIV, human immunodeficiency virus; HTLV, human T-lymphotropic virus.

within 2 to 4 weeks of a viral or other infection (Table 43-5). The condition bears strong similarity to two other conditions: postvaccination encephalomyelitis, which follows immunization (see Chapter 48), and the experimental autoimmune demyelinating disease, experimental allergic encephalomyelitis (EAE).[169,170] Postinfectious encephalomyelitis and postvaccinal encephalomyelitis have been grouped under the common term *acute disseminated encephalomyelitis* (ADEM), which is therefore a final common pathway of autoimmune CNS injury that may be produced by a variety of infectious agents or immunizations.[169,170]

Postinfectious encephalomyelitis is more common in children than in adults and is rare in the elderly. In children, the peak age of onset is 5 to 8 years. The onset of postinfectious encephalomyelitis may be preceded by fever, malaise, headache, nausea, vomiting, or combinations of these symptoms. These prodromal symptoms are followed by the abrupt—at times fulminant—onset of CNS dysfunction. Altered mental state is almost universal and may range from drowsiness to frank coma. Meningeal signs are common. Neurologic examination may reveal unilateral or bilateral corticospinal tract signs, hemiplegia, ataxia, aphasia, sensory loss, visual field defects, or cranial nerve palsies. Focal or generalized seizures occur in up to 70 percent of children under 5 years of age, 80 percent of whom may develop status epilepticus.[171] Occasionally, postinfectious encephalomyelitis may be accompanied by optic neuritis or by involvement of the peripheral nervous system. The simultaneous occurrence of central and peripheral demyelinating events appears to be more common in adults than children.[172] A syndrome of ataxia may be seen in patients following chicken pox or, less frequently, other viral infections.[173]

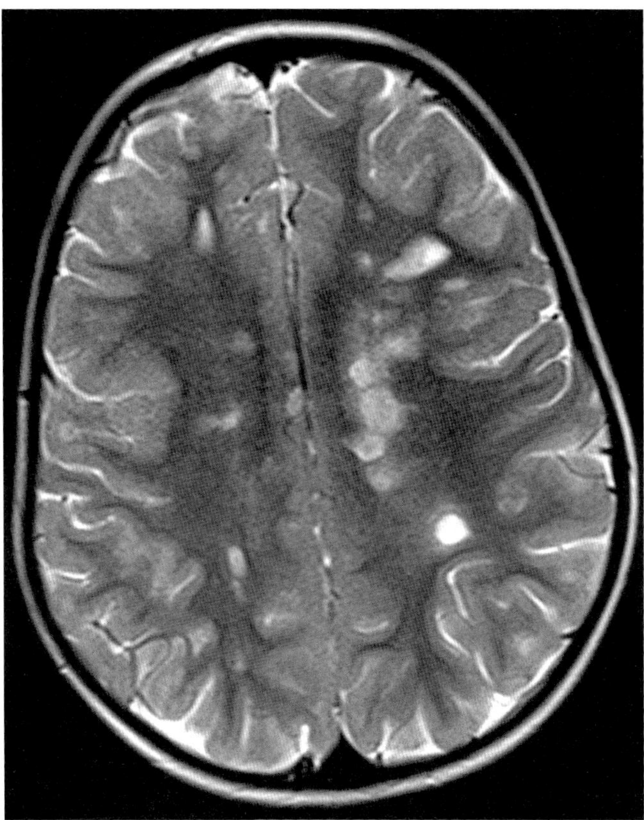

FIGURE 43-7 ■ Acute disseminated encephalomyelitis. T2-weighted MRI showing multifocal areas of increased signal in the white matter. (From Wender M: Acute disseminated encephalomyelitis (ADEM). J Neuroimmunol 231:92, 2011, with permission from Elsevier.)

The presence of multifocal neurologic signs should raise the level of suspicion of ADEM, as should the presence of signs referable to both the CNS and the peripheral nervous system. Excluding active nervous system infection is important. CSF typically shows a lymphocytic pleocytosis; however, roughly 30 percent of patients will have a mixed pleocytosis with neutrophilic predominance.[174] Traditionally, the presence of oligoclonal bands was considered unusual; in one study, however, oligoclonal bands were detected in 20 percent of patients with ADEM.[175] In a longitudinal study, oligoclonal bands were reported in 65 percent of individuals presenting with illnesses initially diagnosed as ADEM, but over 50 percent of these patients were subsequently diagnosed as having multiple sclerosis.[176]

MRI with gadolinium enhancement is the diagnostic study of choice in ADEM. T2 and FLAIR sequences classically show multiple, large, asymmetric, irregularly shaped lesions involving subcortical white matter and the gray-white junction of both cerebral hemispheres (Fig. 43-7).[176] Periventricular white matter may be involved, but lesions confined to the corpus callosum are unusual, in contrast to multiple sclerosis.[172] Gadolinium enhancement is seen in 30 to 100 percent of patients and may vary with stage of the disease.[171] Ring-enhancing lesions are sometimes found but should raise particular concern regarding brain abscess or other active CNS infection.[172] Spinal cord involvement, usually with extensive edema and swelling, may occur in children or adults and has a predilection for the thoracic region.[172] The majority of these lesions will resolve over time.[172]

Acute Hemorrhagic Leukoencephalitis

In roughly 2 percent of children (more rarely in adults), postinfectious encephalitis may present with fulminant hemorrhagic demyelination and cerebral edema, a condition termed "acute hemorrhagic leukoencephalitis," "acute necrotizing hemorrhagic leukoencephalitis," or "Weston Hurst syndrome."[171] MRI demonstrates not only demyelination but also hemorrhage, edema, and at times evidence of ischemia on diffusion-weighted images.[177] In contrast to postinfectious encephalomyelitis, mortality is greater than 50 percent.

Transverse Myelitis

Postinfectious encephalomyelitis may be confined to the spinal cord, resulting in transverse myelitis (Table 43-5).[178] Unlike postinfectious encephalomyelitis, which is more frequent in young children, transverse myelitis is more common in the second decade of life. In the majority of cases, the condition involves the thoracic level of the spinal cord. Onset of symptoms is often abrupt, with rapid progression to maximal deficit; in some patients, however, progression occurs over 1 to 2 weeks. Symptoms typically include fever, back and leg pain, muscle weakness, sensory disturbances, and sphincter dysfunction. Neurologic examination may demonstrate corticospinal tract signs and level-specific sensory loss. The patient may initially exhibit flaccid weakness that progresses over weeks to spasticity. CSF usually shows a lymphocytic or polymorphonuclear pleocytosis with protein levels that may be as high as 500 mg/dl. MRI of the spinal cord often demonstrates focal areas of increased T2 signal. Acute transverse myelitis may represent the first episode of multiple sclerosis or neuromyelitis optica.[179] MRI may have diagnostic value in differentiating these entities from postviral transverse myelitis: partial transverse lesions are more likely to indicate multiple sclerosis, whereas longitudinal involvement of multiple segments is associated with neuromyelitis optica.[180]

Approach to Patients with Postinfectious Neurologic Injury

Initial approach to the patient with suspected Guillain–Barré syndrome involves hospitalization and, if the patient is demonstrating respiratory failure, intubation (see Chapter 59). The major initial step in patients with suspected postinfectious encephalomyelitis is to exclude multifocal CNS infection or, less likely, vasculitis. In patients with transverse myelitis, extrinsic spinal cord compression requiring surgery must be excluded. Lumbar puncture is of diagnostic value in Guillain–Barré syndrome. In contrast, the most valuable diagnostic test in postinfectious encephalomyelitis or transverse myelitis is contrast-enhanced MRI. In Guillain–Barré syndrome, the efficacy of plasma exchange and intravenous immunoglobulin G has been demonstrated in controlled trials, as discussed in Chapter 59. In contrast, the treatment of ADEM is typically based on case reports and observational studies; some evidence exists for the use of methylprednisolone, usually given at a dose of 1 gram daily for 5 days.[154,172–174,181] Plasma exchange (usually five exchanges in total, performed daily or every other day) and intravenous immunoglobulin G, given as a total dose of 2 g/kg over 3 to 5 days, have also been used, either in combination with methylprednisolone or after methylprednisolone failure.[174] A variety of other immunosuppressive agents including cyclophosphamide have been used in individual cases. Initial treatment of acute transverse myelitis typically involves high-dose intravenous methylprednisolone.[181] Although treatment of acute hemorrhagic leukoencephalitis is frequently unsuccessful, occasional patients have survived after early treatment with combinations of methylprednisolone, intravenous immunoglobulin G, plasma exchange, or cyclophosphamide.[172]

ACKNOWLEDGEMENTS

The author thanks Dr. Karen Salzman for assistance in identifying appropriate imaging studies for this chapter. The author is supported by the Neurology and Research Services, Veterans Affairs Medical Center and the Department of Neurology, University of Utah Health Sciences Center.

REFERENCES

1. Whitley RJ, Roizman B: Herpes simplex virus infections. Lancet 357:1513, 2001.
2. Greenlee JE, O'Neill FJ: Polyomaviruses. p. 581. In: Richman DD, Whitley RJ, Hayden FG (eds): Clinical Virology. 3rd ed. ASM Press, Washington DC, 2009.
3. Griffin DE: Alphaviruses. p. 1023. In: Knipe DM, Howley PM (eds): Fields Virology. 5th ed. Lippincott Williams & Wilkins, Philadelphia, 2007.
4. Kinchington PR, Leger AJ, Guedon JM, et al: Herpes simplex virus and varicella zoster virus, the house guests who never leave. Herpesviridae 3:5, 2012.
5. Diamond MS, Shrestha B, Mehlhop E, et al: Innate and adaptive immune responses determine protection against disseminated infection by West Nile encephalitis virus. Viral Immunol 16:259, 2003.
6. Levi ME, Quan D, Ho JT, et al: Impact of rituximab-associated B-cell defects on West Nile virus meningoencephalitis in solid organ transplant recipients. Clin Transplant 24:223, 2010.
7. Greenlee JE: Progressive multifocal leucoencephalopathy in the era of natalizumab: a review and discussion of the implications. Int MS J 13:100, 2006.
8. Rotbart HA: Viral meningitis. Semin Neurol 20:277, 2000.
9. Kupila L, Vuorinen T, Vainionpaa R, et al: Etiology of aseptic meningitis and encephalitis in an adult population. Neurology 66:75, 2006.
10. Michos AG, Syriopoulou VP, Hadjichristodoulou C, et al: Aseptic meningitis in children: analysis of 506 cases. PLoS One 2:e674, 2007.
11. Romero JR, Newland JG: Viral meningitis and encephalitis: traditional and emerging viral agents. Semin Pediatr Infect Dis 14:72, 2003.
12. Koskiniemi M, Rantalaiho T, Piiparinen H, et al: Infections of the central nervous system of suspected viral origin: a collaborative study from Finland. J Neurovirol 7:400, 2001.
13. Centers for Disease Control and Prevention (CDC) West Nile virus disease and other arboviral diseases—United States, 2011. MMWR Morb Mortal Wkly Rep 61:510, 2012.
14. Bode AV, Sejvar JJ, Pape WJ, et al: West Nile virus disease: a descriptive study of 228 patients hospitalized in a 4-county region of Colorado in 2003. Clin Infect Dis 42:1234, 2006.

15. Barton LL, Hyndman NJ: Lymphocytic choriomeningitis virus: reemerging central nervous system pathogen. Pediatrics 105:e35, 2001.
16. de Ory F, Avellon A, Echevarria JE, et al: Viral infections of the central nervous system in Spain: a prospective study. J Med Virol 85:554, 2013.
17. Hubalek Z, Rudolf I: Tick-borne viruses in Europe. Parasitol Res 111:9, 2012.
18. Misra UK, Kalita J: Overview: Japanese encephalitis. Prog Neurobiol 91:108, 2010.
19. Rotbart HA: Enteroviral infections of the central nervous system. Clin Infect Dis 20:971, 1995.
20. Whitley RJ, Roizman B: Herpes simplex virus. p. 409. In: Richman DD, Whitley RJ, Hayden FG (eds): Clinical Virology. 3rd ed. ASM Press, Washington DC, 2009.
21. Bergstrom T, Vahlne A, Alestig K, et al: Primary and recurrent herpes simplex virus type 2-induced meningitis. J Infect Dis 162:322, 1990.
22. Tyler KL: Herpes simplex virus infections of the central nervous system: encephalitis and meningitis, including Mollaret's. Herpes 11(suppl 2):57A, 2004.
23. Dylewski JS, Bekhor S: Mollaret's meningitis caused by herpes simplex virus type 2: case report and literature review. Eur J Clin Microbiol Infect Dis 23:560, 2004.
24. Landry ML, Greenwold J, Vikram HR: Herpes simplex type-2 meningitis: presentation and lack of standardized therapy. Am J Med 122:688, 2009.
25. Aurelius E, Franzen-Rohl E, Glimaker M, et al: Long-term valacyclovir suppressive treatment after herpes simplex virus type 2 meningitis: a double-blind, randomized controlled trial. Clin Infect Dis 54:1304, 2012.
26. Pahud BA, Glaser CA, Dekker CL, et al: Varicella zoster disease of the central nervous system: epidemiological, clinical, and laboratory features 10 years after the introduction of the varicella vaccine. J Infect Dis 203:316, 2011.
27. Klein NC, McDermott B, Cunha BA: Varicella-zoster virus meningoencephalitis in an immunocompetent patient without a rash. Scand J Infect Dis 42:631, 2010.
28. Gilden D, Cohrs RJ, Mahalingam R, et al: Neurological disease produced by varicella zoster virus reactivation without rash. Curr Top Microbiol Immunol 342:243, 2010.
29. Chan CW, Tam KM, To WK, et al: Hypoglycorrhachia in herpes zoster associated encephalitis of an immunocompetent young male: an unusual presentation. J Neurol 252:987, 2005.
30. Habib AA, Gilden D, Schmid DS, et al: Varicella zoster virus meningitis with hypoglycorrhachia in the absence of rash in an immunocompetent woman. J Neurovirol 15:206, 2009.
31. Romero JR, Simonsen KA: Powassan encephalitis and Colorado tick fever. Infect Dis Clin North Am 22:545, 2008.
32. Barton LL: Human infection with lymphocytic choriomeningitis virus. Emerg Infect Dis 16:1046, 2010.
33. Greenlee JE, Carroll KC: Cerebrospinal fluid in central nervous system infections. p. 6. In: Scheld WM, Whitley RJ, Marra CM (eds): Infections of the Central Nervous System. 3rd ed. Lippincott Williams & Wilkins, Philadelphia, 2004.
34. Bonthius DJ: Lymphocytic choriomeningitis virus: a prenatal and postnatal threat. Adv Pediatr 56:75, 2009.
35. Fischer SA, Graham MB, Kuehnert MJ, et al: Transmission of lymphocytic choriomeningitis virus by organ transplantation. N Engl J Med 354:2235, 2006.
36. Macneil A, Stroher U, Farnon E, et al: Solid organ transplant-associated lymphocytic choriomeningitis, United States, 2011. Emerg Infect Dis 18:1256, 2012.
37. Galazka AM, Robertson SE, Kraigher A: Mumps and mumps vaccine: a global review. Bull World Health Organ 77:3, 1999.
38. Stahl JP, Mailles A, Dacheux L, et al: Epidemiology of viral encephalitis in 2011. Med Mal Infect 41:453, 2011.
39. Centers for Disease Control and Prevention (CDC): Mumps outbreak on a university campus—California, 2011. MMWR Morb Mortal Wkly Rep 61:986, 2012.
40. Marra CM: Human immunodeficiency virus. p. 273. In: Scheld WM, Whitley RJ, Marra CM (eds): Infections of the Central Nervous System. 3rd ed. Lippincott Williams & Wilkins, Philadelphia, 2004.
41. Kahn JO, Walker BD: Acute human immunodeficiency virus type 1 infection. N Engl J Med 339:33, 1998.
42. Robinson CC, Willis M, Meagher A, et al: Impact of rapid polymerase chain reaction results on management of pediatric patients with enteroviral meningitis. Pediatr Infect Dis J 21:283, 2002.
43. Davies NW, Brown LJ, Gonde J, et al: Factors influencing PCR detection of viruses in cerebrospinal fluid of patients with suspected CNS infections. J Neurol Neurosurg Psychiatry 76:82, 2005.
44. Gilden DH, Bennett JL, Kleinschmidt-DeMasters BK, et al: The value of cerebrospinal fluid antiviral antibody in the diagnosis of neurologic disease produced by varicella zoster virus. J Neurol Sci 159:140, 1998.
45. Garro AC, Rutman MS, Simonsen K, et al: Prevalence of Lyme meningitis in children with aseptic meningitis in a Lyme disease-endemic region. Pediatr Infect Dis J 30:990, 2011.
46. Tveitnes D, Natas OB, Skadberg O, et al: Lyme meningitis, the major cause of childhood meningitis in an endemic area: a population based study. Arch Dis Child 97:215, 2012.
47. Hopkins S, Jolles S: Drug-induced aseptic meningitis. Expert Opin Drug Saf 4:285, 2005.
48. Nettis E, Calogiuri G, Colanardi MC, et al: Drug-induced aseptic meningitis. Curr Drug Targets Immune Endocr Metabol Disord 3:143, 2003.
49. Davis LE: Acute and recurrent viral meningitis. Curr Treat Options Neurol 10:168, 2008.
50. Steiner I, Budka H, Chaudhuri A, et al: Viral meningoencephalitis: a review of diagnostic methods and guidelines for management. Eur J Neurol 17:999, 2010.

51. Desmond RA, Accortt NA, Talley L, et al: Enteroviral meningitis: natural history and outcome of pleconaril therapy. Antimicrob Agents Chemother 50:2409, 2006.
52. Rotbart HA, Webster AD: Treatment of potentially life-threatening enterovirus infections with pleconaril. Clin Infect Dis 32:228, 2001.
53. Ihanamaki T, Seppanen M, Tiainen M, et al: Echovirus type 4 as a probable cause of meningitis associated with bilateral optic neuritis: a case report. Clin Infect Dis 38:e49, 2004.
54. Waespe N, Steffen I, Heininger U: Etiology of aseptic meningitis, peripheral facial nerve palsy, and a combination of both in children. Pediatr Infect Dis J 29:453, 2010.
55. Lee HY, Chen CJ, Huang YC, et al: Clinical features of echovirus 6 and 9 infections in children. J Clin Virol 49:175, 2010.
56. Munoz-Sellart M, Garcia-Vidal C, Martinez-Yelamos S, et al: Peripheral facial palsy after varicella. Report of two cases and review of the literature. Enferm Infecc Microbiol Clin 28:504, 2010.
57. Sanjay S, Chan EW, Gopal L, et al: Complete unilateral ophthalmoplegia in herpes zoster ophthalmicus. J Neuroophthalmol 29:325, 2009.
58. Heppner PA, Schweder PM, Monteith SJ, et al: Acute hydrocephalus secondary to herpes simplex type II meningitis. J Clin Neurosci 15:1157, 2008.
59. Aydemir C, Eldes N, Kolsal E, et al: Acute tetraventricular hydrocephalus caused by mumps meningoencephalitis in a child. Pediatr Neurosurg 45:419, 2009.
60. Maraite N, Mataigne F, Pieri V, et al: Early decompressive hemicraniectomy in fulminant herpes simplex encephalitis. Bull Soc Sci Med Grand Duche Luxemb 279, 2010.
61. Kumar G, Kalita J, Misra UK: Raised intracranial pressure in acute viral encephalitis. Clin Neurol Neurosurg 111:399, 2009.
62. Glaser CA, Gilliam S, Schnurr D, et al: In search of encephalitis etiologies: diagnostic challenges in the California Encephalitis Project, 1998–2000. Clin Infect Dis 36:731, 2003.
63. Whitley RJ: Herpes simplex encephalitis: adolescents and adults. Antiviral Res 71:141, 2006.
64. Baringer JR, Pisani P: Herpes simplex virus genomes in human nervous sytem tissue analyzed by polymerase chain reaction. Ann Neurol 36:823, 1994.
65. Aurelius E, Johansson B, Skoldenberg B, et al: Encephalitis in immunocompetent patients due to herpes simplex virus type 1 or 2 as determined by type-specific polymerase chain reaction and antibody assays of cerebrospinal fluid. J Med Virol 39:179, 1993.
66. Whitley RJ, Kimberlin DW: Herpes simplex encephalitis: children and adolescents. Semin Pediatr Infect Dis 16:17, 2005.
67. Whitley RJ, Lakeman F: Herpes simplex virus infections of the central nervous system: therapeutic and diagnostic considerations. Clin Infect Dis 20:414, 1995.
68. Tan IL, McArthur JC, Venkatesan A, et al: Atypical manifestations and poor outcome of herpes simplex encephalitis in the immunocompromised. Neurology 79:2125, 2012.
69. Livorsi D, Anderson E, Qureshi S, et al: Brainstem encephalitis: an unusual presentation of herpes simplex virus infection. J Neurol 257:1432, 2010.
70. Booss J, Esiri MM: Herpes simplex encephalitis. p. 41. In: Booss J, Esiri MM (eds): Viral Encephalitis in Humans. ASM Press, Washington DC, 2003.
71. Jubelt B, Mihai C, Li TM, et al: Rhombencephalitis/brainstem encephalitis. Curr Neurol Neurosci Rep 11:543, 2011.
72. Whitley RJ, Soong SJ, Linneman Jr C, et al: Herpes simplex encephalitis. Clinical Assessment. JAMA 247:317, 1982.
73. Taylor SW, Lee DH, Jackson AC: Herpes simplex encephalitis presenting with exclusively frontal lobe involvement. J Neurovirol 13:477, 2007.
74. Al-Shekhlee A, Kocharian N, Suarez JJ: Re-evaluating the diagnostic methods in herpes simplex encephalitis. Herpes 13:17, 2006.
75. Lakeman FD, Whitley RJ: Diagnosis of herpes simplex encephalitis: application of polymerase chain reaction to cerebrospinal fluid from brain-biopsied patients and correlation with disease. National Institute of Allergy and Infectious Diseases Collaborative Antiviral Study Group. J Infect Dis 171:857, 1995.
76. Weil AA, Glaser CA, Amad Z, et al: Patients with suspected herpes simplex encephalitis: rethinking an initial negative polymerase chain reaction result. Clin Infect Dis 34:1154, 2002.
77. Denes E, Labach C, Durox H, et al: Intrathecal synthesis of specific antibodies as a marker of herpes simplex encephalitis in patients with negative PCR. Swiss Med Wkly 140:w13107, 2010.
78. Schulte EC, Sauerbrei A, Hoffmann D, et al: Acyclovir resistance in herpes simplex encephalitis. Ann Neurol 67:830, 2010.
79. Kakiuchi S, Nonoyama S, Wakamatsu H, et al: Neonatal herpes encephalitis caused by a virologically confirmed acyclovir-resistant herpes simplex virus 1 strain. J Clin Microbiol 51:356, 2013.
80. Whitley RJ, Alford CA, Hirsch MS, et al: Factors indicative of outcome in a comparative trial of acyclovir and vidarabine for biopsy-proven herpes simplex encephalitis. Infection 15(suppl 1):S3, 1987.
81. Hjalmarsson A, Blomqvist P, Skoldenberg B: Herpes simplex encephalitis in Sweden, 1990–2001: incidence, morbidity, and mortality. Clin Infect Dis 45:875, 2007.
82. McGrath N, Anderson NE, Croxson MC, et al: Herpes simplex encephalitis treated with acyclovir: diagnosis and long term outcome. J Neurol Neurosurg Psychiatry 63:321, 1997.

83. Gilden D, Mahalingam R, Nagel MA, et al: Review: the neurobiology of varicella zoster virus infection. Neuropathol Appl Neurobiol 37:441, 2011.
84. Bruxelle J, Pinchinat S: Effectiveness of antiviral treatment on acute phase of herpes zoster and development of post herpetic neuralgia: review of international publications. Med Mal Infect 42:53, 2012.
85. Kost RG, Strauss SE: Postherpetic neuralgia—pathogenesis, treatment, and prevention. N Engl J Med 335:32, 1996.
86. Oxman MN, Levin MJ, Johnson GR, et al: A vaccine to prevent herpes zoster and postherpetic neuralgia in older adults. N Engl J Med 352:2271, 2005.
87. Dubinsky RM, Kabbani H, El-Chami Z, et al: Practice parameter: treatment of postherpetic neuralgia: an evidence-based report of the Quality Standards Subcommittee of the American Academy of Neurology. Neurology 63:959, 2004.
88. Gilden D, Cohrs RJ, Mahalingam R, et al: Varicella zoster virus vasculopathies: diverse clinical manifestations, laboratory features, pathogenesis, and treatment. Lancet Neurol 8:731, 2009.
89. Mailles A, Stahl JP: Infectious encephalitis in France in 2007: a national prospective study. Clin Infect Dis 49:1838, 2009.
90. Granerod J, Ambrose HE, Davies NW, et al: Causes of encephalitis and differences in their clinical presentations in England: a multicentre, population-based prospective study. Lancet Infect Dis 10:835, 2010.
91. Booss J, Esiri MM: Varicella-zoster virus: the paradox of immune mediation and immunocmpromize. p. 127. In: Booss J, Esiri MM (eds): Viral Encephalitis in Humans. ASM Press, Washington DC, 2003.
92. Petersen LR, Marfin AA: West Nile virus: a primer for the clinician. Ann Intern Med 137:173, 2002.
93. Solomon T, Whitley RJ: Arthropod-borne viral encephalitides. p. 205. In: Scheld WM, Whitley RJ, Marra CM (eds): Infections of the Central Nervous System. Lippincott Williams & Wilkins, Philadelphia, 2004.
94. Davis LE, DeBiasi R, Goade DE, et al: West Nile virus neuroinvasive disease. Ann Neurol 60:286, 2006.
95. Sejvar JJ, Haddad MB, Tierney BC, et al: Neurologic manifestations and outcome of West Nile virus infection. JAMA 290:511, 2003.
96. Anninger WV, Lomeo MD, Dingle J, et al: West Nile virus-associated optic neuritis and chorioretinitis. Am J Ophthalmol 136:1183, 2003.
97. Leis AA, Stokic DS, Polk JL, et al: A poliomyelitis-like syndrome from West Nile virus infection. N Engl J Med 347:1279, 2002.
98. Tyler KL: West Nile virus infection in the United States. Arch Neurol 61:1190, 2004.
99. Petropoulou KA, Gordon SM, Prayson RA, et al: West Nile virus meningoencephalitis: MR imaging findings. AJNR Am J Neuroradiol 26:1986, 2005.
100. Makhoul B, Braun E, Herskovitz M, et al: Hyperimmune gammaglobulin for the treatment of West Nile virus encephalitis. Isr Med Assoc J 11:151, 2009.
101. Griffin DE: Arboviruses and the central nervous system. Springer Semin Immunopathol 17:121, 1995.
102. Smith DW, Mackenzie JS, Weaver SC: Alphaviruses. p. 1241. In: Richman DD, Whitley RJ, Hayden FG (eds): Clinical Virology. 3rd Ed. ASM Press, Washington DC, 2009.
103. Deresiewicz RL, Thaler SJ, Hsu L, et al: Clinical and neuroradiographic manifestations of eastern equine encephalitis. N Engl J Med 336:1867, 1997.
104. Dobler G, Gniel D, Petermann R, et al: Epidemiology and distribution of tick-borne encephalitis. Wien Med Wochenschr 162:230, 2012.
105. Fishbein DB, Robinson LE: Current concepts: rabies. N Engl J Med 329:1632, 1993.
106. Centers for Disease Control and Prevention (CDC) Imported human rabies in a U.S. Army soldier—New York, 2011. MMWR Morb Mortal Wkly Rep 61:302, 2012.
107. Vetter JM, Frisch L, Drosten C, et al: Survival after transplantation of corneas from a rabies-infected donor. Cornea 30:241, 2011.
108. Maier T, Schwarting A, Mauer D, et al: Management and outcomes after multiple corneal and solid organ transplantations from a donor infected with rabies virus. Clin Infect Dis 50:1112, 2010.
109. Srinivasan A, Burton EC, Kuehnert MJ, et al: Transmission of rabies virus from an organ donor to four transplant recipients. N Engl J Med 352:1103, 2005.
110. Smith JS, Fishbein DB, Rupprecht CE, et al: Unexplained rabies in three immigrants in the United States a virologic investigation. N Engl J Med 324:205, 1991.
111. Jackson AC, Ye H, Phelan CC, et al: Extraneural organ involvement in human rabies. Lab Invest 79:945, 1999.
112. Jogai S, Radotra BD, Banerjee AK: Rabies viral antigen in extracranial organs: a post-mortem study. Neuropathol Appl Neurobiol 28:334, 2002.
113. Mrak RE, Young L: Rabies encephalitis in a patient with no history of exposure. Hum Pathol 24:109, 1993.
114. Laothamatas J, Hemachudha T, Mitrabhakdi E, et al: MR imaging in human rabies. AJNR Am J Neuroradiol 24:1102, 2003.
115. Frenia ML, Lafin SM, Barone JA: Features and treatment of rabies. Clin Pharm 11:37, 1992.
116. Hattwick MAW, Weis TT, Stechschulte CJ, et al: Recovery from rabies. A case report. Ann Intern Med 76:931, 1972.
117. Jackson AC: Current and future approaches to the therapy of human rabies. Antiviral Res 99:61, 2013.
118. Willoughby Jr RE, Tieves KS, Hoffman GM, et al: Survival after treatment of rabies with induction of coma. N Engl J Med 352:2508, 2005.

119. Ooi MH, Wong SC, Lewthwaite P, et al: Clinical features, diagnosis, and management of enterovirus 71. Lancet Neurol 9:1097, 2010.
120. Jang S, Suh SI, Ha SM, et al: Enterovirus 71-related encephalomyelitis: usual and unusual magnetic resonance imaging findings. Neuroradiology 54:239, 2012.
121. Kang SS, McGavern DB: Lymphocytic choriomeningitis infection of the central nervous system. Front Biosci 13:4529, 2008.
122. Douvoyiannis M, Litman N, Goldman DL: Neurologic manifestations associated with parvovirus B19 infection. Clin Infect Dis 48:1713, 2009.
123. Ward KN, Andrews NJ, Verity CM, et al: Human herpesviruses-6 and -7 each cause significant neurological morbidity in Britain and Ireland. Arch Dis Child 90:619, 2005.
124. Yao K, Honarmand S, Espinosa A, et al: Detection of human herpesvirus-6 in cerebrospinal fluid of patients with encephalitis. Ann Neurol 65:257, 2009.
125. Griffin DE: Emergence and re-emergence of viral diseases of the central nervous system. Prog Neurobiol 91:95, 2010.
126. Kleinschmidt-DeMasters BK, Gilden DH: The expanding spectrum of herpesvirus infections of the nervous system. Brain Pathol 11:440, 2001.
127. Majid A, Galetta SL, Sweeney CJ, et al: Epstein-Barr virus myeloradiculitis and encephalomyeloradiculitis. Brain 125:159, 2002.
128. Portegies P, Corssmit N: Epstein-Barr virus and the nervous system. Curr Opin Neurol 13:301, 2000.
129. Quartier P, Foray S, Casanova JL, et al: Enteroviral meningoencephalitis in X-linked agammaglobulinemia: intensive immunoglobulin therapy and sequential viral detection in cerebrospinal fluid by polymerase chain reaction. Pediatr Infect Dis J 19:1106, 2000.
130. Cunningham CK, Bonville CA, Ochs HD, et al: Enteroviral meningoencephalitis as a complication of X-linked hyper IgM syndrome. J Pediatr 134:584, 1999.
131. Ganjoo KN, Raman R, Sobel RA, et al: Opportunistic enteroviral meningoencephalitis: an unusual treatable complication of rituximab therapy. Leuk Lymphoma 50:673, 2009.
132. Ahmed R, Buckland M, Davies L, et al: Enterovirus 71 meningoencephalitis complicating rituximab therapy. J Neurol Sci 305:149, 2011.
133. Anders HJ, Goebel FD: Neurological manifestations of cytomegalovirus infection in the acquired immunodeficiency syndrome. Int J STD AIDS 10:151, 1999.
134. Carrigan DR: Adenovirus infections in immunocompromised patients. Am J Med 102:71, 1997.
135. Clark DA: Human herpesvirus 6 and human herpesvirus 7: emerging pathogens in transplant patients. Int J Hematol 76(suppl 2):246, 2002.
136. Chretien F, Belec L, Hilton DA, et al: Herpes simplex virus type 1 encephalitis in acquired immunodeficiency syndrome. Neuropathol Appl Neurobiol 22:394, 1996.
137. Gray F, Belec L, Lescs MC, et al: Varicella-zoster virus infection of the central nervous system in the acquired immune deficiency syndrome. Brain 117:987, 1994.
138. van de Beek D, Patel R, Daly RC, et al: Central nervous system infections in heart transplant recipients. Arch Neurol 64:1715, 2007.
139. Dewhurst S: Human herpesvirus type 6 and human herpesvirus type 7 infections of the central nervous system. Herpes 11(suppl 2):105A, 2004.
140. Pot C, Burkhard PR, Villard J, et al: Human herpesvirus-6 variant A encephalomyelitis. Neurology 70:974, 2008.
141. Maschke M, Kastrup O, Diener HC: CNS manifestations of cytomegalovirus infections: diagnosis and treatment. CNS Drugs 16:303, 2002.
142. Birnbaum T, Padovan CS, Sporer B, et al: Severe meningoencephalitis caused by human herpesvirus 6 type B in an immunocompetent woman treated with ganciclovir. Clin Infect Dis 40:887, 2005.
143. Perez-Liz G, Del Valle L, Gentilella A, et al: Detection of JC virus DNA fragments but not proteins in normal brain tissue. Ann Neurol 64:379, 2008.
144. Berger JR, Concha M: Progressive multifocal leukoencephalopathy: the evolution of a disease once considered rare. J Neurovirol 1:5, 1995.
145. Palazzo E, Yahia SA: Progressive multifocal leukoencephalopathy in autoimmune diseases. Joint Bone Spine 79:351, 2012.
146. Tavazzi E, Ferrante P, Khalili K: Progressive multifocal leukoencephalopathy: an unexpected complication of modern therapeutic monoclonal antibody therapies. Clin Microbiol Infect 17:1776, 2011.
147. Koralnik IJ, Wuthrich C, Dang X, et al: JC virus granule cell neuronopathy: a novel clinical syndrome distinct from progressive multifocal leukoencephalopathy. Ann Neurol 57:576, 2005.
148. Yousry TA, Pelletier D, Cadavid D, et al: Magnetic resonance imaging pattern in natalizumab-associated progressive multifocal leukoencephalopathy. Ann Neurol 72:779, 2012.
149. Greenlee JE: Progressive multifocal leukoencephalopathy. p. 399. In: Aminoff MJ, Goetz CG (eds): Handbook of Clinical Neurology. Elsevier, Amsterdam, 1998.
150. Marzocchetti A, Di Giambenedetto S, Cingolani A, et al: Reduced rate of diagnostic positive detection of JC virus DNA in cerebrospinal fluid in cases of suspected progressive multifocal leukoencephalopathy in the era of potent antiretroviral therapy. J Clin Microbiol 43:4175, 2005.
151. Aksamit AJ: Treatment of non-AIDS progressive multifocal leukoencephalopathy with cytosine arabinoside. J Neurovirol 7:386, 2001.
152. Tan IL, McArthur JC, Clifford DB, et al: Immune reconstitution inflammatory syndrome in natalizumab-associated PML. Neurology 77:1061, 2011.

153. Vendrely A, Bienvenu B, Gasnault J, et al: Fulminant inflammatory leukoencephalopathy associated with HAART-induced immune restoration in AIDS-related progressive multifocal leukoencephalopathy. Acta Neuropathol (Berl) 109:449, 2005.
154. Tunkel AR, Glaser CA, Bloch KC, et al: The management of encephalitis: clinical practice guidelines by the Infectious Diseases Society of America. Clin Infect Dis 47:303, 2008.
155. Kupersmith MJ, Martin V, Heller G, et al: Idiopathic hypertrophic pachymeningitis. Neurology 62:686, 2004.
156. Zuliani L, Graus F, Giometto B, et al: Central nervous system neuronal surface antibody associated syndromes: review and guidelines for recognition. J Neurol Neurosurg Psychiatry 83:638, 2012.
157. Adamo MA, Deshaies EM: Emergency decompressive craniectomy for fulminating infectious encephalitis. J Neurosurg 108:174, 2008.
158. Sikorska B, Liberski PP: Human prion diseases: from kuru to variant Creutzfeldt-Jakob disease. Subcell Biochem 65:457, 2012.
159. Johnson RT: Prion diseases. Lancet Neurol 4:635, 2005.
160. Prusiner SB: The prion diseases. Brain Pathol 8:499, 1998.
161. Brown P, Brandel JP, Sato T, et al: Iatrogenic Creutzfeldt-Jakob disease, final assessment. Emerg Infect Dis 18:901, 2012.
162. Collins SJ, Sanchez-Juan P, Masters CL, et al: Determinants of diagnostic investigation sensitivities across the clinical spectrum of sporadic Creutzfeldt-Jakob disease. Brain 129:2278, 2006.
163. Geschwind MD, Haman A, Miller BL: Rapidly progressive dementia. Neurol Clin 25:783, 2007.
164. Wieser HG, Schindler K, Zumsteg D: EEG in Creutzfeldt-Jakob disease. Clin Neurophysiol 117:935, 2006.
165. Macfarlane RG, Wroe SJ, Collinge J, et al: Neuroimaging findings in human prion disease. J Neurol Neurosurg Psychiatry 78:664, 2007.
166. Hamlin C, Puoti G, Berri S, et al: A comparison of tau and 14-3-3 protein in the diagnosis of Creutzfeldt-Jakob disease. Neurology 79:547, 2012.
167. Almond JW: Bovine spongiform encephalopathy and new variant Creutzfeldt-Jakob disease. Br Med Bull 54:749, 1998.
168. Zeidler M, Sellar RJ, Collie DA, et al: The pulvinar sign on magnetic resonance imaging in variant Creutzfeldt-Jakob disease. Lancet 355:1412, 2000.
169. Young NP, Weinshenker BG, Lucchinetti CF: Acute disseminated encephalomyelitis: current understanding and controversies. Semin Neurol 28:84, 2008.
170. Wender M: Acute disseminated encephalomyelitis (ADEM). J Neuroimmunol 231:92, 2011.
171. Tenembaum S, Chamoles N, Fejerman N: Acute disseminated encephalomyelitis: a long-term follow-up study of 84 pediatric patients. Neurology 59:1224, 2002.
172. Tenembaum S, Chitnis T, Ness J, et al: Acute disseminated encephalomyelitis. Neurology 68:S23, 2007.
173. van der Maas NA, Bondt PE, de Melker H, et al: Acute cerebellar ataxia in the Netherlands: a study on the association with vaccinations and varicella zoster infection. Vaccine 27:1970, 2009.
174. Sonneville R, Klein I, de Broucker T, et al: Post-infectious encephalitis in adults: diagnosis and management. J Infect 58:321, 2009.
175. de Seze J, Debouverie M, Zephir H, et al: Acute fulminant demyelinating disease: a descriptive study of 60 patients. Arch Neurol 64:1426, 2007.
176. Schwarz S, Mohr A, Knauth M, et al: Acute disseminated encephalomyelitis: a follow-up study of 40 adult patients. Neurology 56:1313, 2001.
177. Mader I, Wolff M, Nagele T, et al: MRI and proton MR spectroscopy in acute disseminated encephalomyelitis. Childs Nerv Syst 21:566, 2005.
178. Borchers AT, Gershwin ME: Transverse myelitis. Autoimmun Rev 11:231, 2012.
179. Fazio R, Radaelli M, Furlan R: Neuromyelitis optica: concepts in evolution. J Neuroimmunol 231:100, 2011.
180. Scott TF, Frohman EM, De Seze J, et al: Evidence-based guideline: clinical evaluation and treatment of transverse myelitis: report of the Therapeutics and Technology Assessment Subcommittee of the American Academy of Neurology. Neurology 77:2128, 2011.
181. Sebire G, Hollenberg H, Meyer L, et al: High dose methylprednisolone in severe acute transverse myelopathy. Arch Dis Child 76:167, 1997.
182. Kappos L, Bates D, Edan G, et al: Natalizumab treatment for multiple sclerosis: updated recommendations for patient selection and monitoring. Lancet Neurol 10:745, 2011.

CHAPTER

44

HIV and Other Retroviral Infections of the Nervous System

MICHAEL J. PELUSO ■ SERENA SPUDICH

Human immunodeficiency virus type 1 (HIV-1) infection involves the central nervous system (CNS) beginning during primary viremia and continuing over the course of untreated infection.[1,2] Although the majority of patients with HIV infection do not present with neurologic symptoms, HIV disease has protean manifestations in the CNS determined largely by host characteristics such as immune status, treatment history, and access and adherence to antiretroviral therapy (ART).

THIRTY YEARS LATER: HIV BEYOND THE IMMUNE SYSTEM

Thirty years after the report of five unexplained cases of *Pneumocystis carinii* pneumonia in men suffering from what would eventually become recognized as the acquired immunodeficiency syndrome (AIDS), HIV infection remains the subject of intense biochemical, molecular, clinical, and epidemiologic investigation. HIV infection is a bloodborne and sexually transmitted disease that impacts both individual and public health and has disproportionately affected vulnerable and marginalized individuals and populations including the poor and underserved, injection drug users, commercial sex workers, and men who have sex with men. The epidemic has also changed in the last decades. What once was largely a disease of young men who have sex with men in urban centers has expanded to affect all populations; the highest route of overall transmission of HIV is currently through heterosexual contact, often in rural areas in individuals unaware of their risk of HIV acquisition.[3]

It is estimated that there are currently 34 million people infected with HIV worldwide and 2.5 million new infections annually. Around 1.7 million individuals die from the disease and its sequelae each year.[4] Although the greatest number of new

Aminoff's Neurology and General Medicine, Fifth Edition.

infections and the worst outcomes occur in the lowest-resource settings in sub-Saharan Africa and Southeast Asia, nearly 50,000 individuals are newly infected in the United States each year, reflecting little change over the course of the epidemic.[5]

A better understanding of the virus's characteristics, including its pathogenesis and transmission patterns, has led to both prophylactic and therapeutic interventions, but many questions about the pathogenesis of HIV infection remain unanswered. An increased focus on the effects of HIV infection beyond the immune system has emerged, including its end-organ effects on the nervous system.

HIV IN THE NERVOUS SYSTEM

HIV is a single-stranded, positive-sense retrovirus of the genus *Lentivirus*. Once transmitted to a new host, the virus uses a reverse transcriptase to transcribe viral RNA into DNA. This DNA is, in turn, integrated into the genome of the host. The stages of HIV infection are divided into the acute phase that immediately follows transmission and includes the $CD4^+$ T-cell nadir, the asymptomatic latent phase characterized by a slow decline in $CD4^+$ T cells, and the symptomatic phase of chronic AIDS.[6] In antiretroviral-naïve patients, it takes approximately 10 years to develop AIDS, although this time may be extended indefinitely with combination ART (cART; Fig. 44-1). Following the development of AIDS, median survival is typically between 1 and 4 years.

It is increasingly recognized that the body's reaction to HIV infection can be as damaging as the activity of the virus itself, and this is particularly true in the nervous system. The inflammatory milieu that is induced by the activity of HIV in invading cells and triggers an immune response has important implications throughout the time course of infection. It is thought that HIV pathogenesis within the CNS is mediated primarily by inflammation induced by both systemic immune activation as well as HIV infection of macrophages, microglia, and astrocytes. It is hypothesized that an indirect toxic injury to neurons results from a cascade of chronic and persistent neuroinflammation, in part fostered by cytokines produced by infected or activated cells

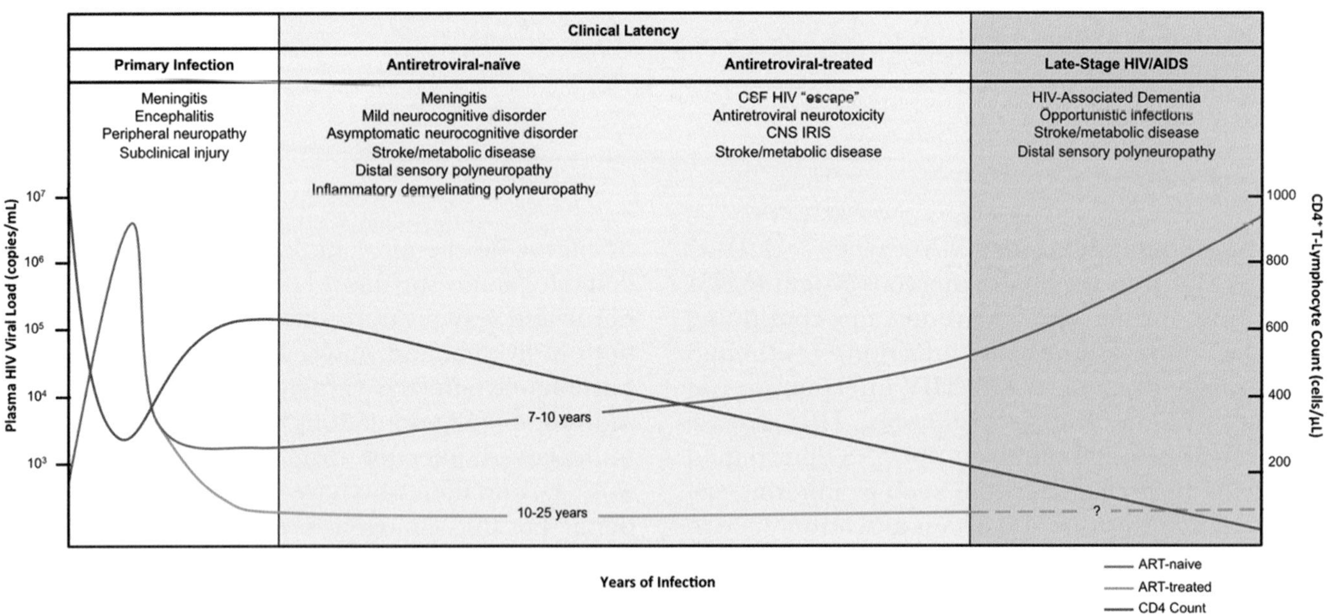

FIGURE 44-1 ▪ Typical time course of HIV-1 infection and characteristic neurologic abnormalities. Primary HIV infection refers to the first year following viral transmission, which includes the acute retroviral syndrome, widespread distribution of the virus, the seeding of lymphoid organs, and the $CD4^+$ T-cell nadir. After a recovery in the $CD4^+$ T-cell count, infected individuals enter a long period of clinical latency in which they experience a slow decline in the $CD4^+$ T-cell population. If treatment is not initiated, the $CD4^+$ T-cell count falls to critically low levels and the patient develops acquired immunodeficiency syndrome (AIDS) after 7 to 10 years. This period is characterized by viral proliferation, acquisition of opportunistic infections, and end-organ damage in a variety of body systems, ultimately leading to death from one or a combination of these causes. If treatment is initiated, clinical latency persists for an undetermined period of time, but patients continue to be at risk of a variety of neurologic complications, including several unique to individuals on therapy.

within the brain.[7] In the earliest stages of infection, the virus crosses the blood–brain barrier for the first time and initiates cytokine release that contributes to breakdown of that barrier. Other effects include a cerebrospinal fluid (CSF) pleocytosis, macrophage and lymphocyte activation, interference with neuronal synthesis and maintenance pathways, and ultimately neuronal injury that can be detected through biomarkers and neuroimaging. Although control of the virus through the initiation of cART can decrease the viral load and supppress the immune response, the CNS remains particularly vulnerable to further insult and may not normalize as well as systemic compartments.[8]

Recent studies of the end-organ effects of HIV beyond the immune system have led to the recognition of a biologic compartmentalization that allows for infection and injury of target tissue, independent evolution of the virus from its counterparts in the plasma, and protection of the virus from systemic therapy.[9] The development of these distinct biologic compartments, such as those in the breast and genital tract, facilitates viral replication, complicates viral eradication, and leads to organ-specific effects.[10,11] Chronic HIV infection is associated with the establishment of a CNS reservoir of infection, as evidenced by the detection of HIV DNA in perivascular brain macrophages, microglial cells, and astrocytes, compartmentalization of HIV quasispecies in CNS tissues, and clinical cases of isolated CNS "escape" from antiretroviral therapy.[12–15] Targeting treatments and strategies towards CNS reservoirs of HIV has become an important aspect of recent efforts to achieve a cure for HIV infection.

NEUROLOGIC DYSFUNCTION IN THE SETTING OF ANTIRETROVIRAL THERAPY

The introduction of cART in the mid-1990s fundamentally altered the landscape of both systemic and neurologic HIV disease. The profound immunodeficiency associated with HIV/AIDS that acted as the substrate for the "classic" neurologic manifestations of the disease itself and the opportunistic infections with which it was associated can now be significantly delayed or prevented, transforming the disease from one that was uniformly fatal into a manageable chronic illness.

In general, antiretroviral therapy suppresses both plasma and CSF viral levels and improves neurologic outcomes in patients with HIV infection.[16] Typically, plasma HIV RNA suppression is paralleled by suppression in the CSF, and the initiation of cART also limits the extent of immune activation in the CSF, as measured by white blood cell count and immunologic markers.[17,18] With systemic control of the virus and improved immune status has come a striking decline in the occurrence of neurologic opportunistic infections over the last two decades, while the attenuation of viral replication and immune activation in the CNS has resulted in a decline in the incidence of the most dramatic forms of HIV-associated neurologic disease.[19] Nevertheless, even individuals with well-controlled HIV infection continue to experience neurologic dysfunction which, although often less pronounced than the illnesses experienced 30 years ago by many patients with AIDS, has the potential to seriously impact productivity and quality of life.[20,21]

HIV-Associated Neurocognitive Disorder

What was previously defined in its most severe form as the AIDS-dementia complex is now represented by a spectrum of disorders reflecting the variability in presentation, outcome, and impact of neurologic disease.

HIV-associated neurocognitive disorder (HAND) comprises a diverse set of neurocognitive diseases, ranging from clinically asymptomatic impairment to severe dementia. HAND is a clinical diagnosis defined by abnormalities identified through neuropsychologic testing and is subdivided into three categories of increasing severity: asymptomatic neurocognitive impairment, mild neurocognitive disorder, and HIV-associated dementia (HAD) (Table 44-1).[22] These diagnoses require the administration of a specific neuropsychologic test battery assessing language, attention, executive functioning, memory (learning and recall), processing speed, visuospatial abilities, and motor skills. While the incidence of the most severe manifestations of HAND has decreased in the setting of widespread access to cART, mild-to-moderate HAND has persisted and has become the most prevalent primary CNS complication of HIV infection.[20]

Asymptomatic Neurocognitive Impairment

The most benign and most common manifestation of HAND is asymptomatic neurocognitive impairment, which has been identified in approximately

TABLE 44-1 ■ Classification of HIV-Associated Neurocognitive Disorder (HAND) in Patients Being Treated with Antiretroviral Therapy

	Asymptomatic Neurocognitive Impairment (ANI)	Mild Neurocognitive Disorder (MND)	HIV-Associated Dementia (HAD)
Neuropsychological Testing Abnormalities	One standard deviation below the age- and education-adjusted mean on two cognitive domains	One standard deviation below the age- and education-adjusted mean on two cognitive domains	Two standard deviations below the age- and education-adjusted mean on two cognitive domains, especially learning, information processing, and attention/concentration
Effect on Everyday Function	None	Mild May be noted by self or others, including impairments in mental acuity, work efficiency, maintenance of home life, social functioning	Marked May be noted by self or others, manifesting as severe difficulty in work, independent maintenance of home life, and social functioning
	Absent	Absent	May be present, but must be absent on at least one prior occasion where dementia was present
Dementia	Absent	Absent	Present Other causes such as opportunistic infection, vascular dementia, severe active drug use must be absent

one-third of HIV-infected patients.[20] It is characterized as a subclinical cognitive decline with decreased performance on neuropsychologic testing in two or more domains not attributable to comorbid conditions (e.g., mood disorders, substance abuse). It specifically requires that no negative impact on everyday functioning is present, distinguishing it from mild neurocognitive disorder.

It is unclear whether asymptomatic neurocognitive impairment predicts more severe neurologic impairment later in the course of HIV, whether it contributes to neuropathologic vulnerability, and whether early intervention with cART at this stage might prevent ongoing deterioration.[23]

Mild Neurocognitive Disorder

A form of mild cognitive impairment is being recognized increasingly in individuals treated with cART, who typically have a relatively reconstituted immune system characterized by high $CD4^+$ T-cell counts and suppressed or undetectable viral loads. As the population of patients with chronic, well-controlled HIV infection continues to grow, so too does the overall prevalence of mild neurocognitive disorder, which may approach 12 percent in some studies.[20]

The diagnosis of mild neurocognitive disorder depends on the detection of abnormalities in neuropsychologic testing in attention, processing speed, memory, and executive function domains. In contrast to those with asymptomatic neurocognitive impairment, patients typically are aware of a subtle impairment in cognitive ability and increased difficulty carrying out activities of daily living. Mild neurocognitive disorder can also affect both pyramidal and extrapyramidal motor systems, producing symptoms such as ataxia, tremor, and incoordination that may worsen over time. It can lead to behavioral symptoms that are independent of those associated with mood disorders concomitant with HIV infection.[24]

HIV-Associated Dementia

The disorder initially described 25 years ago as the AIDS-dementia complex is now known as HIV-associated dementia (HAD), the most dramatic manifestation of HAND. The diagnosis remains a challenge, as there are no diagnostic studies or laboratory tests that are specific for HAD.[22]

The diagnosis of HAD is based on progressive neurocognitive impairment and the exclusion of other conditions that can mimic these symptoms including CNS opportunistic infections and mass lesions such as tumors. HAD is still identified most commonly in patients not taking antiretroviral therapy; the prevalence in treated patients may be as low as 2 percent.[20,25] HAD most typically occurs in patients with slowed cognitive processing in the context of long-standing HIV infection and is often accompanied by motor abnormalities such as slowed movement and spastic gait along with hyperactive muscle

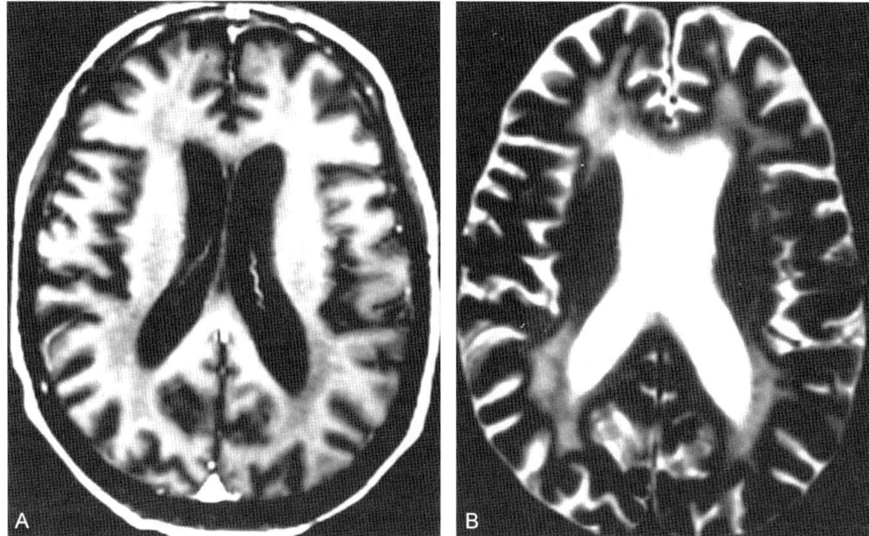

FIGURE 44-2 ■ **A,** T1-weighted magnetic resonance image (MRI) of patient with HIV-associated dementia showing marked cerebral and cortical atrophy. **B,** T2-weighted MRI of the same patient showing extensive hyperintense signal abnormalities in the white matter. (From Berger JR: AIDS and the nervous system. p. 851. In Aminoff MJ (ed): Neurology and General Medicine. 4th Ed. Churchill Livingstone Elsevier, Philadelphia, 2008, with permission.)

stretch reflexes. Evaluation with computed tomography (CT) or magnetic resonance imaging (MRI) of the brain is used to exclude other AIDS-related neurologic conditions, including opportunistic infections and CNS lymphoma. With these diagnoses excluded, diffuse cerebral atrophy and subcortical or periventricular white matter changes are consistent with, although not specific for, HAD.[26]

Etiology

Although the biologic substrate of HAND in the setting of antiretroviral therapy is unknown, one potential mechanism involves injury occurring in the earliest stages of HIV infection. Such injury would begin before treatment is initiated and would continue along a trajectory that may or may not be mitigated by initiation of cART. After several years, a combination of host susceptibility and disease factors may result in the development of symptomatic neurologic disease.

Another possibility is that, due to the compartment-specific nature of CNS HIV infection, neurologic injury is incurred despite the initiation and continuation of systemically suppressive treatment. Even in individuals with no overt signs or symptoms of neurocognitive impairment, the presence of HIV in the CNS may result in constant low-level inflammation and immune activation that may lead to ongoing brain injury. CSF immune activation, brain inflammation detected by magnetic resonance spectroscopy, and microglial activation persist in patients on long-term suppressive antiretroviral therapy.[27]

Diagnosis and Management

Because HAND has no specific diagnostic markers, it is necessary to exclude CNS opportunistic infections, delirium, toxic-metabolic disorders, psychiatric disease, and other neurodegenerative conditions before making the diagnosis. Although traditional neuroimaging is useful in excluding other HIV-associated disease processes, including CNS lymphoma, infections, and inflammatory processes, there are no findings on standard imaging that are specific for HAND (Fig. 44-2). Efforts to use more advanced neuroimaging techniques to identify mild HAND have included brain mapping, high-field structural imaging, functional MRI, and magnetic resonance spectroscopy.[28,29] The utility of these new modalities remains to be determined. Figure 44-3 provides an algorithm for the identification and management of HAND.[30]

Performance on neuropsychologic tests in severe forms of HAND improves with the initiation of cART.[31] The introduction of cART has been associated with decreased incidence and prevalence of HAD despite increases in the prevalence of milder forms of HAND.[25] While initiation of cART significantly improves cognitive performance and

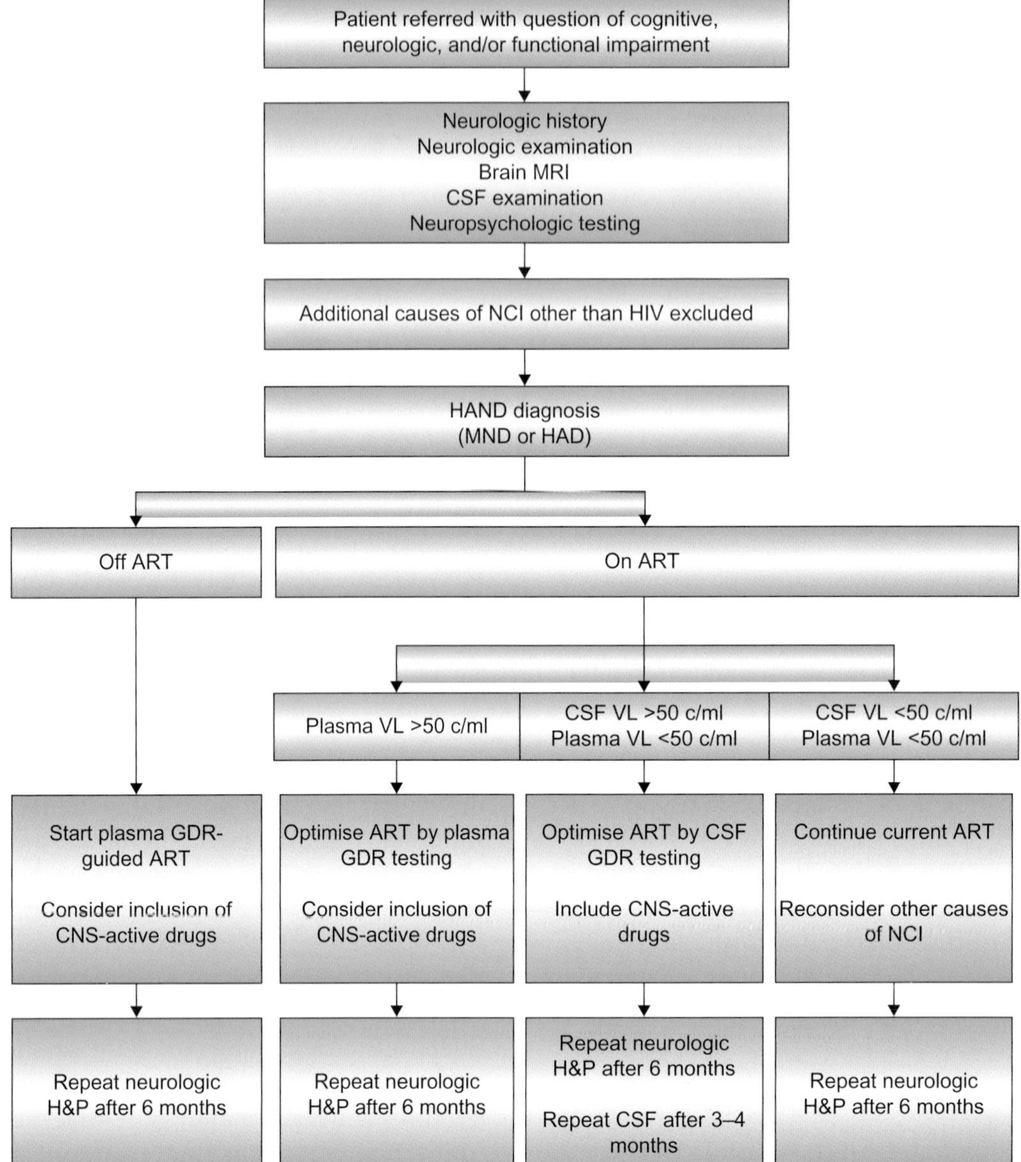

FIGURE 44-3 ■ Diagnostic and management algorithm for HIV-associated neurocognitive disorder. GDR, genotype drug resistance; H&P, history and physical examination; MND, mild neurocognitive disorder; NCI, neurocognitive impairment; VL, viral load. (Adapted from the European AIDS Clinical Society Guidelines, Version 6.1, November 2012.)

neurologic function in antiretroviral naïve patients with HAD, this improvement is frequently incomplete.[32] Furthermore, many patients already taking cART also have HAND.

Treatment

Adjunctive therapies that target the CNS have been studied in an attempt to attenuate the inflammatory events that are postulated in the pathogenesis of HAND. Adjunctive therapies other than with antiretroviral agents, including with memantine, selegiline, and nimodipine, have not been successful.[33] Valproic acid and lithium have been hypothesized to decrease HIV replication and neuroinflammation through their glycogen synthase kinase-3β activity, as have serotonin reuptake inhibitors such as citalopram and paroxetine through an unknown mechanism; no clear improvement in HAND has been demonstrated with these agents.[34] Due to its anti-inflammatory and antiviral effects, the antibiotic minocycline has also been suggested as a potential therapy, but randomized trials have been unsuccessful.[35] Statins, which have widespread

TABLE 44-2 ■ Proposed CNS Penetration-Effectiveness (CPE) Ranks for Commonly Used Antiretroviral Agents, 2010

	CNS Penetration-Effectiveness Score			
Drug Class	**4**	**3**	**2**	**1**
NRT Inhibitor	Zidovudine	Abacavir Emtricitabine	Lamivudine Stavudine	Didanosine Tenofovir Zalcitabine
NNRT Inhibitor	Nevirapine	Delavirdine Efavirenz	Etravirine	–
Protease Inhibitor	Indinavir/r	Darunavir/r Fosamprenavir/r Indinavir Lopinavir/r	Atazanavir Atazanavir/r Fosamprenavir	Nelfinavir Ritonavir Saquinavir Saquinavir/r Tipranavir/r
Entry Inhibitor	Vicriviroc	Maraviroc	–	Enfurvirtide
Integrase Inhibitor	–	Raltegravir	–	–

Adapted from Clifford DB: HIV and the brain: update 2010. International AIDS Society–USA, March 22, 2010, New York, NY.
Higher numbers indicate higher CNS penetration and effectiveness. NRT, nucleoside reverse transcriptase; NNRT, non-nucleoside reverse transcriptase; /r = ritonavir boosted.

anti-inflammatory effects, are under study.[36] Methylphenidate successfully treats fatigue and psychomotor slowing in patients with HAND, but does not alter the course of the disease.[37,38] An alternate treatment strategy using antiretroviral drugs that penetrate into the CNS is discussed later.

Targeted Treatment of CNS HIV Infection

By separating the CNS from the systemic circulation, the blood–brain and blood–CSF barriers affect the ability of antiretroviral agents to access the CNS compartment. In addition, local spontaneous replication of HIV within this viral sanctuary may allow for independent mutations of HIV virions.[9] While the response of CSF HIV RNA levels to cART parallels that in the plasma, the rate of decay in the CSF may be more gradual in some patients, suggesting a compartmentalization characterized by slower cell turnover, extended macrophage release, or attenuated drug entry.[39]

Because of the blood–brain barrier, HIV in the CNS may be protected from the full effect of antiretroviral agents, especially those drugs that are large or hydrophilic. The CNS penetration-effectiveness (CPE) index represents an effort to estimate quantitatively the relative ability of each antiretroviral agent to penetrate the CNS and interfere with CSF HIV replication. Each agent is assigned a CPE score based on presumed CNS exposure and efficacy of the drug in relation to others in its class (Table 44-2).

Some studies have shown that antiretroviral regimens with higher CPE scores tend to be more successful at achieving HIV RNA suppression in the CNS.[40] While more potent HIV RNA suppression in this compartment might be expected to lead to better neurocognitive outcomes, results have been mixed, with some studies showing that regimens with higher CPE scores actually lead to poorer neurocognitive performance or only benefit patients treated with more than the standard cART regimen of three drugs.[41–43]

The inability of antiretroviral therapy to control the potential reservoir of HIV that exists in monocytes has been proposed as one possible explanation for continued neurocognitive impairment in the setting of cART. As a result, a monocyte efficacy (ME) score has been proposed as an alternative means of quantifying the ability of antiretroviral agents to affect neurologic outcomes. Preliminary work has suggested that that the ME score correlates with neurocognitive performance even when CPE score does not.[44]

Progressive Disease Despite Systemic Response

Several new clinical syndromes have been recognized in patients taking systemically suppressive cART, often after a long period of apparently successful treatment. A phenomenon of CSF/plasma viral load discordance in the setting of new neurologic symptoms has been identified in some patients with a well-controlled plasma viral load.[14,15] This discordance syndrome is also known as *symptomatic CSF escape*. Although the virus is controlled or suppressed in the plasma, it is present at a concentration of 1 log greater in the CSF. Patients with symptomatic CSF escape include a broad spectrum of individuals with cART-managed HIV including those persistently suppressed or well-controlled for many years, as well as those with recent spikes in viral load and those beginning to achieve viral control.

The pathogenesis of symptomatic CSF escape is related to the failure of cART to suppress local CNS infection despite peripheral $CD4^+$ T-cell reconstitution. Although detectable CSF HIV in the context of cART is required, it is not sufficient, since asymptomatic CSF escape has been identified as a frequent finding (up to 10%) in asymptomatic individuals undergoing lumbar puncture in the context of HIV research studies.[45] A moderately reconstituted immune system may actually contribute to the symptomatic syndrome by eliciting a symptomatic inflammatory response and providing a substrate for ongoing discordant HIV replication within the CNS. This process may lie on the spectrum of the immune reconstitution inflammatory syndrome (IRIS), but may represent a stable state of antigen and immune response within the CNS, rather than the exaggerated response upon immune reconstitution that occurs in IRIS. Low $CD4^+$ T-cell nadir (i.e., <250 cells/mm^3) may be a risk factor for CSF "escape," suggesting that a history of advanced immunosuppression may confer increased risk of the syndrome.[14,15] In addition to resistance and poor penetration, poor medication adherence might also contribute by leading to insufficient drug concentrations in the CSF and thus to the selection of resistant virus within the CSF.

The clinical features of symptomatic CSF escape include a variety of subacute to acute, progressive neurologic symptoms including cognitive, sensory, and motor impairment resulting in significant debilitation. Diagnosis is achieved through the recognition of plasma/CSF discordance and the exclusion of opportunistic infections including progressive multifocal leukoencephalopathy (PML). Imaging may show white matter hyperintensities on T2-weighted MRI sequences. Resistance genotyping of CSF HIV may demonstrate mutations in the CSF viral subpopulation. The CSF typically shows elevated protein level and white blood cell counts consistent with an inflammatory response beyond that seen in healthy controls without HIV infection and neurologically asymptomatic HIV-infected subjects taking cART.[17] Elevated CSF neopterin and pronounced inflammation with $CD8^+$ T-lymphocyte infiltration are seen on brain biopsy. Some patients with CSF escape demonstrate improvement when the antiretroviral therapy regimen is optimized based upon the results of genotyping and CPE score of the current cART regimen.

Reports of a *CD8 T-cell encephalitis* in subjects taking cART probably reflect a disorder on a similar spectrum.[46,47] This disorder has been considered a form of CNS IRIS related to HIV itself although, as in symptomatic CSF escape, many of these patients developed the syndrome while apparently immunologically stable on cART. Several reports have demonstrated perivascular inflammation and leukoencephalopathy following initiation of cART, which is consistent with previous descriptions of IRIS relating to other pathogens.[48]

Emerging Issues in Neurologic HIV Infection

A number of new concerns regarding neurologic manifestations of HIV have arisen in the era of widespread access to cART; epidemiologic shifts in HIV disease incidence, prevalence, and course; and demographic changes in individuals infected with the virus.

HIV and Hepatitis C Coinfection

HIV and hepatitis C virus (HCV) coinfection occurs in up to 40 percent of individuals, due in many cases to similar routes of transmission.[49] Intravenous drug users are more likely to be coinfected with both pathogens. Patients coinfected with HIV and HCV have more rapid progression of both diseases and worse overall clinical and survival outcomes.[50]

HCV has been detected both in brain tissue and in CSF of HIV and HCV coinfected patients, and HCV core protein has been demonstrated to induce neuronal injury.[51,52] MR spectroscopy has detected reduced cerebral *N*-acetylaspartate in these patients, further suggesting neuronal injury.[53] HIV and HCV coinfected individuals may exhibit a higher prevalence of multiple neurologic disorders than patients infected with HIV alone, including an elevated risk of seizures.[54]

Some studies have indicated that coinfection with HIV and HCV leads to more severe cognitive effects than infection with HIV alone.[55] Others have suggested that while the overall level of neurocognitive deficits is similar, specific impaired cognitive domains may differ.[56,57]

There are many confounding factors related to combined HIV and HCV disease including mood disorders, substance abuse, and socioeconomic influences. HCV management with interferon-α, itself known to cause cognitive abnormalities in uninfected individuals, may result in improved cognitive profiles in the coinfected population.[58,59]

Aging with HIV Infection

With widespread access to cART has come a dramatic increase in life expectancy for people living with HIV infection, with some living with the disease for over 20 years. HIV-associated cognitive deficits, particularly mild HAND, therefore have the opportunity to evolve over time and become confounded by typical age-associated neurocognitive disorders. At the same time, some individuals are beginning to acquire HIV infection at older ages, perhaps resulting in host factors that are different from those that characterized the initial epidemic. By the year 2015, half of the global HIV-infected population will be older than 50 years, and in sub-Saharan Africa nearly 14 percent of the HIV-infected population is already over 50 years old.[60,61]

The normal process of aging involves the development of subtle deficits in neuropsychologic domains that parallel those affected by HAND, including processing speed, memory, and attention.[62,63] Studies have suggested that age has an effect on cognitive impairment in patients infected with HIV and that older age at seroconversion and duration of infection may increase the risk of HAD.[64–66] It is unclear whether there is an additive effect, in which HIV-related cognitive impairment directly compounds age-related impairment, or whether the effect is accelerated, with the combination of age-related and HIV-related impairment resulting in an overall level of impairment significantly worse than the combination.

More recent models suggest that HAND in cART-treated patients may reflect premature aging and an increased likelihood of neurodegeneration.[67] This model takes into consideration the growing evidence for persistent neurodegeneration in patients treated with cART as well as the facilitated expression of separate (i.e., non-HAD) neurodegenerative processes identified through CSF and neuropathologic markers of neurodegeneration.[68,69]

Imaging studies of HIV-infected individuals older than 60 years have shown disruptions in structural networks that exceed that expected with normal aging, even in the setting of access to cART.[70] Individuals predisposed to neurodegeneration by the apolipoprotein E4 allele exhibit even worse neural network disruption.[71] Aging patients with HIV infection display a diminished utilization of brain reserve; while patients without HAND are able to compensate for age-related declines in attention through utilization of brain reserve, individuals with HAND may be unable to do so, leading to worsening cognitive decline.[72] These changes are possibly related to a combination of declines in dopaminergic function and glial activation in the setting of neuronal injury.[73,74]

Stroke

Stroke is under-reported in the HIV-infected population[75]; during the cART era, rates of hospitalization for ischemic stroke in patients with HIV have increased dramatically, whereas those in non-HIV infected persons have declined.[76] In the context of HIV infection, ischemic stroke affects patients who are more likely female, younger, and lack traditional risk factors for cerebrovascular disease.[77] HIV infection is an important risk factor for stroke in the developing world as well.[78]

In the pre-cART era, most cases of stroke in HIV-infected patients were attributed to the intracranial opportunistic infections and tumors associated with advanced immunosuppresion. In the cART era, the pathogenesis of stroke in HIV-infected persons is likely to be due to a multifactorial combination of HIV infection itself and side effects from the activity of antiretroviral agents including dyslipidemia.

HIV itself induces endothelial activation, which can lead to ischemic vascular events in the heart and brain. Cardiac disease has been increasingly recognized in the HIV-infected population and cardioembolic causes of cerebral ischemia are more common than in the pre-cART era. Especially in the late stages of the disease, HIV-infected patients have diastolic dysfunction and HIV-associated dilated cardiomyopathy, which was identified as the cause of stroke in 20 percent of patients in one series.[79] While opportunistic vasculitis was commonly implicated in ischemic stroke in the pre-cART era,[5] a small-vessel vasculopathy related to the virus is increasingly common.[75,80] Hypercoagulability and intracranial aneurysms occur more frequently in this population than the general population and can lead to stroke.[79,81]

Although cART increases life expectancy, it also may allow patients to develop age-related atherosclerotic disease. Longer exposure to the virus itself may exacerbate stroke risk through mechanisms described earlier. In addition, the protease inhibitors used in cART regimens contribute to numerous metabolic abnormalities including lipodystrophy, dyslipidemia, and insulin resistance.[82] However, an uncontrolled HIV viremia may be a greater risk factor for stroke than antiretroviral medications, as suggested by the results of a study in which participants who interrupted therapy to reduce their overall exposure to antiretroviral drugs actually demonstrated increased cardiovascular-related morbidity and death.[83]

Metabolic disorders also worsen neurologic performance outside the context of clinically detectable stroke in patients with HIV infection. Insulin resistance and poor glucose control have been associated with poorer neurocognitive performance.[84,85] Clinical or subclinical carotid artery disease is also significantly associated with neurocognitive decline,[86,87] and central obesity contributes to worse neurocognitive performance in HIV-infected patients.[88]

Central Neurotoxicity of Antiretroviral Agents

The tissue-specific adverse effects of antiretroviral agents outside the nervous system include pancreatitis, lactic acidosis, ototoxicity, and lipodystrophy. In addition to controlling systemic HIV levels, a goal of therapy is to protect the brain from damage related to viral pathogenesis and to eliminate the CNS reservoir of the virus. Although antiretroviral therapy that achieves sufficient penetration into the CSF can successfully control CNS viral replication, there has been growing concern that the therapeutic concentrations needed to achieve effective viral suppression are associated with a risk of neurotoxic adverse effects.

Recent in vitro work has suggested that abacavir, efavirenz, etravirine, nevaripine, and atazanavir have the most neurotoxic potential.[89] The mechanism of antiretroviral toxicity outside the nervous system may relate to inhibition of mitochondrial DNA production, but it is unclear whether this occurs in the CNS.[90] Neurotoxicity may be related not to cell death, but rather associated with reversible dendritic changes.[89]

The adverse reactions associated with efavirenz are the most common and include sleep disturbances (e.g., abnormal dreams, nocturnal awakening, and insomnia), mood disorders, impaired concentration, and, in some cases, suicidal ideation.[91] These reactions typically occur in the days following initiation of treatment and are most common during the first 4 weeks; nearly half of all subjects will experience some form of reaction and the effects can persist for months or years.[92,93] The incidence of these side effects may be related to drug concentration, which demonstrates significant variability between individuals, possibly related to differences in liver metabolism.[94] Although the adverse effects of efavirenz have typically been considered mild, they can also manifest as severe depression, mania, and aggression.[91,95] Neuropsychiatric effects are the primary reason for efavirenz discontinuation, suggesting that they might also have an impact on medication adherence.[96] Abacavir, etravirine, nevaripine, and atazanavir have fewer clinical reports of neurotoxicity but each has been associated with dizziness, fatigue, and rare instances of peripheral neuropathy, although the latter is difficult to separate from the effects of HIV itself, as discussed later.

NEUROLOGIC DYSFUNCTION IN ANTIRETROVIRAL-NAIVE PATIENTS

The advent of antiretroviral therapy has led to a 10-fold decrease in CNS disease.[19] However, in the United States, an estimated 34 percent of patients reach a $CD4^+$ count below 200 cells/μl by the time they are diagnosed with HIV infection.[97] Therefore, some patients still present with the classic complications of AIDS. This decline of neurologic complications in the developed world has not been paralleled in resource-poor settings internationally, where the diagnosis and management of neurologic disease are complicated by a lack of access to HIV diagnostic and neurologic imaging technology, limited treatment programs that often begin late in the disease course, and neurologic coinfections with endemic pathogens including malaria and tuberculosis.

Effects of Primary HIV in the Central Nervous System

The study of neurologic disease in HIV infection has traditionally focused on chronic and late-stage neurocognitive manifestations, but recent work has shown effects of HIV on the CNS much earlier in the disease course, including during primary HIV infection (defined as the first year following transmission of the virus). Primary HIV infection is characterized by a rapid and dramatic rise of HIV RNA levels in the plasma, accompanied by an increase in HIV antibody levels that are detectable within 2 weeks of transmission by fourth-generation enzyme immunosorbent assay (EIA) tests. In at least two-thirds of individuals, the period of seroconversion is accompanied by the acute retroviral syndrome, characterized by vague symptoms of fatigue, malaise, fever, and anorexia. Within a few months of seroconversion, a partially effective immune response causes HIV RNA to stabilize at a reduced, chronic, individual-specific level.[98] This plateau is a result of the increased activity of $CD8^+$ T cells in conjunction with a decreased reservoir of $CD4^+$ T cells available for infection by the virus.

In addition to the acute retroviral syndrome, a subgroup of individuals newly infected with HIV develop neurologic symptoms and signs around the time of seroconversion. HIV can be found in the CSF and brain tissue of patients during the earliest stages of infection, in the weeks to months following viral transmission.[99] Indeed, HIV has been identified in the CSF as early as 8 days after transmission.[1] Immune activation accompanies the presence of HIV virions in the CSF during primary infection, and the elevation in CSF leukocyte count, neopterin, and inflammatory cytokines during the first months of infection suggests that CNS injury can take place during this period.[100] Biomarkers of neuronal injury are elevated in patients with primary HIV infection and correlate with both neuroinflammatory markers and MR spectroscopic evidence of neuronal dysfunction.[101]

One of the first syndromes to be linked with primary HIV infection was aseptic meningitis, characterized by a CSF lymphocytosis with or without clinical signs of meningitis. Other individuals experience varying degrees of encephalopathy in the setting of meningoencephalitis, encephalitis, or encephalomyelitis. Acute neuropathies, including facial nerve paralysis and optic neuritis, also occur frequently with seroconversion and are common in acute HIV infection. Although clinically heterogeneous, these neurologic syndromes associated with primary HIV infection share several common features, including onset 2 to 3 weeks after the symptomatic manifestations of the acute retroviral syndrome, a self-limited course, and evidence of temporally associated HIV seroconversion. The pathogenesis of these syndromes is therefore probably due to a host-mediated autoimmune response in the setting of massive systemic immune activation. Evaluation of patients with these acute neurologic syndromes should include not only HIV antibody testing but also nucleic acid testing for the presence of HIV by polymerase chain reaction (PCR) since antibody responses may be absent or indeterminate during the earliest stages of infection.

Symptomatic seroconversion, also characterized by a variety of non-neurologic symptoms, has been associated with more rapid disease progression.[102] It appears that these early signs of neuroinflammation are related to objective neuronal injury, but it is unclear whether inflammation or injury at this early time-point predicts neurologic outcomes in later stages of the disease, and whether the early initiation of antiretroviral therapy can ameliorate these processes before systemic immunosuppression occurs.

CNS Complications of Longstanding Untreated HIV Infection

Classic HIV-Associated Dementia

The disorder now called HAD was initially described as the AIDS-dementia complex. There are no individual diagnostic studies or laboratory tests that are specific for HAD. Identification of this disorder depends on the recognition of the clinical syndrome and the exclusion of alternative diagnoses. Diagnostic criteria and approach to treatment were described earlier and in Table 44-1. Initiation of antiretroviral therapy is associated in the majority of patients with a dramatic improvement of clinical signs and symptoms over the early weeks to months of treatment.[103] More gradual improvement may be detectable up to 18 months later.[104]

Opportunistic Infections

For the first two decades following the discovery of HIV infection, opportunistic infections were among the most dramatic and dreaded complications of the disease (Table 44-3).[105] The incidence of these complications has declined with the widespread use of cART in the developed world, but HIV-associated opportunistic infections remain a significant cause of morbidity and mortality worldwide, particularly in areas where access and adherence to antiretroviral therapy are limited.[19]

Any individual with advanced HIV infection is at risk of the development of a CNS opportunistic infection, including patients with AIDS who are not on therapy, those with undiagnosed HIV (who may initially present with a CNS opportunistic infection), and those in whom antiretroviral therapy has begun (who in turn might develop IRIS, as described earlier). More rarely, patients on ART may develop CNS opportunistic infections, due either to failure of complete viral suppression or to lack of immunologic restoration on ART.

CNS opportunistic infections should be considered in patients experiencing significant immunosuppression, typically below 200 $CD4^+$ T cells/μl, although some opportunistic disorders (e.g., tuberculosis meningitis, PML) can manifest in individuals with higher T-cell counts. Diagnosis is typically made using a combination of the clinical presentation (including host factors, symptoms, presence of other known active infections, presence or absence of prophylactic medications, and serologies) combined with CSF and imaging studies. In resource-poor settings where investigations are limited, clinicians may be required to rely upon the history and physical findings alone.

A description of the time course and determination of whether focal deficits are present are important elements for determining the identity of a CNS opportunistic infection (Fig. 44-4). Some infections, such as cryptococcal meningitis, cytomegalovirus encephalitis, and toxoplasmosis, manifest acutely over a few days. Others, such as primary CNS lymphoma and PML, follow a subacute course over weeks to months. Focal deficits typically characterize infections that involve mass lesions, such as primary CNS lymphoma or toxoplasmosis, and are also seen in PML. These localizing signs are less frequently present in other opportunistic infections causing meningitis or encephalitis.

Once a particular opportunistic disease process has been identified, antiretroviral therapy should be initiated or modified in conjunction with appropriate antimicrobial therapy. Typically, such treatment is required until immune recovery ($CD4^+$ T-cell count exceeding 200 cells/μl for 6 months) has been achieved. When this is not possible, patients may need to remain on lifelong antimicrobial suppression.

Multiple opportunistic processes coexist in up to 15 percent of these patients.[105] The presence of a concurrent process must be considered in patients who worsen despite apparently adequate treatment for the initial infection.

Toxoplasmosis

The incidence of toxoplasmosis encephalitis in HIV-infected patients has declined substantially since the introduction of cART, but it remains the most common neurologic opportunistic disease associated with HIV infection in many regions.[19] The infection is related to the reactivation of latent toxoplasmic bradyzoites that survive in brain and muscle after the initial ingestion of oocysts and replication of tachyzoites. The immunodeficiency caused by HIV infection results in a loss of the ability of $CD4^+$ T cells to control this latent infection.

Patients with toxoplasmosis present with fever, headache, and focal deficits that may be accompanied by an altered mental state. These symptoms usually present rapidly over a few days to weeks. Brain imaging demonstrates single or multiple ring-enhancing lesions, most often located in the deep gray matter although they can be present anywhere in the brain (Fig. 44-5). A "target sign" of enhancement has been recently recognized to be a hallmark imaging finding.[106] Serum *Toxoplasma* IgG is typically positive, but, as immunity may wane with advanced immunosuppression, treatment for toxoplasmosis is recommended even in those with negative tests when suspected clinically. CSF PCR-based detection of *Toxoplasma* DNA has a reduced sensitivity in patients with AIDS.

Traditionally, toxoplasmosis has been treated with a combination of pyrimethamine, folinic acid, and sulfadiazine. In resource-poor settings, trimethoprim-sulfamathoxazole has been shown to

TABLE 44-3 ■ Presentation and Diagnosis of HIV-Associated Opportunistic Infections of the Central Nervous System

	Cerebral Toxoplasmosis	Primary CNS Lymphoma	Progressive Multifocal Leukoencephalopathy	Cytomegalovirus Encephalitis	Cryptococcal Meningitis	Tuberculous Meningitis
Disease Characteristics						
CD4 Count	<200	<100	<100	<50	<50	Variable
Time Scale	Days	Weeks to months	Weeks to months	Days to weeks	Days to weeks	Days to weeks
Signs/Symptoms						
Alertness	Reduced	Variable	Preserved	Reduced	Variable	Reduced
Fever	+/–	–	–	+/–	+/–	+
Seizures	+	+	–	+	–	–
Headache	+	+	–	–	+	+
Focal Deficits	+	+	+	–	–	+/–
CSF Studies						
WBC	Increased	Increased	Unchanged	Increased	Unchanged	Increased
Protein	Increased	Unchanged/increased	Unchanged/increased	Increased	Increased	Increased
Glucose	Decreased	Unchanged	Unchanged	Unchanged	Decreased	Decreased
Other Tests	Toxoplasma PCR	Epstein–Barr virus PCR	JC virus PCR	Cytomegalovirus PCR	Increased opening pressure; antigen test	Acid-fast bacilli stain; *M. tuberculosis* PCR
Imaging Findings						
Focal Lesions	+	+	+	–	–	–
Number	Multiple	One or few	One or multiple	n/a	n/a	n/a
Mass Effect	+	+	–	–	–	–
Enhancement	+(ring)	+(ring or complete)	–	+(periventricular)	+(meningeal)	+(basilar)
Location	Basal ganglia, cortex	Periventricular, subependymal	Subcortical white matter; brainstem	Periventricular	Basal ganglia	Basal ganglia
Special Features	Eccentric target sign	Ring- or completely enhancing	Dark on T1, bright on T2	n/a	Gelatinous pseudocysts	Tuberculomas, abscesses

PCR, disease-specific polymerase chain reaction test.

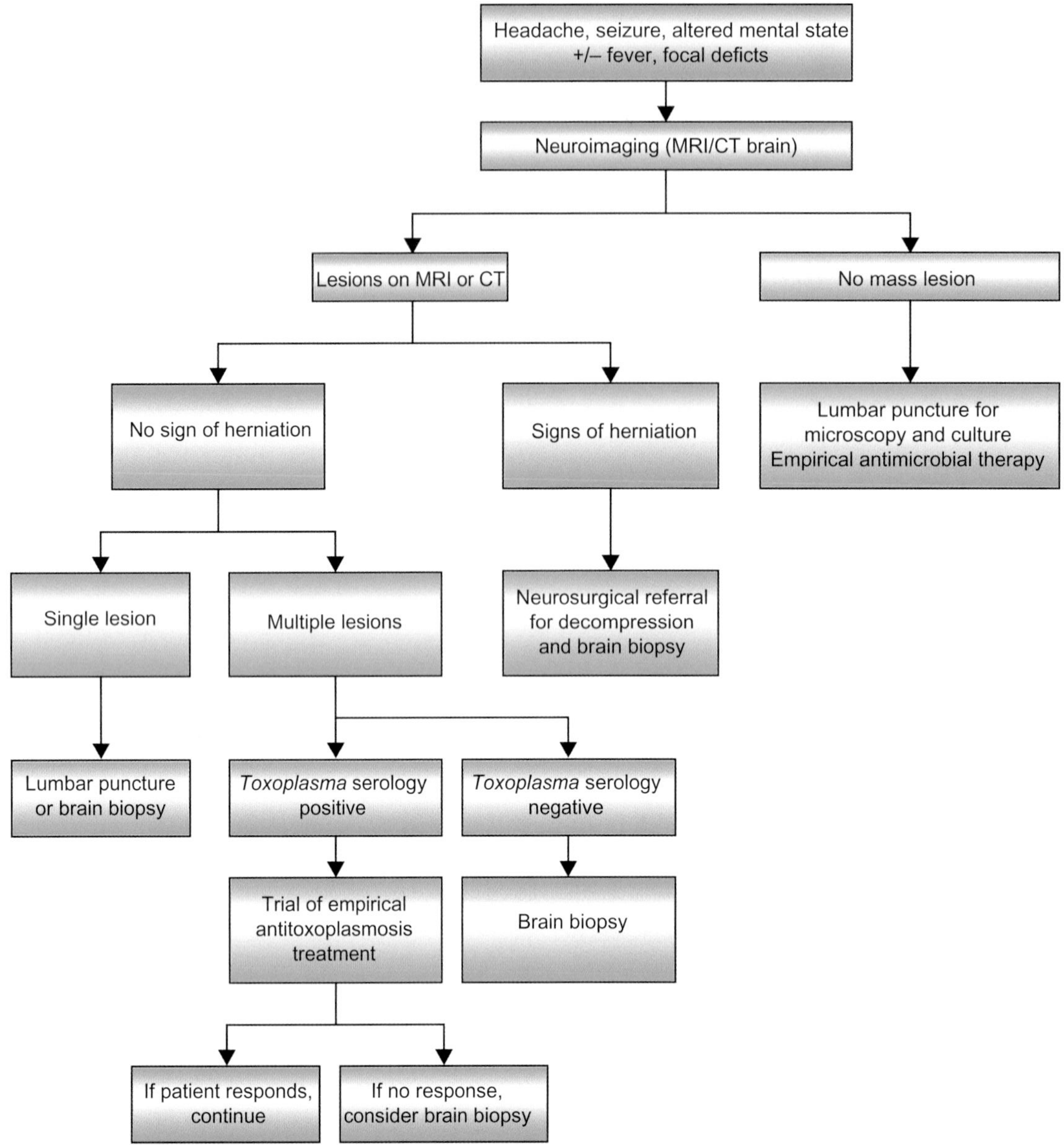

FIGURE 44-4 ■ Algorithm of diagnostic principles for CNS opportunistic infections. (From Tan IL, Smith BR, von Geldern G, et al: HIV-associated opportunistic infections of the CNS. Lancet Neurol 11:605, 2012, with permission.)

be equally effective.[107] Patients typically experience improvement within the first week of initiating therapy, and if there is no response to therapy within 5 days, alternative diagnoses should be considered. After the 6-week induction period, maintenance therapy should continue until the patient's immune system is reconstituted with a $CD4^+$ T-cell count persistently above 200 cells/μl. Compared with other neurologic complications of HIV, there have only been sparse reports of IRIS with toxoplasmosis.[108] In HIV-infected persons, the 1-year mortality associated with toxoplasmosis is as high as 60 percent,[109] though in patients who have immune recovery due to antiretroviral therapy and adherence to anti-toxoplasmosis treatment, recovery is possible, sometimes with little or no clinical sequelae of disease.

Primary CNS Lymphoma

Primary CNS lymphoma is most commonly a multicentric, high-grade, B-cell tumor associated with monocloncal Epstein–Barr virus infection. Patients may experience a nonspecific syndrome of lethargy, altered cognition, headache, and focal abnormalities associated with growth of the mass lesion. Symptoms usually are present for several weeks

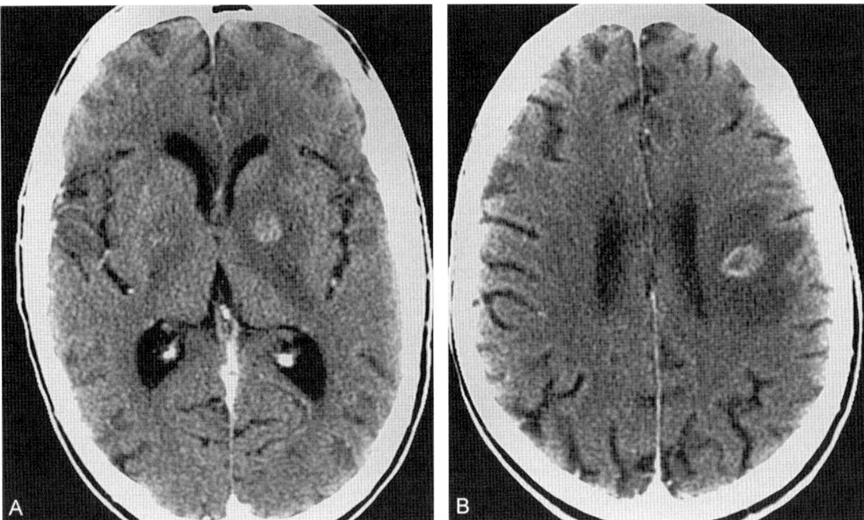

FIGURE 44-5 ■ A 33-year-old HIV-positive man presented with a seizure and right hemiparesis. **A**, Contrast-enhanced CT scan shows edema in the basal ganglia bilaterally, with abnormal central enhancement, more marked on the left than on the right. The ventricles and sulci are excessively prominent for a patient of this age, consistent with the global parenchymal volume loss of HIV dementia. **B**, A more superior image shows a ring-enhancing lesion with surrounding vasogenic edema in the left frontal lobe. The patient's anti-*Toxoplasma* titer was positive, and he responded well to a course of toxoplasmosis-specific therapy, supporting the diagnosis of toxoplasmosis. (Courtesy of Nancy Fischbein, MD, University of California, San Francisco.)

and may be associated with constitutional symptoms such as low-grade fever, weight loss, and night sweats. In some cases, primary CNS lymphoma may present as an infiltrative lesion that resembles an encephalitis or rhombencephalitis, without focal findings or headache.

Classic lesions on MRI are multifocal, supratentorial, and often located along the ependyma. They may demonstrate heterogeneous ring enhancement with contrast, and be accompanied by marked edema and mass effect, leading them to be radiologically indistinguishable from *Toxoplasma* abscesses.[110] More rarely, they may be hypodense on CT or hyperintense on T2-weighted MRI sequences with no enhancement and little mass effect. Patients are often given empiric anti-*Toxoplasma* therapy if radiologically compatible lesions are identified and serum *Toxoplasma* IgG is positive. If no improvement is noted within 5 days, further aggressive evaluation for alternate causes, including primary CNS lymphoma, is warranted. Identification of EBV DNA in the CSF can be a useful test in patients with HIV and suspected CNS lymphoma; although the sensitivity is low, using a cut-off value of 10,000 copies per ml can significantly improve specificity.[111] A positive EBV PCR in CSF combined with a hypermetabolic lesion on positron emission tomography (PET) or single-photon emission computed tomography (SPECT) scan has been considered adequate for initiation of treatment for lymphoma.[112] In some cases a brain biopsy is required for definitive diagnosis.

The prognosis of primary CNS lymphoma has improved dramatically in the cART era. Patients are treated with effective ART, combined with antitumor therapy employed for persons who are not infected with HIV, including radiation and high-dose methotrexate.

Cryptococcal Meningitis

The inhalation of the encapsulated yeast *Cryptococcus neoformans* from soil or pigeon droppings leads to primary, latent, or disseminated disease (see Chapter 46). Although primary infection is typically pulmonary in nature, cryptococcal meningitis can result from reactivation of latent infection in immunocompromised patients. The reactivated yeast forms cerebral "soap-bubble cysts," which are accumulations in the Virchow–Robin spaces surrounding the deep penetrating vessels.

Cryptococcal meningitis often leads to communicating hydrocephalus. More than 15 percent of patients develop increased intracranial pressure, which may present with headache, vomiting, visual and hearing loss, cranial nerve palsy, altered consciousness, and even death.[113] In some cases, hydrocephalus may be asymptomatic.

The organism may be detected in the CSF with either India ink staining or more sensitive and specific cryptococcal antigen assays.[114] Cryptococcal serum and urine antigen has also been demonstrated to be highly sensitive for CNS disease in HIV-infected patients.[115] Neuroimaging may be normal or show hydrocephalus, leptomeningeal enhancement, gelatinous pseudocysts (particularly in the basal ganglia), or, more rarely, enhancing lesions in the parenchyma bordering the CSF spaces, especially in the posterior fossa and occipital lobes.

Management of cryptococcal meningitis, particularly when associated with increased intracranial pressure, prevents blindness, deafness, brain injury, and death. Serial daily lumbar punctures, each removing enough CSF volume to keep the pressure below 20 cmH_2O, can improve symptoms and reduce neurologic morbidity.[116] First-line therapy for cryptococcal meningitis is intravenous amphotericin B with oral flucytosine for 2 weeks, followed by oral fluconazole for 8 weeks. Prophylaxis with fluconazole should be continued at least until the patient's immune system is reconstituted.

Cytomegalovirus Encephalitis

Cytomegalovirus (CMV) is widespread—most individuals worldwide become infected by adulthood. Encephalitis caused by CMV typically occurs only in patients with advanced immunosuppression ($CD4^+$ count <50 cells/μl). Patients typically appear acutely ill, with a rapidly progressive encephalopathy that may be accompanied by seizures and typically involves bilateral subependymal structures, leading to profound amnesia. In addition, patients may experience visual symptoms including central scotoma, loss of peripheral vision, or floaters—signs of CMV retinitis which, if untreated, can lead to blindness and warrant ophthalmologic evaluation. Additionally, concomitant adrenal involvement can lead to hyponatremia.

The diagnosis of CMV encephalitis involves identifying meningeal or periventricular enhancement on MRI. CSF studies reveal a pleocytosis with neutrophils as the predominant cell type and may also show red blood cells and xanthochromia along with a high protein level. CMV PCR in the CSF is highly sensitive and specific for the diagnosis, and quantitative testing can aid in monitoring the response to therapy.

CMV encephalitis in HIV-infected patients should be treated with cART plus an anti-CMV agent such as ganciclovir or valganciclovir. Patients are often left with profound morbidity even when progression of disease is halted. Retinitis can be managed with a sustained-release antiviral intraocular implant and prevented with oral gangciclovir.[117] Other agents, such as foscarnet or cidofovir, can be considered in cases in which leukopenia or resistance is an issue. All patients should continue on prophylaxis with long-term oral therapy until they achieve a persistent $CD4^+$ T-cell count exceeding 200 cells/μl.

Progressive Multifocal Leukoencephalopathy

PML is caused by the JC virus, a common polyomavirus that reactivates in immunosuppresed individuals and occasionally in individuals with high $CD4^+$ T-cell counts. While the sequence of events leading to PML is unclear, it is likely to be related to viral mutations conferring neurovirulence and the subsequent infection of oligodendrocytes and astrocytes.[118,119]

Patients with PML experience subacute to acute progressive focal neurologic deficits. Brain MRI shows one or more subcortical confluent white matter lesions corresponding to the clinical deficits. These lesions have typical qualities of demyelination, including marked hyperintensity on T2-weighted sequences and hypointensity on T1-weighted sequences, with no mass effect and absent or only trace enhancement with contrast.[120] CSF JC virus PCR is highly specific but has a sensitivity of 60 to 80 percent in the current cART era; repeat CSF analysis may be warranted if the test is negative and clinical suspicion high. A CSF pleocytosis is typically absent and a mildly elevated protein concentration is the most common abnormal finding on routine CSF analysis.[120] Rarely, brain biopsy is required to make the diagnosis.

Immune reconstitution induced by cART therapy results in PML remission in the majority of HIV-infected patients; before the cART era, remission was rare.[121] Immune reconstitution with cART in patients with PML increases survival from 10 to 75 percent.[121] PML arrests or remits in approximately 50 percent of patients who are being treated with cART.[122]

There is no effective JC virus–directed antiviral therapy despite studies of cidofovir, mefloquine, and mirtazapine. Paradoxically, neurologic IRIS has been extensively described in the context of PML through recognition that the initiation of cART results in emergence of an unexpected number of PML cases, many of which have atypical features on neuroimaging including avid contrast enhancement.[123] These cases of PML suggest that immune reconstitution leads to an extreme, but localized, inflammatory response in a subset of patients, with JC virus serving as the inciting antigen. Corticosteroids may be beneficial in such cases though recommendations are conflicting.[124]

Tuberculous Meningitis

Nearly one-third of the global population is infected with *Mycobacterium tuberculosis*, a bacillus that is transmitted through aerosolized droplets and controlled by T-cell immunity (see Chapter 41). When this immunity wanes with HIV infection, *M. tuberculosis* disseminates to extrapulmonary sites including the CNS. Within the CNS, granulomas are formed in the subpial and subependymal layers of the brain, and these can expand into abscesses or rupture to cause meningitis. The mortality from tuberculous meningitis in patients with HIV is over 50 percent, and cART initiation does not necessarily improve outcomes.[125,126]

Despite the importance of rapid treatment of tuberculosis infection, definitive diagnosis is often challenging since the tuberculin skin test and interferon-γ release assay are particularly insensitive in patients with $CD4^+$ T-cell counts below 200 cells/μl.[127] The CSF profile typically shows increased lymphocytes, depressed glucose, and normal or mildly elevated protein levels.[105] In many resource-poor settings, the diagnosis of tuberculous meningitis may rely only upon CSF studies without a definitive molecular diagnosis through culture or PCR-based techniques.

Management of tuberculous meningitis begins with a standard quadruple-therapy regimen (rifampin, isoniazid, ethambutol, pyrazinamide) for 2 months, followed by 9 to 12 months of isoniazid and rifampin maintenance therapy. In cases in which the organism is drug-resistant, second-line therapies including fluoroquinolones and injectable aminoglycosides must be used; worse outcomes occur in these individuals.[128]

Antimycobacterial therapy should begin prior to the initiation of cART in patients with tuberculous meningitis, presumably to decrease the risk of IRIS.[126] The use of adjuvant corticosteroids remains controversial in tuberculous meningitis; studies have suggested that dexamethasone decreases mortality but may not improve morbidity in those patients who survive the illness.[129]

SPINAL CORD DISEASE ASSOCIATED WITH HIV INFECTION

The most common spinal cord disorder in patients with AIDS is vacuolar myelopathy, which before the cART era was present in 30 percent of patients at autopsy and closely associated with opportunistic infections.[130,131] Patients present with progressive leg weakness and spasticity along with sensory ataxia and loss of vibratory and joint position sense. Urinary frequency and urgency as well as erectile dysfunction may also occur. There is typically an absence of back pain and no involvement of the upper extremities. A lumbar puncture should be performed to exclude infectious or oncologic causes. Spinal MRI should be performed to exclude space-occupying or compressive spinal cord lesions, but is typically normal. In some cases, cord atrophy or non-enhancing T2-weighted hyperintensities may be present correlating with histopathologic findings of vacuolation.[132]

Management of HIV-associated myelopathy should focus on physical and occupational therapy and symptomatic management, with adjunctive treatments to manage pain, spasticity, and incontinence.

HIV-ASSOCIATED PERIPHERAL NEUROPATHIES

The peripheral nervous system is particularly affected during primary HIV infection, and peripheral neuropathies constitute the most prevalent neurologic problems in patients with AIDS. The most common of these chronic peripheral neuropathies are a distal sensory polyneuropathy and a neuropathy secondary to antiretroviral toxicity.

Distal Sensory Polyneuropathy

Distal sensory polyneuropathy occurs in up to two-thirds of HIV-infected individuals and is most common in older patients with more advanced disease characterized by low $CD4^+$ T-cell counts and high plasma viral loads.[133,134] It is particularly common in individuals with concomitant alcohol use or diabetes, and in those who have used neurotoxic antiretrovirals including stavudine and didanosine.

The distal sensory polyneuropathy may be related to loss of distal unmyelinated fibers in addition to Wallerian degeneration of myelinated fibers. Patients experience progressively worsening parasthesias and dysthesias that begin distally and then slowly spread to more proximal regions. In late disease, the thighs and hands may be affected and distal muscle wasting may occur. The diagnosis can usually be made by the history and a neurologic examination, with decreased ankle reflexes and diminished vibratory, pinprick, and temperature thresholds in the legs. Patients with a coexisting myelopathy may have a mixed picture of proximal hyperreflexia and distal hyporeflexia. Distal sensory polyneuropathy should be considered as a diagnosis of exclusion after other neuropathic processes including diabetes, syphilis, thyroid abnormalities, and vitamin deficiencies are considered. Electromyography and nerve conduction studies demonstrate features of a predominately axonal neuropathy but are usually not necessary to make the diagnosis.[135]

Treatment begins with the discontinuation or dose reduction of neurotoxic antiretroviral drugs, with subsequent resolution in neuropathic symptoms usually taking between 8 and 16 weeks. Following antiretroviral discontinuation, symptoms might actually worsen for 4 to 8 weeks in a phenomenon known as the "coasting period."[136] Symptomatic management involves treatment of neuropathic pain with gabapentin, pregabalin, lamotrigine, or tricyclic antidepressant medications, which are all generally compatible with antiretroviral medications including protease inhibitors.

Inflammatory Polyneuropathies

Inflammatory neuropathies are relatively uncommon in patients with HIV infection. Primary HIV infection may be complicated by an acute inflammatory polyneuropathy; patients experience a rapidly ascending paralysis and loss of reflexes. Unlike typical Guillain–Barré syndrome, albuminocytologic dissociation may not occur in the CSF. Chronic inflammatory demyelinating polyneuropathy progresses more slowly and often relapses.

Since inflammatory neuropathies are thought to be associated with an autoimmune component, it has been suggested that they might respond to immunomodulation with plasmapheresis or intravenous immunoglobulin. In severely immunosuppressed patients with evidence of coexisting CMV infection, therapy with ganciclovir, foscarnet, or cidofovir is recommended.[137]

HIV infection may cause a sensory neuronopathy or rarely a systemic vasculitis. The vasculitis typically occurs in the early symptomatic stage of the disease and may lead to a simple or multiple mononeuropathy or to cranial neuropathies. Nerve biopsy shows a necrotizing vasculitis. Other causes of mononeuropathy, such as herpes zoster, CMV infection, or lymphomatous infiltration of nerve roots, must be excluded; multifocal neuropathies in HIV-infected patients may also arise from neurolymphomatosis and diffuse infiltrative lymphocytosis syndrome (see Chapter 59).

A cauda equina syndrome due to CMV infection may occur with advanced HIV infection or, less commonly, at first presentation. It is characterized by progressive paraparesis and sacral paresthesias, with an ascending sensory loss, areflexia, and sphincter dysfunction. A similar presentation may occur in the upper extremities; this polyradiculitis presents with pain, weakness, and often asymmetric atrophy. The CSF typically shows a polymorphonuclear pleocytosis, and CMV may be detected by culture or DNA PCR assay. In occasional instances, cytomegalic cells may be found in the CSF. Treatment is with ganciclovir, foscarnet, or both.

MUSCLE DISORDERS AND HIV INFECTION

These are discussed in Chapter 59 and are mentioned here only briefly. Several muscle disorders may occur in HIV-infected patients including polymyositis and a syndrome resembling inclusion-body myopathy. A myositis resembling polymyositis also occurs as part of IRIS. Type II muscle fiber atrophy sometimes leads to proximal muscle weakness and wasting, accompanied by a normal serum CK level. Vasculitic processes and opportunistic infections can involve muscle—treatment involves antiretroviral and immunomodulatory agents or specific antimicrobial therapy. Pyomyositis manifesting as localized pain and swelling in a limb is usually associated with *Staphylococcus aureus* infection. Nemaline rod myopathy may occur with or without associated inflammation. High-dose zidovudine treatment may cause a proximal myopathy associated with myalgias in the thighs and calves. Serum CK levels are normal or mildly elevated. Muscle biopsy reveals "ragged red" fibers consistent with mitochondrial toxicity. Discontinuation of the medication usually results in improvement but recovery is sometimes incomplete.

INFECTION WITH HUMAN T-LYMPHOCYTIC VIRUS TYPE I

Worldwide, as many as 20 million people are infected by the human T-lymphocytic virus type I (HTLV-1), a retrovirus endemic to Japan and equatorial regions of the Caribbean, South America, and Africa.[138] In these areas, the prevalence of HTLV-1 can be as high as 2 percent.[139] In the United States, HTLV-1 infection is most common in Native American and African American populations.[140] Like HIV, HTLV-1 is a blood-borne virus that can be transmitted through sexual contact, breastfeeding, intrauterine infection, intravenous drug use, and exposure to contaminated blood products.

The majority of individuals harboring the HTLV-1 virus are asymptomatic carriers. Between 2 and 3 percent of patients develop adult T-cell leukemia (ATL),[141] which in many cases is fatal.[142] Up to 4 percent exhibit a progressive, debilitating myelopathy known as HTLV-associated myelopathy or tropical spastic paraparesis (HAM/TSP).

Although commonly used, the term HAM/TSP is problematic since HTLV-associated disorders are limited neither to myelopathy nor to tropical regions of the world.[143,144] HAM/TSP is best conceptualized as a variety of neurologic syndromes caused by HTLV-1 infection.

Pathogenesis of Neurologic Disorder

The mechanism by which HTLV-1 induces HAM/TSP is uncertain, but may be related to direct glial cell toxicity,[145] autoimmunity resulting from molecular mimicry,[146] or the generation of myelinotoxic metabolites by a neuroinflammatory response within the CNS.[145–147] Genetics may also play a role in determining the magnitude of the immune response, or in affecting the rate of disease progression.[148,149]

Symptoms, Signs, and Course of Infection

HAM/TSP presents as a slow, progressive spastic paraparesis accompanied by bladder dysfunction and sensory abnormalities. The most common symptoms are leg weakness and difficulty walking, sometimes associated with leg and back pain and with parasthesias. Falls are common and result in significant morbidity.[150] Urinary symptoms include nocturia and hyperactive bladder[151]; erectile dysfunction also occurs.[151,152] Patients with HAM/TSP have high rates of coexisting depression.[153]

HAM/TSP is associated with non-neurologic manifestations including pulmonary abnormalities (e.g., centrilobular nodules, thickened bronchovascular bundles, ground-glass opacities, bronchiectasis, intralobular septal thickening), bladder and renal infections, arthritis, and the presence of other autoimmune disorders (e.g., Sjögren syndrome, sarcoidosis). These processes probably result in part from the altered host immune response induced by HTLV-1.

Typical signs in HAM/TSP include a spastic paraparesis with reduced pain sensation, along with bilateral upper-extremity hyperreflexia in the absence of arm weakness. Urodynamic studies demonstrate bladder dysfunction. Less commonly, patients have neuromuscular manifestations including inflammatory myopathy or demonstrate ophthalmologic findings such as uveitis, retinal vasculitis, or lymphomatous eye infiltration.[154]

Progression from mild to severe disability can range from 2 to 10 years.[155] Risk factors for more rapid progression include severe spasticity, diminished vibration sense, and the presence of tremor.[155] Disease progression is more rapid in women than men, particularly in those who are premenopausal.[156]

Proviral load, the number of integrated copies of HTLV-1 expressed as a proportion of peripheral blood mononuclear cells, has also been identified as a marker of disease progression. Whereas the viral load in an untreated patient with HIV infection increases as the disease progresses, the HTLV-1 proviral loads remains relatively stable. Symptomatic individuals have proviral loads at least 10 times greater than asymptomatic individuals and progress more rapidly, possibly due to increased activity of infected lymphocytes in the CNS.[157] Unlike HIV infection, the proviral load is maintained through cell division rather than viral replication, resulting in a slower evolution.[158]

Diagnostic Studies

The diagnosis of HAM/TSP requires the exclusion of other disorders that can cause a chronic, progressive spastic paraparesis including mass lesions within the spinal cord, extrinsic cord compression, multiple sclerosis, amyotrophic lateral sclerosis, vitamin deficiencies (e.g., vitamin B_{12}), syphilis, and HIV vacuolar myelopathy.

In addition to serologic testing for the presence of the virus and determination of the proviral load, the peripheral blood smear in HAM/TSP reveals atypical lymphocytes with convoluted nuclei, known as "flower cells." Further serologic testing may show hypergammaglobulinemia, increased β_2-microglobulin, and an elevated $CD4^+$ T-cell count.

The CSF in patients with HAM/TSP demonstrates a lymphocyte-predominant pleocytosis and elevated CSF protein concentration in the setting of normal glucose levels. The magnitude of these abnormalities declines over the disease course. Oligoclonal bands, inflammatory markers, and HTLV-1–specific antibodies may also be present. A CSF proviral load greater than 10 percent and a ratio with the plasma proviral load of greater than 1:1 may distinguish HAM/TSP from asymptomatic disease.[159]

MRI does not distinguish HAM/TSP from other demyelinating processes; spine MRI is normal most commonly. Brain MRI findings may include T2-weighted hyperintensities in the subcortical, deep, and periventricular white matter. These multifocal white matter lesions are associated with longer duration of disease and increased disability.

Treatment

Treatment options for HAM/TSP is limited due to a combination of factors including a disease burden that is highest in countries where access to care is limited and surveillance data are poor; little financial incentive for drug development for a relatively rare disorder; and difficulty in developing trials due to a limited understanding of disease pathogenesis.[140]

A wide array of interventions that lack efficacy have been tried in HAM/TSP. Corticosteroids are the most commonly prescribed drugs, and there is some evidence for efficacy in the short term.[140,160]

Although associations between inflammatory cytokines and proviral load have been identified, there are few randomized, controlled trials of immunomodulatory drugs.[161] Interferon-α has been tested in small series but the drug also is limited by a severe side-effect profile. The efficacy of other agents such as cyclosporine, azathioprine, and sulphasalazine remains unclear. The utility of treatment with monoclonal antibodies is unclear.[140] Although antiretroviral agents against HTLV-1 are effective in the laboratory, studies have failed to demonstrate a decrease in the proviral load, perhaps due to the lack of continuous replication cycles requiring reverse transcriptase in chronic HTLV-1 carriers.[162]

Due to the lack of effective disease-modifying therapies, symptomatic management is the mainstay of treatment. Spasticity and muscle spasms can be relieved with a combination of physical therapy and muscle relaxants. Neuropathic pain is managed with gabapentin or tricyclic agents. The threshold for testing for and treating urinary tract infections should be low; urine acidification can decrease this risk. Oxybutynin can be used to relieve urinary urgency and frequency arising from bladder spasticity, and stool softeners help manage chronic constipation.

REFERENCES

1. Valcour V, Chalermchai T, Sailasuta N, et al: Central nervous system viral invasion and inflammation during acute HIV infection. J Infect Dis 206:275, 2012.
2. Gisslen M, Fuchs D, Svennerholm B, et al: Cerebrospinal fluid viral load, intrathecal immunoactivation, and cerebrospinal fluid monocytic cell count in HIV-1 infection. J Acquir Immune Defic Syndr 21:271, 1999.
3. De Cock KM, Jaffe HW, Curran JW: The evolving epidemiology of HIV/AIDS. AIDS 26:1205, 2012.
4. UNAIDS: AIDSinfo: Epidemiological Status: World Overview. Unaids.org. Available at: http://www.unaids.org/en/dataanalysis/datatools/aidsinfo. Accessed January 21, 2013
5. Centers for Disease Control and Prevention Estimated HIV Incidence in the United States, 2007–2010. HIV Surveillance Supplemental Report 17:1, 2012.
6. Pantaleo G, Graziosi C, Fauci AS: New concepts in the immunopathogenesis of human immunodeficiency virus infection. N Engl J Med 328:327, 1993.
7. Kaul M: HIV-1 associated dementia: update on pathological mechanisms and therapeutic approaches. Curr Opin Neurol 22:315, 2009.
8. Anthony IC, Ramage SN, Carnie FW, et al: Influence of HAART on HIV-related CNS disease and neuroinflammation. J Neuropathol Exp Neurol 64:529, 2005.
9. Coffin J, Swanstrom R: HIV pathogenesis: dynamics and genetics of viral populations and infected cells. Cold Spring Harb Perspect Med 3:a012526, 2013.

10. Salazar-Gonzalez JF, Salazar MG, Learn GH, et al: Origin and evolution of HIV-1 in breast milk determined by single-genome amplification and sequencing. J Virol 85:2751, 2011.
11. Anderson JA, Ping L-H, Dibben O, et al: HIV-1 populations in semen arise through multiple mechanisms. PLoS Pathog 6:e1001053, 2010.
12. Schnell G, Joseph S, Spudich S, et al: HIV-1 replication in the central nervous system occurs in two distinct cell types. PLoS Pathog 7:e1002286, 2011.
13. Thompson KA, Cherry CL, Bell JE, et al: Brain cell reservoirs of latent virus in presymptomatic HIV-infected individuals. Am J Pathol 179:1623, 2011.
14. Canestri A, Lescure F-X, Jaureguiberry S, et al: Discordance between cerebral spinal fluid and plasma HIV replication in patients with neurological symptoms who are receiving suppressive antiretroviral therapy. Clin Infect Dis 50:773, 2010.
15. Peluso MJ, Ferretti F, Peterson J, et al: Cerebrospinal fluid HIV escape associated with progressive neurologic dysfunction in patients on antiretroviral therapy with well controlled plasma viral load. AIDS 26:1765, 2012.
16. Price RW, Spudich S: Antiretroviral therapy and central nervous system HIV type 1 infection. J Infect Dis 197(suppl 3):S294, 2008.
17. Spudich S, Lollo N, Liegler T, et al: Treatment benefit on cerebrospinal fluid HIV-1 levels in the setting of systemic virological suppression and failure. J Infect Dis 194:1686, 2006.
18. Spudich SS, Nilsson AC, Lollo ND, et al: Cerebrospinal fluid HIV infection and pleocytosis: relation to systemic infection and antiretroviral treatment. BMC Infect Dis 5:98, 2005.
19. d'Arminio Monforte A, Cinque P, Mocroft A, et al: Changing incidence of central nervous system diseases in the EuroSIDA cohort. Ann Neurol 55:320, 2004.
20. Heaton RK, Clifford DB, Franklin DR, et al: HIV-associated neurocognitive disorders persist in the era of potent antiretroviral therapy: CHARTER Study. Neurology 75:2087, 2010.
21. Robertson KR, Smurzynski M, Parsons TD, et al: The prevalence and incidence of neurocognitive impairment in the HAART era. AIDS 21:1915, 2007.
22. Antinori A, Arendt G, Becker JT, et al: Updated research nosology for HIV-associated neurocognitive disorders. Neurology 69:1789, 2007.
23. Heaton RK, Grant I, Butters N, et al: The HNRC 500—neuropsychology of HIV infection at different disease stages. HIV Neurobehavioral Research Center. J Int Neuropsychol Soc 1:231, 1995.
24. Castellon SA, Hinkin CH, Myers HF: Neuropsychiatric disturbance is associated with executive dysfunction in HIV-1 infection. J Int Neuropsychol Soc 6:336, 2000.
25. Heaton RK, Franklin DR, Ellis RJ, et al: HIV-associated neurocognitive disorders before and during the era of combination antiretroviral therapy: differences in rates, nature, and predictors. J Neurovirol 17:3, 2011.
26. Tucker KA, Robertson KR, Lin W, et al: Neuroimaging in human immunodeficiency virus infection. J Neuroimmunol 157:153, 2004.
27. Edén A, Price RW, Spudich S, et al: Immune activation of the central nervous system is still present after >4 years of effective highly active antiretroviral therapy. J Infect Dis 196:1779, 2007.
28. Ragin AB, Du H, Ochs R, et al: Structural brain alterations can be detected early in HIV infection. Neurology 79:2328, 2012.
29. Wright PW, Heaps JM, Shimony JS, et al: The effects of HIV and combination antiretroviral therapy on white matter integrity. AIDS 26:1501, 2012.
30. European AIDS Clinical Society: EACS Guidelines Version 7, 2013. http://www.eacsociety.org/Portals/0/Guidelines_Online_131014.pdf
31. Schmitt FA, Bigley JW, McKinnis R, et al: Neuropsychological outcome of zidovudine (AZT) treatment of patients with AIDS and AIDS-related complex. N Engl J Med 319:1573, 1988.
32. Ferrando S, van Gorp W, McElhiney M, et al: Highly active antiretroviral treatment in HIV infection: benefits for neuropsychological function. AIDS 12:F65, 1998.
33. Uthman OA, Abdulmalik JO: Adjunctive therapies for AIDS dementia complex. Cochrane Database Syst Rev:CD006496, 2008.
34. Ances BM, Letendre SL, Alexander T, et al: Role of psychiatric medications as adjunct therapy in the treatment of HIV associated neurocognitive disorders. Int Rev Psychiatry 20:89, 2008.
35. Sacktor N, Miyahara S, Deng L, et al: Minocycline treatment for HIV-associated cognitive impairment: results from a randomized trial. Neurology 77:1135, 2011.
36. Probasco JC, Spudich SS, Critchfield J, et al: Failure of atorvastatin to modulate CSF HIV-1 infection: results of a pilot study. Neurology 71:521, 2008.
37. Breitbart W, Rosenfeld B, Kaim M, et al: A randomized, double-blind, placebo-controlled trial of psychostimulants for the treatment of fatigue in ambulatory patients with human immunodeficiency virus disease. Arch Intern Med 161:411, 2001.
38. Hinkin CH, Castellon SA, Hardy DJ, et al: Methylphenidate improves HIV-1-associated cognitive slowing. J Neuropsychiatry Clin Neurosci 13:248, 2001.
39. Eggers C, Hertogs K, Stürenburg H-J, et al: Delayed central nervous system virus suppression during highly active antiretroviral therapy is associated with HIV encephalopathy, but not with viral drug resistance or poor central nervous system drug penetration. AIDS 17:1897, 2003.
40. Letendre S, Marquie-Beck J, Capparelli E, et al: Validation of the CNS penetration-effectiveness rank for quantifying antiretroviral penetration into the central nervous system. Arch Neurol 65:65, 2008.

41. Tozzi V, Balestra P, Salvatori MF, et al: Changes in cognition during antiretroviral therapy: comparison of 2 different ranking systems to measure antiretroviral drug efficacy on HIV-associated neurocognitive disorders. J Acquir Immune Defic Syndr 52:56, 2009.
42. Marra CM, Zhao Y, Clifford DB, et al: Impact of combination antiretroviral therapy on cerebrospinal fluid HIV RNA and neurocognitive performance. AIDS 23:1359, 2009.
43. Smurzynski M, Wu K, Letendre S, et al: Effects of central nervous system antiretroviral penetration on cognitive functioning in the ALLRT cohort. AIDS 25:357, 2011.
44. Shikuma CM, Nakamoto B, Shiramizu B, et al: Antiretroviral monocyte efficacy score linked to cognitive impairment in HIV. Antivir Ther 17:1233, 2012.
45. Edén A, Fuchs D, Hagberg L, et al: HIV-1 viral escape in cerebrospinal fluid of subjects on suppressive antiretroviral treatment. J Infect Dis 202:1819, 2010.
46. Gray F, Lescure F-X, Adle-Biassette H, et al: Encephalitis with infiltration by $CD8^+$ lymphocytes in HIV patients receiving combination antiretroviral treatment. Brain Pathol 23:525, 2013.
47. Lescure F-X, Moulignier A, Savatovsky J, et al: CD8 encephalitis in HIV-infected patients receiving cART: a treatable entity. Clin Infect Dis 57:101, 2013.
48. Venkataramana A, Pardo CA, McArthur JC, et al: Immune reconstitution inflammatory syndrome in the CNS of HIV-infected patients. Neurology 67:383, 2006.
49. Jones R, Dunning J, Nelson M: HIV and hepatitis C co-infection. Int J Clin Pract 59:1082, 2005.
50. Anderson KB, Guest JL, Rimland D: Hepatitis C virus coinfection increases mortality in HIV-infected patients in the highly active antiretroviral therapy era: data from the HIV Atlanta VA Cohort Study. Clin Infect Dis 39:1507, 2004.
51. Wilkinson J, Radkowski M, Laskus T: Hepatitis C virus neuroinvasion: identification of infected cells. J Virol 83:1312, 2009.
52. Vivithanaporn P, Maingat F, Lin L-T, et al: Hepatitis C virus core protein induces neuroimmune activation and potentiates human immunodeficiency virus-1 neurotoxicity. PloS One 5:e12856, 2010.
53. Forton DM, Allsop JM, Cox IJ, et al: A review of cognitive impairment and cerebral metabolite abnormalities in patients with hepatitis C infection. AIDS 19(suppl 3):S53, 2005.
54. Vivithanaporn P, Nelles K, DeBlock L, et al: Hepatitis C virus co-infection increases neurocognitive impairment severity and risk of death in treated HIV/AIDS. J Neurol Sci 312:45, 2012.
55. Hinkin CH, Castellon SA, Levine AJ, et al: Neurocognition in individuals co-infected with HIV and hepatitis C. J Addict Dis 27:11, 2008.
56. Clifford DB, Yang Y, Evans S: Neurologic consequences of hepatitis C and human immunodeficiency virus coinfection. J Neurovirol 11(suppl 3):67, 2005.
57. Crystal H, Kleyman I, Anastos K, et al: Effects of hepatitis C and HIV on cognition in women: data from the Women's Interagency HIV Study. J Acquir Immune Defic Syndr 59:149, 2012.
58. Poutiainen E, Hokkanen L, Niemi ML, et al: Reversible cognitive decline during high-dose alpha-interferon treatment. Pharmacol Biochem Behav 47:901, 1994.
59. Thein HH, Maruff P, Krahn MD, et al: Improved cognitive function as a consequence of hepatitis C virus treatment. HIV Med 8:520, 2007.
60. Kirk JB, Goetz MB: Human immunodeficiency virus in an aging population, a complication of success. J Am Geriatr Soc 57:2129, 2009.
61. Negin J, Cumming RG: HIV infection in older adults in sub-Saharan Africa: extrapolating prevalence from existing data. Bull World Health Organ 88:847, 2010.
62. Kramer AF, Madden DJ: Attention. p. 189. In: Craik FIM, Salthouse TA (eds): The Handbook of Aging and Cognition. Psychology Press, New York, 2008.
63. Reger M, Welsh R, Razani J, et al: A meta-analysis of the neuropsychological sequelae of HIV infection. J Int Neuropsychol Soc 8:410, 2002.
64. Valcour V, Shikuma C, Shiramizu B, et al: Higher frequency of dementia in older HIV-1 individuals: the Hawaii Aging with HIV-1 Cohort. Neurology 63:822, 2004.
65. Bhaskaran K, Mussini C, Antinori A, et al: Changes in the incidence and predictors of human immunodeficiency virus-associated dementia in the era of highly active antiretroviral therapy. Ann Neurol 63:213, 2008.
66. Sevigny JJ, Albert SM, McDermott MP, et al: Evaluation of HIV RNA and markers of immune activation as predictors of HIV-associated dementia. Neurology 63:2084, 2004.
67. Brew BJ, Crowe SM, Landay A, et al: Neurodegeneration and ageing in the HAART era. J Neuroimmune Pharmacol 4:163, 2009.
68. Brew BJ, Pemberton L, Blennow K, et al: CSF amyloid beta42 and tau levels correlate with AIDS dementia complex. Neurology 65:1490, 2005.
69. Green DA, Masliah E, Vinters HV, et al: Brain deposition of beta-amyloid is a common pathologic feature in HIV positive patients. AIDS 19:407, 2005.
70. Ances BM, Vaida F, Yeh MJ, et al: HIV infection and aging independently affect brain function as measured by functional magnetic resonance imaging. J Infect Dis 201:336, 2010.
71. Jahanshad N, Valcour VG, Nir TM, et al: Disrupted brain networks in the aging HIV+ population. Brain Connect 2:335, 2012.
72. Chang L, Holt JL, Yakupov R, et al: Lower cognitive reserve in the aging human immunodeficiency virus-infected brain. Neurobiol Aging 34:1240, 2013.
73. Chang L, Wang G-J, Volkow ND, et al: Decreased brain dopamine transporters are related to cognitive deficits in HIV patients with or without cocaine abuse. Neuroimage 42:869, 2008.

74. Chang L, Lee PL, Yiannoutsos CT, et al: A multicenter in vivo proton-MRS study of HIV-associated dementia and its relationship to age. Neuroimage 23:1336, 2004.
75. Rabinstein AA: Stroke in HIV-infected patients: a clinical perspective. Cerebrovasc Dis 15:37, 2003.
76. Ovbiagele B, Nath A: Increasing incidence of ischemic stroke in patients with HIV infection. Neurology 76:444, 2011.
77. Chow FC, Regan S, Feske S, et al: Comparison of ischemic stroke incidence in HIV-infected and non-HIV-infected patients in a US health care system. J Acquir Immune Defic Syndr 60:351, 2012.
78. Heikinheimo T, Chimbayo D, Kumwenda JJ, et al: Stroke outcomes in Malawi, a country with high prevalence of HIV: a prospective follow-up study. PloS One 7:e33765, 2012.
79. Ortiz G, Koch S, Romano JG, et al: Mechanisms of ischemic stroke in HIV-infected patients. Neurology 68:1257, 2007.
80. Connor MD, Lammie GA, Bell JE, et al: Cerebral infarction in adult AIDS patients: observations from the Edinburgh HIV Autopsy Cohort. Stroke 31:2117, 2000.
81. Padayachy V, Robbs JV: Carotid artery aneurysms in patients with human immunodeficiency virus. J Vasc Surg 55:331, 2012.
82. Valcour V, Maki P, Bacchetti P, et al: Insulin resistance and cognition among HIV-infected and HIV-uninfected adult women: the Women's Interagency HIV Study. AIDS Res Hum Retroviruses 28:447, 2012.
83. El-Sadr WM, Lundgren JD, Neaton JD, et al: CD4+ count-guided interruption of antiretroviral treatment. N Engl J Med 355:2283, 2006.
84. Schuur M, Henneman P, van Swieten JC, et al: Insulin-resistance and metabolic syndrome are related to executive function in women in a large family-based study. Eur J Epidemiol 25:561, 2010.
85. Valcour VG, Shikuma CM, Shiramizu BT, et al: Diabetes, insulin resistance, and dementia among HIV-1-infected patients. J Acquir Immune Defic Syndr 38:31, 2005.
86. Becker JT, Kingsley L, Mullen J, et al: Vascular risk factors, HIV serostatus, and cognitive dysfunction in gay and bisexual men. Neurology 73:1292, 2009.
87. Crystal HA, Weedon J, Holman S, et al: Associations of cardiovascular variables and HAART with cognition in middle-aged HIV-infected and uninfected women. J Neurovirol 17:469, 2011.
88. McCutchan JA, Marquie-Beck JA, Fitzsimons CA, et al: Role of obesity, metabolic variables, and diabetes in HIV-associated neurocognitive disorder. Neurology 78:485, 2012.
89. Robertson K, Liner J, Meeker RB: Antiretroviral neurotoxicity. J Neurovirol 18:388, 2012.
90. Divi RL, Einem TL, Fletcher SLL, et al: Progressive mitochondrial compromise in brains and livers of primates exposed in utero to nucleoside reverse transcriptase inhibitors (NRTIs). Toxicol Sci 118:191, 2010.
91. Arribas JR: Efavirenz: enhancing the gold standard. Int J STD AIDS 14(suppl 1):6, 2003.
92. Adkins JC, Noble S: Efavirenz. Drugs 56:1055, 1998.
93. Fumaz CR, Muñoz-Moreno JA, Moltó J, et al: Long-term neuropsychiatric disorders on efavirenz-based approaches: quality of life, psychologic issues, and adherence. J Acquir Immune Defic Syndr 38:560, 2005.
94. Hasse B, Günthard HF, Bleiber G, et al: Efavirenz intoxication due to slow hepatic metabolism. Clin Infect Dis 40:e22, 2005.
95. Gutiérrez F, Navarro A, Padilla S, et al: Prediction of neuropsychiatric adverse events associated with long-term efavirenz therapy, using plasma drug level monitoring. Clin Infect Dis 41:1648, 2005.
96. Leutscher PDC, Stecher C, Storgaard M, et al: Discontinuation of efavirenz therapy in HIV patients due to neuropsychiatric adverse effects. Scand J Infect Dis 45:645, 2013.
97. Centers for Disease Control and Prevention Reported CD4+ T-lymphocyte results for adults and adolescents with HIV infection—37 States, 2005–2007. HIV Surveillance Supplemental Report 16, 2010.
98. Lindbäck S, Karlsson AC, Mittler J, et al: Viral dynamics in primary HIV-1 infection. Karolinska Institutet Primary HIV Infection Study Group. AIDS 14:2283, 2000.
99. Pilcher CD, Shugars DC, Fiscus SA, et al: HIV in body fluids during primary HIV infection: implications for pathogenesis, treatment and public health. AIDS 15:837, 2001.
100. Spudich S, Gisslén M, Hagberg L, et al: Central nervous system immune activation characterizes primary human immunodeficiency virus 1 infection even in participants with minimal cerebrospinal fluid viral burden. J Infect Dis 204:753, 2011.
101. Peluso MJ, Meyerhoff DJ, Price RW, et al: Cerebrospinal fluid and neuroimaging biomarker abnormalities suggest early neurological injury in a subset of individuals during primary HIV infection. J Infect Dis 207:1703, 2013.
102. Lindbäck S, Thorstensson R, Karlsson AC, et al: Diagnosis of primary HIV-1 infection and duration of follow-up after HIV exposure. Karolinska Institute Primary HIV Infection Study Group. AIDS 14:2333, 2000.
103. Sacktor NCN, Lyles RHR, Skolasky RLR, et al: Combination antiretroviral therapy improves psychomotor speed performance in HIV-seropositive homosexual men. Multicenter AIDS Cohort Study (MACS). Neurology 52:1640, 1999.
104. Tozzi V, Balestra P, Galgani S, et al: Positive and sustained effects of highly active antiretroviral therapy on HIV-1-associated neurocognitive impairment. AIDS 13:1889, 1999.
105. Tan IL, Smith BR, von Geldern G, et al: HIV-associated opportunistic infections of the CNS. Lancet Neurol 11:605, 2012.

106. Kumar GGS, Mahadevan A, Guruprasad AS, et al: Eccentric target sign in cerebral toxoplasmosis: neuropathological correlate to the imaging feature. J Magn Reson Imaging 31:1469, 2010.
107. Dedicoat M, Livesley N: Management of toxoplasmic encephalitis in HIV-infected adults (with an emphasis on resource-poor settings). Cochrane Database Syst Rev:CD005420, 2006.
108. Martin-Blondel G, Alvarez M, Delobel P, et al: Toxoplasmic encephalitis IRIS in HIV-infected patients: a case series and review of the literature. J Neurol Neurosurg Psychiatry 82:691, 2011.
109. Antinori A, Larussa D, Cingolani A, et al: Prevalence, associated factors, and prognostic determinants of AIDS-related toxoplasmic encephalitis in the era of advanced highly active antiretroviral therapy. Clin Infect Dis 39:1681, 2004.
110. Utsuki S, Oka H, Abe K, et al: Primary central nervous system lymphoma in acquired immune deficiency syndrome mimicking toxoplasmosis. Brain Tumor Pathol 28:83, 2011.
111. Corcoran C, Rebe K, van der Plas H, et al: The predictive value of cerebrospinal fluid Epstein-Barr viral load as a marker of primary central nervous system lymphoma in HIV-infected persons. J Clin Virol 42:433, 2008.
112. Liu Y: Demonstrations of AIDS-associated malignancies and infections at FDG PET-CT. Ann Nucl Med 25:536, 2011.
113. Chen Y-Y, Lai C-H: Nationwide population-based epidemiologic study of cryptococcal meningitis in Taiwan. Neuroepidemiology 36:79, 2011.
114. Cohen DB, Zijlstra EE, Mukaka M, et al: Diagnosis of cryptococcal and tuberculous meningitis in a resource-limited African setting. Trop Med Int Health 15:910, 2010.
115. Jarvis JN, Percival A, Bauman S, et al: Evaluation of a novel point-of-care cryptococcal antigen test on serum, plasma, and urine from patients with HIV-associated cryptococcal meningitis. Clin Infect Dis 53:1019, 2011.
116. Wijewardana I, Jarvis JN, Meintjes G, et al: Large volume lumbar punctures in cryptococcal meningitis clear cryptococcal antigen as well as lowering pressure. J Infect 63:484, 2011.
117. Biron KK: Antiviral drugs for cytomegalovirus diseases. Antiviral Res 71:154, 2006.
118. Sunyaev SR, Lugovskoy A, Simon K, et al: Adaptive mutations in the JC virus protein capsid are associated with progressive multifocal leukoencephalopathy (PML). PLoS Genet 5:e1000368, 2009.
119. Merabova N, Kaniowska D, Kaminski R, et al: JC virus agnoprotein inhibits in vitro differentiation of oligodendrocytes and promotes apoptosis. J Virol 82:1558, 2008.
120. Berger JR, Aksamit AJ, Clifford DB, et al: PML diagnostic criteria: consensus statement from the AAN Neuroinfectious Disease Section. Neurology 80:1430, 2013.
121. Antinori A, Cingolani A, Lorenzini P, et al: Clinical epidemiology and survival of progressive multifocal leukoencephalopathy in the era of highly active antiretroviral therapy: data from the Italian Registry Investigative Neuro AIDS (IRINA). J Neurovirol 9(suppl 1):47, 2003.
122. De Luca A, Giancola ML, Ammassari A, et al: Potent anti-retroviral therapy with or without cidofovir for AIDS-associated progressive multifocal leukoencephalopathy: extended follow-up of an observational study. J Neurovirol 7:364, 2001.
123. Cinque P, Bossolasco S, Brambilla AM, et al: The effect of highly active antiretroviral therapy-induced immune reconstitution on development and outcome of progressive multifocal leukoencephalopathy: study of 43 cases with review of the literature. J Neurovirol 9(suppl 1):73, 2003.
124. Kaplan JE, Benson C, Holmes KH, et al: Guidelines for prevention and treatment of opportunistic infections in HIV-infected adults and adolescents: recommendations from CDC, the National Institutes of Health, and the HIV Medicine Association of the Infectious Diseases Society of America. MMWR Recomm Rep 58:1, 2009.
125. Simmons CP, Thwaites GE, Quyen NTH, et al: Pretreatment intracerebral and peripheral blood immune responses in Vietnamese adults with tuberculous meningitis: diagnostic value and relationship to disease severity and outcome. J Immunol 176:2007, 2006.
126. Török ME, Yen NTB, Chau TTH, et al: Timing of initiation of antiretroviral therapy in human immunodeficiency virus (HIV)–associated tuberculous meningitis. Clin Infect Dis 52:1374, 2011.
127. Syed Ahamed Kabeer B, Sikhamani R, Swaminathan S, et al: Role of interferon gamma release assay in active TB diagnosis among HIV infected individuals. PloS One 4:e5718, 2009.
128. Török ME, Chau TTH, Mai PP, et al: Clinical and microbiological features of HIV-associated tuberculous meningitis in Vietnamese adults. PloS One 3:e1772, 2008.
129. Thwaites GE, Nguyen DB, Nguyen HD, et al: Dexamethasone for the treatment of tuberculous meningitis in adolescents and adults. N Engl J Med 351:1741, 2004.
130. Petito CK: Review of central nervous system pathology in human immunodeficiency virus infection. Ann Neurol 23(suppl 1):S54, 1988.
131. Dal Pan GJ, Glass JD, McArthur JC: Clinicopathologic correlations of HIV-1-associated vacuolar myelopathy: an autopsy-based case-control study. Neurology 44:2159, 1994.
132. Sartoretti-Schefer S, Blättler T, Wichmann W: Spinal MRI in vacuolar myelopathy, and correlation with histopathological findings. Neuroradiology 39:865, 1997.
133. Letendre SL, Ellis RJ, Everall I, et al: Neurologic complications of HIV disease and their treatment. Top HIV Med 17:46, 2009.

134. Lichtenstein KA, Armon C, Baron A, et al: Modification of the incidence of drug-associated symmetrical peripheral neuropathy by host and disease factors in the HIV outpatient study cohort. Clin Infect Dis 40:148, 2005.
135. Evans SR, Clifford DB, Kitch DW, et al: Simplification of the research diagnosis of HIV-associated sensory neuropathy. HIV Clin Trials 9:434, 2008.
136. Wulff EA, Wang AK, Simpson DM: HIV-associated peripheral neuropathy: epidemiology, pathophysiology and treatment. Drugs 59:1251, 2000.
137. Jacobson MA: Treatment of cytomegalovirus retinitis in patients with the acquired immunodeficiency syndrome. N Engl J Med 337:105, 1997.
138. Proietti FA, Carneiro-Proietti ABF, Catalan-Soares BC, et al: Global epidemiology of HTLV-I infection and associated diseases. Oncogene 24:6058, 2005.
139. Alarcón JO, Alarcón JO, Friedman HB, et al: High endemicity of human T-cell lymphotropic virus type 1 among pregnant women in Peru. J Acquir Immune Defic Syndr 42:604, 2006.
140. Martin F: Prospects for the management of human T-cell lymphotropic virus type 1-associated myelopathy. AIDS 13:161, 2011.
141. Iwanaga M, Watanabe T, Yamaguchi K: Adult T-cell leukemia: a review of epidemiological evidence. Front Microbiol 3:322, 2012.
142. Hisada M, Stuver SO, Okayama A, et al: Persistent paradox of natural history of human T lymphotropic virus type I: parallel analyses of Japanese and Jamaican carriers. J Infect Dis 190:1605, 2004.
143. Araujo A, Silva MTT: The HTLV-1 neurological complex. Lancet Neurol 5:1068, 2006.
144. Roman GC, Navarro-Roman LI: The discovery of HTLV-1 myelitis: 21 years later. Lancet Neurol 6:104, 2007.
145. Höllsberg P, Wucherpfennig KW, Ausubel LJ, et al: Characterization of HTLV-I in vivo infected T cell clones. IL-2-independent growth of nontransformed T cells. J Immunol 148:3256, 1992.
146. Lee SM, Morcos Y, Jang H, et al: HTLV-1 induced molecular mimicry in neurological disease. Curr Top Microbiol Immunol 296:125, 2005.
147. Ijichi S, Izumo S, Eiraku N, et al: An autoaggressive process against bystander tissues in HTLV-I-infected individuals: a possible pathomechanism of HAM/TSP. Med Hypotheses 41:542, 1993.
148. Nagai M, Usuku K, Matsumoto W, et al: Analysis of HTLV-I proviral load in 202 HAM/TSP patients and 243 asymptomatic HTLV-I carriers: high proviral load strongly predisposes to HAM/TSP. J Neurovirol 4:586, 1998.
149. Sabouri AH, Saito M, Usuku K, et al: Differences in viral and host genetic risk factors for development of human T-cell lymphotropic virus type 1 (HTLV-1)-associated myelopathy/tropical spastic paraparesis between Iranian and Japanese HTLV-1-infected individuals. J Gen Virol 86:773, 2005.
150. Facchinetti LD, Araujo AQ, Chequer GL, et al: Falls in patients with HTLV-I-associated myelopathy/tropical spastic paraparesis (HAM/TSP). Spinal Cord 51:222, 2012.
151. Castro NM, Rodrigues Jr W, Freitas DM, et al: Urinary symptoms associated with human T-cell lymphotropic virus type I infection: evidence of urinary manifestations in large group of HTLV-I carriers. Urology 69:813, 2007.
152. Oliveira P, Castro NM, Muniz AL, et al: Prevalence of erectile dysfunction in HTLV-1–infected patients and its association with overactive bladder. Urology 75:1100, 2010.
153. Galvão-Castro AV, Boa-Sorte N, Kruschewsky RA, et al: Impact of depression on quality of life in people living with human T cell lymphotropic virus type 1 (HTLV-1) in Salvador, Brazil. Qual Life Res 21:1545, 2011.
154. Kamoi K, Mochizuki M: HTLV-1 uveitis. Front Microbiol 3:270, 2012.
155. Gotuzzo E, Cabrera J, Deza L, et al: Clinical characteristics of patients in Peru with human T cell lymphotropic virus type 1-associated tropical spastic paraparesis. Clin Infect Dis 39:939, 2004.
156. Lima MASD, Bica RBS, Araújo AQC: Gender influence on the progression of HTLV-I associated myelopathy/tropical spastic paraparesis. J Neurol Neurosurg Psychiatry 76:294, 2005.
157. Takenouchi N, Yamano Y, Usuku K, et al: Usefulness of proviral load measurement for monitoring of disease activity in individual patients with human T-lymphotropic virus type I-associated myelopathy/tropical spastic paraparesis. J Neurovirol 9:29, 2003.
158. Salemi M, Vandamme A-M, Desmyter J, et al: The origin and evolution of human T-cell lymphotropic virus type II (HTLV-II) and the relationship with its replication strategy. Gene 234:11, 1999.
159. Silva MTT, Araujo A: Spinal cord swelling in human T-lymphotropic virus 1-associated myelopathy/tropical spastic paraparesis: magnetic resonance indication for early anti-inflammatory treatment? Arch Neurol 61:1134, 2004.
160. Croda MG, de Oliveira ACP, Vergara MPP, et al: Corticosteroid therapy in TSP/HAM patients: the results from a 10 years open cohort. J Neurol Sci 269:133, 2008.
161. Starling ALB, Martins-Filho OA, Lambertucci JR, et al: Proviral load and the balance of serum cytocines in HTLV-1-asymptomatic infection and in HTLV-1-associated myelopathy/tropical spastic paraparesis (HAM/TSP). Acta Tropica 125:75, 2013.
162. Machuca A, Rodés B, Soriano V: The effect of antiretroviral therapy on HTLV infection. Virus Res 78:93, 2001.

CHAPTER

45

Neurologic Complications of Organ Transplantation and Immunosuppressive Agents

ROY A. PATCHELL

Over the past 60 years, organ transplantation has become the treatment of choice for many otherwise fatal diseases. Advances in tissue matching, improvements in surgical technique, and the development of new immunosuppressive agents have increased both the number and type of transplantations performed. Kidney, bone marrow, heart, lung, liver, and pancreas transplants are now used regularly in the treatment of end-stage disease.

Three types of transplants exist: *syngeneic* (identical twins), *allogeneic* (different genetic origins), and *autologous* (patient's own tissue). Of these, allogeneic transplants are the most common, although autologous transplants of bone marrow have become common in conjunction with chemotherapy. When a new organ is implanted in the same anatomic site as the old one (e.g., liver transplantation), the transplant is said to be *orthotopic*. When the organ is transplanted into a site that was not the original location of the organ being replaced, the transplant is termed *heterotopic*.

Advances in immunology and transplant technique have allowed longer survival for transplant recipients, but long survival has resulted in the emergence of an increased number of neurologic complications. Depending on the type of organ transplanted, 30 to 60 percent of transplant recipients will develop neurologic problems that can be divided into two major categories: (1) those common to all allogeneic transplants, which are due primarily to the effects of long-term immunosuppression, and (2) those specific to particular transplant types, due either to the underlying disease that led to the need for a transplant or to some phenomenon particular to the transplantation technique.[1–8]

NEUROLOGIC COMPLICATIONS COMMON TO ALL TRANSPLANTATION TYPES

Long-Term Effects of Immunosuppressants

Syngeneic and autologous transplants do not require immunosuppression; however, most transplants are allogeneic, and most transplant recipients therefore require some degree of chronic, lifelong immunosuppressive therapy in order to prevent rejection of the transplanted organ. Both immunosuppressive agents themselves and the resulting immunosuppression may affect the nervous system either directly or indirectly. The major neurologic complications of immunosuppression include direct neurotoxic side effects of immunosuppressive drugs, infections, and the development of new malignancies.

DIRECT NEUROLOGIC SIDE EFFECTS

Calcineurin Inhibitors

Cyclosporine and tacrolimus (FK-506) are the most commonly used immunosuppressive drugs in organ transplantation. These agents bind to calcineurin and selectively inhibit both helper and cytotoxic T cells by blocking antigen-induced T-cell activation[9–11]; these drugs also inhibit lymphokine production and release. Renal and hepatic toxicity along with hypertension are the most serious systemic complications of these drugs, although neurologic complications occur in 15 to 40 percent of patients.[9–13]

Calcineurin inhibitors (CNIs) are used for both chronic maintenance immunosuppression and for the treatment of acute organ rejection.[3,11] Cyclosporine and tacrolimus produce almost identical side effects, although some evidence indicates that neurologic side effects are slightly more common with tacrolimus.[14,15]

Although higher blood levels of CNIs are generally associated with side effects, there is no simple correlation between serum levels and the development of any specific neurologic complication. Other factors in combination with CNIs increase the risk of developing neurologic problems including cranial radiation, hypocholesterolemia, hypomagnesemia, β-lactam antibiotic therapy, high-dose corticosteroids, hypertension, and uremia.[9–13]

Tremor is the most common neurologic complication of CNIs and is present in up to 40 percent of patients.[9,11,12] The tremor is usually mild and develops within days of initiation of the medication. It is typically caused by sympathetic activation, but patients with CNI-induced encephalopathy or leukoencephalopathy may also experience tremor, and tremor may be a part of a syndrome of generalized cerebellar dysfunction.[16] Approximately one-third of patients who receive *parenteral* tacrolimus develop headache; oral administration is only rarely associated with headaches.

Most of the serious neurologic toxicity of CNIs is due to their tendency to produce hypertension.[9–13] The hypertension that nearly always complicates CNI use is due in part to renal toxicity and, to a larger extent, to stimulation of the sympathetic nervous system. The encephalopathy of CNI toxicity is better correlated with the rate of change in blood pressure from the patient's baseline level than with serum drug levels.[12,13] CNI neurotoxicity may be thought of as a forme fruste of hypertensive encephalopathy and is characterized by tremor, abnormalities in mental state ranging from mild inattention to akinetic mutism and coma, seizures, and various visual syndromes characteristic of dysautoregulation in the posterior circulation.[12,13] Magnetic resonance imaging shows increased signal on T2-weighted images in the occipital white matter, although the anterior circulation territory and gray matter may be involved. Flow studies such as single-photon emission computed tomography demonstrate increased flow with extravasation of water.[6,9,12,13] These clinical and white matter findings are identical to those found in patients with hypertensive encephalopathy and are termed the posterior reversible encephalopathy syndrome (PRES). The patient's blood pressure need not be very high for occurrence of this syndrome, which appears to be related to the rate of change of blood pressure combined with a loss of cerebral autoregulation. Lowering of the blood pressure by any means, including but not limited to lowering the blood level of the drug, will usually result in resolution of the clinical syndrome and the imaging abnormalities.

CNIs are epileptogenic and cause seizures in 2 to 6 percent of recipients.[9,11,12] The seizures may be focal or generalized and are usually (but not invariably) associated with high serum levels. Hypertension, hypomagnesemia, hypocholesterolemia, aluminum overload, and the concomitant administration of high-dose corticosteroids have been identified as aggravating or precipitating factors.[11,13]

Neuralgia and neuropathy are less common complications of CNIs. Sensory disturbances consisting of paresthesias, dysesthesias, and hyperesthesias of the distal extremities (especially hands) are more common than weakness. Nerve conduction and electromyographic abnormalities are rarely present, although evidence of combined demyelination and axonal damage has been reported.[13,17]

The treatment for all the direct neurotoxic side effects of CNIs is either to decrease the dose or to eliminate the drug entirely, if possible. Nearly all of the direct side effects are usually reversible after drug discontinuation.

mTOR Inhibitors

Sirolimus and everolimus drugs are immunosuppressive drugs that act by inhibiting the mammalian target of rapamycin (mTOR) and ultimately blockading T-cell activation.[11] These agents have similar side effects and cause increases in serum cholesterol and triglycerides. Myelosuppression is also common as are dermatologic problems. These agents have relatively few neurologic side effects but a PRES-like syndrome which resolves on discontinuation of the drug has been reported rarely.

Corticosteroids

Corticosteroids were the first immunosuppressive agents used in transplantation and continue to be used for long-term immunosuppression and for the treatment of acute rejection.[1,11] Corticosteroids affect both cellular and humoral immunity and expose patients to a greater risk of opportunistic infection than do the newer immunosuppressive agents that are relatively T-cell specific. The most common neurologic side effects of corticosteroids are myopathy, steroid psychosis, and problems resulting from corticosteroid withdrawal. The systemic side effects of corticosteroids are not reviewed here.

The exact frequency of corticosteroid myopathy is unknown, but many patients on moderate-dose corticosteroids develop some signs of myopathy 2 to 3 weeks after the start of therapy.[18] The syndrome is characterized by proximal muscle weakness that is most severe in the hip girdle. Treatment is to discontinue the corticosteroids (if possible) or to change to a nonfluorinated corticosteroid (e.g., hydrocortisone) and decrease the dose. The myopathy usually resolves completely in 2 to 8 months after corticosteroid therapy is stopped.[1,18]

Psychiatric complications occur frequently in patients taking corticosteroids. The phrase *steroid psychosis* refers to several psychiatric syndromes that are associated with corticosteroids. Many patients develop mild psychiatric symptoms including anxiety, insomnia, irritability, difficulties with concentration and memory, and mood changes.[1,18] More severe acute psychiatric syndromes occur in about 3 percent of patients including affective disorders, schizophrenia-like syndromes, or delirium.[1,11,18] The treatment of steroid psychosis involves stopping the drug (when possible) or changing over to dexamethasone (the corticosteroid least likely to cause steroid psychosis) and reducing the dose. In addition, affective syndromes may respond to lithium, and schizophrenia-like syndromes are treatable with major tranquilizers.

Withdrawal from corticosteroids also may cause neurologic complications, including myalgias and arthralgias ("steroid pseudorheumatism"), and a syndrome consisting of headache, lethargy, and nausea, with or without a low-grade fever.

Spinal cord or cauda equina compression from epidural lipomatosis caused by corticosteroids has been reported in transplant recipients.[1] This rare complication usually does not occur in patients taking less than the equivalent of 30 mg/day of prednisone. Clinical manifestations can include back pain, myelopathy, and radiculopathy. The usual treatment is surgical decompression, although simply discontinuing corticosteroid therapy occasionally has improved symptoms.

OKT3 Monoclonal Antibody and other Monoclonal Antibodies

OKT3 (Muromonab-CD3) is a monoclonal antibody directed against $CD3^+$ lymphocytes.[10,11,19] Its major neurologic side effect is aseptic meningitis, which occurs in about 5 percent of patients during the first 3 days of exposure. Cerebrospinal fluid analysis shows a lymphocytic pleocytosis with normal glucose and normal or slightly elevated protein concentration. The syndrome is self-limited and benign. Lumbar puncture and culture of the cerebrospinal fluid should be performed to exclude bacterial or fungal meningitis. The meningeal inflammation is probably part of a cytokine release syndrome or an allergic process similar to that which occurs with nonsteroidal anti-inflammatory drugs or intravenous immunoglobulin.[20]

A more severe syndrome with variable degrees of mental status derangement, including seizures, may occur even more rarely.[21] It is associated with neuroimaging evidence of cerebral edema, but it is also self-limited and benign, even if the OKT3 is continued. OKT3 use also predisposes patients to develop lymphoproliferative processes (including lymphoma), a side effect that appears to be dose related.

Antithymocyte and Antilymphoblast Globulins

Antithymocyte globulin (ATG) and antilymphoblast globulin (ALG) are antisera directed against thymocytes or lymphocytes. Rarely, patients develop an aseptic meningitis similar to that seen with OKT3, which is also self-limited and benign.[1,10,11]

Azathioprine

Azathioprine is an antimetabolite that suppresses both cell-mediated and humoral immunity. Although used less frequently now that more specific immunosuppressants are available, the drug is still occasionally used for long-term immunosuppression. There are no direct neurotoxic side effects, although the nervous system may be affected secondary to infection or liver failure.[1,10,11]

Neurologic Infections

Patients who receive long-term immunosuppression are at increased risk of developing infections. Neurologic infections occur in 5 to 15 percent of all transplant recipients, but are important clinically since about half of the central nervous system (CNS) infections that occur in immunocompromised patients result in death.[1,22,23] Nearly every conceivable organism has been reported to infect transplant recipients, but about 75 percent of the cases are due to *Listeria monocytogenes*, *Cryptococcus neoformans*, or *Aspergillus fumigatus*.[22,23]

Transplant recipients are at increased risk of infection for several reasons, the most important of which is the immunosuppression necessary to prevent rejection of the allograft. However, factors other than exogenous immunosuppressive agents also contribute to the risk of infection. After transplantation, patients often have indwelling catheters, endotracheal tubes, and other portals of entry for infection. The patients' underlying diseases and their complications (especially hyperglycemia and uremia) also contribute to the net state of immunosuppression. In addition, certain infections (especially viruses) themselves also cause suppression of the immune system leading to increased susceptibility to other infections.[22,23] The single most important risk factor for developing post-transplantation CNS infection is the magnitude and length of immunosuppression.

CNS infections in immunocompromised hosts may be difficult to recognize. The usual signs of infection, such as fever and meningismus, may be subtle or absent, as these signs depend on a vigorous immune response to the infection. Because the usual signs of CNS infection may be absent and because nearly any organism—bacteria, fungus, parasite, or virus—may be responsible, the clinician should have a high index of suspicion for infectious causes of neurologic deterioration in any transplant recipient.

An infection outside the nervous system should alert the clinician to a possible neurologic infection. Skin lesions may be found to harbor *Cryptococcus*, and lung infection suggests *Aspergillus*, *Nocardia*, or *Cryptococcus*.

Acute meningitis is often due to *L. monocytogenes*, whereas chronic meningitis, often with cranial nerve palsies, suggests tuberculosis or fungal organisms. A progressive syndrome with hemiparesis, visual symptoms, ataxia, dysarthria, and dementia should raise suspicion of progressive multifocal leukoencephalopathy caused by the JC polyomavirus (see Chapter 43). A localized mass lesion (e.g., a brain abscess) is often due to multiple organisms including anaerobes, but the predominant organism in the immunocompromised patient is usually *Aspergillus*, *Nocardia*, or *Toxoplasma*.

Another clue to the causative organism is the time period following transplantation.[1,22,23] In the early period (up to 1 month after transplantation), CNS infections are rare; when infections are present, they usually were acquired before the transplantation or from the donor organ itself, or relate to surgical complications of the transplant including the presence of indwelling catheters. These infections are usually due to common pathogens that are found in the general (nonimmunosuppressed) population. If opportunistic infections occur during the first month after transplantation, there is usually some environmental problem (e.g., *Aspergillus* in the air supply).

In the intermediate period (between 1 and 6 months after transplantation), the net state of immunosuppression is usually at its peak due to prolonged immunosuppressive therapy and the immunomodulatory effect of common viral infections. During this period, the risk of CNS infection is greatest. Two types of infections predominate—viruses and opportunistic organisms. Viral infections (especially cytomegalovirus and Epstein–Barr virus) predispose patients to develop infections with opportunistic organisms, including *Listeria*, *Aspergillus*, and *Nocardia*.[22,23]

Most late infections (more than 6 months after transplantation) fall into three categories: the lingering effects of an infection acquired earlier, opportunistic infections related to long-term immunosuppression, or the return to a pattern of infection similar to that seen in nonimmunosuppressed individuals. Most lingering infections are caused by viruses and include progressive chorioretinitis from cytomegalovirus as well as Epstein–Barr virus–related B-cell lymphoproliferative disease such as CNS lymphoma.[1,22,23]

Opportunistic infections that develop more than 6 months after transplantation tend to occur in patients with chronic allograft rejection who have been maintained on higher than usual doses of long-term immunosuppressive agents (e.g., corticosteroids) and have received additional antirejection therapy (usually with OKT3, antithymocyte globulin, or antilymphoblast globulin). These patients are at the greatest risk of developing opportunistic CNS infections. *Cryptococcus*, *Listeria*, and *Nocardia* species are the most common organisms responsible. Most instances of cryptococcal meningitis that occur in transplant recipients are found in these patients.

Not all patients who survive for longer than 6 months after transplantation are at a substantially increased risk of developing opportunistic infections. Patients who are maintained on minimal long-term immunosuppression and whose post-transplantation courses have been free of chronic viral infections or the need for excessive antirejection therapy have only a slightly increased risk of infection. In these patients, the organisms causing CNS infections are usually the same as those present in the nonimmunosuppressed population.

Lymphoproliferative Disorders

Lymphoproliferative syndromes can occur after prolonged immunosuppression. Early reports identified an increase in non-Hodgkin lymphoma (including CNS lymphoma) in transplant recipients, but many of these apparently malignant lymphomas lacked the histologic and genotypic characteristics of true lymphomas.[1,24] The term *post-transplantation lymphoproliferative disorder* is now used to describe a wide spectrum of abnormal proliferations of B lymphocytes ranging from "benign" diffuse polyclonal lymphoid hyperplasia to malignant monoclonal lymphoma.[1,25] CNS involvement occurs in 15 to 25 percent of patients with post-transplantation lymphoproliferative disorder, and the CNS is the only site of detectable disease in about 85 percent of cases that involve the CNS.[1,24,26,27]

Post-transplantation lymphoproliferative syndromes are strongly associated with Epstein–Barr virus infection (unlike primary CNS lymphoma in immunocompetent patients). These B-cell lymphomas arise deep in the brain with a propensity for the perivascular spaces. CNS lymphoma is distinguished from progressive multifocal leukoencephalopathy by mass effect and enhancement on magnetic resonance imaging (MRI).

Therapy for CNS post-transplantation lymphoproliferative disorder consists of reduction of immunosuppression, antiviral therapy, conventional cytotoxic chemotherapy, radiotherapy, and experimental therapies including anti–B-cell antibodies and interferon-α.[1,24,28] The overall survival rate of patients with the disorder is only about 30 percent.[24,26] Outcome data in large series are not available, but it is clear that CNS involvement makes the prognosis extremely poor.[28]

Seizures

Seizures are a common neurologic complication after organ transplantation, occurring in 6 to 36 percent of patients.[1] The most common causes of seizures are immunosuppressive drugs (especially cyclosporine, tacrolimus, and OKT3), metabolic derangements, and hypoxic-ischemic injury (usually producing seizures in the first weeks after heart, lung, or liver transplantation). Infection, stroke, and tumor are less frequent causes of seizures in these patients. Often, the seizure disorder is transient and requires no treatment other than reduction in the dose of responsible medications, correction of metabolic problems, or treatment of underlying infection.

Long-term treatment with antiepileptic drugs is undesirable in transplant recipients because many of the older anticonvulsants (e.g., phenytoin, phenobarbital, and carbamazepine) interfere with the metabolism of commonly used immunosuppressive agents due to induction of the hepatic cytochrome oxygenase P450 system.[29] Anticonvulsants may lead to a decrease in CNI levels, and the dose of immunosuppresants may need to be adjusted.

Patients who have had only a single seizure should not be started on long-term anticonvulsants. For short-term acute management of status epilepticus, the benzodiazepines are the least likely to interfere with the metabolism of immunosuppressive drugs and can be given either orally or intravenously.

In patients who require long-term treatment with anticonvulsants, the choice should involve agents that have oral and intravenous formulations and do not induce hepatic enzymes, such as valproic acid and levetiracetam. Valproic acid should be avoided in patients with liver transplants, however, because of potential hepatotoxicity.

NEUROLOGIC COMPLICATIONS ASSOCIATED WITH SPECIFIC TRANSPLANTATION TYPES

Renal Transplantation

Since the first successful human renal transplantation in 1954, the procedure has developed into the best therapy for most patients with end-stage renal disease. The kidney is the most frequently transplanted solid organ, and there is now a virtually 100 percent 1-year survival rate, with an approximately 90 percent graft survival rate. The 5-year survival rate for nondiabetic renal transplant recipients exceeds 90 percent.[1,30] Approximately 30 percent of renal transplant recipients develop neurologic complications (Table 45-1).[5–7,31–34]

Renal transplantation is most often performed in patients with glomerulonephritis (membranous or membranoproliferative), diabetes mellitus, or hypertensive renal disease. Other common underlying disorders include polycystic kidney disease, systemic lupus erythematosus, amyloidosis, analgesic nephropathy, and obstructive nephropathy. The toxic effects of pretransplantation uremia may cause subclinical neurologic impairment and leave the nervous system vulnerable to subsequent injury following transplantation. Many underlying diseases, especially diabetes and hypertension, are associated with accelerated atherosclerosis and therefore predispose patients to develop cerebrovascular complications before and after transplantation.[35]

TABLE 45-1 ■ Neurologic Complications of Renal Transplantation

Complication	Percentage Affected
Cerebrovascular events	10
CNS infections	9
Metabolic encephalopathy	10
Seizures	6
Peripheral nerve lesions	5
CNS post-transplantation lymphoproliferative disease	0.3

Based on pooled data from references 1–8, 32–35.
CNS, central nervous system.

Most of the neurologic complications of renal transplantation are due to the underlying disease for which the transplantation was performed.[35] Polycystic kidney disease may be associated with cerebral berry aneurysms, hypertension with ischemic and hemorrhagic stroke, and systemic lupus erythematosus with mental state changes. Rapid correction of hyponatremia may lead to central pontine myelinolysis, a syndrome that can range in severity from mild quadriparesis to deep coma or even death (see Chapter 17).[36]

The renal transplantation procedure itself is relatively benign. Neurologic complications, other than those caused by anesthesia or intraoperative hypotension, consist mainly of peripheral nerve injuries.[35] The most common peripheral nerve injuries involve the femoral and lateral femoral cutaneous nerves due to compressive injury caused by self-retaining retractors.[37,38] In a few patients, the caudal spinal cord is supplied by branches of the internal iliac arteries rather than by intercostal arteries; in these patients, when the iliac artery is used to supply blood to the allograft, spinal cord ischemia may result.[35]

Many renal transplant recipients have some degree of vascular compromise either as a result of their underlying disease (e.g., hypertension, diabetes) or because of emboli associated with underlying atherosclerosis or heart disease.[35] The most common post-transplantation neurologic complications in this patient population are therefore cerebrovascular, occurring in approximately 9 percent of all renal transplant recipients.[1,33,36]

Acute rejection of the renal allograft can produce an encephalopathic syndrome presenting as a nonfocal encephalopathy with headache, altered mental state, and seizures. Systemic manifestations may include fever, weight gain, renal failure, and swelling and tenderness of the graft. This syndrome has been described only in renal transplantations, and the mechanism is unclear; soluble neuroactive immune factors (e.g., cytokines) released during the rejection process may play a role. A similar syndrome occurs as a side effect of OKT3.

Bone Marrow Transplantation

Bone marrow transplantation became a viable treatment option in the late 1960s, and with improvements in tissue matching, immunosuppression, and supportive care, the technique has developed into an important treatment for aplastic anemia, certain inborn errors of metabolism, and a variety of hematologic, lymphoreticular, and solid malignancies.[39] Today, bone marrow transplantation is the second most common type of organ transplantation. Most of the associated neurologic complications occur in allogeneic transplants, which usually require long-term immunosuppression.[40] These neurologic complications occur in 60 to 70 percent of allogeneic bone marrow recipients and are the cause of death in 5 to 10 percent (Table 45-2).[32,33,40–47]

The underlying disorders for which allogeneic bone marrow transplantations are performed may be the cause of neurologic problems following the transplant. Leukemias recur in the CNS in up to 15 percent of patients undergoing transplantation for acute lymphoblastic leukemia and may present with neoplastic meningitis.[4] Patients with malignancies in addition may have also received prior radiation and chemotherapy that may result in neurologic damage (see Chapter 28).

The procedure for bone marrow transplantation is the most benign of all transplantation procedures. No anesthesia or incisions are required, and the donor's bone marrow is infused intravenously, usually with no immediate complications. In the past, toxic myelolethal preparatory regimens often caused neurologic complications, but modern preparatory regimens consisting of alkylating agents (usually cyclophosphamide) with or without small doses ($\leq$2,000 cGy) of total-body irradiation rarely cause acute neurologic problems. However, even the relatively low doses of cranial radiation used may produce permanent cognitive dysfunction in long-term survivors, especially children.[48]

The timetable of infection after bone marrow transplantation differs from that following other types of transplantations.[22,23] Patients are usually more severely immunosuppressed at the time of transplantation because of the underlying disorder (e.g., aplastic anemia, leukemia) and the required myeloablative preparatory regimen. After transplantation, patients are granulocytopenic for about 1 month until the new marrow begins to function. During this period, bacterial (especially gram-negative), viral (especially herpes simplex virus), and fungal infections may occur. Even after apparent hematologic recovery, immunologic abnormalities of both cell-mediated and humoral immunity persist for up to 1 year.[45] After the first month, viral infections (especially cytomegalovirus) and protozoan infections (especially *Toxoplasma gondii*) become more common. Patients usually require less long-term immunosuppressive therapy than patients undergoing other transplantations, and sometimes immunosuppression may be discontinued after successful engraftment if no graft-versus-host disease is present. Perhaps as a consequence, the prevalence of post-transplantation lymphoproliferative disorders with CNS involvement is lower than with other types of transplantations.[24]

A major problem after bone marrow transplantation remains the development of graft-versus-host disease, which occurs in up to 40 percent of patients with human leukocyte antigen (HLA)–matched and 75 percent of HLA-mismatched transplants.[49] This complication results from an attack on host tissue by immunologically competent lymphocytes. Although most frequently associated with bone marrow transplantation, it also occurs occasionally after liver transplantation and, in severely immunosuppressed patients, following lymphocyte-containing blood transfusions.

Acute graft-versus-host disease occurs within 3 months after transplantation and is characterized by rash, diarrhea, and liver dysfunction; no neurologic complications are associated. Chronic graft-versus-host disease develops in 35 to 40 percent of patients undergoing bone marrow transplantation

TABLE 45-2 ■ Neurologic Complications of Bone Marrow Transplantation

Complication	Percentage Affected
Cerebrovascular events	10
CNS infections	12
Metabolic encephalopathy	30
Seizures	10
Peripheral nerve lesions	–
CNS post-transplantation lymphoproliferative disease	0.1

Based on pooled data from references 1–6, 8, 32, 40–47, 56.
CNS, central nervous system.

who survive for longer than 100 days and is characterized by a syndrome that has features in common with some autoimmune disorders (especially scleroderma), with multisystem involvement that includes the nervous system.[49]

Chronic graft-versus-host disease has been implicated in several neuromuscular and CNS complications following bone marrow transplantation.[50] Polymyositis that is clinically indistinguishable from the idiopathic form has been reported. Treatment directed against graft-versus-host disease with immunosuppressive agents usually results in improvement of symptoms. Myasthenia gravis with elevated serum acetylcholine receptor antibody levels has also been described.[50] Acetylcholine receptor antibodies appear to develop as part of the graft-versus-host disease process and are not due to the transfer of active B-cell clones from donor to recipient. Usually, there is a good response to both immunosuppressive agents and cholinesterase inhibitors. Peripheral neuropathies have also been associated with chronic graft-versus-host disease with clinical findings similar to those of chronic inflammatory demyelinating polyneuropathy. Most patients respond to immunosuppressive therapy.

Cerebrovascular complications are a relatively frequent problem after bone marrow transplantation. Infarcts are found in 4 to 13 percent of patients at autopsy, and underlying nonbacterial thrombotic endocarditis or infective endocarditis is often the cause.[41,51–53]

In some autopsy series, nonbacterial thrombotic endocarditis has been present in 4 to 9 percent of patients, after both allogeneic and autologous bone marrow transplantations.[41,51] The reason for this prevalence of nonbacterial thrombotic endocarditis in bone marrow recipients is unknown, although there is an association with disseminated intravascular coagulation and other acquired hypercoagulable states.[54–56] Despite prolonged thrombocytopenia and abnormalities in coagulation, cerebral hemorrhages are relatively rare after bone marrow transplantation.

Cardiac Transplantation

Cardiac transplantation is used to treat medically intractable dilated, hypertrophic, restrictive, and ischemic cardiomyopathies, as well as some cases of rheumatic heart disease. These conditions predispose patients to develop cerebral embolic events, chronic brain hypoperfusion, and hypoxia. Neurologic complications are frequent after cardiac transplantation and occur in up to 60 percent of patients (Table 45-3).[5,6,32,57–64]

The heart transplantation procedure is a major cause of neurologic complications. During transplantation, patients are often on a bypass pump for several hours and may be subjected to long periods of hypotension and hypoxia.[37,65] During the procedure, patients are also at risk of emboli from blood clots or air. Autopsy series have shown that up to 50 percent of patients have focal cerebral infarcts or evidence of diffuse hypoxic-ischemic injury following cardiac transplantation.[32,60–64] Ischemic insults present in the perioperative period as either focal neurologic deficits or as nonfocal encephalopathies (e.g., when a diffuse bilateral shower of emboli is present) and may be accompanied by seizures.

Peripheral nerve injuries are another relatively common complication of the transplantation procedure, occurring in about 13 percent of patients.[61] The most frequently encountered lesions are brachial plexus injuries caused by retraction of the chest wall during surgery or from cardiac catheterization. The phrenic nerve also may be damaged by retraction or by the practice of packing the heart in ice during the transplantation.[66]

Although the pattern and timetable of CNS infections are similar to those in other types of transplantations, the side effects of immunosuppression are more common and severe in cardiac transplant recipients because higher doses of immunosuppressive agents are often used. *Toxoplasma* infections

TABLE 45-3 ■ Neurologic Complications of Cardiac Transplantation

Complication	Percentage Affected
Cerebrovascular events	30
CNS infections	12
Metabolic encephalopathy	5
Seizures	15
Peripheral nerve lesions	13
CNS post-transplantation lymphoproliferative disease	0.75

Based on pooled data from references 1–8, 32, 57–64.
CNS, central nervous system.

account for a higher percentage of CNS infections than in other transplantations, and the source of infection is sometimes the donor organ itself. Post-transplantation lymphoproliferative disorders with CNS involvement are more common after cardiac transplantation (and especially combined heart and lung transplantation) than following other types of transplantation.[1,24]

After transplantation, patients continue to be at risk of stroke due to cardiac emboli, underlying atherosclerosis, and arrhythmias. Syncope may also occur due to arrhythmias and coronary artery spasm.

Pulmonary Transplantation

The first successful lung transplantation was performed in the mid-1980s, and lungs are now transplanted either singly or bilaterally and with or without combined heart transplantation. For transplantation involving lung alone, the 1-year survival rate is around 80 percent.[32] The 5-year survival rate for combined heart and lung transplant recipients is over 80 percent.[32] Neurologic complications are frequent after lung transplantation and occur in 45 to 60 percent of patients (Table 45-4).[22,67]

Lung transplantations are used to treat a variety of end-stage lung diseases including emphysema, other severe chronic obstructive pulmonary diseases, cystic fibrosis, α_1-antitrypsin deficiency, and idiopathic pulmonary fibrosis. Many of the neurologic complications are related to chronic hypoxia or the return of hypoxia following graft failure.[35] Seizures (22 to 27%) and metabolic encephalopathies (including from hypoxia) are the most common neurologic complications.[68,69]

TABLE 45-4 ■ Neurologic Complications of Pulmonary Transplantation

Complication	Percentage Affected
Cerebrovascular events	15
CNS infections	12
Metabolic encephalopathy	7
Seizures	25
Peripheral nerve lesions	5
CNS post-transplantation lymphoproliferative disease	0.8

Based on pooled data from references 1–8, 22, 32, 35, 66–70.
CNS, central nervous system.

The lung transplantation procedure is the cause of several neurologic complications including stroke and diffuse hypoxic-ischemic brain injury. Cerebrovascular complications are found in more than 50 percent of autopsied recipients of lung transplants.[32] Peripheral nerves are also occasionally damaged by the transplantation surgery; phrenic nerve injury (usually unilateral) is found in between 3 and 7 percent of patients.[66,70]

Lung and combined heart and lung transplantations require the largest doses of short- and long-term immunosuppressive agents of any type of transplantation, and therefore complications from these medications are more common than in other transplant recipients. In a large autopsy series, neurologic infections were found in 10 percent of lung transplant recipients and 14 percent of heart/lung patients.[32] Post-transplantation lymphoproliferative disorders involving the CNS have been found in 7 percent of patients at autopsy.[32]

Hepatic Transplantation

Hepatic transplantation is used to treat chronic advanced liver disease due to cholestatic diseases (e.g., primary biliary cirrhosis and sclerosing cholangitis), hepatocellular disorders (e.g., alcoholic or viral hepatitis), vascular diseases (e.g., the Budd–Chiari syndrome), hepatic malignancies (e.g., hepatoma, cholangiocarcinoma, and isolated hepatic metastasis such as in carcinoid tumor), fulminant hepatic failure (e.g., due to viral hepatitis or drug-induced liver damage), and metabolic liver diseases (e.g., α_1-antitrypsin deficiency, Wilson disease, glycogen storage diseases, and protoporphyria).[35,71] Liver transplant recipients frequently suffer neurologic complications, with frequencies ranging from 20 to 30 percent of patients in clinical series to more than 80 percent in autopsy series (Table 45-5).[32,71–76]

Because of organ shortages, patients frequently wait a considerable time for liver transplantation. As a result, by the time of transplantation, patients are often critically ill, with many having some degree of metabolic encephalopathy due to chronic liver failure.[35] The encephalopathy may continue if the transplantation is unsuccessful or may recur if the transplanted organ fails. Prior to transplantation,

TABLE 45-5 ■ Neurologic Complications of Hepatic Transplantation

Complication	Percentage Affected
Cerebrovascular events	30
CNS infections	15
Metabolic encephalopathy	60
Seizures	20
Peripheral nerve lesions	8
Central pontine myelinolysis	12*
CNS post-transplantation lymphoproliferative disease	0.4

Based on pooled data from references 1–8, 32, 67–69, 72–78.
CNS, central nervous system.
*Autopsy data only.

patients often have coagulopathies due to liver failure and are prone to develop CNS hemorrhage in the perioperative period.

The liver transplantation procedure itself is not benign. Because of blood loss during the procedure, patients often require massive replacements of blood and electrolytes and suffer prolonged periods of hypotension, which may cause diffuse hypoxic-ischemic damage to the brain or watershed infarctions.[35] Intraoperative infarctions may also be caused by air embolism or artery-to-artery embolism.

During the transplantation procedure, peripheral nerves may be injured in about 6 percent of patients. Injuries to the brachial plexus may be caused by axillary dissection done for the placement of femoral-axillary venous bypasses. Other neuropathies occur from catheterization injuries, nerve compression, and surgical retraction.[77]

The side effects of immunosuppression after liver transplantation are similar to those seen in other types of transplantations. The frequency of post-transplantation lymphoproliferative disorders with CNS involvement is second only to cardiac and combined heart and lung transplantations. Because liver transplant recipients have more of the factors associated with cyclosporine toxicity (e.g., hypocholesterolemia, hypertension), the direct neurotoxic side effects of CNIs are more common and severe.

An unusual neurologic complication that occurs at an increased rate in liver transplant recipients is central pontine myelinolysis, which is found in 7 to 13 percent of autopsied liver transplant recipients.[32,36,78] During the liver transplantation procedure, patients almost always experience an abrupt increase in serum sodium concentrations caused by the rapid correction of intraoperative blood loss with intravenous fluids and blood products that contain high amounts of sodium.[79,80]

The clinical manifestations of central pontine myelinolysis (discussed further in Chapter 17) such as altered mental state or coma, pseudobulbar palsy, and quadriplegia may be masked following liver transplantation by other neurologic or systemic disturbances. As a result, the diagnosis is often discovered only at autopsy, although the diagnosis can be made antemortem by MRI. There is no specific treatment, although avoidance of rapid changes in serum sodium concentration by using low-sodium intravenous fluids and blood products may help prevent this complication.

Pancreatic Transplantation

Pancreatic transplantations are performed in patients with type 1 diabetes mellitus who have extensive end-organ damage.[81,82] Most pancreas transplantations are done in conjunction with renal transplantations, either simultaneously or in patients who already have a functioning renal transplant.

The major goal of pancreatic transplantation is to prevent or reverse the secondary complications of diabetes by making patients truly euglycemic. Whole-pancreas transplants cause patients to become euglycemic within hours after transplantation, and there is a greater than 90 percent graft survival rate at 1 year.[82] Neurologic complications are relatively frequent and occur in about 60 percent of patients.

All pancreatic transplant recipients have severe diabetes with end-organ involvement, including nephropathy, retinopathy, and peripheral neuropathy. Many patients also have evidence of peripheral vascular disease and stroke. In addition, because most patients have end-stage renal disease secondary to diabetes, they may also have experienced the neurologic complications associated with renal failure. Nearly all patients have some degree of peripheral or autonomic neuropathy at the time of transplantation. Several studies have demonstrated that these neuropathies improve following pancreatic transplantation.[82–85]

Neurologic complications related to the transplantation procedure are rare. However, 26 percent of patients may suffer either stroke or global hypoxic-ischemic events during subsequent surgical procedures unrelated to the transplantation procedure. Pancreatic transplants require a relatively high level of immunosuppression, and complications related to immunosuppression and antirejection agents are similar in frequency to those present in hepatic or cardiac transplantation.

REFERENCES

1. Patchell RA: Neurological complications of organ transplantation. Ann Neurol 36:688, 1994.
2. Wijdicks EFM: Neurologic complications in transplant recipients: a bird's eye view. p. 57. In Wijdicks EFM (ed): Neurologic Complications in Organ Transplant Recipients. Butterworth-Heinemann, Boston, 1999.
3. Padovan CS, Sostak P, Straube A: Neurological complications after organ transplantation. Nervenarzt 71:249, 2000.
4. Bashir RM: Neurologic complications of organ transplantation. Curr Treat Options Neurol 3:543, 2001.
5. Pustavoitau A, Bhardwaj A, Stevens R: Neurological complications of transplantation. J Intensive Care Med 26:209, 2011.
6. Zivković SA, Abdel-Hamid H: Neurologic manifestations of transplant complications. Neurol Clin 28:235, 2010.
7. Senzolo M, Ferronato C, Burra P: Neurologic complications after solid organ transplantation. Transpl Int 22:269, 2009.
8. Fernandez-Ramos JA, Lopez-Laso E, Ordonez-Diaz MD, et al: Complicaciones neurologicas en transplantados de organo solido. Ann Pediatr 78:149, 2013.
9. Graham RM: Cyclosporine: mechanisms of action and toxicity. Cleve Clin J Med 61:308, 1994.
10. Coelho T, Tredger M, Dhawan A: Current status of immunosuppressive agents for solid organ transplantation in children. Pediatr Transplant 16:106, 2012.
11. Taylor AL, Watson CJ, Bradley JA: Immunosuppressive agents in solid organ transplantation: mechanisms of action and therapeutic efficacy. Crit Rev Oncol Hematol 56:23, 2005.
12. Wijdicks EFM: Neurologic manifestations of immunosuppressive agents. p. 127. In Wijdicks EFM (ed): Neurologic Complications in Organ Transplant Recipients. Butterworth-Heinemann, Boston, 1999.
13. Gijtenbeek JMM, van der Bent MJ, Vecht CJ: Cyclosporine toxicity: a review. J Neurol 246:339, 1999.
14. Freise CE, Rowley H, Lake J, et al: Similar clinical presentation of neurotoxicity following FK 506 and cyclosporine in a liver transplant recipient. Transplant Proc 23:3173, 1991.
15. Emiroglu R, Ayvaz I, Moray G, et al: Tacrolimus-related neurologic and renal complications in liver transplantation: a single-center experience. Transplant Proc 38:619, 2006.
16. Scherrer U, Vissing SF, Morgan BJ, et al: Cyclosporine-induced sympathetic activation and hypertension after heart transplantation. N Engl J Med 323:693, 1990.
17. Amato AA, Barohn RJ, Sahenk Z, et al: Polyneuropathy complicating bone marrow and solid organ transplantation. Neurology 43:1513, 1993.
18. Rösener M, Martin E, Zipp F, et al: Neurologic side-effects of pharmacologic corticoid therapy. Nervenarzt 67:983, 1996.
19. Chatenoud L, Ferran C, Legendre C, et al: In vivo cell activation following OKT3 administration. Transplantation 49:697, 1990.
20. Gaston RS, Deierhoi MH, Patterson T, et al: OKT3 first-dose reaction: association with T cell subsets and cytokine release. Kidney Int 39:141, 1991.
21. Shihab FS, Barry JM, Norman DJ: Encephalopathy following the use of OKT3 in renal allograft transplantation. Transplant Proc 25:31, 1993.
22. Tolkoff-Rubin NE, Hovingh GK, Rubin RH: Central nervous system infections. p. 141. In Wijdicks EFM (ed): Neurologic Complications in Organ Transplant Recipients. Butterworth-Heinemann, Boston, 1999.
23. Fishman JA, Rubin R: Infection in organ-transplant recipients. N Engl J Med 338:1741, 1998.
24. Penn I: De novo malignant lesions of the central nervous system. p. 217. In Wijdicks EFM (ed): Neurologic Complications in Organ Transplant Recipients. Butterworth-Heinemann, Boston, 1999.
25. Swerdlow SH: Post-transplant lymphoproliferative disorders: a morphologic, phenotypic and genotypic spectrum of disease. Histopathology 20:373, 1992.
26. Cohen JI: Epstein-Barr virus lymphoproliferative disease associated with acquired immunodeficiency. Medicine (Baltimore) 70:137, 1991.
27. Thomas JA, Allday MJ, Crawford DH: Epstein-Barr virus-associated lymphoproliferative disorders in immunocompromised individuals. Adv Cancer Res 57:329, 1991.
28. Benkerrou M, Durandy A, Fischer A: Therapy for transplant-related lymphoproliferative diseases. Hematol Oncol Clin North Am 7:467, 1993.
29. Lake KD: Management of drug interactions with cyclosporine. Pharmacotherapy 11:110S, 1991.
30. Keown PA, Shackleton CR, Ferguson BM: Long-term mortality, morbidity, and rehabilitation in organ transplant recipients. p. 54. In: Leendert PC, Solez K (eds): Organ Transplantation: Long-Term Results. Marcel Dekker, New York, 1992.
31. Ponticelli C, Campise MR: Neurological complications in kidney transplant recipients. J Nephrol 18:521, 2005.

32. Martinez AJ: The neuropathology of organ transplantation: comparison and contrast in 500 patients. Pathol Res Pract 194:473, 1998.
33. Schwechheimer K, Hashemian A: Neuropathologic findings after organ transplantation: an autopsy study. Gen Diagn Pathol 141:35, 1995.
34. Awan AQ, Lewis MA, Postlethwaite RJ, et al: Seizures following renal transplantation in childhood. Pediatr Nephrol 13:275, 1999.
35. Lee JM, Raps EC: Neurologic complications of transplantation. Neurol Clin 16:21, 1998.
36. Martin RJ: Central pontine and extrapontine myelinolysis: the osmotic demyelination syndromes. J Neurol Neurosurg Psychiatry 75:22, 2004.
37. Junaid I, Kwan JTC, Lord RHH: Femoral neuropathy in renal transplantation. Transplantation 56:240, 1993.
38. Sharma KR, Cross J, Santiago F, et al: Incidence of acute femoral neuropathy following renal transplantation. Arch Neurol 59:541, 2002.
39. Armitage JO: Bone marrow transplantation. N Engl J Med 330:827, 1994.
40. Graus F, Saiz A, Sierra J, et al: Neurologic complications of autologous and allogeneic bone marrow transplantation in patients with leukemia: a comparative study. Neurology 46:1004, 1996.
41. Mohrmann RL, Mah V, Vinters HV: Neuropathologic findings after bone marrow transplantation: an autopsy study. Hum Pathol 21:630, 1990.
42. Diener HC, Ehninger G, Schmidt H, et al: Neurologische Komplikationen nach Knochenmarktransplantation. Nervenarzt 62:221, 1991.
43. Guerrero A, Perez-Simon JA, Gutierrez N, et al: Neurological complications after autologous stem cell transplantation. Eur Neurol 41:48, 1999.
44. Gallardo D, Ferra C, Berlanga JJ, et al: Neurologic complications after allogeneic bone marrow transplantation. Bone Marrow Transplant 18:1135, 1996.
45. Maschke M, Dietrich U, Prumbaum M, et al: Opportunistic CNS infection after bone marrow transplantation. Bone Marrow Transplant 23:1167, 1999.
46. Sostak P, Padovan CS, Yousry TA, et al: Prospective evaluation of neurological complications after allogeneic bone marrow transplantation. Neurology 60:842, 2003.
47. Furlong TG, Gallucci BB: Pattern of occurrence and clinical presentation of neurological complications in bone marrow transplant patients. Cancer Nursing 17:27, 1994.
48. Andrykowski MA, Altmaier EM, Barnett RL, et al: Cognitive dysfunction in adult survivors of allogeneic marrow transplantation: relationship to dose of total body irradiation. Bone Marrow Transplant 6:269, 1990.
49. Ferrara JLM, Deeg HJ: Graft-versus-host disease. N Engl J Med 324:667, 1991.
50. Campellone JV, Lacomis D: Neuromuscular disorders. p. 169. In Wijdicks EFM (ed): Neurologic Complications in Organ Transplant Recipients. Butterworth-Heinemann, Boston, 1999.
51. Kupari M, Volin L, Suokas A, et al: Cardiac involvement in bone marrow transplantation: electrocardiographic changes, arrhythmias, heart failure and autopsy findings. Bone Marrow Transplant 5:91, 1990.
52. Martino P, Micozzi A, Venditti M: Catheter-related right-sided endocarditis in bone marrow transplant recipients. Rev Infect Dis 12:250, 1990.
53. Vukelja SJ, Baker WJ, Jeffreys P, et al: Nonbacterial thrombotic endocarditis clinically mimicking venoocclusive disease of the liver complicating autologous bone marrow transplantation. Am J Clin Oncol 15:500, 1992.
54. Gordon B, Haire W, Kessinger A, et al: High frequency of antithrombin 3 and protein C deficiency following autologous bone marrow transplantation for lymphoma. Bone Marrow Transplant 8:497, 1991.
55. Harper PL, Jarvis J, Jennings I, et al: Changes in the natural anticoagulants following bone marrow transplantation. Bone Marrow Transplant 5:39, 1990.
56. Coplin WM, Cochran MS, Levine SR, et al: Stroke after bone marrow transplantation: frequency, aetiology and outcome. Brain 124:1043, 2001.
57. Andrews BT, Hershon JJ, Calanchini P, et al: Neurologic complications of cardiac transplantation. West J Med 153:146, 1990.
58. Martin AB, Bricker JT, Fishman M, et al: Neurologic complications of heart transplantation in children. J Heart Lung Transpl 11:933, 1992.
59. Jarquin-Valdivia AA, Wijdicks EF, McGregor C: Neurologic complications following heart transplantation in the modern era: decreased incidence, but postoperative stroke remains prevalent. Transplant Proc 31:2161, 1999.
60. Malheiros SM, Almeida DR, Massaro AR, et al: Neurologic complications after heart transplantation. Arq Neuropsiquiatr 60:192, 2002.
61. Mayer TO, Biller J, O'Donnell J, et al: Contrasting the neurologic complications of cardiac transplantation in adults and children. J Child Neurol 17:195, 2002.
62. Perez-Miralles F, Sanchez-Manso JC, Almenar-Bonet L, et al: Incidence of and risk factors for neurologic complications after heart transplantation. Transplant Proc 37:4067, 2005.
63. Zierer A, Melby SJ, Voeller RK, et al: Significance of neurologic complications in the modern era of cardiac transplantation. Ann Thorac Surg 83:1684, 2007.
64. Cemillán CA, Alonso-Pulpón L, Burgos-Lázaro R, et al: Neurological complications in a series of 205 orthotopic heart transplant patients. Rev Neurol 38:906, 2004.
65. Eidelman BH, Obrist WD, Wagner WR, et al: Cerebrovascular complications associated with the use of

artificial circulatory support services. Neurol Clin 11:463, 1993.

66. Dorffner R, Eibenberger K, Youssefzadeh S, et al: Diaphragmatic dysfunction after heart or lung transplantation. J Heart Lung Transplant 16:566, 1997.
67. Goldstein LS, Haug MT, Perl J, et al: Central nervous system complications after lung transplantation. J Heart Lung Transplant 17:185, 1998.
68. Wong M, Mallory GB, Goldstein J, et al: Neurologic complications of pediatric lung transplantation. Neurology 53:1542, 1999.
69. Vaughn BV, Ali II, Olivier KN, et al: Seizures in lung transplant recipients. Epilepsia 37:1175, 1996.
70. Maziak DE, Maurer JR, Kesten S: Diaphragmatic paralysis: a complication of lung transplantation. Ann Thorac Surg 61:170, 1996.
71. Belle SH, Detre KM: Report from the Pitt-UNOS liver transplant registry. Transplant Proc 25:1137, 1993.
72. Stein DP, Lederman RJ, Vogt DP, et al: Neurological complications following liver transplantation. Ann Neurol 31:644, 1992.
73. Moreno E, Gómez SR, Gonzalez I, et al: Neurologic complications in liver transplantation. Acta Neurol Scand 87:25, 1993.
74. Guarino M, Stracciari A, Pazzaglia P, et al: Neurological complications of liver transplantation. J Neurol 243:137, 1996.
75. Blanco K, De Girolami U, Jenkins RI, et al: Neuropathology of liver transplantation. Clin Neuropathol 14:109, 1995.
76. Colombari RC, de Ataíde EC, Udo EY, et al: Neurological complications prevalence and long-term survival after liver transplantation. Transplant Proc 45:1126, 2013.
77. Campellone JV, Lacomis D, Giuliani MJ, et al: Mononeuropathies associated with liver transplantation. Muscle Nerve 21:896, 1998.
78. Ferreiro JA, Robert MA, Townsend J, et al: Neuropathologic findings after liver transplantation. Acta Neuropathol 84:1, 1992.
79. Holt AW, McCall PR, Gutteridge GA, et al: Plasma osmolality changes during liver transplantation. Transplant Proc 23:1986, 1991.
80. Yu J, Zheng SS, Liang TB, et al: Possible causes of central pontine myelinolysis after liver transplantation. World J Gastroenterol 10:2540, 2004.
81. Sutherland DER, Gores PF, Farney AC, et al: Evolution of kidney, pancreas, and islet transplantation for patients with diabetes at the University of Minnesota. Am J Surg 166:456, 1993.
82. Sutherland DE, Gruessner AC, Gruessner RW: Pancreas transplantation: a review. Transplant Proc 30:1940, 1998.
83. Kennedy WR, Navarro X, Goetz FC, et al: Effects of pancreatic transplantation on diabetic neuropathy. N Engl J Med 322:1031, 1990.
84. Müller-Felber W, Landgraf R, Scheuer R, et al: Diabetic neuropathy 3 years after successful pancreas and kidney transplantation. Diabetes 42:1482, 1993.
85. Hathaway D, Abell T, Cardoso S, et al: Improvement in autonomic function following pancreas-kidney versus kidney-alone transplantation. Transplant Proc 25:1306, 1993.

CHAPTER

46

Fungal Infections of the Central Nervous System

JOHN R. PERFECT

Recognition of fungal infections of the central nervous system (CNS) is increasing in frequency due to the growing population of immunocompromised patients and improvements in diagnostic techniques. Published information on the diagnosis and treatment of these diverse infections ranges from extensive to nonexistent. Therefore, a comprehensive survey of the literature coupled with clinical experience informs the diagnosis, pathophysiology, and management of these potentially life-threatening infections. Major recent references are cited here, and earlier references can be found in the previous edition of this work.[1]

PATHOGENS

Fungi that cause CNS infection can be divided into two general groups. The first group consists of primary pathogens including *Cryptococcus neoformans/gattii*, *Coccidioides immitis/posadasii*, *Blastomyces dermatitidis*, *Paracoccidioides brasiliensis*, *Sporothrix schenckii*, *Histoplasma capsulatum*, *Pseudallescheria boydii* (*Scedosporium apiospermum*), and the dematiaceous molds. CNS involvement by these fungi occurs in patients with apparently intact immune systems and, at even higher rates, in immunosuppressed patients. The second group consists of secondary opportunists that cause CNS infection almost exclusively in patients with defective host defenses; this group includes *Candida* species, *Aspergillus* species, and mucormycosis caused by fungi in the order Mucorales. Finally, some fungi for which only a few case reports of CNS involvement exist are mostly common in the environment and include *Alternaria*,[2] *Rhodotorula*, *Aureobasidium*,[3] *Arthrographis*,[4] *Acremonium*,[5] *Clavispora*,[6] *Blastoschizomyces*,[7] *Trichosporon*,[8] *Sepedonium*,[9] *Bipolaris*,[10] *Schizophyllum*,[11] *Paecilomyces*,[12] *Pneumocystis*,[13] and *Ustilago*. Such cases generally have some feature of the history, such as direct trauma or CNS penetration, that explains the presence of the fungus in the CNS. Two examples are the fungal meningitis outbreaks of 2002 with *Exophiala* (Wangiella) *dermatitidis* and of 2012 with *Exserohilum rostratum*; both were associated with injection of compounded, preservative-free corticosteroids.[14–16]

Aminoff's Neurology and General Medicine, Fifth Edition.

Some of the key characteristics of the more common CNS fungal infections are listed in Table 46-1.

HOST FACTORS

Geographic factors are important for certain CNS fungal infections. Several groups of fungi are not geographically restricted and have worldwide distribution including *Candida albicans* and other *Candida* species, *Aspergillus* species, and *Cryptococcus neoformans/ C. gattii.* However, certain mycoses such as histoplasmosis, blastomycosis, coccidioidomycosis, penicillinosis, and paracoccidioidomycosis are largely confined to certain geographic areas, although these lines are blurred with modern travel. It is therefore essential that clinicians evaluating patients with fungal infections acquire an accurate travel history.

The CNS is an immunologically sequestered site, with anatomic barriers that exclude not only invading microorganisms but also some components of the immune system. Host defenses normally are highly effective in excluding fungi from the CNS, but certain conditions can lead to failure of this protective function. Some of these conditions are obvious, such as trauma or the presence of indwelling catheters that allow direct inoculation of organisms into the CNS, immaturity of the blood–brain barrier in neonates, and a high-grade fungemia. In most cases, the fungus enters via the respiratory tract and seeds the CNS hematogenously, but other extracranial origins of CNS infection have been identified such as abscesses, mycotic aneurysms, and meningitis, which can arise from septic emboli associated with endocarditis.[17] Rhinocerebral mucormycosis involves vascular invasion and direct extension into the CNS.

TABLE 46-1 ■ Features of Common Fungal Infections of the Central Nervous System

				Major Pathologic Manifestations		
Pathogen	**Risk Factors**	**CSF Cultures Positive**	**CSF Serologies**	**Meningitis**	**Infarct**	**Abscess or Mass**
Aspergillus spp.	Neutropenia, corticosteroids	Rare	None	+	++++	++
Blastomyces dermatitidis	None known	Rare	Ab	+	-	++
Candida spp.	Neutropenia, corticosteroids, CSF shunts, polymorphonuclear leukocyte defects, prematurity	50%	None	++	-	+++
Coccidioides immitis	AIDS, corticosteroids	25–45%	Ab	++++	+	+
Cryptococcus neoformans	AIDS, corticosteroids	75–85%	An	++++	+	++
Dematiaceous fungi	None	Rare	None	+	-	++++
Histoplasma capsulatum	AIDS, corticosteroids	50%	Ab/An	+++	+	+
Paracoccidioides brasiliensis	None	Rare	None	++	-	+
Pseudallescheria boydii	Corticosteroids, aspiration	Rare	None	++	-	++
Sporothrix schenckii	Alcohol, AIDS?	Rare	Ab	++	-	-
Zygomycetes (Mucorales)	Diabetes, deferoxamine, intravenous drug use	Rare	None	+	++++	+++

Ab, antibody test; An, antigen test; AIDS, acquired immunodeficiency syndrome; CSF, cerebrospinal fluid.

The most important risk factor for the development of CNS fungal infections is suppression of the host immune system, whether due to an underlying disease or to immunosuppressive drugs. Both the etiology of these CNS infections and their response to therapy depend on the type of immune suppression. For instance, administration of immunosuppressive drugs such as systemic corticosteroids is a leading risk factor for development of CNS fungal infections with *C. neoformans* and *Aspergillus* species. Neutropenia due to cancer chemotherapy is associated with CNS infections caused by *Aspergillus* and *Candida* species, and treatment with the iron chelator deferoxamine predisposes to rhinocerebral mucormycosis.[18] Several underlying diseases are associated with an increased incidence of CNS fungal infections. The most important of these associations is the link between the acquired immunodeficiency syndrome (AIDS) and cryptococcal meningitis. Prior to the advent of antiretroviral therapy (ART), rates reported from several cities ranged between 24 and 66 per 1000 AIDS patients, but this incidence has been reduced with effective ART.[19] Cryptococcal meningitis continues to occur early, in some patients who have not received antiretroviral drugs, or later, as viral resistance develops to ART. In 2009, the US Centers for Disease Control estimated that worldwide there were 1 million cases per year of cryptococcosis, with over 600,000 deaths, making it the most deadly invasive fungal infection in the world today.[20] Cryptococcal meningitis accounts for approximately 8 percent of all invasive mycoses among transplant recipients.[21] There have also been several reports of patients infected with human immunodeficiency virus (HIV) who have contracted CNS infections with *Aspergillus* species.[22] These infections have predominantly been manifest as cerebral mass lesions, although cerebral infarctions, meningitis, and spinal cord involvement have also been observed. Patients with advanced HIV infection may also present with disseminated and CNS histoplasmosis, penicillinosis, coccidioidomycosis, blastomycosis, or sportrichosis.

Patients who undergo organ transplantation and receive concomitant immunosuppression are at significant risk of CNS fungal infection. The most common fungal pathogens in this setting are *C. neoformans*, *Aspergillus* species, and *Candida* species. Infection with *C. neoformans* in organ transplant recipients is usually manifested as chronic meningitis occurring 6 months or more after transplantation. Infections with *Aspergillus* and *Candida* species usually occur within the first 2 months after organ transplantation, and CNS involvement is usually manifested by brain abscesses. CNS aspergillosis may be underdiagnosed in organ transplant recipients; in one series of 44 brains from liver transplant recipients examined at autopsy, 9 cases of cerebral aspergillosis were identified, of which only 2 were diagnosed before death.[23]

Other high-risk underlying diseases or conditions associated with CNS fungal infection include malignancies, diabetes mellitus, and prematurity. Poorly controlled diabetic patients with or without ketoacidosis are at increased risk of rhinocerebral mucormycosis. Premature infants are at risk of disseminated infections with *Candida* species, with substantial implications for survival and neurodevelopment issues with CNS involvement.[24]

Infections that arise from direct inoculation of fungi into the CNS are usually seen after head trauma or neurosurgical procedures or as complications of implanted cerebrospinal fluid (CSF) shunts. In patients who have open head injuries, fungi that are ubiquitous in the environment may contaminate the wounds, leading to meningitis and focal brain abscesses. With CSF leaks, the initial infection may be bacterial, but during the use of broad-spectrum antibacterial drugs, superinfection with *Candida* can occur.

CNS fungal infections can be occasionally associated with the presence of a CSF-diverting shunt. The most common fungus associated with CSF shunt infections is *C. albicans*. It appears that infection occurs as a result of either contamination of the shunt apparatus during insertion or subsequent manipulation, or through hematogenous spread. Among the published cases of CSF shunt infections with *C. albicans*, an association exists with recent antibacterial therapy and colonization with *Candida* species at other body sites. Other fungi that have caused CNS infection in the setting of a CSF shunt include *C. neoformans*,[25] *Trichosporon beigelii*,[26] *Candida glabrata*, and *Candida tropicalis*. There is some controversy concerning the origin of cryptococcal shunt infections. In many of the patients with CSF shunts who were subsequently found to have *C. neoformans* infection, the shunts were originally placed for either idiopathic hydrocephalus or chronic culture-negative meningitis; these patients probably had chronic CNS cryptococcal infection before their shunts were inserted.[25]

There are rare reports of fungal infection associated with neurosurgical procedures; among these, *Aspergillus* and *Candida* species account for most cases.[27–29] In some of these patients, infection was attributed to direct extension of the fungus from the paranasal sinuses, and in others it was thought that fungi were introduced with devices inserted during the operative procedure. Many of these patients have additional predisposing conditions such as prior treatment with antibacterial agents or high-dose corticosteroids. The dramatic outbreak of over 500 patients with meningitis, arachnoiditis, and epidural abscesses due to *Exserohilum rostratum* contamination of injectable corticosteroids around the spine emphasizes how fungi can aggressively establish disease and travel through tissue with direct inoculation.[14,16]

Immune Reconstitution Syndrome

While host immunity is critical in the eradication of CNS infections, immunologic recovery can also be detrimental and contribute towards worsening disease expression. This entity of overstimulation of the immune system has been called *immune reconstitution syndrome* (IRS) or *immune reconstitution inflammatory syndrome* (IRIS) and has been described during ART, in transplant recipients, and even in apparently normal hosts with cryptococcal meningitis.[30–35] For example, upon initiation of ART during management of HIV-related cryptococcal meningitis, HIV RNA levels decline rapidly and there is repopulation of the host with memory and naïve $CD4^+$ lymphocytes; within 4 to 6 weeks, an immunologic shift occurs from a Th2 to a Th1 response. IRIS may be manifested by headaches, fever, CSF lymphocytosis, increased intracranial pressure, and evidence of increased inflammation on neuroimaging without evidence of viable yeasts in the CSF. The pathologic finding is that of granuloma formation. Patients who initiated ART within 30 to 60 days of treatment for *C. neoformans* infection are significantly more likely to develop IRIS than those who initiated ART at a later time.[34,35] This observation has led to controversy about when to start ART during the management of cryptococcal meningitis—present guidelines give a generous range of between 2 and 10 weeks for ART initiation after the start of antifungal therapy.

Similarly, in solid organ transplant recipients with cryptococcosis, IRIS was observed in 5 percent of patients within 1 to 2 months after initiation of antifungal therapy and was more common in those receiving potent immunosuppressive regimens and those with graft loss.[32] IRIS can occur in any patient in whom there is a rapid shift in immune reactivity.[33] Since the appearance of IRIS in fungal CNS infections is commonly misconstrued as a treatment failure or relapse of infection that leads to unwarranted or inappropriate changes in specific therapy, its clinical recognition is important. IRIS should be considered when treatment appears to have controlled fungal disease by culture or biomarker data but new signs of inflammation develop clinically or on imaging studies.[30]

Recognition of IRIS is important to the clinical management of CNS fungal infections because overabundance of inflammation leads to clinical worsening. Corticosteroid therapy may be considered to reduce inflammation and cerebral edema.

CRYPTOCOCCUS NEOFORMANS AND *GATTII*

The encapsulated yeast *C. neoformans* is the most common cause of fungal meningitis.[32] The first report of cryptococcal infection in humans was provided by Busse and Buschke in 1894 in a patient with bone infection and probable disseminated disease. The first case of meningeal cryptococcal infection was reported 10 years later, in 1905, and cryptococcosis emerged as a significant CNS infection during the twentieth century. The number of infections with *C. neoformans* rose dramatically in the United States and certain African countries following the onset of the AIDS epidemic. In less-developed countries lacking access to ART, cryptococcal meningitis continues to occur frequently.

This ubiquitous encapsulated saprophytic yeast occupies a wide environmental niche. It is found worldwide in bird excreta, soil, animals, and even humans. It is likely that most infections occur after inhalation of small yeasts or basidiospores leading to a primary pneumonia or a primary lung–lymph node complex in which the yeasts remain dormant for long periods until host defenses become weakened. The reason this yeast has a particular tendency to spread to the CNS remains imprecisely explained. Ligands on *C. neoformans* such as the hyaluronic acid antigen (CPS1) have been associated with the CD44 receptor on brain endothelial cells, perhaps allowing for transcytosis through the blood–brain barrier.[36,37]

CNS infection usually manifests as a meningitis or meningoencephalitis, although mass lesions or torulomas may be seen. There are four serotypes (A to D) based on the type of capsular polysaccharide, which are divided into several species: *C. neoformans* var. *grubii* or *neoformans* (serotypes A and D), and *C. gattii* (serotypes B and C). All serotypes can cause meningitis, but there is some geographic variation in the distribution of disease; most patients with cryptococcal meningitis in the United States and Europe have been infected with either serotype A or D. Infections with *C. gattii* are found more commonly in southern California, Southeast Asia, and Australia; this distribution reflects the natural distribution of certain *Eucalyptus* trees that are likely one of the environmental repositories.[38] A recent outbreak of *C. gattii* infections on Vancouver Island showed that there are other trees, such as firs and oaks, that can contain this fungus, perhaps related to ecologic evolution in the setting of global climate change.[39,40] Despite earlier reports that many patients with cryptococcal meningitis had no known immune deficiency, recent experience suggests that a much higher proportion of patients have some identifiable form of immunosuppression. Probably less than 10 percent of patients with cryptococcal meningitis have no known underlying disease. Most cases occur in those with known defective cell-mediated immunity due to corticosteroid treatment, reticuloendothelial malignancy, organ transplantation, sarcoidosis, collagen vascular diseases, or AIDS. Lymphocyte functions are abnormal in most patients with disseminated cryptococcosis. Most patients with HIV infection have CD4 counts below 100/μl. Recent studies have attempted to determine genetic susceptibility to cryptococcosis.[41] Most patients with AIDS and cryptococcosis present with a particularly high burden of yeasts. India ink examinations of the CSF are positive in over 80 percent of patients, and extraordinarily high titers of cryptococcal polysaccharide antigen in CSF and serum are common, with quantitative viable yeast counts that can exceed 10^6 colony-forming units (CFU)/ml of CSF.[42] The response of some of these patients to infection includes a paucity of CSF leukocytes; approximately two-thirds of patients with AIDS and cryptococcal meningitis have fewer than 20 leukocytes/mm^3 in their CSF on presentation. This combination of a high burden of yeast and a quantitative deficiency in the inflammatory response indicates an impaired immune system and can lead to a poor prognosis despite fungicidal therapy.

Patients with cryptococcal meningitis may present with a wide spectrum of CNS findings, ranging from symptoms of headaches with or without fever to subacute dementia developing over months. The latex agglutination test and enzyme-linked immunosorbent assay are both sensitive (>90%) and specific (>90%) if proper controls are used. Recently, an inexpensive and simple lateral flow assay has been developed and it compares favorably to the other antigen tests.[43,44] Although cases occasionally are difficult to diagnose, with the proper use of CSF culture, India ink studies, and polysaccharide antigen tests, the only limiting factor in the diagnosis of CNS cryptococcosis is usually failure to perform a lumbar puncture because the diagnosis is not considered.

COCCIDIOIDES IMMITIS AND *POSADASII*

Coccidioides immitis and *Coccidioides posadasii* are dimorphic fungi with a natural habitat in semiarid soil, which explains their geographic distribution in the southwestern United States and in parts of Mexico and South America. Because many tourists travel through these areas and may become infected, clinicians outside the organism's natural habitat occasionally encounter coccidioidomycosis. Inhalation of the arthrospores leads to a primary pulmonary infection. Most patients remain asymptomatic, and fewer than 0.2 percent of primary infections disseminate outside the lung. Occasionally, the fungus reaches the meninges, either by hematogenous spread or direct extension from osteomyelitis of the skull or vertebrae; seeding of the CNS usually occurs a few months after the primary infection.

Symptoms of chronic meningitis are most common.[45] There are cases in which brain involvement occurs without meningitis, but this presentation is unusual.[46,47] Spinal arachnoiditis with obstructive hydrocephalus and cerebral vasculitis with infarcts and abscesses also have been reported.[48–50] It appears that patients with coccidioidomycosis involving the facial skin are at higher risk of meningitis than those with skin involvement at more distant body sites.[51]

Diagnosis may be confirmed by culture of the fungus from the CSF, but in endemic areas it is diagnosed in many patients on the basis of a CSF pleocytosis (which demonstrates eosinophilia in up to 70% of cases) and the presence of complement-fixing antibodies (CFA) in the CSF. CFA titers are positive in approximately 70 percent of patients at initial diagnosis, and in almost all patients as meningitis progresses.

It is likely that genetic susceptibility plays an important role as a risk factor for meningitis. Meningitis appears to develop at greater rates in blacks, Filipinos, and possibly other ethnic groups such as Hispanics compared to whites.

Most patients who contract CNS infection with coccidioides have no apparent underlying disease, but immunosuppressed patients are at greater risk of CNS involvement. Corticosteroid treatment has been associated with more severe manifestations of primary infection, as well as with reactivation of latent disease and dissemination to the CNS. There have also been many reported cases of CNS infection with coccidioides in patients with AIDS and in transplant recipients.[52] The natural history of coccidioidal meningitis is such that patients whose only detected extrapulmonary site of infection is the CNS live significantly longer than those with more diffuse disease.[53] White blood cell count in the CSF decreases during the course of both treated and untreated infection, and therefore cannot be used to gauge response to therapy. Lifelong triazole therapy for meningitis is required because of the extremely high rate of relapse.[54]

HISTOPLASMA CAPSULATUM

Histoplasma capsulatum is a dimorphic fungus endemic in certain areas of the Ohio and central Mississippi River Valley in the United States as well as in Latin America. It can be found in bird and bat guano, and in soil contaminated with this guano. Outbreaks of the disease have been attributed to disturbance of contaminated soil, allowing the conidia to become airborne and inhaled. Asymptomatic infection in endemic areas is very common; skin test data indicate that up to 69 percent of the population show evidence of prior infection in endemic areas.[55] Most infected individuals have minimal symptoms, and dissemination occurs only rarely. When dissemination does occur, between 10 and 25 percent of patients develop CNS involvement. Although granulomas and other brain parenchymal lesions have been described, most patients with CNS lesions present with meningitis.

Although *Histoplasma* meningitis can occur in apparently normal hosts, it occurs in immunocompromised populations at a higher rate. Patients with AIDS and solid organ transplant are at high risk of development of disseminated disease, usually due to reactivation of latent infection.[56,57] Because CSF cultures may be positive in only 10 to 30 percent of cases even when large volumes (10 to 20 ml) of CSF are incubated for weeks, it is important to assay CSF serologies. There are occasional serologic cross-reactions with other fungi, which can cause diagnostic confusion.[58] The *Histoplasma* CSF polysaccharide antigen has been found to be positive in 40 percent of patients with histoplasma meningitis and is a reasonable first screening test.

BLASTOMYCES DERMATITIDIS

Blastomyces dermatitidis is a dimorphic fungus endemic in Africa and in certain parts of the lower Mississippi River Valley, North Central states, and mid-Atlantic states in the continental United States. It is presumed that spores are inhaled from a source in the soil, but its natural location in the environment has been identified only occasionally. Most individuals have subclinical disease, and dissemination occurs rarely. Disseminated blastomycosis is characterized by granulomatous and suppurating lesions of the lung, bone, and skin. In some series, blastomycosis has been reported to involve the brain in 6 to 33 percent of disseminated cases. Although patients with CNS blastomycosis usually present with evidence of infection at other sites, occasionally meningitis is the initial presentation without evidence of extraneural disease. CSF cultures are rarely positive, and a chronic neutrophilic pleocytosis is a common finding in blastomycotic meningitis.[59] CNS involvement occasionally presents with a mass lesion (blastomycoma) in the brain parenchyma.

Immunocompromised patients are at increased risk of infection with *B. dermatitidis*. A review of 24 cases of infection with *B. dermatitidis* in a heterogeneous population of immunocompromised patients showed 6 cases of disseminated disease, including 4 with CNS involvement.[60]

PARACOCCIDIOIDES BRASILIENSIS

Paracoccidioides brasiliensis is a dimorphic fungus endemic to subtropical areas of Mexico and Central and South America. The lung is the primary location for initial infection; a few patients present with widely disseminated disease that can involve the

CNS. Small case series report dissemination in 9 to 27 percent of patients, and the infection reportedly involves the CNS in approximately 13 percent.[61]

Meningitis is an unusual manifestation of CNS infection with *P. brasiliensis*, with brain parenchymal involvement more common; patients frequently present with seizures.[62] CNS infection occurs in normal hosts and in those who are immunosuppressed. The host response against this microorganism remains poorly understood.

SPOROTHRIX SCHENCKII

Sporothrix schenckii is a worldwide saprophyte of vegetation, notably sphagnum moss. Sporothricosis presents as a chronic infection of skin and the subcutaneous lymphatic system, developing after a primary inoculation such as a rose-thorn puncture. Pulmonary disease from inhalation of spores is uncommon. Dissemination beyond the skin, lung, and joints is rare; only approximately a dozen cases of *Sporothrix* meningitis have been reported, and most do not have overt extraneural disease at presentation.[63] Diagnosis of this infection with low fungal burden in the CNS can be extremely difficult using traditional culture methods. To reduce delays of up to 6 to 7 months, a test for *Sporothrix* antibodies in the CSF should be performed.

Although meningitis with *S. schenckii* is so uncommon that risk factors cannot be defined accurately, certain patients may be predisposed to dissemination from a local infection including patients with myelodysplastic syndromes, ethanol abusers, or patients taking corticosteroids. Disseminated and CNS sporothricosis has also been described in patients with AIDS.[63]

PENICILLIUM MARNEFFEI

Penicillium marneffei is a dimorphic fungus that is found in the geographic range of bamboo rats, and has become a common cause of opportunistic infection in HIV-infected patients in parts of Southeast Asia. Pathophysiologically, the infection appears similar to histoplasmosis but it has a unique predisposition for producing skin lesions. In one series, 3 of 20 CSF samples were positive for this fungus during disseminated disease. Around 10 percent of patients with disseminated penicilliosis also have concomitant cryptococcal meningitis.

CANDIDA SPECIES

Candida species form part of the normal human microbial flora and rarely cause invasive disease unless host defenses are impaired. The yeast can gain access to the bloodstream and then the CNS via contaminated intravenous catheters or through illicit intravenous drug use.[64] Neonates, neutropenic patients, and those recovering from major surgery are particularly susceptible to invasive candidiasis, including CNS involvement.[65–67] The placement of foreign bodies in the CNS, such as drug wafer implants, can provide an entry for *Candida* infections.[68,69] Based on autopsy studies, *Candida* species are the most common fungi to invade the CNS in the setting of malignancy, and their ability to transverse the immature blood–brain barrier is a dreaded complication of fungemia in neonates with associated neurodevelopmental morbidity.[24,70] *Candida* may cause meningitis, ventriculitis, or parenchymal lesions such as abscesses or granulomas. *C. albicans* is the species implicated in most CNS infections, but other species such as *Candida tropicalis*, *Candida lusitaniae*, and *Candida parapsilosis* occasionally produce CNS disease.[71–75]

In the normal host, *Candida* rarely causes deep-seated infections. Factors that can encourage spread of *Candida* from mucosal surfaces to deeper tissues, such as the subarachnoid space, include prematurity, broad-spectrum antibacterial therapy, hyperalimentation, malignancy, indwelling catheters, treatment with corticosteroids, neutropenia, abdominal surgery, diabetes mellitus, burns, and intravenous drug use. *Candida* invades brain tissue more commonly than the subarachnoid space.

Candida meningitis has been reported in both congenital and acquired immunodeficiency syndromes, emphasizing the importance of the host response. For example, patients with chronic granulomatous disease of childhood and myeloperoxidase deficiency may present with *Candida* meningitis.[76] Several cases of *Candida* meningitis have been reported in patients with the global immune defects caused by severe combined immune deficiency (SCID) and the specific innate immunity defects of chronic mucocutaneous candidiasis.[77,78] Therefore, a specific underlying immune deficiency should be considered in any case of spontaneously occurring *Candida* meningitis, especially in children. Patients with AIDS frequently have mucocutaneous forms of candidiasis such as thrush and esophagitis, but involvement of the CNS has been reported rarely in these patients. *Candida* meningitis has been described as a superinfection of the CNS in patients recovering from bacterial meningitis.[79] *Candida* infection can involve the brain and subarachnoid space by direct extension through trauma, ventriculostomy placement, or ventricular shunts, particularly in the presence of antibacterial use. *Candida* uncommonly can also invade from adjacent paranasal sinuses or bone.[80] The infection may produce intracranial extension through an arteritis and even lead to subarachnoid hemorrhage.[79]

The CSF in *Candida* meningitis can show a predominance of either mononuclear or neutrophilic cells.[81] Only approximately half of routine CSF cultures yield the fungus, despite the fact that *Candida* organisms are easy to grow in the laboratory; a large CSF volume is needed to optimize culture, and better methods of CSF detection need to be validated to detect fungal products such as arabinitol or antigens such as beta-D-glucan or mannan.[82,83] The clinical significance of a positive culture for *Candida* from CSF obtained through an indwelling device such as a ventriculostomy tube may not be clear as the fungus is a frequent contaminant; if a positive culture is found and CSF parameters are normal, another CSF specimen should be obtained from a lumbar puncture.[84] In the absence of symptoms or an abnormal CSF profile, and with a negative follow-up culture, further treatment is probably unnecessary but the device should be removed and, when necessary, replaced.[65,84]

ASPERGILLUS SPECIES

Aspergillus species are ubiquitous in the environment and can be found in the air of most buildings, including hospitals. Both neutrophils and macrophages provide important host defense mechanisms directed against the spores and hyphae of *Aspergillus*. CNS infection with *Aspergillus* species can develop by direct extension from the paranasal sinuses by direct inoculation after head trauma, following surgery, or by hematogenous spread in immunocompromised hosts, particularly those with prolonged neutropenia. This fungus accounts for approximately 5 percent of CNS fungal infections.[70] A clinically important characteristic of *Aspergillus* infections is their predilection to invade arteries, causing thromboses and cerebral infarction or mycotic aneurysm. Less commonly, meningitis and meningoencephalitis can occur, and rhinocerebral disease similar to mucormycosis has been described.[22,85–87]

Most intracranial infections with *Aspergillus* occur in neutropenic patients. The risk of disseminated aspergillosis with subsequent brain parenchymal involvement or meningitis increases with the duration of neutropenia. Most infections manifest as brain parenchymal lesions, but spinal cord lesions may also develop. Occasionally, *Aspergillus* infection involves the vertebrae and eventually the subarachnoid space. Patients with chronic granulomatous disease of childhood with its lack of an oxidative burst by phagocytes are particularly susceptible to this type of infection. The pulmonary alveolar macrophage may be most important in initial control of this ubiquitous fungus in the lungs, but polymorphonuclear leukocytes are probably crucial in defense against CNS invasion.

Diagnosis can be delayed because of insensitivity of cultures, and both CSF polymerase chain reaction and galactomannan antigen tests on CSF are helpful in diagnosing CNS involvement.[88]

MUCORMYCOSIS

Fungi of the order Mucorales are widespread in the environment, and infection is usually due to inhalation of spores. The genus *Rhizopus* is responsible for most human infections. CNS infection in compromised hosts can occur by direct extension from the paranasal sinuses, through hematogenous spread such as with illicit intravenous drug use, or by spread along nerve roots.[89] Mucormycosis commonly is associated with invasion of arteries and thrombosis, with resulting tissue infarction. Presentation involving invasion of the subarachnoid space occurs occasionally, but disease limited to the meninges is unusual. In a large review of 929 cases with mucormycosis, 283 patients had CNS infection, of which 69 percent was rhinocerebral, 16 percent was localized cerebral infection, and 15 percent had hematogenous dissemination from other organs.[90]

Patients with diabetes mellitus (with or without ketoacidosis) or malignancy or those receiving immunosuppressive drugs or prolonged voriconazole therapy are at risk of this disseminated infection. There have been reports of disseminated mucormycosis, including brain involvement, in patients on dialysis receiving the iron chelator deferoxamine; this agent may interfere with the antifungal activity of transferrin, thus allowing for dissemination of the mold.[18] A different iron chelator, deferasirox, cannot be used as a siderophore by the fungus and actually has been evaluated as a treatment of mucormycosis as it competes for essential iron supplies with the fungus.[91]

PSEUDALLESCHERIA BOYDII

Pseudallescheria boydii has a worldwide distribution in soil and contaminated water. This fungus is also known as *Monosporium apiospermum* or *Scedosporium apiospermum* when it is in the asexual state. Although rare, CNS infection can result in brain abscesses or chronic neutrophilic meningitis.[92–94] Classically, CNS infection is associated with aspiration of contaminated water during trauma, or near-drowning in fresh water.[92] Presumably, the fungus penetrates through the cribiform plate during water immersion or establishes a pulmonary focus with later dissemination to the CNS, producing meningitis or brain abscesses. Other risk factors for infection include corticosteroid use and diabetes.

PHAEOHYPHOMYCOSIS

The dematiaceous fungi are a group of common environmental molds that have brown pigment in their walls; diverse genera are linked by their ability to produce melanin. This group of fungi has occasionally caused CNS infection, and for certain species it appears that there is some neurotropism. *Cladosporium trichoides*, also known as *Xylohypha bantiana* and finally renamed as *Cladophialophora bantianum*, is the most common isolate of this class of fungi found in CNS infections, which usually manifest as a brain abscess, although meningitis has been described.[95–97] Meningitis caused by other species of these "black molds" is also occasionally reported, such as with *Rhinocladiella mackenzei*.[98]

CNS infections with these organisms have been caused by contaminated corticosteroid injections around the spine.[2,10] In 2002, *Exophiala dermatitidis* produced four cases of meningitis from contaminated corticosteroids injected epidurally for pain management. Patients presented with headaches, altered mental states, and focal neurologic findings approximately 1 to 3 months after the injections.[99] A larger outbreak of *Exserohilum rostratum* infection in 2012 and 2013 involved over 500 cases; clinical presentations ranged from meningitis with or without stroke to parameningeal infections (e.g., epidural abscess, arachnoiditis with cauda equina syndrome, and vertebral osteomyelitis).[100–103]

Most patients diagnosed with brain abscesses due to one of the dematiaceous fungi have no apparent underlying immune defect, but immunosuppressed patients may be at special risk.[104] The portal of entry for these fungi is not known in most cases, but because of a predilection for abscess formation in the frontal and parietal lobes, at least some of these infections may result from direct extension through the sinuses.

HYALOHYPHOMYCOSIS

Nonpigmented, hyaline filamentous molds cause occasional infections of the CNS. Meningitis and cerebritis have been reported with *Acremonium* and *Paecilomyces* species.[2,105] In severely neutropenic patients, the soil saprophytes, *Fusarium* species, can produce CNS lesions. Because of similar histopathologic features, *Fusarium* infection can be confused with aspergillosis unless cultures are performed. In the growing immunosuppressed population, *Trichosporon* infection, which usually involves only superficial skin or hair shafts, can disseminate to the brain; CNS infections with *T. beigelii* or *T. ashaii* and *Blastoschizomyces capitatus* (*Geotrichum capitatum*) have been reported to cause CNS diseases.[7,8]

DIAGNOSIS

The diagnosis of CNS fungal infections can be very difficult, even in the setting of disseminated fungal infection. Factors that lead to this difficulty include the unusual and varied clinical presentations of patients with CNS fungal infections, difficulty in culturing organisms from the CNS due to a low burden of fungus, and the lack of sensitive serologic tests for most fungi.

In cases of cerebral mass lesions due to fungi, many patients present with nonfocal neurologic symptoms and signs. For instance, many patients present only with altered sensorium or seizures, despite having extensive CNS infection on neuroimaging. Fungal meningitis usually leads to chronic signs and symptoms including a combination of fever, headache, lethargy, confusion, nausea, vomiting, stiff neck, and neurologic deficits. However, the characteristic markers of CNS infection, fever and headache, both may be absent, and patients may present initially only with a subacute dementia. Cases of cryptococcal, coccidioidal, and *Histoplasma* meningitis may be indolent, with symptoms persisting for months to years if untreated; in consequence, the timing of symptoms is not always an accurate guide to diagnosis. In contrast, occasional cases of cryptococcal meningitis present acutely after only several days of symptoms, especially in severely immunocompromised patients and particularly those receiving high doses of corticosteroids or with advanced HIV infection.

Fungal infection is a primary consideration in the differential diagnosis of patients with chronic meningitis, defined as those with meningitis-related CNS abnormalities that either progress or fail to improve during at least 4 weeks of observation. The differential diagnosis of chronic meningitis includes both infectious and noninfectious causes (Table 46-2), but fungal infection should be high in the differential diagnosis. It may be particularly difficult to distinguish infection due to fungi from that caused by certain other subacute or chronic pathogens such as mycobacteria.

The CSF findings in fungal meningitis are well described. In most instances a mononuclear pleocytosis is present, with leukocyte counts ranging between 20 and 500 cells/mm^3. In some cases of fungal meningitis there is a predominance of polymorphonuclear cells. Eosinophilic pleocytosis of the CSF has been described in approximately 70 percent of cases of coccidioidal meningitis and, rarely, in cases of cryptococcal meningitis.[106,107] Very low CSF leukocyte counts ($<10/mm^3$) may occur when patients are severely immunosuppressed; a normal CSF profile has been observed in some cases. CSF protein levels usually are elevated, but if very high protein concentrations ($\geq 1.0\,g/dl$) are present, a subarachnoid block is likely. CSF glucose concentrations may vary from normal to low. The causes of hypoglycorrhachia are listed in Table 46-3. The finding of a low glucose concentration in the CSF favors an infectious disorder and may have prognostic significance in that persistent hypoglycorrhachia after treatment for cryptococcal meningitis without HIV infection raises concern for relapse. Elevated CSF pressures of 250 mmH$_2$O or higher may have prognostic and therapeutic implications, particularly in cryptococcal meningitis.[108]

TABLE 46-2 ■ Differential Diagnosis of Chronic Meningitis

Infectious Causes	Noninfectious Causes
Fungal infections	Chronic benign lymphocytic meningitis
Mycobacterial infections	Subarachnoid hemorrhage
Parameningeal infections	Systemic lupus erythematosus
Syphilis	Granulomatous arteritis
Lyme disease	Carcinomatous meningitis
Brucellosis	Sarcoidosis
Toxoplasmosis	Behçet disease
Nocardiosis	
Actinomycosis	
Leptospirosis	
Helminthic meningitis	
Viral meningitis	

It is unusual to see fungi on direct stains prepared from CSF, except in the case of cryptococcal meningitis. India ink preparations of CSF are positive in only 50 percent of all patients with cryptococcal meningitis, and in 80 percent or more of those who have underlying HIV infection. The number of fungi present in CSF in cases of fungal meningitis is highly variable. In some cases of cryptococcal meningitis, there are at least 10^6 CFU/ml of CSF, whereas the dimorphic fungi often have less than 1 CFU/ml of CSF. Approximately 75 percent of all patients with cryptococcal meningitis yield positive CSF cultures; patients with HIV infection have positive cultures in 90 percent of cases. Unfortunately, in meningitis cases due to fungi other than cryptococci, CSF cultures are often negative, and they are rarely positive in patients with cerebral mass lesions. For example, only one-third to one-half of patients with coccidioidal meningitis yield CSF cultures that are positive. Patients with blastomycotic meningitis rarely yield positive CSF cultures, and in proven *Histoplasma* meningitis it is difficult to find the organisms in the subarachnoid space, even at necropsy. Because the burden of organisms in CSF is so often low, relatively large volumes of CSF (10 to 20 ml) should be obtained and sent for culture in suspected cases.

TABLE 46-3 ■ Differential Diagnosis of Low Cerebrospinal Fluid Glucose Concentration

Acute bacterial meningitis
Mycobacterial meningitis
Fungal meningitis
Subarachnoid hemorrhage
Carcinomatous meningitis
Meningeal cysticercosis/trichinosis
Drug-induced meningitis (nonsteroidal anti-inflammatory agents)
Acute syphilitic meningitis
Chemical meningitis (direct intrathecal injections)
Viral meningitis (rare)
Hypoglycemia
Rheumatoid meningitis
Lupus myelopathy
Amebic meningitis

The laboratory should centrifuge specimens and culture the sediment on appropriate fungal media. *Candida* organisms usually can be identified within a few days; in occasional patients, hypertonic media may be helpful for growing the yeast. In neonates, CSF cultures are important as blood cultures may be negative and CSF parameters may be normal in culture-positive candida meningitis.[109] *Cryptococcus* should be identified within 3 to 10 days in most cases, but the classic dimorphic fungi (e.g., *Histoplasma* or *Coccidioides*) may require longer incubations. The lysis-centrifugation method for isolating *H. capsulatum* from blood and CSF has improved detection compared with routine methods. Blood cultures may also be helpful for identifying the fungus that is causing meningitis in a particular host; *Candida* species or *Cryptococcus* are the fungal organisms most likely to be present on blood cultures. CSF cultures can also be negative simply because the samples were not taken from the localized site of active infection. For example, because fungi commonly cause a basilar meningitis, cisternal or ventricular fluid may occasionally yield organisms when fluid from the lumbar space is sterile.[110]

Serologic tests are important for the diagnosis of many fungal infections in the CNS. For example, the latex agglutination test, ELISA, and lateral flow assay for detection of cryptococcal polysaccharide antigen are the best serologic tests for this agent and can be used with rapidity on serum or CSF. The tests are often positive even when culture is negative. When samples are heated to eliminate rheumatoid factor and proper controls for nonspecific agglutination and interfering substances are used, the antigen tests are more than 90 percent sensitive and specific for cryptococcal infection.[111] If surface condensation from agar plates is added to the assay, false-positive results may occur, which can also be seen with disseminated *T. beigelii* infections and paravertebral bacterial infections. If a positive antigen test occurs in a patient whose clinical presentation is not consistent with cryptococcal meningitis, the laboratory should repeat the test, and if it is still positive, a repeat lumbar puncture is indicated. False-negative results may be due to very low burdens of pathogens, a prozone phenomenon due to antigen excess, or the performance characteristics of various different proprietary antigen detection kits. The value of using cryptococcal antigen titers as prognostic guides is well established; however, titers are less valuable for guiding specific therapeutic decisions.[112]

Detection of the *Histoplasma* polysaccharide antigen in urine and serum is a valuable adjunctive test in the diagnosis of disseminated disease. It is also useful in monitoring therapy and for the early detection of relapsing infection in HIV-positive patients.[113] False-positive results may occur in patients with meningitis due to other fungi. Tests detecting CSF antibodies against *Histoplasma* antigens are also useful, and are positive in approximately 75 percent of patients with CNS infection. Although sensitive, these antibody tests are not highly specific, and positive results may also be found in patients with other fungal infections or with bacterial meningitis. The best way to diagnose CNS *Histoplasma* infections when cultures are negative is to perform both antigen and antibody testing. Empiric treatment for *Histoplasma* infection should be started in patients with chronic meningitis of uncertain etiology when the antigen or antibody assays are positive in the CSF.

In coccidioidomycosis, elevated serum CFA titers above 1:32 to 1:64 are the hallmark of disseminated disease.[114] Some patients with isolated meningitis without extraneural infection may also have low serum CFA titers. In patients with coccidioidal meningitis, CFA titers are present in the CSF in 70 percent of patients initially and in almost 100 percent as the infection progresses. CFA is absent from unconcentrated CSF in the presence of high serum titers due to extraneural disease, unless there is a parameningeal lesion next to the dura. The CFA titers appear to parallel the course of meningeal disease and have been used to guide treatment; titers should decline with successful therapy.

The ability to detect specific antibodies in CSF has been used in the diagnosis of meningitis caused by *S. schenckii.* Waiting for culture data can lead to delays of up to 7 months from the onset of symptoms, and therefore latex agglutination and enzyme immunoassay tests have been used successfully to detect CSF antibodies confirming the diagnosis of *Sporothrix* meningitis. When a titer cut-off of 1:8 or higher is used, there is no cross-reaction with other fungal, bacterial, or viral pathogens.

There is intense interest in developing serologic tests for other fungal infections, especially those due to *Candida* and *Aspergillus.* Detection of unique antigens (beta-D-glucan and mannan) or metabolic products (arabinitol and mannitol) from these fungi in CSF has not yet been extensively validated in the clinical setting of meningitis.[82,83,115] However, it is likely that the galactomannan detection test for *Aspergillus* on CSF will prove useful in diagnosing this rare and difficult-to-detect infection.

Two other approaches for diagnosis of fungal meningitis are detection of host products and the use of molecular amplification. Although not specific for fungi, CSF lactic acid concentrations usually are elevated in fungal meningitis and, in some cases, specific fungal T-cell responses can be detected.[116] It is likely that as further experience accumulates with polymerase chain reaction–based diagnostics for meningitis, fungal sequences will be included in new diagnostic approaches.[117]

Imaging studies can be helpful in the diagnosis and staging of CNS fungal infections. Localization of mass lesions or areas of meningeal inflammation by computed tomography (CT) or magnetic resonance imaging (MRI) can guide the neurosurgeon to areas for biopsy. MRI with contrast enhancement is more sensitive than contrast CT scans. In cases of fungal meningitis, CT and MRI may be unremarkable or show leptomeningeal enhancement, hydrocephalus, infarction (as with mucormycosis), or edema.[118] When meningitis is refractory to conventional diagnostic approaches, meningeal biopsy for histologic study and culture can be considered although false negatives can occur.

TREATMENT

Experience in the treatment of fungal CNS infections is varied. For example, treatment for cryptococcal meningitis has been studied intensively, whereas many fungal CNS infections are so rare that only a few cases have been described. An important adjunct to antifungal therapy is the reversal, if possible, of any immunocompromising conditions. This may include decreasing doses of corticosteroids or the use of immunomodulators to improve host immunity.

Specific Fungal Infections in the Central Nervous System

Cryptococcal Meningitis

Before the availability of amphotericin B, cryptococcal meningitis was uniformly fatal, although occasionally an untreated patient survived for several years. Early treatment trials showed that immunosuppressed patients with cryptococcal meningitis had higher treatment failure rates than immunocompetent patients. Patients with AIDS were found to have low response rates to initial therapy and high relapse rates once therapy was stopped. Because of this important dichotomy in the patient populations with cryptococcal meningitis, the treatments for patients with and without HIV infection are discussed separately. The 2010 Cryptococcal Guidelines of the Infectious Diseases Society of America (IDSA) separated risk groups into those with AIDS, transplant recipients, and non-AIDS, non-transplant patients.[119]

Non-Immunosuppressed Patients

Amphotericin B used alone at daily doses of 0.4 to 0.8 mg/kg per day for 10 weeks provides effective therapy for patients without HIV infection who develop cryptococcal meningitis. The addition of flucytosine to this regimen has been studied in an effort to decrease both the duration of therapy and the total dose of amphotericin B. Following early trial data, experience with amphotericin B plus flucytosine as primary therapy in cryptococcal meningitis has accumulated.[120] This combination usually sterilizes the CSF within 2 weeks and cures many patients within 4 to 6 weeks, with manageable amphotericin B toxicity. Patients with good prognostic features and no known immunosuppressive conditions have been successfully managed with as little as 4 weeks of combined therapy. The regimen nevertheless requires the administration of an intravenous medication for prolonged periods, and some treatment failures (15 to 30%) do occur.

Treatment regimens using oral antifungal agents for cryptococcal meningitis would obviously be attractive, and therefore both itraconazole and fluconazole have been tried.[121] There are no large trials comparing azole antifungals with amphotericin B in patients without HIV infection. Personal experience and data extrapolated from trials with patients with AIDS suggest that fluconazole can be used successfully as monotherapy for patients with cryptococcal meningitis, but it may not be as effective as the combination of amphotericin B plus flucytosine because of reduced fungicidal activity. Therefore, most experts do not recommend use of fluconazole (1200 mg/day) alone for induction therapy of cryptococcal meningitis.[119] Itraconazole has also been used successfully in treating cryptococcal meningitis, but because there is more experience with fluconazole, many physicians consider this the preferred azole.[122] A compromise can be reached in an effort to reduce the amount of time on intravenous therapy by using an induction phase of amphotericin B plus flucytosine followed by prolonged consolidation and maintenance (suppressive) phases with oral fluconazole. This combined drug regimen is recommended in treatment guidelines published by the Infectious Diseases Society of America, and consists of amphotericin B at a dose of 0.7 to 1.0 mg/kg per day plus flucytosine at a dose of 100 mg/kg per day to keep serum levels below 100 μg/ml for 2 weeks, after which the patient is switched to fluconazole at a dose of 400 mg/day, assuming normal renal function, for a minimum of 10 weeks.[119,123] A lumbar puncture should also be considered after 2 weeks; if the CSF culture still yields *C. neoformans*, treatment with amphotericin B and flucytosine should be reinstituted for another 2-week course of induction therapy.[123] If the CSF is sterile after induction amphotericin B plus flucytosine therapy, fluconazole can be continued. The total duration of fluconazole therapy should be tailored to the individual patient, but at least 10 weeks of treatment should be administered, and this should be extended for patients with immunosuppression.[123] Because most relapses of cryptococcal meningitis occur within 6 months to 1 year after stopping therapy, generally a maintenance or suppressive dose of fluconazole 200 to 400 mg/day is given for 6 months to 1 year in patients who do not have HIV infection. Additional and higher doses of fluconazole may be required in patients with brain parenchymal lesions, persistent symptoms, concomitant immunosuppressive therapy, or underlying immunosuppressing diseases.

The need for intraventricular or intrathecal amphotericin B in cryptococcal meningitis remains controversial. Some investigators have used intraventricular amphotericin B with success in cases with a poor prognosis. However, this route of administration is rarely necessary and may have complications. In high-risk patients, it may be better to switch to lipid-based amphotericin B regimens and use doses up to 5 mg/kg per day or possibly higher, rather than risk the side effects of direct injection of amphotericin B into CSF. These lipid formulations are highly recommended in transplant recipients but are more costly.

Once therapy has been started, the frequency of lumbar punctures should be determined by clinical response. As mentioned above, a lumbar puncture performed after the second week of therapy should show that the CSF is sterile if the combination of amphotericin B and flucytosine was used. Once therapy is completed, further lumbar punctures should be performed at intervals, depending on the patient's signs and symptoms. Persistently elevated polysaccharide antigen titers or positive India ink examinations indicate failure of therapy only when the CSF culture is positive or the patient demonstrates neurologic deterioration. There is probably little value in following serial cryptococcal polysaccharide antigen titers to make therapeutic decisions.

Immunosuppressed Patients

The management of cryptococcal meningitis in patients with AIDS presents a major therapeutic challenge. Response to initial therapy in ART-treated cases has improved, and the relapse rate, which was once very high, has been reduced by maintenance or suppressive fluconazole treatment and ART. Recurrence of symptomatic cryptococcal meningitis in patients with AIDS is typically due to the same strain that caused the original infection and it is thought that the prostate or brain parenchyma can serve as a site for persistent residual infection despite sterilization of the CSF.[124]

There is a substantial amount of clinical data to support recommendations for the treatment of AIDS-associated cryptococcal meningitis published by the Infectious Diseases Society of America.[119,123]. Induction therapy includes amphotericin B 0.7-1.0 mg/kg per day with or without flucytosine 100 mg/kg per day for around 2 weeks. The combination regimen is favored because of more rapid CSF sterilization, potentially fewer relapses, and better outcomes.[125] In patients who have significant renal dysfunction, liposomal amphotericin B 4 mg/kg per day or amphotericin B lipid complex 5 mg/kg per day can be substituted for amphotericin B. The induction period usually lasts for 2 weeks but can vary depending on clinical response. Patients are then switched to fluconazole (400 to 800 mg/day) for 10 weeks. Fluconazole alone has been evaluated for primary therapy of cryptococcal meningitis, but clinical experience suggests that it takes longer to sterilize the CSF than amphotericin B and requires higher doses.[42,121,126] Triazoles may be more effective when the burden of yeasts in CSF is lower. It is anticipated that 80 to 90 percent of patients will respond well to this initial course of therapy. The third stage of the treatment plan is the continued use of prolonged fluconazole at a dose of 200 mg/day for prevention of relapses.[127] The high rate of relapse in these patients led to the initial institution of lifelong fluconazole suppressive therapy for all patients with AIDS who respond to initial treatment for cryptococcal meningitis. However, the immune restoration associated with ART has prompted reinvestigation of lifelong suppression; patients who have been treated with antiretroviral therapy and have a sustained immunologic response may be able to safely discontinue maintenance therapy.[123] Appropriate candidates for stopping maintenance therapy are patients who have had at least 2 years of therapy with fluconazole, along with a CD4 count above 100 cells/μl (or more than 10% CD4 cells). These patients should be monitored closely, and fluconazole maintenance reinstituted if the CD4 count falls below 100 cells/μl or below 10 percent CD4 cells or if there is reappearance of serum cryptococcal antigen titers that were previously negative. In one prospective trial, 42 patients who had responded to antifungal therapy for cryptococcal meningitis were randomized to either continue or discontinue maintenance therapy for cryptococcal meningitis once the CD4 count had increased to above 100 cells/μl and the HIV viral load had been below 50 copies/ml for 3 months on ART; over a median follow-up of 48 weeks, no relapses occurred in either group.[128]

Complications

Increased intracranial pressure is a well-described problem in patients being treated for cryptococcal meningitis.[108,129] Symptoms in such patients usually begin shortly after initiating antifungal therapy and include systemic hypertension, increasing headaches, impaired consciousness, visual impairment, and cranial nerve palsies. These symptoms can occur suddenly, and head imaging usually shows no evidence of hydrocephalus or mass lesions. The opening pressure at lumbar puncture can be extremely high ($\geq$250 mmH$_2$O). The pathophysiologic cause of increased intracranial pressure in this setting is uncertain but may well be CSF outflow obstruction.[129] Most patients with AIDS-associated cryptococcal meningitis present with increased intracranial pressure, and up to 70 percent of this patient population will have opening pressures exceeding 200 mmH$_2$O on the initial lumbar puncture. In these patients, symptoms generally respond rapidly to removal of large volumes of CSF, which can be accomplished with CSF drainage. Treatment guidelines published by the Infectious Diseases Society of America recommend that sufficient CSF be removed to achieve a closing pressure either below 200 mmH$_2$O or 50 percent of the opening pressure. Some patients require serial lumbar punctures for relief of severe symptoms and physical findings; for those patients requiring very frequent lumbar punctures, placement of a ventricular shunt should be considered.[108,130] Despite theoretical concerns regarding placement of catheters into infected spinal fluid, experience shows no increased difficulties in clearing the infection. Placement of a lumbar drain is another option, but the relatively frequent complication of bacterial superinfection precludes long-term use. The use of corticosteroids or acetazolamide to decrease raised intracranial pressures in the setting of AIDS-associated cryptococcal meningitis does not appear to be beneficial except when corticosteroids are used in the setting of IRIS.[123,131]

Visual loss in cryptococcal meningitis may not respond to maneuvers aimed at decreasing intracranial pressure. Blindness is usually not due to endophthalmitis and is often bilateral and permanent.[132] Many treatments have been tried unsuccessfully in an effort to restore vision including repeated lumbar punctures, treatment with corticosteroids, fenestration of the optic nerve sheath, and release of perioptic nerve arachnoidal adhesions. The management of IRIS in cyptococcal meningitis is uncertain. First, the diagnosis is imprecise but is considered when CSF cultures are negative and the antigen is stable or decreasing on therapy despite persistent or increasing evidence of inflammation by CSF analysis or neuroimaging. Treatment is not well-studied but clinical response does occur to corticosteroids. When to start ART after the institution of antifungal therapy is not known, and until definitive studies occur, guidelines give a range of 2 to 10 weeks.[119]

There are several major prognostic factors that determine the outcome of patients with cryptococcal meningitis. Control of the underlying disease is the most important factor. The burden of yeasts in the CSF, indicated by positive India ink examinations, high polysaccharide antigen titers, and elevated intracranial pressure, is also predictive. High numbers of yeasts worsen the prognosis, and patients may then need more aggressive individual clinical management. The impact of the host response is also important; patients with a poor CSF inflammatory response, such as those with less than 20 leukocytes/mm^3 on CSF examination, do not respond as well to therapy, and studies suggest that immunomodulators may be of help. Interferon-γ levels in the CSF may help determine clearance of infection, and treatment with recombinant interferon-γ tends to reduce CSF yeast counts faster than otherwise.[133] Clinical symptoms at presentation, such as a decreased sensorium, suggest advanced disease and also a poor prognosis.

CANDIDA *MENINGITIS*

While there are reports of spontaneous cures of meningitis due to *Candida* species, clinical experience suggests that treatment is indicated for all patients. Even with treatment, mortality rates for *Candida* meningitis range between 10 and 20 percent. There is no consensus on the best regimen, but the combination of amphotericin B and flucytosine has synergistic activity against *Candida* in vitro and has resulted in a high cure rate.[134] There is substantial experience with amphotericin B alone, which also can successfully treat *Candida* meningitis.[67] Fluconazole with high CSF penetration can be used in certain cases, although it usually does not sterilize CSF as fast as amphotericin B–containing regimens.[135] Liposomal amphotericin B has been used after failure of conventional amphotericin B and has been combined successfully with flucytosine.[136] In patients with ventriculoperitoneal shunts or ventriculostomies, it is recommended that any prosthetic material or device be replaced during systemic antifungal therapy.[137] Although mortality has improved with treatment, neurodevelopmental disabilities may persist in neonates.[138–140]

COCCIDIOIDAL MENINGITIS

In contrast to meningitis due to other fungi, the primary mode of treatment for coccidioidal meningitis with amphotericin B is not systemic but intraventricular. In these infections, systemic amphotericin B in a total dose of 0.5 to 1.0 g is given mainly to treat undetected foci outside the CNS. Control of the CNS infection is then achieved by intraventricular administration of amphotericin B. Intrathecal therapy is begun with small doses of 0.01 mg/day and increased gradually, as tolerated, up to 0.5 mg/day. The drug can be administered into the lumbar, cisternal, or ventricular space; the latter is preferred. Arachnoiditis, neurotoxicity, and secondary bacterial infections of the CSF can complicate therapy. Recommendations for length of therapy are variable, and because of the poor prognosis for complete cure some patients have been treated indefinitely. The CSF leukocyte count has been used to follow progress and to judge the need for further therapy. Lowering of the CSF antibody titers after treatment is a good prognostic sign. If the patient worsens during treatment, the possibility of hydrocephalus or a superimposed bacterial infection should be considered.

There has been some clinical benefit from treatment with oral azoles. Miconazole and ketoconazole have been tried, but response has been only fair, and therefore these agents are not recommended. More experience has focused on using fluconazole and itraconazole as therapy for coccidioidal meningitis.[141] In one study of 47 patients with coccidioidal meningitis treated with fluconazole 400 mg/day, a positive response to therapy occurred in 37 patients unrelated to the presence of hydrocephalus or HIV infection.[142] Toxicity is minimal in patients treated for long periods. It is therefore reasonable to consider fluconazole as a first-line agent in patients with coccidioidal meningitis; its ease of administration and lack of toxicity compared with intrathecal amphotericin B are important considerations. The optimal dose of fluconazole is not certain and some authorities believe that 800 mg/day of fluconazole should be used as initial treatment. The use of induction therapy with intrathecal amphotericin B followed by long-term azole therapy has also been proposed as a possible treatment option in some cases. It is unclear what role voriconazole or posaconazole will have in treatment of refractory disease.[143] Current treatment strategies consider coccidioidal meningitis to be suppressed rather than cured, thus requiring lifelong therapy. Observational studies suggest that with current treatments, over 70 percent of patients will relapse on discontinuation of treatment.

Other Fungal Infections

Meningitis due to *Histoplasma*, *Sporothrix*, or *Blastomyces* usually responds to prolonged courses of amphotericin B. The role of azole drugs in these infections is not clearly defined, but they are generally used only after aggressive induction treatment most commonly with a lipid amphotericin B formulation.[113,144] *P. boydii* CNS infections may respond to initial therapy with the newer triazoles such as voriconazole.[145] Cotrimoxazole has been used successfully in paracoccidioides meningitis.[61]

Infections of the CNS with *Aspergillus* species are usually fatal despite therapy. However, there are a few cases of successful therapy with high-dose amphotericin B, and extended-spectrum new triazoles such as voriconazole have improved outcome in CNS aspergillosis.[146] Patients with CNS aspergillosis may be considered for combination therapy with voriconazole or posaconazole plus an echinocandin and possibly also the addition of lipid amphotericin B. It also may be helpful to debulk a large abscess surgically.

Mucormycosis of the CNS should be treated initially with high doses (5 mg/kg daily) of lipid formulations of amphotericin B and, if possible, surgical debridement of infarcted tissue. Surgical debulking of fungal masses is even more important in the phaeohyphomycoses, which then may be treated with a combination of a polyene, an azole, and flucytosine.[147]

Surgical Treatment

Neurosurgical procedures can play an important role in the diagnosis and treatment of some CNS fungal infections. Obtaining appropriate CSF or tissue samples for diagnosis using neurosurgical procedures may be required in some cases. The placement of CSF-diverting shunts may be needed in cases of hydrocephalus or increased intracranial pressure even during the period of active drug treatment of infection. The placement of reservoirs to allow for chronic intrathecal administration of antifungals may also be required in certain CNS infections.

Surgical resection of parenchymal lesions has been undertaken to reduce mass effect in some cases of *Histoplasma*, *Cryptococcus*, and *Aspergillus* infection, but for these fungi the presence of parenchymal CNS lesions usually does not routinely indicate the need for neurosurgical excision. In contrast, when black molds such as *Cladophialophora* or *Rhinocladiella* species and other dematiaceous fungi cause mass lesions, surgical resection or debulking is usually required for cure. Rhinocerebral infections due to mucormycosis also require prompt debridement of necrotic tissue in the brain.

Fungal infections of CSF shunts and reservoirs are uncommon and are most often due to *Candida* species. Shunt infections should be treated with removal of the shunt and systemic antifungal therapy when possible. However, there are cases in which shunt removal is not possible or in which shunt placement occurs during periods of active drug treatment of meningitis. It is recommended that in the setting of a CNS fungal infection, the shunt should be removed if it was placed prior to the initiation of antifungal therapy.

REFERENCES

1. Cox GM, Durack DT, Perfect JR: Fungal infections of the nervous system. p. 899. In Aminoff MJ (ed): Neurology and General Medicine. 4th Ed. Churchill Livingstone Elsevier, Philadelphia, 2008.
2. Ohashi Y: On a rare disease due to *Alternaria tenuis* Nees. Tohoku J Exp Med 72:78, 1960.
3. Krcmery V, Spanik S, Denisovicoua A, et al: *Aureobasidium mansosni*, meningitis in a leukemia patient successfully treated with amphotericin B. Chemotherapy 40:70, 1994.
4. Chin-Hong PV, Sutton DA, Roemer M, et al: Invasive fungal sinusitis and meningitis due to *Arthrographis*

kalrae in a patient with AIDS. J Clin Microbiol 39:804, 2001.
5. Papadatos C, Pavlatou M, Alexiou D: Cephalosporium meningitis. Pediatrics 44:749, 1969.
6. Kremery Jr V, Mateicka F, Grausoua S, et al: Invasive infections due to *Clavispora lusitaniae*. FEMS Immunol Med Microbiol 23:75, 1999.
7. Girmenia C, Micozzi A, Venditti M, et al: Fluconazole treatment of *Blastoschizomyces capitatus* meningitis in an allogeneic bone marrow recipient. Eur J Clin Microbiol Infect Dis 10:752, 1991.
8. Santoro F, Afchain D, Pierce R, et al: Serodiagnosis of toxoplasma infection using a purified parasite protein (P30). Clin Expern Immunol 62:262, 1985.
9. Mukerji S, Patwardhan JR, Gadgil RK: Bacterial and mycotic infection of the brain. Indian J Med Sci 25:791, 1971.
10. Fuste FJ, Ajello L, Threlkeld R, et al: *Drechslera hawaiiensis*: causative agent of a fatal fungal meningoencephalitis. Sabouraudia 11:59, 1973.
11. Malassezia AS, Komiyama A, Hasegawa O: Fungal meningitis caused by a *Malassezia* species masquerading as painful ophthalmoplegia. Clin Neurol (Tokyo) 33:462, 1993.
12. Fagerburg R, Suh B, Buckley HR: Cerebrospinal fluid shunt colonization and obstruction by *Paecilomyces varoti*. J Neurosurg 54:257, 1981.
13. Baena Luna MR, Munoz Garcia J, Grancha Bertolin C, et al: *Pneumocystis carinii* en liquido cefalorraguideo. Ann Med Interne 15:265, 1998.
14. Kauffman CA, Pappas PG, Patterson TF: Fungal infections associated with contaminated methylprednisolone injections—preliminary report. N Engl J Med 368:2495, 2012.
15. Pettit AC, Pugh ME: Index case for the fungal meningitis outbreak, United States. N Engl J Med 368:970, 2013.
16. Centers for Disease Control and Prevention (CDC) Multistate outbreak of fungal infection associated with injection of methylprednisolone acetate solution from a single compounding pharmacy—United States, 2012. MMWR Morb Mortal Wkly Rep 61:839, 2012.
17. Takeda S, Wakabayashi K, Yamazaki K, et al: Intracranial fungal aneurysm caused by *Candida endocarditis*. Clin Neuropathol 17:199, 1998.
18. Boelaert JR, Fenves AZ, Coburn JW: Deferoxamine therapy and mucormycosis in dialysis patients: report of an international registry. Am J Kidney Dis 18:660, 1991.
19. Mirza SA, Phelan M, Rimland D, et al: The changing epidemiology of cryptococcosis: an update from population-based active surveillance in 2 large metropolitan areas, 1992-2000. Clin Infect Dis 36:789, 2003.
20. Park BJ, Wannemuehler KA, Marston BJ, et al: Estimation of the current global burden of cryptococcal meningitis among persons living with HIV. AIDS 20:525, 2009.
21. Pappas P, Alexander B, Andes D, et al: Invasive fungal infections among organ transplant recipients: results of the Transplant-Associated Infection Surveillance Network (TRANSNET). Clin Infect Dis 50:1101, 2012.
22. Carrazana EJ, Rossitch Jr E, Morris J: Isolated central nervous system aspergillosis in the acquired immunodeficiency syndrome. Clin Neurol Neurosurg 93:227, 1991.
23. Hagensee M, Bauwens JE, Kjos B, et al: Brain abscess following marrow transplantation: experience at the Fred Hutchinson Cancer Research Center, 1984-1992. Clin Infect Dis 19:402, 1994.
24. Benjamin DK, Stoll BJ, Fanaroff AA, et al: Neonatal candidiasis among extremely low birth weight infants: risk factors, mortality rates, and neurodevelopmental outcomes at 18 to 22 months. Pediatrics 117:84, 2006.
25. Ingram CW, Haywood HB, Morris VM, et al: Cryptococcal ventricular peritoneal shunt infection: clinical and epidemiological evaluation of two closely associated cases. Infect Immun 14:719, 1993.
26. Ashpole RD, Jacobson K, King AT, et al: Cystoperitoneal shunt infection with *Trichosporon beigelii*. Br J Neurosurg 5:515, 1991.
27. Takeshita S, Izawa M, Kubo O: Aspergillotic aneurysm formation of cerebral artery following neurosurgical operation. Surg Neurol 38:146, 1992.
28. Komatsu Y, Narushima K, Kobayashi E, et al: *Aspergillus* mycotic aneurysm–case report. Neurol Med Chir 31:346, 1991.
29. Sharma RR, Gurusinghe NT, Lynch PG: Cerebral infarction due to aspergillus arteritis following glioma surgery. Br J Neurosurg 6:485, 1992.
30. Singh N, Perfect JR: Immune reconstitution syndrome associated with opportunistic mycoses. Lancet Infect Dis 7:395, 2007.
31. Shelburne SA, Visnegarwala F, Darcourt J, et al: Incidence and risk factors for immune reconstitution inflammatory syndrome during highly active antiretroviral therapy. AIDS 19:399, 2005.
32. Singh N, Lortholary O, Alexander BD, et al: An immune reconstitution syndrome-like illness associated with *Cryptococcus neoformans* infection in organ transplant recipients. Clin Infect Dis 40:1756, 2005.
33. Ecevit IZ, Clancy CJ, Schmalfuss IM, et al: The poor prognosis of central nervous system cryptococcosis among nonimmunosuppressed patients: a call for better disease recognition and evaluation of adjuncts to antifungal therapy. Clin Infect Dis 42:1443, 2006.
34. Shelburne III SA, Hamill RJ, Rodriguez-Barradas MC, et al: Immune reconstitution inflammatory syndrome: emergence of a unique syndrome during highly active antiretroviral therapy. Medicine (Baltimore) 81:213, 2002.
35. Lortholary O, Fontanet A, Memain N, et al: Incidence and risk factors of immune reconstitution inflammatory syndrome complicating HIV-associated cryptococcosis in France. AIDS 19:1043, 2005.

36. Jong AWC, Chen HM, Luo F, et al: Identification and characterization of CPS1 as a hyaluronic acid synthase contributing to the pathogenesis of *Cryptococcus neoformans* infection. Eukaryot Cell 6:1486, 2007.
37. Jong AWC, Gonzales-Gomez I, Kwon-Chung KJ, et al: Hyaluronic acid receptor CD44 deficiency is associated with decreased *Cryptococcus neoformans* brain infection. J Biol Chem 287:15298, 2012.
38. Ellis D, Pfeiffer T: The ecology of *Cryptococcus neoformans*. Eur J Epidemiol 8:321, 1992.
39. Kidd SE, Hagen F, Tscharke RL, et al: A rare genotype of *Cryptococcus gattii* caused the cryptococcosis outbreak on Vancouver Island (British Columbia, Canada). Proc Natl Acad Sci USA 101:17258, 2004.
40. MacDougall LKS, Galanis E, Mak S, et al: Spread of *Cryptococcus gattii* in British Columbia, Canada, and detection in the Pacific Northwest, USA. Emerg Infect Dis 13:42, 2007.
41. Hu XP, Wu JQ, Zhu LP, et al: Association of Fcγ receptor IIB polymorphism with cryptococcal meningitis in HIV-uninfected Chinese patients. PLOS One 7:e42439, 2012.
42. Bicanic T, Muzoora C, Brouwer AE, et al: Independent association between rate of clearance of infection and clinical outcome of HIV-associated cryptococcal meningitis: analysis of a combined cohort of 262 patients. Clin Infect Dis 49:702, 2009.
43. Jarvis J, Percival A, Bauman S, et al: Evaluation of a novel point-of-care cryptococcal antigen test on serum, plasma, and urine from patients with HIV-associated cryptococcal meningitis. Clin Infect Dis 53:1019, 2011.
44. Hansen J, Slechta ES, Neary B, et al: Large-scale evaluation of the immuno-mycologics lateral flow and enzyme-linked immunoassays for detection of cryptococcal antigen in serum and cerebrospinal fluid. Clin Vaccine Immunol 20:52, 2013.
45. Mischel PS, Vinters HV: Coccidioidomycosis of the central nervous system: neuropathological and vasculopathic manifestations and clinical correlates. Clin Infect Dis 20:400, 1995.
46. Banuelos AF, Williams PL, Johnson RH, et al: Central nervous system abscesses due to Coccidioides species. Clin Infect Dis 22:240, 1996.
47. Mendel E, Milefchik EN, Amadi J, et al: Coccidioidomycosis brain abscess. Case report. J Neurosurg 81:614, 1994.
48. Winston DJ, Kurtz TO, Fleischmann J, et al: Successful treatment of spinal arachnoiditis due to coccidioidomycosis. Case report. J Neurosurg 59:328, 1983.
49. Williams PL, Johnson R, Pappagianis D, et al: Vasculitic and encephalitic complications associated with *Coccidioides immitis* infection of the central nervous system in humans: report of 10 cases and review. Clin Infect Dis 14:673, 1992.
50. Drake KW, Adam RD: Coccidioidal meningitis and brain abscesses: analysis of 71 cases at a referral center. Neurology 73:1780, 2009.
51. Arsura EL, Kilgore WB, Caldwell JW, et al: Association between facial cutaneous coccidioidomycosis and meningitis. West J Med 169:13, 1998.
52. Ampel NM, Dols CL, Galgiani JN: Coccidioidomycosis during human immunodeficiency virus infection: results of a prospective study in a coccidioidal endemic area. Am J Med 94:235, 1993.
53. Vincent T, Galgiani JN, Huppert M, et al: History of coccidioidal meningitis: VA–Armed Forces cooperative studies. Clin Infect Dis 16:247, 1993.
54. Dewsnup DH, Galgiani JN, Graybill JR, et al: Is it ever safe to stop azole therapy for *Coccidioides immitis* meningitis? Ann Intern Med 124:305, 1996.
55. Leggiadro RJ, Luedtke GS, Convey A, et al: Prevalence of histoplasmosis in a midsouthern population. South Med J 84:1360, 1991.
56. Wheat LJ, Slama TG, Zeckel ML: Histoplasmosis in the acquired immune deficiency syndrome. Am J Med 78:203, 1985.
57. Cuellar-Rodriguez J, Avery RK, Lard M, et al: Histoplasmosis in solid organ transplant recipients: 10 years of experience at a large transplant center in an endemic area. Clin Infect Dis 49:710, 2009.
58. Wheat J, French M, Batteiger B, et al: Cerebrospinal fluid *Histoplasma* antibodies in central nervous system histoplasmosis. Arch Intern Med 145:1237, 1985.
59. Harley WB, Lomis M, Haas DW: Marked polymorphonuclear pleocytosis due to blastomycotic meningitis: case report. Clin Infect Dis 18:816, 1994.
60. Pappas PG, Threlkeld MG, Bedsole GD, et al: Blastomycosis in immunocompromised patients. Medicine (Baltimore) 72:311, 1993.
61. de Almeda SM: Central nervous system paracoccidioidomycosis: an overview. Braz J Infect Dis 9:126, 2005.
62. de Almeda S, Queiroz-Telles F, Teive H, et al: Central nervous system paracoccidioidomycosis: clinical features and laboratorial findings. J Infect 48:193, 2004.
63. Penn CC, Goldstein E, Bartholomew WR: *Sporothrix schenckii* meningitis in a patient with AIDS. Clin Infect Dis 15:741, 1992.
64. del Pozo MM, Bermejo F, Molina JA, et al: Chronic neutrophilic meningitis caused by *Candida albicans*. Neurologia 13:362, 1998.
65. Arisoy ES, Arisoy AE, Dunne Jr WM: Clinical significance of fungi isolated from cerebral fluid in children. Pediatr Infect Dis J 13:127, 1994.
66. Rodriquez-Arrondo F, Aquirrebengoa K, De Arce A, et al: Candidal meningitis in HIV-infected patients: treatment with fluconazole. Scand J Infect Dis 30:417, 1998.
67. Casado JL, Quereda C, Oliva J, et al: Candidal meningitis in HIV-infected patients: analysis of 14 cases. Clin Infect Dis 25:673, 1997.
68. O'Brien D, Stevens NT, Lim CH, et al: *Candida* infection of the central nervous system following neurosurgery: a 12-year review. Acta Neurochir 153:1347, 2011.

69. O'Brien D, Cotter M, Lim CH, et al: *Candida parapsilosis* meningitis associated with Gliadel (BCNU) wafer implants. Br J Neurosurg 25:289, 2011.
70. Mori T, Ebe T: Analysis of cases of central nervous system fungal infections reported in Japan between January 1979 and June 1989. Intern Med 31:174, 1992.
71. Jamjoom A, Jamjoom ZA, Al-Hedaithy S: Ventriculitis and hydrocephalus caused by *Candida albicans* successfully treated by antimycotic therapy and cerebrospinal fluid shunting. Br J Neurosurg 6:501, 1992.
72. Flynn PM, Mariana NM, Rivera GK, et al: *Candida tropicalis* infections in children with aspergillus leukemia. Leuk Lymphoma 10:369, 1993.
73. Goldani LZ, Santos RP: *Candida tropicalis* as an emerging pathogen in *Candida* meningitis: case report and review. Braz J Infect Dis 6:631, 2010.
74. Sarma PS, Buraira P, Padhye AA: *Candida lusitaniae* causing fatal meningitis. Postgrad Med J 69:878, 1993.
75. Faix RG: *Candida parapsilosis* meningitis in a premature infant. Pediatr Infect Dis J 2:462, 1983.
76. Ludviksson BR, Thoraparensen O, Gudnason T, et al: *Candida albicans* meningitis in a child with myeloperoxidase deficiency. Pediatr Infect Dis J 12:162, 1993.
77. Smego RA, Devoe PW, Sampson HA, et al: *Candida* meningitis in two children with severe combined immunodeficiency. J Pediatr 104:902, 1984.
78. Glocker EO, Hennigs A, Nabavi M, et al: A homozygous CARD9 mutation in a family with susceptibility to fungal infections. N Engl J Med 361:1727, 2009.
79. Kupsky RR, Kupsky WJ, Haas JE: Arteritis and fatal subarachnoid hemorrhage complicating occult *Candida* meningitis: unusual presentation in pediatric acquired immunodeficiency syndrome. Arch Pathol Lab Med 122:1030, 1998.
80. Kaji M, Shoji H, Oizumi K: Intractable meningitis and intracranial abscess following sinusitis due to *Candida* species. Kurume Med J 45:279, 1998.
81. Voice RA, Bradley SF, Sangeorzan JA, et al: Chronic candidal meningitis: an uncommon manifestation of candidiasis. Clin Infect Dis 19:60, 1994.
82. Petraitiene R, Petraitis V, Hope WW, et al: Cerebrospinal fluid and plasma $(1\rightarrow3)$-β-D-glucan as surrogate markers for detection and monitoring of therapeutic response in experimental hematogenous *Candida* meningoencephalitis. Antimicrob Agents Chemother 52:4121, 2008.
83. Verduyn Lunel FM, Voss A, Kuijper EJ, et al: Detection of the *Candida* antigen mannan in cerebrospinal fluid specimens from patients suspected of having *Candida* meningitis. J Clin Microbiol 42:867, 2004.
84. Geers TA, Gordon SM: Clinical significance of *Candida* species isolated from cerebrospinal fluid following neurosurgery. Clin Infect Dis 28:1139, 1999.
85. Antinori S, Corbellino M, Meroni L, et al: *Aspergillus* meningitis: a rare clinical manifestation of central nervous system aspergillosis. Case report and review of 92 cases. J Infect 66:218, 2013.
86. Haran RP, Chandy MJ: Intracranial aspergillus granuloma. Br J Neurosurg 7:383, 1993.
87. Breneman E, Colford Jr JM: Aspergillosis of the CNS presenting as aseptic meningitis. Clin Infect Dis 15:737, 1992.
88. Klont RR, Mennink-Kersten MA, Verweij PE: Utility of *Aspergillus* antigen detection in specimens other than serum specimens. Clin Infect Dis 39:1467, 2004.
89. McLean FM, Ginsborg LE, Stanton CA: Perineural spread of rhinocerebral mucormycosis. AJNR Am J Neuroradiol 17:114, 1996.
90. Roden MM, Zaoutis TE, Buchanan WL, et al: Epidemiology and outcome of zygomycosis: a review of 929 reported cases. Clin Infect Dis 41:634, 2005.
91. Spellberg B, Ibrahim AS, Chin-Hong PV, et al: The Deferasirox-AmBisome Therapy for Mucormycosis (DEFEAT Mucor) study: a randomized, double-blinded, placebo-controlled trial. J Antimicrob Chemother 67:715, 2012.
92. Kershaw P, Freeman R, Templeton D, et al: *Pseudallescheria boydii* infection of the central nervous system. Arch Neurol 47:468, 1990.
93. Kantarcioglu AS, Guarro J, de Hoog GS: Central nervous system infections by members of the *Pseudallescheria boydii* species complex in healthy and immunocompromised hosts: epidemiology, clinical characteristics and outcome. Mycoses 51:275, 2008.
94. Marco de Lucas E, Sadaba P, Lastra García-Barón P, et al: Cerebral scedosporiosis: an emerging fungal infection in severe neutropenic patients: CT features and CT pathologic correlation. Eur Radiol 16:496, 2006.
95. Sekhon AS, Galbraith J, Mielke BW, et al: Cerebral phaeohyphomycosis caused by *Xylohypha bantiana*, with a review of the literature. Eur J Epidemiol 8:387, 1992.
96. Tintelnot K, de Hoog GS, Thomas E, et al: Cerebral phaeohyphomycosis caused by an *Exophiala* species. Mycoses 34:239, 1991.
97. Garg N, Devi IB, Vajramani GV, et al: Central nervous system cladosporiosis: an account of ten culture-proven cases. Neurol India 55:282, 2007.
98. Al-Tawfiq JA, Boukhamseen A: Cerebral phaeohyphomycosis due to *Rhinocladiella mackenziei* (formerly *Ramichloridium mackenziei*): case presentation and literature review. J Infect Public Health 4:96, 2011.
99. Centers for Disease Control and Prevention (CDC): Exophiala infection from contaminated injectable steroids prepared by a compounding pharmacy—United States, July-November 2002. MMWR Morb Mortal Wkly Rep 51:1109, 2002.
100. Bell WR, Dalton JB, McCall CM, et al: Iatrogenic *Exserohilum* infection of the central nervous system: mycological identification and histopathological findings. Mod Pathol 26:166, 2013.
101. Smith RM, Schaefer MK, Kainer MA, et al: The Multistate Fungal Infection Outbreak Response

Team. Fungal infections associated with contaminated methylprednisolone injections—preliminary report. N Engl J Med 369:1598, 2013.
102. Kerkering TM, Grifasi ML, Baffoe-Bonnie AW, et al: Early clinical observations in prospectively followed patients with fungal meningitis related to contaminated epidural steroid injections. Ann Intern Med 158:154, 2013.
103. Kainer MA, Reagan DR, Nguyen DB, et al: Tennessee Fungal Meningitis Investigation Team. Fungal infections associated with contaminated methylprednisolone in Tennessee. N Engl J Med 23:2194, 2012.
104. Harrison DK, Moser S, Palmer CA: Central nervous system infections in transplant recipients by *Cladophialophora bantiana*. South Med J 101:292, 2008.
105. Fincher RM, Fisher JF, Lovell RD, et al: Infection due to the fungus *Acremonium* (cephalosporium). Medicine (Baltimore) 70:398, 1991.
106. Weller PF: Eosinophilic meningitis. Am J Med 95:250, 1993.
107. Ragland AS, Arusa E, Ismail Y, et al: Eosinophilic pleocytosis in coccidioidal meningitis: frequency and significance. Am J Med 195:254, 1993.
108. Graybill JR, Sobel J, Saag M, et al: Diagnosis and management of increased intracranial pressure in patients with AIDS and cryptococcal meningitis. Clin Infect Dis 30:47, 2000.
109. Cohen-Wolkowiez M, Smith PB, Mangum B, et al: Neonatal *Candida* meningitis: significance of cerebrospinal fluid parameters and blood cultures. J Perinatol 27:97, 2007.
110. Gonyea EF: Cisternal puncture and cryptococcal meningitis. Arch Neurol 28:200, 1973.
111. Tanner DC, Weinstein MP, Fedorciw B, et al: Comparison of commercial kits for detection of cryptococcal antigen. J Clin Microbiol 32:1680, 1994.
112. Powderly WG, Cloud GA, Dismukes WE, et al: Measurement of cryptococcal antigen in serum and cerebrospinal fluid: value in the management of AIDS-associated cryptococcal meningitis. Clin Infect Dis 18:789, 1994.
113. Wheat LJ, Musial CE, Jenny-Avital E: Diagnosis and management of central nervous system histoplasmosis. Clin Infect Dis 40:844, 2005.
114. Pappagianis D, Zimmer BL: Serology of coccidioidomycosis. Clin Microbiol Rev 3:247, 1990.
115. Liappis AP, Kan VL, Richman NC, et al: Mannitol and inflammatory markers in the cerebral spinal fluid of HIV-infected patients with cryptococcal meningitis. Eur J Clin Microbiol Infect Dis 27:477, 2008.
116. Body BA, Oneson RH, Herold DA: Use of cerebrospinal fluid lactic acid concentration in the diagnosis of fungal meningitis. Ann Clin Lab Sci 17:429, 1987.
117. Binnicker MJ, Popa AS, Catania J, et al: Meningeal coccidioidomycosis diagnosed by real-time polymerase chain reaction analysis of cerebrospinal fluid. Mycopathologia 171:285, 2011.
118. Karam F, Chmel H: Rhino-orbital cerebral mucormycosis. Ear Nose Throat J 69:187, 1990.
119. Perfect JR, Dismukes WE, Pappas PG, et al: Clinical practice guidelines for the management of cryptococcal disease: 2010 update by the Infectious Diseases Society of America. Clin Infect Dis 50:291, 2010.
120. Dromer F, Bernede-Bauduin C, Guillemot D, et al: Major role for amphotericin B-flucytosine combination in severe cryptococcosis. PLoS One 3:e2870, 2008.
121. Saag MS, Powderly WG, Cloud GA, et al: Comparison of amphotericin B with fluconazole in the treatment of acute AIDS-associated cryptococcal meningitis. N Engl J Med 326:83, 1992.
122. Denning DW, Tucker RM, Hanson LH, et al: Itraconazole therapy for cryptococcal meningitis and cryptococcosis. Arch Int Med 149:2301, 1989.
123. Saag MS, Graybill JR, Larsen RA, et al: Practice guidelines for the management of cryptococcal disease. Infectious Disease Society of America. Clin Infect Dis 30:710, 2000.
124. Spitzer ED, Spitzer SG, Freundlich LF, et al: Persistence of initial infection in recurrent *Cryptococcus neoformans* meningitis. Lancet 341:595, 1993.
125. Saag MS, Cloud GA, Graybill JR, et al: A comparison of itraconazole versus fluconazole as maintenance therapy for AIDS-associated cryptococcal meningitis. National Institute of Allergy and Infectious Diseases Mycoses Study Group. Clin Infect Dis 28:291, 1999.
126. Loyse A, Wilson D, Meintjes G, et al: Comparison of the early fungicidal activity of high-dose fluconazole, voriconazole, and flucytosine as second-line drugs given in combination with amphotericin B for the treatment of HIV-associated cryptococcal meningitis. Clin Infect Dis 54:121, 2012.
127. Bozzette SA, Larsen RA, Chin J: A placebo-controlled trial of maintenance therapy with fluconazole after treatment of cryptococcal meningitis in the acquired immunodeficiency syndrome. N Engl J Med 324:580, 1991.
128. Vibhagool A, Sungkanuparph S, Mootsikapun P, et al: Discontinuation of secondary prophylaxis for cryptococcal meningitis in human immunodefiiency virus-infected patients treated with highly active antiretroviral therapy: a prospective, multicenter randomized study. Clin Infect Dis 36:1329, 2003.
129. Denning DW, Armstrong RW, Lewis BH, et al: Elevated cerebrospinal fluid pressures in patients with cryptococcal meningitis and acquired immunodeficiency syndrome. Am J Med 91:267, 1991.
130. Tang LM: Ventriculoperitoneal shunt in cryptococcal meningitis with hydrocephalus. Surg Neurol 33:314, 1990.
131. Johnston SRD, Corbett EL, Foster O: Raised intracranial pressure and visual complications in acquired immunodeficiency syndrome patients with cryptococcal meningitis. J Infect 24:185, 1992.

132. Rex JH, Larsen RA, Dismukes WE, et al: Catastrophic visceral loss due to *Cryptococcus neoformans* meningitis. Medicine (Baltimore) 72:207, 1993.
133. Jarvis JN, Meintjes G, Rebe K, et al: Adjunctive interferon-γ immunotherapy for the treatment of HIV-associated cryptococcal meningitis: a randomized controlled trial. AIDS 26:1105, 2012.
134. Smego RA, Perfect JR, Durack DT: Combined therapy with amphotericin B and 5-fluorocytosine for *Candida* meningitis. Rev Infec Dis 6:791, 1984.
135. Jafari HS, Saez-Llorens X, Severein C, et al: Effects of antifungal therapy on inflammation, sterilization, and histology in experimental *Candida albicans* meningitis. Antimicrob Agents Chemother 38:83, 1994.
136. Houmeau L, Monfort-Gouraud M, Boccara JF, et al: *Candida* meningitis, in a premature infant, treated with liposomal amphotericin B and flucytosine. Arch Fr Pediatr 50:227, 1993.
137. Sanchez-Portocarrero J, Martin-Rabadan P, Saldana CJ, et al: *Candida* cerebrospinal fluid shunt infection. Report of two new cases and review of the literature. Diagn Microbiol Infect Dis 20:33, 1994.
138. Eissenberg LG, Goldman WE, Schlesinger PH: *Histoplasma capsulatum* modulates the acidification of phagolysosomes. J Exp Med 177:1605, 1993.
139. Nguyen MH, Yu VL: Meningitis caused by *Candida* species: an emerging problem in neurosurgical patients. Clin Infect Dis 21:323, 1995.
140. Lee BE, Cheung PY, Robinson JL, et al: Comparative study of mortality and morbidity in premature infants (birth weight, <1.250 g) with candidemia or candidal meningitis. Clin Infect Dis 27:559, 1998.
141. Mathisen G, Shelub A, Truong J, Wigen C: Coccidioidal meningitis: clinical presentation and management in the fluconazole era. Medicine (Baltimore) 89:251, 2010.
142. Galgiani JN, Catanzaro A, Higgs J, et al: Fluconazole therapy for coccidioidal meningitis. Ann Intern Med 119:28, 1993.
143. Kim MM, Vikram HR, Kusne S, et al: Treatment of refractory coccidioidomycosis with voriconazole or posaconazole. Clin Infect Dis 53:1060, 2011.
144. Bariola JR, Perry P, Pappas PG, et al: Blastomycosis of the central nervous system: a multicenter review of diagnosis and treatment in the modern era. Clin Infect Dis 50:797, 2010.
145. Troke P, Aguirrebengoa K, Arteaga C, et al: Global Scedosporium Study Group. Treatment of scedosporiosis with voriconazole: clinical experience with 107 patients. Antimicrob Agents Chemother 52:1743, 2008.
146. Schwartz S, Ruhnke M, Ribaud P, et al: Improved outcome in central nervous system aspergillosis, using voriconazole treatment. Blood 106:2641, 2005.
147. Li DM, de Hoog GS: Cerebral phaeohyphomycosis–a cure at what lengths? Lancet Infect Dis 9:376, 2009.

CHAPTER

47

Parasitic Infections of the Central Nervous System

EDSEL MAURICE T. SALVANA ■ ROBERT A. SALATA ■ CHARLES H. KING

Protozoans and helminths are responsible for a significant burden of human disease, disproportionately affecting resource-limited countries worldwide. These agents are collectively referred to as parasites, implying dependence on an adversely affected host, but in this context are no different from other infectious agents, such as bacteria and viruses.

Protozoan parasites are single-celled, microscopic organisms that characteristically undergo multiplication in the mammalian host. In contrast, helminthic parasites are multicellular, vary tremendously in size, and, in general, are not capable of multiplying within the mammalian or definitive host.

Protozoa and helminths have complex life cycles and have adapted to exist within the hostile environment of one and sometimes several hosts. The distribution of these infectious agents parallels the poor socioeconomic conditions in the developing world. However, with widespread travel, infections due to these agents are being seen more frequently in nonendemic settings. In addition, with the increasing number of immunosuppressed patients (infected with human immunodeficiency virus [HIV], or after transplant or chemotherapy) worldwide, disease manifestations can be more frequent, severe, and aggressive. Central to the clinician's approach to the patient with a central nervous system (CNS) infection with a protozoan or helminthic organism is a thorough travel history, and an increased index of suspicion. Once such an infection is suspected, appropriate workup can be initiated.

The following descriptions are organized to include the disease entities summarized in Table 47-1.

PROTOZOAN INFECTIONS

Cerebral Malaria

Malaria is the most important parasitic infection worldwide. Nearly 3.3 billion people were at risk of malaria in 2010, and an estimated 149 million to 274 million cases were reported. About 655,000 deaths were due to malaria, more than 85 percent of which were in children younger than 5 years of age. Despite a decrease in the prevalence by 17 percent in the last decade, much of this decline was in the European, American, and Western Pacific regions. Currently, 81 percent of cases are from Africa.[1] Prior to intensive worldwide efforts toward malaria control by the United Nations and the Global Fund

Aminoff's Neurology and General Medicine, Fifth Edition.

TABLE 47-1 ■ Parasitic Infections of the Central Nervous System

Organism	Geographic Distribution	Major CNS Syndromes	Mode of Infection	CNS Pathologic Stage
Protozoans				
Plasmodium falciparum	Africa, Haiti, South America, Southeast Asia, Oceania	Encephalopathy, coma, seizures	Mosquito	Merozoite
Toxoplasma gondii	Cosmopolitan	Congenital: retinopathy, intracranial calcification, intellectual developmental disability, seizures Immunocompromised: encephalitis, meningoencephalitis, mass lesions	Fecal-oral	Tachyzoite
Trypanosoma brucei, T. gambiense, T. rhodesiense	Northern and western sub-Saharan Africa, eastern Equatorial Africa	Personality changes, indifference, stupor, and coma in late stages	Tsetse flies	Procyclic form
Naegleria fowleri	Southern United States, Australia, Great Britain, former Czechoslovakia	Acute rapidly progressive meningoencephalitis	Fresh water	Trophozoite
Acanthamoeba species	Cosmopolitan	Subacute, chronic meningoencephalitis	Fresh water, contact lenses and solutions	Trophozoite
Entamoeba histolytica	Africa, Mexico, South America, India, Southeast Asia	Brain abscess	Fecal-oral	Trophozoite
Helminths				
Taenia solium	Cosmopolitan	Neurocysticercosis: seizures, hydrocephalus, chronic meningitis	Fecal-oral	Intermediate tissue cyst
Echinococcus granulosus	Cosmopolitan	CNS hydatidosis	Fecal-oral	Intermediate tissue cyst
Echinococcus multilocularis	Arctic	CNS hydatidosis	Fecal-oral	Intermediate tissue cyst
Spirometra species	Cosmopolitan	Sparganosis	Ingestion of uncooked meat	Intermediate tissue cyst
Strongyloides stercoralis	Tropics, subtropics	Polymicrobial meningitis, encephalitis	Autoinfection	Filariform larvae
Trichinella spiralis	Cosmopolitan	Seizures, meningoencephalitis	Uncooked meat	Cysts of immature larvae
Angiostrongylus cantonensis	Asia, Africa, Pacific, Cuba, Jamaica	Eosinophilic meningitis	Uncooked snails, crustacea	Developing adult
Gnathostoma spinigerum	Asia, India, Israel	Eosinophilic meningitis	Uncooked fish, frog, bird, snake	Developing adult
Toxocara species	Cosmopolitan	Seizures, palsies, retinal mass	Fecal-oral	Developing adult
Onchocerca volvulus	Africa, South America, Central America, Yemen	Retinopathy, keratitis	Black fly	Microfilariae
Loa loa	Africa	Encephalopathy	Deerfly	Microfilariae
Schistosoma species	Africa, Asia, Brazil	Seizures, cerebritis, tumor, spinal cord compression	Exposure to infected fresh water	Eggs
Paragonimus species	Asia, Central and South America	Meningitis, mass lesion, infarction	Uncooked crustacea	Maturing adult

CNS, central nervous system.

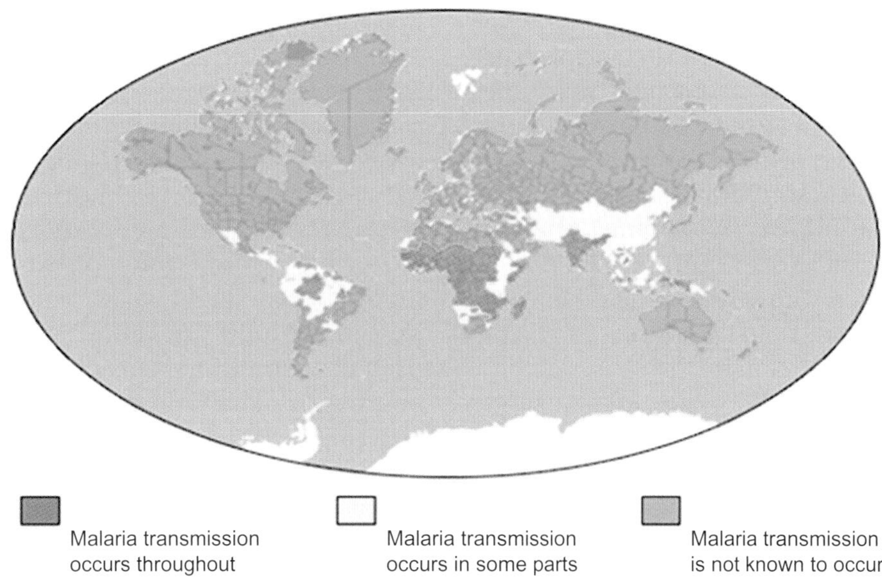

FIGURE 47-1 ■ Global map of malaria transmission. (From the US Centers for Disease Control and Prevention.)

to Fight AIDS, Tuberculosis, and Malaria, malaria was estimated to cost Africa about 12 billion dollars annually.[2]

Malaria infection is widely distributed (Fig. 47-1), with *Plasmodium falciparum* predominating in sub-Saharan Africa, Haiti, New Guinea, Southeast Asia, South America, and Oceania. The majority of cases of malaria in the United States are imported by travelers to and immigrants from malarial areas, with more than 8,000 cases reported from 1999 through 2008.[3]

Five species of malaria infect humans: *P. falciparum*, *Plasmodium vivax*, *Plasmodium ovale*, *Plasmodium malariae*, and *Plasmodium knowlesi*.[2,4] The life cycle of *Plasmodium* is similar across species. The infective sporozoites are injected by female *Anopheles* mosquitoes into subcutaneous tissue or directly into the blood stream, and thereafter circulate to the liver to invade hepatocytes. Parasites multiply, and after 1 to 2 weeks, schizonts rupture and release thousands of merozoites, which then enter the bloodstream to infect erythrocytes. All exoerythrocytic forms of *P. falciparum* rupture at about the same time, and none persists chronically in the liver.

Invasion of erythrocytes by merozoites requires specific surface receptors on the parasite and erythrocyte. In contrast with other *Plasmodium* species, *P. falciparum* uses multiple redundant pathways to invade, including sialic acid–dependent glycophorin pathways, and non-sialic acid–dependent ones. In addition, *P. falciparum* can invade erythrocytes of all ages, and parasitemia can reach high levels. The magnitude of parasitemia was previously thought to relate to the degree of morbidity and mortality, but other factors such as the degree of metabolic stress in nutritionally deficient children, presence of parasitic coinfections, and other less-understood mechanisms may play significant roles in adverse outcomes.[5]

Within the erythrocyte, merozoites eventually develop into schizonts, which rupture to release merozoites capable of infecting new erythrocytes. Only the asexual erythrocytic stages are directly deleterious to the host, and the mechanisms involved in the development of clinical manifestations are related to fever, anemia, and tissue hypoxia, as well as host factors including immunopathologic events.[5,6]

P. falciparum causes the most significant morbidity and mortality. A number of serious complications can occur in *P. falciparum* malaria, including acute renal failure, pulmonary edema, acidosis, hypoglycemia, and cerebral malaria.[2,5]

Cerebral malaria occurs in 0.5 to 1 percent of *P. falciparum* cases, and is associated with a 15 to 20 percent mortality.[7,8] Significant neurologic sequelae develop in 11 percent of cases.[8] Sequestration of parasitized erythrocytes within the capillaries of the cerebral cortex is typically observed, but is likely not the only pathogenic mechanism. While the pathogenesis of cerebral malaria is incompletely understood and remains highly speculative, it is postulated that parasitized red blood cells express parasite-derived variant surface antigens, causing the erythrocytes to adhere to endothelial cells of venules, resulting in microvascular obstruction.[9] Cerebral malaria is associated with specific *var* genes, the gene family that encodes the malarial cytoadherence protein *Plasmodium falciparum* erythrocyte membrane protein 1 (PfEMP1).[10] Specifically, a subset of group A *var* genes containing domain cassettes 8 and 13 of the PfEMP1 were shown to be associated with severe cerebral malaria in children, and encoded the ligand that mediated adhesion to brain endothelium.[11–13]

Endothelial cells are a major site of pathology, particularly in cerebral malaria, as these show signs of activation, including characteristic morphologic changes, upregulation of surface adhesion molecules and antigens, and production of numerous cytokines and other mediators. Proinflammatory cytokines such as tumor necrosis factor α (TNF-α), lymphotoxin, interferon-γ (IFN-γ), and interleukin-1β (IL-1β) may play a role in pathogenesis, as these are increased in cerebral malaria.[9] Nitrous oxide was initially thought to contribute to the development of cerebral malaria, but recent studies have suggested that it plays a critical role in improving survival by modulating the immune response. Two randomized control trials are under way using inhaled nitrous oxide as adjuvant therapy in children with severe malaria to test this hypothesis.[6] Increased intracranial pressure does contribute to morbidity and mortality, and is a marker for poor outcomes. However, opening pressures have not correlated with mortality, and are probably not a critical factor in determining survival.[6,8]

High fever and rigors are the hallmarks of acute malaria. A prodrome may occur with malaise, headache, myalgias, and fatigue that can mimic viral illness. Other manifestations include backache, arthralgias, abdominal pain, nausea, vomiting, cough, tachypnea, lethargy, and delirium. Fever commonly rises to 105°F and may remain elevated between paroxysms of *P. falciparum* infection. On examination, patients frequently have splenomegaly and tender hepatomegaly. Lymphadenopathy is not a feature, and its presence should prompt investigation of an alternative etiology.[14]

The World Health Organization (WHO) defines cerebral malaria as unarousable coma in a person with *P. falciparum* asexual parasitemia, in whom other causes of encephalopathy have been excluded. While this definition is very specific, patients typically manifest a spectrum of disease, and many will need to be treated as cerebral malaria. Presenting features may include seizures (15 to 20% in adults, 80% in children), disturbances of consciousness, acute delirium, meningismus, and, infrequently, focal neurologic abnormalities, including pyramidal signs, cranial nerve abnormalities, or movement disorders.[7] Decorticate posturing or decerebrate posturing is more common in children and may indicate hypoglycemia or increased intracranial pressure. Adults are more likely than children to present with diffuse encephalopathy and no focal neurologic signs. Other causes of CNS infection and encephalopathy must be excluded, and biochemical screening of blood and examination of cerebrospinal fluid (CSF) are mandatory.[15] Hypoglycemia may occur as a complication of severe *P. falciparum* malaria or its treatment, especially in pregnant patients or in association with severe disease, and may be responsible for deteriorating neurologic status.[14]

Cerebral malaria should be suspected in any person with impaired consciousness, fever, and recent travel to or residence in a *P. falciparum*–endemic country.[15] Demonstration of malaria parasites (specifically *P. falciparum*) in thick and thin blood smears establishes the diagnosis. However, sensitivity and specificity of microscopy are operator dependent, and can be problematic in nonendemic countries, where laboratory technicians are not experienced in microscopic evaluation, or in resource-limited settings where diagnostic equipment is substandard or unavailable.[2,15] Methods with similar or greater sensitivity than blood smears are available. These techniques include an enzyme-linked immunosorbent assay (ELISA) for a histidine-rich *P. falciparum* antigen, an immunoassay for species-specific parasite lactate dehydrogenase isoenzymes, and DNA hybridization and amplification of parasite DNA or mRNA using polymerase chain reaction (PCR).[14]

Several point-of-care diagnostics based on these immunoassays have been developed and field-tested. However, these tests are considered complementary to microscopy since thick smears remain more sensitive in expert hands, speciation with antigen tests only distinguishes between falciparum and non-falciparum species, and the test can be persistently positive for a time after clearance of parasitemia. Moreover, point-of-care assay results are qualitative and cannot be used to measure parasite burden.[7,15,16]

A variety of abnormalities in laboratory tests may be observed in cases of falciparum malaria, including a normocytic, normochromic hemolytic anemia, leukopenia, monocytosis, thrombocytopenia, proteinuria, azotemia, elevated liver enzymes, and disseminated intravascular coagulation. With severe *P. falciparum* malaria, lactic acidosis, elevated blood creatinine, and hypoglycemia may be observed.[14]

When cerebral malaria is a consideration, lumbar puncture should be performed to exclude other causes of encephalopathy. In cerebral malaria, CSF examination occasionally reveals elevated protein concentration or mild pleocytosis, especially if seizures have occurred.[7] Hypoglycorrhachia is not a feature and would indicate other causes. Imaging with computed tomography (CT) may show some brain edema in advanced stages. Magnetic resonance imaging (MRI) often shows brain enlargement without edema.[15] Funduscopy should be performed since the presence of malaria retinopathy is the only reliable clinical feature that distinguishes cerebral malaria from other CNS pathologies.[7]

Delay in the diagnosis of *P. falciparum* infection can prove to be fatal because patients, especially children, who appear clinically stable may deteriorate rapidly if not treated. If *P. falciparum* infection is suspected, patients should be hospitalized.[3] Travel history to *P. falciparum*–endemic areas should be elicited, and it should be determined whether the patient took adequate antimalarial prophylaxis. Adults with uncomplicated *P. falciparum* malaria suspected to be chloroquine-resistant, and who are not desperately ill and are capable of taking oral medication, can be treated with oral atovaquone plus proguanil (four 250 mg/100 mg tablets daily for 3 days), with artemether-lumefantrine (four tablets twice a day for 3 days), or with oral quinine (650 mg salt three times daily) plus doxycycline (100 mg twice daily) or clindamycin (20 mg/kg daily in three divided doses) for 7 days. Alternative agents for oral treatment include mefloquine (unless there is concern for resistance if acquired in the regions of Southeast Asia), chloroquine, and hydrochloroquine (if acquired in chloroquine-sensitive areas).[17] Oral quinine may cause cinchonism, characterized by tinnitus, headache, nausea, and visual disturbances.[7]

Severe malaria, including cerebral malaria, should be treated parenterally. Quinidine gluconate is given by continuous intravenous infusion (10 mg/kg loading dose, then 0.02 mg/kg per minute). This is usually continued for 72 hours and stopped sooner if parasitemia decreases to 1 percent or less. Quinidine can be cardiotoxic, and appropriate monitoring must be performed. Once the patient improves and can take oral medication, quinidine can be discontinued and a 7-day course of treatment can be completed with a combination of oral quinine and tetracycline. Intravenous artesunate is available as an investigational new drug from the Centers for Disease Control, and should be administered with either atovaquone–proguanil, doxycycline, clindamycin (in pregnant women), or mefloquine.[17]

After initiation of antimalarial therapy, patients with *P. falciparum* infection must be closely monitored for complications and response to treatment. Seizures should be treated with anticonvulsants, and frequent glucose monitoring is essential to manage hypoglycemia, especially in those treated with quinidine or quinine. Maintaining adequate fluid balance is critical in preventing further morbidity, especially in those with renal failure or pulmonary edema. Blood transfusions can be used to correct anemia, but can lead to significant fluid overload.[7] Despite a lack of clear evidence, the CDC strongly recommends exchange transfusions for severe malaria, including those patients with cerebral malaria, acute respiratory distress syndrome, renal failure, or parasitemia exceeding 10 percent.[18]

Hyperosmolar agents such as mannitol are helpful in patients with increased intracranial pressure. Other adjunctive therapies such as corticosteroids and chelating agents provide little benefit and should be avoided because of deleterious effects.[15] Trials looking at the effect of inhaled nitrous oxide or erythropoetin on cerebral malaria are under way.[6,7]

Cerebral Toxoplasmosis

Toxoplasma gondii is an apicomplexan protozoan that causes a zoonosis which manifests as an encephalitis or a chorioretinitis in humans. Infection may be acute or chronic, symptomatic or asymptomatic, and may affect both normal and immunocompromised hosts.[19,20] The prevalence of *Toxoplasma* infection worldwide is 25 to 30 percent, but varies greatly between 10 and 80 percent depending on location.[19] Infection is typically acquired when oocysts (containing sporozoites) or cysts (containing bradyzoites) are ingested from contaminated soil, water, fruits, vegetables, animal litter, or undercooked meat.[19,21] Other known routes of transmission include congenital infection, accidental inoculation of organisms in laboratory workers, and organ transplantation.[19]

Cats are the definitive hosts of *Toxoplasma*, and are a major zoonotic reservoir. Oocysts or cysts can infect virtually any mammalian host. After these are ingested by cats, *T. gondii* invades the intestinal epithelial cells and begins the definitive life cycle, eventually producing millions of oocysts.[22]

Upon entry into humans, the sporozoite or bradyzoite, depending on the infective stage ingested, transforms into a tachyzoite that disrupts host cells and disseminates via the lymph and blood. The tachyzoite invades host cells and forms a protective parasitophorous vacuole within the cytoplasm. Interestingly, the parasite is able to modify the host cell behavior by commandeering the cell's signaling cascades and other metabolic processes.[20] *T. gondii* enters protected sites such as the brain and cornea, presumably through infected leukocytes, which exhibit increased migration and adhesion.[23,24] Tachyzoite invasion is associated with a robust Th-1 response mediated by IL-12 and IFN-γ secretion by macrophages, neutrophils and dendritic cells, causing the proliferation of $CD4^+$ and $CD8^+$ T-cells.[23] *T. gondii* modulates the host immune response as it shifts from active to latent infection by tightly regulating IL-12 production in order to prevent host death. This ensures that the parasite is able to infect the host chronically and increases the chances of replication and transmission.[20] The tachyzoites eventually transform into bradyzoites, forming cysts that are established in numerous tissues and organs. These elicit little or no inflammatory response but persist as reservoirs for reactivation or transmission (Fig. 47-2).[24]

Approximately 80 percent of primary toxoplasmosis infection is asymptomatic in immunocompetent adults. Nontender cervical adenopathy is most frequently seen among symptomatic individuals, but generalized adenopathy may be present. In some cases, adenopathy is accompanied by fever, night sweats, malaise, sore throat, rash, hepatosplenomegaly, and atypical lymphocytosis. The course of toxoplasmosis is usually benign and self-limited. A minority of patients can develop persistent lymphadenopathy. Rarely, immmunocompetent individuals have progressive disseminated disease with CNS infection.[19]

Chorioretinitis from *T. gondii* occurs mostly in congenital infection, but may occasionally present in acute or reactivation disease.[21] The lesion is a focal, necrotizing retinitis with intense vitreal inflammation, showing a characteristic "headlight in fog" appearance. Relapses of chorioretinitis are frequent, and are evident in the areas around the chorioretinal scars (Fig. 47-3).[22]

Congenital infection is a result of primary infection of the mother during gestation. Chronic infection in

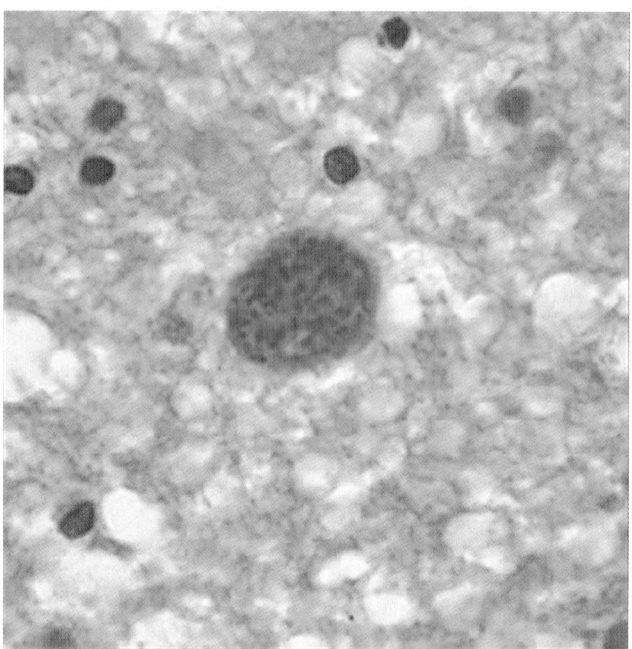

FIGURE 47-2 ■ *Toxoplasma gondii* cyst in brain tissue stained with hematoxylin and eosin. (From the US Centers for Disease Control and Prevention.)

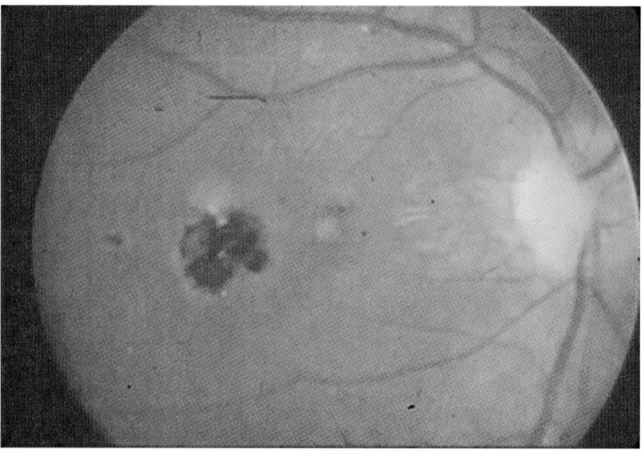

FIGURE 47-3 ■ *Toxoplasma* chorioretinitis: a pale, atrophied lesion containing black pigment. (From the US Centers for Disease Control and Prevention.)

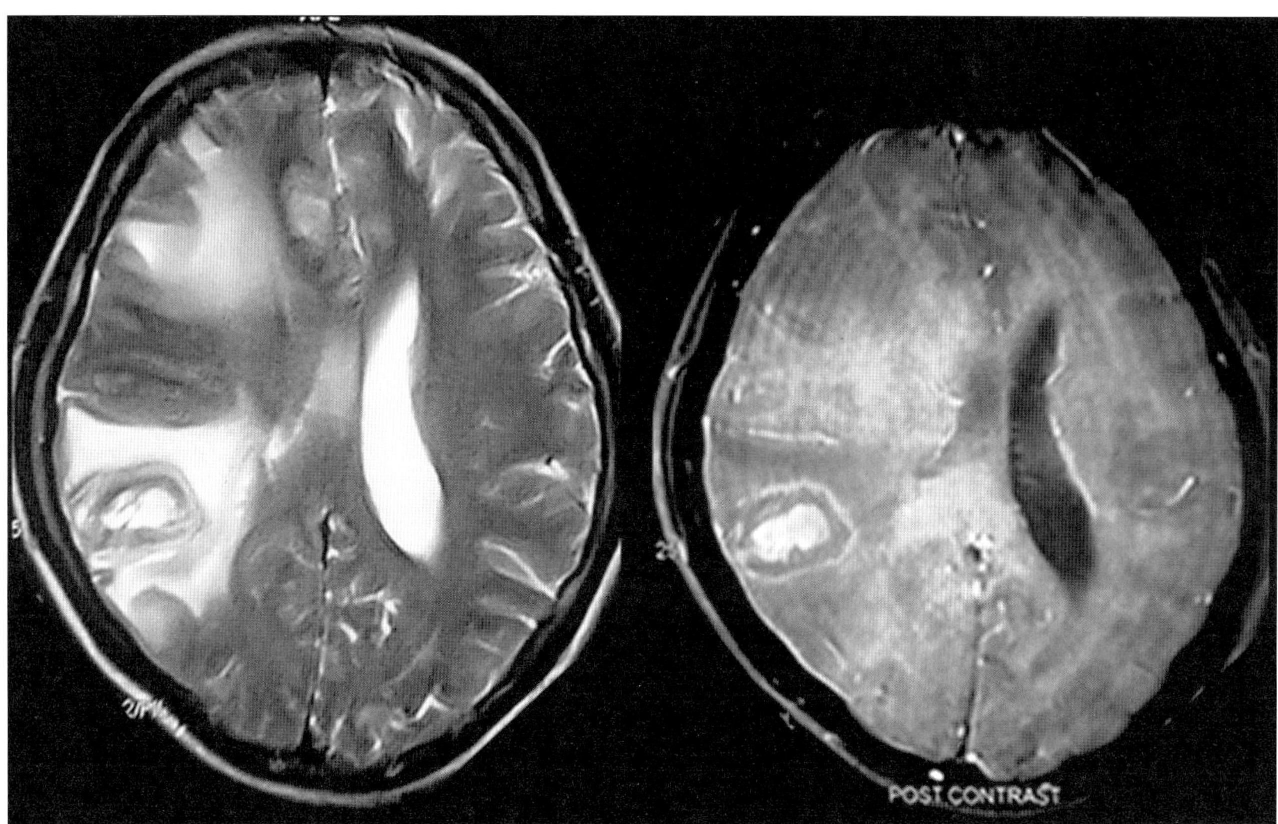

FIGURE 47-4 ■ Magnetic resonance imaging (MRI) with toxoplasmosis in a patient with AIDS. Left image is a T2-weighted MRI showing the lesion with extensive perilesional edema; right image shows T1 contrast-enhancement of toxoplasmosis lesion. (Courtesy of Dr. Nicolette Mariano.)

the immunocompetent mother prior to conception is not transmitted to the fetus, but transmission has been documented with reactivation disease in HIV-infected pregnant women.[21,25] Infection acquired in the first trimester is severe and can be associated with spontaneous abortion. Infection later in pregnancy can be symptomatic and be of variable severity depending on individual factors. In the newborn, the presence of hydrocephalus, retinochoroiditis, or intracranial calcifications is suggestive of congenital toxoplasmosis and should be evaluated accordingly. Most infants are asymptomatic at birth, but may present with overt symptoms, including severe developmental delay later in life.[21]

Severe and often fatal toxoplasmosis has occurred in patients immunocompromised by treatment with corticosteroids or cytotoxic agents, and in those with lymphoreticular malignancies, organ transplantation, or acquired immunodeficiency syndrome (AIDS). In HIV infection, the rate of reactivation toxoplasmosis is highest in those with full-blown AIDS. While most disease in these patients is from reactivation, primary infection may occur. Immunodeficient individuals with toxoplasmosis usually manifest with encephalitis, meningoencephalitis, or mass lesions (Fig. 47-4). Pneumonitis or myocarditis may also develop.[22]

Early in the HIV epidemic, one-third or more of AIDS patients with antibodies to *T. gondii* developed reactivation CNS disease. However, the widespread use of antimicrobial drugs to prevent *Pneumocystis jiroveci* and the advent of potent combination antiretroviral therapy has resulted in decreased toxoplasmosis-associated deaths.[19,26] In HIV-infected persons, *Toxoplasma* encephalitis usually develops when the CD4 count falls below 100/mm^3. These patients most frequently have multifocal abscesses scattered throughout the cerebral hemispheres and present subacutely with focal neurologic deficits. The occurrence of fever, headache, seizures, and alterations in mental state is variable.[14]

The diagnosis of primary toxoplasmosis in immunocompetent hosts, transplant patients, and pregnant women is typically established through serology: with a positive IgM, IgG seroconversion in paired sera, or a twofold increase in IgG titers. Prenatal diagnosis can be confirmed by PCR or mouse assays of amniotic fluid or serology from newborn serum or cord blood. Most disease in immunocompromised hosts is reactivation disease, and so the presence of IgG antibodies is suggestive of the diagnosis. Histology of brain biopsy specimens confirms the diagnosis, but is impractical in most cases. PCR of serum, CSF, and biopsy tissue has been done with varying degrees of success. CSF PCR is very specific, but sensitivity is low (50%) and it may become negative after treatment is started. Mouse assays of these specimens are usually performed only in reference laboratories. For retinochoroiditis, serology of aqueous humor in parallel with serum can help establish the diagnosis, and PCR of these samples can detect the parasite as well.[19,25]

Cranial imaging should be performed in patients with suspected CNS toxoplasmosis. MRI usually reveals multiple ring-enhancing or solid lesions typically located in the basal ganglia (Fig. 47-4). In severe immunosuppression, atypical presentations with either a solitary lesion or lack of enhancement may occur.[22,27] In infants, CT is the method of choice, although ultrasound can be used.[21] Mononuclear pleocytosis, elevated protein, and normal glucose are often reported in the CSF; these are nonspecific, and lumbar puncture may be hazardous in those with large mass lesions.[14]

Definitive diagnosis of toxoplasmosis is made in the presence of a compatible clinical syndrome, consistent findings on MRI, CT, or other imaging modalities, and detection of the protozoan in a clinical sample. Patients with suspected *Toxoplasma* encephalitis, in the context of a positive IgG antibody, are typically started on empiric therapy and monitored for clinical and imaging response for about 3 weeks. Biopsy is reserved for refractory cases, or when alternative diagnoses such as CNS lymphoma cannot be excluded.[22,25]

Immunocompetent patients with lymphadenopathy are usually not treated unless they have severe or persistent disease. Individuals exposed through laboratory accidents or via transfusions can develop severe disease and should receive treatment. These patients should be treated for 2 to 4 weeks with a combination of pyrimethamine, sulfadiazine, and folinic acid and then reassessed.[22]

Suspected cases of ocular toxoplasmosis with documented inflammatory changes on fundoscopy should be started on treatment to prevent progression to blindness. Pyrimethamine, sulfadiazine, and leucovorin are used as therapy, using weight-based dosing for neonates and infants. Clindamycin can be substituted for sulfadiazine in cases of sulfonamide hypersensitivity. Corticosteroids are used adjunctively to decrease inflammation and the risk of complications especially if cerebral edema is present on neuroimaging.[21,22]

Management of infected pregnant women varies between countries and within countries. Confirming a diagnosis of acute infection is essential due to the potential toxicity of the drugs used for treatment and in guiding any decision to terminate the pregnancy. Specific treatment indications and regimens for pregnant women have been reviewed elsewhere.[22]

Acute disseminated infection in immunocompromised patients should always be treated. Treatment is continued for 4 to 6 weeks beyond the resolution of all signs and symptoms. Acute toxoplasmosis is most likely to occur in seronegative transplant patients receiving organs from seropositive donors. Secondary prophylaxis to prevent recurrences is of benefit, and should be continued for life unless the original immunocompromising condition has significantly improved or resolved.[22]

AIDS patients with CD4 counts less than 100 cells/mm^3 are already on primary toxoplasmosis prophylaxis if they are on trimethoprim-sulfamethoxazole for *Pneumocystis* pneumonia (PCP). Patients who usually develop reactivation toxoplasmosis encephalitis are those with a late HIV diagnosis, or who are on alternative PCP prophylaxis without anti-*Toxoplasma* activity. The treatment of *Toxoplasma* encephalitis in HIV patients should always utilize at least two agents. There is evidence that trimethoprim-sulfamethoxazole (15 to 20 mg/kg daily of the trimethoprim component in three divided doses) is better tolerated and may be as effective as the standard pyrimethamine-sulfadiazine combination. This regimen can be utilized as intravenous therapy for severely ill patients. Induction treatment should be continued for at least 6 weeks, followed by maintenance therapy until CD4 counts are above 200 cells/mm^3 for at least 3 months.[22,25]

First-line treatment for toxoplasmosis is usually a combination of pyrimethamine and a sulfonamide. These antifolates are active against tachyzoites and are synergistic in combination. Pyrimethamine is lipid-soluble and readily penetrates the brain parenchyma even in the absence of inflammation.[25] In severe infection in adults, a loading dose of 200 mg is given orally followed by 50 to 75 mg daily for 3 to 6 weeks. Folinic acid (10 to 25 mg/day), during and for 1 week after pyrimethamine treatment has ceased, is added to decrease bone marrow suppression. For adults, sulfadiazine is also given at a dose to 1 to 1.5 g orally every 6 hours. Clindamycin 600 mg orally or intravenously every 6 hours can be substituted for sulfa drugs in case of hypersensitivity. Other agents that have been used include trimethoprim-sulfamethoxazole (see earlier), dapsone, clarithromycin, azithromycin, and atovaquone.[22,25] There are different dosing regimens for children.

African Trypanosomiasis

Human African trypanosomiasis, more commonly known as sleeping sickness, affects 300,000 people in sub-Saharan Africa, with 32,000 new cases occurring every year. Approximately 60 million people living in endemic areas are at risk.[28] The vector, *Glossina*, is also known as the tsetse fly. Two distinct forms exist: western (chronic) sleeping sickness, due to infection by *Trypanosoma brucei gambiense*, and eastern and southern (acute) sleeping sickness, caused by *Trypanosoma brucei rhodesiense*.[29,30]

Trypanosoma brucei gambiense occurs mainly in the northern and western areas of sub-Saharan Africa, and is responsible for the majority of cases. The disorder has a subacute course and is perpetuated mainly through local reservoirs of chronically infected humans. East African trypanosomiasis occurs in the eastern and southern parts of equatorial Africa and is typically acquired from zoonotic sources. It has a more fulminant course, with death occurring within a few weeks after infection, thereby decreasing the possibility of human reservoirs for infection. Most cases in travelers have been due to *T. b. rhodesiense*.[30]

Trypanosoma brucei undergoes several developmental stages in the tsetse fly over a life cycle of about 3 weeks. Upon ingestion with a blood meal, bloodstream trypomastigotes become procyclic trypomastigotes in the insect midgut and divide rapidly. These then leave the midgut and transform into epimastigotes, eventually making their way into the fly's salivary glands. They change into metacyclic trypomastigotes, which are injected into the human or mammalian host with the blood meal. The metacyclic trypanosomes transform into the bloodstream form and invade extracellular spaces, including the blood, lymphatics, tissue fluids, and, eventually, the CNS via the CSF (Fig. 47-5).[14]

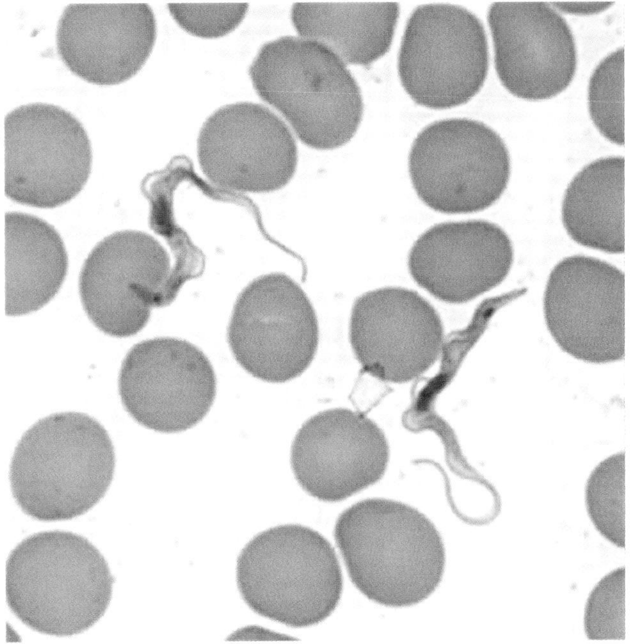

FIGURE 47-5 ▪ African trypanosomes in thin blood smear. (From the US Centers for Disease Control and Prevention.)

Bloodstream trypomastigotes evade the immune system by antigenic variation of their variant surface glycoproteins (VSGs), and through acquisition of resistance to serum lipoprotein-associated trypanolytic factors, a phenomenon specifically observed in pathogenic *T. b. gambiense* and *T. b. rhodesiense* infections of humans. Specific mutations in the apoprotein L-I (*Apo-LI*) gene, which encodes a major trypanolytic factor known as serum resistance-associated (SRA) protein, can overcome the parasite's resistance to this protein, but these protective *Apo-LI* mutations are also strongly associated with risk of adult-onset nephropathy and renal failure, as demonstrated in African American patients.[31,32] In a rare instance, *Apo-LI* mutation has enabled a trypanosome parasite of livestock, *T. evansi*, to infect a human patient.[33,34]

The earliest clinical manifestation in both types of infection is a local, hard, painful lesion (trypanosomal chancre) at the site of the insect bite; this is more common in *T. b. rhodesiense* infection and rare with *T. b. gambiense*. Histologic examination of the chancre shows a lymphocytic infiltrate with dividing trypanosomes. Shortly afterward, widespread dissemination of the organism occurs via the bloodstream and lymphatics. Lymphadenopathy of the subclavicular and cervical regions (Winterbottom sign) is typical, especially in *T. b. gambiense* infection. Signs and symptoms of dissemination include headache, dizziness, fever, tachycardia, and prostration.[29] The systemic phase occurs in recurrent fashion, with each episode lasting 1 to 6 days followed by an asymptomatic period of up to several weeks. These usually represent the emergence of new antigenic variants. With progression of the disease, the systemic episodes decline in severity. As trypanosomes invade the CNS, symptoms consistent with a meningoencephalitis occur, with increasingly severe neurologic manifestations leading to coma and death.[30]

The early systemic stage of Gambian trypanosomiasis lasts from 6 months to 1 year. Neurologic changes are often subtle and include indifference, aimless gazing, inversion of the sleep cycle, tremor, and hyperesthesia. In the late stages there is progressive CNS involvement, with somnolence alternating with insomnia, alterations in thermoregulation, incoordination, hypertonia, abnormal movements and gait, tremor, and hyperreflexia leading to coma and death.[29,30]

With trypanosomiasis due to *T. b. rhodesiense*, signs and symptoms occur within a few days after the tsetse bite. Among travelers, the disease often manifests on the return journey or shortly thereafter. The clinical features are similar to those seen in West African disease, except that they are briefer but more acute. Lymphadenopathy is rare. CNS invasion occurs early, and there is rapid neurologic deterioration, with death occurring in a matter of weeks to months after the onset of symptoms.[29,30]

Blood, CSF, and aspirates of lymph nodes should be examined for trypanosomes in suspected cases. Fresh thick blood smears in the early stages may show motile forms. Microscopic examination of buffy-coat smears of blood stained with Giemsa is highly sensitive. Concentration techniques can increase yield. The card agglutination trypanosomiasis test (CATT) is of value for screening of patients, but usually requires parasitologic confirmation in areas of low prevalence. PCR has been successfully used in veterinary applications, but has not been extensively validated for human infection.[29,35] Loop-mediated DNA amplification assays (LAMP assays) provide low-technology PCR-like amplification of parasite DNA, and may prove useful for early diagnosis in more remote, resource-limited locations.[36]

The CSF examination shows an increased protein concentration, pleocytosis (with morular cells: large, mulberry-like cells), increased IgM, and occasional trypanosomes. Nonspecific laboratory abnormalities may include anemia, monocytosis, and increased serum IgM. CSF markers of brain damage such as IL-10 (or panels of proinflammatory markers) may help make the diagnosis of second-stage disease but their diagnostic performance is still being validated.[30]

Drug treatment is dependent on the stage of illness and the type of trypanosomiasis. For early-stage disease, both forms respond to suramin and pentamidine. Both drugs can have severe side effects, and should be used only with caution in a hospital setting. Suramin in adults is given intravenously initially as a test dose of 100 to 200 mg then increased, as tolerated, to 20 mg/kg (1 g maximum) on days 1, 3, 7, 14, and 21. Transient albuminuria is often observed; heavy proteinuria, shock, febrile reactions, and desquamative rash are less common side effects. Pentamidine is given intramuscularly at 4 mg/kg per day for 10 total doses daily or on alternate days. Hypotension, fever, rash, azotemia, liver enzyme abnormalities, and hypoglycemia may occur.[37]

For advanced stages with CNS involvement, melarsoprol is used for both forms, while elflornithine is most useful against Gambian disease. For Gambian disease, melarsoprol is given as 2.2 mg/kg per day intravenously for 10 days. For Rhodesian infection, melarsoprol is used most widely as a series of three to four daily injections, with a total daily dose of 3.6 mg/kg daily at a maximum of 200 to 500 mg per injection. For patients with severe CNS involvement (higher CSF protein levels and pleocytosis), up to four 3-day courses of arsenical therapy, spaced 7 days apart, may be necessary. Toxic effects of the arsenicals include optic nerve atrophy, rash, and acute encephalopathy. Prednisone, which reduces the risk of encephalopathy by two-thirds and the risk of death by 50 percent, should be used in all melarsoprol-treated patients.[14]

Eflornithine (100 mg/kg every 6 hours IV for 14 days) is a less toxic compound for Gambian disease. Due to treatment failures and high cost, shorter combination treatment regimens using nifurtimox plus eflornithine have been developed which decrease toxicity and cost and improve effectiveness of treatment for second-stage Gambian trypanosomiasis. The schedule is eflornithine 200 mg/kg intravenously twice daily for 7 days, plus nifurtimox 5 mg/kg orally three times daily for 10 days. Further drug combination protocols aimed at decreasing costs with fewer side effects are in development.[37,38]

Primary Amebic Meningoencephalitis and Granulomatous Amebic Encephalitis

Primary amebic meningoencephalitis is an acute, rapidly progressive, necrotizing meningoencephalitis caused by the free-living ameba-flagellate *Naegleria fowleri.* The disease occurs sporadically, and is associated with exposure to fresh water, particularly hot springs, and lake water contaminated with warm effluent from industrial sources.[39]

Infection is acquired when water containing the ameba is accidentally inhaled, usually during swimming or diving. The *Naegleria* trophozoite rapidly invades the olfactory neuroepithelium, gaining access to the brain through sustentacular cells which phagocytose the amebae and transport them through the cribriform plate.[40,41] *Naegleria* infection initially involves the superficial gray matter with eventual extension to the deep matter and cerebellum. Prominent involvement of the frontotemporal areas, olfactory bulbs, and subarachnoid space has been observed. Neutrophil invasion, extensive necrosis, and vascular invasion are typical. The pathogenesis of infection likely involves multiple mechanisms, including secretion of lytic enzymes, elucidation of apoptotic factors, production of membrane pore-forming proteins, and direct feeding by the amoeba, resulting in a marked cytopathic effect.[40]

Patients present acutely within 1 to 7 days from exposure. Common but nonspecific symptoms include severe headache, fever, lethargy, nausea, and vomiting. Olfactory involvement, manifesting as nasal stuffiness or changes in smell, may be a clue to the etiology. Seizures, nuchal rigidity, and confusion, followed by coma, usually develop within days. Focal neurologic signs occur early. The patient then rapidly deteriorates and death occurs within a week. Pulmonary edema and heart failure may complicate the course. Brainstem herniation due to inflammation and increased intracranial pressure is the usual cause of death.[40,41]

Examination of the CSF commonly shows neutrophilic pleocytosis, very low glucose and high protein levels, and red blood cells. Opening pressure is elevated. Motile *Naegleria* trophozoites on wet mount may be identified on phase-contrast microscopy. Giemsa or Wright stain can help differentiate the trophozoite from host cells (Fig. 47-6).[40]

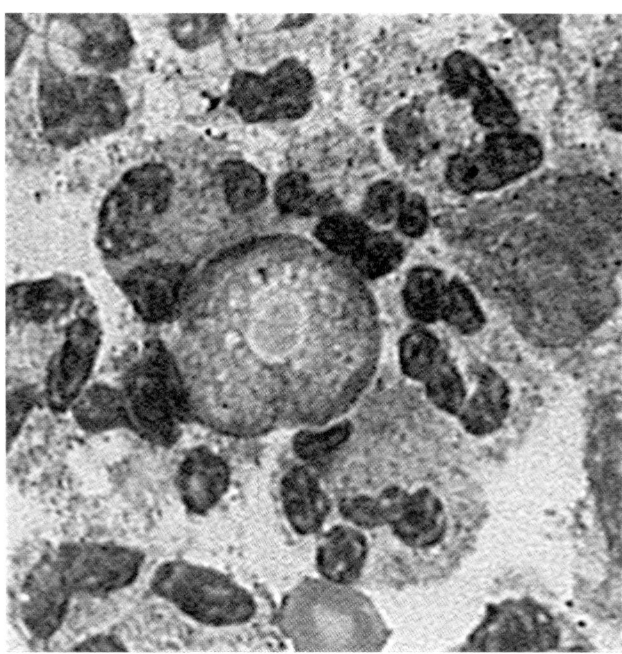

FIGURE 47-6 ■ Primary amebic meningoencephalitis: *Naegleria* trophozoite in CSF. (From the US Centers for Disease Control and Prevention.)

Only a few survivors of primary amebic meningoencephalitis have been reported, likely because of delays in diagnosis and the rapid progression of symptomatic disease. *Naegleria* is highly susceptible to amphotericin B administered both systemically and intrathecally (both initially at 1.5 mg/kg daily). Combination therapy using amphotericin with other agents such as miconazole (350 mg intravenously daily and 10 mg/m^2 body surface area intrathecally) plus rifampin (10 mg/kg) has been successful in one case.[41]

Granulomatous amebic encephalitis is a subacute, indolent, usually fatal meningoencephalitis caused by either of two species of free-living ameba, *Acanthamoeba* spp. or *Balamuthia mandrillaris.* Due to the rarity of the latter, only the *Acanthamoeba* form will be discussed in this chapter.

Acanthamoeba causes two characteristic disease entities in humans: acanthamoebal keratitis and granulomatous amebic encephalitis. *Acanthamoeba* keratitis occurs in immunocompromised and immunocompetent hosts, and is usually associated with contaminated or improperly disinfected contact lenses. It will cause blindness if not diagnosed and treated early in its course. Granulomatous amebic encephalitis typically occurs in immunocompromised hosts, particularly in AIDS patients.[42] It usually starts as a result of either direct olfactory bulb invasion or hematogenous seeding of *Acanthamoeba* from an initial focus in the lungs or skin.[40,43]

Acanthamoeba is a free-living organism that is commonly found in the environment. Unlike *Naegleria*, invasive *Acanthamoeba* disease is most frequently an opportunistic infection and is quite rare, despite the ameba's widespread distribution.[41]

Granulomatous amebic encephalitis has an insidious onset of symptoms, with nonspecific complaints such as headache, nausea, vomiting, nuchal rigidity, fever, seizures, and behavioral changes. Focal neurologic signs eventually emerge, including aphasia, ataxia, and cranial nerve palsies. As the disease progresses, increased intracranial pressure eventually causes lethargy and coma, with death occurring due to brain herniation.[41]

Multiple ring-enhancing lesions are seen on neuroimaging, representing multiple brain abscesses, with a propensity for the temporal and parietal lobes.[40,43] Histopathologic examination shows granuloma formation with white blood cell infiltration, giant cells, vasculitis, mycotic aneurysms, and few neutrophils. Cysts and trophozoites may be seen around and within granulomas, with a characteristic round nucleus and eosinophilic nucleolus. Expression of a mannose-binding protein allows the ameba to adhere to epithelial cell surfaces. It then secretes a metalloproteinase and several serine proteinases that are cytotoxic, degrading the basement membrane and stroma.[42]

CSF typically shows a lymphocytic pleocytosis, increased protein concentration, and slightly low or normal glucose level; amebae are usually not present. Serologic tests are of uncertain value as antibodies can exist in healthy individuals. Histopathology or culture of brain tissue may also establish the diagnosis.[40]

Due to the rarity of the disease and its subacute nature, the diagnosis in most cases of granulomatous amebic encephalitis is established postmortem. Treatment experience is extremely limited. Most patients, especially those with HIV, will die. Successful therapy with different combinations of pentamidine isethionate, sulfadiazine, 5′-flucytosine, fluconazole, itraconazole, and trimethoprim-sulfamethoxazole has been reported. Azithromycin and milfetosine have shown in vitro activity. Use of inert polymers to deliver antimicrobials that would not otherwise penetrate the CSF, such as chitosan and its derivatives packaged in microspheres, shows some promise, but this approach is still in development.[41]

Cerebral Amebiasis Due to *Entamoeba histolytica*

Entamoeba histolytica, the causative agent of amebic dysentery, infects about 10 percent of the world's population, accounting for 50 million symptomatic cases and 100,000 deaths each year.[44] In the United States, amebiasis prevalence is 4 percent; the disorder is seen most commonly in chronically institutionalized individuals, homosexual men, and lower socioeconomic groups in the southeast.[45,46]

Entamoeba histolytica disease was initially thought to occur as either a symptomatic infection or an asymptomatic carrier state. Genetic studies have revealed that *Entamoeba dispar*, a morphologically identical species, is responsible for most carrier states. A nonpathogenic carrier form of *E. histolytica* does occur, but is much less common than *E. dispar*.[46]

Infection occurs by ingestion of cysts in contaminated food or water, or as a sexually transmitted disease through anal-oral contact. Excystation occurs in the small intestine, producing trophozoites. The parasite colonizes the colon where some trophozoites encyst and are passed in the stool to begin the cycle anew. Symptomatic disease occurs when trophozoites invade the colonic mucosa and form flask-shaped ulcers with extensive necrosis.[47]

Invasive disease most frequently presents as inflammatory colitis. Hematogenous spread to extraintestinal sites is rare and most frequently involves the liver. Ectopic sites include the lungs, genitourinary system, skin, and brain. Contiguous spread of infection from liver abscesses into the pleural, pericardial, and peritoneal spaces may also occur.[44,48]

In reported series, 0.6 to 8.1 percent of cases of fatal amebiasis have been complicated by brain abscess. Patients present with focal neurologic signs, seizures, and mental status changes. The areas of the brain most frequently involved are the basal ganglia and frontal lobes. In the few cases in which lumbar puncture has been performed, a mild pleocytosis and increased protein concentration were observed.[44,49]

Cerebral amebiasis is usually associated with a concurrent hepatic abscess. Patients with known hepatic abscesses who develop neurologic symptoms should undergo CT or MRI to rule out CNS disease.[49,50]

Serology, which is up to 90 percent sensitive in invasive disease, does not distinguish between current and past disease and is most useful in travelers and residents of nonendemic areas. Amebae are rarely found in CSF. Stool antigen testing is more sensitive than microscopy and can distinguish between *E. dispar* and *E. histolytica*. Other tests include nucleic acid amplification techniques such as PCR.[50]

Most cases of cerebral amebiasis have been fatal or found at autopsy. Delays in diagnosis likely contribute to the high mortality. Early administration of metronidazole (750 mg three times daily for 7 to 10 days), which has exceptional amebicidal activity and CNS penetration, provides the best chance for cure. Surgical drainage and antiepileptics should be used as needed, in conjunction with medical therapy.[51,52]

TABLE 47-2 ■ Helminths Causing Disease of the Central Nervous System

Class	Species
Cestodes (tapeworms)	*Taenia solium*
	Echinococcus granulosus
	Echinococcus multilocularis
	Spirometra species
Nematodes (roundworms)	*Strongyloides stercoralis*
	Trichinella spiralis
	Angiostrongylus cantonensis
	Toxocara species
	Onchocerca volvulus
	Loa loa
Trematodes (flukes)	*Schistosoma mansoni*
	Schistosoma japonicum
	Schistosoma haematobium
	Paragonimus species

HELMINTHIC INFECTION

Due to their relatively large size (50 µm up to 15 m), parasites pose a distinct problem for host immunity.[53] Helminths causing CNS disease are diverse, with complex life cycles involving both human and nonhuman animal hosts during different stages of their development.[54] In this section, helminths have been grouped by taxonomic class (i.e., as cestodes [tapeworms], nematodes [roundworms], or trematodes [flukes]) because parasites of the same class share common features of development and often produce similar CNS pathology. Table 47-2 summarizes the class distribution of the helminthic species discussed in this chapter.[14]

Cestodes

CYSTICERCOSIS

Cysticercosis is the most common CNS parasitic infection in the world, and is a leading cause of acquired epilepsy.[55] It is highly endemic in developing countries, and in the United States and Canada it is frequently diagnosed among immigrant populations.[56,57] Transmission within the United States has been documented among household contacts of tapeworm-infected immigrants from endemic areas.[58]

Only *Taenia solium* causes neurocysticercosis. Ingestion of tapeworm eggs causes cysticercosis. *Taenia* carriers who handle food can transmit disease through the fecal-oral route and are the major source of infection. Tapeworm eggs in feces can contaminate soil, vegetables, and other food items. Ingestion of viable cysticerci from undercooked pork meat does not cause cysticercosis but results in tapeworm infection (taeniasis) instead.[55,59]

After the eggs are ingested, oncospheres are liberated, penetrate the bowel wall, and enter the bloodstream. These disseminate widely, favoring muscle and subcutaneous tissue. Larval forms develop and mature into cysticerci. Neurocysticercosis occurs when cysticerci develop in the eye, brain, or spinal cord.[60]

A cysticercus is made up of an invaginated scolex surrounded by a vesicular wall. In the brain parenchyma, vesicular cysticerci elicit little or no inflammatory reaction. As the cysticercus involutes, it passes into the colloidal stage characterized by a mononuclear infiltrate surrounding the cysticercus with surrounding edema and gliosis due to the release of parasite antigens. Neurologic symptoms begin to manifest at this point. As further involution occurs (granular and calcific stages), edema decreases but astrocytic changes lead to the formation of granulomas with multinucleated giant cells. Persistence of these abnormal areas of tissue results in foci that can lead to recurrent seizures. The role of calcified cysticerci in recurrent seizures is controversial, but they may continue to serve as a source of worm antigens that can elicit recurrent bouts of inflammation.[55]

While most cases of neurocysticercosis are parenchymal and present with seizures, extraparenchymal disease does occur and can lead to more severe manifestations. Extraparenchymal cysticerci may develop in the subarachnoid, ventricular, or basal cisterns, and can cause hydrocephalus, arachnoiditis, and meningeal inflammation. Subarachnoid cysts may grow abnormally, causing grape-like cystic masses referred to as racemose cysticercosis.[61]

Seizures—focal or generalized—are the primary or sole manifestation in 70 percent of cases. Focal neurologic deficits may occur as well, including stroke-like syndromes.[55] The severity and type of manifestations are dependent on the location and quantity of the lesions, and the host immune response.[59] Spinal cord cysticercosis may lead to compressive myelopathy or a radiculopathy. Ocular disease can cause visual field defects, decreased acuity, and blindness from vitritis, uveitis, or endophthalmitis.[55]

Neurocysticercosis is usually diagnosed by exposure history supported by compatible symptoms, serology, and neuroimaging.[55,56] Travel to endemic areas or previous residence in an area of high prevalence should alert clinicians to the possibility of the disease. Clinical symptoms are nonspecific, and routine laboratory testing does not show any typical abnormalities. Diagnostic criteria have been proposed but are not yet widely used.[55]

Neuroimaging has revolutionized the diagnosis of neurocysticercosis (Fig. 47-7). CT is more useful in detecting calcifications and granulomas, while MRI is better for detecting vesicular cysticerci and extraparenchymal disease.[60] MRI can also demonstrate fine details such as the scolex, and can distinguish between viable and nonviable cysts. Most patients have fewer than 10 cysts, which may be up to 5 cm in diameter. Extraparenchymal disease can cause hydrocephalus; arachnoiditis can manifest as leptomeningeal enhancement.[55,60]

Serology helps establish evidence of exposure but may not distinguish between exposure, the presence of a tapeworm (taeniasis), and cysticercosis. CSF analysis commonly shows monocytic pleocytosis and sometimes the presence of eosinophils.[60]

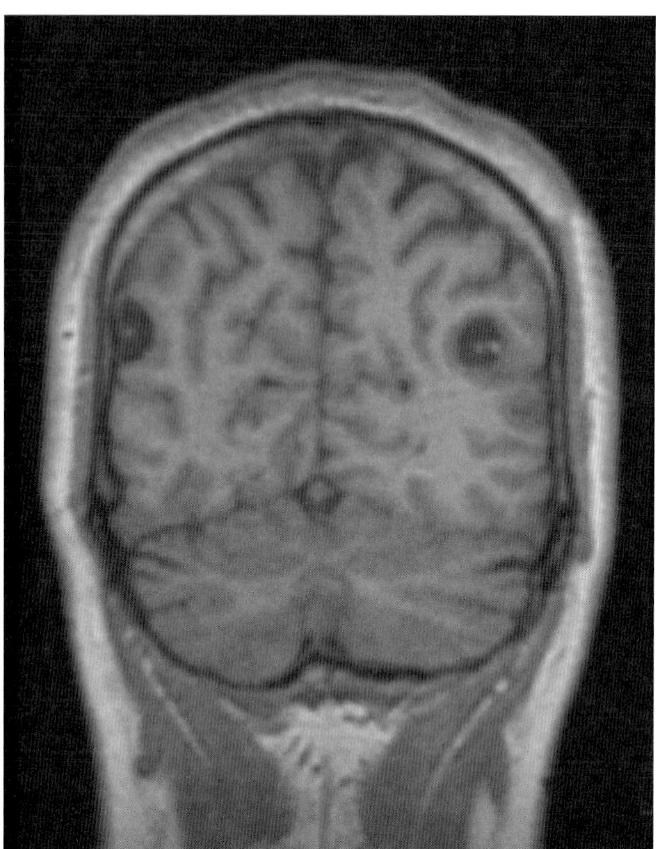

FIGURE 47-7 ■ Coronal T1-weighted MRI showing neurocysticercosis.

Detection of worm antigens and antibodies in the CSF is highly sensitive and specific for neurocysticercosis. Lentil lectin glycoprotein Western blot (LLGP-WB) using CSF is more than 90 percent sensitive and 100 percent specific. ELISAs for cysticercosis antigens have been developed, but may not be specific for neurocysticercosis if performed on serum. Newer methods and antigens in development can detect neurocysticercosis without the need for imaging, and may be particularly useful in resource-limited settings.[62]

Specific antiparasitic therapy is not always indicated for neurocysticercosis. Calcified and granulomatous cysticerci are frequent incidental findings on cranial imaging. However, active parenchymal and extraparenchymal lesions may not be seen on CT, and the calcified cysticerci may be a clue to their presence. Viable cysts are an indication for treatment.[59] Treatment results in faster improvement of colloidal and vesicular cysticerci, decreased seizure recurrence in patients with colloidal cysticerci, and a lower rate of grand mal seizures in those with vesicular cysticerci.[63]

Albendazole, 15 mg/kg daily in two divided doses (maximum 400 mg twice daily by mouth) for 8 to 30 days, is the drug of choice. It is superior to praziquantel, and also destroys subarachnoid and ventricular cysts.[55,59] Praziquantel, 50 mg/kg daily in three divided doses for 2 to 4 weeks, is an effective alternative for parenchymal cysts.[52] A single-day course of praziquantel (three doses in 2-hour intervals) is as effective as the 2-week regimen, which has tremendous implications for resource-limited settings.[59] Some authorities prefer to use the single-day dose regimen for patients with solitary cysts and a longer 15- to 30-day course for patients with multiple cysts.[55]

Corticosteroids are used as adjunctive therapy to decrease pericystic inflammation (which may trigger seizures) or arachnoiditis during treatment. They increase levels of albendazole and decrease levels of praziquantel. Consequently, corticosteroids are co-administered with albendazole and delayed with praziquantel. Prednisone (50 to 100 mg orally daily) or dexamethasone (10 mg intramuscularly or 4 to 6 mg orally daily) is typically used. The duration of treatment is concurrent with the antihelminthic course and is given as needed when manifestations of inflammation occur from the destruction of the cysts.[59]

First-line, single-drug anticonvulsant medication is usually adequate to control seizures. Optimal length of treatment is unclear, and withdrawal is typically followed by recurrence in about half of patients, despite an adequate antihelminthic course. Calcification of cysts may indicate the need for long-term antiseizure medication.[55]

Surgical intervention in conjunction with medical treatment is usually indicated for extraparenchymal neurocysticercosis. Medical therapy alone may cause acute hydrocephalus and exacerbate arachnoiditis, and can lead to infarction and chronic inflammation. Traditionally, open craniotomy and shunt placement have been used to extract cysts and treat hydrocephalus. New endoscopic neurosurgical techniques have decreased the need for open procedures for intraventricular cysts, with the added benefit of a decreased incidence of hydrocephalus needing shunt placement, as compared to medical therapy alone. Infratentorial intraventricular cysts may not be amenable to endoscopic removal. Subarachnoid neurocysticercosis is associated with high (50%) mortality if managed by shunting alone and should be treated with antihelminthics in combination with steroids. The length of treatment and dose of albendazole for subarachnoid cysts has not been adequately established, and some patients may need prolonged or repeated dosing of antiparasitic drugs.[61]

ECHINOCOCCOSIS (HYDATID DISEASE) AND SPARGANOSIS

Other cestodes may cause human CNS tissue injury, including the canine tapeworms *Echinococcus granulosus* and *Echinococcus multilocularis*, and the diphyllobothroid tapeworms of the *Spirometra* genus. Humans are intermediate hosts for these worms.[51]

E. granulosus causes cystic echinococcosis, and is found in all continents, with the highest prevalence occurring in northeast Africa, South America and Eurasia.[64,65] *E. multilocularis*, causing alveolar echinococcosis, is restricted to the Northern hemisphere.[64] Migrating oncospheres rarely encyst in the CNS. However, those that do reach the CNS can induce local inflammation and obstruction, causing meningitis, seizures, and hydrocephalus.[66] Hydatid cysts can also form within vertebral bone, causing compression or spinal dislocation leading to spinal cord damage.[67] CNS hydatid cysts are usually associated with cysts elsewhere in the body (Fig. 47-8).

Eosinophilia or eosinophilic meningitis is not seen consistently. Serologic testing has evolved substantially over the years from the relatively insensitive and nonspecific Cassoni intradermal test, to complement fixation and indirect hemagglutination assays,

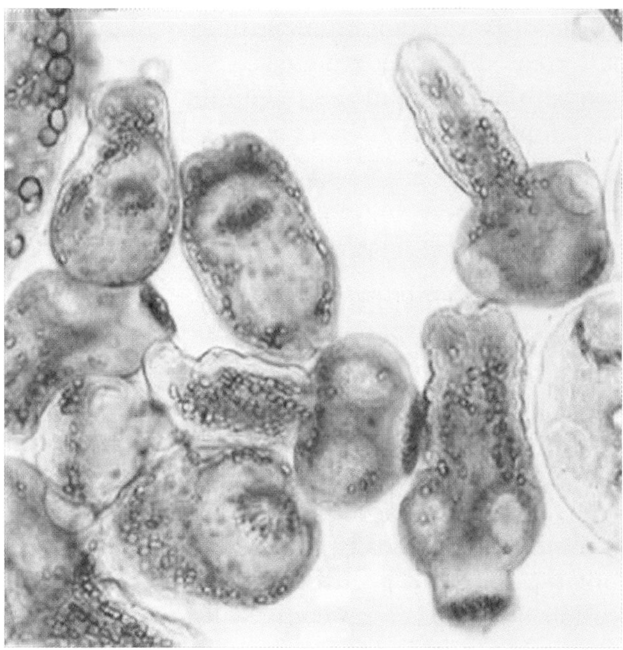

FIGURE 47-8 ▪ *Echinococcus* sp. Protoscoleces. (From the US Centers for Disease Control and Prevention.)

to the more sensitive and specific ELISA, indirect immunofluorescence antibody test, immunoelectrophoresis, and immunoblot assays. Other promising tests in various stages of development include PCR, antigen tests, and a dipstick field test for circulating antigen.[68] Ultrasonography is the main mode of diagnosis for hepatic cysts. In CNS disease, aspiration or excisional surgical biopsy (with precautions for preventing spillage of the cyst contents) may be necessary to establish the diagnosis. Albendazole, 15 mg/kg daily (maximum, 400 mg twice daily by mouth) for 1 to 6 months, is the treatment for cystic echinococcosis, usually with surgical resection. By contrast, alveolar echinococcosis is not amenable to medical treatment alone, and surgery is the only reliable means of cure. Vertebral bone hydatid cysts do not respond well to medical therapy, and surgical excision is the primary treatment.[52,64,65]

Spirometra larvae cause sparganosis. Humans are infected through accidental ingestion of procercoids in copepods from contaminated water, or by cutaneous exposure to, or ingestion of meat from, an infected intermediate host.[51] Symptoms arise from mass effects of cysts in the CNS or may result from cyst invasion in and around the eye.[69,70] Surgery, including stereotactic aspiration or removal techniques, is the treatment of choice, with complete removal of the worm and granuloma as the goal. A few patients with minimal disease manifestations have done well with medical treatment using albendazole or praziquantel, but symptomatic disease is best treated with complete excision in combination with antihelminthics to eliminate any residual infection.[71]

Nematodes

DISSEMINATED STRONGYLOIDIASIS

Strongyloides stercoralis is a gastrointestinal nematode endemic to humid tropical regions, including Southeast Asia, Africa, and Latin America, as well as the southeastern United States and southern Europe. Travel to or migration of patients from these areas accounts for most disease seen in temperate regions.[72] Most infections are asymptomatic and may persist for decades due to the worm's ability to complete its full life cycle within humans.[73] *Strongyloides*, in contrast with other enteric nematodes, is ovoviviparous. In some patients, noninfectious rhabditiform larvae are able to transform into infectious filariform larvae within the intestinal tract and cause autoinfection. In immunosuppressed hosts such as those with AIDS and human T-lymphotropic virus type 1 (HTLV-1) infection, autoinfection with *Strongyloides* may result in overwhelming, sometimes fatal, disease.[72,73]

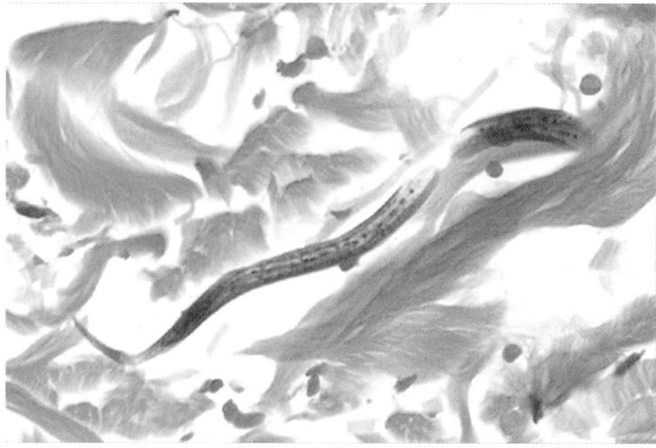

FIGURE 47-9 ■ *Strongyloides stercoralis* larva in tissue (intestine). (From the US Centers for Disease Control and Prevention.)

Disseminated strongyloidiasis occurs when the larvae migrate away from the lungs and gastrointestinal tract into other organs. Large numbers of larvae migrating from the gut carry enteric bacteria into the bloodstream, resulting in polymicrobial infection and septic shock (Fig. 47-9).[73] CNS involvement often results in acute mental status deterioration, with signs of suppurative meningitis, eventually progressing to coma.[74] The process can be subacute, and may be mistaken for cerebritis, chronic meningoencephalitis, or CNS vasculitis.[14] The diagnosis of CNS strongyloidiasis is usually made on finding larvae in stool in patients with a compatible systemic syndrome. Promising tools for diagnosis include PCR, ELISA, and other antibody-based tests.[72] Treatment includes aggressive antibiotic treatment for bacterial superinfection, with antihelminthic therapy using ivermectin or albendazole. While corticosteroids may have a role in decreasing inflammation, these may cause further immunosupression leading to further autoinfection.[74]

In immunosuppressed individuals, it may not be possible to eradicate infection. If immunosuppression is suspended or reduced during antiparasitic therapy, the effectiveness of antihelminthics is improved.[73,74] Disseminated strongyloidiasis may be prevented by screening at-risk patients with a

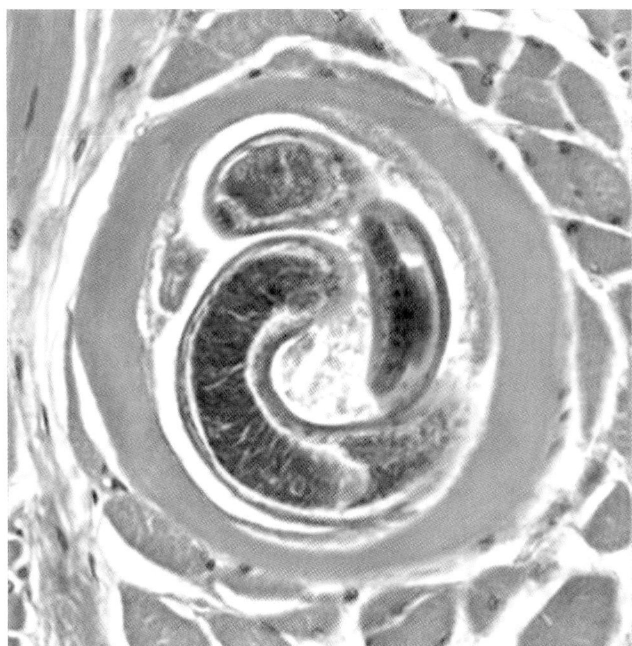

FIGURE 47-10 ■ *Trichinella spiralis:* encysted larva in muscle tissue. (From the US Centers for Disease Control and Prevention.)

stool examination prior to the initiation of immunosuppressive therapy. In AIDS patients, screening and treatment of all stool-positive individuals may be helpful in preventing overwhelming superinfection. Empiric treatment with ivermectin for high-risk individuals has been advocated by some when diagnostic evaluation is unavailable or unreliable, but is of uncertain benefit.[72]

TRICHINOSIS

Trichinella spiralis is a zoonotic infection acquired by ingestion of contaminated undercooked or raw pork or game meat. Infectious cysts in striated muscle tissue are digested, releasing L1 larvae which mature into adults in the small intestine. The adult forms release newborn larvae in a few weeks. The newborn larvae disseminate in lymph and blood and cause symptoms of trichinosis by invading various body tissues. Newborn larvae develop into infective L1 larvae in striated muscle to complete the life cycle (Fig. 47-10).[75,76]

Trichinosis is characterized by fever, diarrhea, headache, myalgia, and facial edema.[77] Neurologic disease occurs due to aberrant larval migration into the CNS. This can lead to diffuse lesions, along with blood-vessel obstruction, leading to infarction and the production of inflammatory exudates. Larvae subsequently may return into the circulation or become trapped and die, causing further inflammation. Mortality is about 17 percent.[78]

A muscle biopsy demonstrating *Trichinella* larvae (Fig. 47-10) is the diagnostic procedure of choice. Neurotrichinellosis should be suspected in patients with infarcts associated with fevers, myalgia, eosinophilia, and periorbital edema. Larvae may be present in CSF in between 8 and 28 percent of patients with neurologic symptoms.[78] CT or MRI scans may reveal multiple infarcts or hemorrhagic lesions, either in areas corresponding to focal motor deficits or throughout the brain.[79] Electroencephalography may show diffuse slowing, but this is nonspecific.[78]

Albendazole (400 mg orally twice daily) or mebendazole (5 mg/kg daily in two divided doses) for 10 to 15 days is the preferred drug for treatment of neurotrichinosis; the second-line drug thiabendazole has antiparasite activity but has more side effects. Corticosteroids decrease signs and symptoms and are recommended, although they may enhance larval dissemination and should be used after starting antihelminthics.[78,80]

EOSINOPHILIC MENINGITIS: ANGIOSTRONGYLIASIS, GNATHOSTOMIASIS, AND VISCERAL LARVA MIGRANS

Human CNS disease can occur following accidental ingestion of infective third-stage larvae of the rat lungworm *Angiostrongylus cantonensis*. Snails, slugs, undercooked prawns, crabs, or vegetables contaminated with larvae are the usual sources of infection.[81]

Neurologic disorders also occur with infection caused by *Gnathostoma* parasites of dogs and cats. Ingested raw or undercooked freshwater fish, poultry, snakes, or frogs which harbor third-stage larvae may cause infection. Humans may also be infected by direct larval penetration of the skin or ingesting water contaminated with *Cyclops* spp. harboring second-stage larvae, which develop further into third-stage larvae in humans.[82]

Angiostrongyliasis is endemic to Southeast Asia and the Pacific islands, but is being reported increasingly worldwide, with snail vectors present in North and South America.[83] Gnathostomiasis is endemic in Southeast Asia, especially Thailand, with increasing infections in Mexico and Central and South America.[82]

With both parasites, CNS involvement is heralded by symptoms occurring between 1 and 4 weeks after exposure, and commonly presents with frontal or bitemporal headache, meningismus, vomiting, and paresthesia. Spinal cord involvement may present as radiculomyeloencephalitis.[82]

CSF examination shows intense eosinophilic pleocytosis (up to 90%), with mildly elevated protein and normal or low-normal glucose levels.[84] Cytology occasionally reveals parasite larvae, but the specific diagnosis is more frequently based on a combination of clinical presentation, exposure history, and serologic evidence. Optimal therapy has not been established.[82] Mebendazole or albendazole with corticosteroids have been used to treat angiostrongyliasis[85]; albendazole and ivermectin with corticosteroids have been used to treat systemic gnathostomiasis. Efficacy of these regimens has not been clearly defined.[82] Both infections are self-limited, although neurologic deficits may persist. Corticosteroids decrease the severity and duration of headaches in angiostrongyliasis.[86]

Visceral larva migrans should be included in the differential diagnosis of eosinophilic meningitis. Infection is acquired by inadvertent ingestion of the eggs of animal roundworms (usually *Toxocara canis* or *Toxocara cati*) from contaminated soil or fomites.[87] Infection is most often seen in children. Eggs hatch within the gut and the resulting second-stage larvae disseminate, occasionally migrating into the CNS or eyes.[88] Neurologic symptoms are rare, but migrating worms may cause seizures, meningitis, vasculitis, encephalitis, optic neuritis, myelitis, radiculitis, and facial nerve involvement.[87] Infection may manifest with fever, hepatomegaly, eosinophilia, and pulmonary symptoms. Diagnosis is made through eliciting a history of animal exposure, and serology using a standardized antigen (TES). However, purely ocular disease may yield only low or nonspecific anti-*Toxocara* titers.[88] A CSF eosinophilic pleocytosis may be present. Corticosteroids are recommended for ocular disease, but their role is less clear for other CNS syndromes. The efficacy of antiparasitic therapy in neurotoxocariasis is unclear, but albendazole is the drug of choice as it penetrates the CNS and has low toxicity.[87]

ONCHOCERCIASIS AND LOIASIS

The filarial nematode parasites *Onchocerca volvulus* and *Loa loa* are transmitted from human to human by biting flies *Simulium* and *Chrysops*, respectively.[89,90] Onchocerciasis is found in sub-Saharan Africa, Central and South America, and Yemen.[91] Loiasis is found in Central Africa, especially in the areas of Cameroon, Central African Republic, Democratic Republic of Congo, Equatorial Guinea, Gabon, and Sudan.[89] In both diseases, developing filarial adults release microfilariae within the body, and the host reaction to these widely distributed larval forms causes CNS disease.

Onchocerciasis is a leading cause of blindness.[90] Microfilaria invade and affect virtually all parts of the eye except the lens, leading to impaired vision and eventually blindness from corneal opacities, optic atrophy, chorioretinal degeneration, and cataracts.[91]

Onchocerciasis can be diagnosed by examination of skin snips for microfilariae. Curative treatment is problematic because drugs such as diethylcarbamazine and suramin cause an exacerbation of ocular inflammation, as well as intense pruritus and systemic symptoms, a phenomenon termed the Mazzotti reaction.[91] This is a result of the massive release of worm antigens and the parasite's *Wolbachia* endosymbiont bacterium.[91,92] Repeated annual administration of ivermectin controls microfilarial load without exacerbating ocular symptoms, but the number of annual doses needed for eradication is unclear.[90] Caution must be used to exclude concurrent loiasis before starting ivermectin.

Loa loa infection is associated with focal areas of angio-edematous skin reactions (Calabar swellings) and the occasional visible passage of worms in subconjunctival tissue.[93] It was previously regarded as a nuisance disease, with few debilitating complications. However, in recent years, treatment of patients with ivermectin for onchocerciasis has precipitated severe adverse events related to *Loa* infection, causing encephalitis and coma sometimes leading to death, especially in those with very high *Loa loa* microfilaremia.[89,93] Efforts to map areas of coendemic onchocerciasis and loiasis are under way to decrease the risk of precipitating these reactions with therapy.[89]

Trematodes

SCHISTOSOMIASIS

Schistosoma spp. are trematode helminthic parasites acquired by contact with fresh water harboring infective larvae (cercariae). Cercariae are released by intermediate snail hosts.[94] There are three major species: *S. mansoni*, endemic to Africa, the Eastern Mediterranean, the Caribbean, and South America; *S. haematobium*, found in the Middle East and Africa; and *S. japonicum*, found in China, Indonesia, and the Philippines. Two minor species, *S. mekongi* and *S. intercalatum*, have limited distribution in Southeast Asia, and Central and West Africa, respectively.[95]

After cercariae penetrate the skin, developing worms migrate to the mesenteric blood vessels (*S. mansoni* and *S. japonicum*) or to the venous system surrounding the ureters, bladder and reproductive organs (*S. haematobium*). Host morbidity results from parasite eggs lodging in surrounding host tissues, with resultant granulomatous inflammation and scar formation.[95,96]

CNS disease (neuroschistosomiasis) is commonly thought to be rare but it is frequently underdiagnosed.[97] Aberrant deposition of eggs within nervous tissues, causing inflammation and fibrosis, manifests with neurologic symptoms in less than 5 percent of cases.[96,98]

Cerebral schistosomiasis occurs mainly with *S. japonicum*, and can present as an acute encephalitis. Headaches, seizures, visual impairment, delirium, motor deficits and ataxia in combination with encephalitis have been described. Myelopathy, including acute transverse myelitis and subacute myeloradiculopathy, is a more common feature of *S. haematobium* or *S. mansoni* neuroschistosomiasis.[96]

Evidence of infection, either through parasitologic methods (eggs in the urine, stool, or rectal or cervical biopsies) or serology (circumoval precipitin test, ELISA, indirect hemagglutination, immunofluorescence, and other methods), coupled with neurologic symptoms and, when available, CT or MRI findings consistent with disease in the brain or spinal cord, is highly suggestive of neuroschistosomiasis. Definitive diagnosis is through the demonstration of eggs in neural tissue, but is highly invasive and is rarely necessary.[95,96]

Treatment goals include the control of symptoms and eradication of worms, and treatment is most effective when started early.[96] Praziquantel (50 mg/kg daily in two divided doses for 5 days) is the usual regimen, although higher doses (60 mg/kg daily for 6 days) are used for chronic *S. japonicum* infection.[98] Alternatives include oxamniquine (for *S. mansoni* only) and metrifonate (for *S. haematobium* only).[96] Corticosteroids are recommended to control inflammation, although there is no consensus on the amount and length of treatment. High daily doses are common: prednisone (1.5–2 mg/kg), dexamethasone (16–32 mg), and methylprednisolone (20 mg/kg) for 3 weeks.[96,98] Praziquantel is contraindicated in neuroschistosomiasis occurring with acute Katayama syndrome, and corticosteroids alone are used during this phase. Artemether in combination with corticosteroids has been proposed for this indication, but no trials have been performed.[96]

Paragonimiasis

Tissue trematodes infect humans who inadvertently ingest larval metacercariae from raw or insufficiently cooked intermediate animal or plant hosts.[99] *Paragonimus* species are endemic in areas of Asia (particularly China and Southeast Asia), sub-Saharan Africa, and South and Central America, and are transmitted through the consumption of crustaceans. Paragonimiasis transmission has also been documented within the United States.[99,100] Disease occurs as maturing larvae migrate through host tissues from the gastrointestinal tract to the lungs.[99,101] CNS disease is rare, and occurs due to aberrant migration into the brain or spinal cord. Presenting CNS symptoms typically include seizures, headache, and visual disturbances. Intellectual deterioration and vomiting may also be noted.[51,101]

Diagnosis depends on a history of exposure, along with parasitologic, serologic, or biopsy evidence of infection. Sputum examination for ova can identify the lung fluke *Paragonimus westermani*, but multiple specimens may be needed.[99] Radiographic examination of the lungs may show typical lesions of paragonimiasis, but may be mistaken for tuberculosis, which is usually coendemic in areas where this fluke is common. Simultaneous tuberculosis and paragonimiasis has been reported.[102] Neuroimaging studies may reveal ventricular dilatation and multiple cystic or calcified lesions within cerebral tissues, with surrounding edema. Peripheral or ring enhancement may be present on MRI.[51]

CNS paragonimiasis seems to benefit from praziquantel treatment, but no controlled studies have been done. Surgical removal of calcified lesions has been performed in some instances, but should be considered on a case-by-case basis.[51]

REFERENCES

1. World Health Organization: World Malaria Report 2011. http://www.who.int/malaria/world_malaria_report_2011/en/index.html. WHO, Geneva, 2011.
2. Greenwood BM, Bojang K, Whitty CJ, et al: Malaria. Lancet 365:1487, 2005.
3. Arguin PM, Mali S: Infectious diseases related to travel: malaria. http://wwwnc.cdc.gov/travel/yellowbook/2012/chapter-3-infectious-diseases-related-to-travel/malaria.htm. In: Centers for Disease Control and Prevention: CDC Health Information for International Travel 2012, Oxford University Press, New York, 2012.
4. Rajahram GS, Barber BE, William T, et al: Deaths due to *Plasmodium knowlesi* malaria in Sabah, Malaysia: association with reporting as *Plasmodium malariae* and delayed parenteral artesunate. Malar J 11:284, 2012.
5. Miller LH, Baruch DI, Marsh K, et al: The pathogenic basis of malaria. Nature 415:673, 2002.
6. Bergmark B, Bergmark R, De Beaudrap P, et al: Inhaled nitric oxide and cerebral malaria: basis of a strategy for buying time for pharmacotherapy. Pediatr Infect Dis J 31:e250, 2012.
7. Mishra SK, Newton CR: Diagnosis and management of the neurological complications of falciparum malaria. Nat Rev Neurol 5:189, 2009.
8. Idro R, Jenkins NE, Newton CR: Pathogenesis, clinical features, and neurological outcome of cerebral malaria. Lancet Neurol 4:827, 2005.
9. Rénia L, Wu Howland S, Claser C, et al: Cerebral malaria: mysteries at the blood-brain barrier. Virulence 3:193, 2012.
10. Pati SS, Mishra SK: Infectious disease: pathogenesis of cerebral malaria – a step forward. Nat Rev Neurol 8:415, 2012.
11. Lavstsen T, Turner L, Saguti F, et al: *Plasmodium falciparum* erythrocyte membrane protein 1 domain cassettes 8 and 13 are associated with severe malaria in children. Proc Natl Acad Sci USA 109:e1791, 2012.
12. Avril M, Tripathi AK, Brazier AJ, et al: A restricted subset of *var* genes mediates adherence of *Plasmodium falciparum*-infected erythrocytes to brain endothelial cells. Proc Natl Acad Sci USA 109:e1782, 2012.
13. Claessens A, Adams Y, Ghumra A, et al: A subset of group A-like *var* genes encodes the malaria parasite ligands for binding to human brain endothelial cells. Proc Natl Acad Sci USA 109:e1772, 2012.
14. Salata RA, King CH: Parasitic infections of the central nervous system. p. 921. In Aminoff MJ (ed): Neurology and General Medicine. 4th Ed. Churchill Livingstone Elsevier, Philadelphia, 2008.
15. Thakur K, Zunt J: Neurologic parasitic infections in immigrants and travelers. Semin Neurol 31:231, 2011.
16. Abba K, Deeks JJ, Olliaro P, et al: Rapid diagnostic tests for diagnosing uncomplicated *P. falciparum* malaria in endemic countries. Cochrane Database Syst Rev 7:CD008122, 2011.
17. Centers for Disease Control and Prevention: Guidelines for treatment of malaria in the United States. http://www.cdc.gov/malaria/resources/pdf/treatmenttable.pdf, 2011.
18. Centers for Disease Control and Prevention: Treatment of malaria: guidelines for clinicians (United States). http://www.cdc.gov/malaria/diagnosis_treatment/clinicians3.html, 2011.
19. Robert-Gangneux F, Dardé ML: Epidemiology of and diagnostic strategies for toxoplasmosis. Clin Microbiol Rev 25:264, 2012.
20. Denkers EY, Bzik DJ, Fox BA, et al: An inside job: hacking into Janus kinase/signal transducer and activator of transcription signaling cascades by the intracellular protozoan *Toxoplasma gondii*. Infect Immun 80:476, 2012.
21. Kaye A: Toxoplasmosis: diagnosis, treatment, and prevention in congenitally exposed infants. J Pediatr Health Care 25:355, 2011.
22. Montoya JG, Liesenfeld O: Toxoplasmosis. Lancet 363:1965, 2004.
23. Feustel SM, Meissner M, Liesenfeld O: *Toxoplasma gondii* and the blood-brain barrier. Virulence 3:182, 2012.
24. Sullivan Jr WJ, Jeffers V: Mechanisms of *Toxoplasma gondii* persistence and latency. FEMS Microbiol Rev 36:717, 2012.
25. Kaplan JE, Benson C, Holmes KH, Centers for Disease Control and Prevention (CDC) National Institutes of Health HIV Medicine Association of the Infectious Diseases Society of America Guidelines for prevention and treatment of opportunistic infections in HIV-infected adults and adolescents: recommendations from CDC, the National Institutes of Health, and the HIV Medicine Association of the Infectious Diseases Society of America. MMWR Recomm Rep 58:1, 2009.
26. Jones JL, Sehgal M, Maguire JH: Toxoplasmosis-associated deaths among human immunodeficiency virus-infected persons in the United States, 1992–1998. Clin Infect Dis 34:1161, 2002.
27. Kastrup O, Wanke I, Maschke M: Neuroimaging of infections. NeuroRx 2:324, 2005.
28. Fèvre EM, Wissmann BV, Welburn SC, et al: The burden of human African trypanosomiasis. PLoS Negl Trop Dis 2:e333, 2008.
29. Malvy D, Chappuis F: Sleeping sickness. Clin Microbiol Infect 17:986, 2011.
30. Blum JA, Neumayr AL, Hatz CF: Human African trypanosomiasis in endemic populations and travellers. Eur J Clin Microbiol Infect Dis 31:905, 2012.
31. Genovese G, Friedman DJ, Ross MD, et al: Association of trypanolytic ApoL1 variants with kidney disease in African Americans. Science 329:841, 2010.
32. Bostrom MA, Kao WH, Li M, et al: Genetic association and gene-gene interaction analyses in African

American dialysis patients with nondiabetic nephropathy. Am J Kidney Dis 59:210, 2012.
33. Vanhollebeke B, Truc P, Poelvoorde P, et al: Human *Trypanosoma evansi* infection linked to a lack of apolipoprotein L-I. N Engl J Med 355:2752, 2006.
34. Gadelha C, Holden JM, Allison HC, et al: Specializations in a successful parasite: what makes the bloodstream-form African trypanosome so deadly? Mol Biochem Parasitol 179:51, 2011.
35. Thumbi SM, McOdimba FA, Mosi RO, et al: Comparative evaluation of three PCR base diagnostic assays for the detection of pathogenic trypanosomes in cattle blood. Parasit Vectors 1:46, 2008.
36. Njiru ZK, Mikosza AS, Armstrong T, et al: Loop-mediated isothermal amplification (LAMP) method for rapid detection of *Trypanosoma brucei rhodesiense*. PLoS Negl Trop Dis 2:e147, 2008.
37. Simarro PP, Franco J, Diarra A, et al: Update on field use of the available drugs for the chemotherapy of human African trypanosomiasis. Parasitology 139:842, 2012.
38. Barrett MP, Boykin DW, Brun R, et al: Human African trypanosomiasis: pharmacological re-engagement with a neglected disease. Br J Pharmacol 152:1155, 2007.
39. De Jonckheere JF: Origin and evolution of the worldwide distributed pathogenic amoeboflagellate *Naegleria fowleri*. Infect Genet Evol 11:1520, 2011.
40. Visvesvara GS, Moura H, Schuster FL: Pathogenic and opportunistic free-living amoebae: *Acanthamoeba* spp., *Balamuthia mandrillaris*, *Naegleria fowleri*, and *Sappinia diploidea*. FEMS Immunol Med Microbiol 50:1, 2007.
41. Visvesvara GS: Amebic meningoencephalitides and keratitis: challenges in diagnosis and treatment. Curr Opin Infect Dis 23:590, 2010.
42. Panjwani N: Pathogenesis of *Acanthamoeba* keratitis. Ocul Surf 8:70, 2010.
43. Khan NA: *Acanthamoeba* and the blood-brain barrier: the breakthrough. J Med Microbiol 57:1051, 2008.
44. Baxt LA, Singh U: New insights into *Entamoeba histolytica* pathogenesis. Curr Opin Infect Dis 21:489, 2008.
45. Ravdin JI: Amebiasis. Clin Infect Dis 20:1453, 1995.
46. Lowther SA, Dworkin MS, Hanson DL: *Entamoeba histolytica/Entamoeba dispar* infections in human immunodeficiency virus-infected patients in the United States. Clin Infect Dis 30:955, 2000.
47. Santi-Rocca J, Rigothier MC, Guillén N: Host-microbe interactions and defense mechanisms in the development of amoebic liver abscesses. Clin Microbiol Rev 22:65, 2009.
48. Bercu TE, Petri WA, Behm JW: Amebic colitis: new insights into pathogenesis and treatment. Curr Gastroenterol Rep 9:429, 2007.
49. Maldonado-Barrera CA, Campos-Esparza Mdel R, Muñoz-Fernández L, et al: Clinical case of cerebral amebiasis caused by *E. histolytica*. Parasitol Res 110:1291, 2012.
50. Fotedar R, Stark D, Beebe N, et al: Laboratory diagnostic techniques for *Entamoeba* species. Clin Microbiol Rev 20:511, 2007.
51. Finsterer J, Auer H: Parasitoses of the human central nervous system. J Helminthol 10:1, 2012.
52. Anonymous: Drugs for parasitic infections. Med Lett Drugs Ther http://secure.medicalletter.org/downloads/PARA_TOC.pdf, 2010.
53. Mulcahy G, O'Neill S, Fanning J, et al: Tissue migration by parasitic helminths—an immunoevasive strategy? Trends Parasitol 21:273, 2005.
54. Hughes AJ, Biggs BA: Parasitic worms of the central nervous system: an Australian perspective. Intern Med J 32:541, 2002.
55. Del Brutto OH: Neurocysticercosis: a review. Scientific World Journal 2012:159821, 2012.
56. Coyle CM, Mahanty S, Zunt JR, et al: Neurocysticercosis: neglected but not forgotten. PLoS Negl Trop Dis 6:e1500, 2012.
57. Del Brutto OH: A review of cases of human cysticercosis in Canada. Can J Neurol Sci 39:319, 2012.
58. Schantz PM, Moore AC, Munoz JL, et al: Neurocysticercosis in an Orthodox Jewish community in New York City. N Engl J Med 327:692, 1992.
59. Sotelo J: Clinical manifestations, diagnosis, and treatment of neurocysticercosis. Curr Neurol Neurosci Rep 11:529, 2011.
60. Takayanagui OM, Odashima NS, Bonato PS, et al: Medical management of neurocysticercosis. Expert Opin Pharmacother 12:2845, 2011.
61. Kelesidis T, Tsiodras S: Extraparenchymal neurocysticercosis in the United States. Am J Med Sci 344:79, 2012.
62. Esquivel-Velázquez M, Ostoa-Saloma P, Morales-Montor J, et al: Immunodiagnosis of neurocysticercosis: ways to focus on the challenge. J Biomed Biotechnol 2011:516042, 2011.
63. Del Brutto OH, Roos KL, Coffey CS, et al: Meta-analysis: cysticidal drugs for neurocysticercosis: albendazole and praziquantel. Ann Intern Med 45:43, 2006.
64. McManus DP, Gray DJ, Zhang W, et al: Diagnosis, treatment, and management of echinococcosis. BMJ 344:e3866, 2012.
65. Brunetti E, White Jr AC: Cestode infestations: hydatid disease and cysticercosis. Infect Dis Clin North Am 26:421, 2012.
66. Turgut M: Intracranial hydatidosis in Turkey: its clinical presentation, diagnostic studies, surgical management, and outcome. A review of 276 cases. Neurosurg Rev 24:200, 2001.
67. Prabhakar MM, Acharya AJ, Modi DR, et al: Spinal hydatid disease: a case series. J Spinal Cord Med 28:426, 2005.
68. Zhang W, Wen H, Li J, et al: Immunology and immunodiagnosis of cystic echinococcosis: an update. Clin Dev Immunol 2012:101895, 2012.

69. Tsai MD, Chang CN, Ho YS, et al: Cerebral sparganosis diagnosed and treated with stereotactic techniques. Report of two cases. J Neurosurg 78:129, 1993.
70. Holodniy M, Almenoff J, Loutit J, et al: Cerebral sparganosis: case report and review. Rev Infect Dis 13:155, 1991.
71. Ou Q, Li SJ, Cheng XJ: Cerebral sparganosis: a case report. Biosci Trends 4:145, 2010.
72. Montes M, Sawhney C, Barros N: *Strongyloides stercoralis*: there but not seen. Curr Opin Infect Dis 23:500, 2010.
73. Mejia R, Nutman TB: Screening, prevention, and treatment for hyperinfection syndrome and disseminated infections caused by *Strongyloides stercoralis*. Curr Opin Infect Dis 25:458, 2012.
74. Keiser PB, Nutman TB: *Strongyloides stercoralis* in the immunocompromised population. Clin Microbiol Rev 17:208, 2004.
75. Ilic N, Gruden-Movsesijan A, Sofronic-Milosavljevic L: *Trichinella spiralis*: shaping the immune response. Immunol Res 52:111, 2012.
76. Bruschi F, Korenaga M, Watanabe N: Eosinophils and *Trichinella* infection: toxic for the parasite and the host? Trends Parasitol 24:462, 2008.
77. Murrell KD, Pozio E: Worldwide occurrence and impact of human trichinellosis, 1986–2009. Emerg Infect Dis 17:2194, 2011.
78. Neghina R, Neghina AM, Marincu I, et al: Reviews on trichinellosis (II): neurological involvement. Foodborne Pathog Dis 8:579, 2011.
79. Gelal F, Kumral E, Vidinli BD, et al: Diffusion-weighted and conventional MR imaging in neurotrichinosis. Acta Radiol 46:196, 2005.
80. Watt G, Saisorn S, Jongsakul K, et al: Blinded, placebo-controlled trial of antiparasitic drugs for trichinosis myositis. J Infect Dis 182:371, 2000.
81. Hochberg NS, Blackburn BG, Park SY, et al: Eosinophilic meningitis attributable to *Angiostrongylus cantonensis* infection in Hawaii: clinical characteristics and potential exposures. Am J Trop Med Hyg 85:685, 2011.
82. Ramirez-Avila L, Slome S, Schuster FL, et al: Eosinophilic meningitis due to *Angiostrongylus* and *Gnathostoma* species. Clin Infect Dis 48:322, 2009.
83. Wang QP, Wu ZD, Wei J, et al: Human *Angiostrongylus cantonensis*: an update. Eur J Clin Microbiol Infect Dis 31:389, 2012.
84. Lo III ReV, Gluckman SJ: Eosinophilic meningitis. Am J Med 114:217, 2003.
85. Chotmongkol V, Sawadpanitch K, Sawanyawisuth K, et al: Treatment of eosinophilic meningitis with a combination of prednisolone and mebendazole. Am J Trop Med Hyg 74:1122, 2006.
86. Thanaviratananich S, Thanaviratananich S, Ngamjarus C: Corticosteroids for parasitic eosinophilic meningitis. Cochrane Database Syst Rev 10:CD009088, 2012.
87. Finsterer J, Auer H: Neurotoxocarosis. Rev Inst Med Trop Sao Paulo 49:279, 2007.
88. Smith H, Holland C, Taylor M, et al: How common is human toxocariasis? Towards standardizing our knowledge. Trends Parasitol 25:182, 2009.
89. Kelly-Hope LA, Bockarie MJ, Molyneux DH: *Loa loa* ecology in central Africa: role of the Congo River system. PLoS Negl Trop Dis 6:e1605, 2012.
90. Basáñez MG, Pion SD, Boakes E, et al: Effect of single-dose ivermectin on *Onchocerca volvulus*: a systematic review and meta-analysis. Lancet Infect Dis 8:310, 2008.
91. Crump A, Morel CM, Omura S: The onchocerciasis chronicle: from the beginning to the end? Trends Parasitol 28:280, 2012.
92. Tamarozzi F, Halliday A, Gentil K, et al: Onchocerciasis: the role of *Wolbachia* bacterial endosymbionts in parasite biology, disease pathogenesis, and treatment. Clin Microbiol Rev 24:459, 2011.
93. Hoerauf A, Pfarr K, Mand S, et al: Filariasis in Africa—treatment challenges and prospects. Clin Microbiol Infect 17:977, 2011.
94. Vale TC, de Sousa-Pereira SR, Ribas JG, et al: *Neuroschistosomiasis mansoni*: literature review and guidelines. Neurologist 18:333, 2012.
95. Salvana EM, King CH: Schistosomiasis in travelers and immigrants. Curr Infect Dis Rep 10:42, 2008.
96. Ross AG, McManus DP, Farrar J, et al: Neuroschistosomiasis. J Neurol 259:22, 2012.
97. Ferrari TC, Moreira PR: Neuroschistosomiasis: clinical symptoms and pathogenesis. Lancet Neurol 10:853, 2011.
98. Carod Artal FJ: Cerebral and spinal schistosomiasis. Curr Neurol Neurosci Rep 12:666, 2012.
99. Keiser J, Utzinger J: Food-borne trematodiases. Clin Microbiol Rev 22:466, 2009.
100. Lane MA, Barsanti MC, Santos CA, et al: Human paragonimiasis in North America following ingestion of raw crayfish. Clin Infect Dis 49:e55, 2009.
101. Fried B, Abruzzi A: Food-borne trematode infections of humans in the United States of America. Parasitol Res 106:1263, 2010.
102. Belizario V, Guan M, Borja L, et al: Pulmonary paragonimiasis and tuberculosis in Sorsogon, Philippines. Southeast Asian J Trop Med Public Health 28(suppl 1):37, 1997.

CHAPTER

48

Neurologic Complications of Vaccination

ALEX C. TSELIS

Yet it was with those who had recovered from the disease that the sick and the dying found most compassion. These knew what it was from experience, and had now no fear for themselves; for the same man was never attacked twice—never at least fatally.

Thucydides, *The Peloponnesian War: Plague of Athens*, 430 BC

Moreover, I have known certain persons who were regularly immune, though surrounded by the plague-stricken, and I shall have something to say about this in its place, and shall inquire whether it is impossible for us to immunize ourselves against pestilential fevers.

Fracastoro, *On Contagion*, 1546

Infectious diseases have historically been the major cause of human morbidity and mortality, and vaccinations have added immeasurably to human health by preventing them. The benefits of vaccinations have not come without some costs, however, and rare adverse effects of vaccines occur. Many important adverse events are neurologic, and these are discussed in this chapter. The US Centers for Disease Control and Prevention (CDC) regularly update and publish useful summaries of vaccine recommendations.[1] Figure 48-1 shows a current schedule for the routine immunization of healthy children and adolescents.

HISTORY OF VACCINES

The idea of vaccination came from the observation that a survivor of "the plague" was unlikely to fall ill from that disease a second time. It had long been known that matter from smallpox lesions, when inoculated into the skin of a naive recipient, often caused a mild form of the disease, yet protected against the full disease. This method, called variolation, was introduced to Europe in 1721; however, variolation occasionally resulted in fully virulent smallpox. In 1798, cowpox inoculation was shown to protect against smallpox, with no possibility of transmitting fully virulent smallpox. This basic strategy of vaccination was employed to generate Louis Pasteur's rabies vaccine, Max Theiler's yellow fever vaccine, and Jonas Salk's and Albert Sabin's polio vaccines. Other important, currently used vaccines include those against influenza, whooping cough (pertussis), diphtheria, tetanus, hepatitis B, measles, mumps, and rubella, and infection with *Haemophilus influenzae* B, meningococcus, human papillomavirus, and varicella zoster. Vaccines are available in Asia to prevent Japanese encephalitis and in central Europe to prevent tick-borne encephalitis.

Aminoff's Neurology and General Medicine, Fifth Edition.

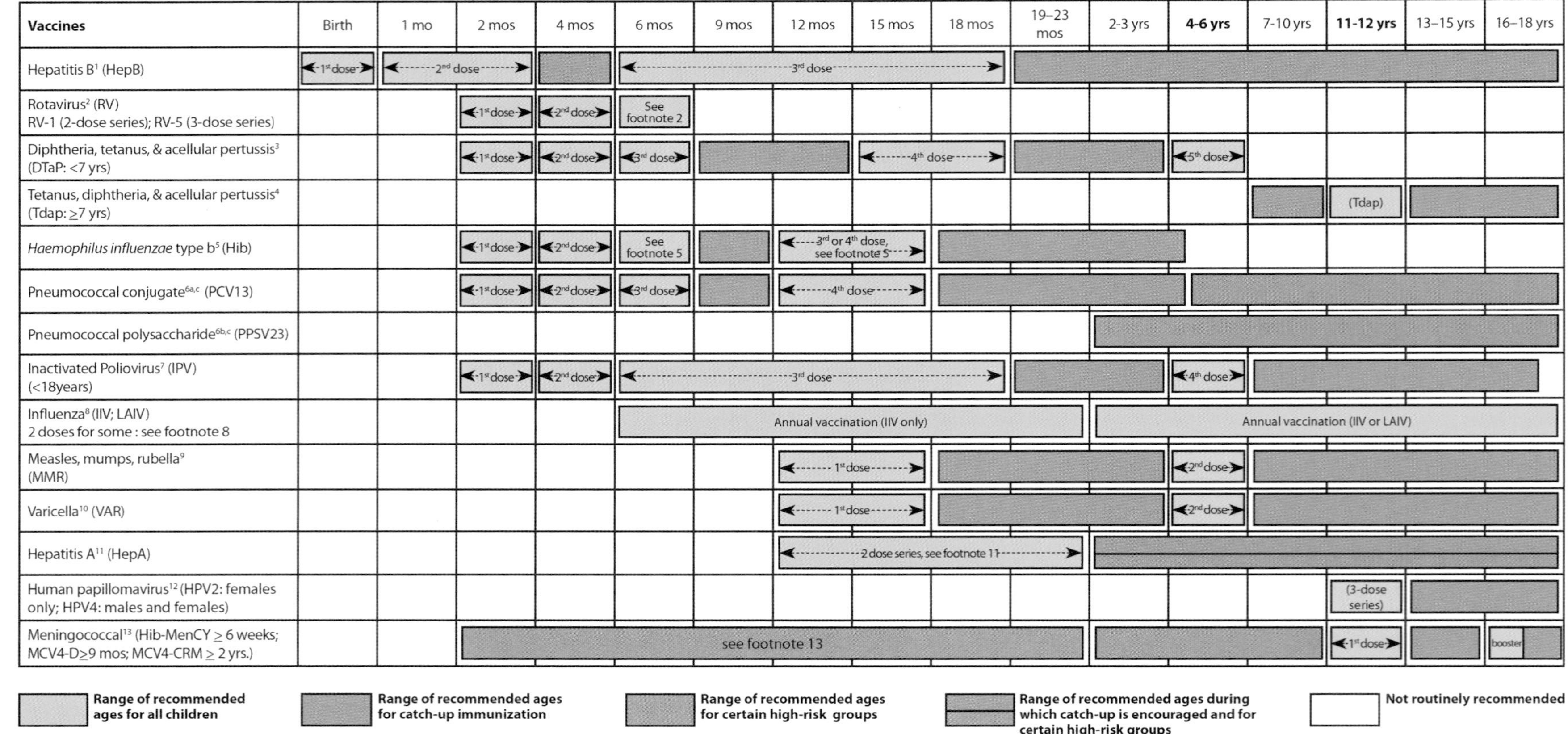

FIGURE 48-1 ■ Recommended immunization schedule for healthy children and adolescents. Recommended schedule for the immunization of persons aged 0 through 18 years by the Advisory Committee on Immunization Practices, 2013. Recommended immunization schedules for both children and adults can be found at the CDC website in various formats, including downloadable charts, and the detailed information contained in the footnotes shown on the illustration is available there. http://www.cdc.gov/vaccines/schedules.

TYPES OF VACCINES

Vaccines are made up of relevant antigens presented to the immune system in a way that generates protective immunity against the fully virulent pathogen without causing disease. Different vaccines have distinct mechanisms of action. These include inactivated, attenuated, subunit, recombinant, component, DNA, and vector vaccines.

Inactivated vaccines consist of pathogens that have been treated by chemical or physical methods so that they are nonviable. These treatments generally modify viral proteins essential to some critical function, such as attachment of the virus to the cell. In successful vaccines, these inactivated organisms still have sufficient antigenicity that protective immunity is achieved without the possibility of causing infection. Examples of inactivated vaccines include influenza vaccine, the Salk polio vaccine, rabies vaccine, and the whole-cell pertussis vaccine.

Attenuated vaccines use a virus (or other pathogen) that has been adapted to replicating in a different host system, such as in tissue culture or in chicken eggs. This is achieved by serially passaging the virulent (or wild-type) pathogen in an alternative host system. The pathogen is now "adapted" to the alternative host system and humans become an "unnatural host." The agent is unable to express its full virulence and therefore causes a mild infection while still stimulating full immunity. An example of an attenuated vaccine is the combined measles, mumps, and rubella (MMR) vaccine.

Subunit vaccines are composed of subunits of a pathogen that are both nontoxic and immunogenic. The older hepatitis B vaccine is an example, as is the acellular pertussis vaccine. The older hepatitis B vaccine consisted of a hepatitis B surface antigen (HBsAg) that was originally purified from the plasma of hepatitis B carriers. Because of concerns about using human-derived material, the gene for the hepatitis B surface antigen was introduced into yeast that then synthesized pure hepatitis B surface antigen.

Viral envelope proteins can self-assemble and form virosomes or "virus-like" particles (VLPs). These virosomes stimulate both cell-mediated and humoral immunity and have been used in the human papillomavirus vaccine.

Component vaccines usually consist of the capsular material of common bacterial pathogens. Antibodies to the capsules allow opsonization of the organism. Examples of component vaccines are those for pneumococcus, meningococcus, and *Haemophilus influenzae* B. These vaccines are often not sufficiently immunogenic in very young infants and have to be specially formulated by conjugation to peptides, which enhances their antigenicity.

Toxoid vaccines are bacterial toxins (e.g., diphtheria, tetanus) that have been rendered nontoxic through chemical treatment, but remain immunogenic.

DNA vaccines are DNA sequences of the gene for an immunogenic antigen that are injected into muscle, where they direct the synthesis of the antigenic peptide. This is then presented to the immune system by the "infected" muscle cell, mimicking a natural infection. DNA vaccines, however, have proved to be poorly immunogenic in humans and none are currently available for human use.

Vector vaccines consist of a nonpathogenic virus that has one of its genes replaced with a gene for an antigen of interest. Such vaccines are being investigated but are not yet available for human use.

Adjuvants

Many vaccines that consist of protein molecules, as opposed to attenuated organisms or multicomponent bacterial cells, may not be very immunogenic, since to attract the attention of the immune system, some damage or injury is required along with the relevant antigen. Often a simple molecule can be added to the vaccine antigen to yield a stronger immune response; such a molecule is known as an adjuvant and probably acts as an agonist to pattern recognition receptors (PRRs) in innate immune cells. Alum salts are an example of a commonly used adjuvant that was first used in the 1930s. Adjuvants have to be carefully formulated since they can lead to severe inflammation. Freund's complete adjuvant is an example that is used in the laboratory, mixed with white matter or purified myelin antigens, to trigger experimental allergic encephalomyelitis (EAE), an inflammatory demyelination of the brain in an animal model of multiple sclerosis. The US Food and Drug Administration (FDA) does not currently approve the use of pure adjuvants outside of a vaccine, and alum salts and ASO4 (a lipid compound) are the only adjuvants approved for use in a vaccine formulation. Several other adjuvants have been approved in Europe.

Reverse Vaccinology

More recently, the methods of "reverse vaccinology" have been exploited to make effective vaccines. The process involves sequencing the genome of a target pathogen and scanning for genes that may be useful for vaccines, such as those encoding for virulence factors or surface proteins. These proteins can then be separately expressed and screened for use in animal models, after which human trials can be organized. The advantage of reverse genetic methods is that all of the proteins are available for testing, rather than only an unsuitable subset expressed by a cell line. An example is that of vaccines against meningococcal meningitis, which are protective to all but one serotype, the capsular polysaccharide of which mimics certain neural antigens and is therefore poorly immunogenic.

COMPLICATIONS OF VACCINATION

The benefits of vaccination are balanced against the adverse effects that vaccinations can cause. Most often, they induce a nonspecific inflammatory reaction with headache, malaise, mild fever, and pain at the injection site. This reaction is self-limited and needs no treatment beyond mild analgesics. More serious adverse effects include contamination of the vaccine with fully virulent virus, reversion of attenuated virus to a fully virulent form, contamination of the vaccine with previously unrecognized agents, the use of inappropriate antigens that cause an aberrant immune response with injurious effects, and induction of an immune response with autoimmune character. Some other adverse effects are of unknown mechanisms.

Some vaccines have inadvertently contained fully virulent virus. In the so-called Cutter incident, inadequate inactivation of the virulent virus during manufacturing occurred shortly after the introduction of the Salk inactivated poliovirus vaccine. Procedures for inactivation of the virus by treatment with formalin were not followed precisely, and as a result some of the virus that went into the vaccine was fully virulent, causing cases of paralytic poliomyelitis.

Reversion to a virulent form occurs rarely with the use of the Sabin vaccine, which is an attenuated poliovirus vaccine. During replication of the virus, mutations that restore pathogenicity may occur in rare instances and result in vaccine-associated paralytic poliomyelitis. In some cases, the virulent vaccine virus spreads to the vaccinated person's contacts, and small outbreaks of polio can result.

Contamination with previously unrecognized agents is an ever-present danger, and there are numerous examples. In World War II, US military personnel serving in the tropics contracted hepatitis after being vaccinated for yellow fever. The yellow fever vaccine, an attenuated vaccine, had human serum added to it for stabilization of the attenuated virus; some of this serum had been obtained from carriers of hepatitis B. Another contaminant of yellow fever vaccine was avian sarcoma leukosis virus, present silently in chicken eggs, which were used for growing virus for vaccine manufacture. The Salk polio vaccine virus was grown in monkey kidney tissue culture, which contained the simian vacuolating virus 40 (SV40) in latent form, thus contaminating the vaccine with this agent. Recently a few rotavirus vaccine lots were found to be contaminated with porcine circovirus, which has never been associated with human infection or disease.[2]

A more ominous example is that of the contamination of louping-ill vaccine, used in animals, with the scrapie agent. The vaccine virus was initially grown in the brains of sheep and processed to vaccine virus. At least one of these sheep had scrapie, and the vaccine was contaminated with infectious prions, causing an outbreak of scrapie in the vaccinated animals. As a consequence of this incident, the FDA requires that any animal protein products used in the manufacture of vaccines are from countries certified to be free of bovine spongiform encephalopathy, which is known to be transmissible to humans.

Inactivation of some viruses may render certain important antigens nonantigenic. For example, the formalin-inactivated measles vaccine used in the 1960s provided short-term protection but in some cases resulted in "atypical measles," an unusually severe form of measles often complicated by pneumonia. These patients were found not to have antibodies to the F (fusion) protein of the measles virus, so that the virus was able to spread by cell-to-cell fusion. It is thought that formalin rendered the F protein nonimmunogenic, so that the spread of wild virulent virus infection was unchecked.

Inappropriate immune responses are well recognized to occur after vaccinations, especially with vaccines made from viruses grown in neural tissue. The classic example is that of the old neurally derived rabies virus, which often resulted in "neuroparalytic accidents" of acute demyelination in either the central or peripheral nervous system. Both acute disseminated encephalomyelitis (ADEM) and Guillain–Barré syndrome (GBS) were observed after the use of these older rabies vaccines. Other vaccines have also been thought to have a causal connection to demyelination. Restricted forms of central demyelination, such as optic neuritis and transverse myelitis, have been described but are rare enough that a causal connection is in doubt. Restricted peripheral forms of demyelination, such as brachial plexopathy, have also been reported.

One potential mechanism of demyelination by vaccines is that of molecular mimicry, in which antigenic epitopes in the vaccine resemble those in myelin. Although this mechanism of mimicry has not clearly been shown to act in central demyelination (except possibly for measles, as discussed later), neurally derived vaccines contain myelin antigens themselves (rather than mimics) and therefore can trigger such disease. Peripheral demyelination is known to occur by this mechanism.

An instructive example of demyelination triggered by a neurally based vaccine is that of rabies vaccine. The idea of using modified infectious material to protect from viral disease was adopted by Pasteur, who used attenuated rabies virus from infected rabbit spinal cord to protect dogs from rabies. His strategy was to take infected rabbit spinal cord and allow it to dry, which attenuated the virus present in the cord. The longer the desiccation, the more attenuated the virus became. Eventually, the virus was sufficiently attenuated that it was innocuous but sufficiently immunogenic that it could prevent infection by fully virulent virus. The vaccine was originally administered as a series of injections of ever less attenuated virus, the idea being to stimulate the immune system with more virulent and therefore antigenic virus. The original Pasteur vaccine was thus rather cumbersome to administer, with multiple painful injections, and frequently gave rise to "neuroparalytic accidents." This phenomenon inspired experiments by Thomas Rivers, who showed that a similar central demyelination could be induced in monkeys by serial injections of sterile white matter; this was the origin of experimental allergic encephalomyelitis, a model now used to study multiple sclerosis.

In order to minimize this complication of neurally based vaccines, vaccines have been made from virus that was grown in myelin-free environments. Fuenzalida first produced a myelin-free vaccine in 1956 by propagating virus in neonatal mouse brains, which still contained neural antigens. The first non-neural tissue-based vaccine was the duck embryo vaccine, in which vaccine virus was propagated in duck eggs. Human cells were used to develop rabies vaccines that were free of animal proteins, and the human diploid cell vaccine, the contemporary standard, was first developed in the early 1960s. Very few "neuroparalytic accidents" have occurred with the current neural antigen–free vaccines. Thus, the more free vaccines are of neural tissue, the lower the risk. In some parts of the world, however, the cheaper neurally based vaccines are still in use.

Some adverse events are of unknown mechanism. For example, rare episodes of intussusception were reported several years ago after the administration of rotavirus vaccine, with 15 cases occurring with administration of 1.5 million doses, leading to withdrawal of that vaccine.[3]

DETECTION OF VACCINE ADVERSE EVENTS

Detection of vaccine adverse events can be difficult as they are uncommon and often manifest as illnesses that are known to occur in the unvaccinated. Many of these illnesses are not reportable to health departments. Health officials, however, will take note of an unusually high incidence of disease and launch an investigation. Surveillance for any unusual disease activity can be active or passive. Active surveillance is when cases are actively sought by sending questionnaires to physicians' offices and hospitals or by systematically examining hospital records. Passive surveillance occurs when physicians or the public send unsolicited information about cases to health department officials. Passive surveillance provides very limited epidemiologic information, as it does not indicate the proportion of those with the complication who were actually reported (no numerator information) and how many were actually exposed to the vaccine (no denominator information); furthermore, the clinical details often are insufficient to make a secure diagnosis.

Case reports and case series of illnesses following a vaccination may be published, but it is difficult to establish causality on this basis and, in fact, such reports may be misleading. The older literature is replete with case reports of illness following vaccination, but in which a causal connection was never made. Certain reports have generated considerable controversies that have led to a decrease in vaccine use and to outbreaks of disease, emphasizing the necessity of performing controlled studies that can address the issue of causality.

Randomized, double-blind, placebo-controlled trials of vaccines are required as part of the FDA approval process and are very reliable, but only common adverse events are detected. The Vaccine Adverse Event Reporting System (VAERS) is a passive surveillance system in which complications are reported to the FDA. Another passive surveillance system consists of the National Vaccine Injury Compensation Program (NVICP), which compensates individuals who have had a serious and permanent adverse effect from a vaccine and who meet other criteria.

The establishment of extensive databases provides a new resource for vaccine safety studies. The CDC is operating a Vaccine Safety Datalink (VSD) project, which links to the databases of eight health maintenance organizations with 6 million members. This database has been used for a number of population-based studies, including vaccine safety studies.[4] General information on vaccinations and reporting of adverse events is available from various internet sites (Table 48-1).

A particularly valuable resource regarding the evaluation of these adverse event reports is a series of reviews published by the Institute of Medicine.[5–7] A committee of experts is convened to review all published and available unpublished reports of adverse events attributed to vaccines. The evidence for and against a vaccine is divided into mechanistic and epidemiologic categories. The former establishes a direct causal relation; thus a case of aseptic meningitis following varicella zoster virus vaccination will be considered to be due to the vaccine only if the vaccine strain virus is present in the cerebrospinal fluid (CSF). This mechanistic evidence must be complemented by epidemiologic data to determine the precise risk of an adverse event.

TABLE 48-1 ■ Vaccine Web Sites

www.vaccine.org	General site of Allied Vaccine Group
www.cispimmunize.org	General information site
Vaers.hhs.gov	Vaccine Adverse Event Reporting System
www.cdc.gov/vaccines/ACIP/index.html	Advisory Committee on Immunization Practices
www.hrsa.gov/vaccinecompensation	National Vaccine Injury Compensation Program

Smallpox

Smallpox (or variola) is a highly contagious disease caused by a double-stranded DNA virus that is airborne.[8] Smallpox is mostly of historic significance at this time, but its potential as a weapon of biowarfare has drawn public health interest in smallpox vaccination issues. The illness begins abruptly with headache, fever, and back pain followed by a characteristic rash that begins on the face, followed by the arms and legs, and finally spreads to the torso. The rash begins with scattered macules and evolves into papules, vesicles, and finally pustules that then dry and crust over. The patient ceases to be contagious after the crusts fall off. There are two broad forms of the disease: the severe form, variola major, which had a mortality rate of about 30 percent, and a milder form, variola minor (alastrim), with a mortality rate of approximately 1 to 5 percent. There are several types of variola major, with the hemorrhagic smallpox form of the disease having a mortality of nearly 100 percent.

The original smallpox vaccination (variolation) involved the transfer of material from smallpox pustules or crusts into a scratch in the skin of the subject to be vaccinated. This method often resulted in a milder form of the disease, presumably because the preparation of the material from the smallpox lesions attenuated the smallpox virus contained therein. Variolation was the first example of an attenuated vaccine. However, the attenuation was often inadequate and some recipients developed full-blown smallpox as well as other diseases such as syphilis. Jennerian vaccination uses an animal poxvirus to induce cross-protective immunity against smallpox. The modern vaccine virus is not cowpox but vaccinia, a related virus; at what point cowpox was replaced by vaccinia or whether the original "cowpox" was some mixture of cowpox and vaccinia viruses is unknown.

Vaccinia is quite reactogenic and has a spectrum of systemic complications including nonspecific malaise and fever, as well as a number of skin reactions including urticaria, erythema multiforme, bacterial infection at the injection site, and progressive vaccinia infection, which occurs in the immunosuppressed and can be fatal.[6] A few cases of mild myopericarditis have been reported in civilian and military vaccinees, with resolution and return to active duty in 7 to 10 days.

Neurologic complications are uncommon, but well reported. In a report from south Wales in which a large population was vaccinated against smallpox as a result of an epidemic in 1962, the risk of any neurologic complications was 5 per 100,000 subjects vaccinated, and the risk of encephalitis-encephalopathy was roughly 2 per 100,000 vaccinations.

More recent series suggest that postvaccinal encephalitis is uncommon, occurring in 2 to 6 per million primary vaccinees, depending on age.[9] The risk in Europe is much higher, perhaps as high as 1 in 4,000, presumably because a different strain of vaccinia virus is used. There have been rare reports of isolation of vaccinia virus in the CSF in cases of encephalitis following vaccination. The overall death rate from all causes following smallpox vaccination is 0.5 to 5 per million vaccinees.

Measles, Mumps, and Rubella

Measles, mumps, and rubella were once common childhood illnesses in the developed world, but they became rare after the introduction of vaccines that prevent them. These vaccines are commonly given together in combination as the MMR vaccine. More recently, polyvalent vaccines have been introduced to minimize the number of injections to which small children are subjected. Formulations containing only some of these have been used in the past: measles (M) vaccine and measles plus rubella (MR).

Measles

Measles is a viral exanthem caused by an enveloped single-stranded RNA virus that is transmitted through the air and initially infects the respiratory epithelium, where it replicates. This replication gives rise to a primary viremia that implants virus in lymphoid tissues. A secondary viremia follows, and the virus is disseminated throughout the body. During measles a significant distortion of the immune system occurs, with paradoxic features. There is a nonspecific systemic immune activation, along with immunosuppression, causing susceptibility to bacterial and viral superinfections that are the main causes of morbidity and mortality and are enhanced by malnutrition, making measles a major cause of death in developing countries. The main complication of measles is pneumonia, due to bacterial superinfection in children and due to direct measles virus infection of the lungs in adults. Pneumonia occurs in roughly 10 percent of patients and causes more than 60 percent of the mortality resulting from the disease. Other complications include otitis media and laryngotracheobronchitis.

The main neurologic complication of measles, occurring in roughly 1 per 1,000 cases, is ADEM, in which multifocal inflammatory demyelination occurs within the central nervous system. ADEM may be due to molecular mimicry, since T cells from measles-associated ADEM patients proliferate upon exposure to myelin basic protein; cells from patients with uncomplicated measles do not. The mortality rate of ADEM is between 10 and 30 percent, and long-term sequelae are common and severe.[10]

Measles virus was first isolated and propagated in tissue culture by Enders and Peebles in 1954, and efforts at making measles vaccine followed shortly thereafter. The first vaccines were made from the Edmonston B strain, which was obtained from the original Edmonston isolate (named after the individual from whom it was first obtained) by serial passage in primary kidney cells (24 passages), primary human amnion cells (28 passages), chicken embryos (6 passages), and then into chicken embryo cells. This vaccine was first introduced in 1963, but the high rate of fever and rash prompted its discontinuation. Other vaccine strains that were less reactogenic were then developed. One of these, the Moraten strain introduced in 1968, was derived from the Edmonston B strain by a further 40 passages in chicken embryo cells. Another strain, the Schwarz strain, was obtained from the Edmonston B strain by a further 85 passages in chicken embryo cells and was used from 1965 to 1976. The Moraten vaccine is the only one used in the United States today, although other vaccine strains are used elsewhere in the world. Before vaccination, 4 million cases of measles occurred annually in the United States, whereas there were only 309 cases in 1995 due to widespread vaccination.

Neurologic complications of measles vaccination have been reported but are uncommon. Case reports of encephalopathies do not, by themselves, provide evidence of causation. In order to better understand the risk of adverse events with measles vaccine, Weibel and co-workers analyzed data from claims of measles vaccine–induced encephalopathy submitted to the National Vaccine Injury Compensation Program.[11] In the years 1970 to 1993, 403 claims of postvaccination encephalopathy were reviewed; inclusion criteria included an acute encephalopathy 2 to 15 days after vaccination (M, MR, MMR) with permanent brain damage or death, with no other known cause that would explain the illness. Of these 403 purported cases, 48 met the criteria. The mean age of the cases was 17.5 months (range, 10 to 49 months).

Three main groups of complications were identified: ataxia, behavioral changes, and seizures. Fever preceded the encephalopathy in most, and one-quarter of the cases had a measles-like rash 1 to 2 weeks after vaccination. CSF was analyzed in most and was abnormal in 40 percent: pleocytosis was present in 70 percent, and protein concentration was elevated in more than one-third. No other viruses were found to be present. When the number of patients with encephalopathy was plotted against the day of onset, a typical epidemic curve was obtained with a peak at 8 to 9 days, suggesting a causal (rather than merely temporal) connection between the vaccination and the neurologic illness. Clinical and pathologic data do not point to any single neurologic disease entity. The risk of neurologic illness can be estimated from the fact that from 1970 to 1993, approximately 75 million children had measles vaccine by age 4 years, based on a 90 percent immunization rate and 83 million births. The limits of risk are, based on 48 claimants meeting criteria and on all 403 claimants, 0.64 to 5.37 cases per million vaccinees.

In a study of 1.8 million Finnish MMR vaccinees, actively surveyed from 1982 to 1996, adverse events included 77 that were neurologic and consisted mostly of febrile seizures with good recovery. One patient later developed Lennox–Gastaut syndrome. Four cases of encephalitis were reported, one of which was found to be due to herpes simplex virus; the others were uncharacterized. Some other neurologic complications were found to be due to other known causes (such as bacterial meningitis). Miscellaneous other neurologic disorders included cases of GBS (two patients, with eventual recovery), transient confusion, and transient ataxia. Interestingly, no cases of autism were found.[12]

In 1998, MMR vaccine was proposed as a cause of autism, a complex and heterogeneous neurobehavioral syndrome. Much discussion has been stimulated by a report of 12 children who developed cognitive problems as well as inflammatory bowel disease a few days to a few months after receiving the MMR vaccine.[13] Questions were raised about the conduct of the study, with improper consent procedures, inconsistent use of data, irreproducibility of some laboratory findings, and failure to declare conflicts of interest. In 2004, the interpretation of the paper as establishing a causal connection between MMR and autism was retracted by 10 of 12 authors who could be contacted. As further irregularities came to light, the paper was retracted in its entirety by the journal.[14]

The ages at which MMR vaccine is given are also the ages when autism manifests clinically; however, the beginnings of this behavioral disease occur much earlier in life.[15,16] A report from the Institute of Medicine reviewed published and unpublished reports concerning the issue of MMR vaccine and concluded that there is no causal connection between the vaccine and autism.[7] Another hypothesis was that autism was caused in especially susceptible subjects by thimerosal, a mercury-containing preservative that was used in inactivated vaccines (but not attenuated vaccines such as MMR). A review of the literature also has shown no clear causal connection between thimerosal and autism, and, in any case, thimerosal is no longer used in childhood vaccines.

Mumps

Mumps is an acute febrile illness caused by rubulavirus, a member of the paramyxovirus group. The clinical illness in children usually is self-limited, with fever, malaise, headache, and often an acute painful parotitis. The disease is complicated occasionally by meningitis and rarely by meningoencephalitis, which may lead to residual deficits. Sensorineural deafness is an uncommon sequela but can be a major cause of deafness in children during epidemics. In adults, mumps has a higher rate of systemic complications such as orchitis in men and oophoritis and mastitis in women, as well as pancreatitis and myocarditis. The main original vaccine virus strains were named the Jeryl Lynn and Urabe strains, after the hosts from which the original unattenuated viruses were isolated. Mumps vaccine was first licensed for use in 1967. The number of cases of mumps in the United States was over 150,000 in 1968 and decreased to less than 3,000 two decades later. The number of cases increased briefly after vaccination rates declined, but decreased again after mumps vaccination was required for school entry.

Aseptic viral meningitis is the main neurologic complication of mumps vaccination and is probably related to natural mumps frequently causing meningitis. The Urabe strain vaccine was discontinued in the United States after it was linked to aseptic meningitis in 1 case in 900 vaccinees in one Japanese series and 1 case in 200,000 vaccinees in another.[17] For the Jeryl Lynn vaccine, the incidence is 1 case in 1.8 million vaccinees; by comparison, aseptic meningitis occurs in approximately 1 in 400 cases of natural mumps.[17] This aseptic meningitis is self-limited and requires no specific therapy.

Rubella

Rubella is a self-limited viral infection in children, characterized by a fever and rash, caused by a single-stranded RNA virus. The virus causes most of its damage through prenatal infection. This congenital rubella syndrome is well described, and the triad of neurologic, eye, and cardiac defects is characteristic. The disease also includes a spectrum of uncommon disorders in all age groups including thrombocytopenic purpura, hepatitis, bone lesions, interstitial pneumonitis, diabetes mellitus, and thyroid problems.[15]

The vaccine has very few complications in children, with rare mild rash and fever. In adults, the most common side effect of the vaccine is polyarthralgias. A few scattered reports of peripheral mononeuropathies and radiculopathy following rubella vaccination have been published, but a review of these could not establish a causal relationship.[18]

Diphtheria, Pertussis, and Tetanus

Diphtheria

Diphtheria is a disease caused by strains of *Corynebacterium diphtheriae*, which produce diphtheria toxin, a binary toxin consisting of two molecular components termed fragments A and B. Fragment B binds to the target cell and allows access of fragment A to the cytoplasm. Fragment A then inactivates elongation factor-2 (EF-2), inhibiting protein synthesis in the cell and leading to necrosis. Usually diphtheria infects the pharyngeal epithelium, where the superficial layers of the mucosa become necrotic and provide an excellent culture medium for the bacteria. These areas of tissue necrosis with exudation form the so-called diphtheritic "membranes." Systemic absorption of diphtheria toxin from the pharynx causes cardiac and neurologic effects. Patients with diphtheritic myocarditis may develop congestive heart failure; pathologic examination shows interstitial inflammation and hyaline degeneration of fibers. Diphtheritic "neuritis" includes several entities, including an isolated paralysis of the soft palate, ocular motor palsies, paralysis of the diaphragm, and a disorder resembling GBS. The pathogenesis of these various disorders is not understood.

In the 1920s, before diphtheria toxoid was introduced, there were approximately 100,000 cases in the United States annually. In the past few decades, no more than a handful of cases have occurred each year. When vaccine coverage decreases, large epidemics of the disease follow, as happened in Russia in the 1990s, when the public health infrastructure could no longer cover the population adequately. The mortality rate of the untreated disease is 30 to 50 percent. After the introduction of antitoxin therapy, the mortality rate declined to 10 to 20 percent; modern intensive care has reduced this rate further to 5 to 10 percent.

Vaccination against diphtheria was originally undertaken by injecting mixtures of toxin and antitoxin. In the early 1920s, it was found that treatment of diphtheria toxin with formalin resulted in a nontoxic immunogenic toxoid. This toxoid was incorporated with tetanus toxoid and inactivated whole-pertussis cells to make the diphtheria-pertussis-tetanus (DPT) vaccine that first became widely available in the mid-1940s.

There have been remarkably few neurologic complications from diphtheria toxoid, although they may be difficult to discern, as the toxoid is usually given in combination with pertussis and tetanus vaccines. Local injection-site reactions can be painful as they are intramuscular; infants may react with prolonged crying, irritability, drowsiness, loss of appetite, and vomiting. Limitation of abduction of the injected arm may occur regardless of age.

Pertussis

Pertussis, or whooping cough, is caused by *Bordetella pertussis*, a commonly circulating bacterium that has multiple antigenic components. The disease begins with a seemingly minor upper respiratory infection, with minimal fever and an intermittent cough, that then becomes severe and progresses to paroxysms in which coughing becomes very vigorous, interfering with breathing and increasing intracranial pressure by continual coughing. This paroxysmal stage lasts between 2 and 6 weeks before resolving.

The disease was commonly lethal in the past. At the beginning of the 1900s, approximately 5 of every 1,000 liveborn infants died of pertussis before 5 years of age. Today, there are fewer than 10 deaths per year in the United States. When vaccine coverage declines, the disease reemerges because pertussis vaccine protects only against bacterial toxins but does not necessarily eliminate the pathogen from the population (unlike smallpox, for example). The pathogenesis of the disease is not completely known, but is probably due to a toxic effect on respiratory epithelium with denudation of respiratory passages.

An important complication of pertussis is pertussis encephalopathy, a vaguely described syndrome of encephalopathy and seizures. In the years 1997 to 2000, pertussis encephalopathy and seizures occurred in 0.1 and 0.8 percent of cases, respectively.[17,18] There appear to be two clinical forms, one with an abrupt onset of seizures and coma and the other with the gradual onset of somnolence progressing to coma. The prognosis appears to be rather poor, with death, permanent cognitive deficits, and recovery each occurring in one-third of cases.[19] The pathologic changes are characterized by vascular congestion and brain petechiae. The pathogenesis probably involves the effects of anoxia and increased venous pressure in the brain caused by the severe cough. Interestingly, intravenous injection of toxin does not appear to cause neurologic complications.

Pertussis vaccine has dramatically decreased the burden of disease in vaccinated populations; it declined from about 200,000 cases in the United States in the mid-1930s to a nadir of 1,010 cases in 1976, with a subsequent increase to about 8,000 cases occurring in 2000 for unclear reasons. The original vaccine consisted of inactivated whole bacterial cells. Whole-cell vaccine is "reactogenic," causing painful local injection-site reactions and fever. The latter can lead to febrile seizures in children, who are especially susceptible. This reaction triggered reports of severe neurologic illnesses following pertussis vaccination which likely were related in many cases to the fever alone.

To ascertain the risk of neurologic illness attributable to pertussis vaccine, an active survey of encephalopathic illnesses was performed in all British children from July 1976 to June 1979 in the National Childhood Encephalopathy Study (NCES).[20] A comparison was made of rates of vaccination in those with or without encephalopathy. A small excess of patients with encephalopathy was found following vaccination. All vaccines with a pertussis component, for example, pure pertussis vaccination, DPT vaccination, and diphtheria-pertussis (DT) vaccination, were counted as pertussis vaccination. The study's methodology has been criticized, and it is likely that other concurrent diseases in part explained the neurologic problems. In particular, some severe epileptic encephalopathies (Dravet syndrome), due to mutations in sodium channels, manifest themselves at the same age that pertussis vaccine is given.[21] Furthermore, there were problems with choice of controls, blinding of investigators, misclassification of cases, and uncertainties regarding the onset of disease. These questions about the conduct of the study have been elaborated in published critiques and these risk estimates are no longer used by the British legal system as a basis for estimating liability.[22,23] A large case-control study was performed in the United States with the intent of avoiding the methodologic difficulites of NCES, and did not find any increased risk of onset of serious acute neurologic illness in the 7 days after DTP vaccine exposure for young children.[24]

A new acellular vaccine consisting only of a subset of antigenic components of the bacterial cell was introduced in 1996 and appears to be much less reactogenic.

TETANUS

Tetanus is a neurologic disease caused by *Clostridium tetani*, which is present ubiquitously in soil. The organism has two toxins carried on a plasmid: tetanospasmin, the neurotoxic component, and tetanolysin, which is a hemolysin. Tetanospasmin is elaborated locally and transported to the CNS in the blood and via local axonal transport. It interferes with release of the presynaptic inhibitory neurotransmitters glycine and γ-aminobutyric acid (GABA), causing inappropriate disinhibition of spinal cord reflex arcs, with resultant greatly increased tone in the muscles and intermittent painful spasms. Respiratory compromise may lead to death. The toxin is very potent, a lethal dose being only 2.5 ng/kg. The case fatality ratio of the untreated disease is 25 to 70 percent overall and 100 percent at the extremes of age; with intensive care, the mortality rate decreases to 10 to 20 percent.

Tetanus toxoid consists of formalin-treated tetanospasmin, which induces an immune response that provides good protection lasting around 10 years. Adverse events are rare and are mostly anecdotal.[25] Brachial plexopathy occurs in 1:100,000 vaccinees within 1 month of vaccination, and there may be a slightly increased risk of GBS (0.4 per million doses). One person had an illness resembling GBS on each of three vaccinations with tetanus toxoid. There is some evidence that tetanus toxoid may decrease the risk of multiple sclerosis.[26]

Influenza

Influenza is an acute, febrile, debilitating viral infection of the upper respiratory tract that causes significant work and school absences each year. It can be complicated by pneumonia and, rarely, by ADEM. In children, the complications of influenza or its treatment include encephalopathies such as Reye syndrome as well as a toxic encephalopathy of unclear nature, possibly related to cytokine production in the course of disease. The virus was first isolated in 1933. In 1935, neutralizing antibodies were detected in subjects given subcutaneous injections of influenza virus. The first trial of an influenza vaccine demonstrated some degree of protection in 1936. The virus at the time was grown in a suspension of mouse lung and then injected into children. Further studies of influenza vaccination using inactivated virus were carried out by the military in the early 1940s with clear benefit, leading to the licensing of influenza vaccines in the United States in 1945. In 1947, a dramatic failure of the vaccine during an influenza epidemic led to the discovery that the vaccine produced immunity to the vaccine virus but not to the epidemic strain as a result of antigenic change in influenza virus. Such change can be of two types: (1) antigenic drift, in which the accumulation of mutations in the genes coding for the surface antigens of the virus renders it sufficiently different from the previous strains so that it can cause disease despite exposure to the previous virus, and (2) antigenic shift, in which there is reassortment of genes coding for the surface proteins from viruses circulating between birds and pigs. This experience led to the establishment of worldwide sentinel centers by the World Health Organization, which monitor for new strains of influenza virus every year so that the new strains can be incorporated into the updated vaccine. The recent circulation of the H5N1 strain in Southeast Asia is of great concern because of the highly lethal nature of the disease and its potential for human-to-human transmission.

Current vaccines are of two types. An inactivated vaccine uses two strains of influenza A and one influenza B virus, all grown in embryonated chicken eggs and inactivated with β-propiolactone. A cold-adapted attenuated vaccine, containing two influenza A and one influenza B attenuated strains, has been introduced and is given as a nasal spray.

In 1975, a fatal case of swine flu in a military recruit prompted the institution of a national swine flu vaccination program because of the fear that the outbreak would resemble the 1918 influenza epidemic that caused such widespread mortality. The vaccine was produced, and 45 million doses were administered by mid-December 1976. In late November and early December 1976, cases of GBS were reported to local health departments and prompted an investigation of the relationship to the flu vaccine. The results of an active surveillance of all such cases reported during the period of vaccination, prompted by reports of a possible causal connection and requested by a court in which a lawsuit had been filed, uncovered 1,300 possible cases, of which 944 could be evaluated.[27] There were 504 cases in vaccinees and 440 cases in nonvaccinees. Although the data were insufficient to diagnose GBS definitively, the cases could be classified by the extent of involvement into "extensive" and "limited" paresis. When the distribution of cases was plotted as a function of time since vaccination, the "extensive" cases followed a typical log-normal epidemic curve, whereas cases of limited paresis did not, implying a causal relationship between vaccination and GBS in a small number of cases. The effect of the vaccine lasted 6 to 8 weeks, and the actual risk of GBS attributable to vaccine was 4.8 to 5.9 per million vaccinees. Interestingly, no such increased risk was found in England and the Netherlands, as well as in 1.7 million US military personnel who received a double dose.[6,28] Furthermore, there was no increased risk of GBS following influenza vaccination in other subsequent seasons.[29–31] The threat of severe influenza pandemics remains, and antigenic shifts are likely to challenge us with high-morbidity pandemics.

In the late 1990s, an H5N1 outbreak among chickens in Hong Kong led to a number of human deaths, although the virus was not easily transmissible to humans. Since then, the virus has appeared in many other countries but has not led to many human infections, which is fortunate since the case fatality rate is high in both humans and birds.

Despite a theoretical concern for the safety of influenza vaccines in patients with a history of multiple sclerosis and central demyelination, it appears to be quite safe. There was no increase in the onset or relapses of multiple sclerosis in a retrospective study following swine flu vaccine.[32] There were also no increases in relapse rate in a double-blind trial involving 66 patients with multiple sclerosis.[33] Non–swine influenza vaccines are safe to use in multiple sclerosis, and a case-control study of influenza vaccine performed by the Vaccine Safety Datalink Study Group demonstrated no association with either multiple sclerosis or optic neuritis.[34] The same study also showed no association between vaccination against hepatitis B, tetanus, measles, or rubella and either multiple sclerosis or optic neuritis. The Immunization Safety Review Committee of the Institute of Medicine concluded that there was sufficient evidence to reject any causal relationship between such relapses and influenza vaccination.[6]

Hepatitis B

Hepatitis B is caused by a hepadnavirus, a partially double-stranded DNA virus, which is endemic worldwide, especially in sub-Saharan Africa and Southeast Asia. The virus is present in blood and semen and can thus be transmitted sexually and through inadequately processed blood products. The disease is usually self-limited in adults, with a clinical spectrum of asymptomatic infection to severe disease, followed by resolution and clearance of virus. However, in infants and children (80 to 90% of those infected before 1 year) as well as in some adults (approximately 5% of those infected), the acute infection is often asymptomatic but evolves into a chronic active hepatitis, with progression to cirrhosis and possibly hepatocellular cancer. In highly endemic areas such as sub-Saharan Africa and Southeast Asia, this is one of the most common cancers, leading to significant mortality.

In 1991, two cases of central demyelination were reported after receipt of the recombinant hepatitis B vaccine, one being in a patient with preexisting multiple sclerosis.[35] A report of eight patients with disseminated central demyelination with persistent activity on imaging studies caused much controversy in France.[36] After other cases were subsequently reported, calculations of the expected number of new cases of multiple sclerosis (1 to 3 per 100,000 annually) showed that the disease incidence in the vaccinees (0.65 per 100,000 annually) was actually less than would have been expected.[37] A population-based retrospective cohort study of 134,698 persons compared the rate of CNS demyelination in hepatitis B vaccinees with that in nonvaccinees and found no difference.[38] In a case-control study from British Columbia, the rates of development of multiple sclerosis in adolescents vaccinated against hepatitis B in the years 1992 to 1998 (after universal hepatitis B vaccination became standard) were compared with those not vaccinated in the years 1986 to 1992 (before the vaccine was available); no statistically significant difference was found between the two groups.[39] A multicenter hospital-based study in France also found no evidence of an association between central demyelination and receipt of hepatitis B vaccine.[40] There is therefore no evidence of causality between hepatitis B vaccination and multiple sclerosis. Other studies have found no evidence that hepatitis B vaccine triggers relapses in patients with established multiple sclerosis.[41]

Poliomyelitis

Poliomyelitis, caused by poliovirus type 1, 2, or 3, usually is asymptomatic or consists of a mild febrile illness in early childhood. In older children, adolescents, or adults, the febrile illness may be accompanied by damage to the anterior horn cells in the spinal cord. The disease is spread by fecal-oral contact and caused considerable morbidity before vaccination became widely available.

Early attempts at vaccination in the 1930s were disastrous—inadequate attenuation of the virulent virus led to polio in recipients (there was no test for attenuation of viruses), different serotypes were unknown and therefore not protected against, and there were no safety precautions against injecting neurally derived material. In the Cutter incident, which was associated with the Salk inactivated vaccine, 260 vaccinees and contacts contracted polio.

These cases were thought to be related to the vaccine because they occurred in just a few western states, all were injected by vaccine supplied by a single manufacturer (Cutter Laboratories), the injected extremities were disproportionately affected, and the cases were traced to lots that were found to be inadequately attenuated.

The Sabin oral vaccine consists of attenuated virus that replicates in the gut and induces immunity in both the vaccinee and contacts (because the vaccinee sheds vaccine virus). Rarely, however, the virus reverts to a virulent form and may cause vaccine-associated paralytic poliomyelitis (VAPP) in 1 per 1 million doses in vaccinees or their contacts. Because the only polio seen in North America was vaccine associated, the Sabin vaccine was withdrawn from use in 1994. It is still in use in other parts of the world and has occasionally caused small epidemics of paralytic disease, with a recently reported outbreak occurring in China in 2004.

EMERGING VIRUSES

The global burden of viral disease is increasing. Arboviruses (arthropod-borne viruses) play an important role due to climate factors that encourage the growth of arthropod populations, greater access to various means of transportation, and exploration of previously isolated areas. Some of the most important of these viruses result in dengue fever, Japanese encephalitis, tick-borne encephalitis, and West Nile fever. These viruses have achieved prominence because of an increasing number of infections and disease with an increasing geographic spread.

Dengue, for instance, has not only reached a very high incidence rate but has become more severe, resulting in dengue hemorrhagic fever and dengue shock syndrome. Some dengue encephalitis cases have also been reported. Dengue hemorrhagic fever and dengue shock syndrome occur in areas where more than one (of four) serotypes co-circulate. Infection with one serotype confers protection against that serotype but enhances the effects of other serotypes. The implications for vaccine design are obvious. A phase 2 trial of an attenuated tetravalent vaccine in 3,673 participants, given at 0, 6 and 12 months, demonstrated that a safe vaccine against dengue was possible.[42]

Another important threat to public health is enterovirus 71, which can cause an undifferentiated febrile illness, hand-foot-and-mouth disease, and has been associated with a brainstem encephalitis in children with a high case fatality rate (see Chapter 43). Already vaccines against enterovirus 71 are in phase 3 trials after demonstration of efficacy and safety in a 1,200-participant phase 2 trial.[43]

THERAPEUTIC VACCINATION

Other potential uses for vaccines that are evolving include therapeutic vaccines, meant to modify or abolish an already established disease process, rather than to prevent the disease from beginning. Such a strategy has been attempted in the treatment of Alzheimer disease in which a β-amyloid fragment was used to immunize patients against disease-causing β-amyloid. Unfortunately, despite success in rodent models, several patients developed an immune-mediated encephalitis.[44] A similar strategy may be useful in prion disease, if an appropriate antigen can be identified. A vaccine that could cause an immune deviation from a Th2 to a Th1 response may be useful in chronic intracellular infections that stimulate a humoral immune response (Th2) rather than the more effective cell-mediated immunity (Th1). Cancer vaccines have also been investigated and at least two are in clinical trials for prostate adenocarcinoma and melanoma.

REFERENCES

1. Akinskaya-Beysolow I, Jenkins R, Meissner H, et al: Advisory Committee on Immunization Practices (ACIP) recommended immunization schedule for persons ages 0 through 18 years—United States, 2013. MMWR Surveill Summ 62(suppl 1):2, 2013.
2. Rotavirus WHO: vaccines. WHO position paper—January 2013. Wkly Epidemiol Rec 88:49, 2013.
3. Rennels M: The rotavirus vaccine story: a clinical investigator's view. Pediatrics 106:123, 2000.
4. Chen R, DeStefano F, Davis R, et al: The Vaccine Safety Datalink: immunization research in health maintenance organizations in the USA. Bull World Heath Organ 78:186, 2000.
5. Institute of Medicine: Adverse Effects of Vaccines. Evidence and Causality. National Academies Press, Washington DC, 2012.
6. Institute of Medicine: Influenza Vaccines and Neurological Complications. Immunization Safety Review. National Academies Press, Washington DC, 2004.
7. Institute of Medicine: Vaccines and Autism. Immunization Safety Review. National Academies Press, Washington DC, 2004.

8. Brennan J, Henderson D: The diagnosis and management of smallpox. N Engl J Med 346:1300, 2002.
9. Fulginiti V, Papier A, Lane J, et al: Smallpox vaccination: a review, part II. Adverse events. Clin Infect Dis 37:251, 2003.
10. Tselis A, Lisak R: Acute disseminated encephalomyelitis. p. 147. In: Antel J, Birnbaum G, Hartung H (eds): Clinical Neuroimmunology. Oxford University Press, New York, 2005.
11. Weibel R, Casarta V, Benor D, et al: Acute encephalopathy followed by permanent brain injury or death associated with further attenuated measles vaccines: a review of claims submitted to the National Vaccine Injury Compensation Program. Pediatrics 101:383, 1998.
12. Patja A, Davidkin I, Kurki T, et al: Serious adverse events after measles-mumps-rubella vaccination during a fourteen year prospective followup. Pediatr Infect Dis J 19:1127, 2000.
13. Wakefield A, Murch S, Anthony A, et al: Ileal-lymphoid-nodular hyperplasia, nonspecific colitis and pervasive developmental disorder in children. Lancet 351:637, 1998.
14. Editors of the Lancet: Retraction of ileal-lymphoid-nodular-hyperplasia, nonspecific colitis and pervasive developmental disorder. Lancet 375:445, 2010.
15. Halsey N, Hyman S: Measles-mumps-rubella vaccine and autistic spectrum disorder: report from the New Challenges in Childhood Immunizations Conference convened in Oak Brook, Illinois, June 12-13, 2000. Pediatrics 107:E84, 2001.
16. Taylor B: Vaccines and the changing epidemiology of autism. Child Health Dev 232:511, 2006.
17. Plotkin S, Wharton M: Mumps vaccine. p. 267. In: Plotkin S, Orenstein W (eds): Vaccines. WB Saunders, Philadelphia, 1999.
18. Institute of Medicine Adverse Effects of Pertussis and Rubella Vaccines. National Academies Press, Washington DC, 1991.
19. Zellweger H: Pertussis encephalopathy. Arch Pediatr 76:381, 1959.
20. Miller D, Ross E, Alderslade R, et al: Pertussis immunization and serious acute neurological illness in children. BMJ 282:1595, 1981.
21. Berkovic S, Harkin L, McMahon JM, et al: De-novo mutations of the sodium channel gene SCN1A in alleged vaccine encephalopathy: a retrospective study. Lancet Neurol 3:488, 2006.
22. McIntosh A, McMahon J, Dibbens L, et al: Effects of vaccination on onset and outcome of Dravet syndrome: a retrospective study. Lancet Neurol 9:592, 2010.
23. Griffith A: Permanent brain damage and pertussis vaccination: is the end of the saga in sight? Vaccination 7:199, 1989.
24. Gale JL, Thapa PB, Wassilak SG, et al: Risk of severe acute neurologic illness after immunization with diphtheria-tetanus-pertussis vaccine. A population-based case-control study. JAMA 271:37, 1994.
25. Schlenska G: Unusual neurological complications following tetanus toxoid administration. J Neurol 215:299, 1977.
26. Hernan M, Alonso A, Hernandez-Dias S: Tetanus vaccination and risk of multiple sclerosis. A systematic review. Neurology 67:212, 2006.
27. Langmuir A, Bregman D, Kurland L, et al: An epidemiologic and clinical evaluation of Guillain-Barré syndrome reported in association with the administration of swine influenza vaccines. Am J Epidemiol 119:841, 1984.
28. Ropper A, Victor M: Influenza vaccination and the Guillain-Barré syndrome. N Engl J Med 339:1845, 1998.
29. Hurwitz E, Schonberger L, Nelson D, et al: Guillain-Barré syndrome and the 1979-1980 influenza vaccine. N Engl J Med 304:1557, 1981.
30. Kaplan J, Katona P, Hurwitz E, et al: Guillain-Barré syndrome in the United States, 1979–1980 and 1980–1981. Lack of an association with influenza vaccination. JAMA 248:698, 1982.
31. Lasky T, Terracciano G, Magder L, et al: The Guillain-Barré syndrome and the 1992–1993 and 1993–1994 influenza vaccines. N Engl J Med 339:1797, 1998.
32. Kurland L, Molgaard C, Kurland E, et al: Swine flu vaccine and multiple sclerosis. JAMA 251:2672, 1984.
33. Myers L, Ellison G, Lucia M, et al: Swine influenza virus vaccination in patients with multiple sclerosis. J Infect Dis 136:2672, 1977.
34. DeStefano F, Verstraeten T, Jackson L, et al: Vaccinations and risk of central nervous system demyelinating diseases in adults. Arch Neurol 60:504, 2003.
35. Herroelen L, De Keyser J, Ebinger G: Central nervous system demyelination after immunization with recombinant hepatitis B vaccine. Lancet 338:178, 1991.
36. Tourbah A, Gout O, Liblau R, et al: Encephalitis after hepatitis B vaccination. Recurrent disseminated encephalitis or MS? Neurology 53:396, 1999.
37. Monteyne P, Andre F: Is there a causal link between hepatitis B vaccination and multiple sclerosis? Vaccine 18:1994, 2000.
38. Zipp F, Weil J, Einhaupl K: No increase in demyelinating diseases after hepatitis B vaccination. Nat Med 5:1999, 1999.
39. Sadovnick A, Scheifele D: School-based hepatitis B vaccination programme and adolescent multiple sclerosis. Lancet 355:549, 2000.
40. Touze E, Fourrier A, Rue-Fenouche C, et al: Hepatitis B vaccination and first central nervous system demyelinating event: a case-control study. Neuroepidemiology 21:180, 2002.

41. Confavreux C, Suissa A, Saddier P, et al: Vaccinations and the risk of relapse in multiple sclerosis. N Engl J Med 344:319, 2001.
42. Sabchareon A, Wallace D, Sirivichayakul K, et al: Protective efficacy of the recombinant live-attenuated CYD tetravalent dengue vaccine in Thai schoolchidren: a randomized, controllled phase 2b trial. Lancet 380:1559, 2012.
43. Zhu F, Liang L, Ge H, et al: Immunogenicity and safety of an enterovirus 71 vaccine in healthy Chinese children and infants: a randomized, double blind, placebo-controlled phase 2 clinical trial. Lancet 381:1037, 2013.
44. Ogogorzo J, Gilman S, Dartigues J, et al: Subacute meningoencephalitis in a subset of patients with AD after Abeta42 immunization. Neurology 61:46, 2003.

CHAPTER

49

Sarcoidosis of the Nervous System

ALLAN KRUMHOLZ ■ BARNEY J. STERN

Sarcoidosis was first described in 1877 by Sir Jonathan Hutchinson as a disease of the skin.[1,2] At the turn of the century, Caesar Boeck termed the disease *multiple benign sarkoid*, because of its histologic similarity to sarcoma, and from this is derived the modern term *sarcoidosis*.[3] Boeck also demonstrated the unifying pathologic feature of sarcoidosis as epithelioid cell granulomas that could involve different organs. Sarcoidosis is today recognized as a multisystem granulomatous disorder of unknown etiology. Typical presentations include bilateral hilar adenopathy, pulmonary infiltration, and skin and eye lesions.[4]

Neurologic involvement in sarcoidosis was first reported in the early 1900s by Heerfordt, who described patients with cranial nerve palsies.[5] Varied neurologic manifestations of sarcoidosis are now recognized to occur in 5 to 15 percent of patients.[6,7] Neurosarcoidosis manifests in diverse ways, including with cranial neuropathies, aseptic meningitis, mass lesions, encephalopathy-vasculopathy, seizures, hypothalamic–pituitary disorders, hydrocephalus, myelopathy, peripheral neuropathy, and myopathy.[8–13] Because its neurologic manifestations are so diverse, its etiology is unknown, and confirmative laboratory tests are lacking, neurosarcoidosis poses a clinical challenge. The diagnosis of neurosarcoidosis is usually based on the identification of a characteristic neurologic presentation in an individual with systemic sarcoidosis; however, neurologic manifestations are the presenting feature for approximately 50 percent of patients with sarcoidosis.[6,7] Optimal management of patients with neurosarcoidosis requires an understanding of the broad clinical spectrum of the disorder, the best methods of confirming the diagnosis, and the full range of treatment options.

SARCOIDOSIS

The first internationally accepted definition of sarcoidosis remains of value today: "sarcoidosis is a multisystem granulomatous disorder of unknown

Aminoff's Neurology and General Medicine, Fifth Edition.

TABLE 49-1 ■ Frequency of Organ Involvement in Sarcoidosis

Manifestation	Frequency (%)
Intrathoracic	87
Hilar nodes	72
Lung parenchyma	46
Upper respiratory tract	6
Dermatologic	
Skin	18
Erythema nodosum	15
Ocular	15
Lacrimal gland	3
Parotid gland	6
Splenomegaly	10
Peripheral lymphadenopathy	28
Bone	3
Cardiac	3
Hepatomegaly	10
Hypercalcemia	13
Neurologic	5–15
Hematologic, endocrinologic, gastrointestinal, and genitourinary	Rare

etiology, most commonly affecting young adults and presenting most frequently with bilateral hilar adenopathy, pulmonary infiltration, skin or eye lesions. The diagnosis is established most securely when clinical and radiographic findings are supported by histologic evidence of widespread noncaseating epithelioid-cell granulomas in more than one organ."[14] Sarcoidosis usually presents between the ages of 20 and 40 years but can occur in children[15] as well as in older populations. Its clinical manifestations are similar in all age groups. Intrathoracic structures are most commonly affected, followed by lymph node, skin, and ocular disease (Table 49-1). Although a diagnosis of sarcoidosis is most secure when it is based on histologic confirmation, in around 30 percent of patients the diagnosis is based solely on clinical and radiologic findings.[16]

Involvement of any organ by sarcoidosis is possible and may occur with or without symptoms. It is estimated that 20 to 40 percent of patients are asymptomatic at presentation, their disease being discovered by routine chest radiography.[16] In fewer than 10 percent of patients, the onset of symptoms is neither systemic nor pulmonary.[17,18] Neurologic presentations of sarcoidosis are in this category.

Many laboratory abnormalities have been described in sarcoidosis, but no specific or highly sensitive diagnostic test is available. Active sarcoidosis may cause an elevation in serum angiotensin-converting enzyme (ACE), which can then serve as a marker of systemic disease activity,[7–10] but serum ACE is nonspecific, and often elevated in patients with other conditions such as liver disease, diabetes mellitus, hyperthyroidism, systemic infection, malignancy, and Gaucher disease.

Most patients with systemic sarcoidosis have a good prognosis. For approximately two-thirds, the disease resolves spontaneously without major difficulties. This benign course is most common in asymptomatic patients with only hilar adenopathy on chest radiographs, who have a 70 to 80 percent chance of spontaneous remission.[16,19] However, for one-third of patients, symptoms persist or the disease progressively worsens. Pulmonary dysfunction is the major issue for most patients with a persistent or progressive clinical course.[3,16,18,19] Mortality in systemic sarcoidosis is reported as below 5 percent. Deaths are most often due to respiratory failure; neurologic and cardiac involvement is also associated with a relatively high risk of death.[16,18,19]

The basis of therapy for all forms of sarcoidosis is corticosteroids.[4] However, debate continues as to the precise indications for treatment, because many patients are asymptomatic at the time of presentation and the rate of spontaneous resolution of sarcoidosis is high. In addition, the clinical presentations and course are so varied that treatment studies—particularly large, well-controlled studies—are not available. Corticosteroid treatment seems most clearly indicated for patients with significant functional impairment in any organ system, particularly with major pulmonary, cardiac, ocular, or central nervous system (CNS) involvement.[16,18,19] Alternative immunosuppressive treatment options are discussed in detail later.[20]

PATHOPHYSIOLOGY

Although the precise etiology of sarcoidosis remains unknown, major strides have been made in understanding its pathogenesis. There is strong evidence that sarcoidosis is caused by heightened immune

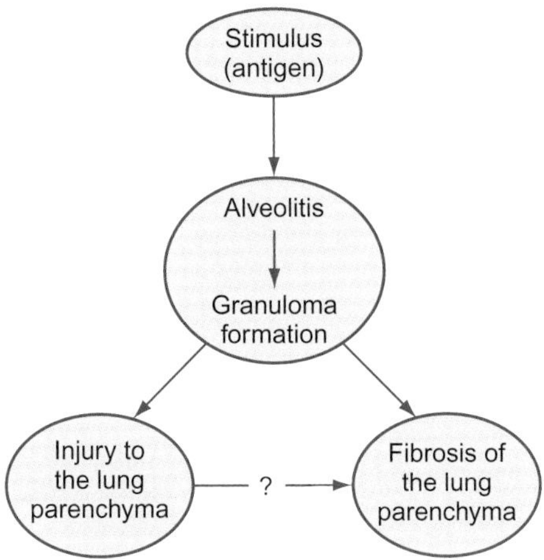

FIGURE 49-1 ■ Postulated mechanisms of pulmonary damage in sarcoidosis.

processes at sites of disease activity.[16,21–30] This contrasts sharply with earlier concepts that had related sarcoidosis to impaired immunity and to generalized anergy.[3]

Current understanding of the immunopathology of sarcoidosis derives largely from studies of pulmonary sarcoidosis. The initial lesion in pulmonary sarcoidosis is an alveolitis, an inflammation of the alveolar structures of the lung (Fig. 49-1). Undoubtedly, processes similar to those in the lung underlie the pathogenesis of other forms of sarcoidosis, including neurosarcoidosis (Fig. 49-2).

Sarcoidosis can be thought of as an inflammatory response to an as yet unidentified foreign antigen.[16,23,24] The central pathologic hallmark of sarcoidosis, the granuloma, consists of macrophages, macrophage-derived epithelioid cells, and multinucleated giant cells that secrete cytokines (Fig. 49-3).[25] Surrounding this central core are $CD4^+$ and $CD8^+$ T lymphocytes, B lymphocytes, plasma cells, and fibroblasts.[22,23,25,26,]

Unfortunately, the inciting antigen or antigens remain unknown. Among the suspected causes have been infectious agents, organic agents such as pine pollen, and inorganic substances.[16,26,30] Of the various possible infectious causes, mycobacterial infections have received the most attention.[27–30] More recently, *Propionibacterium* species have also been implicated.[16,31]

In reaction to an antigen, monocytes and macrophages form granulomas, and ultimately irreversible obliterative fibrosis can develop. Small foci of ischemic necrosis occur, probably as a consequence of in situ thrombosis due to perivascular

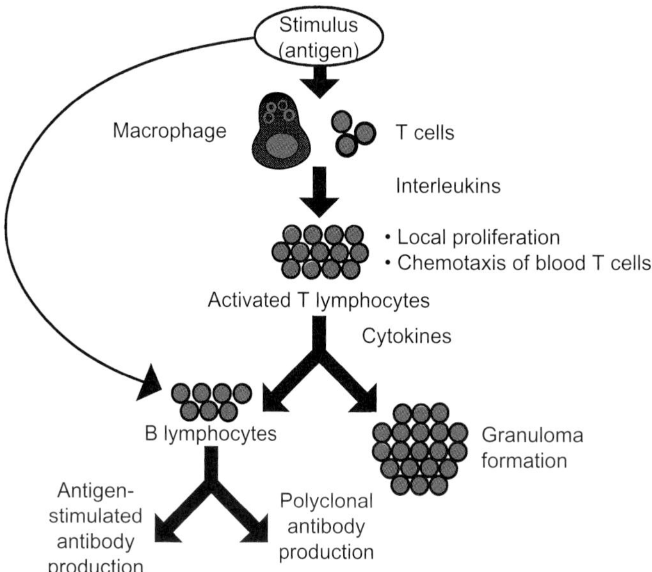

FIGURE 49-2 ■ Immunologic mechanisms active in the pathogenesis of granulomatous inflammation in neurosarcoidosis.

inflammation. Importantly, granulomas are not specific for sarcoidosis, and nearly identical lesions occur in a variety of other conditions that must be excluded before a diagnosis of sarcoidosis can be made.[26]

The pathology of neurosarcodosis is characterized by noncaseating granulomas and the accompanying diffuse mononuclear cell infiltrates that can be found in any part of the neuraxis, including peripheral nerve or muscle. The most common site of inflammation is the meninges, especially in the basal region of the brain (Figs. 49-4 and 49-5).[8–10] Sarcoid granulomas may be widely distributed or concentrated in one or more areas to form a mass lesion. Although sarcoidosis is not usually considered to be a primary vasculitis, arteriolar and venous infiltration can occur and may lead to infarction.[8–11] The granulomatous inflammation found pathologically may correlate directly with clinical deficits or may be subclinical.[8–11]

Inflammation affecting primarily the leptomeninges may spread along Virchow–Robin perivascular spaces to invade the brain or spinal cord, or it may remain more localized, involving the cranial nerves. Inflammation can also extend to the cerebrospinal fluid (CSF)-containing spaces, leading to hydrocephalus. Brain or spinal cord disease may appear as discrete granulomatous mass lesions or a diffuse encephalopathy-vasculopathy. The hypothalamic

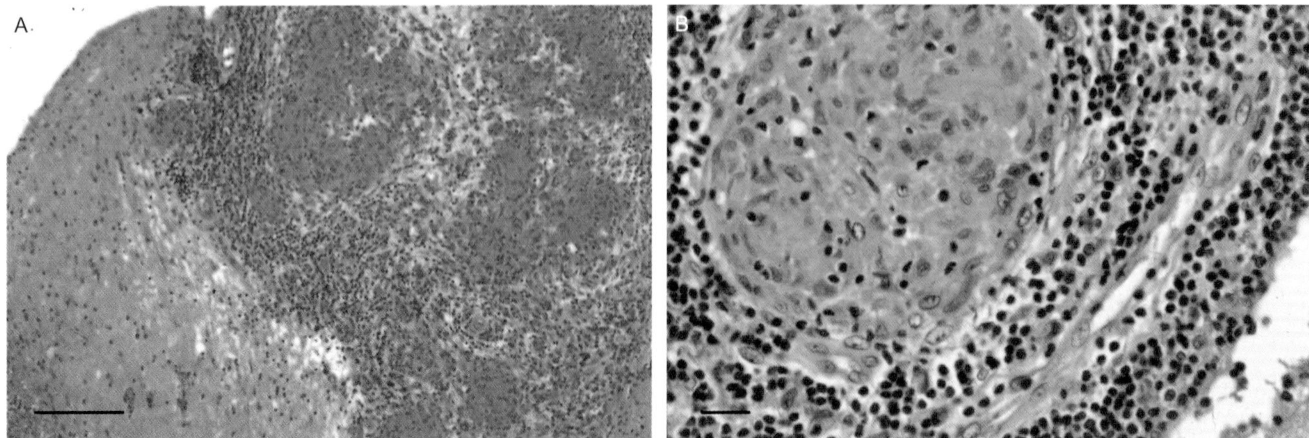

FIGURE 49-3 ■ Brain-biopsy section stained with hematoxylin and eosin. **A**, Low magnification photomicrograph showing dense granulomatous inflammation involving leptomeninges, with underlying gliotic cerebral cortex in a patient with neurosarcoidosis (scale bar, 50 μm). **B**, High magnification photomicrograph showing Virchow–Robin space involvement by a collection of epithelioid histiocytes (granulomatous inflammation) and lymphocytes in a patient with neurosarcoidosis (scale bar, 20 μm).

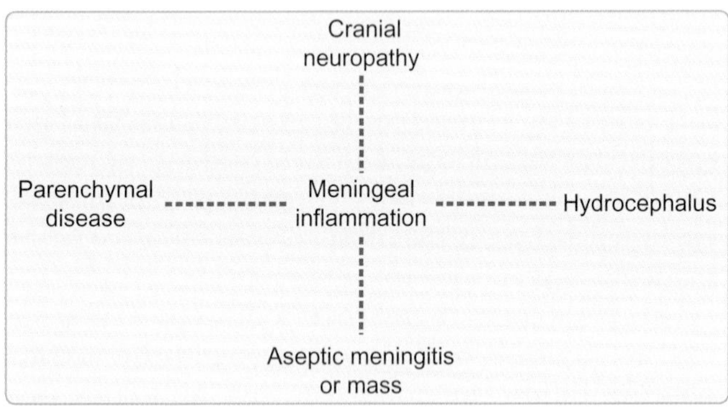

FIGURE 49-4 ■ Central nervous system (CNS) sarcoidosis: clinicopathologic relationships.

region is the most common site of parenchymal disease.

Granulomas can also be found in the epineurium and perineurium of peripheral nerves. The endoneurium may contain a mononuclear cell infiltrate. Perivascular and vascular inflammation may be seen in the epineurial and perineurial vessels. Nerve fibers of all sizes can be affected; a predominantly axonal neuropathy is usual, with only minor segmental demyelination.[8–10]

Muscle pathology is common in sarcoidosis. Muscle biopsy of symptomatic patients reveals typical noncaseating granulomas. More diffuse inflammation can occur, with muscle fiber degeneration along with regeneration and fibrosis.[8–10] Asymptomatic noncaseating granulomas are found in as many as one-half of all patients with systemic sarcoidosis undergoing muscle biopsy.[8–10]

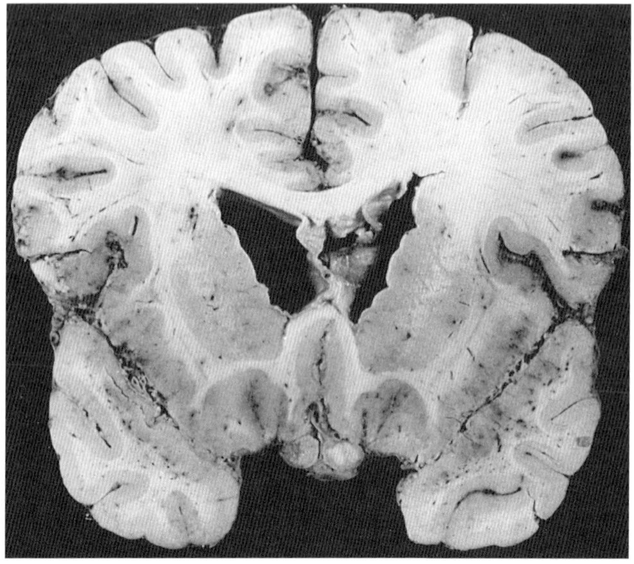

FIGURE 49-5 ■ Coronal midfrontal pathologic section of the brain of a patient with neurosarcoidosis, showing thickening and inflammatory changes of the basal meninges and optic chiasmal region.

EPIDEMIOLOGY

The prevalence of sarcoidosis is estimated to be on the order of 60 per 100,000 population, with an annual incidence of approximately 11 per 100,000 population. However, the exact prevalence and incidence are difficult to validate because there is no single confirmatory diagnostic test.[16] Sarcoidosis can occur at any age, although its peak is found in the third and fourth decades.

Population differences for sarcoidosis have been described. In the United States, its incidence is increased in blacks compared with whites; the disease also seems to be more severe in blacks.[14,16] Certain areas of the world, such as Sweden, have a higher incidence of sarcoidosis, whereas it is quite rare in other areas, such as China or Southeast Asia.[18] These observations raise the possibility of a genetic predisposition to the development of sarcoidosis, which does seem to occur with greater likelihood in some families.[32] As yet, no well-defined genetic pattern has emerged and no consistent mode of inheritance is recognized.[14,16] An increasing number of studies address candidate genes that may predispose to the development of sarcoidosis.[32–34]

TABLE 49-2 ■ Complications of Neurosarcoidosis

Clinical Manifestation	Approximate Frequency (%)
Cranial neuropathy	50–75
Facial palsy	25–50
Aseptic meningitis	10–20
Hydrocephalus	10
Parenchymal disease	
Endocrinopathy	10–15
Mass lesion(s)	5–10
Encephalopathy-vasculopathy	5–10
Seizures	5–10
Myelopathy	5
Neuropathy	5–10
Myopathy	10

NEUROLOGIC MANIFESTATIONS

Neurologic symptoms are the presenting feature of sarcoidosis in around 50 percent of individuals with neurosarcoidosis.[6,7] Some three-fourths of patients with neurologic disease present within 2 years of developing symptomatic systemic sarcoidosis. The approximate frequency of the various neurologic complications is presented in Table 49-2. Only rarely do patients with neurosarcoidosis have no evidence of even asymptomatic disease in other organ systems, such as the lungs.[6,8–10,17,35] One-third to one-half of patients with neurosarcoidosis will develop more than one neurologic manifestation of their disease.

Cranial Neuropathy

The most frequent neurologic complication of sarcoidosis is cranial neuropathy, occurring in approximately three-quarters of patients with neurosarcoidosis.[6–10] Any cranial nerve can be affected. More than one-half of patients will have involvement of multiple cranial nerves.[6,7]

Olfactory nerve dysfunction may occur secondary to meningeal sarcoidosis involving the subfrontal region. However, anosmia or hyposmia may also result from local nasosinus granulomatous invasion. *Optic nerve* involvement is much less frequent than other ocular manifestations of sarcoidosis such as uveitis. Optic neuropathy can present with visual loss that is acute, subacute, or chronic and can be painful or painless.[36] The visual loss may be due to bulbar or retrobulbar invasion of the optic nerve by granulomas, compression of the optic nerve by a granulomatous mass, or optic atrophy. Optic disc edema may be secondary to papilledema from sarcoidosis-induced increased intracranial pressure or result from direct local invasion by sarcoid. A chiasmal syndrome also has been reported.[36]

Disorders of ocular motility may follow involvement of the *oculomotor, trochlear,* or *abducens nerves.*[6,7] Typically, these nerves are damaged in their extra-axial course in the subarachnoid space as they traverse the meninges. However, they may also be involved in local orbital disease, and rarely the brainstem nuclei and eye movement pathways can be affected.[6–10] Occasionally, pupillary dysfunction is seen.[7] Uncommonly, disordered ocular motility is due to sarcoidosis involving the extraocular muscles themselves.[7]

Trigeminal nerve disease may present as facial numbness or, rarely, trigeminal neuralgia.[6] Headache may also represent trigeminal nerve dysfunction intracranially. Involvement of the muscles of mastication is unusual.

Of the cranial nerve syndromes, peripheral *facial nerve* palsy is the most common, and it is also the single most frequent neurologic manifestation of sarcoidosis. It develops in 25 to 50 percent of all patients with neurosarcoidosis. Although the condition is usually unilateral, bilateral facial palsy can occur, presenting with either simultaneous or sequential paralysis. More than half of all patients with facial palsy also have other forms of nervous system involvement. In patients with an isolated facial palsy, the spinal fluid typically is normal, but when other manifestations of neurosarcoidosis are present, the CSF is abnormal in 80 percent of patients. The specific cause of facial nerve palsy in sarcoidosis is variable. Rarely, the facial palsy is caused by parotid inflammation. More commonly, the nerve is compromised as it traverses the meninges and subarachnoid space, or facial paresis is due to intra-axial inflammation of the facial nerve. In general, the prognosis for the facial palsy is good, with more than 80 percent of patients having recovery of function.[6,7,12]

Eighth cranial nerve involvement is the second most common cranial neuropathy occurring in sarcoidosis. Inflammation may involve the auditory or vestibular portions of the nerve.[7,37] Loss of hearing or vestibular dysfunction may be sudden or insidious and often fluctuates over time. If hearing loss occurs, it is typically of the sensorineural type. As with facial nerve palsy, bilateral eighth nerve disease may occur, and either bilateral seventh or eighth nerve dysfunction is suggestive of neurosarcoidosis.[6–10]

Glossopharyngeal and *vagus nerve* involvement causes dysphagia and dysphonia. Hoarseness is more commonly due to laryngeal nerve dysfunction from intrathoracic disease than CNS inflammation involving the vagus nerve.[38]

Eleventh and *twelfth cranial nerve* disease may occur but seems to be rare.

Meningeal Disease

Meningeal disease occurs in approximately 10 to 20 percent of patients with neurosarcoidosis and can present as aseptic meningitis or, less commonly, as a meningeal or dural-based mass lesion. Aseptic meningitis is characterized by headache, meningismus, and sterile CSF with usually a mononuclear pleocytosis that can be recurrent.[39] Hypoglycorrhachia, or low CSF glucose concentration, is occasionally found, and there is often an elevation of the CSF protein concentration. It is not uncommon for there to be asymptomatic chronic meningitis within the context of other CNS manifestations of sarcoidosis. When meningeal sarcoid mass lesions occur, they may mimic intracranial tumors, such as meningiomas (Fig. 49-6).[40,41]

Hydrocephalus

Hydrocephalus is noted in about 10 percent of neurosarcoidosis patients and may have fatal consequences. Patients with acute hydrocephalus may die suddenly of increased intracranial pressure, and even patients with chronic hydrocephalus have the potential for acute decompensation. Patients with hydrocephalus characteristically present with headache, altered mentation or consciousness, and impaired gait. On examination, papilledema or other signs of raised intracranial pressure may be found. Acute decompensating hydrocephalus is a medical emergency that necessitates prompt diagnosis and treatment. Once clinically suspected, the diagnosis of hydrocephalus is best substantiated with imaging studies, such as cranial computed tomography (CT) or magnetic resonance imaging (MRI). A diagnostic lumbar puncture has been associated with sudden neurologic deterioration in some patients with hydrocephalus.[42]

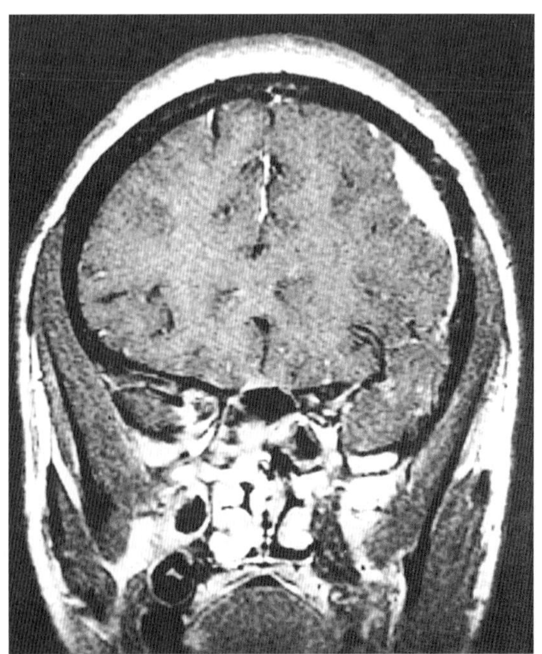

FIGURE 49-6 ■ Cranial magnetic resonance imaging (MRI), coronal section, T1-weighted image with gadolinium, demonstrating an enhancing convexity sarcoid mass lesion that was initially mistaken for a meningioma.

Chronic basilar meningitis with obliteration of subarachnoid CSF flow is a major cause of communicating hydrocephalus. In addition, infiltration of the ventricular system by granulomas, granulomatous compression of the aqueduct, or outlet obstruction of the fourth ventricle by granulomas may cause noncommunicating hydrocephalus.[43]

Parenchymal Disease

Parenchymal brain disease is reported in about 50 percent of patients with neurosarcoidosis and can present in several forms. Hypothalamic dysfunction is the most common manifestation of CNS parenchymal disease.

Endocrine Disorders

Any of the neuroendocrinologic systems can be affected by sarcoidosis due to either a hypothalamic or pituitary granulomatous mass or a more diffuse local encephalopathy.[44–46] Given the predilection of sarcoidosis for the basal meninges (Fig. 49-7), the relative frequency of such endocrinologic disturbances is not surprising.[47] Potential endocrinologic manifestations include thyroid disorders, disorders of cortisol metabolism, and sexual dysfunction. An elevated serum prolactin level, found in 3 to 32 percent of patients with sarcoidosis, may be an indication of hypothalamic dysfunction. Because neuroendocrinologic involvement is relatively common in individuals with CNS neurosarcoidosis, patients with more than just an isolated facial palsy probably merit a thorough evaluation with specific attention to hypothalamic hypothyroidism, hypocortisolism, and hypogonadism.

Hypothalamic disorders vary in their effect on vegetative functions. A disorder of thirst is the most common hypothalamic disorder related to neurosarcoidosis and is attributed to a change in the hypothalamic osmostat. More rarely, the syndrome of inappropriate secretion of antidiuretic hormone or diabetes insipidus occurs.[7,46] Neurosarcoidosis-induced disruptions of hypothalamic function can also cause disorders of appetite, libido, temperature control, weight regulation, and sleep.[6,7,46] Similar manifestations may occur from pituitary involvement.

Mass Lesions

An intraparenchymal lesion due to sarcoidosis may present as an isolated mass (Fig. 49-8) or masses in any cerebral area or as multiple cerebral nodules.[6–10]

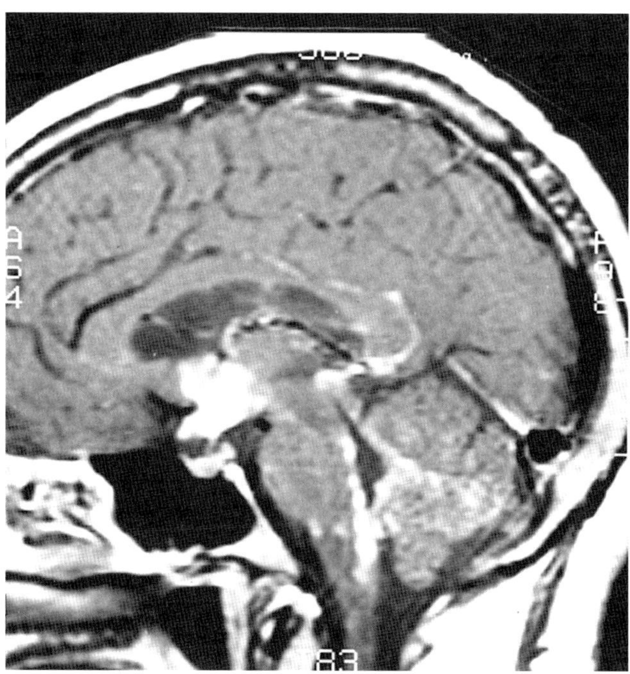

FIGURE 49-7 ■ Cranial MRI, sagittal section, T1-weighted image with gadolinium, showing hypothalamic and pituitary involvement by sarcoidosis.

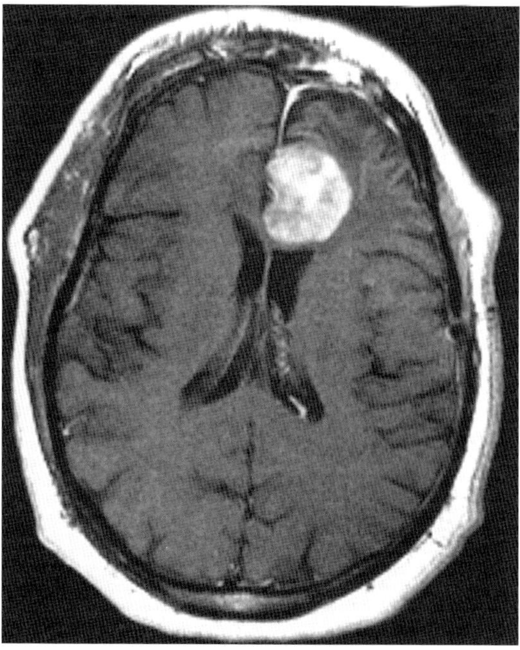

FIGURE 49-8 ■ Cranial MRI, axial section, T1-weighted image with gadolinium, demonstrating a frontal intracerebral mass that was proven by biopsy to be neurosarcoidosis.

Such nodules may represent an inflammatory reaction in the Virchow–Robin spaces. Subdural plaque-like masses may also occur and are discussed later. Calcifications may be seen, mimicking infection or tumor. Although intraparenchymal mass lesions were historically considered rare, CT and MRI have shown parenchymal disease to be more frequent. The symptoms and signs in individual cases depend on the location of the lesion.

ENCEPHALOPATHY-VASCULOPATHY

The diffuse encephalopathy and vasculopathy associated with neurosarcoidosis are not well understood. It is often difficult, both clinically and pathologically, to differentiate clearly between these entities and they frequently coexist. It is best therefore to consider them as a single overlapping entity, while recognizing that in individual patients, one form or the other may predominate.[6–11]

The diffuse encephalopathy-vasculopathy found in neurosarcoidosis can involve the cerebral hemispheres or posterior fossa. Patients may experience delirium, personality change, or isolated memory disturbance as a result of focal or diffuse parenchymal inflammation (Fig. 49-9).[6–11,48] Clinical findings correlate with the extent of enhancement on imaging studies including hyperintensity on T2-weighted or fluid-attenuated inversion recovery (FLAIR) MRI sequences.

Encephalopathic patients may have perivascular inflammation or granulomas infiltrating both arteries and veins, extending into the brain parenchyma. Several investigators have observed granulomatous arteritis in patients with neurosarcoidosis, involving small or large vessels (Fig. 49-10).[49,50–53] Veins can also be involved, producing venous infarctions.[50,51] Dural sinus obstruction may occur, causing intracranial hypertension.[7] Although the disease is rarely evident on angiography, changes suggestive of vasculitis as well as an ill-defined occlusive process may occur.[50,51]

Transient ischemic attack and ischemic stroke due to neurosarcoidosis are described.[50–52] Ischemic stroke usually is the consequence of inflammation and thrombosis of large or small arteries, but other causes include compressive perivascular mass lesions and emboli from sarcoidosis-associated cardiomyopathy or resultant cardiac arrhythmias. Caplan and co-workers have emphasized arterial and venous involvement of the meninges and parenchyma in the angiitic form of sarcoidosis and related this condition to perivascular lesions in the optic fundus.[52]

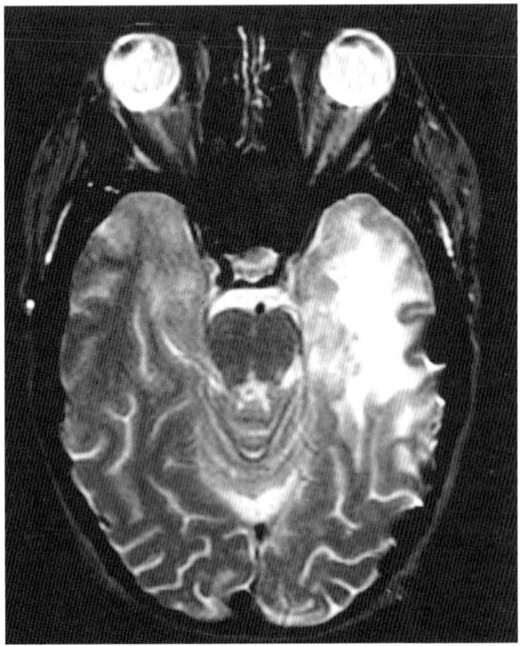

FIGURE 49-9 ■ Cranial MRI, axial section, T2-weighted image, showing a large area of hyperintensity in the temporal lobe that was proven by biopsy to be sarcoidosis manifesting with a focal encephalopathy-vasculopathy.

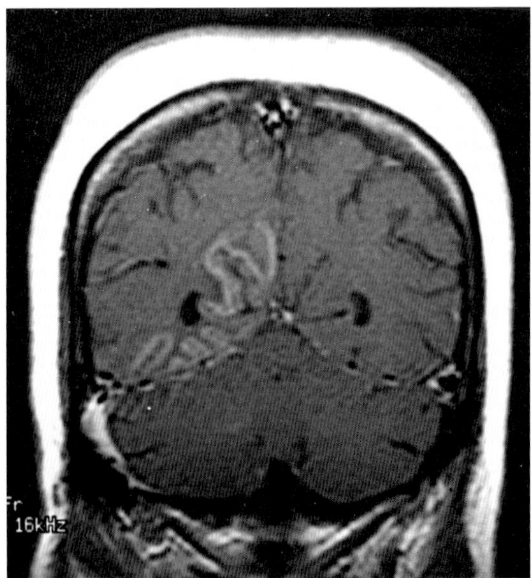

FIGURE 49-10 ■ Cranial MRI, coronal section, T1-weighted image with gadolinium, showing gyral enhancement in the distribution of a posterior cerebral artery branch stroke.

SEIZURES

Seizures may be a manifestation of CNS parenchymal disease due to neurosarcoidosis They may be focal or generalized and portend a relatively poorer prognosis than otherwise, reflecting the concurrence of severe CNS parenchymal disease or hydrocephalus.[13] Seizures in patients with neurosarcoidosis are relatively easy to control when the underlying CNS inflammatory process is treated effectively.[13,53]

MYELOPATHY

Spinal cord sarcoidosis may manifest as intramedullary, intradural but extramedullary, or extradural granulomatous masses.[54,55] Intramedullary spinal cord disease can present with a myelitis that is analogous to the cerebral encephalopathy-vasculopathy described earlier. Intraspinal mass lesions due to sarcoidosis present with a nonspecific imaging appearance, though associated leptomeningeal enhancement suggests sarcoidosis in the proper circumstances (Fig. 49-11). In addition, sarcoidosis may present as a radiculopathy, polyradiculopathy, or cauda equina syndrome. Spinal arachnoiditis sometimes occurs. Spinal cord sarcoidosis may appear in late stages as focal spinal cord atrophy.[54,55]

Peripheral Neuropathy

Although sarcoidosis commonly affects cranial nerves, peripheral neuropathy is described less frequently. It may take the form of a chronic sensorimotor, pure motor, or pure sensory polyneuropathy, mononeuritis multiplex, or an acute demyelinating polyneuropathy.[56–60] Historically, the most common form is a chronic sensorimotor polyneuropathy of axonal type.[56] Sarcoid neuropathy typically begins months to years following an initial diagnosis, but in some instances, symptoms precede the discovery of systemic disease. The neuropathy is usually mild and classically manifests with distal paresthesias, decreased vibration appreciation and proprioception, and reduced ankle reflexes.[56] Neuropathy has been attributed to epineurial and perineurial granulomas and an associated granulomatous vasculitis, producing axonal degeneration with associated demyelination. Endoneurial granulomas may also occur and are associated with primary

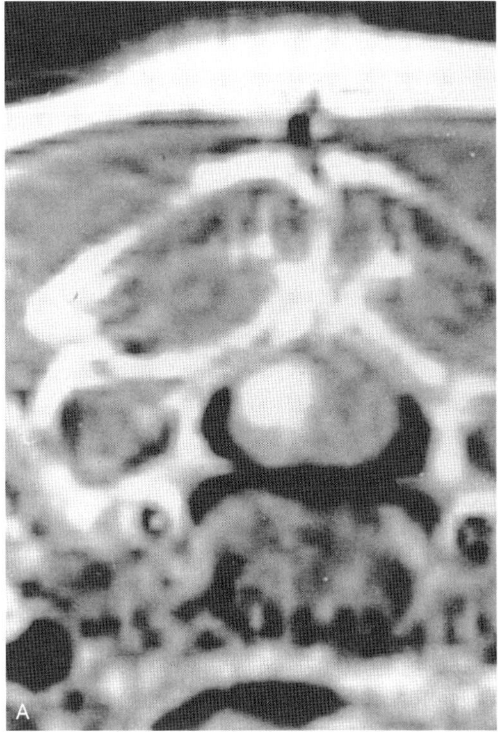

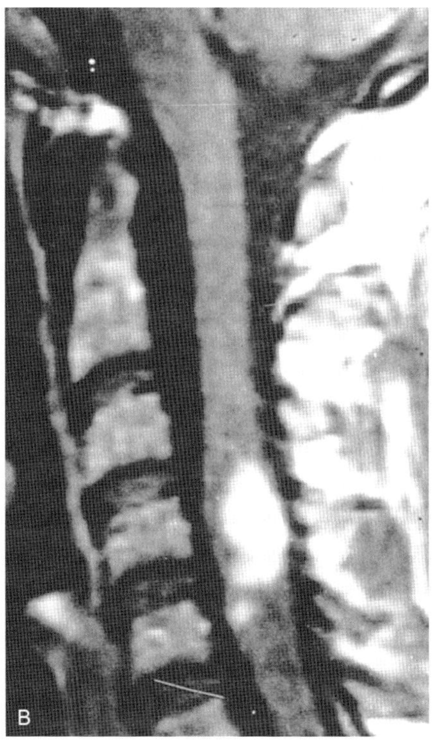

FIGURE 49-11 ▪ Spinal MRI. **A,** Axial view. **B,** Sagittal view, with gadolinium, demonstrating an enhancing intraspinal mass due to sarcoidosis.

segmental demyelination in patients with sensorimotor neuropathy. Nerve damage may be due to granulomatous vasculitis, the compressive effects of granulomas, or local effects of inflammation.

A sarcoidosis-associated small-fiber sensory neuropathy manifests with uncomfortable paresthesias distally in the extremities, associated with impaired pain and temperature appreciation and autonomic dysfunction.[57] Initially patients can experience multiple painful sensory mononeuropathies.[58] The pathophysiology of this process is poorly understood as granulomas are not found on skin biopsy. It is possible that the neuropathy is a response to inflammatory mediators, especially tumor necrosis factor alpha (TNF-α).[7,60]

Myopathy

Manifestations of sarcoid myopathy include acute, subacute, or chronic weakness; fatigue; muscle pain; and palpable muscle nodules. Severe muscle disease can result in fibrosis and contractures. Sarcoidosis may also manifest with myositis, muscle atrophy, or occasional pseudohypertrophy. Muscle involvement by noncaseating granulomas can be demonstrated with muscle biopsy, and incidental granulomas have been found in as many as 50 percent of patients with sarcoidosis but no clinical evidence of muscle disease. Differentiating between sarcoid myopathy, polymyositis or dermatomyositis, and granulomatous myopathy may be difficult, and it is important to evaluate other organ systems carefully for evidence of sarcoidosis.[6,7,61]

DIFFERENTIAL DIAGNOSIS

Diagnostically, two common clinical situations occur with neurosarcoidosis. In the first, a patient without established sarcoidosis has a clinical picture suggestive of neurosarcoidosis; the major goal is then to establish the presence of systemic sarcoidosis. In the second, a patient with already established systemic sarcoidosis develops neurologic symptoms, and it is then necessary to confirm that the neurologic problem is due to neurosarcoidosis rather than another cause.

Presence of Systemic Sarcoidosis

When a patient without documented systemic sarcoidosis develops a clinical syndrome suggestive of neurosarcoidosis, histologic evidence of sarcoidosis should be sought in other organ systems (Table 49-1). Sarcoidosis most frequently affects the intrathoracic structures (87% of patients), followed by lymph node, skin, and ocular involvement. Since corticosteroid therapy may mask signs of systemic disease, treatment should be postponed, if possible, while a search for systemic disease is initiated.[7,62]

Pulmonary involvement is so common in sarcoidosis that this possibility should be considered first when attempting to establish the presence of systemic sarcoidosis unless there is obvious skin disease or palpable lymphadenopathy. Evidence to support pulmonary involvement can be obtained from chest radiographs or CT scans and pulmonary function testing, including lung diffusion capacity. When these studies suggest pulmonary or intrathoracic lymph node involvement, transbronchial or mediastinal biopsy can be used to confirm the diagnosis.

Other sites of involvement of systemic disease can be considered for biopsy on the basis of clinical assessments including the nasosinus mucosa, conjunctiva, lacrimal gland, liver, and muscle.

A thorough ocular examination is indicated to search for uveitis, retinal periphlebitis, or superficial lesions for biopsy. Other ocular findings in sarcoidosis include iritis, retinal lesions (vascular sheathing, granulomas, vascular occlusions, and chorioretinitis), and optic disc pathology (edema, granulomatous nodules, and atrophy).[7,62]

Gallium-67 scanning has previously been promoted as a valuable imaging method for the detection of systemic sarcoidosis,[63] but recent experience indicates that fluorodeoxyglucose positron emission tomography (PET) scanning is more sensitive for highlighting regions of increased metabolic activity due to sarcoidosis.[64] Although increased activity on PET scans can represent neoplasia or infection as well as granulomatous inflammation, when used in the proper context, PET scanning can be a valuable tool for targeting biopsy.

Various laboratory measures may be abnormal in sarcoidosis including increased serum ACE level; increased serum gamma globulins; hematologic abnormalities such as anemia, leukopenia, and thrombocytopenia; and metabolic derangements, such as hypercalcemia, hypercalciuria, and hepatic and renal dysfunction. None is highly specific for sarcoidosis, but the most specific is the serum ACE level. Serum ACE is thought to be produced by alveolar macrophages and epithelioid giant cells and, in effect, reflects the "granulomatous load" of a patient. Serum ACE is neither highly sensitive, with just 50 to 60 percent of patients with active sarcoidosis showing abnormalities, nor very specific, because it is also often elevated in patients with other conditions.[7–10,65–67]

Diagnosis of Neurosarcoidosis

Patients with well-documented systemic sarcoidosis who develop neurologic disease merit careful appraisal to exclude causes other than sarcoidosis for their neurologic problem. Neurosarcoidosis can be confused with many other neurologic diseases and, because it is often not possible or judicious to biopsy affected tissue from the nervous system, the diagnosis may need to be made on purely clinical grounds.

Consideration must be given to disease entities that may mimic neurosarcoidosis, particularly infection and neoplasia. Once such disorders have been excluded, treatment for neurosarcoidosis can be instituted. When the response to treatment is disappointing, the diagnosis of neurosarcoidosis should be reviewed and a more extensive evaluation, including biopsy, contemplated to exclude other causes of symptoms and signs.

Brain imaging studies can be particularly helpful in neurosarcoidosis, and MRI with contrast is the preferred technique.[68] T1-weighted sequences provide less useful information than T2-weighted and FLAIR sequences where areas of hyperintensity can be better appreciated, especially in a periventricular distribution. Administration of contrast demonstrates leptomeningeal enhancement (Fig. 49-12) as well as parenchymal abnormalities (Figs. 49-7 and 49-8). Enhancement presumably reflects a breakdown of the blood–brain barrier and implies active inflammation. MRI changes in neurosarcoidosis may involve the white matter and mimic those seen in multiple sclerosis (Fig. 49-13).[7,69] Spinal MRI may reveal intramedullary disease, which appears as an enhancing fusiform enlargement, focal or diffuse enhancement, or atrophy (Fig. 49-11).[54,55] Enhancing nodules or thickened or matted nerve roots may be appreciated in the cauda equina.

CSF analysis may be helpful, and more than 50 percent of patients with CNS sarcoidosis have some CSF abnormality.[6,7,65,70] Reported abnormalities include an elevated CSF pressure, a high protein level, hypoglycorrhachia, and a usually predominantly mononuclear pleocytosis, with up to several hundred cells per mm^3. In addition, some patients have oligoclonal bands in the CSF or an elevated immunoglobulin G (IgG) index. None of these abnormalities is specific for neurosarcoidosis.[70]

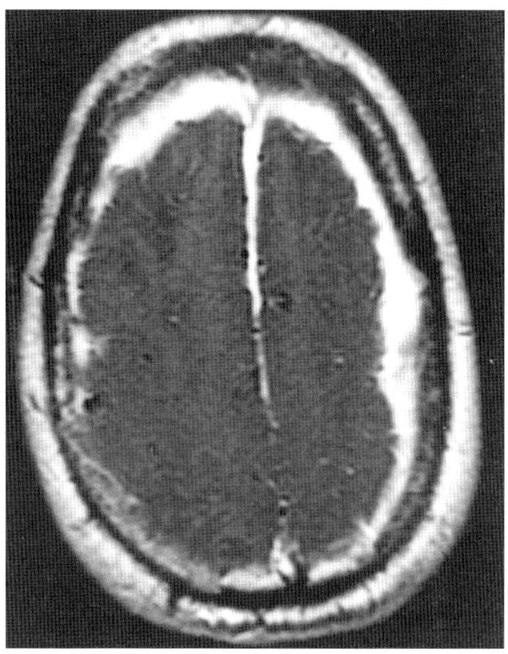

FIGURE 49-12 ▪ Cranial MRI, axial view, T1-weighted image, with gadolinium, demonstrating marked dural enhancement due to sarcoidosis.

The CSF level of ACE activity tends to be raised in some 50 percent of untreated patients with CNS sarcoidosis, although abnormalities are also seen in the presence of infection and malignancy.[7,65,66,67] CSF ACE is thought to be produced by CNS granulomas, especially those near the meninges. A normal CSF ACE assay, however, does not exclude the diagnosis of neurosarcoidosis.[7–10,65] Because of limited sensitivity and specificity, assay of CSF ACE activity is not recommended.[67]

Evoked potentials may be useful in evaluating some patients with neurosarcoidosis. Visual evoked potentials (VEPs) can reveal abnormalities of the anterior visual pathways. They are often abnormal in patients with symptomatic optic nerve disease and may be abnormal in some patients with CNS sarcoidosis but no clinical evidence of optic nerve dysfunction.[7,71] Similarly, brainstem auditory evoked potentials (BAEPs) are often abnormal in patients with brainstem or eighth nerve symptoms and may be abnormal in neurologically

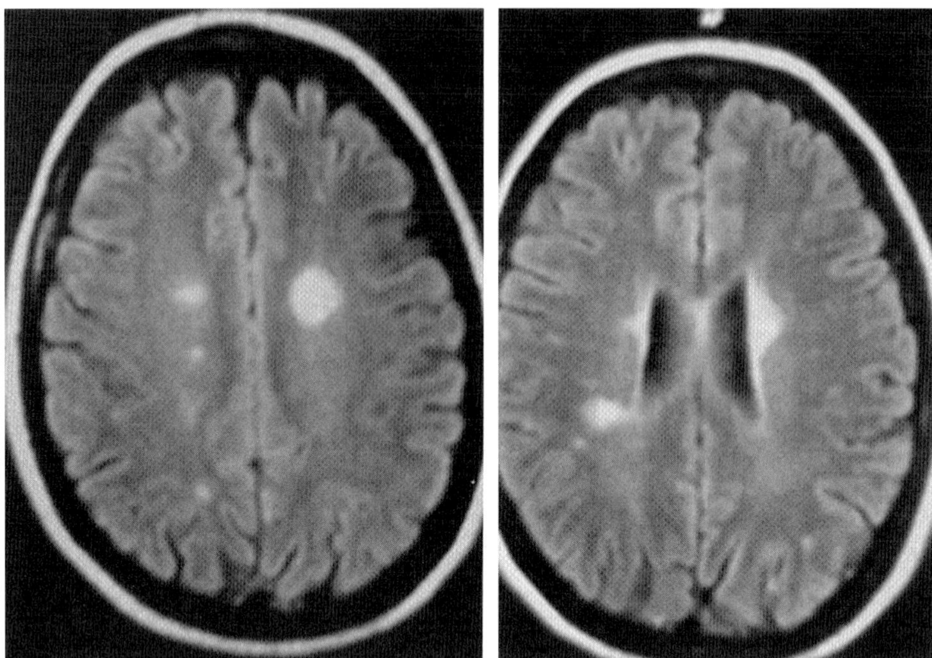

FIGURE 49-13 ▪ MRI findings of multifocal white matter–type changes in neurosarcoidosis. (From Scott TF, Yandora K, Kunschere LJ, et al: Neurosarcoidosis mimicry of multiple sclerosis: clinical, laboratory, and imaging characteristics. Neurologist 16:386, 2010, with permission.)

ill patients without overt disease in these areas.[7,72] Somatosensory evoked potentials (SSEPs) have not been comprehensively studied in the assessment of patients with sarcoidosis; preliminary evidence suggests that their clinical utility is similar to that of visual and brainstem auditory evoked potentials in confirming the involvement of a specific sensory system.[7,73]

Nerve conduction studies in patients with sarcoidosis-associated neuropathy usually reveal changes compatible with an axonal neuropathy, although slowing is sometimes more pronounced and suggestive of demyelination.[7,74] Electromyography may show denervation in patients with a neuropathy or radiculopathy and myopathic changes in patients with a symptomatic myopathy.[7,61] MRI of muscles may show a characteristic "star-shaped" pattern seen with sarcoid muscle nodules.[75] Muscle or nerve biopsy can be informative and muscle biopsy can be targeted to areas of MRI enhancement.[7]

Patients with sarcoidosis-associated small-fiber neuropathy typically have normal nerve conduction velocities but may have abnormalities on quantitative sensory and autonomic testing and a decreased number of small fibers in cutaneous nerves on skin biopsy of the extremities.[7,59]

The diagnosis of sarcoidosis is most secure when it is based on pathology and when more than one organ system is involved. However, since tissue from the nervous system is difficult to secure for pathologic analysis and other tests are not diagnostic of neurosarcoidosis, the diagnosis must sometimes remain tentative despite all efforts. In considering a diagnosis of neurosarcoidosis, it is useful to grade its likelihood.[43] We have found the following categories useful, as adapted from Zajicek and co-workers[35,62]:

Possible neurosarcoidosis: the clinical syndrome and diagnostic evaluation suggest neurosarcoidosis. Infection and malignancy are not excluded *or* there is no pathologic confirmation of systemic sarcoidosis.

Probable neurosarcoidosis: the clinical syndrome and diagnostic evaluation suggest neurosarcoidosis. Alternative diagnoses are excluded. There is pathologic confirmation of systemic sarcoidosis.

Definite neurosarcoidosis: the clinical presentation is suggestive of neurosarcoidosis, other diagnoses are excluded, and there is supportive nervous system pathology *or* the criteria for "probable" neurosarcoidosis are met and the patient has had a beneficial response to immunotherapy over a 6- to 12-month observation period.

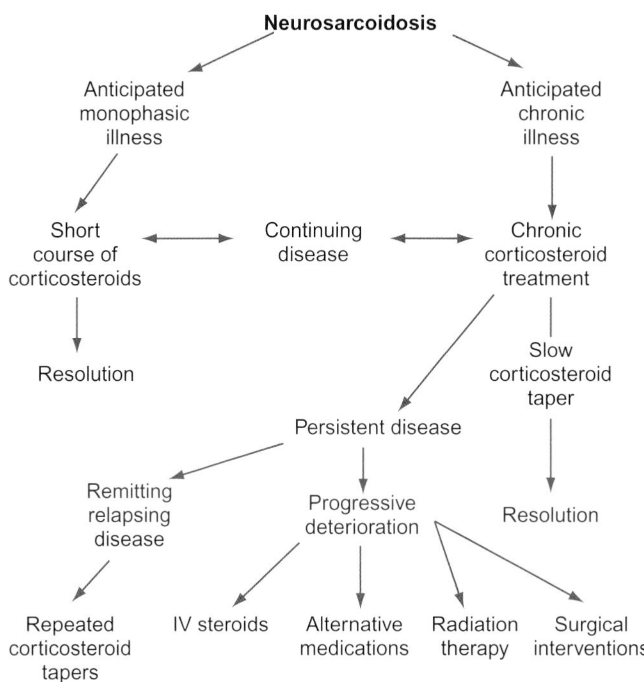

FIGURE 49-14 ■ Treatment paradigm for patients with neurosarcoidosis. IV, intravenous.

TREATMENT

No rigorous studies compare the various treatments for neurosarcoidosis. Although corticosteroid therapy is the mainstay of treatment, decisions regarding the optimal therapeutic dose and duration of therapy are made on an individual basis. A suggested treatment paradigm is shown in Figure 49-14.

Treatment with corticosteroids is widely accepted and recommended for all forms of neurosarcoidosis. Many individual case reports and series provide evidence that on a short-term basis it can produce impressive responses and alleviate symptoms. However, it is not fully established that treatment changes the natural history and long-term course of neurosarcoidosis. A major theoretical goal for long-term treatment with corticosteroids is to diminish the irreversible fibrosis that can develop and to minimize tissue ischemia from perivascular inflammation. Once treatment with corticosteroids or other immunomodulating or immunosuppressive agents is begun, it need not continue indefinitely, particularly at extremely high doses. The inflammatory process can recede, allowing therapy to be withdrawn gradually. Recommended treatment regimens for various specific manifestations of neurosarcoidosis are detailed.

Cranial Neuropathy

Peripheral Facial Palsy

Facial weakness may improve without any specific treatment, and the long-term prognosis for patients seems favorable. A controlled trial of treatment has not been performed; however, it seems reasonable to give a short course (2 to 4 weeks) of prednisone. For the first week, the recommended dosing is in the range of 0.5 to 1.0 mg/kg daily, or 40 to 60 mg daily. This is followed by a gradual reduction leading to discontinuation of prednisone over the subsequent weeks. General supportive care including protection from corneal abrasions, as for any patient with a peripheral facial palsy, should be provided.

Other Cranial Nerve Palsies

Patients with other cranial neuropathies may be managed with a corticosteroid protocol similar to that for peripheral facial palsy. However, often more than 2 weeks of therapy is needed. In particular, patients with optic neuropathy or dysfunction of the eighth cranial nerve may need more prolonged, aggressive therapy, which may not prevent irreversible nerve damage.

Aseptic Meningitis

Acute aseptic meningitis may respond to a short (2- to 4-week) course of prednisone. The goal of therapy for chronic aseptic meningitis is not complete clearing of an asymptomatic CSF pleocytosis. Attempts to completely normalize the CSF expose patients to the adverse side effects of corticosteroids or other therapeutic agents without evidence of benefit in patients who are otherwise asymptomatic.

Hydrocephalus

Asymptomatic ventricular enlargement usually does not require therapy. Mild, symptomatic hydrocephalus may respond to corticosteroid treatment; prolonged therapy is often appropriate. Life-threatening or corticosteroid-resistant hydrocephalus requires ventricular shunting or external ventricular drainage. Unfortunately, mild hydrocephalus may evolve to severe, life-threatening disease quite rapidly; therefore, patients and care-providers should be well educated as to the symptoms of acute progressive hydrocephalus and know to obtain prompt emergency care. High-dose intravenous corticosteroid therapy (methylprednisolone 20mg/kg per day for 3 days) sometimes stabilizes a patient with life-threatening hydrocephalus, but urgent ventricular drainage is usually necessary. Shunt placement is not without risk in this patient population, which is the reason that "prophylactic" shunting in asymptomatic patients with hydrocephalus is not advocated. Shunt obstruction is common, and placement of a foreign object in the CNS of an immunosuppressed host predisposes to infection. To further complicate management, there are case reports of patients with relatively modest hydrocephalus who, following a diagnostic lumbar puncture, develop marked neurologic deterioration, sometimes with a fatal outcome.[7]

Parenchymal Disease

Corticosteroid therapy may improve patients with a diffuse encephalopathy-vasculopathy or CNS mass lesion. Only rarely, however, does immunosuppressive treatment improve neuroendocrine dysfunction or vegetative symptoms.

Corticosteroid treatment of CNS parenchymal disease and other severe neurologic manifestations of sarcoidosis usually starts with prednisone, 1.0 to 1.5mg/kg daily. Critically ill patients may require high-dose intravenous corticosteroid therapy.[7,76] A short course of methylprednisolone, 20mg/kg daily intravenously for 3 days, followed by prednisone, 1.0 to 1.5mg/kg daily for 2 to 4 weeks, is a typical regimen. These higher intravenous doses are used in patients with particularly severe disease. Such patients often require more prolonged therapy, and prednisone should thus be tapered slowly, for example, by 5-mg decrements every 2 weeks as the clinical course is monitored. Neurosarcoidosis may worsen at a prednisone dose of 10mg or less daily.

Once a daily prednisone dose of approximately 10mg is achieved, the patient should be evaluated for evidence of worsening disease. Clinical disease can be monitored by symptoms and examination, but surveillance of subclinical disease of the CNS involves neuroimaging. Intense enhancement in the meninges, for example, suggests that neurosarcoidosis is active, and further decreases in the corticosteroid dose may lead to a clinical exacerbation. Other manifestations of neurosarcoidosis can be evaluated for subclinical deterioration on an individualized basis (e.g., by evaluating nerve conduction studies or serum creatine kinase level), but persistent mild CSF abnormalities are usually not an indication for continuing or escalating corticosteroid therapy. If neurosarcoidosis appears quiescent, a low daily prednisone dose of about 10mg can be tapered further by 1mg every 2 to 4 weeks. If a patient has a clinical relapse, the dose of prednisone should be doubled unless the dose is very modest, in which case a prednisone dose of 10 to 20mg daily can be prescribed; the patient should then be observed for approximately 4 weeks before another taper is contemplated. Patients may require multiple cycles of higher and lower corticosteroid dosing during attempts to taper medications. Since the disease may become quiescent, patients may be needlessly exposed to the harmful side effects of long-term, high-dose corticosteroids if attempts are not made to withdraw medication.

Seizures are generally not a major limiting problem and can usually be well controlled with antiepileptic medications if the underlying CNS inflammatory reaction is treated effectively. Seizures are an indication of, or marker for, the presence of parenchymal involvement of the brain.[12,13]

In patients with a CNS mass lesion that is unresponsive to high-dose corticosteroids, surgical resection may be considered, especially in life-threatening situations.

Peripheral Neuropathy and Myopathy

Patients with peripheral neuropathy or myopathy may respond to a several-week course of corticosteroids, usually beginning with oral prednisone, 1mg/kg per day (or approximately 60mg/day). Here, too, prolonged treatment may be indicated, and corticosteroids should be tapered slowly, as discussed earlier.

GENERAL SUPPORTIVE CARE

Patients with neurosarcoidosis, and particularly those receiving treatment with immunosuppressive agents, require close attention to their general medical well-being, including monitoring for potential adverse effects of treatment. Formal, prescribed exercise and dietary programs are often beneficial in helping patients avoid the weight gain associated with high-dose and long-term corticosteroid treatment. Rehabilitation services should be utilized as appropriate. Depression is not uncommon, and treatment is often helpful. Sleep disorders, especially sleep apnea, should be considered as a cause of fatigue or cognitive decline.

Therapy for endocrinologic disturbances is important. In particular, hypothyroidism, especially hypothalamic hypothyroidism, and hypogonadism are major problems in neurosarcoidosis that often require therapy. Patients receiving protracted, low-dose corticosteroid regimens require supplemental doses of corticosteroids during periods of intercurrent illness or stress. Hyperglycemia is a potential side effect of long-term, high-dose corticosteroid treatment but usually is not associated with ketoacidosis. Exercise and dietary programs are useful in managing hyperglycemia, but oral hypoglycemic agents or insulin therapy may occasionally be needed.[77]

Patients with sarcoidosis are at risk of osteoporosis, especially from corticosteroid therapy. The treatment of osteoporosis in this context is a challenge because sarcoidosis may cause hypercalcemia and hypercalciuria. Management requires reduction of corticosteroid dosage when possible, cautious use of supplements of calcium and vitamin D, hormonal treatment, and use of other bone-building agents.[78] Screening and serial measurements of bone density may be particularly useful.

Patients with refractory neurosarcoidosis are at risk from both the sarcoidosis-associated inflammatory process and the complications of various therapies. If a patient is not doing well, not only should the original diagnosis of sarcoidosis be questioned, but the patient should also be evaluated for intercurrent complications such as infection and malignancy.

ALTERNATIVE TREATMENTS

Treatment alternatives to corticosteroids are increasingly considered for patients with neurosarcoidosis (Fig. 49-14).[7–10,79] Indications for their use include contraindications to corticosteroids as initial therapy, serious chronic adverse effects of corticosteroids, an anticipated chronic course requiring high doses of corticosteroids, and progressive disease activity despite aggressive corticosteroid therapy. Medication alternatives to corticosteroids that have been used include immunosuppressive agents such as mycophenolate mofetil,[80–82] azathioprine, methotrexate,[82,83] cyclophosphamide, cyclosporine,[72] chlorambucil, and the purine analogue cladribine (2-chlorodeoxyadenosine).[7–10,77,84] Experience with these agents is limited, and they have not been studied in a scientifically controlled manner against placebos or comparable treatments.

Alternative therapy may allow a gradual decrease in corticosteroid dosage to prevent or minimize corticosteroid complications, often without deterioration in the patient's clinical status. Rarely, however, can corticosteroids be eliminated completely, and some patients may continue to deteriorate despite combination therapy.[6–10,78] The potential adverse effects of the therapy and extent of systemic disease should determine the choice of alternative treatment. It is wise to choose an agent whose adverse effects spare an organ or organ system that may already be compromised. In general, the side effects of these medications are limited, predictable, and respond to withdrawal of the offending agent. It may even be possible to restart the medication in some cases, without recurrent side effects.

Because TNF-α is implicated in the pathogenesis of granulomatous inflammation, TNF-α antagonists such as infliximab (Remicade)[81,85–88] and adalimumab (Humira)[88] have been used with success for refractory neurosarcoidosis.[7–10,20,79,81,85–89] Infliximab has been used in conjunction with corticosteroids and mycophenolate to treat severe CNS disease and adalimumab or intravenous immunoglobulin therapy may be beneficial for patients with small-fiber neuropathy.[90] Rituximab (a monoclonal antibody directed against B cells) has been beneficial in some case reports.[91]

Another option for some patients with refractory CNS sarcoidosis is radiation therapy. The small number of reported patients treated in this manner precludes definitive conclusions about efficacy. Some case reports suggest a beneficial response, especially if total nodal and craniospinal irradiation is performed.[92] A total dose of 19.5 Gy with daily fractionation of 1.5 Gy has been suggested. It appears that although radiation therapy is sometimes of benefit, continued immunosuppressive therapy is usually necessary.

Although it is not possible to predict with absolute certainty which patients with neurosarcoidosis will have disease refractory to conventional corticosteroid treatment, certain patients may have a particularly high-risk clinical profile. Patients with an optic neuropathy or CNS parenchymal disease (e.g., mass lesions or extensive encephalopathy-vasculopathy) are at especially high risk. Such patients might benefit from the prompt use of adjunctive alternative treatment if they either become refractory to corticosteroids or develop intolerable side effects. If a patient is stable for several months on low-dose prednisone and an alternative treatment, slow tapering of one of the drugs can be attempted.

PROGNOSIS

The clinical course and prognosis for neurosarcoidosis vary, but are somewhat predictable.[12,92] Some two-thirds of patients will have a monophasic neurologic illness; the remainder have a chronically progressive or remitting-relapsing course. Those with a monophasic illness typically have an isolated cranial neuropathy, most often involving the facial nerve, or an episode of aseptic meningitis. Those with a chronic course usually have CNS parenchymal disease, hydrocephalus, multiple cranial neuropathies (especially involving the optic or vestibulocochlear nerve), peripheral neuropathy, or myopathy.[12] Patients with CNS parenchymal disease or hydrocephalus are at highest risk of death, from either the inflammatory process itself or complications of therapy. Historically, mortality with neurosarcoidosis has been reported as approximately 5 to 10 percent, but more recent experience with new advances in treatment suggest that the mortality is in the lower range of that estimate.[6–10,12,13,93]

Because most patients with neurosarcoidosis are treated with immunosuppressive agents, it is impossible to determine the natural history of the untreated disorder.[6,7,12] Although therapy can certainly improve patients in the short term, it is not clear that the ultimate outcome of the disease is changed.[90] Even in severely ill or impaired patients, the inflammatory process may spontaneously subside over time. Other patients with remitting-relapsing or progressive disease can become severely incapacitated even with aggressive treatment.

In monitoring the response to treatment, a target measure, such as a specific clinical sign, symptom, functional assessment, or neurodiagnostic test, should be sought. For instance, a timed walk can be used for clinical assessment in some patients with gait disturbance from myopathy or spinal cord involvement; in patients with an intracranial mass, contrast-enhanced MRI is a helpful measure. This type of focused approach can be used to judge a response over a relatively short period of time.

REFERENCES

1. James DG, Williams WJ: Sarcoidosis and Other Granulomatous Disorders. WB Saunders, Philadelphia, 1985.
2. Burns TM: Neurosarcoidosis. Arch Neurol 60:1166, 2003.
3. Lieberman J, Kataria YP, Young JRL: Historical perspective of sarcoidosis. p. 1. In Lieberman J (ed): Sarcoidosis. Grune & Stratton, Orlando, FL, 1985.
4. Johns CJ, Michele TM: The clinical management of sarcoidosis: a 50-year experience at the Johns Hopkins Hospital. Medicine (Baltimore) 78:65, 1999.
5. Heerfordt C: Uber eine 'Febrid uveo-parotidea subchronica' an den Glandula parotis und der Uvea des Auges lokalisiert und haufig mit Paresencerebrospinaler Nerven kompliziert. Albrecht v. Graefes. Arch Ophthalmol 70:254, 1909.
6. Stern BJ, Krumholz A, Johns C, et al: Sarcoidosis and its neurological manifestations. Arch Neurol 42:909, 1985.
7. Krumholz A, Stern BJ: Neurological manifestations of sarcoidosis. p. 463. In: Aminoff MJ, Goetz CG (eds): Handbook of Clinical Neurology, Vol 71: Systemic Diseases (Part III). Elsevier, Amsterdam, 1998.
8. Terushkin V, Stern BJ, Judson MA, et al: Neurosarcoidosis: presentations and management. Neurologist 16:2, 2010.
9. Pawate S, Moses H, Sriram S: Presentations and outcomes of neurosarcoidosis: a study of 54 cases. QJM 102:449, 2009.
10. Joseph FG, Scolding NJ: Sarcoidosis of the nervous system. Pract Neurol 7:234, 2007.
11. Younger DS, Hays AP, Brust JC, et al: Granulomatous angiitis of the brain: an inflammatory reaction of diverse etiology. Arch Neurol 45:514, 1988.
12. Luke RA, Stern BJ, Krumholz A, et al: Neurosarcoidosis: the long-term clinical course. Neurology 37:461, 1987.
13. Krumholz A, Stern BJ, Stern EG: Clinical implications of seizures in neurosarcoidosis. Arch Neurol 48:842, 1991.
14. James DG, Turlaf J, Hosoda Y, et al: Description of sarcoidosis: report of the subcommittee on classification and definition. Ann NY Acad Sci 278:742, 1976.
15. Weinberg S, Bennett H, Weinstock I: CNS manifestations of sarcoidosis in children. Clin Pediatr 22:447, 1983.
16. Iannuzzi MC, Rybicki BA, Teirstein AS, Sarcoidosis. N Engl J Med 357:2153, 2007.
17. Nozaki K, Scott TF, Sohn M, Judson MA: Isolated neurosarcoidosis: case series in 2 sarcoidosis centers. Neurologist 18:373, 2012.
18. Tanoue LT, Zitnik R, Elias JA: Systemic sarcoidosis. p. 745. In: Baum GL, Wolinsky E (eds): Textbook of Pulmonary Diseases. Little, Brown, Boston, 1994.
19. Hoitsma E, Drent M, Sharma OP: A pragmatic approach to diagnosing and treating sarcoidosis in the 21st century. Curr Opin Pulm Med 16:472, 2010.

20. Agbogu BN, Stern BJ, Swell C, et al: Therapeutic considerations in patients with refractory neurosarcoidosis. Arch Neurol 52:875, 1995.
21. James DG: State-of-the art lecture: etiology of sarcoidosis. p. 43. In Sharma OP (ed): Proceedings of the Fourteenth International Conference on Sarcoidosis and Other Granulomatous Disorders. Edizioni Bongraf, Milan, 1994.
22. Semenzato G, Agostinit C: State-of-the art lecture: immunopathologies of sarcoidosis. p. 59. In Sharma OP (ed): Proceedings of the Fourteenth International Conference on Sarcoidosis and Other Granulomatous Disorders. Edizioni Bongraf, Milan, 1994.
23. Weissler JC: Southwestern internal medicine conference: sarcoidosis: immunology and clinical management. Am J Med Sci 307:233, 1994.
24. Moller DR: Cells and cytokines involved in the pathogenesis of sarcoidosis. Sarcoidosis Vasc Diffuse Lung Dis 16:25, 1999.
25. Myatt N, Coghill GK, Morrison K, et al: Detection of tumour necrosis factor in sarcoidosis and tuberculosis granulomas using situ hybridization. J Clin Pathol 47:423, 1994.
26. Thomas PD, Hunninghake GW: Current concepts of the pathogenesis of sarcoidosis. Am Rev Respir Dis 135:747, 1987.
27. Joyce-Brady M: Tastes great, less filling: the debate about mycobacteria and sarcoidosis. Am Rev Respir Dis 145:986, 1992.
28. Popper HH, Winter E, Hofler G: DNA of *Mycobacterium tuberculosis* in formalin-fixed, paraffin-embedded tissue in tuberculosis and sarcoidosis detected by polymerase chain reaction. Am J Clin Pathol 101:738, 1994.
29. Ghossein RA, Ross DG, Salomon RN, et al: A search for mycobacterial DNA in sarcoidosis using the polymerase chain reaction. Am J Clin Pathol 101:733, 1994.
30. Muller-Quernheim J: Sarcoidosis: immunopathogenic concepts and their clinical application. Eur Respir J 112:716, 1998.
31. Ishige I, Usui Y, Takemura T, et al: Quantitative PCR of mycobacterial and propionibacterial DNA in lymph nodes of Japanese patients with sarcoidosis. Lancet 354:120, 1999.
32. Rybicki BA, Iannuzzi MC, Frederick MM, et al: Familial aggregation of sarcoidosis: a case-control etiologic study of sarcoidosis (ACCESS). Am J Resp Crit Care Med 164:2085, 2001.
33. Hofmann S, Franke A, Fischer A, et al: Genome-wide association study identifies ANXA11 as a susceptibility locus for sarcoidosis. Nat Genet 40:1103, 2008.
34. Smith G, Brownel I, Sanchez M, Prystowsky S: Advances in the genetics of sarcoidosis. Clin Genet 73:401, 2008.
35. Zajicek JP, Entzian P, Dalhoff K, et al: Central nervous system sarcoidosis—diagnosis and management. QJM 92:103, 1999.
36. Graham EM, Ellis CJK, Sanders MD: Optic neuropathy in sarcoidosis. J Neurol Neurosurg Psychiatry 49:756, 1986.
37. Colvin IB: Audiovestibular manifestations of sarcoidosis: a review of the literature. Laryngoscope 116:75, 2006.
38. Tobias JK, Santiago SM, Williams AJ: Sarcoidosis as a cause of left recurrent laryngeal nerve palsy. Arch Otolaryngol Head Neck Surg 116:971, 1990.
39. Plotkin GR, Patel BR: Neurosarcoidosis presenting as chronic lymphocytic meningitis. Pennsylvania Med 89:36, 1986.
40. Osenbach RK, Blumenkopf BH, Ramirez Jr H, et al: Meningeal neurosarcoidosis mimicking convexity en-plaque meningioma. Surg Neurol 26:387, 1986.
41. Sethi KD, El Gammal T, Patel BR, et al: Dural sarcoidosis presenting with transient neurologic symptoms. Arch Neurol 43:595, 1986.
42. Scott TF: Cerebral herniation after lumbar puncture in sarcoid meningitis. Clin Neurol Neurosurg 102:26, 2000.
43. Schlitt M, Duvall ER, Bonnin J, et al: Neurosarcoidosis causing ventricular loculation, hydrocephalus, and death. Surg Neurol 26:67, 1986.
44. Capellan JI, Cuellar Olmedo L, Martinez Martin J, et al: Intrasellar mass with hypopituitarism as a manifestation of sarcoidosis. J Neurosurg 73:283, 1990.
45. Missler U, Mack M, Nowack G: Pituitary sarcoidosis. Klin Wochenschr 68:342, 1990.
46. Bihan H, Christozova V, Dumas J-L: Sarcoidosis: clinical hormonal, and magnetic imaging (MRI) manifestations of hypothalamic-pituitary disease in 9 patients and review of the literature. Medicine (Baltimore) 86:259, 2007.
47. Chapelon C, Ziza JM, Piette JC, et al: Neurosarcoidosis: signs, course and treatment in 35 confirmed cases. Medicine (Baltimore) 69:261, 1990.
48. Cordingley G, Navarro C, Brust JCM: Sarcoidosis presenting as senile dementia. Neurology 31:1148, 1981.
49. Meyer J, Foley J, Campagna-Pinto D: Granulomatous angiitis of the meninges in sarcoidosis. Arch Neurol 69:587, 1953.
50. Brown MM, Thompson AJ, Wedzicha JA, et al: Sarcoidosis presenting with stroke. Stroke 20:400, 1989.
51. Corse AM, Stern BJ: Neurosarcoidosis and stroke. Stroke 21:152, 1990.
52. Caplan L, Corbett J, Goodwin J, et al: Neuro-ophthalmologic signs in the angiitic form of neurosarcoidosis. Neurology 33:1130, 1983.
53. Joseph FG, Scolding NJ: Neurosarcoidosis: a study of 30 new cases. J Neurol Neurosurg Psychiatry 80:297, 2008.
54. Junger SS, Stern BJ, Levin E: Intramedullary spinal sarcoidosis: clinical and magnetic resonance imaging characteristics. Neurology 43:333, 1993.
55. Olek M, Jaitly R, Kuta A: Sarcoidosis and spinal cord atrophy. Neurologist 1:240, 1995.
56. Zuniga G, Ropper AH, Frank J: Sarcoid peripheral neuropathy. Neurology 41:1558, 1991.
57. Hoitsma E, Marziniak M, Faber CG, et al: Small fiber neuropathy in sarcoidosis. Lancet 359:2085, 2002.

58. Dreyer M, Vucic S, Cros DP, et al: Multiple painful sensory mononeuropathies (MPSM), a novel pattern of sarcoid neuropathy. J Neurol Neurosurg Psychiatry 75:1645, 2004.
59. Judson MA: Small fiber neuropathy in sarcoidosis: something beneath the surface. Respir Med 105:1, 2011.
60. Bakkers M, Merkies ISJ, Lauria G, et al: Intraepidermal nerve fiber density and its application in sarcoidosis. Neurology 3:1142, 2009.
61. Ando DG, Lynch III JP, Fantone CJ: III: Sarcoid myopathy with elevated creatine phosphokinase. Am Rev Respir Dis 131:298, 1985.
62. Judson MA, Baughman RP, Teirstein AS, et al: Defining organ involvement in sarcoidosis: the ACCESS proposed instrument. Sarcoidosis Vas Diffuse Lung Dis 16:15, 1999.
63. Savolaine ER, Schlembach PJ: Gallium scan diagnosis of sarcoidosis in the presence of equivocal radiographic and CT findings: value of lacrimal gland biopsy. Clin Nucl Med 15:198, 1990.
64. Dubey N, Miletich RS, Wasay M, et al: Role of fluorodeoxyglucose positron emission tomography in the diagnosis of neurosarcoidosis. J Neurol Sci 205:77, 2002.
65. Chan Seem CP, Norfolk G, Spokes EG: CSF angiotensin-converting enzyme in neurosarcoidosis. Lancet 1:456, 1985.
66. Tahmoush AJ, Amir MS, Connor WW, et al: CSF-ACE activity in probable neurosarcoidosis. Sarcoidosis Vasc Diffuse Lung Dis 19:191, 2002.
67. Dale JC, O'Brien JF: Determination of angiotensin-converting enzyme levels in cerebrospinal fluid is not a useful test for the diagnosis of neurosarcoidosis. Mayo Clin Proc 74:535, 1999.
68. Sherman JL, Stern BJ: Sarcoidosis of the CNS: comparison of unenhanced and enhanced MR images. Am J Neuroradiol 11:915, 1990.
69. Scott TF, Yandora K, Kunschere LJ, et al: Neurosarcoidosis mimicry of multiple sclerosis: clinical, laboratory, and imaging characteristics. Neurologist 16:386, 2010.
70. Reske D, Petereit H-F, Heiss W-D: Difficulties in the differentiation of chronic inflammatory diseases of the central nervous system—value of cerebrospinal fluid analysis and immunological abnormalities in the diagnosis. Acta Neurol Scand 112:207, 2005.
71. Streletz LJ, Chambers RA, Bae SH: Visual evoked potentials in sarcoidosis. Neurology 31:1545, 1981.
72. Oksanen V, Salmi T: Visual and auditory evoked potentials in the early diagnosis and follow-up of neurosarcoidosis. Acta Neurol Scand 74:38, 1986.
73. Stern BJ, Schonfeld SA, Sewell C, et al: The treatment of neurosarcoidosis with cyclosporine. Arch Neurol 49:1065, 1992.
74. Challenor YB, Felton CP, Brust JCM: Peripheral nerve involvement in sarcoidosis: an electrodiagnostic study. J Neurol Neurosurg Psychiatry 47:1219, 1984.
75. Otake S, Banno T, Ohaba S: Muscular sarcoidosis: findings at MR imaging. Radiology 176:145, 1990.
76. Soucek D, Prior C, Loef G: Successful treatment of spinal sarcoidosis by high-dose intravenous methylprednisolone. Clin Neuropharmacol 16:464, 1993.
77. Keenan GF: Management of complications of glucocorticoid therapy. Clin Chest Med 18:507, 1997.
78. Schneyer CR: Abnormal bone metabolism in a neurological setting. Neurologist 1:259, 1995.
79. Scott TF, Yandora K, Valeri A, et al: Aggressive therapy for neurosarcoidosis: long-term follow-up of 48 treated patients. Arch Neurol 64:691, 2007.
80. Androdias G, Mailler D, Marignier R, et al: Mycophenolate mofetil may be effective in CNS sarcoidosis but not in sarcoid myopathy. Neurology 76:1168, 2011.
81. Moravan M, Segal BM: Treatment of CNS sarcoidosis with infliximab and myocphenolatemofetil. Neurology 72:338, 2009.
82. Lower EE, Baughman RP: The use of low-dose methotrexate in refractory sarcoidosis. Am J Med Sci 299:153, 1990.
83. Lower EE, Baughman RP: Prolonged use of methotrexate for sarcoidosis. Arch Intern Med 155:846, 1995.
84. Lower EE, Broderick JP, Brott TG, et al: Diagnosis and management of neurological sarcoidosis. Arch Intern Med 157:1864, 1997.
85. Katz JM, Bruno MK, Winterkorn JMS, et al: The pathogenesis and treatment of optic disc swelling in neurosarcoidosis: a unique therapeutic response to infliximab. Arch Neurol 60:426, 2003.
86. Pettersen JA, Zochodne DW, Bell RB, et al: Refractory neurosarcoidosis responding to infliximab. Neurology 59:1660, 2002.
87. Kobylecki C, Shaunak S: Refractory neurosarcoidosis responsive to infliximab. Pract Neurol 7:112, 2007.
88. Santos E, Shaunak S, Renowden S, et al: Treatment of refractory neurosarcoidosis with infliximab. J Neurol Neurosurg Psychiatry 81:241, 2010.
89. Heffernan MP, Smith DI: Adalimumab for treatment of cutaneous sarcoidosis. Arch Dermatol 142:17, 2006.
90. Parambil JG, Tavee JO, Zhou L, et al: Efficacy of intravenous immunoglobulin for small fiber neuropathy associated with sarcoidosis. Respir Med 105:101, 2011.
91. Bomprezzi R, Pati S, Chansakul C, et al: A case of neurosarcoidosis successfully treated with rituximab. Neurology 75:568, 2010.
92. Ahmad K, Kim YH, Spitzer AR, et al: Total nodal radiation in progressive sarcoidosis. Am J Clin Oncol 15:311, 1992.
93. Ferriby D, de Seze J, Stojkovic T, et al: Long-term follow-up of neurosarcoidosis. Neurology 57:927, 2001.

CHAPTER

50

Connective Tissue Diseases, Vasculitis, and the Nervous System

RICHARD B. ROSENBAUM

Aminoff's Neurology and General Medicine, Fifth Edition.

The diseases discussed in this chapter are linked by their inflammatory mechanisms and the diversity of their effects on the nervous system. They often present diagnostic challenges. After reviewing each disease, the differential diagnosis of some specific neurologic syndromes is explored.

CONNECTIVE TISSUE DISEASES

Systemic Lupus Erythematosus

SYSTEMIC DISEASE

Systemic lupus erythematosus (SLE) is an inflammatory autoimmune disease characterized by the presence of a broad spectrum of autoantibodies, including antinuclear antibodies (ANAs). It is protean in its neurologic and systemic manifestations. Its severity varies from relatively mild skin problems and arthralgias to life-threatening multiorgan failure. The American College of Rheumatology (ACR) classification criteria are helpful for assessing the possibility of SLE and for understanding its diversity (Table 50-1). These criteria were designed for classification purposes for research studies and must be used cautiously for diagnosis as many are nonspecific. The criteria are also insensitive, and some patients have SLE even though they meet fewer than four criteria. The prevalence of SLE is 100 per million; 90 percent of patients are women, and the disease is more prevalent in blacks than whites. Peak age at onset is 15 to 25 years old.

SLE usually causes systemic symptoms such as fatigue, malaise, and fever. Perhaps 80 percent of patients have skin manifestations, such as sun sensitivity or the classic malar rash, and arthralgias or nondeforming arthritis. Other systemic manifestations include pericarditis, pleuritis, renal disease (ranging from asymptomatic proteinuria or hematuria to severe glomerulonephritis), anemia (classically autoimmune hemolytic anemia), thrombocytopenia, leukopenia, or lymphopenia. Inflammation can affect nearly any part of the body, including the lungs, gastrointestinal tract, and eyes.

Autoantibodies are present universally in patients with SLE. ANAs are present in nearly all lupus patients but also occur in about 10 percent of the general population, usually at a low titer, and in many other inflammatory diseases including rheumatoid arthritis (RA), Sjögren syndrome, systemic sclerosis, polymyositis, and multiple sclerosis. Patients with SLE often have other antibodies against more specific nuclear antigens, such as extractable nuclear antigen (anti-ENA), anti-Ro (SSA), anti-La (SSB), anti-Sm (anti-Smith, not to be confused with anti-SM, which is anti–smooth muscle), and antiribonucleoprotein (anti-RNP). Anti-Ro is often positive in the rare lupus patient who lacks ANA. Anti-dsDNA (double-stranded DNA) is also strongly suggestive of SLE. Depressed levels of complement components C3 and C4 are common in patients with lupus, especially during flares of inflammation, and suggest immune-complex deposition, classically glomerulonephritis.

TABLE 50-1 ■ American College of Rheumatology Classification Criteria for Systemic Lupus Erythematosus

1. Malar rash
2. Discoid rash
3. Photosensitive rash
4. Oral ulcers
5. Nonerosive arthritis in two or more joints
6. Pleuritis or pericarditis
7. Glomerulonephritis or proteinuria
8. Seizures or psychosis
9. Hemolytic anemia, leukopenia, lymphopenia, or thrombocytopenia
10. Immunologic laboratory abnormality, such as antibodies to double-stranded DNA or the SM antigen or a false-positive serologic test for syphilis
11. Positive antinuclear antibody test that is not caused by a medication

Patients are considered to have lupus if they meet four criteria and have no alternative diagnostic explanation for the abnormalities.

Modified from Tan EM, Cohen AS, Fries JF, et al: The 1982 revised criteria for the classification of systemic lupus erythematosus. Arthritis Rheum 25:1271, 1982.

Many patients with SLE have serum antiphospholipid antibodies; the most commonly assayed antibody is directed against cardiolipin. Some of these antibodies may prolong the partial thromboplastin time and are referred to as lupus anticoagulants. However, antiphospholipid antibodies rarely cause bleeding and paradoxically are frequently associated with thrombosis. Antiphospholipid antibodies may also be responsible for false-positive nontreponemal serologic tests for syphilis Most people with antiphospholipid antibodies do not have lupus or other autoimmune disease. Antiphospholipid antibodies may be present transiently, especially after acute viral infections, and may occur in many other systemic illnesses (Table 50-2).

The antiphospholipid antibody syndrome is defined as the persistence of moderate to high titers of antiphospholipid antibodies combined with a clinical episode of thrombosis or of

TABLE 50-2 ■ Conditions in Which Antiphospholipid Antibodies May Be Found

Behçet syndrome
Human immunodeficiency virus infection
Juvenile rheumatoid arthritis
Lyme disease
Malignant atrophic papulosis
Myasthenia gravis
Neuroleptic drug use
Rheumatic fever
Rheumatoid arthritis
Sarcoidosis
Sjögren syndrome
Syphilis
Systemic sclerosis
Temporal arteritis
Viral infection

Adapted from Rosenbaum RB, Campbell SM, Rosenbaum JT: Clinical Neurology of Rheumatic Diseases. Butterworth Heinemann, Stoneham, 1996.

pregnancy morbidity.[1] This syndrome is associated with thrombosis, especially deep venous thrombosis, pulmonary embolism, nonbacterial thrombotic endocarditis, and stroke and may accompany failures of pregnancy, including miscarriage, fetal death, premature birth due to placental insufficiency, pre-eclampsia, or eclampsia. Other phenomena that occur in antiphospholipid antibody syndrome include livedo reticularis, arthralgias, cardiac valve abnormalities, hemolytic anemia, thrombocytopenia, pulmonary hypertension, and Raynaud phenomenon. The antiphospholipid antibody syndrome may occur in patients with SLE or in isolation, in which case it is called primary antiphospholipid antibody syndrome. Patients with SLE who have antiphospholipid antibodies are more likely to develop neurologic manifestations including stroke and nonischemic syndromes such as headache and less common syndromes, such as chorea or myelitis.[2] Further discussion of the antiphospholipid antibody syndrome is provided in Chapters 11 and 25.

A variety of autoantibodies, including antibodies against endothelium, neurofilament, glial fibrillary acidic protein, neurons, microtubule-associated protein 2, lymphocytes, ribosomal P protein, NMDA receptor subtype 2, and gangliosides, occur in some patients with neurologic manifestations of lupus.[3] None of these has proven pathogenic action or diagnostic value.

Central Nervous System Disease

The central nervous system (CNS) manifestations of SLE vary tremendously in their symptoms, severity, mechanisms, and treatment. Although at times they are referred to collectively as neuropsychiatric lupus, they are best analyzed as a number of separate syndromes (Table 50-3). Depending on diagnostic criteria used, between 12 and 95 percent of patients with SLE have one of these symptoms during the course of their illness, and many patients will have more than one.[4] Neurologic events may be due to factors other than the direct effects of inflammatory disease (e.g., hypertension, uremia, other metabolic derangements, drug toxicity, opportunistic infections, coincident illnesses); in one series, more than 40 percent of neurologic syndromes in patients with lupus were not directly due to lupus affecting the nervous system.[5]

Cognitive dysfunction affects up to 80 percent of patients with SLE at some time during the illness.[6] The cognitive difficulties can be relatively mild and transient; irreversible deficits and dementia are much less common.

Migraine or tension headaches occur in patients with lupus, but whether they are more common in these patients is unclear.[7] When patients with lupus develop a new headache pattern, the differential diagnosis includes meningitis, stroke, posterior reversible encephalopathy syndrome, or pseudotumor cerebri.

More than one-tenth of patients with SLE seize at some time during the course of their illness.[8] Seizures can be one-time events, particularly if related to reversible conditions, such as metabolic derangements, drug toxicity, posterior reversible encephalopathy syndrome, or infections. However, SLE may also cause recurrent focal or generalized seizures, particularly in patients who have antiphospholipid or anti-Sm antibodies, stroke, or other focal brain lesions.

Patients with SLE are at increased risk of ischemic and hemorrhagic stroke via a variety of mechanisms, including cardiogenic emboli (in patients with myocardial infarction, atrial fibrillation, or nonbacterial endocarditis), atherosclerosis of large or small vessels, thrombosis associated with antiphospholipid

TABLE 50-3 ■ Central Nervous System Syndromes Observed in Systemic Lupus Erythematosus

Aseptic meningitis
Cerebrovascular disease (ischemic or hemorrhagic)
Demyelinating disease
Headache
Movement disorder (chorea)
Myelopathy
Seizure disorder (focal or generalized)
Acute confusional state
Anxiety disorder
Cognitive dysfunction
Mood disorder
Psychosis

Modified from ACR Ad Hoc Committee on Neuropsychiatric Lupus Syndromes: The American College of Rheumatology nomenclature and case definitions of neuropsychiatric lupus syndromes. Arthritis Rheum 42:599, 1999.

antibodies, and rarely, vasculitis. Patients with lupus are more than twice as likely as matched controls to develop carotid plaque.[9] All lupus patients need aggressive primary stroke prevention with attention to well-known risk factors such as smoking, hypertension, hyperlipidemia, and diabetes. When a patient does have a stroke, brain imaging is usually supplemented with a thorough evaluation of cardiac sources of emboli, vascular imaging of the head and neck, and measurement of antiphospholipid antibodies to clarify the etiology of the stroke and plan secondary stroke prevention.

Chorea occurs in perhaps 1 percent of patients with lupus. The movement disorder can be unilateral or bilateral, evolve slowly, and remit spontaneously; it may be the first clinical sign of lupus or appear later in the disease.[10] The chorea is often sensitive to variations in female steroid hormones. Patients with chorea often have increased levels of antiphospholipid antibodies but rarely have evidence of focal cerebral ischemia. Other movement disorders, such as cerebellar ataxia or reversible parkinsonism, are rare.[11]

Acute or subacute transverse myelopathy occurs in 1 to 2 percent of patients with SLE, sometimes as the initial presentation. Some patients evolve within 24 hours a flaccid, hyporeflexic paraplegia with urinary retention; these patients often have nausea, vomiting, fever, and active systemic disease. Their prognosis for neurologic recovery is poor.[12] Other patients evolve over days a spastic hyperreflexic paraparesis. They are usually afebrile and do not have active systemic disease; they may recover, or have recurrent episodes. Patients with optic neuritis or recurrent episodes of myelopathy may have neuromyeltitis optica with aquaporin-4 spectrum autoimmunity.[13]

Magnetic resonance imaging (MRI) of the spinal cord often shows T2 intramedullary signal extending over many spinal segments. Spinal fluid commonly shows a mild pleocytosis and elevated protein concentration and occasionally contains oligoclonal bands that are not present in the serum.

Acute episodes of aseptic meningitis occur in less than 1 percent of patients with SLE.[14] Spinal fluid studies are necessary to exclude an infectious cause, particularly in immunosuppressed patients. In patients with aseptic meningitis, spinal fluid usually shows a mononuclear pleocytosis, normal glucose, variable protein levels, and no evidence of a causative organism by culture, polymerase chain reaction, or serology. Drug-induced meningitis is an important consideration in the differential diagnosis. The aseptic meningitis of lupus can be self-limited or corticosteroid-responsive but is sometimes recurrent.

Patients with lupus commonly experience depression, anxiety, and other affective disorders. Perhaps one-fifth of patients will experience major depression during their lives, and many more will have difficulty with mood or anxiety. These disorders do not correlate with brain inflammation and are treated with routine psychiatric drugs, such as selective serotonin reuptake inhibitors and benzodiazepines, rather than with immunosuppressive therapy.

Patients with lupus are at risk of psychosis, delirium, or acute confusional states. When these occur, the differential diagnosis includes a wide variety of causes of encephalopathy, such as CNS inflammation directly from lupus, hypertensive encephalopathy, uremia, other metabolic derangements, drug toxicity, or seizures. Patients with hypertension, renal failure, or taking drugs such as corticosteroids or cyclosporine may develop the posterior reversible encephalopathy syndrome.[15] In psychotic patients on corticosteroids, differentiating lupus psychosis from steroid psychosis is important to plan therapy.[16]

The focal neurologic syndromes of SLE may mimic many clinical features of multiple sclerosis. The ACR classification (Table 50-3) refers to these as demyelinating syndromes, but a more general description is that of multifocal white matter lesions. Like the lesions of multiple sclerosis, these lesions are often associated with relapsing-remitting focal syndromes involving areas such as the optic nerve, brainstem, and spinal cord. In patients with lupus, MRI of the brain often shows areas of T2 signal in the cerebral white matter, including periventricular lesions. Occasionally patients with lupus have oligoclonal bands in the cerebrospinal fluid (CSF) that are not present in serum or increased intrathecal immunoglobulin G synthesis. Conversely, some patients with MS have systemic autoantibodies such as ANAs or antiphospholipid antibodies.

Peripheral Nervous System Disease

The peripheral nervous system is also affected in SLE (Table 50-4). Carpal tunnel syndrome is probably the most common manifestation, occurring in up to 30 percent of patients in different series. Patients occasionally have other compression neuropathies. A number of patients develop a distal symmetric axonal sensory or sensorimotor peripheral neuropathy, which is usually relatively mild. Patients with mild neuropathy rarely need nerve biopsy or aggressive immunosuppression, even though the nerve, if biopsied, might show some epineurial vasculitis. Findings of autonomic neuropathy, such as abnormal pupillary responses, impaired sweating, loss of cardiovascular reflexes, and impaired gastrointestinal mobility, can also occur in lupus patients, regardless of whether they have sensory neuropathy.[17]

Acute demyelinating polyneuropathy, clinically and electrodiagnostically similar to Guillain–Barré syndrome, affects up to 1 percent of patients with lupus, depending on the series. This is higher than in the general population. The differential diagnosis of acute motor neuropathy in patients with lupus includes vasculitic neuropathy, particularly if the presentation is asymmetric; however, this is uncommon. Patients with lupus also have increased risk of chronic inflammatory demyelinating polyneuropathy, myasthenia gravis, and possibly neuralgic amyotrophy.

Less than 2 percent of patients with lupus develop cranial mononeuropathies, most often of the facial nerve.

TABLE 50-4 ■ Peripheral Nervous System Syndromes in Patients with Systemic Lupus Erythematosus

Syndrome	Prevalence
Sensory or sensorimotor distal neuropathy	7.5%
Mononeuropathy	1.5%
Cranial neuropathy	1.7%
Mononeuritis multiplex	0.6%
Guillain–Barré syndrome	0.1%
Chronic inflammatory demyelinating polyneuropathy	0.3%
Autonomic neuropathy	0
Myasthenia gravis	0
Neuropathies not directly attributable to SLE	5.3%

The prevalence rates are from the University of Toronto SLE database, based on following 1,533 patients with lupus; mean disease duration was 8.3 years at time of diagnosis of neuropathy.[97]
Prevalence rates differ in different series.

Treatment

Treatment of SLE, with or without neurologic involvement, must be individualized based on the organ systems involved and the severity of involvement. Thus, mild arthralgias might be treated with nonsteroidal anti-inflammatory drugs (NSAIDs), whereas severe renal or other visceral disease often justifies aggressive immunosuppression with cyclophosphamide or mycophenolate mofetil. Many of the neurologic manifestations of SLE can be treated symptomatically. Examples include recurrent headache, mood and anxiety disorders, carpal tunnel syndrome, and length-dependent peripheral neuropathy. Cognitive dysfunction usually requires no specific therapy; behavioral approaches to cognitive therapy deserve exploration.

All patients with SLE should attend to factors for stroke prevention. Those who have had a stroke associated with atrial fibrillation or some other cardiac sources are often treated with warfarin. The appropriate treatment (anticoagulation versus antiplatelet medications) for patients with stroke and antiphospholipid antibodies is debated, as discussed in Chapter 11.

Patients with lupus psychosis can be managed with antipsychotic drugs, and, once corticosteroid-induced psychosis has been excluded, with steroids. Patients with Guillain–Barré syndrome or myasthenia can be treated with intravenous immunoglobulin (IVIg) or plasmapheresis; however, some patients do not respond to these but appear responsive to corticosteroids combined with cyclophosphamide. Patients with focal CNS inflammatory syndromes such as myelopathy, optic neuritis, or focal cerebral white matter lesions are sometimes treated with corticosteroids alone, but prognosis is better if this is combined with immunosuppressives such as cyclophosphamide.

Sjögren Syndrome

Systemic Disease

Sjögren syndrome is a chronic autoimmune disorder that causes inflammation in many organs but particularly in the exocrine glands, primarily the salivary and lacrimal glands, leading to dry mouth (xerostomia) and dry eyes (xerophthalmia) that can be severe enough to damage the conjunctiva or cornea (keratoconjunctivitis sicca).[18] In many cases, Sjögren syndrome is associated with other rheumatic diseases such as rheumatoid arthritis, SLE, or systemic sclerosis. Sjögren syndrome occurring without another connective tissue disease is known as primary Sjögren syndrome, which is the focus in the following discussion. Most (90%) patients with Sjögren syndrome are women, usually middle-aged. The prevalence is difficult to determine because of varying definitions, but in the United States it may exceed 1,000 cases per million. The European classification criteria are listed in Table 50-5.

TABLE 50-5 ■ European Diagnostic Criteria for Sjögren Syndrome

1. Ocular dryness, daily, for more than 3 months
2. Oral dryness for more than 3 months
3. Objective evidence of keratoconjunctivitis sicca, such as a positive Schirmer I test (<5 mm in 5 minutes) or an increased Rose Bengal score
4. Histopathology with a focus score of 1 in a minor salivary gland biopsy specimen
5. Objective evidence of reduced salivary flow (salivary flow rate [<1.5 ml in 15 minutes], salivary scintigraphy, or parotid sialography)
6. Autoantibodies including anti-Ro (SSA) or La (SSB), ANA, or rheumatoid factor

Probable Sjögren syndrome: presence of three or more items

Definite Sjögren syndrome: presence of four or more items

Modified from Vitali C, Bombardieri S, Moutsopoulos HM, et al: Assessment of the European classification criteria for Sjögren's syndrome in a series of clinically defined cases: results of a prospective multicentre study. The European Study Group on Diagnostic Criteria for Sjögren's syndrome. Ann Rheum Dis 55:116, 1996.

In addition to dry eyes and dry mouth, Sjögren syndrome may cause dysfunction of other exocrine glands, resulting in dry skin, vagina, or upper respiratory tract. Patients commonly have systemic symptoms such as arthralgias, myalgias, or fatigue, and less often weight loss or fever. They may have palpable purpura due to small-vessel vasculitis, but inflammation of larger arteries is uncommon. Sjögren syndrome may also cause renal (interstitial nephritis, renal tubular acidosis), thyroid (thyroiditis, hypothyroidism), gastrointestinal (atrophic gastritis, dysphagia), pulmonary (interstitial pneumonitis), and liver disease (biliary cirrhosis, sclerosing cholangitis). Liver, spleen, or lymph nodes may be enlarged. Patients have an increased risk of developing lymphoma.

The common symptoms of dry eyes or dry mouth have numerous alternative causes including drugs, aging, or the local effects of contact lenses. In patients with sicca, parotid enlargement, systemic symptoms, and neurologic findings, sarcoidosis is often prominent in the differential diagnosis.

The pathogenesis of Sjögren syndrome is unknown. The pathologic changes in exocrine glands are lymphocytic infiltrates. Patients with Sjögren syndrome commonly have serologic evidence of autoimmunity including ANAs (present in perhaps three-fourths of patients). The anti-Ro (SSA) and anti-La (SSB) antibodies are more specific to Sjögren syndrome but are also sometimes present in patients with SLE and other autoimmune disease and have limited sensitivity, occurring in between one-fourth and three-fourths of patients. Blood studies may also show rheumatoid factor, anemia, lymphopenia, and hypergammaglobulinemia; monoclonal gammopathy occurs less frequently.

Central Nervous System Disease

The prevalence of CNS disease in patients with Sjögren syndrome is unclear, with wide-ranging estimates. Part of this discrepancy is because the most common CNS problems are mild and nonspecific, such as subtle cognitive dysfunction, headache, or affective disorders.[19] Probably 10 percent or less of patients with Sjögren syndrome have serious neurologic complications, such as focal brain lesions, which may present abruptly, simulating a stroke, or more gradually.[20] The cerebral hemispheres or the brainstem can be affected; white matter syndromes are more common than gray matter syndromes. Neuropathologic examination of the focal brain lesions shows mononuclear infiltrates of veins, venules, and, less commonly, small arteries or arterioles. The surrounding brain tissue may show focal infarcts, which are usually microscopic. Meningeal vessels are often involved. Syndromes clinically associated with gray matter disease, such as seizures, may occur but are less common.

Even though the pathologic process in patients with Sjögren syndrome often includes the meninges, clinical meningitis is not common; however, instances of aseptic meningitis do occur and at times become chronic or recurrent. The CSF typically shows mild mononuclear pleocytosis, occasional elevation of protein level, and, less frequently, oligoclonal bands that are not present in the serum or evidence of increased intrathecal IgG synthesis.

Lesions localized to the spinal cord are one of the most common focal CNS findings in Sjögren syndrome. The myelopathy may evolve slowly or rapidly, be generalized or localized, with presentations as varied as transverse myelopathy or Brown-Séquard syndrome. Some patients also have episodes of optic neuritis. In most cases, spinal MRI shows T2-hyperintense intramedullary lesions spanning multiple spinal segments. Sometimes the cord appears swollen, and some lesions enhance with gadolinium. Patients with optic neuritis or longitudinally extensive myelopathy may be part of the spectrum of neuromyelitis optica and often have aquaporin 4 antibodies.

The CNS lesions of Sjögren syndrome can evolve with a relapsing-remitting course that approximates that of multiple sclerosis. When Sjögren syndrome causes optic neuritis, focal paresthesias, brainstem syndromes such as internuclear ophthalmoplegia, or myelopathy, the diagnosis may erroneously be that of multiple sclerosis.

Peripheral Nervous System Disease

In patients with Sjögren syndrome, peripheral nervous disease is more common than CNS disease, and can be the presenting manifestation.[21] The peripheral neuropathies of Sjögren syndrome can be separated into a number of clinical syndromes, but many patients have overlapping features (Table 50-6).

Distal sensory or sensorimotor neuropathy, clinically evident in up to one-fifth of patients with Sjögren syndrome, is the most common peripheral neuropathy. Other patients will have asymptomatic neuropathy detectable by nerve conduction studies. The typical presentation is a chronic distal axonal neuropathy including small and large sensory fibers. Distal motor involvement is less common. Nerve biopsy specimen usually shows nonspecific axonal loss rather than vasculitis. Some patients with otherwise idiopathic axonal neuropathy will meet diagnostic criteria for Sjögren syndrome.[22] However, if neuropathy patients have dry eyes or a dry mouth but no other objective supportive findings, they are unlikely later to develop systemic manifestations of Sjögren syndrome.

TABLE 50-6 ■ Peripheral Nervous System Syndromes in Patients with Sjögren Syndrome

Sensory neuronopathy (sensory ataxic neuropathy)
Painful sensory neuropathy
Autonomic neuropathy
Trigeminal neuropathy
Mononeuritis multiplex
Multiple cranial neuropathy
Radiculoneuropathy

Data from Mori K, Iijima M, Koike H, et al: The wide spectrum of clinical manifestations in Sjögren's syndrome–associated neuropathy. Brain 128:2518, 2005.

Sensory neuronopathy presents acutely or indolently as asymmetric dysfunction of large and small sensory fibers. Patients often have impaired distal or proximal cutaneous touch, pain, temperature, and joint position senses. They may have pseudoathetosis and sensory ataxia with depressed tendon reflexes.[23] Many patients also have trigeminal or autonomic neuropathy. On electrodiagnostic studies, most patients have some low-amplitude or unobtainable sensory nerve action potentials and somatosensory evoked potentials. Spinal cord MRI often shows T2-hyperintense signal in the posterior columns.[24] Sensory nerve biopsy shows axonal loss of large and small myelinated fibers and of unmyelinated fibers, but few biopsy specimens show vasculitic changes or lymphocytic infiltrates. Pathologic findings in the dorsal root ganglia may include neuronal destruction and lymphocytic infiltration. In addition to dry eyes and dry mouth, these patients often fully meet diagnostic criteria for Sjögren syndrome, including objective evidence of xerophthalmia and xerostomia and abnormal lip biopsy samples; however, they usually do not have other systemic manifestations.

Trigeminal neuropathy impairs sensation, usually in the mandibular or maxillary divisions, unilaterally or bilaterally, with acute or subacute evolution, but causes no trigeminal motor dysfunction. Electrodiagnostic studies suggest abnormality of the trigeminal ganglion with impaired blink reflexes but normal masseteric reflexes.

Mild autonomic neuropathy, with manifestations such as Adie pupil, orthostatic hypotension, impaired sweating, constipation or diarrhea, and abnormal cardiac reflexes, often accompanies the other neuropathies of Sjögren syndrome. In an occasional patient, more severe autonomic dysfunction, sometimes accompanied by antibodies against the ganglionic acetylcholine receptor, is the predominant neurologic problem.[25]

Mononeuritis multiplex or multiple cranial neuropathies may also occur. In contrast to trigeminal sensory neuropathy, the multiple cranial neuropathies may also affect motor function and can include nerves III, V, VI, VII, IX, X, and XII. Biopsy of an involved peripheral nerve is likely to show epineurial vasculitis.

Other neuropathic presentations occasionally found in patients with Sjögren syndrome include painful asymmetric sensory neuropathy, proximal radiculoneuropathy, Guillain–Barré syndrome, and lower motor neuronopathy. Predominantly motor neuropathy is less common in patients with Sjögren syndrome. Motor neuron disease is only linked to Sjögren syndrome by case reports. Carpal tunnel syndrome occurs in some patients with Sjögren syndrome.

Treatment

Treatment varies greatly depending on the organs involved and the severity of disease.[26] Dry eyes may be treated with artificial tears or topical approaches; arthralgias may be controlled with nonsteroidal anti-inflammatory drugs or with antimalarials such as hydroxychloroquine. There is no specific cure for some neurologic syndromes, such as mild cognitive impairment, trigeminal neuropathy, or distal sensory neuropathy. Myelopathy or symptomatic focal brain lesions are often treated with corticosteroids, sometimes in conjunction with cyclophosphamide. Mononeuritis multiplex or multiple cranial neuropathies also appear responsive to corticosteroids, sometimes with cyclophosphamide added. A minority of patients with sensory neuronopathy improve after treatment with corticosteroids, IVIg, or other immunosuppressants.[27]

Systemic Sclerosis

Systemic sclerosis causes a noninflammatory vasculopathy and fibrosis in multiple organs. The pathogenesis is unknown, but the combination of microvascular ischemia and fibrosis causes the bulk of clinical manifestations of systemic sclerosis. Strictly speaking, "scleroderma" refers to the typical skin thickening of systemic sclerosis; however, patients may have purely cutaneous scleroderma alone without having systemic sclerosis, and scleroderma limited to the skin is not associated with the neurologic complications discussed later. Estimated prevalence in the United States is between 100 and 300 cases per million population, with an annual incidence about one-tenth of the prevalence; the disease affects women more than men, and blacks more than whites.

Systemic Disease

Scleroderma with visceral involvement is called systemic sclerosis; this is further divided into limited cutaneous systemic sclerosis and diffuse cutaneous systemic sclerosis. Patients with limited cutaneous systemic sclerosis may have "CREST syndrome": subcutaneous calcinosis, Raynaud phenomenon, esophageal dysfunction, sclerodactyly (tight digital skin), and telangiectasia. The esophageal disease often causes dysphagia. Some patients have only CREST and no other systemic disease; however, systemic sclerosis can also cause pulmonary fibrosis, renal or cardiac involvement, especially with hypertension, hypothyroidism, sicca syndrome, arthralgias, and tenosynovitis. Almost all patients with systemic sclerosis have some serologic evidence of autoimmunity, including ANAs and antibodies directed against antigens such as centromeres, topoisomerase, U1-RNP, RNA polymerase III, U3-RNP, and Th/To.[28] These antibodies have some prognostic value: for example, patients with anti-centromere antibodies usually have the CREST syndrome, are at risk of pulmonary hypertension, but usually do not develop more diffuse systemic disease. Perhaps those with anti-U1-RNP or anti-Scl-70 are more prone to neurologic complications.

Central Nervous System Disease

CNS disease is not particularly common in patients with systemic sclerosis, so whether reported cases represent true pathogenic associations is often problematic. For example, nearly one-third of patients with systemic sclerosis have migraine, but a pathologic association has not been proven. Case reports link systemic sclerosis to intracerebral vasculopathy, presenting with transient ischemic attacks (TIAs), ischemic strokes, or intracranial hemorrhages. Other case reports link systemic sclerosis to multiple sclerosis, optic neuropathy, memory impairment, or affective disorders.

About one-third of patients with systemic sclerosis, compared to less than one-tenth of control patients, have basal ganglia calcification visible by computed tomography (CT) scan. Patients with SLE may also have an increased prevalence of basal ganglia calcification.

Peripheral Nervous System Disease

Patients with systemic sclerosis probably are at increased risk of developing carpal tunnel syndrome. Trigeminal sensory neuropathy, similar to that described in Sjögren syndrome, affects 1 percent or more of patients with systemic sclerosis. Distal symmetric axonal neuropathy, plexopathies, and mononeuritis multiplex occur infrequently.

Many forms of autonomic dysfunction affect patients with systemic sclerosis, including abnormal sympathetic skin responses, even in nonsclerodermatous skin, abnormal cardiovascular reflexes, impaired urodynamics, erectile dysfunction, and abnormal pupillary responses to sympathetic or parasympathetic stimuli.[29] With the exception of erectile dysfunction, these autonomic changes are usually asymptomatic.

Treatment

Data on the treatment of neurologic disease in patients with systemic sclerosis are scant. Trigeminal neuropathy or mild distal neuropathy is usually not specifically treated. Case reports suggest a possible benefit of cyclosporine in patients with cerebral vasculopathy.[30]

Rheumatoid Arthritis

Rheumatoid arthritis is a chronic disease characterized by symmetric joint inflammation, particularly of the small distal joints such as the metacarpophalangeal, proximal interphalangeal, wrist, and metatarsophalangeal joints. Rheumatoid arthritis has a prevalence of between 10,000 and 20,000 cases per million population, affecting women more often than men. More than four-fifths of those with rheumatoid arthritis have autoimmune serologic changes, particularly the presence of rheumatoid factor, which is nonspecific and present in many other inflammatory conditions and in a small percentage of the population. Autoantibodies to cyclic citrullinated peptide (anti-CCP) are more specific than rheumatoid factor for the diagnosis of rheumatoid arthritis.

Systemic Disease

Patients with rheumatoid arthritis can develop systemic manifestations such as subcutaneous rheumatoid nodules, sicca syndrome, Felty syndrome of hypersplenism, amyloidosis, scleritis or episcleritis, lung or heart involvement, anemia of chronic disease, eosinophilia, and thrombocytosis. A rare but serious complication is widespread rheumatoid vasculitis, with neurologic complications such as those of other medium-vessel vasculitides (discussed later). A community-based survey of rheumatoid arthritis found extra-articular manifestation in nearly one-half of patients over 30 years of follow-up; important neurologic manifestations were cervical myelopathy in 2 percent, neuropathy in 2 percent, and major organ vasculitis in less than 1 percent.[31]

Central Nervous System Disease

Patients with rheumatoid arthritis are probably at increased risk of headache and neck ache but rarely develop serious or focal cerebral disease. Strokes due to rheumatoid vasculitis are quite infrequent. Pachymeningitis caused by rheumatoid nodules or pannus is a rare complication of chronic rheumatoid arthritis. The lesions are visible by contrast-enhanced MRI, which can demonstrate focal or irregular dural thickening.[32] Clinical manifestations can be absent, focal (e.g., optic neuropathy, spinal cord compression), or nonfocal (e.g., headache, mental status changes).

Cervical myelopathy caused by atlantoaxial subluxation and by soft-tissue pannus is a feared late complication of rheumatoid arthritis due to the laxity of inflamed ligaments. Subluxation is usually anterior but can be in any direction. It is rare in the first years of rheumatoid arthritis but develops in more than one-fourth of those who have had the disease for more than 15 years.[33] The subluxation is usually asymptomatic; however, the risk of cord compression increases as subluxation increases, particularly in those with a small spinal canal. Signs of myelopathy (quadriparesis, spasticity, sensory loss, sphincter disturbance) may evolve slowly or worsen suddenly. Patients with high cervical instability are at particular risk of spinal cord injury during intubation.

Vertical atlantoaxial subluxation can lead to brainstem compression; possible symptoms, in addition to those of cervical myelopathy, include bulbar palsy, trigeminal or high cervical sensory loss, ophthalmoparesis, nystagmus, drop attacks, hydrocephalus, and sleep apnea. A rare presentation is vertebral arterial stroke due to the subluxed neck.

Cervical collars can decrease neck ache or headache due to atlantoaxial subluxation; however, a halo and cervical traction are needed if neck stabilization is required. Surgical stabilization in patients with myelopathy or brainstem compression can prevent further neurologic loss but often does not improve existing neurologic deficits.[34]

Peripheral Nervous System Disease

Carpal tunnel syndrome is the most common neurologic manifestation of rheumatoid arthritis. Estimates of its prevalence vary; careful questioning of patients with rheumatoid arthritis reveals median-distribution sensory symptoms in more than half. Patients are more likely than age-matched controls to develop carpal tunnel syndrome, especially when they have hand flexor tenosynovitis. The carpal tunnel syndrome can improve with successful treatment of the arthritis or after carpal tunnel surgery, occasionally supplemented by tenosynovectomy.

Ulnar nerve compression at the ulnar groove, radial or posterior interosseus nerve compression, compression of the fibular or posterior tibial nerves by a Baker cyst in the popliteal region, tarsal tunnel syndrome, and digital neuropathies may affect patients with rheumatoid arthritis.

Mild length-dependent symmetric sensory neuropathy is a potential late effect of rheumatoid arthritis, especially in those with more severe disease. If a nerve biopsy is performed, the specimen may show vasculitic changes, but this is not indicative of systemic vasculitis and is not an indication for immunosuppressive treatment. Patients may also have autonomic neuropathy with impaired sweating or abnormal postural and cardiovascular reflexes, even in the absence of sensory neuropathy. Patients who develop rheumatoid vasculitis are at risk of developing a mononeuritis multiplex.

Myopathies in Connective Tissue Disease

The classic inflammatory myopathies are dermatomyositis (DM), polymyositis (PM), and inclusion-body myositis (IBM).[35] Both DM and PM cause subacute, predominantly proximal, weakness, sparing the face and eyes. Serum creatine kinase (CK) is elevated up to 50 times normal. Electromyography (EMG) shows brief, low-amplitude, easily recruited motor unit potentials, often accompanied by fibrillation potentials or positive sharp waves. Antisynthetase autoantibodies are present in up to one-fourth of patients with DM or PM; anti-Jo is the most common of these and is associated with interstitial lung disease. Despite these similarities, DM and PM differ in their pathology, immunopathogenesis, and relation to other connective tissue diseases.

DM can affect either children or adults. It is usually accompanied by characteristic skin changes: heliotrope upper eyelid discoloration with swelling and an erythematous rash on the face, neck, anterior chest, back and shoulders, and extensor surfaces of extremity joints. On the fingers, a papular, reddish purple keratotic rash can involve the knuckles but spare the phalanges (Grottron rash). Fingernails may show dilated capillaries under the bases and distorted cuticles. In DM, inflammatory changes concentrate around blood vessels and in the perifascicular connective tissue. Perifascicular atrophy of myocytes is characteristic. The inflammatory cells are predominantly $CD4^+$. DM affects about one-eighth of patients with systemic sclerosis.[36,37] Furthermore, DM and Sjögren syndrome may occur together.[38]

PM rarely occurs before the age of 18 years. Weakness develops insidiously and is not associated with rash. Muscle biopsy sample shows inflammatory infiltrates, predominantly $CD8^+$ lymphocytes, invading muscle fibers. PM occurs in 5 to 8 percent of patients with SLE and has a lower prevalence in patients with rheumatoid arthritis or Sjögren syndrome. Given the vagaries of diagnostic definition and the multiplicity of overlaps among the connective tissue diseases, the division among diseases associated with DM or PM can hardly be absolute.

Sporadic IBM usually begins after age 50, particularly in men, and is the most common progressive muscle disease in older adults. It causes a distinct pattern of weakness, favoring the quadriceps, gluteus maximus, and forearm flexors and extensors. Biceps and triceps weakness and foot drop are often present. A muscle biopsy specimen shows vacuoles, intracellular protein aggregates, or mitochondrial pathology; mononuclear cell infiltrates, mainly with $CD4^+$ and $CD8^+$ T cells, concentrate in the endomysium.[39] IBM is linked to the autoimmune connective tissue diseases by a few case reports.[40]

Immune-mediated necrotizing myopathy is a more recently recognized form of inflammatory myopathy, characterized by proximal weakness that can be severe, very high serum CK levels, and paucity of inflammatory infiltrates on muscle biopsy. Some patients have autoantibodies against signal recognition protein or against 3-hydroxy-3-methylglutaryl-coenzyme A reductase. There may be an association between necrotizing myopathy and SLE.[41]

More details on the inflammatory myopathies are available in Chapter 59.

Myositis is not the only form of muscle dysfunction seen in those with connective tissue diseases. Patients with advanced rheumatoid arthritis often have diffuse weakness with a normal EMG and serum CK. Muscle biopsy shows type II atrophy, the same pattern that can be seen with disuse. Similarly, patients with Sjögren syndrome may have mild weakness with normal serum CK levels. Severe hypokalemia due to distal renal tubular acidosis is a rare cause of weakness in patients with Sjögren syndrome. More than half of patients with systemic sclerosis have mild proximal muscle weakness. Inflammatory myopathy is uncommon; more common is "nonspecific" myopathy with normal or mildly elevated serum muscle enzymes, normal or slightly decreased duration of motor units on EMG, and normal spontaneous activity. Muscle biopsy can show intimal proliferation in endomysial and perimysial blood vessels, increase in connective tissue, or atrophy of type II muscle fibers, but no inflammation other than occasional perivascular infiltrates.

Drug toxicity is another cause of muscle disease in patients being treated for connective tissue diseases. Corticosteroid myopathy is a common cause of proximal weakness, especially in patients on high doses or chronic therapy. Treatment with cyclosporine or chloroquine may rarely cause myalgias and weakness. Penicillamine can cause myositis.

VASCULITIS

The vasculitides are a diverse group of illnesses characterized by inflamed blood vessels. They can be subdivided based on the size and type of blood vessels that are inflamed, details of pathology, and areas of the body involved. Most vasculitis is systemic, with involvement of multiple organ systems. However, there are two classic forms of vasculitis in which the principal manifestations are neurologic: primary angiitis of the CNS and nonsystemic vasculitic neuropathy.

Primary Vasculitis of the Nervous System

Primary Angiitis of the Central Nervous System

Primary angiitis of the CNS (PACNS) is a clinical challenge: a rare disease that causes common syndromes such as headache, encephalopathy, or stroke, is potentially fatal but potentially treatable, and is difficult to diagnose, even with cerebral angiography and brain biopsy.[42,43] Synonyms include cerebral granulomatous angiitis, giant cell granulomatous angiitis of the CNS, and isolated angiitis of the CNS. PACNS is pathologically defined by transmural, predominantly monocytic, infiltrates of small to medium (<200 μm in diameter) vessels in the leptomeninges or cerebral cortex.[44] The vessel walls show fibrinoid necrosis, sometimes with granulomas. Parenchymal brain tissue may show ischemic or hemorrhagic infarction. Alternative diagnoses such as systemic vasculitis or infection must be excluded.

PACNS usually presents with headache and change in mental status. Patients less frequently have a stroke or multiple strokes; about one-third of patients have focal neurologic findings at presentation and another one-sixth develop focal findings later in their illness. Symptoms usually evolve gradually, and most patients have been symptomatic for more than 1 month before the diagnosis is made. Myelitis is an uncommon presentation of PACNS. Systemic symptoms such as fever or weight loss affect only a minority of patients. More than 80 percent of patients with PACNS have an elevated CSF protein level, usually over 100 mg/dl, and most have CSF pleocytosis, oligoclonal bands, or an elevated IgG index; CSF glucose concentration is usually normal. Patients may have anemia, peripheral leukocytosis, or elevated erythrocyte sedimentation rate.

Brain CT scans or MRIs typically show multiple ischemic infarcts or more diffuse confluent lesions. Focal brain hemorrhage may occur. However, a normal MRI brain scan does not completely exclude CNS vasculitis.

Cerebral angiographic findings of vasculitis are multifocal vessel narrowing, poststenotic dilatations, and focal variations of blood flow, usually involving multiple vessels. These findings are neither sensitive nor specific; for example, similar vessel changes can occur in meningitis, after subarachnoid hemorrhage, with atherosclerosis, or with other noninflammatory vasculopathies. Reversible cerebral vasospasm syndrome (RCVS) is another cause of multifocal vessel narrowing which can cause acute headache, especially in young women.[45] At first, MRI or CT brain scan is usually normal, but focal hemorrhages or ischemic changes may develop later. Another brain imaging pattern can be that of posterior reversible encephalopathy syndrome. The angiographic changes are reversible in RCVS, resolving usually within 3 months. The CSF is usually normal or shows minimal elevation of protein.

The diagnosis of PACNS is definite only when confirmed by brain biopsy, which should include both cortex and meninges and can be done at a site that is abnormal by MRI or at the nondominant frontal lobe or tip of the nondominant temporal lobe. In one series of patients with suspected PACNS, the biopsy specimen confirmed PACNS in 36 percent, established an alternative diagnosis in 39 percent, and was not diagnostic in 25 percent.

Patients with PACNS are typically treated with corticosteroids, often supplemented by other immunosuppressants. Although there are many anecdotal examples of treatment response, there are no controlled data on treatment. Among a group of patients with suspected PACNS and nondiagnostic brain biopsies, about one-half had a good outcome 1 year later regardless of whether they were treated with immunosuppressants, emphasizing that the diagnosis should be established pathologically whenever possible prior to initiating therapy.[46]

Nonsystemic Vasculitic Neuropathy

Mononeuritis multiplex is the most common clinical presentation of nonsystemic vasculitic neuropathy (NSVN), also called primary angiitis of the peripheral nervous system.[47] Inflammation of individual nerves causes acute or subacute pain and sensory or sensorimotor deficit in the territory of the inflamed nerves. In some patients, discrete involvement of a few nerves is evident; in others, there is an asymmetric neurologic deficit including the territories of many nerves; least commonly, the overlap is so extensive that the deficit fits a distal symmetric pattern. The neurologic deficit is usually worse distally, but many patients have some proximal weakness. Leg nerves, particularly the fibular, are more often affected than arm nerves, and inflammation often affects the proximal nerve trunk rather than traditional sites for compressive neuropathies. Infrequently, a cranial nerve, most commonly the facial nerve, is involved.

Patients with NSVN may have some manifestations of systemic illness including weight loss, fever, elevated erythrocyte sedimentation rate, positive ANA or rheumatoid factor, anemia, peripheral leukocytosis, or thrombocytosis. CSF protein concentration is occasionally elevated. Less common findings are a serum monoclonal gammopathy or mild CSF pleocytosis.

In more than 90 percent of patients with vasculitic neuropathy, electrodiagnostic studies are consistent with an asymmetric axonal neuropathy; some patients show partial motor conduction block.[48]

The definitive pathologic changes of vasculitic neuropathy are inflammatory cells infiltrating the walls of epineurial and perineurial arterioles, usually accompanied by fibrinoid necrosis, disruption of endothelial cells or the internal elastic lamina, or hemorrhage into the vessel wall. The involved arterioles are usually 75 to 200 μm in diameter. Typically, a pure sensory nerve, such as the sural or superficial fibular, is biopsied. Patients may also have vasculitis of muscle, especially in the perimesial arterioles, even though they have no clinical evidence of myopathy and no direct inflammation of myocytes. Biopsy of the peroneus brevis muscle at the time of nerve biopsy increases the diagnostic sensitivity for vasculitis. About 60 percent of patients with a confirmed diagnosis of vasculitis by clinical criteria show definite vasculitis by nerve or muscle biopsy. When vasculitis affects the nerve proximal to the biopsy site, nerve biopsy may show less-specific findings such as vessel thickening, narrowing, or thrombosis, epineurial capillary proliferation, periadventitial hemosiderin, asymmetric nerve fiber loss, or Wallerian-like degeneration.[49]

Based on uncontrolled clinical experience, treatment of NSVN involves corticosteroids, starting, for example, with prednisone 1 mg/kg daily, and then tapering the dose and changing to alternate-day dosing. More aggressive immunosuppression with agents such as cyclophosphamide or methotrexate is typically added if patients do not respond to prednisone. Occasional patients with mild and stable presentations are not treated. The nerve inflammation of NSVN leads to fascicular nerve infarction and axonal interruption; recovery of individual nerves can occur, but recovery of neurologic function takes many months. Many patients regain motor function and sensory perception but have chronic pain.[50] Patients should be followed closely when therapy is tapered; nearly one-half of patients relapse despite initial responses to therapy. If patients with NSVN have no systemic features and do not have hepatitis B infection, the risk of later developing vasculitis in major organs is low.

Systemic Vasculitis

Systemic Disease

Systemic vasculitis of medium (0.2- to 2.0-mm diameter) and small blood vessels (arterioles, capillaries, postcapillary venules) is a spectrum of diseases including polyarteritis nodosa (PAN), Churg–Strauss syndrome, microscopic polyangiitis, granulomatosis with polyangiitis (formerly Wegener granulomatosis), and Kawasaki disease. All can cause CNS disease, especially strokes, or disease of the peripheral nervous system, especially vasculitic neuropathy, to variable degrees. Differentiating among the systemic necrotizing vasculitides is challenging; patients often overlap diagnostic categories.[51] Most forms of systemic vasculitis can cause systemic illness, necrotizing skin lesions, inflammation of the gastrointestinal tract, involvement of joints and muscles, and renal disease. A 2-year study at a British hospital serving 415,000 people found 56 cases of granulomatosis with polyangiitis, 23 cases of microscopic polyangiitis, 18 cases of Churg–Strauss syndrome, and 2 cases of PAN.[52]

PAN is the prototypic systemic vasculitis with inflammation of medium-sized arteries but is becoming less frequently diagnosed, with an annual incidence in developed countries of 9 or fewer per million. Chronic hepatitis B infection can cause PAN, so incidence is higher where hepatitis B is endemic. Patients with PAN are almost always systemically ill, with fever, weight loss, malaise, fatigue, and myalgias. Inflammation of medium-sized subcutaneous vessels can lead to livedo reticularis, subcutaneous nodules (to be distinguished from the palpable purpura of small-vessel vasculitis), skin ulcerations, and digital ischemia. One half of patients have gastrointestinal involvement, often with abdominal pain. Renal inflammation may cause renal infarcts, hypertension, proteinuria, hematuria, or elevated blood urea nitrogen and creatinine, but glomerulonephritis is not a feature of classic PAN. Abdominal angiography often shows multiple mesenteric or renal microaneurysms. Coronary arteriolar vasculitis can cause patchy areas of myocardial necrosis, congestive heart failure, and tachycardia; infarcts in the full territory of a coronary artery are less common. Vasculitis may extend to many other organs, including the brain, but classic PAN does not affect the lungs.

Churg–Strauss syndrome can resemble PAN in its effects on skin, gastrointestinal tract, heart, muscle, nerve, and brain. Renal disease is less common than in PAN. However, Churg–Strauss syndrome is remarkable for its striking, almost universal, lung pathology with asthma and pulmonary infiltrates and for eosinophilia; all are rare in PAN. The ACR classification criteria for Churg–Strauss syndrome require that the patient have at least four of the following six findings: asthma, blood eosinophil count greater than 10 percent, mononeuropathy or polyneuropathy, pulmonary infiltrates, abnormal paranasal sinuses, and biopsy evidence of extravascular eosinophilia.

Granulomatosis with polyangiitis is characterized by granulomas and small- and medium-vessel vasculitis of the upper respiratory tract, lungs, and kidneys. The mucosal inflammation can cause necrotic ulcers of the sinuses, pharynx, or ears, and lung findings, ranging from transient infiltrates to severe pulmonary hemorrhage. The renal disease is typically glomerulonephritis, whether mild proliferative or necrotizing crescentic. The ACR classification criteria that distinguish granulomatosis with polyangiitis from other forms of vasculitis require any two of the following four features: nasal or oral inflammation, abnormal chest radiograph, microhematuria or red cell casts in the urine sediment, and pathologic granulomatous inflammation in or around the wall of an artery or arteriole. The disease evolves over months and can also cause inflammatory eye disease, myalgias, joint disease, skin lesions (either palpable purpura or the lesions of medium-vessel vasculitis), pericarditis, and neuropathy.

Microscopic polyangiitis causes vasculitis of medium and small vessels. Necrotizing glomerulonephritis is common, which distinguishes it from PAN. The diagnosis of microscopic angiitis is excluded if patients meet criteria for either Churg–Strauss syndrome or granulomatosis with polyangiitis.

Kawasaki disease occurs predominantly in children and, aside from aseptic meningitis, infrequently causes neurologic syndromes.[53]

Vasculitis can accompany a number of other systemic diseases, including SLE, Sjögren syndrome, sarcoidosis, and rheumatoid arthritis. Patients with hepatitis C infection may have vasculitis associated with type 2 cryoglobulinemia, and vasculitis may accompany many other viral infections, such as with human immunodeficiency virus, hepatitis B virus, cytomegalovirus, and herpes zoster virus; syphilis, Lyme disease, and fungal, rickettsial, and mycobacterial infections may also be responsible. Cerebral vasculitis can complicate bacterial meningitis or be part of a paraneoplastic syndrome.[54]

Antineutrophil cytoplasmic antibodies (ANCAs) can be helpful in the diagnosis of systemic vasculitides, particularly in patients with renal disease, but must be interpreted with caution. There are two antibody patterns. The c-ANCA pattern on immunofluorescence is usually associated with antibodies to proteinase-3, which can be detected by an enzyme-linked immunosorbent assay (ELISA). The combination of the c-ANCA and antiproteinase 3 is sensitive for granulomatosis with polyangiitis but may be negative, particularly if the disease spares the kidney. c-ANCA/antiproteinase 3 may also be present in PAN, Churg–Strauss syndrome, and microscopic polyangiitis, usually associated with renal involvement. The p-ANCA pattern is a much less specific finding and can be positive in a variety of inflammatory diseases. However, when the p-ANCA pattern is associated with antibodies to myeloperoxidase (anti-MPO on ELISA), the combination relatively strongly suggests glomerulonephritis associated with systemic necrotizing vasculitis such as microscopic polyangiitis, Churg–Strauss syndrome, localized necrotizing glomerulonephritis, or granulomatosis with polyangiitis.

Central Nervous System Disease

CNS syndromes in patients with systemic vasculitis are varied. The approximate prevalences of CNS complications of PAN are stroke 11 percent, altered mental status 10 percent, and seizures 4 percent. Similar presentations of cerebral vasculitis can occur in the other systemic vasculitides, perhaps less frequently in microscopic polyangiitis.[55] Arteritis can affect arterioles and small arteries in the meninges and cerebrum. Strokes can be single or multiple, affecting small vessels at any place in the brain. TIAs are less frequent, and intracranial hemorrhages or extracranial arterial dissections are uncommon events in patients with systemic vasculitis. Psychometric testing in patients with systemic vasculitis sometimes shows mild cognitive impairment.[56]

Patients with granulomatosis with polyangiitis have a similar incidence of strokes, seizures, and other focal cerebral syndromes. In addition, granulomatous disease can cause hypertrophic pachymeningitis or pituitary disease.[57]

Peripheral Nervous System Disease

More than half of patients with PAN and an even higher proportion of patients with Churg–Strauss syndrome have peripheral neuropathy. The classic form is ischemic mononeuropathy or mononeuritis multiplex, which is a common presenting manifestation of necrotizing vasculitis. Other patients have mild patches of cutaneous dysesthesias or paresthesias due to cutaneous mononeuropathies. Another clinical pattern of vasculitic neuropathy is a mild distal symmetric sensorimotor neuropathy. Similar neuropathies occur in patients with granulomatosis with polyangiitis or microscopic polyangiitis, but the clinical prevalence is lower, and neuropathy is less likely to be a presenting symptom. However, if patients with granulomatosis with polyangiitis are studied with EMG and nerve conduction studies, nearly one-third have some evidence of distal axonal neuropathy.[58]

The clinical presentations and pathologic findings of neuropathy in patients with systemic vasculitis are similar to those described for NSVN. Exceptional findings are limitation of inflammation to vessels less than 40 μm in diameter in some cases of microscopic polyangiitis or the occasional appearance of epineurial granulomas in granulomatosis with polyangiitis.

A rare manifestation of systemic vasculitis is an acute ascending paralysis, clinically similar to Guillain–Barré syndrome, but distinguished on electrodiagnostic studies by results favoring axonal rather than demyelinating pathology and on nerve biopsy by evidence of vasculitis.

Cranial neuropathies can occur in patients with systemic vasculitis; cranial nerves III, V, VI, VII, and most frequently VIII in PAN. Single or multiple cranial neuropathies are even more frequent in patients with granulomatosis with polyangiitis where granulomatous disease in the ear, sinuses, or orbit can lead to focal nerve inflammation or compression and to hearing loss.

Treatment

Glucocorticoids and cyclophosphamide are mainstays in the treatment of systemic vasculitis, but there are no rigid rules for their use. Some patients with mild disease improve when treated only with high-dose corticosteroids. Cyclophosphamide or rituximab should be added if patients do not respond to corticosteroids or if they have major organ involvement, such as gastrointestinal bleeding, perforation, or infarction; pancreatitis; severe glomerulonephritis or renal failure; cardiomyopathy; or CNS disease.[59] PAN and Churg–Strauss vasculitis may respond to corticosteroids alone; most patients with granulomatosis with polyangiitis and microscopic polyangiitis require additional therapy.

Polymyalgia Rheumatica and Temporal Arteritis

Temporal arteritis (TA) is the most common vasculitis of large elastic arteries, characterized pathologically by granulomatous arterial inflammation with giant cells, usually located between the media and intima. Giant cell arteritis is often used as a synonym for TA, even though there are other forms of arteritis, such as Takayasu arteritis, that are also characterized pathologically by giant cells in arteries. Polymyalgia rheumatica (PMR) is a chronic idiopathic systemic inflammatory illness that is intimately related to TA.[60]

Systemic Disease

Polymyalgia is a chronic disease that causes pain and stiffness in patients older than 50 years. It is common, affecting nearly 1 percent of those older than 50, women more than men, and reaching peak prevalence in the eighth decade of life.[61] The pain typically affects proximal joints symmetrically, shoulders more than hips or neck, with prominent morning stiffness; it is often described as myalgic, but the cause is synovitis, and actual muscle weakness is not part of the syndrome. Symptoms can start abruptly or evolve slowly; ACR diagnostic criteria require that symptoms last for more than 1 month. Systemic symptoms can include fatigue, fever, malaise, anorexia, or weight loss. About half of patients with PMR have distal asymmetric synovitis that can cause arthralgias and tenderness of the knees, wrists, ankles, or dorsal feet.

TA is a systemic vasculitis that shares the time course, systemic symptoms, and epidemiologic characteristics of PMR. About one-half of patients with TA have polymyalgia and one-sixth or more of patients with PMR have TA. The average annual incidence of TA in Olmstead County, Minnesota, in those older than 50 years is 188 cases per million population.[62] Characteristics of TA are headache, jaw claudication, and risk of sudden blindness and stroke. Patients with TA usually have scalp pain, ranging from nonlocalized tenderness to enlarged, nodular, painful scalp arteries, particularly the temporal artery. Patients can have other manifestations of large-artery inflammation, such as asymmetric pulses or blood pressure, limb claudication, aortic aneurysm or dissection, aortic valve insufficiency, myocardial infarction, intestinal ischemia, or Raynaud phenomenon.

PMR and TA are usually associated with an elevated erythrocyte sedimentation rate and C-reactive protein (CRP). Other laboratory abnormalities can include anemia, mild leukocytosis or thrombocytosis, and mild elevations of liver enzymes, especially of alkaline phosphatase, and, occasionally, of antiphospholipid antibodies.

The diagnosis of TA can be proven by temporal artery biopsy, but the arterial giant-cell inflammation can be patchy. Ideally, the biopsy includes a portion of the artery that is abnormal to palpation. The biopsy should sample at least 0.5 cm of artery, and multiple sections should be reviewed.[63] If the findings from the first biopsy specimen are negative on frozen sections, biopsy should be performed on the contralateral temporal artery; the biopsy specimen can still be positive after corticosteroid therapy has started and treatment should be immediately initiated while biopsy is being arranged.[64]

Temporal artery color Doppler ultrasound can be sensitive and specific for temporal arteritis when done by the best ultrasonographers; however, less experienced ultrasonographers may give less valuable results.[65] Patients with temporal arteritis are at increased risk of aortic aneurysms and dissections.[66]

Central Nervous System Disease

Headache is characteristic of TA and is the presenting symptom in about one-third of patients. The headache has no pathognomonic features, so TA should be considered in everyone older than 50 years who develops new or different headache.

Sudden visual loss is one of the most serious manifestations of TA. The usual mechanism is occlusion of the posterior ciliary artery causing arteritic anterior ischemic optic neuropathy. Monocular blindness may be sudden or evolve over a few days. Some patients have had a preceding episode of amaurosis fugax. Examination shows a relative afferent pupillary defect. Within a day or two, the optic disc swells and has chalky white coloration that distinguishes it from nonarteritic anterior ischemic optic neuropathy; some patients have cotton wool spots or flame-shaped hemorrhages. TA infrequently causes central retinal artery occlusion or retrobulbar optic neuritis.

Stroke or TIA can occur in patients with TA, and focal cerebral ischemia may even be the initial manifestation of TA. However, stroke affects probably less than 5 percent of patients with TA. Strokes are typically embolic from effects on the extradural carotid or, more commonly, vertebral arteries. Intracranial arteries, which lack internal elastic lamina, are rarely affected by TA.

Peripheral Nervous System Disease

TA may affect the peripheral nervous system as well. Ophthalmoparesis occurs in as many as 6 percent of patients: in TA, the differential diagnosis of abnormal eye movement includes brainstem stroke, isolated cranial neuropathy, and ischemic necrosis of extraocular muscles. Patients may develop other ischemic cranial neuropathies. Peripheral neuropathy patterns may be of distal symmetric polyneuropathy, mononeuropathy, or mononeuropathy multiplex. Carpal tunnel syndrome is the most common focal neurologic manifestation of PMR and is often among the presenting symptoms.

Treatment

Corticosteroids are the initial treatment for TA or PMR. For patients with TA, the initial prednisone dose is at least 40 mg daily; many clinicians start at 60 mg daily or more. Given the risks of major neurologic complications, corticosteroids should be introduced without delay in patients in whom the diagnosis of TA is likely on clinical grounds, without waiting for the results of biopsy; if the biopsy results are negative, the decision to continue corticosteroids must be made on clinical grounds. Patients with sudden visual loss must be treated with urgency because the contralateral eye can be affected within days. Patients with acute visual loss can be treated with intravenous methylprednisolone, 1 g daily, for the first 3 days before switching to oral therapy. Daily corticosteroids are more effective than alternate-day treatment. In a randomized, double-blind, placebo-controlled trial comparing corticosteroids alone to corticosteroids plus methotrexate, the relapse rate or cumulative steroid requirements were not reduced with the addition of methotrexate.[67] Retrospective data suggest that patients with TA are less likely to have ischemic visual loss or stroke if treated with antiplatelet or anticoagulation drugs.[68]

Patients who have PMR without TA usually respond dramatically to lower doses of prednisone (10 to 20 mg daily).[69] Occasionally PMR patients with mild symptoms can be treated only with nonsteroidal anti-inflammatory drugs.

Takayasu Arteritis

Systemic Disease

Takayasu arteritis, also called pulseless disease, is an idiopathic large-vessel vasculitis that involves the aorta, its major branches, and sometimes the pulmonary artery.[70] It affects adults, almost always before the age of 40, women more than men, and is more common in those of Asian descent. Early symptoms of the disease can include headache, fever, malaise, myalgias, nausea, vomiting, anorexia, weight loss, and irregular menses. Patients may have erythema nodosum, objective evidence of synovitis, an elevated erythrocyte sedimentation rate or C-reactive protein, mild anemia, or peripheral leukocytosis. These systemic inflammatory findings often precede vascular stenosis or occlusion by weeks, but some patients present with acute ischemic events. Typical manifestations of impaired flow in large vessels include arm or leg claudication, decreased peripheral pulses or an asymmetry of blood pressure between the arms, or arterial bruits. Patients may develop hypertension, often associated with renal artery stenosis. Angina, Raynaud phenomenon, and tenderness over inflamed arteries are

TABLE 50-7 ■ Differential Diagnosis of Aortic and Great-Vessel Disease

Inflammatory Aortitis
Syphilis
Tuberculosis
Systemic lupus erythematosus
Rheumatoid arthritis
Spondyloarthropathies
Buerger disease
Behçet syndrome
Cogan syndrome
Kawasaki syndrome
Temporal arteritis
Inflammatory bowel disease
Developmental Abnormalities
Marfan syndrome
Ehlers–Danlos syndrome
Neurofibromatosis
Aortic coarctation
Acquired Abnormalities
Ergotism
Radiation fibrosis
Atherosclerosis
Fibromuscular hyperplasia

From Rosenbaum RB, Campbell SM, Rosenbaum JT: Clinical Neurology of Rheumatic Diseases. Butterworth Heinemann, Stoneham, 1996.

less common findings. Aortic valve insufficiency can develop due to inflammation of the aortic root. The initial systemic symptoms and laboratory manifestations of inflammation usually recede spontaneously, leaving residual findings due to stenosed or occluded major arteries.

Arteriography is needed to define the extent of arterial disease. The subclavian artery is the most commonly involved, but the aorta, common carotid, vertebral, renal, coronary, iliac, mesenteric, and pulmonary arteries are at risk. Many other illnesses merit consideration in the differential diagnosis of disease of the aorta and major arteries (Table 50-7). Biopsy of an involved artery can confirm the diagnosis of Takayasu arteritis by showing arterial inflammation microscopically identical to the changes of giant cell arteritis.

Central Nervous System Disease

Takayasu arteritis may cause ischemic stroke due to carotid or vertebral artery inflammation, stenosis, or occlusion.[71] Among patients with Takayasu arteritis perhaps two-fifths have carotid artery stenoses and nearly one-fifth have vertebral artery stenoses. In addition to stroke and TIA, patients are at increased risk of cardiogenic embolus if they have aortic valve disease or myocardial infarction. Takayasu arteritis does not affect the intracranial arteries, but hypertension increases the risk of ischemic or hemorrhagic stroke.

Peripheral Nervous System Disease

Takayasu arteritis does not usually affect the peripheral nervous system.

Treatment

Takayasu arteritis is resistant to sustained remission.[72] Corticosteroids are standard initial treatment, but many patients do not improve or relapse when these are tapered. In small series, treatment was successful with methotrexate, azathioprine, cyclophosphamide, or anti–tumor necrosis factor agents. Stenotic arterial lesions are sometimes bypassed surgically or treated endovascularly with angioplasty, perhaps with stenting, but these lesions often recur.[73] The optimal antiplatelet or anticoagulant therapy for Takayasu arteritis is unproven.

Behçet Syndrome

Systemic Disease

Behçet syndrome is a multifocal systemic inflammatory disease. Characteristic manifestations are oral and genital ulcers and uveitis; patients may also have asymmetric oligoarticular arthritis, skin lesions (erythema nodosum, pseudofolliculitis, papulopustular lesions, or acneiform nodules), CNS disease, epididymitis, intestinal inflammation or ulcers, thrombophlebitis, and even arterial occlusions or aneurysms. A widely used diagnostic criteria set for Behçet syndrome requires recurrent oral ulcerations plus two of the following: recurrent genital ulcerations, eye lesions (anterior uveitis or retinal vasculitis), and skin lesions. These criteria must be used with care since many of the manifestations, such as oral ulcerations or acneiform rashes, are common in the general population. The median age at disease onset is the late 20s, and males are affected more often than females. Behçet syndrome is most common in the so-called Silk Route countries, lying in a band across Asia from Japan to Turkey. The prevalence varies from more than 3,000 patients per million in some surveys in Turkey to fewer than 10 patients per million in parts of Europe and the United States. There is no specific laboratory test for Behçet syndrome. The erythrocyte sedimentation rate or C-reactive protein is often elevated. The skin pathergy test, performed by pricking the skin with a sterile needle and watching for development of a sterile papulopustular reaction in 24 to 48 hours, is positive in many patients but is nonspecific. Behçet syndrome is often classified as a vasculitis because pathology includes inflammation of venules, but there are no diagnostic pathologic findings.

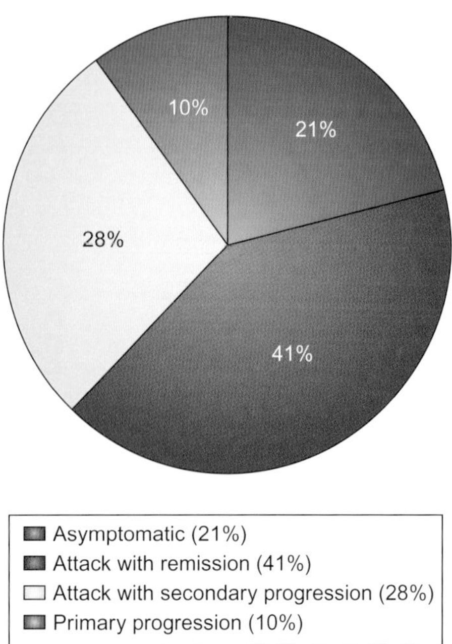

FIGURE 50-1 ■ Patterns of symptoms in patients with neuro-Behçet syndrome and cerebral focal lesions. (Data from Akman-Demir G, Serdaroglu P, Tasçi B, et al: Clinical patterns of neurological involvement in Behçet's disease: evaluation of 200 patients. Brain 122:2171, 1999.)

Central Nervous System Disease

About 5 to 15 percent of patients have CNS inflammatory disease.[74,75] Headache is common, and if patients with headache but no other neurologic findings are counted, the prevalence of CNS disease appears much higher.

Among patients with Behçet syndrome, men are at higher risk than women of neurologic disease. The neurologic manifestations are most likely to appear a few years after the systemic manifestations, so the median age at onset of neuro-Behçet syndrome is the early 30s, although it can be the presenting form of the illness.

There are two distinct patterns of inflammatory brain disease, which rarely coexist.[76,77] The more common is focal brain inflammation that typically affects the brainstem or basal ganglia. Other possible sites of inflammation are the cerebral hemispheres or the spinal cord. Patients usually have signs of bilateral pyramidal dysfunction, hemiparesis, headache, or sphincter dysfunction. Many have behavioral changes such as apathy or disinhibition. Less common findings include ophthalmoplegia, bulbar signs, sensory impairment, meningismus, and fever. Focal neurologic syndromes that are seen infrequently include seizures, psychiatric disturbance, hearing loss, cerebellar syndromes, optic neuropathy, hemianopia, aphasia, aneurysmal subarachnoid hemorrhage, and stroke.

Focal brain inflammation in patients with Behçet syndrome is sometimes asymptomatic, discovered at autopsy or by MRI. When neurologic symptoms develop, they usually evolve over a few days and sometimes remit, but they may proceed in a relapsing progressive or primary progressive pattern (Fig. 50-1).

Brain MRI in those with focal brain disease shows lesions that are hyperintense on T2-weighted sequences and absent or hypointense on T1-weighted images. Acute lesions may have restricted diffusion.[78] The lesions sometimes enhance and may have mass effect; they are more often multiple than single, are most prevalent in the brainstem or basal ganglia, and can be reversible. The CSF in patients with focal brain inflammation often shows an elevated protein level or a pleocytosis, which may be mononuclear or neutrophilic; oligoclonal bands are present infrequently but are absent in the blood. The neuropathology of neuro-Behçet syndrome includes chronic lymphocytic meningoencephalitis and perivenular infiltrates of lymphocytes, neutrophils, eosinophils, or plasmacytes.

The second distinct, less common, CNS syndrome in patients with Behçet syndrome is increased intracranial pressure, usually associated with dural sinus thrombosis rather than focal parenchymal brain inflammation. Most patients with this presentation have headache and papilledema. Unilateral or bilateral sixth cranial nerve palsy sometimes occurs but other lateralizing neurologic findings are less common. CSF examination shows increased spinal fluid pressure. Pleocytosis, subarachnoid hemorrhage, and elevated protein level are unusual findings. In many patients with this presentation, parenchymal lesions are absent.

Peripheral Nervous System Disease

Disease of the peripheral nervous system is unusual in patients with Behçet syndrome; however, case reports document instances of associated peripheral neuropathy or focal or generalized myositis.

Treatment

There is no class I evidence for efficacy of treatment of neuro-Behçet syndrome. Evaluation of therapy is complicated because attacks of brain inflammation may remit spontaneously. Experienced clinicians recommend treating attacks of focal CNS inflammation with prednisone or intravenous methylprednisolone.[76] Some add other forms of immunosuppression. There is anecdotal evidence of efficacy of anti–tumor necrosis factor agents in patients with severe Behçet syndrome.[79] Many patients with venous sinus thrombosis are also treated with heparin or low-molecular-weight heparin.[76,77]

DIFFERENTIAL DIAGNOSIS

The neurologic complications of vasculitis or connective tissue diseases are sporadic manifestations of uncommon illnesses, much less common than the conditions that a neurologist sees daily, such as stroke, seizures, and headache. However, since these inflammatory diseases are often treatable they merit consideration in the differential diagnosis of many neurologic presentations. Diagnosis is further complicated because the classification criteria used for identification of rheumatic diseases were developed and validated in groups of patients with known systemic inflammatory disease and are insensitive to mild or early presentations. Often a thorough systemic medical history, general physical examination, and basic systemic laboratory work, such as a complete blood count, urinalysis, erythrocyte sedimentation rate, and serum metabolic panel, provide the first clues that a patient with a neurologic presentation actually has a systemic illness.

Central Nervous System Syndromes

Meningitis

Acute, recurrent, or chronic meningitis is an infrequent complication of SLE, Sjögren syndrome, Behçet syndrome, PACNS, and systemic necrotizing vasculitis. The CSF usually shows a mild mononuclear pleocytosis, normal or elevated protein level, and normal or slightly depressed glucose concentration. Patients with Behçet or Sjögren syndrome occasionally have more neutrophils in the CSF. In all patients with inflammatory diseases and meningitis, a high priority is excluding infectious causes, especially in patients vulnerable to opportunistic infections. Drug-induced meningitis is another important diagnostic consideration.

Pachymeningitis is visible on MRI as thickened, gadolinium-enhancing dura.[80] Patients may be asymptomatic or have headache, cranial neuropathies, focal brain dysfunction, or seizures. If the dural enhancement is diffuse and smooth, pachymeningitis must be distinguished from intracranial hypotension. Pachymeningitis is a rare late complication of rheumatoid arthritis.[32] It has also occurred in patients with granulomatosus with polyangiitis, Behçet syndrome, Sjögren syndrome, and TA.[81] Some cases of pachymeningitis are idiopathic, but infections and neoplasia must be excluded.

Cerebrovascular Disease

The diseases discussed in this chapter can cause strokes through a wide range of mechanisms. Patients with SLE or with primary antiphospholipid antibody syndrome are prone to nonbacterial endocarditis. Patients with vasculitis may develop myocardial infarction leading to secondary mural thrombosis or arrhythmia. TA or Takayasu arteritis may lead to vertebral or carotid artery stroke. A very unusual cause of vertebral artery stroke is arterial distortion due to cervical ligamentous laxity in a patient with long-standing rheumatoid arthritis. Intracranial arteriolar disease may arise from secondary hypertension, cerebral vasculopathy (e.g., in SLE), or cerebral vasculitis (e.g., in PACNS). Patients with antiphospholipid antibodies have an increased stroke risk.

In patients presenting with a first stroke, the cause is unlikely to be one of the diseases discussed in this chapter. Among 891 first ischemic strokes recorded in a registry, 4 patients had PACNS, 3 had lupus, 1 had systemic vasculitis, and 1 had TA. Intracranial hemorrhage, with varied underlying mechanisms, is an unusual complication of SLE, Behçet syndrome, PACNS, systemic vasculitis, Sjögren syndrome, or large-vessel vasculitis. Further discussion of this topic is provided in Chapter 11.

RELAPSING-REMITTING MULTIFOCAL DISEASE

SLE, primary antiphospholipid antibody syndrome, and Sjögren syndrome may cause relapsing-remitting multifocal CNS syndromes that might be confused with multiple sclerosis. When patients with these conditions have myelopathy or optic neuropathy, their illness often fits the spectrum of neuromyelitis optica, which can follow a relapsing-remitting course.[13] Neuro-Behçet syndrome can also have episodic recurrences and, rarely, primary angiitis of the CNS follows a relapsing-remitting course.[82] The potential for confusion is increased because patients with multiple sclerosis sometimes have antinuclear, antiphospholipid, anti-Ro, or anti-La antibodies. Clues that favor one of the systemic inflammatory diseases over multiple sclerosis are non-neurologic systemic findings, associated peripheral neuropathy, a spinal MRI showing lesions that span more than two spinal segments, or a brain MRI that is atypical for multiple sclerosis, with gray matter lesions or sparing of the corpus callosum. In Behçet syndrome, the MRI often shows large confluent lesions involving the brainstem or basal ganglia. Oligoclonal bands in the CSF but not serum, or increased intrathecal IgG synthesis are sometimes seen in SLE, neuro-Behçet syndrome, or Sjögren syndrome. However, they are present in 90 percent of patients with multiple scelerosis and their absence should lead to consideration of an alternative diagnosis.

HEADACHE

Connective tissue diseases or vasculitis may cause headache through several mechanisms (Table 50-8). When patients have chronic recurrent headache consistent with migraine or tension headache, treatment is often symptomatic and no specific evaluation or anti-inflammatory treatment may be needed.

TABLE 50-8 ■ Selected Causes of Headache in Rheumatic Diseases

Mechanism	Disease
Meningitis	Behçet syndrome
Structural disease of the cervical spine	Rheumatoid arthritis
	Spondyloarthropathies
	Cervical spondylosis and degenerative arthritis
Systemic inflammation	Systemic lupus erythematosus
	Vasculitis
Migraine	Sjögren syndrome
	Systemic sclerosis
	Systemic lupus erythematosus
Extracranial arteritis	Temporal arteritis
Cerebral venous thrombosis	Behçet syndrome
Intracranial arteritis	Primary angiitis of the CNS
Fibromyalgia	Systemic lupus erythematosus
Orbital or sinus granulomas	Granulomatosis with polyangiitis

Adapted from Rosenbaum RB, Campbell SM, Rosenbaum JT: Clinical Neurology of Rheumatic Diseases. Butterworth Heinemann, Stoneham, 1996.

Evaluation is more complex when patients have a new or different headache. TA should be considered in the differential diagnosis of new headache patterns occurring in those older than 50 years. Patients with systemic inflammatory disease and acute headache may warrant assessment for CNS structural lesions or meningitis. There are reported associations of intracranial hypertension and Behçet syndrome, SLE, or Sjögren syndrome; in these patients, cerebral sinus thrombosis must be excluded.[83,84]

MOVEMENT DISORDERS

The best-known association between movement disorders and systemic inflammatory disease is the chorea that can occur in SLE or primary antiphospholipid antibody syndrome.[10] In addition, chorea may occur rarely in Sjögren syndrome, Behçet syndrome, or vasculitis.[26,85] Parkinsonism or cerebellar ataxia due to vasculitis or connective tissue disease, often mediated by cerebral infarction, is also well described but uncommon.[11] Some cases of inflammatory parkinsonism are responsive to dopaminergic therapy, yet reversible with anti-inflammatory treatment.[86] This topic is discussed further in Chapter 58.

Myelopathy

Acute or subacute myelopathy is a rare occurrence in SLE, antiphospholipid antibody syndrome, Sjögren syndrome, Behçet syndrome, and vasculitis. Especially in patients with large-vessel vasculitis, anterior spinal artery infarction is sometimes responsible. However, a more common presentation is as an inflammatory transverse myelitis. In a survey of patients with acute myelitis, 6 percent were associated with SLE, 1 percent with antiphospholipid antibody syndrome, and 9 percent with Sjögren syndrome, compared to 43 percent caused by multiple sclerosis.[87] Patients with systemic inflammatory disease usually have a CSF pleocytosis and mild protein elevation. The spinal MRI is often helpful in distinguishing the myelitis of systemic inflammatory disease from the myelitis of multiple sclerosis, because in the former but not the latter intramedullary lesions often span two or more spinal segments. The clinical variations in myelopathies and their relation to neuromyelitis optica were discussed earlier.

Every patient with myelopathy needs imaging to exclude spinal cord compression. Patients with rheumatoid arthritis and atlantoaxial joint dissociation are especially vulnerable to compression of the high cervical spinal cord.

Seizures

Patients with systemic inflammatory disease or vasculitis are at increased risk of seizures, ranging from single episodes, often attributable to secondary metabolic derangements, posterior reversible encephalopathy syndrome, or infection, to recurrent focal or generalized seizures in patients with focal brain lesions.

A number of anticonvulsants, including phenytoin, carbamazepine, valproic acid, and lamotrigine, can cause drug-induced lupus; however, drug-induced lupus rarely causes CNS disease. The use of these drugs is probably not contraindicated in patients with SLE.

Acute Confusional State

Delirium and other manifestations of encephalopathy can complicate a number of diseases featured in this chapter. Sometimes the pathogenesis is directly related to the inflammatory disease through stroke or focal brain lesions. However, a number of other mechanisms, such as electrolyte disturbance, hepatic or renal failure, hypertensive encephalopathy, seizures, hypoxia, opportunistic infections, or drug toxicity, must be considered, as each requires specific treatment.

Some unusual causes of encephalopathy also require specific management. Posterior reversible encephalopathy syndrome, which can cause headache, confusion, seizures, visual or motor deficits, and characteristic white matter changes on neuroimaging, can be precipitated by severe hypertension, renal failure, or medications such as cyclosporine, cyclophosphamide, and corticosteroids and has affected patients with a variety of connective tissue disorders.[88,89] Treatment includes blood pressure control and discontinuing offending drugs. SLE can be complicated by thrombotic thrombocytopenic purpura, which is characterized by encephalopathy, fever, renal failure, microangiopathic hemolytic anemia, and thrombocytopenia. Thrombotic thrombocytopenic purpura may also present in patients with systemic vasculitis, systemic sclerosis, rheumatoid arthritis, or Sjögren syndrome. Primary treatment is with plasmapheresis and high-dose corticosteroids.[90]

Progressive multifocal leukoencephalopathy may affect patients treated with corticosteroids or other immunosupressants for vasculitis or connective tissue disease and is likely to cause insidious rather than acute changes in mental status.[91] In addition, patients often have visual, motor, sensory, or speech deficits.

Cognitive Dysfunction

Waxing and waning cognitive dysfunction is frequent in patients with SLE or Sjögren syndrome and also affects patients with systemic vasculitis.[56] More severe cognitive dysfunction may occur in these illnesses, as well as with Behçet syndrome. In TA, cognitive dysfunction may improve with corticosteroid therapy.

Affective or Psychotic Disorders

SLE is an example of a systemic inflammatory disease that can cause depression, anxiety, or psychosis. Depression is also common in patients with rheumatoid arthritis, systemic sclerosis, or Sjögren syndrome.[92–94] Depression can be a prominent aspect of PMR. There is ongoing debate on the relative roles of organic brain disease and of reaction to serious illness as the cause of affective disorders in these patients.

Peripheral Nervous System Syndromes

CRANIAL NEUROPATHY

The ACR list of neurologic syndromes (Table 50-4) places cranial neuropathy under syndromes of the peripheral nervous system, even though optic neuropathy and nuclear cranial neuropathies are CNS lesions.

Optic neuritis occurs uncommonly in patients with SLE, antiphospholipid antibody syndrome, Behçet syndrome, Sjögren syndrome, systemic sclerosis, and systemic vasculitis. When optic neuritis occurs in patients with autoimmune connective tissue diseases, it may be a manifestation of neuromyelitis-spectrum autoimmunity. Clinically, the visual findings do not distinguish systemic inflammatory cases from idiopathic or demyelinating optic neuritis. MRI shows enlargement and enhancement of segments of the optic nerve in some cases, but this finding may be seen in idiopathic optic neuritis. In some patients, vision improves after treatment with high-dose corticosteroids or occasionally with more aggressive immunosuppression.

Patients with vasculitis, particularly those with TA, risk sudden visual loss from acute anterior ischemic optic neuropathy. Cases have also been reported associated with rheumatoid arthritis or antiphospholipid antibody syndrome. Patients with granulomatosis with polyangiitis can also develop optic neuropathy from compression.

Ophthalmoparesis is an exceptional event in patients with systemic inflammatory diseases, but when it occurs, detailed neuro-ophthalmologic and imaging examinations may be necessary to identify the neuroanatomic localization and cause (Table 50-9).

TABLE 50-9 ■ Ophthalmoparesis in Connective Tissue Diseases or Vasculitis

Cause of Ophthalmoparesis	Underlying Disease
Internuclear ophthalmoplegia	SLE, vasculitis
Cranial nerve III, IV, or VI palsy	SLE, Behçet syndrome, Sjögren syndrome, granulomatosis with polyangiitis, and other vasculitidites
Cranial nerve VI palsy	Any cause of meningitis or increased intracranial pressure
Orbital inflammation, orbital pseudotumor	Granulomatosis with polyangiitis, and others
Ischemic extraocular muscle necrosis	Temporal arteritis
Myasthenia gravis	Rheumatoid arthritis, SLE
Miller Fisher syndrome	SLE
Brown syndrome (superior oblique tendinitis)	Rheumatoid arthritis, Sjögren syndrome, SLE

SLE, systemic lupus erythematosus.

Trigeminal sensory neuropathy, unilateral or bilateral, especially in the maxillary and mandibular divisions, is particularly associated with Sjögren syndrome and systemic sclerosis. Ischemic cranial mononeuropathies, especially of the facial nerve, are unusual complications of SLE or vasculitis. The annual incidence of Bell palsy is far higher than the prevalence of SLE, and cranial neuropathies occur in less than 1 percent of lupus patients. Most patients with isolated cranial mononeuropathies do not need extensive evaluation for vasculitis or connective tissue disease, unless there are other clues to suggest systemic illness. However, in patients with painless, purely sensory neuropathy of the lower face, connective tissue disease deserves more consideration.

ACUTE INFLAMMATORY DEMYELINATING NEUROPATHY

Literature review suggests that patients with SLE or rheumatoid arthritis have an increased incidence of Guillain–Barré syndrome. An association is plausible because of the tendency of autoimmune diseases to overlap, but there are few data on whether this reflects a true association or publication bias. Antiphospholipid antibodies can appear transiently in patients with Guillain–Barré syndrome and are not by themselves diagnostic of antiphospholipid antibody syndrome. An alternative but uncommon explanation for acute ascending paralysis in patients with lupus or vasculitis is fulminant vasculitic neuropathy. Chronic inflammatory demyelinating polyneuropathy is also linked to systemic inflammatory diseases by case reports.

DYSAUTONOMIA

Autonomic neuropathy, with or without sensory neuropathy or neuronopathy, may complicate a number of connective tissue diseases, including rheumatoid arthritis, SLE, Sjögren syndrome, and systemic sclerosis. In these illnesses autonomic deficits are more likely to be found on physiologic testing than to be symptomatic.

MONONEUROPATHY MULTIPLEX

Vasculitis is a common cause of mononeuritis multiplex. About one-fourth of patients with mononeuropathy multiplex have nonsystemic vasculitic neuropathy and another one-fourth have some form of systemic vasculitis.[48] Vasculitis of the nerve can also be secondary to other systemic diseases, such as rheumatoid arthritis, infections (especially in association with hepatitis B, hepatitis C, and human immunodeficiency virus), sarcoidosis,[95] or paraneoplastic syndromes (especially in association with T-cell lymphomas).[54] Diabetic amyotrophy, diabetic radiculopathy, and other manifestations of multifocal asymmetric diabetic neuropathy are often associated with vasculitis in the affected nerves, a pattern that is unusual in diabetics whose neuropathy is limited to the more common distal symmetric pattern.[96] Mononeuritis multiplex is unusual in patients with SLE or Sjögren syndrome. Other causes of asymmetric multiple neuropathies include Lewis–Sumner syndrome, multifocal motor neuropathy with conduction block, neuralgic amyotrophy, compression neuropathies superimposed on more symmetric neuropathies especially in patients with hereditary liability to pressure palsies, amyloidosis, neoplastic nerve infiltration, Lyme disease, porphyria, and leprosy.

MYASTHENIA GRAVIS

Patients with myasthenia gravis have an increased incidence of other autoimmune diseases. The prevalence of rheumatoid arthritis in patients with myasthenia gravis may be 2 to 4 percent, and the prevalence of SLE is also increased. Case reports link SLE and Lambert–Eaton syndrome. Myasthenia may occur as a toxic effect of penicillamine or chloroquine used to treat connective tissue disorders.

POLYNEUROPATHY

Distal symmetric axonal polyneuropathy may accompany many of the illnesses discussed in this chapter, including perhaps one-fifth of patients with SLE or Sjögren syndrome. Distal sensory neuropathy may be a late finding in rheumatoid arthritis. Vasculitic neuropathy in nonsystemic vasculitic neuropathy or systemic necrotizing vasculitis sometimes causes a distal, relatively symmetric clinical pattern. Neuropathy occurs much less frequently in patients with systemic sclerosis, Behçet syndrome, or TA. Some of the drugs used in treatment of inflammatory diseases, including gold, chloroquine, colchicine, and penicillamine, can cause neuropathy. In patients with multifocal CNS disease, concomitant peripheral neuropathy does not exclude multiple sclerosis but may alert the clinician to check carefully for SLE, Sjögren syndrome, and vasculitis among a number of other systemic illnesses (Table 50-10).

TABLE 50-10 ■ Acquired Combined Peripheral and Central Nervous System Disease

Chronic renal failure
Diabetes mellitus complicated by stroke and neuropathy
Epstein–Barr virus infection
Granulomatosis with polyangiitis
Human immunodeficiency virus infection
Lyme neuroborreliosis
Metastatic and paraneoplastic syndromes
Neurologic complications of alcohol abuse
Neurolymphomatosis or intravascular lymphomatosis
Neurosyphilis
Polyarteritis nodosa
Sarcoidosis
Sjögren syndrome
Systemic lupus erythematosus
Vitamin deficiencies: B_1, B_2, B_6, B_{12}
Whipple disease

From Rosenbaum RB, Campbell SM, Rosenbaum JT: Clinical Neurology of Rheumatic Diseases. Butterworth Heinemann, Stoneham, 1996.

SENSORY NEURONOPATHY

Sensory neuronopathy can occur in Sjögren syndrome; other causes include toxins, like cisplatinin or high doses of pyridoxine, paraneoplastic sensory neuronopathy, and acute or chronic idiopathic sensory neuronopathy.

THERAPEUTIC CHOICES

There is a paucity of class I data on treatment of the neurologic manifestations of connective tissue disease or vasculitis. The rarity and diversity of these syndromes make it difficult to design prospective, randomized, controlled treatment trials. Therefore, the more extensive experience in treating systemic manifestations of SLE or vasculitis is often extrapolated to treating neurologic disease. Glucocorticoids and cyclophosphamide are the therapeutic mainstays. Other immunosuppressants such as azathioprine, methotrexate, or cyclosporine are used at times. Newer approaches to immunomodulation, such as anti–tumor necrosis factor agents or rituxamab, are sometimes tried. The choice of neurologic therapy depends more on the severity of the neurologic complication than on underlying systemic diagnosis. Thus, mononeuritis multiplex, myelitis, symptomatic focal brain lesions, or optic neuritis often warrant aggressive immunosuppression. In contrast, mild peripheral neuropathy, recurrent headache, or subtle cognitive problems might be treated symptomatically. Syndromes such as myasthenia gravis and Guillain–Barré syndrome, in which antibodies play a direct pathogenic role, often respond to plasmapheresis or IVIg. For conditions causing stroke, the mechanism of ischemia determines the appropriate treatment. These are complex therapeutic decisions that emphasize the challenges and rewards of treating patients who have the diseases discussed in this chapter.

ACKNOWLEDGMENT

The author thanks Stephen M. Campbell, MD, for his thoughtful critique of this chapter.

REFERENCES

1. Lim W, Crowther MA, Eikelboom JW: Management of antiphospholipid antibody syndrome. A systematic review. JAMA 295:1050, 2006.
2. Sanna G, D'Cruz D, Cuadrado MJ: Cerebral manifestations of the antiphospholipid (Hughes) syndrome. Rheum Dis Clin North Am 32:465, 2006.
3. Hanly JG, Urowitz MB, Siannis F, et al: Autoantibodies and neuropsychiatric events at the time of systemic lupus erythematosus diagnosis: results from an international inception cohort study. Arthritis Rheum 58:843, 2008.
4. Unterman A, Nolte JE, Boaz M, et al: Neuropsychiatric syndromes in systemic lupus erythematosus: a meta-analysis. Semin Arthritis Rheum 41:1, 2011.
5. Hanly JG, McCurdy G, Fougere L, et al: Neuropsychiatric events in systemic lupus erythematosus: attribution and clinical significance. J Rheumatol 31:2156, 2004.
6. Hanly JG, Harrison MJ: Management of neuropsychiatric lupus. Best Pract Res Clin Rheumatol 19:799, 2005.
7. Mitsikostas DD, Sfikakis PP, Goadsby PJ: A meta-analysis for headache in systemic lupus erythematosus: the evidence and the myth. Brain 127:1200, 2004.
8. Appenzeller S, Cendes F, Costallat LTL: Epileptic seizures in systemic lupus erythematosus. Neurology 63:1808, 2004.
9. Roman MJ, Shanker BA, Davis A, et al: Prevalence and correlates of accelerated atherosclerosis in systemic lupus erythematosus. N Engl J Med 349:2399, 2003.
10. Reiner P, Galanaud D, Leroux G, et al: Long-term outcome of 32 patients with chorea and systemic lupus erythematosus or antiphospholipid antibodies. Mov Disord 26:2422, 2011.
11. Baizabal-Carvallo JF, Jankovic J: Movement disorders in autoimmune diseases. Mov Disord 27:935, 2012.
12. Birnbaum J, Petri M, Thompson R, et al: Distinct subtypes of myelitis in systemic lupus erythematosus. Arthritis Rheum 60:3378, 2009.
13. Pittock SJ, Lennon VA, de Seze J, et al: Neuromyelitis optica and non organ-specific autoimmunity. Arch Neurol 65:78, 2008.
14. Baizabal-Carvallo JF, Delgadillo-Marquez G, Estanol B, et al: Clinical characteristics and outcomes of the meningitides in systemic lupus erythematosus. Eur Neurol 61:143, 2009.
15. Leroux G, Sellam J, Costedoat-Chalumeau N, et al: Posterior reversible encephalopathy syndrome during systemic lupus erythematosus: four new cases and review of the literature. Lupus 17:139, 2008.
16. Pego-Reigosa JM, Isenberg DA: Psychosis due to systemic lupus erythematosus: characteristics and long-term outcome of this rare manifestation of the disease. Rheumatology (Oxford) 47:1498, 2008.
17. Shalimar, Handa R, Deepak KK, et al: Autonomic dysfunction in systemic lupus erythematosus. Rheumatol Int 26:837, 2006.
18. Fox RI: Sjögren's syndrome. Lancet 366:321, 2005.
19. Harboe E, Tjensvoll AB, Maroni S, et al: Neuropsychiatric syndromes in patients with systemic lupus erythematosus and primary Sjögren syndrome: a comparative population-based study. Ann Rheum Dis 68:1541, 2009.
20. Massara A, Bonazza S, Castellino G, et al: Central nervous system involvement in Sjögren's syndrome: unusual, but not unremarkable–clinical, serological characteristics and outcomes in a large cohort of Italian patients. Rheumatology (Oxford) 49:1540, 2010.

21. Mori K, Iijima M, Koike H, et al: The wide spectrum of clinical manifestations in Sjögren's syndrome-associated neuropathy. Brain 128:2518, 2005.
22. Gorson KC, Ropper AH: Positive salivary gland biopsy, Sjögren syndrome, and neuropathy: clinical implications. Muscle Nerve 28:553, 2003.
23. Chad DA, Stone JH, Gupta R: Case records of the Massachusetts General Hospital. Case 14-2011. A woman with asymmetric sensory loss and paresthesias. N Engl J Med 364:1856, 2011.
24. Hermisson M, Klein R, Schmidt F, et al: Myelopathy in primary Sjögren's syndrome: diagnostic and therapeutic aspects. Acta Neurol Scand 105:450, 2002.
25. Kondo T, Inoue H, Usui T, et al: Autoimmune autonomic ganglionopathy with Sjögren's syndrome: significance of ganglionic acetylcholine receptor antibody and therapeutic approach. Auton Neurosci 146:33, 2009.
26. Delalande S, de Seze J, Fauchais AL, et al: Neurologic manifestations in primary Sjögren's syndrome. A study of 82 patients. Medicine (Baltimore) 83:280, 2004.
27. Font J, Valls J, Cervera R, et al: Pure sensory neuropathy in patients with Sjögren's syndrome: clinical, immunological, and electromyographic findings. Ann Rheum Dis 49:775, 1990.
28. Steen VD: Autoantibodies in systemic sclerosis. Semin Arthritis Rheum 35:35, 2005.
29. Bertinotti L, Bracci S, Nacci F, et al: The autonomic nervous system in systemic sclerosis. A review. Clin Rheumatol 23:1, 2004.
30. Terajima K, Shimohata T, Watanabe M, et al: Cerebral vasculopathy showing moyamoya-like changes in a patient with CREST syndrome. Eur Neurol 46:163, 2001.
31. Turesson C, O'Fallon WM, Crowson CS, et al: Extra-articular manifestations in rheumatoid arthritis: incidence trends and risk factors over 46 years. Ann Rheum Dis 62:722, 2003.
32. Servioli MJ, Chugh C, Lee JM, et al: Rheumatoid meningitis. Front Neurol 2:84, 2011.
33. Naranjo A, Carmona L, Gavrila D, et al: Prevalence and associated factors of anterior atlantoaxial luxation in a nation-wide sample of rheumatoid arthritis patients. Clin Exp Rheumatol 22:427, 2004.
34. Krauss WE, Bledsoe JM, Clarke MJ, et al: Rheumatoid arthritis of the craniovertebral junction. Neurosurgery 66:83, 2010.
35. Ernste FC, Reed AM: Idiopathic inflammatory myopathies: current trends in pathogenesis, clinical features, and up-to-date treatment recommendations. Mayo Clin Proc 88:83, 2013.
36. Hall S, Hanrahan P: Muscle involvement in mixed connective tissue disease. Rheum Dis Clin North Am 31:509, 2005.
37. Vianna MAAG Borges CTL, Borba EF, et al: Myositis in mixed connective tissue disease. A unique syndrome characterized by immunohistopathologic elements of both polymyositis and dermatomyositis. Arq Neuropsiquiatr 62:923, 2004.
38. Ohno A, Mitsui T, Endo I, et al: Dermatomyositis associated with Sjögren's syndrome: VEGF involvement in vasculitis. Clin Neuropathol 23:178, 2004.
39. Pestronk A: Acquired immune and inflammatory myopathies: pathologic classification. Curr Opin Rheumatol 23:595, 2011.
40. Derk CT, Vivino FB, Kenyon L, et al: Inclusion body myositis in connective tissue disorders: case report and review of the literature. Clin Rheumatol 22:324, 2003.
41. Ellis E, Ann Tan J, Lester S, et al: Necrotizing myopathy: clinicoserologic associations. Muscle Nerve 45:189, 2012.
42. Salvarani C, Brown Jr RD, Calamia KT, et al: Primary central nervous system vasculitis: analysis of 101 patients. Ann Neurol 62:442, 2007.
43. Birnbaum J, Hellmann DB: Primary angiitis of the central nervous system. Arch Neurol 66:704, 2009.
44. Kadkhodayan Y, Alreshaid A, Moran CJ, et al: Primary angiitis of the central nervous system at conventional angiography. Radiology 233:878, 2004.
45. Singhal AB, Hajj-Ali RA, Topcuoglu MA, et al: Reversible cerebral vasoconstriction syndromes: analysis of 139 cases. Arch Neurol 68:1005, 2011.
46. Alreshaid AA, Powers WJ: Prognosis of patients with suspected primary CNS angiitis and negative brain biopsy. Neurology 61:831, 2003.
47. Collins MP, Dyck PJ, Gronseth GS, et al: Peripheral Nerve Society Guideline on the classification, diagnosis, investigation, and immunosuppressive therapy of non-systemic vasculitic neuropathy: executive summary. J Peripher Nerv Syst 15:176, 2010.
48. Collins MP, Periquet MI: Non-systemic vasculitic neuropathy. Curr Opin Neurol 17:587, 2004.
49. Collins MP, Mendell JR, Periquet MI, et al: Superficial peroneal nerve/peroneus brevis muscle biopsy in vasculitic neuropathy. Neurology 55:636, 2000.
50. Collins MP, Periquet MI, Mendell JR, et al: Nonsystemic vasculitic neuropathy: insights from a clinical cohort. Neurology 61:623, 2003.
51. Stone JH: Polyarteritis nodosa. JAMA 288:1632, 2002.
52. Lane SE, Watts RA, Shepstone L, et al: Primary systemic vasculitis: clinical features and mortality. QJM 98:97, 2005.
53. Newburger JW, Takahashi M, Gerber MA, et al: Diagnosis, treatment, and long-term management of Kawasaki disease: a statement for health professionals from the Committee on Rheumatic Fever, Endocarditis, and Kawasaki Disease, Council on Cardiovascular Disease in the Young, American Heart Association. Pediatrics 114:1708, 2004.
54. Younger DS: Vasculitis of the nervous system. Curr Opin Neurol 17:317, 2002.
55. Pagnoux C, Seror R, Henegar C, et al: Clinical features and outcomes in 348 patients with polyarteritis nodosa: a systematic retrospective study of patients

diagnosed between 1963 and 2005 and entered into the French Vasculitis Study Group Database. Arthritis Rheum 62:616, 2010.

56. Mattioli F, Capra R, Rovaris M, et al: Frequency and patterns of subclinical cognitive impairment in patients with ANCA-associated small vessel vasculitides. J Neurol Sci 195:161, 2002.
57. Seror R, Mahr A, Ramanoelina J, et al: Central nervous system involvement in Wegener granulomatosis. Medicine (Baltimore) 85:54, 2006.
58. de Groot K, Schmidt DK, Arlt AC, et al: Standardized neurologic evaluations of 128 patients with Wegener granulomatosis. Arch Neurol 58:1215, 2001.
59. Gayraud M, Guillevin L, le Toumelin P, et al: Long-term followup of polyarteritis nodosa, microscopic polyangiitis, and Churg-Strauss syndrome. Arthritis Rheum 44:666, 2001.
60. Borchers AT, Gershwin ME: Giant cell arteritis: a review of classification, pathophysiology, geoepidemiology and treatment. Autoimmun Rev 11:A544, 2012.
61. Salvarani C, Cantini F, Boiardi L, et al: Polymyalgia rheumatica and giant-cell arteritis. N Engl J Med 347:261, 2002.
62. Salvarani C, Crowson CS, O'Fallon WM, et al: Reappraisal of the epidemiology of giant cell arteritis in Olmsted county, Minnesota, over a fifty-year period. Arthritis Rheum 51:264, 2004.
63. Mahr A, Saba M, Kambouchner M, et al: Temporal artery biopsy for diagnosing giant cell arteritis: the longer, the better? Ann Rheum Dis 65:826, 2006.
64. Younge BR, Cook Jr BE, Bartley GB, et al: Initiation of glucocorticoid therapy: before or after temporal artery biopsy? Mayo Clinic Proc 79:483, 2004.
65. Arida A, Kyprianou M, Kanakis M, et al: The diagnostic value of ultrasonography-derived edema of the temporal artery wall in giant cell arteritis: a second meta-analysis. BMC Musculoskelet Disord 11:44, 2010.
66. Prieto-Gonzalez S, Arguis P, Garcia-Martinez A, et al: Large vessel involvement in biopsy-proven giant cell arteritis: prospective study in 40 newly diagnosed patients using CT angiography. Ann Rheum Dis 71:1170, 2012.
67. Hoffman G, Cid M, Hellmann D, et al: A multicenter, randomized, double-blind, placebo-controlled trial of adjuvant methotrxate treatment for giant cell arteritis. Arthritis Rheum 46:1309, 2002.
68. Lee MS, Smith SD, Galor A, et al: Antiplatelet and anticoagulant therapy in patients with giant cell arteritis. Arthritis Rheum 54:3306, 2006.
69. Salvarani C, Cantini F, Boiardi L, et al: Polymyalgia rheumatica. Best Pract Res Clin Rheumatol 18:705, 2004.
70. Park MC, Lee SW, Park YB, et al: Clinical characteristics and outcomes of Takayasu's arteritis: analysis of 108 patients using standardized criteria for diagnosis, activity assessment, and angiographic classification. Scand J Rheumatol 34:284, 2005.
71. Li-xin Z, Jun N, Shan G, et al: Neurological manifestations of Takayasu arteritis. Chin Med Sci J 26:227, 2011.
72. Maksimowicz-McKinnon K, Clark TM, Hoffman GS: Limitations of therapy and a guarded prognosis in an American cohort of Takayasu arteritis patients. Arthritis Rheum 56:1000, 2007.
73. Liang P, Hoffman GS: Advances in the medical and surgical management of Takayasu arteritis. Curr Opin Rheumatol 17:16, 2004.
74. Al-Araji A, Sharquie K, Al-Rawi Z: Prevalence and patterns of neurological involvement in Behçet's disease: a prospective study from Iraq. J Neurol Neurosurg Psychiatry 74:608, 2003.
75. Siva A, Saip S: The spectrum of nervous system involvement in Behçet's syndrome and its differential diagnosis. J Neurol 256:513, 2009.
76. Haghighi AB, Pourmand R, Nikseresht AR: Neuro-Behçet's disease. A review. Neurologist 11:80, 2005.
77. Siva A, Altintas A, Saip S: Behçet's syndrome and the nervous system. Curr Opin Rheumatol 17:347, 2004.
78. Kang DW, Chu K, Cho JY, et al: Diffusion weighted magnetic resonance imaging in neuro-Behçet's disease. J Neurol Neurosurg Psychiatry 70:412, 2001.
79. Ribi C, Sztajzel R, Delavelle J, et al: Efficacy of TNF α blockade in cyclophosphamide resistant neuro-Behçet disease. J Neurol Neurosurg Psychiatry 76:1733, 2005.
80. Kupersmith MJ, Martin V, Heller G, et al: Idiopathic hypertrophic pachymeningitis. Neurology 62:686, 2004.
81. Bruggemann N, Gottschalk S, Holl-Ulrich K, et al: Cranial pachymeningitis: a rare neurological syndrome with heterogeneous aetiology. J Neurol Neurosurg Psychiatry 81:294, 2010.
82. Ropper AH, Ayata C, Adelman L: Vasculitis of the spinal cord. Arch Neurol 60:1791, 2003.
83. Stanescu D, Bodaghi B, Huong DL, et al: Pseudotumor cerebri associated with Sjögren's syndrome. Graefes Arch Clin Exp Ophthalmol 241:339, 2003.
84. Sbeiti S, Kayed DM, Majuri H: Pseudotumour cerebri presentation of systemic lupus erythematosus: more than an association. Rheumatoloy (Oxford) 42:808, 2003.
85. Kuriwaka R, Kunishige M, Nakahira H, et al: Neuro-Behçet's disease with chorea after remission of intestinal Behçet diseae. Clin Rheumatol 23:364, 2004.
86. Lee PH, Joo US, Bang OY, et al: Basal ganglia hyperperfusion in a patient with systemic lupus erythematosus-related parkinsonism. Neurology 63:395, 2004.
87. de Seze J, Stojkovic T, Breteau G, et al: Acute myelopathies. Clinical, laboratory and outcome profiles in 79 cases. Brain 124:1509, 2001.
88. Shin KC, Choi HJ, Bae Y, et al: Reversible posterior leukoencephalopathy syndrome in systemic lupus

erythematosus with thrombocytopenia treated with cyclosporine. J Clin Rheumatol 11:164, 2005.

89. Min L, Zwerling J, Ocava LC, et al: Reversible posterior leukoencephalopathy in connective tissue diseases. Semin Arthritis Rheum 35:388, 2006.

90. Allford SL, Hunt BJ, Rose P, et al: Guidelines on the diagnosis and management of the thrombotic microangiopathic haemolytic anemias. Br J Haematol 122:518, 2003.

91. Warnatz K, Peter HH, Schumacher M, et al: Infectious CNS disease as a differential diagnosis in systemic rheumatic diseases: three case reports and a review of the literature. Ann Rheum Dis 62:50, 2003.

92. Covic T, Tyson G, Spencer D, et al: Depression in rheumatoid arthritis patients: demographic, clinical, and psychological predictors. J Psychosom Res 60:469, 2006.

93. Legendre C, Allanore Y, Ferrand I, et al: Evaluation of depression and anxiety in patients with systemic sclerosis. Joint Bone Spine 72:408, 2005.

94. Hanly JG, Fisk JD, McCurdy G, et al: Neuropsychiatric syndromes in patients with systemic lupus erythematosus and rheumatoid arthritis. J Rheumatol 32:1459, 2005.

95. Said G, Lacroix C, Planté-Bordneuve V, et al: Nerve granulomas and vasculitis in sarcoid peripheral neuropathy. A clinicopathological study of 11 patients. Brain 125:264, 2002.

96. Said G, Lacroix C, Lozeron P, et al: Inflammatory vasculopathy in multifocal diabetic neuropathy. Brain 126:376, 2003.

97. Florica B, Aghdassi E, Su J, et al: Peripheral neuropathy in patients with systemic lupus erythematosus. Semin Arthritis Rheum 41:203, 2011.

SECTION

XII

Sleep and Its Disorders

CHAPTER

51

Neurologic Aspects of Sleep Medicine

RENEE MONDERER ■ SHELBY HARRIS ■ MICHAEL THORPY

Aminoff's Neurology and General Medicine, Fifth Edition.

Sleep disorders commonly occur in patients who present to neurologists. At times, symptoms are obvious, such as insomnia or excessive daytime sleepiness. However, some patients have serious sleep disorders, such as sleep apnea, that are often not readily apparent to the patient or physician and can exacerbate a neurologic disorder. Established links exist between sleep apnea and stroke, epilepsy, and migraine, between certain sleep behavior disorders and neurodegenerative diseases, and between circadian rhythm disorders and dementia. In light of these links, it is important that neurologists become familiar with sleep disorders and incorporate sleep diagnosis and treatment into daily practice, and that sleep specialists and internists gain wider appreciation of the impact of sleep disorders on neurologic function and disease. This chapter reviews key aspects of sleep medicine and their association with clinical neurology.

SLEEP PHYSIOLOGY

Sleep is defined by behavioral and physiologic changes that include postural recumbence, behavioral quiescence, eye closure, and specific physiologic parameters based on electroencephalography (EEG), electrooculography (EOG), and electromyography (EMG). Sleep is further subdivided into non–rapid eye movement (NREM) and rapid eye movement (REM) sleep.

The normal adult brain enters sleep first through NREM stages followed by REM sleep approximately 90 minutes later. NREM and REM sleep then alternate through four to six cycles lasting 90 to 110 minutes each. The first third of sleep is dominated by NREM sleep and the last third of the night is dominated by REM sleep. NREM sleep is further divided into three stages (N1, N2, N3).[1]

Sleep Stages

The staging of sleep is based on the recordings of the EEG, chin EMG and EOG made during polysomnography (PSG). The PSG is scored by assigning a sleep stage to each 30-second epoch recorded. The characteristics of the various sleep stages are summarized in Figure 51-1.

Stage Wake

Stage wake can occur when the subject is alert with eyes open or relaxed with eyes closed. When the eyes are open, the EEG shows low-amplitude, fast mixed-frequency activity. The EOG tracing consists of eye movements and eye blinks, and the EMG chin activity is increased. Once the eyes are closed, alpha rhythms (8 to 13 Hz) predominate on the EEG and are most prominent in the occipital leads. This alpha activity attenuates with concentration or with eye opening. Stage W is scored when 50 percent of the epoch shows alpha activity in the occipital region. The normal adult spends less than 5 percent of the night in this stage.

Stage N1

Stage N1 sleep is characterized by light sleep or drowsiness. It is identified by less than 50 percent of the epoch being occupied by alpha activity on the EEG. The EEG also shows low-voltage, mixed-frequency activity predominantly in the theta frequency (4 to 7 Hz). The EOG channel often shows slow rolling eye movements, and EMG activity is diminished. Vertex sharp waves may appear in the central EEG leads in the later part of stage N1. In the normal adult, stage N1 should occupy 2 to 5 percent of sleep, but patients with excessive sleep fragmentation such as those with sleep apnea often have a larger percentage of stage N1 sleep.

Stage N2

Stage N2 sleep is defined by the presence of K-complexes or sleep spindles on the EEG. The background EEG shows low-amplitude, mixed-frequency activity. The EOG typically shows no eye movements, but slow rolling eye movements may persist from stage N1. EMG activity is reduced from stage N1 and wake. Stage N2 generally constitutes 45 to 55 percent of sleep in adults.

Stage N3

Stage N3 sleep, also referred to as slow-wave sleep, represents the deepest sleep stage. Slow-wave sleep was initially divided into stages 3 and 4; however, because of the physiologic similarities between these stages, they have been combined into a single stage. Stage N3 is defined by the presence of high-amplitude slow waves with a frequency of 0.5 to 2 Hz and an amplitude of 75 μV. Slow-wave activity must occupy at least 20 percent of the epoch to meet criteria for stage N3. The EMG is active but diminished compared to stages W and N1, and there are no eye

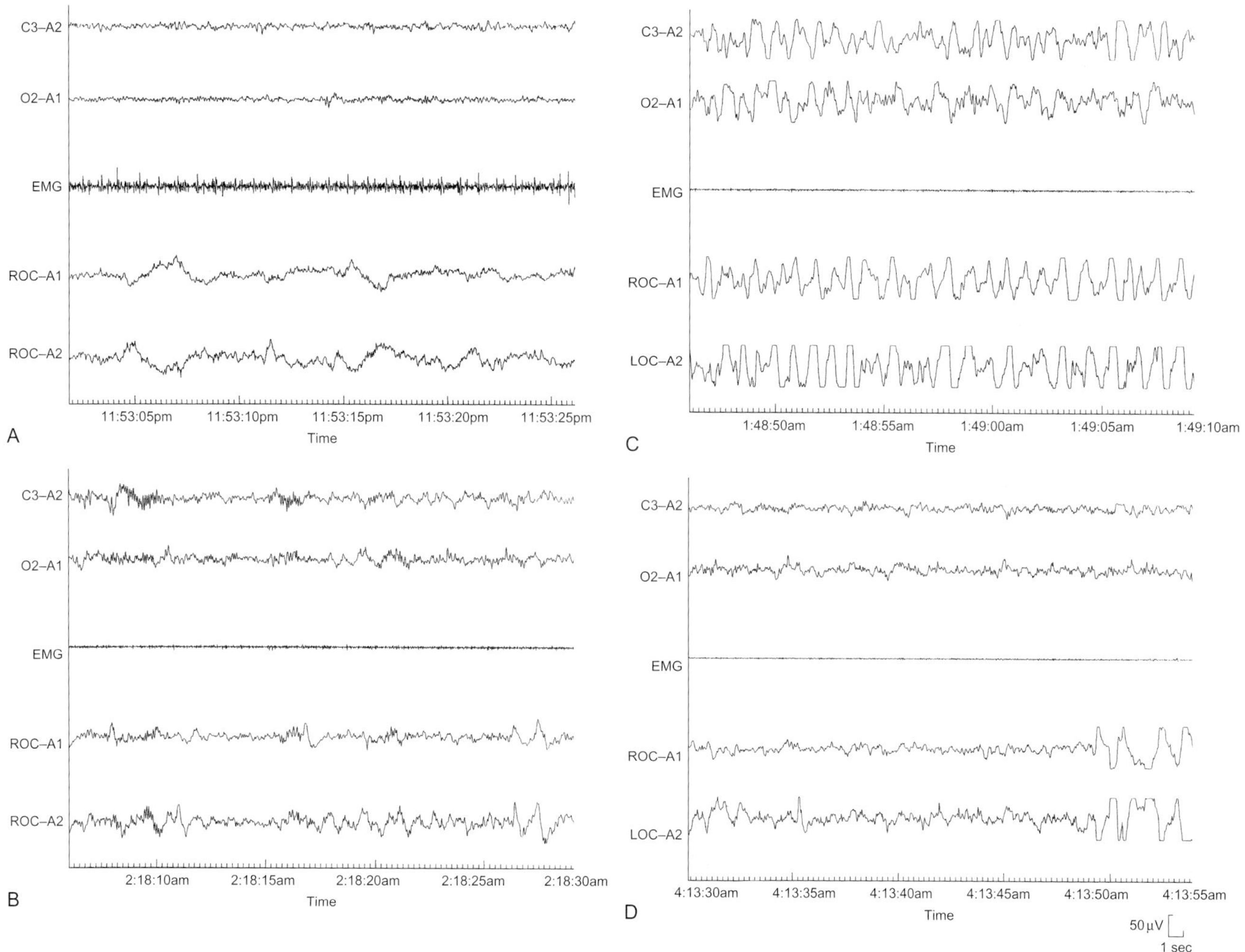

FIGURE 51-1 ■ The stages of sleep. **A,** Stage N1. There is low-voltage mixed-frequency electrocerebral activity with ongoing muscle activity and slow, rolling eye movements. **B,** Stage N2 sleep showing sleep spindles. K-complexes are also classically present but are not clearly shown in this epoch. **C,** Stage N3 sleep, with high-amplitude, low-frequency delta activity in the electroencephalogram (EEG). The eye-movement channels reflect the EEG. **D,** Stage REM. The EEG is of low amplitude and mixed frequency and is accompanied by muscle atonia and rapid eye movements. (Adapted from Abad VC, Guilleminault C: Polysomnographic evaluation of sleep disorders. p. 727. In Aminoff MJ (ed): Aminoff's Electrodiagnosis in Clinical Neurology. 6th Ed. Elsevier Saunders, Oxford, 2012.)

movements. Stage N3 occupies 15 to 25 percent of sleep in healthy adults.

Stage REM

REM sleep is characterized by a highly active brain with loss of muscle tone. The EEG shows a low-voltage, mixed-frequency pattern with sawtooth waves. The chin EMG tone is markedly diminished, and the EOG shows rapid eye movements. There is a cessation of K complexes, sleep spindles, and high-amplitude waves. REM sleep accounts for 20 to 25 percent of total sleep time in healthy adults.

Sleep Patterns Across the Human Lifespan

Sleep patterns change markedly throughout the human lifespan. The most pronounced changes occur during the first year of life. Newborns enter sleep through REM sleep (called "active sleep" in the newborn), and then sleep alternates between REM and NREM in 50- to 60-minute intervals rather than the 90-minute cycles of adults. During the first year of life, EEG patterns develop to allow distinction between different stages of NREM sleep.[2]

Stage N3 sleep is most prominent in childhood and decreases by almost 40 percent in the second decade of life. It further declines with age and is almost absent by the age of 60, especially in men, perhaps due to a decline in the amplitude of EEG waves from reduced synaptic activity.[3]

REM sleep occupies 50 percent of sleep in the first year of life. By 6 years of age, REM sleep time is reduced to 20 to 25 percent of sleep and is maintained at this percentage into old age. REM sleep markedly declines with organic brain dysfunction.

Arousals and episodes of awakening from sleep increase dramatically with age and may correlate with an underlying sleep disorder, medical condition, or neurologic disease. The percentage of stage N1 sleep also increases with age, signifying more transitions between wake and sleep.[4]

Sleep requirements change with age. A newborn sleeps about 16 hours per day. This falls to about 11 hours in children 3 to 5 years of age. Adolescents between 9 and 10 years of age require approximately 10 hours of sleep.[5] Adults average 7.5 to 8 hours of sleep; although this duration remains steady into healthy old age, the ability to consolidate sleep into one a single continuous sleep period declines. Elderly individuals may revert to a biphasic sleep pattern with increased daytime napping.

CIRCADIAN NEUROBIOLOGY

The sleep-wake cycle is regulated by two opposing processes, the circadian rhythm and the homeostatic drive for sleep. The circadian rhythm is set by the suprachiasmatic nucleus of the hypothalamus, which regulates the sleep-wake cycle. The suprachiasmatic nucleus projects to the pineal gland to release melatonin, which promotes sleep. The nucleus is synchronized by external cues known as *zeitgebers*, of which the strongest is light. Light inhibits the release of melatonin from the pineal gland and in this way sleep is influenced by the day-night cycle.

The homeostatic process refers to an increased propensity for sleepiness with longer periods of being awake. Adenosine is a byproduct of the waking brain, and levels rise with prolonged periods of wake, increasing the tendency for sleep. Caffeine is an adenosine antagonist and is used to promote wakefulness.

In the morning, the suprachiasmatic nucleus output is low. The homeostatic drive increases over the day and is opposed by increased output from the suprachiasmatic nucleus. By the end of the day, suprachiasmatic nucleus output is decreased through inhibition by melatonin, and the homeostatic drive is increased, resulting in the onset of sleep.

The circadian rhythm of sleep becomes clinically relevant when the sleep-wake cycle is changed such as in shift work or jet lag. Adaptation becomes difficult both because of sleep loss and increased homeostatic drive for sleep and because the circadian rhythm continues on its own established schedule. Elderly individuals who have difficulty consolidating sleep and those with neurodegenerative diseases often have disruption of the normal cycling of sleep consistent with circadian rhythm disorders. Light therapy can be a useful tool to help reset the circadian rhythm and establish a normal sleep-wake cycle.

NEUROANATOMY OF SLEEP

Changes between wake, NREM, and REM sleep are produced through modulation of neurotransmitters and neuromodulaters interconnecting the neuronal system that regulates sleep.

The ascending arousal system is important in maintaining wakefulness. It is composed of a cholinergic branch and a monoaminergic branch. The cholinergic branch includes the pedunculopontine and laterodorsal tegmental nuclei, which project to the thalamic reticular nucleus in order to activate the cerebral cortex. Acetylcholine excites the thalamic and cortical neurons maximally during wake and REM sleep.

The monoaminergic branch includes the locus coeruleus, dorsal and median raphe nuclei, tuberomammilary nuclei, and ventral periaqueductal gray matter. Histamine, norepinephrine, and serotonin are released from these various nuclei, which are also maximally active during wakefulness in order to activate the cerebral cortex. The monoaminergic system is quiet in NREM sleep and turned off in REM sleep. Hypocretin neurons in the lateral hypothalamus augment this activation of the cortex during wakefulness.

Dopamine is elevated during periods of wakefulness, and dopaminergic neurons modulate cortical activation indirectly through regulatory activity of the globus pallidus and the thalamus.

Sleep onset is associated with a rapid deactivation of both the monoaminergic and cholinergic branches of the arousal system. GABAergic neurons in the preoptic hypothalamus promote sleep onset. The ventrolateral preoptic nucleus sends descending inhibitory projections to multiple arousal systems during sleep.

The homeostatic process and the circadian clock determine the activity of the ventrolateral preoptic nucleus. In NREM sleep, this nucleus inhibits both the cholinergic and monoaminergic branches of the ascending arousal system to induce sleep. In REM sleep, only the monoaminergic nuclei are inhibited, but the cholinergic nuclei are active.

REM sleep is driven by cholinergic neurons in the pons. Descending cholinergic projections produce muscle atonia by activating neurons in the pontine reticular formation and ventral reticular formation that then project to the spinal cord. Glycine is the essential neurotransmitter in these pathways.

The monoaminergic nuclei also inhibit the ascending arousal system during wakefulness, resulting in a system of reciprocal inhibition. This has been termed the "sleep switch." [6,7] Both sides of the switch strongly inhibit each other, resulting in a feedback loop with only two possible states: sleep and wakefulness.

Hypocretin is the stabilizer of this switch. In wakefulness, hypocretin reinforces the arousal system to avert unwanted switches into sleep. Narcolepsy with cataplexy is a disorder of low levels of hypocretin, causing a lack of stability in the "sleep switch," resulting in frequent and unwanted transitions between sleep and wakefulness.

APPROACH TO THE PATIENT WITH SLEEP DISORDERS

Clinical Evaluation

Complaints related to sleep and wakefulness are pervasive in the general population. Approximately 30 percent of adults report one or more symptoms of insomnia including difficulty falling asleep, staying asleep, awakening too early, or nonrestorative sleep.[8] It is estimated that 4 to 21 percent experience excessive daytime sleepiness at least 3 days per week.[9,10] Only 6 percent of patients with sleep complaints see a physician specifically for a sleep problem, and many others resort to over-the-counter medications or self-remedies.[11]

Sleep disorders are associated with significant morbidity and mortality. Insomnia, for example, is associated with impairment of all aspects of quality of life including physical functioning, bodily pain, social functioning, and mental health.[12] Obstructive sleep apnea increases the risk of cardiovascular and cerebrovascular disease as well as causing motor vehicle accidents.[13]

Individuals with sleep disturbances present with any of four main complaints. The first is insomnia, which may be described as difficulty in falling asleep or staying asleep, having an insufficient amount of sleep, or poor quality of sleep. The second is excessive daytime sleepiness (EDS), which may manifest as feelings of lack of energy or tiredness associated with naps, falling asleep at inappropriate times, or difficulty with concentration or memory. The most common cause of EDS is insufficient time for sleep. The third complaint is of abnormal sleep behavior, usually described by a bed partner. The fourth is of an inability to sleep at the desired time. A single sleep disorder may be associated with multiple complaints.

It is important to understand the motivation of patients in seeking treatment. For example, insomnia may impact job performance and cause a concern for loss of employment. A complaint of snoring may present only after a person is forced to sleep in a separate room to prevent disturbing a bed partner. The International Classification of Sleep Disorders (ICSD) has helped unify the approach to sleep complaints by classifying over 80 sleep disorders.

Patients should fill out a sleep questionnaire and a 1- to 2-week sleep diary. The questionnaire should address the patients' usual sleep hours, nocturnal awakenings, daytime napping, work hours, snoring, daytime functioning, sleep environment, movements in sleep (e.g., leg movements), abnormal behaviors in sleep (e.g., sleepwalking), lifestyle factors (e.g., caffeine intake), weight changes, past medical history, social history, medications, family history of sleep disorders, and other sleep symptoms (e.g., cataplexy or sleep paralysis). A sleep diary should record the time of getting in and out of bed, sleep onset time, awakenings, naps, exercise, sleep medication, and caffeine intake. There are several scales used to assess the degree of daytime sleepiness in a person, such as the Epworth Sleepiness Scale, that can help with diagnosis.

In addition to general medical and neurologic examinations, the physical examination should include the patients' weight, height, body mass index, blood pressure, and neck circumference.

The upper airway should be inspected for pharyngeal narrowing, tonsillar enlargement, uvula enlargement or edema, a large tongue, low-lying palate, and micrognathia, all of which are risk factors for sleep apnea.

Laboratory Testing

Polysomnography

The PSG is the most useful diagnostic tool in sleep medicine. Several physiologic variables are recorded during the PSG, including EEG, EMG of the chin and legs, EOG, electrocardiogram, airflow through the nose and mouth, respiratory effort, and oxygen saturation.

The EEG is usually performed using six channels: two frontal leads, two central leads, and two occipital leads. Various stages of sleep are better identified using particular leads, such as identifying delta waves primarily in the frontal leads. A full EEG montage is sometimes used to differentiate parasomnias from epileptiform activity. The EMG of the chin is important in identifying the reduction in muscle tone seen during REM sleep. The EMG of both legs helps capture periodic limb movements in sleep. The EOG is used to identify characteristic eye movements, such as occur during REM sleep. A thermistor or nasal cannula records airflow by monitoring temperature changes. The nasal cannula is attached to a pressure transducer and is more accurate in detecting respiratory changes such as hypopneas. Respiratory effort is recorded using piezoelectric belts around the chest and abdomen in order to differentiate obstructive from central apneas, which are characterized by a complete lack of respiratory effort. A pulse oximeter is usually worn on the finger to monitor oxygen saturation.

The PSG should also include videography to record behavioral changes in sleep, a body position monitor, and snore recording. Sleep is recorded in 30-second intervals termed epochs.

PSG is useful for the diagnosis of sleep-related breathing disorders, narcolepsy, periodic limb movement disorder, and REM sleep behavior disorder. When a patient is diagnosed with sleep apnea, the PSG is also used to determine the optimal positive airway pressure (PAP) for treatment; titration can be performed on two separate nights or, alternatively, a split-night study can be performed. During the split-night study, the patient is observed for the first 2 to 3 hours for signs of sleep apnea and, if it is detected, the technician will interrupt the study and begin titration. Certain sleep disorders do not require PSG, such as insomnia, restless legs syndrome, and circadian rhythm disorders, unless a concomitant breathing disorder is suspected.

Multiple Sleep Latency Test

The multiple sleep latency test (MSLT) is used to document pathologic daytime sleepiness and to make a diagnosis of narcolepsy or idiopathic hypersomnia. It consists of five nap opportunities each 2 hours apart beginning 2 hours after the termination of the nocturnal PSG. The recording montage consists of the EEG, chin EMG, EOG, and electrocardiogram. Each nap is terminated either 20 minutes after starting (if the patient does not fall asleep) or 15 minutes after the first 30-second epoch of sleep.

The average latency to sleep onset across all five naps is calculated. A mean sleep latency of 8 minutes or less with at least two sleep-onset REM periods strongly suggests a diagnosis of narcolepsy. It is important that the MSLT is performed after at least 6 hours of total sleep time because sleep deprivation can mimic narcolepsy.

Maintenance of Wakefulness Test

The maintenance of wakefulness test, a variation of the MSLT, measures a person's ability to stay awake in the daytime. It is useful in determining the effects of treatment on daytime sleepiness and consists of four trials of remaining awake while sedentary every 2 hours, beginning 2 hours after the patient has awakened from nighttime sleep. Each trial is terminated after 40 minutes if the patient remains awake or after the first three consecutive epochs of stage N1 sleep or the first epoch of any other stage of sleep. The mean sleep latency across all four naps is calculated. This test is often used to assess the ability of commercial drivers to remain awake at work.

Actigraphy

Actigraphy is used to objectively assess the patient's sleep-wake schedule in the normal environment for a 1- to 2-week period. The actigraph is worn on the nondominant wrist and detects small movements to establish periods of rest and activity which equate with wake and sleep. It is most useful in patients with circadian rhythm disorders or insomnia.

Home Sleep Studies

A home sleep study is a simplified version of a PSG that usually focuses exclusively on respiratory parameters, without measurement of sleep stages. There are various versions, but all should include nasal airflow, respiratory effort, and an oximeter. According to guidelines, home sleep studies should only be used in patients with a high pretest probability of having obstructive sleep apnea.[14] In practice, it is used in patients with suspected severe uncomplicated obstructive sleep apnea to confirm the diagnosis. The home sleep study is not clinically useful for patients with suspected insomnia, narcolepsy, circadian rhythm disorders, parasomnias, or nocturnal movement disorders.

INSOMNIA

Standardized Definitions

Insomnia is one of the most prevalent health complaints, with 30 to 50 percent of the population reporting transient insomnia. When even more specific diagnostic criteria are utilized, the rates still range between 5 percent and 20 percent.[15,16]

Criteria for insomnia differ somewhat between the three main classification systems: International Classification of Diseases, 10th edition (ICD); Diagnostic and Statistical Manual, Treatment Revision, 4th edition (DSM-IV-TR); and International Classification of Sleep Disorders, 2nd edition (ICSD-2).[17] The ICSD-2 describes 11 subtypes of insomnia that all have as a hallmark symptom a sleep disturbance defined as difficulty initiating sleep, difficulty maintaining sleep, early morning awakenings, or sleep that is of poor quality or nonrestorative.[17] The DSM-IV requires a prominent complaint similar to the ICSD-2, but has a time cut-off, requiring symptoms to be present for at least 1 month. The ICD-10 requires that sleep disturbance must occur at least 3 nights per week.

For many years, insomnia was thought of as a symptom of another underlying condition. Classification symptoms all distinguish between forms of "primary" (insomnia occurring without any comorbidities) and "secondary" insomnia (insomnia due to another disorder). Clinical practice has traditionally been to treat the "cause" first, with the belief that insomnia would remit after the underlying condition was addressed. A major shift in this line of thought has taken place in recent years, with a significant amount of research negating the view of primary and secondary insomnia.[18] The relationship between sleep and psychiatric disorders appears to be bidirectional, and causative factors can be extremely difficult to separate from the insomnia itself. The symptom of "nonrestorative" sleep has also been called into question as it is typically related to another sleep disorder that impairs sleep quality.

Risk Factors and Common Comorbidities

Insomnia is most commonly seen in women, older adults, populations with lower socioeconomic status, those with divorce or marital separation, and in those with comorbid psychiatric or medical disorders. Insomnia is commonly observed in neurologic disorders, particularly Parkinson disease, Alzheimer disease, epilepsy, stroke, multiple sclerosis, and traumatic brain injury.[19] Patients with medical conditions such as pain disorders and heart disease are all at increased risk of insomnia.[20]

Consequences

Insomnia is a risk factor for the development of anxiety, depression, substance use, and suicidality.[21–23] It is also associated with poor attention and concentration, increased work absenteeism, higher medical costs, increased rates of motor vehicle accidents, more falls in the elderly, and reduced overall quality of life.[24–26]

Clinical Assessment and Diagnosis

The history should focus on symptoms, chronology, exacerbating and alleviating factors, social, medical, and psychiatric precipitants and comorbidities, as well as previous therapies and their success. Symptoms of insomnia range from difficulty in falling or staying asleep to early morning awakenings, or a combination of these symptoms.

Understanding a patient's typical sleep-wake periods (on weekdays and weekends) and what the patient does both during the day (including work

TABLE 51-1 ■ Medications and Substances Commonly Associated With Insomnia

Alcohol
Caffeine
Nicotine
Antidepressants
Decongestants
Corticosteroids
Bronchodilators
β-Adrenergic antagonists
Stimulants
Statins

TABLE 51-2 ■ Medical Conditions Commonly Comorbid with Insomnia

Neurologic: stroke, Parkinson disease, neuropathy, traumatic brain injury
Pulmonary: chronic obstructive pulmonary disease, asthma
Endocrine: diabetes, hypertension
Renal: chronic renal failure
Rheumatologic: rheumatoid arthritis, fibromyalgia, osteoarthritis
Cardiovascular: congestive heart failure, coronary artery disease
Gastrointestinal: gastroesophageal reflux

schedule, napping, and exercise) and in the hours leading up to bedtime and throughout the night is important. A detailed analysis of the patient's thoughts and attitudes about sleep and maladaptive behavioral strategies is crucial to design effective treatment. Symptoms of any other sleep disorders that might impact sleep quality should be assessed, such as snoring, restless legs, apnea, pain, and parasomnias. A medication (prescription and over-the-counter) and substance use history (including time of day taken) is important and should include any caffeine, alcohol, or tobacco use. Table 51-1 lists medications and substances commonly associated with insomnia and Table 51-2 summarizes common comorbid medical conditions.

The most common assessment tools for insomnia include a sleep diary and questionnaires such as the Insomnia Severity Index and the Pittsburgh Sleep Quality Index. Overnight PSG may be warranted in cases in which a comorbid additional sleep disorder is considered or when treatment for insomnia has been unsuccessful. Actigraphy can be useful for establishing circadian disturbances that may be contributory as well as for tracking sleep-wake times and treatment response.[27]

Pathophysiology

Insomnia is considered a disorder of hyperarousal, with patients demonstrating higher levels of cortisol, increased basal metabolic rates, and the presence of excessive beta or gamma activity on EEG.

The 3P model describes the development and maintenance of chronic insomnia.[28] This model suggests that individuals may be vulnerable to developing insomnia based on predisposing factors that may be biologic (e.g., a diagnosis of chronic pain), psychologic (e.g., a family history of anxiety), or social (e.g., working shifts). Precipitating factors (e.g., a divorce or cancer diagnosis) may start an acute insomnia episode that is followed by behaviors that perpetuate a chronic insomnia, including worrying about sleep or consequences of poor sleep, spending more time in bed in an attempt to catch up on sleep, napping, and using more caffeine, alcohol, or over-the-counter medications.

Treatment

Treatment for insomnia generally involves nonpharmacologic and pharmacologic approaches. Unless a main, obvious underlying cause is found, treatment should focus on insomnia as a separate diagnosis to any other medical or psychiatric issues that may present simultaneously. Nonpharmacologic treatment is always preferred as a first-line intervention, though for many patients a combination of both behavioral and pharmacologic methods may be most beneficial.

Cognitive Behavioral Therapy

Cognitive behavioral therapy (CBT) is regarded as a highly effective first-line treatment for insomnia. CBT is as effective as the newer benzodiazepine receptor agonists and appears to be more effective in the long term than pharmacologic methods.[29–31] CBT is as effective in patients with or without

TABLE 51-3 ■ Common Sleep Hygiene Recommendations

1. Keep the same bedtime and wake time every day.
2. Limit liquids, heavy meals, tobacco, and alcohol within 3 hours of bedtime.
3. Limit caffeine at least 8 hours before bedtime.
4. Exercise regularly, but not within 3 hours of bedtime.
5. Wind down for at least 1 hour before bed in dim lights. Engage in something quiet, calm, and relaxing.
6. Keep the bedroom quiet, cool, and dark.
7. Take a hot shower or bath 1.5 to 2 hours before bedtime, not right before bed.
8. Limit any screen time (TV, tablets, phone, computer) within an hour of bedtime and during the nighttime hours.

comorbid pain, cancer, depression, and anxiety.[32,33] It improves sleep onset latency, sleep quality, number of awakenings, and total sleep time. It has also been used to help taper off hypnotics; CBT and pharmacotherapy may be started together acutely and then CBT alone may be used chronically following initial gains.[34]

CBT treatments can vary from as few as two 30- to 60-minute sessions to as many as 12 sessions. The core treatment interventions include stimulus control, sleep restriction and sleep hygiene, relaxation training, light therapy, and cognitive therapy.

Stimulus control instructs the patient to use the bed only for sleep and sex, therefore allowing the bed to become conditioned only for those two behaviors. Patients are told to go to bed only when sleepy and to get out of bed if unable to sleep and only return to bed when sleepy again. When out of bed, patients should engage in behaviors that are calm, quiet, and relaxing—all done in dim light without any screen time (e.g., television, cell phones, computers).

Sleep restriction is aimed at minimizing the gap between the amount of time the patient spends in bed and the actual amount of time they are asleep. Patients are advised to select the same awakening time daily (using an alarm) and to allow for a sleep window that approximates the average total sleep time over the past week, but never limiting this to less than 4.5 hours. Sleep hygiene aims to eliminate sleep-incompatible behaviors as described in Table 51-3.

Cognitive therapy teaches patients to challenge maladaptive thoughts and beliefs about sleep, including minimizing worry regarding sleep time and its consequences, and to think realistically about their concerns. Relaxation therapy is helpful for some patients and may include deep breathing or muscle relaxation. Though not routinely used as a part of CBT, strategic use of bright light in the morning or before bedtime may help with some patients who may have a circadian component to their insomnia.

TABLE 51-4 ■ Medications Commonly Used for Treatment of Insomnia

FDA-Approved Pharmacologic Treatments

Drug	Dose (mg)	Half-Life (hrs)	Insomnia Type
Zolpidem	5–10	1.5–2.4	Sleep onset/ maintenance
Zolpidem CR	6.25–12.5	1.6–4.5	Sleep onset/ maintenance
Zolpidem tartrate	1.75–3.5	1.4–3.6	Sleep maintenance
Eszopiclone	1–3	6	Sleep onset/ maintenance
Zaleplon	5–20	1	Sleep onset
Ramelteon	8	1–2.6	Sleep onset
Doxepin	3–6	10–30	Sleep onset
Temazepam	7.5–30	8–15	Sleep maintenance
Estazolam	1–2	10–24	Sleep maintenance
Flurazepam	15–30	48–120	Sleep maintenance
Quazepam	7.5–15	39–73	Sleep maintenance
Triazolam	0.125–0.25	2–6	Sleep onset

Common Off-Label Pharmacologic Treatments

Drug	Half-Life (hrs)	Side Effects
Amitriptyline	12–24	Dry mouth, dizziness, weight gain
Trazodone	3–14	Dizziness, daytime sedation, constipation
Mirtazipine	13–40	Weight gain, constipation
Quetiapine	6	Elevated liver enzymes, agitation
Olanzapine	20–54	Weight gain, orthostasis
Gabapentin	5–7	Dizziness, ataxia, nausea

Pharmacologic Interventions

Benzodiazepine Receptor Agonists.

The US Food and Drug Administration (FDA) approved medications for insomnia (Table 51-4) include the benzodiazepines (e.g., temazepam, flurazepam, estazolam, quazepam, triazolam) and nonbenzodiazepine hypnotics (e.g., zaleplon, zolpidem, and eszopiclone). All of the benzodiazepine receptor agonists have been shown to be efficacious and reduce sleep latency with an increase in overall sleep time. There is no single medication that is preferable to any other FDA-approved medication; the pros and cons of each (half-life, cost, past response to treatment) need to be considered with each patient.

These medications are all absorbed rapidly but vary in their half-life. Medications with a longer half-life may be more beneficial for a patient with sleep maintenance and early morning awakening insomnia, whereas a shorter half-life may be preferred for a patient with prolonged sleep-onset latency. Long-acting medications also have a greater risk of daytime somnolence and impaired cognitive functioning, especially in older adults. Newer medications such as zaleplon, zolpidem, and eszopiclone have fewer daytime side effects.

Longer-term efficacy and safety trials with newer nonbenzodiazepines in patients with insomnia have shown continued efficacy with increasing total sleep time and decreasing sleep latency, with overall improvement in daytime functioning and no development of physiologic tolerance. Zaleplon has a short half-life (1 hour) and is best for sleep-onset problems. Zolpidem can increase total sleep time, but the extended-release form also reduces wake time following sleep onset. A newer form of zolpidem (zolpidem tartrate) is fast-acting and aimed at middle of the night awakenings when the patient has at least 4 hours remaining before awakening; taken sublingually, it rapidly dissolves and helps the patient return to sleep. Dosages of this formulation differ based on gender (1.75 mg for women, 3.5 mg for men). Eszopiclone has been found to be effective for both sleep onset and maintenance issues.

Common side effects of benzodiazepines include residual sedation, impaired psychomotor performance, falls, and an increased risk of motor vehicle accidents. Tolerance, abuse, and dependence (especially with benzodiazepines), rebound insomnia, and anterograde amnesia are also concerns. Since these medications can reduce ventilatory drive, caution should also be used in patients with chronic obstructive pulmonary disease or untreated sleep-related breathing disorders.

The newer nonbenzodiazepines do not tend to have physiologic dependence as a concern, though psychologic dependence can develop. These medications most commonly have drowsiness, dizziness, and headaches as reported side effects. Though less commonly reported, amnesia and complex sleep-related behaviors such as sleepwalking or sleep eating have been reported.

Melatonin Receptor Agonists

Ramelteon is the only FDA-approved nonbenzodiazepine receptor agonist medication to treat sleep-onset insomnia. It is not a scheduled substance and does not act on the GABA receptors. Rather, it is a selective melatonin agonist that binds to the melatonin receptors MT1 and MT2 in the suprachiasmatic nucleus. Particularly helpful in older adult populations, ramelteon has been shown to help increase total sleep time and reduce sleep latency. Potential side effects include drowsiness, fatigue, nausea, dizziness, and headache. It has also been studied in patients with mild-to-moderate obstructive sleep apnea, with no increase in apneic episodes.

Antidepressant Medications

Low-dose doxepin (3 to 6 mg) has recently been FDA approved as a treatment for sleep-maintenance insomnia. It is particularly useful for increasing total sleep time and sleep efficiency in patients with primary insomnia. Given their sedating properties, other antidepressants are commonly used (in much lower dosages than for depression treatment). Although limited evidence exists demonstrating efficacy in the treatment of insomnia, practitioners commonly prescribe trazodone, mirtazapine, and amitriptyline because they are perceived as safer than benzodiazepines with a lower potential for dependence. Many patients also have coexisting depression, anxiety, or both, and prescribing physicians feel that these medications may help with both mood and sleep disturbance. Side effects include drowsiness, weight gain, increased suicidal ideation in young adults, dizziness, cardiac arrhythmias, and priapism (with trazodone in particular).

Alternative Medications

Although many patients resort to over-the-counter medications as sleep aids (particularly those that contain diphenhydramine), these medications are not advised in the treatment of chronic insomnia. Atypical antipsychotics (especially quetiapine and olanzapine) are often used off-label to treat both primary insomnia and insomnia comorbid with psychiatric conditions. Case studies have reported effectiveness, particularly with older adults. However, there is a black-box warning regarding the use of antipsychotics in the elderly due to an increased risk of death. Other side effects commonly include weight gain, orthostasis, daytime sedation, agitation, and elevated liver enzymes.

Antiepileptic medications, particularly gabapentin, have also been used to treat insomnia particularly in patients with comorbid conditions (especially with generalized anxiety disorder, epilepsy, and chronic pain). Side effects include daytime sedation, dizziness, mood changes, and cognitive impairment.

The effects of melatonin taken before bedtime have not been routinely demonstrated, although some reports have suggested decreases in sleep onset latency. Generally well-tolerated by patients, melatonin is not regulated by the FDA and over-the-counter preparations can vary greatly. It is not considered a standard treatment for insomnia and appears to be better suited for treatment of circadian rhythm disorders.

HYPERSOMNIAS

EDS has many implications, including an increased risk of injury at work or home, impaired alertness, increased risk of motor vehicle accidents, and lower overall productivity. EDS can also cause psychologic stress with family, friends, and coworkers.

Narcolepsy

Narcolepsy is a disorder of EDS that is usually associated with cataplexy and other REM phenomena such as sleep paralysis and hypnagogic hallucinations. Sleep regulation and wakefulness are disrupted with rapid transitions between wakefulness and REM sleep, thereby resulting in fragmented sleep and EDS.

Although onset can occur at any age, narcolepsy most commonly begins in the second decade of life with a second peak seen around 35 years of age.[35] There is a prolonged latency of about 10 years from the time of symptom onset to diagnosis, although improved awareness is shortening this interval. Narcolepsy is usually a sporadic disease with only 1 to 4 percent of cases being autosomal-dominantly inherited.[36]

Clinical Features

Excessive Daytime Sleepiness

EDS is the hallmark symptom seen in all patients with narcolepsy and is characterized by a constant baseline sleepiness along with lapses into sleep throughout the day. Short naps are refreshing, but sleepiness returns within a few hours. Sleep attacks (sudden onset of sleep or the irresistible urge to sleep) can occur throughout the day. Activities that are passive increase the likelihood that sleep will occur, but in severe cases sleep attacks can occur during activities such as talking, standing, eating, or driving. Automatic behaviors (activities where the patient is functionally capable but without recall of the events) are also seen in some patients. For example, a patient can drive to a location without remembering the process of getting there.

Cataplexy

Cataplexy is defined as a sudden loss of muscle tone associated with emotion. It is pathognomonic for narcolepsy, although some patients with narcolepsy do not have cataplexy. Patients often describe knee buckling, head dropping, facial twitching, jaw dropping, or weakness of the arms. Emotions that elicit cataplexy are usually positive, such as laughter, excitement, or joy; they can also be negative, such as anger or frustration. If all striated muscles are involved, patients may fall. However, several seconds of build-up often precede a full attack, so most patients are able to sit down to prevent a fall. Patients may avoid emotional situations, such as social events where cataplexy may occur, affecting quality of life.

Sleep Paralysis

Sleep paralysis is a temporary state of involuntary immobility occurring in transitions between REM sleep and wakefulness. Patients are unable to make gross body movements or speak, but they can open their eyes and are aware of their surroundings. Episodes may last a few minutes and abate either spontaneously or when interrupted by noise or other external stimuli. Sleep paralysis can be frightening, especially when first experienced.

Often sleep paralysis is accompanied by hypnagogic hallucinations. About 20 to 50 percent of patients with narcolepsy experience sleep paralysis, but sleep paralysis is also common in the general population.

Hypnagogic Hallucinations

Hypnagogic hallucinations are vivid visual, auditory, tactile, or even kinetic perceptions that, like sleep paralysis, occur during the transitions between wakefulness and REM sleep. Examples include a sensation of impending threat, feelings of suffocation, and sensations of floating, spinning, or falling. Hypnagogic hallucinations occur in 40 to 80 percent of patients with narcolepsy and cataplexy. They are easy to distinguish from the hallucinations occurring in psychiatric disease because patients with narcolepsy usually recognize the events as not real. Psychiatric hallucinations also occur at any time of day, whereas hypnagogic hallucinations surround the sleep period.

Disturbed Nocturnal Sleep

Because narcolepsy is a disorder of EDS, disturbed nocturnal sleep is often overlooked. Patients with narcolepsy typically fall asleep quickly, but have difficulty in maintaining sleep. Frequent arousals are often reported along with difficulty in falling back to sleep. The total amount of sleep in a 24-hour period is the same as in normal individuals; however, it is distributed throughout the day and night, causing daytime sleep attacks and fragmented nocturnal sleep.

Associated Symptoms

Disturbances in memory, concentration, and attention are common in narcolepsy, probably secondary to EDS. REM sleep behavior disorder and periodic limb movements may occur as well. Patients with narcolepsy also report more depressive ideation.

Patients with narcolepsy with cataplexy often have a high body mass index or obesity, attributed to metabolic changes resulting from hypocretin loss.[37] A high body mass index may also predispose patients to developing obstructive sleep apnea; at least 25 percent of patients with narcolepsy have both conditions, which together can worsen EDS, mood, and cognition.[38]

TABLE 51-5 ■ Differential Diagnosis of Excessive Daytime Sleepiness

Sleep apnea
Behaviorally induced insufficient sleep time
Idiopathic hypersomnia
Recurrent hypersomnia (Kleine–Levin syndrome)
Circadian rhythm disorder, shift work disorder
Metabolic encephalopathy
Drug intoxication or withdrawal
Depression
Epilepsy
Malingering

Diagnosis

The differential diagnosis of EDS is shown in Table 51-5. The diagnosis of narcolepsy with cataplexy can be made based on a clear history of EDS and cataplexy. The diagnosis should be confirmed by nocturnal PSG followed by an MSLT. The diagnosis of narcolepsy without cataplexy can be more difficult and requires a PSG and MSLT.

Nocturnal PSG shows a shortened REM latency in 50 percent of patients. Sleep efficiency is often reduced, with multiple awakenings and an increased percentage of stage N1 sleep. The MSLT should show a mean sleep latency of 8 minutes or less along with two or more sleep-onset REM periods in the setting of sufficient nocturnal sleep.

A less commonly used, but very specific and sensitive method to make the diagnosis is through measurement of cerebrospinal fluid (CSF) hypocretin-1 level, which has been shown to be less than 110 pg/ml in 90 percent of patients with narcolepsy with cataplexy.[39] Hypocretin loss is now recognized to be the cause of human narcolepsy with cataplexy, and symptoms begin when the majority of hypocretin cells have degenerated.[40,41]

Pharmacologic Treatments

There is no cure for narcolepsy. Treatment goals are to improve quality of life, EDS, and cataplexy as well as other bothersome REM phenomena. A variety of medications can be used to treat these symptoms (Table 51-6).

TABLE 51-6 ■ Medications Typically Prescribed for Narcolepsy

Drug Name	Dose	Clinical Use	Side Effects
Modafinil (Provigil)	200–400 mg daily in divided dose	EDS	Headache, nausea
Armodafinil (Nuvigil)	150–250 mg daily	EDS	Same as modafinil
Sodium oxybate (Xyrem)	4.5–9 g daily in divided doses	Cataplexy, EDS, broken nighttime sleep	Nausea, vomiting, dizziness
Dextroamphetamine (Dexedrine)	15–60 mg daily	EDS	Irritability, sweating, headaches, tremors
Methylphenidate (Ritalin)	20–60 mg daily in divided doses	EDS	Same as dextroamphetamine
Paroxetine (Paxil)	10–60 mg daily	Cataplexy	Sedation, insomnia, irritability
Phenylzine (Nardil)	15–60 mg daily in divided doses	Cataplexy	Impotence, weight gain, hypertension

EDS, excessive daytime sleepiness.

Excessive Daytime Sleepiness

Modafinil, armodafinil, and sodium oxybate are often used to treat EDS. The various forms of modafinil are effective wake-promoting agents with good safety and tolerability measures and a low abuse potential. Women of childbearing age taking oral contraceptives should use alternative contraception when taking modafinil or armodafinil, as the metabolism of ethinylestradiol may be increased. In the past, amphetamines were the main treatment for excessive daytime sleepiness; dextroamphetamine, methamphetamine, and combinations of amphetamine salts are helpful with improving daytime alertness, but side effects limit their use.

Cataplexy

Sodium oxybate is effective in reducing cataplexy as well as EDS. It also reduces other REM phenomena such as sleep paralysis and hypnagogic hallucinations. Due to its sedative properties, it is commonly given in divided doses at sleep onset and then 2 to 4 hours later. Common side effects include nausea, vomiting, dizziness, and nocturnal enuresis. If used as recommended, sodium oxybate is safe and has a low risk of dependence or tolerance.

Tricyclic antidepressants were initially the treatment of choice for cataplexy. Medications such as protrityline and clomipramine are effective, but side effects can be limiting. Newer norepinephrine reuptake inhibitors, such as venlafaxine and atomoxetine, may be more effective and have a more favorable side-effect profile. Selective serotonin reuptake inhibitors (SSRIs) and monoamine-oxidase inhibitors can also be used for cataplexy but are generally less effective.

Disturbed Nocturnal Sleep

Sodium oxybate increases slow-wave sleep and allows patients to sleep more continuously through the night. Newer nonbenzodiazepines such as zolpidem have also been used to consolidate nighttime sleep, but few studies have tested this approach.

Nonpharmacologic Treatments

Scheduling naps, shifting work periods to times of alertness, avoiding sugar, calculated caffeine use, and following basic sleep hygiene can all benefit patients with narcolepsy. The patient should be advised against driving, bathing, swimming, and using any heavy machinery or household appliances during times of sleepiness. Psychotherapeutic strategies for the management of stressful situations, depression, and anxiety are recommended.

Idiopathic Hypersomnia

Idiopathic hypersomnia is generally less common than narcolepsy, with symptoms beginning in teenagers or young adults. It is typically under-recognized and often a diagnosis made by excluding other causes of EDS.

The primary symptom of idiopathic hypersomnia is EDS despite a full night of sleep and normal sleep architecture; idiopathic hypersomnia includes forms with and without a long sleep time. Patients with long sleep times have at least 10 hours of sleep at night, rarely awaken during nocturnal sleep, have significant difficulty in getting up in the morning, and, unlike patients with narcolepsy, do not find naps to be refreshing. Patients usually report "sleep drunkenness"—difficulty in achieving full alertness upon awakening after a full night of sleep. Patients without long sleep times have less than 10 hours of sleep at night and are less likely to report sleep drunkenness with their EDS. The differential diagnosis of idiopathic hypersomnia is similar to that of narcolepsy.

Nocturnal PSG is routinely performed to exclude other causes of daytime sleepiness and to determine the length of sleep time. An MSLT is also performed, demonstrating EDS with a mean sleep latency of less than 8 minutes and fewer than two sleep onset REM periods (to rule out possible narcolepsy).

Treatment of idiopathic hypersomnia is similar to that of EDS in patients with narcolepsy, focusing on stimulants and wake-promoting agents, especially modafinil and armodafinil. Positive pharmacologic responses are difficult to achieve. Sleep hygiene, proper diet, and strategic use of caffeine should be utilized. Planned naps and increasing time in bed have not been found to be helpful.[42]

Kleine–Levin Syndrome

Kleine–Levin syndrome is a rare disorder with an estimated prevalence of 1 to 2 cases per million people. Patients are mostly adolescent boys; mean age of onset is 15 years, with some rare cases beginning as early as age 9.[43] Rare familial cases have been reported, with Ashkenazi Jews in the United States and Israel particularly affected. In a majority of cases, the first episode is triggered by a high fever or infection. Disease course typically lasts 8 to 14 years with spontaneous remission in adulthood.

The hallmark symptom of Kleine–Levin syndrome is episodic hypersomnia, with sleep time increasing to over 12 hours per day. Cognitive impairment, apathy, confusion, slowness, derealization, and amnesia are typically seen. Though not reported by all patients, hypersexuality, depressed mood, and hyperphagia may occur. Between episodes, functioning returns to normal with regard to sleep needs, cognitive functioning, and appetite.[43]

Medically based differential diagnoses include alcohol and drug use, multiple sclerosis, temporal lobe seizures, stroke, tumor, Lyme disease, and encephalitis. Typical psychiatric differential diagnoses include depression, bipolar disease, and psychotic disorders. Many patients with Kleine–Levin syndrome first present for psychiatric evaluation.

No standard treatment has been adopted for Kleine–Levin syndrome. When given at the beginning of an episode, amantadine may help to shorten or stop an event. Lithium, lamotrigine, and valproic acid may also be beneficial. Stimulants have shown limited efficacy and may worsen behavioral and cognitive symptoms. Risperidone may help with severe cognitive changes. Family supervision is paramount during episodes. Between episodes, the patient should keep a regular sleep-wake schedule and alcohol and nicotine should be avoided.

SLEEP-RELATED BREATHING DISORDERS

Epidemiology

The estimated prevalence of sleep apnea in the general population is approximately 5 percent[44]; however, depending on how obstructive sleep apnea (OSA) is defined, the estimated prevalence may be as high as 20 percent.[45] Sleep apnea is associated with increasing age, male gender, and obesity. It is most common in men over the age of 40 years; the incidence in women increases after menopause. Obesity is present in approximately 70 percent of OSA patients.[5] Many nonobese patients have apnea because of the anatomy of their airway. Nonobese patients are probably underdiagnosed.

Definitions

OSA occurs when there are repetitive episodes of complete or near-complete cessation of airflow during sleep, with continued respiratory effort against a closed airway. These events may cause either a decline in oxygen saturation or a cortical arousal from sleep. Partial reduction in airflow with preserved respiratory effort is defined as a hypopnea.

Obstructive events can occur in any stage of sleep but are most severe during REM sleep, when muscle atonia is present. The pathophysiologies of obstructive apneas and hypopneas are similar and result in the same physiologic consequences. Thus, by PSG they are combined in a single measure known as the apnea-hypopnea index (AHI).

The diagnosis of OSA in adults is made when the AHI is 5 or greater. An index of 5 to 14 is considered to indicate mild OSA; between 15 and 29, moderate OSA; and 30 and above is severe OSA.[1] Generally, the magnitude of the AHI reflects symptom severity; however, some patients may have minimal symptoms but severe sleep apnea on PSG.

Symptoms

Symptoms of OSA are present during both the night and day. Nocturnal symptoms include snoring, gasping or choking, cessation of breathing, frequent arousals, nocturia, excessive movement in sleep, and hyperhidrosis. However, snoring can be the only symptom, and patients are often unaware of any symptoms; it is therefore helpful to interview the bed partner or a family member. Upon awakening, patients often report having a dry mouth, nasal congestion, headaches, or heartburn.

In the daytime, excessive daytime sleepiness is usually present as a result of respiratory events causing disturbed nighttime sleep. Patients report dozing off when sedentary and have difficulty with concentration and attention, which puts them at increased risk of motor vehicle accidents. Individuals with sleep apnea have a motor vehicle accident rate that is approximately threefold higher than the general population.[46] OSA is particularly concerning in commercial drivers and pilots.

Predisposing Factors

It has been shown in many studies that obesity, particularly truncal obesity, increases the likelihood of sleep apnea.[47,48] An increase of body mass index by 1 standard deviation is associated with a fourfold increase in OSA prevalence.

The prevalence of sleep apnea increases with age, with the steepest increase during the transition from middle to older age. In those older than 65, the prevalence of a sleep-related disorder of breathing ranges from 30 to 70 percent, compared to 2 to 4 percent in middle-aged adults.[49,50] The ratio of sleep apnea in men and women is about 2 to 1; however, disease prevalence triples in postmenopausal women, even when corrected for body mass index.[51,52]

There may be a genetic predisposition to sleep apnea. The relative risk is between 3 and 5 when parents have OSA and is independent of lifestyle habits.[53,54] This risk may be due to craniofacial size and shape as well as soft tissue structures and may explain the higher prevalence found in certain ethnic groups, including Asians and African-Americans.[55] Other structural factors that predispose to OSA include chronic nasal congestion, allergies, deviated nasal septum, tonsillar or adenoid hyperplasia or both, retrognathia or micrognathia, dental mandibular crowding, macroglossia, high-arched palate, enlarged uvula, vocal cord paralysis, increased pharyngeal length, and hereditary craniofacial syndromes such as Pierre Robin syndrome or Treacher Collins syndrome. Additional factors include smoking,[56] alcohol intake,[57] chronic nasal congestion,[58] Down syndrome, acromegaly,[59] hypothyroidism,[60] polycystic ovary syndrome,[61] and neuromuscular diseases.

Physiologic Consequences

During an obstructive apnea or hypopnea, tidal volume and oxygen saturation decline, and carbon dioxide levels rise. Sympathetic tone increases with each event, causing vasoconstriction and often tachycardia that results in increased blood pressure. Other physiologic responses include increased release of inflammatory mediators,[62] elevation of leptin levels,[63] increases in platelet adhesiveness, and raised fibrinogen levels.[64,65] Generalized endothelial damage also likely occurs.[66]

Pathophysiologic effects of OSA contribute to increases in morbidity and mortality. Several large studies have shown a dose-dependent relationship between sleep apnea and hypertension.[67,68] Refractory hypertension is a known comorbidity of sleep apnea, and treatment of OSA may lower blood pressure in these patients.[69,70]

Sleep apnea is also a risk factor for atrial fibrillation[71] and results in a 50 percent reduction in post-cardioversion maintenance of normal sinus rhythm after ablation.[72] Studies have shown that untreated sleep apnea increases the risk of coronary artery disease, myocardial infarction, heart failure, cardiovascular mortality, and pulmonary hypertension.[73–77]

The risk of stroke increases in patients with sleep apnea.[78–81] This association is most robust in those with moderate or severe sleep apnea. Sleep apnea is also common in patients after stroke, its prevalence ranging from 50 to 75 percent.[82,83] In this context,

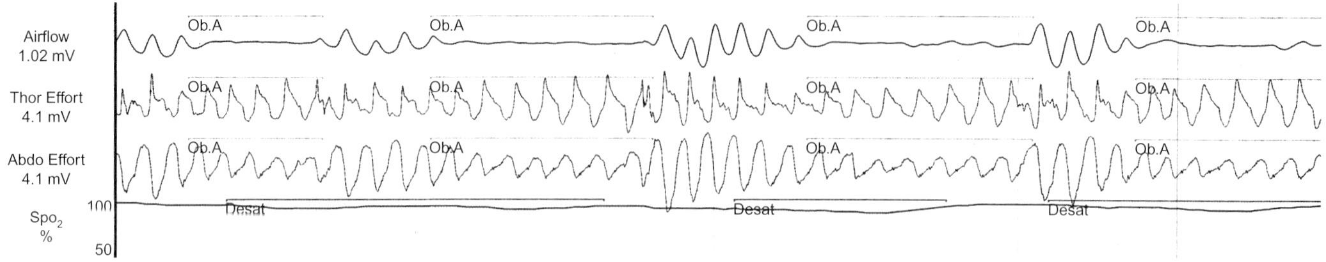

FIGURE 51-2 ■ Obstructive apnea. This 2-minute screen shows complete cessation of airflow for at least 10 seconds, accompanied by persisting respiratory efforts of the thoracic (Thor Effort) and abdominal muscles (Abdo Effort). The associated oxygen desaturation (Desat) is not essential for the events to be scored as obstructive apnea (Ob.A). (From Avidan A, Barkoukis T: Review of Sleep Medicine. 3rd Ed. Elsevier, Philadelphia, 2012.)

central sleep apnea predominates initially but eventually obstructive events persist.[84] Sleep apnea after stroke has been shown to worsen cognitive and motor ability.[85]

Clinical Evaluation

PSG should be performed if sleep apnea is suspected. Obstructive apneas are defined as a 90 percent reduction in air flow lasting for at least 10 seconds, with continued inspiratory effort in thoracic and abdominal muscles (Fig. 51-2). This is in contrast to a central apnea, in which there is complete absence of inspiratory effort. An apnea can also be mixed, characterized by initial cessation of both flow and effort, followed by the appearance of effort without flow.

A hypopnea is defined as a reduction of 30 percent or more in flow for at least 10 seconds, associated with a 3 percent oxygen desaturation (Fig. 51-3). Apneas and hypopneas are combined to calculate the AHI.

A respiratory effort-related arousal is characterized by a series of breaths lasting for at least 10 seconds, with flattening of the nasal pressure waveform leading to an arousal from sleep. If esophageal pressure is measured by manometry, it will show progressively more negative pressures preceding the arousal. On PSG the respiratory disturbance index is calculated by combining the total number of apneas, hypopneas, and respiratory effort-related arousals per hour of sleep. Respiratory effort-related arousals are used to identify patients with upper airway resistance syndrome in whom recurrent arousals from sleep occur without clear apneas or hypopneas on PSG. Patients with this syndrome respond to the same treatments as those with OSA.

Treatment

Positive Airway Pressure Therapy

Continuous positive airway pressure (CPAP) is the treatment of choice for obstructive sleep apnea. CPAP acts as a pneumatic splint to keep the airway

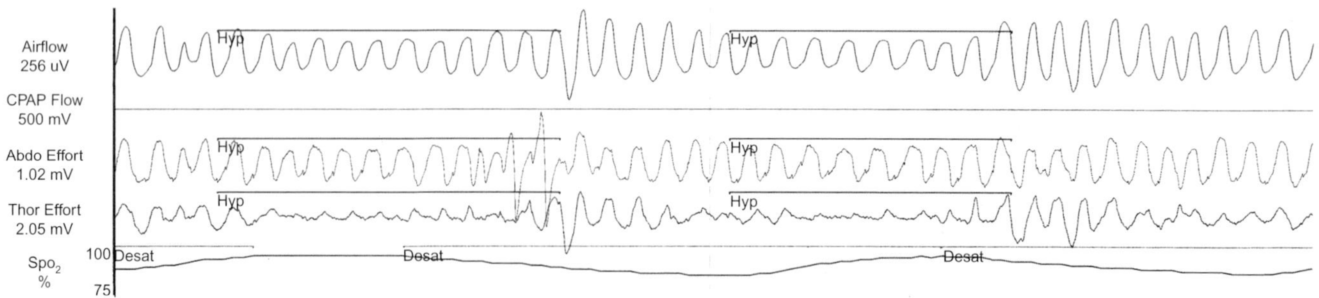

FIGURE 51-3 ■ Obstructive hypopnea (Hyp). This 2-minute screen shows airflow reduced by about 50 percent from baseline. There are persisting respiratory efforts of the thoracic (Thor Effort) and abdominal muscles (Abdo Effort), and a decline of more than 3 pecent in oxygen saturation. CPAP, continuous positive airway pressure; Desat, desaturation. (From Avidan A, Barkoukis T: Review of Sleep Medicine. 3rd Ed. Elsevier, Philadelphia, 2012.)

open, thereby preventing obstruction during sleep. It is effective in ameliorating daytime sleepiness, reducing respiratory events, and normalizing oxygen saturation.

Ideally, an in-laboratory CPAP titration should be performed to determine the optimal pressure. CPAP pressures may need to be increased in REM sleep, when the patient is in the supine position, or after ingestion of sedative medications or alcohol. When high pressures are required, bilevel positive airway pressure (BiPAP) is often used so that patients can exhale against a lower pressure. It is also used in patients who are unable to tolerate CPAP or in those with an element of central hypoventilation.

More recently, auto-CPAP devices have been developed to select the optimal positive airway pressure without in-laboratory titration. Additionally, auto-CPAP devices can deliver the lowest pressure needed regardless of changes in body position, sleep stage, or weight. Different auto-CPAP algorithms are used depending on the manufacturer. Limitations of these devices include erroneously increased pressure due to leakage and the inability to differentiate between central and obstructive respiratory events. Studies to date have shown similar outcomes with CPAP and auto-CPAP therapy.[86,87]

Surgery

Young patients with enlarged tonsils, adenoids, or both respond well to surgical intervention. Uvulopalatopharyngoplasty is the most common surgery performed for OSA and includes resection of the uvula, any redundant retroglossal soft tissue, and palatine tonsillar lymphoid tissue. Unfortunately, success—defined as normalization of AHI to less than 10—only occurs in about 30 percent of patients.[88] Approximately 50 percent of patients have a reduction in apneas by more than 50 percent; however, patients with severe sleep apnea are often left with mild to moderate sleep apnea. The most common side effect of the surgery is nasopharyngeal regurgitation of fluid.

Other surgeries that are performed for sleep apnea include septoplasty, rhinoplasty, nasal turbinate reduction, nasal polypectomy, tongue reduction, palatal implants (Pillar procedure), genioglossal advancement or shortening, and maxillomandibular advancement. Relative contraindications to upper airway surgery include morbid obesity and decompensated respiratory or cardiac conditions. In practice, surgery is recommended when patients are unable to tolerate positive airway pressure therapy. Surgery is most successful in patients with a low body mass index and low AHI.

Oral Appliances

Oral appliances are dental devices made to maintain patency of the upper airway during sleep. Mandibular advancement devices protrude the mandible forward to increase the luminal area of the airway. Tongue-retaining devices, in contrast, keep the tongue in place, preventing occlusion of the upper airway. Some devices combine these two mechanisms.

Most studies have shown that oral appliances reduce snoring and decrease the number of respiratory events, but do not necessarily normalize them to an AHI less than 5.[89,90] The most common adverse effects reported with oral appliances include dental discomfort, temporomandibular joint pain, bruxism, gingival irritation, and hypersalivation. These effects are usually mild and self-limited. Contraindications to oral appliances include an inadequate number of teeth (at least 6 to 10 per arch are needed), severe temporomandibular joint problems, inadequate mandibular protrusive ability, and significant bruxism.

Oral appliances are most effective in mild to moderate OSA, in patients with a body mass index less than 30, and in patients with supine-dependent OSA.[91]

Behavioral Modifications

The most effective behavioral modification for OSA is weight loss. Lifestyle and dietary modifications, pharmacologic therapy, and bariatric surgery can all be effective in achieving this goal. Studies have shown a 50 percent reduction in AHI with a mean weight loss of 9 percent.[92] Other behavioral interventions include smoking cessation, alcohol avoidance, and increasing time of sleep. Positional therapy (avoiding a supine position during sleep) can be used for patients with supine-dependent OSA. To date, no pharmacologic treatment has been effective for OSA.

CIRCADIAN RHYTHM DISORDERS

Circadian rhythm disorders develop when there is a persistent or recurrent pattern of sleep disturbance

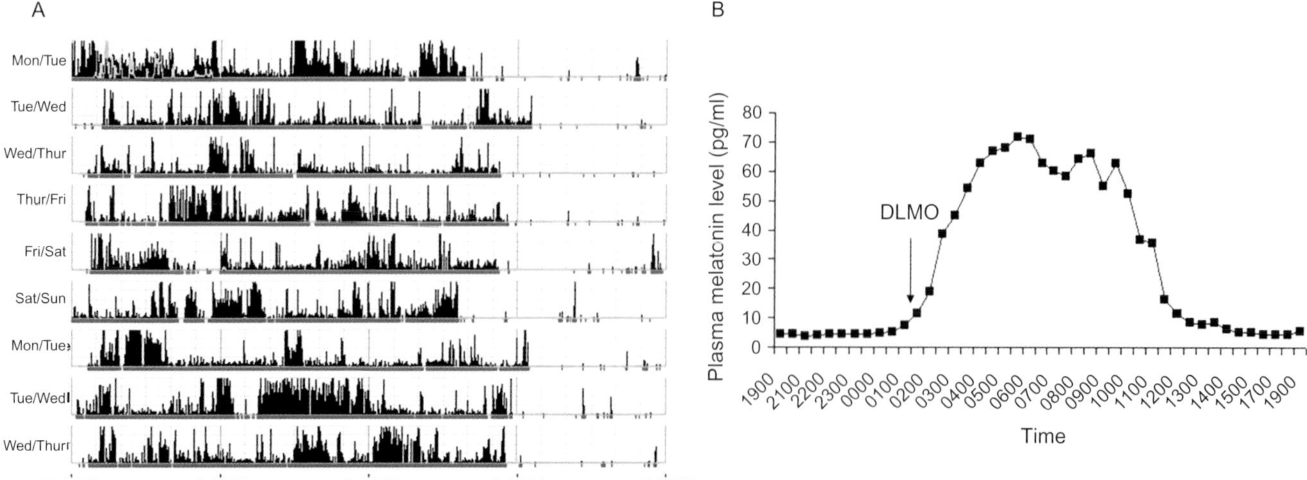

FIGURE 51-4 ■ Actogram of a patient with severe delayed sleep phase disorder (DSPD). **A,** Actogram derived from actigraphy data obtained over 9 days. The yellow lines depict light exposure. The high-amplitude dense bars are representative of wakefulness, and time with little or no activity represents sleep. The average sleep onset is at 5 to 6 A.M. and wake time is from noon to 1 P.M. Note the stable delay of the sleep-wake rhythm in relation to the conventional sleep time and wake-up time. **B,** The 24-hour rhythm of plasma melatonin levels in this patient. The dim-light melatonin onset (DLMO) was defined as an absolute threshold at 10 pg/ml. The DLMO of this patient is delayed, at 1:23 A.M. (which is approximately 5 hours later than expected in nondelayed persons).

because of alterations in the circadian clock or a misalignment between the endogenous circadian rhythm and the external environment imposed by social or work cycles. The sleep disturbances that arise include insomnia, EDS, or both, and lead to impairments in occupational, social, or other aspects of daily functioning.

Various tools are used to make a diagnosis of a circadian rhythm disorder including the history of sleep and wake patterns, a sleep diary, and actigraphy. Other diagnostic tools that are used more in research than clinical practice include assessment of core body temperature and melatonin levels, the latter increasing approximately 2 to 2.5 hours before sleep onset. The nadir of the core body temperature occurs about 2 hours before habitual wake time.

Delayed Sleep Phase Disorder

Delayed sleep phase disorder is characterized by an inability to fall asleep at the appropriate time at night and an inability to awaken in the morning. This results in a delay of the major sleep period relative to the required sleep-wake time (Fig. 51-4). The patient reports symptoms of sleep-onset insomnia and EDS. If the patient is allowed to sleep at the preferred time, sleep quality and duration are normal and stable.

The prevalence of delayed sleep phase disorder is 0.17 percent in the general population.[93] It occurs most often in adolescence, with a prevalence of 7 to 16 percent.[94] It is estimated that 5 to 10 percent of patients with chronic insomnia in a sleep clinic have delayed sleep phase disorder.

Polymorphisms in the clock genes *hPer3* and *hCLOCK* have been associated with delayed sleep phase disorder.[95,96] Additionally, a polymorphism of arylalkylamine *N*-acetyltransferase and an increased frequency of HLA-DR1 are significantly more prevalent in these patients, which may explain the positive family history of such disorder in 40 percent of patients.[97,98] Environmental factors, such as exposure to bright lights in the evening and lack of light in the morning, can intensify the delayed sleep phase.

Treatment often requires a combination of behavioral techniques, light therapy, chronotherapy, and possibly pharmacologic treatments. Behavioral therapy includes maintaining a regular sleep-wake schedule and proper sleep hygiene. Bright light of 2000 to 2500 lux for 2 hours in the biologic morning along with avoidance of bright light in the biologic evening can help achieve earlier sleep and wake times.

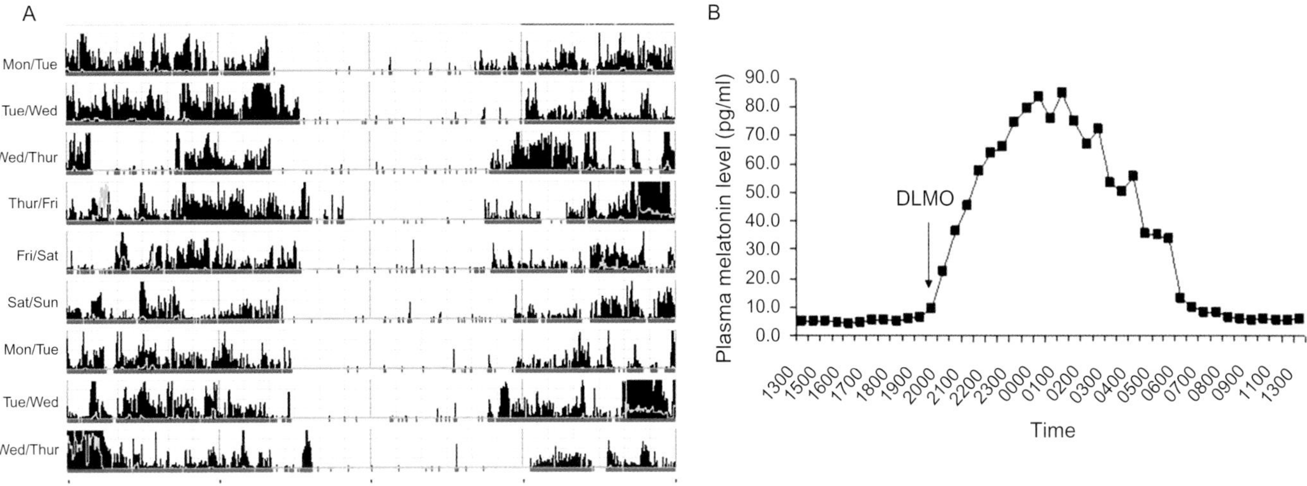

FIGURE 51-5 ■ Actogram of a patient with severe advanced sleep phase disorder. **A,** Actogram derived from actigraphy data obtained over 9 days. The yellow lines depict light exposure. The high-amplitude dense bars are representative of wakefulness, and time with little or no activity time represents sleep. The average sleep onset is 8 to 9 P.M. and wake time is from 4 to 5 A.M. Note the stable advance of the sleep-wake rhythm in relation to the conventional sleep and wake-up times. **B,** The 24-hour plasma melatonin level rhythm of this patient. The DLMO was defined as an absolute threshold at 10 pg/ml. The DLMO of this patient is advanced, at 7:30 P.M. (which is approximately 2–3 hours earlier than expected in nonadvanced persons).

Chronotherapy is a technique that involves progressively changing the sleep time by several hours each night until the desired sleep time is reached. It is a highly effective treatment for delayed sleep phase disorder. Compliance is often difficult, however, because it requires individuals to have a flexible schedule. Vacation time is often the best time to try this approach.

Melatonin taken in the early evening decreases sleep latency, increases sleep duration, and improves daytime functioning in patients with delayed sleep phase disorder.[99,100] Individuals are advised to take 0.3 to 3 mg about 6 hours before their sleep time. Rarely, hypnotics are used to treat delayed sleep phase disorder.

Advanced Sleep Phase Disorder

Advanced sleep phase disorder is a stable advance in the sleep-wake period relative to the desired time. Patients tend to fall asleep early in the night, typically between 6 and 9 P.M., and awaken early in the morning, between 2 and 5 A.M. (Fig. 51-5). Individuals with advanced sleep phase disorder report sleepiness in the early evening making it difficult to participate in activities at that time. Additionally, early morning insomnia can result in EDS. If patients are allowed to sleep at their endogenous circadian period, their sleep time and quality is normal for age.

Advanced sleep phase disorder is more common in middle-aged and older adults, with an estimated prevalence of about 1 percent.[93] Familial forms of advanced sleep phase disorder exist and should be suspected in younger patients. Mutations in the clock genes *hPer2* and *CSK1D* have been identified.[101,102]

Treatment recommendations include a combination of bright light exposure in the evening, adhering to a planned sleep-wake schedule, and good sleep hygiene.[99] Studies have shown that bright lights between 7 and 9 P.M. can phase-delay the circadian clock and improve sleep efficiency.[103,104] Early morning melatonin can theoretically delay the circadian rhythm, but there are no published studies on its efficacy for advanced sleep phase disorder.

Shift Work Disorder

Shift work disorder is a common condition that remains under-recognized and undertreated. It is estimated that 10 percent of shift workers have the disorder. As about 20 percent of the workforce in industrialized countries is employed in some kind of shift work, the prevalence must be high.[105]

Shift work disorder develops when the work schedule occurs during the normal sleep period, resulting in either EDS, insomnia, or both. Difficulty in sleeping occurs when the circadian alerting signal is high, and EDS results from being awake when the circadian alerting signal is low. Additionally, shift workers are often chronically sleep deprived. Night workers sleep between 1 and 4 hours less per night than day workers.[106] Night work and early morning (before 6 A.M.) start times are associated with the most sleep deprivation and greatest wake-time impairments.

Shift work disorder is associated with impairments in performance at work that can have safety consequences, for example, in bus drivers, machine operators, and train conductors. Additional symptoms include chronic fatigue, mood disorders, gastrointestinal problems, as well as disruptions of social and family life. The risk of alcohol or drug abuse, weight gain, hypertension, cardiovascular disease, and breast and endometrial cancer is increased in shift work disorder.[105]

The goals of treatment include realigning the endogenous circadian rhythm with the work schedule and alleviating the insomnia or daytime sleepiness. To achieve circadian realignment, various behavioral interventions can be utilized. The first step includes bright light exposure during the first half of the shift followed by avoidance of bright light about 2 hours before the end of the shift.[107,108] In addition, wearing dark sunglasses in the morning on the way home from work can improve adaptation. It is important that the room for sleeping is dark and quiet, with a comfortable temperature setting, and that no disturbances occur to interrupt sleep.

To help improve alertness on the job, a short 1- to 2-hour nap about 2 to 3 hours before work can decrease sleepiness. Modafinil and armodafinil are FDA-approved for treatment of excessive sleepiness in shift work disorder and significantly improve performance; caffeine is another alerting agent that is frequently used.[109,110]

Melatonin before bedtime in night shift-workers has been shown to improve sleep duration, but it does not significantly improve alertness.[111] Short-acting hypnotics can also improve symptoms of insomnia associated with shift work disorder.

Jet Lag Disorder

Jet lag develops when there is temporary desynchronization between the internal circadian rhythm and external time cues, resulting in insomnia, daytime sleepiness, and general malaise. Factors that increase the severity of symptoms include the number of time zones traveled and the direction of travel. It is generally more difficult to travel eastward than westward. Symptoms usually resolve within 7 days. Frequent flyers can develop functional impairment requiring treatment.

The goal of treatment is to accelerate realignment of the circadian clock to the new time zone. Circadian adaptation to eastward travel necessitates advancing the circadian rhythm, whereas westward travel requires phase delay. Timed light exposure and exogenous melatonin are recommended (Fig. 51-6). Other behavioral interventions include attempted adjustment to the new time zone before leaving the existing one; avoidance of alcohol, caffeine, and dehydration during travel; and timed naps. Hypnotic agents, such as ramelteon and zolpidem, and agents promoting wakefulness, such as modafinil and armodafinil, improve symptoms of insomnia and excessive daytime sleepiness, respectively, in jet lag.[112,113]

Irregular Sleep-Wake Disorder

Irregular sleep-wake disorder is characterized by multiple short sleep and wake periods without a single distinct sleep period. Diagnostic criteria require at least three sleep periods of varying duration in a 24-hour period; however, total sleep time per 24-hour period is normal for age. This results in symptoms of insomnia, excessive EDS, or both. Voluntary maintenance of an irregular sleep-wake schedule must be distinguished from irregular sleep-wake disorder.

This disorder is most commonly seen among institutionalized residents such as those with dementia, mental retardation, and traumatic brain injury.[114] These individuals often lack exposure to external synchronizing cues such as light, activity, and a social schedule. Additionally, neurodegeneration or injury to the central circadian clock system can result in this temporally disorganized sleep-wake schedule.

The goal of treatment for irregular sleep-wake disorder is consolidation of the sleep period, which is

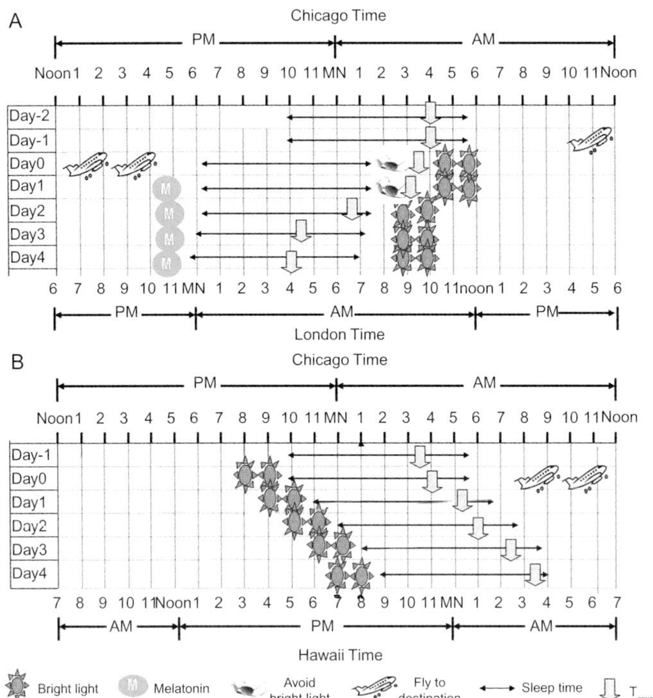

FIGURE 51-6 ■ Strategies to accelerate circadian adaptation to jet lag. **A,** An example of a treatment strategy for jet lag associated with an eastward flight over six time zones (from Chicago to London). Adjustment requires an equal number of hours of phase advance. On arrival, the traveler should avoid bright light in the early-morning hours (before 9 A.M.) for the first 2 days so that light does not decrease before nadir of the core body temperature (which will induce a phase delay), and exposure to bright light after 9 A.M. to induce phase advances. In addition, melatonin, 1 to 5 mg taken at 6 P.M. local time on the departure day and at local bedtime (10 to 11 P.M.) on arrival for 4 days is helpful. **B,** Treatment strategy for jet lag associated with a westward flight over five time zones (from Chicago to Hawaii). The subject should be exposed to as much as light as possible in the late afternoon and early evening at the destination, which will result in the required phase delay.

best achieved with combination therapy consisting of bright light exposure in the daytime, increased structured activities during the day, avoidance of daytime naps, exogenous melatonin in the evening, reduction of noise and light at night, and institution of a bedtime routine.[115] Melatonin alone has not been shown to help nursing home residents; however, it is effective in children with cognitive problems and irregular sleep-wake disorder.[116]

Free-Running Disorder

Free-running disorder is characterized by a sleep-wake pattern that is not entrained to the 24-hour environmental cycle, usually leading to a delay, over time, of sleep onset and wake times. A lack of synchronization between the endogenous circadian clock and the 24-hour light–dark cycle is the cause. Individuals report complaints of insomnia, EDS, and inability to meet social and occupational obligations.

Free-running disorder is seen in 50 percent of blind people and is relatively rare in sighted people.[117] Blind individuals with absence of light perception do not receive photic input to the circadian pacemaker, leading to free-running disorder. The etiology in sighted people is unclear, but predisposing risk factors include a long circadian period that is beyond the range of entrainment to a 24-hour cycle, psychiatric disorders, and neurodegenerative diseases such as dementia.

Treatment is aimed at establishing stable entrainment of the sleep-wake pattern to the 24-hour external cycle. For patients without light perception, combination therapy is helpful and involves creation of structured social and occupational schedules, maintenance of good sleep hygiene, and low-dose melatonin 1 hour before the preferred sleep time.[118] For sighted patients or those with visual impairment but preserved light perception, timed bright light and melatonin along with the above behavioral interventions are effective.

SLEEP-RELATED MOVEMENT DISORDERS

Sleep-related movement disorders are a category of conditions that involve simple, usually stereotyped, movements that affect sleep. The primary disorders that present to the clinician include restless legs syndrome and periodic limb movement disorder.

Restless Legs Syndrome

Restless legs syndrome (RLS) is characterized by a compelling urge to move the limbs that is worse during rest, relieved by movement, and is most prominent in the evening or night. The urge to move is associated with distressing sensations in the limbs that are described as creeping, crawling, tingling, burning, or aching. The symptoms most often occur in the legs, but may involve the arms or other parts of the body as well. Approximately 80 to 90 percent of patients with RLS also have periodic limb movements (PLMS). The condition often has a profound impact on quality of life because of sleep disruptions, including difficulty in initiating and maintaining sleep. The pathophysiology of RLS is not fully understood, but iron deficiency and central dopaminergic system dysfunction have been implicated.

The estimated prevalence of RLS ranges from 3 to 15 percent; however, the prevalence of clinically significant RLS requiring treatment is 1.6 to 2.8 percent.[119,120] The female to male ratio is roughly 2:1. Prevalence increases with age, and treatment is often not sought until after age 40. Familial aggregation is common in primary RLS, with a three- to sixfold greater risk for first-degree relatives of patients with RLS. There is also a high concordance rate (83%) in monozygotic twins. At least five different chromosomes (12q, 2p, 14q, 9p, 22p) have been linked to RLS.[5]. Secondary RLS is associated with many different medical and neurologic conditions (Table 51-7).[121]

TABLE 51-7 ■ Secondary Causes of Restless Legs Syndrome

Medical
Iron-deficiency anemia
End-stage renal disease
Rheumatologic disorders
Diabetes
Obstructive sleep apnea
Liver disease
Chronic obstructive pulmonary disease
Celiac disease
Gastric bypass surgery
Crohn disease
Neurologic
Neuropathy
Parkinson disease
Spinocerebellar ataxia types 1, 2, 3
Multiple sclerosis
Migraines
Myelopathies
Medications
Antihistamines
Neuroleptics
Metoclopramide
Proton pump inhibitors
Selective serotonin reuptake inhibitors (SSRIs)
Serotonin-norepinephrine reuptake inhibitors (SNRIs)
Lithium
Mirtazapine
Lifestyle
Sleep restriction
Smoking
Alcohol
Caffeine
Too little or too much physical activity

Treatment should begin with behavioral modifications such as improving sleep hygiene with regular sleep-wake times, avoiding caffeine and alcohol, and moderate daily exercise. Iron deficiency is a common cause of RLS; therefore, serum iron and ferritin levels should be checked before any medication is initiated. Iron replacement should occur when serum ferritin is below 20 ng/ml.[122]

Dopaminergic agents are the first-line pharmacologic agents for RLS and PLMS (Table 51-8). Levodopa was initially the treatment of choice before the development of dopamine agonists; however, its use is limited by rebound, tolerance, and augmentation (the occurrence of more severe symptoms that develop earlier in the evening).

Dopamine agonists alleviate the symptoms of RLS in 70 to 90 percent of patients with low doses and have less risk of augmentation.[123] Pramipexole is a nonergot-derived D3 and D2 receptor agonist that has proven efficacy for RLS at daily doses of 0.25 to 1 mg.[124] Ropinirole is another nonergot-derived D3 and D2 receptor agonist that is effective for RLS at a mean dose of 2 mg daily.[125] Plasma concentrations of ropinirole and pramipexole peak almost 2 hours after ingestion; therefore, it is important to dose them several hours before symptom onset. Ergot-derived dopamine agonists are not considered first-line treatment because of the risk of pulmonary fibrosis and valvular heart disease. Adverse effects associated with dopamine agonists include nausea, headache, somnolence, and dizziness.

Transdermal dopamine agonists have been approved as an alternative treatment of RLS.

Rotigotine, in patch form, has good long-term safety and efficacy data.[126] The rationale for continuous drug administration is to maintain a more steady plasma level, thus benefiting patients with daytime symptoms of RLS.

Gabapentin and its derivatives (pregabalin and gabapentin enacarbil) have also proved to be effective treatments for RLS and PLMS. Gabapentin can be particularly helpful in patients with painful RLS or those with concomitant neuropathic pain. The mean effective daily dose of gabapentin is around 1800 mg/day, divided into two daily doses; however, doses up to 2400 mg/day may be necessary.[127] Pregabalin has been shown to be effective for RLS as well at a mean effective dose of around 125 mg/day.[128] Gabapentin enacarbil, at a single dose of 600 mg/day, has been shown to have superior absorption and longer duration of action when compared to gabapentin.[129]

Other medications that have shown some efficacy in relieving symptoms of RLS include oxycodone, tramadol, clonazepam, and zolpidem.[130] The side-effect profiles of these medications limit usage; however, they should be considered when first-line therapy fails or as adjunct therapy.

TABLE 51-8 ■ Pharmacologic Therapy for Restless Legs Syndrome

Drug	Dose	Cautions
Dopaminergic Agents		
Levodopa	100–200 mg	Augmentation, rebound, tolerance
Pramipexole	0.25–1 mg	Sleepiness, impulse control impairment
Ropinirole	0.25–2 mg	Sleepiness, impulse control impairment
Rotigotine patch	0.5 mg	Augmentation, skin reaction
Gabapentin and Derivatives		
Gabapentin	600–2400 mg	Somnolence, renal impairment
Pregabalin	75–300 mg	Angioedema, renal impairment
Gabapentin enacarbil	600 mg	Somnolence, renal impairment
Other		
Oxycodone	5–20 mg	Abuse potential, dependence
Tramadol	50–200 mg	Augmentation, withdrawal
Clonazepam	0.25–1 mg	Withdrawal, dependence
Zolpidem	5–10 mg	Complex sleep-related behaviors

Periodic Limb Movements

PLMS are repetitive stereotyped limb movements occurring during sleep. PLMS usually occur in the lower extremities but can involve the arms. The stereotyped movements frequently consist of extension of the big toe with partial flexion of the knee and ankle. Movements may cause an autonomic or cortical arousal or an awakening.

Patients are often asymptomatic, with only the bed partner reporting the abnormal movements. PLMS can be present in many sleep disorders, such as RLS and narcolepsy. Often they are an asymptomatic finding during a sleep study.

Periodic limb movement disorder is characterized by the presence of PLMS along with sleep disruption not otherwise caused by another sleep disorder. Sleep disruption from PLMS can present as daytime sleepiness or insomnia.

If PLMS are found to be part of another sleep disorder, such as RLS, then the primary sleep disorder should be treated. PLMS must be differentiated from periodic limb movement disorder in order to discern whether treatment is needed. The same medications that are used for RLS have been shown to alleviate PLMS.

PARASOMNIAS

Parasomnias are disorders characterized by abnormal behavioral or physiologic events, or both, that accompany sleep-specific sleep stages, or sleep-wake transitions.[17,131,132] These events typically occur because of inappropriate timing of the sleep cycles. Physiologic and behavioral manifestations include activation of the central nervous system, with skeletal muscle activity and associated autonomic changes, resulting in undesirable or unwanted motor or verbal phenomena during sleep. Parasomnias can lead to disrupted sleep, poor health outcomes, psychosocial problems, and even cause physical harm in more severe cases. They are typically classified based on the state in which they occur—REM sleep, NREM sleep, or both sleep states.

NREM Parasomnias

Disorders of arousal during NREM sleep include sleepwalking, sleep terrors, and confusional arousals. Thought to occur due to the instability of slow-wave sleep, arousal disorders are built on the premise that the arousals are not an all-or-none phenomenon, but rather a continuum of reestablishment of full alertness, orientation, judgment, and control over behavior; a rapid alteration of sleep and waking states; or both.[133]

Sleepwalking (Somnambulism)

Sleepwalking refers to a series of multifaceted motor behaviors that are initiated during slow-wave sleep and result in walking during a state of altered consciousness within the first third of the sleep period. Most prevalent in children between 5 and 10 years old and less common in older groups, sleepwalking episodes range from subdued to sophisticated, including unlocking doors, texting, dressing, and driving. They range in duration from 15 seconds to 30 minutes, and recall may be limited or absent. The walker's eyes are open and behaviors may be clumsy. When awakened, the walkers typically respond with simple responses ("had to take a shower"). Sleepwalking in adults can be dangerous as it can be associated with violent or dangerous activity. Sleepwalking patients are generally neurologically normal, but other sleep disorders should be excluded.

Confusional Arousals

Confusional arousals are brief, impaired, and incomplete arousals that typically begin during slow-wave sleep. The individual typically looks confused, especially in the early part of the night. Confusional arousals differ from sleepwalking in that the affected patient does not leave the bed. Most commonly seen during the first third of the night in slow-wave sleep, such arousals can also occur in other NREM sleep stages or the later part of the night. Common examples include sitting up in bed with simple vocalization or picking at bedclothes.

Anxiety, sleep deprivation, fever, and endocrine factors (e.g., pregnancy) may increase the frequency of episodes. Other precipitating factors include alcohol or hypnotic consumption, antihistamines, and lithium. Primary sleep disorders (e.g., apnea or periodic leg movements) may also exacerbate confusional arousals.

Sleep Terrors

Sleep terrors (night terrors, pavor nocturnus) are less common than sleepwalking, beginning with an incomplete arousal from slow-wave sleep. Often associated with a frightening image and autonomic activation, a typical event might terrify the patient, who often emits an abrupt piercing scream and has autonomic and behavioral manifestations of intense fear. Usually associated with agitation, sweating, tachycardia, and hyperpnea, sleep terrors are more common in children than adults. Episodes occur in the first third of the night, with the patient having no or very little recall of the event the next morning. Witnesses tend to be more distressed by the events than patients. Children who present with sleep terrors often grow out of them, but events may continue to be precipitated by alcohol use, stress, sleep deprivation, and shift work. Adults presenting with sleep terrors should be assessed for psychiatric disorders.

Treatment of Arousal Disorders

Management of arousal disorders should involve reassurance and education, especially in children. Symptoms generally do not require intervention and events will usually minimize with time (in children). Although stress or psychiatric issues may be a factor, it should not be the clinician's first assumption as to etiology. Proper clinical management involves the recommendation of sleep hygiene including avoidance of alcohol and drugs, maintenance of a consistent sleep-wake schedule, and reduction of bedroom light and noise. Sleep deprivation should be avoided. The environment should be kept safe to avoid injuries from arousals.

It is often difficult to arouse individuals from slow-wave sleep episodes. When aroused, patients may be confused or even aggressive, with subsequent amnesia for the episode. Scheduled awakenings (awakening the patient 15 minutes before each usual arousal on a regular basis) have been effective.[134]

Stress-management skills, psychotherapy, and hypnosis have also been found useful. Pharmacologic treatment is necessary when events are frequent, put the family or patient at risk of being harmed, or disturb family life (Table 51-9). Benzodiazepines

TABLE 51-9 ■ Pharmacologic Treatment Of Parasomnias

Medication	Effective Dose Range (mg)	Appropriate Patient Population
Non-REM Parasomnias		
Clonazepam	0.5–2.0	First-line treatment
Triazolam	0.125–0.5	First-line treatment
Paroxetine	20–40	Alternative treatment
Zolpidem	5–10	Alternative treatment
Sleep-Related Eating Disorders		
Clonazepam	0.5–2.0	First-line treatment
Lorazepam	1.0–2.0	Side effects with clonazepam
Pramipexole	0.5–1.0	Unresponsive to benzodiazepines, history of substance abuse
Melatonin	3–15	Unresponsive to benzodiazepines, history of substance abuse
REM-Related Parasomnias		
Clonazepam	0.5–2.0	First-line treatment for RBD
Melatonin	3–12	May be effective in RBD
Prazosin	5–15	Nightmares in PTSD
SSRI (e.g., Sertraline)	50–200	History of daytime eating, mood, anxiety disorder
Pramipexole	0.18–0.36	RBD with Parkinson disease
Topiramate	25–400	Binge eating disorder, insomnia

RBD, REM-sleep behavior disorder; PTSD, post-traumatic stress disorder.

(used continuously or as needed), tricyclic antidepressants, and SSRIs (such as paroxetine) have been successfully used in treatment, though controlled trials are sparse.

REM Parasomnias

NIGHTMARES

Nightmares are unpleasant dreams that awaken the individual from REM sleep and are often associated with strong emotions such as fear, anger, sadness, or embarrassment. Although they may occur at any part of the night, they predominantly occur during the final third, when REM sleep is more prominent. Recall is generally vivid and detail oriented. Nightmare disorder can be idiopathic or related to an underlying condition, with recurrent nightmares often linked to psychologic trauma or psychiatric disorders (e.g., post-traumatic stress disorder, affective disorders). Frequent nightmares can lead to disturbed sleep-onset latency, awakenings, restless sleep, insomnia, and a lower overall quality of life.

Although usually seen in children, adults may also experience nightmares that are recurrent, frequent, or both, with causes typically related to stress, post-traumatic stress disorder, antidepressant or antihypertensive medications, withdrawal from alcohol or drugs, narcolepsy, and sleep-related breathing disorders.

Patients should be told to avoid alcohol, drugs, and heavy meals at least 3 hours before bedtime. Clinicians should also assess for any medications or other sleep disorders (e.g., sleep apnea) that might exacerbate nightmares. Though more commonly used to treat hypertension, prazosin is effective as a routine treatment, particularly in post-traumatic nightmares.[135] Imagery rehearsal therapy has shown promising results for nightmare treatment. Patients are taught to "change the dream in any way they wish" and imagine the new dream for 5 to 20 minutes daily.[136]

REM SLEEP BEHAVIOR DISORDER

REM sleep behavior disorder is characterized by forceful motor activity that typically occurs during REM sleep in the absence of the usual muscle atonia. It often involves behaviors dangerous to self or the bed partner, along with unpleasant images or dreams. REM sleep behavior disorder is more frequent in men than women and typically occurs in the middle-aged or elderly. The prevalence is estimated as 0.5 percent.[137] PSG can exclude seizure activity and confirm the presence of increased EMG tone during REM sleep. REM sleep behavior disorder can be idiopathic or related to underlying neurologic conditions (e.g., synucleinopathies), and patients should undergo a thorough physical examination seeking any comorbidities that might interrupt REM sleep.[138] In some patients, REM sleep behavior disorder precedes the development of a synucleinopathy such as Parkinson disease by many years. Acute REM sleep behavior disorder can be induced by medications (e.g., monoamine oxidase inhibitors, SSRIs), benzodiazepine withdrawal, and alcohol.

Measures should be taken to keep the sleep environment safe. The patient should sleep in a separate bed from their partner until events are controlled. Patients usually respond well to clonazepam (0.5 to 2.0 mg). Melatonin, hypnotics, and dopaminergic medications may also be effective in some cases.

Other Parasomnias

Sleep-Related Eating Disorder

Sleep-related eating disorder involves partial arousals from sleep where patients engage in involuntary eating and drinking. It has a higher prevalence in patients with a history of eating disorders or sleepwalking, and can be linked to medications (e.g., zolpidem, anticholinergics, and lithium). Patients may have unexplained weight gain and morning anorexia. They have limited or no memory of events, and foods consumed can even be toxic, inedible, or peculiar such as coffee grounds, frozen or uncooked products, cake mix, eggshells, or cleaning materials. Patients should be evaluated for comorbid sleep disorders such as periodic limb movements and OSA. Topiramate and dopaminergic medications have been effective in some patients.

Sexsomnia

Sexsomnia is characterized by abnormal sexual behaviors during sleep, with patients having little to no memory of the event. Sexual arousal may be accompanied by autonomic activation (e.g., nocturnal penile tumescence, nocturnal emission, vaginal lubrication, and dream orgasm). Many patients have a history of sleepwalking; comorbid sleep disorders should be evaluated. Patients are advised to optimize proper sleep hygiene.

Forensic Implications

Violent behaviors may occur during sleep without conscious awareness, leading to important forensic implications. Behaviors such as murder, assault, or apparent suicide can be linked to disorders of arousal, REM sleep behavior disorder, psychogenic dissociative states, and sleep-related seizures. These sleep-related episodes have been reported in 2 percent of the population,[139] but more prevalence and treatment studies are needed.

Exploding Head Syndrome

Occurring during the switch from wakefulness to sleep, patients may be awakened by the sensation of a loud, explosion-like bursting in the head. Most are usually painless, but patients occasionally note a small stab of pain accompanying the sound. Sleep deprivation and stress often worsen these events, and optimizing sleep hygiene and reassurance that these events are benign are all that is required for treatment.

SLEEP DISORDERS IN PATIENTS WITH NEUROLOGIC DISORDERS

Sleep complaints are common in patients with neurologic disorders. Untreated sleep conditions often worsen neurologic symptoms and increase morbidity and mortality. Neurologists can play a central role in diagnosing these disorders and thereby improve the care of these patients.

Parkinson Disease

Sleep disturbances are common in Parkinson disease, affecting as many as 60 to 98 percent of patients.[140] Common symptoms include difficulty in falling asleep and staying asleep, abnormal movements in sleep, and EDS. Sleep disturbances develop for multiple reasons including: (1) degeneration of the cortical sleep centers that regulate the sleep-wake cycle; (2) side effects of dopaminergic and anticholinergic medications; (3) rigidity, bradykinesia, and dystonia resulting in difficulty in shifting positions during sleep, leading to frequent arousals and sometimes pain; (4) depression and anxiety resulting in insomnia; (5) altered muscle tone in the upper airway facilitating sleep apnea; and (6) dream enactment behavior such as REM sleep behavior disorder. The severity of Parkinson disease is directly related to the severity of the sleep disturbances.

It is helpful to interview the patient in the presence of a close friend or family member when screening for sleep disorders as patients often lack insight into their sleep disturbances. Clinical tools such as the Parkinson Disease Sleepiness Scale or the Epworth Sleepiness Scale can assess need for and response to therapy. Multiple treatment strategies are often needed including medication adjustments, behavioral modifications, and therapy of specific sleep disorders.

Alzheimer Disease

Sleep disturbances are common in dementia and may worsen cognitive function and mood.

Additionally, sleep disruption can worsen caregiver burden and serve as a primary reason for institutionalization. Treatment of sleep disorders can improve cognitive functioning in these patients.

Irregular sleep-wake disorder is the most common sleep problem in Alzheimer disease and typically presents with insomnia at night and EDS.[141] The etiology involves degeneration of the suprachiasmatic nucleus in the hypothalamus and dysregulation of the pineal gland and its melatonin output. Although melatonin levels are lower in Alzheimer disease patients than age-matched controls, studies have not shown a benefit of melatonin supplementation in these patients.[142]

A major factor in the development of irregular sleep-wake disorder in Alzheimer disease is lack of appropriate zeitgebers, such as light and physical activity, which are essential for establishing a regular circadian rhythm. Dementia patients, especially those in nursing homes, frequently lack proper light exposure and physical activity. Behavioral interventions include ensuring adequate activity and light during the daytime and minimizing stimulation and disruptions at night.

Sundowning, defined as agitated behavior that appears in the late afternoon or early evening, is common in Alzheimer disease and other forms of dementia. The exact cause is unknown, but it may be due to changes in melatonin secretion, alterations in the cholinergic projections from the nucleus basalis of Meynert, delay in the body temperature rhythm, or degeneration of the suprachiasmatic nucleus. Behavioral interventions, such as maintaining a regular schedule in a known environment with familiar caregivers, can minimize sundowning. Eliminating delirium-provoking medications is also important.

The presence of other primary sleep disorders such as OSA should be assessed. Treatment of OSA can improve cognitive functioning and sleep disturbances in patients with Alzheimer disease. Patients with dementia are generally able to tolerate CPAP therapy as well as other patients.[143]

Epilepsy

The relationship between sleep and epilepsy is bidirectional. Epilepsy and some of the medications used in its treatment can disturb nocturnal sleep and daytime alertness. Additionally, sleep deprivation and sleep disorders can increase the likelihood of having seizures in a predisposed individual, highlighting the need for proper sleep hygiene in patients with epilepsy.

Patients are often unaware of seizures that occur during sleep. They may report daytime sleepiness, difficulty with concentration, or awakenings, which may be misinterpreted as insomnia. Patients with epilepsy have more sleep fragmentation and sleep stage shifts than those without seizures.[144] Antiepileptic medications such as carbamazepine, levetiracetam, phenytoin, phenobarbital, and topiramate can produce hypersomnolence.

Sleep also influences EEG activity, with increased expression of ictal and interictal discharges during NREM sleep. During NREM sleep, the EEG shows synchronous oscillation of cortical neurons that generate sleep spindles, K complexes, and slow waves that promote seizure propagation.[145] As a result, some patients with epilepsy only have seizures during sleep. Conversely, REM sleep is characterized by EEG desynchronization that inhibits epileptiform discharges.

There is a higher prevalence of OSA in patients with epilepsy, especially in those with medically refractory seizures.[146] OSA likely increases the frequency of seizures due to a combination of recurrent oxygen desaturation, sleep fragmentation, and sleep deprivation.[147] Treatment of sleep apnea tends to improve seizure control, cognitive performance, and quality of life in these patients.

Parasomnias can be difficult to differentiate from certain types of epilepsy such as nocturnal frontal lobe epilepsy. Additionally, these two disorders may coexist in the same patient, highlighting the need for overnight video-EEG and PSG to make a definitive diagnosis. Recent studies have found NREM parasomnias to be more frequent in sporadic and familial forms of nocturnal frontal lobe epilepsy, perhaps due to the two disorders sharing underlying genetic mutations.[148]

Stroke

Sleep apnea is an independent risk factor for hypertension and cardiovascular and cerebrovascular disease. This link is thought is be secondary to increased sympathetic activity in sleep which influences heart rate and blood pressure. Additionally, proinflammatory vascular risk factors, oxidative stress, and endothelial damage are increased in

OSA. Studies also suggest that sleep apnea is a risk factor for new-onset atrial fibrillation, and increases the chance of postablation failure. Other studies have suggested that sleep apnea increases the risk of stroke upon awakening in those with a patent foramen ovale.[149]

Sleep apnea may lead to cognitive decline by increasing small-vessel disease due to systemic chronic hypoxia and sympathetic stress.[150] CPAP treatment may help to prevent cognitive decline in these circumstances.[151]

Sleep apnea is common in patients after stroke and is associated with poorer functional outcome, cognitive functioning, and performance of activities of daily living, along with depressed mood.[152] Preliminary data have shown benefit from CPAP use following stroke in those with OSA.[153]

Headache

Studies have established a strong association between sleep disorders and most primary headache types including migraine, tension, cluster, hypnic, and morning headaches.[154] Conversely, sleep dysregulation caused by most sleep disorders, including insomnia, sleep apnea, hypersomnia, and circadian rhythm disorders, increases the risk of chronic daily headaches. Insomnia is the most common sleep disorder found in patients with migraine and tension-type headaches, and depression and anxiety may be associated. Headache histories should therefore always include a screen for sleep disorders.

Headaches that emerge out of sleep have been linked to sleep apnea. OSA increases the relative risk of chronic headache two- to threefold, and the risk of cluster headache eightfold.[154,155] Studies have shown headache improvement with CPAP use.[156]

Both oversleeping and sleep deprivation are known triggers for migraines. Sleep duration of less than 6 hours and more than 8.5 hours has been associated with increased headache intensity.[157] The optimal sleep duration to reduce headaches in these patients is likely around 7 to 8 hours.

REFERENCES

1. Berry R, Brooks R, Gamaldo CE, et al: The AASM Manual for the Scoring of Sleep and Associated Events: Rules, Terminology and Technical Specifications, Version 2.0. www.aasmnet.org, American Academy of Sleep Medicine, Darien, IL, 2012.
2. Carskadon MA, Dement WC: Normal human sleep: an overview. p. 13. In: Kryger MH, Roth T, Dement C (eds): Principles and Practice of Sleep Medicine. 4th Ed. Elsevier Saunders, Philadelphia, 2005.
3. Redline S, Kirchner HL, Quan SF, et al: The effects of age, sex, ethnicity and sleep disordered breathing on sleep architecture. Arch Intern Med 164:406, 2004.
4. Hirshkowitz M, Moore CA, Hamilton CR, et al: Polysomnography of adults and elderly: sleep architecture, respiration and leg movements. J Clin Neurophysiol 9:56, 1992.
5. Chokroverty S: Sleep and sleep disorders. Ind J Med Res 131:126, 2010.
6. Saper C, Chou T, Scammell T: The sleep switch: hypothalamic control of sleep and wakefulness. Trends Neurosci 24:726, 2001.
7. Saper C, Scammell T, Lu J: Hypothalamic regulation of sleep and circadian rhythms. Nature 437:1257, 2005.
8. Ancoli-Israel S, Roth T: Characteristics of insomnia in the United States: results of the 1991 National Sleep Foundation Survey. I. Sleep 22(suppl 2):S347, 1999.
9. Ohayon MM, Roth T: What are the contributing factors for insomnia in the general population? J Psychom Res 51:745, 2001.
10. Ohayon MM: From wakefulness to excessive sleepiness: what we know and still need to know. Sleep Med Rev 12:129, 2008.
11. National Sleep Foundation: Sleep in America: A National Survey of U.S. Adults. The Gallup Organization, Princeton, NJ, 1995.
12. Katz DA, McHorney CA: The relationship between insomnia and health-related quality of life in patients with chronic illness. J Fam Pract 51:229, 2002.
13. Calvin AD, Somers VK: Obstructive sleep apnea and cardiovascular disease. Curr Opin Cardiol 24:411, 2009.
14. Collop NA, Tracy SL, Kapur V, et al: Obstructive sleep apnea devices for out-of-center (OOC) testing: technology evaluation. J Clin Sleep Med 7:531, 2011.
15. Ohayon MM: Epidemiology of insomnia: what we know and what we still need to learn. Sleep Med Rev 6:97, 2002.
16. Roth T, Coulouvrat C, Hajak G, et al: Prevalence and perceived health associated with insomnia based on DSM-IV-TR; international statistical classification of diseases and realated health problems, tenth revision; and research diagnostic criteria/international classification of sleep disorders, second edition criteria: results from the America Insomnia Survey. Biol Psychiatry 69:592, 2011.
17. AASM: The International Classification of Sleep Disorders, Diagnostic and Coding Manual. 2nd Ed. American Academy of Sleep Medicine, Westchester, IL, 2005.
18. Lichstein KL: Secondary insomnia: a myth dismissed. Sleep Med Rev 10:3, 2006.

19. Mayer G, Jennum P, Reimann D, et al: Insomnia in central neurologic diseases: occurrence and management. Sleep Med Rev 15:369, 2011.
20. Morgan K, Kucharcyzk E, Gregory P: Insomnia: evidence-based approaches to assessment and management. Clin Med 11:278, 2011.
21. Breslau N, Roth T, Rosenthal L, et al: Sleep disturbance and psychiatric disorders: a longitudinal epidemiological study of young adults. Biol Psychiatry 39:411, 1996.
22. Chang PP, Ford DE, Mead A, et al: Insomnia in young men and subsequent depression: the Johns Hopkins Precursors Study. Am J Epidemiol 146:105, 1997.
23. Brower KJ, Aldrich MS, Robinson EA, et al: Insomnia, self-medication and relapse to alcoholism. Am J Psychiatry 158:399, 2001.
24. Powell NB, Schechtman KB, Riley RW, et al: Sleepy driving: accidents and injury. Otolaryngol Head Neck Surg 126:217, 2002.
25. Brassington GS, King AC, Bliwise DL: Sleep problems as a risk factor for falls in a sample of community-dwelling adults aged 64–99 years. J Am Geriatr Soc 48:1234, 2000.
26. Leger D, Scheuermaier K, Philip P, et al: SF-36 evaluation of quality of life in severe and mild insomniacs compared with good sleepers. Psychosom Med 64:49, 2001.
27. Morgenthaler T, Alessi C, Friedman L, et al: Practice parameters for the use of actigraphy in the assessment of sleep and sleep disorders: an update for 2007. Sleep 30:519, 2007.
28. Spielman AJ, Caruso LS, Glovinsky PB: A behavioral perspective on insomnia treatment. Psychiatr Clin North Am 10:541, 1987.
29. Morin CM, Culbert JP, Schwartz SM: Nonpharmacological interventions for insomnia: a meta-analysis of treatment efficacy. Am J Psychiatry 151:1172, 1994.
30. Murtag DR, Greenwood KM: Identifying effective psychological treatments for insomnia: a meta-analysis. J. Consult Clin Psychol 63:79, 1995.
31. Smith MT, Perlis ML, Park A, et al: Behavioral treatment vs pharmacotherapy for insomnia—a comparative meta-analysis. Am J Psychiatry 159:5, 2002.
32. Edinger JD, Olsen KM, Stechuchak KM, et al: Cognitive behavioral therapy for patients with primary insomnia or insomnia associated predominantly with mixed psychiatric disorders: a randomized clinical trial. Sleep 32:499, 2009.
33. Savard J, Simard S, Ivers H, et al: A randomized study on the efficacy of cognitive-behavioral therapy for insomnia secondary to breast cancer: I—sleep and psychological effects. J Clin Oncol 23:6083, 2005.
34. Morin CM, Bastien C, Guay B, et al: Randomized clinical trial of supervised tapering and cognitive behavior therapy to facilitate benzodiazepine discontinuation in older adults with chronic insomnia. Am J Psychiatry 161:332, 2004.
35. Dauvilliers Y, Montplaisir J, Molinari N, et al: Age at onset of narcolepsy in two large populations of patients in France and Quebec. Neurology 57:2029, 2001.
36. Peyerson C, Faraco J, Rogers W, et al: A mutation in a case of early onset narcolepsy and a generalized absence of hypocretin peptides in human narcoleptic brains. Nat Med 6:991, 2000.
37. Hara J, Beuchmann C, Nambu T, et al: Genetic ablation of orexin neurons in mice results in narcolepsy, hypophagia, and obesity. Neuron 30:345, 2001.
38. Sansa G, Iranzo A, Santamaria J: Obstructive sleep apnea in narcolepsy. Sleep Med 11:93, 2010.
39. Mignot E, Lammers G, Ripley B, et al: The role of cerebrospinal fluid hypocretin measurement in the diagnosis of narcolepsy and other hypersomnias. Arch Neurol 59:1553, 2002.
40. Nishino S, Ripley B, Overeem S, et al: Hypocretin (orexin) deficiency in human narcolepsy. Lancet 355:39, 2000.
41. Thannickal T, Siegal J, Nienhuis R, et al: Pattern of hypocretin (orexin) soma and axon loss, and gliosis, in human narcolepsy. Brain Pathol 13:340, 2003.
42. Bassetti C, Aldrich MS: Idiopathic hypersomnia. A series of 42 patients. Brain 120:1423, 1997.
43. Arnulf I, Lin L, Gadoth N, et al: Kleine-Levin syndrome: a systematic study of 108 patients. Ann Neurol 63:482, 2008.
44. Caples SM, Gami AS, Somers VK: Obstructive sleep apnea. Ann Intern Med 142:187, 2005.
45. Young T, Peppard PE: Risk factors for obstructive sleep apnea. JAMA 291:2013, 2004.
46. Findley LJ, Fabrizio M, Thommi G, et al: Severity of sleep apnea and automobile crashes. N Engl J Med 320:868, 1989.
47. Newman AB, Nieto FJ, Guidry U, et al: Relation of sleep-disordered breathing to cardiovascular disease risk factors: the Sleep Heart Health Study. Am J Epidemiol 154:50, 2001.
48. Olson LG, King MT, Hensley MJ, et al: A community study of snoring and sleep-disordered breathing. Prevalence. Am J Respir Crit Care Med 152:711, 1995.
49. Bixler EO, Vgontzas AN, Ten Have T, et al: Effects of age on sleep apnea in men: I. Prevalence and severity. Am J Respir Crit Care Med 157:144, 1998.
50. Ancoli-Israel S, Kripke DF, Klauber MR, et al: Sleep-disordered breathing in community-dwelling elderly. Sleep 14:486, 1991.
51. Young T, Finn L, Austin D, et al: Menopausal status and sleep-disordered breathing in Wisconsin Sleep Cohort Study. Am J Respir Crit Care Med 167:1181, 2003.
52. Bixler EO, Vgontzas AN, Lin HO, et al: Prevalence of sleep disordered breathing in women: effects of gender. Am J Respir Crit Care Med 166:1388, 2003.
53. Pillar G, Lavie P: Assessment of the role of inheritance in sleep apnea syndrome. Am J Respir Crit Care Med 151:688, 1995.

54. Redline S, Tishler PV, Tosteson TD, et al: The familial aggregation of obstructive sleep apnea. Am J Respir Crit Care Med 151:682, 1995.
55. Young T, Skatrud J, Peppard PE: Risk factors for obstructive sleep apnea in adults. JAMA 291:2013, 2004.
56. Wetter DW, Young TB, Bidwell TR, et al: Smoking as a risk factor for sleep-disordered breathing. Arch Intern Med 154:2219, 1994.
57. Scanlan MF, Roebuck T, Little PJ, et al: Effect of moderate alcohol upon obstructive sleep apnoea. Eur Respir J 16:909, 2000.
58. Young T, Finn L, Kim H: Nasal obstruction as a risk factor for sleep-disordered breathing. The University of Wisconsin Sleep and Respiratory Research Group. J Allergy Clin Immunol 99:S757, 1997.
59. Grunstein RR, Ho KY, Sullivan CE: Sleep apnea in acromegaly. Ann Intern Med 115:527, 1991.
60. Lanfranco F, Motta G, Minetto MA, et al: Neuroendocrine alterations in obese patients with sleep apnea syndrome. Int J Endocrinol 2010:474, 2010.
61. Fogel RB, Malhotra A, Pillar G, et al: Increased prevalence of obstructive sleep apnea syndrome in obese women with polycystic ovary syndrome. J Clin Endocrinol Metab 86:1175, 2001.
62. Terramoto S, Yamamoto H, Yamaguchi Y, et al: Obstructive sleep apnea causes systemic inflammation and metabolic syndrome. Chest 127:1074, 2005.
63. Phillips BG, Kato M, Narkiewicz K, et al: Increases in leptin levels, sympathetic drive and weight gain in obstructive sleep apnea. Am J Physiol Heart Circ Physiol 279:H234, 2000.
64. Hui DS, Ko FW, Fok JP, et al: The effects of nasal continuous positive airway pressure on platelet activation in obstructive sleep apnea syndrome. Chest 125:1768, 2004.
65. von Kanel R, Dimsdale JE: Hemostatic alterations in patients with obstructive sleep apnea and the implications for cardiovascular disease. Chest 124:1956, 2003.
66. Ip MS, Tse HF, Lam B, et al: Endothelial function in obstructive sleep apnea and responses to treatment. Am J Respir Crit Care Med 169:348, 2004.
67. Niento FJ, Young TB, Lind BK, et al: Association of sleep-disordered breathing, sleep apnea, and hypertension in a large community-based study. Sleep Heart Health Study. JAMA 283:1829, 2000.
68. Peppard PE, Young T, Palta M, et al: Prospective study of the association between sleep-disordered breathing and hypertension. N Engl J Med 342:1378, 2000.
69. Logan AG, Perlikowski SM, Mente A, et al: High prevalence of unrecognized sleep apnea in drug-resistant hypertension. J Hypertens 19:2271, 2001.
70. Dernaika TA, Kinasewitz GT, Tawk MM: Effects of nocturnal continuous positive airway pressure therapy in patients with resistant hypertension and obstructive sleep apnea. J Clin Sleep Med 5:103, 2009.
71. Gami AS, Hodge DO, Herges RM, et al: Obstructive sleep apnea, obesity, and the risk of incident atrial fibrillation. J Am Coll Cardiol 49:565, 2007.
72. Kangala R, Murali NS, Friedman PA, et al: Obstructive sleep apnea and the recurrence of atrial fibrillation. Circulation 107:2589, 2003.
73. Marrone O, Bonsignore MR: Pulmonary haemodynamics in obstructive sleep apnoea. Sleep Med Rev 6:175, 2002.
74. Leineweber C, Kecklund G, Janszky I, et al: Snoring and progression of coronary artery disease: the Stockholm Female Coronary Angiography Study. Sleep 27:1344, 2004.
75. Shahar F, Whitney CW, Redline S, et al: Sleep-disordered breathing and cardiovascular disease: cross-sectional results of the Sleep Heart Health Study. Am J Respir Crit Care Med 163:19, 2001.
76. Young T, Finn L, Peppard PE, et al: Sleep disordered breathing and mortality: eighteen-year follow-up of Wisconsin sleep cohort. Sleep 31:1071, 2008.
77. Gottlieb DJ, Yenokyan G, Newman AB, et al: Prospective study of obstructive sleep apnea and incident coronary heart disease and heart failure: the sleep heart health study. Circulation 122:352, 2010.
78. Yaggi HK, Concato J, Kernan WN, et al: Obstructive sleep apnea as a risk factor for stroke and death. N Engl J Med 353:2034, 2005.
79. Munoz R, Duran-Cantolla J, Martinez-Vila E, et al: Severe sleep apnea and risk of ischemic stroke in the elderly. Stroke 37:2317, 2006.
80. Artz M, Young T, Finn L, et al: Association of sleep-disordered breathing and the occurrence of stroke. Am J Respir Crit Care Med 172:1447, 2005.
81. Redline S, Yenokyan G, Gottlieb DJ, et al: Obstructive sleep apnea-hypopnea and incident stroke: the Sleep Heart Health Study. Am J Respir Crit Care Med 182:269, 2010.
82. Dyken ME, Im KB: Obstructive sleep apnea and stroke. Chest 136:1668, 2009.
83. Yaggi H, Mohsenin V: Obstructive sleep apnea and stroke. Lancet Neurol 3:333, 2004.
84. Parra O, Arboix A, Bechich S, et al: Time course of sleep-related breathing disorders in first-ever stroke or transient ischemic attack. Am J Respir Crit Care Med 161:375, 2001.
85. Kaneko Y, Hajek VE, Zivanovic V, et al: Relationship of sleep apnea to functional capacity and length of hospitalization following stroke. Sleep 26:293, 2003.
86. Fietz I, Glos M, Moebus I, et al: Automatic pressure titration with APAP is as effective as manual titration with CPAP in patients with obstructive sleep apnea. Respiration 74:279, 2007.
87. Nussbaumer Y, Bloch KE, Genser T, et al: Equivalence of autoadjusted and constant continuous positive airway pressure in home treatment of sleep apnea. Chest 129:638, 2006.

88. Walker-Engstrom ML, Tegelberg A, Wilhelmsson B, et al: 4-Year follow-up of treatment with dental appliance or uvulopalatopharyngoplasty in patients with obstructive sleep apnea: a randomized study. Chest 121:739, 2002.
89. Gotsopoulos H, Chen C, Qian J, et al: Oral appliance therapy improves symptoms in obstructive sleep apnea: a randomized, controlled trial. Am J Respir Crit Care Med 166:743, 2002.
90. Cistulli PA, Gotsopoulos H, Marklund M, et al: Treatment of snoring and obstructive sleep apnea with mandibular repositioning appliances. Sleep Med Rev 8:443, 2004.
91. Ferguson K, Cartwright R, Rogers R, et al: Oral appliances for snoring and obstructive sleep apnea: a review. Sleep 29:244, 2006.
92. Schwartz AR, Gold AR, Schubert N, et al: Effect of weight loss on upper airway collapsibility in obstructive sleep apnea. Am Rev Respir Dis 144:494, 1997.
93. Schrader H, Bovim G, Sand T: The prevalence of delayed and advanced sleep phase syndromes. J Sleep Res 2:51, 1993.
94. Regestein QR, Monk TH: Delayed sleep phase syndrome: a review of its clinical aspects. Am J Psychiatry 152:602, 1995.
95. Archer SN, Carpen JD, Gibson M, et al: Polymorphism in the PER3 promoter associates with diurnal preference and delayed sleep phase disorder. Sleep 33:695, 2010.
96. Katzenberg D, Young T, Finn L, et al: A CLOCK polymorphism associated with human diurnal preference. Sleep 21:569, 1998.
97. Hohjoh H, Takahashi Y, Hatta Y, et al: Possible association of human leucocyte antigen DR1 with delayed sleep phase syndrome. Psychiatry Clin Neurosci 53:527, 1999.
98. Hohjoh H, Takasu M, Shishikura K, et al: Significant association of *arylalkylamine N-acetyltransferase* (*AA-NAT*) gene with delayed sleep phase syndrome. Neurogenetics 4:151, 2003.
99. Morgenthaler TI, Lee-Chiong T, Alessi C, et al: Practice parameters for the clinical evaluation and treatment of circadian rhythm sleep disorders. An American Academy of Sleep Medicine report. Sleep 30:1445, 2007.
100. Nagtegaal JE, Kerkhof GA, Smits MG, et al: Delayed sleep phase syndrome: a placebo-controlled crossover study on the effects of melatonin administered five hours before the individual dim light melatonin onset. J Sleep Res 7:135, 1998.
101. Toh KL, Jones CR, He Y, et al: An h*Per2* phosphorylation site mutation in familial advanced sleep phase syndrome. Science 291:1040, 2001.
102. Xu Y, Padiath QS, Shapiro RE, et al: Functional consequences of a *CKIδ* mutation causing familial advanced sleep phase syndrome. Nature 434:640, 2005.
103. Lack L, Wright H: The effect of evening bright light in delaying the circadian rhythms and lengthening the sleep of early morning awakenings in insomniacs. Sleep 16:436, 1993.
104. Campbell SS, Dawson D, Anderson MW: Alleviation of sleep maintenance insomnia with timed exposure to bright light. J Am Geriatr Soc 41:829, 1993.
105. Drake CL, Roehrs T, Richardson G, et al: Shift work sleep disorder: prevalence and consequences beyond that of symptomatic day workers. Sleep 27:1453, 2004.
106. Akerstedt T: Work hours, sleepiness and the underlying mechanism. J Sleep Res 4:15, 1995.
107. Crowley SJ, Lee C, Tseng CY, et al: Combinations of bright light, scheduled dark, sunglasses, and melatonin to facilitate circadian entrainment to night shift work. J Biol Rhythms 18:513, 2003.
108. Boivin DB, James FO: Circadian adaptation to night shift-work by judicious light and darkness exposure. J Biol Rhythms 17:556, 2002.
109. Czeisler C, Walsh J, Roth T, et al: Modafinil for excessive sleepiness associated with shift-work sleep disorder. N Engl J Med 353:476, 2005.
110. Czeisler C, Walsh J, Wesnes K, et al: Armodafinil for treatment of excessive sleepiness associated with shift work disorder: a randomized controlled study. Mayo Clin Proc 11:958, 2009.
111. Bjorvatn B, Strangenes K, Oyane N, et al: Randomized placebo-controlled field study of the effects of bright light and melatonin in adaptation to night work. Scand J Work Environ Health 33:204, 2007.
112. Rosenberg RP, Bogan RK, Tiller JM, et al: A phase 3, double-blind, randomized, placebo-controlled study of armodafinil for excessive sleepiness associated with jet lag disorder. Mayo Clin Proc 85:630, 2010.
113. Zee PC, Wang-Weigand S, Wright Jr KP, et al: Effects of ramelteon on insomnia symptoms induced by rapid, eastward travel. Sleep Med 11:525, 2010.
114. Pollack CP, Stokes PE: Circadian rest-activity rhythms in demented and nondemented older community residents and their caregivers. J Am Geriatr Soc 45:446, 1997.
115. Dowling GA, Burr RL, Van Somersen EJ, et al: Melatonin and bright-light treatment for rest-activity disruption in institutionalized patients with Alzheimer's disease. J Am Geriatr Soc 56:239, 2008.
116. Pillar G, Shahar E, Peled N, et al: Melatonin improves sleep-wake patterns in psychomotor retarded children. Pediatr Neurol 23:225, 2000.
117. Sack RL, Lewy AJ, Blood ML, et al: Circadian rhythm abnormalities in totally blind people: incidence and clinical significance. J Clin Endocrinol Metab 75:127, 1992.
118. Lewy AJ, Bauer VK, Hasler BP, et al: Capturing the circadian rhythms of free-running circadian blind people with 0.5 mg melatonin. Brain Res 918:96, 2001.
119. Hening W, Walters A, Allen R, et al: Impact, diagnosis, and treatment of restless legs syndrome (RLS) in

a primary care population: the REST (RLS epidemiology, symptom and treatment) primary care study. Sleep Med 5:237, 2004.

120. Allen RP, Walters AS, Montplaisir J, et al: Restless legs syndrome prevalence and impact: REST general population study. Arch Intern Med 165:1286, 2005.
121. Rye DB, Trotti LM: Restless legs syndrome and periodic leg movements of sleep. Neurol Clin 30:1137, 2012.
122. Silber M, Ehrenberg B, Allen R, et al: An algorithm for the management of restless legs syndrome. Sleep Med Rev 10:169, 2006.
123. Happe S, Trenkwalder C: Role of dopamine receptor agonists in the treatment of restless legs syndrome. CNS Drugs 18:27, 2004.
124. Winkelman JW, Sethi KD, Kushida CA, et al: Efficacy and safety of pramipexole in restless legs syndrome. Neurology 67:1034, 2006.
125. Walter AS, Ondo WG, Dreykluft T, et al: Ropinirole is effective in the treatment of restless legs syndrome. TREAT RLS 2: a 12-week, double-blind, randomized, parallel-group, placebo-controlled study. Mov Disord 19:1414, 2004.
126. Oertel W, Trenkwalder C, Benes H, et al: Long-term safety and efficacy of rotigotine transdermal patch for moderate-to-severe idiopathic restless legs syndrome: a 5-year open-label extension study. Lancet Neurol 10:710, 2011.
127. Garcia-Borreguero D, Larrosa O, de la Llave Y, et al: Treatment of restless legs syndrome with gabapentin: a double-blind, cross-over study. Neurology 59:1573, 2002.
128. Allen R, Chen C, Soaita A, et al: A randomized, double-blind, 6-week, dose-ranging study of pregabalin in patients with restless legs syndrome. Sleep Med 11:512, 2010.
129. Lee DO, Ziman RB, Perkins AT, et al: A randomized, double-blind, placebo-controlled study to assess the efficacy and tolerability of gabapentin enacarbil in subjects with restless legs syndrome. J Clin Sleep Med 7:282, 2011.
130. Trenkwalder C, Hening WA, Montagna P, et al: Treatment of restless legs syndrome: an evidence-based review and implications for clinical practice. Mov Disord 23:2267, 2008.
131. American Psychiatric Association: Diagnostic and Statistical Manual of Mental Disorders. 4th Ed. Text Revision. Washington DC, American Psychiatric Association, 2000.
132. Hublin C, Kaprio J: Genetic aspects and genetic epidemiology of parasomnia. Sleep Med Rev 7:413, 2003.
133. Mahowald MW, Schenck CH: Non-rapid eye movement sleep parasomnias. Neurol Clin 23:1077, 2005.
134. Frank NC, Spirito A, Stark L, et al: The use of scheduled awakenings to eliminate childhood sleepwalking. J Pediatr Psychol 22:345, 1997.
135. Krakow B, Zadra A: Clinical management of chronic nightmares: imagery rehearsal therapy. Behav Sleep Med 4:45, 2006.
136. Lancee J, Spoormaker VI, Krakow B, et al: A systematic review of cognitive-behavioral treatment for nightmares: toward a well-established treatment. J Clin Sleep Med 4:475, 2008.
137. Ohayon MM, Caulet M, Priest RG: Violent behavior during sleep. J Clin Psychiatry 58:369, 1997.
138. Ferini-Strambi L, Fantini ML, Zucconi M, et al: REM sleep behavior disorder. Neurol Sci 26:S186, 2005.
139. Mahowald MW, Schenck CH: Violent parasomnias: Forensic medicine issues. p. 960. In: Kryger MH, Roth T, Dement C (eds): Principles and Practice of Sleep Medicine. 4th Ed. Elsevier Saunders, Philadelphia, 2005.
140. Monderer R, Thorpy M: Sleep: disorders and daytime sleepiness in Parkinson's disease. Curr Neurol Neurosci Rep 9:173, 2009.
141. Roth HL: Dementia and sleep. Neurol Clin 30:1213, 2012.
142. Gehrman PR, Connor DJ, Martin JL, et al: Melatonin fails to improve sleep or agitation in double-blind randomized placebo controlled trial of institutionalized patients with Alzheimer's disease. Am J Geriatr Psychiatry 17:166, 2009.
143. Ancoli-Israel S, Baron WP, Cooke JR, et al: Cognitive effects of treating obstructive sleep apnea in Alzheimer's disease: a randomized controlled study. J Am Geriatr Soc 56:2076, 2008.
144. Touchon J, Baldy-Moulinier M, Billiard M, et al: Sleep organization and epilepsy. Epilepsia 2:73, 1991.
145. Dinner DS: Effect of sleep on epilepsy. J Clin Neurophysiol 19:504, 2002.
146. Manni R, Terzaghi M, Arbasino C, et al: Obstructive sleep apnea in a clinical series of adult patients: frequency and features of the comorbidity. Epilepsia 44:836, 2003.
147. Malow BA, Levy K, Maturen K, et al: Obstructive sleep apnea is common in medically refractory epilepsy patients. Neurology 55:1002, 2000.
148. Bisulli F, Naldi I, Vignatelli L, et al: Paroxysmal motor phenomena during sleep: study of the frequency of parasomnias in patients with nocturnal frontal lobe epilepsy and their relatives. Epilepsia 46(suppl 66):284, 2005.
149. Ciccone A, Nobil L, Roccatagliata DV, et al: Causal role of sleep apnea and patent foramen ovale in wake-up stroke. Neurology 76(suppl 4):A170, 2011.
150. Yaffe K, Laffan AM, Harrison SL, et al: Sleep-disordered breathing, hypoxia, and risk of mild cognitive impairment and dementia in older women. JAMA 306:613, 2011.
151. Matthews EE, Aloia MS: Cognitive recovery following positive airway pressure (PAP) in sleep apnea. Prog Brain Res 190:71, 2011.

152. Sandberg O, Franklin KA, Bucht G, et al: Sleep apnea, delirium, depressed mood, cognition, and ADL ability after stroke. J Am Geriatr Soc 49:391, 2001.
153. Ryan CM, Bayley M, Green R, et al: Influence of continuous positive airway pressure on outcomes of rehabilitation in stroke patietns with obstructive sleep apnea. Stroke 42:1062, 2011.
154. Raines JC, Poceta JS, Penzien DB: Sleep and headaches. Curr Neurol Neurosci Rep 8:167, 2008.
155. Nobre ME, Leal AJ, Fiho PM: Investigation into sleep disturbance of patients suffering from cluster headache. Cephalalgia 25:488, 2005.
156. Nath Zallek S, Chervin RD: Improvement in cluster headache after treatment for obstructive sleep apnea. Sleep Med 1:135, 2000.
157. Houle TT, Butschek RA, Turner DP: Stress and sleep predict headache severity in chronic headache sufferers. Pain 153:2432, 2012.

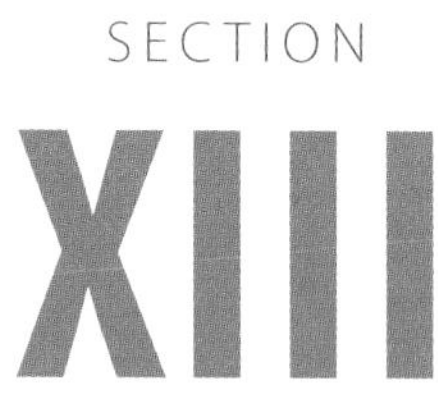

Psychogenic Disorders

CHAPTER

52

Functional Neurologic Symptom Disorders

VICTOR I. REUS

The assessment, treatment, and understanding of patients with neurologic symptoms that remain unexplained after appropriate medical investigation continue to be a source of controversy and confusion. This is so despite the general consensus that they have a high prevalence in neurologic practice and often involve disproportionate usage of medical resources, with possible attendant iatrogenic complications.[1,2] As many as 30 percent of patients seen in an outpatient neurologic practice are found to have unexplained medical illness, 10 percent of whom present with functional neurologic symptomatology.[3,4] Although epidemiologic estimates are somewhat inconsistent because of variations in case definition and differences in ascertainment, the incidence of "conversion disorder" is generally agreed to be on the order of 4 to 12 cases per 100,000 population in a given year, with a prevalence derived from case registries of 50 per 100,000 population.

A variety of diagnostic terms have been applied to such individuals historically, with distinctions made on the number, type, and breadth of somatic symptoms claimed, the degree of associated distress, and the extent to which antecedent psychopathologic mechanisms are present. In the Diagnostic and Statistical Manual of Mental Disorders (DSM-IV),[5] patients presenting with predominant neurologic symptoms of unexplained origin were assessed most commonly as having a conversion disorder, one of a family of somatoform disorders that also included somatization disorder, which required sexual and gastrointestinal symptoms in addition to neurologic and pain complaints, pain disorder, and hypochondriasis. Continuing research on these diagnostic categories, however, failed to support their predictive validity and reliability and has identified extensive comorbidities that resulted in distinctions between disorders that were more theoretical than real. In the recently released, revised edition, DSM-5,[6] these specific diagnoses have been replaced by a simplified category entitled "Somatic Symptom Disorder." Most saliently, the requirement for the existence of "medically unexplained symptoms" has been removed, with additional emphasis placed on the disproportionate thoughts, feelings, and behaviors associated with the somatic symptoms.

Most neurologic patients to be discussed in this chapter would likely qualify for the more specific term of "functional neurologic symptom disorder" if their symptoms did not conform with evidence for a recognized medical or neurologic condition

Aminoff's Neurology and General Medicine, Fifth Edition.

TABLE 52-1 ■ Conversion Disorder (Functional Neurological Symptom Disorder)

Diagnostic Criteria

A. One or more symptoms of altered voluntary motor or sensory function.
B. Clinical findings provide evidence of incompatibility between the symptom and recognized neurological or medical conditions.
C. The symptom or deficit is not better explained by another medical or mental disorder.
D. The symptom or deficit causes clinically significant distress or impairment in social, occupational, or other important areas of functioning or warrants medical evaluation.

Coding note: The ICD-9-CM code for conversion disorder is **300.11**, which is assigned regardless of the symptom type. The ICD-10-CM code depends on the symptom type (see below).

Specify symptom type:

(F44.4) With weakness or paralysis

(F44.4) With abnormal movement (e.g., tremor, dystonic movement, myoclonus, gait disorder)

(F44.4) With swallowing symptoms

(F44.4) With speech symptom (e.g., dysphonia, slurred speech)

(F44.5) With attacks or seizures

(F44.6) With anesthesia or sensory loss

(F44.6) With special sensory symptom (e.g., visual, olfactory, or hearing disturbance)

(F44.7) With mixed symptoms

Specify if:

Acute episode: Symptoms present for less than 6 months.

Persistent: Symptoms occurring for 6 months or more.

Specify if:

With psychological stressor *(specify stressor)*

Without psychological stressor

and if significant distress or impairment in social, occupational or other important areas of functioning were present or medical evaluation was required (Table 52-1). Although the classic presentation of the patient with conversion disorder has long been associated with an affect that seems disconnected with the degree of symptomatology and physical signs observed ("la belle indifference"), such emotional presentations are relatively rare and nonspecific; many patients with conversion disorder will, in fact, be quite concerned about their symptoms and associated functional deficits. The diagnosis continues to require the elimination of alternative explanations for illness behavior, such as malingering, in which symptoms are fabricated for material gain, and factitious disorder, in which symptoms are feigned in order to assume the sick role in the absence of other external incentives. Associated features include onset after stress or trauma, although this is not always present, and dissociative symptoms, such as depersonalization, derealization, and dissociative amnesia. A history of childhood abuse or neglect is sometimes obtained, but no specific genetic risk factors have as yet been identified. Shorter duration of symptoms and acceptance of possible psychological causation are indicators of a positive prognosis, whereas the presence of a comorbid personality disorder or documented physical illness or secondary financial gain are indicative of a worse course.

A persistent concern of clinicians is the possibility of misdiagnosis and the consequence of litigation or sanction if an organic etiology is excluded by definition through usage of a diagnosis of conversion disorder. This concern, however, appears to be misplaced, in that numerous studies have found that the misdiagnosis rate is quite low, remaining at approximately 4 percent over many decades and seemingly unaffected by the introduction of newer and more sensitive diagnostic technologies, such as neuroimaging.

The term "functional neurologic symptom disorder" offers no new insight into etiology or treatment selection, but benefits from being less pejorative and stigmatizing than the terms "hysteria"or "hypochondriasis" and is more mechanistically agnostic than diagnoses employing the terms "psychogenic" or "psychosomatic." Because much of the research done to date utilizes varying terminology, many of these terms are used interchangeably in this review.

Although conversion disorder or functional neurologic symptom disorder was originally conceptualized as involving neurologic mechanisms by Charcot, subsequent formulations by Janet and Freud chose to emphasize psychologic processes of dissociation and conversion following a traumatic experience in the production of somatic symptoms. Hysteria, or more specifically "neurosis," the term preferred by Charcot, was a heterogeneous entity encompassing a variety of symptomatic presentations, ranging from convulsions to paralyses and dystonias to hallucinations and dissociative reactions. The essential element of the disorder, in addition to its protean nature, was that no organic lesion could be recognized. This, however, did not mean that rules and laws regarding its symptomatic presentation could not be elicited through careful observation, and one-third of the lectures that Charcot delivered upon assuming his position as Chair of Nervous Diseases in the Faculty of Medicine in Paris were devoted to the subject. Although Charcot's focus in his lectures on diagnosis and potential mechanisms was predominantly on central nervous system pathology, he came to accept the possibility of unconscious psychologic causation. Regardless of etiology, and in contrast to the views of other prominent neurologists such as S. Weir Mitchell, who thought conscious deception was involved, patients were to be viewed as having a true medical illness and fully deserving of therapeutic support and societal acceptance.

The classic hysterical attack took the form of psychogenic seizures, perhaps because of the role of suggestion and the housing at the Salpêtrière hospital of psychologically vulnerable and impressionable neurotic patients with those subject to true grand mal seizures. According to Charcot, three distinct stages could be observed. The first, the epileptoid, would last a few minutes and was associated with a variety of prodromes: a tightness in the head or the feeling of an obstruction in the throat, a cough or yawn, and pain in the abdomen, particularly over the ovaries in a woman. The patient would then fall, with apparent loss of consciousness and diminished breathing. In the second stage, the tonic phase, the patient would extend the arms and legs and go through a series of short and violent jerking movements alternating with periods of muscle relaxation. This would be followed by disordered random movements ("clownism"; Fig. 52-1) and the classic l'arc de cercle ("the hysterical arch"), with the patient arching their body backwards, resting only on their head and heels. Variations in contorted movements might also follow. In the third stage, the "attitudes passionelles," more dramatic and profound emotional evocation was manifest, with the patients engaging in expressive mimicry of strongly felt past experiences, often yelling, crying, or engaging in complex reenactments of traumatic events. The episode at this point would end or repeat itself in a similar fashion. In some cases an extended post-episode confusional state might exist for several hours or, in some cases, days.

Complete presentations in the manner described were not common in Charcot's day and quickly became even rarer, to the point of being primarily of historical interest today. What is important, however, is that many of the individual component parts persist as core elements of the varying functional nervous system disorders discussed in this chapter. Charcot's contributions to treatment likewise provide the basis for the standard elements of psychotherapeutic intervention today. In essence, physicians should try to act psychologically, through exerting their powers of persuasion in as positive a manner as possible. The condition should be accepted by the physician, but only with the patient agreeing that the condition can be cured and only if the patient will join in the therapeutic work to be done. Reeducation, various forms of gradual increases in physical activity, and rudimentary techniques of muscle relaxation were tried and found to be helpful. Isolation of the patient to prevent social reinforcement of pathologic symptomatology was also recognized as important.

Evidence exists that many neurologists, although adept in differential diagnosis, remain uncomfortable in their management of such individuals and often erroneously believe them to be feigning or somehow deceptive in their presentation, even though Charcot himself stressed that this was not the case and that true hysteria could be distinguished from simulation and malingering.[7] An in-depth interview of a representative sample of neurologists has found that the concept of conversion disorder is recognized and seen frequently in a normal clinician's workload. The possibility of a functional condition was often recognized early in the clinical encounter but was not reported to limit the scope of the examination or subsequent laboratory evaluation. Patients themselves were viewed as difficult to deal with, and as more disabled and requiring more effort on the part of the clinician. Most neurologists thought a psychologic formulation of the condition was relevant to understanding the patient and treatment, but they themselves did not feel competent to construct one. Most felt that feigning and conversion disorders existed on a continuum and that deception could not be excluded. Given the prevalence of functional nervous system disorders and the degree to which clinicians remain discomforted by their presentation, an expanded

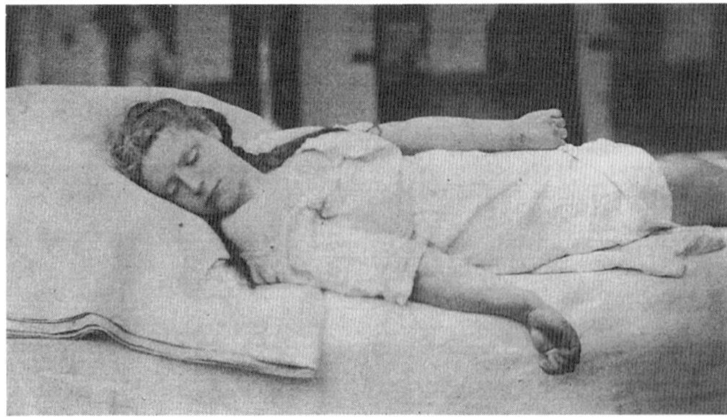

FIGURE 52-1 ■ A case of psychogenic nonepileptic seizure at the Salpêtrière. The patient is exhibiting what Charcot termed the stage of "clownism." (From Desire-Magloire Bourneville D-M, Regnard P: Icononographie Photographique de la Salpêtrière, Paris, 1877-80.)

research effort directed towards better characterization of patients, the development of more effective treatment options, and a more extensive educational outreach to treating physicians would seem warranted. This chapter reviews the most common types of functional neurologic symptom disorders and current approaches to their differential diagnoses, as well as possible treatment approaches.

CLINICAL ASSESSMENT PRINCIPLES

As noted by Stone and Carson,[8] it is essential to build rapport with patients through acceptance of their concern regarding their physical symptomatology, as well as through elicitation of their belief system regarding possible etiology and prognosis, and a systematic probing of their presenting symptoms and associated functional status. Clinicians are encouraged to emphasize the mechanisms of symptoms rather than their cause and to detail how the diagnosis was made, emphasizing reversibility, the absence of other conditions, and the importance of self-help. The presence of strong denial, prominent depression and anxiety, dissociative symptoms, or delusional thoughts is an indication for psychiatric referral and appropriate psychopharmacologic intervention. Given the high incidence of comorbid depression and anxiety, it is important to screen for the requisite symptoms of both and their associated physiologic correlates, which include loss of interest in pleasurable activities, diminished energy, alterations in sleep patterning and duration, psychomotor slowing or activation, change in appetite and weight, impaired cognition, feelings of guilt or worthlessness and morbid thoughts of death or suicide. Patients with predominant anxiety may express their concern through excessively exaggerating their condition and may have experienced episodes of panic, in which short-lived periods of shortness of breath, tremor, perspiration, heart palpitations, gastrointestinal symptoms, and lightheadedness are accompanied by a feeling of doom and loss of control. Cultural factors may also help to shape the experience of the patient and the presentation to the clinician.[9]

The diagnosis of a functional neurologic symptom disorder should be based on positive findings from the clinical and laboratory examination that contradict the known pathophysiology of neurologic disease, and not simply on an absence of corroborating data.[10,11] Such findings include changes in tremor when the patient is distracted ("tremor entrainment test"), the observation of closed eyes with resistance to opening during an observed seizure, and the "Hoover sign," when weakness of hip extension is diminished during contralateral hip flexion against resistance. Communication of the diagnosis to the patient should incorporate these principles as well, and may require considerable tact and skill (Table 52-1). Many of the conditions to be considered in a proper differential diagnosis evolve episodically over time and may present initially in an amorphous fashion, with nonspecific or evanescent symptoms, requiring the clinician to resist arriving at a diagnosis and disposition prematurely.

SPECIFIC FUNCTIONAL DISORDERS

Psychogenic Nonepileptic Seizures

Psychogenic nonepileptic seizures are defined as sudden paroxysmal events associated with apparently involuntary changes in motor behavior, sensation, cognition, or autonomic function that are not accompanied by comparable electroencephalographic changes (Fig. 52-2).[11–13] The condition is relatively uncommon and, despite increased use of telemetry, relatively hard to diagnose, as exemplified by an average delay in diagnosis of up to 7 years, a usual past history of failed response to extensive trials of antiepileptic drugs, and the incurring of significant medical costs before the correct diagnosis is achieved.[14–17]

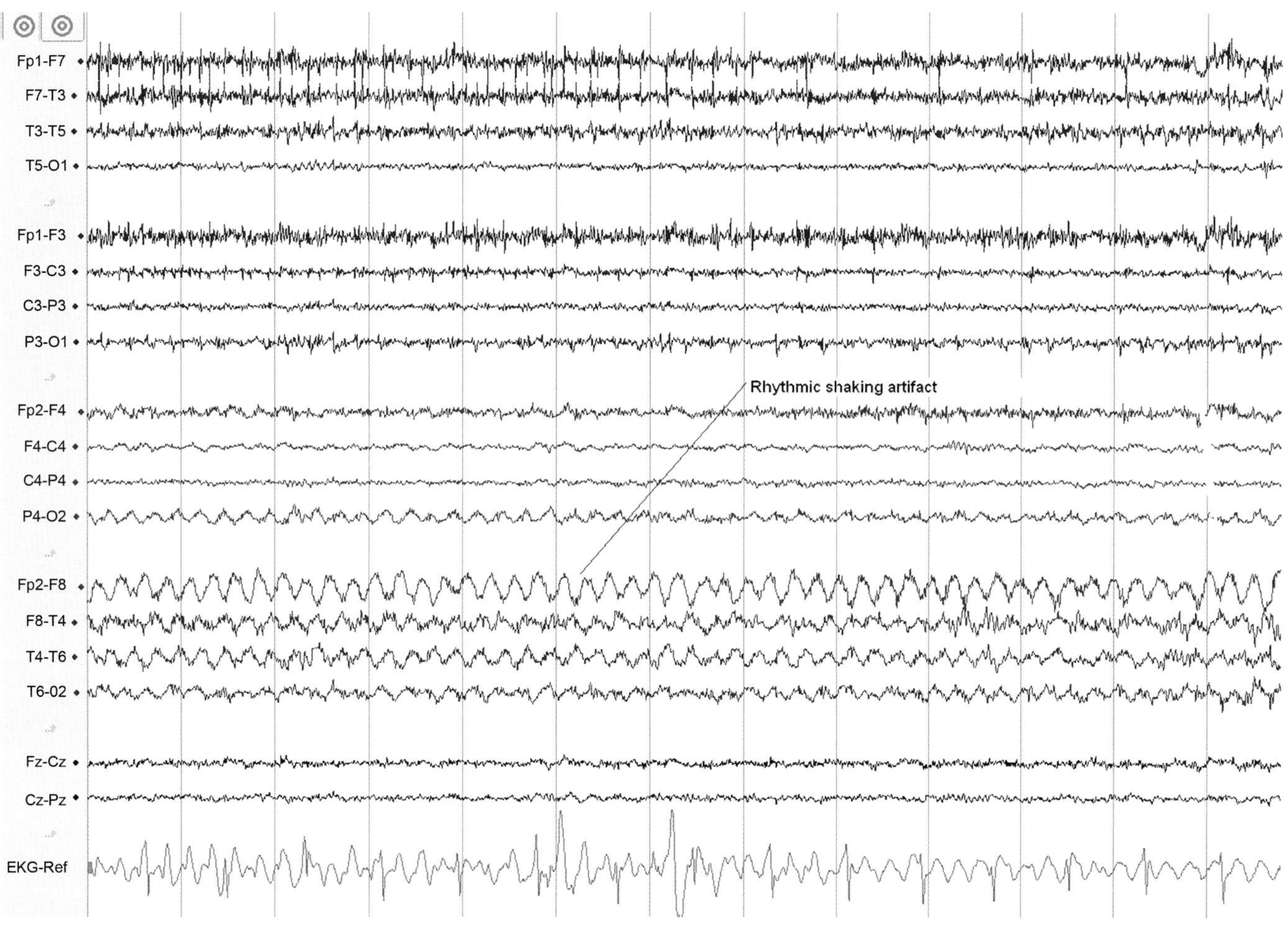

FIGURE 52-2 ■ Ten-second page of digital EEG recorded during video-EEG telemetry in a 55-year-old woman with psychogenic nonepileptic seizures characterized by asynchronous limb shaking and unresponsiveness. (Courtesy of Tina Shih, MD, University of California, San Francisco.)

The majority of patients are female and are adolescent to young adult in age, although presentation after 60 years of age can occur as well.[18] Predisposing factors include a past history of sexual, physical, or emotional abuse in a majority of subjects,[13] and comorbid psychiatric conditions, such as mood and anxiety disorders, post-traumatic stress disorder, and dissociative disorders.[16] Such patients are also more likely to experience chronic pain and to have an associated Cluster A or Cluster B personality disorder. The presence of alexithymia, which is defined as deficits in the processing and description of emotional states, has not proven useful in discriminating patients with psychogenic causation from those with organic etiology. Complicating matters even more, some individuals have an antecedent history of head trauma or neuropsychiatric deficit and may even have clear evidence of independently documented and established epileptic seizures. Patients with late-onset psychogenic nonepileptic seizures have been found to have high rates of comorbid serious medical illness and associated health-related anxiety. Psychogenic seizures are frequently brought on by psychosocial stressors, but can also be elicited by photic stimulation, hyperventilation, and loud noises.[13] A variety of characteristic signs and symptoms have been observed in association with psychogenic seizures (Table 52-2), but objective evidence of oral laceration, urinary incontinence and cyanosis is rare. Compared to nonpsychogenic events, psychogenic seizures are usually longer in duration and associated with a shorter postictal state that is often dramatic in its behavioral presentation. Although clinical history

TABLE 52-2 ■ Salient Clinical Features of Psychogenic Nonepileptic Seizures

Head and Neck
Ictal eye closure
Forceful eye closure
Geotropic eye movements
Preserved pupillary reflexes
Closed mouth
Midline tongue protrusion
Ictal weeping with tears
Motor
Undulating/fluctuating movements
Rhythmic pelvic movements
Bicycling movements
Injury
Lack of objective evidence of injury
Autonomic
Lack of cardiorespiratory compromise with prolonged generalized seizures
No ictal tachycardia or ictal tachycardia <30% of baseline
Seizure Duration
Prolonged, often >2 minutes
Postictal State
Rapid recovery
Postictal whispering
Partial motor response
Telegraphic speech
Baby talk
Shallow, rapid soft breathing
Frequent "Status"/PNES "Status"

(From: Sahaya, K, Dholakia S, Sahota P: Psychogenic non-epileptic seizures: a challenging entity. J Clin Neurosci 18:1602, 2011, with permission.)
PNES, psychogenic nonepileptic seizures.

and observation may be suggestive of the diagnosis, the gold standard remains video electroencephalography, with postictal assessment of changes in serum prolactin sometimes being a useful adjunct. Naturalistic monitoring in anticipation of an observed event is preferable, but various factitious induction techniques are sometimes employed, albeit at the risk of endangering therapeutic trust and the patient's willingness to engage in future treatment recommendations.

Differential diagnosis should include consideration of "pseudo-pseudoseizures," in which organic etiologies may cause unusual motor activity and disturbances of consciousness in the absence of epileptiform activity on monitored EEG.[19] Such cases usually are diagnosed eventually by the persistence of abnormal laboratory findings or by the progression of the etiologic condition. Clinical cases in the literature include presentations stemming from limbic encephalitis, convulsive syncope, transient ischemic attacks, paroxysmal dyskinesias, and frontal lobe epilepsy. Consideration of additional diagnostic procedures involving the recording of electrocerebral activity by sphenoidal or other nonstandard electrodes, antibody testing, tilt-table testing with cardiac monitoring, carotid ultrasound, and genetic profiling may be warranted, depending on the history in a given case.[20–25] Linguistic techniques involving conversation analysis of the ways in which patients with psychogenic seizures differ from those with epilepsy in talking about their attacks have also been found to discriminate reliably between patient groups.

Once diagnostic confidence is achieved, it is essential to present the results of the assessment in a noncritical manner, stressing the positive prognosis, the involuntary nature of the episodes, and the identification of key elements to be pursued, such as a history of abuse or trauma. Although randomized controlled trials are lacking, interventions directed towards decreasing the positive reinforcement associated with the patient's assumption of the sick role and the social attention directed to it, as well as efforts focused on diminishing possible cognitive distortions and the emotional distress derived from past psychologic traumas, are frequently beneficial.[26] A variety of modalities have been reported to be effective, including cognitive–behavioral therapy, family and group therapy, reassurance, physical therapy, hypnosis, and transcranial magnetic stimulation.[27] Psychopharmacotherapy may be indicated when comorbid mood or anxiety disorders are present. A significant majority of patients with psychogenic seizures will improve after such interventions, but one-quarter of responders may relapse or develop novel conversion symptoms.[28] Employment status is a key positive indicator of prognosis.

Despite symptomatic improvement, a number of patients will remain disabled with incomplete resolution of symptoms, depending on the degree to which the individual is able to develop an improved self-image and optimism about their functional abilities.[29,30] Recent outcome studies ranging from 1 to 10 years in length have indicated that only approximately one-third of patients will become completely free of attacks. In some cases, however, it may be sufficient to simply discontinue antiepileptic drugs and tell the patient the diagnosis; such an intervention has been shown to dramatically decrease health-care utilization even if the attacks are not eliminated completely. The pathophysiology of psychogenic seizures remains unclear despite functional imaging studies that have implicated specific frontal subcortical pathways and the regional cerebral blood flow and neuroimaging studies that are discussed later.[31–35]

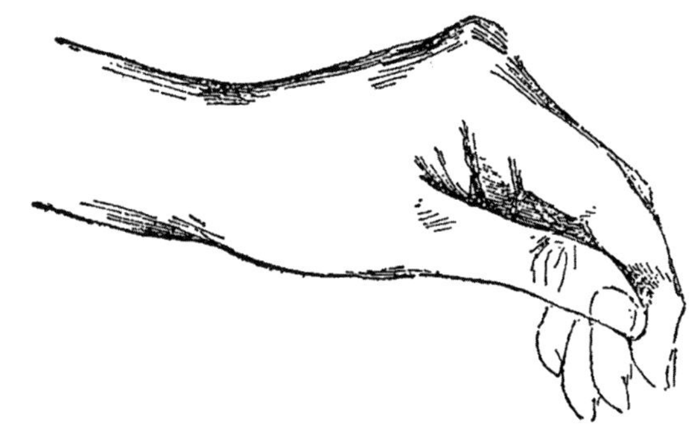

FIGURE 52-3 ■ Charcot's drawing of a "hysterical" contracture. The contracture would be maintained during sleep, but relax or disappear under chloroform anesthesia. (Charcot J-M: Clinical Lectures on the Diseases of the Nervous System (III). New Sydenham Society, London, 1889.)

Functional Motor, Movement, and Gait Disorders

Weakness and Gait Disorders

Psychogenic disorders with weakness or abnormal movements are common, but estimates of their prevalence vary widely in different series, as do the criteria used for making the diagnosis.[36–38] Women are more affected than men, usually presenting in young to mid-adulthood.

Functional weakness often presents in sudden fashion, usually unilaterally. The annual incidence has been reported to be 3.9 per 100,000 in the general population, and is frequently associated with comorbid psychiatric disorders, most commonly major depression, generalized anxiety disorder, and panic disorder. It may occur in the context of other functional complaints, but also may be a concomitant of true injury, with the weakness described in ego dystonic terms. Inconsistency in presentation and proximal flexor and distal extensor weakness may be observed, along with other signs. Patients often deny stress as a possible contributor to their illness and frequently are as disabled as patients with weakness of comparable duration due to neurologic disease.

In complaints of limb weakness, the examined limb is often diffusely weak, but an inverse of pyramidal weakness may also be observed, with weaker flexors in the arms and extensors in the legs. Inconsistency in the examination findings may occur as well, with the patient able to walk normally or stand on tiptoes, but unable to lift up the leg or flex the ankle when asked. A dragging gait, with the hip internally or externally rotated in the presence of unilateral leg weakness, and "give way" weakness, in which the patient can initially contract an arm or leg, for example, against the examiner, but then suddenly "gives way" and can offer no further resistance, may be observed. Similar give-way weakness may also occur from pain or in patients with myasthenia gravis.

Exaggerated slowness may be observed, as well as weakness or paralysis without associated atrophy and with nonanatomic associated sensory loss. Spontaneous remissions may occur. Psychogenic paralysis may simulate either an upper or lower motor neuron lesion and may be associated with either pseudocontracture or flaccidity (Figs. 52-3 and 52-4). Observation of posture can sometimes be informative; in cases of true hemiplegia, for example, the upper extremity is flexed, adducted, and pronated whereas the lower extremity is extended. Psychogenic hemiplegia will usually not follow this pattern and—in addition—may demonstrate sparing of the face.

Gait abnormalities are not uncommon. Astasia-abasia is a particularly dramatic, albeit uncommon, presentation in which patients complain of being unable to walk normally and fall when they try to stand, even though they can be shown to move their legs normally when in a lying or sitting position.

The pathophysiology of psychogenic paralysis has been explored using transcranial magnetic stimulation. Motor system excitability is normal at rest but appears to decrease in patients with psychogenic movement disorders, whereas it increases in normal

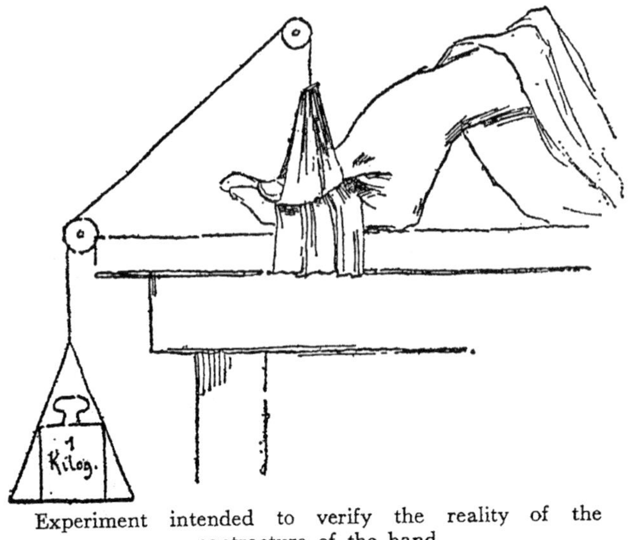

FIGURE 52-4 ■ Charcot's method of demonstrating the difference between a consciously willed and an involuntary "hysterical" contracture. In a case of hysteria, the thumb, under traction, would rise, but return to its original position without fatigue upon release of the weight. (Charcot J-M: Clinical Lectures on the Diseases of the Nervous System (III). New Sydenham Society, London, 1889.)

volunteers when subjects are asked to imagine moving their affected limb. Curiously, seeing another individual move that same limb results in parallel motor activation in both groups, suggesting that deficits in movement control may not carry over to the function of mirror neurons. Functional imaging investigations employing single-photon emission computed tomography (SPECT), positron emission tomography (PET), and functional magnetic resonance imaging (fMRI) have implicated abnormalities of executive inhibition functions in prefrontal neural circuits and their projections to motor areas. The importance of emotional state in the production of functional motor symptoms is suggested by abnormal correlations between amygdala and motor system activation in the performance of simple motor tasks involving the affected limbs. Patients with functional tremor have also been shown to have lower functional connectivity between the right temporoparietal junction and sensorimotor cortices and cerebellum, suggesting a deficit in generation of sensory prediction during motor preparation.

Functional neuroimaging studies of conversion disorder have implicated neural circuits involving frontal and subcortical pathways, specifically, the orbitofrontal cortex, regulating input from the thalamus, amygdala, and cortex, and the anterior cingulate cortex.[31,32] Measurement of regional cerebral blood flow in patients directed to move the affected as opposed to the nonaffected limbs has shown a unique activation of the appropriate lateral anterior cingulate cortex and orbitofrontal cortex, with absent activation of motor and premotor cortex, suggesting inhibition of mechanisms involved in the normal initiation of movement.[33] More elaborate models, involving neuroanatomic networks active in alexithymia, dissociation, and avoidance behaviors, and incorporating the nucleus accumbens and parietal cortex, have also been put forward.[12] More recently, it has been suggested that the unconscious and dissociative "unawareness" aspects of psychogenic neurologic disorders involve possible inferior parietal and temporoparietal cortex dysfunction.[34] Neuroimaging studies of patients with individually distinct psychogenic motor abnormalities have implicated specific deficits in prefrontal inhibition of primary motor-sensory cortex, attentional dysregulation, intentional disturbances, impaired action authorship and awareness of self-agency (i.e., the perception that an action is the consequence of one's own intention).[35]

Movement Disorders

Psychogenic movement disorders frequently demonstrate abrupt onset and disability out of proportion to the physical examination, and findings may worsen during the clinical evaluation.

Observing the effects of distraction, and of ballistic and entrainment maneuvers, as well as noting frequency and amplitude variability, limb coherence, and the presence of agonist–antagonist coactivation can be useful in the differential diagnosis of suspected psychogenic tremor, while simultaneous electromyographic (EMG) and electroencephalographic (EEG) measurement of muscle contraction burst length, antagonist muscle pattern, and readiness potential changes on the EEG can be useful in discriminating functional myoclonus from nonpsychogenic myoclonus. Patients with psychogenic myoclonus will usually have an EMG burst length greater than 50 msec and a variable EMG antagonist pattern. The Bereitschaftpotential or readiness potential is a small change in cerebral potential that develops a second before voluntary movement and can be reliably demonstrated in patients with functional myoclonus.

In the entrainment test, the patient is asked to make a rhythmic tapping movement with one hand at approximately 3 Hz or to attempt to copy the movement exhibited by the examiner. In patients with functional tremor, the tremor in this limb will either stop or begin to follow the same rhythm as the examiner's, or they will be unable to duplicate the examiner's movement in their limb without apparent awareness of why they have failed. False-negative results can occur if the tremors are long-standing or dependent on mechanics. Functional tremors can sometimes be abolished by asking the subject to make a ballistic movement with their unaffected hand or through attempted immobilization of the affected limb. When they occur in more than one limb, they are usually found to have the same frequency, whereas organic tremors in different limbs often have somewhat different rhythms. Psychogenic parkinsonism may be present in 0.5 percent of patients presenting with parkinsonism. Although it has been suggested that imaging dopamine transporter uptake in the striatum may discriminate between organic and psychogenic etiologies, some patients with early or preclinical Parkinson disease or with vascular or drug-induced parkinsonism may have normal dopamine imaging, making longitudinal assessments and additional ancillary data essential before a final diagnosis is reached.

The distinction of psychogenic from nonpsychogenic dystonia may be particularly difficult. Neurophysiological assessment of short and long intracortical inhibition, cortical silent period, and reciprocal inhibition may not discriminate between them. Spasmodic torticollis, a dystonic hand with clenched fist, or an inverted plantarflexed ankle is encountered most commonly, occurring suddenly, sometimes after a minor trauma, and in association with expressed pain and functional weakness.

TREATMENT

Treatment approaches are similar to those for patients with psychogenic nonepileptic seizures and hinge upon collaborative neurologic and psychiatric efforts.[37] In delivering the diagnosis, the physician should acknowledge the real suffering and distress associated with weakness or movement disorder and avoid statements that perpetuate a mind–body dualism; referral to a psychiatrist for treatment can be made specifically to treat identified comorbidities, but also to initiate interventions that address the hypothesized impaired neural circuitry through enhanced patient autonomy and diminished iatrogenic risk. The tenor of the discussion should be on empiricism and practicality, to do "what works best" on the expressed targets of motor dysfunction. Manual-based cognitive behavioral therapy directed towards identifying possible internal states or external environmental influences on motor dysfunction and to increasing personal mastery over motor function have been reported to be effective, as has pharmacotherapy with citalopram or paroxetine, and venlafaxine for nonresponders, in the only prospective treatment trial yet published.[37,38] Recently, studies of functional paralysis have reported significant efficacy from repetitive transcranial magnetic stimulation to the motor cortex, although the numbers of patients studied were small and no placebo controls were employed. Complementary and alternative medical treatments for psychogenic movement disorders include acupuncture, hypnosis, and EMG biofeedback, with limited supportive evidence available.

Functional Visual Loss

Medically unexplained visual loss is dramatic but less common than psychogenic motor dysfunction or psychogenic seizures, occurring in only 2 of 45 consecutive children with functional symptoms in one reported case series.[39,40] Both eyes are involved in up to 65 percent of cases, with decreased acuity and constricted visual fields being the most common complaints.[41] It is usually more marked in one eye than the other, with the smaller field being on the hemianesthetic side, most often the left, in cases where additional sensory disturbances are present. Often the visual field deficit becomes progressively smaller and smaller during the course of the examination, either as a result of fatigue or secondary to suggestion, with the resulting perimeter outline acquiring a spiral shape. In cases of psychogenic blindness in one eye, diplopia may be produced through the use of prisms. As is the case in psychogenic seizures and motor disturbances, true organic deficits, such as pseudotumor cerebri, may exist concurrently with those having psychogenic causation. The presence of a central scotoma is usually indicative of an organic etiology. An additional eye condition that may mimic the signs of functional visual loss is central serous choreoretinopathy, with a majority of patients reporting the experience of disturbing psychologic events shortly before visual loss.

Associated conditions include hysterical blepharospasm and hysterical pseudomyopia, involving spasm of the ciliary muscle and an alteration in accommodation that appears to require significant adjustment in refraction; when atropine is administered, the refraction will normalize. Patients with functional blepharospasm can be reliably distinguished from those with essential blepharospasm by assessment of blink reflex recovery, which is normal in psychogenic blepharospasm but significantly disinhibited in those with essential blepharospasm.[42] Micropsia and macropsia are rarer psychogenic complaints and need to be distinguished from true lesions of the visual cortex.

Identification of functional visual loss requires demonstration of better visual function than that claimed by the patient, and is usually accomplished by a series of assessments that test the patient's often erroneous presumptions regarding performance. These include tests of stereopsis and "fogging" of the unaffected eye in claimed monocular visual loss, tests of tangent screen and coordination for claimed constriction of the visual fields, and binocular perimetry testing in claimed monocular field deficits. Steroacuity requires visual acuity in both eyes, with binocular fusion, and is incompatible with a report of monocular vision loss. A complaint of constricted visual fields may be clinically evaluated in the office when the patient is told that they are being tested for finger-to-nose coordination when in fact their peripheral vision is being assessed. Obstacle courses, observation of stereotypies, and optokinetic-drum testing may be employed in cases involving severe visual loss or blindness (as described in detail elsewhere[39]). In cases of severe visual loss or total blindness, patients may exhibit a number of ancillary behaviors that should not be specifically affected, such as an inability to write their name clearly or a tendency to look away from the examiner, even when engaged in conversation. In optokinetic-drum testing, the presence of nystagmus indicates that at least 20/400 vision exists. More intensive technologic methods, such as optical coherence tomography and the recording of visual evoked potentials, may also be helpful in particularly difficult cases.

Treatment approaches may involve psychiatric referral, if additional behavioral symptomatology or history is elicited, or be limited to reassurance or hypnosis, but the absence of controlled studies makes specific recommendations problematic.[43]

Functional Dysphonia and Aphonia

Functional dysphonia is identified as a disturbance in the quality of, or loss of, the voice in the absence of structural laryngeal or neurologic pathology. It ranges widely in severity and associated distress. Recognized by Charcot as "hysterical mutism,"[44] functional dysphonia has been reported to be present in 10 to 40 percent of cases seen in tertiary-care voice clinics,[45–49] occurring principally in women, often after respiratory tract infections or surgery.[49,50] A lifetime prevalence of 29 percent and a point prevalence of 7.5 percent have been reported in a survey of primary-care patients. Sometimes psychogenic mutism is combined with psychogenic deafness and, in other cases, it may be followed by a period of stammering upon resolution of the original presentation. In psychogenic aphonia the patient will often talk in a whisper, sometimes with unusual articulation of specific words. Laryngoscopic examination sometimes reveals adductor weakness of the vocal cords.

As noted with other functional neurologic symptom disorders, comorbidity with depression, anxiety, and other somatization symptoms is common, as are personality traits of introversion and neuroticism, which have been hypothesized by Roy and Bless[49] to be associated with conditioned laryngeal inhibitory responses to specific environmental triggers in stressful circumstances. A family history of dysphonia and professional voice use has been reported to be a significant predictor of risk as well.[51] Regardless of the etiologic formulation, however, functional dysphonia has proved to be responsive to a number of voice therapies directed at decreasing laryngeal muscle tension. These may include cognitive–behavioral therapy, electromyographic feedback, progressive relaxation, vocal function exercises, laryngeal massage, resonance voice therapy, and transcricothyroid membrane lidocaine injections, but controlled trials with active comparators are lacking, as is evidence of long-term effectiveness.[52] Voice function exercises have been shown to result in positive changes in specific acoustic measures such as jitter, shimmer, and harmonic-to-noise ratio, as well as in self-report and laryngoscopic findings. Manual massage of the larynx has also been found to be of use, sometimes after only one session, with evidence of improved acoustic measures and reduced severity and frequency of vocal tract discomfort. In general, however, most patients require at least 30 to 40 sessions of voice therapy for lasting benefit. Deficits in emotional processing have been hypothesized to be central to many cases of functional dysphonia, giving rise to interventions that involve explication of the metaphorical meaning of loss of speech in order to give "voice" to the hypothesized repressed emotion. Whether this formulation is useful in selection of the treatment modality likely depends on unique aspects of an individual presentation. A recent Cochrane review found that a combination of direct and indirect voice therapy improved both self- and observer-rated as well as instrumentally evaluated vocal functioning, compared to no intervention, with benefits lasting at least 14 weeks.[53] No prophylactic effectiveness in preventing voice dysfunction could be shown, however. Critical evaluation of voice therapy trials is complicated by the fact that the treatment cannot be adequately blinded and that, by necessity, it has to be calibrated uniquely to the individual and lacks elements of generalizability.

Nondermatomal Somatosensory Deficits

Nondermatomal somatosensory deficits, which often occur after minor injury, may be seen in 25 to 50 percent of a population with chronic pain, sometimes in association with litigation or Workmen's Compensation claims.[54,55] Onset is usually gradual, in concert with increasing complaints of diffuse and spreading pain, and waxing and waning changes in pain intensity. Abrupt presentations may also occur, however, usually immediately after a precipitating event, and the pain is often described as "burning" or "deep aching" in nature. The sensory deficits frequently accompany parallel and unusual alterations in motor function, and are primarily elicited as deficits in pinprick sensation or insensitivity to deep tissue pressure (or both) that may increase or decrease in association with changes in pain intensity. Contradictory responses to repetitive stimulation are often present, with increasing or decreasing intensity noted by the patient, and sometimes with impairment of vibratory sense. A classic sign in hemilateral anesthesia is loss of vibration sense over one side of the sternum, which is impossible with a truly organic etiology. A quadratomal or hemibody distribution ipsilateral to the chronic pain is most typical; unilateral deficits usually do not cross the midline. Certain areas sometimes retain normal sensation on the side of claimed anesthesia, particularly in areas involving the head, nipple, or genitals (Fig. 52-5). In certain classic cases, the unilateral anesthesia affected a portion of a limb, stopping abruptly in a transverse fashion in a manner similar to when a sock or glove is worn. The specific border of the anesthesia may be shown to vary, depending upon the direction that test stimuli are applied and whether they follow a linear or zig-zag pattern. Subjectively, the patient is often more concerned about the associated pain than the accompanying sensory deficit.[54]

Standardized assessment protocols incorporating documentation by body maps of subjective complaints and objective responses to light touch, pinprick, temperature, vibration, and deep-tissue pressure, and changes over the course of the evaluation, are useful in establishing a baseline and improvement over time. In laboratory settings, quantitative sensory testing may be employed. In the "Yes-No" test the patient is instructed to close the eyes and say yes every time a touch is felt and no when it is not felt; on initial presentations, the patient will usually say yes every time he has been touched on the normal side of his body but also will say no every time he has been touched on the anesthetic side. Interestingly, patients with claimed anesthesia in critical areas usually showed no disturbance in functional performance. Complex delicate movements can continue even with the loss of presumed proprioceptive feedback in completely anesthetic hands, and self-injury, such as cuts or burns, does not usually occur.

Psychogenic hyperesthesia, in which the patient is hypersensitive to touch in specific areas, may also occur. Mannkopf sign refers to a change in pulse rate of the order of 10 to 30 beats per minute when pressure is applied to a painful spot. Patients who are malingering reportedly show no alteration in pulse rate. The tender spots are usually limited to one side of the body and are most often situated over the vertebral spine or inguinal regions. In some individuals, application of pressure to these areas may, in fact, trigger a more profound behavioral or emotional reaction.

The pathophysiology of these nondermatomal sensory deficits is incompletely understood and

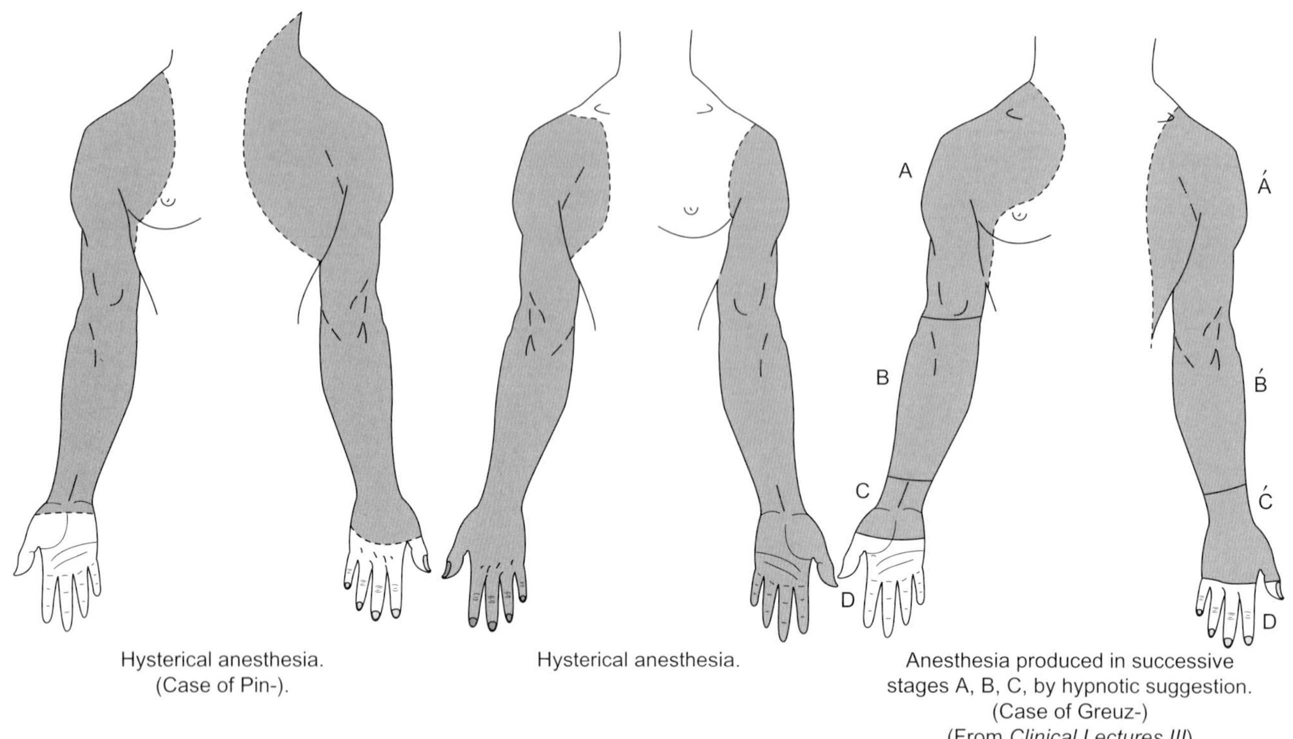

FIGURE 52-5 ■ Charcot's demonstration of "hysterical" anesthesia, including "glove-and-sleeve" anesthesia occurring in geometric segments. The shading has been improved from the original for clarity. (Charcot J-M: Clinical Lectures on the Diseases of the Nervous System (III). New Sydenham Society, London, 1889.)

current hypotheses derive primarily from empiric animal studies rather than from clinical populations. Babinski believed that psychogenic anesthesia was almost always the result of suggestion on the part of the examining clinician, but others have postulated that the phenomenon is more likely to be due to autosuggestion. Neuroimaging studies have implicated hypometabolism in the somatosensory cortex which, in the context of ongoing nociceptive, idiopathic, and neuropathic pain, results in a maladaptive inhibition of all sensory input, much akin to "deafferentiation pain."[54]

Treatment of the associated pain will often result in transient improvement of the sensory disturbance, but relapse is common. Addressing a comorbid psychiatric disorder through pharmacotherapy, cognitive–behavioral therapy, or relaxation training can be helpful, as can sodium amytal and sodium pentobarbital infusions, both in deciding the diagnosis and in facilitating neurorehabilitation.[56] Intravenous administration of sodium amytal usually produces significant pain relief, as well as a reduction in the area and severity of the anesthetic symptoms. Anesthesia secondary to organic etiology, such as that observed in peripheral nerve injury or spinal cord damage, remains unchanged but, again, in some individuals, both functional and organically derived symptoms may be present. No specific personality type or psychiatric condition has, however, been found to be specifically associated with the disorder.[55]

Nonorganic Hearing Loss

The prevalence of nonorganic hearing loss has been estimated to be less than 2 percent of the general population, but it is somewhat higher in children (7%), and markedly increased (10 to 50%) when compensation is sought.[57] Typical mean age of onset in children is between 10 and 12 years, with only rare cases occurring before age 7. Various definitions have been put forward, but reserving the term for abnormal responses to audiometry that are greater than can be explained by organic pathology recognizes that many patients may, in fact, have both organic and nonorganic components involved in the expressed deficit. Austen and Lynch suggest that the majority of cases involve either malingering or factitious disorder and that true cases of nonorganic hearing loss secondary to conversion disorder are relatively rare, although somewhat more common in clinics offering cochlear implants.[57] Paradoxically, in comparison with other functional nervous system disorders, patients with nonorganic hearing loss secondary to conversion disorder have been found to exhibit more consistency in audiological testing than patients with malingering or factitious etiologies. In terms of lifestyle, patients with nonorganic hearing loss who are malingering tend to live as hearing people and only present their dysfunction when being examined or when secondary gain is present; patients who suffer from conversion disorder often desire to live entirely as a deaf person, avoiding activities that are more directed to hearing individuals and often seeking whatever medical interventions might help them to deal with their deficit. Psychiatric referral is usually indicated, after a straightforward and therapeutically hopeful explication of the audiometric results and their positive prognostic value. Conversion deafness is considered to be the most psychologically pathologic of the varying subgroups, although within the subgroup itself there is a marked variation in psychologic well-being.

Nonspecific Functional Neurologic Symptom Disorders

CHRONIC SUBJECTIVE DIZZINESS

Approximately 20 percent of primary-care patients seek medical evaluation of dizziness at some point in their lives, with 30 percent reporting chronic or recurrent symptoms.[58] Of these, approximately one-third will have no specific physical etiology, whereas 10 percent will report being functionally impaired. Symptoms may be preceded by medical or psychologic conditions that have caused an acute disturbance of balance or dizziness, but persist long after the original causation has ended. In addition to the primary complaint, patients may describe a hypersensitivity to motion and discomfort with complex visual stimuli or demanding visual tasks, such as a computer game. Sensory loss is sometimes described. Ataxia and falls are rare, despite a subjective sense of imbalance while standing or walking. The neurologic examination, including specific assessment of vestibular function and balance, is usually normal, but exaggerated responses and falls may be observed on one-legged stance and tandem Romberg tests. A comprehensive laboratory evaluation would include a head MRI; audiologic assessment; tests of basic balance function, including oculomotor, positional, caloric, and rotary-chair testing; recording of vestibular evoked myogenic potentials; and sensory organization testing utilizing computerized dynamic posturography.

Treatment approaches parallel those recommended for other manifestations of conversion disorder and include both dynamic and cognitive–behavioral psychotherapeutic approaches tailored toward patient acceptance and historical elements unique to a given case. Despite the absence of organic etiology, vestibular balance and rehabilitation therapy may also be effective in improving balance problems and any associated sensory and motor symptoms in patients with functional chronic dizziness. The aims of such therapy are to reduce patients' hypersensitivity to motion cues and increase their confidence in maintaining balance by presenting them with motion stimuli of increasing complexity, incorporating both external objects as well as their own movements. Support for graduated increases in physical exercise and educational input regarding fall prevention and balance control can also be helpful in communicating an acceptance of the patient's phenomenology, and in encouraging them to assume self-control, while also diminishing avoidance behaviors that impair function. Selective serotonin reuptake inhibitors are sometimes beneficial as well.

CHRONIC HEADACHES

Psychologic factors are present to some degree in most cases of primary headache, but may be predominant in a select cohort of patients whose headaches do not conform to standard episodic description but are chronic, subjectively severe, and associated with a disproportionate impairment of function.[59] Psychogenic headaches may be either diffuse or localized, but are most commonly described in terms of a specific sharp pain at one particular point in the skull. Such patients seem to have an ingrained intense anticipation and expectation of disabling headache pain and engage in "catastrophizing" the experience and its consequent effects. Feelings of helplessness are conspicuous. The subjective intensity of pain experienced is a function of expectation as well as actual stimulus intensity; neuroimaging studies have found that the anterior insula and dorsal anterior cingulate cortex are particularly involved in regulating the subjective components, while more objective sensory analysis of the pain stimulus resides in the posterior insula, thalamus, and somatosensory cortex. Therapeutic interventions are most commonly directed towards treatment of associated accompanying conditions, such as depression, and to identification and diminishment of stressful precipitants and perpetuating factors. Behavioral interventions designed to increase self-mastery and confidence in the prevention and amelioration of pain are most effective.[60] Patients often erroneously use effortful focusing to try to suppress their pain but in so doing increase the salience of the stimulus; teaching the patient to accept their pain so that the emotional energy can be redirected towards more meaningful goals is often an effective cognitive reframing technique. Recent research has suggested that the subjective experience of chronic pain in the context of ongoing emotional distress can induce neuroplastic changes in somatosensory neural networks that may be long-lasting, but has also shown that psychologic and psychopharmacologic therapeutics may be as successful in amelioration of symptomatology as psychologic trauma was in its genesis.[61]

Psychogenic Amnesia and Fugue

The term *psychogenic amnesia* has historically been used to describe an episode of anterograde or retrograde memory dysfunction that appears to be preceded by psychologic stress or trauma in the absence of definable brain damage.[62] Psychiatric diagnostic manuals have most commonly placed such presentations in the category of dissociative disorders, along with dissociative identity disorder and dissociative fugue, but less encompassing and severe memory loss may also appear in the context of acute or post-traumatic stress disorders and in somatic symptom disorders in general. Cases of dissociative fugue, in which the individual with psychogenic amnesia leaves their usual environment in a precipitous fashion, are rare and usually brief in duration.

Clinically, the content of the memory loss usually involves information of a personal nature that is integrally interwoven with the experience of psychologic trauma. Although conceptually the dissociated state may serve to protect other core aspects of identity, the degree of functional and social impairment can be severe. Retrograde amnesia of autobiographic episodic memory, with preservation of somatic memory and of new autobiographic episodic memory learning capacity, is most characteristic; the loss of memory may sometimes be content specific or limited to specific periods in past life. Anterograde memory deficits may sometimes also be present and, in rare cases, individuals have preserved retrograde autobiographical episodic memory and yet are unable to acquire any new knowledge in these domains. Objective evidence of loss of procedural skill memory is rare. In some cases of functional memory loss, no clear psychologic precipitant can be ascertained. Although evidence of structural neurologic damage is, by definition, absent, recent research involving functional neuroimaging has identified state-dependent decreases in prefrontal cortex and right temporal frontal metabolism in patients with psychogenic amnesia that normalized with memory recovery following psychologic treatment.[62] Hypometabolism in the insula, which seems involved in the ability to project oneself in time, has also been observed in patients with psychogenic amnesia. Such data may serve to support the conceptualization of psychogenic amnesia as a brain-based "disconnection syndrome"[63] and facilitate therapeutic interventions that are humane and psychologically supportive in nature. Areas of the brain integral in the formation of autobiographic memory and emotional processing such as the hippocampus, amygdala, and prefrontal cortex are highly sensitive to the neuropathologic effects of stressful and traumatic experiences, such as child abuse and neglect, suggesting a possible etiologic role for such events in the genesis of functional amnesia.

The described deficits have led some observers to conceptualize unilateral functional nervous system motor and somatosensory disorders as similar in nature to the neglect syndrome seen with lesions of the right hemisphere and involving frontal-parietal cortical circuits, and cortical-subcortical pathways when motor neglect is observed. As described by Perez and colleagues,[34] dysfunction in the perigenual anterior cingulate cortex leads to impaired motivated behavior, motor control, and affect regulation, whereas dysfunction in the posterior parietal cortex and its connections is associated with impaired spatial and perceptual awareness, including motor intention awareness and self agency.

Other connections between these regions and the dorsolateral prefrontal cortex are hypothesized to regulate awareness and intentional control, which appear to be deficient in these patients.

ETHICAL DILEMMAS IN FUNCTIONAL NEUROLOGIC SYMPTOM DISORDERS

Functional neurologic symptom disorders that are true conversion disorders, with minimal evidence of malingering or feigning, can be chronic in nature and resistant to timely resolution. Physicians and clinic staff frequently resent such patients, viewing them as unfairly utilizing limited medical resources and erroneously seeing their behaviors as under conscious volition, even when such evidence is absent. Such patients themselves may reject psychologic interpretations as irrelevant to their symptomatology and angrily resist any suggested behavioral treatments as insensitive to their complaints and stigmatizing. The desire to avoid such interactions has led some physicians to advocate therapeutic deception, either in the delivery of the diagnosis or in the selection of treatment.[64] Ultimately, however, such approaches are indefensible on moral grounds and unlikely to be successful in the long term. Neurorehabilitation may indeed be helpful to a given individual, but the referral should be based on a faithful and truthful communication between physician and patient that delivers the diagnostic findings in the context of the hypothesized psychologic etiology. The treatment decisions themselves, however, may be pragmatic and incorporate both physical and psychologic components, to the degree that the patient is accepting of them. Referral to free self-help websites (www.neurosymptoms.org) may be helpful in educating patients and provide a cognitive framework for them to understand their symptoms and the types of therapeutic interventions that might be of benefit.

REFERENCES

1. Dinwiddie SH: Somatization disorder: past, present and future. Psychiatr Ann 43:78, 2013.
2. Carson AJ, Brown R, David AS, et al: Functional (conversion) neurological symptoms: research since the millennium. J Neurol Neurosurg Psychiatry 83:842, 2012.
3. Stone J: Functional neurological symptoms. Clin Med 13:80, 2013.
4. Nicholson TR, Stone J, Kanaan RA: Conversion disorder: a problematic diagnosis. J Neurol Neurosurg Psychiatry 82:1267, 2011.
5. American Psychiatric Association Diagnostic and Statistical Manual of Mental Disorders, Fourth Edition (DSM-IV). American Psychiatric Association, Washington DC, 1994.
6. American Psychiatric Association Diagnostic and Statistical Manual of Mental Disorders, Fifth Edition (DSM 5). American Psychiatric Association, Washington DC, 2013.
7. Kanaan R, Armstrong D, Barnes P, et al: In the psychiatrist's chair: how neurologists understand conversion disorder. Brain 132:2889, 2009.
8. Stone J, Carson A: Functional neurological symptoms: assessment and management. Neurol Clin 29:1, 2011.
9. Brown RJ, Lewis-Fernandez R: Culture and conversion: implications for DSM 5. Psychiatry 74:187, 2011.
10. Browning M, Fletcher P, Sharpe M: Can neuroimaging help us to understand and classify somatoform disorders? A systematic and critical review. Psychosom Med 73:173, 2011.
11. Garcia-Campayo J, Fayed N, Serrano-Blanco A, et al: Brain dysfunction behind functional symptoms: neuroimaging and somatoform, conversive and dissociative disorders. Curr Opin Psychiatry 22:224, 2009.
12. Baslet G: Psychogenic non-epileptic seizures: a model of their pathogenic mechanism. Seizure 20:1, 2011.
13. Sahaya K, Dholakia SA, Sahota PK: Psychogenic nonepileptic seizures: a challenging entity. J Clin Neurosci 18:1602, 2011.
14. Reuber M, Fenandez G, Bauer J, et al: Diagnostic delay in psychogenic nonepileptic seizures. Neurology 58:493, 2002.
15. Mostacci B, Bisulli F, Alvisi L, et al: Ictal characteristics of psychogenic nonepileptic seizures: what we have learned from video/EEG recordings—a literature review. Epilepsy Behav 22:144, 2011.
16. Siket MS, Merchant RC: Psychogenic seizures: a review and description of pitfalls in their acute diagnosis and management in the emergency department. Emerg Med Clin North Am 29:73, 2011.
17. Martin RC, Gilliam FG, Kilgore M, et al: Improved health care resource utilization following video-EEG-confirmed diagnosis of nonepileptic psychogenic seizures. Seizure 7:385, 1998.
18. Behrouz R, Heriaud L, Benbadis SR: Late-onset psychogenic nonepileptic seizures. Epilepsy Behav 8:649, 2006.
19. Caplan JP, Binius T, Lennon VA, et al: Pseudopseudoseizures: conditions that may mimic psychogenic nonepileptic seizures. Psychosomatics 52:501, 2011.
20. Foster AR, Caplan JP: Paraneoplastic limbic encephalitis. Psychosomatics 50:108, 2009.
21. Kung DH, Qiu C, Kass JS: Psychiatric manifestations of anti-NMDA receptor encephalitis in a man without tumor. Psychosomatics 52:82, 2011.

22. Kellinghaus C, Luders HO: Frontal lobe epilepsy. Epileptic Disord 6:223, 2004.
23. Ozkara C, Metin B, Kucukoglu S: Convulsive syncope: a condition to be differentiated from epilepsy. Epileptic Disord 11:315, 2009.
24. Ali S, Khan MA, Khealani B: Limb-shaking transient ischemic attacks: case report and review of the literature. BMC Neurol 6:5, 2006.
25. van Rootselaar AF, Schade van Westrum S, Velis DN, et al: The paroxysmal dyskinesias. Pract Neurol 9:102, 2009.
26. LaFrance Jr WC, Barry JJ: Updates on treatments of psychological nonepileptic seizures. Epilepsy Behav 7:364, 2005.
27. Goldstein LH, Deale AC, Mitchell-O'Malley SJ, et al: An evaluation of cognitive behavioral therapy as a treatment for dissociative seizures: a pilot study. Cogn Behav Neurol 17:41, 2004.
28. Stonnington CM, Barry JJ, Fisher RS: Conversion disorder. Am J Psychiatry 163:1510, 2006.
29. Ettinger AB, Devinsky O, Weisbrot DM, et al: A comprehensive profile of clinical, psychiatric and psychosocial characteristics of patients with psychogenic nonepileptic seizures. Epilepsia 40:1292, 1999.
30. Pestana E, Foldvary-Schaefer N, Marsilio D: Quality of life in patients with psychogenic seizures. Neurology 60(suppl):A355, 2003.
31. Spence SA, Crimlisk HL, Cope H, et al: Discrete neurophysiologic correlates in prefrontal cortex during hysterical and feigned disorder of movement. Lancet 355:1243, 2000.
32. Halligan PW, Athwal BS, Oakley DA, et al: Imaging hypnotic paralysis: implications for conversion hysteria. Lancet 355:986, 2000.
33. Vuilleumier P, Chicherio C, Assal F, et al: Functional neuroanatomic correlates of hysterical sensorimotor loss. Brain 124:1077, 2001.
34. Perez DL, Barsky AJ, Daffner K, et al: Motor and somatosensory conversion disorder: a functional unawareness syndrome? J Neuropsychiatry Clin Neurosci 24:141, 2012.
35. Stone J, Warlow C, Sharpe M: The symptom of functional weakness: a controlled study of 107 patients. Brain 133:1537, 2010.
36. Czarnecki K, Hallett M: Functional (psychogenic) movement disorders. Curr Opin Neurol 25:507, 2012.
37. Kranick S, Gorrindo T, Hallett M: Psychogenic movement disorders and motor conversion: a roadmap for collaboration between neurology and psychiatry. Psychosomatics 52:109, 2011.
38. Ellenstein A, Kranick SM, Hallett M: An update on psychogenic movement disorders. Cur Neurol Neurosci Rep 11:396, 2011.
39. Pula J: Functional vision loss. Curr Opin Ophthalmol 23:460, 2012.
40. Bain KE, Beatty S, Lloyd C: Non-organic visual loss in children. Eye 14:770, 2000.
41. Lim SA, Siatkowski RM, Farris BK: Functional visual loss in adults and children: patient characteristics, management, and outcomes. Ophthalmology 112:1821, 2005.
42. Schwingenschuh P, Katschnig P, Edwards MJ, et al: The blink reflex recovery cycle differs between essential and presumed psychogenic blepharospasm. Neurology 76:610, 2011.
43. Ruddy R, House A: Psychosocial interventions for conversion disorder. Cochrane Database Syst Rev:CD005331, 2005.
44. Shuster JP, Mouchabac S, Le Strat Y, et al: Hysterical mutism. Encephale 37:339, 2011.
45. Roy N: Functional dysphonia. Curr Opin Otolaryngol Head Neck Surg 11:144, 2003.
46. Bridger MW, Epstein R: Functional voice disorders: a review of 109 patients. J Laryngol Otol 97:1145, 1983.
47. Koufman J, Blalock P: Functional voice disorders. Otolaryngol Clin North Am 24:1059, 1991.
48. Schalen L, Andersson K: Differential diagnosis and treatment of psychogenic voice disorder. Clin Otolaryngol 17:225, 1992.
49. Roy N, Bless DM: Toward a theory of the dispositional bases of functional dysphonia and vocal nodules: exploring the role of personality and emotional adjustment. p. 461. In: Kent R, Ball M (eds): Voice Quality Measurement. Singular Publishing Group, San Diego, 2000.
50. Ng KO, Lee JF, Mui WC: Aphonia induced by conversion disorder during a Cesarian section. Acta Anaesthesiol Taiwan 50:138, 2012.
51. Deary V, Miller T: Reconsidering the role of psychosocial factors in functional dysphonia. Curr Opin Otolaryngol Head Neck Surg 19:150, 2011.
52. Bos-Clark M, Carding P: Effectiveness of voice therapy in functional dysphonia: where are we now? Curr Opin Otolaryngol Head Neck Surg 19:160, 2011.
53. Routsalainen JH, Sellman J, Lehto L, et al: Interventions for treating functional dysphonia in adults. Cochrane Database Syst Rev:CD006373, 2007.
54. Mailis-Gagnon A, Nicholson K: On the nature of nondermatomal somatosensory deficits. Clin J Pain 27:76, 2011.
55. Egloff N, Maecker F, Stauber S, et al: Nondermatomal somatosensory deficits in chronic pain patients: are they really hysterical? Pain 153:1847, 2012.
56. Nichols LL, Zasler ND, Martelli M: Sodium amobarbital: historical perspectives and neurorehabilitation clinical caveats. NeuroRehabilitation 31:95, 2012.
57. Austen S, Lynch C: Non-organic hearing loss redefined: understanding, categorizing and managing non-organic behaviour. Int J Audiol 43:449, 2004.
58. Honaker JA, Gilbert JM, Staab JP: Chronic subjective dizziness versus conversion disorder: discussion of clinical findings and rehabilitation. Am J Audiol 19:3, 2010.
59. Borkum JM: Chronic headaches and the neurobiology of somatization. Curr Pain Headache Rep 14:55, 2010.

60. Holdroyd KA, Labus JS, Carlson B: Moderation and mediation in the psychological and drug treatment of chronic tension-type headache: the role of disorder severity and psychiatric comorbidity. Pain 143:213, 2009.
61. Brody AL, Saxena S, Stoessel P, et al: Regional brain metabolic changes in patients with major depression treated with either paroxetine or interpersonal therapy. Archiv Gen Psychiatry 58:631, 2001.
62. Staniloiu A, Markowitsch HJ, Brand M: Psychogenic amnesia—a malady of the constricted self. Conscious Cogn 19:778, 2010.
63. MacDonald K, MacDonald T: Peas, please: a case report and neuroscientific review of dissociative amnesia and fugue. J Trauma Dissociation 10:420, 2009.
64. Kirschner KL, Smith GR, Antiel RM, et al: Why can't I move, Doc? Ethical dilemmas in treating conversion disorders. PM R 4:296, 2012.

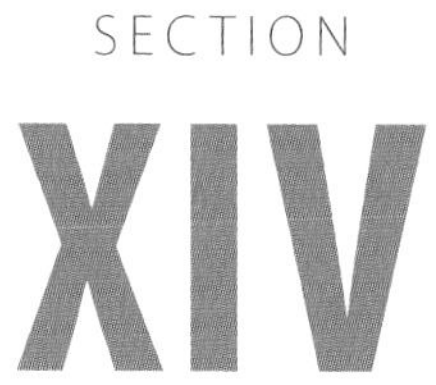

SECTION XIV

Imaging and Perioperative Care

CHAPTER

53

Neurologic Complications of Imaging Procedures

WILLIAM P. DILLON ■ CHRISTOPHER F. DOWD

Neurologic complications of imaging procedures are varied and largely related to either local complications of an invasive procedure or complications arising from the systemic use of intravenous contrast agents. This chapter provides a summary of neurologic complications related to those imaging procedures that are commonly performed in modern radiologic practices. Some historical perspective is presented as well, and the reader must be aware that changes in the practice of radiologic procedures affect the kinds of complications and their incidence over time.

COMPLICATIONS OF INTRAVENOUS INJECTION OF CONTRAST MATERIAL

Radiographic contrast agents have been in use for over 70 years and are employed in approximately 10 million radiographic procedures annually in the United States. They find wide use in the evaluation of disease processes both within the central nervous system (CNS) and throughout the body. Contrast material helps define normal vascular anatomy as well as pinpoint patterns of abnormal contrast enhancement indicative of pathologic processes. Most patients tolerate radiographic contrast with few or no side effects.

Iodinated Contrast Media

Iodinated contrast medium is currently available in ionic and nonionic, water-soluble formulations. Ionic contrast media are less expensive but are associated with a higher incidence of adverse reactions than nonionic contrast agents; approximately 4 to 12 percent of patients receiving ionic media experience some hypersensitivity reaction within minutes or after several hours compared with 1 to 3 percent of patients receiving nonionic contrast media.[1] Nonionic contrast agents have largely replaced ionic contrast media for intravascular use throughout the body and should be used exclusively in children younger than 2 years, patients at risk of allergic reactions, and those with renal failure, diabetes, cardiopulmonary disease, or serious illnesses. Another advantage of nonionic agents is their isotonicity, which markedly reduces the sensation of heat and flushing.[1]

Aminoff's Neurology and General Medicine, Fifth Edition.

Prior allergic-like reaction to intravenous contrast material is the most substantial risk factor for a recurrent allergic-like adverse event. Although such a history is not an absolute predictor, the reported incidence of recurrent reactions ranges up to 35 percent.[2] Atopic individuals (particularly those with multiple severe allergies) and asthmatics are also at increased risk of allergic-like contrast reactions.

The toxicity of ionic contrast media is well documented and is related to the tonicity, ionic charge, and chemical toxicity of the agents, as well as allergic/anaphylactic phenomena.[2] Idiosyncratic allergic reactions may occur on first or subsequent contrast administration and range from hives to more severe reactions such as pulmonary or cerebral edema, laryngospasm, bronchospasm, and cardiovascular collapse. Dose-related effects of tonicity and chemical toxicity mainly affect the heart, lungs, and kidneys and include cardiovascular depression and renal failure. Secondary neurologic symptoms and signs may result when significant cardiorenal dysfunction occurs. Life-threatening reactions occur in approximately 0.05 to 0.16 percent of ionic contrast media injections and 0.03 percent with nonionic contrast materials; the death rate, however, is similar with both types of agents, occurring in approximately 1 to 3 per 100,000 injections.[1,3,4]

The most common major neurologic complication ascribed to ionic contrast media is a seizure, which occurs primarily in patients with primary or metastatic tumors.[5] Seizures and parkinsonian symptoms as well as cortical blindness have also been reported after the use of ionic media during cardiac or vertebral angiographic procedures.[6,7] The cortical blindness is usually transient and has been associated with abnormal retention of contrast medium within the occipital cortex. It has been postulated that a time- and dose-related breakdown of the blood–brain barrier leads to subsequent direct neuronal toxicity. Aggravation of myasthenia gravis is a potential risk of intravenous ionic contrast administration but appears to be somewhat less frequent with the nonionic formulations.[8] These complications are now rarely seen because low osmolality, nonionic contrast media have largely replaced ionic media for intravascular use.

Regardless of the type of contrast medium used, extravasation into the soft tissues of the arm at the time of injection may lead to local tissue injury, including skin necrosis. The risk of severe soft-tissue injury is greatest with extravasation of ionic contrast agents that have been injected by power injectors.[9] Swelling, which attends severe extravasation injuries, can also lead to compartment syndromes and therefore to injury of the peripheral nervous system. Automated power injectors, which are used in daily practice, may result in the extravasation of large volumes of contrast material, leading to severe tissue damage. Infants, young children, and unconscious and debilitated patients (e.g., diabetics, patients receiving chemotherapy) are particularly at risk of extravasation.[10]

Contrast Media for Magnetic Resonance Imaging

Contrast media for magnetic resonance imaging (MRI) have a lower toxicity profile and much higher patient tolerance than iodinated contrast media. Most magnetic resonance contrast agents are variations of chelates of gadolinium, a lanthanide metal. Gadolinium is toxic in its free form, but through chelation with DTPA or other moieties is safely distributed and then eliminated from the body by renal clearance. Both ionic and nonionic formulations of gadolinium are available. Gadolinium-based contrast media are safe and well tolerated by the vast majority of patients; the incidence of complications is less than 0.5 percent.[11–13] Minor side effects, including headache, nausea, and vomiting, are sometimes noted, but the risk of anaphylaxis is extremely low, on the order of 1 per several 100,000 injections.[14] Nonetheless, severe reactions and death secondary to gadolinium administration have been reported.[15] Li and associates showed that among 45 patients who developed reactions to gadolinium, only 3 (6.7%) had prior adverse reactions to iodinated contrast, 3 had prior reactions to a different gadolinium-based compound, and 10 had prior food or drug allergies (9) or asthma (1).[11]

Gadolinium agents cross the placenta, with undetermined effects on developing fetuses, and are seen in small amounts in the breast milk of lactating mothers; therefore, they are not recommended for use in pregnant women unless absolutely necessary.[16] It is unlikely that the small amount of gadolinium absorbed by a nursing infant's gastrointestinal tract will be harmful but, if concern exists, the nursing mother can be advised to discard her breast milk for 24 hours after gadolinium administration.

Nephrogenic systemic fibrosis, characterized by fibrosis of skin and other organs, has been documented following gadolinium administration in patients with renal failure. For this reason, gadolinium administration is not advised in patients with glomerular filtration rate of less than 30 ml/min per $1.73\,m^2$.[17] Macrocyclic gadolinium contrast agents appear to decrease the availability of free gadolinium and thus of nephrogenic systemic fibrosis in those with renal failure. Dialysis immediately following gadolinium administration is recommended to minimize this possible complication.[18,19]

Other novel MRI contrast agents are also now available for limited clinical applications. The superparamagnetic iron chelates work on the basis of reducing signal within normal tissues such as lymph nodes and liver and thus provide contrast for nonenhancing abnormal tissues.[20–22] Chelates of manganese are also approved for liver imaging. Free manganese has a theoretical risk of parkinsonian complications, but the chelated compound caused no serious side effects during phase 2 clinical trials.[12] Intravascular contrast agents are being evaluated and promise to improve magnetic resonance angiography and perfusion of brain tumors.

Deleterious effects of MR imaging exposure on pregnant women or the developing fetus have not been shown. Nevertheless, it is recommended that women of reproductive age be screened for pregnancy before entering the MR environment. The clinician should confer with the radiologist and document that the information cannot be acquired by other nonionizing means (e.g., ultrasonography), that the data are needed to effect the care of the patient or fetus during the pregnancy, and that it is not prudent to wait until the patient is no longer pregnant to obtain these data.[23]

Miscellaneous Complications of Contrast Media

Reflux of ionic x-ray contrast medium has been reported into the abdominal port of a ventriculoperitoneal shunt after bladder rupture sustained during voiding cystourethrography. This extravasated contrast medium then tracked up the ventriculoperitoneal shunt, causing seizures and ventriculitis.[24]

Venous air embolism has been documented during infusion of contrast medium, due to either scalp vein malposition or inadvertent trapping of air within power injectors or tubing.[25,26] Venous air embolism can cause stroke, especially in infants with patent cardiac foramen ovale or other right-to-left shunts. The presence of iatrogenic air in the venous sinuses is important to recognize and distinguish from infectious causes.

Acetazolamide, a vasodilator of the cerebral circulation, is now occasionally administered before perfusion MR and computed tomography (CT) studies. Comparison of studies before and after acetazolamide allows determination of the cerebral vascular reserve. Acetazolamide, although well tolerated, has minor side effects such as nausea and headache. It is a diuretic, so adequate hydration and satisfactory serum potassium levels must be ensured, particularly in those already receiving diuretics for medical reasons. Acetazolamide is probably not indicated in the setting of acute stroke because its diuretic effect may reduce cerebral perfusion.

NONINVASIVE IMAGING PROCEDURES

Computed Tomography

Neurologic complications of x-ray CT are usually related to complications of sedation, contrast administration, or other mishaps that incidentally attend the procedure. There is a small risk of radiation-induced cataracts, leukemia, and other tumors following multiple CT studies, especially in children.[27] This concern has increased with recent technologic advances: helical-mode scanners are now used routinely in CT angiography and CT perfusion studies to scan rapidly large regions of the body. Multiple scans during infusions of contrast material may result in additional radiation exposure. For this reason, MRI and ultrasound are better methods for following patients who require repeated imaging procedures, as long as their diagnostic benefit is equivalent to or better than that of CT.

Magnetic Resonance Imaging

MRI has rapidly gained wide acceptance in the imaging of the CNS as well as for musculoskeletal and many cardiac and general body applications. Images are produced by placing a patient in an extremely strong static magnetic field (on the order of 15,000 to 30,000 times the Earth's magnetic field) and then probing the magnetic relaxation properties of water protons in the body using radiofrequency pulses; computer mathematical manipulation allows the production of images.

Because of the need for a very strong continuous magnetic field, the presence of metal objects in or around the imaging environment can be hazardous, since they can accelerate as missiles, harming patients and staff. Patients, staff, and others coming into proximity of the magnet are therefore routinely screened for ferromagnetic objects. The major contraindications to MRI examinations include the prior placement of ferromagnetic aneurysm clips or cardiac pacemakers, intraocular metallic foreign bodies, certain types of prosthetic cardiac valves, electronic or magnetically activated medical devices, and any other large, potentially ferromagnetic foreign body.[28,29] Pacemakers have long been considered an absolute contraindication to MRI, but recent literature suggests that these studies can be safely performed in some patients as long as precautions are taken before, during, and after the MR study and the benefit of MR outweighs the risk of pacemaker malfunction or harm to the patient.[30] Implanted cardiac defibrillators likewise have long been considered an absolute contraindication to MRI, but Junttila and colleagues showed no adverse events from repetitive MRI at 1.5 T in 10 patients with implanted defibrillators.[31]

The hazard of aneurysm clips deserves special attention. Most currently manufactured aneurysm clips have few if any ferromagnetic properties, as judged by lack of deflection within a magnetic field when tested in vitro.[32] At least one instance of fatal clip movement in a patient has, however, been reported, and in that case was due to inaccurate information supplied during the screening process.[33] The performance of MRI in patients with aneurysm clips is therefore a matter of controversy; newer nonferromagnetic clips, such as titanium alloys, appear to be safe at 1.5 T, but discretion is always advised.[34,35] At higher field strengths, such as 3 T, titanium alloy clips are preferred if MR is necessary, but care must be taken while moving patients through the opening of the bore toward the center of the magnet, as the largest torque forces occur during this maneuver.[36] The potential information to be gained from the procedure must be carefully balanced against the potential danger of clip movement. Although the metal from the clip may cause significant artifact on the examination, useful information can often still be gleaned by appropriately tailoring the examination.

The potential risks of metallic stents and endovascular detachable coils also merit consideration. A new generation of MRI scanners, including at 3.0 T, with shorter lengths and wider apertures (e.g., 70 cm diameter and about 160 cm length), results in much larger gradients. Larger magnetic susceptibility of the employed material, larger mass, higher magnetic field, and larger gradient will increase the magnetic force on the metallic implant upon entering the MRI magnet.[37]

These devices produce ferromagnetic artifacts, and thus the local anatomy is distorted on MRI.[38–40] MRI is safe at 1.5 T for patients who have recently had placement of a coronary stent.[41] Some monitoring devices are potentially dangerous because looped metallic wires may acquire induced currents, resulting in burns to the skin attachment sites. For this reason, all physiologic monitoring equipment and other devices must be carefully screened and approved specifically for use during MRI.[42–44] Exposure of electrically conductive leads or wires to the RF transmitted power during MR scanning should be performed with caution and appropriate steps taken to ensure that lead or tissue heating does not result. Patients who require EKG monitoring and who are unconscious, sedated, or anesthetized should be examined after each MR imaging sequence and repositioning of the EKG leads and any other electrically conductive material with which the patient is in contact should be considered.[23] Extensive testing and safety information about specific devices is available from MRIsafety.com as well as from Shellock and associates.[45]

Screening of patients referred for MRI is essential prior to the examination. If patients are unable to fill out a questionnaire or are unconscious and their family is not present or unable to provide the required information, they should be thoroughly examined by medical personnel with attention to surgical scars. If these are present, a radiograph is suggested prior to MRI.[23] When in doubt, the presence of a specific medical device must be documented precisely and in writing before entry of the patient into the magnet. This information can be checked against the known magnetic deflection properties of the device, as appropriate. In patients with a history of possible metallic ocular foreign body, plain radiography of the orbit or low-dose orbital CT can be used to exclude the presence of significant metal fragments, as these can move in the magnetic field and result in ocular injury and blindness.[41–49]

Another potential hazard related to the static magnetic field required for MRI is that of missile injury, mentioned earlier. The missile effect is perhaps the most serious potential hazard because many clinicians entering the MR environment are not aware that the magnet is always "on." Paper clips, scissors, vacuum cleaners, oxygen tanks, anesthetic equipment and other ferromagnetic metallic items have been rapidly pulled into the bore of a magnet when inappropriately brought close to it, sometimes with fatal results.[48,50] Proper introduction to safety precautions for visitors is important. The American College of Radiology recommends that zones of access be created and labeled to inform the public as they get closer to the magnet room itself.[23]

The rapid switching of the gradient coils used in MRI may result in induced voltage and current in implanted wires, such as cardiac leads or brain-implanted electrodes, as well as thermal injuries. These gradients may also cause a loud vibration or banging noise that can result in hyperacusis or tinnitus. Both temporary and permanent instances of hearing loss have also been reported; for these reasons, the use of earplugs is mandatory during MR examination for all patients as well as accompanying parents or visitors within the magnet room. These are especially recommended in cases requiring very rapid switching of gradients coils, as with most magnetic resonance angiography sequences and ultrafast techniques such as fast spin-echo and echo-planar techniques (e.g., diffusion and perfusion imaging and functional MRI).[51] Tissue heating is also a potential but to date insignificant complication of MRI. The US Food and Drug Administration (FDA) limits the specific absorption rate (SAR), which is the radiofrequency energy deposition, to 0.4 W/kg averaged over the body. In animal studies, levels at 10 times this rate over a 75-minute period raise the skin and eye temperature of a sheep by only 1.5°C, with no observed side effects. Nonetheless, the FDA has determined limits, particularly for small infants and children.

SPINAL PROCEDURES

Myelography and Intrathecal Injections of Contrast Media

The number of myelographic procedures has diminished dramatically since the introduction of MRI and CT. MRI has clearly been established as superior to myelography in the evaluation of lumbar disc disease,[52] discitis and vertebral osteomyelitis,[53] myelopathy, and extradural and intradural spinal mass lesions.[54] Compared with CT and MRI, myelography is limited as a single investigation of lumbar disc disease because of its insensitivity to extraforaminal, paraspinous, and lateral disc disease.

When myelography is recommended, it is almost invariably performed in conjunction with CT. CT myelography is preferred to plain-film myelography for evaluating the thecal sac in those patients who cannot tolerate MRI because of severe claustrophobia or because of other contraindications to the magnetic environment, discussed previously. Many patients with severe spondylitic disease of the spine or failed-back syndrome may benefit from CT myelography. In such instances, a lumbar puncture is performed for instillation of 5 to 8 ml of iodinated contrast before thin-section CT scanning is performed. In many patients, CT myelography may complement MRI, especially in patients who have bony osteophytes that may be difficult to distinguish on MR.

Few indications remain for traditional plain-film (high-dose) myelography. Those with suspected cerebrospinal fluid (CSF) loculations or arachnoid cysts may still benefit from myelography because the septations separating these CSF-filled structures can be difficult to detect on MRI and the dynamic nature of myelography can be useful. In addition, myelography in combination with CT is required occasionally to locate precisely the site of a spinal CSF leak. Myelography is also indicated for the evaluation of patients with back pain after orthopedic instrumentation because CT and MRI are compromised by metallic artifacts.

The reduction in myelograms performed at teaching institutions has reduced the exposure of trainees in radiology to this procedure. As with any procedure, the incidence of complications associated with a procedure relates to the experience of the practitioner. In the case of myelography, it is our impression that the rate of complications is on the rise because of the decrease in experience of recent trainees. It is therefore appropriate to review the neurologic complications of myelography and intrathecal injections of contrast material despite their decline in use.

TERMINOLOGY

Myelography entails plain-film examination of the spine following intrathecal instillation of iodinated contrast media through either a lumbar puncture or a cervical puncture at the C1–C2 level, posterior to the spinal cord. Water-soluble, nonionic contrast agents are used exclusively. Using a tilt-table and fluoroscopy, the contrast is positioned by gravity into the area of interest. Cervical, thoracic, and lumbar myelography as well as "total" myelography can be accomplished through a single needle puncture. Before MRI, the choice of a lumbar or C1–C2 puncture was largely determined on the basis of clinical symptomatology. Low-dose (lower than routinely administered for plain-film myelography) injections before CT scanning, so-called *CT myelography*, has replaced formal plain-film myelography. Current multidetector high-speed CT scanners are capable of high-resolution, less than 1-mm contiguous scans through the entire spinal canal in less than 30 seconds and from these, superb tomographic re-formations in the sagittal and coronal planes are possible. Occasionally contrast must be positioned intracranially to opacify the CSF cisterns. MRI has now largely replaced CT cisternography, but it is still used occasionally to evaluate for CSF leak and the presence of intracranial arachnoid cyst.

TECHNIQUE

Several approaches are used to perform intrathecal injections. Typically, a 22-gauge or smaller spinal needle is positioned with fluoroscopic guidance in the lumbar subarachnoid space. This requires topical and subcutaneous anesthesia and is contraindicated in those with bleeding disorders. If required, a C1–C2 puncture may be safely performed using lateral fluoroscopy so that the needle can be placed posterior to the spinal cord without moving the patient and the flow of the contrast material can be monitored. The needle enters the lateral neck just below the mastoid tip and is fluoroscopically positioned in the posterior aspect of the cervical subarachnoid space, which is usually rather capacious, behind the cervical spinal cord.

As discussed later, C1–C2 puncture carries a risk of cervical cord puncture, and efforts must be taken to avoid this by proper positioning of the patient and careful technique. The procedure now is frequently performed using CT guidance, which is safer than fluoroscopic guidance. Often, low-dose injection of contrast medium via the lumbar route is adequate to examine the cervical spine and is associated with fewer potential complications than the C1–C2 route. CT is performed immediately after instillation of contrast medium. Delayed CT was used in the past to evaluate for syringomyelia, but MRI now best evaluates this condition.

Cisternal puncture in the suboccipital region is rarely if ever performed. The authors have never performed this procedure themselves and see little indication for its use in the current era of MRI.

COMPLICATIONS OF INTRATHECAL PUNCTURE

The neurologic complications of myelography and intrathecal injections can be separated according to those related to intrathecal needle puncture itself and those related to the presence of intrathecal contrast material.

Vasovagal Response

Vasovagal syncope occurs infrequently during lumbar puncture. Its occurrence can be anticipated by communication with the patient and by noting the initial appearance of diaphoresis. This usually occurs during head elevation and can be countered by prompt lowering of the patient's head.

Headache

Headache and associated nausea and vomiting are the most frequent complications of lumbar puncture and myelography.[55–57] The incidence of headache after myelography decreased with the development of nonionic, water-soluble contrast agents, but remains between 6 and 40 percent. The etiology of the headache is often obscure and may be related to neurotoxic effects of the contrast agent, persistent CSF leak at the puncture site, and psychologic factors. The incidence of post–dural puncture headache can be reduced by the use of a small-gauge lumbar-puncture needle. Other factors that have been identified include gender (11.1% female vs. 3.6% male), age (11.0% 31 to 50 years of age vs. 4.2% others), previous history of post-puncture headache (26.4% positive vs. 6.2% negative), and needle bevel orientation (16.1% perpendicular vs. 5.7% parallel to the spinal axis). The latency between lumbar puncture and headache onset ranges from 6 to 72 hours and the duration from 3 to 15 days. In 34 of 48 (71%) patients with post–lumbar puncture headache, at least one of the following was present: neck stiffness, tinnitus, hypoacusia, photophobia, or nausea.[58]

The condition is usually self-limiting; caffeine alleviates the symptoms and reduces the course of the illness. When bed rest and caffeine prove ineffective, an autologous epidural blood patch at the site of puncture works well for the majority of patients.[59]

After myelography, it is common practice to keep patients in a supine position, with the head elevated approximately 25 to 45 degrees. Short-duration (1 hour) is as effective as long-duration (4 hours) supine recumbency in preventing post–lumbar puncture headache.[60] Oral hydration is also encouraged.

Hearing Loss

Hearing loss has been described as an adverse reaction after lumbar puncture as well as myelography. Michel and Brusis reported nine cases of hearing loss after myelography, lumbar puncture, and spinal anesthesia.[61–63] In six of the nine patients, bilateral impairment was present; recovery of normal hearing occurred in six patients. They speculated that alteration in the pressure equilibrium between CSF and perilymph in the setting of a patent cochlear aqueduct results in the release of perilymphatic fluid into the subarachnoid space; alternatively, a direct toxic effect of contrast material on the inner ear may be a factor in hearing loss. They recommended the use of small-gauge spinal needles to reduce the leakage of CSF through the dural puncture. The use of nonionic myelographic agents is now standard, and these agents have been shown to be safer than ionic formulations.

Epidermoid Tumors

Iatrogenic intraspinal epidermoid tumors have been reported as sequelae of lumbar puncture.[64–66] It is believed that implantation of epithelial cells from the skin into the thecal sac or epidural space during lumbar puncture may allow this benign tumor to grow gradually. The incidence of iatrogenic epidermoid tumors is exceedingly rare, but up to 40 percent of those occurring in the lumbar spine are thought to relate to prior lumbar puncture. The time from LP to tumor presentation is typically from 2 to 8 years. Epidermoid tumors appear on MRI as masses with signal characteristics similar to CSF, but with reduced apparent diffusion coefficient derived from diffusion-weighted images. The presence of this rare tumor should arouse suspicion of possible iatrogenic causes, and a history of prior lumbar puncture should be sought.

Hemorrhage

Intracranial hemorrhages secondary to myelography have been well documented.[67,68] It is likely that this complication relates to persistent CSF leakage and low intracranial CSF pressure, which then result in the production of subdural hematomas or intracranial hemorrhages. Direct laceration of a vessel is rare.[54,69] Acute epidural hematoma complicating myelography in a normotensive patient with normal blood coagulability is rare but has been reported by Stevens and colleagues.[70]

Spinal punctures should not be performed in the setting of abnormal coagulation factors. In patients receiving systemic anticoagulants, there is an increased risk of epidural hematoma at the site of puncture.[71] The Society of Interventional Radiology published consensus guidelines in 2009 for the management of coagulation status prior to image-guided procedures.[72] It recommends that prior to spinal procedures such as lumbar puncture, vertebroplasty, and nerve blocks or epidural injections, an INR above 1.5 and platelet count below 50,000/µl be corrected, and that clopidogrel (Plavix) be stopped for 5 days and low-molecular-weight heparin for 1 day prior to the procedure.

Puncture of the Spinal Cord

Although uncommon, puncture of the spinal cord has been described.[73] This complication can be avoided by restricting lumbar punctures to below the L2 level. A low-lying conus or tethered cord will increase the risk of cord puncture, and it is therefore important to review the MR or other spinal imaging studies prior to lumbar puncture.

Complications of C1–C2 Puncture

Complications related to the C1–C2 approach have been well documented in the literature and include direct puncture of the spinal cord, laceration of epidural and vertebral venous and arterial structures, and spinal cord compression related to neck hyperextension during the procedure.[74] Spinal cord and blood vessel punctures are the most serious complications and occur primarily because of incorrect positioning of the patient's neck and misdirection of the x-ray beam. The indications for C1–C2 puncture are infrequent. In those patients who cannot undergo MRI but who require cervical myelography, low-dose CT myelography through a lumbar puncture usually suffices. This route of administration has been associated with a slightly higher incidence of headache, nausea, and vomiting than with the C1–C2 puncture; however, the use of low-dose, nonionic, water-soluble agents has reduced these complications to an acceptable level. Therefore, in our view, there are few indications for the C1–C2 approach in current neuroradiologic practice. Rarely a patient who cannot undergo MRI may require C1–C2 puncture to determine the upper margin of a spinal block.

The injection of contrast material into the spinal cord may be associated with hemorrhagic necrosis of the gray matter and acute neurologic decline.[75] Acute and permanent trigeminal dysesthesias and quadriparesis are reported complications of C1–C2 injections. These may be ameliorated by prompt administration of high-dose corticosteroids.[75] The important factor in avoiding this complication is proper patient positioning. A free flow of CSF should be documented before contrast injection. The patient should experience no pain during the initial instillation of a small amount of contrast medium. If there *is* pain, the procedure should be terminated immediately and the cause of the pain assessed.

Katoh and associates documented three cases of epidural injection during a C1–C2 puncture, a complication we have also seen in our practice.[74] Injection into the epidural venous plexus and intra-arterial injection into an aberrant vertebral artery have also been documented. In approximately 2 percent of patients, the vertebral artery swings inferiorly into the posterior C1–C2 interspace; in such cases, an approach by lateral C1–C2 puncture may then inadvertently lacerate or puncture it. Rogers reported the death of a patient after C1–C2 myelography due to acute subdural hemorrhage as a consequence of laceration of an anomalous intraspinal vertebral artery.[76]

Robertson and Smith documented 68 major complications of cervical myelography.[77] Two-thirds of the complications were attributed to cervical spine hyperextension during the procedure and one-third to lateral C1–C2 puncture. The narrow sagittal diameter of the spinal canal and severe cervical spondylosis were frequent contributing factors to hyperextension injury of the cervical spinal cord. These complications are now rare as MRI is the study of choice in patients with suspected spinal canal stenosis, severe spondylosis, or myelopathy of any cause. Should cervical CT myelography be required, it is our recommendation that it be performed via a low-dose lumbar injection followed by thin-section CT rather than C1–C2 puncture.

Complications from Intrathecal Administration of Contrast Agents

Neurologic complications related to the intrathecal administration of contrast agents range from aseptic meningitis to encephalopathy and seizures. Other reported complications include hyperthermia, hallucinations, depression and anxiety states, and headache. The development of nonionic, water-soluble contrast agents has reduced these neurotoxic side effects significantly. On occasion, intrathecal gadolinium has been used to perform MR myelography in search of a CSF leak. A small amount (0.3 ml) of gadolinium is administered intrathecally and MR scans are performed following this with fat-suppressed T1-weighted images. An inadvertent overdose of 6 ml of intrathecal gadolinium in one patient reportedly resulted in transient neurotoxic manifestations, including a decreased level of consciousness, global aphasia, rigidity, and visual disturbance.[78]

Meningitis

Both aseptic and bacterial meningitis are reported complications of myelography.[79] Bacterial meningitis, which is characterized by the abrupt onset of fever, usually within 24 hours after the intrathecal instillation of contrast, must always be excluded when it is a clinical possibility. Use of facemasks by physicians performing lumbar puncture has been advocated to reduce the possibility of oral contamination.[80–82] In aseptic meningitis, transient CSF pleocytosis (neutrophils and lymphocytes) and elevated protein concentrations accompany symptoms and signs that are similar to those of bacterial meningitis. Once a bacterial infection has been excluded, the use of corticosteroids may be helpful in relieving symptoms of aseptic meningitis. Persistent leakage of CSF at the puncture site must also be considered in patients with postural headache and pleocytosis, since the clinical picture may be confused with aseptic meningitis.

Seizures

Intrathecal contrast material may cause other, less frequent but potentially serious complications. Encephalopathy, seizures, and focal neurologic deficits have all been reported after myelography, presumably owing to reflux of contrast material into the subarachnoid space about the brain.[83] The risk of seizures is on the order of 0.1 to 0.3 percent with the nonionic, water-soluble contrast agent iopamidol. Increased risk of seizures is present when the total dose of iodine is greater than 4,500 mg, there is a preexisting seizure disorder, a cervical route of injection is chosen, or the patient is concurrently taking a drug known to lower the seizure threshold.

Inadvertent administration of ionic contrast media used for urography or angiography during myelography causes convulsions that probably arise within the spinal cord itself as well as the brain.[84] These water-soluble, ionic contrast agents are visually indistinguishable from the nonionic contrasts used for myelography; therefore, care must be taken in identifying by their label those indicated for myelography.

Arachnoiditis

Arachnoiditis, or inflammation of the leptomeninges, has also been ascribed to the use of contrast agents for myelography.[85] Iophendylate (Pantopaque), an oil-soluble contrast agent no longer used in clinical practice, was first noted to cause arachnoiditis, especially when accompanied by subarachnoid blood (i.e., after a traumatic tap). Water-soluble contrast agents reduced the incidence of arachnoiditis and were proven safe in the setting of subarachnoid hemorrhage.[86] In many cases it is difficult to ascribe this syndrome with confidence to the contrast agent because confounding variables such as trauma, surgery, infection, or bleeding may have occurred within the spinal subarachnoid space and these have also been associated with arachnoiditis. The issue is further complicated by the observation that arachnoiditis can be induced by intrathecal corticosteroid injections.[87] Clinically, patients usually have symptoms of constant low back pain aggravated by movement. Evidence of multifocal radiculopathy is found on examination. On repeat myelography or MRI, the nerve roots of the cauda equina appear thickened, clumped, and adherent to the periphery of the thecal sac. Enhancement of the roots may occur following intravenous contrast administration. Arachnoiditis is now rarely seen with the use of water-soluble, nonionic contrast agents.

Discography

The value of discography is primarily as a provocative test that attempts to recreate the patient's back pain syndrome, with the goal of isolating the generator of pain. A needle is placed in the nucleus pulposus of a lumbar or cervical disc and water-soluble contrast agent is injected while observing the patient's response. CT can be performed after discography for added spatial resolution. Horton and Daftari found that although MRI and discography correlated in many instances, MRI could not reliably predict which disc was the cause of a patient's pain.[88]

Discography is a controversial procedure.[89–92] Johnson found no evidence that diagnostic discography injured normal discs,[93] but two reports have demonstrated exacerbation of preexisting herniated disc material by discography.[94,95] Carragee and associates found that discography resulted in accelerated disc degeneration, disc herniation, loss of disc height and signal and the development of reactive endplate changes compared to match-controls.[96]

Complications with discography are mainly related to either septic or aseptic discitis. Antibiotics are often added to the contrast media used for discography, but evidence of benefit for their routine use is lacking.[97] Care must be taken to prevent intrathecal instillation of antibiotic-contrast solutions. The incidence of discitis may be related to the length of the procedure, the use of a single needle rather than coaxial technique, and breaks in sterile technique.

Epidural and Transforaminal Anesthetic Neural Block

Patients with back or neck pain often benefit from local anesthetic blockade either to confirm the location of the pain generator or to reduce pain, or both. Diagnostic and therapeutic nerve root blocks involve the local injection of anesthetics such as 0.75 percent bupivacaine with or without steroid compounds around exiting nerves or into the epidural space of patients suffering from local or radicular back or neck pain. Injections are administered via a 22- to 25-gauge needle placed into the area of interest using fluoroscopic or CT guidance. Direct injections are made into the epidural compartment of the spine, facet joints, or focally around an exiting nerve near the neural foramen. Complications of these procedures include spinal cord or cerebellar infarction secondary to injection into or spasm of the vertebral or radiculomedullary arteries, inadvertent injection into the spinal cord or nerve root itself, infection, and rare allergic or other side effects related to the injected agents. Botwin and co-workers reviewed the incidence of complications of fluoroscopically guided lumbar epidural injections in 207 patients and found a 9.6 percent incidence of minor complications ranging from transient headache, back pain, leg pain, facial flushing, vasovagal reaction, and increased blood sugar levels, most likely induced by systemic absorption of corticosteroid.[98] Serious complications such as epidural hematoma, spinal cord injection, and paraplegia or quadriplegia secondary to inadvertent injection into the spinal or vertebral artery have been reported following transforaminal epidural nerve block.[99–101] An outbreak of fungal meningitis caused by contaminated steroid mixtures occurred in 2012.[102,103]

ANGIOGRAPHY

Angiography is essential in the diagnostic evaluation of many patients with vascular disease, but it carries the greatest risk of morbidity among diagnostic imaging procedures. This risk is generated by the necessity of inserting a catheter into a blood vessel, directing the catheter to the required location, injecting contrast material to visualize the vessel, and removing the catheter while maintaining hemostasis. Skill, experience, and judgment are elements that help reduce the risk of this invasive procedure, but risk cannot be eliminated completely. Moreover, therapeutic transcatheter procedures (embolizations) have become important definitive and adjunctive therapies in patients with cerebrovascular, visceral, and peripheral vascular disease. The decision to undertake a diagnostic or therapeutic angiographic procedure requires sober assessment of the goals of the investigation and its risks.

Neurologic complications of angiography or embolization are the most feared because of the relative permanence of the deficit, which can profoundly impair the patient. Neurologic sequelae are encountered most often in angiographic procedures undertaken to evaluate or treat the vessels of the brain and spinal cord, but they can result from procedures undertaken to evaluate vascular disease elsewhere.

Cerebral and Aortic Angiography

Most aortic arch, carotid, and vertebral arteriograms are carried out by transfemoral arterial access. A common femoral arterial puncture provides retrograde access through the aorta to the aortic arch and great vessels. Selective catheterization of the carotid or vertebral arteries can be accomplished with a wide variety of catheter–guide wire combinations.

The most feared complication of cerebral angiography is stroke. Thrombus can form on or inside the tip of the catheter, especially if the catheter is not flushed properly with heparinized saline at regular intervals. Atherosclerotic intimal plaque may be present along the arterial wall, especially at the common carotid bifurcation. This thrombus or plaque can embolize distally into the cerebral circulation by force of injection or from dislodgment of plaque by the catheter or guide wire. The duration and extent of the resulting ischemic neurologic deficit depend on the size and length of the embolus, its composition (fresh thrombus is thought to fragment more readily), its location, and the available collateral circulation. Identified risk factors for ischemic complications include lack of experience on the part of the angiographer,[104] atherosclerosis, vasospasm, low cardiac output, decreased oxygen-carrying capacity, and advanced age. The risk of a neurologic complication has been estimated by many authors and is variable. Hankey and colleagues reviewed eight prospective and seven retrospective studies involving over 8,000 patients with known ischemic cerebrovascular disease and estimated the risk of cerebral angiography at 4 percent for transient ischemic attack and stroke, 1 percent for permanent deficit, and very low (<0.1%) for death.[105]

Bendszus and colleagues assessed the incidence of clinically silent embolism after angiography with diffusion-weighted MRI.[106] The frequency of lesions was significantly higher in patients with a history of vasculopathy or with vessels difficult to probe. Fluoroscopy time, amount of contrast used, and use of additional catheters were also correlated with the appearance of lesions.

Ischemic complications can also result from intimal dissection of the carotid or vertebral artery by direct trauma from the tip of the catheter or guide wire, allowing thrombus to form underneath a dissected intima and increasing the possibility of a thromboembolic complication. Catheter-induced spasm of an artery also raises the potential for neurologic complication. Although usually temporary, this phenomenon can result in a transient deficit if the spasm prevents adequate blood flow distally, or if a dissection results from further contrast injections within a spastic arterial segment.

Intravascular contrast material injected into the cerebral vasculature may have a toxic effect on the brain. In particular, patients with dolichoectasia of the basilar artery may sustain reversible brainstem dysfunction and acute short-term memory loss after multiple contrast injections into the vertebrobasilar system. Limiting contrast reduces the occurrence of this phenomenon.

Rarely, an intracranial aneurysm ruptures during an angiographic contrast injection, causing subarachnoid hemorrhage.[107,108] This is reported to result from the force of the injection, although this theory is not accepted universally.

Before catheter insertion into the common femoral artery, the local soft tissues must be infiltrated with an anesthetic agent, usually lidocaine. If the anesthetic agent is inadvertently injected into the femoral nerve, this may cause transient dysesthesias along the course of the nerve, which lies medial to the common femoral artery in the inguinal space.

In decades past, common practice dictated the use of a direct carotid artery puncture for the performance of cerebral angiography. Although this technique is now outmoded, rare circumstances might require its use. Administration of local anesthesia for such a procedure may result in direct intracarotid injection of lidocaine, which can cause generalized seizures. Moreover, intimal damage may occur at the puncture site from the puncture needle or from subintimal contrast or saline injection, the most common cause of a neurologic deficit occurring during direct carotid angiography. Poor hemostatic control of the carotid puncture site may cause an expanding hematoma.

Spinal Angiography

Spinal angiography may be indicated to evaluate vascular malformations and tumors and to identify the artery of Adamkiewicz before aortic aneurysm repair. Although the procedure requires the use of relatively large volumes of contrast and is tedious and lengthy compared with most other angiographic procedures, the incidence of complications is low. Forbes and colleagues evaluated 134 consecutive spinal angiograms prospectively and found neurologic complications in only 3 patients (2.2%), 2 of whom recovered fully within 24 hours and 1 within 1 week. The adverse events included paraparesis, subjective visual blurring, and speech changes.[109]

Peripheral Angiography

Peripheral (noncerebral-noncardiac) angiography also uses a transfemoral approach where possible. Although the cerebral vasculature is not examined per se, there is a risk of producing a cerebral embolic event if the subclavian or axillary arteries require examination because of the adjacent origins of the vertebral and carotid arteries.

Many patients undergo peripheral angiography to evaluate atherosclerotic disease of the abdominal aorta and iliofemoral system, which itself may preclude the use of a femoral artery puncture. If transfemoral access is not possible because of severe atherosclerosis, the axillary or brachial routes may be used. Each has its own set of risks. An axillary puncture is performed with the arm abducted. The axillary artery is palpated, and the puncture is made as deep into the axilla as possible. The left axilla is chosen for most examinations of the descending aorta and its branches; the right axilla is preferred for studies of the carotid and vertebral arteries. For peripheral angiography, an axillary approach carries a twofold to fourfold greater risk of neurologic complications than a transfemoral approach.[110] Stroke can result from dislodgement of atherosclerotic plaque at the origin of the vertebral artery during catheter passage to the aorta. Hemostasis at the puncture site is a much more crucial issue than with a femoral puncture: the axillary artery is more difficult to compress after removal of the catheter, and an expanding hematoma may injure the brachial plexus. The rate of infection related to catheterization is quite small. In one retrospective review of over 2,900 procedures only 3 patients had an infection and all were at the groin puncture site.[111]

Brachial artery access requires the use of a smaller-diameter catheter because of the smaller size of the artery. Risks of cerebral thromboemboli exist as with the transaxillary route. The median nerve can be damaged by needle puncture or by compression from a developing hematoma.[110]

EMBOLIZATION AND STENTING PROCEDURES

The development of new materials and techniques has advanced the field of interventional neuroradiology, providing new therapeutic options for patients with difficult neurovascular problems. A variety of procedures is available, including detachable coil, stent-supported coil, or flow diverter therapy for aneurysms[112]; particulate or liquid adhesive embolization of arteriovenous malformations (AVMs)[113,114]; balloon angioplasty or stenting of stenosis or vasospasm; transarterial or transvenous embolization of dural arteriovenous fistulas; coil occlusion of carotid-cavernous and vertebral fistulas[115,116]; endovascular treatment of vein of Galen malformations; preoperative embolization of tumors; and thrombolysis and thrombectomy of acute arterial or venous thrombosis.[117,118] Many of these diseases place the patient at high risk of cerebral hemorrhage, stroke, or death. These endovascular treatments have their own risks, and therapy should be tailored to the disease risk of individual patients.

The highest complication rates are found predictably with therapies geared to treating the highest-risk diseases. Among potential complications of endovascular aneurysm therapy are aneurysmal rupture and stroke from thromboemboli. The advent of the electrolytically detachable coil reduced these rates compared to prior balloon techniques.[119–121] Several studies have evaluated the risks of surgery compared to endovascular coiling.[122,123] The International Subarachnoid Aneurysm Trial compared outcomes after endovascular and surgical therapy for ruptured aneurysms, and demonstrated a benefit for endovascular therapy at 1 year.[124,125]

Endovascular treatment of AVMs is frequently used as a preoperative adjunct to surgical resection or stereotactic radiosurgery. Embolic materials include liquid adhesives, polyvinyl alcohol particles, and fibered coils. Therapeutic risks include AVM rupture with intracerebral hemorrhage; inadvertent embolization of normal arteries, causing stroke; and gluing of the catheter into the embolized artery.[126–128] In separate studies using different embolic agents (liquid adhesives and polyvinyl alcohol particles) for AVM embolization, the permanent neurologic complication rate was 8 percent in each.[129,130]

Endovascular therapy is also applicable to vascular problems involving the spinal cord. In the treatment of intramedullary AVMs, which often present with hemorrhage, embolization may provide definitive, palliative, or adjunctive therapy. The major risk is occlusion of normal spinal arteries with the embolic material. Casasco and colleagues estimated the risk of a permanent therapy-related neurologic deficit at 5.7 percent.[131] The spinal dural arteriovenous fistula represents a shunt between a dural artery on the nerve root sleeve and an adjacent radicular vein that drains toward the spinal cord, resulting in a venous engorgement syndrome. The risk involved in endovascular treatment of this dural process is lower because spinal arteries are not involved directly.

Stents are being used increasingly in the treatment of diseases of the supra-aortic vessels. The technique has been evaluated in comparison to carotid endarterectomy within several clinical trials.[132–134] This technique can be complicated by transient or permanent neurologic deficits secondary to emboli, dissection, or occlusion of the vessel. The risk of neurologic deficits has decreased as experience has accumulated and newer stent systems have been developed, but it has been estimated as high as 10 to 15 percent.[135] Other complications of carotid artery stenting include transient bradycardia, hypotension, and those related to femoral artery catheterization.[136–138]

Although advances in imaging capabilities, catheters, and embolic materials will advance endovascular capabilities, the knowledge, judgment, and experience of the angiographer will have the greatest effect in diminishing the risks of endovascular therapy.

REFERENCES

1. Cochran ST: Anaphylactoid reactions to radiocontrast media. Curr Allergy Asthma Rep 5:28, 2005.
2. American College of Radiology: ACR Manual on Contrast Media Version 8. 2012. www.hnxtbook.com/nxtbooks/acr/contrastmediamanual2012/.

3. Bush WH, Swanson DP: Acute reactions to intravascular contrast media: types, risk factors, recognition, and specific treatment. AJR Am J Roentgenol 157:1153, 1991.
4. Katayama H, Yamaguchi K, Kozuka T, et al: Adverse reactions to ionic and nonionic contrast media. A report from the Japanese Committee on the Safety of Contrast Media. Radiology 175:621, 1990.
5. LoZito JC: Convulsions: a complication of contrast enhancement in computerized tomography. Arch Neurol 34:649, 1977.
6. May EF, Ling GS, Geyer CA, et al: Contrast agent overdose causing brain retention of contrast, seizures and parkinsonism. Neurology 43:836, 1993.
7. Kinn RM, Breisblatt WM: Cortical blindness after coronary angiography: a rare but reversible complication. Cathet Cardiovasc Diagn 22:177, 1991.
8. Eliashiv S, Wirguin I, Brenner T, et al: Aggravation of human and experimental myasthenia gravis by contrast media. Neurology 40:1623, 1990.
9. Memolo M, Dyer R, Zagoria RJ: Extravasation injury with nonionic contrast material. AJR Am J Roentgenol 160:203, 1993.
10. Bellin MF, Jakobsen JA, Tomassin I, et al: Contrast medium extravasation injury: guidelines for prevention and management. Eur Radiol 12:2807, 2002.
11. Li A, Wong CS, Wong MK, et al: Acute adverse reactions to magnetic resonance contrast media–gadolinium chelates. Br J Radiol 79:368, 2006.
12. Oksendal AN, Hals PA: Biodistribution and toxicity of MR imaging contrast media. J Magn Reson Imaging 3:157, 1993.
13. Hunt CH, Hartman RP, Hesley GK: Frequency and severity of adverse effects of iodinated and gadolinium contrast materials: retrospective review of 456,930 doses. AJR Am J Roentgenol 193:1124, 2009.
14. Shellock FG, Hahn HP, Mink JH, et al: Adverse reaction to intravenous gadoteridol. Radiology 189:151, 1993.
15. Takebayashi S, Sugiyama M, Nagase M, et al: Severe adverse reaction to iv gadopentetate dimeglumine. AJR Am J Roentgenol 160:659, 1993.
16. Webb JA, Thomsen HS, Morcos SK: The use of iodinated and gadolinium contrast media during pregnancy and lactation. Eur Radiol 15:1234, 2005.
17. Thomsen HS, Morcos SK, Almen T, et al: Nephrogenic systemic fibrosis and gadolinium-based contrast media: updated ESUR Contrast Medium Safety Committee guidelines. Eur Radiol 23:307, 2013.
18. Grobner T, Prischl FC: Patient characteristics and risk factors for nephrogenic systemic fibrosis following gadolinium exposure. Semin Dial 21:135, 2008.
19. Gibson SE, Farver CF, Prayson RA: Multiorgan involvement in nephrogenic fibrosing dermopathy: an autopsy case and review of the literature. Arch Pathol Lab Med 130:209, 2006.
20. Schnorr J, Wagner S, Abramjuk C, et al: Focal liver lesions: SPIO-, gadolinium-, and ferucarbotran-enhanced dynamic T1-weighted and delayed T2-weighted MR imaging in rabbits. Radiology 240:90, 2006.
21. Anzai Y: Superparamagnetic iron oxide nanoparticles: nodal metastases and beyond. Top Magn Reson Imaging 15:103, 2004.
22. Tanimoto A, Kuribayashi S: Application of superparamagnetic iron oxide to imaging of hepatocellular carcinoma. Eur J Radiol 58:200, 2006.
23. Kanal E, Barkovich AJ, Bell C, et al: ACR guidance document on MR safe practices: 2013. J Magn Reson Imaging 37:501, 2013.
24. Dalkin B, Franco I, Reda EF, et al: Contrast-induced central nervous system toxicity after radiographic evaluation of the lower urinary tract in myelodysplastic patients with ventriculoperitoneal shunts. J Urol 148:120, 1992.
25. Peled N, Blaser SI, Moore A, et al: Computerized tomography appearance of accidental infusion of air into the venous sinuses. Pediatr Neurosurg 17:251, 1991.
26. Adams M, Quint DJ, Eldevik OP: Iatrogenic air in the cavernous sinus. AJR Am J Roentgenol 159:189, 1992.
27. Pearce MS, Salotti JA, Little MP, et al: Radiation exposure from CT scans in childhood and subsequent risk of leukaemia and brain tumours: a retrospective cohort study. Lancet 380:499, 2012.
28. Teitelbaum GP, Lin MC, Watanabe AT, et al: Ferromagnetism and MR imaging: safety of carotid vascular clamps. AJNR Am J Neuroradiol 11:267, 1990.
29. Shellock FG, Curtis JS: MR imaging and biomedical implants, materials, and devices—an updated review. Radiology 180:541, 1991.
30. Zikria JF, Machnicki S, Rhim E, et al: MRI of patients with cardiac pacemakers: a review of the medical literature. Am J Roentgenol 196:390, 2011.
31. Junttila MJ, Fishman JE, Lopera GA, et al: Safety of serial MRI in patients with implantable cardioverter defibrillators. Heart 97:1852, 2011.
32. Kanal E, Shellock FG: MR imaging of patients with intracranial aneurysm clips. Radiology 187:612, 1993.
33. Klucznik RP, Carrier DA, Pyka R, et al: Placement of a ferromagnetic intracerebral aneurysm clip in a magnetic-field with a fatal outcome. Radiology 187:855, 1993.
34. Dujovny M, Alp MS, Dujovny N, et al: Aneurysm clips: magnetic quantification and magnetic resonance imaging safety – technical note. J Neurosurg 87:788, 1997.
35. Pride Jr GL, Kowal J, Mendelsohn DB, et al: Safety of MR scanning in patients with nonferromagnetic aneurysm clips. J Magn Reson Imaging 12:198, 2000.
36. Kakizawa Y, Seguchi T, Horiuchi T, et al: Cerebral aneurysm clips in the 3-tesla magnetic field. J Neurosurg 113:859, 2010.

37. Lopic N, Jelen A, Vrtnik S, et al: Quantitative determination of magnetic force on a coronary stent in MRI. J Magn Reson Imaging 37:391, 2013.
38. Nehra A, Moran CJ, Cross 3rd DT, et al: MR safety and imaging of neuroform stents at 3T. AJNR Am J Neuroradiol 25:1476, 2004.
39. Hug J, Nagel E, Bornstedt A, et al: Coronary arterial stents: safety and artifacts during MR imaging. Radiology 216:781, 2000.
40. Shellock FG, Shellock VJ: Metallic stents: evaluation of MR imaging safety. AJR Am J Roentgenol 173:543, 1999.
41. Porto I, Selvanayagam J, Ashar V, et al: Safety of magnetic resonance imaging one to three days after bare metal and drug-eluting stent implantation. Am J Cardiol 96:366, 2005.
42. Nakamura T, Fukuda K, Hayakawa K, et al: Mechanism of burn injury during magnetic resonance imaging (MRI)—simple loops can induce heat injury. Front Med Biol Eng 11:117, 2001.
43. Liu CY, Farahani K, Lu DS, et al: Safety of MRI-guided endovascular guidewire applications. J Magn Reson Imaging 12:75, 2000.
44. Kim LJ, Sonntag VK, Hott JT, et al: Scalp burns from halo pins following magnetic resonance imaging. Case illustration. J Neurosurg 99:186, 2003.
45. Shellock FG: Reference Manual for Magnetic Resonance Safety, Implants, and Devices. Biomedical Research Publishing Group, Los Angeles, 2006.
46. Murphy KJ, Brunberg JA: Orbital plain films as a prerequisite for MR imaging: is a known history of injury a sufficient screening criterion? AJR Am J Roentgenol 167:1053, 1996.
47. Hatfield M, Eschbach J: Metallic foreign bodies and MR imaging. AJR Am J Roentgenol 167:1597, 1996.
48. Boutin RD, Briggs JE, Williamson MR: Injuries associated with MR imaging: survey of safety records and methods used to screen patients for metallic foreign bodies before imaging. AJR Am J Roentgenol 162:189, 1994.
49. Otto PM, Otto RA, Virapongse C, et al: Screening test for detection of metallic foreign objects in the orbit before magnetic resonance imaging. Invest Radiol 27:308, 1992.
50. Archibald RC: Hospital details failures leading to M.R.I. fatality. New York Times, August 22, 2001.
51. Price DL, De Wilde JP, Papadaki AM, et al: Investigation of acoustic noise on 15 MRI scanners from 0.2 T to 3 T. J Magn Reson Imaging 13:288, 2001.
52. Modic MT, Masaryk T, Boumphrey F, et al: Lumbar herniated disk disease and canal stenosis: prospective evaluation by surface coil MR, CT, and myelography. AJR Am J Roentgenol 147:757, 1986.
53. Modic MT, Feiglin DH, Piraino DW, et al: Vertebral osteomyelitis: assessment using MR. Radiology 157:157, 1985.
54. Dillon WP, Norman D, Newton TH, et al: Intradural spinal cord lesions: Gd-DTPA-enhanced MR imaging. Radiology 170:229, 1989.
55. Urso S, Giannini S, Migliorini A, et al: The incidence of postural headache in in- and outpatients following lumbar myelography (needles of different gauges and headache). Radiol Med (Torino) 77:165, 1989.
56. Tourtellotte WW, Henderson WG, Tucker RP, et al: A randomized, double-blind clinical trial comparing the 22 versus 26 gauge needle in the production of the post-lumbar puncture syndrome in normal individuals. Headache 12:73, 1972.
57. Sand T: Which factors affect reported headache incidences after lumbar myelography? A statistical analysis of publications in the literature. Neuroradiology 31:55, 1989.
58. Amorim JA, Gomes de Barros MV, Valenca MM: Postdural (post-lumbar) puncture headache: risk factors and clinical features. Cephalalgia 32:916, 2012.
59. Wilton NC, Globerson JH, de Rosayro AM: Epidural blood patch for postdural puncture headache: it's never too late. Anesth Analg 65:895, 1986.
60. Kim SR, Chae HS, Yoon MJ, et al: No effect of recumbency duration on the occurrence of post-lumbar puncture headache with a 22 G cutting needle. BMC Neurol 12:1, 2012.
61. Michel O, Brusis T: Hearing disorders following spinal anesthesia. Reg Anaesth 14:92, 1991.
62. Michel O, Brusis T: Hearing loss as a sequel of lumbar puncture. Ann Otol Rhinol Laryngol 101:390, 1992.
63. Michel O, Brusis T, Loennecken I, et al: Inner ear hearing loss following cerebrospinal fluid puncture: a too little appreciated complication? HNO 38:71, 1990.
64. Issaivanan M, Cohen S, Mittler M, et al: Iatrogenic spinal epidermoid cyst after lumbar puncture using needles with stylet. Pediatr Hematol Oncol 28:600, 2011.
65. Per H, Kumandas S, Gumus H, et al: Iatrogenic epidermoid tumor: late complication of lumbar puncture. J Child Neurol 22:332, 2007.
66. Baba H, Wada M, Tanaka Y, et al: Intraspinal epidermoid after lumbar puncture. Int Orthop 18:116, 1994.
67. Van de Kelft E, Bosmans J, Parizel PM, et al: Intracerebral hemorrhage after lumbar myelography with iohexol: report of a case and review of the literature. Neurosurgery 28:570, 1991.
68. Manji H, Birley H: Subdural haematoma–a complication of myelography in a patient with AIDS. Aids 4:698, 1990.
69. Rando TA, Fishman RA: Spontaneous intracranial hypotension: report of two cases and review of the literature. Neurology 42:481, 1992.
70. Stevens JM, Kendall BE, Gedroyc W: Acute epidural haematoma complicating myelography in a normotensive patient with normal blood coagulability. Br J Radiol 64:860, 1991.

71. Ruff RL, Dougherty Jr JH: Complications of lumbar puncture followed by anticoagulation. Stroke 12:879, 1981.
72. Malloy PC, Grassi CJ, Kundu S, et al: Consensus guidelines for periprocedural management of coagulation status and hemostasis risk in percutaneous image-guided interventions. J Vasc Interv Radiol 20:S240, 2009.
73. Boon JM, Abrahams PH, Meiring JH, et al: Lumbar puncture: anatomical review of a clinical skill. Clin Anat 17:544, 2004.
74. Katoh Y, Itoh T, Tsuji H, et al: Complications of lateral C1-2 puncture myelography. Spine 15:1085, 1990.
75. Simon SL, Abrahams JM, Sean Grady M, et al: Intramedullary injection of contrast into the cervical spinal cord during cervical myelography: a case report. Spine 27:E274, 2002.
76. Rogers LA: Acute subdural hematoma and death following lateral cervical spinal puncture. Case report. J Neurosurg 58:284, 1983.
77. Robertson HJ, Smith RD: Cervical myelography: survey of modes of practice and major complications. Radiology 174:79, 1990.
78. Park KW, Im SB, Kim BT, et al: Neurotoxic manifestations of an overdose intrathecal injection of gadopentetate dimeglumine. J Korean Med Sci 25:505, 2010.
79. Bender A, Elstner M, Paul R, et al: Severe symptomatic aseptic chemical meningitis following myelography: the role of procalcitonin. Neurology 63:1311, 2004.
80. Moen V: Meningitis is a rare complication of spinal anesthesia. Good hygiene and face masks are simple preventive measures. Lakartidningen 95:628, 1998.
81. Gelfand MS, Cook DM: Streptococcal meningitis as a complication of diagnostic myelography: medicolegal aspects. Clin Infect Dis 22:130, 1996.
82. Jorbeck H: Good hygiene prevents meningitis after lumbar puncture. The best insurance is using face masks. Lakartidningen 95:596, 1998.
83. Singh S, Rajpal C, Nannapeneni S, et al: Iopamidol myelography-induced seizures. MedGenMed 7:11, 2005.
84. McClennan BL: Contrast media alert. Radiology 189:35, 1993.
85. Gnanalingham KK, Joshi SM, Sabin I: Thoracic arachnoiditis, arachnoid cyst and syrinx formation secondary to myelography with Myodil, 30 years previously. Eur Spine J 15(suppl 5):661, 2006.
86. Johansen JG, Barthelemy CR, Haughton VM, et al: Arachnoiditis from myelography and laminectomy in experimental animals. AJNR Am J Neuroradiol 5:97, 1984.
87. Roche J: Steroid-induced arachnoiditis. Med J Aust 140:281, 1984.
88. Horton WC, Daftari TK: Which disc as visualized by magnetic resonance imaging is actually a source of pain? A correlation between magnetic resonance imaging and discography. Spine 17(suppl):S164, 1992.
89. Carragee EJ, Alamin TF: Discography. A review. Spine J 1:364, 2001.
90. Carragee EJ, Barcohana B, Alamin T, et al: Prospective controlled study of the development of lower back pain in previously asymptomatic subjects undergoing experimental discography. Spine 29:1112, 2004.
91. Carragee EJ, Hannibal M: Diagnostic evaluation of low back pain. Orthop Clin North Am 35:7, 2004.
92. Carragee EJ, Tanner CM, Khurana S, et al: The rates of false-positive lumbar discography in select patients without low back symptoms. Spine 25:1373, 2000.
93. Johnson RG: Does discography injure normal discs? An analysis of repeat discograms. Spine 14:424, 1989.
94. Poynton AR, Hinman A, Lutz G, et al: Discography-induced acute lumbar disc herniation: a report of five cases. J Spinal Disord Tech 18:188, 2005.
95. Smith MD, Kim SS: A herniated cervical disc resulting from discography: an unusual complication. J Spinal Disord 3:392, 1990.
96. Carragee EJ, Don AS, Hurwitz EL, et al: 2009 ISSLS Prize Winner: Does discography cause accelerated progression of degeneration changes in the lumbar disc: a ten-year matched cohort study. Spine 34:2338, 2009.
97. Willems PC, Jacobs W, Duinkerke ES, et al: Lumbar discography: should we use prophylactic antibiotics? A study of 435 consecutive discograms and a systematic review of the literature. J Spinal Disord Tech 17:243, 2004.
98. Botwin KP, Gruber RD, Bouchlas CG, et al: Complications of fluoroscopically guided transforaminal lumbar epidural injections. Arch Phys Med Rehabil 81:1045, 2000.
99. Tiso RL, Cutler T, Catania JA, et al: Adverse central nervous system sequelae after selective transforaminal block: the role of corticosteroids. Spine J 4:468, 2004.
100. Houten JK, Errico TJ: Paraplegia after lumbosacral nerve root block: report of three cases. Spine J 2:70, 2002.
101. Suresh S, Berman J, Connell DA: Cerebellar and brainstem infarction as a complication of CT-guided transforaminal cervical nerve root block. Skeletal Radiol 36:449, 2007.
102. Roos K: Fungal meningitis due to contaminated epidural steroid injections. Continuum 18:e1, 2012.
103. Kerkering TM, Grifasi ML, Baffoe-Bonnie AW, et al: Early clinical observations in prospectively followed patients with fungal meningitis related to contaminated epidural steroid injections. Ann Intern Med 158:154, 2013.
104. McIvor J, Steiner TJ, Perkin GD, et al: Neurological morbidity of arch and carotid arteriography in cerebrovascular disease. The influence of contrast medium and radiologist. Br J Radiol 60:117, 1987.

105. Hankey GJ, Warlow CP, Sellar RJ: Cerebral angiographic risk in mild cerebrovascular disease. Stroke 21:209, 1990.
106. Bendszus M, Koltzenburg M, Burger R, et al: Silent embolism in diagnostic cerebral angiography and neurointerventional procedures: a prospective study. Lancet 354:1594, 1999.
107. Ohi Y, Ueki S, Isoda H: [Rupture of a giant aneurysm of the internal carotid artery during cerebral angiography (author's transl)]. Rinsho Hoshasen 24:953, 1979.
108. Allcock JM: Aneurysms. p. 2474. In Newton TH Potts DG, editors. Radiology in the Skull and Brain Vol 2. Angiography. CV Mosby, St. Louis, 1974.
109. Forbes G, Nichols DA, Jack Jr CR, et al: Complications of spinal cord arteriography: prospective assessment of risk for diagnostic procedures. Radiology 169:479, 1988.
110. Molnar W, Paul DJ: Complications of axillary arteriotomies. An analysis of 1,762 consecutive studies. Radiology 104:269, 1972.
111. Kelkar PS, Fleming JB, Walters BC, et al: Infection risk in neurointervention and cerebral angiography. Neurosurgery 72:327, 2013.
112. Becske T, Kallmes DF, Saatci I, et al: Pipeline for uncoilable or failed aneurysms: results from a multicenter clinical trial. Radiology 267:858, 2013.
113. Strauss I, Frolov V, Buchbut D, et al: Critical appraisal of endovascular treatment of brain arteriovenous malformation using Onyx in a series of 92 consecutive patients. Acta Neurochir (Wien) 155:611, 2013.
114. Jagadeesan BD, Grigoryan M, Hassan AE, et al: Endovascular balloon-assisted embolization of intracranial and cervical arteriovenous malformations using dual lumen co-axial balloon microcatheters and Onyx: initial experience. Neurosurgery, in press, 2013.
115. Luo CB, Teng MM, Chang FC, et al: Transarterial detachable coil embolization of direct carotid-cavernous fistula: immediate and long-term outcomes. J Chin Med Assoc 76:31, 2013.
116. Williamson RW, Ducruet AF, Crowley RW, et al: Transvenous coil embolization of an intraorbital arteriovenous fistula: case report and review of the literature. Neurosurgery 72:E130, 2013.
117. Saver JL, Jahan R, Levy EI, et al: SOLITAIRE with the intention for thrombectomy (SWIFT) trial: design of a randomized, controlled, multicenter study comparing the SOLITAIRE Flow Restoration device and the MERCI Retriever in acute ischaemic stroke. Int J Stroke, in press, 2012.
118. Nogueira RG, Lutsep HL, Gupta R, et al: Trevo versus Merci retrievers for thrombectomy revascularisation of large vessel occlusions in acute ischaemic stroke (TREVO 2): a randomised trial. Lancet 380:1231, 2012.
119. Guglielmi G: Embolization of intracranial aneurysms with detachable coils and electrothrombosis. p. 63. In: Viñuela F, Halbach VV, Dion JE (eds): Interventional Neuroradiology. Endovascular Therapy of the Central Nervous System. Raven Press, New York, 1992.
120. Guglielmi G, Viñuela F, Sepetka I, et al: Electrothrombosis of saccular aneurysms via endovascular approach. Part 1: electrochemical basis, technique, and experimental results. J Neurosurg 75:1, 1991.
121. Guglielmi G, Viñuela F, Dion J, et al: Electrothrombosis of saccular aneurysms via endovascular approach. Part 2: Preliminary clinical experience. J Neurosurg 75:8, 1991.
122. International Study of Unruptured Intracranial Aneurysms Investigators: Unruptured intracranial aneurysms–risk of rupture and risks of surgical intervention. International Study of Unruptured Intracranial Aneurysms Investigators. N Engl J Med 339:1725, 1998.
123. Wiebers DO, Whisnant JP, Huston 3rd J, et al: Unruptured intracranial aneurysms: natural history, clinical outcome, and risks of surgical and endovascular treatment. Lancet 362:103, 2003.
124. Molyneux A, Kerr R, Stratton I, et al: International Subarachnoid Aneurysm Trial (ISAT) of neurosurgical clipping versus endovascular coiling in 2143 patients with ruptured intracranial aneurysms: a randomised trial. Lancet 360:1267, 2002.
125. Molyneux AJ, Kerr RS, Yu LM, et al: International subarachnoid aneurysm trial (ISAT) of neurosurgical clipping versus endovascular coiling in 2143 patients with ruptured intracranial aneurysms: a randomised comparison of effects on survival, dependency, seizures, rebleeding, subgroups, and aneurysm occlusion. Lancet 366:809, 2005.
126. Viñuela F: Functional evaluation and embolization of intracranial arteriovenous malformations. p. 77. In: Viñuela F, Halbach VV, Dion JE (eds): Interventional Neuroradiology. Endovascular Therapy of the Central Nervous System. Raven Press, New York, 1992.
127. Lee JI, Choi CH, Ko JK, et al: Retained microcatheter after onyx embolization of intracranial arteriovenous malformation. J Korean Neurosurg Soc 51:374, 2012.
128. Newman CB, Park MS, Kerber CW, et al: Over-the-catheter retrieval of a retained microcatheter following Onyx embolization: a technical report. J Neurointerv Surg 4:e13, 2012.
129. Fournier D, TerBrugge KG, Willinsky R, et al: Endovascular treatment of intracerebral arteriovenous malformations: experience in 49 cases. J Neurosurg 75:228, 1991.
130. Purdy PD, Samson D, Batjer HH, et al: Preoperative embolization of cerebral arteriovenous malformations with polyvinyl alcohol particles: experience in 51 adults. AJNR Am J Neuroradiol 11:501, 1990.
131. Casasco AE, Houdart E, Gobin YP, et al: Embolization of spinal vascular malformations. Neuroimaging Clin North Am 2:337, 1992.

132. Brown MM, Rogers J, Bland JM: Endovascular versus surgical treatment in patients with carotid stenosis in the Carotid and Vertebral Artery Transluminal Angioplasty Study (CAVATAS): a randomised trial. Lancet 357:1729, 2001.
133. Yadav JS: Carotid stenting in high-risk patients: design and rationale of the SAPPHIRE trial. Cleve Clin J Med 71(suppl 1):S45, 2004.
134. Brott TG, Hobson 2nd RW, Howard G, et al: Stenting versus endarterectomy for treatment of carotid-artery stenosis. N Engl J Med 363:11, 2010.
135. Leisch F, Kerschner K, Hofman R, et al: Carotid stenting: acute results and complications. Z Kardiol 88:661, 1999.
136. Lovblad KO, Pluschke W, Remonda L, et al: Diffusion-weighted MRI for monitoring neurovascular interventions. Neuroradiology 42:134, 2000.
137. Higashida RT, Meyers PM, Connors JJ, et al: Intracranial angioplasty & stenting for cerebral atherosclerosis: a position statement of the American Society of Interventional and Therapeutic Neuroradiology, Society of Interventional Radiology, and the American Society of Neuroradiology. J Vasc Interv Radiol 16:1281, 2005.
138. Higashida RT, Meyers PM: Intracranial angioplasty and stenting for cerebral atherosclerosis: new treatments for stroke are needed! Neuroradiology 48:367, 2006.

CHAPTER

54

Preoperative and Postoperative Care of Patients with Neurologic Disorders

JOHN P. BETJEMANN ■ S. ANDREW JOSEPHSON

INTRODUCTION

Perioperative care of the patient with neurologic disease provides practitioners with a number of unique challenges ranging from timing of surgery, administration of medications, and anesthetic choices, to postoperative care. This chapter focuses on common neurologic disorders and the perioperative considerations that accompany them.

MOVEMENT DISORDERS

The incidence of Parkinson disease among all ages approximates 14 per 100,000 and increases to a median of 160 per 100,000 in persons over age 70 years.[1] Therefore, thousands of parkinsonian patients will undergo various surgical procedures each year, and many will experience unique perioperative and surgical challenges related to their underlying disorder.

A key factor in caring for parkinsonian patients in any setting is establishing their specific medication regimen and the timing of these medications. Antiparkinsonian medications are almost exclusively oral, making challenging the "nil by mouth" (NPO) status prior to surgery and the timing and administration of perioperative medications. The patient's typical medication regimen should be continued on the day of surgery as close as possible to the time of anesthesia. Levodopa has a short half-life, on the order of 1 to 3 hours; if the planned duration of surgery is long and general anesthesia is being employed, consideration should be given to placing a nasogastric tube and continuing levodopa intraoperatively.[2] Missed doses may precipitate a parkinsonian crisis resulting in severe rigidity and akinesia, leading to prolonged intubation and recovery time. The possibility of resting or orthostatic hypotension, which is common in Parkinson disease and a side effect of many medications used to treat it, should

Aminoff's Neurology and General Medicine, Fifth Edition.

also be considered, and anesthetic agents that commonly cause hypotension should be avoided.

When a patient is unable to take dopaminergic medications orally in the perioperative period, one strategy is to switch patients to a transdermal dopamine agonist, rotigotine, with a half-life of approximately 24 hours.[3] However, this may be challenging for patients taking a complex oral regimen as conversion between various dopaminergic formulations varies widely from patient to patient.

Regional anesthesia has the added benefit of minimizing postoperative nausea and vomiting, which will allow for the timely resumption of oral medications. If general anesthesia is necessary, halothane should be avoided in patients taking levodopa as it sensitizes the heart to catecholamines.[4] Propofol has been associated with worsening dyskinesias but has also been observed to improve tremor; it is often avoided in patients undergoing deep brain stimulation (DBS) surgery.[4] Antiemetics are commonly administered intraoperatively and postoperatively, but dopamine antagonists such as prochlorperazine and metoclopramide can worsen parkinsonism and block the effects of levodopa therapy; therefore, they should be avoided in favor of ondansetron and domperidone.[5]

Extubation of parkinsonian patients may be complicated. Up to one-third of patients have an obstructive ventilatory pattern related to upper airway dysfunction including laryngeal dysmotility and retained secretions.[4] This dysfunction places parkinsonian patients at increased risk of aspiration. Parkinsonian patients are also at a substantially increased risk of developing postoperative confusion and hallucinations, in some cases due to underlying diffuse Lewy body pathology; therefore these patients must be monitored carefully in the postoperative setting and strategies to prevent delirium should be planned in advance.[6] An elevated risk of urinary tract infections, aspiration pneumonias, and bacterial infections has been demonstrated in parkinsonian patients, leading to an increased length of hospital stay and increased perioperative morbidity.[7] Improved surgical outcomes occur when medication regimens are optimized by a neurologist; with early mobilization; when postoperative complications are carefully monitored; and when conversations regarding long-term care and prolonged rehabilitation occur early in the hospitalization.[8]

Special Considerations for Deep Brain Stimulation

DBS is now a well-accepted treatment for medication-resistant Parkinson disease. Given the potential risk of intracerebral hemorrhage with insertion of DBS leads, all antiplatelet medications should be discontinued for 7 to 10 days prior to surgery.[9] Typically, antiparkinsonian medications are discontinued the night before surgery. General anesthesia is avoided so that the patient is awake and parkinsonian symptoms can be monitored intraoperatively. Postoperatively, patients should be kept normotensive to minimize the risk of hemorrhage, and antiparkinsonian medications should be resumed immediately.

Movement-Disorder Emergencies in the Perioperative Period

Perioperative movement-disorder emergencies commonly occur because a patient's usual medication regimen is discontinued or because of new medications introduced in the perioperative period. Diagnosis requires a detailed knowledge of the patient's preexisting conditions and a careful review of preoperative, intraoperative, and postoperative medications. Patients with Parkinson disease who have their levodopa discontinued suddenly for several days may experience parkinsonism-hyperpyrexia, characterized by fever, severe rigidity, autonomic instability, and an elevated serum creatine kinase level.[10] Treatment includes restoration of dopaminergic therapy, and the management strategies discussed later.

Somewhat clinically similar to the parkinsonism-hyperpyrexia syndrome, neuroleptic malignant syndrome results from dopamine receptor blockade. Commonly implicated medications include neuroleptics, antiemetics (e.g., metoclopramide and prochlorperazine), and droperidol, which should be withdrawn promptly. In these syndromes, symptoms may last for days and be life-threatening. Treatment often requires care in the intensive care unit, with aggressive hydration and cooling. Dantrolene, bromocriptine, or amantadine is typically initiated, but the evidence for their efficacy is derived mainly from case reports.

A third and clinically distinct disorder, serotonin syndrome, results from excessive serotonin activity.

It may occur as a consequence of drug interactions, overdose of certain medications, or therapeutic (or recreational) drug use. Manifestations may include hypertension, tachycardia, hyperthermia, diaphoresis, myoclonus, tremulousness, hyperreflexia, confusion, agitation, and even coma.[10] Treatment involves discontinuation of offending agents and often requires care in the ICU, control of the blood pressure, and management with cyproheptadine or benzodiazepines. A final related condition, discussed later, is malignant hyperthermia, a rare genetic disorder triggered by inhalational anesthetics or succinylcholine.

MULTIPLE SCLEROSIS

Anesthetic and surgical complications related to multiple sclerosis (MS) are relatively rare, but certain preoperative, intraoperative, and postoperative considerations are important. There is not abundant evidence to suggest that anesthesia or surgery consistently leads to disease exacerbations, but physiologic stress is commonly considered a cause of exacerbations and is heightened in the perioperative period. Accordingly, patients should be counseled about the potential risk of MS exacerbation with surgery and monitored for such postoperatively.

Disease-modifying therapies (such as β-interferons, glatiramer acetate, fingolimod, dimethyl fumarate, and teriflunomide) aimed at reducing the frequency and severity of MS exacerbations should be continued in the perioperative period.[11] In patients with low medullary and high cervical demyelinating lesions, ventilatory dysfunction should be anticipated, as respiratory effort may be impaired.[12]

Consideration should also be given to choice of anesthetic and anesthetic technique in patients with MS. Systemic administration of certain local anesthetics (e.g., lidocaine) may unmask clinically silent MS plaques or transiently worsen preexisting symptoms.[13] The presumed mechanism involves partial sodium channel blockade exacerbating preexisting conduction block across demyelinated plaques. The findings in a small case series suggested that spinal anesthesia is associated with a higher relapse rate in MS compared to general anesthesia, though the exact underlying mechanism is unknown.[14] A larger, more recent retrospective study of 139 patients with various CNS diseases (including but not limited to MS) found no increase in neurologic relapses following neuraxial anesthesia.[15] Epidural anesthesia may have a lesser risk than intradural anesthesia due to decreased concentrations of anesthetics penetrating the thecal sac. The American Society of Regional Anesthesia and Pain Medicine concluded that the evidence for neuraxial anesthesia affecting neurologic function in patients with preexisting CNS disorders is not definitive and that individual risk–benefit analysis should be employed when selecting a method of anesthesia.[16]

Although general anesthesia has been linked to MS exacerbations, it has often been used successfully, and there is no evidence to suggest that any single intravenous or inhalational anesthetic is preferable to another.[17] If a patient experiences an MS relapse in the immediate postoperative period, the intraoperative temperature recordings should be checked as hyperthermia may cause MS pseudoexacerbations (Uhthoff phenomenon, i.e., symptoms that are not caused by new MS lesions and improve with a return to normothermia).

Caution should also be exercised in patients with MS receiving intrathecal baclofen for spasticity, as abrupt withdrawal may precipitate a potentially life-threatening syndrome characterized by seizures, hallucinations, and autonomic instability.[18] Management includes resumption of baclofen as soon as possible and treatment with high-dose benzodiazepines in the interim.

Patients with MS should be monitored closely in the postoperative period. The appearance of new demyelinating plaques or increased neurologic deficits related to existing plaques may result from the stress of surgery or infection. Such exacerbations may result in impaired respiratory function and in autonomic dysfunction causing labile blood pressure.[17] Baseline neurologic dysfunction in patients with MS combined with the stress of surgery may result in longer recovery times and necessitate rehabilitation upon discharge, even in the absence of any clinical deterioration.

DELIRIUM AND DEMENTIA

Delirium

Delirium is a complex entity characterized by the relatively acute onset of disorientation and attentional deficits that follow a fluctuating course. The incidence of postoperative delirium in the elderly

TABLE 54-1 ■ Incidence of Postoperative Delirium in the Elderly by Surgical Type

Type of Surgery	Incidence Range (%)
Cataract	1–3
General	10–14
Orthopedic (mainly hip)	32–55
Open heart	32–79

ranges from 10 to 60 percent and varies somewhat with the type of surgery performed (Table 54-1).[19] Due to its variable forms—hyperactive, hypoactive, and mixed—delirium is often under-recognized. Hyperactive delirium involves agitation, combativeness, and hypervigilance, as is commonly seen in alcohol withdrawal. This form is easily recognized by clinicians. The hypoactive form, which may present with lethargy, stupor, or even coma, is sometimes difficult to recognize, as patients are less obtrusive and do not seek care or attention. It is not uncommon for these patients to be misdiagnosed with severe depression or for their cognitive dysfunction to be unrecognized.

Research has focused mainly on identifying baseline characteristics that predispose to the development of postoperative delirium and on iatrogenic risks of developing delirium, with relatively less emphasis until recently on the management and the long-term consequences of postoperative delirium. Nearly 98 percent of cases of postoperative delirium occur within 3 days of surgery.[19] An early study of patients undergoing repair of femoral neck fractures showed no difference in the incidence of postoperative confusion when comparing epidural to halothane anesthesia.[20] A more recent meta-analysis compared anesthetic types and supported the notion that general anesthesia was not more likely to be linked with postoperative delirium than regional anesthetic techniques.[21] However, the type of anesthesia does become relevant when considering the timing of a postoperatively altered mental status. Patients receiving regional anesthesia tend to maintain or recover cognitive function more quickly than those receiving general anesthesia. Especially in the first 24 to 48 hours, it is important to consider which type of anesthesia the patient received as this may account for differences in mentation.[19]

Factors that are associated with the development of delirium are well-established (Table 54-2). It is important to recognize the possibility of postoperative delirium in elderly patients and those with baseline cognitive impairment ranging from mild cognitive impairment to frank dementia. In patients undergoing elective surgery, it is especially important to obtain an accurate history of substance use as both intoxication and withdrawal may manifest as delirium following surgery. Even mild pre- to postoperative electrolyte shifts, such as subtle hypo- or hypernatremia, may result in postoperative delirium. Postoperative pain management poses a particular challenge. Both untreated pain and analgesic use may worsen delirium. There remains a tendency to utilize physical restraints postoperatively to prevent patients from disrupting their wounds; such restraints may increase the risk of delirium and therefore should be discontinued as soon as possible.

Postoperative delirium has been associated with a number of poor outcomes. Length of stay, postoperative complications, and mortality are known to increase in the setting of postoperative delirium.[20,22,23] Such patients are more likely to be discharged to a rehabilitation or long-term nursing facility than those without delirium. Postoperative delirium has also been associated with an increased risk of developing dementia in elderly patients with no known baseline cognitive dysfunction, suggesting that delirium may in itself cause long-term neurologic damage.[24]

Treatment of postoperative delirium involves early identification and exclusion of other potential causes of an altered mental state. This workup usually includes neuroimaging to assess for stroke, hemorrhage, or mass lesion; an electroencephalogram to evaluate for seizures; and possibly a lumbar puncture to evaluate for evidence of a cerebral inflammatory or infectious disorder. Treatment depends on identification and reversal of the underlying cause. In the postoperative period, delirium precautions should be instituted, including frequent reorientation, opening blinds to allow for natural light to enter, and maintaining normal sleep–wake cycles. Physical restraints should be discontinued as soon as is safe and replaced with close monitoring from nursing staff, sitters, or family members to ensure patient safety. Unnecessary lines and tubes, particularly urinary catheters, should be discontinued. Early postoperative mobilization, even range-of-motion exercises

TABLE 54-2 ■ Factors Commonly Associated with Delirium

Risk Factors	
Advanced age	Iatrogenic
Baseline cognitive impairment	Poor sleep hygiene
Infection	Physical restraints
Urinary tract infection	Urinary catheters
Pneumonia	Multiple surgical procedures
Toxic derangements	Untreated pain
Intoxication	Medications
Withdrawal (alcohol, benzodiazepines)	Anticholinergics
Poor baseline nutritional status (low serum albumin)	Benzodiazepines
	Barbiturates
Metabolic derangements	Opiates
Hepatic encephalopathy	Corticosteroids
Uremic encephalopathy	Muscle relaxants
Dehydration	Antibiotics (cephalosporins and fluoroquinolones)
Hypoxia and hypercarbia	
Electrolytes: hyponatremia/ hypernatremia, hypercalcemia, hypermagnesemia, hypophosphatemia	

for bedbound patients, and simple acts such as making patients' eyeglasses and hearing aids available are important in treating as well as preventing delirium. Psychoactive medications, particularly anticholinergics, should be discontinued whenever possible. Postoperative pain control should be with minimum levels of analgesics required for relief. If these nonpharmacologic interventions are insufficient, pharmacologic treatment should be considered only if patients pose a risk of direct harm to themselves or the staff, while taking care to avoid the benzodiazepine class of medications, which has a particularly poor cognitive side-effect profile. Common practice is to consider using a low dose of an antipsychotic medication, such as quetiapine, at bedtime.

Dementia

Patients with dementia who undergo surgery require special consideration. It is crucial to establish the patient's preoperative baseline cognitive and physical function with family and caregivers in order to assess accurately their postoperative level of functioning. Patients with dementia are often elderly and have numerous medical comorbidities as well as a poor nutritional status, dehydration, and baseline electrolyte abnormalities. These conditions should be optimized or corrected preoperatively in order to maximize recovery and shorten length of hospital stay. Acetylcholinesterase inhibitors used to treat dementia should be continued throughout the perioperative period, although this class of medications may prolong the effects of succinylcholine.

Patients with dementia are at an increased risk of numerous postoperative complications. In particular, they are at higher risk of postoperative renal failure, pneumonia, urinary tract infections, sepsis, and strokes compared to age-matched controls.[25] They also have an increased risk of postoperative delirium related to their baseline cognitive impairment and comorbidities.

Postoperative care for patients with dementia mostly revolves around the prevention and treatment of delirium. Although surgery alone may be sufficient to precipitate delirium in a patient with dementia, other triggers should still be investigated. Patients with Alzheimer disease, and probably many other neurodegenerative conditions, are at increased risk of seizures, emphasizing the need to obtain an electroencephalogram for those with an unexplained altered mental state postoperatively. Postoperative pain control can be challenging as patients with severe dementia may not be able to verbalize whether they are in pain. Pharmacologic management of delirium in patients with dementia should be used as infrequently as possible. Benzodiazepines in particular should be avoided, and low-dose antipsychotics should be used sparingly—a US Food and Drug Administration black box warning links antipsychotics to increased mortality among elderly patients. In patients with Lewy body dementia, antipsychotics should be avoided due to their profound sedating and extrapyramidal effects, which may be irreversible. Patients with dementia and their families should be counseled early regarding the possibility of a prolonged postoperative hospital course and the potential for discharge to a rehabilitation or nursing facility; in the setting of elective surgeries, these considerations may impact the decision to proceed.

TABLE 54-3 ■ Common Warning Features Associated with Secondary Headaches

Subjective	Physical Examination
New headache after age 50	Focal neurologic deficit
Change in character of prior headache	Fever
Worsens with Valsalva, exertion, cough, or sneezing	Hypertension
Awakens patient from sleep or typically occurs in the morning	Altered mental status
Associated seizure	Papilledema
Associated diplopia	Meningismus
Positional component	Scalp tenderness (especially over temporal artery)
Thunderclap in onset	
Immunocompromised state	
Jaw claudication	

HEADACHE

A detailed headache history is important when evaluating patients with postoperative headaches, as preexisting primary headache disorders, such as migraine and tension headache, are common and often exacerbated by the stress of surgery and the dehydration that accompanies the NPO status. There are numerous warning features in the history and physical examination that signal the possibility of a secondary headache phenomenon related to a structural brain injury (Table 54-3).

Migraine

Patients with migraine should have their prophylactic medications continued in the perioperative period. Their migraine-abortive agents should also be continued postoperatively, though caution should be exercised when prescribing triptan medications after vascular surgeries given their vasoactive properties. Intravenous hydration with normal saline and administration of antiemetics such as prochlorperazine may be useful for attacks even when the migraine is not accompanied by significant nausea and vomiting. A brief course of a nonsteroidal anti-inflammatory drug (e.g., naproxen or intravenous ketorolac) may be used in refractory cases.

Medication Overuse

As many as 4 percent of the population overuse analgesics for the treatment of pain including headache, and it is estimated that up to 1 percent of the general population have medication-overuse headache.[26] While postoperative pain may require narcotics, treatment of headaches with short-acting narcotics sometimes exacerbates the primary headache disorder and prolongs the period of recovery. Nearly all agents given to abort headache may be associated with medication-overuse headache. Treatment for this condition is gradual discontinuation of the medication; however, symptoms of opiate withdrawal including headache, nausea, vomiting, tachycardia, and insomnia are common, and therefore these medications are best weaned outside the perioperative period.[26]

Caffeine Withdrawal

Due to the high frequency of consumption, caffeine withdrawal has become a widely recognized source of headache. Cessation of caffeine intake in people with low-to-moderate daily caffeine consumption (235 mg, approximately 2.5 cups of coffee) was associated with high depression scores, fatigue, and headache in a controlled trial.[27] Headaches from caffeine withdrawal may begin 24 hours after cessation and last up to 5 or 6 days.[28] In patients with postoperative headache, a careful caffeine history should be taken and—when caffeine withdrawal is responsible—resumption of normal caffeine intake permitted.

Intracranial Hypotension

Dural puncture with resultant intracranial hypotension remains a common cause of perioperative headache with an incidence ranging from 2 to 36 percent after spinal anesthesia and as high as 85 percent after accidental dural puncture with a large-bore needle during epidural anesthesia.[29] Among such headaches, 90 percent will begin within 72 hours of the puncture and 66 percent within 48 hours.[30] A headache immediately following the procedure should raise suspicion of an alternate etiology. The headache of intracranial hypotension is typically located in the frontal and occipital regions, is exacerbated by an upright posture, and is

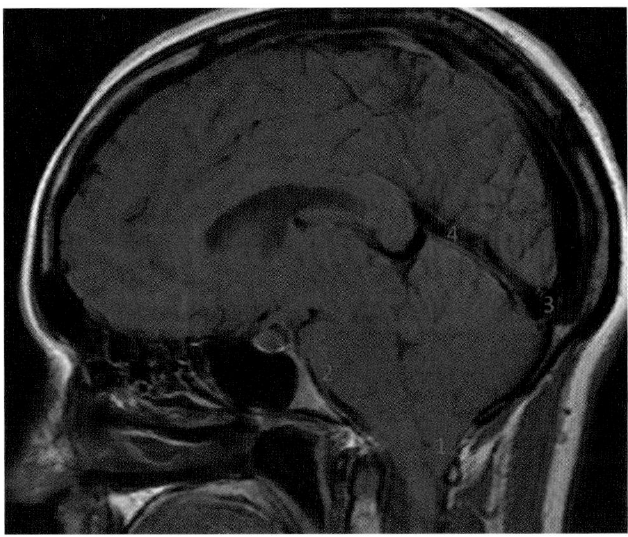

FIGURE 54-1 ■ Noncontrast sagittal T1 magnetic resonance image of a patient with cerebrospinal fluid leak and resultant intracranial hypotension. Image demonstrates downward descent of the cerebellar tonsils (1), effacement of the prepontine cistern with the pons apposed to the clivus (2), and prominent venous vasculature including the torcula (3) and straight sinus (4).

alleviated by recumbency. Accompanying symptoms may include nausea, vomiting, tinnitus, vertigo, paresthesias, diplopia, and cranial nerve palsies.[30] MRI findings of intracranial hypotension include diffuse pachymeningeal enhancement, subdural fluid collections, engorged cerebral venous sinuses, and descent of the cerebellar tonsils (Fig. 54-1).[31]

Prevention of post–dural puncture headache involves using a smaller gauge or noncutting needle. Caffeine, gabapentin, theophylline, and hydrocortisone have some efficacy in the treatment of such headache.[32] Epidural blood patch remains the mainstay of treatment; in a study of 504 patients, complete relief was noted in 75 percent, incomplete relief in 18 percent, and failure to relieve symptoms in only 7 percent.[33] If the initial blood patch does not relieve symptoms, a second blood patch should be administered, often with an extended period of lying supine following the procedure.

SEIZURES AND EPILEPSY

Epilepsy has a cumulative incidence of approximately 3 percent in the general population and is therefore commonly encountered in the perioperative period.[34] Perioperative seizures directly related to general anesthesia occur in only 2 percent of epileptic patients.[35] A large retrospective study demonstrated that recent (within 1 week) preoperative seizures were associated with a significantly higher likelihood of postoperative seizures.[36] Patients with epilepsy should be advised to take their antiepileptic medications on the morning of surgery, and these medications should be resumed as soon as possible postoperatively. Preferably, these drugs should be administered orally, although intravenous preparations of phenytoin, sodium valproate, levetiracetam, phenobarbital, lacosamide, and benzodiazepines are an alternative for those with limited oral intake. Oral and intravenous dosages are largely equivalent, but the frequency of administration may vary from one preparation to another, and some extended-release formulations may not be easily converted to an intravenous dose.

Both phenytoin and fosphenytoin can precipitate hypotension and arrhythmias with rapid intravenous infusion; however, fosphenytoin can generally be infused at a faster rate and with a lower risk of local adverse effects following extravasation, and therefore is the intravenous phenytoin preparation of choice.[37] Phenytoin can be administered via feeding tube, but levels are altered by enteral feedings, making the intravenous preparation preferable in such instances.[38]

Antiepileptic drug levels should not be checked routinely in the perioperative period unless there has been a recent change in seizure frequency or concern for drug toxicity. Antiepileptic medications have many drug interactions, particularly in the case of the cytochrome P450–inducing agents phenytoin, carbamazepine, phenobarbital, and primidone, which can result in decreased levels of many medications including some antibiotics, immunosuppressants, analgesics, and neuromuscular blocking agents.[39]

It is widely believed that some general anesthetics can have both pro- and anticonvulsant properties depending on the dose and clinical situation. Enflurane, sevoflurane, and etomidate induce epileptiform activity on the electroencephalogram and should generally be avoided in patients with epilepsy.[40,41] Concurrent administration of nitrous oxide may decrease the epileptogenic potential of sevoflurane.[41] Intravenous anesthetics including barbiturates and propofol are used for the treatment of status epilepticus, but at induction have been reported to be excitatory and can rarely precipitate a seizure.[42] Some opioids, particularly meperidine and to a lesser extent fentanyl, have been linked to seizures, especially with intrathecal use.[42] Propofol and opioids can also cause myoclonus and tremulousness that may clinically mimic seizures. Neuromuscular blocking agents have not been linked to seizures; however, if seizures are suspected while these drugs are being administered, continuous electroencephalographic monitoring is required as clinical manifestations of seizures will be masked.

Evidence regarding the epileptic potential of local anesthetics is conflicting, although they likely can cross the blood–brain barrier.[42] Studies investigating regional blockade in patients with epilepsy have concluded that perioperative seizures were not increased in frequency.[36]

Postoperative seizures should be considered as an etiology for delayed awaking after anesthesia. A relatively high frequency of seizures has been found in patients with altered mental state or "spells" both in the intensive care unit and in general medical wards.[43,44] If possible, an extended electroencephalogram should be obtained to exclude nonconvulsive seizures, but this should not delay treatment in cases where the suspicion of seizures is high.

NEUROMUSCULAR DISORDERS

Neuromuscular diseases present the neurologist, surgeon, and anesthesiologist with some important general considerations common to this group of disorders as well as challenges inherent to specific diseases. All patients with severe neuromuscular disease are at risk of increased ventilatory complications due to respiratory weakness, and preoperative pulmonary assessment with forced vital capacity and maximal inspiratory force should be performed. Complications in patients with respiratory weakness include an increased sensitivity to respiratory depression from opioids, barbiturates, and benzodiazepines, as well as difficulty in weaning from the ventilator. Patients with some neuromuscular disorders including the muscular dystrophies have an increased risk of life-threatening cardiac dysrhythmias along with depressed cardiac contractility, warranting a preoperative assessment with electrocardiography and echocardiography.[45] Depolarizing neuromuscular blockers such as succinylcholine can lead to hyperkalemia and resultant cardiac dysfunction in these patients and should be avoided.

Motor Neuron Disease

The timing of surgical procedures and anesthetic choice in patients with amyotrophic lateral sclerosis is important given an often profound progressive underlying respiratory weakness. Procedures such as percutaneous endoscopic gastrostomy should be undertaken when the forced vital capacity is still more than 50 percent of the predicted value.[46] There are reports of nondepolarizing neuromuscular blockade precipitating severe weakness in patients with amyotrophic lateral sclerosis.[47] The underlying mechanism may involve defective neuromuscular transmission in new nerve sprouts reaching previously denervated muscles. However, due to the previously described effects of succinylcholine in many neuromuscular disorders, low doses of nondepolarizing blockers are preferred when neuromuscular blockade is necessary.

A relationship between spinal anesthesia and worsening of symptoms in amyotrophic lateral sclerosis had previously been suggested.[48] More recent reports indicate that epidural anesthesia may be used safely in these patients without exacerbating neurologic symptoms.[49,50] Given the potential complications and prolonged recovery times following anesthesia and surgery, a multidisciplinary preoperative approach with cardiac and pulmonary screening is warranted, with appropriate preoperative counseling of the patient and family members regarding these risks.

Peripheral Nerve Disorders

The prevalence of diabetic autonomic neuropathy, a complication of both type 1 and type 2 diabetes, ranges from 7.7 percent in newly diagnosed diabetics to 90 percent in those awaiting pancreatic transplant.[51] Poor glycemic control and duration of disease are felt to be risk factors for the development and progression of the neuropathy.[51,52] These patients are at increased risk of significant bradycardia during induction of anesthesia as well as intraoperative hypotension requiring vasopressor support.[53,54] Although there are no specific guidelines for anesthetic choice, etomidate and opioids may minimize hemodynamic instability while thiopental and propofol may carry a higher risk of hypotension.[55]

Charcot–Marie–Tooth disease, the most common hereditary motor and sensory polyneuropathy, has also been associated with autonomic dysfunction.[56] Additionally, respiratory muscle weakness is found in a minority of patients. In a review of 86 patients with Charcot–Marie–Tooth disease undergoing surgery, few complications were seen.[57] Although succinylcholine was previously felt to be contraindicated, Antognini did not find a significantly increased risk of poor outcomes with this drug but still recommended avoidance if at all possible on theoretical grounds.[57]

Case series describe surgery as a potential trigger for acute inflammatory demyelinating polyradiculoneuropathy (AIDP; Guillain–Barré syndrome), a relatively common cause of acute paralysis. A recent retrospective analysis of 63 patients with AIDP found that 9.5 percent had undergone surgery within the prior 6 weeks and that the relative risk of developing AIDP in the 6-week postoperative period was 13 times higher than the baseline incidence in the population.[58] The precise mechanism for this association is unknown, but one theory is that surgery alters the immune system, igniting a pathway leading to molecular mimicry against peripheral nerve components, perhaps in the setting of postoperative infection.

With both AIDP and chronic inflammatory demyelinating polyradiculoneuropathy (CIDP), perioperative forced vital capacity and maximal inspiratory force should be monitored serially to provide some indication as to whether a patient can be extubated safely. Patients with AIDP and CIDP are sensitive to nondepolarizing muscle relaxants, which may necessitate prolonged postoperative ventilation when administered.[49,59] Reports of worsening neurologic function in patients with AIDP following epidural anesthesia exist.[60] Local anesthesia has been linked to hypotension, bradycardia, and cardiac complications in patients with AIDP, presumably due to involvement of the autonomic nervous system.[61] There are no firm recommendations regarding the preferred anesthetic technique for patients with AIDP and CIDP.

Myopathies

Patients with muscular dystrophies including Duchenne, Becker, and Emery–Dreifuss often undergo a series of surgeries in their lifetime involving tendon releases and correction of scoliosis. Due to the systemic nature of these disorders, a multidisciplinary perioperative approach involving a neurologist, pulmonologist, cardiologist, and anesthesiologist is often warranted. Many of these disorders are associated with cardiomyopathy and disorders of cardiac conduction.[62] Respiratory function is often compromised because of ventilatory muscle weakness as well as poor mechanics secondary to skeletal abnormalities. For patients with Duchenne muscular dystrophy, the American College of Chest Physicians recommends a thorough preoperative pulmonary evaluation including measurement of forced vital capacity, maximal inspiratory force, and peak cough flow.[63] Patients found to have a forced vital capacity of less than 50 percent of the predicted value should be considered for preoperative training of noninvasive positive pressure ventilation, given the risk of ventilatory compromise following surgery. Most muscular dystrophies are not linked to an increased incidence of malignant hyperthermia. Inhaled anesthetics such as halothane have been associated with rhabdomyolysis in the absence of succinylcholine in patients with elevated serum creatinine kinase levels at baseline.

Patients with other myopathies face similar risks associated with surgery and anesthesia. Reports of hyperkalemic cardiac arrest in children undergoing anesthesia have been linked to previously unrecognized myopathies.[64] Central core myopathy, an autosomal dominant disorder, has been closely linked to malignant hyperthermia, via a common mutation in the ryanodine receptor gene (*RYR1*).[65] The prevalence of malignant hyperthermia has been estimated at 1 per 100,000 hospital discharges in all patients.[66] This rare genetic condition is triggered by exposure to inhalational anesthetics or succinylcholine in susceptible individuals and is characterized by muscle rigidity, tachycardia, hyperthermia, hypercapnea, and metabolic acidosis. Malignant hyperthermia or a malignant hyperthermia-like syndrome has been described in a variety of myopathies and channelopathies (e.g., periodic paralysis).[62] The mainstay of treatment for malignant hyperthermia other than supportive care remains dantrolene, which decreases skeletal muscle calcium release, thereby inhibiting muscle contraction. If anesthesia is required in patients with myotonic dystrophy, depolarizing muscle relaxant drugs should be avoided because they may cause myotonic spasm, and nondepolarizing drugs are given in reduced dosage to patients who are taking quinine for their myotonia.

Myasthenia Gravis

Myasthenia gravis (MG) is the most common neuromuscular junction disorder, and consequently most of the research into the perioperative care of patients with such disorders has focused on MG. The preoperative care of patients with MG begins with appropriate counseling of the patient and family, emphasizing that the stress associated with elective surgery may temporarily worsen the disease, necessitate postoperative care in the intensive care unit, and lead to prolonged intubation. Since thymectomy is a treatment for MG, this surgery provides a natural avenue to study the perioperative care of patients with MG. A study of risk stratification of patients with MG undergoing thymectomy demonstrated that disease duration of greater than 6 years, a history of respiratory disease, daily pyridostigmine dose exceeding 750 mg, and a forced vital capacity of less than 2.9 liters predicted the need for postoperative ventilation.[67] This predictive tool may not apply to patients with MG undergoing surgeries other than thymectomy.[68] A preoperative neurologic examination focusing on facial strength, dysarthria, dysphagia, neck flexion, and formal pulmonary function testing, especially in those patients with bulbar weakness, allows for anticipation of postoperative ventilatory compromise and pulmonary complications including aspiration.

Numerous studies have investigated the effects of pyridostigmine on neuromuscular blockade in the perioperative period.[69–73] There is not sufficient evidence to conclude that changing a patient's pyridostigmine dose prior to surgery significantly impacts neuromuscular blockade or the duration of ventilation and thus the general recommendation is to continue the patient's usual preoperative regimen.[74] Most immunosuppressants in patients with MG do not interact with anesthetics; however, azathioprine extends the effect of succinylcholine and inhibits nondepolarizing neuromuscular blockers.[75]

Elective surgeries should be undertaken when respiratory function is stable and patients are on the lowest possible doses of corticosteroids. In the case of more urgent surgery, presurgical plasma exchange should be considered as it decreases the duration of postoperative ventilation and stay in the intensive care unit in patients undergoing thymectomy.[76] Intravenous immunoglobulin remains another option if plasma exchange is unavailable.

When possible, regional anesthesia is preferable to general anesthesia in patients with MG, as it minimizes the need for neuromuscular blockade and ventilation. Patients with MG have a decreased number of functional acetylcholine receptors and thus their response to neuromuscular blockade may be abnormal during general anesthesia.[77] Patients may have a prolonged blockade when either succinylcholine or nondepolarizing neuromuscular blockers are used.[75] The dosing of neuromuscular blockade should be individualized based on the severity of the patient's myasthenia; however, 50 percent of a routine dose is likely adequate and an extended recovery time should still be anticipated.[71,72,78,79]

Postoperative recovery in patients with MG may be prolonged. Electrolytes, particularly potassium, should be monitored closely, as hypokalemia may worsen weakness in MG. Whenever possible, postoperative analgesia should be minimized and opioids, benzodiazepines, and barbiturates should be avoided if possible due to their respiratory depressant effects. Patients with MG should have their medications reviewed frequently to ensure that they are not receiving drugs that may worsen weakness, such as aminoglycosides. If pyridostigmine cannot be given orally, the parenteral dose should be administered at roughly one-thirtieth of the enteral dose.[19] Atropine should be given before or concurrent with intravenous pyridostigmine to prevent bradycardia and excessive bronchial secretions. Although no precise clinical criteria can determine the timing of extubation, clinical examination including evaluation of neck flexor strength can guide the decision. After extubation, aggressive pulmonary toilet and use of incentive spirometry should be encouraged. Early mobilization shortens the duration of recovery.

Postoperative myasthenic crisis is not uncommon in patients with MG, with an incidence ranging from 12 to 34 percent following thymectomy.[80] The likelihood of postoperative crisis has been related to a prior history of myasthenic crisis, preoperative bulbar weakness, preoperative serum acetylcholine receptor antibody levels of greater than 100 nmol/L, and intraoperative blood loss of greater than 1 liter.[80] Management should involve

TABLE 54-4 ■ Incidence of Perioperative Stroke

Type of Surgery	Incidence (%)
General (no prior history of stroke)[81,82]	0.1–0.07
General (prior history of stroke)[83]	2.9
CABG[84]	3.8
Head and neck[85]	4.8
Cardiac valve[84]	4.8–8.8
CABG plus cardiac valve[84]	7.4
Aortic[86]	8.7
Multiple cardiac valves[84]	9.7

CABG, coronary artery bypass graft.

emergent assessment of the patient's respiratory status, recognizing that intubation is usually necessary. Effective treatment options include prompt initiation of plasma exchange or intravenous immunoglobulin.

PERIOPERATIVE STROKE

Incidence

The incidence of perioperative stroke varies with the type of surgery being performed (Table 54-4).[81–86] The incidence is relatively low among general surgeries but increases in those with prior stroke. Cardiac and aortic surgeries are associated with the highest risk of perioperative stroke, and this incidence increases with a number of operative factors. Aortic manipulation in the setting of known ascending aortic atherosclerosis increases stroke risk.[87] Long duration of cardiopulmonary bypass time (greater than 2 hours) is also an independent risk factor for stroke, probably secondary to multiple emboli as well as to hypoperfusion.[84,87,88] Additional discussion regarding stroke after cardiac surgery in children can be found in Chapter 3. The risk of perioperative stroke following carotid endarterectomy for symptomatic carotid stenosis has not changed significantly over time from the combined risk of 7 percent found in the European Carotid Surgery Trial and the North American Symptomatic Carotid Endarterectomy Trial.[89] Although the type of anesthesia has not been shown definitively to affect the perioperative stroke risk in patients undergoing carotid endarterectomy, regional anesthesia may be preferred and has been shown to limit a wide range of other perioperative complications in this population.[85,90]

Pathophysiology and Timing

The majority of perioperative strokes are ischemic, and a significant proportion demonstrate multiple areas of infarction, suggesting an embolic etiology.[91,92] A study aimed at elucidating the mechanism of perioperative stroke following coronary artery bypass graft surgery found that only 1 percent of strokes were hemorrhagic, and of the ischemic strokes, 62 percent were likely embolic.[93] A review of perioperative strokes found that a minority (5.8 to 16%) occurred during the procedure itself.[91,94] A study of 388 patients with perioperative stroke following coronary artery bypass graft demonstrated that 41.7 percent occurred on postoperative day 1, with an additional 20.4 percent presenting on the second postoperative day.[93] Early embolic strokes in the postoperative period have been attributed to physical manipulation of the heart or aorta during surgery leading to unstable plaque that can break off in the coming days, while more delayed embolic strokes may result from atrial fibrillation or decreased cardiac output in the postoperative period.[85–87] Notably, intraoperative hypoperfusion does not appear to be a common etiology for perioperative stroke but should be considered in the setting of deep watershed infarcts ipsilateral to carotid stenosis.[85]

Risk Factors

Both preoperative and postoperative risk factors can be identified. The most important preoperative risk factor is the presence of a prior stroke or transient ischemic attack.[84,87,91] A history of hypertension, diabetes, chronic obstructive pulmonary disease, peripheral vascular disease, decreased cardiac output, atrial fibrillation, aortic atherosclerosis, and female sex all serve as independent preoperative stroke risk factors.[84,87,88,91,95] Additional likely preoperative risk factors include myocardial infarction in the previous 6 months, current tobacco use, acute renal failure, and increased age.[82] Carotid stenosis and discontinuation of antithrombotic therapies are discussed separately.

Postoperative risk factors for stroke include the combination of low cardiac output and atrial fibrillation. Studies also suggest that blood loss (intraoperative or postoperative), hypotension, and dehydration may contribute to a hypercoagulable state leading to an increased risk of postoperative stroke.[81,84]

Risk Factor Modification and Postoperative Stroke Care

In patients with recent stroke or transient ischemic attack, it is important preoperatively to determine the etiology and whether it was treated appropriately. In cases of possible or known aortic atherosclerosis, the extent of the atherosclerotic plaque can be assessed preoperatively with transesophageal echocardiography, since some surgical techniques may need to be modified in order to minimize the risk of plaque rupture. Some patients with otherwise unexplained stroke will be found to have atrial fibrillation with extended cardiac telemetry.

New-onset atrial fibrillation following cardiac surgery occurs in 30 to 50 percent of patients.[85] The peak incidence occurs on postoperative days 2 to 4, and consideration should be given for postoperative cardiac telemetry monitoring. Patients with known atrial fibrillation should have their antiarrhythmic and rate-controlling medications continued throughout the perioperative period.[85] Volume status should be closely monitored. Although is it not common practice, there is some evidence that prophylactic use of amiodarone and beta-blockers in those not already taking these medications reduces the risk of postoperative atrial fibrillation.[96] There are no controlled trials assessing the utility of anticoagulation for the prevention of stroke in the setting of postoperative atrial fibrillation.

The duration of surgery, particularly the amount of time spent on cardiopulmonary bypass, should be minimized to decrease the perioperative stroke risk. Care should be taken to avoid manipulation of plaque in patients with aortic atheromas. There is a lack of data to suggest an optimal intraoperative blood pressure range. A randomized trial of patients undergoing coronary artery bypass grafting found that cardiac and neurologic complications were lower in patients with a high intraoperative mean arterial pressure (80 to 100 mmHg) compared with low pressure (50 to 60 mmHg).[97] A follow-up study examined the same high mean arterial pressure compared to a customized mean arterial pressure based on each patient's preoperative blood pressure and found no significant difference in cardiac or neurologic outcomes.[98] Intraoperative hyperglycemia has been linked to an excess risk of postoperative atrial fibrillation, but a trial of intense intraoperative glucose control using an insulin infusion found that—for uncertain reasons—these patients were actually at higher risk of postoperative stroke and death than those receiving conventional glucose control.[99,100]

Stroke care in the postoperative period differs in some respects from stroke care in other circumstances. Preoperative statin use, regardless of cholesterol levels, decreases a variety of postoperative cardiac and cerebrovascular events (e.g., death from cardiac causes, myocardial infarction, unstable angina, and stroke) in patients undergoing vascular surgery.[101] Intravenous tissue plasminogen activator is contraindicated following major surgery but many reports document the safety of intra-arterial thrombolysis or thrombectomy for perioperative stroke.[102–104]

Antithrombotics and Anticoagulation in the Perioperative Period

While randomized prospective trials examining the use of antiplatelet agents and anticoagulants in the perioperative period are lacking, there is some evidence to guide clinical decisions. Perioperative stroke risk is increased with discontinuation of antiplatelet medications and anticoagulants.[105–107] A large retrospective study of 2,197 patients with ischemic stroke found that 114 (5.2%) of strokes occurred within 60 days of discontinuing oral antithrombotics.[108] Of these 114 ischemic strokes, 71 (62%) were first-ever strokes and 47 percent of these occurred after medications were stopped in the periprocedural period.

Early postoperative aspirin administration is associated with a 50 percent decrease in the rate of perioperative stroke following coronary artery bypass graft procedures.[109] Compared with aspirin, less is known about the use of clopidogrel in the perioperative period. Studies demonstrate a decreased risk of myocardial infarction but increased transfusion requirements and reoperation rates in patients receiving clopidogrel within 5 days of surgery.[110,111] A recent retrospective study compared three groups: continuation of clopidogrel throughout the perioperative period; replacement of clopidogrel with a different bridging antithrombotic such as aspirin; and discontinuation of clopidogrel without a bridging agent.[112] Although the patients who continued clopidogrel had higher rates of transfusions, there was no difference in postoperative myocardial infarction, stroke, or mortality found between the three groups.

A number of studies have examined the safety and efficacy of anticoagulation in the perioperative period. A large review of patients receiving long-term oral anticoagulation who underwent surgery or other invasive procedures showed that the rate of stroke was 0.4 percent if oral anticoagulation was continued, 0.6 percent if oral anticoagulation was discontinued and intravenous heparin was not used as a bridge, and 0 percent when oral anticoagulation was used with intravenous heparin bridging.[105] The rates of major bleeding in those who continued their preoperative anticoagulation was 0.2 percent for dental procedures and was 0 percent for arthrocentesis, cataract surgery, endoscopy, and colonoscopy (with or without biopsy), identifying a subset of procedures where anticoagulation can likely be continued. Another study of select patients at risk of thromboembolism demonstrated that moderate-intensity anticoagulation (target International Normalized Ratio of 1.5–2.0) was safe and adequate to minimize stroke risk.[113] Less is known about the perioperative risk associated with the newer anticoagulants including the direct thrombin inhibitor dabigitran and the factor Xa inhibitors rivaroxiban and apixaban.

The American College of Chest Physicians has published recent evidence-based guidelines regarding the use of antithrombotics and anticoagulants in the perioperative period.[114] Patients at high risk of thromboembolism who require interruption of oral anticoagulation should receive bridging anticoagulation and should have oral anticoagulation resumed within 12 to 24 hours postoperatively. In patients taking aspirin who are at moderate to high risk of cardiovascular events, the recommendation is to continue aspirin throughout the perioperative period. Among those patients at low risk of cardiovascular events, aspirin should be stopped 7 to 10 days prior to surgery.

Timing of Elective Surgery Following a Stroke

There are few data to guide the timing of elective surgery under general anesthesia following a stroke. Recent stroke patients need a thorough evaluation of stroke etiology prior to being considered for elective surgery. This should include evaluation of the carotid arteries as carotid endarterectomy may be warranted prior to elective surgery for symptomatic disease. Delaying elective surgery following a stroke is based on the theoretical risk of recurrent stroke due to changes in cerebral autoregulation and ongoing inflammation as the brain heals. Accordingly, delaying elective surgery for 4 weeks appears to be sufficient to allow for elimination of this added risk.[115]

Perioperative Considerations Pertaining to Carotid Disease

Discovery of a carotid bruit is not uncommon as part of the preoperative clinical evaluation. An asymptomatic carotid bruit is a marker of general vascular disease and has been associated with the presence of aortic atheromas.[116] However, a prospective study of patients with asymptomatic carotid bruits demonstrated that only 50 percent of patients were found to have carotid stenosis of greater than 50 percent.[117] Therefore, determining which patients with a carotid bruit should undergo carotid imaging is difficult. Patients with symptoms of a stroke or transient ischemic attack over the past 6 months to suggest that the stenosis is symptomatic should undergo imaging, but those without symptoms likely should not unless a surgery is planned with a high risk of hypotension, as unilateral asymptomatic stenosis alone does not increase perioperative stroke risk.

The decision to recommend carotid endarterectomy prior to another surgery depends on whether the patient's carotid stenosis is symptomatic or asymptomatic. A review of carotid artery disease in patients undergoing coronary artery bypass grafting yielded the following stroke rates in asymptomatic carotid stenosis: 1.8 percent in patients without significant carotid stenosis, 3.2 percent in patients with unilateral 50 to 99 percent stenosis, 5.2 percent in patients with bilateral 50 to 99 percent stenosis, and 7 to 11 percent in patients with unilateral carotid occlusion.[118] The risk of perioperative stroke related to unilateral carotid stenosis may be overestimated as many studies do not account for whether the observed stroke occurred in the hemisphere ipsilateral to the stenosis. A study of 358 consecutive patients with varying degrees of asymptomatic and symptomatic carotid stenosis undergoing cardiac or vascular surgeries found that none of the patients with asymptomatic stenosis experienced a perioperative stroke, allowing the authors to conclude that the low risk of perioperative stroke in patients with asymptomatic carotid stenosis does not justify prophylactic carotid endarterectomy.[119] In patients with recently symptomatic severe carotid stenosis who require routine or elective cardiac or vascular surgery, the recommendation is to perform carotid endarterectomy within 2 weeks of the cerebrovascular event for nondisabling stroke or transient ischemic attack and to delay elective surgeries until after the endarterectomy.

Patients with concomitant symptomatic carotid and cardiac disease requiring more urgent cardiac surgery are complicated. Studies have examined a staged approach where carotid endarterectomy is performed prior to cardiac surgery compared with performing the two procedures simultaneously. A 10-year review demonstrated no significant differences in mortality or neurologic complications between the two approaches and demonstrated that the staged procedure was associated with a higher overall complication rate and increased hospital costs.[120] A 2005 evidence-based review published by the American Academy of Neurology concluded that there is insufficient evidence to suggest whether preoperative or concurrent carotid revascularization is superior prior to coronary artery bypass grafting.[121]

REFERENCES

1. Hirtz D, Thurman DJ, Gwinn-Hardy K, et al: How common are the "common" neurologic disorders? Neurology 68:326, 2007.
2. Furuya R, Hirai A, Andoh T, et al: Successful perioperative management of a patient with Parkinson's disease by enteral levodopa administration under propofol anesthesia. Anesthesiology 89:261, 1998.
3. Wüllner U, Kassubek J, Odin P, et al: Transdermal rotigotine for the perioperative management of Parkinson's disease. J Neural Transm 117:855, 2010.
4. Nicholson G, Pereira AC, Hall GM: Parkinson's disease and anaesthesia. Br J Anaesth 89:904, 2002.
5. Brennan KA, Genever RW: Managing Parkinson's disease during surgery. BMJ 341:c5718, 2010.
6. Golden WE, Lavender RC, Metzer WS: Acute postoperative confusion and hallucinations in Parkinson disease. Ann Intern Med 111:218, 1989.
7. Pepper PV, Goldstein MK: Postoperative complications in Parkinson's disease. J Am Geriatr Soc 47:967, 1999.
8. Aminoff MJ, Christine CW, Friedman JH, et al: Management of the hospitalized patient with Parkinson's disease: current state of the field and need for guidelines. Parkinsonism Relat Disord 17:139, 2011.
9. Machado A, Rezai AR, Kopell BH, et al: Deep brain stimulation for Parkinson's disease: surgical technique and perioperative management. Mov Disord 21(suppl 14):S247, 2006.
10. Frucht SJ: Movement disorder emergencies in the perioperative period. Neurol Clin 22:379, 2004.
11. Perumal J, Khan O: Emerging disease-modifying therapies in multiple sclerosis. Curr Treat Options Neurol 14:256, 2012.
12. Smeltzer SC, Skurnick JH, Troiano R, et al: Respiratory function in multiple sclerosis. Utility of clinical assessment of respiratory muscle function. Chest 101:479, 1992.
13. Sakurai M, Mannen T, Kanazawa I, et al: Lidocaine unmasks silent demyelinative lesions in multiple sclerosis. Neurology 42:2088, 1992.
14. Bamford C, Sibley W, Laguna J: Anesthesia in multiple sclerosis. Can J Neurol Sci 5:41, 1978.
15. Hebl JR, Horlocker TT, Schroeder DR: Neuraxial anesthesia and analgesia in patients with preexisting central nervous system disorders. Anesth Analg 103:223, 2006.
16. Neal JM, Bernards CM, Hadzic A, et al: ASRA practice advisory on neurologic complications in regional anesthesia and pain medicine. Reg Anesth Pain Med 33:404, 2008.
17. Dorotta IR, Schubert A: Multiple sclerosis and anesthetic implications. Curr Opin Anaesthesiol 15:365, 2002.
18. Coffey RJ, Edgar TS, Francisco GE, et al: Abrupt withdrawal from intrathecal baclofen: recognition and management of a potentially life-threatening syndrome. Arch Phys Med Rehabil 83:735, 2002.
19. Rubino FA: Perioperative management of patients with neurologic disease. Neurol Clin 22:261, 2004.
20. Berggren D, Gustafson Y, Eriksson B, et al: Postoperative confusion after anesthesia in elderly patients with femoral neck fractures. Anesth Analg 66:497, 1987.
21. Mason SE, Noel-Storr A, Ritchie CW: The impact of general and regional anesthesia on the incidence of post-operative cognitive dysfunction and post-operative delirium: a systematic review with meta-analysis. J Alzheimers Dis 22(suppl 3):67, 2010.
22. Robinson TN, Raeburn CD, Tran ZV, et al: Postoperative delirium in the elderly: risk factors and outcomes. Ann Surg 249:173, 2009.
23. Marcantonio ER, Goldman L, Mangione CM, et al: A clinical prediction rule for delirium after elective noncardiac surgery. JAMA 271:134, 1994.

24. Wacker P, Nunes PV, Cabrita H, et al: Post-operative delirium is associated with poor cognitive outcome and dementia. Dementia Geriatr Cognit Disord 21:221, 2006.
25. Hu CJ, Liao CC, Chang CC, et al: Postoperative adverse outcomes in surgical patients with dementia: a retrospective cohort study. World J Surg 36:2051, 2012.
26. Diener HC, Limmroth V: Medication-overuse headache: a worldwide problem. Lancet Neurol 3:475, 2004.
27. Silverman K, Evans SM, Strain EC, et al: Withdrawal syndrome after the double-blind cessation of caffeine consumption. N Engl J Med 327:1109, 1992.
28. Fennelly M, Galletly DC, Purdie GI: Is caffeine withdrawal the mechanism of postoperative headache? Anesth Analg 72:449, 1991.
29. Olsen KS: Epidural blood patch in the treatment of post-lumbar puncture headache. Pain 30:293, 1987.
30. Turnbull DK, Shepherd DB: Post-dural puncture headache: pathogenesis, prevention and treatment. Br J Anaesth 91:718, 2003.
31. Mokri B: Headaches caused by decreased intracranial pressure: diagnosis and management. Curr Opin Neurol 16:319, 2003.
32. Basurto Ona X, Martinez García L, Solà I, et al: Drug therapy for treating post-dural puncture headache. Cochrane Database Syst Rev 8:CD007887, 2011.
33. Safa-Tisseront V, Thormann F, Malassiné P, et al: Effectiveness of epidural blood patch in the management of post-dural puncture headache. Anesthesiology 95:334, 2001.
34. Hauser WA, Annegers JF, Kurland LT: Incidence of epilepsy and unprovoked seizures in Rochester, Minnesota: 1935-1984. Epilepsia 34:453, 1993.
35. Benish SM, Cascino GD, Warner ME, et al: Effect of general anesthesia in patients with epilepsy: a population-based study. Epilepsy Behav 17:87, 2010.
36. Kopp SL, Wynd KP, Horlocker TT, et al: Regional blockade in patients with a history of a seizure disorder. Anesth Analg 109:272, 2009.
37. Browne TR, Kugler AR, Eldon MA: Pharmacology and pharmacokinetics of fosphenytoin. Neurology 46(suppl 1):S3, 1996.
38. Au Yeung SC, Ensom MH: Phenytoin and enteral feedings: does evidence support an interaction? Ann Pharmacother 34:896, 2000.
39. Patsalos PN, Perucca E: Clinically important drug interactions in epilepsy: interactions between antiepileptic drugs and other drugs. Lancet Neurol 2:473, 2003.
40. Voss LJ, Sleigh JW, Barnard JP, et al: The howling cortex: seizures and general anesthetic drugs. Anesth Analg 107:1689, 2008.
41. Iijima T, Nakamura Z, Iwao Y, et al: The epileptogenic properties of the volatile anesthetics sevoflurane and isoflurane in patients with epilepsy. Anesth Analg 91:989, 2000.
42. Perks A, Cheema S, Mohanraj R: Anaesthesia and epilepsy. Br J Anaesth 108:562, 2012.
43. Kamel H, Betjemann JP, Navi BB, et al: Diagnostic yield of electroencephalography in the medical and surgical intensive care unit. Neurocrit Care 19:336, 2013.
44. Betjemann JP, Nguyen I, Santos-Sanchez C, et al: Diagnostic yield of electroencephalography in a general inpatient population. Mayo Clin Proc 88:326, 2013.
45. Lieb K, Selim M: Preoperative evaluation of patients with neurological disease. Semin Neurol 28:603, 2008.
46. Miller RG, Rosenberg JA, Gelinas DF, et al: Practice parameter: the care of the patient with amyotrophic lateral sclerosis. (An evidence-based review). Muscle Nerve 22:1104, 1999.
47. Rosenbaum KJ, Neich JL, Strobel GE: Sensitivity to nondepolarizing muscle relaxants in amyotrophic lateral sclerosis: report of two cases. Anesthesiology 35:638, 1971.
48. Dripps RD, Vandam LD: Exacerbation of pre-existing neurologic disease after spinal anesthesia. N Engl J Med 255:843, 1956.
49. Hara K, Sakura S, Saito Y, et al: Epidural anesthesia and pulmonary function in a patient with amyotrophic lateral sclerosis. Anesth Analg 83:878, 1996.
50. Kochi T, Oka T, Mizuguchi T: Epidural anesthesia for patients with amyotrophic lateral sclerosis. Anesth Analg 68:410, 1989.
51. Vinik AI, Maser RE, Mitchell BD, et al: Diabetic autonomic neuropathy. Diabetes Care 26:1553, 2003.
52. Vinik AI, Ziegler D: Diabetic cardiovascular autonomic neuropathy. Circulation 115:387, 2007.
53. Maser RE, Lenhard MJ: Cardiovascular autonomic neuropathy due to diabetes mellitus: clinical manifestations, consequences, and treatment. J Clin Endocrinol Metab 90:5896, 2005.
54. Burgos LG, Ebert TJ, Asiddao C, et al: Increased intraoperative cardiovascular morbidity in diabetics with autonomic neuropathy. Anesthesiology 70:591, 1989.
55. Oakley I, Emond L: Diabetic cardiac autonomic neuropathy and anesthetic management: review of the literature. J Am Assoc Nurse Anesth 79:473, 2011.
56. Shankar V, Markan S, Gandhi SD, et al: Perioperative implications of Charcot-Marie-Tooth disease during coronary artery bypass graft surgery. J Cardiothorac Vasc Anesth 21:567, 2007.
57. Antognini JF: Anaesthesia for Charcot-Marie-Tooth disease: a review of 86 cases. Can J Anaesth 39:398, 1992.
58. Gensicke H, Datta AN, Dill P, et al: Increased incidence of Guillain-Barré syndrome after surgery. Eur J Neurol 19:1239, 2012.
59. Brooks H, Christian AS, May AE: Pregnancy, anaesthesia and Guillain-Barré syndrome. Anaesthesia 55:894, 2000.

60. Wiertlewski S, Magot A, Drapier S, et al: Worsening of neurologic symptoms after epidural anesthesia for labor in a Guillain-Barré patient. Anesth Analg 98:825, 2004.
61. Perel A, Reches A, Davidson JT: Anaesthesia in the Guillain-Barré syndrome. A case report and recommendations. Anaesthesia 32:257, 1977.
62. Bertorini TE: Perisurgical management of patients with neuromuscular disorders. Neurol Clin 22:293, 2004.
63. Birnkrant DJ, Panitch HB, Benditt JO, et al: American College of Chest Physicians consensus statement on the respiratory and related management of patients with Duchenne muscular dystrophy undergoing anesthesia or sedation. Chest 132:1977, 2007.
64. Larach MG, Rosenberg H, Gronert GA, et al: Hyperkalemic cardiac arrest during anesthesia in infants and children with occult myopathies. Clin Pediatr (Philadelphia) 36:9, 1997.
65. Quane KA, Healy JM, Keating KE, et al: Mutations in the ryanodine receptor gene in central core disease and malignant hyperthermia. Nat Genet 5:51, 1993.
66. Brady JE, Sun LS, Rosenberg H, et al: Prevalence of malignant hyperthermia due to anesthesia in New York State, 2001–2005. Anesth Analg 109:1162, 2009.
67. Leventhal SR, Orkin FK, Hirsh RA: Prediction of the need for postoperative mechanical ventilation in myasthenia gravis. Anesthesiology 53:26, 1980.
68. Grant RP, Jenkins LC: Prediction of the need for postoperative mechanical ventilation in myasthenia gravis: thymectomy compared to other surgical procedures. Can Anaesth Soc J 29:112, 1982.
69. Eisenkraft JB, Book WJ, Papatestas AE: Sensitivity to vecuronium in myasthenia gravis: a dose-response study. Can J Anaesth 37:301, 1990.
70. Nilsson E, Meretoja OA: Vecuronium dose-response and maintenance requirements in patients with myasthenia gravis. Anesthesiology 73:28, 1990.
71. Sanfilippo M, Fierro G, Cavalletti MV, et al: Rocuronium in two myasthenic patients undergoing thymectomy. Acta Anaesthesiol Scand 41:1365, 1997.
72. Baraka A, Siddik S, Kawkabani N: Cisatracurium in a myasthenic patient undergoing thymectomy. Can J Anaesth 46:779, 1999.
73. Baraka A, Taha S, Yazbeck V, et al: Vecuronium block in the myasthenic patient. Influence of anticholinesterase therapy. Anaesthesia 48:588, 1993.
74. Dillon FX: Anesthesia issues in the perioperative management of myasthenia gravis. Semin Neurol 24:83, 2004.
75. Blichfeldt-Lauridsen L, Hansen BD: Anesthesia and myasthenia gravis. Acta Anaesthesiol Scand 56:17, 2012.
76. d'Empaire G, Hoaglin DC, Perlo VP, et al: Effect of prethymectomy plasma exchange on postoperative respiratory function in myasthenia gravis. J Thorac Cardiovasc Surg 89:592, 1985.
77. Baraka A: Anaesthesia and myasthenia gravis. Can J Anaesth 39:476, 1992.
78. Paterson IG, Hood JR, Russell SH, et al: Mivacurium in the myasthenic patient. Br J Anaesth 73:494, 1994.
79. Sungur Ulke Z, Senturk M: Mivacurium in patients with myasthenia gravis undergoing video-assisted thoracoscopic thymectomy. Br J Anaesth 103:310, 2009.
80. Wendell LC, Levine JM: Myasthenic crisis. Neurohospitalist 1:16, 2011.
81. Kam PC, Calcroft RM: Peri-operative stroke in general surgical patients. Anaesthesia 52:879, 1997.
82. Mashour GA, Shanks AM, Kheterpal S: Perioperative stroke and associated mortality after noncardiac, nonneurologic surgery. Anesthesiology 114:1289, 2011.
83. Landercasper J, Merz BJ, Cogbill TH, et al: Perioperative stroke risk in 173 consecutive patients with a past history of stroke. Arch Surg 125:986, 1990.
84. Bucerius J, Gummert JF, Borger MA, et al: Stroke after cardiac surgery: a risk factor analysis of 16,184 consecutive adult patients. Ann Thorac Surg 75:472, 2003.
85. Selim M: Perioperative stroke. N Engl J Med 356:706, 2007.
86. McKhann GM, Grega MA, Borowicz LM, et al: Stroke and encephalopathy after cardiac surgery: an update. Stroke 37:562, 2006.
87. Hogue CW, Murphy SF, Schechtman KB, et al: Risk factors for early or delayed stroke after cardiac surgery. Circulation 100:642, 1999.
88. Likosky DS, Caplan LR, Weintraub RM, et al: Intraoperative and postoperative variables associated with strokes following cardiac surgery. Heart Surg Forum 7:E271, 2004.
89. Bond R, Rerkasem K, Shearman CP, et al: Time trends in the published risks of stroke and death due to endarterectomy for symptomatic carotid stenosis. Cerebrovasc Dis 18:37, 2004.
90. Schechter MA, Shortell CK, Scarborough JE: Regional versus general anesthesia for carotid endarterectomy: the American College of Surgeons National Surgical Quality Improvement Program perspective. Surgery 152:309, 2012.
91. Limburg M, Wijdicks EF, Li H: Ischemic stroke after surgical procedures: clinical features, neuroimaging, and risk factors. Neurology 50:895, 1998.
92. Restrepo L, Wityk RJ, Grega MA, et al: Diffusion- and perfusion-weighted magnetic resonance imaging of the brain before and after coronary artery bypass grafting surgery. Stroke 33:2909, 2002.
93. Likosky DS, Marrin CA, Caplan LR, et al: Determination of etiologic mechanisms of strokes secondary to coronary artery bypass graft surgery. Stroke 34:2830, 2003.
94. Ng JL, Chan MT, Gelb AW: Perioperative stroke in noncardiac, nonneurosurgical surgery. Anesthesiology 115:879, 2011.
95. Larsen SF, Zaric D, Boysen G: Postoperative cerebrovascular accidents in general surgery. Acta Anaesthesiol Scand 32:698, 1988.

96. Crystal E, Connolly SJ, Sleik K, et al: Interventions on prevention of postoperative atrial fibrillation in patients undergoing heart surgery; a meta-analysis. Circulation 106:75, 2002.
97. Gold JP, Charlson ME, Williams-Russo P, et al: Improvement of outcomes after coronary artery bypass: a randomized trial comparing intraoperative high versus low mean arterial pressure. J Thorac Cardiovasc Surg 110:1302, 1995.
98. Charlson ME, Peterson JC, Krieger KH, et al: Improvement of outcomes after coronary artery bypass II: a randomized trial comparing intraoperative high versus customized mean arterial pressure. J Card Surg 22:465, 2007.
99. Gandhi GY, Nuttall GA, Abel MD, et al: Intraoperative hyperglycemia and perioperative outcomes in cardiac surgery patients. Mayo Clin Proc 80:862, 2005.
100. Gandhi GY, Nuttall GA, Abel MD, et al: Intensive intraoperative insulin therapy versus conventional glucose management during cardiac surgery: a randomized trial. Ann Intern Med 146:233, 2007.
101. Durazzo AE, Machado FS, Ikeoka DT, et al: Reduction in cardiovascular events after vascular surgery with atorvastatin: a randomized trial. J Vasc Surg 39:967, 2004.
102. Chalela JA, Katzan I, Liebeskind DS, et al: Safety of intra-arterial thrombolysis in the postoperative period. Stroke 32:1365, 2001.
103. Fukuda I, Imazuru T, Osaka M, et al: Thrombolytic therapy for delayed, in-hospital stroke after cardiac surgery. Ann Thorac Surg 76:1293, 2003.
104. Moazami N, Smedira NG, McCarthy PM, et al: Safety and efficacy of intraarterial thrombolysis for perioperative stroke after cardiac operation. Ann Thorac Surg 72:1933, 2001.
105. Dunn AS, Turpie AG: Perioperative management of patients receiving oral anticoagulants: a systematic review. Arch Intern Med 163:901, 2003.
106. Blacker DJ, Wijdicks EF, McClelland RL: Stroke risk in anticoagulated patients with atrial fibrillation undergoing endoscopy. Neurology 61:964, 2003.
107. Maulaz AB, Bezerra DC, Michel P, et al: Effect of discontinuing aspirin therapy on the risk of brain ischemic stroke. Arch Neurol 62:1217, 2005.
108. Broderick JP, Bonomo JB, Kissela BM, et al: Withdrawal of antithrombotic agents and its impact on ischemic stroke occurrence. Stroke 42:2509, 2011.
109. Mangano DT: Aspirin and mortality from coronary bypass surgery. N Engl J Med 347:1309, 2002.
110. Vorobcsuk A, Aradi D, Farkasfalvi K, et al: Outcomes of patients receiving clopidogrel prior to cardiac surgery. Int J Cardiol 156:34, 2012.
111. Biancari F, Airaksinen KE, Lip GY: Benefits and risks of using clopidogrel before coronary artery bypass surgery: systematic review and meta-analysis of randomized trials and observational studies. J Thorac Cardiovasc Surg 143:665, 2012.
112. Paul S, Stock C, Chiu YL, et al: Management and outcomes of patients on preoperative Plavix (clopidogrel) undergoing general thoracic surgery. Thorac Cardiovasc Surg 61:489, 2013.
113. Larson BJ, Zumberg MS: Kitchens CS. A feasibility study of continuing dose-reduced warfarin for invasive procedures in patients with high thromboembolic risk. Chest 127:922, 2005.
114. Douketis JD, Spyropoulos AC, Spencer FA, et al: Perioperative management of antithrombotic therapy: antithrombotic therapy and prevention of thrombosis, 9th ed: American College of Chest Physicians evidence-based clinical practice guidelines. Chest 141(suppl 2):e326S, 2012.
115. Blacker DJ, Flemming KD, Link MJ, et al: The preoperative cerebrovascular consultation: common cerebrovascular questions before general or cardiac surgery. Mayo Clin Proc 79:223, 2004.
116. Katz ES, Tunick PA, Rusinek H, et al: Protruding aortic atheromas predict stroke in elderly patients undergoing cardiopulmonary bypass: experience with intraoperative transesophageal echocardiography. J Am Coll Cardiol 20:70, 1992.
117. Mackey AE, Abrahamowicz M, Langlois Y, et al: Outcome of asymptomatic patients with carotid disease. Neurology 48:896, 1997.
118. Naylor AR, Mehta Z, Rothwell PM, et al: Carotid artery disease and stroke during coronary artery bypass: a critical review of the literature. Eur J Vasc Endovasc Surg 23:283, 2002.
119. Gerraty RP, Gates PC, Doyle JC: Carotid stenosis and perioperative stroke risk in symptomatic and asymptomatic patients undergoing vascular or coronary surgery. Stroke 24:1115, 1993.
120. Gopaldas RR, Chu D, Dao TK, et al: Staged versus synchronous carotid endarterectomy and coronary artery bypass grafting: analysis of 10-year nationwide outcomes. Ann Thorac Surg 91:1323, 2011.
121. Chaturvedi S, Bruno A, Feasby T, et al: Carotid endarterectomy - an evidence-based review: report of the Therapeutics and Technology Assessment Subcommittee of the American Academy of Neurology. Neurology 65:794, 2005.

CHAPTER

55

Neurologic Disorders and Anesthesia

ALEJANDRO A. RABINSTEIN

Current rates of anesthetic complications are low regardless of the type of anesthesia (general, regional, or local). Yet among the complications that may occur, those affecting the nervous system are perhaps the most feared (Table 55-1). This chapter reviews anesthetic-related perioperative neurologic problems as well as perioperative complications that are not caused by anesthesia but are often erroneously attributed to it. Considerations regarding the challenges of anesthesia in patients with established neurologic disease are considered but are discussed in more detail in Chapter 54.

PERIOPERATIVE MENTAL STATUS CHANGES

Postoperative Coma and Delayed Awakening

Failure to arouse and delayed awakening are the most common early neurologic problems following general anesthesia. True prolonged postoperative coma is relatively uncommon, with estimates ranging from 0.005 to 0.08 percent following general surgery, but with higher rates reported after cardiac surgery.[1–4] Advanced age, urgent surgery, preexisting brain disorders, perioperative hypotension, postoperative organ failure, and sepsis are independently associated with postoperative coma.[3,5]

Delayed emergence from anest hesia is the most common cause of early failure to regain alertness after surgery; although this situation is benign, more serious alternative causes include stroke, anoxic-ischemic brain injury, and status epilepticus. Sepsis and multiorgan failure may produce severe encephalopathy and prolong unresponsiveness, sometimes for days after their resolution. The main causes of impairment of consciousness following surgery are found in Table 55-2.

When a neurologist is asked to evaluate an unresponsive patient following surgery, the principal goal is to determine whether any form of severe acute neurologic disease is responsible. It is therefore important to obtain a detailed history of the patient's preoperative status, review pertinent intraoperative information, and clarify the condition of the patient since surgery. In these situations, direct communication with the anesthesia and surgical teams may provide additional relevant information, such as the presence of clinical

Aminoff's Neurology and General Medicine, Fifth Edition.

TABLE 55-1 ■ Major Neurologic Complications of Different Types of Anesthesia

General Anesthesia
Postoperative coma and delayed awakening
Postoperative delirium
Postoperative cognitive dysfunction
Seizures
Malignant hyperthermia
Worsening or relapse of preexisting neurologic disease
Ischemic optic neuropathy
Regional Anesthesia
CNS toxicity
Postoperative cognitive dysfunction
Seizures
Headache after dural puncture
Epidural hematoma
Epidural abscess
Neuropathy
Transient pain in buttocks and legs
Worsening or relapse of preexisting neurologic disease
Ischemic optic neuropathy
Transient hypoacusis
Cranial nerve palsies
Local Anesthesia
Neuropathy

From Rabinstein AA, Keegan MT: Neurologic complications of anesthesia: a practical approach. Neurology Clin Pract 3:295, 2013, with permission.

features suggesting seizure occurrence or a history of immediate awakening followed by unconsciousness, suggesting cerebral embolism or seizures. It should be determined whether the patient became hypoxemic, hypotensive, or had marked lability of blood pressure; profuse blood loss; poor hemostasis; or cardiac arrhythmias during or immediately after surgery. Intraoperative hypotension and fluctuations in hemodynamic parameters are common in patients with postoperative coma after cardiovascular surgery.[4,6]

General clinical examination is important. A slow respiratory pattern and darkened skin color raises the possibility of CO_2 narcosis. An irregular pulse may signify atrial fibrillation and its increased risk of postoperative stroke. Splinter hemorrhages in the conjunctiva or nail bed suggest fat embolism after long-bone fracture surgery. The neurologic examination should focus on the assessment of level of consciousness, brainstem reflexes, gaze (conjugate versus dysconjugate, presence of skew deviation), eye movements (roving, ocular dipping or bobbing, nystagmoid jerks), muscle tone, response to central (sternal or supraorbital) and peripheral (limb) pain, and presence of adventitious movements. The presence of lateralizing signs requires brain imaging. Brainstem findings or bilateral focal signs should raise suspicion of basilar thromboembolism, prompting vessel imaging. Subtle abnormal movements of the eyes, facial muscles, or fingers may be the only manifestations of underlying status epilepticus and necessitate urgent electroencephalography (EEG). Drug toxicity should be suspected in patients with rigidity, hyperreflexia, and tremors, with or without concurrent fever. Myoclonus may occur with any toxic or metabolic encephalopathy, but can also follow severe global brain anoxia. Asterixis may be a sign of hyperammonemia but also occurs in other metabolic encephalopathies and as a side effect of medications. In patients lacking motor responses after pharmacologic neuromuscular blockade, it must be determined—sometimes by electrophysiologic nerve-stimulation studies—whether blockade is continuing; when paralysis is persistent, administration of an antidote may require consideration.

Additional testing is directed by the history and physical findings. If reassuring and nonfocal, further investigations can be postponed. Brain imaging is indicated in patients with new focal deficits. Computerized tomography (CT) scan is reliable for the detection of acute hemorrhage and can document territorial ischemic infarctions and massive brain edema. Magnetic resonance imaging (MRI) may be necessary to diagnose an embolic shower and subtle manifestations of global anoxic-ischemic injury such as early cortical injury.[4] In patients with brainstem signs, MRI of the brain can be combined with MR angiography to exclude vertebrobasilar occlusion. EEG should be reserved for those with suspected seizures, and the use of continuous monitoring then may increase the diagnostic yield. Lumbar puncture is rarely necessary in patients with postoperative encephalopathy unless central nervous system (CNS) infection is a possible cause. Serum studies should be used judiciously, including

TABLE 55-2 ■ Common Etiologies of Postoperative Impairment of Consciousness

Prolonged Anesthetic and Analgesic Effect
Advanced age
Decreased metabolism and clearance
Toxic Encephalopathy
Perioperative drugs (e.g., benzodiazepines, opiates, serotoninergic agents)
Drug interactions
Metabolic Encephalopathy
Renal failure
Liver failure
Hypercapnia and hypoxia
Hypoglycemia
Hyponatremia and other electrolyte abnormalities
Hyperosmolality
Acidemia
Septic encephalopathy
Acute stroke
Ischemic
Thromboembolism
Fat embolism
Air embolism
Hemodynamic hypoperfusion
Hemorrhagic
Seizures and status epilepticus (convulsive and nonconvulsive)
Anoxic/ischemic global brain injury

arterial blood gas to exclude CO_2 retention, and serum glucose, sodium, creatinine and blood urea nitrogen, and ammonia to exclude various metabolic disturbances.

A history of delayed arousal after a previous surgery makes a diagnosis of delayed emergence from anesthesia more likely. Older age and renal and hepatic insufficiency may compromise drug metabolism and clearance, increasing the risk of delayed arousal. Review of the anesthesia course may guide the use of naloxone (for reversal of opioid effect), flumazenil (to reverse benzodiazepines), and physostigmine (to reverse neuromuscular blockade) in appropriate cases.

The prognosis of patients with postoperative coma varies markedly depending on etiology. Although the prognosis is favorable in patients with reversible toxic or metabolic causes, the mortality may exceed 80 percent in patients with multifocal infarctions revealed by brain MRI.[4] In survivors of prolonged postoperative coma, long-term functional outcome is frequently poor.[7]

Postoperative Delirium

Postoperative delirium is common, with a reported incidence as high as 40 to 60 percent of patients.[8–10] Delirium can occur immediately following anesthesia or after some interval from a seemingly normal recovery from the anesthetic. The latter is more commonly persistent and often multifactorial in etiology. The risk of delirium is increased in the elderly and in patients with previous cognitive impairment, a history of substance use (including alcohol), and those receiving polypharmacy before surgery and narcotics or benzodiazepines perioperatively.[8,9,11] A previous episode of postoperative delirium predicts recurrence.[11] Perioperative hypoxemia and hemodynamic instability, profuse intraoperative blood loss, and postoperative organ failure may also increase the risk of postoperative delirium.[11]

There is limited evidence that the type and route of anesthesia influence the risk of postoperative delirium, with higher rates following general anesthesia. Deeper intraoperative levels of sedation with propofol increase the risk of postoperative delirium in elderly patients undergoing surgery for hip fracture.[12] Direct alteration of brain function by the anesthetic agent may be responsible.[12]

Evaluation of patients with postoperative delirium begins by considering risk factors for its development (see Table 54-2 in Chapter 54). Time should be spent reviewing the medications that the patient was taking prior to surgery, and those administered during and after the operation. Toxic and metabolic factors are the most frequent causes. Exclusion of acute structural brain injury, seizures, and meningoencephalitis (an exceptional cause of perioperative coma) is the primary responsibility of the consulting neurologist. Primary neurologic diagnoses to be considered include ischemic infarctions (often bilateral or in the brainstem), intracranial hemorrhage (intraparenchymal, subdural, or rarely subarachnoid), nonconvulsive status epilepticus, and posterior reversible encephalopathy syndrome.

TABLE 55-3 ■ Complications Attributed to Spinal or Epidural Block by Patients and Legal Advisers and Reported to Swedish Patient Insurance Database During 1980–1984

	Type of Anesthesia			
Complication	Epidural Block	Intrathecal Block	Caudal Block	Block and General Anesthesia in Combination
Death	1	–	–	–
Brain damage	1	–	–	1
Symptoms of cauda equina lesions	12	20	2	5
Spinal/epidural hematoma	2	–	–	–
Subdural hematoma	–	2	–	–
Subarachnoid hemorrhage	1	–	–	–
Significant paresis	10	7	–	–
Purulent meningitis	–	2	–	–
Deep local infection	–	1	–	–
Somatosensory disturbances	18	21	–	4
Chronic back pain	7	8	1	2

From Puke M, Arnér S, Norlander O: Complications of regional anaesthesia, with special reference to epidural, spinal and caudal anaesthesia. p. 1106. In Nunn JF, Utting JE, Brown BR Jr (eds): General Anaesthesia. 5th Ed. Butterworth, London, 1989, with permission.

Management of the delirium depends on its cause. Discontinuation of sedatives and narcotics is often the only intervention required. When agitation is present and patients may harm themselves or others, oral quetiapine, olanzapine, or, in more severe cases, intravenous haloperidol may be necessary. Dexmedetodimine, a central α_2-adrenergic agonist, is particularly useful for additional sedation or when agitation is accompanied by sympathetic hyperactivity. Benzodiazepines may worsen delirium and therefore should be reserved for specific indications, such as alcohol withdrawal.

In most cases, postoperative delirium is transient and reversible. Complications sometimes stemming from it include aspiration, self-removal of the endotracheal tube or indwelling catheters, and delays in mobilization that, in turn, result in an increased risk of thromboembolism, infections, and deconditioning. In addition, the occurrence of postoperative delirium is related to a greater risk of postoperative cognitive dysfunction, particularly during the first few months following surgery.[11,13]

POSTOPERATIVE NEUROLOGIC DEFICITS

Cognitive Dysfunction

Postoperative cognitive dysfunction occurs more often in older patients and in those with postoperative delirium.[10,13] Its incidence is greatest after major cardiovascular surgery, ranging from 30 to 80 percent during the first few weeks after surgery and 10 to 60 percent after 3 to 6 months.[14] Additional risk factors include alcohol abuse, lower educational level, and previous stroke.[15,16] Patients affected by this complication, even when transient, may have worse long-term cognitive outcomes, greater disability (particularly in the elderly), and a higher mortality.[17] Perhaps surprisingly, there is no definitive evidence that the choice of anesthetic regimen (such as general or regional anesthesia) or the depth of anesthesia alters the risk of postoperative cognitive dysfunction, which has been related to a dysregulated neuroinflammatory response.[18] Maintenance of physiologic homeostasis during and after surgery may minimize the risk of this complication.[19]

Paraparesis

Epidural hematoma is probably the most feared complication of spinal and epidural anesthesia (Table 55-3). Although it is rare, patients at higher risk include those with advanced age, alcoholism, anatomic abnormalities of the vertebral column leading to difficulties with needle placement, and, most importantly, coagulopathy due to a bleeding diathesis or anticoagulant effect.[20,21]

Symptoms of epidural hematoma typically present within the first few hours after the surgery.[21] Attributing them to anesthetic effects may delay the diagnosis and decrease the chances of recovery after surgical evacuation. The neurologist should contact the anesthesiologist to clarify the anesthetic approach used, the effects of the drugs administered, and the expectation of the duration of their effect. In the acute phase, it may be difficult to differentiate between a compressive epidural hematoma and spinal cord ischemia. Preservation of posterior column sensation is expected with an anterior spinal artery infarction. Spinal CT scan allows visualization of the hematoma in most cases, but its sensitivity is suboptimal when hardware is present. Therefore, MRI of the spine should be obtained urgently if possible. Urgent surgical evacuation of the hematoma may result in excellent functional recovery when undertaken promptly.[21]

The American Society of Regional Anesthesia and Pain Medicine has published recommendations for the management of patients receiving antithrombotics who require regional anesthesia.[20] Warfarin should be discontinued 5 days before planned regional anesthesia, and anticoagulation with warfarin should be reversed until the international normalized ratio (INR) is 1.5 or less before urgent interventions. Patients at high risk of thromboembolism should receive bridging with unfractionated heparin (to be stopped 4 hours before surgery) or low-molecular-weight heparin (reduced to half of the usual daily dose and stopped 24 hours before surgery). After surgery, warfarin can be resumed on the first day and heparin products restarted after 24 hours following minor surgeries or 48 to 72 hours after major surgeries. Although continuation of aspirin is acceptable if necessary, clopidogrel should be discontinued 5 to 10 days before the surgery and can be restarted 24 hours after it. These recommendations do not provide guidance for patients receiving any of the newer anticoagulants (e.g., dabigatran, rivaroxaban, apixaban). Depending on the estimated bleeding risk, it is prudent to discontinue dabigatran 3 to 5 days before the procedure. The factor Xa inhibitors rivaroxaban and apixaban should be discontinued 1 to 3 days before the intervention depending on the estimated bleeding risk.

TABLE 55-4 ■ Patterns of Onset and Resolution of Four Neurologic Syndromes Occurring in Rare Patients Following Spinal or Epidural Block

Neurological Syndrome	Onset of Symptoms	Resolution of Symptoms
Aseptic meningitis	<24 hours	<7–10 days
Cauda equina syndrome	Immediate or several days' delay	Permanent or temporary
Adhesive arachnoiditis	Weeks after block	Permanent
Epidural abscess	Days to months after block	Permanent or temporary

Epidural abcess can also cause postoperative paraparesis, but its presentation is usually delayed (at least for days after surgery), and cases exclusively related to neuroaxial blockade are rare (Table 55-4).[22]

Neuropathy

The incidence of neuropathy has been estimated to be less than 0.04 percent after neuroaxial blockade and less than 3 percent following peripheral blockade.[23] Neurologic symptoms and deficits are typically transient. Although prospective studies with blinded assessment are lacking, persistent postoperative neuropathy after regional anesthesia is quite infrequent.[23,24]

Neuropathies can occur due to various mechanisms, some of which are not strictly related to anesthesia. Mechanical stress from stretch or compression of nerves as a result of malpositioning during surgery is a common cause; neuropathies are more likely to occur after prolonged surgeries. Other risk factors include male gender, diabetes mellitus, smoking, hypertension, vascular disease, obesity or extremely thin body habitus, and preexisting clinical or subclinical nerve dysfunction.[25,26] Some of these associations suggest that ischemic and metabolic insults play a role in pathogenesis.

The most frequently affected nerves in the upper extremities are the ulnar nerve and brachial plexus and in the lower extremities the sciatic, femoral, and fibular (peroneal) nerves and the lumbosacral

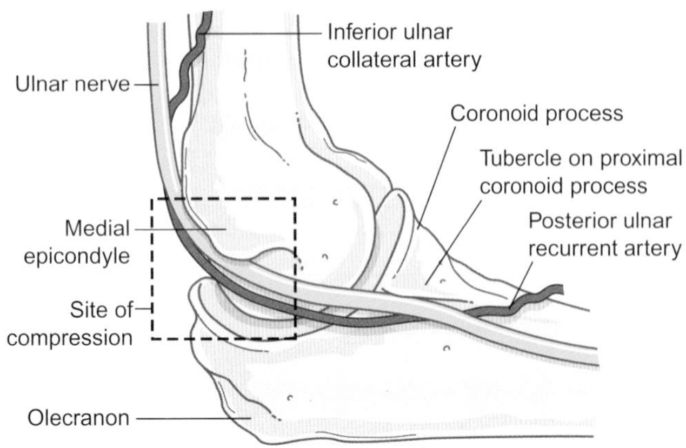

FIGURE 55-1 ■ Typical anatomic site of ulnar nerve compression during surgery.

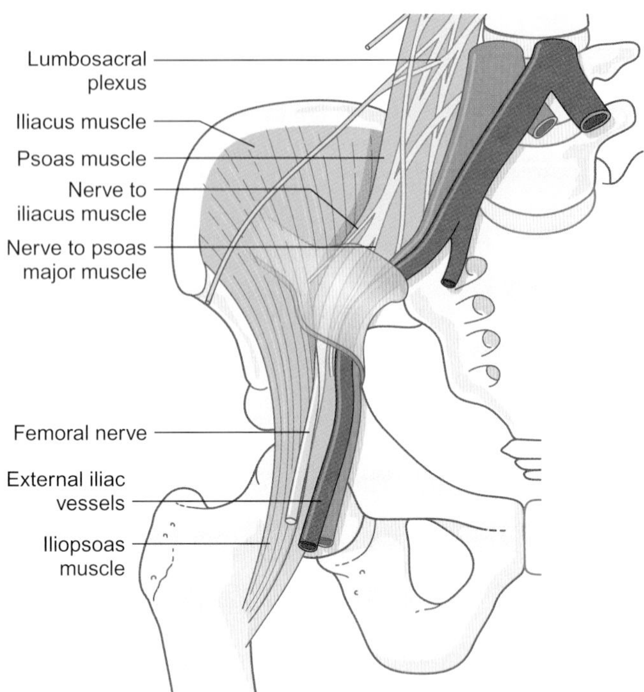

FIGURE 55-2 ■ Illustration of the common mechanism of compression of the femoral nerve through pressure applied with the surgical separator.

plexus. The predisposition of these particular nerves probably relates to their susceptibility to stretch and compression. The most common deficits that result are pure sensory and sensorimotor disturbances.[25,26] Positioning strategies to reduce the risk of each of these peripheral neuropathies have been outlined.[27] Avoidance of arm abduction beyond 90 degrees in supine patients diminishes stretch of the brachial plexus. Minimizing pressure over the ulnar groove, avoidance of excessive flexion of the elbow (Fig. 55-1), and use of protective elbow padding are recommended to reduce ulnar nerve injuries. Restricting stretch of the hamstring muscle and the degree of hip flexion when the patient is in the lithotomy position lessens the risk of sciatic neuropathy. Perioperative fibular (peroneal) neuropathies can be averted through careful avoidance of prolonged pressure over the fibular head and the use of protective padding. Limb position and external compression play a lesser role in the pathogenesis of perioperative femoral neuropathies, which are attributed most often to damage from inappropriate retractor placement (Fig. 55-2).[25]

Cauda equina syndrome is a rare complication of spinal anesthesia, attributed speculatively to maldistribution of the local anesthetic into the subarachnoid space.[28] Most reported cases have occurred after continuous spinal anesthesia, and the predominant manifestations are related to the S1 nerve roots, presumably because of their more posterior location.[29]

Full recovery from these neuropathies is often seen after days to weeks, but some patients suffer persistent disability. There is insufficient information to guide prognostication, except that electrodiagnostic evidence of demyelination (conduction block) rather than axonal loss implies a better prognosis than otherwise.

Transient Neurologic Symptoms

A syndrome known to anesthesiologists as *transient neurologic symptoms* is characterized by early postoperative pain in the buttocks and legs after spinal anesthesia. The pain, which may be severe, typically develops after an initial asymptomatic period of a few hours and is frequently bilateral. The syndrome resolves spontaneously within 2 to 5 days. The risk of this complication is higher with lidocaine and mepivacaine than with other local anesthetics and is not influenced by the dose or concentration of the drug.[30] The main differential diagnoses include cauda equina syndrome, aseptic meningitis, adhesive arachnoiditis, and epidural hematoma or abscess. Imaging reveals no structural abnormality that can explain the symptoms, and the etiology remains uncertain.

Visual Loss

Posterior ischemic optic neuropathy is a rare complication of complex spine surgeries that require prolonged prone positioning, associated with intraoperative blood loss and hemodynamic instability.[31] The performance of staged surgeries, a more liberal intraoperative transfusion strategy, avoidance of intraoperative hypotension, and maintenance of the head at or above the level of the heart have each been recommended, but the etiology of the condition is unclear and the value of these strategies is unproven.[32] Although the visual impairment can be transient, it is often severe and bilateral and may be permanent in some cases. Cardiac surgeries also may be complicated in rare instances by visual loss, typically due to anterior ischemic optic neuropathy or retinal embolism.[33] Anesthesia technique does not appear to be associated with the risk of perioperative visual loss.[32,33]

Hearing Loss

Ear blockage may occur after general anesthesia with nitrous oxide in patients susceptible to eustachian tube obstruction. Presumably mucosal edema facilitates the development of the condition. Prognosis is favorable, with resolution over hours to a few days.

Transient hypoacusis, typically subtle, may follow spinal anesthesia.[34] The proposed mechanism is a decrease in cerebrospinal fluid volume reducing perilymphatic pressure and leading to endolymphatic hydrops. The hypoacusis is frequently, but not always, associated with headache. Use of smaller-diameter spinal needles may reduce the risk.[34,35]

Cranial Nerve Palsies

Abducens nerve palsy has been described after spinal anesthesia, and it can be unilateral or, rarely, bilateral. Typically accompanied by positional headache, it occurs in cases with substantial cerebrospinal fluid loss. The risk is related to the diameter of the spinal needle.[36]

Pupillary changes may follow neuroaxial blocks. Horner syndrome sometimes occurs after epidural anesthesia, typically after labor; the condition lasts only for the duration of the anesthetic block.[37] It can also occur transiently after brachial plexus blockade. Anisocoria found after surgery should not be attributed to anesthetic blockade except when the patient is fully lucid and the examination clearly reveals an isolated Horner syndrome.

Bilateral pupillary dilatation in the immediate perioperative period may be caused by "total" spinal anesthesia, a condition provoked by the unintentional injection of the anesthetic drug into the subarachnoid space. Marked mydriasis and unconsciousness are common, and the problem is typically recognized in the operating room.

Exceptional cases of unilateral and transient trigeminal and facial nerve dysfunction have also been reported after epidural anesthesia for women in labor.[38]

PERIOPERATIVE RIGIDITY

The differential diagnosis of a febrile and rigid patient includes serotonin syndrome, neuroleptic malignant syndrome, and malignant hyperthermia. Serotonin syndrome is most common in the postoperative period, and any patient receiving serotonergic drugs, especially in combination, is at risk of this disorder. Commonly used serotonergic medications include antidepressants, mood stabilizers, antihistamines, triptans, muscle relaxants, and amphetamines, and those prescribed frequently after surgery include opiates (particularly fentanyl), tramadol, and antiemetics.[39] Diagnosis is based on the presence of alterations in consciousness (sometimes with agitation), signs of neuromuscular irritability (hyperreflexia, clonus, rigidity, tremors, myoclonus), and features of autonomic instability (fever, tachycardia, hypertension, diaphoresis).[40] Patients often have mydriasis and hyperactive bowel sounds with diarrhea. The predominance of the rigidity in the lower limbs compared with the upper limbs is distinctive. In severe cases, pronounced ridigity is associated with fever and muscle injury. Recovery follows prompt discontinuation of all serotonergic drugs, usually over hours to days. Cyproheptadine or chlorpromazine may accelerate recovery in more severe cases. Induced neuromuscular paralysis may be necessary in patients with extreme rigidity, fever, and rhabdomyolysis.

The neuroleptic malignant syndrome is uncommon. It presents 1 to 3 days after exposure to an antidopaminergic drug, with clinical features that include extreme rigidity, fever, dyasutonomia, and an elevated serum creatine kinase level.[41] Bradykinesia, lead-pipe rigidity without leg predominance, hyporeflexia, and normal bowel sounds distinguish it from the serotonin syndrome. When the diagnosis of neuroleptic malignant syndrome is suspected, antidopaminergic medications should be stopped and patients should be monitored for dysautonomic complications. Bromocriptine, a dopamine agonist, may diminish the rigidity; severe cases are treated with dantrolene, a potent muscle relaxant.

Malignant hyperthermia occurs in the operating room upon anesthesia induction and neuromuscular paralysis, or within minutes of anesthesia cessation.[42] It is caused by mutations affecting receptors that control the transport of calcium from the sarcoplasmic reticulum to the cytoplasm. Exposure to inhalational anesthetics, especially when succinylcholine is administered, results in excessive availability of calcium in the cytoplasm which, in turn, provokes sustained muscle contraction. A hypermetabolic crisis follows, manifest by hypercapnia, hyperthermia, and mixed acidosis. Severe rhabdomyolysis and cardiac arrhythmias may occur if the diagnosis is delayed. Immediate discontinuation of the anesthetic agent and administration of dantrolene are extremely effective in reversing the syndrome.

PERIOPERATIVE SEIZURES

Surgery—with the exeption of neurosurgery—does not predispose to seizures in general. Some anesthetics have antiepileptic properties while others lower the seizure threshold (Table 55-5). Seizures following anesthesia are uncommon overall.[43] Risk factors include a history of epilepsy (especially in children), previous structural brain injury, and substance abuse.

When postoperative seizures occur in patients with epilepsy, they are generally related to poor preoperative control of the epilepsy and not to the anesthetic.[44] In patients with epilepsy, drugs known to lower the seizure threshold should be avoided.[45] Epileptic seizures should be differentiated from seizure-like movements (including myoclonus, often seen upon propofol withdrawal) and psychogenic nonepileptic seizures.

Postoperative seizures in patients without a history of epilepsy should lead to evaluation of a structural brain lesion, such as an acute stroke, more commonly seen after cardiovascular surgery. Old cortical strokes may also serve as a substrate for postoperative seizures, usually occurring with some delay after the surgery and not precipitated by anesthesia itself.

TABLE 55-5 ■ Anesthetics and Analgesics Reported to Cause or Suppress Seizure Activity in Humans

Proconvulsants	*Anticonvulsants*
Nitrous oxide	Halothane
Halothane	Enflurane
Enflurane	Isoflurane
Isoflurane	Thiopental
Morphine	Etomidate
Meperidine	Diazepam
Fentanyl	Lorazepam
Sufentanil	Midazolam
Methohexital	Ketamine
Etomidate	Propofol
Diazepam	Local anesthetics
Ketamine	
Propofol	
Local anesthetics	

Modified from Modica PA, Tempelhoff R, White PF: Pro- and anticonvulsant effects of anesthetics. Part 1. Anesth Analg 70:303, 1990, with permission.

Postcraniotomy seizures are more frequent and vary depending on the type of surgery. Seizures can occur, albeit rarely, even after operations in the posterior fossa. The value of prophylactic antiseizure medications is unclear.[46]

PERIOPERATIVE HEADACHE

Although there are many causes of postoperative headache (Table 55-6), those most directly related to anesthesia follow regional anesthesia. Dural puncture can cause a persistent leak of cerebrospinal fluid and the ensuing intracranial hypotension manifests with orthostatic headaches (i.e., they are worsened when the patient is upright and ameliorated by recumbency). This complication is more common in thin young women.[47] It sometimes occurs in obstetric patients when inadvertent dural puncture occurs during epidural anesthesia. Use of smaller needle size and good technique (e.g., bevel inserted parallel to the plane of the dural fibers, use of a single pass) decrease the incidence of this type of headache.

TABLE 55-6 ■ Causes of Perioperative Headache

Exacerbation of preexistent primary headache disorder
Myofascial headache
Caffeine withdrawal
Post-dural puncture headache
Closed air-space headache (e.g., effects of nitrous oxide on inflamed sinus or middle ear)
Trigeminal branch neuropathy
Structural intracranial lesion
CNS Infection

An arbitratry period of recumbency following dural puncture does not decrease the incidence of headache,[47] and early ambulation may actually be preferable. Caffeine is often recommended for treatment and seems to work in practice but its value, or that of nonsteroidal anti-inflammatory agents, has not been demonstrated conclusively. Morphine, cosyntropin, and aminophylline are the agents best supported by evidence of efficacy,[48] but they are rarely prescribed for the headaches that follow dural puncture. Epidural blood patch is the best treatment for this type of headache, and it is effective in more than three-quarters of patients. Its efficacy may be lower if placed more than 4 days after the puncture.[49]

Another cause of headache directly related to anesthesia is sinus or middle ear block in patients receiving nitrous oxide. As the gas equilibrates with the air contained in these cavities, pressure may mount in patients with mucosal inflammation.

Compression of the supraorbital or infraorbital branches of the trigeminal nerve from a tight face mask used during anesthesia may also be a rare cause of severe headache after surgery.

ANESTHESIA IN PATIENTS WITH NEUROLOGIC DISEASE

Neurologists are often asked by patients with chronic neurologic disease or their families whether exposure to anesthesia during surgery can exacerbate their underlying condition. The answer depends on the disease in question, the type of surgery, and the condition of the patient.

There are no studies comparing the safety of regional to general anesthesia in patients with preexisting neurologic disease. It has been postulated that techniques of regional anesthesia may exacerbate previous neurologic injury by inducing a secondary insult, particularly in patients with preexisting peripheral neuropathies. However, the results from most studies indicate that anesthesia can generally be used safely in patients with various neurologic diseases.[24]

Alzheimer Disease

Anesthetic drugs, especially inhalational agents, have the potential to induce or accelerate the neurodegenerative changes characteristic of Alzheimer disease.[50,51] Potential mechanisms include neuronal calcium dysregulation, increased amyloid beta production and aggregation, increased tau phosphorylation, and activation of apoptotic pathways in the predisposed brain exposed to isoflurane. The evidence for these effects comes from experimental models, and there is no conclusive clinical data associating anesthetic exposure with a greater risk of Alzheimer disease[50]; indeed, some epidemiologic studies appear to refute any such association.[52,53] Various anesthetic gases may have different effects. Isoflurane, but not desflurane, has been associated with an increase in Aβ40 protein levels in human cerebrospinal fluid 24 hours after surgery compared with control patients undergoing spinal anesthesia.[54]

Many general anesthetics decrease central acetylcholine release and depress cholinergic transmission in the basal forebrain, a condition that mimics changes found in Alzheimer disease.[55] Most anesthetic agents also interact with muscarinic and nicotinic receptors in the brain, typically in a dose-dependent manner.[55] Propofol and remifentanil interfere less with cholinergic function than inhalational drugs and other opioids.[55]

Observational studies indicate that presurgical cognitive impairment and dementia are associated with postoperative cognitive decline, poor functional recovery, and an increased risk of death.[9] Whether adjustments in the anesthetic regimen (such as the use of propofol instead of inhalational agents) can decrease this risk remains unclear. Hypnotics, opioids, inhalational drugs, and neuromuscular blocking agents produce more variable responses with advanced age and should be used prudently in patients with documented cognitive impairment.[56]

Parkinson Disease

For patients with Parkinson disease who require surgery, the main problem relates to transient discontinuation of their antiparkinsonian regimen. These medications should be continued to as close to the beginning of anesthesia as possible, and restarted as soon after surgery as feasible to minimize parkinsonian complications. In prolonged surgeries, intraoperative administration of levodopa via a nasogastric tube can be considered. During the early postoperative period, patients with Parkinson disease have an increased risk of postextubation respiratory failure and aspiration pneumonia due to upper airway dysfunction, as well as hemodynamic instability from impairment of autonomic control.[57] Delirium is also common postoperatively in patients with Parkinson disease.

Succinylcholine may be unsafe in patients with Parkinson disease who are very rigid because of an increased risk of inducing severe hyperkalemia; nondepolarizing muscle relaxants can be used safely instead. Inhalational anesthetics should be administered cautiously due to a greater risk of inducing hypotension and cardiac arrhythmia. Ketamine use may be associated with an excessive sympathetic response. Thiopental can theoretically decrease striatal dopamine release, but is probably safe. Propofol is generally the preferred induction agent for these patients.[58]

Antidopaminergic drugs should be avoided, including various antiemetics commonly prescribed in the recovery room (e.g., droperidol, metoclopramide). Meperidine should not be used in patients who have taken selegiline or rasagiline in the preceding 2 weeks because this combination can result in severe hypertension or hypotension, respiratory depression, convulsions, malignant hyperthermia, excitation, peripheral vascular collapse, coma, and death. Tramadol, methadone, tapentadol, and propoxyphene must also be avoided for the same reason. When fentanyl is administered, greater rigidity can be expected, and occasionally opioids of all types can cause severe acute dystonia responsive to naloxone.[59]

Functional neurosurgery (deep brain stimulation) for the treatment of Parkinson disease represents a particular challenge because—depending on technique—patients are kept awake to allow for adequate monitoring and targeting of deep brain structures during lead insertion. The advantages of awake craniotomy need to be balanced against the risk of operative complications such as intracranial hemorrhage, which may increase when patients are uncomfortable and not fully cooperative.[60] When trying to preserve patient cooperation, dexmedetomidine can be helpful in providing mild sedation.[61] Propofol is also a good agent as it does not affect electrophysiologic monitoring.[62]

Epilepsy

The risk of perioperative seizures is very small in patients with epilepsy undergoing general anesthesia, and epileptic patients do not appear to have an increased risk of other perioperative adverse effects.[43] Children with epilepsy may be more susceptible than adults to develop seizures associated with anesthesia.[43,63] Regional blockade can be performed safely.[64]

Many anesthetic agents produce complex effects on brain electrical activity and may have proconvulsant and anticonvulsant properties depending on the dose and concentration (Table 55-5).[45] Although most anesthetic regimens are safe for patients with epilepsy, some agents should be used cautiously because of their proconvulsant potential at usual doses, including etomidate[65] and intravenous lidocaine.[66] Sevoflurane is more epileptogenic than the other inhaled anesthetics,[45] and short-acting opioids (e.g., alfentanil, sulfentanil, remifentanil) increase epileptiform activity during intraoperative electrocorticography for epilepsy surgery.[67] Propofol, barbiturates, benzodiazepines, and other volatile agents (especially isoflurane and desflurane) conversely have antiepileptic effects and are the preferred options in patients with epilepsy.[45]

Other Chronic Diseases of the CNS

Patients with multiple system atrophy and an accompanying dysautonomia may develop dangerous hemodynamic instability in the perioperative period. General anesthesia can be used safely in these patients, but agents that lead to hypotension should be avoided; spinal anesthesia may be preferable.[68]

Patients with amyotrophic lateral sclerosis are particularly susceptible to the effects of muscle relaxants. Succinylcholine should be avoided in all patients with severe neuromuscular disease because it can induce hyperkalemia.[69] When muscle relaxation is deemed indispensable, nondepolarizing blocking agents should be administered in low doses using nerve stimulator monitoring. A regimen of propofol and remifentanil without muscle relaxation is safe in these patients.[70] In patients with amyotrophic lateral sclerosis requiring gastrostomy tube placement, opiates may decrease the ventilatory drive, precipitating respiratory failure.

Worsening myelopathic symptoms following spinal anesthesia have been reported rarely in patients with multiple sclerosis, but a large case series of patients with multiple sclerosis, amyotrophic lateral sclerosis, and postpolio syndrome revealed no instances of severe exacerbation of preoperative neurologic deficits after spinal or epidural anesthesia.[71]

Patients with Huntington disease may need close monitoring due to their underlying movement disorder, but can receive anesthesia safely.[72] Responses to muscle relaxants, induction agents, volatile anesthetics, benzodiazepines, and opioids are usually normal.

Neuromuscular Disorders

Severe neurologic complications were rare (0.4%) in a large series of patients with diabetic and nondiabetic peripheral neuropathy who underwent surgery under regional anesthesia.[73] The risk of cauda equina syndrome may be increased in patients with spinal stenosis.[74]

The surgical planning of patients with myasthenia gravis should incorporate input from the treating neurologist. Preoperative treatment with plasma exchange or intravenous immunoglobulin can reduce the risk of postoperative myasthenic crisis. After surgery, early weaning from mechanical ventilation and prompt reinstitution of aceylcholinesterase inhibitors are advisable. Various medications may worsen myasthenia gravis, including muscle relaxants and certain antibiotics (such as the aminoglycosides).

The risk of malignant hyperthermia may be increased in patients with muscular dystrophies, although the degree of this risk is not well defined.[75] Succinylcholine is contraindicated in patients with muscular dystrophies and metabolic myopathies because of the danger of life-threatening hyperkalemia and rhabdomyolysis.[75,76]

ANESTHESIA IN THE NEUROCRITICAL CARE UNIT

Anesthetic drugs are commonly prescribed in the intensive care unit (ICU) for sedation, control of intracranial hypertension, and treatment of refractory seizures. The prolonged administration and high doses used for some of these indications may provoke complications not encountered with regular perioperative use.

Prolonged sedation in the ICU is associated with a greater incidence of delirium. Daily sedative interruption in patients receiving mechanical ventilation decreases the duration of mechanical ventilation and length of stay in the ICU.[77] This practice should be combined with daily monitoring for signs of delirium employing validated scores, such as the Confusion Assessment Method for the intensive care unit (CAM-ICU).[78] Dexmedetomidine, a central α_2-agonist, is associated with reduced rates of delirium when compared with benzodiazepines such as lorazepam or midazolam.[79,80] Propofol infusion syndrome is a potentially life-threatening complication caused by the prolonged administration of high doses of this drug (usually exceeding 4 to 5 mg/kg per hour for more than 48 hours).[81] Initially recognized in children, who appear to be at higher risk, it also can occur in adults and presents with lactic acidosis, rhabdomyolysis, hyperlipidemia hyperkalemia, renal failure, and refractory bradycardia with cardiac failure.[82] In the most severe cases, cardiac arrest may occur.[83] Uncoupling of the respiratory chain causing impaired mitochondrial free fatty acid metabolism is involved in the pathogenesis of this disorder.[84,85] Propofol infusion syndrome has been reported during the treatment of refractory status epilepticus[83] and in severe traumatic brain injury patients with refractory intracranial hypertension.[86] Since other options exist for control of refractory seizures or recalcitrant intracranial hypertension, it is advisable to avoid using large doses of propofol for these indications.

Patients with prolonged refractory status epilepticus are commonly treated with anesthetics; in addition to propofol, options include high-dose midazolam, barbiturates, and less commonly ketamine and inhalational anesthetics such as isoflurane.[87] Continuous infusion of high-dose lorazepam may produce severe acidosis from propylene glycol toxicity and therefore its use should be discouraged.[88] Midazolam is safe and effective, but tachyphylaxis develops over time. Hence, the most refractory cases require induction of coma by other anesthetics. Complications from barbiturate coma include hypotension from myocardial depression, ileus, hepatotoxicity, and increased susceptibility to infections (particularly pneumonia). Isoflurane can be effective in aborting seizures and does not cause prolonged coma after its discontinuation (in contrast to barbiturates), but may induce neurotoxicity.[89,90] Ketamine, an *N*-methyl-D-aspartate antagonist, may be an alternative agent for the treatment of refractory status epilepticus, but reported experience has been mixed thus far in regard to efficacy.[91,92] It has a good safety profile even in critically ill patients, and concerns about its potential for increasing intracranial pressure are probably exaggerated.

REFERENCES

1. Arbous MS, Meursing AE, van Kleef JW, et al: Impact of anesthesia management characteristics on severe morbidity and mortality. Anesthesiology 102:257, 2005.
2. Moller JT, Johannessen NW, Espersen K, et al: Randomized evaluation of pulse oximetry in 20,802 patients: II. Perioperative events and postoperative complications. Anesthesiology 78:445, 1993.
3. Newman J, Blake K, Fennema J, et al: Incidence, predictors and outcomes of postoperative coma: an observational study of 858606 patients. Eur J Anaesthesiol 30:476, 2013.
4. Gootjes EC, Wijdicks EF, McClelland RL: Postoperative stupor and coma. Mayo Clin Proc 80:350, 2005.
5. Anastasian ZH, Ornstein E, Heyer EJ: Delayed arousal. Anesthesiol Clin 27:429, 2009.
6. Ganushchak YM, Fransen EJ, Visser C, et al: Neurological complications after coronary artery bypass grafting related to the performance of cardiopulmonary bypass. Chest 125:2196, 2004.
7. Rodriguez RA, Nair S, Bussière M, et al: Long-lasting functional disabilities in patients who recover from coma after cardiac operations. Ann Thorac Surg 95:884, 2013.
8. Dyer CB, Ashton CM, Teasdale TA: Postoperative delirium. A review of 80 primary data-collection studies. Arch Intern Med 155:461, 1995.
9. Robinson TN, Raeburn CD, Tran ZV, et al: Postoperative delirium in the elderly: risk factors and outcomes. Ann Surg 249:173, 2009.
10. Rudolph JL, Marcantonio ER, Culley DJ, et al: Delirium is associated with early postoperative cognitive dysfunction. Anaesthesia 63:941, 2008.
11. Deiner S, Silverstein JH: Postoperative delirium and cognitive dysfunction. Br J Anaesth 103(suppl 1):i41, 2009.
12. Sieber FE, Zakriya KJ, Gottschalk A, et al: Sedation depth during spinal anesthesia and the development of postoperative delirium in elderly patients undergoing hip fracture repair. Mayo Clin Proc 85:18, 2010.
13. Saczynski JS, Marcantonio ER, Quach L, et al: Cognitive trajectories after postoperative delirium. N Engl J Med 367:30, 2012.
14. Rasmussen LS: Postoperative cognitive dysfunction: incidence and prevention. Best Pract Res Clin Anaesthesiol 20:315, 2006.
15. Hudetz JA, Iqbal Z, Gandhi SD, et al: Postoperative cognitive dysfunction in older patients with a history of alcohol abuse. Anesthesiology 106:423, 2007.
16. Monk TG, Weldon BC, Garvan CW, et al: Predictors of cognitive dysfunction after major noncardiac surgery. Anesthesiology 108:18, 2008.
17. Steinmetz J, Christensen KB, Lund T, et al: Long-term consequences of postoperative cognitive dysfunction. Anesthesiology 110:548, 2009.
18. Vacas S, Degos V, Feng X, et al: The neuroinflammatory response of postoperative cognitive decline. Br Med Bull 106:161, 2013.
19. Steinmetz J, Funder KS, Dahl BT, et al: Depth of anaesthesia and post-operative cognitive dysfunction. Acta Anaesthesiol Scand 54:162, 2010.
20. Horlocker TT, Wedel DJ, Rowlingson JC, et al: Regional anesthesia in the patient receiving antithrombotic or thrombolytic therapy: American Society of Regional Anesthesia and Pain Medicine Evidence-Based Guidelines (Third Edition). Reg Anesth Pain Med 35:64, 2010.
21. Amiri AR, Fouyas IP, Cro S, et al: Postoperative spinal epidural hematoma (SEH): incidence, risk factors, onset, and management. Spine J 13:134, 2013.
22. Cook TM, Counsell D, Wildsmith JA: Royal College of Anaesthetists Third National Audit Project: Major complications of central neuraxial block: report on the Third National Audit Project of the Royal College of Anaesthetists. Br J Anaesth 102:179, 2009.
23. Brull R, McCartney CJ, Chan VW, et al: Neurological complications after regional anesthesia: contemporary estimates of risk. Anesth Analg 104:965, 2007.
24. Neal JM, Bernards CM, Hadzic A, et al: ASRA practice advisory on neurologic complications in regional

anesthesia and pain medicine. Reg Anesth Pain Med 33:404, 2008.

25. Warner MA: Perioperative neuropathies. Mayo Clin Proc 73:567, 1998.
26. Welch MB, Brummett CM, Welch TD, et al: Perioperative peripheral nerve injuries: a retrospective study of 380,680 cases during a 10-year period at a single institution. Anesthesiology 111:490, 2009.
27. American Society of Anesthesiologists Task Force on Prevention of Perioperative Peripheral Neuropathies: Practice advisory for the prevention of perioperative peripheral neuropathies: an updated report by the American Society of Anesthesiologists Task Force on prevention of perioperative peripheral neuropathies. Anesthesiology 114:741, 2011.
28. Rigler ML, Drasner K, Krejcie TC, et al: Cauda equina syndrome after continuous spinal anesthesia. Anesth Analg 72:275, 1991.
29. Schneider M, Ettlin T, Kaufmann M, et al: Transient neurologic toxicity after hyperbaric subarachnoid anesthesia with 5% lidocaine. Anesth Analg 76:1154, 1993.
30. Zaric D, Pace NL: Transient neurologic symptoms (TNS) following spinal anaesthesia with lidocaine versus other local anaesthetics. Cochrane Database Syst Rev 2:CD003006, 2009.
31. Ho VT, Newman NJ, Song S, et al: Ischemic optic neuropathy following spine surgery. J Neurosurg Anesthesiol 17:38, 2005.
32. Postoperative Visual Loss Study Group: Risk factors associated with ischemic optic neuropathy after spinal fusion surgery. Anesthesiology 116:15, 2012.
33. Roth S: Perioperative visual loss: what do we know, what can we do? Br J Anaesth 103(suppl 1):i31, 2009.
34. Cosar A, Yetiser S, Sizlan A, et al: Hearing impairment associated with spinal anesthesia. Acta Otolaryngol 124:1159, 2004.
35. Erol A, Topal A, Arbag H, et al: Auditory function after spinal anaesthesia: the effect of differently designed spinal needles. Eur J Anaesthesiol 26:416, 2009.
36. Thömke F, Mika-Grüttner A, Visbeck A, et al: The risk of abducens palsy after diagnostic lumbar puncture. Neurology 54:768, 2000.
37. Biousse V, Guevara RA, Newman NJ: Transient Horner's syndrome after lumbar epidural anesthesia. Neurology 51:1473, 1998.
38. Carrero EJ, Agustí M, Fábregas N, et al: Unilateral trigeminal and facial nerve palsies associated with epidural analgesia in labour. Can J Anaesth 45:893, 1998.
39. Boyer EW, Shannon M: The serotonin syndrome. N Engl J Med 352:1112, 2005.
40. Dunkley EJ, Isbister GK, Sibbritt D, et al: The Hunter Serotonin Toxicity Criteria: simple and accurate diagnostic decision rules for serotonin toxicity. QJM 96:635, 2003.
41. Strawn JR, Keck Jr PE, Caroff SN: Neuroleptic malignant syndrome. Am J Psychiatry 164:870, 2007.
42. Denborough M: Malignant hyperthermia. Lancet 352:1131, 1998.
43. Benish SM, Cascino GD, Warner ME, et al: Effect of general anesthesia in patients with epilepsy: a population-based study. Epilepsy Behav 17:87, 2010.
44. Niesen AD, Jacob AK, Aho LE, et al: Perioperative seizures in patients with a history of a seizure disorder. Anesth Analg 111:729, 2010.
45. Voss LJ, Sleigh JW, Barnard JP, et al: The howling cortex: seizures and general anesthetic drugs. Anesth Analg 107:1689, 2008.
46. Pulman J, Greenhalgh J, Marson AG: Antiepileptic drugs as prophylaxis for post-craniotomy seizures. Cochrane Database Syst Rev 2:CD007286, 2013.
47. Kuntz KM, Kokmen E, Stevens JC, et al: Post-lumbar puncture headaches: experience in 501 consecutive procedures. Neurology 42:1884, 1992.
48. Basurto Ona X, Uriona Tuma SM, Martínez García L, et al: Drug therapy for preventing post-dural puncture headache. Cochrane Database Syst Rev 2:CD001792, 2013.
49. Safa-Tisseront V, Thormann F, Malassiné P, et al: Effectiveness of epidural blood patch in the management of post-dural puncture headache. Anesthesiology 95:334, 2001.
50. Baranov D, Bickler PE, Crosby GJ, et al: Consensus statement: First International Workshop on Anesthetics and Alzheimer's disease. Anesth Analg 108:1627, 2009.
51. Tang J, Eckenhoff MF, Eckenhoff RG: Anesthesia and the old brain. Anesth Analg 110:421, 2010.
52. Bohnen NI, Warner MA, Kokmen E, et al: Alzheimer's disease and cumulative exposure to anesthesia: a case-control study. J Am Geriatr Soc 42:198, 1994.
53. Gasparini M, Vanacore N, Schiaffini C, et al: A case-control study on Alzheimer's disease and exposure to anesthesia. Neurol Sci 23:11, 2002.
54. Zhang B, Tian M, Zheng H, et al: Effects of anesthetic isoflurane and desflurane on human cerebrospinal fluid Aβ and tau level. Anesthesiology 119:52, 2013.
55. Fodale V, Quattrone D, Trecroci C, et al: Alzheimer's disease and anaesthesia: implications for the central cholinergic system. Br J Anaesth 97:445, 2006.
56. Funder KS, Steinmetz J, Rasmussen LS: Anaesthesia for the patient with dementia undergoing outpatient surgery. Curr Opin Anaesthesiol 22:712, 2009.
57. Nicholson G, Pereira AC, Hall GM: Parkinson's disease and anaesthesia. Br J Anaesth 89:904, 2002.
58. Kalenka A, Schwarz A: Anaesthesia and Parkinson's disease: how to manage with new therapies? Curr Opin Anaesthesiol 22:419, 2009.
59. Iselin-Chaves IA, Grotzsch H, Besson M, et al: Naloxone-responsive acute dystonia and parkinsonism following general anaesthesia. Anaesthesia 64:1359, 2009.

60. Seijo FJ, Alvarez-Vega MA, Gutierrez JC, et al: Complications in subthalamic nucleus stimulation surgery for treatment of Parkinson's disease. Review of 272 procedures. Acta Neurochir (Wien) 149:867, 2007.
61. Rozet I, Muangman S, Vavilala MS, et al: Clinical experience with dexmedetomidine for implantation of deep brain stimulators in Parkinson's disease. Anesth Analg 103:1224, 2006.
62. Lefaucheur JP, Gurruchaga JM, Pollin B, et al: Outcome of bilateral subthalamic nucleus stimulation in the treatment of Parkinson's disease: correlation with intra-operative multi-unit recordings but not with the type of anaesthesia. Eur Neurol 60:186, 2008.
63. Ren WH: Anesthetic management of epileptic pediatric patients. Int Anesthesiol Clin 47:101, 2009.
64. Kopp SL, Wynd KP, Horlocker TT, et al: Regional blockade in patients with a history of a seizure disorder. Anesth Analg 109:272, 2009.
65. Reddy RV, Moorthy SS, Dierdorf SF, et al: Excitatory effects and electroencephalographic correlation of etomidate, thiopental, methohexital, and propofol. Anesth Analg 77:1008, 1993.
66. DeToledo JC: Lidocaine and seizures. Ther Drug Monit 22:320, 2000.
67. Wass CT, Grady RE, Fessler AJ, et al: The effects of remifentanil on epileptiform discharges during intraoperative electrocorticography in patients undergoing epilepsy surgery. Epilepsia 42:1340, 2001.
68. Konarzewski WH, Knorr C: Spinal anaesthesia and Shy Drager syndrome. Anaesthesia 52:1020, 1997.
69. Brambrink AM, Kirsch JR: Perioperative care of patients with neuromuscular disease and dysfunction. Anesthesiol Clin 25:483, 2007.
70. Onders RP, Carlin AM, Elmo M, et al: Amyotrophic lateral sclerosis: the Midwestern surgical experience with the diaphragm pacing stimulation system shows that general anesthesia can be safely performed. Am J Surg 197:386, 2009.
71. Hebl JR, Horlocker TT, Schroeder DR: Neuraxial anesthesia and analgesia in patients with preexisting central nervous system disorders. Anesth Analg 103:223, 2006.
72. Kivela JE, Sprung J, Southorn PA, et al: Anesthetic management of patients with Huntington disease. Anesth Analg 110:515, 2010.
73. Hebl JR, Kopp SL, Schroeder DR, et al: Neurologic complications after neuraxial anesthesia or analgesia in patients with preexisting peripheral sensorimotor neuropathy or diabetic polyneuropathy. Anesth Analg 103:1294, 2006.
74. Moen V, Dahlgren N, Irestedt L: Severe neurological complications after central neuraxial blockades in Sweden 1990–1999. Anesthesiology 101:950, 2004.
75. Gurnaney H, Brown A, Litman RS: Malignant hyperthermia and muscular dystrophies. Anesth Analg 109:1043, 2009.
76. Benca J, Hogan K: Malignant hyperthermia, coexisting disorders, and enzymopathies: risks and management options. Anesth Analg 109:1049, 2009.
77. Kress JP, Pohlman AS, O'Connor MF, et al: Daily interruption of sedative infusions in critically ill patients undergoing mechanical ventilation. N Engl J Med 342:1471, 2000.
78. Ely EW, Inouye SK, Bernard GR, et al: Delirium in mechanically ventilated patients: validity and reliability of the confusion assessment method for the intensive care unit (CAM-ICU). JAMA 286:2703, 2001.
79. Pandharipande PP, Pun BT, Herr DL, et al: Effect of sedation with dexmedetomidine vs lorazepam on acute brain dysfunction in mechanically ventilated patients: the MENDS randomized controlled trial. JAMA 298:2644, 2007.
80. Riker RR, Shehabi Y, Bokesch PM, et al: Dexmedetomidine vs midazolam for sedation of critically ill patients: a randomized trial. JAMA 301:489, 2009.
81. Kam PC, Cardone D: Propofol infusion syndrome. Anaesthesia 62:690, 2007.
82. Fong JJ, Sylvia L, Ruthazer R, et al: Predictors of mortality in patients with suspected propofol infusion syndrome. Crit Care Med 36:2281, 2008.
83. Iyer VN, Hoel R, Rabinstein AA: Propofol infusion syndrome in patients with refractory status epilepticus: an 11-year clinical experience. Crit Care Med 37:3024, 2009.
84. Jorens PG, Van den Eynden GG: Propofol infusion syndrome with arrhythmia, myocardial fat accumulation and cardiac failure. Am J Cardiol 104:1160, 2009.
85. Mehta N, DeMunter C, Habibi P, et al: Short-term propofol infusions in children. Lancet 354:866, 1999.
86. Cremer OL, Moons KG, Bouman EA, et al: Long-term propofol infusion and cardiac failure in adult head-injured patients. Lancet 357:117, 2001.
87. Rabinstein AA: Management of status epilepticus in adults. Neurol Clin 28:853, 2010.
88. Arroliga AC, Shehab N, McCarthy K, et al: Relationship of continuous infusion lorazepam to serum propylene glycol concentration in critically ill adults. Crit Care Med 32:1709, 2004.
89. Mirsattari SM, Sharpe MD, Young GB: Treatment of refractory status epilepticus with inhalational anesthetic agents isoflurane and desflurane. Arch Neurol 61:1254, 2004.
90. Fugate JE, Burns JD, Wijdicks EF, et al: Prolonged high-dose isoflurane for refractory status epilepticus: is it safe? Anesth Analg 111:1520, 2010.
91. Rosati A, L'Erario M, Ilvento L, et al: Efficacy and safety of ketamine in refractory status epilepticus in children. Neurology 79:2355, 2012.
92. Shorvon S, Ferlisi M: The treatment of super-refractory status epilepticus: a critical review of available therapies and a clinical treatment protocol. Brain 134:2802, 2011.

SECTION

XV

Critical Illness and General Medical Disorders

CHAPTER

56

Neurologic Complications in Critically Ill Patients

JOHN A. MORREN ■ EDWARD M. MANNO

Injury to other organ systems may have direct or remote neurologic effects. Hepatic, cardiac, pulmonary, pancreatic, and renal dysfunction can directly impact neurologic function through a variety of mechanisms outlined elsewhere in this book. This chapter examines the immediate and long-term effects of critical illness on both the central and peripheral nervous systems (CNS and PNS).

SEPTIC ENCEPHALOPATHY

Septic encephalopathy is a nebulous term used to describe an encephalopathy encountered in critically ill patients that cannot be explained by either direct neurologic injury, indirect effects of other failing organ systems, or exogenous toxins. It is a diagnosis of exclusion. Septic encephalopathy is defined as "altered brain function due to the presence of microorganisms or toxins in the blood," but this definition is incomplete since bacteremia is rare and exogenous substances are not mentioned.[1] Sepsis-associated encephalopathy and sepsis-associated delirium have been proposed as more descriptive terms but are not widely used.[2]

Epidemiology

Encephalopathy during critical illness is common. It is estimated that between 9 and 71 percent of critically ill patients become confused. The higher estimates in this range are more accurate when more sensitive tests are employed and as physicians have become more aware of the diagnosis.[1–4] The presence and severity of this encephalopathy have significant impact on both immediate mortality and long-term cognitive capabilities.[3]

Overview of the Mechanisms of Sepsis

A response to an infection is initiated when pattern-recognizing receptors on macrophages bind cellular components of microbial cell walls. Binding of these receptors initiates a signaling cascade, via the nuclear factor-κB system, to release cytosolic factors that translocate to the nucleus, activating gene transcription for a variety of proteins including proinflammatory cytokines (tumor necrosis factor and interleukin 1), chemokines, intercellular adhesion molecule 1, vascular cell adhesion molecule 1, and

Aminoff's Neurology and General Medicine, Fifth Edition.

nitric oxide. These factors subsequently attract polymorphonuclear leukocytes to the site of the injury and these release local substances that account for the cutaneous changes occurring with inflammation (e.g., erythema, edema, warmth).[5]

Inflammation is subsequently regulated through a balance between proinflammatory cytokines released by macrophages and anti-inflammatory factors released by polymorphonuclear leukocytes. This balance typically leads to local infection control. Sepsis occurs when the response to an infection generalizes beyond local boundaries to affect remote organ systems.[6] The systemic inflammatory response syndrome (SIRS) reflects a similar process that is initiated by conditions other than acute infection. Systemic release of proinflammatory cytokines can become self-sustaining, leading to a cycle of systemic inflammation, complement activation, and stimulation of both coagulation and fibrinolytic cascades. Various single nucleotide polymorphisms increase susceptibility to sepsis on a genetic basis.[5,7]

Sepsis affects organ systems primarily through its effect on the endothelium of vascular tissue. Sepsis induces both vasodilation (most likely through nitric oxide) and myocardial depression, which leads to significant hypotension.[8] Regional circulation is altered, affecting the distribution of blood to ischemic organs. Endothelial dysfunction also leads to increased vascular permeability with subsequent tissue edema. Decreased functional capillaries at the microcirculatory level may be due to either extrinsic compression from tissue edema or intravascular coagulation. Red cell deformability is decreased in sepsis, further inhibiting oxygen delivery.[9]

Oxygen utilization at the mitochondrial level is affected directly by proinflammatory mediators, which cause mitochondrial dysfunction through direct inhibition of respiratory chain enzymatic function. Oxidative stress–induced damage is believed to account for an increase in mitochondrial breakdown products, and cell death may be attributed to cellular inability to utilize oxygen.[10]

Secondary cell death through apoptosis is actually decreased in sepsis. However, septic mediators and proinflammatory cytokines also delay apoptosis in macrophages and neutrophils, leading to a net effect of prolonged inflammatory physiology.[11]

Pathogenesis of the Encephalopathy

The endothelial and microvascular effects of sepsis affect all organs. The subsequent hypoxia from pulmonary failure, uremia from renal failure, and alterations in amino acid metabolism from hepatic failure may contribute to the encephalopathy commonly encountered in septic patients. However, an encephalopathy may also develop early in the course of sepsis or SIRS that precedes the development of secondary organ failure.[12] Although the exact mechanism of this neurologic dysfunction is unknown, it is generally believed that septic mediators, primarily the proinflammatory cytokines and complement factors, gain access to the brain neuropil, leading to functional disruption of neurologic transmission and eventual cell damage and death.[13]

How these factors gain access to the brain has been an area of considerable study. Animal models have supported a direct toxic effect of some mediators on the integrity of the blood–brain barrier. Neonatal kittens exposed to *E. coli* lipopolysaccharide develop diffuse cerebral white matter disruption with noted extravasation of Evans blue dye throughout the brain. Similarly, horseradish peroxidase is transported into the septic rat neuropil in a retrograde fashion, disrupting the blood–brain barrier.[14] Lipopolysaccharide exposures have been linked to direct transport of cytokines across the blood–brain barrier in mice.[15] Inflammatory mediators in the cerebrospinal fluid (CSF) may also gain access to the brain through the circumventricular organs located around the midline ventricular system.

Blood–brain barrier disruption may not be necessary for leukocyte-induced inflammatory mediators to gain access to the brain. Tissue necrosis factor and interferon-γ directly increase the permeability of cerebral endothelial cells through increased pinocytosis without immediate disruption of the blood–brain barrier's intercellular tight junctions.[12,16] Radiolabeled amino acids and albumin have been detected in the brains of septic rats.[17] The CSF profile in septic patients is generally acellular, but protein concentration may be increased.

Once inflammatory mediators have gained access to the brain parenchyma, the effects are similar to those seen in other organs. Localized cerebral edema can occur due to endothelial damage.

Cerebral blood flow and metabolism are depressed in septic patients and cerebral autoregulation is disturbed.[18] The resulting cerebral hypoperfusion may contribute to encephalopathy. These vascular changes may result from direct neural involvement of inflammatory mediators. Astrocytes contain receptors for these inflammatory mediators and damage to their end foot processes has been demonstrated in animal models of sepsis, leading to poor blood flow coupling.[19] Decreased cerebral blood flow during sepsis may also be the direct result of mitochondrial dysfunction or a response to decreased cerebral metabolism. Direct mitochondrial dysfunction from endotoxemia is probably mediated through nitric oxide.[20]

Cerebral ischemia is present in many cases of sepsis. Dead neurons have been identified in septic pigs with maintained cerebral perfusion, and microvascular lesions are commonly found in humans at pathology and on neuroimaging.[19,21,22] Neuronal apoptosis in the setting of ischemia is presumably due to mitochondrial dysfunction.[23] Postmortem studies have shown inducible nitric oxide synthase leading to apoptosis in the hippocampus.[24]

The parasympathetic nervous system may in part mediate the inflammatory response as increased vagal tone appears to decrease inflammation and improve mortality in animal models of sepsis.[25]

Presentation and Evaluation

The encephalopathy associated with sepsis and SIRS may present acutely or subtly with a slow progression. Disorientation, impaired cognition, and inattentiveness can progress to agitation, delirium, stupor, and coma. The pupils are typically small and minimally reactive. Brainstem reflexes are generally maintained until late in the course. Focal signs are rare but may occur.[26]

The diagnosis remains one of exclusion. The patient should be evaluated for meningitis and encephalitis of infectious and autoimmune or paraneoplastic origin. Similarly, encephalopathies secondary to failure of other organ systems (e.g., hepatic, renal, pulmonary, and pancreatic) should be considered and treated. Clearance and metabolism of sedative medications commonly employed to treat critically ill patients may be delayed in multiorgan failure, complicating evaluation. Direct cerebral hypoperfusion from cardiac failure may also contribute to encephalopathy.

Serum levels of neuron specific enolase and S-100B are markers of neuronal and astrocytic damage; both have been shown to increase with septic encephalopathy and correlate with a worse outcome, but typically are not useful in clinical practice.[27] The electroencephalogram (EEG) may be normal but becomes slower with increasing encephalopathy, progressing from theta to delta activity and finally to a burst-suppression pattern (Fig. 56-1). Mortality correlates with worsening EEG findings.[28] Nonconvulsive status epilepticus is probably under-recognized; continuous EEG monitoring may be helpful in its detection.[29] Magnetic resonance imaging (MRI) is most sensitive to the changes that can occur during sepsis. Microhemorrhages and small ischemic lesions are detected in approximately 10 percent of patients, white matter changes are common, and cortical atrophy may occur in severe cases.[22] The utility of somatosensory evoked potentials, functional MRI, and positron emission tomography (PET) requires more study.

Pathologically, small ischemic lesions are found in most autopsy samples. Additional findings include microhemorrhages in approximately 25 percent, microthrombi in 9 percent, white matter damage in 9 percent, and microabscesses in less than 5 percent.[26,30]

Management and Future Studies

Unfortunately, there are no specific treatments for the encephalopathy associated with sepsis and SIRS. Early recognition and treatment of the underlying illness is the most effective therapy.

The multitude of inflammatory mediators that are believed to be involved in the development of the encephalopathy make specific targets for treatment difficult to ascertain. Inhibitors of nitric oxide synthase have been disappointing in animal studies, but inhibitors of glutamate, antioxidants, and complement factors have shown some promise.[31–33]

NEUROMUSCULAR CONDITIONS IN CRITICALLY ILL PATIENTS

Critically ill patients may have neuromuscular signs due to many possible etiologies that affect the CNS as well as the PNS (Table 56-1). Lesion localization is particularly challenging to the clinician faced with multiple confounding factors in the setting of critical illness, including the frequent inability to obtain a history from patients, given mental status changes and physical impediments (e.g., endotracheal and orogastric tubes). In the modern intensive care unit (ICU), the multiplicity of invasive lines, tubings, electrodes and wiring for monitoring equipment, limb splints, restraints, occlusive dressings, and bandages all represent formidable physical obstructions to the clinical examination. Neuromuscular diagnoses are often delayed in

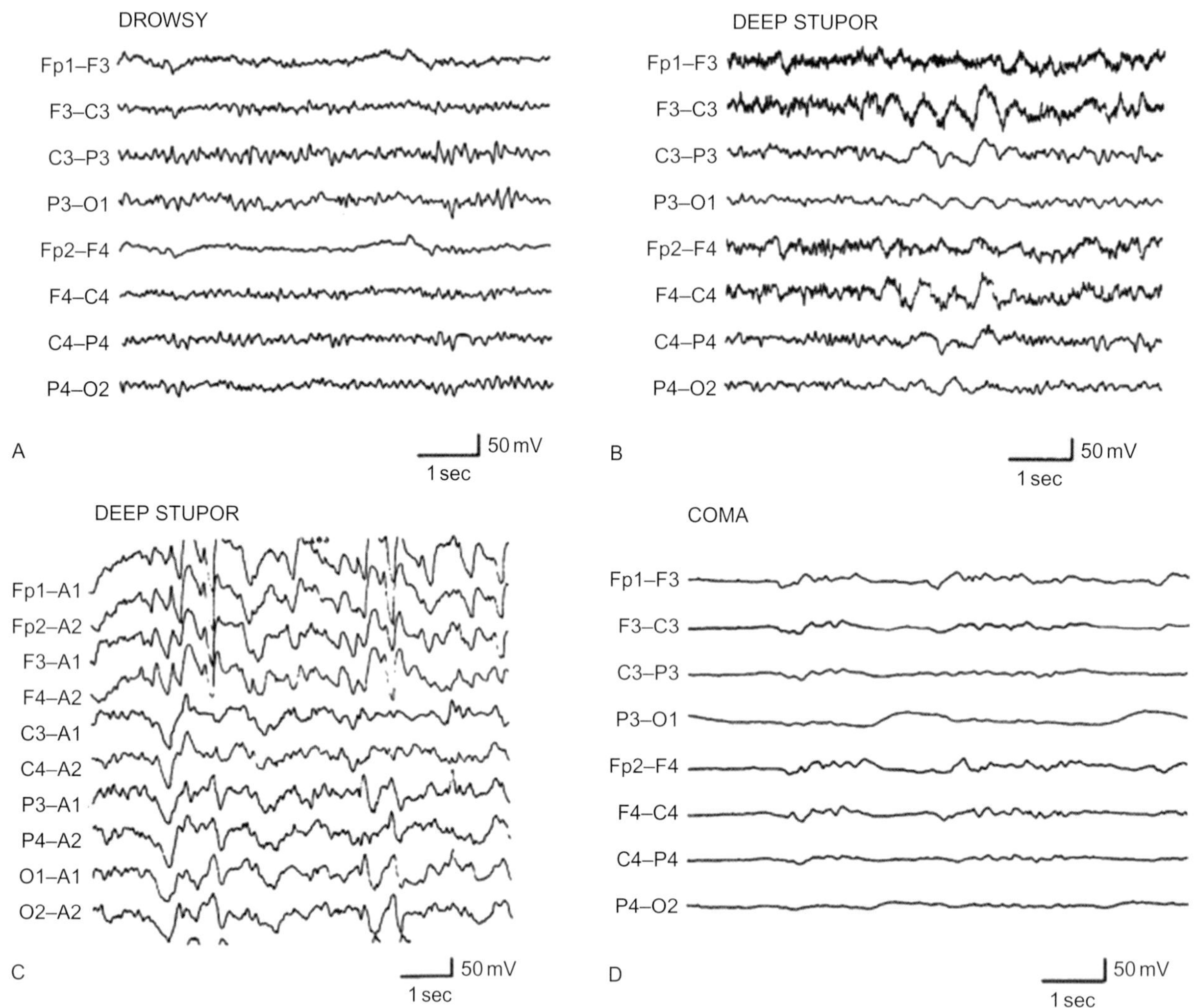

FIGURE 56-1 ■ Electroencephalograms (EEGs) from patients with septic encephalopathy. **A,** Patient with mild encephalopathy. The EEG shows a mild excess of low-voltage 6- to 7-Hz theta rhythms in both left (odd-numbered electrode placements) and right (even-numbered placements) hemispheres. **B** to **D,** Severely encephalopathic patients. **B,** Bilateral intermittent rhythmic delta (<3 Hz) waves on a background of mild slowing. **C,** Triphasic waves. **D,** Burst-suppression pattern. (From Bolton CF, Young GB. Neurological complications in critically ill patients. p. 981. In Aminoff MJ (ed): Neurology and General Medicine. 4th Ed. Churchill Livingstone Elsevier, Philadelphia, 2008, with permission.)

critically ill patients due to the severity of underlying illness. Many primary critical care conditions will present with respiratory dysfunction and motor impairment that can be difficult to separate from primary neurologic conditions.

Electrodiagnostic testing is an important part of the routine evaluation of critically ill patients with unexplained neuromuscular deficits. These investigations, however, are also significantly hampered by ICU conditions including electric interference, cool and edematous limbs, restricted access to sites of stimulation and recording due to physical barriers, and limited patient cooperation.

Critical illness polyneuropathy and myopathy are important conditions, but in diagnosing them, the clinician should be diligent in excluding the other disorders listed in Table 56-2. Electrodiagnostic studies are ordered to support a clinical diagnosis such as Guillain–Barré syndrome and myasthenia gravis. The more extensive use of electrodiagnostic testing has allowed for the diagnosis of relatively uncommon neuromuscular conditions including Lambert–Eaton myasthenic syndrome and primary motor neuron disease, which may also be "unmasked" by intercurrent critical illness.

TABLE 56-1 ■ Differential Diagnosis of Neuromuscular Signs in Critically Ill Patients

Encephalopathy	*Neuromuscular Transmission Defects*
Septic	Neuromuscular blocking agents
Anoxic-ischemic	Aminoglycoside toxicity
Other	Myasthenia gravis
Myelopathy	Lambert–Eaton myasthenic syndrome
Anoxic-ischemic	Hypocalcemia
Traumatic	Hypomagnesemia
Other	Organophosphate poisoning
Neuropathy	Wound botulism
Critical illness polyneuropathy	Tick-bite paralysis
Thiamine deficiency	*Myopathy*
Vitamin E deficiency	Critical illness (myosin-deficient) myopathy
Nonspecific nutritional deficiency	Cachexia
Pyridoxine abuse	Acute rhabdomyolysis
Hypophosphatemia	Acute necrotizing myopathy of intensive care
Aminoglycoside toxicity	Electrolyte disturbances: potassium, phosphate, calcium, magnesium
Penicillin toxicity	Corticosteroid myopathy
Guillain–Barré syndrome	Muscular dystrophy
Motor neuron disease	Polymyositis
Porphyria	Acid maltase deficiency
Carcinomatous polyneuropathy	
Compression neuropathy	
Diphtheria	

From Bolton CF, Young GB. Neurological complications in critically ill patients. p. 981. In Aminoff MJ (ed): Neurology and General Medicine. 4th Ed. Churchill Livingstone Elsevier, Philadelphia, 2008, with permission.

Muscle biopsies are increasingly employed in critically ill patients with clinical suspicion of myopathy and the need to distinguish between inflammatory (e.g., dermatomyositis, polymyositis) and noninflammatory (e.g., corticosteroid- or statin-related) etiologies.

Disorders of Nerve

CRITICAL ILLNESS POLYNEUROPATHY

Critical illness polyneuropathy (CIP) was first diagnosed in the 1980s. It may affect one-half to three-quarters of ICU patients,[34–38] and may cause both limb and respiratory muscle weakness. The major risk factors for critical illness polyneuropathy include SIRS, sepsis, multiorgan failure, and hyperglycemia.[39] Definite associations with drug treatments like corticosteroids remain controversial.

Failure to wean from mechanical ventilation is a common presenting feature and may be the only sign of the condition. This cause of failure to wean is important to differentiate from other etiologies in the ICU including encephalopathy-related central drive failure, phrenic nerve trauma, neuromuscular junction dysfunction, and myopathies. Decreased maximal inspiratory and expiratory pressures and vital capacities correlate with limb muscle weakness and are associated with delayed extubation, prolonged ventilation, and unplanned readmission to the ICU.[40,41]

The facial muscles are typically spared in critical illness polyneuropathy. This feature allows for the recognition of a fairly specific pattern of preserved facial

TABLE 56-2 ■ Generalized Neuromuscular Conditions Associated With Critical Illness

Condition	Incidence	Clinical Features	Electrophysiologic Findings	Serum Creatine Kinase Level	Muscle Biopsy	Prognosis
Polyneuropathy						
Critical illness polyneuropathy	Common	Flaccid limbs and respiratory weakness	Axonal degeneration of motor and sensory fibers	Nearly normal	Denervation atrophy	Variable
Neuromuscular Transmission Defect						
Transient neuromuscular blockade	Common with neuromuscular blocking agents	Flaccid limbs and respiratory weakness	Abnormal repetitive nerve stimulation studies	Normal	Normal	Good
Critical Illness Myopathy						
Thick-filament myosin loss	Common with steroids, neuromuscular blocking agents, and sepsis	Flaccid limbs and respiratory weakness	Abnormal spontaneous activity	Mildly elevated	Loss of thick (myosin) filaments	Good
Rhabdomyolysis	Rare	Flaccid limbs and myoglobinuria	Near normal	Markedly elevated (myoglobinuria)	Normal or mild necrosis	Good
Necrotizing myopathy of intensive care	Rare	Flaccid weakness and myoglobinuria	Severe myopathy	Markedly elevated (myoglobinuria)	Marked necrosis	Poor
Disuse (cachectic) myopathy	Common?	Muscle wasting	Normal	Normal	Normal or type II fiber atrophy	Good
Combined polyneuropathy and myopathy	Common	Flaccid limbs and respiratory weakness	Indicate combined polyneuropathy and myopathy	Variable	Denervation atrophy and myopathy	Variable

From Bolton CF, Young GB. Neurological complications in critically ill patients. p. 981. In Aminoff MJ (ed): Neurology and General Medicine. 4th Ed. Churchill Livingstone Elsevier, Philadelphia, 2008, with permission.

grimacing with flaccid or absent limb movements in response to deep nail-bed pressure. Typically, there is loss of previously preserved muscle stretch reflexes. If the patient is cooperative, muscle strength can be tested using the Medical Research Council (MRC) scale or handgrip dynamometry. An "MRC sum score" of less than 48 establishes ICU-acquired paresis and is associated with protracted mechanical ventilation, prolonged length of stay in the ICU, increased mortality, and reduced quality of life in survivors.[40,42–46] Although predominantly a motor problem, loss of pain, temperature, proprioception, and vibration sensation may be noted occasionally. In some circumstances weakness may be generalized rather than length-dependent. Although most patients improve, the degree of residual disability after discharge from the acute care setting is variable and depends heavily upon the electrodiagnostic findings.

Laboratory findings may be consistent with SIRS, sepsis, and multiorgan failure. Lumbar puncture is not usually required but will typically show a normal CSF protein concentration without albuminocytologic dissociation such as occurs in Guillain–Barré syndrome.

The pattern of electrodiagnostic abnormalities seen in critical illness polyneuropathy is consistent with a length-dependent, sensorimotor, axonal polyneuropathy. The initial changes are marked by a reduction in the amplitude of sensory nerve and compound muscle action potentials, predominantly in the lower extremities. In keeping with an axonal neuropathy, distal latencies and conduction velocities are typically normal or minimally abnormal (Fig. 56-2). Additionally, some have argued that for a diagnosis of "definite" critical illness polyneuropathy, repetitive nerve stimulation testing should be performed to demonstrate the absence of a decremental response as occurs in myasthenia gravis.[47] Technical difficulties including edema and other cutaneous factors (which increase impedance

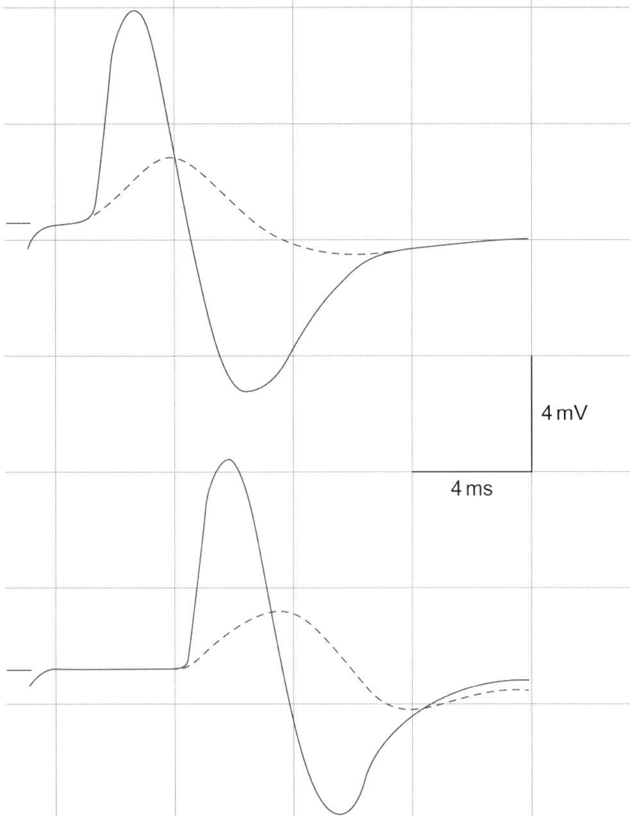

FIGURE 56-2 ■ Compound muscle action potential recording from the thenar muscle on stimulation of the median nerve at the wrist (*upper panel*) and elbow (*lower panel*), at the onset of sepsis (*solid line*) and 3 weeks later (*dotted line*). Note the marked drop in amplitude and mild but definite increase in duration without a change in latency. (From Latronico N, Bolton CF. Critical illness polyneuropathy and myopathy: a major cause of muscle weakness and paralysis. Lancet Neurol 10:931, 2011, with permission.)

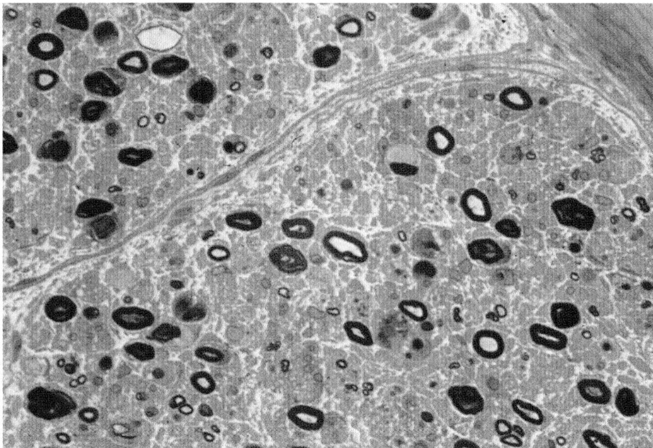

FIGURE 56-3 ■ Transverse section of the superficial fibular (peroneal) nerve showing severe axonal degeneration and loss of myelinated fibers. (Toluidine blue; original magnification 773 ×.) (Modified from Zochodne DW, Bolton CF, Wells GA, et al: Critical illness polyneuropathy: a complication of sepsis and multiple organ failure. Brain 110:819, 1987, with permission. Courtesy of Douglas Zochodne, MD.)

and produce spuriously low recordings) are often encountered in critical care patients and should raise concern when interpreting the electrophysiologic findings.

There is some evidence that compound muscle action potential duration may be slightly prolonged, a change typically seen in critical illness myopathy due to muscle fiber membrane dysfunction.[47] This finding may implicate a subtle component of overlapping pathophysiologies.

It may not be possible to elicit motor unit potentials when consciousness is depressed as voluntary activation of muscles is required. If present, they can be normal or mildly myopathic. It typically takes 2 to 3 weeks after the initial nerve injury for the emergence of abnormal spontaneous activity including positive sharp waves and fibrillation potentials, by which time further reduction of the sensory nerve and compound muscle action potentials may have occurred due to ongoing axon loss. Even in severe cases, axonal changes predominate without evidence of a concomitant demyelinating process. As recovery occurs, spontaneous activity tends to subside and, by about 2 months, motor unit potentials are longer and larger than normal, and many are polyphasic.

It has been suggested that patients at risk of critical illness polyneuropathy should be monitored in the ICU with serial fibular (peroneal) motor nerve conduction studies to identify the process early in its course.[48]

The specific clinical and electrodiagnostic features of CIP usually obviate the need for tissue diagnosis. However, distal-predominant motor and sensory nerve fiber degeneration has been demonstrated on nerve and muscle biopsies as well as on autopsy findings in patients with critical illness polyneuropathy (Figs. 56-3 and 56-4).[49,50] Histopathologic examination reveals acute denervation atrophy of muscle (both type I and type II fibers) with scattered, angulated fibers (Fig. 56-5). As the process advances, some degree of reinnervation occurs, as evidenced by fiber-type grouping; group atrophy has also been described.[51] Inflammation in either nerve or muscle is conspicuously absent. The CNS is generally

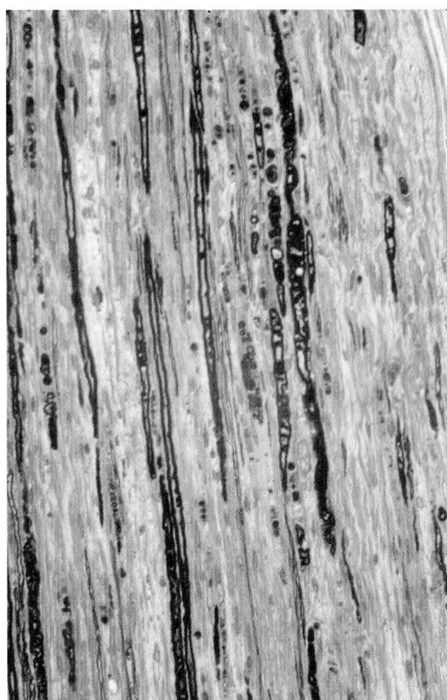

FIGURE 56-4 ■ Longitudinal section of the deep fibular (peroneal) nerve demonstrating axonal degeneration and loss of myelinated fibers. (Toluidine blue; original magnification 778 ×.) (Modified from Zochodne DW, Bolton CF, Wells GA, et al: Critical illness polyneuropathy: a complication of sepsis and multiple organ failure. Brain 110:819, 1987, with permission. Courtesy of Douglas Zochodne, MD.)

devoid of changes except for chromatolysis of the anterior horn cells secondary to distal motor axonal injury.[52] Intercostal and phrenic nerves undergo a similar process of motor axon loss, resulting in denervation atrophy of respiratory muscles, explaining the associated respiratory compromise.

A component of potentially reversible functional disruption precedes structural degeneration of nerves in critical illness polyneuropathy.[50] Such a phenomenon is mirrored simultaneously in multiple failing organs and is likely a result of shared microcirculatory, cellular, and metabolic pathophysiologic mechanisms.[53] The basis of this reversible peripheral nerve dysfunction may lie in abnormal nerve excitability due to an induced channelopathy. The evidence points to a shift in the voltage dependence of sodium channel fast inactivation towards a more negative potential so that affected peripheral nerves tend to remain in the depolarized state.[54]

This early functional disruption may be the basis for electrophysiologic changes in peripheral nerves and muscles that are rapid in onset (often within hours) and may be reversible, corresponding to the rapid onset of clinical deficits. These patients generally have a better prognosis than those already developing axonal degeneration.[54]

Apart from systemic and microcirculatory factors that promote peripheral nerve ischemia, there is evidence for mitochondrial dysfunction with reduced ATP biosynthesis and energy generation (cytopathic hypoxia).[55,56] Metabolic disruptions include an increase in the production of cytokines, nitric oxide, and stress hormones that can lead to hyperglycemia from increased insulin resistance.[53] Decreased metabolic demands reduce hormonal stimulation, which, in conjunction with direct mitochondrial inhibition from nitrogen and oxygen reactive species, leads to mitochondrial ATP generation failure.[53] Impairment in axonal transport systems due to energy failure may be responsible for the distal-predominant pattern of nerve fiber involvement.[51]

In patients with critical illness polyneuropathy, the vascular endothelium of epineurial and endoneurial vessels has increased expression of E-selectin, a marker of endothelial cell activation.[57] As a consequence, activated leukocytes within the endoneurial space produce local cytokines that increase microvascular permeability. The subsequent endoneurial edema compromises the blood–nerve barrier. Such deleterious fluid dynamics are enhanced by hyperglycemia and hypoalbuminemia.[58] The peripheral axon which is exposed to this process is then further susceptible to circulating toxins in the setting of sepsis.

Recommendations for patient management include the prevention and aggressive treatment of sepsis and related multiple organ failure. Although malnutrition is not clearly implicated in the pathogenesis of critical illness polyneuropathy, benefits are likely when nutritional status is optimized by the timely use of total parenteral or enteral nutrition. Early intervention with rehabilitative exercises should be encouraged.

There is no evidence to support the use of intravenous immunoglobulin or other agents (e.g., antioxidants, hormones) thought to abort the septic cascade.[46,59–61] Insulin therapy to maintain euglycemia reduces the incidence of critical illness polyneuropathy and the duration of mechanical ventilation in critically ill patients.[62,63] Studies have demonstrated a 20 to 44 percent reduction in the incidence of neuromuscular dysfunction in patients receiving intensive treatment for hyperglycemia.[64,65] However, intensive insulin therapy to maintain strict blood glucose control also increases

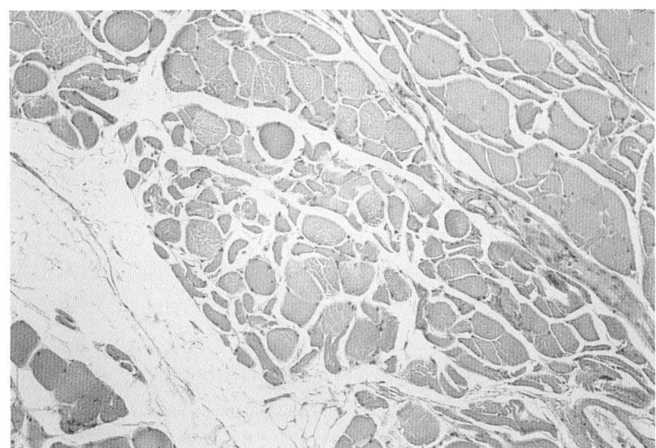

FIGURE 56-5 ■ Transverse section of intercostal muscle showing variation in muscle fiber size and scattered and grouped atrophic fibers consistent with denervation atrophy. (Hematoxylin and eosin; original magnification 195 ×.) (Modified from Zochodne DW, Bolton CF, Wells GA, et al: Critical illness polyneuropathy: a complication of sepsis and multiple organ failure. Brain 110:819, 1987, with permission. Courtesy of Douglas Zochodne, MD.)

mortality in adult ICU patients so the optimum glycemic target remains unclear for these patients.[66,67]

The underlying systemic condition is responsible for a mortality rate of up to 50 percent in patients with critical illness polyneuropathy.[68] A study of long-term outcomes demonstrated that 21 percent of patients with critical illness polyneuropathy still had severe residual disability 1 year after the acute illness.[34]

Motor Neuropathy and Neuromuscular Blocking Agents

Competitive (nondepolarizing) neuromuscular blocking agents including pancuronium and vecuronium have been associated with electrophysiologic evidence of long-term neuromuscular junction dysfunction and polyneuropathy.[46] These agents traditionally have been used for muscular relaxation during mechanical ventilation. Discontinuation after prolonged use is associated with difficulty in weaning the patient from the ventilator, often accompanied by limb weakness.

Under these circumstances, injury appears to occur at multiple sites. A myopathic component is suggested by a mild-to-moderate elevation in serum creatine kinase level. Postsynaptic deficits in transmission at the neuromuscular junction can be demonstrated by low-frequency repetitive nerve stimulation. Motor-predominant axon-loss changes are detected on nerve conduction studies and supported by needle electromyography.

It is unclear whether denervation occurs as a primary or secondary process. In some circumstances there may be no actual axonal disruption. Electrodiagnostic findings may thus be the result of profound and prolonged neuromuscular junction blockade producing a "functional denervation" in affected muscles that may manifest varying degrees of denervation atrophy and muscle necrosis.

Zifko and colleagues suggested a major role for sepsis in the pathogenesis of this condition and that, if various systemic complications can be treated successfully, spontaneous improvement and rapid recovery may ensue.[69] It is generally recommended that the dose and duration of neuromuscular blocking agents be judiciously minimized as a reasonable preventive measure.

Fortunately, the routine use of pancuronium and vecuronium for ventilated, critically ill patients has become less common. When neuromuscular blockade is required, the use of alternative nondepolarizing agents is recommended; data suggest that cisatracurium besylate improves survival and decreases mechanical ventilation time in patients with acute respiratory distress syndrome with fewer apparent deleterious effects on muscle function.[70]

Chronic Polyneuropathies

On occasion, the neuropathy found in critically ill patients represents an exacerbation or worsening of a long-standing chronic polyneuropathy. This neurologic decompensation may manifest as sensorimotor deficits in the limbs as well as respiratory muscle weakness. Patients who may be affected in this manner include those with chronic inflammatory demyelinating polyneuropathy (CIDP) or diabetic polyneuropathy.

These cases are best confirmed with electrodiagnostic studies including phrenic nerve conduction studies and diaphragmatic needle electrode examination (optimally, in conjunction with neuromuscular ultrasound).

Neuromuscular Transmission Disorders and Myopathies

Features of preexisting neuromuscular junction disorders and myopathies are difficult to differentiate from the myriad of possible causes of muscle weakness in the critical care setting. A fatigable pattern of weakness with prominent oculobulbar findings should raise suspicion of a neuromuscular junction disorder. These disorders as well as myopathies may transiently worsen with intercurrent illness. In patients with central core disease, malignant hyperthermia is a significant risk (see Chapter 55). Succinylcholine and volatile anaesthetics should be strictly avoided in these patients. Electrodiagnostic studies with repetitive nerve stimulation and (rarely) muscle biopsy may be employed to establish a specific diagnosis.

Transient Neuromuscular Junction Blockade

In cases where neuromuscular junction blocking agents are used for muscle relaxation in mechanically ventilated patients, normal liver and kidney function facilitates rapid metabolism and clearance of the drug. However, in critical illness, renal and hepatic function may be compromised, and neuromuscular junction blocking agents may remain active long after discontinuation due to the protracted half-life in these patients.[71] This prolonged blockade may augment some of the injuries to the peripheral nervous system attributed to sepsis itself, and convalescence may require weeks to months. Electrodiagnostic evaluation with repetitive nerve stimulation may help in the confirmation and quantification of this deficit.

Critical Illness Myopathy

While critical illness polyneuropathy was being characterized in the 1980s, clinicians were also appreciating an acute myopathy in severely ill patients treated for conditions such as status asthmaticus and organ transplantation.[72–82] Various terms have marked the condition's etymologic evolution including acute quadriplegic myopathy, critical care myopathy, acute necrotizing myopathy of intensive care, thick filament myopathy, and pancuronium-associated myopathy. Eventually, the term "critical illness myopathy" was accepted for standard reference to this disorder.[83]

Although critical illness myopathy may occur independently of critical illness polyneuropathy, these conditions most often coexist.[84,85] Difficulty with differentiation has led to the nonspecific but frequent reference to "polyneuromyopathy" in the literature. There is a strong correlation between the severity of critical illness and sepsis and the early onset and severity of critical illness polyneuropathy and myopathy.[86] Patients at particular risk of critical illness myopathy specifically include those with status asthmaticus, among whom up to one-third may be affected.[77] It may also be seen in up to 7 percent of patients after orthotopic liver or heart transplantation.[78,82] A predisposition for myopathy in transplant populations with coexisting renal failure has also been demonstrated.[78] Other risk factors include exposure to corticosteroids and neuromuscular junction blockers, especially when pathologic examination shows myosin loss.[72,74,87–90]

The exact time course is often difficult to determine in the context of septic encephalopathy and administration of sedating medications and neuromuscular blocking agents. The most prominent clinical feature is generalized flaccid weakness affecting the appendicular, truncal, and cranial musculature. There is usually no myalgia or muscle tenderness. An important manifestation is neck flexor weakness, which correlates well with diaphragmatic weakness and difficulty in weaning from mechanical ventilation.[91] Although a pupil-sparing ophthalmoparesis may be present, ocular muscle involvement should prompt exclusion of a neuromuscular junction transmission disorder.[92] The loss of muscle stretch reflexes is a variable finding, although in most cases they are depressed.

In the laboratory evaluation, serum creatine kinase levels are usually mildly increased in at least 50 percent of patients.[68] This is in contrast to patients with critical illness polyneuropathy, who typically have normal serum creatine kinase levels.[48] More marked elevation should raise suspicion of other myopathies listed in Table 56-2. The highest serum creatine kinase levels are seen with necrotizing myopathies and rhabdomyolysis, in which there is often concomitant myoglobinuria. Patients receiving corticosteroids may have at least a 10-day delay in serum creatine kinase elevation related to critical illness myopathy.[93]

In critical illness myopathy, typical findings on nerve conduction studies are low-amplitude compound muscle action potentials, which are often increased in duration to more than twice normal, most pronounced in the lower limbs.[94–96] Slowing of muscle fiber conduction has been a proposed explanation for this finding.[94,96–98] Sensory nerve action potentials are expected to be normal but may be technically difficult to obtain due to skin conditions and tissue edema; this difficulty may be minimized by the use of near-nerve recordings.

The needle electrode examination often shows evidence of abnormal spontaneous activity including fibrillation potentials and positive sharp waves. Activation typically reveals short-duration, low-amplitude motor unit potentials, an increased number of polyphasic potentials, and normal or early recruitment. In unresponsive patients, some authors have suggested recording from the tibialis anterior, employing reflexive activation after plantar stimulation. Alternatively, direct muscle stimulation may be used and, although technically challenging, can demonstrate reduced muscle membrane excitability. This occurs when the compound muscle action potential amplitude after direct muscle stimulation is less than 3 mV and the ratio of the amplitude after nerve stimulation to that after direct muscle stimulation is more than 0.5.[99,100] Since a response to direct muscle stimulation but not nerve stimulation is seen in critical illness polyneuropathy, this test may be helpful in differentiating between these two related conditions, although it is less helpful when both disorders coexist.[101,102] Repetitive nerve stimulation testing should be performed to demonstrate the absence of a decremental response as occurs with defects of neuromuscular transmission. In patients with critical illness myopathy and respiratory impairment, the findings on phrenic nerve conduction studies and needle electrode examination of the diaphragm may be similar to those in critical illness polyneuropathy.[103] Motor unit potentials occurring during attempted inspiration or sniffing usually have a myopathic appearance regardless of the underlying diagnosis.

Typical muscle biopsy findings include type II–predominant fiber atrophy with myofibrillar disorganization. There may be variable degrees of both necrosis and myofiber regeneration. Thick-filament myosin loss is the most characteristic feature and may be related to a decreased transcription rate or loss of myosin messenger RNA.[104]

The underlying pathophysiology of critical illness myopathy includes muscle inexcitability due to a shift in the voltage dependence of sodium channel fast inactivation similar to that seen in critical illness polyneuropathy.[105–109] This process seems to be augmented by sepsis. Evidence also supports muscle perfusion deficits at the capillary level.[110,111] Muscle wasting is primarily due to degradation of myofibrillar proteins, which comprise 60 to 70 percent of total muscle protein; as a consequence, there is prominent loss of myosin filaments with sarcomeric disorganization.[112] Similar to critical illness polyneuropathy and other organ failure during sepsis, there is muscle fiber bioenergetic failure due to mitochondrial dysfunction. Toxicity appears to be mediated by ATP depletion, intracellular antioxidant diminution, and nitric oxide production.[113]

Thick-Filament Myosin Loss

This feature of critical illness myopathy has been specifically associated with the term "acute quadriplegic myopathy" and is also referred to as "myosin-deficient" myopathy (see Chapter 55). Classically, cases occur in severe asthmatic and post-transplant patients who are mechanically ventilated after receiving high-dose corticosteroids and neuromuscular blocking agents. There may be a slight elevation in serum creatine kinase levels, and muscle biopsy shows selective loss of thick (myosin) filaments. Although these changes can be appreciated on light microscopy, they are better seen on electron microscopy along with varying degrees of muscle necrosis (Fig. 56-6).

In the absence of any specific treatment, it is recommended that corticosteroids and neuromuscular blocking agents be avoided or limited as much as possible. With recovery, there is a gradual reduction in myonecrosis and reappearance of thick myosin filaments.

Rhabdomyolysis

Rhabdomyolysis is another muscular complication that can occur in the context of critical illness with corticosteroid and neuromuscular blocking agent use.[114] It may have many causes and presents with myalgia and muscle tenderness, weakness, and possible swelling. It is associated with hyperkalemia and hypocalcemia, placing the patient at risk of cardiac arrhythmias. There is also a significant risk of acute renal failure especially from marked myoglobinuria. In contrast with usual forms of critical illness myopathy, extensive myolysis results in serum creatine kinase levels that frequently exceed 10,000 IU/L.

The electrodiagnostic findings are consistent with an acute myopathy with typically normal motor and sensory nerve conduction studies. Electromyography usually reveals normal motor unit morphology with scant fibrillation potentials.[115]

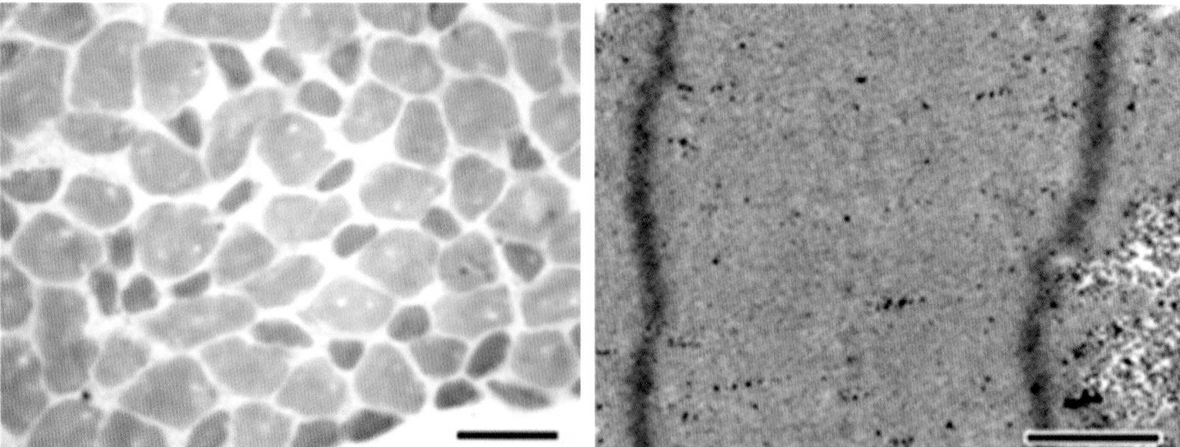

FIGURE 56-6 ■ Critical illness myopathy. **A,** ATPase enzyme histochemistry at pH 9.8 shows atrophy of type II (dark) fibers. Scale bar, 100 µm. **B,** Electron micrograph demonstrating loss of thick filaments. Scale bar, 0.5 µm. (Courtesy of Susan M. Staugaitis, M.D., Ph.D., Cleveland Clinic.)

A muscle biopsy is usually not required for diagnosis, but, when obtained, typically shows a variable degree of myonecrosis without inflammation or any other specific pathologic features. Rarely in bacteremic patients, muscle biopsy may confirm coexisting microabscesses (mostly seen in tropical countries or in children).[46] With appropriate supportive therapy to avoid renal failure and treatment of the underlying condition, patients with rhabdomyolysis usually have a good functional prognosis.

Acute Necrotizing Myopathy of Intensive Care

This condition is considered a more severe variant of rhabdomyolysis. Serum creatine kinase levels are greatly elevated and there is florid myoglobinuria. Biopsy demonstrates extensively severe myonecrosis. In severe cases, the prognosis is poor as significant muscle weakness may persist.[116]

Cachectic Myopathy

In cachectic myopathy, muscle weakness and atrophy are related to extensive disuse or catabolic predisposition in patients with starvation and malnutrition. Patients at particular risk include those with anorexia nervosa or those who have undergone gastric bypass surgery.[117,118] Cachectic myopathy is not uncommon in the ICU, and is characterized by normal serum creatine kinase levels and electrodiagnostic findings. The only abnormality on muscle biopsy may be type II fiber atrophy. The prognosis is variable and is related to the underlying disorder.

Management of Critical Illness Myopathy

The recognition of the clinical features, laboratory abnormalities, and electrodiagnostic findings of critical illness myopathy obviates the need for biopsy in many cases. Biopsy is most helpful when another myopathic process (e.g., inflammatory) needs to be excluded.

Evidence now supports the early initiation of rehabilitative exercises, without waiting for patients to be deemed clinically stable or "medically optimized," despite previous recommendations.[119] Serial muscle biopsies have demonstrated that repeated daily passive mobilization prevents muscle atrophy.[120,121] Although muscle strength is not greatly improved, early physical and occupational therapy while patients are in the ICU improves functional independence, minimizes delirium, and increases the number of ventilator-free days compared with standard care.[121] When possible, the use of a bedside ergometer for daily cycle sessions following ICU admission improves functional exercise capacity, quadriceps muscle strength, and functional status.[122]

Consistent with current practice trends, the use of paralytic agents in the mechanically ventilated patient should be minimized. The duration of mechanical ventilation, coma, and overall ICU and hospital length of stay may be reduced with a protocol of coordinated daily interruption of sedation and trials of spontaneous breathing.[123] With such an approach, there is improvement in 1-year survival with a number needed to treat of 7 patients.[123]

Mixed Critical Illness Polyneuropathy and Myopathy

The precise incidence of critical illness polyneuropathy and myopathy is difficult to ascertain due to wide variability in study populations, risk factors, and the timing of assessments. In patients mechanically ventilated for 4 to 7 days or those with multiorgan failure, the reported incidence is 25 to 33 percent based on clinical assessment[43,45,86] and 30 to 58 percent when electrodiagnostic techniques are used.[43,45,86,124,125] A systematic review of published data showed that critical illness polyneuropathy and myopathy were present in 46 percent of adult ICU patients who had prolonged mechanical ventilation, sepsis, or multiorgan failure.[126] Prospective studies have identified independent risk factors including, severity of illness, multiple ($\geq$2) organ dysfunction, duration of vasopressor support, duration of ICU stay, hyperglycemia, female sex, renal failure and renal replacement therapy, hyperosmolality, parenteral nutrition, low serum albumin, and CNS dysfunction.[127] Aminoglycoside antibiotics, neuromuscular junction blocking agents, and corticosteroids have been implicated as risk factors as well.[48,59,62,63,128]

Incidence estimates are further complicated by difficulty in separating critical illness polyneuropathy from critical illness myopathy. Most cases of neuromuscular weakness in the ICU likely have a component of both. Accordingly, there may be overlapping clinical, laboratory, electrodiagnostic, and biopsy findings.

Both critical illness polyneuropathy and critical illness myopathy cause limb and diaphragm weakness that persists for months or years after resolution of critical illness. Nearly one-third of these patients with either or both of these conditions do not recover independent ambulation or spontaneous ventilation.[129] Critical illness polyneuropathy has been identified as the main contributor to persistent disability while critical illness myopathy is more frequently, but not always, associated with complete recovery.[130]

Patients with either or both conditions are likely to benefit from fastidious treatment of infection, optimized nutrition, correction of underlying metabolic and electrolyte disturbances, deep vein thrombosis prophylaxis, chest physiotherapy and pulmonary toilet, frequent turning and pressure-point padding, orthotics use, and a proactive physical therapy regimen as discussed above.[131]

Electrodiagnostic Studies of the Respiratory System

Phrenic nerve conduction studies and diaphragmatic electromyography (with or without neuromuscular ultrasound) have proved quite useful in establishing a neuromuscular basis for respiratory impairment in critically ill patients. These diagnostic modalities may also indirectly implicate impairment of "central drive," when the deficit is due to injury to the autonomic centers of respiration (see Chapter 1). This electrodiagnostic testing often complements other tests of respiratory function including vital capacity and maximum inspiratory and expiratory force, and may help with decisions regarding the need for intubation and ventilatory support.[132] It may also be helpful for long-term prognostication by quantifying the degree of demyelination or denervation affecting the phrenic nerves.

REFERENCES

1. Young GB, Boulton CB, Austin TW, et al: The encephalopathy associated with septic illness. Clin Invest Med 13:297, 1990.
2. Ebersoldt M, Sharshar T, Annane D: Sepsis-associated delirium. Intensive Care Med 33:941, 2007.
3. Sprung CL, Peduzzi PN, Shatney CH, et al: Impact of encephalopathy on mortality in the sepsis syndrome. The Veterans Administration Systemic Sepsis Cooperative Study Group. Crit Care Med 18:801, 1990.
4. Eidelman LA, Putterman D, Spring CL: The spectrum of septic encephalopathy. Definitions, etiologies, and mortalities. JAMA 275:470, 1996.
5. Neviere R: Pathophysiology of sepsis. www.UptoDate.com, 2013.
6. Bone RC: Immunologic dissonance: a continuing evolution in our understanding of the systemic inflammatory response syndrome (SIRS) and the multiple organ dysfunction syndrome (MODS). Ann Intern Med 125:680, 1996.
7. Frantz S, Ertl G, Bauersachs J: Mechanisms of disease: Toll-like receptors in cardiovascular disease. Nat Clin Pract Cardiovasc Med 4:444, 2007.
8. Price S, Anning PB, Mitchel JA, et al: Myocardial dysfunction in sepsis: mechanisms and therapeutic implications. Eur Heart J 20:715, 1999.
9. De Backer D, Creteur J, Preiser JC, et al: Microvasular blood flow is altered in patients with sepsis. Am J Respir Crit Care Med 166:98, 2002.
10. Harris A, Huet D, Duranteau J: Alteration of mitochondrial function in sepsis and critical illness. Curr Opin Anaesthesiol 22:143, 2009.

11. Coopersmith CM, Stromberg PE, Dunne WM, et al: Inhibition of intestinal epithelial apotosis and survival in a murine model of pneumonia induced sepsis. JAMA 287:1716, 2002.
12. Papadopoulos MC, Davies C, Moss RF, et al: Pathophysiology of septic encephalopathy: a review. Crit Care Med 28:3019, 2000.
13. Manno EM: Evaluation and treatment of the patient with toxic-metabolic encephalopathies. p. 259. In: Batjer H, Loftus C (eds): Textbook of Neurological Surgery. Lippincott-Raven, Philadelphia, 2002.
14. Manno EM: Neurological complications of medical illness: critical illness neuropathy and myopathy. p. 182. In Manno EM (ed): Emergency Management in Neurocritical Care. Wiley-Blackwell, Oxford, 2012.
15. Pan W, Hsuchou H, Yu C, et al: Permeation of blood borne IL1 across the blood brain barrier and the effects of LPS. J Neurochem 106:313, 2008.
16. Huynh HK, Dorovini-Zis K: Effects of interferon-gamma on primary cultures of human brain endothelial cells. Am J Pathol 142:1265, 1993.
17. Deng X, Wang X, Andersson R: Endothelial barrier resistance in multiple organs after septic challenges in the rat. J Appl Physiol 78:2052, 1995.
18. Maekawa T, Fujii Y, Sadamitsu D, et al: Cerebral circulation and metabolism in patients with septic encephalopathy. Am J Emerg Med 9:139, 1991.
19. Papadoupoulos MC, Moss RF, Lamb FJ, et al: Faecal peritonitis causes oedema and neuronal injury in pig cerebral cortex. Clin Sci 96:461, 1999.
20. Fink M: Cytopathic hypoxia in sepsis. Acta Anaesth Scand 110:87, 1997.
21. Sharshar T, Annane D, de la Grandmaison GL, et al: The neuropathology of septic shock. Brain Pathol 14:21, 2004.
22. Sharshar T, Carlier R, Bernard F, et al: Brain lesions in septic shock: a magnetic resonance imaging study. Intensive Care Med 33:798, 2007.
23. Chuang YC, Tsai JL, Chang AY, et al: Dysfunction of the mitochondrial respiratory chain in the rostral ventral medulla during experimental endotoxemia in the rat. J Biomed Sci 9:542, 2002.
24. Sahrshar T, Gray F, Lorin de la Grandmaison G, et al: Apoptosis of neurons in cardiovascular autonomic centers triggered by inducible nitric oxide synthetase after death from septic shock. Lancet 362:1799, 2003.
25. Bordovikova LV, Ivanoya S, Zhang M, et al: Vagus nerve stimulation attenuates the systemic inflammatory response to endotoxin. Nature 405:458, 2000.
26. Ebersoldt M, Sharshar T, Annane D: Sepsis-associated delirium. Intensive Care Med 33:941, 2007.
27. Hsu AA, Fenton K, Weinstein S, et al: Neurological injury markers in children with septic shock. Pediatric Crit Care 9:245, 2008.
28. Young GB, Bolton CF, Archibald YM, et al: The electroencephalogram in sepsis-associated encephalopathy. J Clin Neurophysiol 9:145, 1992.
29. Towne AR, Waterhouse EJ, Boggs JG, et al: Prevalence of nonconvulsive status in comatose patients. Neurology 54:340, 2000.
30. Pytel P, Alexander JJ: Pathogenesis of septic encephalopathy. Curr Opin Neurol 22:283, 2009.
31. Lopez A, Lorente JA, Steingrub J, et al: Multicenter, randomized, placebo controlled, double-blinded trial of the nitric oxide inhibitor 546C88: effect on survival in patients with septic shock. Crit Care Med 32:21, 2004.
32. Barenchello T, Machado RA, Constantino L, et al: Antioxidant treatment prevented late memory impairment in an animal model of sepsis. Crit Care Med 35:2186, 2007.
33. Umgelter A, Reindl W, Lutz J, et al: Treatment of septic patients with an arginine based endotoxin adsorber column improves hemodynamics and reduces oxidative stress: results of a feasibility study. Blood Purif 26:333, 2008.
34. Leijten FS, De Weerd AW, Poortvliet DC: Critical illness polyneuropathy in multiple organ dysfunction syndrome and weaning from the ventilator. Intensive Care Med 22:856, 1996.
35. Druschky A, Herkert M, Radespiel-Troger M, et al: Critical illness polyneuropathy: clinical findings and cell culture assay of neurotoxicity assessed by a prospective study. Intensive Care Med 27:686, 2001.
36. Garnacho-Montero J, Madrazo-Osuna J, Garcıa-Garmendia JL, et al: Critical illness polyneuropathy: risk factors and clinical consequences. A cohort study in septic patients. Intensive Care Med 27:1288, 2001.
37. Tepper M, Rakic S, Haas JA, et al: Incidence and onset of critical illness polyneuropathy in patients with septic shock. Neth J Med 56:211, 2000.
38. Thiele RI, Jakob H, Hund E, et al: Sepsis and catecholamine support are the major risk factors for critical illness polyneuropathy after open heart surgery. Thorac Cardiovasc Surg 48:145, 2000.
39. American College of Chest Physicians/Society of Critical Care Medicine Consensus Conference: Definitions for sepsis and organ failure and guidelines for the use of innovative therapies in sepsis. Crit Care Med 20:864, 1992.
40. De Jonghe B, Bastuji-Garin S, Durand MC, et al; for the Groupe de Reflexion et d'Etude des Neuromyopathies en Reanimation: Respiratory weakness is associated with limb weakness and delayed weaning in critical illness. Crit Care Med 35:2007, 2007.
41. Latronico N, Guarneri B, Alongi S, et al: Acute neuromuscular respiratory failure after ICU discharge. Report of five patients. Intensive Care Med 25:1302, 1999.
42. Herridge MS, Cheung AM, Tansey CM, et al; for the Canadian Critical Care Trials Group: One-year outcomes in survivors of the acute respiratory distress syndrome. N Engl J Med 348: 683, 2003.

43. Herridge MS, Tansey CM, Matte A, et al: Functional disability 5 years after acute respiratory distress syndrome. N Engl J Med 364:1293, 2011.
44. De Jonghe B, Bastuji-Garin S, Sharshar T, et al: Does ICU-acquired paresis lengthen weaning from mechanical ventilation? Intensive Care Med 30:1117, 2004.
45. Ali NA, O'Brien Jr JM, Hoffmann SP, et al; for the Midwest Critical Care Consortium: Acquired weakness, handgrip strength, and mortality in critically ill patients. Am J Respir Crit Care Med 178:261, 2008.
46. De Jonghe B, Sharshar T, Lefaucheur JP, et al; for the Groupe de Reflexion et d'Etude des Neuromyopathies en Reanimation: Paresis acquired in the intensive care unit: a prospective multicenter study. JAMA 288:2859, 2002.
47. Bolton CF: Neuromuscular manifestations of critical illness. Muscle Nerve 32:140, 2005.
48. Latronico N, Bertolini G, Guarneri B, et al: Simplified electrophysiological evaluation of peripheral nerves in critically ill patients: the Italian multicentre CRIMYNE study. Crit Care 11:R11, 2007.
49. Witt NJ, Zochodne DW, Bolton CF, et al: Peripheral nerve function in sepsis and multiple organ failure. Chest 99:176, 1991.
50. Latronico N: Muscle weakness during critical illness. Eur Crit Care Emerg Med 2:61, 2010.
51. Latronico N, Recupero D, Candiani A, et al: Critical illness myopathy and neuropathy. Lancet 347:1579, 1996.
52. Zochodne DW, Bolton CF, Wells GA, et al: Critical illness polyneuropathy. A complication of sepsis and multiple organ failure. Brain 110:819, 1987.
53. Singer M, De Santis V, Vitale D, et al: Multiorgan failure is an adaptive, endocrine-mediated, metabolic response to overwhelming systemic inflammation. Lancet 364:545, 2004.
54. Novak KR, Nardelli P, Cope TC, et al: Inactivation of sodium channels underlies reversible neuropathy during critical illness in rats. J Clin Invest 119:1150, 2009.
55. Sibbald WJ, Messmer K, Fink MP: Roundtable conference on tissue oxygenation in acute medicine. Brussels, Belgium, 14–16 March 1998. Intensive Care Med 26:780, 2000.
56. Fink MP, Evans TW: Mechanisms of organ dysfunction in critical illness: report from a Round Table Conference held in Brussels. Intensive Care Med 28:369, 2002.
57. Fenzi F, Latronico N, Refatti N, et al: Enhanced expression of E-selectin on the vascular endothelium of peripheral nerve in critically ill patients with neuromuscular disorders. Acta Neuropathol 106:75, 2003.
58. Latronico N, Peli E, Botteri M: Critical illness myopathy and neuropathy. Curr Opin Crit Care 11:126, 2005.
59. Hermans G, De Jonghe B, Bruyninckx F, et al: Interventions for preventing critical illness polyneuropathy and critical illness myopathy. Cochrane Database Syst Rev 1:CD006832, 2009.
60. Wijdicks EF, Fulgham JR: Failure of high dose intravenous immunoglobulins to alter the clinical course of critical illness polyneuropathy. Muscle Nerve 17:1494, 1994.
61. Mohr M, Englisch L, Roth A, et al: Effects of early treatment with immunoglobulin on critical illness polyneuropathy following multiple organ failure and gram-negative sepsis. Intensive Care Med 23:1144, 1997.
62. Hermans G, Wilmer A, Meersseman W, et al: Impact of intensive insulin therapy on neuromuscular complications and ventilator dependency in the medical intensive care unit. Am J Respir Crit Care Med 175:480, 2007.
63. Van den Berghe G, Schoonheydt K, Becx P, et al: Insulin therapy protects the central and peripheral nervous system of intensive care patients. Neurology 64:1348, 2005.
64. Van den Berghe G, Wilmer A, Hermans G, et al: Intensive insulin therapy in the medical ICU. N Engl J Med 354:449, 2006.
65. Van den Berghe G, Wouters P, Weekers F, et al: Intensive insulin therapy in critically ill patients. N Engl J Med 345:1359, 2001.
66. Qaseem A, Humphrey LL, Chou R, et al: Use of intensive insulin therapy for the management of glycemic control in hospitalized patients: a clinical practice guideline from the American College of Physicians. Ann Intern Med 154:260, 2011.
67. Finfer S, Chittock DR, Su SY, et al: Intensive versus conventional glucose control in critically ill patients. N Engl J Med 360:1283, 2009.
68. Lacomis D: Neuromuscular disorders in critically ill patients: review and update. J Clin Neuromuscul Dis 12:197, 2011.
69. Zifko UA, Zipko HT, Bolton CF: Clinical and electrophysiological findings in critical illness polyneuropathy. J Neurol Sci 159:186, 1998.
70. Papazian L, Forel JM, Gacouin A, et al: for the ACURASYS Study Investigators: Neuromuscular blockers in early acute respiratory distress syndrome. N Engl J Med 363:1107, 2010.
71. Segredo V, Caldwell JE, Matthay MA, et al: Persistent paralysis in critically ill patients after long-term administration of vecuronium. N Engl J Med 327:524, 1992.
72. Shee CD: Risk factors for hydrocortisone myopathy in acute severe asthma. Respir Med 84:229, 1990.
73. Blackie JD, Gibson P, Murree-Allen K, et al: Acute myopathy in status asthmaticus. Clin Exp Neurol 30:72, 1993.
74. Griffin D, Fairman N, Coursin D, et al: Acute myopathy during treatment of status asthmaticus with

corticosteroids and steroidal muscle relaxants. Chest 102:510, 1992.
75. Leatherman JW, Fluegel WL, David WS, et al: Muscle weakness in mechanically ventilated patients with severe asthma. Am J Respir Crit Care Med 153:1686, 1996.
76. Road J, Mackie G, Jiang TX, et al: Reversible paralysis with status asthmaticus, steroids, and pancuronium: clinical electrophysiological correlates. Muscle Nerve 20:1587, 1997.
77. Douglass JA, Tuxen DV, Horne M, et al: Myopathy in severe asthma. Am Rev Respir Dis 146:517, 1992.
78. Campellone JV, Lacomis D, Kramer DJ, et al: Acute myopathy after liver transplantation. Neurology 50:46, 1998.
79. Miró O, Salmerón JM, Masanés F, et al: Acute quadriplegic myopathy with myosin-deficient muscle fibres after liver transplantation: defining the clinical picture and delimiting the risk factors. Transplantation 67:1144, 1999.
80. Subramony SH, Carpenter DE, Raju S, et al: Myopathy and prolonged neuromuscular blockade after lung transplant. Crit Care Med 19:1580, 1991.
81. Chetaille P, Paut O, Fraisse A, et al: Acute myopathy of intensive care in a child after heart transplantation. Can J Anaesth 47:342, 2000.
82. Perea M, Picón M, Miró O, et al: Acute quadriplegic myopathy with loss of thick (myosin) filaments following heart transplantation. J Heart Lung Transplant 20:1136, 2001.
83. Lacomis D, Zochodne DW, Bird SJ: Critical illness myopathy. Muscle Nerve 23:1785, 2000.
84. Koch S, Spuler S, Deja M, et al: Critical illness myopathy is frequent: accompanying neuropathy protracts ICU discharge. J Neurol Neurosurg Psychiatry 82:287, 2011.
85. Bednarik J, Lukas Z, Vondracek P: Critical illness polyneuromyopathy: the electrophysiological components of a complex entity. Intensive Care Med 29:1505, 2003.
86. de Letter MA, Schmitz PI, Visser LH, et al: Risk factors for the development of polyneuropathy and myopathy in critically ill patients. Crit Care Med 29:2281, 2001.
87. Lacomis D, Smith TW, Chad DA: Acute myopathy and neuropathy in status asthmaticus: case report and literature review. Muscle Nerve 16:84, 1993.
88. Danon MJ, Carpenter S: Myopathy with thick filament (myosin) loss following prolonged paralysis with vecuronium during steroid treatment. Muscle Nerve 14:1131, 1991.
89. Hirano M, Ott BR, Raps EC, et al: Acute quadriplegic myopathy: a complication of treatment with steroids, nondepolarizing blocking agents, or both. Neurology 42:2082, 1992.
90. Waclawik AJ, Sufit RL, Beinlich BR, et al: Acute myopathy with selective degeneration of myosin filaments following status asthmaticus treated with methylprednisolone and vecuronium. Neuromuscul Disord 2:19, 1992.
91. Dhar R: Neuromuscular respiratory failure. Continuum (Minneap Minn) 15:40, 2009.
92. Sitwell LD, Weinshenker BG, Monpetit V, et al: Complete ophthalmoplegia as a complication of acute corticosteroid- and pancuronium-associated myopathy. Neurology 41:921, 1991.
93. Hanson P, Dive A, Brucher JM, et al: Acute corticosteroid myopathy in intensive care patients. Muscle Nerve 20:1371, 1997.
94. Park EJ, Nishida T, Sufit RL, et al: Prolonged compound muscle action potential duration in critical illness myopathy: report of nine cases. J Clin Neuromuscul Dis 5:176, 2004.
95. Goodman BP, Harper CM, Boon AJ: Prolonged compound muscle action potential duration in critical illness myopathy. Muscle Nerve 40:1040, 2009.
96. Allen DC, Arunachalam R, Mills KR: Critical illness myopathy: further evidence from muscle-fiber excitability studies of an acquired channelopathy. Muscle Nerve 37:14, 2008.
97. Trojaborg W: Electrophysiologic techniques in critical illness-associated weakness. J Neurol Sci 242:83, 2006.
98. Case Records of the Massachusetts General Hospital Weekly clinicopathological exercises. Case 11—1997. A 51-year-old man with chronic obstructive pulmonary disease and generalized muscle weakness. N Engl J Med 336:1079, 1997.
99. Rich MM, Bird SJ, Raps EC, et al: Direct muscle stimulation in acute quadriplegic myopathy. Muscle Nerve 20:665, 1997.
100. Rich MM, Teener JW, Raps EC, et al: Muscle is electrically inexcitable in acute quadriplegic myopathy. Neurology 46:731, 1996.
101. Bird SJ: Myopathies and disorders of neuromuscular transmission. p. 1507. In: Brown W, Bolton C, Aminoff MJ (eds): Neuromuscular Function and Disease. WB Saunders, Philadelphia, 2002.
102. Lefaucheur JP, Nordine T, Rodriguez P, et al: Origin of ICU acquired paresis determined by direct muscle stimulation. J Neurol Neurosurg Psychiatry 77:500, 2006.
103. Bolton C, Chen R, Wijdicks E, et al: Diseases of the peripheral nervous system. p. 165. In Bolton CF, Chen R, Wijdicks EFM, et al (eds): Neurology of Breathing. Butterworth-Heinemann Elsevier, Philadelphia, 2004.
104. Larsson L, Li X, Edstrom L, et al: Acute quadriplegia and loss of muscle myosin in patients treated with nondepolarizing neuromuscular blocking agents and corticosteroids: mechanisms at the cellular and molecular levels. Crit Care Med 28:34, 2000.
105. Rich MM, Pinter MJ, Kraner SD, et al: Loss of electrical excitability in an animal model of acute quadriplegic myopathy. Ann Neurol 43:171, 1998.

106. Rich MM, Pinter MJ: Crucial role of sodium channel fast inactivation in muscle fibre inexcitability in a rat model of critical illness myopathy. J Physiol 547:555, 2003.
107. Filatov GN, Rich MM: Hyperpolarized shifts in the voltage dependence of fast inactivation of Nav1.4 and Nav1.5 in a rat model of critical illness myopathy. J Physiol 559:813, 2004.
108. Khan J, Harrison TB, Rich MM: Mechanisms of neuromuscular dysfunction in critical illness. Crit Care Clin 24:165, 2008.
109. Rossignol B, Gueret G, Pennec JP, et al: Effects of chronic sepsis on the voltage-gated sodium channel in isolated rat muscle fibers. Crit Care Med 35:351, 2007.
110. Piper RD, Pitt-Hyde M, Li F, et al: Microcirculatory changes in rat skeletal muscle in sepsis. Am J Respir Crit Care Med 154:931, 1996.
111. Neviere R, Mathieu D, Chagnon JL, et al: Skeletal muscle microvascular blood flow and oxygen transport in patients with severe sepsis. Am J Respir Crit Care Med 153:191, 1996.
112. Callahan LA, Supinski GS: Sepsis-induced myopathy. Crit Care Med 37(suppl 10):S354, 2009.
113. Brealey D, Brand M, Hargreaves I, et al: Association between mitochondrial dysfunction and severity and outcome of septic shock. Lancet 360:219, 2002.
114. Bird SJ, Rich MM: Critical illness myopathy and polyneuropathy. Curr Neurol Neurosci Rep 2:527, 2002.
115. Al-Jaberi M, Katirji B: The value of EMG in rhabdomyolysis. Muscle Nerve 18:1043, 1995.
116. Zochodne DW, Ramsay DA, Saly V, et al: Acute necrotizing myopathy of intensive care: electrophysiological studies. Muscle Nerve 17:285, 1994.
117. Hsia AW, Hattab EM, Katz JS: Malnutrition-induced myopathy following Roux-en-Y gastric bypass. Muscle Nerve 24:1692, 2001.
118. McLoughlin DM, Spargo E, Wassif WS, et al: Structural and functional changes in skeletal muscle in anorexia nervosa. Acta Neuropathol 95:632, 1998.
119. Centre for Clinical Practice at NICE (UK). Rehabilitation After Critical Illness. NICE Clinical Guideline No. 83. London: National Institute for Health and Clinical Excellence (UK); 2009. Available from: http://www.ncbi.nlm.nih.gov/books/NBK11653/ (accessed March 30, 2013).
120. Griffiths RD, Palmer TE, Helliwell T, et al: Effect of passive stretching on the wasting of muscle in the critically ill. Nutrition 11:428, 1995.
121. Schweickert WD, Pohlman MC, Pohlman AS, et al: Early physical and occupational therapy in mechanically ventilated, critically ill patients: a randomised controlled trial. Lancet 373:1874, 2009.
122. Burtin C, Clerckx B, Robbeets C, et al: Early exercise in critically ill patients enhances short-term functional recovery. Crit Care Med 37:2499, 2009.
123. Girard TD, Kress JP, Fuchs BD, et al: Efficacy and safety of a paired sedation and ventilator weaning protocol for mechanically ventilated patients in intensive care (Awakening and Breathing Controlled trial): a randomised controlled trial. Lancet 371:126, 2008.
124. Leijten FS, Harinck-de Weerd JE, Poortvliet DC, et al: The role of polyneuropathy in motor convalescence after prolonged mechanical ventilation. JAMA 274:1221, 1995.
125. Garnacho-Montero J, Amaya-Villar R, García-Garmendía JL, et al: Effect of critical illness polyneuropathy on the withdrawal from mechanical ventilation and the length of stay in septic patients. Crit Care Med 33:349, 2005.
126. Stevens RD, Dowdy DW, Michaels RK, et al: Neuromuscular dysfunction acquired in critical illness: a systematic review. Intensive Care Med 33:1876, 2007.
127. Latronico N, Bolton CF: Critical illness polyneuropathy and myopathy: a major cause of muscle weakness and paralysis. Lancet Neurol 10:931, 2011.
128. Nanas S, Kritikos K, Angelopoulos E, et al: Predisposing factors for critical illness polyneuromyopathy in a multidisciplinary intensive care unit. Acta Neurol Scand 118:175, 2008.
129. Latronico N, Shehu I, Seghelini E: Neuromuscular sequelae of critical illness. Curr Opin Crit Care 11:381, 2005.
130. Guarneri B, Bertolini G, Latronico N: Long-term outcome in patients with critical illness myopathy or neuropathy: the Italian multicentre CRIMYNE study. J Neurol Neurosurg Psychiatry 79:838, 2008.
131. Apte-Kakade S: Rehabilitation of patients with quadriparesis after treatment of status asthmaticus with neuromuscular blocking agents and high-dose corticosteroids. Arch Phys Med Rehabil 72:1024, 1991.
132. Zifko U, Chen R, Remtulla H, et al: Respiratory electrophysiological studies in Guillain-Barré syndrome. J Neurol Neurosurg Psychiatry 60:191, 1996.

CHAPTER

57

Seizures and General Medical Disorders

SIMON M. GLYNN ■ JACK M. PARENT ■ MICHAEL J. AMINOFF

Seizures commonly arise as a symptom of neurologic dysfunction in various general medical disorders. The occurrence of epileptic seizures in medically ill patients often carries significant implications regarding the treatment and prognosis of the primary disease. In addition, the treatment of epilepsy due to primary disturbances of central nervous system (CNS) function, or of seizures caused by general medical disorders, may be complicated or influenced by factors associated with systemic disease. The occurrence and management of seizures in common medical conditions that may either produce acute or recurrent seizures, or exacerbate an existing epilepsy syndrome, are discussed in this chapter. Attention is also directed at certain uncommon medical diseases in which seizures are a relatively frequent complication, and at the treatment of preexisting epilepsy in patients with medical conditions that might complicate management. Selected therapeutic agents and recreational drugs that may cause seizures are reviewed.

Some general points are worthy of emphasis. First, in persons with epilepsy, seizures often occur in the context of medical illness. Second, "acute symptomatic seizures" do not necessitate a diagnosis of epilepsy. This term was introduced in the 1970s to differentiate seizures occurring in the context of an acute illness from epileptic seizures and is defined as "a clinical seizure occurring at the time of a systemic insult or in close temporal association with a documented brain insult."[1] This term, then, includes seizures due to disorders that may be reversible (e.g., alcohol intoxication) as well as seizures occurring in the acute phase after an irreversible brain injury (e.g., stroke) that may subsequently lead to development of epileptic seizures. Different neurophysiologic mechanisms are probably responsible for acute symptomatic seizures and later unprovoked (epileptic) seizures, despite the fact that both may relate to the same injury. Conceptual advances in understanding this process of epileptogenesis are

Aminoff's Neurology and General Medicine, Fifth Edition.

outside the scope of this chapter and are reviewed elsewhere.[2,3] Finally, acute symptomatic seizures in comatose or critically ill patients may have subtle or no clinical manifestations and may be detected by electroencephalography (EEG), as discussed in a later section.

RENAL FAILURE

Seizures are common in acute uremia, typically developing between 7 and 10 days after the onset of renal failure, while the patient is anuric or oliguric.[4] Generalized convulsive seizures are most common; partial seizures or even epilepsia partialis continua may also occur. Seizures are relatively unusual in chronic renal insufficiency, occurring in less than 10 percent of cases and usually only when a significant encephalopathy is present or at a preterminal stage.[4] Generalized tonic-clonic seizures are the most common seizure type, but partial and myoclonic seizures also may be seen.[4] Treatment requires the correction of metabolic abnormalities and renal failure, and antiseizure medications. Status epilepticus occurs rarely and acute management is the same as when it occurs in other contexts. Phenytoin, valproic acid, and phenobarbital are all effective for seizures in renal failure. Newer antiepileptic drugs (AEDs) should be used cautiously in patients with renal impairment, given their extensive renal clearance.

Risk factors for acute symptomatic seizures in renal failure include hypertensive encephalopathy, metabolic disturbances, and altered renal clearance of proconvulsant medications such as penicillin. Hypocalcemia and hypomagnesemia may be seen in renal disease, and seizures in this context present an increased risk of convulsive status epilepticus.

Dialysis also increases the risk of generalized convulsive seizures, usually during the end of or the first several hours after a hemodialysis session (termed *dialysis disequilibrium syndrome*). Fluid shifts may be responsible, leading to cerebral edema from increased brain osmolality in the uremic state.[5] Improved dialysis techniques have reduced the incidence of seizures. The dialysis encephalopathy syndrome of myoclonus, asterixis, a distinctive speech disorder, psychiatric disturbances, and seizures due to increased aluminum levels in the brain has largely disappeared in response to removing aluminum from the dialysate.

Prominent myoclonus that may or may not be epileptic occurs in renal failure. Cephalosporins,[6] levetiracetam,[7] amlodipine,[8] and verapamil, diltiazem, and nifedipine may induce acute myoclonic jerking without convulsive seizures. Metformin in the presence of end-stage renal disease[9] and pregabalin[10] may also induce myoclonus in patients receiving hemodialysis. Valproate may be especially helpful for myoclonic seizures.

Use of Antiepileptic Drugs in Renal Disease

Several points require emphasis. First, loading doses for AEDs are determined by their respective volumes of distribution; AEDs with large volumes are lipophilic, and less available for dialysis. This volume is independent of renal clearance and usually is not modified in renal impairment.[11]

Second, protein binding of drugs is affected in renal disease. The fraction of drug that is protein bound does not exert any pharmacologic effect, and many AEDs bind extensively to serum albumin (Table 57-1). Patients with chronic renal disease are hypoalbuminemic, so protein binding is decreased; a larger amount of free drug is therefore available to exert a pharmacologic effect. Uremic molecules may also bind to plasma proteins, displacing drugs.[11] For these reasons, the free serum level—where available—should guide therapy.

Third, uremic molecules downregulate the expression of cytochrome P450 enzymes, so decreasing hepatic metabolism and increasing drug half-life and the risk of drug toxicity for AEDs that are hepatically metabolized (Table 57-1).[12,13]

Fourth, depending on the dialysis technique and the AED, some drugs are cleared by dialysis. As protein binding increases and the volume of distribution increases, the fraction removed declines (Table 57-1).[11] The advent of dialysis membranes with larger surface areas and pore size enables more drugs to be dialyzed than previously.[12,13] For example, post-dialysis seizures resulted from decreased serum levels of phenytoin after the introduction of improved dialysis membranes.[14] For this reason, AEDs that are cleared significantly by hemodialysis should be taken after the dialysis session or supplemental doses prescribed.

Fifth, newer AEDs tend to be rapidly and completely absorbed when given orally, have linear kinetics, and fewer drug–drug interactions. Renal clearance is important for the newer AEDs, which

TABLE 57-1 ■ Selected Pharmacokinetics of Antiepileptic Drugs

		Volume of Distribution (V_d L/kg) (0.6 = V_d for H_2O)	Renal Elimination	Hepatic Metabolism	Molecular Weight (Hemodialysis More Effective If Low)
First- and Second-Generation AEDs					
Minimal or no protein binding	Ethosuximide*	0.6 to 0.7	Minimal	High	141
	Primidone	0.4 to 1.0	Minimal	High	218
Moderate protein binding	Phenobarbital	0.5 to 1.0	Minimal	High	232
High protein binding	Benzodiazepines, including clobazam	1.4 to 1.8 (CLZ), 1.1 to 3.4 (DZP), 1.3 (LZP)	Minimal	High	300 (CLZ), 284 (DZP), 321 (LZP)
	Carbamazepine	0.8 to 2.0	Minimal	High	236
	Phenytoin	0.5 to 1.0	Minimal	High	252
	Valproic acid	0.14 to 0.23	Minimal	High	144
Third- and Fourth-Generation AEDs					
Minimal or no protein binding	Eslicarbazepine		Minimal	High	296
	Felbamate	0.7 to 1.0	Moderate	Moderate	238
	Gabapentin*	0.8 to 1.8	High	None	171
	Lacosamide	0.6	Minimal	Moderate	250
	Levetiracetam*	0.7	Moderate	None	170
	Pregabalin*	0.5	High	Minimal	159
	Rufinamide	0.7	Minimal	High	238
	Topiramate	0.6 to 0.8	Moderate	Moderate	339
	Vigabatrin*	1.1	High	None	129
Moderate protein binding	Lamotrigine	0.9 to 1.3	Minimal	High	256
	Oxcarbazepine[†]	0.7	Minimal	High	252
	Zonisamide	0.8 to 1.6	Minimal	Moderate	212
High protein binding	Ezogabine	2 to 3	High	High	303
	Stiripentol[‡]	–	Minimal	High	234
	Tiagabine	–	Minimal	High	412

*Is not protein bound.
†The active metabolite 10-*OH*-carbamazepine is 40% bound (minimal–moderate).
‡Approved in Europe for SMEI (Dravet syndrome).
CLZ, clobazam; DZP, diazepam; LZP, lorazepam.
Data from: Israni RK, Kasbekar N, Haynes K. et al: Use of antiepileptic drugs in patients with kidney disease. Semin Dial 19:408, 2006; Diaz A, Deliz B, Benbadis SR: The use of newer antiepileptic drugs in patients with renal failure. Expert Rev Neurother 12:99, 2012; Johannessen Landmark C, Patsalos PN: Drug interactions involving the new second- and third-generation antiepileptic drugs. Expert Rev Neurother 10:119, 2010; and individual product monographs in Micromedex Healthcare Series (Internet database). Thomson Reuters (Healthcare) Inc, Greenwood Village, CO (updated periodically).

usually require dose adjustments in the setting of reduced renal function.

There are few data or systematic reviews on the use of AEDs in renal failure, including patients on dialysis.[11,15] Data for the pharmacokinetics of individual AEDs and recommended dosing adjustments for newer antiepileptic medicines are summarized in Tables 57-1 and 57-2, respectively.

TABLE 57-2 ■ Dose Adjustments for Selected Newer AEDs in Renal Disease

	AED dose				
	GFR 60–90 ml/min	**GFR 30–60 ml/min**	**GFR 15–30 ml/min**	**GFR ≤15 ml/min**	**Hemodialysis**
Third- and Fourth-Generation AEDs					
Gabapentin	300–1200 mg t.i.d.	200–700 mg b.i.d.	200–700 mg/day	100–300 mg/day	Plus 125–350 mg after HD
Levetiracetam	500–1000 mg b.i.d.	250–750 mg b.i.d.	250–500 mg b.i.d.	500–1000 mg/day	Plus 250–500 mg after HD
Topiramate	50% decrease for ≤ 70 ml/min	50% decrease	50% decrease		Plus 50–100 mg after HD
Zonisamide	100–400 mg/day	100–400 mg/day			
Oxcarbazepine	300–600 mg b.i.d.	300–600 mg b.i.d.	300 mg/day (starting dose)		
Felbamate	None	50% decrease			
Lamotrigine*	None	None	None	None	
Tiagabine	None	None	None	None	None
Vigabatrin	25% decrease	50% decrease	75% decrease		
Rufinamide	None	None	None		Plus 30% of dose after HD
Lacosamide	None	None	300 mg/day		Plus ≤50% replacement dose
Ezogabine	None	50–200 mg t.i.d.	50–200 mg t.i.d.		
Eslicarbazepine	None	400–600 mg/day	400–600 mg/day		
Clobazam	None	None	None		None
Pregabalin	None	50% decrease	25–150 mg/day	25–75 mg/day	Plus 25–150 mg after HD

*The product monograph for Lamictal XR recommends reduced maintenance doses in patients with significant renal impairment, and caution in patients with severe renal impairment. Lamotrigine pharmacokinetics were essentially unchanged in a study comparing 10 subjects with renal failure (estimated creatine clearance of 10 to 25 ml/min) to that of 11 healthy subjects. (Wootton R, Soul-Lawton J, Rolan PE, et al: Comparison of the pharmacokinetics of lamotrigine in patients with chronic renal failure and healthy volunteers. Br J Clin Pharmacol 43:23, 1997.)

Blanks indicate inadequate data; individual AEDs should be used with caution or avoided in these circumstances. "None" indicates no change in dose is recommended. HD, hemodialysis; b.i.d., 2 times daily; t.i.d., 3 times daily.

Data from: Israni RK, Kasbekar N, Haynes K. et al: Use of antiepileptic drugs in patients with kidney disease. Semin Dial 19:408, 2006; Diaz A, Deliz B, Benbadis SR: The use of newer antiepileptic drugs in patients with renal failure. Expert Rev Neurother 12:99, 2012; and individual product monographs in the Micromedex Healthcare Series (Internet database). Thomson Reuters (Healthcare) Inc, Greenwood Village, CO (updated periodically).

HEPATIC DISEASE

Seizures are relatively uncommon in patients with acute hepatic encephalopathy, at least when seizures related to alcohol withdrawal are excluded. Either focal or generalized seizures may occur, usually in severe hepatic encephalopathy. Treatment involves management of the hepatic dysfunction and hepatic encephalopathy. Anticonvulsant therapy often is not required except when an underlying cause of epilepsy (e.g., prior cerebral trauma) is present.

Chronic liver disease does not usually cause convulsions.[16] The occurrence of seizures in alcoholics with hepatic cirrhosis is usually related to prior trauma, intracranial hemorrhage, or alcohol withdrawal. Seizures are common in Reye syndrome and rare in Wilson disease. Convulsions in patients with acute hepatic necrosis are frequently associated with severe hypoglycemia.

Gabapentin, vigabatrin and levetiracetam are the only AEDs not hepatically metabolized. Certain AEDs, including selected newer agents, undergo extensive hepatic metabolism (Table 57-1) but unless hepatic dysfunction is severe, the effect of hepatic dysfunction on anticonvulsant pharmacokinetics is difficult to predict. The free fraction of highly protein-bound AEDs may increase due to hypoalbuminemia, and serum free drug levels should be followed (if available). Lamotrigine metabolism is reduced in patients with significant liver disease, necessitating a decrease in dosage.[17] Dosage reduction is required also in patients with unconjugated hyperbilirubinemia (Gilbert syndrome). Barbiturates, benzodiazepines, and other sedatives or CNS depressant drugs may unmask hepatic encephalopathy in patients with compensated liver disease and are relatively contraindicated.[18] Valproic acid is potentially hepatotoxic and should be used with care—if at all—in patients with established liver disease.

Drug-induced liver injury by first- and second-generation AEDs seems independent of dose (except in children younger than 2 years, taking valproic acid). In most cases, these reactions are reversible by stopping the AED. Infrequently, acute hepatic failure may necessitate transplantation. AEDs (as a class) were the third most common cause (phenytoin, n=10; valproic acid, n=10) of acute drug-induced liver failure requiring liver transplantation in the United States between 1990 and 2002 (n=270).[19] Two types of injury are described.

First, an immune-mediated hypersensitivity syndrome characterized by fever, rash, and hepatic involvement may occur several weeks after starting an AED. A prime example of this reaction is the acute hepatic injury caused by phenytoin, and in perhaps 30 percent of persons with acute hepatic injury on carbamazepine.[20] The risk of hypersensitivity reactions is 1 to 10 per 10,000 for phenytoin, carbamazepine, phenobarbital, and lamotrigine; the risk probably is similar for zonisamide, based on its class (sulfonamide).[21]

Second, AEDs may cause a hepatocellular injury pattern as a direct effect of hepatic metabolism, and not as a hypersensitivity syndrome. This is exemplified by the hepatic injury induced by valproic acid (and, frequently, carbamazepine).[20] Presentation is with fatigue, nausea, vomiting, and weakness; the combination of high serum aminotransferases and jaundice, if present, predicts a mortality of 10 to 50 percent in these patients.[20] The incidence of hepatic injury on valproic acid is very high, perhaps 1 in 800 for children less than 2 years old, and the drug is relatively contraindicated in this population.

Hyperammonemia may occur with normal liver function tests in the majority of persons on valproic acid, with no associated clinical symptoms. This seems unrelated to the dose (except in children less than 2 years old). Topiramate may increase the risk of hyperammonemic encephalopathy and hepatic injury from valproic acid. For felbamate, concern for acute hepatic failure (as well as aplastic anemia) has limited the use of this AED; frequent monitoring of hepatic function is required, although the usefulness of this is not clear.[22]

CARDIAC DISEASE

Cardiac disease may lead to seizures from cardioembolic stroke and focal ischemia or from global cerebral ischemia after cardiac arrest. Seizures may also infrequently complicate coronary bypass surgery.[23]

Cardiovascular disease and epilepsy may coexist, especially in the elderly, persons with congenital cardiac disease, and persons with alcohol or polysubstance use. This complicates treatment of acute seizures and status epilepticus. Intravenous benzodiazepines may cause hypotension in medically ill or elderly patients. Phenytoin and fosphenytoin may cause hypotension or cardiac arrhythmias with intravenous infusions. Fosphenytoin, a water-soluble prodrug of phenytoin that does not require propylene glycol as a diluent, is generally preferred for treating status epilepticus as its infusion rate is faster and there is a lesser risk of arrhythmia than with phenytoin.[24] If fosphenytoin is not available, valproic acid, levetiracetam, or lacosamide are alternatives in these patient populations.

AEDs that affect sodium channels may influence cardiac excitability and conduction, but long-term AED use has been associated only rarely with significant cardiovascular complications. Prolonged PR interval is seen in patients on lacosamide and carbamazepine. Symptomatic arrhythmias have been reported in patients receiving lacosamide and carbamazepine in therapeutic dosages, but underlying cardiac abnormalities or multiple sodium-channel AEDs usually (but not always) have been present.[25,26] Shortening of the QT interval is seen in patients on rufinamide. Routine electrocardiograms should probably be obtained in all patients started on these AEDs and in all patients with pre-existing cardiac disease. Epilepsy patients as a group have lower heart-rate variability than normal—this is a marker of impaired vagal activity and predicts arrhythmias and mortality in cardiac patients.[27,28] This may be relevant to the phenomenon of sudden unexplained death in epilepsy (SUDEP); if correct, the effect of AEDs on these measures may be important, but this has not yet been demonstrated.[28]

Anticonvulsant agents may also interact with certain cardiac medications. The concomitant use of phenytoin and quinidine may increase ectopy in patients with ventricular arrhythmias. The metabolism of quinidine, digoxin, lidocaine, and mexiletine may be increased by phenytoin and phenobarbital because of induction of hepatic microsomal enzymes. Amiodarone increases phenytoin levels, and calcium-channel blocking agents, such as verapamil, may increase serum carbamazepine concentrations. For these reasons, serum AED levels and cardiovascular function should be followed closely when either antiepileptic or cardiac medications are introduced or altered.

SEIZURES IN CRITICALLY ILL PATIENTS

General Considerations

Seizures are among the most common neurologic complications of severe medical illnesses treated in the ICU. In one study, neurologic complications occurred in 217 (12.3%) of a total of 1,758 patients admitted to an ICU with a non-neurologic primary diagnosis.[29] Seizures occurred in 61 cases (28.1%) and were the most frequent neurologic complication after metabolic encephalopathy. Seizures most commonly resulted from vascular lesions, but infection, metabolic derangement, mass lesion, hypoxia, and a variety of other causes were found. Approximately two-thirds of patients experienced focal-onset seizures, and the remainder had seizures of presumed generalized onset. Status epilepticus occurred in six cases, two of which were refractory and required management by pentobarbital-induced coma. Neurologic complications were associated with increased mortality rates and longer lengths of stay in the ICU and hospital.

More aggressive AED therapy of discrete seizures is often warranted, given the increased risk of seizure-related complications, in patients who are already compromised by severe illness such as multi-organ system failure. However, anticonvulsants are ineffective in controlling seizures caused by various metabolic derangements such as severe hypoglycemia or hyperglycemia, hyponatremia, and hypocalcemia. In these instances, therapy should be directed at correcting the underlying metabolic abnormality. When AED treatment is necessary, the increased potential for complex drug interactions in patients receiving numerous other medications, altered pharmacokinetics due to factors such as renal or hepatic impairment, and adverse systemic effects must be considered. For example, in the hypoalbuminemic patient, it may be necessary to monitor free anticonvulsant drug levels when using an AED, such as phenytoin, that exhibits significant serum protein binding. Treatment may also be further complicated by the requirement for parenteral administration in patients with gastrointestinal dysfunction.

Nonconvulsive Status Epilepticus

Nonconvulsive seizures and nonconvulsive (i.e., absence or complex partial) status epilepticus may occur in critically ill patients.[30] Although its incidence is not known, nonconvulsive status epilepticus is probably under-recognized based on studies of patients in neurologic ICUs using continuous EEG monitoring.[31,32] This condition should be suspected in any critically ill patient with altered mental status of unknown cause. Subtle motor activity, such as rhythmic twitching of fingers or eye movements, should raise suspicion of seizure activity in this setting. Diagnosis depends on prolonged EEG recordings. Quantitative EEG techniques have been helpful to detect electrographic seizures in these patients in context with other changes on the EEG (Fig. 57-1). Prompt recognition and treatment are essential because delay is associated with a poor outcome.[32]

Seizures Caused by Anoxic-Ischemic Encephalopathy

Seizures resulting from global anoxic-ischemic cerebral damage occur acutely after resuscitation from cardiopulmonary arrest in 15 to 44 percent of survivors.[33] They typically commence within 24 hours of cardiopulmonary arrest and may consist of generalized tonic-clonic, tonic, myoclonic, or partial seizures, as well as tonic-clonic or myoclonus status epilepticus. Electrographic status epilepticus with restricted clinical manifestations (usually limited solely to extraocular or facial muscles) is also well

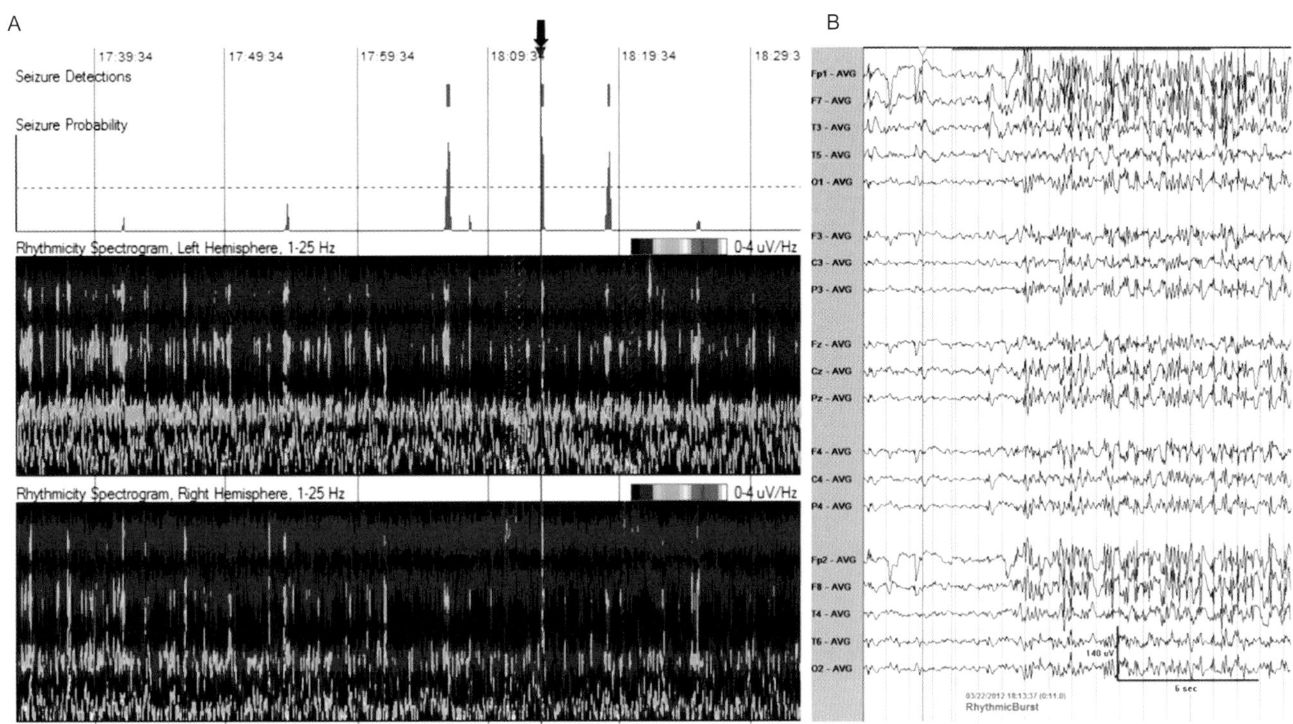

Figure 57-1 ■ **A,** Quantitative EEG. EEG for 1 hour in a young man intubated for respiratory failure with symptomatic generalized epilepsy and subtle tonic seizures. The upper two panels use a proprietary algorithm to calculate the probability of seizures over time (Persyst seizure detection, Persyst Corporation, San Diego, CA). The lower two panels show time along the x-axis, frequency on the y-axis (0–25 Hz) and EEG on a color scale. Most power is in the delta range for most of the tracing. There is an asymmetry in faster frequencies, increased over the left hemisphere. Intermittent bursts of power in higher frequencies represent brief electrographic seizures, with subtle or no clinical correlate on video. **B,** EEG recorded using an average reference and corresponding to arrow in **A**.

described after cardiopulmonary arrest, but may be difficult to recognize.[34]

The occurrence of seizures or even generalized tonic-clonic status epilepticus does not influence the eventual clinical outcome of patients in postanoxic coma. However, myoclonic status epilepticus, that is, continuous myoclonus for at least 30 minutes with or without other seizure types, does suggest a poor prognosis after global cerebral hypoxic-ischemic insult. It may begin at any time within approximately 5 days after cardiopulmonary arrest, most often within 24 hours Generalized myoclonus may be synchronous or asynchronous, but sometimes involves the facial muscles predominantly. The EEG typically reveals generalized spike-wave or polyspike-wave bursts on an abnormal background or a burst-suppression pattern; a diffuse unreactive alpha-frequency pattern is sometimes found. Neuropathologic examination shows diffuse anoxic-ischemic damage involving cerebral cortex, hippocampus, cerebellar Purkinje cells, thalamus, basal ganglia, and, to a lesser extent, the brainstem and spinal cord.

Myoclonus status epilepticus is poorly responsive to anticonvulsant therapy and may well represent a marker of severe anoxic-ischemic brain injury that rarely permits survival.[33] Treatment decisions in these settings should be individualized based on the clinical examination and neurophysiologic studies.

CONNECTIVE TISSUE DISEASES

The connective tissue diseases are discussed in detail in Chapter 50. Of these, systemic lupus erythematosus (SLE) probably has the highest incidence of neurologic or psychiatric manifestations. Among these, seizures are the most frequent neuropsychiatric manifestation, both at time of diagnosis and during disease flares, seen in 40 to 85 percent of persons with SLE.[35] The prevalence of epilepsy in the

SLE population is also increased, variably reported in larger series to be from 3 to 29 percent.[36,37]

Generalized convulsive seizures are the most common seizure type and may reflect direct brain involvement or may be due to a hypertensive or metabolic encephalopathy, especially in the context of lupus nephritis and uremia or as a complication of immunosuppressive therapy. Focal seizures and status epilepticus are relatively rare. Occasionally, seizures or other neuropsychiatric manifestations are the initial features of SLE, and systemic manifestations may not develop for many years.[38] Neuropsychiatric manifestations imply a poorer prognosis for SLE than otherwise, but the presence of seizures or psychosis without other neurologic features or significant renal disease does not reduce survival.[39]

Various antibodies have been implicated in the pathogenesis of neuropsychiatric SLE. Of these, antiphospholipid antibodies are important as these can lead to arterial or venous thrombosis and also may have a direct neuromodulatory effect.[40] The frequency of seizures and epilepsy may correlate with the presence of these antibodies, although this is not clear.[41,42] Cerebral microinfarcts and, less often, subarachnoid and intracerebral hemorrhages are found on pathologic examination and may relate to an immunologically mediated vasculopathy.[43]

Treatment of CNS lupus is discussed in Chapter 50. The treatment of an isolated seizure during an SLE flare does not necessarily require anticonvulsant therapy. However, AEDs are frequently started for a limited time (e.g., 3 months) while immunosuppression is used to treat the SLE flare. Although a drug-induced lupus may occur with various AEDs (including phenytoin, carbamazepine, valproic acid, and lamotrigine), there is no evidence that AEDs exacerbate idiopathic SLE, and anticonvulsant treatment should not be withheld from patients with SLE when it is required for seizure control.

Cerebral vasculopathy from other causes may lead to seizures. Antiphospholipid antibody syndrome may be seen without SLE. In Sjögren or Behçet syndrome, convulsions may be associated with a disease flare. Seizures rarely are described due to cerebral involvement in rheumatoid arthritis, scleroderma, or mixed connective tissue disease. The one exception to this is linear scleroderma with hemifacial atrophy of the face, or Parry–Romberg syndrome, in which intractable epilepsy can be part of the spectrum of disease.[44]

TABLE 57-3 ■ Antigens for Autoantibodies Associated With Seizures

Intracellular Antigens
ANNA-1, CRMP5, GAD65, Ma2
Extracellular (Cell Surface or Synapse) Antigens
AMPA receptor, GABA(B) receptor, ganglionic AChR, NMDA receptor, VGKC complex (Caspr2; Lgi1)

AChR, acetylcholine receptor; ANNA-1, antineuronal nuclear antibody-type 1; Caspr2, contactin-associated protein-like 2; CRMP5, collapsin response-mediator protein 5; GABA(B), γ-aminobutyric acid subtype B; GAD65, glutamic acid decarboxylase 65; Lgi1, leucine-rich glioma inactivated 1; NMDA, *N*-methyl-D-aspartate; VGKC, voltage-gated potassium channel antibody.

INFLAMMATORY AND AUTOIMMUNE DISEASES

Systemic autoimmune diseases with neurologic manifestations including seizures may occur in the context of systemic cancer or immune-mediated medical illnesses, including thyroid disease and inflammatory bowel disease.

Limbic encephalitis is the prototype for neurologic presentations of autoimmune disease. Clinical features include impaired short-term memory, hallucinations, and sleep disturbance; patients are anxious, irritable, or paranoid. Partial and secondarily generalized seizures are seen in nearly all cases, and often do not respond to AEDs. Diagnosis is by autoantibodies to intracellular antigens, or extracellular (cell surface) antigens involved in synaptic transmission (Table 57-3). Paraneoplastic etiologies for limbic encephalitis must be excluded. These syndromes are discussed in detail in Chapter 27.

Hashimoto encephalopathy is a relapsing encephalopathy occurring in association with Hashimoto thyroiditis, with high titers of antithyroid peroxidase antibodies (anti-TPO), antithyroid microsomal antibodies, and antithyroglobulin antibodies. Thyroid hormone levels are usually decreased (hypothyroid), but 30 percent of persons may be euthyroid or hyperthyroid. Seizures occur in the majority of these patients. Many patients respond to intravenous methylprednisolone (termed steroid-responsive encephalopathy associated with autoimmune thyroiditis, or SREAT).[45] AEDs are required for acute seizures; seizures tend to remit as the encephalopathy improves. The disorder is discussed in detail in Chapter 18.

Inflammatory bowel diseases, including ulcerative colitis and Crohn disease, are chronic relapsing inflammatory diseases of the gut. Both conditions are associated with neurologic and systemic complications, possibly including an increased incidence of epilepsy, but this is not quite clear.[46] The epidemiologic association of celiac disease with epilepsy is clearer, seen in between 3.5 and 5.5 percent of patients with celiac disease.[47,48]

Occasionally, seizures are the first presentation of multiple sclerosis.[49] On balance the incidence in multiple sclerosis is quite low, varying in different series from no change from baseline risk of seizures[50] to 7.8 percent.[51] Focal seizures as well as generalized convulsive seizures may occur. One-third of seizures occur in the context of an acute flare of the disease, and occasionally present as focal status epilepticus.[52] Seizures usually stop with disease remission. The reason for the occurrence of seizures (a cortical disturbance) in demyelinating disease is not clear, but specialized magnetic resonance imaging sequences do demonstrate intracortical lesions in patients with seizures.[53]

HEPATIC PORPHYRIAS

Porphyrias are caused by deficiencies in enzymes of the heme biosynthetic pathway that lead to the accumulation of heme precursors (porphyrins). The inherited conditions are classified into the acute porphyrias (hepatic porphyrias) and cutaneous (erythropoetic) porphyrias, reflecting the location of the accumulation of porphyrins. Three of the acute porphyrias may present with epilepsy and neuropsychiatric symptoms: acute intermittent porphyria (AIP), hereditary coproporphyria, and variegate porphyria.

Acute intermittent porphyria is the commonest hepatic porphyria, and the one most frequently associated with seizures and epilepsy. The clinical features of variegate porphyria are identical to AIP, except for cutaneous photosensitivity seen in 30 percent. Persons are asymptomatic until exposed to circumstances that demonstrate the deficiency, including infection, hormonal cycles, diet, or medications. Symptoms are due to an acute neuropathy and evolve over hours or days. These include abdominal pain, nausea, vomiting, weakness, and severe neuropathic pain. Laboratory studies demonstrate increased δ-aminolevulinic acid (ALA) and porphobilinogen in the urine.

Encephalopathy, coma, or seizures are seen in 5 to 20 percent of persons during acute attacks, and may be the presenting feature in AIP.[54] Seizures may be partial or generalized convulsive seizures[55,56] and, rarely, status epilepticus.[56] These seizures may reflect a direct neurologic effect of ALA binding to GABA receptors.[56] Defects in hepatic heme synthesis may also alter brain levels of neurotransmitters.[57] Seizures may also be symptomatic of metabolic disturbances from excessive vomiting or inappropriate antidiuretic hormone secretion.

All the enzyme-inducing antiepileptic drugs, valproic acid, and benzodiazepines may exacerbate or precipitate attacks by stimulating hepatic ALA synthase activity, and these drugs should be avoided.[55,56,58] Experimental studies suggest that lamotrigine, felbamate, topiramate, or tiagabine use will exacerbate hepatic porphyrias.[59,60] These studies are supported clinically in the case of lamotrigine.[61]

Gabapentin, pregabalin and levetiracetam are probably safe, and gabapentin[62] and levetiracetam[63] have been used successfully for acute seizures and status epilepticus. The use of intravenous benzodiazepines seems relatively safe but this is debated.[58] If seizures are medically refractory, magnesium sulfate may be infused intravenously to keep serum magnesium concentrations between 2.5 and 7.5 mmol/L.[56]

Long-term pharmacotherapy of recurrent seizures in patients with hepatic porphyria is difficult. Clonazepam may be safe in the chronic treatment of patients with hepatic porphyria[58] despite evidence that clonazepam is porphyrinogenic.[55] The preferred AED is probably gabapentin, pregabalin, or levetiracetam.[62,63] Urine ALA and porphobilinogen levels must be monitored closely during therapy.

SEIZURES IN TRANSPLANT RECIPIENTS

The neurologic complications of organ transplantation are summarized in Chapter 45. Transplant recipients are at high risk of seizures that may relate to their underlying illness, irradiation or chemotherapy, and perioperative metabolic abnormalities or complications such as cerebral ischemia. After surgery, the effects of immunosuppression, therapeutic agents, and rejection are also important causes. The approximate percentage incidence of seizures varies depending on the transplanted organ (Chapter 45). Children in general appear to be at greater risk than adults of post-transplantation seizures.[64,65]

Immunosuppressive agents, especially cyclosporine, have been associated with seizures. Such seizures may occur with serum levels of cyclosporine within or exceeding the therapeutic range and may relate to a cyclosporine metabolite.[66] Various metabolic and systemic abnormalities, as well as other therapeutic agents, have been reported to potentiate them. These factors include concomitant methylprednisolone therapy, hypertension, hypomagnesemia, hypocholesterolemia, microangiopathic hemolytic anemia,[67,68] and (after renal transplantation) aluminum overload.

Other immunosuppressive agents may also cause post-transplantation seizures. Tacrolimus (FK506) has neurologic complications similar to cyclosporine, including seizures and encephalopathy,[69,70] and the antirejection agent muromonab-CD3 (OKT3) can cause seizures as part of a cytokine encephalopathy.[71] Sirolimus (rapamycin), one of the newer immunosuppressive agents, did not cause seizures or other neurotoxicity in at least one series consisting of kidney and liver transplant recipients.[72] In bone marrow recipients, busulfan, either alone or in combination with cyclophosphamide, may cause seizures.[73]

Seizures may also result from CNS infections or relate to noninfectious structural and metabolic abnormalities that require specific treatment. Cerebral ischemia or hemorrhage, hyponatremia with central pontine myelinolysis, hyperosmolar states, hypoglycemia, delayed malignancy related to prior treatment, or multiorgan system failure may be responsible. Finally, transplant rejection may lead to an encephalopathy syndrome that includes seizures, sometimes as the first manifestation of rejection.[74]

The treatment of seizures in transplant recipients may be difficult. When seizures are self-limited and caused by correctable abnormalities that are not recurrent, anticonvulsant therapy is not required. Prolonged seizures or those placing the patient at high risk of complications should be controlled with intravenous benzodiazepines. Long-term anticonvulsant therapy is required for recurrent seizures. An antiseizure agent is selected, bearing in mind the type of transplantation procedure undergone by the patient and the immunosuppressive drugs in use. Valproic acid is best avoided in liver recipients because of its potential hepatotoxicity; low-dose levetiracetam (500 mg twice daily) is a reasonable alternative, although experience is limited.[75,76] Carbamazepine should not be used in bone marrow recipients because it may cause myelosuppression. Bone marrow engraftment occurs 2 to 6 weeks after transplantation, and phenytoin, phenobarbital and valproic acid are best avoided over this period in favor of a newer agent.

The enzyme-inducing AEDs may have an effect on immunosuppressive agents metabolized by the liver. Thus, the clearance of cyclosporine and corticosteroids is increased by phenobarbital, phenytoin, and carbamazepine,[77] necessitating increased dosages of corticosteroids by 25 to 30 percent and of cyclosporine depending on serum cyclosporine levels. The use of valproic acid avoids such pharmacokinetic interactions. Oxcarbazepine add-on therapy led to decreased serum cyclosporine and sodium concentrations in a single report involving a renal transplant patient, but the abnormalities reversed with reduction in the dose of oxcarbazepine.[78] Levetiracetam does not appear to influence immunosuppressive drug levels, has been used successfully in liver transplant recipients, and therefore may be a good initial choice for AED therapy in the overall transplant population. The lack of hepatic enzyme–inducing activity of pregabalin and gabapentin suggests that they also may be useful in this context.

HUMAN IMMUNODEFICIENCY VIRUS INFECTION AND SEIZURES

Seizures occur in perhaps 10 percent of persons infected with human immunodeficiency virus (HIV).[79] They may occur at any stage of HIV infection or acquired immunodeficiency syndrome (AIDS) and are sometimes the presenting symptom of HIV infection.[79] Involvement of the nervous system is present at autopsy in 85 percent of persons with HIV infection.[80] The introduction of combination antiretroviral treatment (cART) using protease inhibitors has reduced brain involvement by opportunistic infections in these autopsy series, but also corresponds to an increase in HIV encephalopathy from 34 to 60 percent, perhaps reflecting the dramatic improvement of survival in HIV infection.[80] Variants of HIV encephalitis with intense perivascular inflammation have also emerged, presumably due to an exaggerated response from a newly reconstituted immune system.[80]

In nearly half of the patients with HIV/AIDS seen for seizures, no cause except HIV infection is found and in these persons direct cerebral HIV infection seems the correct explanation.[79] Other important CNS disorders that may be responsible and are associated with HIV/AIDS include CNS toxoplasmosis, cryptococcal meningitis, neurotuberculosis, progressive multifocal leukoencephalopathy, and CNS lymphoma. Systemic illness, drug or alcohol use (especially cocaine), and even antiretroviral agents are also important causes of symptomatic seizures.[81] A detailed diagnostic evaluation is therefore required when HIV-infected patients experience the new onset of seizures.

The risk of subsequent seizures following a first seizure is relatively high in HIV-infected persons, and for this reason AEDs are usually started following a first seizure.[79] Monotherapy with one of the newer antiepileptic agents that do not induce hepatic enzymes is preferable as first-line therapy. On balance, the older enzyme-inducing antiepileptic agents are best avoided in patients with HIV/AIDS, because of concerns about hypoalbuminemia, hypergammaglobulinemia (which may predispose to AED hypersensitivity reactions), and potential drug–drug interactions.[82] For example, phenytoin interacts with protease inhibitors, affecting viral load, and may cause intoxication in patients treated concurrently with fluconazole, commonly prescribed in AIDS patients.[83]

SEIZURES ASSOCIATED WITH SYSTEMIC CANCER

Seizures are an important complication of systemic cancer. The number of persons who develop seizures varies by series and seizure type, from 12 to 35 percent.[84] Seizures are a more common neurologic complication of systemic cancer in children and were the second most common reason for pediatric neurology referrals (18 percent of referrals) in one series, compared to only 5 percent in adults.[85]

Different potential etiologies must be considered when seizures occur in patients with cancer. First, seizures may be due to direct brain effects including parenchymal metastasis in 10 to 20 percent of persons with systemic cancer.[86] These lesions deafferent the adjacent cortex and may alter the immediate microenvironment by distortion, ischemia, or hemorrhage. All of these factors contribute to epileptogenesis in the adjacent cortical tissue and subsequent seizures that arise in these circumstances. Metastases are especially frequent for melanoma, lung, breast, renal cell, gastrointestinal, and germ cell tumors, as well as when leptomeningeal seeding occurs by malignant tumor cells (carcinomatous meningitis).[87]

Second, seizures may be symptomatic of an associated diagnosis or condition occurring in systemic cancers. For example, they may result from cerebrovascular events due to hypercoagulable states or nonbacterial thrombotic endocarditis associated with cancer. CNS infections, including fungal or parasitic abscesses, may result from immunosuppression after chemotherapy and produce seizures. Convulsions are an uncommon complication of chemotherapy, but may be seen with etoposide, L-asparaginase, alkylating agents such as chlorambucil or busulfan, immunotherapies, methotrexate, and cytosine arabinoside.[87] Other causes include cancer-induced metabolic disturbances, paraneoplastic encephalitis, and drugs used to treat cancer complications, such as pain medications or antibiotics.

Guidelines for the treatment of patients with single metastatic lesions recommend surgery (if possible) followed by whole-brain radiation therapy.[88] In patients not presenting with seizures, AEDs may be given perioperatively for 7 days and then discontinued.[89] Phenytoin is frequently used in this circumstance, although patients receiving whole-brain cranial irradiation have an increased risk of Stevens–Johnson syndrome, and levetiracetam is preferred for this reason. AEDs are not indicated for persons with metastatic disease who have not had seizures.

Once a seizure has occurred, AEDs are recommended. There are no recommendations for the type of AED, dose, or length of therapy.[88] Chemotherapeutic agents used to treat systemic cancers complicate the selection of an AED. Drug interactions may occur. For example, corticosteroids are indicated for patients with symptoms secondary to elevated intracranial pressure. Phenobarbital and phenytoin shorten the half-life of corticosteroids, and increased or decreased serum concentrations of phenytoin have been described in patients receiving corticosteroids.[90] A second concern is that many chemotherapeutic agents undergo hepatic metabolism or induce or interfere with hepatic enzymes. Consequently, AEDs that induce hepatic enzymes or are metabolized hepatically may lower the effectiveness of cancer chemotherapy, interfere with seizure control, or induce anticonvulsant toxicity.[91] Because of the potential for drug–drug interactions, AEDs that do not induce hepatic enzymes, including levetiracetam, gabapentin, pregabalin, or lacosamide, are preferred in individuals undergoing cancer chemotherapy.

ENDOCRINE OR METABOLIC DISORDERS

Disorders of Glucose Metabolism

Both focal motor and generalized seizures may occur in patients with hypoglycemia; seizure flurries or convulsive status epilepticus may also occur. Other neurologic abnormalities include depressed level of consciousness, behavioral changes, tremor, and hemiparesis. These deficits correlate poorly with level of hypoglycemia, although in symptomatic patients levels are usually below 40mg/dl. Hypoglycemia must be considered as a possible cause in any patient with seizures; it is treated by intravenous administration of dextrose and correction of any other metabolic abnormalities. Patients usually do well but are best hospitalized for observation because hypoglycemia may recur hours after initial treatment.

Seizures are relatively common in nonketotic hyperglycemia and may be of any type. Partial motor seizures or epilepsia partialis continua may be the presenting feature. The range of glucose elevation is broad and may be associated with only mild elevation of serum osmolarity. Seizures are refractory to AEDs but respond to correction of hyperglycemia with insulin and intravenous fluid replacement. Associated focal neurologic abnormalities are usually transient, and recovery is typically complete if treatment is initiated before coma occurs. Anticonvulsant therapy is not required for seizures related to nonketotic hyperglycemia. Phenytoin must specifically be avoided because it can exacerbate hyperglycemia by inhibiting insulin release.

Thyroid Disease

Seizures are not uncommon in hypothyroidism, are usually generalized, and remit with treatment of the hypothyroidism. Anticonvulsant drugs, such as phenytoin and carbamazepine, may reduce serum thyroxine and triiodothyronine measurements because of competition for serum-binding proteins; however, patients remain clinically euthyroid because free thyroxine and triiodothyronine fractions are increased.[92]

Seizures are uncommon in thyrotoxicosis, but hyperthyroidism or excess thyroxine may occasionally cause seizures or exacerbate preexisting epilepsy. Both partial and generalized seizures may occur in hyperthyroid patients and in those receiving thyroxine for hypothyroidism. In addition, worsening of both partial and generalized epilepsies may occur with increased thyroxine levels.[93] When seizures occur in the setting of thyrotoxicosis, the hyperthyroid state should be corrected; anticonvulsants usually are not required except occasionally in the acute setting.

Disorders of Sodium Homeostasis

A full account of the neurologic manifestations is provided in Chapter 17. Hyponatremic encephalopathy relates to an osmotic imbalance between the extracellular fluid and brain cells, and the effects of a compensatory loss of intracellular cations. Neurologic symptoms reflect the rate of development of hyponatremia rather than absolute serum sodium levels, and chronic hyponatremia is surprisingly well tolerated. Seizures are usually seen in the context of acute hyponatremia with concentrations less than 115 mEq/L, but seizures may occur at higher levels if the decrease is very rapid.[94] Children are at high risk of cerebral edema in hyponatremia.[95] Both partial and generalized seizures may occur.

Seizures require treatment using intravenous hypertonic (3%) saline. This should be given at a controlled rate so that increases in serum sodium concentration do not exceed 1 mmol/L (1 mEq/L) per hour; treatment can be stopped once the patient is asymptomatic. The correction should not exceed 12mmol/L (12mEq/L) over the first 24 hours and 25mmol/L (25mEq/L) in the initial 48 hours.[96,97] More rapid correction of hyponatremia may cause osmotic demyelination (previously termed pontine and extrapontine myelinolysis), as well as seizures.[98]

Hypernatremia indicates a relative deficit of body water related to body sodium content. As a consequence, water shifts from the intracellular to extracellular compartment. If severe (>160 mEq/L), this causes an encephalopathy. The aim of treatment is to replace body water. Partial or generalized seizures may occur, especially during rehydration. Cautious correction of hypernatremia with half-isotonic saline may lower the risk of convulsions during treatment.[97]

Calcium and Magnesium Imbalance

The causes and clinical features of hypocalcemia are reviewed in Chapter 17. Altered sensorium and seizures are common neurologic manifestations of hypocalcemia. Hypocalcemic seizures are usually generalized, but partial seizures occur in 20 percent of patients and may include motor or sensory phenomenology. Between 30 and 70 percent of patients with hypoparathyroidism experience seizures, often accompanied by an altered sensorium and tetany, although tetany is occasionally absent. Treatment of hypocalcemic seizures involves correction of serum calcium levels and treatment of any underlying cause.

Multifocal and generalized seizures may also be provoked by hypomagnesemia, especially when the serum magnesium concentration decreases below 0.8 mEq/L (see Chapter 17). Convulsions in such circumstances are treated with magnesium salts administered by slow intravenous bolus after the adequacy of renal function has been determined; calcium gluconate should be available to counteract transient hypermagnesemia.

Hypercalcemia infrequently causes seizures. Seizures are not seen in hypermagnesemia.

SEIZURES RELATED TO ALCOHOL, MEDICATIONS, AND RECREATIONAL DRUG USE

Alcohol

Seizures are a common consequence of alcohol abuse, as discussed in Chapter 33. Alcohol potentiates the activity of $GABA_A$ receptors, and alcohol dependence seems to result in a compensatory downregulation of these receptors. As a consequence, when alcohol and its effect on the $GABA_A$ receptors are withdrawn, there is decreased neuronal inhibition and seizures.[99] Alcohol-related seizures are usually self-limited generalized convulsions that occur within 48 hours after stopping alcohol, often accompanied by other signs and symptoms of alcohol withdrawal. Seizures may be isolated or occur in flurries and are usually due to acutely declining ethanol levels in long-standing heavy drinkers.[100] Convulsive status epilepticus may result uncommonly from alcohol withdrawal.[101] The brain substrates responsible for these seizures are largely in the brainstem, and perhaps for this reason AEDs effective for generalized epilepsies seem to be helpful.[99] In the United States, benzodiazepines are preferred to treat alcohol withdrawal and to prevent seizures.

Patients with seizures solely in the setting of alcohol or drug abuse do not, by definition, have epilepsy. Because seizures are self-limited, long-term AED therapy is not indicated. However, approximately 2 to 4 percent of patients with alcohol-related seizures have preexisting epilepsy.[100] These patients should be advised against chronic alcohol use or binge drinking.[102]

Cocaine and other Recreational Drugs

Seizures may be induced by acute intoxication with recreational drugs, especially cocaine[103] and other stimulants, or, less frequently, may appear as a withdrawal phenomenon. Seizures are typically isolated convulsions that are self-limited and do not require acute or long-term treatment with AEDs. Between 2 and 8 percent of patients presenting with cocaine toxicity exhibit seizures, usually an isolated generalized convulsive seizure.[103] This risk is highest with rapid administration (intravenous or inhaled crack cocaine) and may reflect a direct CNS stimulant effect through blockage of neurotransmitter reuptake at dopaminergic and noradrenergic nerve terminals, perhaps a kindling effect with chronic use, cerebrovascular or systemic effects, or a terminal event in massive cocaine overdose.[100,103]

Seizures are infrequent in intoxication with other recreational drugs. Amphetamine is an uncommon cause of generalized convulsions, which occur more commonly after intravenous use and administration of high doses. Seizures are also uncommon with phencyclidine. Heroin use has been associated with convulsions, although this may relate to anoxia and chemical adulterants rather than to a convulsant effect of heroin itself.[104] Complications of intravenous drug abuse that may cause seizures, including infectious endocarditis and HIV infection, should be sought in patients with convulsions associated with the use of heroin or other intravenous drugs. Marijuana is often used concurrently with heroin and other recreational drugs but seems independently to lower the risk of a first seizure.[104]

Medications

ANTIDEPRESSANT DRUGS

The most commonly implicated drugs in causing seizures are the tricyclic antidepressants (TCAs) and bupropion. The relative risk of TCAs at usual therapeutic doses is actually quite low, but on overdose TCAs may cause seizures due to their effect on $GABA_A$ receptors, decreasing inhibition. Compared to other drugs, overdose with TCAs is also associated with high mortality.[105] Bupropion is a monocyclic inhibitor of dopamine and has a clear dose-related risk of seizures, with a seizure incidence of 0.4 percent at doses of 450 mg/day or less, increasing to 2.2 percent at doses exceeding 450 mg/day.[106] Conversely, the selective serotonin reuptake inhibitors (SSRIs) appear to have low epileptogenic potential even in overdose, with no seizures in a series of 234 cases of fluoxetine overdose.[107] The seizure risk with SSRIs is generally quoted as 0.2 percent, based on premarketing data for sertraline.[108] Importantly, antidepressants as a class may actually reduce the risk of seizures compared to placebo,[109] consistent with the observation that low levels of pre/post-serotonergic transmission in depressed persons may be a risk factor for seizures.[110]

Antipsychotics and Lithium

Clozapine, an atypical antipsychotic, demonstrates a clear dose-related risk of seizures of 0.9 percent for doses less than 600 mg/day and 1.5 percent for higher doses,[111] and has the highest seizure risk of all the antipsychotic medications.[109] An increased risk of seizures has also been reported with olanzapine and quetiapine, but the other atypical antipsychotics (ziprasidone, aripiprazole, and risperidone) as a group do not seem to be associated with an increased incidence of seizures.[109] Seizures with lithium intoxication are common when levels exceed 3.0 mEq/L although seizures have been reported in patients on lithium at therapeutic levels.[109]

Antibiotics

Seizures have been reported for penicillins, cephalosporins, carbapanems (β-lactam antibiotics), and fluoroquinolones. They are believed to be due to direct or indirect binding to $GABA_A$ receptors.[112] Of these antibiotics, the risk is highest for imipenem, from 0.2 to 0.9 percent, although acute seizures were seen in one series in 11 of 200 patients on imipenem.[113,114] Risk is increased in the very young or very old and with renal insufficiency, focal neurologic deficits, and severity of illness, and when given intravenously or intrathecally.[112]

Other Agents

Tramadol is a weak μ-opioid receptor agonist that also induces serotonin release and inhibits the reuptake of norepinephrine. Seizures have been reported with tramadol at therapeutic doses, but are very frequent at supratherapeutic levels, occurring in 14 percent of overdoses in one series.[115,116]

Isoniazid is a common cause of drug-induced seizures, particularly in intentional overdose, believed to be due to inhibition of pyridoxine (vitamin B_6) metabolism that is required to synthesize GABA.[117] For this reason, isoniazid-induced seizures may be refractory to AEDs and should be treated with intravenous pyridoxine.[112]

Seizures may result from certain antiasthmatic medications and especially theophylline. This is most likely due to the inhibition of phosphodiesterase, which may reduce adenosine-mediated CNS inhibition.[118] Status epilepticus may be seen in acute overdose; it does not respond to AEDs and requires hemodialysis or hemoperfusion therapy.[118,119] Theophylline is best avoided in persons with epilepsy for these reasons.

Seizures have been reported with the anesthetic agents propofol, sevolfurane, and lidocaine.[113] Propofol, which acts on the $GABA_A$ receptors and is used in the treatment of refractory status epilepticus, has also been associated with seizures during induction or recovery from anesthesia.[120] Seizures can occur in the setting of abruptly stopping benzodiazepines and barbiturates, and also baclofen, which may cause nonconvulsive status epilepticus.[121]

CEREBRAL TRAUMA, SEIZURES, AND EPILEPSY

Traumatic brain injuries (TBI) are an important cause of seizures and epilepsy, especially in young adults, and may also worsen seizures in persons with preexisting epilepsy.[122,123] Post-traumatic seizures may present across the spectrum of simple to complex seizures, including generalized and secondarily generalized seizures and (infrequently) status epilepticus.

Seizures caused by TBI are classified as immediate (at the moment of injury, or within minutes), early (within the first 7 days), and late (beyond the first week after injury).[124] The incidence of immediate seizures following TBI is 1 to 4 percent[125,126]; they are usually generalized convulsions and do not imply that the patient will develop epilepsy.[127]

Early seizures developing more than 1 hour after injury do present an increased risk of post-traumatic epilepsy. These seizures are symptomatic for the physics of the initial brain injury including shearing injury to fiber tracts and blood vessels, bleeding, and brain swelling.[128] The incidence for early seizures (within the first 7 days) is 2 to 9 percent, depending on the severity of the brain injury. Most early seizures are generalized convulsions; for late post-traumatic seizures, seizure types are more variable.[129]

The latency from the initial brain injury to a first unprovoked seizure can be up to several years.[124] Approximately 80 percent of individuals with post-traumatic epilepsy experience their first seizure within the first 12 months after injury and more than 90 percent do so before the end of the second year.[130] However, the risk still is increased more than 10 years after the traumatic event.[131] The presence of early seizures is the most important risk factor for the development of late seizures and epilepsy, and the incidence of late seizures in persons with early seizures is high, from 25 to 75 percent.[132,133] Other risk factors include open or penetrating brain injury, focal lesions (hematoma, contusion) or neurologic signs, and prolonged coma or amnesia.[134,135]

The precise mechanisms of epileptogenesis that leads to late seizures are poorly understood. Secondary epileptogenesis may also occur—the initial epileptogenic focus causes the emergence of a second distant and perhaps ultimately independent seizure focus in the hippocampal formation, especially in children.[136]

The EEG is disappointing as a predictor of the risk of development of post-traumatic epilepsy, as many patients who eventually develop post-traumatic epilepsy have normal recordings early after injury.[135] Magnetic resonance imaging of the brain is the imaging modality of choice, and has shown some promise for improving prediction of post-traumatic seizure risk.[137]

Treatment of early-onset seizures is imperative, as they may lead to secondary brain damage as a result of increased metabolic demand, raised intracranial pressure, and excess neurotransmitter release. However, although AEDs decrease early seizures, prospective clinical trials have failed to demonstrate that preventing early seizures using AEDs affects mortality, morbidity, or the development of late epilepsy.[138] These include randomized or quasi-randomized monotherapy studies using phenytoin, phenobarbital, carbamazepine, and valproic acid.[139–141] Glucocorticoids also appear to have no benefit in preventing the development of seizures after traumatic brain injury.[142]

REFERENCES

1. Beghi E, Carpio A, Forsgren L, et al: Recommendation for a definition of acute symptomatic seizure. Epilepsia 51:671, 2010.
2. Goldberg EM, Coulter DA: Mechanisms of epileptogenesis: a convergence on neural circuit dysfunction. Nat Rev Neurosci 14:337, 2013.
3. Pitkanen A, Lukasiuk K: Mechanisms of epileptogenesis and potential treatment targets. Lancet Neurol 10:173, 2011.
4. Bolton C, Young G: Neurological Complicaions of Renal Disease. Butterworth, Boston, 1990.
5. Fraser CL, Arieff AI: Nervous system complications in uremia. Ann Intern Med 109:143, 1988.
6. Grill MF, Maganti R: Cephalosporin-induced neurotoxicity: clinical manifestations, potential pathogenic mechanisms, and the role of electroencephalographic monitoring. Ann Pharmacother 42:1843, 2008.
7. Vulliemoz S, Iwanowski P, Landis T, et al: Levetiracetam accumulation in renal failure causing myoclonic encephalopathy with triphasic waves. Seizure 18:376, 2009.
8. Wallace EL, Lingle K, Pierce D, et al: Amlodipine-induced myoclonus. Am J Med 122:e7, 2009.
9. Jung EY, Cho HS, Seo JW, et al: Metformin-induced encephalopathy without lactic acidosis in a patient with contraindication for metformin. Hemodial Int 13:172, 2009.
10. Yoo L, Matalon D, Hoffman RS, et al: Treatment of pregabalin toxicity by hemodialysis in a patient with kidney failure. Am J Kidney Dis 54:1127, 2009.
11. Diaz A, Deliz B, Benbadis SR: The use of newer antiepileptic drugs in patients with renal failure. Expert Rev Neurother 12:99, 2012.
12. Verbeeck RK, Musuamba FT: Pharmacokinetics and dosage adjustment in patients with renal dysfunction. Eur J Clin Pharmacol 65:757, 2009.
13. Cervelli M, Russ G: Principles of drug therapy, dosing, and prescribing in chronic kidney disease and renal replacement therapy. p. 871. In: Floege J, Johnson RJ, Feehally J (eds): Comprehensive Clinical Nephrology. Elsevier Saunders, Philadelphia, 2010.
14. Frenchie D, Bastani B: Significant removal of phenytoin during high flux dialysis with cellulose triacetate dialyzer. Nephrol Dial Transplant 13:817, 1998.
15. Johannessen Landmark C, Patsalos PN: Drug interactions involving the new second- and third-generation antiepileptic drugs. Expert Rev Neurother 10:119, 2010.

16. Lockwood A: Hepatic encephalopathy. p. 167. In: Arieff A, Griggs R (eds): Metabolic Brain Dysfunction in Systemic Disorders. Little, Brown, Boston, 1992.
17. Marcellin P, de Bony F, Garret C, et al: Influence of cirrhosis on lamotrigine pharmacokinetics. Br J Clin Pharmacol 51:410, 2001.
18. Plum F, Heinfelt B: The neurological complications of liver disease. In: Vinken P, Bruyn G (eds): Handbook of Clinical Neurology Vol 27. Elsevier, Amsterdam, 1986.
19. Russo MW, Galanko JA, Shrestha R, et al: Liver transplantation for acute liver failure from drug induced liver injury in the United States. Liver Transpl 10:1018, 2004.
20. Bjornsson E: Hepatotoxicity associated with antiepileptic drugs. Acta Neurol Scand 118:281, 2008.
21. Krauss G: Current understanding of delayed anticonvulsant hypersensitivity reactions. Epilepsy Curr 6:33, 2006.
22. O'Neil MG, Perdun CS, Wilson MB, et al: Felbamate-associated fatal acute hepatic necrosis. Neurology 46:1457, 1996.
23. Roach GW, Kanchuger M, Mangano CM, et al: Adverse cerebral outcomes after coronary bypass surgery. Multicenter study of perioperative ischemia research group and the ischemia research and education foundation investigators. N Engl J Med 335:1857, 1996.
24. Ramsay RE, DeToledo J: Intravenous administration of fosphenytoin: options for the management of seizures. Neurology 46:S17, 1996.
25. Kenneback G, Bergfeldt L, Vallin H, et al: Electrophysiologic effects and clinical hazards of carbamazepine treatment for neurologic disorders in patients with abnormalities of the cardiac conduction system. Am Heart J 121:1421, 1991.
26. Chinnasami S, Rathore C, Duncan JS: Sinus node dysfunction: an adverse effect of lacosamide. Epilepsia 54:e90, 2013.
27. Thayer JF, Yamamoto SS, Brosschot JF: The relationship of autonomic imbalance, heart rate variability and cardiovascular disease risk factors. Int J Cardiol 141:122, 2010.
28. Lotufo PA, Valiengo L, Bensenor IM, et al: A systematic review and meta-analysis of heart rate variability in epilepsy and antiepileptic drugs. Epilepsia 53:272, 2012.
29. Bleck TP, Smith MC, Pierre-Louis SJ, et al: Neurologic complications of critical medical illnesses. Crit Care Med 21:98, 1993.
30. Delanty N, Vaughan CJ, French JA: Medical causes of seizures. Lancet 352:383, 1998.
31. Jordan KG: Continuous EEG and evoked potential monitoring in the neuroscience intensive care unit. J Clin Neurophysiol 10:445, 1993.
32. Young GB, Jordan KG, Doig GS: An assessment of nonconvulsive seizures in the intensive care unit using continuous EEG monitoring: an investigation of variables associated with mortality. Neurology 47:83, 1996.
33. Wijdicks EF, Parisi JE, Sharbrough FW: Prognostic value of myoclonus status in comatose survivors of cardiac arrest. Ann Neurol 35:239, 1994.
34. Simon RP, Aminoff MJ: Electrographic status epilepticus in fatal anoxic coma. Ann Neurol 20:351, 1986.
35. Spinosa MJ, Bandeira M, Liberalesso PB, et al: Clinical, laboratory and neuroimage findings in juvenile systemic lupus erythematosus presenting involvement of the nervous system. Arq Neuropsiquiatr 65:433, 2007.
36. Avcin T, Benseler SM, Tyrrell PN, et al: A followup study of antiphospholipid antibodies and associated neuropsychiatric manifestations in 137 children with systemic lupus erythematosus. Arthritis Rheum 59:206, 2008.
37. Yu HH, Lee JH, Wang LC, et al: Neuropsychiatric manifestations in pediatric systemic lupus erythematosus: a 20-year study. Lupus 15:651, 2006.
38. Tola MR, Granieri E, Caniatti L, et al: Systemic lupus erythematosus presenting with neurological disorders. J Neurol 239:61, 1992.
39. Brown M, Swash M: Systemic lupus erythematosus. In: Toole F (ed): Handbook of Clinical Neurology Vol 55. Elsevier, Amsterdam, 1989.
40. Cimaz R, Meroni PL, Shoenfeld Y: Epilepsy as part of systemic lupus erythematosus and systemic antiphospholipid syndrome (Hughes syndrome). Lupus 15:191, 2006.
41. Appenzeller S, Cendes F, Costallat LT: Epileptic seizures in systemic lupus erythematosus. Neurology 63:1808, 2004.
42. Ranua J, Luoma K, Peltola J, et al: Anticardiolipin and antinuclear antibodies in epilepsy–a population-based cross-sectional study. Epilepsy Res 58:13, 2004.
43. Hanly JG, Walsh NM, Sangalang V: Brain pathology in systemic lupus erythematosus. J Rheumatol 19:732, 1992.
44. Kister I, Inglese M, Laxer RM, et al: Neurologic manifestations of localized scleroderma: a case report and literature review. Neurology 71:1538, 2008.
45. Castillo P, Woodruff B, Caselli R, et al: Steroid-responsive encephalopathy associated with autoimmune thyroiditis. Arch Neurol 63:197, 2006.
46. Lossos A, River Y, Eliakim A, et al: Neurologic aspects of inflammatory bowel disease. Neurology 45:416, 1995.
47. Bushara KO: Neurologic presentation of celiac disease. Gastroenterology 128:S92, 2005.
48. Labate A, Gambardella A, Messina D, et al: Silent celiac disease in patients with childhood localization-related epilepsies. Epilepsia 42:1153, 2001.
49. Gambardella A, Valentino P, Labate A, et al: Temporal lobe epilepsy as a unique manifestation of multiple sclerosis. Can J Neurol Sci 30:228, 2003.

50. Nyquist PA, Cascino GD, McClelland RL, et al: Incidence of seizures in patients with multiple sclerosis: a population-based study. Mayo Clin Proc 77:910, 2002.
51. Sokic DV, Stojsavljevic N, Drulovic J, et al: Seizures in multiple sclerosis. Epilepsia 42:72, 2001.
52. Thompson AJ, Kermode AG, Moseley IF, et al: Seizures due to multiple sclerosis: seven patients with MRI correlations. J Neurol Neurosurg Psychiatry 56:1317, 1993.
53. Calabrese M, De Stefano N, Atzori M, et al: Extensive cortical inflammation is associated with epilepsy in multiple sclerosis. J Neurol 255:581, 2008.
54. Bylesjo I, Forsgren L, Lithner F, et al: Epidemiology and clinical characteristics of seizures in patients with acute intermittent porphyria. Epilepsia 37:230, 1996.
55. Bonkowsky HL, Sinclair PR, Emery S, et al: Seizure management in acute hepatic porphyria: risks of valproate and clonazepam. Neurology 30:588, 1980.
56. Sadeh M, Blatt I, Martonovits G, et al: Treatment of porphyric convulsions with magnesium sulfate. Epilepsia 32:712, 1991.
57. Lavandera JV, Fossati M, Azcurra J, et al: Glutamatergic system: another target for the action of porphyrinogenic agents. Cell Mol Biol (Noisy-Le-Grand) 55:23, 2009.
58. Suzuki A, Aso K, Ariyoshi C, et al: Acute intermittent porphyria and epilepsy: safety of clonazepam. Epilepsia 33:108, 1992.
59. Hahn M, Gildemeister OS, Krauss GL, et al: Effects of new anticonvulsant medications on porphyrin synthesis in cultured liver cells: potential implications for patients with acute porphyria. Neurology 49:97, 1997.
60. Krijt J, Krijtova H, Sanitrak J: Effect of tiagabine and topiramate on porphyrin metabolism in an in vivo model of porphyria. Pharmacol Toxicol 89:15, 2001.
61. Gregersen H, Nielsen JS, Peterslund NA: Acute porphyria and multiple organ failure during treatment with lamotrigine. Ugeskr Laeger 158:4091, 1996.
62. Krauss GL, Simmons-O'Brien E, Campbell M: Successful treatment of seizures and porphyria with gabapentin. Neurology 45:594, 1995.
63. Paul F, Meencke HJ: Levetiracetam in focal epilepsy and hepatic porphyria: a case report. Epilepsia 45:559, 2004.
64. Martin AB, Bricker JT, Fishman M, et al: Neurologic complications of heart transplantation in children. J Heart Lung Transplant 11:933, 1992.
65. Vaughn BV, Ali II, Olivier KN, et al: Seizures in lung transplant recipients. Epilepsia 37:1175, 1996.
66. Cilio MR, Danhaive O, Gadisseux JF, et al: Unusual cyclosporin related neurological complications in recipients of liver transplants. Arch Dis Child 68:405, 1993.
67. Ghany AM, Tutschka PJ, McGhee Jr RB, et al: Cyclosporine-associated seizures in bone marrow transplant recipients given busulfan and cyclophosphamide preparative therapy. Transplantation 52:310, 1991.
68. Reece DE, Frei-Lahr DA, Shepherd JD, et al: Neurologic complications in allogeneic bone marrow transplant patients receiving cyclosporin. Bone Marrow Transplant 8:393, 1991.
69. Eidelman BH, Abu-Elmagd K, Wilson J, et al: Neurologic complications of FK 506. Transplant Proc 23:3175, 1991.
70. Freise CE, Rowley H, Lake J, et al: Similar clinical presentation of neurotoxicity following FK 506 and cyclosporine in a liver transplant recipient. Transplant Proc 23:3173, 1991.
71. Shihab F, Barry JM, Bennett WM, et al: Cytokine-related encephalopathy induced by OKT3: incidence and predisposing factors. Transplant Proc 25:564, 1993.
72. Maramattom BV, Wijdicks EF: Sirolimus may not cause neurotoxicity in kidney and liver transplant recipients. Neurology 63:1958, 2004.
73. De La Camara R, Tomas JF, Figuera A, et al: High dose busulfan and seizures. Bone Marrow Transplant 7:363, 1991.
74. Gross ML, Pearson RM, Kennedy J, et al: Rejection encephalopathy. Lancet 2:1217, 1982.
75. Chabolla DR, Harnois DM, Meschia JF: Levetiracetam monotherapy for liver transplant patients with seizures. Transplant Proc 35:1480, 2003.
76. Glass GA, Stankiewicz J, Mithoefer A, et al: Levetiracetam for seizures after liver transplantation. Neurology 64:1084, 2005.
77. Soto Alvarez J, Sacristan Del Castillo JA, Alsar Ortiz MJ: Effect of carbamazepine on cyclosporin blood level. Nephron 58:235, 1991.
78. Rosche J, Froscher W, Abendroth D, et al: Possible oxcarbazepine interaction with cyclosporine serum levels: a single case study. Clin Neuropharmacol 24:113, 2001.
79. Wong MC, Suite ND, Labar DR: Seizures in human immunodeficiency virus infection. Arch Neurol 47:640, 1990.
80. Neuenburg JK, Brodt HR, Herndier BG, et al: HIV-related neuropathology, 1985 to 1999: rising prevalence of HIV encephalopathy in the era of highly active antiretroviral therapy. J Acquir Immune Defic Syndr 31:171, 2002.
81. Dal Pan G, McArthur J, Harrison M: Neurological symptoms in HIV infection. p. 141. In: Berger J, Levy R (eds): AIDS and the Nervous System. 2nd Ed. Lippincott-Raven, Philadelphia, 1997.
82. Romanelli F, Jennings HR, Nath A, et al: Therapeutic dilemma: the use of anticonvulsants in HIV-positive individuals. Neurology 54:1404, 2000.
83. Cadle RM, Zenon 3rd GJ, Rodriguez-Barradas MC, et al: Fluconazole-induced symptomatic phenytoin toxicity. Ann Pharmacother 28:191, 1994.

84. Villemure JG, de Tribolet N: Epilepsy in patients with central nervous system tumors. Curr Opin Neurol 9:424, 1996.
85. Clouston PD, DeAngelis LM, Posner JB: The spectrum of neurological disease in patients with systemic cancer. Ann Neurol 31:268, 1992.
86. Del Maestro R, Sabbagh A, Lary A, et al: Metastatic disease. p. 459. In: Shorvon S, Andermann F, Guerini R (eds): The Causes of Epilepsy. Cambridge University Press, Cambridge, 2011.
87. Stein DA, Chamberlain MC: Evaluation and management of seizures in the patient with cancer. Oncology (Williston Park) 5:33, 1991.
88. Kalkanis SN, Kondziolka D, Gaspar LE, et al: The role of surgical resection in the management of newly diagnosed brain metastases: a systematic review and evidence-based clinical practice guideline. J Neurooncol 96:33, 2010.
89. Mikkelsen T, Paleologos NA, Robinson PD, et al: The role of prophylactic anticonvulsants in the management of brain metastases: a systematic review and evidence-based clinical practice guideline. J Neurooncol 96:97, 2010.
90. Maschio M, Dinapoli L, Zarabia A, et al: Issues related to the pharmacological management of patients with brain tumours and epilepsy. Funct Neurol 21:15, 2006.
91. Vecht CJ, Wagner GL, Wilms EB: Interactions between antiepileptic and chemotherapeutic drugs. Lancet Neurol 2:404, 2003.
92. Surks MI, DeFesi CR: Normal serum free thyroid hormone concentrations in patients treated with phenytoin or carbamazepine. A paradox resolved. JAMA 275:1495, 1996.
93. Su YH, Izumi T, Kitsu M, et al: Seizure threshold in juvenile myoclonic epilepsy with Graves disease. Epilepsia 34:488, 1993.
94. Boggs JG: Seizures in medically complex patients. Epilepsia 38(suppl 4):S55, 1997.
95. Castilla-Guerra L, del Carmen Fernández-Moreno M, López-Chozas JM, et al: Electrolytes disturbances and seizures. Epilepsia 47:1990, 2006.
96. Kucharczyk J, Fraser C, Arieff A: Central nervous system manifestations of hyponatremia. p. 55. In: Arieff A, Griggs R (eds): Metabolic Brain Dysfunction in Systemic Disorders. Little, Brown, Boston, 1992.
97. Adrogue HJ, Madias NE, Hypernatremia. N, Engl J: Med 342:1493, 2000.
98. Lin CM, Po HL: Extrapontine myelinolysis after correction of hyponatremia presenting as generalized tonic seizures. Am J Emerg Med 26:632.e5, 2008.
99. Rogawski MA: Update on the neurobiology of alcohol withdrawal seizures. Epilepsy Curr 5:225, 2005.
100. Earnest MP: Seizures. Neurol Clin 11:563, 1993.
101. Lowenstein DH, Alldredge BK: Status epilepticus at an urban public hospital in the 1980s. Neurology 43:483, 1993.
102. Mattson R: Alcohol-related seizures. p. 143. In: Porter R, Mattson R, Cramer J (eds): Alcohol and Seizures. FA Davis, Philadelphia, 1990.
103. Pascual-Leone A, Dhuna A, Altafullah I, et al: Cocaine-induced seizures. Neurology 40:404, 1990.
104. Ng SK, Brust JC, Hauser WA, et al: Illicit drug use and the risk of new-onset seizures. Am J Epidemiol 132:47, 1990.
105. Olson KR, Kearney TE, Dyer JE, et al: Seizures associated with poisoning and drug overdose. Am J Emerg Med 12:392, 1994.
106. Davidson J: Seizures and bupropion: a review. J Clin Psychiatry 50:256, 1989.
107. Borys DJ, Setzer SC, Ling LJ, et al: Acute fluoxetine overdose: a report of 234 cases. Am J Emerg Med 10:115, 1992.
108. Pfizer Inc: Product information: ZOLOFT(R) oral tablets, concentrate, sertraline hydrochloride oral tablets, concentrate. 2009.
109. Alper K, Schwartz KA, Kolts RL, et al: Seizure incidence in psychopharmacological clinical trials: an analysis of Food and Drug Administration (FDA) summary basis of approval reports. Biol Psychiatry 62:345, 2007.
110. Jobe PC, Browning RA: The serotonergic and noradrenergic effects of antidepressant drugs are anticonvulsant, not proconvulsant. Epilepsy Behav 7:602, 2005.
111. Pacia SV, Devinsky O: Clozapine-related seizures: experience with 5,629 patients. Neurology 44:2247, 1994.
112. Wallace KL: Antibiotic-induced convulsions. Crit Care Clin 13:741, 1997.
113. Ruffmann C, Bogliun G, Beghi E: Epileptogenic drugs: a systematic review. Expert Rev Neurother 6:575, 2006.
114. Fink MP, Snydman DR, Niederman MS, et al: Treatment of severe pneumonia in hospitalized patients: results of a multicenter, randomized, double-blind trial comparing intravenous ciprofloxacin with imipenem-cilastatin. The Severe Pneumonia Study Group. Antimicrob Agents Chemother 38:547, 1994.
115. Kahn LH, Alderfer RJ, Graham DJ: Seizures reported with tramadol. JAMA 278:1661, 1997.
116. Marquardt KA, Alsop JA, Albertson TE: Tramadol exposures reported to statewide poison control system. Ann Pharmacother 39:1039, 2005.
117. Wills B, Erickson T: Chemically induced seizures. Clin Lab Med 26:185, 2006.
118. Bahls FH, Ma KK, Bird TD: Theophylline-associated seizures with "therapeutic" or low toxic serum concentrations: risk factors for serious outcome in adults. Neurology 41:1309, 1991.
119. Scheuer M: Medical patients with epilepsy. p. 557. In: Resor S, Kutt H (eds): The Medical Treatment of Epilepsy. Marcel Dekker, New York, 1992.

120. Walder B, Tramer MR, Seeck M: Seizure-like phenomena and propofol: a systematic review. Neurology 58:1327, 2002.
121. Zak R, Solomon G, Petito F, et al: Baclofen-induced generalized nonconvulsive status epilepticus. Ann Neurol 36:113, 1994.
122. Bruns Jr J, Hauser WA: The epidemiology of traumatic brain injury: a review. Epilepsia 44 (suppl 10):2, 2003.
123. Jensen FE: Introduction. Posttraumatic epilepsy: treatable epileptogenesis. Epilepsia 50(suppl 2):1, 2009.
124. Lowenstein DH: Epilepsy after head injury: an overview. Epilepsia 50(suppl 2):4, 2009.
125. Annegers JF, Hauser WA, Coan SP, et al: A population-based study of seizures after traumatic brain injuries. N Engl J Med 338:20, 1998.
126. Asikainen I, Kaste M, Sarna S: Early and late posttraumatic seizures in traumatic brain injury rehabilitation patients: brain injury factors causing late seizures and influence of seizures on long-term outcome. Epilepsia 40:584, 1999.
127. McCrory PR, Bladin PF, Berkovic SF: Retrospective study of concussive convulsions in elite Australian rules and rugby league footballers: phenomenology, aetiology, and outcome. BMJ 314:171, 1997.
128. Gupta YK, Gupta M: Post traumatic epilepsy: a review of scientific evidence. Indian J Physiol Pharmacol 50:7, 2006.
129. Haltiner AM, Temkin NR, Dikmen SS: Risk of seizure recurrence after the first late posttraumatic seizure. Arch Phys Med Rehabil 78:835, 1997.
130. da Silva AM, Vaz AR, Ribeiro I, et al: Controversies in posttraumatic epilepsy. Acta Neurochir Suppl (Wien) 50:48, 1990.
131. Christensen J, Pedersen MG, Pedersen CB, et al: Long-term risk of epilepsy after traumatic brain injury in children and young adults: a population-based cohort study. Lancet 373:1105, 2009.
132. Aarabi B, Taghipour M, Haghnegahdar A, et al: Prognostic factors in the occurrence of posttraumatic epilepsy after penetrating head injury suffered during military service. Neurosurg Focus 8:e1, 2000.
133. Frey LC: Epidemiology of posttraumatic epilepsy: a critical review. Epilepsia 44(suppl 10):11, 2003.
134. Pagni CA: Posttraumatic epilepsy. Incidence and prophylaxis. Acta Neurochir Suppl (Wien) 50:38, 1990.
135. da Silva AM, Nunes B, Vaz AR, et al: Posttraumatic epilepsy in civilians: clinical and electroencephalographic studies. Acta Neurochir Suppl (Wien) 55:56, 1992.
136. Diaz-Arrastia R, Agostini MA, Frol AB, et al: Neurophysiologic and neuroradiologic features of intractable epilepsy after traumatic brain injury in adults. Arch Neurol 57:1611, 2000.
137. Kumar R, Gupta RK, Rao SB, et al: Magnetization transfer and T2 quantitation in normal appearing cortical gray matter and white matter adjacent to focal abnormality in patients with traumatic brain injury. Magn Reson Imaging 21:893, 2003.
138. Beghi E: Overview of studies to prevent posttraumatic epilepsy. Epilepsia 44(suppl 10):21, 2003.
139. Temkin NR, Dikmen SS, Wilensky AJ, et al: A randomized, double-blind study of phenytoin for the prevention of post-traumatic seizures. N Engl J Med 323:497, 1990.
140. Temkin NR, Dikmen SS, Anderson GD, et al: Valproate therapy for prevention of posttraumatic seizures: a randomized trial. J Neurosurg 91:593, 1999.
141. Chang BS, Lowenstein DH: Quality Standards Subcommittee of the American Academy of Neurology: Practice parameter: antiepileptic drug prophylaxis in severe traumatic brain injury: report of the Quality Standards Subcommittee of the American Academy of Neurology. Neurology 60:10, 2003.
142. Watson NF, Barber JK, Doherty MJ, et al: Does glucocorticoid administration prevent late seizures after head injury? Epilepsia 45:690, 2004.

CHAPTER

58

Movement Disorders Associated with General Medical Diseases

CHADWICK W. CHRISTINE ■ MICHAEL J. AMINOFF

Movement disorders may complicate a variety of general medical diseases. Evaluation of patients with involuntary movements or postures requires a detailed history, including an account of perinatal events, ethnicity, parental consanguinity, psychiatric disorders, past medications, exposure to infectious agents, immunologic status, substance abuse, and exposures to toxins. The age of onset and pattern of progression further direct the evaluation. Clinical examination should be directed at determining the character and distribution of the abnormal movements and excluding non-neurologic causes.

CHOREA AND DYSTONIA

Dystonia or chorea occurs in a wide variety of medical disorders. Although chorea is typically a more fluid, "dance-like" undulation of a limb, and dystonia is a slower movement or a sustained abnormal posture of a limb or the trunk, it is sometimes difficult to distinguish between them. Approximately 25 percent of dystonias and most choreas are symptomatic or secondary to a neurodegenerative disorder, hereditary metabolic defect, or systemic medical disorder. Responsible neurodegenerative or inherited metabolic disorders are reviewed elsewhere.[1,2]

Aminoff's Neurology and General Medicine, Fifth Edition.

In a series of 51 cases of chorea from Italy, vascular causes were identified in 40 percent, drug-induced causes in 14 percent, acquired immunodeficiency syndrome (AIDS)–related causes in 10 percent, Huntington disease in 10 percent, hyperglycemia in 4 percent, and hyponatremia in 4 percent; single cases (2 percent each) of borreliosis (Lyme disease), Sydenham chorea, and acanthocytosis were also identified.[3] The epidemiology will differ in regions where AIDS or other infectious conditions are more prevalent. Chorea is usually associated with dysfunction of the thalamus or basal ganglia. In most cases, the physiologic effect of the disorder reduces inhibitory input from the globus pallidus interna to the motor thalamus, resulting in excessive thalamocortical motor facilitation.[4]

Dystonia is characterized by impaired inhibition at multiple levels of the central nervous system, and altered levels of several neurotransmitters have been reported in various diencephalic nuclei, as well as the putamen, globus pallidus, red nucleus, and subthalamic nucleus. Nonetheless, the generation of dystonia remains poorly understood.[1]

Hypoxic-Ischemic Disorders

Chorea and dystonia due to hypoxia-ischemia may result from global or focal cerebral hypoperfusion as well as cellular hypoxia, such as in mitochondrial toxicity. Hypoxia-ischemia causes a decrease in the levels of inhibitory neurotransmitters, with hypoxic-ischemic necrosis of medium-sized inhibitory striatal spiny neurons (GABA-ergic) and enkephalinergic putamenal projections to the external pallidum. In contrast, the striatal cholinergic system becomes upregulated after hypoxia-ischemia, and it is therefore interesting that anticholinergic agents often reduce dystonic movements. Onset of a movement disorder is often delayed after hypoxic injury. This may reflect the time required for remyelination, inflammatory changes, ephaptic transmission, oxidation reactions, maturational or aberrant synaptic reorganization, trans-synaptic neuronal degeneration, or denervation supersensitivity to occur.

Stroke may cause a variety of movement disorders depending on the location of the lesion and age of the patient. In a series of 1,500 patients with stroke, Alarcon and colleagues found that movement disorders occurred in about 4 percent of these patients; chorea occurred in 36 percent, whereas dystonia, tremor, and parkinsonism were less common, occurring in 28, 25, and 10 percent, respectively.[5] The average age at onset of chorea was 75 years, whereas that for dystonia was 48. *Hemichorea* occurred most commonly with contralateral thalamic strokes but also occurred with other lesions of the basal ganglia (putamen and subthalamic nucleus), white matter tracts (corona radiata, internal and external capsule), and pons. Like hemichorea, *hemiballism* is most often caused by a lesion of the contralateral subthalamic nucleus but may occur with lesions of the frontal and parietal lobes or the corona radiata. Putamenal strokes caused *focal-* or *hemidystonia* most frequently, although lesions of the pons or globus pallidus and larger strokes of the frontal lobe were also sometimes responsible. The time to onset of the movement disorder was shorter for chorea—usually within 1 week of the stroke—whereas dystonia and tremor developed 2 to 3 weeks after stroke. Most patients who develop chorea or dystonia after a stroke improve over time.[4]

Chorea or dystonia resulting from global hypoxic-ischemic injury differs in infants, children, and adults. In infants and children, the interval before the movement disorder develops is longer and abnormal movements are more likely to generalize. In adults, chorea or dystonia becomes manifest as any hemiparesis resolves and it usually remains localized. Only in young children with postpump chorea and adults with post-thalamotomy syndrome does the movement disorder commonly begin within a week of injury. Such differences may relate to differences in neuroplasticity or variability in the metabolic response of the brain to injury.[6]

What determines whether global cerebral hypoxia-ischemia causes dystonia or parkinsonism? Marsden and colleagues have noted that, at the time of anoxia, the mean age of patients developing the akinetic-rigid syndrome was 41 years, whereas for those developing pure dystonia it was 13.5 years, suggesting that there is an age-dependent difference in the effect of cerebral hypoxia. Moreover, injury to the putamen is more likely to cause dystonia, whereas lesions of the globus pallidus are usually associated with parkinsonism.[7] Perinatal hypoxic-ischemic injury may lead to any pattern of dystonia, often after a long interval. At onset the dystonia is focal or, rarely, segmental, and commonly spreads over a period of 6 months to 28 years, resulting in segmental dystonia, hemidystonia, or generalized dystonia.[6]

Postoperative encephalopathy with chorea, also known as *postpump chorea*, consists of chorea, athetosis, or ballismus, episodic eye deviations, and hypotonia (Chapter 4). It occurs in infants or children within 12 days of cardiac surgery involving hypothermia, cardiopulmonary bypass, and often complete circulatory arrest, and may be severe. Although this surgical complication was previously common, occurring in up to 20 percent of children, current techniques have drastically reduced its incidence.[8] Risk factors include age at time of surgery (higher risk between 6 months and 5 years), rapid cooling during cardiopulmonary bypass, lower body temperature, and the duration of hypothermic circulatory arrest. Infants younger than 6 weeks are less susceptible; in older infants, the chorea is often mild and reversible. The pathophysiology is poorly understood, although it seems likely that hypoxic-ischemic mechanisms secondary to surgical technique (including deep hypothermia) play a role.[8]

Children and young adults sustaining acute hypoxic injury may also develop dystonia. They usually have focal or unilateral findings clinically and on imaging studies, despite the global insult. Dystonia may develop after 1 week to 3 years[7] and typically generalizes over the following months (up to 5 to 10 years); imaging shows abnormalities especially in the putamen.

Polycythemic chorea occurs for uncertain reasons.[9] Polycythemia rubra vera has a male predominance, but polycythemic chorea is more common in women. Neurologic manifestations of polycythemia are common, occurring in 50 to 80 percent of patients, and include headache, vertigo, stroke, visual symptoms, tinnitus, and paresthesias. Chorea is a rare complication, occurring in 0.5 to 5 percent of patients.[9] Examination may also show a plethoric complexion and splenomegaly. The chorea may be the presenting symptom of polycythemia and may begin suddenly or gradually, is sometimes episodic, and typically becomes generalized but affects particularly the facial, lingual, and brachial muscles. The limbs are hypotonic, with pendular patellar tendon reflexes. The chorea may persist for up to several years, with spontaneous remissions and recurrences. Treatment is of the underlying polycythemia but additional symptomatic control with dopamine-depleting or dopamine-blocking agents may be necessary.

Toxins

Exposure to certain gases and heavy metals is a rare cause of encephalopathy, parkinsonism, and dystonia, probably as a result of cellular hypoxia from mitochondrial dysfunction or the generation of free radicals. *Carbon monoxide* toxicity appears to result from a combination of tissue hypoxia and direct cellular toxicity. After initial recovery, about 10 percent of survivors will develop parkinsonism several weeks to months later; approximately 80 percent recover within 6 months.[10] Imaging often reveals focal injury particularly to the pallidum and diffuse white matter changes, and the findings on magnetic resonance spectroscopy of white matter lesions are consistent with demyelination.[11] Treatment with levodopa and anticholinergic agents usually is unhelpful.[10]

Cyanide poisoning commonly results in death, but may cause parkinsonism and dystonia.[12,13] The movement abnormalities may initially improve, only to worsen days to months later, followed by stabilization and gradual but incomplete recovery. Cyanide reacts with cytochrome *c* oxidase, causing cellular hypoxia. Imaging studies show lesions in the caudate and lentiform nuclei, precentral cortex, and cerebellum. Functional imaging shows reduced dopamine transporter uptake suggestive of nigral neuronal loss.[13]

Ingestion of *methanol* results in the production of formaldehyde by the liver; the liver and erythrocytes synthesize formic acid, which inhibits cytochrome *c* oxidase and, thus, mitochondrial electron transport and tissue adenosine triphosphate production. Metabolic acidosis injures the retina and optic nerves and leads to necrosis of the putamen, subcortical white matter, cerebellum, brainstem, and spinal cord, resulting in parkinsonism, bradykinetic dystonia, tremor, and blindness.[14,15] Initial treatment relies on correction of the metabolic acidosis with ethanol and elimination of methanol with hemodialysis. Gradual improvement may occur with time, and treatment with amantadine and dopaminergic medications sometimes helps.[14]

Manganese toxicity may occur as an occupational exposure (e.g., in miners of the ore or with chronic exposure to metal alloys, batteries, paint, varnish, enamel, or colored glass), or as a consequence of liver failure. Manganese increases free radical formation, inhibits antioxidant function, may reduce mitochondrial energy production, and perhaps increases glutamate neurotoxicity. In addition to foot dystonia, parkinsonism, early freezing of gait, a distinct gait disturbance (cock gait), hyperreflexia, and Babinski signs may occur.[16,17] Remission may occur in mild cases if further exposure is prevented, but the course is otherwise progressive. There are reports of improvement after chelation.[18] Pathologic examination reveals damage to the globus pallidus and substantia nigra pars reticulata (which are downstream from the nigrostriatal dopaminergic pathway), consistent with the failure to respond to levodopa.[17] Magnetic resonance imaging (MRI) may show hyperintensity of the putamen on T1-weighted images. A similar syndrome (with elevated serum manganese and putamen T1 hyperintensity) has been described in methcathinone (ephedrine) users when the drug was produced using potassium permanganate oxidation of ephedrine or pseudoephedrine.[19]

Organic *mercury* poisoning, as seen formerly with the ingestion of certain fungicides and shellfish (Minamata disease), causes visual loss, ataxia, paresthesias, and cognitive dysfunction. Choreoathetosis, parkinsonism, and tremor also occur, and dystonic posturing is occasionally seen. Inorganic mercury poisoning, seen in glass blowers, hatters, and battery workers, produces a psychotic encephalopathy and tremor.[20]

Dystonia secondary to copper accumulation occurs in *Wilson disease*. If hepatic damage is mild, significant improvement follows chelation therapy with penicillamine or trientine and zinc, which reduces dietary absorption of copper. Liver transplantation may be required for nonresponders and patients with severe liver dysfunction.[21] The movement disorder may respond to trihexyphenidyl, levodopa, dopamine agonists, or amantadine.

Cellular and global hypoxia-ischemia have been implicated in *disulfiram* overdose in adults and children.[22,23] In one such case, psychomotor slowing and parkinsonism were evident several days after awakening from coma, and over 10 years progressed to include dystonia of a lower limb, the eyelids, and speech. Brain computed tomography (CT) shows hypodense lesions, and MRI shows hyperintense lesions in the pallidum and inferior putamen.[22] Chorea has also been described as a consequence of toluene (glue sniffing) and thallium exposures.[24]

Drug-Induced Dystonia and Chorea

Medications may cause dystonia (Chapter 32) and chorea (Table 58-1). Acute iatrogenic dystonic reactions are idiosyncratic, reversible, and common. They may occur almost immediately (minutes to hours) after the first dose of a medication, or days to weeks later. For dystonia, the most common offenders include antipsychotics (both typical and atypical), benzodiazepines, anticonvulsants, dopamine agonists, and tricyclic antidepressants.[25] Reactions have been encountered less often with calcium-channel blockers, propranolol, histamine blocking drugs (cimetidine, ranitidine, cetirizine), and substituted benzamides (metoclopramide, sulpiride, clebopride, and domperidone). Dystonia may occur soon after starting antidepressants or develop after chronic use. Many agents (and medication classes) including tetracyclics (trazodone and amoxipine), tricyclics (clomipramine, amitriptyline, and imipramine), selective serotonin reuptake inhibitors (including fluoxetine, paroxetine, fluvoxamine, escalopram, citalopram, and sertraline), and serotonin-norepinephine reuptake inhibitor (duloxetine) have been associated with development of dystonia.[25,26] Patients with AIDS dementia complex are particularly sensitive to neuroleptic-related acute dystonic reactions because of underlying dopaminergic dysfunction.[27]

If dystonia develops acutely, treatment involves discontinuation of the offending agent and administration of an anticholinergic, or benzodiazepine. Diphenhydramine, benztropine mesylate, chlorpheniramine, diazepam, or lorazepam may be given orally or intravenously; treatment for several days is sometimes necessary, especially if the causal agent was taken regularly or in depot form. If dystonia is mild or develops slowly, gradual down-titration of the medication is appropriate.

Chorea has been reported secondary to a variety of medications including anticonvulsants (phenytoin, carbamazepine, valproate, and gabapentin), stimulants (amphetamine, cocaine, methylphenidate, pemoline), benzodiazepines, estrogens, lithium, levodopa (with or without catechol-*O*-methyltransferase [COMT] inhibitors), dopamine agonists, tricyclic antidepressants, and antihistamines, as well as other agents such as baclofen, cimetidine, thyroxine, cyclosporine, and aminophylline.[25] Azar and colleagues reported chorea and encephalopathy associated with ciprofloxacin[28]; another case associated with 4-aminopyridine overdose has also been reported.[29] Disulfiram overdose or poisoning (discussed earlier) may present clinically with encephalopathy, ketotic hyperglycemia, and dystonia.[22]

Tardive syndromes develop after the introduction of the provoking medication, usually a dopamine

TABLE 58-1 ■ Selected Drugs and Toxins Inducing Chorea and Dystonia

Drug or Toxin	Chorea	Dystonia
Anticholinergics	Benzhexol, trihexyphenidyl	–
Antiepileptics	Carbamazepine, felbamate, gabapentin, lamotrigine, phenytoin, valproic acid	–
Anti-infectious agents	Ciprofloxacin	–
Antidepressants and anxiolytics	Tricyclic agents	Selective serotonin reuptake inhibitors, tricyclic agents, benzodiazepines
Cardiac medications	Flecainide	Flecainide
Calcium-channel blockers	–	Cinnarizine, flunarizine, verapamil
Dopamine agonists and levodopa	Apomorphine, bromocriptine, pergolide, pramipexole, ropinirole, lisuride, cabergoline, levodopa	Apomorphine, bromocriptine, pergolide, pramipexole, ropinirole, lisuride, cabergoline, levodopa
Dopamine-receptor blocking drugs	Antipsychotics, metoclopramide, antiemetics	Antipsychotics, metoclopramide, antiemetics
Histamine-receptor blocking drugs	Cyproheptadine	Cimetidine, ranitidine, cetirizine
Hormones	Oral contraceptives, estrogens, thyroxine	–
Immunosuppressants	Corticosteroids, cyclosporine	–
Stimulants	Amphetamine, cocaine, methylphenidate, pemoline	–
Serotonin receptor antagonists	Ondansetron	Ondansetron
Miscellaneous drugs	Baclofen, digoxin, lithium, theophylline, 4-aminopyridine	Clebopride, disulfiram, domperidone, metoclopramide, sulpiride
Toxins/metals	Mercury, thallium, toluene	Carbon monoxide, cyanide, disulfiram, manganese, methanol, mercury, thallium

receptor blocking drug. Most patients have been on the medication for at least 3 months; the disorder may first manifest after the causal agent has been discontinued, but typically does so within 6 months of withdrawal. The syndrome may involve dyskinesias, typically repetitive orolingual facial movements or repetitive movements of the head, trunk, and extremities. Older patients seem more susceptible than young persons. A tardive syndrome also may take the form of dystonia, chorea, akathisia, tremor, or myoclonus.

A number of medications have been associated with the development of tardive dyskinesia. In a series of 434 patients, 44 percent were considered secondary to haloperidol, 39 percent to metoclopramide, 20 percent to amitriptyline/perphenazine, and 16 percent to thioridazine. Although "atypical" antipsychotic agents are thought to be less likely to cause tardive dyskinesia, a similar incidence and prevalence was found in one study of patients treated with typical and atypical antipsychotics when clozapine was excluded.[30] Other dopamine-blocking agents such as the antiemetics prochlorperazine and promethazine may cause tardive syndromes. Less commonly, certain calcium-channel blockers (especially cinnarizine and flunarizine) and rarely serotonin reuptake inhibitors have been associated with the development of tardive dyskinesia. The causal agent should be discontinued if feasible; the withdrawal of dopamine-blocking agents may initially exacerbate the dyskinesia, but the movement disorder ultimately decreases or disappears in up to 50 percent of patients, persisting unchanged in the remainder. Dopamine-depleting agents (reserpine, tetrabenazine) are the most useful adjunctive treatments, followed by benzodiazepines and by dopamine agonists and GABA agonists; anticholinergic drugs may exacerbate the syndrome.[31]

Tardive dystonia may be indistinguishable from idiopathic dystonia and may respond to sensory tricks. It may be focal, segmental, or generalized; however, the head and neck region are most commonly affected, resulting in torticollis, blepharospasm, or oromandibular dystonia.[31] Orobuccal-lingual dyskinesia or other tardive movements may occur in tardive dystonia, unlike in idiopathic dystonia. The onset is insidious, typically after several years of antipsychotic use, but may occur with exposures shorter than 1 year. Tapering the antipsychotic occasionally produces gradual or partial remission of tardive dystonia, often after an initial worsening. An increase in dose of the antipsychotic or its continuation may lead to temporary benefit, but probably worsens the long-term outlook. If treatment with an antipsychotic is necessary, replacement of the original neuroleptic with clozapine or sometimes quetiapine has been helpful. Approximately 50 percent of patients benefit from dopamine-depleting or -blocking agents and anticholinergic treatment.[31] For patients with focal or segmental dystonia, botulinum toxin injections are beneficial. Stereotactic surgery, including pallidotomy and pallidal deep brain stimulation, has been successful for severe tardive dystonia unresponsive to other measures.[32]

Some medications appear to cause chorea in the setting of preexisting basal ganglia injury. For example, dose-related dyskinesias develop in a large proportion of parkinsonian patients taking carbidopa-levodopa. Similarly, many patients who develop chorea while taking oral contraceptives have had striatal abnormalities on imaging studies or have a past history of Sydenham chorea, chorea gravidarum, or chorea with Henoch–Schönlein purpura.[33]

Among illicit drugs, cocaine and amphetamines (Chapter 34) have been most frequently associated with dyskinesias. Both influence central dopaminergic mechanisms, and cocaine also decreases serotonin turnover and degradation. Both may lead to choreoathetoid movements of the extremities, less often the head or trunk, or buccolingual dyskinesias within 24 hours of use; these typically resolve without treatment in 2 to 6 days. However, in chronic users, chorea persisting for more than 1 year after discontinuation of these stimulants has been described.[34]

Infectious Disorders

Infections may cause the full spectrum of movement disorders (Table 58-2). Movement abnormalities usually develop during the acute illness and are transient, but abnormal movements sometimes begin or persist after the infection has cleared. One mechanism is vasculitic ischemia of the basal ganglia, although direct neuronal injury by the organism or a toxin, and autoimmune cross-reactivity with basal ganglia epitopes are also postulated to play a role.

Bacterial Infections

Sydenham chorea is a transient chorea that develops in about 26 percent of patients with rheumatic fever. It is the most common cause of acute chorea in children, and typically affects children between ages 7 and 12 (with a range of 3 to 17 years).[35] After 10 years of age, it is more common in girls. The chorea is usually generalized (80% of cases), and may be the presenting feature of rheumatic fever. An encephalopathy occurs in 10 percent.[35] Dysarthria and behavioral abnormalities are common; a recent study found obsessive-compulsive disorder and attention deficit and hyperactivity in about 25 percent of patients.[36] The pathogenesis of Sydenham chorea may be related to the development of antineuronal antibodies.[37] Although the condition usually improves over months, residual chorea has been observed in 50 percent of patients 2 years after onset, and behavioral abnormalities may persist. Symptomatic treatment with valproic acid or carbamazepine may be considered in those with severe chorea.[35] Dopamine-receptor blocking drugs are reserved for those who do not respond to these anticonvulsants. In about half of affected patients, chorea recurs within 2 years of the initial episode in the absence of infection. Prophylaxis with penicillin should be considered to avert further rheumatologic injury. Neuroimaging studies may be normal or show contralateral or bilateral striatal abnormalities that resolve as the chorea settles. Positron emission tomography (PET) scanning shows reversible striatal hypermetabolism.

Tuberculous meningitis may cause dystonia or chorea. Brain imaging may be normal or show ischemic or hemorrhagic infarcts. Direct infection or infarction of the basal ganglia may account for the development of the movement disorder. Treatment is with antituberculous therapy. Most patients improve over several weeks.[38]

Mycoplasma pneumoniae causes pneumonia but also affects the central nervous system (CNS) in approximately 5 percent of patients requiring hospitalization. Aseptic meningitis, cranial neuritis,

TABLE 58-2 ■ Movement Disorders Produced by Various Infectious Agents

Infectious Agent	Chorea	Dystonia	Myoclonus	Tremor	Parkinsonism
Arboviruses	X				X
Cytomegalovirus	X	X		X	
Enteroviruses	X				X
Epstein–Barr virus	X				
Herpes simplex viruses	X				
Herpes zoster virus			X	X	X
HIV	X		X	X	X
HIV plus *Toxoplasma gondii*	X	X		X	X
HIV plus herpes zoster			X		
HIV plus *Mycobacterium tuberculosis*	X				
HIV plus *Treponema pallidum*	X				
Influenza viruses	X	X		X	
Japanese encephalitis virus	X	X		X	X
Lassa virus				X	
Machupo virus (Bolivian hemorrhagic fever)				X	
Measles virus	X		X		X
Paramyxovirus (mumps)	X		X		
Rubella virus	X			X	
African trypanosomiasis				X	X
Corynebacterium diphtheriae	X				
Lyme borreliosis			X		
Legionella species	X				
Mycoplasma pneumoniae	X	X			X
Salmonella species	X		X	X	X
Group A *Streptococcus*	X	X			X
Mycobacterium tuberculosis	X	X	X	X	X
Treponema pallidum	X				
Plasmodium falciparum	X	X	X	X	X
Schistosoma mansoni			X (segmental)		
Tropheryma whipplei			X	X	X
Taenia solium (neurocysticercosis)	X	X	X	X	X
Cryptococcal meningoencephalitis			X		X
Prions			X		X

Adapted from Alarcón F, Giménez-Roldán S: Systemic diseases that cause movement disorders. Parkinsonism Relat Disord 11:1, 2005.

transverse myelitis, or encephalitis may occur, and neurologic symptoms may precede pulmonary ones. Generalized choreoathetosis and dystonia have been described.[39,40] Cerebral imaging may be unremarkable or show abnormalities in the caudate, putamen, and globus pallidus. The cerebrospinal fluid (CSF) is normal or exhibits a mild lymphocytosis with elevated protein concentration. The diagnosis is made by respiratory cultures and tests for serum and CSF complement-fixing and cold agglutinin antibodies.

In Legionnaire disease (*Legionella pneumophila*), high fevers and pulmonary involvement may be accompanied in approximately 20 percent of cases by headache and, rarely, by chorea.[41] The CSF and head CT scan are normal, and the diagnosis is made by serologic studies. The chorea may persist for up to 2 years.

Chorea has also been reported uncommonly in patients with Lyme encephalitis[3] or neurosyphilis[42] and rarely with other infections.

Viral Infections

Viral encephalitis (including Japanese encephalitis, West Nile, St. Louis, herpes simplex, dengue, mumps, and measles) may be accompanied by movement disorders. Japanese encephalitis, endemic to much of Asia, causes dystonia or parkinsonism several weeks after infection. Brain MRI typically shows abnormalities in the thalamus, globus pallidus or putamen.[43] Varicella has been associated with transient chorea and dystonia.[44] Chorea can be an early feature of herpes simplex encephalitis but more frequently signals a relapse.[45] In adults, human immunodeficiency virus (HIV) infection may present with hemichorea-hemiballism or with generalized chorea, usually in the presence of dementia. Most AIDS-related cases are secondary to toxoplasmosis but may also relate to HIV encephalitis, cryptococcal infection, or progressive multifocal leukoencephalopathy.[27]

Fungal and Parasitic Infections

In HIV-seropositive patients, cerebral toxoplasmosis is the most common cause of dyskinesia. *Toxoplasma* abscesses in various diencephalic structures have been associated with contralateral limb ballism, choreoathetosis, and dystonia.[27] Treatment of the infection is usually successful, but improvement in the dyskinesia is seen in only approximately 25 percent of instances, suggesting irreversible injury to the basal ganglia. Improvement of the dyskinesia may occur with dopamine-blocking agents or dopamine depleters such as tetrabenazine. Hemichorea and hemiballismus have been reported only rarely in cryptococcal meningitis and may respond to antifungal treatment.[46]

Autoimmune, Inflammatory, and Paraneoplastic Disorders

In systemic lupus erythematosus (SLE), choreoathetosis develops in 1 to 2 percent of patients and may be the presenting feature.[47,48] In most, the chorea occurs before the age of 30 years and tends to manifest during a lupus flare. It may be generalized or lateralized and is usually transient, lasting for a few days up to 3 years; recurrence occurs in approximately 25 percent of cases. Rarely, the chorea is permanent. The chorea may be self-limited or respond to corticosteroid or symptomatic treatment. Imaging studies may be abnormal, but the location of any lesions does not usually explain the chorea.

Patients with SLE and chorea may possess antiphospholipid antibodies (lupus anticoagulant or anticardiolipin antibody) that predispose to endovascular thrombosis and cerebral infarction.[49] Approximately 30 percent of patients with SLE with these antibodies have thrombotic events. Laboratory studies reveal that whole-blood clotting time is prolonged, and the prothrombin time and the Russell viper venom time may be abnormal. Chorea in several patients with SLE and antiphospholipid antibodies has improved within days on aspirin therapy or warfarin, consistent with a vascular mechanism. Thus, chorea in SLE may result from autoimmune vasculitic cerebral microthrombosis or direct antibody-mediated basal ganglia dysfunction, or both.[49]

The antiphospholipid syndrome may occur in the absence of SLE or other autoimmune conditions, the so-called primary antiphospholipid syndrome. Clinically and pathophysiologically, this condition is indistinguishable from that associated with SLE. In addition to lupus anticoagulant and an immunoglobulin (IgG) anticardiolipin antibody, many patients have a low titer of antinuclear antibody, 30 percent have a false-positive Venereal Disease Research Laboratory (VDRL) test, and some have antithyroid antibodies. Chorea (either lateralized or generalized) has been the most frequently reported movement disorder, occurring in 1 to 4 percent of patients with primary or secondary antiphospholipid syndrome, although tics, dystonia, myoclonus, and corticobasal syndrome may occur.[50] Brain MRI shows lesions of the basal ganglia in 6 to 16 percent of patients; labeled glucose PET imaging has revealed increased uptake contralateral to the hemichorea.[49] For patients with no vascular events, treatment may consist of discontinuation of estrogen or progesterone (if applicable) and immunosuppressant treatment. For patients who have had a vascular event, anticoagulation is recommended to reduce the risk of recurrent thrombosis.[51]

Chorea is a rare complication of polyarteritis nodosa and isolated angiitis of the CNS. Patients with Behçet syndrome (recurrent oral and genital ulcers, uveitis, and skin lesions) may present with chorea,[52] jaw-opening dystonia,[53] or paroxysmal dystonia.[54] Typically, these patients have had an increased CSF protein concentration and lymphocytosis. They respond to immunosuppression but may require other agents to control movements. Chorea may also develop in Churg–Strauss syndrome.

Chorea may occur in Hashimoto thyroiditis. The CSF protein concentration is usually elevated, and some samples have oligoclonal bands or a mononuclear pleocytosis. Characteristically, the electroencephalogram (EEG) shows epileptiform activity, and transient or permanent areas of increased T2 signal are seen on brain MRI, particularly in the frontal and temporal lobes. Patients respond to prednisone, with a slow taper once improvement is stable. Complete remissions can be anticipated, although relapses sometimes occur or a deficit remains. Spontaneous remissions are rare.[55]

Dystonia and tremor[56] or chorea[57] may be part of a movement disorder associated with celiac disease. Abdominal pain, ataxia, diarrhea, and myoclonus may also occur. Diagnosis is supported by demonstration of gliadin antibodies and characteristic findings on small bowel biopsy. The condition may respond to a gluten-free diet.[57]

Chorea and dystonia are rare complications of paraneoplastic syndromes. In a series of 979 patients with paraneoplastic diseases, 9 presented with chorea and 3 had dystonia or dyskinesia.[58] Most had small-cell cancer of the lung, and 1 each had non–small-cell lung cancer, renal cancer, and colon cancer. Most of these patients had CV2/ collapsing response-mediator protein (CRMP)-5 antibodies, but ANNA-1 (anti-Hu) antibodies were found in 4. In many patients, chorea was the initial symptom. CSF was abnormal in some patients. Brain imaging was abnormal in 4 of the 9 patients, with diffuse hyperintensity of the white matter in T2-weighted MRI; 2 showed basal ganglia hyperintensity. Improvement may occur with cancer treatment or symptomatic medications (dopamine-blocking medications or benzodiazepines). Laryngospasm, jaw-opening dystonia, and cervical dystonia have been described in paraneoplastic syndromes associated with antineuronal antibody type 2 (ANNA-2, also known as anti-Ri antibodies).[59] Although patients with anti-NMDA receptor encephalitis usually present with behavioral changes and seizures, dyskinesias involving the face, trunk, abdomen, and extremities develop in 80 percent; orobuccolingual dyskinesias are most common.[60]

Metabolic Disorders

The association between thyrotoxicosis and choreoathetosis or dystonic posturing was recognized by Gowers in 1893, particularly in young women, but patients of either sex may be affected. Chorea occurs in about 1 to 2 percent of those with *hyperthyroidism* and its course usually parallels that of the thyroid disorder.[61] Abnormal movements typically involve the limbs, sometimes unilaterally, and are most conspicuous distally; the neck and face may also be affected. Paroxysmal (rather than more continuous) choreoathetosis may occur in rare instances; paroxysmal and kinesigenic choreoathetosis have also been reported with iatrogenic hyperthyroidism. No cerebral lesions have been noted on MRI or at autopsy. Treatment consists primarily in normalization of thyroid function (antithyroid drugs, radioiodine, or thyroidectomy). Chorea may respond to dopamine receptor blockers or propranolol even before hyperthyroidism has resolved. Altered dopamine turnover or increased dopamine receptor sensitivity may be responsible for the dyskinesia. Since chorea may occur in both hyperthyroidism secondary to Graves disease and iatrogenic thyrotoxicosis, it is hypothesized that the disorder results from a direct effect of thyroxine on the basal ganglia, perhaps by increasing dopamine receptor sensitivity.[61]

Hypocalcemia from idiopathic hypoparathyroidism rarely may cause dystonia or choreoathetosis.[62] The abnormal movements may be the presenting complaint, may be asymmetric, are usually paroxysmal, and rarely are kinesigenic. Patients are usually younger than 30 years, with calcium levels of 4 to 6 mg/dl, elevated serum phosphorus levels (5 to 12 mg/dl), and low serum magnesium. Brain imaging frequently reveals basal ganglia calcification that persists after treatment of hypocalcemia and resolution of chorea or dystonia.

Generalized chorea or hemiballism-hemichorea may occur in *nonketotic hyperosmolar hyperglycemia*.[63] Brain CT may show high-density lesions, and MRI often shows high T1 signal and hypoperfusion in the caudate or putamen contralateral to the side involved clinically. These imaging findings are considered to be a consequence of hyperviscosity and cytotoxic edema, not petechial hemorrhage.[64] The chorea may resolve with correction of hyperglycemia; however, dopamine-depleting agents or dopamine-blocking agents may be useful treatments until the condition resolves. Severe *hypoglycemia* may be accompanied by either generalized chorea or hemichorea that resolves as blood glucose normalizes.[65]

Dystonia or chorea has rarely been noted in hypernatremic dehydration, hyponatremia, and hypomagnesemia and also after central pontine myelinolysis.[66]

Other Causes

Post traumatic focal and hemidystonia may occur rarely as a long-term consequence of severe head injury.[67]

Approach to Diagnosis

The evaluation of patients with involuntary movements or postures requires a detailed history, as outlined earlier. Characterization of the movement disorder and its distribution, together with findings such as organomegaly, skin lesions, retinal or optic nerve disease, or neurologic deficits, narrows the differential diagnosis. The relaxed patient must be observed carefully while lying, sitting, standing, and walking to determine whether any abnormality is exacerbated by movement or rest. The patient should perform tasks that are particularly impaired because certain movement disorders are solely task specific.

The age of onset and the pattern of involvement and progression vary with the etiology. Focal or task-specific dystonias, often associated with a dystonic or essential-type tremor, onset in adulthood, a benign history, and no other abnormalities on examination are usually idiopathic. Limb dystonia beginning as action dystonia is usually idiopathic, whereas dystonia beginning at rest is sometimes symptomatic. Dystonia with onset in the legs is usually idiopathic in children but symptomatic in adults. Chorea or dystonia of acute or subacute onset or having a rapidly progressive course is more likely to be symptomatic. Hemidystonia at any age suggests a secondary etiology, and approximately 75 percent of patients have contralateral basal ganglia abnormalities on imaging, a history of hemiparesis, or both. One-third of hemidystonic patients have infarction or hemorrhage of the contralateral basal ganglia, especially the putamen. Generalized dystonia beginning at an early age may be idiopathic or symptomatic, but it is more often symptomatic when onset is in adulthood. Childhood-onset dystonias tend to become generalized, whereas those commencing in adulthood often remain focal or segmental. Similarly, tardive dystonia may be generalized in children, but it usually remains focal or multifocal in adults. Thus, dystonia of sudden onset, rapid progression, onset in infancy, cranial onset in children, lower-extremity onset in adults, or hemidystonia at any age is more likely symptomatic and requires full evaluation.

A large number of factors contribute to decision-making in the evaluation of chorea and dystonia. Brain MRI has a high yield, and basic laboratory studies include a complete blood count and blood electrolytes, calcium, phosphorus, uric acid, and liver and thyroid function tests. Any patient with chorea or dystonia younger than 40 years must be evaluated for Wilson disease. Evaluation for vascular disease, a hypercoagulable state, connective tissue disorders, and antiphospholipid antibodies may be required. Serum antistreptolysin O or antihyaluronidase titers and an electrocardiogram are useful when Sydenham chorea is suspected. Neurodegenerative and hereditary metabolic disorders require a separate battery of studies, which are described elsewhere.[1,2]

Treatment

The treatment of secondary dystonia or chorea is difficult. In symptomatic cases, the underlying pathologic process should be treated first, as discussed earlier. General therapeutic measures may provide symptomatic benefit when specific treatments of the underlying lesion have failed to temper the movement disorder satisfactorily. Anticholinergics, dopaminergics, antidopaminergics, benzodiazepines, anticonvulsants, and certain other medications (discussed later) are used, based on patient age, tolerance, coexisting medical illnesses, and interactions with other medications taken concomitantly. All of these medications are disappointingly variable in their efficacy. Unfortunately, there is a paucity of adequate trials demonstrating therapeutic benefit or comparative efficacy because patient numbers are small, common side effects make double-blinding difficult, and nonspecific effects such as sedation can diminish abnormal movements. Moreover, spontaneous remissions, partial or complete, and transient or permanent, may occur unpredictably.

Anticholinergic medication, of which trihexyphenidyl is the best studied, is more effective in mild dystonia and in younger patients. Approximately one-third of patients with secondary dystonia benefit, and up to 50 percent of those with perinatal hypoxic injury improve.[68] The selected agent is started at a low dose, which is increased slowly, depending on response and tolerance. (A particular daily dose may take several weeks to produce maximal benefit.) Side effects can be dose-limiting, particularly with advancing age. Tricyclic antidepressants and diphenhydramine are also sometimes used for their anticholinergic effects.

The useful antidopaminergic medications include dopamine depleters (reserpine, tetrabenazine) or dopamine receptor antagonists. Both reserpine and tetrabenazine are helpful for tardive dystonia.[69] Tetrabenazine has been the most useful single agent, particularly in tardive dyskinesia, tardive dystonia, Huntington chorea, and idiopathic generalized dystonia.

Dopaminergic supplementation using levodopa is singularly effective in patients with dopamine-responsive dystonia, which may be present in 5 to 10 percent of patients with childhood-onset hereditary dystonia beginning in the legs, with or without diurnal fluctuations. It is less useful in treating symptomatic dystonias. In some instances, levodopa may actually worsen symptomatic dystonia, whereas improvement occurs with dopamine agonists or amantadine.[70]

Anticonvulsants have been tried, usually with disappointing results. For example, in a study of 67 patients with dystonia, only 11 percent obtained moderate or greater benefit from carbamazepine.[68] Baclofen, a presynaptic γ-aminobutyric acid agonist, is also frequently tried and occasionally is effective, either orally or intrathecally.[71] Other medications that have been tried alone or in combination, with variable benefit, include benzodiazepines, particularly clonazepam (27% with secondary dystonia may benefit[68]), muscle relaxants, cyproheptadine, and lithium. Adult-onset cranial or focal limb dystonias are best treated with intramuscular botulinum toxin.[71]

Surgical approaches are sometimes warranted. Deep brain stimulation of the globus pallidus is effective for primary dystonia, myoclonus dystonia, and tardive dystonia.[32] Selective peripheral denervation is sometimes successful for blepharospasm and cervical dystonia, but is now generally reserved for cases refractory to botulinum toxin.[72] The use of deep brain stimulation for refractory chorea is being explored.[73]

MYOCLONUS

Myoclonus is an acute, brief, involuntary jerk caused by a sudden muscle contraction (positive myoclonus) or relaxation (negative myoclonus). It can be classified by distribution, the location of the generator, or the underlying etiology. It may recur in the same muscle groups (focal or segmental myoclonus) or asynchronously and asymmetrically in different muscle groups (multifocal or generalized myoclonus), and it may occur at rest (spontaneous), on movement (action or intentional myoclonus), or in response to specific stimuli (reflex myoclonus).

Myoclonus occurs in healthy individuals (hiccups, hypnic jerks) or as a movement disorder with an idiopathic (essential), epileptic, or symptomatic etiology. Symptomatic myoclonus is the most common variety and may be due to primary neurologic causes, but it is more commonly seen in a general medical setting, to which this section is devoted. Myoclonus may be generated from spinal, subcortical, or cortical circuits and involves the somatotopically organized dorsal column/lemniscal and corticospinal systems superimposed on the spinoreticular and reticulospinal circuits.[74]

Hypoxia-Ischemia

Posthypoxic action myoclonus may occur in survivors of cardiopulmonary arrest. Two forms of myoclonus are recognized in this context: acute posthypoxic myoclonus, which develops soon after hypoxia and is characterized by generalized myoclonus, and chronic posthypoxic myoclonus, which begins after a delay and is characterized by action myoclonus.[75] Multifocal myoclonus begins as the patient regains consciousness and is aggravated by voluntary motor activity. Cerebellar ataxia and cognitive impairment are often associated. Typically these signs improve with time, although some positive myoclonus and gait difficulty due to negative myoclonus may persist, resulting in falls.

Acute posthypoxic myoclonus is characterized by severe, generalized myoclonus in comatose patients.[75] The jerk-like movements develop within the first day after hypoxia and are characterized by violent flexion movements. If myoclonus persists for more than 30 minutes or for most of the resuscitation day, it is often called myoclonus status epilepticus, despite the lack of evidence that the myoclonus is epileptic in nature. Wijdicks and associates found that in over 95 percent of patients with posthypoxic myoclonus, an EEG performed on the first hospital day demonstrated a burst-suppression pattern, alpha-pattern coma, or polyspike-wave activity.[76] Myoclonus status epilepticus occurs in 30 to 40 percent of comatose adult survivors of cardiopulmonary resuscitation, is difficult to control, and has a poor prognosis. A meta-analysis of 134 patients with myoclonus status epilepticus found that 89 percent died, 8 percent remained in a persistent vegetative state, and 3 percent survived (two patients are described as having had a good outcome).[77] It is uncertain whether a similar outcome occurs in patients treated with hypothermia.

Chronic posthypoxic myoclonus (Lance–Adams syndrome) occurs within days to weeks after hypoxic injury, usually while the patient is still in coma. The myoclonus predominantly involves the limbs and is precipitated by active or passive movement; it occasionally spreads to other portions of the body. It may be stimulus sensitive, and negative myoclonus may also occur, predisposing patients to falls. Treatment of chronic posthypoxic myoclonus is not satisfactory. However, clonazepam, valproate, and piracetam are often helpful. Treatment with 5-hydroxytryptophan (often with carbidopa to limit nausea), levetiracetam, and sodium oxybate may also be helpful.[78] Other agents such as baclofen, diazepam, ethanol, and methysergide are sometimes worthwhile.[75]

Metabolic Disorders

Metabolic disorders are commonly associated with mental status changes and negative myoclonus (asterixis), which is usually of brainstem reticular origin. Renal failure and its treatment may both be associated with neurologic dysfunction. Generalized and multifocal positive and negative myoclonus occur in *uremic encephalopathy* (Chapter 16). It may occur at rest, with movement, or in response to a stimulus. Myoclonus also occurs in patients with *dialysis dementia* (Chapter 16). The myoclonus is exacerbated during and after dialysis and is most prominent in the face and upper limbs.

In *hepatic insufficiency* of any cause, asterixis is typical, but multifocal positive myoclonus also occurs. Treatment requires addressing the underlying disorder. In rare instances, Wilson disease may present with progressive myoclonus.[21]

Hyperglycemia is the most common metabolic disturbance causing focal motor phenomena. In nonketotic hyperglycemia, severe hyperglycemia, hyperosmolality, and dehydration are accompanied by segmental or generalized myoclonic seizures in up to 20 percent of patients.[79] Asterixis or negative myoclonus is also seen. EEG shows diffuse slowing, sometimes with a spike-wave pattern. The glucose level is typically over 600 mg/dl and osmolality above 300 mOsm/kg H_2O, with mild or absent ketoacidosis. The myoclonus resolves with treatment of the hyperosmolality, and not with anticonvulsants, but therapy should be gradual, repleting approximately half the fluid deficit in the first 12 hours and the remainder over the next 24 hours because faster rates may precipitate CNS hyperglycemia and cerebral edema.

Vitamin B_{12} deficiency may cause myoclonus in children[80] and adults.[81] The myoclonus resolves after treatment with vitamin B_{12}. Myoclonus may also occur after intramuscular vitamin B_{12} administration.

Pellagra (niacin deficiency) is characterized by the triad of myoclonus, altered mental status, and generalized hypertonicity; a dermatitis is sometimes present. It typically occurs in alcoholism but can be seen in malabsorption conditions and after treatment with certain medications (5-fluorouracil, isoniazid, pyrazinamide, ethionamide, 6-mercaptopurine, hydantoins, phenobarbital, and chloramphenicol). In one series of 230 patients with suspected Creutzfeldt–Jakob disease, 5 were found at autopsy to have pathologic features of pellagra and 4 of the 5 had had myoclonus.[82] Early replacement of niacin is required. Hypernatremic dehydration has also been associated with transient myoclonus and chorea in chronic alcoholism.

Autoimmune and Inflammatory Disorders

Myoclonus occurs in about 40 percent of patients with *Hashimoto encephalopathy* (also called encephalopathy associated with autoimmune thyroid disease).[83] Any combination of cognitive impairment, encephalopathy, psychosis, transient neurologic deficits, myoclonus or tremor, seizures, somnolence, or coma develops and fluctuates over weeks to months. The myoclonus may be generalized or multifocal and spontaneous or reflex-evoked, and is without EEG correlates. Patients are clinically euthyroid, with elevated antithyroid antibodies, the levels of which correlate poorly with the clinical state.[83] Further clinical and laboratory details are provided in Chapter 18.

Myoclonus has been described in the *antiphospholipid syndrome*.[50] Nonvasculitic *autoimmune inflammatory meningoencephalitis* may present with the rapid onset of dementia, parkinsonism, and myoclonus. In a single case, the EEG pattern consisted of persistent periodic sharp waves suggestive of Creutzfeldt–Jakob disease; dramatic clinical improvement occurred with corticosteroids.[84]

A myoclonic syndrome often accompanied by ataxia may occur in *celiac disease*, despite normal vitamin B_{12} and E levels.[85] Typically, patients have a gastrointestinal syndrome that may include chronic diarrhea and abdominal pain, although gastrointestinal complaints may be subtle (only nausea and vomiting episodes during infection in one report).[86] Action or reflex myoclonus may occur in patients with established celiac disease, but whether this relates to inadequate dietary restriction or poor compliance is uncertain. The myoclonus initially may be focal but usually becomes multifocal; generalized convulsions may develop. The jerks are usually preceded by a time-locked polyspike EEG discharge, supporting a cortical origin. In some cases improvement occurs after a gluten-free diet is instituted. Anticonvulsant or benzodiazepine therapy is commonly required but is incompletely effective. Opsoclonus-myoclonus has also been described in a child with celiac disease and responded to a gluten-free diet.[87]

Drug- and Toxin-Induced Myoclonus

Neuroleptic malignant syndrome may complicate neuroleptic treatment but also occurs with dopamine-depleting agents and on withdrawal of dopaminergic treatments. It is primarily due to functional dopamine deficiency, which leads to disinhibition of cortical and subcortical excitatory pathways; norepinephrine and serotonin may also be involved. Its incidence is 0.2 percent of patients exposed to neuroleptic agents.[88] The disorder occurs within a month of starting the neuroleptic agent. Fever, rigidity, and an elevated serum creatine kinase (CK) (the major criteria) and tachycardia, labile blood pressure, tachypnea, diaphoresis (autonomic instability), altered mental status, and leukocytosis (the minor criteria) develop over 24 to 72 hours.[88] Altered mental status and rigidity are often the first signs and are each present in over 95 percent of instances. The presence of all three major or two major and four minor criteria is highly predictive of the syndrome. The movement disorder is primarily an axial rigidity with tremor, choreoathetosis, dystonia, or myoclonus in the limbs. Rhabdomyolysis, renal insufficiency, respiratory failure, adult respiratory distress syndrome, disseminated intravascular coagulation, myocardial infarction, pulmonary embolism, and coma may complicate the picture.

Treatment involves discontinuing the offending drug (or reinstituting dopaminergic medication) and supportive therapy (including cooling if warranted); it may require administering the muscle excitation–contraction uncoupler dantrolene sodium at 2 to 8 mg/kg four times daily (maximum 10 mg/kg per dose) and the dopamine agonist bromocriptine at 5 mg four times daily (up to 50 mg/day) or other dopamine agonists, or carbidopa-levodopa. Dopaminergic treatment should continue for 7 to 10 days, which is the usual duration of the disorder. Rhabdomyolysis and renal failure are the greatest predictors of poor outcome. Survivors almost always achieve complete recovery.

The *serotonin syndrome* is a potential complication of treatment with antidepressants and related medications that increase cerebral serotonin neurotransmission. It is characterized by mental status changes, autonomic hyperactivity and neuromuscular abnormalities.[88] The prerequisite is a recent increase in the dosage of a serotonergic agent or the addition of a new one. Cognitive and behavioral changes include confusion, hypomania, and agitation, and myoclonus, ataxia, hyperreflexia, or tremor may also be present. Autonomic disturbances include nausea, vomiting, diarrhea, labile blood pressure, fever, shivering, and diaphoresis. Seizures may occur. The symptoms may begin as early as 2 hours after the medication is taken and usually resolve within 24 hours on discontinuation of the offending agent. When severe, serotonin syndrome may be indistinguishable from neuroleptic malignant syndrome and has a similar risk of multiple organ failure and death. Treatment requires discontinuation of precipitating drugs, supportive care, treatment for hyperthermia using benzodiazepines or neuromuscular paralysis, and administration of a 5-HT_{2A} antagonist such as cyproheptadine (4 to 8 mg, followed by 4 mg six times daily to a total of 0.5 mg/kg daily) or chlorpromazine (50 to 100 mg intramuscularly).[88]

Of the non-neuroleptic psychiatric medications capable of causing myoclonus, *lithium* toxicity is well described. A variety of presentations occur including action, spontaneous, or stimulus-sensitive myoclonus, sometimes with opsoclonus. The myoclonus is of cortical origin but is not associated with epileptiform abnormalities.[89] Vomiting and a decreased level of consciousness may also be present; in rare instances the presence of cognitive changes and characteristic EEG findings suggests the erroneous diagnosis of Creutzfeldt–Jakob disease. Full recovery is usual. Overdose with *tricyclic antidepressants* may result in myoclonus because of their ability to inhibit reuptake of serotonin and norepinephrine.[90] Myoclonus may occur with *levodopa* treatment.[91] Reducing the levodopa dosage may diminish the myoclonus.

Tardive myoclonus due to neuroleptic medications is the least common of the tardive syndromes. It usually affects the face, neck, or upper limbs and responds to withdrawal of the neuroleptic treatment, but the movements may take several months to resolve. Benzodiazepines are sometimes useful.[31]

A number of other medications and toxins have occasionally been associated with myoclonus and are summarized in Table 58-3. A recent pharmocovigilance study in 423 patients found drug-induced myoclonus was associated with anti-infectious agents (15%), antidepressants (15%), anxiolytics (14%), opiate agents (12%), antiparkinsonian medications (7%), and neurolepics (12%).[92]

Among illicit drugs, *cocaine* most commonly causes movement disorders. Myoclonus can be seen in the setting of a cocaine-induced disorder resembling neuroleptic malignant syndrome[34] or as multifocal rest and action myoclonus together with opsoclonus and ataxia.

Myoclonus may develop in *gasoline sniffers* as a result of lead toxicity; it may be segmental or generalized and occurs spontaneously, with movement, or in response to an external stimulus.[93] The condition may respond to chelation treatment with dimercaprol and calcium disodium edetate, although repeated exposures may result in a permanent encephalopathy. High serum levels of *bismuth*, used for treatment of certain gastrointestinal symptoms, may result in confusion followed by severe myoclonus, truncal ataxia, dysarthria, tremor, and sometimes generalized convulsions and coma.[94] The syndrome can evolve slowly over months or acutely over days and has sometimes been confused with Creutzfeldt–Jakob disease or rapid-onset Alzheimer disease. The myoclonus may be multifocal or a massive generalized movement, and may occur spontaneously, on action, and in response to stimuli. Recovery over 3 to 12 weeks is the rule when the bismuth intake is discontinued early; chelation with dimercaprol may enhance renal clearance but has been associated with clinical deterioration in one patient.[94] Diazepam, clonazepam, or valproic acid may reduce myoclonus.

Paraneoplastic Disorders

Multifocal myoclonus with opsoclonus is most commonly seen as a paraneoplastic syndrome. In children, 50 percent have an underlying neuroblastoma, whereas in adults it is more frequently associated with breast, ovarian, or small-cell lung cancers.[95] The most common antibody associated with paraneoplastic myoclonus is anti-Ri (antineuronal nuclear autoantibody type 2 or ANNA-2) but myoclonus has also been associated with anti-Ma2, anti-Hu and antiamphiphysin antibodies. PET with CT may be useful if initial radiologic screening is negative and early detection and treatment of the tumor appears to be useful.[96] Occasionally the myoclonus improves with treatment of the underlying malignancy or prednisone, rarely with plasmapheresis, intravenous immunoglobulin, cyclophosphamide, or immunoadsorption therapy with a protein A column. Myoclonus may respond to antiepileptic drugs.[97]

Action and postural myoclonus has been reported in the setting of carcinomatous meningitis.[98] It has also been described with rare tumors; in one child with a cerebellar ganglioglioma. The myoclonus resolved with successful removal of the tumor.[99]

Infections

Viral encephalopathies are the most common infectious cause of myoclonus (Table 58-2). In subacute sclerosing panencephalitis, myoclonus is time-locked to generalized bursts of high-voltage slow waves (periodic complexes) occurring approximately

TABLE 58-3 ■ Drugs and Toxins Inducing Myoclonus

Anesthetics
Etomidate, enflurane, chloralose, methohexital, propofol, thiopental, spinal anesthesia
Anticonvulsants
Carbamazepine, gabapentin, phenytoin, lamotrigine, primidone, topiramate, valproic acid, vigabatrin
Antihistamines
Promethazine, omeprazole, oxatomide
Anti-infectious Agents
Carbenicillin, cephalosporins, ciprofloxacin, cefmetazole, gatifloxacin, imipenem, isoniazid, pefloxacin, piperazine, penicillin, (quinolones), ticarcillin, trimethoprim-sulfamethoxazole
Cardiac Medications
Diltiazem, flecainide, propafenone
Chemotherapeutic Agents
Busulfan, chlorambucil, ifosfamide, prednimustine
Dopaminergic Agents
Levodopa, bromocriptine, pergolide
Miscellaneous Medications
Amantadine, carisoprodol, cimetidine, metoclopramide, opiates, physostigmine, L-tryptophan
Narcotics
Diamorphine, fentanyl, hydrocodone, hydromorphone, methadone, meperidine, morphine, tramadol
Nonsteroidal Anti-inflammatory Drugs
Diclofenac
Psychiatric Medications
Antipsychotic medications, tricyclic antidepressants, lithium, monoamine oxidase inhibitors, selective serotonin reuptake inhibitors, clozapine, buspirone, lorazepam, methaqualone, midazolam, mirtazapine, sedative-hypnotics
Solvents and Gases
Acetone, carbon disulfide, ethyl benzene, methanol, ethylene oxide, formaldehyde, hydrogen sulfide, nitrous oxide, methyl chloride, methyl ethyl ketone, toluene
Heavy Metals
Aluminum, arsenic, bismuth salts, lead, manganese, organic mercury, thallium
Illicit Drugs
Cocaine, marijuana, methaqualone (Quaalude), methylenedioxymethamphetamine (MDMA)
Miscellaneous Agents and Toxins
Carbon monoxide poisoning, dichloroethane (used in dry cleaning), intrathecal water-soluble contrast media, tetraethyl lead
Pesticides
Aldrin, chlordane, chlordecone, cyclodienes, DDT, lindane, methyl bromide, organophosphate compounds, pyrethroids
Withdrawal Syndromes
Benzodiazepines, carbamazepine, dopaminergics

every 5 to 15 seconds on EEG. The myoclonus is relatively resistant to treatment, but sodium valproate, phenobarbital, carbamazepine, clonazepam, or levetiracetam may be tried. Herpes simplex virus encephalitis and postviral acute demyelinating encephalomyelopathy may also cause myoclonus. Segmental spinal myoclonus has occurred as a late complication of herpes myelitis.[100]

Myoclonus occurs rarely with HIV infection. In a study of 2,460 inpatients with HIV infection, only

4 had myoclonus (2 with spinal myoclonus and 2 with generalized myoclonus).[101] Evaluation suggested four different causes: toxoplasmosis, HIV encephalopathy, tuberculous radiculomyelopathy, and herpes zoster. The myoclonus tends to be most prominent in the face, trunk, and proximal limbs and may be spontaneous or stimulated. Rarely, the myoclonus occurs with seroconversion, but usually the affected patients are significantly ill, often taking multiple medications. Treatment depends on the underlying cause; in some cases, myoclonus has resolved with antimicrobial treatment for opportunistic infections, retroviral therapy, or additional symptomatic medications. Other rare viral causes of myoclonus include mumps,[102] chickenpox,[103] parainfluenza virus type 3, coxsackievirus B3, poliovirus, St. Louis encephalitis, JC virus causing progressive multifocal leukoencephalitis, and encephalitis lethargica. Opsoclonus-myoclonus may also be the presenting symptom of West Nile virus infection.[104]

Bacterial infections associated with myoclonus are less common than viral infections. Spinal myoclonus and opsoclonus-myoclonus have been reported in Lyme neuroborreliosis[105] and in typhoid (enteric fever).[106] Opsoclonus-myoclonus has also been described as a sequela of group A β-hemolytic streptococcal infection, and responds to corticosteroid treatment.[107] Multifocal myoclonus may be a rare feature of tuberculous meningitis or cerebral tuberculomas.[108,109] Approximately 25 percent of patients with Whipple disease (discussed in Chapter 13) due to the gram-positive bacillus *Tropheryma whipplei* have myoclonus, although oculofacial and occulomasticatory myorrhythmias are the most characteristic movement disorders described.[110,111]

Multifocal myoclonus may occur in the postmalaria neurologic syndrome, which also includes encephalopathy, tremor, and ataxia, beginning days to weeks after treatment of malaria. It responds rapidly to corticosteroids.[112] Multifocal and oculopalatal myoclonus have also been reported in neurocysticercosis.[113]

Injury by Physical Agents

Spinal myoclonus may develop as a late complication of spine irradiation for cancer.[114] The high-pressure neurologic syndrome, which occurs on diving beyond a depth of 100 meters, consists of cognitive impairment and hyperkinesis.[115] Myoclonus occurs at a depth of 300 to 500 meters or 50 to 60 atmospheres. Segmental myoclonus has been reported in the setting of electrical injury.[116] Finally, myoclonus may occur as a long-term consequence of severe head injury.[67]

Approach to Diagnosis

As mentioned earlier, the clinical approach to evaluation of myoclonus requires a detailed history and full neurologic and general medical examination. If the myoclonus is considered pathologic and no offending drug or toxin is appreciated, screening blood studies may include a complete blood count and erythrocyte sedimentation rate; determination of electrolyte and glucose levels; thyroid, renal and hepatic function tests; and drug and toxin testing. An EEG to exclude an epileptic basis and brain and spine MRI to exclude structural causes are important. Paraneoplastic antibody testing may also be helpful.

Treatment

When possible, myoclonus should be treated by addressing the underlying medical disorder. Immunotherapy may help when postinfectious or paraneoplastic causes are responsible.[117] The location of the generator of the myoclonus can guide treatment. Cortical myoclonus responds best to anticonvulsants, particularly sodium valproate (0.6 to 3 g daily), clonazepam (0.5 to 12 mg daily), levetiracetam (1,000 to 3,000 mg daily), primidone (50 to 1,000 mg daily), and piracetam (2 to 20 g daily).[74] Reticular reflex myoclonus and spinal myoclonus may respond to clonazepam. Other medications that have been anecdotally useful include anticholinergic agents, baclofen, tetrabenazine, acetazolamide, and opiates; γ-aminobutyric acid receptor agonists may also be effective. Combinations of two or three medications may be more effective than monotherapy.[74]

TREMOR

Tremor is the most common of all involuntary movements and is defined as an involuntary, rhythmic oscillation of a body part. It can be physiologic (normal) or pathologic, and is characterized by its frequency, amplitude, and distribution, and the position in which it occurs. Tremor is most easily classified as rest or action tremor.

Some forms of tremor are generated primarily by a central oscillator, as in essential tremor, and others, such as physiologic tremor, are mainly mechanical in origin. Central tremor is generated in the cerebellothalamocortical and dentatorubro-olivary pathways, with a poorly understood contribution from basal ganglia circuits. Rest tremor is characteristic of *parkinsonism*, which itself may occur secondary to a variety of causes. Such rest tremor is often accompanied by rigidity, bradykinesia, or postural instability, but may occur in isolation. Mechanical tremors decrease in amplitude and frequency with a load, whereas centrally generated tremors decrease only in amplitude.

Stroke

Tremor may occur as a consequence of stroke. The most common lesions involve the thalamus, mesencephalon, rubro-olivary tract, and cerebellar tracts. Limb tremor may occur with lesions of the cerebral cortex.[5]

Medications

Medications can cause the full spectrum of tremor subtypes (rest, postural, or kinetic), although postural tremor is most common (Table 58-4).[118] Intention tremor refers to the subtype of kinetic tremor that becomes more prominent as the limb approaches the target. Commonly used medications such as adrenergic agonists, including all β-agonists, lithium, caffeine, corticosteroids, tricyclic antidepressants, cyclosporine, and thyroid excess usually cause postural tremor. Dopaminergic and anticonvulsant medications also cause an enhanced

TABLE 58-4 ■ Drugs and Toxins Causing Tremor

Drug or Toxin	Kinetic or Postural Tremor	Intention Tremor	Rest Tremor
Anticonvulsants	Carbamazepine, felbamate, lamotrigine, phenytoin, tiagabine, topiramate, valproate, vigabatrin	–	Valproate
Antidepressants and mood stabilizers	Amitriptyline, lithium, MAOIs, SSRIs, valproate	Lithium	Lithium, SSRIs, valproate
Anti-infectious agents	Trimethoprim-sulfamethoxazole	Vidarabine	Trimethoprim-sulfamethoxazole, amphotericin
β-Adrenergic agonists	Salbutamol, salmeterol	Salbutamol, salmeterol	
Cardiac medications	Amiodarone, mexiletine, procainamide		
Chemotherapy	Cytarabine, ifosfamide, tacromilus, vincristine	Cytarabine, ifosfamide	Thalidomide
Dopamine-blocking and -depleting agents	Cinnarizine, haloperidol, metoclopramide, thioridazine, reserpine, tetrabenazine	–	Cinnarizine, metoclopramide, neuroleptics (e.g., haloperidol, thioridazine), reserpine, tetrabenazine
Recreational agents	Cocaine, ethanol, MDMA, nicotine	–	Cocaine, ethanol, MDMA, MPTP
Hormone treatments	Calcitonin, sex steroids, thyroxine, (medroxy)progesterone, tamoxifen	Epinephrine	(Medroxy)progesterone
Immunosuppressants	Cyclosporine, tacrolimus, interferon-α	Cyclosporine, tacrolimus	Cyclosporine
Metals	Arsenic, cyanide, lead, mercury	–	Lead, manganese, mercury
Miscellaneous agents	Metoclopramide, cimetidine, theophylline, caffeine	–	Metoclopramide
Toxins	–	–	Methanol
Withdrawal syndromes	Cannabis, ethanol	–	–

MAOI, monoamine oxidase inhibitor; MDMA, methylenedioxymethamphetamine; MPTP, 1-methyl-4-phenyl-1,2,3,6-tetrahydropryidine; SSRI, selective serotonin reuptake inhibitor.

physiologic tremor. Lithium- or valproic acid–induced tremor is present at rest and enhanced with posture or action. The antiarrhythmic amiodarone may cause a postural and terminal movement tremor in 20 to 30 percent of patients. Central cholinergic agonists such as nicotine, anticholinesterases, and aminopropanols are also tremorgenic.

Central monoaminergic stimulation by neuroleptics, phenylethylamines, and indoles may result in a parkinsonian rest tremor and a postural tremor. Specifically, tremor is seen in neuroleptic malignant syndrome and serotonin syndrome (see p. 1191). Dopamine receptor–blocking drugs and dopamine-depleting agents such as tetrabenazine and reserpine may also trigger a rest tremor.

Toxins and Recreational Agents

A variety of toxins cause tremor directly or as part of a withdrawal syndrome (Table 58-4). Tremor may occur with acute cocaine intoxication, and persists in abstinent cocaine-, alcohol-, and opiate-dependent subjects for months after the last use; rest tremor is reportedly more common in those with prior cocaine use.[34] Alcohol and other drug withdrawal states enhance, sometimes asymmetrically, postural physiologic tremor, which decreases with time but can be treated with propranolol or benzodiazepines. The intention tremor of chronic alcohol abuse, however, is the result of cerebellar injury by alcohol. With cannabis use, withdrawal symptoms may occur after as little as 7 days of use and include tremor, irritability, restlessness, anorexia, fever, and other sympathetic effects.[34]

Intoxication with heavy metals and organic compounds may produce a rest or action tremor, and improvement after withdrawal of the toxin depends on the severity and duration of exposure.

Metabolic Disorders

Almost any metabolic derangement may be associated with tremor. Thyrotoxicosis is the most common, producing an enhanced physiologic tremor. It affects any age group and responds to treatment of the underlying disorder, but it can also be ameliorated by propranolol. Tremor is one of the first and most prevalent signs of hypoglycemia and may be seen in nonketotic hyperglycemia along with myoclonus, chorea, and dystonia. In renal insufficiency, a postural and action tremor is often evident before asterixis develops, and may foreshadow encephalopathy. The tremor in Wilson disease may be postural, kinetic, or at rest. A coarser movement of the upper limb ("wing beating" tremor) also occurs.[21] It is present in the proximal arms and occasionally the head in the flexion-extension plane, and is due to thalamocapsular and cerebellar system pathologic processes. Chelation therapy and liver transplantation can reverse the neuropathologic process, but there is no effective symptomatic treatment.[21] Hemochromatosis is associated with tremor, parkinsonism, and dementia due to iron deposits in the basal ganglia; progression may be forestalled by phlebotomy or liver transplantation.[119] Variegate porphyria and the hyperadrenergic state associated with pheochromocytoma may also cause tremor, as can striatal injury in the setting of hypoxic-ischemic encephalopathy.[6]

Hypomagnesemia and hypocalcemia may lead to tremor, muscle twitching, and irritability, and a severe, movement-associated, distal flapping tremor may occur in hypercalcemia due to hyperparathyroidism. Tremor has been reported with hyponatremia and its correction.[120] Severe vitamin E deficiency may cause tremor in addition to spinocerebellar findings and peripheral neuropathy, and tremors may respond to vitamin E supplementation.[121] In infants, vitamin B_{12} deficiency can produce a generalized tremor syndrome and mental retardation, which are partially reversible with supplementation, although the abnormal movements may transiently increase with treatment before resolving.[80]

Infections

Viral encephalitides are probably the most common infections to cause tremor (Table 58-2). Generalized tremors have also been described with poliovirus infection, St. Louis encephalitis, and the rhombencephalitis that sometimes complicates hand-foot-and-mouth disease (due to enterovirus 71). Respiratory syncytial virus encephalitis[122] and mumps,[102] with a predilection for the cerebellum, manifest as intention tremor and ataxia. Echovirus 21 encephalitis[123] and Japanese encephalitis[124] result in tremor through basal ganglia and cerebellar involvement. Herpes zoster–related vasculitis affecting the midbrain may result in an ipsilateral cerebellar syndrome with intention tremor.[125] Congenital cytomegalovirus infection and rubella[126] and adult tick-borne meningoencephalitis[127] result in long-lasting neurologic dysfunction, including tremor. The encephalopathy sometimes present with Lassa fever may be accompanied by tremor, seizures, and coma.[128] Meningoencephalitic involvement with flaviviruses may cause tremor in addition to the typical dengue hemorrhagic fever.[129] A similar picture is seen in Bolivian hemorrhagic fever caused by Machupo virus (family Arenaviridae), which responds to ribavirin.[130]

Tremor disorders occur rarely in early HIV infection but occur in 5 to 44 percent of those with HIV-associated dementia. Tremor may be part of a parkinsonian syndrome or may occur in isolation. Typically, there is a symmetric postural tremor but there may be a rest component; kinetic components are rare. Holmes (rubral) tremor, in which rest, postural, and kinetic components are present, has been reported in AIDS and often results from opportunistic infections such as tuberculosis or toxoplasmosis. In addition to drug-induced tremor from dopamine-blocking drugs such as neuroleptics and antiemetics, AIDS patients may develop a reversible rest or postural tremor from trimethoprim-sulfamethoxazole.[131] Treatment of tremor in HIV infection depends on etiology; drug-induced tremor and tremor secondary to opportunistic infection may be reversible.[27]

Tremor occurs in up to 17 percent of those with tuberculous meningitis[108] and 30 percent of those with tuburculomas[109] and is usually of the postural variety. It may respond to antituberculous therapy over several weeks; if not, symptomatic treatment may be considered.

Recovery from *Plasmodium falciparum* malaria is occasionally followed by a corticosteroid-responsive encephalopathy with postural tremor, cerebellar ataxia, myoclonus, seizures, and motor aphasia.[132] In neurocysticercosis, tremor and parkinsonism are the most frequent movement disorders.[38] Tremor is also seen in typhoid, together with altered bowel habits.[133] Unilateral postural, kinetic, and Holmes tremor have been reported with thalamic toxoplasmosis in HIV-positive patients.[134]

Immune Disorders

CNS lupus may include tremor among its many features. Waldenström macroglobulinemia has been associated with an asymmetric tremor and peripheral neuropathy.[135] Basal ganglia and brainstem involvement in Behçet syndrome may result in postural tremor, and pyramidal and extrapyramidal findings.[52] Tremor may occur as a complication of celiac disease.[56]

In Hashimoto encephalopathy, in which myoclonus and seizures are common, 80 percent of patients have postural tremor.[136] In patients older than 50 years with cerebellar degeneration, the etiology is paraneoplastic in about half. Intention tremor, ataxia, and dysarthria are particularly associated with anti-Yo antibodies in gynecologic cancers and anti-Hu antibodies in small-cell lung cancers.[137]

Some immune-mediated polyneuropathies, particularly those associated with IgM monoclonal gammopathy, are accompanied by a distally predominant action and postural tremor. In a recent case-control study, 29 percent of subjects with IgM monoclonal gammopathy of undetermined significance had tremor compared to 9 percent of controls; among the 60 with tremor, 49 had postural and kinetic tremor, 8 had rest tremor, and 3 had mixed rest and action tremor.[138] The tremor sometimes responds to immunosuppressive therapy or propranolol. A postural and kinetic tremor may follow Guillain–Barré syndrome and occur in chronic inflammatory demyelinating polyneuropathy.[139]

Other Causes of Tremor

Cerebral radiation and gamma-knife treatments rarely cause postural or Holmes tremor.[140] A postural and intention tremor may develop during compression during dives to depths greater than 100 meters as part of the high-pressure neurologic syndrome.[115] It usually remits on decompression but occasionally persists for several months.

Approach to Diagnosis

Rapid onset (over days to months) of tremor is atypical for essential tremor but may occur when drug induced or related to an underlying medical disorder. If no offending drug or toxin is recognized, screening blood studies should include determination of electrolyte and glucose concentrations as well as thyroid, renal, and hepatic function tests. Testing for serum cortisol, parathyroid hormone, and ceruloplasmin; 24-hour urinary copper excretion; and toxicology assays may also be necessary in individual instances. Brain MRI may be required to exclude structural causes, particularly when there are other neurologic findings or the tremor is asymmetric.

Treatment

In all cases of tremor, an underlying disorder should be sought and treated while symptomatic treatment is contemplated. Action tremor, and particularly aggravated physiologic tremor, usually responds to adrenergic blockade or primidone. Other agents, including alprazolam, atenolol, gabapentin, sotolol, and topiramate, are also useful. Other treatments showing some benefit include nadolol, nimodipine, clonazepam, botulinum toxin A, deep brain stimulation, thalamotomy and gamma-knife thalamotomy.[141] Pregabalin is sometimes helpful.[139] Rest tremor is treated by anticholinergic agents, amantadine, and dopaminergic medications; deep brain stimulation of the globus pallidus or subthalamic nucleus may be used in patients with severe tremor that is refractory to medications.[142]

Cerebellar tremor is the most difficult to treat and only occasionally improves with the treatments described above.[143] Holmes (rubral) tremor is poorly responsive to treatment but sometimes improves with levodopa, dopamine agonists, trihexyphenidyl, or some of the medications used for essential tremor; in other instances, deep brain stimulation may be necessary.[143]

PARKINSONISM

Parkinson disease is the most common cause of parkinsonism, but there are a number of other causes that relate to systemic disease and therefore merit discussion here.

Vascular Causes

An akinetic-rigid syndrome may occur acutely or may develop in a delayed manner, months to years after focal, multifocal, or global ischemic events and is called vascular parkinsonism. Unlike classic Parkinson disease, it usually occurs later in life (in the seventh or eighth decade) and symptoms develop more rapidly. It is usually symmetric, with limb rigidity or spasticity, and postural instability.[144] Rest tremor is uncommon but postural tremor may occur. Brain imaging shows bilateral lesions sometimes involving the basal ganglia. Treatment with levodopa should be attempted but is often disappointing. Other vascular events such as a midbrain hemorrhage, subdural hematoma, cortical venous thrombosis, and giant cerebral artery aneurysm may cause parkinsonism.

Medications and Bone Marrow Transplantation

Drug-induced parkinsonism is common; one population-based study found that parkinsonism was likely drug-induced in 20 percent of cases.[145] Drug-induced parkinsonism differs from Parkinson disease in that symptom onset may be rapid, often over weeks, bradykinesia is more symmetric, and tremor and postural instability are less common.[146] However, individual cases may be clinically indistinguishable from Parkinson disease. Drug-induced parkinsonism occurs most often in patients treated with D2 dopamine receptor blockers (e.g., antipsychotics and metoclopramide), monoamine depleters (reserpine or tetrabenazine), and certain calcium-channel blockers (especially cinnarizine and flunarizine). A French pharmacovigilance center reported 155 cases of drug-induced or -worsened parkinsonism between 1993 and 2009. About 70 percent of the cases were observed in the first 3 months after introduction of the suspect drug, whereas 30 percent occurred after 1 year. Rigidity was the most common symptom. Antipsychotic treatment (including haloperidol, risperidone, and olanzapine) was cited in 113 cases, diazepines in 15, selective serotonin reuptake inhibitors in 12, calcium-channel blockers (flunarizine, cinnarizine, verapamil and diltiazem) in 13, H1 antihistamines in 12, valproate in 10, metoclopramide in 9, and lithium in 4. Improvement occurred after stopping the medication in 89 percent of cases (Table 58-4). Abrupt discontinuation of dopamine-blocking medications should be avoided. In our experience, reversal of symptoms may take months or even up to a year.

Acute or subacute parkinsonism has developed from disulfiram treatment or overdose. Encephalopathy, hyperglycemia, ketosis, bradykinesia, and rest tremor may develop and may improve after disulfiram is discontinued and with supportive therapy. CT may show hypodensity and MRI shows increased T2 signal in the putamen and globus pallidus.[147]

After bone marrow or organ transplantation, parkinsonism developed in several patients after starting cyclosporine and resolved after discontinuing it.[148]

Toxins

Since the recognition that 1-methyl-4-phenyl-1,2,3,6-tetrahydropryidine (MPTP) caused rapid-onset parkinsonism, a great deal of research has shown that factors adversely affecting energy metabolism and disposal of damaged proteins in dopaminergic neurons may cause parkinsonism. In most epidemiologic studies, prolonged exposure to pesticides (particularly insecticides and herbicides) is a risk factor for Parkinson disease.[149]

Other toxins that have been associated with parkinsonism include polychlorinated biphenyls (PCBs), carbon monoxide, cyanide,[12,150] some metals (mercury and manganese), and some organic solvents (carbon disulfide, trichloroethylene, and methanol).[151] A disorder similar to manganism may follow intravenous methcathinone use for recreational purposes (discussed on p. 1182).[19] Carbon monoxide toxicity results from a combination of tissue hypoxia and direct cellular toxicity especially affecting the basal ganglia.[152] After initial recovery, about 10 percent of survivors will develop parkinsonism (hypomimia, rigidity, bradykinesia but without rest tremor) several weeks to months later that does not respond to antiparkinsonian medications. Approximately 80 percent of those who develop parkinsonism will recover within 6 months.[10]

Methanol poisoning may cause an acute parkinsonian state but has also been associated with the development of parkinsonism with chronic exposure. Acute intoxication may cause coma. Upon recovery, visual impairment, hypophonia, rigidity, and bradykinesia develop and may respond to dopaminergic agents. Brain imaging shows hypointensity of the putamen on CT scan and hyperintense lesions of the putamen on T2-weighted MRI.[153] Occupational exposure to manganese, such as in welding, is not associated with the development of Parkinson disease,[154] but manganese exposure alone or in combination with liver failure may cause parkinsonism. Brain MRI often shows increased signal in the globus pallidus on T1-weighted images.[155] In some cases there is improvement after chelation therapy.[18] This form of parkinsonism is poorly responsive to dopaminergic treatment.[156]

Metabolic Disorders

Several metabolic conditions may mimic Parkinson disease including hypothyroidism, extrapontine myelinolysis, chronic liver failure, hemochromatosis,[119] and Wilson disease. In Wilson disease rigidity, bradykinesia, hypophonic speech, and tremor as well as autonomic disturbances may occur.[21] Parkinsonism has been described in liver failure from other causes. In a prospective study, 21 percent of patients with liver failure being considered for liver transplantation had parkinsonism.[157] Clinical features included rapid progression over months, symmetric akinetic-rigid syndrome, postural but not rest tremor, and early gait impairment. Serum and CSF manganese levels were elevated, and MRI showed hyperintensities involving the globus pallidus and substantia nigra resembling that seen in patients with manganese exposure (Fig. 58-1). Some of these patients responded to levodopa.[157]

Although Goswami and colleagues found that idiopathic hypoparathyroidism was associated with basal ganglia calcifications in 107 of 145 patients, parkinsonism occurred in only 2.[62] Treatment with calcium, parathyroid hormone, and levodopa may be helpful, but treatment with vitamin D is also sometimes required.[158] In rare instances, parkinsonism has developed in patients with hyperparathyroidism and resolved after surgery.

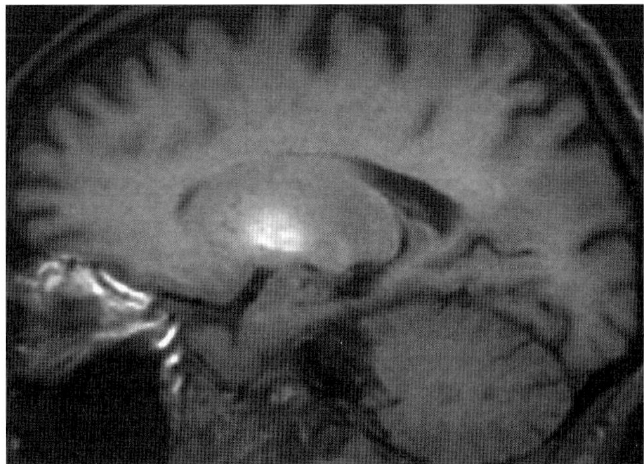

FIGURE 58-1 ■ Sagittal T1-weighted magnetic resonance image (MRI) showing increased signal in the globus pallidus in a 39-year-old man with advanced liver disease due to hepatitis with a 1-year history of a gait disturbance and intermittent tremulousness. Examination showed subtle tremulousness and slowing of rapid repetitive movements in all limbs. Laboratory evaluation revealed elevated serum manganese.

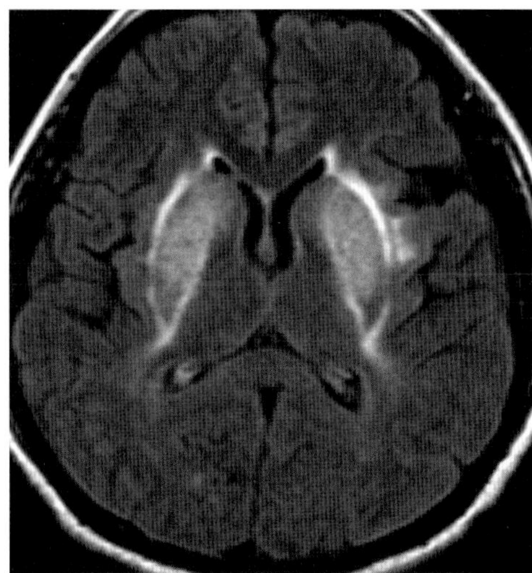

FIGURE 58-2 ▪ This axial fluid-attenuated inversion recovery (FLAIR)–weighted MRI was obtained from a 41-year-old woman with a long history of diabetes and dialysis-dependent renal failure with rapid-onset encephalopathy, dysarthria, tremor, rigidity, and bradykinesia. It shows increased signal in the putamen and globus pallidus bilaterally. Her condition improved with dialysis.

Acute parkinsonism has been described in patients with diabetes and uremia requiring dialysis. Cognitive impairment, dysarthria, bradykinesia, and rigidity develop over days to weeks. There is typically an elevated serum creatinine, uremia, and a metabolic acidosis. Brain CT shows hypodense lenticular nuclei, and MRI shows T1 hypointense and T2 hyperintense lesions in the putamen and globus pallidus[159] (Fig. 58-2). The condition and imaging abnormalities may resolve with hemodialysis. Developmentof this syndrome has been related to the occurrence of preceding hypoglycemia.[160]

Infections

Various infections may cause parkinsonism acutely or as a long-term complication (Table 58-2). Viral infections that have been associated with this phenotype include herpes simplex, HIV, Japanese encephalitis, coxsackie B, influenza A, measles (and related subacute sclerosing panencephalitis), mumps, polio, Western equine encephalitis, and St. Louis encephalitis.[161] Japanese encephalitis, prevalent in most Southeast Asian countries, is estimated to be the most common viral cause of parkinsonism. Parkinsonism or other movement disorders develop 1 to 4 weeks after the acute phase and may persist for months to years.

HIV infection may cause parkinsonism by direct injury to the basal ganglia or as a consequence of immunodeficiency. AIDS-associated parkinsonism is characterized by symmetric bradykinesia, rigidity, postural instability and gait impairment; tremor is often absent.[27] Mirsattari and colleagues found a 5 percent incidence of parkinsonism in a cohort of 115 HIV-infected patients, all of whom had severe immunosuppression with a mean CD4 count of 14 cells/mm^3.[162] Postural and gait instability may occur early. The parkinsonism may be secondary to opportunistic infection, drug induced, or related more directly to the HIV infection. There is evidence of early involvement of the basal ganglia in HIV infection: anatomic neuroimaging reveals selective basal ganglia atrophy, and functional imaging shows relative hypermetabolism in the basal ganglia and thalamus. Neuropathologic examination frequently shows evidence of HIV infection with microglial nodule encephalitis affecting the putamen and caudate nuclei. Both lymphoma and opportunistic infections with *Toxoplasma* and *Cryptococcus* show an affinity for the basal ganglia.[27]

Progressive multifocal leukoencephalopathy caused by JC virus in immunosuppressed individuals may also cause parkinsonism.[162] Perhaps because of the early involvement of the basal ganglia, HIV-infected patients develop drug-induced parkinsonism at lower doses of antipsychotic treatments.[27] One patient has been described who developed parkinsonism while being treated with a protease inhibitor (ritonavir) and buspirone.[163]

When evaluating patients with HIV-related parkinsonism, opportunistic infection and drug-induced causes require exclusion. Treatment with dopaminergic medications may help. In some AIDS patients, parkinsonism has improved after initiation of combination antiretroviral therapy.[164] Another patient, whose initial presentation was parkinsonism with supranuclear gaze paresis and postural instability and who did not have an AIDS-defining diagnosis but had a CD4 count of 266, improved on treatment with combined antiretroviral therapy after obtaining no benefit with levodopa.[165]

Since the epidemic of 1916 to 1927, only sporadic cases of parkinsonism following encephalitis lethargica have been described.[166] CSF shows a lymphocytic pleocytosis and oligoclonal bands, but bacterial and viral studies are unrevealing. Brain imaging may show inflammatory changes in the basal ganglia or brainstem. Dale and colleagues found elevated basal ganglia antibodies in 20 patients who developed parkinsonism, a sleep disorder, dyskinesia, and neuropsychiatric symptoms that were attributed to encephalitis lethargica. In 65 percent, antistreptolysin-O titers were elevated and 95 percent had basal ganglia antibodies, raising the possibility that encephalitis lethargica is an autoimmune condition possibly triggered by bacterial infection such as in Sydenham chorea.[166] In a subsequent study in children with clinical features of encephalitis lethargica, NMDA receptor antibodies were found in those with dyskinesias, agitation, and seizures but not in those with parkinsonism and somnolence.[167] In another case series with similar observations, abnormal basal ganglia glucose metabolism was found in 7 of 8 patients.[168] There are anecdotal reports of improvement with methylprednisolone with or without intravenous immunoglobulin.[166,168]

Tuberculous meningitis is a rare cause of parkinsonism.[108] Infection with *Mycoplasma pneumoniae* is another rare cause of parkinsonism. The condition begins with a flu-like illness, and bradykinesia follows; T2-weighted MRI shows increased signal of the basal ganglia, which resolves several months after treatment of the infection.[169] Reversible parkinsonism has been reported in Lyme disease. Other infections associated with parkinsonism, generally in association with other neurologic abnormalities, include prion disease and neurosyphilis.[170]

Malaria and neurocysticercosis (both parasitic conditions) may cause parkinsonism and tremor. In neurocysticercosis, improvement may occur with albendazole and, when hydrocephalus is present, placement of a CSF shunt.[38]

Autoimmune and Paraneoplastic Disorders

Parkinsonism may occur as a complication of systemic lupus erythematosus; rigidity and akinesia is more common than tremor, and pyramidal signs may be present.[171] In a case series of 41 patients with CNS lupus, 2 presented with parkinsonism and responded to immunosuppressant (but not dopaminergic) treatment.[47] In addition to the common findings of recurrent oral and genital ulcerations, bilateral posterior uveitis and retinal vasculitis, skin papules, parkinsonism, and postural tremor have been observed in Behçet syndrome.[52] Nonvasculitic autoimmune inflammatory meningoencephalitis may present with rapidly progressive myoclonus, dementia, and parkinsonism that improves with high-dose corticosteroids. The EEG may show persistent periodic sharp waves reminiscent of Creutzfeldt–Jakob disease.[84] Parkinsonism has been described as a rare complication of the antiphospholipid antibody syndrome. The brain MRI shows periventricular white matter changes and the condition responds poorly to levodopa.[172]

Paraneoplastic parkinsonism (with bradykinesia, rigidity, and tremor) has been described in patients with anti-Ma2 antibodies, which are often associated with paraneoplastic limbic or brainstem encephalitis.[173] Parkinsonism has been reported in association with the collapsin response-mediator protein (CRMP)-5 antibody[174] (although chorea was more common) and the anti-neuronal nuclear autoantibody type 2.[175] Finally, parkinsonism occurred in 8 of 77 with voltage-gated potassium channel antibodies.

Trauma

Development of parkinsonism after a single head injury is rare; it typically follows severe injury with loss of consciousness.[67] Symptoms may develop over several months after injury. Neuroimaging usually demonstrates a lesion of the globus pallidus or substantia nigra.[176] Parkinsonism may be secondary to chronic subdural hematoma,[177] typically developing within weeks of the causal injury. Complete or near-complete remission of parkinsonism often follows drainage of the hematoma.

Parkinsonism may occur after repeated head injury, as in boxing. A variable spectrum of signs and symptoms may be present, including behavioral changes, dementia, and corticospinal and cerebellar deficits; dysarthria is especially common, and parkinsonism occurred in 18 of 48 subjects with recurrent head injury in a recent series.[178] Pathologic examination has revealed atrophy of the cerebral hemispheres, medial temporal lobe, thalamus, mammillary bodies, and brainstem. Histologic examination revealed extensive tau-immunoreactive neurofibrillary tangles, astrocytic tangles, and spindle-shaped neuritis. The disorder was distinguished from other tauopathies by its patchy distribution and the preferential involvement of the superficial cortical layers.[178] Patients often respond to dopaminergic treatment. The relationship of nonrepetitive remote head trauma to Parkinson disease is controversial and unsettled.[179,180]

Other Causes of Parkinsonism

Some aspects of parkinsonism may be simulated by communicating or noncommunicating hydrocephalus or a subdural hematoma and may resolve after ventricular peritoneal shunting.[177] In normal-pressure hydrocephalus, gait abnormalities predominate.[181] Mass lesions are rare causes of parkinsonism. Parkinsonism resulting from focal irradiation of the brain or brainstem may respond to dopaminergic treatment and is sometimes partially reversible.[182]

Approach to Diagnosis

Rapid onset of parkinsonism over days to months is atypical of Parkinson disease but occurs when drug induced, after infection, due to a structural brain injury (subdural hematoma, stroke, or hydrocephalus), or secondary to an underlying medical condition. If no offending drug or toxin can be identified, screening blood tests should be performed (blood electrolyte and glucose levels, erythrocyte sedimentation rate, and antinuclear antibody, as well as thyroid, renal, and hepatic function tests). Testing for 24-hour urinary copper excretion and serum ceruloplasmin determination should be considered in patients younger than 40 years. Toxicologic screening tests may be necessary in individuals for whom no cause is found. Brain imaging, particularly MRI, may be helpful.

Treatment

The management of secondary parkinsonism depends on the cause but generally includes symptomatic measures. The most common cause is medication related. When possible, the offending medication should be tapered to prevent worsening of any underlying psychiatric disorder for which it may have been prescribed and also to reduce the risk of precipitating a tardive movement disorder. When a behavioral disorder requires a dopamine-blocking agent, it is sometimes possible to switch to an antipsychotic medication with less affinity for the D2 receptor, such as clozapine or quetiapine. It may take weeks to many months for the full effect of a dopamine-blocking drug such as haloperidol to resolve.

In other cases of secondary parkinsonism, management of the underlying medical disorder may take precedence. In many cases, however, treatment of the primary disorder is inadequate and symptomatic therapy is appropriate. In general, treatment of parkinsonism with levodopa, dopamine agonists, or both, may improve bradykinesia, rigidity, or tremor. The effectiveness of dopaminergic treatment varies considerably between conditions. Other agents that may be particularly useful for tremor include amantadine and anticholinergic agents.[183] Deep brain stimulation of the globus pallidus or subthalamic nucleus may be considered in selected patients who are refractory to medications.

REFERENCES

1. Phukan J, Albanese A, Gasser T, et al: Primary dystonia and dystonia-plus syndromes: clinical characteristics, diagnosis, and pathogenesis. Lancet Neurol 10:1074, 2011.
2. Walker RH: Differential diagnosis of chorea. Curr Neurol Neurosci Rep 11:385, 2011.
3. Piccolo I, Defanti CA, Soliveri P, et al: Cause and course in a series of patients with sporadic chorea. J Neurol 250:429, 2003.
4. Bejot Y, Giroud M, Moreau T, et al: Clinical spectrum of movement disorders after stroke in childhood and adulthood. Eur Neurol 68:59, 2012.
5. Alarcon F, Zijlmans JC, Duenas G, et al: Post-stroke movement disorders: report of 56 patients. J Neurol Neurosurg Psychiatry 75:1568, 2004.
6. Khot S, Tirschwell DL: Long-term neurological complications after hypoxic-ischemic encephalopathy. Semin Neurol 26:422, 2006.
7. Bhatt MH, Obeso JA, Marsden CD: Time course of postanoxic akinetic-rigid and dystonic syndromes. Neurology 43:314, 1993.
8. Przekop A, McClure C, Ashwal S: Postoperative encephalopathy with choreoathetosis. Handb Clin Neurol 100:295, 2011.
9. Marvi MM, Lew MF: Polycythemia and chorea. Handb Clin Neurol 100:271, 2011.
10. Choi IS: Parkinsonism after carbon monoxide poisoning. Eur Neurol 48:30, 2002.
11. Sohn YH, Jeong Y, Kim HS, et al: The brain lesion responsible for parkinsonism after carbon monoxide poisoning. Arch Neurol 57:1214, 2000.
12. Rosenow F, Herholz K, Lanfermann H, et al: Neurological sequelae of cyanide intoxication—the patterns of clinical, magnetic resonance imaging, and positron emission tomography findings. Ann Neurol 38:825, 1995.
13. Zaknun JJ, Stieglbauer K, Trenkler J, et al: Cyanide-induced akinetic rigid syndrome: clinical, MRI, FDG-PET, beta-CIT and HMPAO SPECT findings. Parkinsonism Relat Disord 11:125, 2005.

14. Davis LE, Adair JC: Parkinsonism from methanol poisoning: benefit from treatment with anti-Parkinson drugs. Mov Disord 14:520, 1999.
15. Blanco M, Casado R, Vazquez F, et al: CT and MR imaging findings in methanol intoxication. AJNR Am J Neuroradiol 27:452, 2006.
16. Huang CC, Chu NS, Lu CS, et al: The natural history of neurological manganism over 18 years. Parkinsonism Relat Disord 13:143, 2007.
17. Cersosimo MG, Koller WC: The diagnosis of manganese-induced parkinsonism. Neurotoxicology 27:340, 2006.
18. Herrero Hernandez E, Discalzi G, Valentini C, et al: Follow-up of patients affected by manganese-induced Parkinsonism after treatment with $CaNa_2EDTA$. Neurotoxicology 27:333, 2006.
19. Stepens A, Logina I, Liguts V, et al: A Parkinsonian syndrome in methcathinone users and the role of manganese. N Engl J Med 358:1009, 2008.
20. Clarkson TW, Magos L, Myers GJ: The toxicology of mercury—current exposures and clinical manifestations. N Engl J Med 349:1731, 2003.
21. Pfeiffer RF: Wilson's disease. Semin Neurol 27:123, 2007.
22. Krauss JK, Mohadjer M, Wakhloo AK, et al: Dystonia and akinesia due to pallidoputaminal lesions after disulfiram intoxication. Mov Disord 6:166, 1991.
23. Mahajan P, Lieh-Lai MW, Sarnaik A, et al: Basal ganglia infarction in a child with disulfiram poisoning. Pediatrics 99:605, 1997.
24. Miyasaki JM: Chorea caused by toxins. Handb Clin Neurol 100:335, 2011.
25. Zesiewicz TA, Sullivan KL: Drug-induced hyperkinetic movement disorders by nonneuroleptic agents. Handb Clin Neurol 100:347, 2011.
26. Madhusoodanan S, Alexeenko L, Sanders R, et al: Extrapyramidal symptoms associated with antidepressants—a review of the literature and an analysis of spontaneous reports. Ann Clin Psychiatry 22:148, 2010.
27. Tse W, Cersosimo MG, Gracies JM, et al: Movement disorders and AIDS: a review. Parkinsonism Relat Disord 10:323, 2004.
28. Azar S, Ramjiani A, Van Gerpen JA: Ciprofloxacin-induced chorea. Mov Disord 20:513, 2005.
29. King AM, Menke NB, Katz KD, et al: 4-aminopyridine toxicity: a case report and review of the literature. J Med Toxicol 8:314, 2012.
30. Woods SW, Morgenstern H, Saksa JR, et al: Incidence of tardive dyskinesia with atypical versus conventional antipsychotic medications: a prospective cohort study. J Clin Psychiatry 71:463, 2010.
31. Fernandez HH, Friedman JH: Classification and treatment of tardive syndromes. Neurologist 9:16, 2003.
32. Vidailhet M, Jutras MF, Grabli D, et al: Deep brain stimulation for dystonia. J Neurol Neurosurg Psychiatry 84:1029, 2013.
33. Miranda M, Cardoso F, Giovannoni G, et al: Oral contraceptive induced chorea: another condition associated with anti-basal ganglia antibodies. J Neurol Neurosurg Psychiatry 75:327, 2004.
34. Brust JC: Substance abuse and movement disorders. Mov Disord 25:2010, 2010.
35. Cardoso F: Sydenham's chorea. Handb Clin Neurol 100:221, 2011.
36. Maia DP, Teixeira Jr AL, Quintao Cunningham MC, et al: Obsessive compulsive behavior, hyperactivity, and attention deficit disorder in Sydenham chorea. Neurology 64:1799, 2005.
37. Dale RC, Brilot F: Autoimmune basal ganglia disorders. J Child Neurol 27:1470, 2012.
38. Alarcon F, Gimenez-Roldan S: Systemic diseases that cause movement disorders. Parkinsonism Relat Disord 11:1, 2005.
39. Beskind DL, Keim SM: Choreoathetotic movement disorder in a boy with *Mycoplasma pneumoniae* encephalitis. Ann Emerg Med 23:1375, 1994.
40. Green C, Riley DE: Treatment of dystonia in striatal necrosis caused by *Mycoplasma pneumoniae*. Pediatr Neurol 26:318, 2002.
41. Bamford JM, Hakin RN: Chorea after legionnaire's disease. Clin Res Br Med J 284:1232, 1982.
42. Ozben S, Erol C, Ozer F, et al: Chorea as the presenting feature of neurosyphilis. Neurol India 57:347, 2009.
43. Misra UK, Kalita J: Spectrum of movement disorders in encephalitis. J Neurol 257:2052, 2010.
44. Gollomp SM, Fahn S: Transient dystonia as a complication of varicella. J Neurol Neurosurg Psychiatry 50:1228, 1987.
45. Rathi N, Rathi A: Relapse of herpes simplex encephalitis presenting as choreoathetosis. Indian J Pediatr 77:901, 2010.
46. Teive HA, Troiano AR, Cabral NL, et al: Hemichorea-hemiballism associated to cryptococcal granuloma in a patient with AIDS: case report. Arq Neuropsiquiatr 58:965, 2000.
47. Joseph FG, Lammie GA, Scolding NJ: CNS lupus: a study of 41 patients. Neurology 69:644, 2007.
48. Baizabal-Carvallo JF, Jankovic J: Movement disorders in autoimmune diseases. Mov Disord 27:935, 2012.
49. Peluso S, Antenora A, De Rosa A, et al: Antiphospholipid-related chorea. Front Neurol 3:150, 2012.
50. Martino D, Chew NK, Mir P, et al: Atypical movement disorders in antiphospholipid syndrome. Mov Disord 21:944, 2006.
51. Ruiz-Irastorza G, Crowther M, Branch W, et al: Antiphospholipid syndrome. Lancet 376:1498, 2010.
52. Joseph FG, Scolding NJ: Neuro-Behçet's disease in Caucasians: a study of 22 patients. Eur J Neurol 14:174, 2007.
53. Revilla FJ, Racette BA, Perlmutter JS: Chorea and jaw-opening dystonia as a manifestation of NeuroBehçet's syndrome. Mov Disord 15:741, 2000.

54. Pellecchia MT, Cuomo T, Striano S, et al: Paroxysmal dystonia in Behçet's disease. Mov Disord 14:177, 1999.
55. Mijajlovic M, Mirkovic M, Dackovic J, et al: Clinical manifestations, diagnostic criteria and therapy of Hashimoto's encephalopathy: report of two cases. J Neurol Sci 288:194, 2010.
56. Fung VS, Duggins A, Morris JG, et al: Progressive myoclonic ataxia associated with celiac disease presenting as unilateral cortical tremor and dystonia. Mov Disord 15:732, 2000.
57. Pereira AC, Edwards MJ, Buttery PC, et al: Choreic syndrome and coeliac disease: a hitherto unrecognised association. Mov Disord 19:478, 2004.
58. Vigliani MC, Honnorat J, Antoine JC, et al: Chorea and related movement disorders of paraneoplastic origin: the PNS EuroNetwork experience. J Neurol 258:2058, 2011.
59. Pittock SJ, Parisi JE, McKeon A, et al: Paraneoplastic jaw dystonia and laryngospasm with antineuronal nuclear autoantibody type 2 (anti-Ri). Arch Neurol 67:1109, 2010.
60. Panzer J, Dalmau J: Movement disorders in paraneoplastic and autoimmune disease. Curr Opin Neurol 24:346, 2011.
61. Docherty MJ, Burn DJ: Hyperthyroid chorea. Handb Clin Neurol 100:279, 2011.
62. Goswami R, Sharma R, Sreenivas V, et al: Prevalence and progression of basal ganglia calcification and its pathogenic mechanism in patients with idiopathic hypoparathyroidism. Clin Endocrinol (Oxf) 77:200, 2012.
63. Oh SH, Lee KY, Im JH, et al: Chorea associated with non-ketotic hyperglycemia and hyperintensity basal ganglia lesion on T1-weighted brain MRI study: a meta-analysis of 53 cases including four present cases. J Neurol Sci 200:57, 2002.
64. Kandiah N, Tan K, Lim CC, et al: Hyperglycemic choreoathetosis: role of the putamen in pathogenesis. Mov Disord 24:915, 2009.
65. Lai SL, Tseng YL, Hsu MC, et al: Magnetic resonance imaging and single-photon emission computed tomography changes in hypoglycemia-induced chorea. Mov Disord 19:475, 2004.
66. de Souza A, Desai PK: Delayed chorea after recovery from a symmetric parkinsonian syndrome due to striatal myelinolysis. J Clin Neurosci 19:1165, 2012.
67. Krauss JK, Trankle R, Kopp KH: Post-traumatic movement disorders in survivors of severe head injury. Neurology 47:1488, 1996.
68. Greene P, Shale H, Fahn S: Experience with high dosages of anticholinergic and other drugs in the treatment of torsion dystonia. Adv Neurol 50:547, 1988.
69. Kang UJ, Burke RE, Fahn S: Tardive dystonia. Adv Neurol 50:415, 1988.
70. Rilstone JJ, Alkhater RA, Minassian BA: Brain dopamine-serotonin vesicular transport disease and its treatment. N Engl J Med 368:543, 2013.
71. Albanese A, Barnes MP, Bhatia KP, et al: A systematic review on the diagnosis and treatment of primary (idiopathic) dystonia and dystonia plus syndromes: report of an EFNS/MDS-ES Task Force. Eur J Neurol 13:433, 2006.
72. Jankovic J: Treatment of hyperkinetic movement disorders. Lancet Neurol 8:844, 2009.
73. Edwards TC, Zrinzo L, Limousin P, et al: Deep brain stimulation in the treatment of chorea. Mov Disord 27:357, 2012.
74. Caviness JN, Truong DD: Myoclonus. Handb Clin Neurol 100:399, 2011.
75. Frucht S, Fahn S: The clinical spectrum of posthypoxic myoclonus. Mov Disord 15(suppl 1):2, 2000.
76. Wijdicks EF, Parisi JE, Sharbrough FW: Prognostic value of myoclonus status in comatose survivors of cardiac arrest. Ann Neurol 35:239, 1994.
77. Hui AC, Cheng C, Lam A, et al: Prognosis following postanoxic myoclonus status epilepticus. Eur Neurol 54:10, 2005.
78. Frucht SJ, Houghton WC, Bordelon Y, et al: A single-blind, open-label trial of sodium oxybate for myoclonus and essential tremor. Neurology 65:1967, 2005.
79. Stahlman GC, Auerbach PS, Strickland WG: Neurologic manifestations of non-ketotic hyperglycemia. J Tenn Med Assoc 81:77, 1988.
80. Ozdemir O, Baytan B, Gunes AM, et al: Involuntary movements during vitamin B_{12} treatment. J Child Neurol 25:227, 2010.
81. Wu MS, Hsu YD, Lin JC, et al: Spinal myoclonus in subacute combined degeneration caused by nitrous oxide intoxication. Acta Neurol Taiwan 16:102, 2007.
82. Kapas I, Majtenyi K, Toro K, et al: Pellagra encephalopathy as a differential diagnosis for Creutzfeldt-Jakob disease. Metab Brain Dis 27:231, 2012.
83. de Holanda NC, de Lima DD, Cavalcanti TB, et al: Hashimoto's encephalopathy: systematic review of the literature and an additional case. J Neuropsychiatry Clin Neurosci 23:384, 2011.
84. Hoffman Snyder C, Mishark KJ, Caviness JN, et al: Nonvasculitic autoimmune inflammatory meningoencephalitis imitating Creutzfeldt-Jakob disease. Arch Neurol 63:766, 2006.
85. Bhatia KP, Brown P, Gregory R, et al: Progressive myoclonic ataxia associated with coeliac disease. The myoclonus is of cortical origin, but the pathology is in the cerebellum. Brain 118:1087, 1995.
86. Hanagasi HA, Gurol E, Sahin HA, et al: Atypical neurological involvement associated with celiac disease. Eur J Neurol 8:67, 2001.
87. Deconinck N, Scaillon M, Segers V, et al: Opsoclonus-myoclonus associated with celiac disease. Pediatr Neurol 34:312, 2006.
88. Robottom BJ, Weiner WJ, Factor SA: Movement disorders emergencies. Part 1: Hypokinetic disorders. Arch Neurol 68:567, 2011.

89. Caviness JN, Evidente VG: Cortical myoclonus during lithium exposure. Arch Neurol 60:401, 2003.
90. Vandel P: Antidepressant drugs in the elderly—role of the cytochrome P450 2D6. World J Biol Psychiatry 4:74, 2003.
91. Fahn S: The spectrum of levodopa-induced dyskinesias. Ann Neurol 47:S2, 2000.
92. Brefel-Courbon C, Gardette V, Ory F, et al: Drug-induced myoclonus: a French pharmacovigilance database study. Neurophysiol Clin 36:333, 2006.
93. Goodheart RS, Dunne JW: Petrol sniffer's encephalopathy. A study of 25 patients. Med J Aust 160:178, 1994.
94. Teepker M, Hamer HM, Knake S, et al: Myoclonic encephalopathy caused by chronic bismuth abuse. Epileptic Disord 4:229, 2002.
95. Dalmau J, Rosenfeld MR: Paraneoplastic syndromes causing movement disorders. Handb Clin Neurol 100:315, 2011.
96. Titulaer MJ, Soffietti R, Dalmau J, et al: Screening for tumours in paraneoplastic syndromes: report of an EFNS task force. Eur J Neurol 18:19, 2011.
97. Vedeler CA, Antoine JC, Giometto B, et al: Management of paraneoplastic neurological syndromes: report of an EFNS Task Force. Eur J Neurol 13:682, 2006.
98. Valldeoriola F, Gonzalez J, Vila N, et al: Action myoclonus as an early clinical sign of carcinomatous meningitis. Mov Disord 11:223, 1996.
99. Koh KN, Lim BC, Hwang H, et al: Cerebellum can be a possible generator of progressive myoclonus. J Child Neurol 25:728, 2010.
100. Estraneo A, Saltalamacchia AM, Loreto V: Spinal myoclonus following herpes zoster radiculitis. Neurology 68:E4, 2007.
101. Mattos JP, Rosso AL, Correa RB, et al: Movement disorders in 28 HIV-infected patients. Arq Neuropsiquiatr 60:525, 2002.
102. Ichiba N, Miyake Y, Sato K, et al: Mumps-induced opsoclonus-myoclonus and ataxia. Pediatr Neurol 4:224, 1988.
103. Bhatia K, Thompson PD, Marsden CD: "Isolated" postinfectious myoclonus. J Neurol Neurosurg Psychiatry 55:1089, 1992.
104. Alshekhlee A, Sultan B, Chandar K: Opsoclonus persisting during sleep in West Nile encephalitis. Arch Neurol 63:1324, 2006.
105. Peter L, Jung J, Tilikete C, et al: Opsoclonus-myoclonus as a manifestation of Lyme disease. J Neurol Neurosurg Psychiatry 77:1090, 2006.
106. Khosla SN, Srivastava SC, Gupta S: Neuro-psychiatric manifestations of typhoid. J Trop Med Hyg 80:95, 1977.
107. Dassan P, Clarke C, Sharp DJ: A case of poststreptococcal opsoclonus-myoclonus syndrome. Mov Disord 22:1490, 2007.
108. Alarcon F, Duenas G, Cevallos N, et al: Movement disorders in 30 patients with tuberculous meningitis. Mov Disord 15:561, 2000.
109. Alarcon F, Maldonado JC, Rivera JW: Movement disorders identified in patients with intracranial tuberculomas. Neurologia 26:343, 2011.
110. Revilla FJ, de la Cruz R, Khardori N, et al: Teaching NeuroImage: oculomasticatory myorhythmia: pathognomonic phenomenology of Whipple disease. Neurology 70:e25, 2008.
111. Fenollar F, Puechal X, Raoult D: Whipple's disease. N Engl J Med 356:55, 2007.
112. Lawn SD, Flanagan KL, Wright SG, et al: Postmalaria neurological syndrome: two cases from the Gambia. Clin Infect Dis 36:e29, 2003.
113. Puri V, Chowdhury V, Gulati P: Myoclonus: a manifestation of neurocysticercosis. Postgrad Med J 67:68, 1991.
114. Loscher WN, Trinka E: Late delayed postradiation spinal myoclonus or psychogenic movement disorder? Mov Disord 18:346, 2003.
115. Talpalar AE: High pressure neurological syndrome. Rev Neurol 45:631, 2007.
116. Lim EC, Seet RC: Segmental dystonia following electrocution in childhood. Neurol Sci 28:38, 2007.
117. Klaas JP, Ahlskog JE, Pittock SJ, et al: Adult-onset opsoclonus-myoclonus syndrome. Arch Neurol 69:1598, 2012.
118. Morgan JC, Sethi KD: Drug-induced tremors. Lancet Neurol 4:866, 2005.
119. Costello DJ, Walsh SL, Harrington HJ, et al: Concurrent hereditary haemochromatosis and idiopathic Parkinson's disease: a case report series. J Neurol Neurosurg Psychiatry 75:631, 2004.
120. Ellis SJ: Severe hyponatraemia: complications and treatment. QJM 88:905, 1995.
121. Garcia Ruiz PJ, Mayo D, Hernandez J, et al: Movement disorders in hereditary ataxias. J Neurol Sci 202:59, 2002.
122. Hirayama K, Sakazaki H, Murakami S, et al: Sequential MRI, SPECT and PET in respiratory syncytial virus encephalitis. Pediatr Radiol 29:282, 1999.
123. Freund A, Zass R, Kurlemann G, et al: Bilateral oedema of the basal ganglia in an echovirus type 21 infection: complete clinical and radiological normalization. Dev Med Child Neurol 40:421, 1998.
124. Misra UK, Kalita J: Movement disorders in Japanese encephalitis. J Neurol 244:299, 1997.
125. Keswani P, Gupta R, Singh KP, et al: Unilateral ataxia following herpes zoster of spinal C4 segment. J Assoc Physicians India 41:178, 1993.
126. Riikonen R: Infantile spasms: infectious disorders. Neuropediatrics 24:274, 1993.
127. Gunther G, Haglund M, Lindquist L, et al: Tick-borne encephalitis in Sweden in relation to aseptic meningo-encephalitis of other etiology: a prospective

study of clinical course and outcome. J Neurol 244:230, 1997.
128. Cummins D, Bennett D, Fisher-Hoch SP, et al: Lassa fever encephalopathy: clinical and laboratory findings. J Trop Med Hyg 95:197, 1992.
129. Vasconcelos PF, da Rosa AP, Coelho IC, et al: Involvement of the central nervous system in dengue fever: three serologically confirmed cases from Fortaleza Ceara, Brazil. Rev Inst Med Trop Sao Paulo 40:35, 1998.
130. Kilgore PE, Ksiazek TG, Rollin PE, et al: Treatment of Bolivian hemorrhagic fever with intravenous ribavirin. Clin Infect Dis 24:718, 1997.
131. Floris-Moore MA, Amodio-Groton MI, Catalano MT: Adverse reactions to trimethoprim/sulfamethoxazole in AIDS. Ann Pharmacother 37:1810, 2003.
132. van der Wal G, Verhagen WI, Dofferhoff AS: Neurological complications following *Plasmodium falciparum* infection. Neth J Med 63:180, 2005.
133. Kumar A: Movement disorders in the tropics. Parkinsonism Relat Disord 9:69, 2002.
134. Lekoubou A, Njouoguep R, Kuate C, et al: Cerebral toxoplasmosis in acquired immunodeficiency syndrome (AIDS) patients also provides unifying pathophysiologic hypotheses for Holmes tremor. BMC Neurol 10:37, 2010.
135. Klein CJ, Moon JS, Mauermann ML, et al: The neuropathies of Waldenstrom's macroglobulinemia (WM) and IgM-MGUS. Can J Neurol Sci 38:289, 2011.
136. Castillo P, Woodruff B, Caselli R, et al: Steroid-responsive encephalopathy associated with autoimmune thyroiditis. Arch Neurol 63:197, 2006.
137. Mehta SH, Morgan JC, Sethi KD: Paraneoplastic movement disorders. Curr Neurol Neurosci Rep 9:285, 2009.
138. Ahlskog MC, Kumar N, Mauermann ML, et al: IgM-monoclonal gammopathy neuropathy and tremor: a first epidemiologic case control study. Parkinsonism Relat Disord 18:748, 2012.
139. Coltamai L, Magezi DA, Croquelois A: Pregabalin in the treatment of neuropathic tremor following a motor axonal form of Guillain–Barré syndrome. Mov Disord 25:517, 2010.
140. Chiou TS, Tsai CH, Lee YH: Unilateral Holmes tremor and focal dystonia after gamma knife surgery. J Neurosurg 105(suppl):235, 2006.
141. Zesiewicz TA, Elble RJ, Louis ED, et al: Evidence-based guideline update: treatment of essential tremor: report of the Quality Standards Subcommittee of the American Academy of Neurology. Neurology 77:1752, 2011.
142. Jimenez MC, Vingerhoets FJ: Tremor revisited: treatment of PD tremor. Parkinsonism Relat Disord 18(suppl 1):S93, 2012.
143. Elble RJ: Tremor: clinical features, pathophysiology, and treatment. Neurol Clin 27:679, 2009.
144. Gupta D, Kuruvilla A: Vascular parkinsonism: what makes it different? Postgrad Med J 87:829, 2011.
145. Wenning GK, Kiechl S, Seppi K, et al: Prevalence of movement disorders in men and women aged 50-89 years (Bruneck Study cohort): a population-based study. Lancet Neurol 4:815, 2005.
146. Bondon-Guitton E, Perez-Lloret S, Bagheri H, et al: Drug-induced parkinsonism: a review of 17 years' experience in a regional pharmacovigilance center in France. Mov Disord 26:2226, 2011.
147. Laplane D, Attal N, Sauron B, et al: Lesions of basal ganglia due to disulfiram neurotoxicity. J Neurol Neurosurg Psychiatry 55:925, 1992.
148. Lima MA, Maradei S, Maranhao Filho P: Cyclosporine-induced parkinsonism. J Neurol 256:674, 2009.
149. Kieburtz K, Wunderle KB: Parkinson's disease: evidence for environmental risk factors. Mov Disord 28:8, 2013.
150. Di Filippo M, Tambasco N, Muzi G, et al: Parkinsonism and cognitive impairment following chronic exposure to potassium cyanide. Mov Disord 23:468, 2008.
151. Caudle WM, Guillot TS, Lazo CR, et al: Industrial toxicants and Parkinson's disease. Neurotoxicology 33:178, 2012.
152. Prockop LD, Chichkova RI: Carbon monoxide intoxication: an updated review. J Neurol Sci 262:122, 2007.
153. Reddy NJ, Lewis LD, Gardner TB, et al: Two cases of rapid onset Parkinson's syndrome following toxic ingestion of ethylene glycol and methanol. Clin Pharmacol Ther 81:114, 2007.
154. Mortimer JA, Borenstein AR, Nelson LM: Associations of welding and manganese exposure with Parkinson disease: review and meta-analysis. Neurology 79:1174, 2012.
155. Josephs KA, Ahlskog JE, Klos KJ, et al: Neurologic manifestations in welders with pallidal MRI T1 hyperintensity. Neurology 64:2033, 2005.
156. Koller WC, Lyons KE, Truly W: Effect of levodopa treatment for parkinsonism in welders: a double-blind study. Neurology 62:730, 2004.
157. Burkhard PR, Delavelle J, Du Pasquier R, et al: Chronic parkinsonism associated with cirrhosis: a distinct subset of acquired hepatocerebral degeneration. Arch Neurol 60:521, 2003.
158. Tambyah PA, Ong BK, Lee KO: Reversible parkinsonism and asymptomatic hypocalcemia with basal ganglia calcification from hypoparathyroidism 26 years after thyroid surgery. Am J Med 94:444, 1993.
159. Wang HC, Cheng SJ: The syndrome of acute bilateral basal ganglia lesions in diabetic uremic patients. J Neurol 250:948, 2003.
160. Jurynczyk M, Rozniecki J, Zaleski K, et al: Hypoglycemia as a trigger for the syndrome of acute bilateral basal ganglia lesions in uremia. J Neurol Sci 297:74, 2010.
161. Jang H, Boltz DA, Webster RG, et al: Viral parkinsonism. Biochim Biophys Acta 1792:714, 2009.

162. Mirsattari SM, Power C, Nath A: Parkinsonism with HIV infection. Mov Disord 13:684, 1998.
163. Clay PG, Adams MM: Pseudo-Parkinson disease secondary to ritonavir-buspirone interaction. Ann Pharmacother 37:202, 2003.
164. Kobylecki C, Silverdale MA, Varma A, et al: HIV-associated parkinsonism with levodopa-induced dyskinesia and response to highly-active antiretroviral therapy. Mov Disord 24:2441, 2009.
165. Jang W, Kim JS, Ahn JY, et al: Reversible progressive supranuclear palsy-like phenotype as an initial manifestation of HIV infection. Neurol Sci 33:1169, 2012.
166. Dale RC, Church AJ, Surtees RA, et al: Encephalitis lethargica syndrome: 20 new cases and evidence of basal ganglia autoimmunity. Brain 127:21, 2004.
167. Dale RC, Irani SR, Brilot F, et al: N-methyl-D-aspartate receptor antibodies in pediatric dyskinetic encephalitis lethargica. Ann Neurol 66:704, 2009.
168. Lopez-Alberola R, Georgiou M, Sfakianakis GN, et al: Contemporary encephalitis lethargica: phenotype, laboratory findings and treatment outcomes. J Neurol 256:396, 2009.
169. Zambrino CA, Zorzi G, Lanzi G, et al: Bilateral striatal necrosis associated with *Mycoplasma pneumoniae* infection in an adolescent: clinical and neuroradiologic follow up. Mov Disord 15:1023, 2000.
170. Spitz M, Maia FM, Gomes HR, et al: Parkinsonism secondary to neurosyphilis. Mov Disord 23:1948, 2008.
171. Khubchandani RP, Viswanathan V, Desai J: Unusual neurologic manifestations (I): Parkinsonism in juvenile SLE. Lupus 16:572, 2007.
172. Huang YC, Lyu RK, Chen ST, et al: Parkinsonism in a patient with antiphospholipid syndrome—case report and literature review. J Neurol Sci 267:166, 2008.
173. Dalmau J, Graus F, Villarejo A, et al: Clinical analysis of anti-Ma2-associated encephalitis. Brain 127:1831, 2004.
174. Yu Z, Kryzer TJ, Griesmann GE, et al: CRMP-5 neuronal autoantibody: marker of lung cancer and thymoma-related autoimmunity. Ann Neurol 49:146, 2001.
175. Pittock SJ, Lucchinetti CF, Lennon VA: Anti-neuronal nuclear autoantibody type 2: paraneoplastic accompaniments. Ann Neurol 53:580, 2003.
176. Bhatt M, Desai J, Mankodi A, et al: Posttraumatic akinetic-rigid syndrome resembling Parkinson's disease: a report on three patients. Mov Disord 15:313, 2000.
177. Gelabert-Gonzalez M, Serramito-Garcia R, Aran-Echabe E: Parkinsonism secondary to subdural haematoma. Neurosurg Rev 35:457, 2012.
178. McKee AC, Cantu RC, Nowinski CJ, et al: Chronic traumatic encephalopathy in athletes: progressive tauopathy after repetitive head injury. J Neuropathol Exp Neurol 68:709, 2009.
179. Noyce AJ, Bestwick JP, Silveira-Moriyama L, et al: Meta-analysis of early nonmotor features and risk factors for Parkinson disease. Ann Neurol 72:893, 2012.
180. Goldman SM, Kamel F, Ross GW, et al: Head injury, alpha-synuclein Rep1, and Parkinson's disease. Ann Neurol 71:40, 2012.
181. Stolze H, Kuhtz-Buschbeck JP, Drucke H, et al: Comparative analysis of the gait disorder of normal pressure hydrocephalus and Parkinson's disease. J Neurol Neurosurg Psychiatry 70:289, 2001.
182. Voermans NC, Bloem BR, Janssens G, et al: Secondary parkinsonism in childhood: a rare complication after radiotherapy. Pediatr Neurol 34:495, 2006.
183. Lees AJ, Hardy J, Revesz T: Parkinson's disease. Lancet 373:2055, 2009.

CHAPTER

59

Neuromuscular Complications of General Medical Disorders

JEFFREY W. RALPH ■ MICHAEL J. AMINOFF

Diagnosis of disorders of the neuromuscular system involves localizing the lesion anatomically and then weighing the validity of specific diagnostic hypotheses. Symmetry and rapidity of the disease process are major diagnostic considerations. Pure motor syndromes localize to the anterior horn cells, neuromuscular junctions, or muscles, though, rarely, neuropathies can also produce pure motor deficits. Combinations of motor and sensory deficits suggest radiculopathy, plexopathy, or neuropathy.

A diagnostic strategy complementary to the aforementioned approach employs pattern matching. Neuromuscular diseases present with one of five basic patterns (Table 59-1).[1] Weakness is usually a more prominent feature of demyelinating than axonal neuropathies.

In general, electromyography (EMG) and nerve conduction studies (NCSs) are essential for confirming the anatomic localization, differentiating axonal from demyelinating neuropathies, and making prognostic statements. Decisions concerning the need for muscle or nerve biopsies should be deferred until electrodiagnostic testing is completed.

TABLE 59-1 ■ Classification of Neuromuscular Diseases by Presentation Patterns

Acute Generalized Weakness
Guillain–Barré Syndrome
Botulism
Necrotizing myopathy
Tick paralysis
Severe electrolyte imbalance
Periodic paralysis
Subacute or Chronic Generalized Weakness
Amyotrophic lateral sclerosis
Demyelinating motor neuropathies
Myopathy
Myasthenia gravis
Slowly Progressive, Generalized Weakness More Than Numbness
Demyelinating polyneuropathy
Slowly Progressive, Distal Numbness More Than Weakness
Axonal polyneuropathy
Numbness, Weakness, or Pain Limited to One Limb
Radiculopathy
Plexopathy
Entrapment neuropathy
Initial nerve involved by vasculitic neuropathy

Adapted from McCarthy RJ, Olney RK: Neuromuscular disease. p. 287. In Corey-Bloom J (ed): Diagnosis-Based Adult Neurology. Mosby, St. Louis, 1997.

DISORDERS OF THE MOTOR NEURON

Amyotrophic lateral sclerosis (ALS) is the most common and prototypic motor neuron disease. It presents with flaccid weakness and atrophy of muscles without associated pain or sensory disturbances. Degeneration of upper motor neurons also occurs, producing spasticity and hyperreflexia in wasted limbs. Most cases are sporadic, but approximately 10 percent are inherited in autosomal-dominant or -recessive patterns. The pathogenesis of ALS is not known, but it is possible that multiple pathogenic mechanisms are at play, including impaired cellular handling of oxidative stress, neuroinflammation, neurotrophic factor deficiency, glutamate-induced excitotoxicity, and defects in protein metabolism and autophagy. There is no cure for ALS, although riluzole modestly slows progression of disease.[2] Noninvasive ventilation, careful nutritional monitoring and supplementation, and multidisciplinary care can improve the quality of life.[3] A sporadic clinical variant characterized by solely lower motor neuron involvement (progressive muscular atrophy) is managed similarly.

Hereditary anterior horn cell diseases include spinal muscular atrophy, Kennedy syndrome, and hexosaminidase A deficiency. Kennedy syndrome (spinal and bulbar muscular atrophy) is an X-linked disease characterized by proximal muscle weakness, muscle atrophy, and fasciculations, especially periorally. Affected individuals often have gynecomastia and testicular atrophy with reduced fertility. Expansion of a CAG repeat in the androgen receptor gene is responsible.[4]

Compression of the spinal cord may result in segmental loss of anterior horn cells. In cervical spondylosis, combined injury to both the anterior horn cells and descending corticospinal tracts may occur, leading to atrophy and weakness in the hands combined with spastic paraparesis; such a presentation mimics that of ALS.

Many viruses have central nervous system (CNS) tropism, but only a few strains cause acute and selective loss of anterior horn cells. Poliovirus is an enterovirus spread via a fecal-hand-oral route. Most patients are either asymptomatic or develop only mild constitutional symptoms. More severe signs and symptoms may occur in nonparalytic poliomyelitis, and the cerebrospinal fluid (CSF) findings are often indicative of aseptic meningitis. Individuals developing acute paralytic poliomyelitis experience constitutional symptoms but also develop rapidly progressive weakness over the course of one to a few days. Weakness is often focal and asymmetric in the limbs or bulbar muscles, but may be symmetric or generalized. It frequently improves over several weeks to months. Rarely, the live-attenuated oral poliovirus vaccine can cause paralytic poliomyelitis.

Postpolio syndrome consists of slowly progressive new or worsened weakness, together with fatigue or pain in the muscles or joints, typically occurring many years after acute paralytic poliomyelitis in about 20 to 40 percent of individuals. The pathogenesis may involve late denervation of previously reinnervated muscle fibers or musculoskeletal abnormalities.[5]

Viruses other than poliovirus, such as West Nile virus (WNV), echovirus, coxsackievirus, herpes zoster virus, and Epstein–Barr virus may also cause loss of motor neurons.[6–9] Only about 20 percent of WNV infections are symptomatic, usually manifesting as a febrile illness. A maculopapular rash is common. About 1 percent of infected individuals develop neurologic symptoms that may include meningoencephalitis, flaccid paralysis, or both.[10] As in poliovirus infection, the weakness is often proximal and asymmetric, with no significant sensory abnormalities. The CSF shows a lymphocytic or neutrophilic pleocytosis (30 to 150 cells/mm^3) and high protein content. CSF and serum should be screened for IgM antibodies to WNV. Treatment is supportive. Rarely, WNV may present with brachial plexopathy,[11] rhabdomyolysis, or a predominantly demyelinating polyneuropathy similar to Guillain–Barré syndrome.[12]

Paraneoplastic lower motor neuron involvement may occur rarely with lymphoproliferative disorders, thymoma, and various cancers (bronchial, ovarian, renal, and prostate).[13–16] Patients may have anti-Hu (ANNA-1) and anti-Yo (PCA-1) antibodies, CSF protein is often elevated, and there is a variable CSF pleocytosis. The weakness may improve after treatment of the cancer.

RADICULOPATHY

Pain or numbness in a dermatomal pattern accompanied by weakness in a segmental pattern suggests a radiculopathy. External compression is the most frequent cause of nerve root injury, by either intervertebral disc herniation or spondylosis. Radiculopathy resulting from degenerative spine disease is discussed further in Chapter 22. Other causes of radiculopathy may include gouty spine disease, Paget disease, Tarlov cysts, and methylacrylate extrusion during spine surgery. Extradural tumors such as schwannomas, neurofibromas, and meningiomas may also produce a radiculopathy. A radiculopathy may result from epidural or spinal anesthesia; the injury may result from direct trauma to the nerve or from chemical injury related to the injected substance.

Diabetic thoracoabdominal radiculopathy (diabetic truncal neuropathy) is a common cause of noncompressive radiculopathy. Patients present with pain and hyperalgesia in a region along the chest or abdomen. The pattern of involvement may be clearly dermatomal, but often the changes span more than one segment. Segmental weakness may manifest as an outpouching of the abdominal wall. The pathophysiology is unclear, but an inflammatory vasculopathy may be responsible.

Compression of multiple lumbosacral nerve roots produces a cauda equina syndrome, which may lead to permanent urinary and fecal incontinence and lower extremity weakness and numbness and thus constitutes a neurosurgical emergency. The usual cause is a large, midline disc herniation. Chronic cauda equina syndrome may be caused by a developmental anomaly, such as a tethered spinal cord.

Spondylosis is the most common cause of polyradiculopathy, although metastatic spinal disease should also be considered. Cancers of the breast, lung, prostate, or kidney, or multiple myeloma metastasize most frequently to the spine. Polyradiculopathy results from direct tumor compression or from leptomeningeal infiltration of the roots by tumor cells (neoplastic meningitis). Treatment of spinal bony metastases often involves external beam irradiation, although decompressive surgery may be necessary in radiation-resistant tumors.

Carcinomatous meningitis often affects the caudal roots first. Cranial neuropathies, meningeal signs and symptoms, and a myelopathy may be associated features. CSF analysis typically shows a pleocystosis, hypoglycorrhachia, elevated protein level, and malignant cells on cytologic analysis. The yield of positive cytology for malignant cells is increased significantly by repeating the lumbar puncture. Treatment is usually palliative and includes radiation therapy and intrathecal chemotherapy. The median survival of patients with leptomeningeal metastases is 4 months.

Infectious causes of polyradiculopathy include cytomegalovirus (CMV), *Borrelia burgdorferi* (Lyme disease), Epstein–Barr virus, herpes simplex virus, *Mycobacterium tuberculosis*, and *Treponema pallidum*. CMV polyradiculopathy usually presents as a late complication of acquired immunodeficiency syndrome (AIDS), but it can be a presenting manifestation of human immunodeficiency virus (HIV) infection.[17] The onset of flaccid paraparesis, lower extremity numbness, and urinary retention may be acute or subacute.[18,19] A neutrophilic pleocytosis on CSF analysis is a clue to the diagnosis; the diagnosis is confirmed by a culture or CMV DNA polymerase chain reaction (PCR) assay on CSF. Treatment includes ganciclovir, foscarnet, or both.

Arachnoiditis is a nonspecific term for inflammation of the spinal leptomeninges. Historically, arachnoiditis has been associated with tuberculous and syphilitic meningitis and with obsolete oil-based contrast agents for myelography. Currently, the term often refers to the appearance of thickened meninges and clumping of the nerve roots on magnetic resonance imaging (MRI) of the spine, usually in patients who have undergone lumbar spine surgery. There is controversy about the association of the imaging findings, clinical findings, and symptoms.[20] Arachnoiditis has also been described in association with toxoplasmosis[21] and subarachnoid hemorrhage[22]; sometimes the cause is not known.

DISORDERS OF POSTERIOR ROOT GANGLIA

Diffuse or regional impairment of tactile sensation or gait ataxia without weakness suggests degeneration of posterior root ganglia cells (sensory neuronopathy). Patients may also have facial numbness and autonomic involvement, manifesting as gastroparesis, orthostatic hypotension, sexual impairment, and Adie pupils. EMG and nerve conduction studies differentiate sensory neuronopathies from more common distal sensory axonal polyneuropathies. Sensory neuronopathies may be acquired (Table 59-2) or hereditary.[23]

Paraneoplastic sensory neuronopathy (see Chapter 27) is commonly associated with small-cell lung cancer but also occurs with breast or ovarian cancer, Hodgkin lymphoma, neuroendocrine tumors, and sarcoma.[24–26] Symptom onset is generally subacute. Antibodies to the Hu antigen (ANNA-1) are usually present, but their absence does not exclude the possibility of paraneoplastic sensory neuronopathy. Antibodies to the collapsin response-mediator protein5 (CRMP5) have also been described in some patients with small-cell lung cancer.[27] Sensory neuronopathy may occur with other paraneoplastic syndromes. Management is directed to the diagnosis and treatment of the underlying cancer. Treatment of the paraneoplastic condition with IVIg, plasmapheresis, or other immunosuppressive therapies is often disappointing.[28]

Autoimmune or inflammatory conditions associated with sensory neuronopathy (sometimes as the initial manifestation) include Sjögren syndrome and autoimmune hepatitis.[29] Most of the patients described by Griffin and colleagues also had sicca symptoms, positive serologic tests for connective tissue disease, and positive Schirmer tests at the time of presentation to the neurology clinic.[30]

TABLE 59-2 ■ Disorders of Posterior Root Ganglia

Autoimmune
Autoimmune chronic active hepatitis
Paraneoplastic syndrome
Sjögren syndrome
Idiopathic
Infectious
Epstein–Barr virus infection
Human immunodeficiency virus infection
Rickettsia conorii infection
Varicella zoster infection
Nutritional
Nicotinic acid deficiency
Pyridoxine deficiency
Vitamin E deficiency
Toxic
? Antibiotic-related
Cisplatin
Pyridoxine
Thalidomide

The posterior root ganglia of patients are infiltrated by T lymphocytes. IVIg and plasmapheresis have benefited some patients.[31,32]

An acute sensory neuronopathy syndrome characterized by the acute onset of widespread sensory symptoms, areflexia, impaired vibratory sensation, and gait ataxia has developed 4 to 12 days after initial antibiotic treatment for a febrile illness.[33] The underlying pathogenesis in such cases may be infectious, postinfectious, or toxic (related to antibiotic use).

Infectious causes of sensory neuronopathy are shown in Table 59-2. HIV infection may cause a sensory neuronopathy. T-cell infiltration of dorsal root ganglia has been found in patients with end-stage AIDS. Many of these patients also had pallor of the cervical portion of the gracile tract at autopsy, suggesting that a "dying-back" axonopathy occurs along with sensory neuron loss.[34]

Latent infection of the dorsal root ganglia occurs following primary varicella zoster virus infection. When cell-mediated immunity is compromised, reactivation of viral replication causes the clinical syndrome of herpes zoster. The elderly, transplant recipients, and HIV-positive patients are particularly vulnerable. The prodromal stage of herpes zoster includes fevers, dysesthesias, and malaise. Several days later, a vesicular eruption appears in a dermatomal distribution. Pathologically, there is intense inflammation of the dorsal root ganglia. Once the lesions become encrusted, they are no longer infectious. Approximately 3 percent of patients develop segmental paresis, perhaps from spread of the virus to the anterior horn cells. Most patients recover muscle strength with time.[35] Treatment during the early stages of infection includes acyclovir, valacyclovir, or famcyclovir. Postherpetic neuralgia may occur, particularly in the elderly. Tricyclic drugs or anticonvulsants are effective treatments, as discussed in Chapter 43.

A number of toxins and vitamin deficiencies cause sensory neuronopathy. Because many of these also cause an axonopathy, they are discussed later (pp. 1224–1225).

Hereditary sensory neuronopathy (hereditary sensory and autonomic neuropathy [HSAN]) is both genetically and phenotypically heterogeneous; some forms present with predominantly small-fiber involvement, whereas others have mixed small- and large-fiber involvement. There is variable involvement of the autonomic nervous system. Commercial genetic testing is available for some types.

PLEXOPATHY

Trauma and compression, including at childbirth, cause most plexus injuries; other causes include tumor infiltration, postirradiation injury, and infection. An autoimmune monophasic neuritis, often idiopathic but sometimes associated with diabetes mellitus, may involve portions of either the brachial or lumbosacral plexus.

Sports, motorcycle, and industrial accidents cause traction injury to the brachial plexus. If the arm is located at the side of the patient at the time of impact or is distracted away from the torso, the upper roots and plexus are preferentially injured. If the arm is elevated above the head, the lower trunks and roots are most vulnerable. Compression injury of the brachial or lumbosacral plexus may occur during surgery or coma or from mass lesions such as a hematoma or tumor.

Immune brachial plexopathy (brachial plexus neuritis, neuralgic amyotrophy, Parsonage–Turner syndrome) is an acute monophasic neuropathy that presents with severe shoulder pain accompanied by muscle weakness and atrophy. Both sporadic and hereditary forms exist. Proximal muscle groups are more commonly affected than distal ones; involvement may be either unilateral or bilateral. Sensory loss is mild. Ipsilateral diaphragmatic weakness sometimes occurs from phrenic nerve involvement. Nerve biopsy specimens have revealed perineurial thickening and perivascular inflammatory infiltrates.[36] Corticosteroids or IVIg, or both, have been used in treatment with anecdotally reported success, but controlled studies are needed.[37] Aggressive treatment to control pain is important. The prognosis is excellent, with 60 percent of patients recovering completely within 1 year and 80 percent within a few years.

Nondiabetic lumbosacral radiculoplexus neuropathy refers to a similar disorder that affects the lower extremities. As with immune brachial plexus neuropathy, pain is often the initial symptom. It may occur in the back, buttock, thigh, or leg. Proximal weakness is more common than distal weakness. In time, however, the weakness often becomes more diffuse in the limb, and bilateral involvement is common. Clinically, sensory deficits (despite the pain) tend to be relatively mild. Nerve biopsies have shown evidence of ischemic injury and epineurial perivascular inflammatory collections.[38] Some improvement in strength occurs with time but long-standing motor deficits are common. Case reports suggest a potential benefit of corticosteroids, plasmapheresis, or IVIg therapy, but no positive controlled trials have been published.[39] Diabetic lumbosacral radiculoplexopathy (proximal diabetic neuropathy; diabetic amyotrophy) is discussed in Chapter 19.

Breast and lung cancers are the two most common secondary neoplasms to infiltrate the brachial plexus. Gastrointestinal and genitourinary cancers, melanomas, and lymphomas may also metastasize to the brachial plexus. Colorectal cancer is the most common neoplasm to infiltrate the lumbosacral plexus, but uterine, prostate, and ovarian cancer may also do so; other neoplasms may spread to the lumbosacral plexus metastatically.

Radiation therapy that includes the plexus in the field (as for breast cancer) may produce delayed weakness, dysesthesias, and numbness in the affected limb (Chapter 28). Irradiation causes marked fibrosis of the nerve fibers, loss of myelin, and destruction of the vascular supply.[40] The period between the radiation treatment and onset of symptoms ranges from a few weeks to more than 30 years.[41] Paresthesias in the median-innervated digits are a common initial symptom. Subsequently, weakness of the intrinsic hand muscles develops. Prominent limb pain and a Horner syndrome suggest tumor involvement rather than radiation-induced injury, whereas the presence of fasciculation potentials and myokymia on needle EMG suggests radiation injury. Distinction of these two disorders is aided by MRI.

Patients with radiation-induced lumbosacral plexopathy have generally been treated for lymphoreticular, testicular, uterine, or ovarian cancer. Patients usually present with slowly progressive distal weakness; numbness or paresthesia is less common. Mild pain occurs in 50 percent of patients. The CSF protein concentration may be elevated. As with radiation-induced brachial plexopathy, the condition may stabilize, but patients are often disabled.

Finally, a lower motor neuron syndrome affecting the legs, with relatively intact sensation, may also occur following irradiation of the distal spinal cord and cauda equina. Patients generally received more than 40 Gy.[42] Pathologic examination of the cauda equina shows a vasculopathy of the proximal nerve roots. Although the condition eventually stabilizes, patients are usually left with significant disabilities. There is no treatment.

Neurogenic thoracic outlet syndrome occurs when an anomalous fibrous band between the first thoracic rib and a cervical rib or elongated transverse process on the seventh vertebral body exerts pressure on the first thoracic nerve root or the lower trunk of the brachial plexus. This leads to wasting and atrophy of the hand muscles, particularly of the thenar eminence, and intermittent pain and paresthesias of the inner arm and medial hand, including the fourth and fifth digits. Electrodiagnostic studies confirm the diagnosis. A chest x-ray may show the cervical rib or an elongated transverse process (Fig. 59-1); the fibrous band shows up as a radiolucency. MRI may be helpful in showing and localizing plexus involvement (Fig. 59-2). Treatment is surgical.

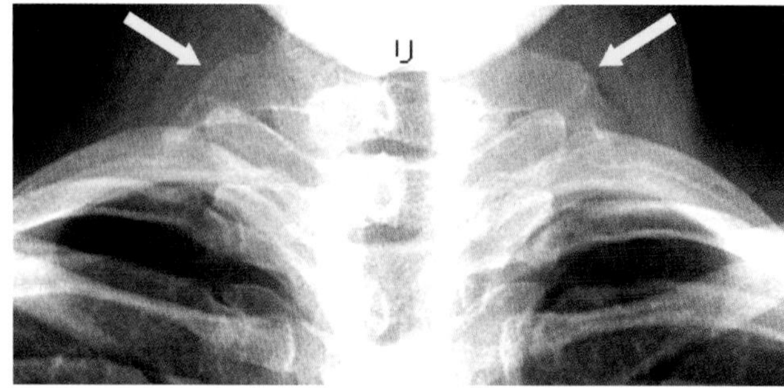

FIGURE 59-1 ▪ Chest radiograph of a 31-year-old right-handed woman with slowly progressive wasting and weakness of the left hand and numbness along the medial left forearm and hand. Bilateral cervical ribs are present (*arrows*). This finding may be associated with the neurogenic thoracic outlet syndrome. A fibrous band originating from the cervical rib compresses the inferior elements of the brachial plexus, leading to a wasted hand.

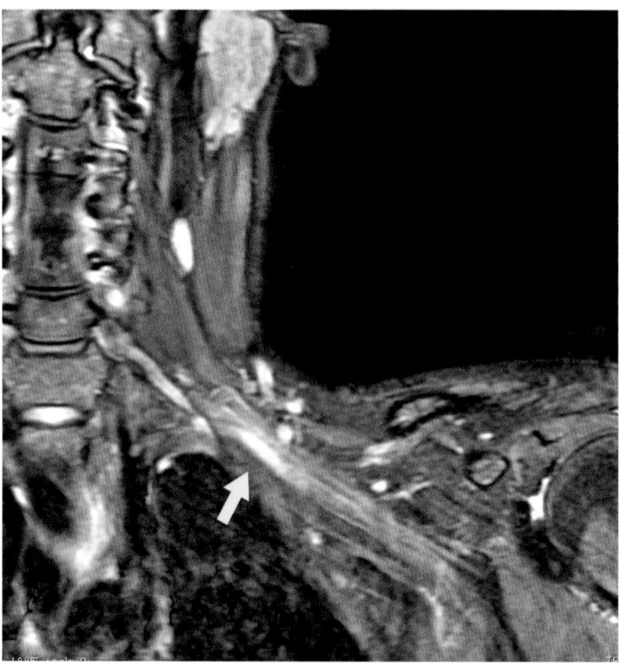

FIGURE 59-2 ▪ Coronal T2-weighted magnetic resonance image (MRI) of the left brachial plexus from the same patient as in Figure 59-1. There is increased signal in the left lower trunk (*arrow*), illustrating the usefulness of MRI for localizing nerve trunk lesions.

PERIPHERAL NEUROPATHY

The distribution of findings may suggest either a focal, multifocal, or generalized/symmetric pattern of nerve involvement. For the multifocal and generalized neuropathies in particular, identifying the relative involvement of motor and sensory fibers (Tables 59-3, 59-4, and 59-5) narrows the differential diagnosis. Sensory neuropathies may be further subdivided according to whether predominantly large- or small-diameter fibers are affected (Tables 59-4 and 59-5). Knowing whether the pathogenesis is predominantly axonal or demyelinating (Tables

TABLE 59-3 ■ Causes of Acquired Peripheral Neuropathy with Predominantly Motor Involvement

Inflammatory and Infectious
Chronic inflammatory demyelinating polyradiculoneuropathy
Guillain–Barré syndrome
Infectious mononucleosis
Multifocal motor neuropathy
Metabolic
Diabetic lumbosacral radiculoplexopathy (diabetic amyotrophy)
Porphyria
Neoplastic
Lymphoma
Toxic
Dapsone
Lead
Mercury
Nitrofurantoin
Organophosphates

TABLE 59-4 ■ Causes of Acquired Peripheral Neuropathy with Predominantly Large-Fiber Sensory Loss

Connective tissue disorder (especially Sjögren syndrome, systemic lupus erythematosus)
Diabetes mellitus
Monoclonal gammopathy
Nutritional
Vitamin B_{12} deficiency
Vitamin E deficiency
Pyridoxine deficiency
Paraneoplastic (associated with anti-Hu antibody)
Renal failure
Toxic
Cisplatin
Pyridoxine
Nitrous oxide
Glutethimide

59-6 and 59-7) also refines the diagnostic search. Generally, patients with axonal neuropathies present with predominantly sensory signs and symptoms, whereas patients with demyelinating neuropathies

TABLE 59-5 ■ Causes of Acquired Peripheral Neuropathy with Predominantly Small-Fiber Sensory Loss

Metabolic
Amyloidosis
Early diabetic polyneuropathy
Fabry disease
Renal failure
Tangier disease
Infective
Human immunodeficiency virus infection
Leprosy
Toxic
Arsenic
Chloramphenicol
Metronidazole
Thallium
Other
Sensory neuritis of Wartenberg
Sensory perineuritis

have more significant weakness. Given the exceptions to this rule, however, nerve conduction studies must be performed to distinguish between these two possibilities. Finally, the time course of symptom onset has important implications for pathogenesis (Table 59-8). Discussion here focuses on those peripheral neuropathies associated with systemic diseases.

Focal Neuropathy

A focal neuropathy may occur wherever ischemia, trauma, compression, injection, infection, or tumor infiltration affects the nerve. Focal *ischemic neuropathies* are uncommon following brief acute arterial occlusion. An exception to this rule is acute ischemic fibular (peroneal) neuropathy after thrombosis or embolism of the superficial femoral or popliteal arteries. The patient presents with a cool, pulseless distal lower extremity, sudden pain in the calf or foot, and footdrop. The nerve's susceptibility is related to the common occurrence of a single arterial feeder at the lateral aspect of the knee. Once circulation is restored, recovery may take weeks but is often good. Arterial insufficiency may lead to chronic ischemic

TABLE 59-6 ■ Acquired Symmetric Length-Dependent Axonal Polyneuropathy Associated with Systemic Disease

Drugs
Amiodarone
Chemotherapeutic agents (Adriamycin doxorubicin., Taxol paclitaxel., vincristine)
Dapsone
Disulfiram
Hydralazine
Isoniazid
Metronidazole
Nitrofurantoin
Phenytoin
Tricyclic antidepressants
Endocrine
Acromegaly
Diabetes mellitus
Hypothyroidism
Infectious
Hepatitis B
HIV infection
Lyme disease
Mononucleosis
Tick paralysis
Metabolic
Critical illness
Hyperglycemia
Hypoglycemia
Hypophosphatemia
Renal failure
Neoplastic and Paraneoplastic
Amyloidosis
Leukemia
Lymphoma
Monoclonal gammopathy
Small-cell lung cancer
Nutritional
Deficiency of vitamin B_1, B_6, B_{12}, or E or of copper
Vitamin B_6 intoxication
Toxins
Acrylamide
Alcohol
Arsenic
Carbon disulfide
Industrial toxins
Lead
Mercury
Methylbutyl ketone
Thallium
Triorthocresylphosphate
Trauma
Cold
Mechanical
Radiation

TABLE 59-7 ■ Acquired Demyelinating Neuropathy Associated with Systemic Diseases

Acute
Acute arsenic poisoning
Diphtheria
Guillain–Barré syndrome
Subacute and Chronic
Chronic inflammatory demyelinating polyradiculoneuropathy
Monoclonal gammopathy
Monoclonal gammopathy of undetermined significance
Multiple myeloma
Cryoglobulinemia
Waldenström macroglobulinemia
POEMS syndrome (osteosclerotic myeloma)
Lymphoma
Lymphoproliferative disorder
After allogenic stem-cell transplant for malignancy
Toxins
n-Hexane
Tacrolimus

neuropathies. Brachial artery to cephalic vein shunts placed for hemodialysis have been associated with median, ulnar, and radial neuropathies. A vascular steal syndrome seems to be a major mechanism of nerve injury, but direct compression of nerves and distal limb edema may also play a role.

Benign *tumors* of nerves (schwannomas and meningiomas) usually present as sporadic, solitary tumors with or without neurologic signs or symptoms. In a patient with multiple such lesions, however, neurofibromatosis should be suspected. An enlarging lesion or the development or progression of neurologic signs should raise suspicion of malignant transformation.

The common *entrapment* neuropathies—median neuropathy at the wrist, ulnar neuropathy at the elbow, and fibular (peroneal) neuropathy at the fibular head—share anatomic factors that increase the susceptibility of the nerve to injury; these factors include superficial nerve location, adjacent bony structures, and enclosure by nonelastic connective tissues. External compression of nerves generally causes focal demyelination before significant axonal loss.

Various medical conditions contribute to carpal tunnel syndrome (CTS; median nerve entrapment

TABLE 59-8 ■ Cause of Peripheral Neuropathy in Relation to Onset and Time Course

Acute Onset (Hours to Days)
Compression
Diphtheria
Guillain–Barré syndrome
HIV infection
Ischemia
Lyme disease
Porphyria
Tick paralysis
Toxic (e.g., arsenic)
West Nile virus infection
Subacute Onset (Weeks to Months)
Infectious
Inflammatory and immune disorders
Metabolic
Nutritional
Paraneoplastic
Toxic
Chronic (Years)
Amyloidosis
Chronic inflammatory demyelinating polyradiculoneuropathy
Diabetes mellitus
Hereditary neuropathy
Monoclonal gammopathy
Monophasic
Guillain–Barré syndrome
Herpes zoster
Inflammatory ganglionopathy
Single toxic exposure
Relapsing
Hereditary neuropathy with liability to pressure palsy
Inflammatory and immune disorders (chronic inflammatory demyelinating polyradiculoneuropathy, monoclonal gammopathy, connective tissue disorders)
Porphyria
Refsum disease
Repeated toxic exposure

at the wrist), the most common compressive neuropathy. Diabetes mellitus is a major risk factor, with one study showing a morbidity ratio of 2.5 for diabetic men and 2.3 for diabetic women.[43] The pathogenesis of CTS in this context may relate to chronic endoneurial hypoxia and changes in the connective tissues of the nerve sheath or transverse carpal ligament.[44] Hypothyroidism and acromegaly are also associated with CTS. In acromegaly, edema of synovial tissues may cause nerve compression. In pregnancy (Chapter 31), edema and weight gain contribute to increased pressure in the carpal tunnel. Rheumatoid arthritis is the most important inflammatory condition associated with CTS. Rheumatoid nodules, wrist deformity, and tenosynovitis are all contributory factors. When CTS accompanies a distal symmetric polyneuropathy in a nondiabetic patient, amyloidosis should be considered. If such patients undergo carpal tunnel surgery, fat and ligament tissue should be sent to pathology for analysis for possible amyloid deposition. Other risk factors for CTS include female gender, ganglion cysts, lipomas, nonspecific tenosynovitis, gout, sarcoidosis, multiple myeloma, aromatase inhibitors, and hereditary neuropathy with liability to pressure palsies. Repetitive hand motions in certain occupations may also be contributory. Conservative management of CTS includes the nocturnal use of wrist splints to prevent wrist flexion or extension (which reduces pressure within the carpal tunnel) or oral or injected corticosteroids. For severe neuropathies or for those in whom conservative measures have failed, surgical release of the carpal tunnel is effective.

The evaluation and management of the other common entrapment neuropathies are discussed in standard neurologic texts.

Multifocal Neuropathy

Most multifocal neuropathies are immune mediated or infectious (Table 59-9). The immune-mediated forms may be idiopathic, triggered by an infection or toxin/medication, or associated with diabetes mellitus. The most severe presentation is the acute and catastrophic appearance of multiple mononeuropathies (mononeuritis multiplex) caused by systemic vasculitis.

Vasculitic Neuropathy

Vasculitic neuropathy is an ischemic neuropathy caused by obliteration of the nerve's nutrient blood

TABLE 59-9 ■ Causes of Multifocal Neuropathy

Infection
Diffuse infiltrative lymphocytosis syndrome
Herpes zoster
Human immunodeficiency virus infection
Leprosy
Lyme disease
Syphilis
Tuberculosis
Ischemia
Vasculitic neuropathy
Systemic necrotizing vasculitis
Vasculitis associated with connective tissue diseases (rheumatoid arthritis, Sjögren syndrome, systemic lupus erythematosus)
Vasculitis associated with infections (hepatitis B and C, HIV)
Medication-induced vasculitis
Nonsystemic vasculitic neuropathy
Diabetes mellitus (diabetic lumbosacral radiculoplexus neuropathy, diabetic mononeuropathies)
Idiopathic Immune-Mediated Neuropathy
Idiopathic brachial plexopathy
Graft-versus-host disease
Multifocal acquired demyelinating sensory and motor neuropathy (Lewis–Sumner syndrome)
Multifocal motor neuropathy
Sarcoidosis
Sensory neuritis of Wartenberg
Sensory perineuritis
Multiple Compressions and Entrapments
Amyloidosis
Neurolymphomatosis
Rheumatologic conditions
Trauma
Tumors
Genetic Conditions
Hereditary neuropathy with liability to pressure palsy
Porphyria

vessels by inflammatory infiltrates. It usually presents as a subacutely evolving, asymmetric, painful sensory or sensorimotor neuropathy. Often, the deficits are in the distribution of multiple individual nerves (mononeuropathy multiplex). Nerves in the lower extremities are often affected first, but any nerve may be involved. Over time in untreated patients, as additional nerves become injured, motor and sensory deficits may become confluent, thereby mimicking a polyneuropathy. Sometimes, as in the case of cryoglobulinemic vasculitic neuropathy, the initial presentation of a vasculitic neuropathy is symmetric.

Neuropathy may occur with primary vasculitis, in which the underlying cause is not known, or secondary vasculitis, in which the causative factor is identified. The primary systemic vasculitides are classified according to size of the damaged blood vessels, organs involved, and the suspected immunopathologic mechanisms at play. Polyarteritis nodosa, microscopic polyangiitis, Wegener granulomatosis, and Churg–Strauss syndrome are the primary systemic vasculitides most commonly associated with vasculitic neuropathies.[45,46] The most common vasculitic neuropathy is an idiopathic form similar to polyarteritis nodosa and microscopic polyangiitis but without overt systemic involvement, called nonsystemic vasculitic neuropathy.[47] Because these patients do not have a defined connective tissue or other systemic disease, the diagnosis is established by nerve biopsy. Most of these patients have an elevated erythrocyte sedimentation rate, and a minority are anemic with peripheral leukocytosis and thrombocytosis. Secondary vasculitis may be associated with connective tissue diseases, infections, neoplasms, medications, or toxins.

Given the broad differential diagnosis of vasculitic neuropathy, the laboratory evaluation is extensive and often includes a complete blood count and erythrocyte sedimentation rate; examination for antinuclear antibodies, rheumatoid factor, antineutrophil cytoplasmic antibodies, complement levels, and hepatitis B and C serologies; urinalysis with microscopic analysis; and renal and hepatic function tests. The work-up may also include an HIV antibody test, chest x-ray, and Lyme antibody studies. An electrodiagnostic study is essential to document the multifocal nature of the axon loss. A nerve biopsy is often necessary for diagnosis. For the systemic vasculitides, the diagnostic yield is increased if biopsy is performed on both the nerve and muscle.[48,49]

The systemic vasculitides are often fatal if untreated, so aggressive immunosuppression with combined corticosteroids and cyclophosphamide is usually indicated. When vasculitis is caused by drugs, removal of the offending agent often leads to benefit. For vasculitis associated with chronic viral infections, treatment often includes antiviral therapy or removal of viral antigens by plasmapheresis.

Hepatitis B

Approximately one-third of cases of polyarteritis nodosa are associated with hepatitis B infection.[50] More than 80 percent of patients with hepatitis B–associated polyarteritis nodosa have a neuropathy.[50] Although the clinical features may be indistinguishable from classic polyarteritis nodosa, the disease manifestations of hepatitis B–associated vasculitis may be more severe. Immune complex deposition is thought to be the main immunopathologic mechanism.

Treatment of hepatitis B–related vasculitic neuropathy is specialized. Although immunosuppressive therapies lead to increased viral replication, two retrospective studies suggest that a short course of corticosteroids is beneficial.[51] Following the steroid therapy, either interferon-α or lamivudine may be used for at least 6 months. Plasma exchanges are usually given concurrently over a 10-week period to clear the immune complexes. Relapses are uncommon.

Hepatitis C

A minority of patients with hepatitis C virus (HCV) infection develop a peripheral neuropathy, sometimes associated with cryoglobulinemia. As cryoglobulinemia can cause a vasculitic neuropathy with more severe neurologic deficits, the following discussion focuses on it.

HCV is the most common cause of essential mixed cryoglobulinemia, which occurs in about one-third of patients with HCV; a cryoglobulinemic neuropathy only occurs in 2 to 3 percent of patients.[52,53] Other manifestations of cryoglobulinemia include edema, palpable purpura, and membranoproliferative glomerulonephritis. The cryoglobulinemia results from an oligoclonal expansion of B-lymphocytes.[54] Most cryoglobulinemic neuropathies are distal, axonal, and symmetric with predominantly sensory deficits. Mononeuropathies, either single or multiple, may also occur. Rarely, patients with cryoglobulinemia may develop demyelinating polyneuropathies associated with IgM binding to myelin.[55]

The best treatment strategy for HCV-associated cryoglobulinemic neuropathy is not known but mild neuropathies are often treated with pegylated interferon-α2b (INF-α) plus ribavirin. The INF-α may occasionally exacerbate a vasculitic neuropathy or produce a new multifocal neuropathy.[56] For severe neuropathies refractory to INF-α, immunosuppression with corticosteroids combined with cyclophosphamide or plasmapheresis should be considered. Another treatment option for patients refractory to INF-α is administration of monoclonal anti-CD20 antibodies (rituximab).[57]

Other Infections

Any organism can produce a vasculitis if it elicits either circulating or in situ immune complexes.[58] CMV and herpes zoster are the only two infections known to infect endothelial cells of peripheral nerve blood vessels.[59,60]

HIV infection (Chapter 44) may rarely cause a systemic vasculitis.[61] It usually occurs in the early symptomatic stage of the disease. Multiple patterns of nerve involvement have been described, including mononeuropathy, mononeuritis multiplex, cranial neuropathies, distal symmetric polyneuropathy, and asymmetric polyneuropathy. The possibility of CMV vasculitis must be excluded in this patient population. In CMV-negative cases, nerve biopsy samples show a necrotizing vasculitis that may involve the endoneurial vessels in addition to the epineurial vessels. Other causes of multifocal neuropathies in HIV patients include neurolymphomatosis and diffuse infiltrative lymphocytosis syndrome.[62]

Idiopathic Immune-Mediated Multifocal Neuropathy

Immune-mediated multifocal neuropathies exist in which the target of the immunologic attack is the myelin or axon rather than the blood vessels. These entities include multifocal motor neuropathy, Lewis–Sumner syndrome (or multifocal acquired demyelinating sensory and motor neuropathy [MADSAM]), sensory perineuritis, and migratory sensory neuropathy of Wartenberg. In some cases, there is overlap between these neuropathies and Guillain–Barré syndrome (GBS) and chronic inflammatory demyelinating polyneuropathy (CIDP). Because GBS and CIDP are usually associated with generalized weakness, however, they are discussed separately in a later section.

Multifocal motor neuropathy is important to recognize because it can superficially mimic motor neuron disease, and attention here is focused on this disorder. Patients typically present with painless wasting, weakness, and sometimes fasciculations of the distal upper-extremity muscle groups, although any muscle group may be affected, even the tongue.[63] Careful examination reveals that weakness occurs in a peripheral nerve rather than segmental pattern. Upper motor neuron signs are not present. Patients may complain of mild sensory symptoms such as numbness or paresthesia, but the sensory examination is typically normal. Reflexes tend to be depressed only in regions of weakness. Nerve conduction studies usually reveal conduction block in motor nerves along with normal sensory nerve conduction responses.[64,65] Many patients have elevated titers to GM1 ganglioside.[66]

IVIg is the most effective therapy for multifocal motor neuropathy, with approximately 80 percent of patients responding to it. Its efficacy has been confirmed by multiple randomized, placebo-controlled trials. Other agents that may improve or stabilize the disease include subcutaneous immunoglobulin,[67] cyclophosphamide, azathioprine, rituximab, and interferon-β.[68] Mycophenolate mofetil did not have an IVIg-sparing effect in a randomized, controlled trial.[69] Although a few patients have been reported to respond to prednisone, it is usually ineffective or may cause an exacerbation of weakness. Plasmapheresis is usually not effective.

SARCOIDOSIS

Neurosarcoidosis is discussed in Chapter 49, to which the reader is referred.

INFECTIOUS NEUROPATHY

Lyme disease and leprosy are important causes of multifocal neuropathy and are discussed separately in Chapters 40 and 42.

Polyneuropathy

The medical disorders discussed in this section cause generalized and symmetric neuropathies. In axonal neuropathies, the sensory and motor deficits are usually length dependent such that the deficits are most severe in the feet. With long-term disease, a classic stocking-glove neuropathy occurs, with or without autonomic involvement. In demyelinating polyneuropathies, however, the weakness may involve proximal and distal muscle groups more equally.

ENDOCRINE NEUROPATHY

Diabetic Polyneuropathy

As discussed in Chapter 19, diabetes mellitus may be associated with both generalized and focal neuropathies. The focal neuropathies include lumbosacral radiculoplexus neuropathy (diabetic amyotrophy; proximal diabetic neuropathy), thoracolumbar neuropathy, entrapment neuropathies, and cranial neuropathies. The generalized neuropathies include distal symmetric sensory or sensorimotor polyneuropathy, acute painful neuropathy, autonomic neuropathy, and acute motor neuropathy.

Approximately 50 percent of diabetics develop a distal symmetric sensorimotor polyneuropathy.[70] Risk factors for polyneuropathy include degree of hyperglycemia, duration of diabetes, age, hypertension, hypertriglyceridemia, and smoking. The association between prediabetes and polyneuropathy is a subject of active debate. A number of investigators have found an increased prevalence of impaired glucose tolerance in patients with idiopathic neuropathy.[71] However, a careful controlled case-control study of patients with idiopathic neuropathy did not show a significant association between prediabetes and neuropathy.[72]

Early symptoms include distal numbness, burning dysesthesias, and allodynia in the feet or toes. Although discomfort is present throughout the day, it often worsens at night or with rest. Cramps are common in the calves and foot muscles. Treatment consists of tight glycemic control, which helps to prevent and slow the progression of the polyneuropathy.[73] Large-scale controlled trials of aldose reductase inhibitors and nerve growth factor in the treatment of diabetic neuropathy have yielded disappointing results.[74,75] Controlled trials of intravenous and oral preparations of the antioxidant α-lipoic acid have demonstrated its benefit on neuropathy signs and pain.[76,77]

Other Neuropathies

Hypothyroidism is a common cause of median neuropathy at the wrist (CTS). Myxedematous tissue beneath the flexor retinaculum is thought to cause median nerve compression. Hypothyroidism may also cause a polyneuropathy that presents with distal dysesthesias and stocking-and-glove sensory loss. Reflexes may be diminished with a delayed relaxation phase. Electrodiagnostic and pathologic studies have shown mixed axonal and demyelinating features. Considerable improvement may occur in both CTS and hypothyroid polyneuropathy following replacement therapy.

Acromegaly may cause entrapment neuropathies due to connective tissue hyperplasia and bony overgrowth. A sensorimotor polyneuropathy may also occur associated with hypertrophic, sometimes palpable, nerves.

INFECTIOUS NEUROPATHY

HIV Neuropathy

As discussed in Chapter 44, HIV infection is associated with both acute and chronic, multifocal or generalized polyneuropathies. These include mononeuritis multiplex from vasculitic neuropathy, GBS, CIDP, and distal sensory polyneuropathy. Of all these neuropathies, distal sensory polyneuropathy is by far the most common, occurring in at least 50 percent of patients with advanced HIV.[78] In the era before combination antiretroviral therapy, reduced $CD4^+$ lymphocyte cell counts and increased HIV viral loads increased the risk and severity of HIV polyneuropathy. Dideoxynucleoside antiretrovrials also increase the risk of neuropathy, possibly because of toxicity to mitochondria. A polyneuropathy (usually symmetric) may occur as part of the diffuse infiltrative lymphomatosis syndrome.[62]

Patients typically present with burning dysesthesia in feet and ankles, often with prominent allodynia. On examination, small-fiber sensory modalities are affected predominantly. Weakness related to the neuropathy is uncommon, even in advanced cases. There is no specific treatment, although a number of symptomatic treatments for neuropathic pain, including gabapentin, amitriptyline, tramadol, and lamotrigine, are effective.

Other Neuropathies

HCV infection and leprosy may cause generalized and symmetric peripheral nerve involvement, as is discussed earlier in this chapter and elsewhere in this volume.

IMMUNE-MEDIATED NEUROPATHY

Guillain–Barré Syndrome

Once used interchangeably with the label *acute inflammatory demyelinating polyneuropathy*, GBS now encompasses any acute, idiopathic inflammatory polyneuropathy producing progressive muscle weakness and areflexia, regardless of whether the underlying neuropathy is demyelinating or axonal. In many cases, a respiratory or gastrointestinal illness precedes the onset of neurologic symptoms by 1 to 3 weeks. Often paresthesias in the distal limbs herald the onset of the neuropathy. Pain similar to sciatica, myalgia, or a cramp may also occur. Rapidly progressive, symmetric weakness soon follows. Typically the weakness starts in the legs, but it may begin in the arms or face. Symptoms may progress acutely over just a few days or subacutely over as long as 4 weeks. The degree of weakness at the nadir of the progressive phase is highly variable, from mild weakness to quadriplegia with respiratory failure. Maximum deficits occur within 1 month, followed by a plateau lasting for days to weeks and rarely months. Gradual improvement occurs after the plateau phase. Prognosis is good, with a 5 percent mortality rate. Permanent disabilities remain in 5 to 10 percent of patients, mild deficits in 65 to 75 percent, and no deficit in 15 percent. The annual incidence is 1 to 2 cases per 100,000 population.

The initial assessment of GBS patients should include measurements of respiratory capacity and inspiratory force. Patients with a vital capacity of less than 20 ml/kg or a maximum inspiratory pressure less than 30 cmH_2O are likely to require mechanical ventilation.[79] These measurements are much more sensitive than arterial blood gas analysis for predicting incipient neuromuscular respiratory failure. Admission to the intensive care unit (ICU) is warranted for any patient with rapidly progressive disease, significant bulbar or facial weakness, or autonomic dysfunction. Motor findings typically outweigh sensory deficits. One-third of patients may develop facial diplegia. Stretch reflexes are hypoactive or absent.

Blood tests and a lumbar puncture should be undertaken to evaluate for other causes of acute polyneuropathy or polyradiculopathy. In 50 percent of patients, an initial CSF sample will reveal an elevated protein concentration; with subsequent analysis, 90 percent of samples show increased protein, with values ranging from 55 to 250 mg/dl. The CSF is usually acellular with normal pressure. If more than 10 white cells/mm^3 are present, alternative diagnoses should be considered. Nerve conduction studies commonly show evidence of a polyneuropathy, usually demyelinating, but are sometimes normal when the patient first presents.

In Western societies, GBS is usually a demyelinating polyradiculoneuropathy. A number of infections may trigger GBS, including CMV, Epstein–Barr virus, herpesvirus, *Campylobacter jejuni*, *Mycoplasma pneumoniae*, and HIV. Rabies and swine flu vaccinations, recent surgery, and pregnancy have also been implicated as triggers for GBS. Both humoral immune responses and T-cell activation are thought to play roles in the pathogenesis. Pathologically, there is the early appearance of lymphocytes surrounding nerve vessels. This is followed by demyelination. Secondary "bystander" axonal degeneration may also occur.

In northern China, the most common GBS subtype is an *acute motor axonal neuropathy* (AMAN) associated with *C. jejuni* infection. These patients often have antibodies to gangliosides, including GM1, GD1a, and GD1b. The strains of *C. jejuni* associated with AMAN have GM1-like epitopes in their lipopolysaccharide membranes that contain a Gal(b1–3) GalNac moiety.[80] Terminal motor axon branches and the internode axonolemma also contain a high concentration of this moiety. Because of molecular mimicry between these bacterial and axon antigens, those portions of the motor axons appear to be the initial targets in the autoimmune attack.

There are several other variants of GBS. The most common, the *Miller Fisher syndrome*, accounts for about 5 percent of all cases of GBS. Patients develop the triad of ophthalmoplegia, ataxia, and areflexia, with varying degrees of limb weakness. Almost all cases of Miller Fisher syndrome are associated with IgG antibodies to GQ1b. Other variants include weakness without paresthesias or sensory loss, pharyngeal-cervical-brachial weakness, paraparesis, facial paresis with distal paresthesias, pure ataxia, acute pandysautonomia, and acute motor-sensory axonal neuropathy (AMSAN). All variants have in common absent or diminished stretch reflexes, elevated CSF protein concentrations, and electrodiagnostic abnormalities.

For severe cases, treatment includes support in the ICU and immune-modulatory therapy. Plasmapheresis or IVIg is effective in improving short- and long-term neurologic function.[81,82] The costs of plasmapheresis and IVIg are similar, and the relapse rate for IVIg is no different from that for plasmapheresis. Compared with plasmapheresis, IVIg is associated with fewer complications (e.g., hemodynamic fluctuations), is easier to administer, and is usually available in community hospitals where plasmapheresis may not be accessible. A combination of plasmapheresis followed immediately by IVIg does not lead to significantly better outcomes.[83]

Corticosteroids are not beneficial.[80]

Chronic Inflammatory Demyelinating Polyradiculoneuropathy

CIDP is a chronic neuropathy characterized by symmetric weakness, sensory loss, and depressed stretch reflexes. Weakness usually affects both proximal and distal muscle groups. The cranial nerves are rarely involved, but cranial neuropathies may be a presenting feature. A small percentage of patients have papilledema. The weakness must progresses beyond 2 months in order to meet an arbitrary criterion for the diagnosis of CIDP. The clinical course may be relapsing, progressive, or stepwise. There are a number of clinical variants of CIDP manifesting with either pure motor or sensory involvement or with evidence of only distal demyelination. CIDP may occur with certain medical disorders, including monoclonal gammopathies, inflammatory bowel disease, thyroid disease, HIV infection, diabetes mellitus, Charcot–Marie–Tooth neuropathies, and CNS demyelination.

The electrodiagnostic and pathologic features are similar to those of GBS. Lumbar puncture typically reveals an acellular CSF with an elevated protein level, but other laboratory tests are unremarkable. Nerve conduction studies confirm impaired nerve conduction velocities or the presence of conduction block caused by demyelination. Nerve biopsy is occasionally performed, and the findings include endoneurial perivascular inflammation with demyelination, remyelination (onion bulb formations), and secondary axonal degeneration.

Randomized, controlled trials have demonstrated the benefit of corticosteroids, plasmapheresis, and IVIg.[84–87] A crossover study demonstrated that plasmapheresis and IVIg are about equally effective.[88] The efficacy of IVIg for CIDP has also been confirmed. Azathioprine, cyclosporine, mycophenolate, and cyclophosphamide are sometimes reported to be beneficial but have not been tested in controlled clinical trials. Overall, most patients respond to treatment, but relapses are common. Only a minority of patients achieve a complete remission. Aggressive and early treatment is warranted because unchecked disease may eventually lead to axon loss and muscle atrophy for which there is no specific treatment.

Polyneuropathy Associated with Monoclonal Gammopathy of Undetermined Significance

A monoclonal gammopathy of undetermined significance (MGUS) may present as a symmetric sensorimotor polyneuropathy with variable proportions of axonal or myelin injury. The prevalence of MGUS is 1 to 3 percent in people older than 50 years. Only a minority of those with MGUS ever develop a clinically significant neuropathy, the precise number varying in different series and depending on which heavy chain is involved. Compared with neuropathy patients having IgA and IgG MGUS, patients with IgM MGUS have more sensory ataxia and more evidence of demyelination on electrodiagnostic studies. Specific antibodies can sometimes be found to myelin-specific proteins. The CSF is acellular but the protein concentration is often elevated.

Generally, neuropathies associated with MGUS respond less well to immunosuppressive or immunomodulatory therapy than idiopathic CIDP. IgG and IgA MGUS neuropathies respond better than IgM MGUS neuropathies to plasmapheresis. Improvement has also been documented with rituximab, fludarabine, and alkylating agents.[89] Some patients have responded to IFN-α and IVIg. Long-term studies to determine the relationship between between specific immunologic markers and disease recurrence will help to develop targeted therapies.[90]

Critical Illness Polyneuropathy

More than 50 percent of critically ill patients with sepsis and multiorgan disease fail to wean from ventilatory support. Examination in moderately advanced cases reveals flaccid, symmetric weakness, depressed or absent tendon reflexes, and impaired distal sensation. Other causes of weakness in the ICU setting include prolonged neuromuscular blockade from drugs, critical illness myopathy, and cervical myelopathy. CSF protein level is normal or only mildly elevated. Electrodiagnostic studies confirm the presence of a sensorimotor polyneuropathy. Treatment is supportive. The prognosis is variable, depending on the degree of axon loss. A more complete account of this disorder is provided in Chapter 56.

Uremic Neuropathy

Uremic polyneuropathy presents as restless legs, weakness, cramps, and distal paresthesias and dysesthesias in patients with end-stage renal disease (serum creatinine levels of 5 mg/dl or higher). The prevalence among patients undergoing hemodialysis treatment is 50 to 60 percent. Electrodiagnostic studies typically show evidence of distal axon loss with some evidence of demyelination. Usually the neuropathy is slowly progressive, but rapidly progressive uremic neuropathy with prominent demyelinating features has been described.[91] Renal transplantation is the best treatment for uremic polyneuropathy. Further details are provided in Chapter 16.

Neoplastic and Paraneoplastic Neuropathies

Monoclonal Gammopathy

Multiple myeloma, Waldenström macroglobulinemia, osteosclerotic myeloma (POEMS syndrome of polyneuropathy, organomegaly, endocrinopathy, M protein, and skin changes), lymphoma, and leukemia are associated with a monoclonal gammopathy. Generally, symptoms and signs are similar to those of polyneuropathy related to an MGUS. Frequently, these neuropathies are associated with significant distal weakness and some demyelinating features on nerve conduction studies.[92]

Amyloidosis

Amyloidosis causes a slowly progressive distal sensorimotor polyneuropathy. Distal lower-extremity pain and paresthesias are common presenting symptoms. On examination, there is usually greater impairment of small- than large-fiber sensory function. Autonomic neuropathy frequently occurs, leading to orthostatic lightheadedness, diarrhea, bladder dysfunction, and impotence. CTS is also common.

In primary amyloidosis, the amyloid fibrils consist of portions of monoclonal immunoglobulin light chains (Bence Jones protein). In almost all these patients, a monoclonal protein may be detected in either the serum or urine. Diagnosis depends on identifying amyloid deposition in tissues. An abdominal fat aspirate is probably the best initial step for establishing the diagnosis; the diagnostic yield is more than 70 percent. If this is negative, a rectal or nerve biopsy may be considered. By suppressing monoclonal light-chain production, alkylating agents extend survival in patients with primary amyloidosis. Autologous peripheral blood stem-cell transplantation is also available, but has a high morbidity and mortality. In familial amyloidosis, the fibrils are usually composed of mutant transthyretin. Molecular genetic testing for transthyretin mutations is a sensitive diagnostic test. Orthotopic liver transplantation is an effective treatment.

Paraneoplastic Neuropathy

Patients with anti-Hu (ANNA-1) antibodies usually present with a sensory neuropathy, but about 25 percent of patients present with a subacute sensorimotor polyneuropathy.[25,28,93] Rarely, the associated neuropathy is acute, thereby mimicking GBS. Most of these patients have small-cell lung carcinoma.

Peripheral neuropathy occurs as a feature of paraneoplastic syndromes associated with anti-CV2 antibody in about 50 percent of cases.[94] Usually it is a mixed axonal and demyelinating sensorimotor polyneuropathy, but a pure sensory neuropathy may also occur. Rarely, sensorimotor neuropathies have been described with anti-Ri (ANNA-2) and anti-Yo (PCA-1) antibodies.

NUTRITIONAL NEUROPATHY

Vitamin B_1 (Thiamine) Deficiency

Thiamine deficiency is uncommon in industrialized countries. Inadequate consumption may occur in the context of chronic alcohol abuse, total parenteral nutrition, prolonged vomiting, and bariatric surgery. Initial neuropathic symptoms (dry beriberi) include burning dysesthesias in the feet with mild sensory loss. Fatigue, muscle aches, and cramps in the lower extremities are common. Although progression is usually subacute to chronic, the neuropathy sometimes develops over a few days. In severe cases, there may be significant weakness of ankle dorsiflexion and finger and wrist extension in addition to stocking-glove sensory deficits. The recurrent laryngeal nerve may become involved, causing hoarseness. With thiamine supplementation, the neuropathy typically improves, albeit modestly. Further details are provided in Chapter 15.

Vitamin B_6 (Pyridoxine) Deficiency

Deficiency of vitamin B_6 (pyridoxine) causes a distal axonal sensorimotor polyneuropathy. It is a known complication of taking the prescription medications isoniazid and hydralazine. If these medications are prescribed, oral supplementation of vitamin B_6 at daily doses of 50 to 100 mg is advised. Vitamin B_6 deficiency may also occur with chronic peritoneal dialysis or alcoholism.[95]

Overdosing with vitamin B_6 may cause an ataxic sensory neuronopathy associated with degeneration of posterior root ganglia neurons. Stretch reflexes are hypoactive or globally absent. Most patients have numbness, paresthesia, and gait ataxia. Daily ingestion of as little as 200 mg per day has been associated with the development of a peripheral neuropathy in some instances.

Vitamin B_{12} (Cobalamin) Deficiency

The classic neurologic presentation of vitamin B_{12} deficiency is combined degeneration of the dorsal and lateral columns of the spinal cord. Patients present with distal numbness, paresthesias, and, occasionally, dysesthesias. Compared with patients with idiopathic distal polyneuropathy, patients with vitamin B_{12} deficiency are more likely to have concomitant involvement of the upper and lower extremities, initial symptom onset in the hands, and a sudden onset of symptoms.[96] In more advanced cases, paraparesis occurs with extensor plantar responses. Malabsorption is the cause of most cases; it may be due to pernicious anemia, gastric or bowel surgery, or inflammatory bowel disease. Neurologic manifestations of vitamin B_{12} deficiency may occur without anemia or elevated mean corpuscular volume. Testing for elevations of serum homocysteine and methylmalonic acid is helpful when the vitamin B_{12} level is borderline low. With early treatment, the paresthesias may improve, but loss of large-fiber sensory axons is often permanent. Traditionally, vitamin B_{12} is supplemented with weekly to monthly intramuscular injections. Because individuals with pernicious anemia still absorb small amounts of vitamin B_{12}, oral supplementation at a dose of 1,000 to 2,000 μg daily may be equally effective.[97]

Vitamin E Deficiency

Vitamin E deficiency presents as a spinocerebellar ataxia with polyneuropathy. It usually results from lipid malabsorption; errors of vitamin E absorption or transport are less common causes.[98] Pathologically, there is degeneration of sensory axons, posterior root ganglia, posterior columns, and spinocerebellar tracts. The diagnosis is made by measuring serum α-tocopherol levels. Proper supplementation depends on the underlying cause of the deficiency.

Copper Deficiency

Copper deficiency has been associated with a myeloneuropathy characterized clinically by limb paresthesia and spastic paraparesis.[99,100] Patients have deficits of large-fiber sensation, and many have extensor plantar responses. Often patients have microcytic anemia and neutropenia. Many patients have had prior gastric surgery. Some cases have been linked to excessive zinc levels, which are known to cause copper deficiency. Following copper supplementation, some patients show neurologic improvement.

Toxic Neuropathy

Alcoholic Neuropathy

A distal axonal polyneuropathy is a common complication of chronic alcoholism, occurring in approximately 10 to 50 percent of patients, depending on the study and diagnostic criteria.[101,102] Superficial sensation is principally impaired and dysesthesias are common. Pathologically, there is loss of sensory and motor axons. The pathophysiology is not fully understood but may involve direct toxicity of alcohol on peripheral nerves; vitamin deficiencies, including thiamine deficiency, are probable contributing factors. Treatment involves abstinence and vitamin supplementation. Prognosis is good for mild to moderate neuropathy after 3 to 5 years of abstinence. Further details are provided in Chapter 33.

Neuropathies Associated with Heavy Metal Exposure

Severe lead poisoning produces a subacute, asymmetric, predominantly motor neuropathy that preferentially affects the wrist and finger extensors. Footdrop is another common manifestation. Prognosis for recovery is good if the lead exposure is eliminated. Abdominal pain, anemia, encephalopathy, and mild sensory deficits may also occur.

Arsenic ingestion typically causes acute abdominal pain followed in 5 to 10 days by dysesthesias in the hands and feet. This is followed by an axonal polyneuropathy presenting as symmetric ascending weakness. The weakness may progress over several weeks. Recovery depends on the degree of axonal loss.

Additional details about the neurologic complications of heavy metal exposure are given in Chapter 35.

Medications and other Chemicals

Medications and chemicals generally cause a subacutely progressive symmetric, distal, and length-dependent neuropathy, with sensory and motor axonal degeneration. A careful review of occupational exposures to toxins as well as exposures related to hobbies usually leads to candidate toxins. If the exposure is terminated, the neuropathy may continue to worsen for days to weeks ("coasting") before its course is arrested. A number of toxins have been incriminated (Table 59-6 and Chapter 35).

Hereditary Neuropathy

Hereditary neuropathy typically presents with slowly progressive distal weakness and numbness. Examination of the feet may reveal pes cavus and hammertoes, features reflecting long-standing atrophy and weakness of the intrinsic foot muscles. Only those hereditary neuropathies with prominent systemic manifestations are discussed here.

Adrenomyeloneuropathy

Adrenomyeloneuropathy is a milder phenotype of adrenoleukodystrophy, the X-linked disease associated with degeneration of white matter and the adrenal cortex caused by mutations of the *ABCD1* gene. Adrenomyeloneuropathy may present from childhood to middle age, usually in men, but occasionally in women. Patients present with a spastic paraparesis, sphincter abnormalities, and sexual dysfunction with or without symptomatic adrenal insufficiency or cognitive problems. The neuropathy is responsible for weakness and depressed ankle reflexes. Nerve conduction studies typically have shown a mixed axonal and demyelinating polyneuropathy. Testing for very-long-chain fatty acids is the initial diagnostic test for both males and females. Bone marrow transplantation is an effective treatment for those with MRI evidence of brain involvement and minimal neuropsychologic findings. Reduction of hexacosanoic acid by Lorenzo's oil remains an investigational therapeutic approach for adrenoleukodystrophy.[103]

Fabry Disease

Fabry disease is an X-linked recessive disorder of the gene encoding α-galactosidase A. Deficiency of this lysosomal enzyme causes widespread accumulation of globotriaosylceramide (GL-3) in cells throughout the body. Males present in adolescence with crises of severe pain in the extremities, vascular cutaneous lesions (angiokeratomas), hypohidrosis, corneal and lenticular opacities, and proteinuria. Renal function gradually deteriorates over time, leading to end-stage renal disease. In middle age, cardiovascular and cerebrovascular disease is another cause of significant morbidity and mortality. Patients have a distal small-fiber polyneuropathy with normal nerve conduction velocities.[104] Pain may respond to phenytoin, carbamazepine, or gabapentin.[105] The diagnosis is usually made by demonstration of deficient α-galactosidase A activity in plasma, leukocytes, or cultured cells. Hemodialysis or renal transplantation is often necessary. An expert panel has recommended that enzyme replacement therapy be initiated as early as possible for all males and for females with significant disease.[106]

Porphyria

Inherited defects in the hepatic enzymes responsible for heme synthesis—the hepatic porphyrias—may be associated with acute episodes of CNS and peripheral nervous system dysfunction. These disorders include acute intermittent porphyria, hereditary coproporphyria, and variegate porphyria. The erythropoietic porphyrias are associated with photosensitivity but not neurologic disease. Between attacks, patients with hepatic porphyrias are normal. An attack is typically triggered by a drug that activates the hepatic cytochrome P-450 system, although hypoglycemia and hormonal factors may also contribute.

Clinically, patients present with acute, severe colicky abdominal pain accompanied by psychiatric disturbances. Often, medications used to treat pain and anxiety only exacerbate the attack by inducing certain hepatic enzymes. A painful, often asymmetric axonal neuropathy typically appears 2 to 3 days after the onset of abdominal pain. The weakness frequently begins in the upper extremities. Proximal or distal muscle groups may be involved. Reflexes are usually lost in proportion to weakness, unlike the early areflexia typically seen in GBS. Despite the pain, sensory deficits are usually mild and patchy. The combination of abdominal pain and neuropathy makes the clinical presentation similar to heavy metal intoxication.

Screening for the hepatic porphyrias involves an analysis of the heme precursors in urine. The results of the urinalysis may be normal in asymptomatic carriers. Treatment includes stopping all medications that could potentially exacerbate the attack and infusing heme. Although recovery from the psychiatric disturbances is typically rapid, recovery of the peripheral nerves depends on the severity and extent of the axon loss; ultimate recovery of the peripheral nervous system is generally good.

Refsum Disease

Refsum disease is an autosomal-recessive disorder characterized by anosmia, retinitis pigmentosa, deafness, ataxia, ichthyosis and neuropathy. Symptoms may begin at any age. Over 90 percent of cases are associated with mutations of the phytanoyl-CoA hydroxylase gene[107]; less than 10 percent are associated with mutations of the *PEX7* gene. The consequence of these mutations is a build-up of phytanic acid in various tissues. The presence of high levels of serum phytanic acid (>200 μmol/L) establishes the diagnosis. Phytanic acid deposition in Schwann cells and the endoneurial space leads to a distal, symmetric sensorimotor neuropathy. Reduction of phytanic acid concentrations by dietary restriction, plasmapheresis, or lipid apheresis improves ichthyosis, sensory neuropathy, and ataxia but may not benefit the retinitis pigmentosa, anosmia, and deafness.

Tangier Disease

Tangier disease is a rare autosomal-recessive disorder caused by mutations in both alleles of the adenosine triphosphate–binding cassette A1 gene (*ABCA1*). The protein deficiency causes decreased lipid removal from cells, widespread tissue accumulation of cholesteryl esters, and the absence of plasma high-density lipoproteins (HDLs).[108] Absent high-density lipoproteins with normal triglyceride level and the presence of enlarged orange tonsils differentiates Tangier disease from other lipoprotein disorders. Patients may develop corneal opacities or hypersplenism. Despite the high-density lipoprotein deficiency, atherosclerosis does not develop earlier than normal. Polyneuropathy may take one of three forms: asymmetric, relapsing-remitting sensorimotor mononeuropathies, usually associated with normal conduction velocities; symmetric, slowly progressive distal polyneuropathy; and a slowly progressive neuropathy affecting the face and upper limbs with distal hand weakness and facial diplegia and accompanied by dissociative sensory loss that may mimic the presentation of a syrinx. There is currently no specific treatment for Tangier disease.

NEUROMUSCULAR JUNCTION DISORDERS

In disorders of the neuromuscular junction (Table 59-10), patients present with weakness but not numbness. The congenital myasthenic syndromes are discussed elsewhere.

Botulism

Botulism is an acute paralytic illness caused by a toxin produced by *Clostridium* bacteria. Botulism results from (1) ingestion of the preformed toxin with absorption through the intestines, accounting for the vast majority of cases of adult food-borne botulism; (2) ingestion of clostridial spores that colonize the intestines and produce the toxin, accounting for virtually all forms of infant botulism and occurring rarely in adults with altered intestinal flora; or (3) infection of a wound, with local production and absorption of the toxin ("wound botulism").[109,110] Improperly preserved food is the most common cause of food-borne botulism. In California, wound botulism has become a recognized complication of intravenous "black tar" heroin use.[111] Botulism may occur in rare instances among patients treated with botulinum toxin for dystonia or other movement disorders.[112]

TABLE 59-10 ■ Disorders of the Neuromuscular Junction

Botulism
Congenital myasthenic syndromes
Lambert–Eaton myasthenic syndrome
Myasthenia gravis
Medications
Anesthetics (e.g., ether, isoflurane, lidocaine, methoxyflurane, procaine, succinylcholine)
Antibiotics (e.g., aminoglycosides, ampicillin, fluoroquinolone, lincosamides, macrolides, polymyxins, tetracyclines)
Anticonvulsants (e.g., phenytoin, trimethadione)
Cardiac drugs (e.g., β-adrenergic blockers, bretylium, calcium-channel blockers, lidocaine, procainamide, quinidine, trimethaphan)
Hormones (e.g., adrenocorticotropic hormone, corticosteroids, thyroid hormone)
Psychiatric drugs (e.g., lithium, phenelzine, phenothiazines)
Rheumatoid arthritis drugs (e.g., chloroquine, D-penicillamine)
Other medications (e.g., anticholesterol drugs, anticholinesterase toxicity, any respiratory depressant, aprotinin, botulinum toxin, carnitine, citrate, curare and its derivatives, ergonovine, eyedrops aminoglycosides, β-adrenergic blockers, corticosteroids., gadolinium, interferon-α and -β, intravenous radiographic contrast media, methimazole, oxytocin, quinine, tetanus antitoxin)
Electrolyte disturbances
Calcium
Magnesium
Toxins (e.g., cocaine, carbamate insecticides, organophosphate insecticides, black widow spider venom, scorpion venom, snake venom, tick neurotoxin)

Adult food-borne botulism is characterized by rapidly progressive cranial nerve palsies, descending weakness, and autonomic dysfunction.[110] The most common symptoms and signs include dysphagia, hypoactive gag reflex, dry mouth, diplopia, ptosis, extraocular movement abnormalities, fixed or dilated pupils, bulbar or limb weakness (especially proximally), constipation, nausea, and vomiting. Stretch reflexes are usually hypoactive or absent but may be normal. Mental status, sensation, and CSF are usually normal. There is usually no response to edrophonium chloride (Tensilon). Atypical symptoms, signs, and ancillary test results are not uncommon and do not exclude the diagnosis. The symptoms and signs in infant botulism are similar to those in adults, with the additional features of hypotonia, poor suck, and failure to thrive. Symptoms usually begin 18 to 36 hours after ingestion of the spores and progress rapidly over 2 to 4 days; recovery begins within a few weeks.

Eight toxin types have been described (A, B, C1, C2, D, E, F, and G), but human botulism is associated only with types A, B, and E and, rarely, with F and G. In all forms of botulism, the toxin initially becomes disseminated via the systemic circulation before uptake by the terminals of peripheral cholinergic axons. Once the toxin is inside the nerve terminals, essential proteins for acetylcholine release are cleaved. Subsequently, both muscarinic and nicotinic nerve terminals degenerate. Recovery from botulism, therefore, requires regrowth of axon terminals and restoration of the neuromuscular junction.

The diagnosis of botulism is usually confirmed by the detection of the toxin in the serum, stool, or wound. In addition, the wound and stool specimens are cultured to identify the offending organism. Electrodiagnostic studies are also helpful in showing impaired neuromuscular transmission.

Treatment consists of early antitoxin administration and supportive care. For adults, an equine trivalent antitoxin is effective against the type A, B, and E toxins. An effective human antitoxin (BabyBIG) is available specifically for infants and has a much lower risk of anaphylaxis than the equine product.[113]

Wound debridement and antibiotics are indicated for wound botulism but should probably be delayed until the antitoxin is given. Prognosis is usually excellent with proper supportive and respiratory care. Recovery may take several weeks to months, depending on the degree of nerve end-terminal destruction.

Lambert–Eaton Myasthenic Syndrome

Lambert–Eaton myasthenic syndrome (LEMS) is an autoimmune disorder in which antibodies directed against presynaptic voltage-gated calcium channels cause proximal limb and trunk weakness. Significant ptosis and bulbar weakness are uncommon. A striking clinical feature of LEMS is that strength often improves following brief exertion. Autonomic symptoms such as a dry mouth, constipation, and urinary retention are frequent. Tendon reflexes are usually hypoactive or absent but may improve after brief exercise.

Approximately 50 to 60 percent of patients with LEMS have an associated small-cell lung cancer. Approximately 3 percent of patients with small-cell lung cancer develop LEMS.[114] Nonparaneoplastic LEMS also occurs, particularly in younger individuals.

Marked post-tetanic facilitation of the compound muscle action potential establishes the diagnosis. Detecting the presence of calcium-channel antibodies also confirms the diagnosis.

Survival in paraneoplastic LEMS depends on the treatment of the underlying neoplasm. Anticholinesterase drugs alone may modestly benefit strength. More effective is the orphan drug 3,4-diaminopyridine, which blocks potassium channels and thereby prolongs the activation of voltage-gated calcium channels. The increased concentrations of calcium in the axon terminals facilitate acetylcholine release presynaptically. Other treatments that may be effective include plasmapheresis, IVIg, prednisone, and azathioprine.

Myasthenia Gravis

There are two clinical forms of myasthenia gravis: ocular and generalized. In the ocular form, weakness is restricted to the eyelids and extraocular muscles. Individuals with generalized myasthenia frequently also have weakness of those muscles plus variable weakness of bulbar, respiratory, or limb muscles.

About 50 percent of patients present with ptosis or diplopia. Of these, about half will progress to generalized myasthenia gravis. A number of autoimmune diseases may be associated, including autoimmune thyroid disease and, more rarely, rheumatoid arthritis and systemic lupus erythematosus (SLE).

Approximately 75 percent of myasthenics have thymic abnormalities. Thymic hyperplasia is the most common abnormality; about 15 percent of patients have a thymoma, usually a noninvasive cortical thymoma. Approximately one-third of patients with a thymoma develop myasthenia gravis.[115] Because of the risks of thymoma, MRI or CT of the mediastinum is necessary for all newly diagnosed myasthenic patients. Thymectomy is generally recommended for all patients with thymomatous myasthenia gravis. In rare instances, myasthenia gravis has been associated with small-cell lung cancer and Hodgkin disease. Rarely, a medication such as D-penicillamine can induce the onset of autoimmune myasthenia gravis, possibly through antigenic mimicry.

The diagnosis is made by the history, examination, presence of acetylcholine receptor antibodies (present in up to 90% of cases of generalized disease), edrophonium chloride test, and electrophysiologic studies. Approximately 35 to 50 percent of patients testing negative for acetylcholine receptor antibodies have antibodies to the muscle-specific receptor tyrosine kinase (MuSK).[116] It is rare for patients to have antibodies both to the acetylcholine receptor and to MuSK. Most patients with MuSK antibodies are women, and many have prominent bulbar, neck, and respiratory weakness.[117,118] Standard electrodiagnostic tests for myasthenia gravis may be normal or only mildly abnormal in patients with MuSK-seropositive myasthenia. Treatment of myasthenia gravis consists of anticholinesterases, immunomodulation, thymectomy, or some combination of these approaches. The first major prospective, multicenter trial on the benefit of thymectomy for seropositive, nonthymomatous generalized myasthenia gravis is currently in progress.[119]

Medications and Toxins

A number of medications (Chapter 32) and toxins impair neuromuscular transmission. These are summarized in Table 59-10.

MYOPATHY

Myopathies usually present with symmetric, proximal weakness. Involvement of the neck flexors and extensors and the facial muscles is not uncommon, but weakness of the extraocular muscles is rare. Muscle atrophy and depressed stretch reflexes occur in advanced cases. The common causes of myopathy are listed in Table 59-11. The congenital and genetic myopathies are beyond the scope of this discussion and are covered in general neurology textbooks. Although myalgia may occur with certain myopathies, most myopathies (including the inflammatory myopathies) are painless. Exercise intolerance and exercise-induced muscle cramps are clues to one of the metabolic myopathies.

The evaluation for a suspected myopathy begins with measurement of serum creatine kinase (CK) activity. Increased serum CK levels usually imply sarcolemmal injury. Normal serum CK levels may

TABLE 59-11 ■ Acquired Myopathies

Endocrine
Acromegaly
Corticosteroids
Hyperparathyroidism
Hyperthyroidism
Hypothyroidism
Infectious
Cysticercosis
Human immunodeficiency virus
Toxoplasmosis
Trichinosis
Viral myositis (e.g., adenovirus, influenza)
Inflammatory
Dermatomyositis
Inclusion-body myositis
Polymyalgia rheumatica
Polymyositis
Polymyositis or dermatomyositis associated with
Scleroderma
Mixed connective tissue disease
Systemic lupus erythematosus
Rheumatoid arthritis
Sjögren syndrome
Systemic vasculitis
Sarcoidosis
Medication-Related
Chloroquine
Colchicine
Corticosteroids (see endocrine causes)
Fibric acid derivatives (clofibrate, gemfibrozil, and others)
3-Hydroxy-3-methylglutaryl coenzyme A (HMG-CoA) reductase inhibitors (lovastatin, simvastatin, and others)
Malignant hyperthermia (usually from general anesthetics)
Vincristine
Zidovudine
Metabolic and Toxic
Alcohol
Critical illness
Hyperkalemia
Hypokalemia
Uremia

occur with disuse atrophy, corticosteroid myopathy, mitochondrial myopathies, and critical illness myopathy associated with thick-filament loss. Many of the metabolic myopathies are associated with normal serum CK levels between attacks. Mild to moderate serum elevations of CK are generally seen with the inflammatory myopathies, toxic myopathies, and adult-onset muscular dystrophies. High serum CK levels are associated with severe toxic/necrotizing myopathies (related to medications or severe electrolyte disturbances) and muscular dystrophy presenting in childhood. Needle EMG supports the clinical diagnosis and excludes the possibility of a neuropathy. The electromyographer may also advise the best target for a muscle biopsy, which is often required for a definitive diagnosis.

Endocrine-Related Myopathy

Acromegaly

Slowly progressive proximal weakness not associated with muscle atrophy occurs in about half of acromegalic patients. Many patients have decreased exercise tolerance. Serum CK levels may be mildly elevated. When growth hormone levels normalize, the myopathy usually resolves.

Corticosteroid Myopathy

Corticosteroid myopathy may occur with either excessive exogenous or endogenous corticosteroids and is characterized by the insidious onset of proximal limb weakness. Patients who develop weakness usually have other stigmata of long-term corticosteroid use, including a moon facies, suprascapular fat pad, and fragile skin. Old age and cancer are risk factors for corticosteroid myopathy.[120] Myalgias may occur. Serum CK levels are typically normal.

The dose and duration of corticosteroid treatment associated with the development of a myopathy vary widely, but most patients have received therapy for at least 4 weeks. With high-dose corticosteroids, however, the weakness may occur within 2 weeks of starting therapy. The fluorinated corticosteroids, including triamcinolone, betamethasone, and dexamethasone, are particularly likely to cause myopathy. Pathologically, there is selective atrophy of the type 2, glycolytic muscle fibers without muscle degeneration or inflammation. The pathogenesis probably relates to impairment of muscle protein and carbohydrate metabolism. The goal of treatment is to lower the corticosteroid dose to as low a level as possible. Recovery may take weeks to months but is usually excellent.

A severe, acute necrotizing myopathy can result from large doses of intravenous corticosteroids combined with a neuromuscular blocking agent, usually in the setting of treatment for status asthmaticus.[121–123] There is probably overlap between this condition and critical illness myopathy (Chapter 56).

Hyperparathyroidism and Osteomalacia

Proximal muscle weakness may be associated with primary and secondary hyperparathyroidism, vitamin D deficiency, and other disorders of vitamin D metabolism.

Patients with primary hyperparathyroidism often complain of weakness and fatigue, but objective loss of muscle power is uncommon. Proximal weakness may be associated with discomfort on movement. Muscle stretch reflexes tend to be brisk. Serum CK levels are normal. Pathologically, atrophy of type II muscle fibers is a consistent feature. Secondary parathyroidism usually occurs in the setting of renal failure. The myopathy associated with uremia is discussed later.

Osteomalacia presents with proximal weakness and bone pain. Nutritional deficiency of vitamin D is the leading cause of osteomalacia worldwide, but gastrectomy and celiac sprue are responsible for most of the cases in the United States. Renal tubular acidosis and anticonvulsant therapy may also cause osteomalacia by interfering with vitamin D metabolic pathways. Vitamin D deficiency may lead to secondary hyperparathyroidism; it may then be difficult to determine which factor is more important in the pathogenesis of the weakness. When vitamin D–deficient patients are supplemented with vitamin D, the response is variable and any improvement occurs over many weeks.

Hyperthyroidism and Hypothyroidism

Approximately 50 percent of thyrotoxic patients develop weakness. The pattern of weakness is typically proximal; patients frequently complain of fatigue and breathlessness. Myalgia is common. Usually the onset is insidious, although the onset may be more rapid in severe hyperthyroidism. In fact, rhabdomyolysis with myoglobinuric renal failure may occur in the setting of a thyroid storm. In general, however, severe generalized weakness in thyrotoxic patients should raise the suspicion of concomitant myasthenia gravis. Serum CK levels are usually normal. The EMG reveals small, short, polyphasic motor units without abnormal spontaneous activity. In addition to nonspecific myopathic findings, muscle biopsies may reveal a lower proportion of type I fibers. Following treatment, the proportion of type I fibers increases. Prognosis for recovery is excellent once a euthyroid state is achieved.

Thyrotoxic periodic paralysis is characterized by recurrent attacks of generalized weakness lasting for minutes to days. The weakness may be provoked by a carbohydrate meal, cold, or rest after exercise. It is usually seen in young Asian or Native American adults. The paralytic attacks are not related to the duration or severity of the thyrotoxicosis. Treatment of acute paralytic attacks includes potassium supplements. The paralytic attacks disappear once the patient is maintained in a euthyroid state.

Hypothyroidism causes a myopathy characterized by proximal weakness, fatigue, slowed movements and reflexes, cramps, stiffness, myoedema, and muscle enlargement.[124] The serum CK level is elevated even in asymptomatic hypothyroid patients and is frequently elevated more than 10 times the upper limit of normal in symptomatic patients. The EMG findings may be normal. Nonspecific myopathic findings are seen on muscle biopsy. After thyroid supplementation, recovery is excellent.

Infectious Myopathies

Human Immunodeficiency Virus Infection

As discussed in Chapter 44, several different types of myopathy have been associated with HIV infection. First, an inflammatory myopathy resembling polymyositis (PM) both clinically and pathologically may occur. Although it may present at any stage of HIV infection, it is usually a complication of AIDS. Patients present with slowly progressive proximal arm and leg weakness. Serum CK levels are elevated, often more than 10 times the upper limit of normal. Pathologically, the findings are similar to idiopathic PM. Viral particles have not been identified in muscle cells. Most cases respond to corticosteroid therapy. Second, a nemaline rod myopathy may occur with or without associated inflammation in HIV patients.[125,126] Third, inclusion-body myositis (IBM) has been described in HIV patients. It is clinically and pathologically indistinguishable from sporadic IBM, except that the age at onset is earlier. Fourth, muscle atrophy and weakness occur in the HIV wasting syndrome. Pathologically, there is atrophy of the type II muscle fibers. Tumor necrosis factor α (TNF-α) is implicated in the pathogenesis of this syndrome. Fifth, myoglobinuria (sometimes recurrent) may occur at any stage of HIV infection.[127] Multiple factors, including concomitant medication use, probably contribute to its pathogenesis. Sixth, a pyomyositis manifesting as localized pain and swelling in a limb may occur. It is usually associated with *Staphylococcus aureus* infection.[128] Seventh, a proximal myopathy associated with myalgias in the thighs and calves may occur with high-dose zidovudine (AZT) treatment.[129] Serum CK levels may be normal or mildly elevated. Pathologically, many fibers reveal "ragged red" features consistent with mitochondrial toxicity. Discontinuation of the medication usually results in improvement but sometimes not full recovery.

Viral Myositis

Viruses implicated with causing a myopathy include adenovirus, coxsackievirus A and B, echovirus, influenza A and B, Epstein–Barr virus, adenovirus, echovirus, parvovirus, parainfluenza virus, paramyxovirus, CMV, hepatitis B, herpes simplex virus, herpes zoster, human T-lymphotropic virus 1 (HTLV-1), and HIV. Myalgia is the most common neuromuscular symptom associated with viral illness. After the viral illness, swollen muscles and sometimes rhabdomyolysis with myoglobinuria occur. For many of the virus strains mentioned here, there is no clear evidence that the virus actually infects or replicates within human muscle tissue. In such cases, the pathogenesis of the muscle injury is uncertain.

Other Infections

The three most common parasitic infections of muscle are toxoplasmosis, cysticercosis, and trichinosis.

Toxoplasmosis is the most common protozoan infection to cause a myositis, the others being sarcocystis, trypanosomiasis, microsporidiosis, and malaria. *Toxoplasma gondii* is transmitted to humans by ingestion of undercooked meats and by contact with cat feces. Patients present with a fever accompanied by any one of multiple possible systemic features, including lymphadenopathy, pericarditis, hepatosplenomegaly, meningoencephalitis, and myositis. The myositis associated with toxoplasmosis resembles idiopathic PM and dermatomyositis (DM). Pathologically, cysts containing bradyzoites may be seen in muscle fibers or near inflammatory infiltrates. Prognosis for a full recovery is excellent following treatment.

Cestode (tapeworm) infections resulting in myopathy include cysticercosis, echinococcosis, coenurosis, and sparganosis. Cysticercosis caused by *Taenia solium* infection may result from eating uncooked infected meat (particularly pork) and by the fecal-oral route. Patients may present with enlarged yet weak muscles (pseudohypertrophy). Myalgia and muscle tenderness are common.

Nematode (roundworm) infections associated with a myopathy include trichinosis, toxocariasis, cutaneous larva migrans, and dracontiasis. Trichinosis occurs after ingestion of inadequately cooked meat. Following a prodrome of abdominal cramps and diarrhea, patients develop generalized weakness that may be accompanied by the classic cutaneous stigmata of DM. Serum CK levels are elevated and eosinophilia is present.[130]

Inflammatory Myopathies

DM, PM, and IBM present with subacute to chronic, symmetric proximal limb weakness with sparing of the ocular muscles. All share evidence of lymphocytic infiltration of the muscle, but important differences exist among these diseases, particularly in mechanisms of pathogenesis and response to treatment. Autoimmune necrotizing myopathies present in a similar fashion but lack lymphocytic infiltrates.

Dermatomyositis and Polymyositis

The annual incidence of DM and PM in the general population is 0.1 to 1 per 100,000. Women are affected more often than men. Most patients present with a several-month history of subacute proximal weakness, usually without significant muscle atrophy. Typically, the onset of the weakness cannot be precisely recalled. Other symptoms may include dysphagia, nasal regurgitation, or aspiration from weakness of oropharyngeal muscles or the upper esophagus. Myalgias and muscle tenderness occur in 25 to 50 percent of cases but tend to be mild. Muscle pain is more prominent in viral or bacterial myositis, the inherited metabolic myopathies, polymyalgia rheumatica, and fibromyalgia.

In DM, various cutaneous manifestations may precede or accompany the onset of weakness. These include Gottron sign (scaly, erythematous rash over the extensor surfaces of the metacarpophalangeal and interphalangeal joints; a similar rash may occur over the extensor surfaces of the elbows and knees), diffuse flat erythema in the anterior neck and chest and other sun-exposed areas, swelling and reddish violaceous discoloration of the upper eyelids (heliotrope rash), periungual erythema, dilated nailbed capillary loops, and rough, cracked skin at the fingertips (so-called mechanic's hands). Of note, patients with DM and SLE often share the same 308A polymorphism of the TNF-α promoter region, which suggests that ultraviolet light–induced production of TNF-α may contribute to light sensitivity in both diseases.[131]

Interstitial lung disease is an important complication of PM and DM. Particularly for PM, the presence of interstitial lung disease is associated with antibodies to the histidyl-transfer RNA (histidyl-tRNA) synthetase (anti–Jo-1). The lung disease may precede the myopathy or accompany it in 5 to 40 percent of patients with DM and PM and may present acutely with a nonproductive cough, dyspnea, hypoxemia, and lung infiltrates or chronically with dyspnea. Sometimes it is discovered in asymptomatic patients on screening chest radiographs. The presence of interstitial lung disease is a poor prognostic factor for long-term survival.[132] Patients with DM and PM may have cardiac involvement, which may manifest as supraventricular arrhythmias, atrioventricular conduction blocks, and bundle branch block. Congestive heart failure has also been described.

Malignancies are seen in 6 to 45 percent of DM patients and in 0 to 28 percent of PM patients.[133] A wide variety of cancers are associated with DM including ovarian, lung, pancreatic, stomach, and colorectal cancer, and non-Hodgkin lymphoma. Non-Hodgkin lymphoma, and lung and bladder cancers have been associated with PM. Age-appropriate cancer screening tests should be performed in all patients; in those over age 65 years, CT scans of the chest, abdomen, and pelvis are recommended. Pelvic ultrasonography and transvaginal ultrasound are advocated by some experts. Full laboratory screening studies are also important.

PM and DM may overlap with scleroderma, SLE, and, rarely, rheumatoid arthritis and Sjögren syndrome. In scleroderma, a bland myopathy with mild to absent elevations of serum CK levels is common. In a few patients, severe proximal muscle weakness occurs with significant serum CK elevations. Overall, the incidence of myositis in scleroderma ranges from 5 to 17 percent. In North American patients, the anti–PM-Scl antibody is a marker for scleroderma-myositis. PM and DM also occur in association with SLE. The presence of autoantibodies against nuclear components helps distinguish a PM-SLE overlap syndrome from idiopathic PM. In a cohort of 330 patients with SLE, 10 had a myositis.[134] Serum CK levels are usually elevated in PM and DM and generally reflect the disease activity; levels are generally higher in PM than DM and may even be normal in active DM.

Serum antibody tests to nuclear and cytoplasmic components help support the clinical diagnosis of PM or DM, assist the diagnosis of overlap syndromes, and categorize subgroups of inflammatory myopathies. Muscle-specific antibodies have specific associations with HLA haplotypes and certain disease manifestations. These include antibodies to aminoacyl transfer RNA synthetases, components of the signal recognition particle (SRP), and nuclear helicase/adenosine triphosphatase Mi-2. About 50 to 75 percent of those with antibodies to cytoplasmic transfer RNA synthetases (including anti–Jo-1) have interstitial lung disease. Patients with anti-SRP antibodies often have acute-onset severe myositis without an associated rash or lung disease. Patients with anti–Mi-2 antibodies usually have a florid rash and an abrupt onset of weakness.[135]

MRI shows evidence of inflammation in muscles and subcutaneous fat, fibrosis, and calcification. Because MRI is noninvasive, it can be performed serially to assess disease progression and monitor response to treatment; it may also be used to identify a site for biopsy.

EMG typically reveals increased insertional activity and fibrillation potentials with myopathic (low-amplitude, short-duration, polyphasic) motor unit potentials. Ideally, a muscle biopsy should be performed on a superficial muscle with abnormal findings on EMG of the homologous contralateral muscle.

Pathologically, the inflammation in PM is perivascular, perimysial, and endomysial. There is no evidence of damage to the capillaries. There is invasion of non-necrotic muscle fibers ubiquitously expressing major histocompatibility complex (MHC)-1 by cytotoxic $CD8^+$ T cells. These findings support the hypothesis that the cytotoxic T cells recognize an antigen bound to major histocompatibility complex-1. The identity and origin of this putative antigen are not known. Major histocompatibility complex-1 is normally not expressed on the surface of muscle fibers.

In DM, the inflammation is predominantly in the perivascular or interfascicular space and less so in the endomysium. The inflammatory infiltrate is primarily composed of B cells and $CD4^+$ T cells. Unlike PM, the immune attack appears to be primarily directed against the vascular endothelium. The sequence of events is thought to include antibody deposition on the endothelial cells, followed by complement activation, and, finally, membrane attack complex (MAC)–mediated microvascular injury.[136] Chronic ischemia is thought to produce perifascicular atrophy, a hallmark pathologic feature of DM.

Corticosteroids are widely recognized as first-line treatment for PM. The typical daily dose is 1 to 1.5 mg/kg. This dose is continued until strength improves and then a careful, slow taper is started. A number of agents, including azathioprine, methotrexate, cyclosporine, tacrolimus, or mycophenolate mofetil, may be used concurrently or subsequently for a corticosteroid-sparing effect. Patients taking prednisone plus azathioprine have a better functional outcome and need a lower prednisone maintenance dose than those taking prednisone alone. For refractory cases of DM and PM, IVIg appears to be effective.[137,138] Results from a large randomized controlled trial of rituximab in myositis failed to meet the primary endpoint.[139] Anti–tumor necrosis factor agents have shown mixed results in small randomized clinical trials. Plasmapheresis did not show a benefit in a double-blind, placebo-controlled trial.[140]

Inclusion-Body Myositis

IBM is a slowly progressive, debilitating myopathy of unknown cause. It is the most common myopathy in patients older than 50 years.[141,142] Early involvement of the finger flexors, wrist flexors, knee extensors, and ankle dorsiflexors is common. Dysphagia may occur, which may be treated with a cricopharyngeal myotomy. A wide variety of autoimmune diseases have been described in association with IBM.

Hyporeflexia is common; some patients have clinical and electrodiagnostic evidence of a peripheral neuropathy.[143]

The serum CK level can be normal or up to 10-fold above the upper limit of normal. The EMG findings are similar to those of DM and PM, except that long-duration motor unit potentials are commonly observed and do not exclude the diagnosis of IBM.

Pathologically, there is endomysial inflammation with a $CD8^+$ T-lymphocyte predominance, basophil-rimmed vacuoles with eosinophilic inclusions, and intracellular amyloid deposits detected by fluorescence microscopy of Congo red–stained sections or electron microscopy demonstrating 15- to 18-nm tubulofilaments.[144] The vacuoles contain various products of muscle degradation including myeloid bodies, membrane fragments, and debris. In addition, numerous proteins also expressed in Alzheimer disease are found in muscle fibers. This has led to the notion that IBM is a degenerative disease associated with aging. There is generally no effective immunomodulating treatment, although individual patients have responded to corticosteroids, IVIg[145,146] and mycophenolate mofetil.[147]

Autoimmune Necrotizing Myopathy

Necrotizing myopathies are usually toxin-induced and resolve with removal of the toxin; rarely, they are immune mediated and chronic. Patients present with progressive, symmetric proximal muscle weakness of acute or subacute onset. Some patients have distal weakness, and many have dysphagia. Serum CK levels can be elevated markedly (over 20 times the upper limit of normal). The autoimmune disorder may be idiopathic or, rarely, relates to malignancies or use of statin drugs. Paraneoplastic necrotizing myopathy may occur with gastrointestinal tumors, small-cell lung cancer, and breast cancer. Other patients with autoimmune necrotizing myopathy, usually without malignancies, have antibodies to the signal recognition particle (anti-SRP antibodies). An endomysial microangiopathy leading to capillary loss occurs in anti-SRP myopathy. Rarely, statin drugs may cause an autoimmune necrotizing myopathy that persists despite discontinuation of the drug.

Sarcoidosis

Granulomatous inflammation of muscle is usually associated with sarcoidosis but can also be seen in infectious disease,[148] inflammatory bowel disease, foreign body reactions,[149] thymoma,[150] lymphoma,[151] and myasthenia gravis. It may also occur without any evidence of systemic disease.

Asymptomatic involvement of the muscle occurs in 50 to 80 percent of cases of sarcoidosis. Symptomatic involvement occurs in less than 3 percent of cases. Most patients with sarcoid myopathy present with slowly progressive, proximal weakness.[152] Rarely, patients present with acute myositis[153] or a palpable nodular type of myopathy. The response to corticosteroid therapy is unpredictable. Compared with sarcoid myopathy, patients with isolated granulomatous myopathy have milder, predominantly distal weakness, and the response to corticosteroids tends to be better.[154,155]

Polymyalgia Rheumatica

Polymyalgia rheumatica presents with achiness and morning stiffness in the shoulder and hip girdles in patients older than 50 years. Malaise, fever, and anorexia with weight loss are common. There is an association with temporal arteritis and rheumatoid arthritis. The erythrocyte sedimentation rate is almost always increased. There is no weakness. Although muscle biopsy specimens are generally normal, MRI or ultrasonography of the shoulders consistently reveals evidence of bursitis.[156,157] The symptoms usually respond to low-dose corticosteroids.

Critical Illness Myopathy

Patients with critical illness may develop an acute, acquired myopathy associated with exposure to high-dose corticosteroids and neuromuscular blocking agents (Chapter 56).[158] Critical illness myopathy may be suspected first when patients fail to wean from mechanical ventilation. Patients have flaccid, diffuse weakness that affects the limbs, neck flexors, and diaphragm. Tendon reflexes are usually depressed. Approximately one-third of ICU patients treated for status asthmaticus develop critical illness myopathy.[123] Other risk factors include severe medical illness, renal failure, and hyperglycemia.[159] Patients with critical illness myopathy may also have clinical and electrodiagnostic features of critical illness polyneuropathy. Critical illness myopathy should be distinguished from rhabdomyolysis with myoglobinuria, which can also occur in the ICU setting. Electrodiagnostic testing helps to clarify the diagnosis. Needle EMG reveals fibrillation potentials in limb muscles of some but not all patients. Short, small, polyphasic motor unit potentials are seen. Electrical inexcitability of the muscle to direct needle stimulation occurs in this entity but not in polyneuropathy.[160] Most patients have elevations of serum CK levels, but a normal level does not exclude the diagnosis. Pathologically, there is muscle-fiber atrophy with evidence of a disrupted intramyofibrillar network. Loss of thick filaments (myosin) is a characteristic feature. The pathogenesis is uncertain but may involve glucocorticoid-induced proteolysis of contractile proteins in the setting of muscle-fiber denervation. There is no specific treatment for critical illness myopathy, but corticosteroids and neuromuscular blocking agents should be limited, if possible. Neurologic recovery is usually excellent, assuming that the patient recovers from the underlying medical illness.[161]

Metabolic and Toxic Myopathies

Alcohol

Alcoholics may develop an acute necrotizing or chronic myopathy. The acute form presents as an attack of pain and swelling in a limb, usually the calf or thigh. In severe cases, myoglobinuria occurs. The attack usually occurs in the course of a heavy drinking binge. If probed, patients may recall prior bouts of pain and swelling in the limbs associated with earlier drinking binges. Serum CK levels are often markedly elevated. Recovery usually occurs over 1 to 2 weeks, but patients are prone to have subsequent episodes of acute myopathy if drinking is resumed.

The chronic form presents as chronic limb-girdle weakness with preserved reflexes. Serum CK levels are usually normal but may be elevated. Muscle biopsy specimen abnormalities are usually mild and include type II fiber atrophy.

Hyperkalemia or Hypokalemia

Hyperkalemia causes acute generalized weakness and cardiac arrhythmias. The weakness typically begins in the legs and then generalizes over hours to days. Respiratory failure occurs in about 50 percent of cases. Painful dysesthesias may precede the onset of weakness. Reflexes are usually absent. In most cases, the serum potassium level exceeds 7.5 mEq/L. Paralysis only occurs in patients with some degree of chronic hyperkalemia. Electrodiagnostic testing has shown slowing of nerve conduction velocities and low compound muscle action potential amplitudes.[162] The immediate treatment goal is to prevent a cardiac arrhythmia, which can be achieved with an infusion of calcium gluconate.

Hypokalemia may be associated with acute paralysis or subacute myopathy. Acute hypokalemic paralysis occurs in patients with chronic potassium depletion. The onset of weakness occurs over hours to days. Once it starts, the weakness tends to accelerate. In mild cases, weakness may be limited to the legs, but in severe cases quadriplegia with neuromuscular respiratory failure may occur. Extraocular muscles are spared. The potassium level is always below 3.0 mEq/L. The subacute myopathy associated with hypokalemia is characterized by the onset of proximal limb weakness over weeks to months. Serum CK levels are elevated, sometimes markedly. Pathologically, there is muscle-fiber necrosis with multiple vacuoles in some muscle fibers. Occasionally, the course may be more rapid, associated with myalgia, tenderness, and myoglobinuria. Once the hypokalemia is corrected, recovery is rapid and complete.

Uremia

Uremic myopathy, characterized by proximal weakness, limited endurance, and rapid fatigability, occurs in patients with end-stage renal disease. It usually only occurs with glomerular filtration rates below 25 ml/min.[163] Approximately 50 percent of dialysis patients have this condition. Often, the weakness is mild, and EMG and serum CK levels are normal. Pathologically, there is atrophy of type II muscle fibers. A number of metabolic derangements may contribute to this condition, including secondary hyperparathyroidism, impaired vitamin D metabolism, carnitine deficiency, and reduced clearance of toxic "middle molecules." Insulin resistance,[164] alterations of mitochondrial metabolism, and anemia may also have roles in pathogenesis. Although there is currently no specific treatment for uremic myopathy, an emphasis should be placed on preventing secondary hyperparathyroidism and improving the patient's nutritional status. Carnitine supplementation may be considered.[165] Renal transplantation offers the best chance of improvement.

Medication-Induced Myopathy

Many different medications cause a myopathy (Chapter 32). Most of these cause a necrotizing myopathy that presents clinically with the acute to subacute onset of generalized weakness. In severe cases, myoglobinuria occurs. Myalgias may occur. Serum CK values are usually elevated. Pathologically, necrosis and regeneration of muscle fibers occur, with myophagocytosis. Statins (3-hydroxy-3-methylglutaryl-CoA reductase inhibitors), fibric acid derivatives (clofibrate, gemfibrozil, and others), organophosphates, α-aminocaproic acid, and hypervitaminosis E are all associated with a necrotizing myopathy. Any medication that lowers potassium levels, including diuretics, licorice, and laxatives, may produce a myopathy. Chronic hydroxychloroquine or colchicine use can cause vacuolar myopathy; impaired renal function significantly increases the risk of colchine-induced myopathy. A few medications (e.g., zidovudine) cause a mitochondrial myopathy. Once the offending medication is discontinued, most patients make a rapid and full recovery.

Statin-Induced Myopathy

Statins rarely cause a necrotizing myopathy with hyperCKemia.[166] In most patients, the myopathy reverses in weeks to months after withdrawal of the statin, and the serum CK levels normalize. In a subset of patients, however, the myopathy persists despite drug discontinuation. Evidence for an autoimmune basis for this myopathy includes: (1) expression of MHC-1 antigen on non-necrotic muscle fibers, (2) the presence of autoantibodies against muscle 3-hydroxy-3-methylglutaryl-CoA reductase (HMGCR), and (3) improvement with immunosuppressive therapies such as prednisone.[167,168] High levels of HMGCR in regenerating muscle fibers may be responsible for triggering or perpetuating the immune response.[168]

RHABDOMYOLYSIS AND MYOGLOBINURIA

Any cause of muscle injury leads to an increase in serum concentration of myoglobin. Urine dipstick tests are positive when urine concentrations of myoglobin reach 0.5 to 1 mg/dl. If the concentration of

TABLE 59-12 ■ Acquired Causes of Myoglobinuria and Rhabdomyolysis

Trauma or Infarction	
Compartment syndromes	
Crush injuries	
Immobilization	
Infections	
Viral	
Adenovirus influenza A and B	Epstein–Barr virus
Coxsackievirus	Herpes simplex virus
Cytomegalovirus	HIV
Enterovirus	Varicella-zoster
Bacterial	
Francisella tularensis	*Neisseria*
Clostridium	*Staphylococcus aureus*
Legionella	*Streptococcus pneumoniae*
Leptospira	*Salmonella typhi*
Nontraumatic Overexertion	
Exercise	
Prolonged dystonia or chorea	
Delirium	
Status epilepticus	
Extremes of Body Temperature	
Burns	
Fevers	
Hypothermia	
Drugs and Toxins	
Drugs	
Antidepressants (all classes)	Miscellaneous
Depolarizing neuromuscular blockers (succinylcholine)	Azathioprine
	Colchicine
HMG-CoA reductase inhibitors	Gemfibrozil
Inhaled anesthetics (halothane)	Pentamidine
Neuroleptic medications	Pyrazinamide
Nonsteroidals	Zidovudine
Toxins	
Amphetamines	Ethanol
Arsenic	Ethylene glycol
Carbon monoxide	Haff disease
Cocaine	Strychnine
Ecstasy	Venoms (bee, hornet, snake, spider, and parrotfish)
Metabolic Abnormalities	
Diabetic ketoacidosis	Hypophosphatemia
Hypokalemia	Hypothyroidism
Hyper- or hyponatremia	
Inflammatory Myopathy	
Dermatomyositis	
Polymyositis	

myoglobin in the urine surpasses 250 μg (normal is less than 5 ng/ml), the urine will have a cola-color tinge. This reflects destruction of more than 100 g of muscle.

Recognition of myoglobinuria is important because of the potentially life-threatening complication of acute tubular necrosis. Management includes hydration with alkaline fluids and induced diuresis with hyperosmolar agents such as mannitol. Electrolyte imbalances, such as hyperkalemia or hypocalcemia, may cause cardiac arrhythmias and require prompt reversal. The prognosis for neurologic recovery is usually excellent given the tremendous regenerative capacity of skeletal muscle.

Rhabdomyolysis leading to myoglobinuria may occur when there is direct injury to the sarcolemma or when energy failure occurs. In addition to pigmenturia, presenting symptoms include myalgia, weakness, and muscle swelling. The many causes of myoglobinuria are outlined in Table 59-12.[169]

It should be noted that vigorous exercise (e.g., military physical fitness training) elevates serum CK values in most people (commonly exceeding five times the upper limit of normal), but visible myoglobinuria or muscle weakness are rare.[170,171] Polymorphisms in the myosin light chain kinase, α-actin 3, and creatine kinase MM genes have all been associated with higher serum CK elevations after exercise and may be risk factors for exertional myoglobinuria.[172,173]

Recurrent myoglobinuria, regardless of whether it is associated with exercise, should prompt an investigation into a metabolic myopathy. Glycogen storage diseases, fatty acid oxidation disorders, and mitochondrial cytopathies have all been associated with recurrent myoglobinuria. Diagnosis of these disorders usually requires the analysis of specific enzyme activities in muscle biopsies.

REFERENCES

1. McCarthy RJ, Olney RK: Neuromuscular diseases. p. 287. In Corey-Bloom J (ed): Diagnosis-Based Adult Neurology. Mosby, St. Louis, 1997.
2. Lacomblez L, Bensimon G, Leigh PN, et al: Dose-ranging study of riluzole in amyotrophic lateral sclerosis. Amyotrophic Lateral Sclerosis/Riluzole Study Group II. Lancet 347:1425, 1996.
3. Forshew DA, Bromberg MB: A survey of clinician's practice in the symptomatic treatment of ALS. Amyotroph Lateral Scler Other Motor Neuron Disord 4:258, 2003.
4. La Spada AR, Wilson EM, Lubahn DB, et al: Androgen receptor gene mutations in X-linked spinal and bulbar muscular atrophy. Nature 352:77, 1991.
5. Windebank AJ, Litchy WJ, Daube JR, et al: Lack of progression of neurologic deficit in survivors of paralytic polio: a 5-year prospective population-based study. Neurology 46:80, 1996.
6. Sejvar JJ, Haddad MB, Tierney BC, et al: Neurologic manifestations and outcome of West Nile virus infection. JAMA 290:510, 2003.
7. Dietz V, Andrus J, Olive JM, et al: Epidemiology and clinical characteristics of acute flaccid paralysis associated with non-polio enterovirus isolation: the experience in the Americas. Bull World Health Organ 73:597, 1995.
8. Wong M, Connolly AM, Noetzel MJ: Poliomyelitis-like syndrome associated with Epstein-Barr virus infection. Pediatr Neurol 20:235, 1999.
9. Nash D, Mostaahsari F, Fine A, et al: The outbreak of West Nile virus infection in the New York City area in 1999. N Engl J Med 344:1807, 2001.
10. Peterson LR, Narfin AA: West Nile virus: a primer for the clinician. Ann Intern Med 137:173, 2002.
11. Almhanna K, Palanichamy N, Sharma M, et al: Unilateral brachial plexopathy associated with West Nile virus meningoencephalitis. Clin Infect Dis 36:1629, 2003.
12. Ahmed S, Libman R, Wesson K, et al: Guillain-Barré syndrome: an unusual presentation of West Nile virus infection. Neurology 55:144, 2000.
13. Verma A, Berger JR, Snodgrass S, et al: Motor neuron disease: a paraneoplastic process associated with anti-Hu antibody and small-cell lung carcinoma. Ann Neurol 40:112, 1996.
14. Forsyth PA, Dalmau J, Graus F, et al: Motor neuron syndromes in cancer patients. Ann Neurol 41:722, 1997.
15. Khwaja S, Sripathi N, Ahmad BK, et al: Paraneoplastic motor neuron disease with type 1 Purkinje cell antibodies. Muscle Nerve 21:943, 1998.
16. Ferracci F, Fassetta G, Butler MH, et al: A novel antineuronal antibody in a motor neuron syndrome associated with breast cancer. Neurology 53:852, 1999.
17. Anders HJ, Goebel FD: Cytomegalovirus polyradiculopathy in patients with AIDS. Clin Infect Dis 27:345, 1998.
18. So YT, Olney RK: Acute lumbosacral polyradiculopathy in acquired immunodeficiency syndrome: experience in 23 patients. Ann Neurol 35:53, 1994.
19. Anders HJ, Goebel FD: Neurological manifestations of cytomegalovirus infection in the acquired immunodeficiency syndrome. Int J STD AIDS 10:151, 1999.
20. Petty PG, Hudgson P, Hare WSC: Symptomatic lumbar spinal arachnoiditis: fact or fallacy? J Clin Neurosci 7:395, 2000.
21. Coan ET, Kabukcuglu S, Arslantas A, et al: Spinal toxoplasmic arachnoiditis associated with osteoid

formation: a rare presentation of toxoplasmosis. Spine 26:1726, 2001.

22. Kok AJM, Verhagen WIM, Bartels RHMA, et al: Spinal arachnoiditis following subarachnoid haemorrhage: report of two cases and review of the literature. Acta Neurochir (Wien) 142:795, 2000.
23. Sghirlanzoni A, Pareyson D, Lauria G: Sensory neuron diseases. Lancet Neurol 4:349, 2005.
24. Dalmau J, Furneaux HM, Gralla RJ, et al: Detection of the anti-Hu antibody in the serum of patients with small cell lung cancer—a quantitative Western blot analysis. Ann Neurol 27:544, 1990.
25. Lucchinetti CF, Kimmel DW, Lennon VA: Paraneoplastic and oncologic profiles of patients seropositive for type 1 antineuronal nuclear autoantibodies. Neurology 50:652, 1998.
26. Camessanché JP, Antoine JC, Honnorat J, et al: Paraneoplastic peripheral neuropathy associated with anti-Hu antibodies: a clinical and electrophysiological study of 20 patients. Brain 125:166, 2002.
27. Yu Z, Kryzer TJ, Griesmann GE: CRMP-5 neuronal autoantibody: marker of lung cancer and thymoma-related autoimmunity. Ann Neurol 49:146, 2001.
28. Sillevis Smitt P, Grefkens J, de Leeuw B, et al: Survival and outcome in 73 anti-Hu positive patients with paraneoplastic encephalomyelitis/sensory neuronopathy. J Neurol 249:745, 2002.
29. Merchut MP, Adams EM, Morrissey MM: Sensory neuronopathy in autoimmune chronic active hepatitis. Neurology 43:2410, 1993.
30. Griffin JW, Cornblath DR, Alexander E, et al: Ataxic sensory neuropathy and dorsal root ganglionitis associated with Sjögren's syndrome. Ann Neurol 27:304, 1990.
31. Chen WH, Yeh JH, Chiu HC: Plasmapheresis in the treatment of ataxic sensory neuropathy associated with Sjögren's syndrome. Eur Neurol 45:270, 2001.
32. Takahashi Y, Takata T, Hoshino M, et al: Benefit of IVIG for long-standing ataxic sensory neuronopathy with Sjögren's syndrome. Neurology 60:503, 2003.
33. Sterman AB, Schaumburg HH, Asbury AK: The acute sensory neuronopathy syndrome: a distinct clinical entity. Ann Neurol 7:354, 1980.
34. Scaravilli F, Sinclair E, Arango JC, et al: The pathology of the posterior root ganglia in AIDS and its relationship to the pallor of the gracile tract. Acta Neuropathol (Berl) 84:163, 1992.
35. Elliott KJ: Other neurological complications of herpes zoster and their management. Ann Neurol 35(suppl): S57, 1994.
36. Dyck PJB, Englestad J, Suarez G, et al: Biopsied upper limb nerves provide information about distribution and mechanisms in immune brachial plexus neuropathy abstract.. Neurology 56:A395, 2001.
37. Johnson NE, Petraglia AL, Huang JH, et al: Rapid resolution of severe neuralgic amyotrophy after treatment with corticosteroids and intravenous immunoglobulin. Muscle Nerve 44:304, 2011.
38. Dyck PJB, Engelstad J, Norell J, et al: Microvasculitis in non-diabetic lumbosacral radiculoplexus neuropathy (LSRPN): similarity to the diabetic variety (DLSRPN). J Neuropathol Exp Neurol 59:525, 2000.
39. Thaisetthawatkul P, Dyck PJ: Treatment of diabetic and nondiabetic lumbosacral radiculoplexus neuropathy. Curr Treat Options Neurol 12:95, 2010.
40. Wilbourn AJ: Brachial plexus lesions. p. 1362. In: Dyck PJ, Thomas PK (eds): Peripheral Neuropathy. 4th Ed. Elsevier Saunders, Philadelphia, 2005.
41. Olsen NK, Pfeiffer P, Johannsen L, et al: Radiation-induced brachial plexopathy: neurological follow-up in 161 recurrence-free breast cancer patients. Int J Radiat Oncol Biol Phys 26:43, 1993.
42. Bowen J, Gregory R, Squier M, et al: The post-irradiation lower motor neuron syndrome. Neuronopathy or radiculopathy? Brain 119:1429, 1996.
43. Stevens JC, Beard CM, O'Fallon WM, et al: Conditions associated with carpal tunnel syndrome. Mayo Clin Proc 67:541, 1992.
44. Dyck PJ, Giannini C: Pathologic alterations in the diabetic neuropathies of humans: a review. J Neuropathol Exp Neurol 55:1181, 1996.
45. Moore PM, Richardson B: Neurology of the vasculitides and connective tissue diseases. J Neurol Neurosurg Psychiatry 65:10, 1998.
46. Langford CA, Vasculitis J: Allergy Clin Immunol 111:S602, 2003.
47. Said G, LaCroix-Ciaudo C, Fujimura H, et al: The peripheral neuropathy of necrotizing arteritis: a clinicopathological study. Ann Neurol 23:461, 1988.
48. Claussen GC, Thomas TD, Goyne C, et al: Diagnostic value of nerve and muscle biopsy in suspected vasculitis cases. J Clin Neuromuscul Dis 1:117, 2000.
49. Collins MP, Mendell JR, Periquet MI, et al: Superficial peroneal nerve/peroneus brevis muscle biopsy in vasculitic neuropathy. Neurology 55:636, 2000.
50. Guillevin L, Mahr A, Callard P, et al: Hepatitis B virus-associated polyarteritis nodosa: clinical characteristics, outcome, and impact of treatment in 115 patients. Medicine (Baltimore) 84:313, 2005.
51. Guillevin L, Lhote F, Cohen P, et al: Corticosteroids plus pulse cyclophosphamide and plasma exchange versus corticosteroids plus pulse cyclophosphamide alone in the treatment of polyarteritis nodosa and Churg-Strauss syndrome patients with factors predicting poor prognosis. Arthritis Rheum 38:1638, 1995.
52. Santoro F, Manganelli F, Briani C, et al: Prevalence and characteristics of peripheral neuropathy in hepatitis C virus population. J Neurol Neurosurg Psychiatry 77:626, 2006.
53. Ferri C, Zignego AL, Giuggioli D, et al: HCV and cryoglobulinemic vasculitis. Cleve Clin J Med 69(suppl 2): SII20, 2002.

54. De Vita S, De ReV, Gasparotto D, et al: Oligoclonal non-neoplastic B cell expansion is the key feature of type II mixed cryoglobulinemia. Arthritis Rheum 43:94, 2000.
55. Thomas FP, Lovelace RE, Ding XS, et al: Vasculitic neuropathy in a patient with cryoglobulinemia and anti-MAG IgM monoclonal gammopathy. Muscle Nerve 15:891, 1992.
56. Pateron D, Fain I, Sehonnou J, et al: Severe necrotizing vasculitis in a patient with hepatitis C virus infection treated with interferon. Clin Exp Rheumatol 14:79, 1996.
57. Sansonno D, De ReV, Lauletta G, et al: Monoclonal antibody treatment of mixed cryoglobulinemia resistant to interferon alpha with an anti-CD20. Blood 101:2818, 2003.
58. Collins MP, Kissel JT: Neuropathies with systemic vasculitis. p. 2348. In: Dyck PJ, Thomas PK (eds): Peripheral Neuropathy. 4th Ed. Elsevier Saunders, Philadelphia, 2005.
59. Said G, Lacroix C, Chemouilli P, et al: Cytomegalovirus neuropathy in acquired immunodeficiency syndrome: a clinical and pathological study. Ann Neurol 29:139, 1991.
60. Chretien F, Gray F, Lescs MC, et al: Acute varicella-zoster virus ventriculitis and meningo-myelo-radiculitis in acquired immunodeficiency syndrome. Acta Neuropathol (Berl) 86:659, 1993.
61. Chetty R: Vasculitides associated with HIV infection. J Clin Pathol 54:275, 2001.
62. Moulignier A, Authier FJ, Baudrimont M, et al: Peripheral neuropathy in human immunodeficiency virus infected patients with the diffuse infiltrative lymphocytosis syndrome. Ann Neurol 41:438, 1997.
63. Kaji R, Shibasaki H, Kimura J: Multifocal demyelinating motor neuropathy: cranial nerve involvement and immunoglobulin therapy. Neurology 42:506, 1992.
64. Chaudhry V, Corse AM, Cornblath DR, et al: Multifocal motor neuropathy: electrodiagnostic features. Muscle Nerve 17:198, 1994.
65. Katz J, Wolfe G, Bryan W, et al: Electrophysiologic findings in multifocal motor neuropathy. Neurology 48:700, 1997.
66. Pestronk A, Choksi R: Multifocal motor neuropathy: serum IgM anti-GM1 ganglioside antibodies in most patients detected using covalent linkage of GM1 to ELISA plates. Neurology 49:1289, 1997.
67. Harbo T, Andersen H, Hess A, et al: Subcutaneous versus intravenous immunoglobulin in multifocal motor neuropathy: a randomized, single-blinded cross-over trial. Eur J Neurol 16:631, 2009.
68. Vlam L, van der Pol WL, Cats EA, et al: Multifocal motor neuropathy: diagnosis, pathogenesis and treatment strategies. Nat Rev Neurol 8:48, 2011.
69. Piepers S, Van den Berg-Vos R, Van der Pol WL, et al: Mycophenolate mofetil as adjunctive therapy for MMN patients: a randomized, controlled trial. Brain 130:2004, 2007.
70. Dyck PJ, Kratz KM, Karnes JL, et al: The prevalence by staged severity of various types of diabetic neuropathy, retinopathy, and nephropathy in a population-based cohort: the Rochester Diabetic Neuropathy Study. Neurology 43:817, 1993.
71. Smith AG: Impaired glucose tolerance and metabolic syndrome in idiopathic neuropathy. J Peripher Nerv Syst 17(suppl 2):15, 2012.
72. Hughes RA, Umapathi T, Gray IA, et al: A controlled investigation of the cause of chronic idiopathic axonal polyneuropathy. Brain 127:1723, 2004.
73. The Diabetes Control and Complications Trial Research Group: The effect of intensive treatment of diabetes on the development and progression of long-term complications in insulin-dependent diabetes mellitus. N Engl J Med 329:977, 1993.
74. Nicolucci A, Carinci F, Cavaliere D, et al: A meta-analysis of trials on aldose reductase inhibitors in diabetic peripheral neuropathy. Diabet Med 13:1017, 1996.
75. Yuen EC, Mobley WC: Therapeutic potential of neurotrophic factors for neurological disorders. Ann Neurol 40:346, 1996.
76. Ametov AS, Barinov A, Dyck PJ, et al: The sensory symptoms of diabetic polyneuropathy are improved with alpha-lipoic acid: the SYDNEY trial. Diabetes Care 26:770, 2003.
77. Ziegler D, Ametov A, Barinov A, et al: Oral treatment with alpha-lipoic acid improves symptomatic diabetic polyneuropathy: the SYDNEY 2 trial. Diabetes Care 29:2365, 2006.
78. Simpson DM, Kitch D, Evans SR, et al: HIV neuropathy natural history cohort study: assessment measures and risk factors. Neurology 66:1679, 2006.
79. Lawn ND, Fletcher DD, Henderson RD, et al: Anticipating mechanical ventilation in Guillain-Barré syndrome. Arch Neurol 58:893, 2001.
80. Yuki N, Hartung HP: Guillain-Barré syndrome. N Engl J Med 366:2294, 2012.
81. Raphaël JC, Chevret S, Hughes RA, et al: Plasma exchange for Guillain-Barré syndrome. Cochrane Database Syst Rev 7:CD001798, 2012.
82. Hughes RA, Swan AV, van Doorn PA: Intravenous immunoglobulin for Guillain-Barré syndrome. Cochrane Database Syst Rev 7:CD002063, 2012.
83. Plasma Exchange/Sandoglobulin Guillain-Barré Syndrome Trial Group: Randomised trial of plasma exchange, intravenous immunoglobulin, and combined treatments in Guillain-Barré syndrome. Lancet 349:225, 1997.
84. Hughes RA, Donofrio P, Bril V, et al: Intravenous immune globulin (10% caprylate-chromatography purified) for the treatment of chronic inflammatory demyelinating polyradiculoneuropathy (ICE study): a randomised placebo-controlled trial. Lancet Neurol 7:136, 2008.

85. Mehndiratta MM, Hughes RA: Plasma exchange for chronic inflammatory demyelinating polyradiculoneuropathy. Cochrane Database Syst Rev 9:CD003906, 2012.
86. Van den Bergh PY, Hadden RD, Bouche P, et al: European Federation of Neurological Societies/Peripheral Nerve Society guideline on management of chronic inflammatory demyelinating polyradiculoneuropathy: report of a joint task force of the European Federation of Neurological Societies and the Peripheral Nerve Society—first revision. Eur J Neurol 17:356, 2010.
87. Hughes RA, Mehndiratta MM: Corticosteroids for chronic inflammatory demyelinating polyradiculoneuropathy. Cochrane Database Syst Rev 8:CD002062, 2012.
88. Dyck PJ, Litchy WJ, Kratz KM, et al: A plasma exchange versus immune globulin infusion trial in chronic inflammatory demyelinating polyradiculoneuropathy. Ann Neurol 36:838, 1994.
89. Dyck PJ, Low PA, Windebank AJ, et al: Plasma exchange in polyneuropathy associated with monoclonal gammopathy of undetermined significance. N Engl J Med 325:1482, 1991.
90. Ramchandren S, Lewis RA: An update on monoclonal gammopathy and neuropathy. Curr Neurol Neurosci Rep 12:102, 2012.
91. Ropper AH: Accelerated neuropathy of renal failure. Arch Neurol 50:536, 1993.
92. Sung JY, Kuwabara S, Ogawara K, et al: Patterns of nerve conduction abnormalities in POEMS syndrome. Muscle Nerve 26:189, 2002.
93. Camdessanche JP, Antoine JC, Honnorat J, et al: Paraneoplastic peripheral neuropathy associated with anti-Hu antibodies. A clinical and electrophysiological study of 20 patients. Brain 125:166, 2002.
94. Antoine JC, Honnorat J, Camdessanche JP, et al: Paraneoplastic anti-CV2 antibodies react with peripheral nerve and are associated with a mixed axonal and demyelinating peripheral neuropathy. Ann Neurol 49:214, 2001.
95. Moriwaki K, Kanno Y, Nakamoto H, et al: Vitamin B6 deficiency in elderly patients on chronic peritoneal dialysis. Adv Perit Dial 16:308, 2000.
96. Saperstein DS, Wolfe GI, Gronseth GS, et al: Challenges in the identification of cobalamin-deficiency polyneuropathy. Arch Neurol 60:1296, 2003.
97. Kuzminski AM, Del Giacco EJ, Allen RH, et al: Effective treatment of cobalamin deficiency with oral cobalamin. Blood 92:1191, 1998.
98. Jackson CE, Amato AA, Barohn RJ: Isolated vitamin E deficiency. Muscle Nerve 19:1161, 1996.
99. Kumar N, Gross JB, Ahlskog JE: Myelopathy due to copper deficiency. Neurology 61:273, 2003.
100. Kumar N, McEnvoy KM, Ahlskog JE: Myelopathy due to copper deficiency following gastrointestinal surgery. Arch Neurol 60:1782, 2003.
101. Koike H, Sobue G: Alcoholic neuropathy. Curr Opin Neurol 19:481, 2006.
102. Vittadini G, Buonocore M, Colli G, et al: Alcoholic polyneuropathy: a clinical and epidemiological study. Alcohol Alcohol 36:393, 2001.
103. Moser HW, Raymond GV, Lu SE, et al: Follow-up of 89 asymptomatic patients with adrenoleukodystrophy treated with Lorenzo's oil. Arch Neurol 62:1073, 2005.
104. Scott LJ, Griffin JW, Luciano C, et al: Quantitative analysis of epidermal innervation in Fabry disease. Neurology 52:1249, 1999.
105. Ries M, Mengel E, Kutschke G, et al: Use of gabapentin to reduce chronic neuropathic pain in Fabry disease. J Inherit Metab Dis 26:413, 2003.
106. Eng CM, Germain DP, Banikazemi M, et al: Fabry disease: guidelines for the evaluation and management of multi-organ system involvement. Genet Med 8:539, 2006.
107. Jansen GA, Wanders RJ, Watkins PA, et al: Phytanoyl-coenzyme A hydroxylase deficiency—the enzyme defect in Refsum's disease. N Engl J Med 337:133, 1997.
108. Rust S, Rosier M, Funke H, et al: Tangier disease is caused by mutations in the gene encoding ATP-binding cassette transporter 1. Nat Genet 22:352, 1999.
109. Maselli RA, Ellis W, Mandler RN, et al: Cluster of wound botulism in California: clinical, electrophysiologic, and pathologic study. Muscle Nerve 20:1284, 1997.
110. Cherington M: Clinical spectrum of botulism. Muscle Nerve 21:701, 1998.
111. Passaro DJ, Werner SB, McGee J, et al: Wound botulism associated with black tar heroin among injecting drug users. JAMA 279:859, 1998.
112. Bhatia KP, Munchau A, Thompson PD, et al: Generalised muscular weakness after botulinum toxin injections for dystonia: a report of three cases. J Neurol Neurosurg Psychiatry 67:90, 1999.
113. Arnon SS, Schechter RN, Maslanka SE, et al: Human botulism immune globulin for the treatment of infant botulism. N Engl J Med 354:462, 2006.
114. Elrington GM, Murray NM, Spiro SG, et al: Neurological paraneoplastic syndromes in patients with small cell lung cancer: a prospective survey of 150 patients. J Neurol Neurosurg Psychiatry 54:764, 1991.
115. Morgenthaler TI, Brown LR, Colby TV, et al: Thymoma. Mayo Clin Proc 68:1110, 1993.
116. Hoch W, McConville J, Helms S, et al: Auto-antibodies to the receptor tyrosine kinase MuSK in patients with myasthenia gravis without acetylcholine receptor antibodies. Nat Med 7:365, 2001.
117. Sanders D, El-Salem K, Massey J, et al: Clinical aspects of MuSK antibody positive seronegative MG. Neurology 60:1978, 2003.

118. Evoli A, Tonali P, Padua L, et al: Clinical correlates with anti-MuSK antibodies in generalized seronegative myasthenia gravis. Brain 126:2304, 2003.
119. Wolfe GI, Kaminski HJ, Jaretzki III A, et al: Development of a thymectomy trial in nonthymomatous myasthenia gravis patients receiving immunosuppressive therapy. Ann NY Acad Sci 998:473, 2003.
120. Batchelor TT, Taylor LP, Thaler HT, et al: Steroid myopathy in cancer patients. Neurology 48:1234, 1997.
121. Hirano M, Ott BR, Raps EC, et al: Acute quadriplegic myopathy: a complication of treatment with steroids, nondepolarizing blocking agents, or both. Neurology 42:2082, 1992.
122. Griffin D, Fairman N, Coursin D, et al: Acute myopathy during treatment of status asthmaticus with corticosteroids and steroidal muscle relaxants. Chest 102:510, 1992.
123. Douglass JA, Tuxen DV, Horne M, et al: Myopathy in severe asthma. Am Rev Respir Dis 146:517, 1992.
124. Duyff RF, Van den Bosch J, Laman DM, et al: Neuromuscular findings in thyroid dysfunction: a prospective clinical and electrodiagnostic study. J Neurol Neurosurg Psychiatry 68:750, 2000.
125. Feinberg DM, Spiro AJ, Weidenheim KM: Distinct light microscopic changes in human immunodeficiency virus-associated nemaline myopathy. Neurology 50:529, 1998.
126. Simpson DM, Bender AN: Human immunodeficiency virus-associated myopathy: analysis of 11 patients. Ann Neurol 24:79, 1988.
127. Chariot P, Ruet E, Authier FJ, et al: Acute rhabdomyolysis in patients infected by human immunodeficiency virus. Neurology 44:1692, 1994.
128. Vassilopoulos D, Chalasani P, Jurado RL, et al: Musculoskeletal infections in patients with human immunodeficiency virus infection. Medicine (Baltimore) 76:284, 1997.
129. Dalakas MC, Illa I, Pezeshkpour GH, et al: Mitochondrial myopathy caused by long-term zidovudine therapy. N Engl J Med 322:1098, 1990.
130. Santos Duran-Ortiz J, Garcia-de la Torre I, Orozco-Barocio G, et al: Trichinosis with severe myopathic involvement mimicking polymyositis: report of a family outbreak. J Rheumatol 19:310, 1992.
131. Werth VP, Callen JP, Ang G, et al: Associations of tumor necrosis factor alpha and HLA polymorphisms with adult dermatomyositis: implications for a unique pathogenesis. J Invest Dermatol 119:617, 2002.
132. Selva-Ocallaghan A, Labrador-Horrillo M, Munoz-Gall X, et al: Polymyositis/dermatomyositis-associated lung disease: analysis of a series of 81 patients. Lupus 14:534, 2005.
133. Hill CL, Zhang Y, Sigurgeirsson B, et al: Frequency of specific cancer types in dermatomyositis and polymyositis: a population-based study. Lancet 357:96, 2001.
134. Dayal NA, Isenberg DA: SLE/myositis overlap: are the manifestations of SLE different in overlap disease? Lupus 11:293, 2002.
135. Love LA, Leff RL, Fraser DD, et al: A new approach to the classification of idiopathic inflammatory myopathy: myositis-specific autoantibodies define useful homogeneous patient groups. Medicine (Baltimore) 70:360, 1991.
136. Emslie-Smith AM, Engel AG: Microvascular changes in early and advanced dermatomyositis: a quantitative study. Ann Neurol 27:343, 1990.
137. Dalakas MC, Illa I, Dambrosia JM, et al: A controlled trial of high-dose intravenous immune globulin infusions as treatment for dermatomyositis. N Engl J Med 329:1993, 1993.
138. Cherin P, Pelletier S, Teixeira A, et al: Results and long-term followup of intravenous immunoglobulin infusions in chronic, refractory polymyositis: an open study with thirty-five adult patients. Arthritis Rheum 46:467, 2002.
139. Oddis CV, Reed AM, Aggarwal R, et al: Rituximab in the treatment of refractory adult and juvenile dermatomyositis and adult polymyositis: a randomized, placebo-phase trial. Arthritis Rheum 65:314, 2013.
140. Miller FW, Leitman SF, Cronin ME, et al: A randomized double-blind controlled trial of plasma exchange and leukopheresis in patients with polymyositis and dermatomyositis. N Engl J Med 326:1380, 1992.
141. Griggs RC, Askanas V, DiMauro S, et al: Inclusion body myositis and myopathies. Ann Neurol 38:705, 1995.
142. Amato AA, Gronseth GS, Jackson CE, et al: Inclusion body myositis: clinical and pathological boundaries. Ann Neurol 40:581, 1996.
143. Lindberg C, Oldfors A, Hedstrom A: Inclusion body myositis: peripheral nerve involvement. Combined morphological and electrophysiological studies on peripheral nerves. J Neurol Sci 99:327, 1990.
144. Mendell JR, Sahenk Z, Gales T, et al: Amyloid filaments in inclusion body myositis. Novel findings provide insight into nature of filaments. Arch Neurol 48:1229, 1991.
145. Soueidan SA, Dalakas MC: Treatment of inclusion-body myositis with high-dose intravenous immunoglobulin. Neurology 43:876, 1993.
146. Nakayama T, Horiuchi E, Watanabe T, et al: A case of inclusion body myositis with benign monoclonal gammopathy successfully responding to repeated immunoabsorption. J Neurol Neurosurg Psychiatry 68:230, 2000.
147. Mowzoon N, Sussman A, Bradley WG: Mycophenolate (CellCept) treatment of myasthenia gravis, chronic inflammatory polyneuropathy and inclusion body myositis. J Neurol Sci 185:119, 2001.

148. Pearl GS, Sieger B: Granulomatous *Pneumocystis carinii* myositis presenting as an intramuscular mass. Clin Infect Dis 22:577, 1996.
149. Vogel H: Pathologic findings in nerve and muscle biopsies from 47 women with silicone breast implants. Neurology 53:293, 1999.
150. Herrmann DN, Blaivas M, Wald JJ, et al: Granulomatous myositis, primary biliary cirrhosis, pancytopenia, and thymoma. Muscle Nerve 23:1133, 2000.
151. Nakamura Y, Kurihara N, Sato A, et al: Muscle sarcoidosis following malignant lymphoma: diagnosis by MR imaging. Skeletal Radiol 31:702, 2002.
152. Prayson RA: Granulomatous myositis: clinicopathologic study of 12 cases. Am J Clin Pathol 112:63, 1999.
153. Ost D, Yeldandi A, Cugell D: Acute sarcoid myositis with respiratory muscle involvement: case report and review of the literature. Chest 107:879, 1995.
154. Mozaffar T, Lopate G, Pestronk A: Clinical correlates of granulomas in muscle. J Neurol 245:519, 1998.
155. Le Roux K, Streichenberger N, Vial C, et al: Granulomatous myositis: a clinical study of thirteen cases. Muscle Nerve 35:171, 2007.
156. Salvarani C, Cantini F, Olivieri I, et al: Proximal bursitis in active polymyalgia rheumatica. Ann Intern Med 127:27, 1997.
157. Cantini F, Salvarani C, Olivieri I, et al: Shoulder ultrasonography in the diagnosis of polymyalgia rheumatica: a case-control study. J Rheumatol 28:1049, 2001.
158. Lacomis D, Zochodne DW, Bird SJ: Critical illness myopathy. Muscle Nerve 23:1785, 2000.
159. Hund E: Myopathy in critically ill patients. Crit Care Med 27:2544, 1999.
160. Rich MM, Bird SJ, Raps EC, et al: Direct muscle stimulation in acute quadriplegic myopathy. Muscle Nerve 20:665, 1997.
161. Latronico N, Fenzi F, Recupero D, et al: Critical illness myopathy and neuropathy. Lancet 347:1579, 1996.
162. Evers S, Engelien A, Karsch V, et al: Secondary hyperkalaemic paralysis. J Neurol Neurosurg Psychiatry 64:249, 1998.
163. Campistol JM: Uremic myopathy. Kidney Int 62:1901, 2002.
164. Mak RH, DeFronzo RA: Glucose and insulin metabolism in uremia. Nephron 61:377, 1992.
165. Ahmad S, Robertson HT, Golper TA, et al: Multicenter trial of L-carnitine in maintenance hemodialysis patients. II. Clinical and biochemical effects. Kidney Int 38:912, 1990.
166. Shanahan RL, Kerzee JA, Sandhoff BG, et al: Low myopathy rates associated with statins as monotherapy or combination therapy with interacting drugs in a group model health maintenance organization. Pharmacotherapy 25:345, 2005.
167. Needham M, Fabian V, Knezevic W, et al: Progressive myopathy with up-regulation of MHC-I associated with statin therapy. Neuromuscul Disord 17:194, 2007.
168. Mammen AL, Chung T, Christopher-Stine L, et al: Autoantibodies against 3-hydroxy-3-methylglutaryl-coenzyme A reductase in patients with statin-associated autoimmune myopathy. Arthritis Rheum 63:713, 2011.
169. Warren JD, Blumbergs PC, Thompson PD: Rhabdomyolysis: a review. Muscle Nerve 25:332, 2002.
170. Clarkson PM, Kearns AK, Rouzier P, et al: Serum creatine kinase levels and renal function measures in exertional muscle damage. Med Sci Sports Exerc 38:623, 2006.
171. Kenney K, Landau ME, Gonzalez RS, et al: Serum creatine kinase after exercise: drawing the line between physiological response and exertional rhabdomyolysis. Muscle Nerve 45:356, 2012.
172. Clarkson PM, Hoffman EP, Zambraski E, et al: ACTN3 and MLCK genotype associations with exertional muscle damage. J Appl Physiol 99:564, 2005.
173. Heled Y, Bloom MS, Wu TJ, et al: CK-MM and ACE genotypes and physiological prediction of the creatine kinase response to exercise. J Appl Physiol 103:504, 2007.

CHAPTER

60

Disorders of Consciousness in Systemic Diseases

J. CLAUDE HEMPHILL III

Consciousness is a complex and elusive concept that has been the subject of extensive thought and speculation by philosophers, theologians, and scientists since antiquity. The fact that consciousness may mean different things depending on the context (philosophy, religion, science) demonstrates the importance that understanding normal and disordered consciousness holds across a wide variety of fields of study. In medicine, disorders of consciousness are pervasive among the effects of systemic diseases on the nervous system. Because alterations in consciousness may have important diagnostic, therapeutic, and prognostic implications, a pragmatic approach using the neurologic principle of localization and the medical approach of differential diagnosis is useful. The spectrum of consciousness, from wakefulness to coma to brain death, has an anatomic and biologic substrate.

CONSCIOUSNESS

Historical Perspective

Ever since the Greek physician Galen (130 to 200 A.D.) recognized that a wound of the brain could affect the mind, the roles of consciousness and thought as manifestations of brain injury and impairment have held a special role. During the Renaissance, the philosopher Descartes (1596 to 1650) focused on the "mind–brain problem." He thought that the pineal gland was the seat of the soul, and this structure therefore played a special role in his concept of consciousness, although contemporaries granted this honor to the corpus callosum. Late nineteenth and early twentieth century efforts such as William James's "stream of consciousness" focused on psychologic, not anatomic, mechanisms.[1] Although the effect of systemic diseases on consciousness has been recognized since Hippocrates in the fifth century B.C. described "madness on account of bile," the ability to ascribe testable anatomic and biologic correlates to consciousness is distinctly modern.[2] The two main advances that have made this possible are (1) development of an operational definition of consciousness that has practical applicability and (2) understanding of the anatomic substrate of consciousness.

Definition of Consciousness

In medicine, consciousness can be defined as awareness of self and the environment. Thus, decreased

Aminoff's Neurology and General Medicine, Fifth Edition.

TABLE 60-1 ■ Spectrum and Components of Consciousness

Spectrum of Arousal
Alert
Confused
Lethargic
Obtunded
Stuporous
Comatose
Components of Content
Cognition (thought)
Awareness of environment
Memory
Language
Visuospatial integration

consciousness involves impairment of this state of awareness, with coma being its absence. Consciousness and conscious behavior have two basic components: arousal and content.[3] Arousal is behaviorally related to the level of alertness or wakefulness. Content describes the complex range of cognitive functions, including thought, memory, and language. As described later, a simplified anatomic model of consciousness gives arousal and content distinct anatomic localizations. Arousal and content may be independent but are frequently interdependent. For content to be present or at least to be assessed clinically, some degree of arousal must be present. Conversely, if decreased arousal (e.g., from sedative drug intoxication) is overcome by a noxious stimulus, content may be seen to be largely normal until arousal fades again.[3] A description of the state of consciousness of an individual must take into account both level of arousal and quality of content. Different diseases and neuroanatomic sites may be implicated, depending on the specifics of the state of consciousness. The term *level of consciousness* usually refers to level of arousal (Table 60-1).

Anatomy of Consciousness

Although somewhat of an oversimplification, the two different components of consciousness are mediated by two distinct neuroanatomic systems (Fig. 60-1). Arousal is mediated by the ascending reticular activating system (RAS). The RAS is located in the brainstem and is a loosely arranged column of neurons extending from the upper third of the pons to the diencephalic structures of the thalamus and hypothalamus.[4] Projections via subcortical relay nuclei, primarily in the thalamus, integrate RAS-mediated arousal with more diffuse cerebral cortical functions. Experimental studies have demonstrated that stimulation of the RAS in a sleeping animal results in immediate behavioral arousal, but when the RAS is destroyed, no amount of sensory stimulation reverses coma, even with subcortical and cortical structures intact.

The content of consciousness is localized more broadly throughout the cerebral cortex. Certain cognitive functions are diffusely localized throughout both cerebral hemispheres, whereas other functions may have more narrow localization. Receptive language and expressive language are principally localized to the superior temporal lobe or posterior frontal lobe, respectively, of the dominant hemisphere. Although various aspects of memory may be stored diffusely, the mesial temporal lobes and mamillary bodies are important for storage of new short-term memory.[5] Conversely, processes such as thought, orientation, attention, and planning are localized diffusely, especially among both frontal lobes.[6] Because a severe impairment of receptive language is likely to alter the state of awareness of self or environment (as far as can be deduced by examination), some may consider it an altered state of consciousness.[7] Others place more emphasis on impairment of bihemispheric dysfunction, evidenced by decreased attention, concentration, and coherent thought, as defining altered content of consciousness.[6] The important lesson is that different aspects of the content of consciousness may have different anatomical localizations and that global impairment of cognitive function implies bilateral cerebral hemispheric dysfunction or disease.

Implications for Systemic Diseases

Coma, or unconsciousness, is a state of unresponsiveness in which the subject has closed eyes and cannot be aroused appropriately with stimuli.[3] For coma to be present, one of two general anatomic conditions must be satisfied: there must be significant impairment of either the RAS or both cerebral hemispheres (Table 60-2). Structural lesions usually

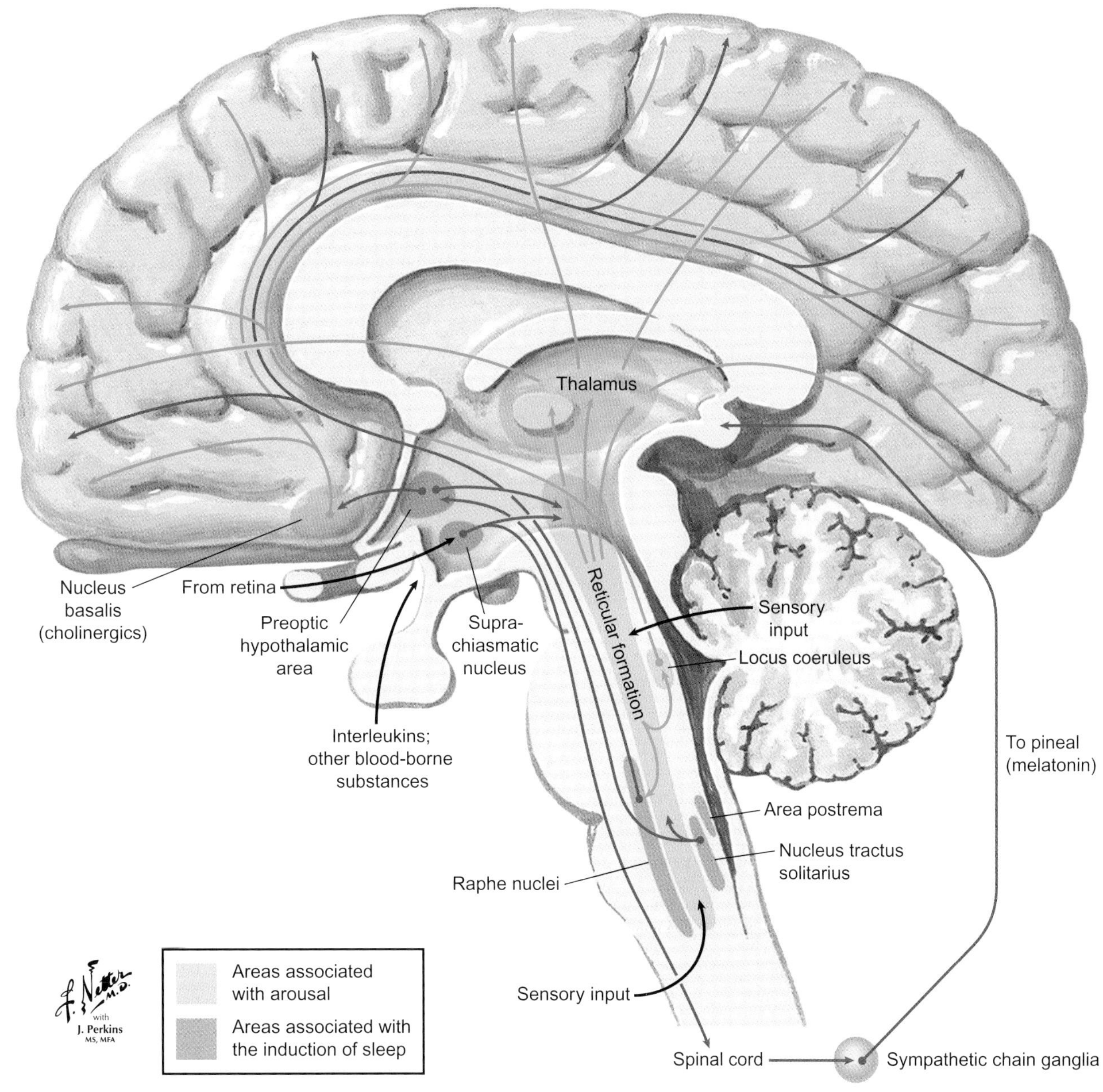

FIGURE 60-1 ▪ Neuroanatomy of consciousness. The reticular formation (also known as the reticular activating system [RAS]) is a loosely arranged column of neurons located in the brainstem. Arousal is largely mediated by the RAS through projections to the cerebral cortex through the thalamus. The content of consciousness is localized more diffusely throughout the cerebral cortex. The reticular formation is distinguished from other brain structures associated with induction of sleep. (Netter illustration from www.netterimages.com.)

cause coma through direct brainstem involvement or through brainstem displacement or compression with subsequent RAS involvement.[3,8] The underlying pathologic processes are often primary neurologic disorders such as intracerebral hemorrhage, traumatic brain injury, subdural hematoma, brain tumors or abscesses, or large cerebral infarctions with mass effect.[9–14] Transtentorial herniation because of a supratentorial mass, direct brainstem impingement from an infratentorial lesion, or direct parenchymal brainstem involvement from hemorrhagic or ischemic stroke are common examples.[15] Less commonly, subfalcine herniation or bihemispheric mass lesions may lead to coma with an intact brainstem due to diencephalic injury. Metabolic disturbances, by contrast, usually cause coma from

TABLE 60-2 ■ Neuroanatomic Localization of Coma

Brainstem (RAS)
Brainstem compression
Transtentorial herniation from supratentorial mass lesion
Subdural hematoma
Intracerebral hemorrhage
Post-traumatic cerebral edema
Large hemispheric infarction with mass effect
Brain tumor or abscess
Acute hydrocephalus
Infratentorial mass lesion
Cerebellar hematoma
Cerebellar infarct
Cerebellar tumor
Intrinsic brainstem involvement
Pontine hemorrhage
Basilar artery occlusion
Metabolic brainstem involvement
Severe hypoxic-ischemic injury
Anesthetic agents (?)
Severe organ failure (?)
Bilateral Cerebral Hemispheres
Subfalcine (cingulate) herniation
Brain tumor or abscess (with edema)
Large hemispheric infarction with mass effect
Bilateral structural hemispheric involvement
Widely metastatic cancer
Primary brain tumor (crossing corpus callosum)
Metabolic encephalopathy
Organ failure
Medications (drugs)
Hypoxic-ischemic injury

RAS, reticular activating system.

diffuse bihemispheric involvement, which presumably results in disconnection between the RAS (and subcortical thalamic relay nuclei) and the hemispheres. The neurologic examination of the comatose patient is an important key in distinguishing the cause and anatomic basis of coma, specifically the presence or absence of other brainstem and cranial nerve abnormalities such as pupillary or extraocular movement dysfunction. The cause of lesser degrees of impaired level of consciousness can also be assessed by determining whether bihemispheric or brainstem dysfunction is responsible.

Sleep should be considered as a separate and distinct entity. Externally, patients in coma initially appear asleep, but sleeping individuals can be roused and then respond to the environment. Normal sleep has several stages that have distinct electroencephalographic (EEG) patterns as discussed in Chapter 51.[16,17] The EEG findings in coma may vary, depending on the cause, but, in general, do not resemble those of sleep.[18] Altered consciousness in systemic disease is a pathologic state in contrast to sleep, which is a necessary and normal function.

MECHANISMS OF IMPAIRED CONSCIOUSNESS IN SPECIFIC DISEASES

A practical approach to determining the cause of impaired consciousness in systemic disease requires an understanding of the mechanisms by which primary neurologic disorders as well as systemic diseases may affect the central nervous system (CNS). The neuroanatomic localization of consciousness implies that both focal and global, or diffuse, processes may alter the level or content of consciousness. Structural causes are intuitively easier to understand than many metabolic or diffuse causes. Compression, distortion, or infarction of the brainstem and RAS are processes for which urgent interventions, such as neurosurgical evacuation of a mass lesion or thrombolysis of an occluded artery, may be indicated.[19,20] In contrast, metabolic encephalopathies cause impaired consciousness (either content or arousal) by interfering diffusely with the functions of the brain on a biochemical level; however, some metabolic encephalopathies can be considered "structural" on a microscopic level when they result in direct cellular brain injury.[21–23] Although the mechanisms by which systemic diseases cause alteration in consciousness are diverse, they can be divided into three broad categories: metabolic encephalopathies, focal neurologic manifestations of systemic disorders, and primary neurologic disorders caused by systemic disease.

Metabolic Encephalopathies

Metabolic encephalopathy is the most frequent cause of disordered consciousness in systemic diseases, and is defined as an alteration in consciousness caused by diffuse or global brain dysfunction from impaired cerebral metabolism. The list of metabolic encephalopathies is extensive and includes such disparate conditions as hypoxic-ischemic encephalopathy, hepatic encephalopathy, drug overdose, bacterial meningitis, and the postseizure state. The principal reason for grouping together this wide variety of disorders is that the neurologic examination may appear quite similar regardless of the underlying etiology. Nevertheless, the cause of the metabolic encephalopathy is the fundamental determinant of treatment and prognosis. Thus, considering the biochemistry of metabolic encephalopathies is of prime importance in their differentiation.

Two common themes emerge with regard to presumptive etiologies of metabolic encephalopathies in systemic disease: impaired substrate delivery (glucose or oxygen) to the brain or release by a systemic disease of a circulating substance that crosses the blood–brain barrier (or enters through a broken blood–brain barrier) and causes neuronal and cellular dysfunction (Table 60-3). The former, implicated in hypoxic-ischemic encephalopathy and hypoglycemia, may result in irreversible brain injury.[24,25] The latter, implicated in most metabolic encephalopathies associated with organ system dysfunction (e.g., hepatic, renal) or with systemic infection, may be largely reversible if the underlying disorder is treated.[26–29] Although there are exceptions, this mechanistic differentiation can be of great importance in determining treatment and prognosis.

TABLE 60-3 ■ Mechanisms of Metabolic Encephalopathies

Impaired Substrate Delivery
Hypoxia-ischemia
Hypoglycemia
Organ Failure
Hepatic encephalopathy
Renal failure
Pancreatic encephalopathy
Carbon dioxide narcosis
Circulating Cytokines (Putative)
Sepsis
Multisystem organ failure
Meningitis
Electrolyte Abnormalities
Hyponatremia
Hypernatremia
Hypercalcemia
Diffuse Brain Infection
HIV infection
Syphilis
Lyme disease
Autoantibodies
Paraneoplastic syndromes
Collagen vascular diseases
Diffusely Decreased Cerebral Metabolism
Medications/anesthesia/sedative drugs
Hypothermia

HIV, human immunodeficiency virus.

When substrate delivery to the brain is globally reduced, encephalopathy and eventually coma may result. Hypoxia, and especially hypoxia-ischemia, may result in permanent cerebral damage diffusely or in selectively vulnerable areas such as the hippocampus, cerebellum, and thalamus. The degree and duration of hypoxia or decreased cerebral blood flow determine the severity and irreversibility of damage. Hypoxic-ischemic encephalopathy most commonly results from severe hypotension or cardiac arrest and is mediated by the neuronal ischemic injury cascade, which includes release of excitatory amino acids, intracellular calcium influx, lipid peroxidation, and cell breakdown.[30] Two clinical trials have demonstrated a beneficial effect of immediate treatment of comatose survivors of cardiac arrest with mild hypothermia (33°C for 12 to 24 hours after out-of-hospital cardiac arrest from ventricular fibrillation or pulseless ventricular tachycardia), and this treatment is part of standard resuscitation guidelines as discussed in Chapter 9.[31–33] Hypoglycemic encephalopathy is potentially reversible, but permanent damage may occur if it is not treated early. Hypertensive encephalopathy may be due to disordered cerebral autoregulation, elevated cerebral vascular resistance, and subsequent globally decreased cerebral blood flow.[34,35] These substrate-delivery encephalopathies have altered cerebral oxygen and glucose delivery as a common pathway, regardless of cause, and may result in severe permanent neurologic damage if not treated urgently.

In contrast, systemic organ failure is a common cause of metabolic encephalopathy and carries a different prognosis than the substrate-delivery encephalopathies. Kidney (uremia) and liver failure are common causes.[36–38] Carbon dioxide narcosis from pulmonary failure and, rarely, pancreatic failure can also cause encephalopathy.[39,40] The biochemical mechanism of uremic encephalopathy is not known precisely, but decreased ability to utilize adenosine triphosphate by the uremic brain and elevated calcium content in the cerebral cortex and hypothalamus have been suggested.[41] In hepatic encephalopathy, endogenous benzodiazepine-like substances may play a role, as suggested by animal studies and from experience in humans with improvement after administration of flumazenil.[42] In hepatic failure, elevated levels of α-ketoglutaramate in the cerebrospinal fluid (CSF) correlate with systemic elevations in ammonia as well as depth of coma.[43] Patients with fulminant hepatic failure may also have severe diffuse cerebral edema,[44] and the acutely increased intracranial pressure provides a structural basis for the coma in this situation. Abnormal function of endocrine organs may cause encephalopathy through primary mechanisms (e.g., myxedema coma,[45] thyrotoxicosis,[46] hypocortisolemia) or through changes in electrolytes or the cerebral acid-base environment (e.g., hypercalcemia in hyperparathyroidism).

Encephalopathy frequently accompanies sepsis, especially when associated with multisystem organ failure.[47,48] Critically ill patients may have multiple reasons for encephalopathy including primary organ failure (especially of kidneys and liver), electrolyte abnormalities, and concurrent use of sedative agents to facilitate interventions such as mechanical ventilation.[49] However, sepsis itself is associated with a metabolic encephalopathy. Although proposed mechanisms of septic encephalopathy range from multiple microabscesses throughout the brain to alterations in cerebral blood flow mediated by nitric oxide, circulating cytokines that cross the blood–brain barrier and are released during sepsis or the systemic inflammatory response syndrome are likely to be implicated.[50] In contrast to substrate-delivery metabolic encephalopathies, these alterations in consciousness are generally thought to be reversible if the underlying organ pathologic process or sepsis is reversed.

Electrolyte and acid-base disturbances are a common cause of encephalopathy. Among these, hyponatremia, hypernatremia, and hypercalcemia are most commonly associated with a decreased level of consciousness.[51] In most circumstances, these encephalopathies are reversible, although rapid correction of hyponatremia should be avoided to decrease the potential of osmotic demyelination (central pontine myelinolysis).[52]

A global decrease in the cerebral metabolic rate of oxygen consumption may occur during profound hypothermia and following sedative drug overdose.[53,54] This is reversible if substrate delivery is maintained. Thus, general anesthesia itself can be viewed as a cause of reversible metabolic encephalopathy or coma. Metabolic encephalopathy, often without a markedly decreased level of consciousness, may be caused by numerous prescription medications and may be mistaken for dementia in the elderly.[55,56] Encephalopathy may also be a manifestation of collagen vascular disease (e.g., systemic lupus erythematosus, SLE), or systemic cancer.[57,58] Although the latter may be mediated by electrolyte disturbances in the setting of the syndrome of inappropriate secretion of antidiuretic hormone or through paraneoplastic antibodies[59] or circulating cytokines, these disorders may also cause alterations in consciousness from focal processes related specifically to the underlying cancer or collagen vascular disease.

The term *delirium* refers to a state of globally disturbed consciousness in which a subject has decreased attention and an altered sensorium, usually developing over hours to days and often with fluctuating symptoms.[60] Agitation and hallucinations may be present but are not required for the diagnosis. Delirium has historically been a general descriptive term akin to metabolic encephalopathy and distinguished from dementia by its fairly abrupt onset, altered sensorium, and association with other medical conditions. However, within the past decade, delirium has been used specifically to describe a state of fluctuating confusion in hospitalized patients, often in those who are critically ill.[19,61] The presence of delirium has been associated with worsened clinical outcome in these patients, and some studies have suggested that delirium is itself an independent condition with a pathophysiology and treatment distinct from the many other systemic diseases known to cause metabolic encephalopathy. The neurotransmitter acetylcholine is particularly implicated in delirium.[62] Predisposing factors include older age, dementia, sensory impairment, sleep deprivation, and the use of sedative medications.[63,64] Inflammatory serum markers and genetic polymorphisms of the apolipoprotein E gene have also been suggested as predictors of presence or duration of delirium.[65,66] In the intensive care unit, the use of the sedative medication dexmedetomidine has been associated with less delirium than benzodiazepine infusions.[63] Long-term cognitive impairment has been associated with delirium in acutely hospitalized patients, especially those with preexisting cognitive impairment.[67] It is distinctly uncommon, however, for delirium to lead to a chronic vegetative or minimally conscious state. It remains controversial whether delirium is principally an indicator of the need for aggressive treatment of underlying medical problems and minimization of sedative usage in the hospital.[68]

Systemic Disorders with Focal Neurologic Manifestations

A variety of systemic disorders may cause alteration of consciousness through either infiltration of the CNS or the presence of discrete lesions. Occasionally, patients may appear clinically to have a diffuse encephalopathy, but close examination reveals focal neurologic signs. In this setting, the distinction between metabolic encephalopathy and diffuse multifocal cerebral disease may be clinically difficult and appear to be only a matter of semantics. Pathologically, however, the processes are quite different, with the latter representing more than just an alteration in substrate delivery or a global process related to circulating systemic factors. The three categories of systemic disease that most often manifest in this manner are collagen vascular diseases, systemic malignancies, and diffuse infections.

Neuropsychiatric complications are frequent clinical manifestations of SLE.[69] Neuropathologic findings in these patients vary from normal to the presence of diffuse microinfarcts. Lupus cerebritis commonly manifests as a focal process with pathologic findings of a bland, and occasionally necrotizing, vasculopathy with perivascular inflammatory infiltrates.[70] There is debate whether this represents a "true" vasculitis or a more infiltrative process surrounding, rather than invading, the vessels. Particular neurologic manifestations depend on lesion location, and aphasia due to focal lesions in the language regions or abulia due to bifrontal lesions are common. Neurosarcoidosis most often manifests as meningeal inflammation or focal cranial neuropathies but can occur as a large cerebral or brainstem mass lesion that affects consciousness.[71]

Systemic cancer affects consciousness in a variety of ways. Cancer may cause metabolic problems related to electrolyte disturbances and primary organ dysfunction.[51] Focal neurologic manifestations in patients with cancer more likely suggest metastatic disease to the CNS, as discussed in Chapter 26. Metastatic brain tumors are much more common than primary brain tumors. Most commonly occurring supratentorially, mass effect from metastases may cause cerebral herniation with brainstem compression or bihemispheric dysfunction.[72] Meningeal carcinomatosis often spares consciousness, except when so extensive that intracranial vessels at the base of the brain are affected, leading to stroke.[73] Cancer treatments themselves may have effects on consciousness. Metabolic encephalopathy may be caused by certain chemotherapeutic agents, and cranial irradiation may result in focal necrosis that is initially difficult to differentiate from recurrent tumor.[74]

Infection may also cause focal or global neurologic disturbances of consciousness. Brain abscess, meningitis, or encephalitis may occur in otherwise normal individuals or in those with compromised immune systems due to a variety of systemic diseases.[75] Several systemic infections are particularly associated with focal processes or infiltration of the nervous system including human immunodeficiency virus (HIV) infection, syphilis, and Lyme disease. Direct infection of neurons by HIV may result in HIV encephalopathy.[76] Although described as a diffuse encephalopathy, it is probably a "microscopic structural" process related to global infection and infiltration. Progressive multifocal leukoencephalopathy (PML) occurs from infection with the JC papovavirus and manifests principally as cerebral white matter lesions that may involve altered consciousness.[77] Patients immunocompromised from HIV infection are also at risk of a myriad of CNS problems, including primary CNS lymphoma, toxoplasmosis, and other opportunistic infections, discussed further in Chapter 44. Syphilis may have a variety of CNS manifestations; consciousness may be affected by strokes in meningovascular syphilis, and dementia occurs in tertiary syphilis.[78] Lyme neuroborreliosis may cause generalized confusion that has been mistaken for psychiatric disease.[79] Like a number of other systemic disorders including SLE, sarcoidosis, PML, and syphilis, Lyme disease may have the neuroimaging appearance of diffuse cerebral white matter (or demyelinating) lesions, and therefore, may mimic multiple sclerosis.

Systemic Diseases Presenting as Primary Neurologic Disorders

Seizures, stroke, and acute mass lesions are primary neurologic disorders that may occur secondary to systemic diseases. Generalized seizures, by definition, result in alteration or loss of consciousness. Stroke and acute mass lesions may cause alterations in consciousness depending on their location. Although systemic diseases such as hypertension and diabetes are implicated in the genesis of stroke, cancer is implicated in metastatic CNS disease, and many systemic disorders cause seizures,[80,81] certain conditions have primary neurologic diagnoses as their principal manifestation.

Large-vessel ischemic strokes may occur from either embolic or thrombotic causes. Infective endocarditis or marantic endocarditis (as in SLE or cancer) may result in embolic infarction that may alter consciousness depending on stroke location and size, as discussed in Chapter 6.[82,83] Hypercoagulable states may occur in cancer or autoimmune disorders and cause thrombotic large-vessel occlusion of the cerebral arterial circulation. Hypercoagulability may also lead to thrombosis of the cerebral venous sinuses; alterations in factors V and VIII as well as proteins C and S during an ulcerative colitis flare are a potentially underrecognized cause.[84] Leukemia with white blood cell counts in excess of 100,000/μl, polycythemia vera with hematocrit greater than 55 percent, and essential thrombocythemia with a platelet count above 1,000,000/μl may each increase blood viscosity leading to thrombotic occlusion. Small-vessel or lacunar infarcts rarely result in alterations in consciousness. Cerebral vasculitis, however, is often associated with confusion and alteration in behavior and the content of consciousness due either to large-vessel stroke or, more commonly, to widespread mid-size and small-vessel infarction. Although cerebral vasculitis may occur in isolation (e.g., granulomatous angiitis of the nervous system), numerous connective tissue disorders, including polyarteritis nodosa and Churg–Strauss syndrome, may be implicated (see Chapter 50).[85,86]

Cerebral mass lesions that lead to a decrease in the level of consciousness usually develop rapidly. Primary and secondary brain tumors may manifest in this manner, but acute intracranial hemorrhage is the most common responsible lesion. Hypertension is the most common cause of intracerebral hemorrhage.[87] Coagulopathy in the setting of liver failure, disseminated intravascular coagulation, or thrombotic thrombocytopenic purpura may precipitate a spontaneous intracerebral, subdural, or epidural hematoma.[88] Mild head trauma, which would otherwise be well tolerated, may lead to severe intracranial bleeding with subdural or intraparenchymal hematoma formation if a concomitant coagulopathy is present.

APPROACH TO PATIENTS WITH DISORDERED CONSCIOUSNESS

The fundamental goal of evaluation of patients with disorders of consciousness is to distinguish processes that may cause ongoing brain injury from those that are reversible if concurrent systemic diseases are treated adequately. The manifestations of systemic diseases in the CNS are protean, and "benign" and "malignant" causes of altered consciousness may appear clinically similar. Thus, an orderly approach to the evaluation of patients is essential for timely and accurate diagnosis, which can direct focused treatment. The approach should combine clinical neurologic assessment with judicious use of other diagnostic studies including neuroimaging, electrophysiologic evaluation, CSF analysis, and other laboratory tests.

Neurologic History and Examination

The neurologic findings in patients with altered consciousness and the time course of onset are the principal components of patient assessment. All supporting studies, regardless of their nature, must be interpreted within the context of the neurologic examination. The neuroanatomy of consciousness forms the underpinning for neurologic assessment, and it is this localization that allows the formation of a differential diagnosis. The first step is to define whether the primary disturbance is of content or arousal.

When content of consciousness is impaired in patients who are alert and without marked decrease in the level of consciousness, neurologic assessment focuses on higher cortical function. Abnormalities of language, visuospatial orientation, and visual fields suggest a focal cerebral cortical lesion. Disordered attention, concentration, and short-term memory usually suggest a more global process involving both cerebral hemispheres. In the former case, stroke, tumor, a demyelinating process, or focal abscess should be considered, and neuroimaging may be diagnostic. In disorders of global cerebral content, a diffuse process is implicated; depending on the history and associated medical and neurologic findings, a primary neurologic process such as Alzheimer disease or a global metabolic encephalopathy from organ dysfunction, medications, or postictal state may be responsible.

The more urgent circumstance occurs in patients with decreased level of arousal, especially coma. Processes, either structural or metabolic, that develop acutely tend to involve a disproportionately decreased level of consciousness compared with those that develop over much longer periods of time.[3] The initial focus of the neurologic examination of the stuporous or comatose patient should be in defining the anatomic localization of the process, distinguishing between brainstem (RAS) and bihemispheric disease. This is also often the distinction between structural (usually RAS) and metabolic (usually bihemispheric) causes of coma. A notable exception is the locked-in state, in which a structural lesion, usually a stroke, involves the brainstem but spares the RAS.[89,90] Patients who are "locked in" are not comatose and may have intact consciousness; motor function in the form of eye opening and blinking is usually retained, whereas ocular movements and appendicular motor function are typically absent. Thus, the first step in clinical evaluation of the apparently comatose patient is to exclude the possibility of the locked-in syndrome, which is suggested by the observation that the patient can open their eyes and blink to command.

Once coma is established, assessment of brainstem and motor function can proceed. Abnormalities of pupillary function, ocular motility, corneal and gag reflexes, and respiratory function help distinguish an intact from an impaired brainstem. Preserved pupillary function is a hallmark for distinguishing between metabolic and structural causes of coma.[3] Reflexive ocular movements (oculocephalic reflexes tested with "doll's eyes" or "cold caloric" maneuvers) are typically preserved in metabolic coma. Occasionally, however, odd conjugate downgaze, skew deviation, and loss of ocular reflexes are found in deep coma caused by metabolic disorders, especially liver failure or sedative drug overdose.[91] Unilateral absence of the corneal or gag reflex suggests structural brainstem impairment. Motor function is symmetric in coma of metabolic origin. Depth of coma, regardless of cause, may determine whether purposeful response to pain is present. Gross asymmetry of purposeful or reflex motor response to pain suggests a structural process. Patients in deep coma of metabolic cause, especially from sedative drug overdose, may exhibit symmetric flexor or extensor posturing, with retained brisk pupillary reflexes and intact brainstem reflexes.

Neuroimaging

Findings on clinical examination direct the need for, and type of, neuroimaging required. Most patients without a history of head trauma who are somnolent with a global alteration in cognitive function and intact brainstem reflexes have a metabolic encephalopathy. When a known systemic cause of metabolic encephalopathy, such as uremia, liver failure, or sedative or other drug use, is present, neuroimaging may not be necessary. Conversely, all patients with coma of unknown etiology require urgent head imaging.

The principal value of early neuroimaging is to evaluate for structural processes. Computerized tomography (CT) is particularly effective at demonstrating acute intracranial hemorrhage and in most centers is more easily obtained in neurologically impaired patients than magnetic resonance imaging (MRI); therefore noncontrast CT is the best first option for neuroimaging in patients with acute alteration or loss of consciousness.[92,93] CT in acute stroke (within the first 12 hours) may be normal or show only subtle abnormalities such as loss of gray-white differentiation or mild edema. CT is greater than 91 percent sensitive for subarachnoid hemorrhage following aneurysm rupture,[94] and nearly always shows acute intraparenchymal or extra-axial processes such as hemorrhage and mass lesions that are causing cerebral herniation. By contrast, head CT in metabolic encephalopathy is usually negative or nondiagnostic.

MRI is much better than CT at delineating specific anatomic structures, especially in the posterior fossa. It is usually not necessary in the emergency setting when CT has been performed. An important exception is when cerebral venous sinus thrombosis is suspected; CT with contrast demonstrates a sign known as the "empty delta" in approximately 30 percent of cases; this represents clot in the torcula, where the superior sagittal sinus meets the paired transverse sinuses.[95] However, MRI with contrast, especially when done with magnetic resonance venography, is highly sensitive and specific for thrombosis of the sagittal sinus or other intracranial venous sinus that might be the cause of coma.[96] For patients in whom altered consciousness or coma is not acute, MRI may be preferable to CT because it is more likely to reveal cerebral metastases, subtle signs of infection or cerebral swelling, or changes that are sometimes seen in certain metabolic conditions, such as basal ganglia abnormalities in liver disease or posterior white matter changes in hypertensive encephalopathy or eclampsia.[97] Newer tools such as magnetic resonance spectroscopy can provide a more direct measure of cerebral metabolism in regions of interest, but its role in routine evaluation remains unclear.[98]

Electrophysiologic Studies

EEG and evoked potentials are the major electrophysiologic modalities of diagnostic use in patients with altered consciousness. They are used mainly to exclude seizures (especially nonconvulsive status epilepticus), to confirm the diagnosis of certain metabolic encephalopathies that may have characteristic EEG patterns, and to provide a guide to prognosis in irreversible cerebral injuries, especially hypoxic-ischemic encephalopathy.[99,100] EEG is indicated in patients with coma of unknown etiology, especially those who have nondiagnostic head imaging studies.

Nonconvulsive status epilepticus is a disorder in which generalized seizures continue without gross motor manifestations of convulsions.[101] This may occur in patients who present with clinically apparent seizures and then continue to seize even after clinical evidence of convulsions ceases. It includes patients with frequent complex partial seizures or absence status (spike-wave stupor).[102] Subclinical electrographic seizures may be identified in up to 20 percent of patients with significant primary neurologic injuries (such as stroke or traumatic brain injury) who undergo continuous EEG monitoring in the neurologic intensive care unit.[103,104] In two studies of inpatients with primarily medical illness outside the intensive care unit, electrographic seizures were found in 7 to10 percent of those monitored with EEG.[105,106] Although this form of status epilepticus as the sole reason for decreased level of consciousness is uncommon, the diagnosis cannot be made without an EEG. Overt status epilepticus, especially myoclonus or nonconvulsive status, after a hypoxic-ischemic cerebral insult carries a poor prognosis.[107]

Metabolic encephalopathies have a relatively uniform pattern on EEG, with diffuse bilateral slowing of the background rhythm. As metabolic coma deepens, amplitude may decrease. Triphasic waves may be found in hepatic encephalopathy but are nonspecific and present in other metabolic encephalopathies, including uremic and septic encephalopathies.[108] In patients with hepatic encephalopathy who are receiving flumazenil as a diagnostic or therapeutic maneuver, EEG monitoring can demonstrate return of more normal background rhythms concurrent with improvement in level of consciousness.[109]

Evoked potential monitoring is usually reserved for the evaluation of comatose patients. Short-latency somatosensory evoked potentials are typically preserved in reversible metabolic encephalopathies.[18] However, in conditions that cause neuronal death, they may be abnormal and of prognostic value. In hypoxic-ischemic encephalopathy, bilateral absence of the N20 component of the somatosensory evoked potential (SSEP) to median nerve stimulation is strongly predictive of a very poor neurologic outcome (see Chapter 9).[110] However, timely availability and variable expertise in interpretation remain shortcomings to widespread implementation.[111]

Cerebrospinal Fluid and Other Laboratory Studies

Prior to the development of CT and MRI, lumbar puncture was a standard part of the investigation of patients with alterations in consciousness. Lumbar puncture is currently performed selectively when meningitis and encephalitis are diagnostic possibilities or when the etiology of coma remains elusive despite clinical evaluation, laboratory testing, and neuroimaging. In comatose patients, neuroimaging should be performed before lumbar puncture because of the rare but potential risk of precipitating transtentorial herniation.[112]

Lumbar puncture may be of particular diagnostic utility in patients with an altered level of consciousness related to unsuspected cerebral venous sinus thrombosis from a hypercoagulable state, in which an elevated opening pressure may be the first diagnostic clue of increased intracranial pressure due to venous outflow obstruction.[113] Analysis of the CSF may also be helpful for evaluation for suspected neurosyphilis, Lyme disease, and neurosarcoidosis. In other conditions such as HIV encephalopathy, CSF cell counts may be mildly elevated. A CSF pleocytosis may rarely be present after seizures, even when no apparent CNS infection is present, but this is uncommon and remains a diagnosis of exclusion.[114]

Laboratory testing of serum electrolytes and of renal and liver function is a fundamental part of the evaluation of all patients with alterations in consciousness. It is important that metabolic derangements found on laboratory testing match the neuroanatomic localization of the patient's syndrome; otherwise, further laboratory, neuroimaging, electrophysiologic, and CSF testing may be required. For example, a patient with liver failure, unilateral impairment of ocular reflexes, and a hemiparesis requires urgent neuroimaging to rule out an intracranial mass lesion such as an acute hematoma, especially because patients with liver failure often have concurrent coagulopathy. Also, when the degree of electrolyte abnormality does not correlate with the depth of alteration in consciousness (e.g., deep coma with a mildly depressed serum sodium concentration), more extensive neurodiagnostic testing should occur.

Diagnosis and Treatment: Coordinated Clinical Approach

The major concern in the management of patients with altered consciousness is preservation or restoration of brain function. The resuscitation principles of maintaining the airway, breathing, and circulation should always be attended to first.[115] By ensuring oxygenation, ventilation, and adequate brain and tissue perfusion, impaired substrate delivery to the brain may be restored and secondary brain injury limited. Neurologic examination should then proceed. Urgent hematologic and biochemical screening tests, including renal and possibly hepatic function studies, should be performed concurrently with neuroimaging, usually CT scanning. Based on these results, EEG and lumbar puncture can be considered. If alteration in consciousness is mild or of relatively long standing, investigation can proceed less urgently.

PROGNOSIS

Prognostication of outcome gives physicians, patients, and families reasonable expectations that can aid in decisions to proceed with, or limit, medical care. It is essential that the prognosticator keep in mind the continuum of prognosis and outcome, recognizing that what would be considered a poor prognosis to some may be acceptable to others.

Coma is one of the most compelling neurologic conditions in which prognostication is often sought. The most important overall determinant of prognosis in coma is the cause of the coma, especially whether the coma is caused by injury to the brain (e.g., from trauma, hypoxia-ischemia, prolonged hypoglycemia) or is secondary to systemic factors (e.g., sedative drug overdose, liver failure, sepsis). In the latter case, prognosis is linked more to the severity of the underlying disease than to the coma itself, although coma in organ failure or sepsis is usually a marker of grave illness that often carries with it a poor prognosis.

There are, however, some general principles to prognostication in coma that may apply across illnesses. There is more information regarding prognosis for hypoxic-ischemic encephalopathy after cardiac arrest than for any other cause of altered consciousness in systemic diseases (see Chapter 9).[36] Specific aspects of the clinical examination performed at different times after cardiac arrest and resuscitation are important predictors of long-term functional outcome, at least in general terms. In an often-cited study performed long before the routine use of hypothermia in comatose cardiac arrest survivors, Levy and associates found that of 70 patients who did not have a withdrawal response or better to painful stimulation in the limbs at 3 days, 93 percent had no recovery or developed a persistent vegetative state, and 7 percent showed some recovery but had severe long-term disability at 1 year; no patients showed moderate or good recovery.[116] Conversely, of 26 patients with withdrawal response (or better) and orienting spontaneous eye movements at 3 days, 77 percent showed moderate to good recovery at 1 year. Recent case series have found that these early clinical examination predictors may be less reliable in patients who are treated with therapeutic hypothermia, with the 3-day motor response having a false-positive rate of approximately 10 percent in predicting a very poor outcome.[117] Thus, a longer duration of observation is prudent in patients who have been treated with therapeutic hypothermia after cardiac arrest. Oculovestibular (cold caloric) reflexes may be an important determinant of severe brainstem damage.

Predictors, either clinical or laboratory-based, for outcome from other causes of metabolic coma are much less available. In a series in which recovery from various forms of coma was assessed, Levy and associates found that 35 percent of patients with hepatic coma and 34 percent of patients with coma caused by renal failure regained independent function, whereas only 12 percent of patients comatose from hypoxia did so.[116] In another study, it was found that only 8 percent of patients with coma of diverse causes recovered fully or with minimal disability when oculovestibular reflexes were absent.[116] The mortality rate in patients with coma from septic encephalopathy and multisystem organ failure approaches 40 percent; this is, however, similar to the mortality rate of multisystem organ failure itself, suggesting that the underlying critical illness, not the presence of coma, defines prognosis in this circumstance. The presence of intact brainstem reflexes (pupils and ocular movements) suggests a more favorable outcome than otherwise in metabolic coma; presumably, these metabolic causes of coma do not cause permanent cerebral damage at least sufficient to cause neuronal death. Most patients who recover from their underlying illness recover completely from coma of metabolic origin. This is not always the case, however, and suggests that some patients with severe critical illness from acute respiratory distress syndrome, sepsis, or electrolyte disturbances may acquire secondary brain injury from either impaired substrate delivery or mechanisms yet to be elucidated.[118]

BRAIN DEATH

The diagnosis of brain death has medical, legal, and ethical implications. In the United States and most other countries, brain death is a prerequisite to most organ donation, although donation following cardiac death is now being used in certain circumstances.[119] Brain death is equivalent to circulatory death (defined by absence of cardiac and respiratory functions) as a medical and legal definition of death, and the time of determination of brain death is considered the time of death.[120] The Uniform Determination of Death Act states that "an individual who has sustained either (1) irreversible cessation of circulatory and respiratory functions or (2) irreversible cessation of all functions of the entire brain, including the brainstem, is dead. A determination of death must be made in accordance with accepted medical standards." Despite ample medical and legal precedent for the concept and importance of brain death, several surveys have indicated lack of knowledge and consistent application of clinical definitions and diagnostic criteria.[121,122] The Quality Standards Subcommittee of the American Academy of Neurology has developed standardized criteria for the determination of brain death in adults, and these form a reasonable, currently accepted medical standard.[123]

The determination of brain death is based primarily on clinical criteria (Tables 60-4 and 60-5), with use of supportive diagnostic tests when necessary. Several prerequisites must be met. It is essential that there be a diagnosis of a CNS catastrophe that is compatible with brain death. These include neurologic disorders (e.g., subarachnoid hemorrhage) and systemic diseases (e.g., hypoxic-ischemic encephalopathy, massive brain edema from fulminant hepatic failure). Complicating conditions that may confound the neurologic examination must be excluded, such as hypothermia ($\leq$36°C), hypotension (systolic blood pressure $\leq$90 mmHg), drug effects such as from neuromuscular blocking agents or sedatives, and facial or cervical trauma that makes it impossible to perform the neurologic examination.

The three clinical features of brain death, all of which must be demonstrated, are cerebral unresponsiveness, absence of brainstem reflexes, and apnea. Cerebral unresponsiveness is demonstrated by absence of cerebral motor response to painful stimulus (supraorbital and nail-bed pressure in all extremities). Brainstem reflexes that must

TABLE 60-4 ■ Conditions to Be Excluded in Using Clinical Criteria for Brain Death

Hypothermia–i.e., temperature ≤36°C
Hypotension/shock–i.e., systolic blood pressure ≤90 mmHg
Hypoxia–i.e., Pa_{O_2} ≤60 mmHg
Sedative drug effects–e.g., high-dose barbiturates
Neuromuscular blocking agents–check peripheral nerve stimulator (for "train-of-four" twitches)
Severe facial trauma–inability to check pupillary or ocular movement function
Severe cervical trauma–high cervical injury interferes with assessment of apnea

TABLE 60-5 ■ Clinical Criteria for Diagnosis of Brain Death

Diagnosis compatible with brain death (e.g., head trauma, stroke, hypoxic-ischemic encephalopathy)
All confounding conditions excluded (see Table 60-4)
Cerebral unresponsiveness: no response to central painful stimulus (supraorbital pressure, temporomandibular joint) in all extremities
Absence of brainstem reflexes
No pupillary reflexes (≤4 mm in size)
No ocular movement (absent doll's eyes or absent response to cold caloric testing)
No facial sensation and motor response (absent corneal reflex)
No pharyngeal response (absent gag and cough reflexes)
Apnea: no clinical evidence of respiratory effort when the Pa_{CO_2} is documented to rise above 60 mmHg or 20 mmHg above a normal baseline
Independent confirmation by a second physician

be demonstrated as absent include pupillary light reflex (usually ≥4 mm in size), ocular movement (absent oculocephalic response or "doll's eyes" and absent response to cold caloric testing), facial sensation and motor response (absent corneal reflex), and pharyngeal response (absent gag and cough reflexes). Apnea is confirmed when the Pa_{CO_2} is documented to rise, following ventilator discontinuation, above 60 mmHg (or 20 mmHg above a normal baseline) without clinical evidence of respiratory effort, indicating absence of function of central respiratory chemoreceptors and neurons located in the medulla. Independent confirmation by a second physician is required for the clinical diagnosis of brain death.

Several confirmatory laboratory tests may be used in the determination of brain death but do not supersede the clinical examination. The use of confirmatory tests is not required and is usually reserved for patients in whom clinical examination cannot be reliably performed because all conditions that may confound the clinical neurologic assessment cannot be excluded. In patients who have received significant doses of sedative agents (e.g., high-dose barbiturates for treatment of elevated intracranial pressure), clinical examination is unreliable for the diagnosis of brain death. In this circumstance, a cerebral blood-flow study demonstrating absence of blood flow to the brain is sufficient for the diagnosis of brain death. Formerly, conventional angiography was performed, but currently a nuclear medicine technetium-99m brain scan is often used.[124] Transcranial Doppler ultrasonography (TCD) (Fig. 60-2) can also be used provided that adequate insonation windows can be obtained.[125] In the absence of sedative medications and hypothermia, EEG performed according to certain specific technical standards can be used when a confirmatory test is necessary.[123]

Some ethical issues remain with regard to brain death.[126,127] Legally, "irreversible cessation of all functions of the entire brain, including the brainstem" indicates brain death, but it has been left to the medical community to decide how to demonstrate this.[123,128] When the accuracy of these stated clinical criteria has been reviewed, the diagnosis of brain death has been considered secure.[120,129] Some have suggested that prolonged unconsciousness or a persistent vegetative state is similar to brain death because purposeful consciousness cannot be regained; although these latter circumstances have been supported in terms of withdrawal of medical support and care due to medical futility, they do not meet the medical or legal definitions of brain death and should not be considered equivalent. Some individuals and cultures do not accept the notion of brain death as equivalent to circulatory death, which can present challenges regarding ongoing medical care and the medical–legal interface.

PERSISTENT VEGETATIVE AND MINIMALLY CONSCIOUS STATES

Brain death could be considered the ultimate loss of consciousness. The neuroanatomy of brain

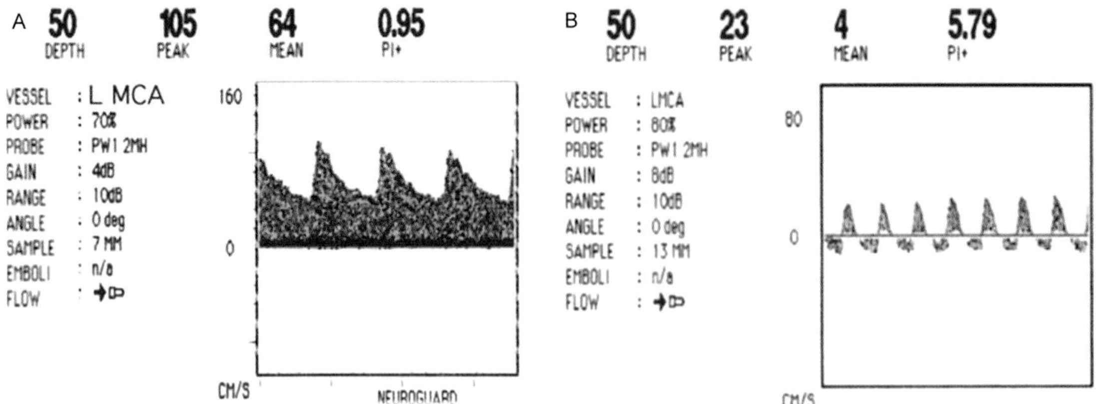

FIGURE 60-2 ■ Diagnosis of brain death by transcranial Doppler ultrasonography (TCD). **A**, Normal blood flow velocity and direction in the left middle cerebral artery (LMCA). **B**, Findings in brain death. Direction of flow is reversed during diastole, indicating cerebral circulatory arrest. For the use of transcranial Doppler ultrasonography as a confirmatory test in brain death, these findings must be present in both anterior circulations as well as in the posterior circulation.

death requires the loss of function of both cerebral hemispheres and the RAS, although it may not be possible clinically to determine cortical function when the RAS and entire brainstem have been completely destroyed. There are, however, circumstances of permanent loss of consciousness other than brain death. It is uncommon for a sleep-like coma state (eyes closed) to persist for more than 2 to 4 weeks.[3] After this time, patients with permanently disordered consciousness usually evolve to a chronically unresponsive state with eyes open. When subjects exhibit this eyes-open unconsciousness with no awareness of self or the environment for more than 1 to 3 months, the definition of a *persistent vegetative state* is met.[130] This state may result from a variety of insults, including acute conditions such as traumatic brain injury, hypoxic-ischemic encephalopathy, and encephalitis, as well as being an end result of chronic neurodegenerative disorders such as Alzheimer disease.[131] Clinically, the vegetative state appears to involve an intact brainstem and absent cerebral cortical function. Autopsy results have largely confirmed this neuroanatomy, showing extensive cortical and hippocampal damage after hypoxic-ischemic encephalopathy and subcortical diffuse axonal injury after trauma. Occasional reports have demonstrated severe brainstem damage, but not in isolation.[131]

A review of the autopsy of Karen Ann Quinlan, who was the subject of dramatic moral and legal debates in 1975 over withdrawal of medical support of patients in a persistent vegetative state, suggested an alternate view of the neuroanatomy of the vegetative state. Quinlan sustained severe hypoxic-ischemic encephalopathy after cardiopulmonary arrest and evolved into a persistent vegetative state after a prolonged coma. Postmortem examination demonstrated severe bilateral damage to the thalamus, out of proportion to any damage found in the cortex or brainstem, suggesting that the thalamus is important for cognition and that severing the connections between the RAS and cerebral cortex may be sufficient to impair consciousness, perhaps permanently.[132] Thus, different neuroanatomic lesions may lead to the clinical picture of a persistent vegetative state and perhaps even the clinical diagnosis of brain death.

It is now clearly recognized that some patients evolve to a clinical state in which they remain severely impaired and unable to perform functionally useful activity and self-care, despite demonstrating evidence of behavioral consciousness and interaction with their environment. This state is known as the *minimally conscious state* and, in contrast to the vegetative state, patients in this state may follow occasional commands, reach for objects, localize noxious stimuli, or demonstrate contingent vocalization, smiling, or crying.[133] Because these activities may be only partially present and able to be performed only intermittently, distinguishing the vegetative and minimally conscious states may be clinically challenging. However, this clinical distinction is important as—while patients who meet the definition of permanent vegetative state are exceedingly unlikely to improve—some patients in a prolonged minimally conscious state do show delayed improvement, especially if traumatic brain injury is the initial cause.[79] Unfortunately most of these patients still remain in a state of severe disability.

The concept of distinguishing vegetative from minimally conscious states may additionally be of ethical importance as minimally conscious patients are awake, may perceive pain, and may raise concerns among families and caregivers regarding patient-level communication and long-term care goals.[134] The best way to distinguish these states is through prolonged and multiple neurologic examinations by different examiners who can objectively document their findings. Interestingly, several recent studies have examined functional neuroimaging using functional MRI or positron emission tomography (PET) in these two patient groups.[85,135] In one study including 54 patients, 5 patients (4 diagnosed clinically as vegetative and 1 as minimally conscious, all as a result of trauma) were able to willfully modulate brain activity seen on functional MRI in response to verbal questions, with activity primarily seen in the supplementary motor area or the parahippocampal gyrus, depending on whether the directions were related to motor or sensory imagery.[85] No patient in a vegetative state or minimally conscious state from hypoxic-ischemic brain injury in this study demonstrated willful modulation of brain activity. A single-patient study, in which a patient in a minimally conscious state 6 years after traumatic brain injury underwent thalamic stimulation with an implantable deep brain stimulator, found improvement in arousal and motor control.[136] The use of brain–computer interfaces to help patients in minimally conscious states interact with their environment is an area of evolving research.[137]

REFERENCES

1. Schooler JW: Introspecting in the spirit of William James: comment on Fox, Ericsson, and Best (2011). Psychol Bull 137:345, 2011.
2. Fins JJ: The ethics of measuring and modulating consciousness: the imperative of minding time. Prog Brain Res 177:371, 2009.
3. Posner JB, Saper CB, Schiff ND, et al: Plum and Posner's Diagnosis of Stupor and Coma. Oxford University Press, New York, 2007.
4. Goldfine AM, Schiff ND: Consciousness: its neurobiology and the major classes of impairment. Neurol Clin 29:723, 2011.
5. Aggleton JP, O'Mara SM, Vann SD, et al: Hippocampal-anterior thalamic pathways for memory: uncovering a network of direct and indirect actions. Eur J Neurosci 31:2292, 2010.
6. Miller EK, Cohen JD: An integrative theory of prefrontal cortex function. Annu Rev Neurosci 24:167, 2001.
7. Farah MJ, Feinberg TE: Consciousness of perception after brain damage. Semin Neurol 17:145, 1997.
8. Fisher CM: Brain herniation: a revision of classical concepts. Can J Neurol Sci 22:83, 1995.
9. Daley ML, Leffler CW, Czosnyka M, et al: Intracranial pressure monitoring: modeling cerebrovascular pressure transmission. Acta Neurochir Suppl 96:103, 2006.
10. Feske SK: Coma and confusional states: emergency diagnosis and management. Neurol Clin 16:237, 1998.
11. Frank JI: Large hemispheric infarction, deterioration, and intracranial pressure. Neurology 45:1286, 1995.
12. Kase CS: Intracerebral haemorrhage. Baillieres Clin Neurol 4:247, 1995.
13. Servadei F: Prognostic factors in severely head injured adult patients with acute subdural haematoma's. Acta Neurochir 139:279, 1997.
14. Shahzadi S, Lozano AM, Bernstein M, et al: Stereotactic management of bacterial brain abscesses. Can J Neurol Sci 23:34, 1996.
15. Ferbert A, Bruckmann H, Drummen R: Clinical features of proven basilar artery occlusion. Stroke 21:1135, 1990.
16. Hirshkowitz M, Sharafkhaneh A: Clinical and technologic approaches to sleep evaluation. Neurol Clin 23:991, 2005.
17. Keenan SA: Normal human sleep. Respir Care Clin N Am 5:319, 1999.
18. Chiappa KH, Hill RA: Evaluation and prognostication in coma. Electroencephalogr Clin Neurophysiol 106:149, 1998.
19. Amar AP: Controversies in the neurosurgical management of cerebellar hemorrhage and infarction. Neurosurg Focus 32:E1, 2012.
20. Lindsberg PJ, Sairanen T, Strbian D, et al: Current treatment of basilar artery occlusion. Ann NY Acad Sci 1268:35, 2012.
21. Auer RN: Hypoglycemic brain damage. Metab Brain Dis 19:169, 2004.
22. Kristian T: Metabolic stages, mitochondria and calcium in hypoxic/ischemic brain damage. Cell Calcium 36:221, 2004.
23. Zheng J, Gendelman HE: The HIV-1 associated dementia complex: a metabolic encephalopathy fueled by viral replication in mononuclear phagocytes. Curr Opin Neurol 10:319, 1997.
24. Edgren E, Hedstrand U, Kelsey S, et al: Assessment of neurological prognosis in comatose survivors of

cardiac arrest. BRCT I Study Group. Lancet 343:1055, 1994.
25. McCall AL: The impact of diabetes on the CNS. Diabetes 41:557, 1992.
26. Levy D: Prognosis of metabolic coma. p. 21. In: Arieff A, Griggs R (eds): Metabolic Brain Dysfunction in Systemic Disorders. Little, Brown, Boston, 1992.
27. Young GB, Austin TW, Archibald YM, et al: The encephalopathy associated with septic illness. Clin Invest Med 13:297, 1990.
28. Khungar V, Poordad F: Hepatic encephalopathy. Clin Liver Dis 16:301, 2012.
29. Seifter JL, Samuels MA: Uremic encephalopathy and other brain disorders associated with renal failure. Semin Neurol 31:139, 2011.
30. Buchan A: Advances in cerebral ischemia: experimental approaches. Neurol Clin 10:49, 1992.
31. The Hypothermia after Cardiac Arrest Study Group: Mild therapeutic hypothermia to improve the neurologic outcome after cardiac arrest. N Engl J Med 346:549, 2002.
32. Bernard SA, Gray TW, Buist MD, et al: Treatment of comatose survivors of out-of-hospital cardiac arrest with induced hypothermia. N Engl J Med 346:557, 2002.
33. Peberdy MA, Callaway CW, Neumar RW, et al: Part 9: post-cardiac arrest care: 2010 American Heart Association Guidelines for Cardiopulmonary Resuscitation and Emergency Cardiovascular Care. Circulation 122:S768, 2010.
34. Paulson OB, Strandgaard S, Edvinsson L: Cerebral autoregulation. Cerebrovasc Brain Metab Rev 2:161, 1990.
35. Bartynski WS: Posterior reversible encephalopathy syndrome, part 2: controversies surrounding pathophysiology of vasogenic edema. AJNR Am J Neuroradiol 29:1043, 2008.
36. Brouns R, De Deyn PP: Neurological complications in renal failure: a review. Clin Neurol Neurosurg 107:1, 2004.
37. Hazell AS, Butterworth RF: Hepatic encephalopathy: an update of pathophysiologic mechanisms. Proc Soc Exp Biol Med 222:99, 1999.
38. Moe SM, Sprague SM: Uremic encephalopathy. Clin Nephrol 42:251, 1994.
39. Bartha P, Shifrin E, Levy Y: Pancreatic encephalopathy—a rare complication of a common disease. Eur J Intern Med 17:382, 2006.
40. Ding X, Liu CA, Gong JP, et al: Pancreatic encephalopathy in 24 patients with severe acute pancreatitis. Hepatobiliary Pancreat Dis Int 3:608, 2004.
41. Fraser CL, Arieff AI: Metabolic encephalopathy as a complication of renal failure: mechanisms and mediators. New Horiz 2:518, 1994.
42. Basile AS, Hughes RD, Harrison PM, et al: Elevated brain concentrations of 1,4-benzodiazepines in fulminant hepatic failure. N Engl J Med 325:473, 1991.
43. Lockwood A: Hepatic encephalopathy. p. 167. In: Arieff A, Griggs R (eds): Metabolic Brain Dysfunction in Systemic Disorders. Little, Brown, Boston, 1992.
44. Herrera JL: Management of acute liver failure. Dig Dis 16:274, 1998.
45. Pittman CS, Zayed AA: Myxedema coma. Curr Ther Endocrinol Metab 6:98, 1997.
46. Li Voon Chong JS, Lecky BR, Macfarlane IA: Recurrent encephalopathy and generalised seizures associated with relapses of thyrotoxicosis. Int J Clin Pract 54:621, 2000.
47. Bolton CF, Young GB, Zochodne DW: The neurological complications of sepsis. Ann Neurol 33:94, 1993.
48. Adam N, Kandelman S, Mantz J, et al: Sepsis-induced brain dysfunction. Expert Rev Anti Infect Ther 11:211, 2013.
49. Hemphill J, Gress D: Neurologic complications of critical illness involving multi-organ failure. p. 525. In: Aminoff MJ, Goetz C (eds): Systemic Diseases, Part III. Handbook of Clinical Neurology. Elsevier, Amsterdam, 1998.
50. Tanaka K, Gotoh K, Gomi S, et al: Inhibition of nitric oxide synthesis induces a significant reduction in local cerebral blood flow in the rat. Neurosci Lett 127:129, 1991.
51. Spinazze S, Schrijvers D: Metabolic emergencies. Crit Rev Oncol Hematol 58:79, 2006.
52. Kumar S, Fowler M, Gonzalez-Toledo E, et al: Central pontine myelinolysis, an update. Neurol Res 28:360, 2006.
53. Croughwell N, Smith LR, Quill T, et al: The effect of temperature on cerebral metabolism and blood flow in adults during cardiopulmonary bypass. J Thorac Cardiovasc Surg 103:549, 1992.
54. Mirski MA, Muffelman B, Ulatowski JA, et al: Sedation for the critically ill neurologic patient. Crit Care Med 23:2038, 1995.
55. Meador KJ: Cognitive side effects of medications. Neurol Clin 16:141, 1998.
56. Boparai MK, Korc-Grodzicki B: Prescribing for older adults. Mt Sinai J Med 78:613, 2011.
57. Clouston PD, DeAngelis LM, Posner JB: The spectrum of neurological disease in patients with systemic cancer. Ann Neurol 31:268, 1992.
58. Miguel EC, Pereira RM, Pereira CA, et al: Psychiatric manifestations of systemic lupus erythematosus: clinical features, symptoms, and signs of central nervous system activity in 43 patients. Medicine (Baltimore) 73:224, 1994.
59. Dalmau J, Graus F, Rosenblum MK, et al: Anti-Hu–associated paraneoplastic encephalomyelitis/sensory neuronopathy. A clinical study of 71 patients. Medicine (Baltimore) 71:59, 1992.
60. Stevens RD, Nyquist PA: Types of brain dysfunction in critical illness. Neurol Clin 26:469, 2008.
61. Hall RJ, Meagher DJ, MacLullich AM: Delirium detection and monitoring outside the ICU. Best Pract Res Clin Anaesthesiol 26:367, 2012.

62. Hughes CG, Patel MB, Pandharipande PP: Pathophysiology of acute brain dysfunction: what's the cause of all this confusion? Curr Opin Crit Care 18:518, 2012.
63. Khan BA, Zawahiri M, Campbell NL, et al: Delirium in hospitalized patients: implications of current evidence on clinical practice and future avenues for research—a systematic evidence review. J Hosp Med 7:580, 2012.
64. Weinhouse GL, Schwab RJ, Watson PL, et al: Bench-to-bedside review: delirium in ICU patients —importance of sleep deprivation. Crit Care 13:234, 2009.
65. Ely EW, Girard TD, Shintani AK, et al: Apolipoprotein E4 polymorphism as a genetic predisposition to delirium in critically ill patients. Crit Care Med 35:112, 2007.
66. Girard TD, Ware LB, Bernard GR, et al: Associations of markers of inflammation and coagulation with delirium during critical illness. Intensive Care Med 38:1965, 2012.
67. MacLullich AM, Beaglehole A, Hall RJ, et al: Delirium and long-term cognitive impairment. Int Rev Psychiatry 21:30, 2009.
68. Nozaki K, Scott TF, Sohn M, et al: Isolated neurosarcoidosis: case series in 2 sarcoidosis centers. Neurologist 18:373, 2012.
69. Hanly JG: Neuropsychiatric lupus. Rheum Dis Clin North Am 31:273, 2005.
70. Janssen B, Bruyn G: Nervous system involvement in systemic lupus erythematosus, including the antiphospholipid syndrome. p. 36. In: Aminoff MJ, Goetz C (eds): Systemic Diseases, Part III. Handbook of Clinical Neurology. Elsevier, Amsterdam, 1998.
71. Nozaki K, Judson MA: Neurosarcoidosis: clinical manifestations, diagnosis and treatment. Presse Med 41:e331, 2012.
72. Lu-Emerson C, Eichler AF: Brain metastases. Continuum (Minneap Minn) 18:295, 2012.
73. Balm M, Hammack J: Leptomeningeal carcinomatosis. Presenting features and prognostic factors. Arch Neurol 53:626, 1996.
74. Newton HB: Neurological complications of chemotherapy to the central nervous system. Handb Clin Neurol 105:903, 2012.
75. Pruitt AA: CNS infections in patients with cancer. Continuum (Minneap Minn) 18:384, 2012.
76. Price RW: Neurological complications of HIV infection. Lancet 348:445, 1996.
77. Steiner I, Berger JR: Update on progressive multifocal leukoencephalopathy. Curr Neurol Neurosci Rep 12:680, 2012.
78. Ghanem KG: Neurosyphilis: a historical perspective and review. CNS Neurosci Ther 16:e157, 2010.
79. Fallon BA, Levin ES, Schweitzer PJ, et al: Inflammation and central nervous system Lyme disease. Neurobiol Dis 37:534, 2010.
80. Chang CW, Bleck TP: Status epilepticus. Neurol Clin 13:529, 1995.
81. Lowenstein DH, Alldredge BK: Status epilepticus at an urban public hospital in the 1980s. Neurology 43:483, 1993.
82. Borowski A, Ghodsizad A, Cohnen M, et al: Recurrent embolism in the course of marantic endocarditis. Ann Thorac Surg 79:2145, 2005.
83. Hart RG, Foster JW, Luther MF, et al: Stroke in infective endocarditis. Stroke 21:695, 1990.
84. Chiarantini E, Valanzano R, Liotta AA, et al: Hemostatic abnormalities in inflammatory bowel disease. Thromb Res 82:137, 1996.
85. Salvarani C, Brown Jr RD, Hunder GG: Adult primary central nervous system vasculitis. Lancet 380:767, 2012.
86. Moore P: Neurologic manifestations of the systemic vasculitides. p. 149. In: Aminoff MJ, Goetz C (eds): Systemic Diseases, Part III. Handbook of Clinical Neurology. Elsevier, Amsterdam, 1998.
87. Adams RE, Powers WJ: Management of hypertension in acute intracerebral hemorrhage. Crit Care Clin 13:131, 1997.
88. del Zoppo GJ, Mori E: Hematologic causes of intracerebral hemorrhage and their treatment. Neurosurg Clin N Am 3:637, 1992.
89. Dollfus P, Milos PL, Chapuis A, et al: The locked-in syndrome: a review and presentation of two chronic cases. Paraplegia 28:5, 1990.
90. Laureys S, Pellas F, Van Eeckhout P, et al: The locked-in syndrome: what is it like to be conscious but paralyzed and voiceless? Prog Brain Res 150:495, 2005.
91. Averbuch-Heller L, Meiner Z: Reversible periodic alternating gaze deviation in hepatic encephalopathy. Neurology 45:191, 1995.
92. Connolly Jr ES, Rabinstein AA, Carhuapoma JR, et al: Guidelines for the management of aneurysmal subarachnoid hemorrhage: a guideline for healthcare professionals from the American Heart Association/American Stroke Association. Stroke 43:1711, 2012.
93. Morgenstern LB, Hemphill III JC, Anderson C, et al: Guidelines for the management of spontaneous intracerebral hemorrhage: a guideline for healthcare professionals from the American Heart Association/American Stroke Association. Stroke 41:2108, 2010.
94. Edlow JA, Samuels O, Smith WS, et al: Emergency neurological life support: subarachnoid hemorrhage. Neurocrit Care 17(suppl 1):S47, 2012.
95. Wasay M, Azeemuddin M: Neuroimaging of cerebral venous thrombosis. J Neuroimaging 15:118, 2005.
96. Dormont D, Anxionnat R, Evrard S, et al: MRI in cerebral venous thrombosis. J Neuroradiol 21:81, 1994.
97. Hinchey J, Chaves C, Appignani B, et al: A reversible posterior leukoencephalopathy syndrome. N Engl J Med 334:494, 1996.
98. Wartenberg KE, Patsalides A, Yepes MS: Is magnetic resonance spectroscopy superior to conventional diagnostic tools in hypoxic-ischemic encephalopathy? J Neuroimaging 14:180, 2004.

99. Crepeau AZ, Rabinstein AA, Fugate JE, et al: Continuous EEG in therapeutic hypothermia after cardiac arrest: prognostic and clinical value. Neurology 80:339, 2013.
100. Cloostermans MC, van Meulen FB, Eertman CJ, et al: Continuous electroencephalography monitoring for early prediction of neurological outcome in postanoxic patients after cardiac arrest: a prospective cohort study. Crit Care Med 40:2867, 2012.
101. Fagan KJ, Lee SI: Prolonged confusion following convulsions due to generalized nonconvulsive status epilepticus. Neurology 40:1689, 1990.
102. Walsh GO, Delgado-Escueta AV: Status epilepticus. Neurol Clin 11:835, 1993.
103. Claassen J, Mayer SA, Kowalski RG, et al: Detection of electrographic seizures with continuous EEG monitoring in critically ill patients. Neurology 62:1743, 2004.
104. Vespa PM, O'Phelan K, Shah M, et al: Acute seizures after intracerebral hemorrhage: a factor in progressive midline shift and outcome. Neurology 60:1441, 2003.
105. Betjemann JP, Nguyen I, Santos-Sanchez C, et al: Diagnostic yield of electroencephalography in a general inpatient population. Mayo Clin Proc 88:326, 2013.
106. Oddo M, Carrera E, Claassen J, et al: Continuous electroencephalography in the medical intensive care unit. Crit Care Med 37:2051, 2009.
107. Wijdicks EF, Parisi JE, Sharbrough FW: Prognostic value of myoclonus status in comatose survivors of cardiac arrest. Ann Neurol 35:239, 1994.
108. Young GB: Metabolic and inflammatory cerebral diseases: electrophysiological aspects. Can J Neurol Sci 25:S16, 1998.
109. Pomier-Layrargues G, Giguere JF, Lavoie J, et al: Flumazenil in cirrhotic patients in hepatic coma: a randomized double-blind placebo-controlled crossover trial. Hepatology 19:32, 1994.
110. Zandbergen EG, Hijdra A, Koelman JH, et al: Prediction of poor outcome within the first 3 days of postanoxic coma. Neurology 66:62, 2006.
111. Wijdicks EF, Hijdra A, Young GB, et al: Practice parameter: prediction of outcome in comatose survivors after cardiopulmonary resuscitation (an evidence-based review): report of the Quality Standards Subcommittee of the American Academy of Neurology. Neurology 67:203, 2006.
112. Evans RW: Complications of lumbar puncture. Neurol Clin 16:83, 1998.
113. Friedman DI, Jacobson DM: Idiopathic intracranial hypertension. J Neuroophthalmol 24:138, 2004.
114. Frank LM, Shinnar S, Hesdorffer DC, et al: Cerebrospinal fluid findings in children with fever-associated status epilepticus: results of the consequences of prolonged febrile seizures (FEBSTAT) study. J Pediatr 161:1169, 2012.
115. Wijdicks E: Neurologic Catastrophes in the Emergency Department. Butterworth-Heinemann, Boston, 1999.
116. Levy DE, Caronna JJ, Singer BH, et al: Predicting outcome from hypoxic-ischemic coma. JAMA 253:1420, 1985.
117. Bouwes A, Binnekade JM, Kuiper MA, et al: Prognosis of coma after therapeutic hypothermia: a prospective cohort study. Ann Neurol 71:206, 2012.
118. Mikkelsen ME, Christie JD, Lanken PN, et al: The adult respiratory distress syndrome cognitive outcomes study: long-term neuropsychological function in survivors of acute lung injury. Am J Respir Crit Care Med 185:1307, 2012.
119. Ates E, Erkasap S, Ihtiyar E, et al: A concept for expanding the donor pool for renal transplantation: non-heart beating donor 1-year retrospective evaluation. Nephrol Dial Transplant 14:1048, 1999.
120. Beresford HR: Brain death. Neurol Clin 17:295, 1999.
121. Payne K, Taylor RM, Stocking C, et al: Physicians' attitudes about the care of patients in the persistent vegetative state: a national survey. Ann Intern Med 125:104, 1996.
122. Youngner SJ: Defining death. A superficial and fragile consensus. Arch Neurol 49:570, 1992.
123. Wijdicks EF, Varelas PN, Gronseth GS, et al: Evidence-based guideline update: determining brain death in adults: report of the Quality Standards Subcommittee of the American Academy of Neurology. Neurology 74:1911, 2010.
124. Yatim A, Mercatello A, Coronel B, et al: ^{99m}Tc-HMPAO cerebral scintigraphy in the diagnosis of brain death. Transplant Proc 23:2491, 1991.
125. Purkayastha S, Sorond F: Transcranial Doppler ultrasound: technique and application. Semin Neurol 32:411, 2012.
126. Laureys S: Science and society: death, unconsciousness and the brain. Nat Rev Neurosci 6:899, 2005.
127. Shewmon DA: Brain death: can it be resuscitated? Issues Law Med 25:3, 2009.
128. Haupt WF, Rudolf J: European brain death codes: a comparison of national guidelines. J Neurol 246:432, 1999.
129. Wijdicks EF: Determining brain death in adults. Neurology 45:1003, 1995.
130. The Quality Standards Subcommittee of the American Academy of Neurology: Practice parameters: assessment and management of patients in the persistent vegetative state (summary statement). The Quality Standards Subcommittee of the American Academy of Neurology. Neurology 45:1015, 1995.
131. The Multi-Society Task Force on PVS: Medical aspects of the persistent vegetative state (1). N Engl J Med 330:1499, 1994.
132. Kinney HC, Korein J, Panigrahy A, et al: Neuropathological findings in the brain of Karen

Ann Quinlan. The role of the thalamus in the persistent vegetative state. N Engl J Med 330:1469, 1994.

133. Eichler AF, Kuter I, Ryan P, et al: Survival in patients with brain metastases from breast cancer: the importance of HER-2 status. Cancer 112:2359, 2008.

134. Jox RJ, Kuehlmeyer K: Introduction: reconsidering disorders of consciousness in light of neuroscientific evidence. Neuroethics 6:1, 2013.

135. Bruno MA, Majerus S, Boly M, et al: Functional neuroanatomy underlying the clinical subcategorization of minimally conscious state patients. J Neurol 259:1087, 2012.

136. Steinert RF, Post Jr CT, Brint SF, et al: A prospective, randomized, double-masked comparison of a zonal-progressive multifocal intraocular lens and a monofocal intraocular lens. Ophthalmology 99:853, 1992.

137. Salvarani C, Brown Jr RD, Hunder GG: Adult primary central nervous system vasculitis: an update. Curr Opin Rheumatol 24:46, 2012.

CHAPTER

61

Dementia and Systemic Disease

VANJA C. DOUGLAS ■ S. ANDREW JOSEPHSON

Dementia is a common problem among the elderly and is associated with a number of important systemic complications. Epidemiologic studies estimate the prevalence of dementia in the United States to be approximately 5 percent over age 70, 25 percent over age 80, and 37 percent over age 90, which ensures that nearly every physician will encounter patients with dementia.[1] Alzheimer disease, the most common form of dementia, is the sixth leading cause of death in the United States and continues to increase in prevalence with an aging population.[2] The purpose of this chapter is to review the causes of dementia and the systemic problems that result in order to arm practitioners with the tools necessary to effectively care for this vulnerable patient population.

CAUSES OF DEMENTIA

Most dementias are the result of progressive neurodegenerative diseases such as Alzheimer disease (Table 61-1). These conditions usually lead to death within 5 to 10 years of clinical onset.[3,4] Patients may also acquire dementia after a temporally isolated event such as a severe traumatic brain injury or encephalitis. In such cases, the dementia is not progressive, and some recovery or adaptation can be expected over time. Dementia may also be reversible when caused by certain treatable systemic conditions. These cases are especially important to recognize, diagnose, and treat.

Alzheimer Disease

Alzheimer disease is the most common cause of dementia in the elderly.[2] The disorder almost invariably begins with insidiously progressive short-term memory loss followed by diminished cognitive function in a range of domains that most often include language, visuospatial ability, and praxis. Memory loss is often initially misattributed to normal aging, often leading to a delay in diagnosis. Symptoms reflect the relative density of neuropathology in different regions of the brain: the highest density of β-amyloid plaques and tau neurofibrillary tangles is usually found in the medial temporal lobes, regions critical for the formation of new memories.[5] Other frequently involved areas include the parietal lobes, which are involved in visuospatial processing. The course is relentlessly progressive and universally

TABLE 61-1 ■ Common Causes of Dementia

	Pathogenesis	Disease
Neurodegenerative Diseases		
	β-Amyloid, tau	Alzheimer disease
	Tauopathy	Frontotemporal lobar degeneration Progressive supranuclear palsy Corticobasal degeneration
	Synucleinopathy	Dementia with Lewy bodies Parkinson disease Multiple system atrophy
	Chronic ischemia	Vascular dementia
Treatable Causes of Dementia		
	Infectious	Chronic meningitis (e.g., mycobacterial, fungal) HIV infection Neurosyphilis (general paresis)
	Metabolic	Hypothyroidism Vitamin B_{12} deficiency Obstructive sleep apnea
	Psychiatric	Depression
	Structural	Hydrocephalus Chronic subdural hematoma Brain tumor

fatal, leading to death within a few years (median, 5 years) from the time of diagnosis.[6] Death is often from aspiration pneumonia or other complications of the bed-bound end-stage of the illness. While social graces are usually preserved early in the course of the illness, behavioral problems such as aggression, agitation, and episodic delirium often emerge in later stages and are particularly problematic for caretakers. Falls are also common when patients develop postural instability later in the disease course.

Risk factors for Alzheimer disease include age, having a first-degree relative with the disease, diabetes, hypertension, obesity, hypercholesterolemia, tobacco use, low educational attainment, traumatic brain injury, and the APOE ε4 allele.[7–9] Factors associated with reduced rates of the disease include regular exercise and higher educational attainment.[10,11] Less than 1 percent of cases are inherited in an autosomal dominant pattern and these are mainly caused by mutations in the genes encoding amyloid precursor protein, presenilin 1, and presenilin 2.[2] There is no treatment that halts the progression of the disease. Centrally acting acetylcholinesterase inhibitors such as donepezil, rivastigmine, and galantamine, and the *N*-methyl-D-aspartate receptor antagonist memantine will boost cognition at various stages of the illness and may as a result temporarily improve quality of life or delay nursing home placement, although clinical effects are marginal.[12] Ongoing efforts to develop novel treatments have focused on early stages of the disease when pathology is present but obvious clinical symptoms have not yet appeared.

Vascular Dementia

Cerebrovascular disease carves several paths to dementia. The accumulation of multiple large territory infarctions in the setting of atrial fibrillation, intracranial atherosclerosis, or other causes of recurrent large-vessel ischemic stroke results in dementia with cognitive deficits referable to the infarcted brain territories. Because dementia progresses with each successive stroke, patients may demonstrate a stepwise decline in function. However, these patients rarely present to medical care with unexplained cognitive complaints because they are already known to have suffered multiple infarctions.

More common among patients presenting with memory or cognitive dysfunction is dementia resulting from the accumulation of innumerable ischemic lesions in the subcortical and periventricular white matter due to chronic small-vessel disease. The clinical syndrome is one of slowly progressive frontal lobe dysfunction, with problems in working memory and executive function. Involvement of the basal ganglia may result in a shuffling gait and postural instability that resembles parkinsonism. Pathologic examination reveals chronic ischemia with arteriolosclerosis and often amyloid angiopathy of small arterioles.[13] Vascular dementia is the second most common cause of dementia in North America and Europe, accounting for up to 20 percent of cases.[14]

The incidence of vascular dementia increases with age, and patients are more likely to have hypertension, diabetes, hyperlipidemia, atrial fibrillation, or a history of tobacco use.[15] Obesity is also a significant risk factor.[16] Vascular dementia is associated with chronic kidney disease, coronary artery disease, and peripheral vascular disease, although these associations may be mediated by common risk factors.[15] No treatment is known to slow its progression, but physical activity may be protective against the development of vascular dementia.[17] It is not known whether aspirin, smoking cessation, or treatment of vascular risk factors prevents or slows the progression of dementia, but these are all standard aspects of secondary stroke prevention and are therefore often a part of the treatment plan for patients with vascular dementia.[15] The acetylcholinesterase inhibitors donepezil and galantamine have a modest benefit in vascular dementia similar to their effect on cognitive function in Alzheimer disease.[18]

Synucleinopathies

The synucleinopathies include dementia with Lewy bodies, Parkinson disease, and multiple system atrophy. The pathologic hallmark of all synucleinopathies is the Lewy body, composed primarily of insoluble α-synuclein aggregates. These aggregates are not common in normal aging; α-synuclein itself is a normally soluble neuronal protein with uncertain function. The role of Lewy bodies and α-synuclein in the pathogenesis of disease is also not well understood.

Parkinsonism is a prominent early feature of most synucleinopathies and describes a clinical syndrome consisting of rigidity, bradykinesia, postural instability, and resting tremor. Rapid eye movement (REM) sleep behavior disorder, in which brainstem projections to the spinal cord that induce atonia during REM sleep are disrupted, causing patients to act out their dreams in dramatic fashion, is another symptom common to the synucleinopathies.[19] REM sleep behavior disorder can precede the onset of parkinsonism in the synucleinopathies by many years.[20]

Dementia with Lewy Bodies

Dementia with parkinsonism is the hallmark of dementia with Lewy bodies. This diagnosis is likely when cognitive dysfunction manifests prior to or within 12 months after the onset of parkinsonism. Other core features include well-formed visual hallucinations (often of animals) and fluctuations in alertness and cognition.[21] Periodic unresponsiveness is often mistaken for syncope or seizure. Cognitive dysfunction consists of impaired visuospatial ability, attention, and executive function, with relatively preserved memory early in the disease course. Patients are exquisitely sensitive to dopamine antagonists and can develop prolonged encephalopathy and rigidity after exposure to relatively small doses of neuroleptics. Donepezil and rivastigmine are effective at ameliorating the cognitive symptoms and are often titrated to higher doses than those used for Alzheimer disease.[22,23] The rate of progression is similar in both diseases although survival after diagnosis may be slightly shorter in Lewy body dementia.[24]

Parkinson Disease

Parkinson disease is a slowly progressive motor disorder in which dementia is usually a late feature. It is due to degeneration of dopaminergic neurons in the substantia nigra pars compacta in the midbrain. The prevalence of dementia in patients with this disease is approximately 30 percent, and it usually manifests a decade or more into the illness.[25,26] Clinical features may echo those of Lewy body dementia, although memory dysfunction is sometimes more prominent.

Multiple System Atrophy

Multiple system atrophy is categorized into two subtypes based on the predominant motor features: parkinsonian (MSA-P, previously known as striatonigral degeneration) and cerebellar (MSA-C, previously olivopontocerebellar atrophy). Both are characterized by progressive decline in multiple neurologic systems and include autonomic dysfunction manifested by urinary incontinence, erectile dysfunction, orthostatic hypotension, and central sleep apnea; bulbar dysfunction manifested by dysphagia; and either prominent cerebellar ataxia or parkinsonism. Dementia is a rare feature of multiple system atrophy, occurring in less than 20 percent of patients.[27] When it does occur, it tends to feature executive and visuospatial dysfunction.[27] The course is typically more rapid than that of Parkinson disease and similar to Lewy body dementia and Alzheimer disease.[28,29]

Tauopathies

The tauopathies are a group of neurodegenerative diseases associated with an abnormal aggregation of tau protein in the brain. The most common is Alzheimer disease, considered separately above.

Frontotemporal Dementia

Frontotemporal dementia is a clinically, pathologically, and genetically diverse disorder. On neuropathologic examination, many cases are associated with inclusions containing tau, a microtubule stabilizing protein.[30] The neuropathology in other cases with similar clinical phenotypes demonstrates inclusions containing TAR DNA-binding protein of 43 kDa (TDP-43) and no tau staining; others are tau negative and TDP-43 negative but positive for the protein fused in sarcoma; and still others are tau negative, TDP-43 negative, fused in sarcoma negative, and ubiquitin positive.[31] Because of overlap between clinical and pathologic subtypes, it is difficult to predict an individual patient's pathology with certainty using current diagnostic techniques, but in general the clinical syndromes associated with tau inclusions are behavioral variant frontotemporal dementia, progressive nonfluent aphasia, progressive supranuclear palsy, and corticobasal syndrome. Semantic dementia, a variant of frontotemporal dementia with progressive impairment in naming and single-word comprehension, is usually associated with TDP-43 pathology. Many TDP-43 positive cases have comorbid motor neuron disease. There are no specific treatments.

The average age of onset is between 50 and 60 years; the incidence does not increase with age.[31] Frontotemporal dementia accounts for a significant proportion of dementia cases in people aged 45 to 65. The time between onset of symptoms and death is slightly shorter than that in Alzheimer disease.[32] The behavioral variant presents with personality changes, apathy or impulsivity, emotional blunting, loss of empathy and social awareness, lack of insight, mental rigidity, change in eating habits, and poor personal hygiene, all reflecting degeneration predominantly of the non-dominant frontal and temporal lobes (Fig. 61-1).[33] When the pathologic process affects the dominant hemisphere, progressive nonfluent aphasia is the typical phenotype and is associated with fewer behavioral changes and more prominent language difficulties.[31]

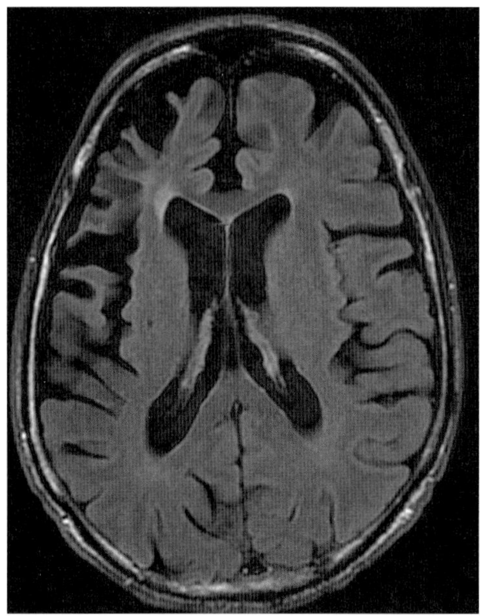

FIGURE 61-1 ■ Frontotemporal dementia. T1-weighted magnetic resonance image (MRI) of the brain demonstrates atrophy of the non-dominant (right) frontal lobe out of proportion to other areas.

Progressive Supranuclear Palsy

Falls are often the earliest symptom in patients with this disorder because of axial rigidity and vertical gaze palsy, the combination of which results in significant postural instability. Cognitive dysfunction is characterized by a frontal lobe syndrome with executive dysfunction and deficits in working memory, judgment, multitasking and cognitive processing speed.[27] Neuropsychiatric symptoms also include apathy, disinhibition, dysphoria, and anxiety.[34] Patients are often first misdiagnosed with Parkinson disease, but the diagnosis becomes clear due to the lack of rest tremor, development of a vertical gaze palsy, relatively rapid progression (the median time from onset to death is approximately 8 years), and poor response to dopamine.[35]

Corticobasal Degeneration

The term corticobasal degeneration is reserved for patients with a specific pathologic diagnosis, the hallmark of which is tau inclusions. In life, corticobasal degeneration is clinically heterogeneous; patients may present with behavioral variant frontotemporal dementia, progressive nonfluent aphasia, or a more classic corticobasal syndrome that includes asymmetric dystonia and rigidity, apraxia, neglect, alien limb phenomenon, and dementia with features similar to progressive supranuclear palsy.[36] Conversely, some patients diagnosed in life with corticobasal syndrome are found to have

Alzheimer disease, progressive supranuclear palsy, or TDP-43 pathology at autopsy.[36]

Systemic Diseases Causing Dementia

A number of systemic disorders may cause cognitive decline and mimic Alzheimer disease or other neurodegenerative diseases. These disorders are of importance because they are often treatable. Cognitive decline in most of these conditions is chronic, although occasionally patients present subacutely. Subacute cognitive decline, also referred to as rapidly progressive dementia, has a much wider differential diagnosis that is beyond the scope of this chapter.

Cognitive dysfunction is an increasingly recognized neurologic complication of *human immunodeficiency virus (HIV) infection,* discussed in Chapter 44. Previously known by such terms as AIDS dementia complex and HIV encephalopathy, the currently accepted terminology is HIV-associated neurocognitive disorder, with three stages of disease based on neuropsychologic testing: asymptomatic neurocognitive impairment, mild neurocognitive disorder, and HIV-associated dementia. Cognitive impairment is described as subcortical, with impaired information-processing speed, multitasking, decision-making, working memory, and verbal fluency. While the incidence of HIV-associated dementia has declined in the era of antiretroviral therapy, the milder subtypes continue to be common, with 33 percent of patients having asymptomatic neurocognitive impairment and 12 percent mild neurocognitive disorder in a large cohort, raising concern that HIV-associated neurocognitive disorder may represent the effect of a reservoir of viral replication sequestered behind the blood–brain barrier.[37] Current research is aimed at investigating the effect of antiretroviral drugs with high CSF penetration on the prevention of HIV-associated neurocognitive disorder.[38] According to guidelines from the United States Preventive Services Task Force, HIV screening should be a routine part of health care maintenance and, by extension, testing is reasonable in any patient presenting with cognitive symptoms.

Public health efforts directed at screening and treatment have led to a decline in the prevalence of the neurologic complications of *syphilis* (Chapter 40). Tertiary syphilis is therefore a less important cause of dementia than in the past. General paresis, or the dementia caused by syphilis, is a result of direct infection of neural tissue by *Treponema pallidum* and occurs decades after the primary infection. Patients develop progressive memory loss and personality change. Because non-treponemal tests such as the rapid plasma reagin (RPR) and Venereal Disease Research Laboratory (VDRL) can be negative in late syphilis, a treponemal test such as the fluorescent treponemal antigen absorption and a lumbar puncture should be performed when the disease is suspected. Lymphocyte count and protein concentration are usually elevated in the spinal fluid.

Rarely, *chronic meningitis* such as that caused by *Mycobacterium tuberculosis* (Chapter 41) or *Cryptococcus neoformans* (Chapter 46) may lead to chronic cognitive decline. Usually the dementia in these cases is accompanied by systemic symptoms of chronic infection such as weight loss, night sweats, and occasional fever. Cognitive symptoms typically have features of delirium including waxing and waning levels of alertness and attention. These conditions are readily distinguished from neurodegenerative diseases with a lumbar puncture demonstrating inflammatory spinal fluid.

In addition to fatigue, cold intolerance, hair loss, myxedema, and weakness, *hypothyroidism* is associated with cognitive dysfunction. The symptoms are usually slowed cognitive processing, impaired learning, and depression.[39] The disorder is readily diagnosed by checking serum levels of thyroid-stimulating hormone.

Deficiency of vitamin B_{12} is associated with an increased risk of developing Alzheimer disease, vascular dementia, and Parkinson disease, but there is no compelling evidence that treatment of the deficiency prevents the development of dementia or improves outcomes in patients who have already developed it.[40,41] However, there are rare cases of patients presenting with dementia and vitamin B_{12} deficiency who have demonstrated sustained recovery after vitamin supplementation, and therefore a trial of this benign treatment is a reasonable approach to these patients.[42]

Structural lesions such as a chronic subdural hematoma, tumors, and hydrocephalus may also lead to dementia. It is for this reason that brain imaging is part of the standard workup for dementia; brain imaging will reveal an abnormal finding that was otherwise unsuspected in 5 percent of cases.[43] Although subdural hematoma may present with seizures or focal neurologic deficits, in some cases the hematoma expands slowly and causes only cognitive symptoms, with subtle or no motor signs. Similarly, brain tumors can mimic neurodegenerative disease, with slow-growing low-grade tumors more likely to do so than glioblastomas or metastases. Symptoms depend on the location of the tumor. Frontal tumors may cause behavioral symptoms such as apathy, loss of insight and judgment, and difficulty with working memory and executive function. Temporal lesions may result in progressive aphasia and memory loss.

Communicating hydrocephalus is associated classically with the triad of dementia, incontinence, and gait disorder, but patients often present with only one of these symptoms. The dementia is typically characterized by frontal lobe dysfunction with symptoms similar to those seen in vascular dementia, although descriptions of large series with robust cognitive testing are lacking. The gait disorder is typically a gait initiation failure, often described as a magnetic gait, where the feet appear stuck to the floor. Treatment is placement of a ventriculoperitoneal shunt. When the diagnosis is suspected after careful correlation between the history, neurologic findings, and brain imaging demonstrating ventriculomegaly out of proportion to sulcal atrophy (Fig. 61-2), a lumbar puncture should be performed. Because hydrocephalus with elevated intracranial pressure can lead to an identical clinical presentation, measurement of the opening pressure is critical. A good response to ventriculoperitoneal shunt is predicted if the patient's symptoms improve after a large volume (30 to 50 ml) of cerebrospinal fluid is removed. Importantly, many cases of so-called normal-pressure hydrocephalus will turn out to be early presentations of a neurodegenerative condition; this possibility should be excluded.

Screening for *depression* should be performed during the evaluation of all patients with cognitive symptoms or complaints both because patients with depression may present with memory complaints and because patients with neurodegenerative disease frequently have comorbid depression that contributes to poor cognition. In contrast to patients with neurodegenerative disease who often lack insight into their forgetfulness and frequently confabulate, patients with depression are frequently concerned about memory loss. In depression, bedside neuropsychologic testing classically reveals deficits in memory retrieval with associated mild deficits in attention, in addition to an affective disorder.[44]

Obstructive sleep apnea is another important cause of cognitive disturbances. The excessive daytime sleepiness that occurs reduces the ability to focus sustained attention and results in executive and memory dysfunction.[45] In addition, sleep apnea is a risk factor for cerebrovascular disease and stroke, which can augment cognitive decline over time.[46] Treating sleep apnea in patients with Alzheimer disease may improve cognitive function.[47] Effective screening for the sleep disorder includes asking bed partners about snoring and querying the patient about daytime sleepiness; positive screening should trigger a referral for overnight polysomnography.

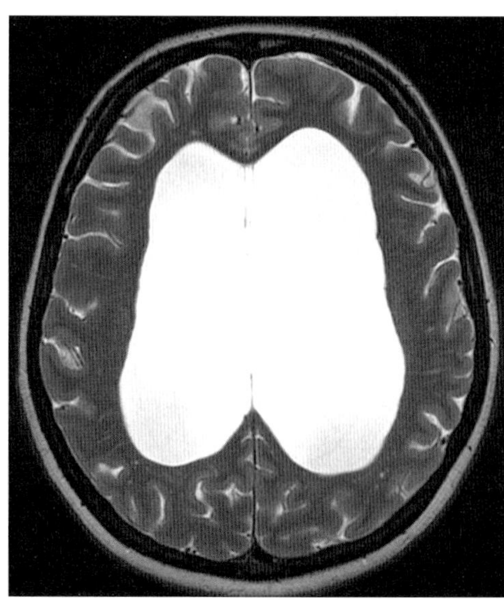

FIGURE 61-2 ■ Communicating hydrocephalus. T2-weighted MRI of the brain showing ventriculomegaly out of proportion to sulcal atrophy.

SYSTEMIC COMPLICATIONS OF DEMENTIA

Patients with dementia are vulnerable to a number of systemic complications (Table 61-2). These complications, especially aspiration leading to pneumonia and falls resulting in hip fracture, are often the ultimate cause of death in patients with advanced dementia. Familiarity with these complications of dementia will help providers caring for this population of patients anticipate and in some cases prevent these problems.

Dysphagia and Aspiration

Dysphagia occurs in 45 percent of patients institutionalized with dementia.[48] In the setting of

TABLE 61-2 ■ Systemic Complications of Dementia and Neurodegenerative Disease

Neurodegenerative Disease	Common Systemic Complications
Alzheimer disease	Agitation/delirium Dysphagia/aspiration Falls
Vascular dementia	Falls Depression
Parkinson disease	Dysphagia/aspiration Falls Orthostatic hypotension Excessive daytime sleepiness Fatigue Constipation Depression
Dementia with Lewy bodies	As with Parkinson disease, plus: Agitation/delirium Hallucinations and sensitivity to antipsychotics
Multiple system atrophy	As with Parkinson disease, plus: Urinary incontinence Sleep-disordered breathing (sleep apnea, stridor, central hypoventilation)
Frontotemporal dementia	Motor neuron disease
Progressive supranuclear palsy	Falls
Corticobasal syndrome	Falls

dementia, the neuroanatomic basis of dysphagia is complex and poorly understood.[49] It tends to occur at earlier stages in the synucleinopathies and Alzheimer disease than in frontotemporal dementia.[50,51] Dysphagia results in decreased oral intake, malnutrition, dehydration, and is a significant risk factor for aspiration of oral contents and resultant pneumonia, which is the most common cause of death among the demented elderly.[52,53] This raises two important questions: can aspiration and aspiration pneumonia be prevented, and how should families of demented patients be counseled regarding the risk and outcome of recurrent aspiration?

Aspiration occurs when food or saliva penetrates the trachea beyond the level of the true vocal folds due to incomplete or delayed closing of the epiglottis during the act of swallowing. During swallowing, the hyoid muscles contract and elevate the larynx, causing the epiglottis to seal the opening to the trachea and allowing oral contents to pass safely into the esophagus. Neurologic disease can cause aspiration due to lesions in the cortex, brainstem, cranial nerves, neuromuscular junction, or muscle that results in incoordination, slowness, or weakness of the swallowing mechanism. In dementia, one theory is that dysphagia is due to disruption of the cortical control of swallowing, causing apraxia and tactile-oral agnosia.[50] Synucleinopathies may also disrupt brainstem swallowing networks and cause dysphagia; in some cases, Lewy bodies themselves may be seen in the esophagus in biopsy specimens, suggesting a more local effect.[54,55] Dysphagia and aspiration occur more typically with liquids than with solids in neurologic disease because liquids enter the posterior oropharynx more quickly and require more complete closure of the trachea and a more rapid swallow mechanism.

Patients with dementia should be routinely screened for symptoms of dysphagia not only to predict and prevent aspiration, but also to assess nutritional status and quality of life with respect to eating. Clinical signs of dysphagia that are most predictive of aspiration include dysphonia and a wet voice or cough after a trial of swallowing 10 ml or 3 oz of thin liquid.[56] An episode of pneumonia in a nursing-home patient is a likely indication of dysphagia and aspiration.[57] When aspiration is suspected, patients should be referred to a speech and swallow therapist to assess the risk of aspiration through a formal dysphagia evaluation that could include a videofluoroscopic swallowing examination or a flexible endoscopic evaluation of swallowing. In addition, the therapist can recommend dietary modifications or swallowing techniques that may lessen the risk of aspiration.

Dietary modifications to reduce the frequency of aspiration consist of thickening liquids to a nectar- or honey-thick consistency to allow the poorly coordinated swallowing mechanism time to function effectively by slowing the passage of oral contents from the posterior oropharynx into the esophagus.[49] The honey-thick consistency is more effective than nectar-thick consistency in reducing aspiration risk compared with thin liquids, but neither reduces the incidence of pneumonia in patients with dementia and Parkinson disease.[58,59] The chin-tuck, in which patients swallow with their chin touching their chest, also reduces the risk of aspiration but not pneumonia, and, while less effective than thickened liquids, it is preferred by patients.[58] Practical challenges to these interventions include the supervision required to remind patients with dementia about proper swallowing technique and an increased risk of dehydration with thickened liquids.[59]

Observational studies have not shown percutaneous enteral feeding tubes to reduce rates of pneumonia or prolong survival in patients with dementia, although no randomized trials have been conducted.[60] There are even more limited data on the effect of nasogastric feeding tubes on quality of life.[61] Patients with dementia in whom tube feeding is considered are often at the end stages of their disease; among nursing home residents with advanced dementia, the 1-year mortality after feeding tube insertion was 64 percent in a recent study of United States Medicare and Medicaid beneficiaries; in another study, median survival after feeding tube insertion was 177 days.[60,62] In the absence of disease-modifying treatment or a clear benefit of tube feeding, the utility of this intervention in patients with dementia has been questioned. Despite this, approximately one-third of nursing home residents with dementia in the United States have feeding tubes.[63]

Tube feeding may not alter the risk of aspiration pneumonia and mortality in part because dysphagia is not the only risk factor for pneumonia among frail elderly patients. Restricting patients' oral intake does not prevent aspiration of saliva or regurgitated stomach contents. In addition to dementia, other risk factors for pneumonia include preexisting lung disease, congestive heart failure, diabetes, malnutrition, bad oral health, and poor functional status.[52,64] Proton pump inhibitors and histamine receptor antagonists are also risk factors for development of pneumonia.[65]

Placement of an enteral feeding tube therefore requires careful discussion with patients and their caregivers, with all parties having a full understanding of the intervention's uncertain benefit in patients with dementia. Because patients with dementia in whom a decision about enteral feeding is being made often lack decision-making capacity, the responsibility for the decision may fall on surrogate decision-makers who struggle with a perceived dichotomy of providing or withholding nutrition. If patients have not made their wishes clear in advance, this can be a difficult position for surrogates. Reframing the decision to include the option of comfort feeding, which consists of hand feeding with the goal of comfort only, can provide caregivers with an acceptable option in which feedings are still being provided despite the risks of aspiration, but the potential harms of a feeding tube are avoided.[66]

Agitation and Delirium

Demented patients sometimes display aggressive or irrational behavior. Because of the practical challenges in managing such behavior and the emotional burden of seeing a loved one act in a manner incongruent with their usual personality, this can be one of the biggest challenges faced by caregivers of demented patients. Agitation may occur in the setting of delirium or it may be a feature of the dementia itself. Delirium is an acute alteration in mental status with a fluctuating course, impaired attention, and disorganized thinking or an altered level of consciousness in which patients are sometimes somnolent and relatively docile but can also be hypervigilant, impulsive, difficult to redirect, and combative. Delirium is a common complication of dementia in hospitals, nursing homes, and the community. At least 50 percent of patients with dementia become delirious when hospitalized, and the prevalence of delirium superimposed on dementia is 17 percent among nursing home residents and 13 percent in the community.[67–69]

Although delirium superimposed on dementia may occur without a specific trigger, there are a number of iatrogenic, metabolic, and systemic derangements that can precipitate an episode of delirium. In such cases, the delirium will not resolve until the underlying problem is diagnosed and treated. Medications are perhaps the most frequent iatrogenic precipitants of delirium. Polypharmacy as well as specific medication classes such as opiates, benzodiazepines, and anticholinergics have been implicated.[70] For this reason, the first step in the treatment of delirium is a thorough review of the patient's medication list, including prescription, nonprescription, and alternative medicines. Attention should be given to reducing doses, minimizing polypharmacy, and replacing neurologically active medications with alternatives. Systemic infections such as cystitis or pneumonia are also common causes of delirium in patients with dementia, as are uremia, hepatic disease, electrolyte and glucose disturbances, hip fracture, and major surgery.[71,72] Indeed, delirium may be the first sign of a metabolic problem or infection and should trigger a laboratory and infectious workup.

Among patients with dementia, agitation and delirium often peak in the afternoon and evening, a phenomenon known as sundowning. The pathophysiologic basis of sundowning is not clear. Current theories propose that degeneration of neurons involved in circadian rhythms in both the suprachiasmatic nucleus and the basal forebrain underlie the development of this time-dependent behavior.[73]

Strategies to prevent delirium differ slightly between the hospital and the nursing home or community setting. In the hospital, two nonpharmacologic interventions have been demonstrated in randomized trials to lower the incidence of delirium. The first is a multicomponent intervention called the Hospital Elder Life Program targeted at specific patient risk factors.[74] Patients with cognitive impairment are frequently reoriented, and visits with volunteers and family members involve structured reminiscence. Sleep deprivation is limited by minimizing night-time interruptions for vital signs and diagnostic tests, avoiding daytime naps, and keeping the hospital ward quiet at night. When applied to medical patients older than 70 years, this intervention resulted in a reduction of delirium incidence from 15 to 9.9 percent.[74]

A second nonpharmacologic intervention effective in preventing delirium is the proactive involvement of a geriatrician in elderly patients admitted with hip fracture. This was demonstrated in a study where patients over age 65 with hip fracture were randomized to usual care or a geriatrics consultation within 24 hours of surgery.[75] The geriatrician ensured adequate hydration, oxygenation, early mobilization, prompt removal of urinary catheters, and early detection and treatment of urinary tract infections. The incidence of delirium in the group receiving the intervention was 32 percent, compared with 50 percent in the usual care group.[75] Based on these studies, current guidelines recommend implementation of multicomponent delirium prevention strategies among hospitalized patients.[76]

When delirium does occur in the hospital setting, the initial focus should be on diagnosing and treating the underlying cause, if found. The same nonpharmacologic measures effective in preventing delirium should be employed to treat it. Pharmacotherapy should be reserved for situations in which patients poses a danger to themselves or to hospital staff. If medications must be administered, the initial choice should be an antipsychotic because this class of medications has the best level of supporting evidence.[77] However, these agents must be used with caution because they are associated with an increased risk of death in the elderly and are not approved by the US Food and Drug Administration for this indication. Antipsychotics are also especially dangerous in dementia with Lewy bodies and should be avoided due to the possibility of precipitating a rapid and sometimes permanent encephalopathy and rigid state, even in low doses.

Outside the hospital setting, agitated and aggressive behavior is less often the result of an acute metabolic or infectious problem and more often the result of the neurodegenerative process itself or sundowning. In this setting, interventions are aimed at reducing the incidence and severity of agitated outbursts and de-escalating aggressive behavior. Both pharmacologic and nonpharmacologic measures have been studied.

Atypical antipsychotics are the most widely studied medications for the prevention of agitation in patients with dementia. A recent meta-analysis of randomized controlled trials found risperidone and olanzapine effective in reducing psychotic symptoms and aggression in Alzheimer disease.[78] There were insufficient data to draw conclusions about other atypical antipsychotics. Risperidone and olanzapine also reduced caregiver burden.[79] Of concern, however, is the finding that atypical antipsychotics increase the risk of death in patients with dementia, likely mediated by an increased incidence of cardiovascular and cerebrovascular events and pneumonia.[78] Antipsychotics also increase the risk of extrapyramidal side effects and accelerate cognitive decline.[80] The use of atypical antipsychotics for behavioral modification in dementia is not approved by regulatory agencies and should be reserved for cases where agitation poses a risk to the safety of the patient or caregiver. In such cases, careful documentation of the consent process is important. Cholinesterase inhibitors are not effective for prevention of agitation in Alzheimer disease, but are helpful in dementia with Lewy bodies.[23,81]

Nonpharmacologic prevention of agitation at home and in the nursing home setting focuses on behavioral techniques aimed at anticipating and avoiding triggers, meeting unmet needs, diffusing aggressive behavior, and minimizing caregiver upset. Several randomized trials have examined caregiver training and support strategies and some have demonstrated improvement in problem behaviors and caregiver well-being.[82,83] One randomized trial of a comprehensive unmet needs intervention in nine nursing homes, dubbed Treatment Routes for Exploring Agitation, resulted in a clinically and statistically significant reduction in physical and verbal agitation.[84] While these types of interventions show promise and lack the risks of pharmacotherapy for agitation in dementia, nonpharmacologic methods require significant investment in human resources without a clear financial incentive and have received less attention and research funding to date.

Depression and other Mood Disorders

Comorbid mood disorders are highly prevalent among patients with dementia. It is estimated that 30 to 50 percent of patients with Alzheimer disease have comorbid depression.[85,86] Approximately 60 percent of patients with Parkinson disease will screen positive for depression and 11 percent will have severe depression.[87] Anxiety is also common in neurodegenerative disease, with prevalence rates of 10 percent and 34 percent in Alzheimer and Parkinson diseases, respectively.[88,89]

Depression has also been identified as a risk factor for dementia in multiple cohort studies, but it is not clear from the data whether depression represents a prodromal phase of dementia, the consequence of dementia, or a modifiable risk factor.[90] Several studies finding a two- to fourfold increased risk of developing dementia later in life among patients with depression in their youth or middle age support the hypothesis that early or mid-life depression is a potentially modifiable risk factor.[90]

Among patients with dementia, data regarding treatment of depression are limited. A Cochrane review updated in 2005 identified only four studies involving 137 subjects with sufficiently detailed efficacy data to use in a meta-analysis.[91] While results from one study were positive, they were limited to a depression rating scale not used in the other three studies and the reviewers therefore concluded that there was only weak evidence that treatment of depression is effective in patients with dementia. Studies of psychosocial methods for treatment of depression in patients with dementia are equally limited.[92]

Falls

Falls are an early feature of some dementias and a late feature of others. The parkinsonian syndromes are all characterized by early falls due to axial rigidity and loss of postural reflexes resulting in postural instability. In progressive supranuclear palsy, the inability to look down because of the supranuclear gaze palsy from which the disease's name is derived is an additional exacerbating factor. In other dementias, while postural instability due to the neurodegenerative disease may contribute to falls, the cause is often multifactorial, with additional risk factors including dizziness, lower-extremity weakness, visual impairment, polypharmacy, orthostatic hypotension, and a home environment that is not optimized for elder living.[93]

Falls are a dangerous and much-feared event for patients with dementia and their caregivers. A fall leading to a broken hip often leads to the end of independent living and carries a high mortality rate.[94] It is estimated that the probability of falling within 1 year among patients older than 65 years is 19 to 36 percent; this probability is likely higher in patients with dementia.[93] For this reason, fall prevention is an important part of the care of elderly demented patients.

The most important factor that predicts future falls in older adults is a prior fall within the past year, with positive likelihood ratios of 2.3 to 2.8.[93] Among patients who have not fallen, subjective and objective assessment of gait and balance is likely the most efficient means of screening for those at highest risk. A self-perceived mobility problem has a positive likelihood ratio of 1.7 to 2.0; objective assessments revealing an inability to stand for 10 seconds while keeping the heel of one foot touching the toe of the other, an inability to tandem walk, and taking more than 13 seconds to walk 10 meters, each have positive likelihood ratios of 2.0 to 2.4.[93] For inpatients, the risk of falls can be assessed using one of several tools, including the St. Thomas Risk Assessment Tool in Falling Elderly Inpatients, the Morse Fall Scale, and the Hednrich Fall Risk Model.[95] Factors predictive of inpatient falls using these tools include a history of recent falls, agitation, visual impairment, the need for frequent toileting, requirement of an aid for ambulation, and gait impairment.[95]

Patients at risk of falls are likely to benefit from multifactorial prevention interventions. A meta-analysis of 159 trials assessing exercise and multifactorial fall prevention programs among community-dwelling older adults found a significant reduction in the risk and rate of falling with exercise programs (risk ratio 0.85 and rate ratio 0.71, respectively); multifactorial fall prevention programs were found to only reduce the rate of falling (rate ratio 0.76).[96] The multifactorial interventions studied in these trials typically include a risk assessment that reviews medications; assessment of basic and instrumental activities of daily living; measurement of orthostatic blood pressure and visual acuity; evaluation of gait, balance, and cognition; and a detailed assessment of home safety. The risk assessment is followed by targeted interventions that may include elimination of high-risk medications (such as antipsychotics and other potentially sedating medications), a physical therapy or exercise program, education of patients and caregivers, and home safety improvements. Multifactorial interventions to reduce falls in the inpatient setting have been proposed but data regarding their effectiveness are inconclusive.[97]

Orthostatic Hypotension

Postural hypotension is a common complication of certain dementias, especially synucleinopathies. Patients with these disorders should be assessed for this condition when presenting with low blood pressure, dizziness, or falls. Assessment and treatment of postural hypotension is discussed in Chapter 8.

Sleep Disorders

Disturbances of sleep are common among patients with dementia. Some disorders, such as sundowning and insomnia, are common to all forms of dementia, whereas others appear unique to the synucleinopathies. This predilection may be due to the predisposition of α-synuclein aggregates to affect brainstem neurons and interrupt projections involved in arousal and modulation of tone during sleep.[98]

REM sleep behavior disorder is a condition in which patients act out their dreams during REM sleep. During REM sleep, pathways descending from the lower brainstem to the spinal cord normally cause atonia.[99] It is hypothesized that degeneration of these descending fibers allows uninhibited flow of cortical signals generated during dreams to cause muscle activation. The movements associated with REM sleep behavior disorder are dramatic; often patients have to stop sleeping with their bed partner in consequence. The sleep disorder may precede the development of other manifestations of a synucleinopathy by many years: approximately 50 to 65 percent of patients with REM sleep behavior disorder will develop a synucleinopathy within 10 years.[100] Clonazepam taken 30 minutes before bedtime is often effective in treating REM sleep behavior disorder but may cause excessive daytime sleepiness, sleep apnea, behavioral disorders, and unsteadiness, especially in demented patients; melatonin at doses of 3 to 9 mg in the evening has also been helpful in non-randomized studies.[101]

Large cohort studies suggest 40 to 50 percent of patients with Parkinson disease suffer from excessive daytime sleepiness, with smaller studies finding similar rates among patients with dementia with Lewy bodies.[102–104] Daytime sleepiness can be exacerbated by the use of the dopamine agonists ropinirole and pramipexole, but it occurs in Parkinson disease independently of medications as well.[105] Fatigue is also a common symptom in Parkinson disease and is more highly correlated with depression than sleepiness, but can occur independently of both.[106] The degree of daytime sleepiness can be assessed using the Epworth Sleepiness Scale. Treatment for excessive daytime sleepiness should start with education on sleep hygiene in order to reduce insomnia. Patients should be screened for sleep apnea and referred for a sleep study if appropriate. Unfortunately, studies of stimulants such as modafenil, methyphenidate, and caffeine have not demonstrated efficacy in reducing either excessive daytime sleepiness or fatigue in Parkinson disease.[107,108]

Excessive daytime sleepiness occurs at a similar frequency in multiple system atrophy as in Parkinson disease, but it is correlated with a higher incidence of sleep-disordered breathing.[109] Sleep-disordered breathing in multiple system atrophy manifests as obstructive sleep apnea, nocturnal stridor, and central hypoventilation and is an important condition for clinicians caring for these patients to recognize.[110] These disorders may also occur in other synucleinopathies but do so less frequently. Stridor is due to dystonia of the vocal cords and can result in airway obstruction; it is a risk factor for shortened survival in multiple system atrophy.[111,112] Treatment with continuous positive airway pressure or botulinum toxin injections to the vocal folds, guided by EMG, may be successful.[113] Tracheostomy may be necessary in cases where stridor occurs during wakefulness or continuous positive airway pressure is not tolerated, although sudden death may still occur due to central hypoventilation.[112]

Gastrointestinal and Genitourinary Complications

Although α-synuclein inclusions were discovered 25 years ago in the enteric nervous system of patients with Parkinson disease, interest in this phenomenon has resurfaced. In a case-control study, Lewy bodies were detected in colonic biopsies from 72 percent of such patients but in no age-matched controls.[114,115] This appears to be a finding present even in early Parkinson disease and holds promise as a biomarker for the illness.[116] Involvement of the enteric nervous system by α-synuclein pathology is a likely explanation for constipation, which is a prominent feature of the synucleinopathies.[115,117]

Incontinence is common in end-stage dementia. In most dementias, the mechanism of incontinence is one of impaired central inhibition, due to involvement of either pontine or forebrain micturition centers, resulting in urge incontinence.[118] This is in contrast to multiple system atrophy, in which a neurogenic bladder with large post-void residuals and overflow incontinence is the rule as part of a more systemic autonomic neuropathy.[119] There are few studies of nonpharmacologic management of urinary incontinence in dementia; among these, timed and prompted voiding may be of benefit.[120] Anticholinergic medications should be used with caution given the risk of precipitating delirium in elderly patients with dementia. Bladder catheters should be avoided because they increase the chance of infection and provide a tether to the patient's bed, thereby decreasing mobility and increasing the risk of delirium.

REFERENCES

1. Plassman BL, Langa KM, Fisher GG, et al: Prevalence of dementia in the United States: the aging, demographics, and memory study. Neuroepidemiology 29:125, 2007.
2. Thies W, Bleiler L; Alzheimer's Association: 2013 Alzheimer's disease facts and figures. Alzheimers Dement 9:208, 2013.
3. Xie J, Brayne C, Matthews FE: Survival times in people with dementia: analysis from population based cohort study with 14 year follow-up. BMJ 336:258, 2008.
4. Wolfson C, Wolfson DB, Asgharian M, et al: A reevaluation of the duration of survival after the onset of dementia. N Engl J Med 344:1111, 2001.
5. Braak H, Braak E: Neuropathological stageing of Alzheimer-related changes. Acta Neuropathol 82:239, 1991.
6. Larson EB, Shadlen MF, Wang L, et al: Survival after initial diagnosis of Alzheimer disease. Ann Intern Med 140:501, 2004.
7. Reitz C, Brayne C, Mayeux R: Epidemiology of Alzheimer disease. Nat Rev Neurol 7:137, 2011.
8. Stern Y, Gurland B, Tatemichi TK, et al: Influence of education and occupation on the incidence of Alzheimer's disease. JAMA 271:1004, 1994.
9. Plassman BL, Havlik RJ, Steffens DC, et al: Documented head injury in early adulthood and risk of Alzheimer's disease and other dementias. Neurology 55:1158, 2000.
10. Larson EB, Wang L, Bowen JD, et al: Exercise is associated with reduced risk for incident dementia among persons 65 years of age and older. Ann Intern Med 144:73, 2006.
11. Roe CM, Xiong C, Miller JP, et al: Education and Alzheimer disease without dementia: support for the cognitive reserve hypothesis. Neurology 68:223, 2007.
12. Raina P, Santaguida P, Ismaila A, et al: Effectiveness of cholinesterase inhibitors and memantine for treating dementia: evidence review for a clinical practice guideline. Ann Intern Med 148:379, 2008.
13. Deramecourt V, Slade JY, Oakley AE, et al: Staging and natural history of cerebrovascular pathology in dementia. Neurology 78:1043, 2012.
14. Lobo A, Launer LJ, Fratiglioni L, et al: Prevalence of dementia and major subtypes in Europe: a collaborative study of population-based cohorts. Neurologic Diseases in the Elderly Research Group. Neurology 54:S4, 2000.
15. Gorelick PB, Scuteri A, Black SE, et al: Vascular contributions to cognitive impairment and dementia: a statement for healthcare professionals from the American Heart Association/American Stroke Association. Stroke 42:2672, 2011.
16. Whitmer RA, Gunderson EP, Barrett-Connor E, et al: Obesity in middle age and future risk of dementia: a 27 year longitudinal population based study. BMJ 330:1360, 2005.
17. Ravaglia G, Forti P, Lucicesare A, et al: Physical activity and dementia risk in the elderly: findings from a prospective Italian study. Neurology 70:1786, 2008.
18. Kavirajan H, Schneider LS: Efficacy and adverse effects of cholinesterase inhibitors and memantine in vascular dementia: a meta-analysis of randomised controlled trials. Lancet Neurol 6:782, 2007.
19. Boeve BF, Silber MH, Ferman TJ, et al: Clinicopathologic correlations in 172 cases of rapid eye movement sleep behavior disorder with or without a coexisting neurologic disorder. Sleep Med 14:754, 2013.
20. Schenck CH, Boeve BF, Mahowald MW: Delayed emergence of a parkinsonian disorder or dementia in 81% of older males initially diagnosed with idiopathic REM

sleep behavior disorder (RBD): 16 year update on a previously reported series. Sleep Med 14:744, 2013.
21. McKeith IG, Dickson DW, Lowe J, et al: Diagnosis and management of dementia with Lewy bodies: third report of the DLB Consortium. Neurology 65:1863, 2005.
22. McKeith I, Del Ser T, Spano P, et al: Efficacy of rivastigmine in dementia with Lewy bodies: a randomised, double-blind, placebo-controlled international study. Lancet 356:2031, 2000.
23. Mori E, Ikeda M, Kosaka K: Donepezil for dementia with Lewy bodies: a randomized, placebo-controlled trial. Ann Neurol 72:41, 2012.
24. Williams MM, Xiong C, Morris JC, et al: Survival and mortality differences between dementia with Lewy bodies vs Alzheimer disease. Neurology 67:1935, 2006.
25. Aarsland D, Zaccai J, Brayne C: A systematic review of prevalence studies of dementia in Parkinson's disease. Mov Disord 20:1255, 2005.
26. Aarsland D, Andersen K, Larsen JP, et al: Prevalence and characteristics of dementia in Parkinson disease: an 8-year prospective study. Arch Neurol 60:387, 2003.
27. Brown RG, Lacomblez L, Landwehrmeyer BG, et al: Cognitive impairment in patients with multiple system atrophy and progressive supranuclear palsy. Brain 133:2382, 2010.
28. Schrag A, Wenning GK, Quinn N, et al: Survival in multiple system atrophy. Mov Disord 23:294, 2008.
29. Watanabe H, Saito Y, Terao S, et al: Progression and prognosis in multiple system atrophy: an analysis of 230 Japanese patients. Brain 125:1070, 2002.
30. Drubin DG, Kirschner MW: Tau protein function in living cells. J Cell Biol 103:2739, 1986.
31. Seelaar H, Rohrer JD, Pijnenburg YA, et al: Clinical, genetic and pathological heterogeneity of frontotemporal dementia: a review. J Neurol Neurosurg Psychiatry 82:476, 2011.
32. Roberson ED, Hesse JH, Rose KD, et al: Frontotemporal dementia progresses to death faster than Alzheimer disease. Neurology 65:719, 2005.
33. Liu W, Miller BL, Kramer JH, et al: Behavioral disorders in the frontal and temporal variants of frontotemporal dementia. Neurology 62:742, 2004.
34. Litvan I, Mega MS, Cummings JL, et al: Neuropsychiatric aspects of progressive supranuclear palsy. Neurology 47:1184, 1996.
35. O'Sullivan SS, Massey LA, Williams DR, et al: Clinical outcomes of progressive supranuclear palsy and multiple system atrophy. Brain 131:1362, 2008.
36. Lee SE, Rabinovici GD, Mayo MC, et al: Clinicopathological correlations in corticobasal degeneration. Ann Neurol 70:327, 2011.
37. Heaton RK, Clifford DB, Franklin Jr DR, et al: HIV-associated neurocognitive disorders persist in the era of potent antiretroviral therapy: CHARTER Study. Neurology 75:2087, 2010.
38. Kranick SM, Nath A: Neurologic complications of HIV-1 infection and its treatment in the era of antiretroviral therapy. Continuum (Minneap Minn) 18:1319, 2012.
39. Davis JD, Tremont G: Neuropsychiatric aspects of hypothyroidism and treatment reversibility. Minerva Endocrinol 32:49, 2007.
40. Moore E, Mander A, Ames D, et al: Cognitive impairment and vitamin B_{12}: a review. Int Psychogeriatr 24:541, 2012.
41. Malouf R, Areosa Sastre A: Vitamin B_{12} for cognition. Cochrane Database Syst Rev:CD004326, 2003.
42. Blundo C, Marin D, Ricci M: Vitamin B_{12} deficiency associated with symptoms of frontotemporal dementia. Neurol Sci 32:101, 2011.
43. Knopman DS, DeKosky ST, Cummings JL, et al: Practice parameter: diagnosis of dementia (an evidence-based review). Report of the Quality Standards Subcommittee of the American Academy of Neurology. Neurology 56:1143, 2001.
44. Mesholam-Gately RI, Giuliano AJ, Zillmer EA, et al: Verbal learning and memory in older adults with minor and major depression. Arch Clin Neuropsychol 27:196, 2012.
45. Tulek B, Atalay NB, Kanat F, et al: Attentional control is partially impaired in obstructive sleep apnoea syndrome. J Sleep Res 22:422, 2013.
46. Loke YK, Brown JW, Kwok CS, et al: Association of obstructive sleep apnea with risk of serious cardiovascular events: a systematic review and meta-analysis. Circ Cardiovasc Qual Outcomes 5:720, 2012.
47. Ancoli-Israel S, Palmer BW, Cooke JR, et al: Cognitive effects of treating obstructive sleep apnea in Alzheimer's disease: a randomized controlled study. J Am Geriatr Soc 56:2076, 2008.
48. Sura L, Madhavan A, Carnaby G, et al: Dysphagia in the elderly: management and nutritional considerations. Clin Interv Aging 7:287, 2012.
49. Alagiakrishnan K, Bhanji RA, Kurian M: Evaluation and management of oropharyngeal dysphagia in different types of dementia: a systematic review. Arch Gerontol Geriatr 56:1, 2013.
50. Easterling CS, Robbins E: Dementia and dysphagia. Geriatr Nurs 29:275, 2008.
51. Ikeda M, Brown J, Holland AJ, et al: Changes in appetite, food preference, and eating habits in frontotemporal dementia and Alzheimer's disease. J Neurol Neurosurg Psychiatry 73:371, 2002.
52. Langmore SE, Skarupski KA, Park PS, et al: Predictors of aspiration pneumonia in nursing home residents. Dysphagia 17:298, 2002.
53. Brunnstrom HR, Englund EM: Cause of death in patients with dementia disorders. Eur J Neurol 16:488, 2009.
54. Alfonsi E, Versino M, Merlo IM, et al: Electrophysiologic patterns of oral-pharyngeal swallowing in parkinsonian syndromes. Neurology 68:583, 2007.

55. Beach TG, Adler CH, Sue LI, et al: Multi-organ distribution of phosphorylated alpha-synuclein histopathology in subjects with Lewy body disorders. Acta Neuropathol 119:689, 2010.
56. McCullough GH, Rosenbek JC, Wertz RT, et al: Utility of clinical swallowing examination measures for detecting aspiration post-stroke. J Speech Lang Hear Res 48:1280, 2005.
57. Cogen R, Weinryb J: Aspiration pneumonia in nursing home patients fed via gastrostomy tubes. Am J Gastroenterol 84:1509, 1989.
58. Logemann JA, Gensler G, Robbins J, et al: A randomized study of three interventions for aspiration of thin liquids in patients with dementia or Parkinson's disease. J Speech Lang Hear Res 51:173, 2008.
59. Robbins J, Gensler G, Hind J, et al: Comparison of 2 interventions for liquid aspiration on pneumonia incidence: a randomized trial. Ann Intern Med 148:509, 2008.
60. Teno JM, Gozalo PL, Mitchell SL, et al: Does feeding tube insertion and its timing improve survival? J Am Geriatr Soc 60:1918, 2012.
61. Sampson EL, Candy B, Jones L: Enteral tube feeding for older people with advanced dementia. Cochrane Database Syst Rev:CD007209, 2009.
62. Kuo S, Rhodes RL, Mitchell SL, et al: Natural history of feeding-tube use in nursing home residents with advanced dementia. J Am Med Dir Assoc 10:264, 2009.
63. Mitchell SL, Teno JM, Roy J, et al: Clinical and organizational factors associated with feeding tube use among nursing home residents with advanced cognitive impairment. JAMA 290:73, 2003.
64. van der Maarel-Wierink CD, Vanobbergen JN, Bronkhorst EM, et al: Risk factors for aspiration pneumonia in frail older people: a systematic literature review. J Am Med Dir Assoc 12:344, 2011.
65. Eom CS, Jeon CY, Lim JW, et al: Use of acid-suppressive drugs and risk of pneumonia: a systematic review and meta-analysis. CMAJ 183:310, 2011.
66. Palecek EJ, Teno JM, Casarett DJ, et al: Comfort feeding only: a proposal to bring clarity to decision-making regarding difficulty with eating for persons with advanced dementia. J Am Geriatr Soc 58:580, 2010.
67. Boorsma M, Joling KJ, Frijters DH, et al: The prevalence, incidence and risk factors for delirium in Dutch nursing homes and residential care homes. Int J Geriatr Psychiatry 27:709, 2012.
68. Fick DM, Agostini JV, Inouye SK: Delirium superimposed on dementia: a systematic review. J Am Geriatr Soc 50:1723, 2002.
69. Fick DM, Kolanowski AM, Waller JL, et al: Delirium superimposed on dementia in a community-dwelling managed care population: a 3-year retrospective study of occurrence, costs, and utilization. J Gerontol A Biol Sci Med Sci 60:748, 2005.
70. Alagiakrishnan K, Wiens CA: An approach to drug induced delirium in the elderly. Postgrad Med J 80:388, 2004.
71. Francis J, Martin D, Kapoor WN: A prospective study of delirium in hospitalized elderly. JAMA 263:1097, 1990.
72. Marcantonio ER, Goldman L, Mangione CM, et al: A clinical prediction rule for delirium after elective noncardiac surgery. JAMA 271:134, 1994.
73. Bedrosian TA, Herring KL, Weil ZM, et al: Altered temporal patterns of anxiety in aged and amyloid precursor protein (APP) transgenic mice. Proc Natl Acad Sci USA 108:11686, 2011.
74. Inouye SK, Bogardus Jr ST, Charpentier PA, et al: A multicomponent intervention to prevent delirium in hospitalized older patients. N Engl J Med 340:669, 1999.
75. Marcantonio ER, Flacker JM, Wright RJ, et al: Reducing delirium after hip fracture: a randomized trial. J Am Geriatr Soc 49:516, 2001.
76. O'Mahony R, Murthy L, Akunne A, et al: Synopsis of the National Institute for Health and Clinical Excellence guideline for prevention of delirium. Ann Intern Med 154:746, 2011.
77. Lonergan E, Britton AM, Luxenberg J, et al: Antipsychotics for delirium. Cochrane Database Syst Rev:CD005594, 2007.
78. Ballard C, Waite J: The effectiveness of atypical antipsychotics for the treatment of aggression and psychosis in Alzheimer's disease. Cochrane Database Syst Rev:CD003476, 2006.
79. Mohamed S, Rosenheck R, Lyketsos CG, et al: Effect of second-generation antipsychotics on caregiver burden in Alzheimer's disease. J Clin Psychiatry 73:121, 2012.
80. Vigen CL, Mack WJ, Keefe RS, et al: Cognitive effects of atypical antipsychotic medications in patients with Alzheimer's disease: outcomes from CATIE-AD. Am J Psychiatry 168:831, 2011.
81. Howard RJ, Juszczak E, Ballard CG, et al: Donepezil for the treatment of agitation in Alzheimer's disease. N Engl J Med 357:1382, 2007.
82. Ayalon L, Gum AM, Feliciano L, et al: Effectiveness of nonpharmacological interventions for the management of neuropsychiatric symptoms in patients with dementia: a systematic review. Arch Intern Med 166:2182, 2006.
83. Gitlin LN, Winter L, Dennis MP, et al: Targeting and managing behavioral symptoms in individuals with dementia: a randomized trial of a nonpharmacological intervention. J Am Geriatr Soc 58:1465, 2010.
84. Cohen-Mansfield J, Thein K, Marx MS, et al: Efficacy of nonpharmacologic interventions for agitation in advanced dementia: a randomized, placebo-controlled trial. J Clin Psychiatry 73:1255, 2012.
85. Lyketsos CG, Lopez O, Jones B, et al: Prevalence of neuropsychiatric symptoms in dementia and mild cognitive impairment: results from the cardiovascular health study. JAMA 288:1475, 2002.
86. Starkstein SE, Mizrahi R, Power BD: Depression in Alzheimer's disease: phenomenology, clinical correlates and treatment. Int Rev Psychiatry 20:382, 2008.

87. Starkstein S, Dragovic M, Jorge R, et al: Diagnostic criteria for depression in Parkinson's disease: a study of symptom patterns using latent class analysis. Mov Disord 26:2239, 2011.
88. Starkstein SE, Jorge R, Petracca G, et al: The construct of generalized anxiety disorder in Alzheimer disease. Am J Geriatr Psychiatry 15:42, 2007.
89. Leentjens AF, Dujardin K, Marsh L, et al: Anxiety rating scales in Parkinson's disease: a validation study of the Hamilton anxiety rating scale, the Beck anxiety inventory, and the hospital anxiety and depression scale. Mov Disord 26:407, 2011.
90. Byers AL, Yaffe K: Depression and risk of developing dementia. Nat Rev Neurol 7:323, 2011.
91. Bains J, Birks JS, Dening TR: The efficacy of antidepressants in the treatment of depression in dementia. Cochrane Database Syst Rev:CD003944, 2002.
92. Verkaik R, van Weert JC, Francke AL: The effects of psychosocial methods on depressed, aggressive and apathetic behaviors of people with dementia: a systematic review. Int J Geriatr Psychiatry 20:301, 2005.
93. Ganz DA, Bao Y, Shekelle PG, et al: Will my patient fall? JAMA 297:77, 2007.
94. Baker NL, Cook MN, Arrighi HM, et al: Hip fracture risk and subsequent mortality among Alzheimer's disease patients in the United Kingdom, 1988–2007. Age Ageing 40:49, 2011.
95. Cumbler EU, Simpson JR, Rosenthal LD, et al: Inpatient falls: defining the problem and identifying possible solutions. Part I: an evidence-based review. Neurohospitalist 3:135, 2013.
96. Gillespie LD, Robertson MC, Gillespie WJ, et al: Interventions for preventing falls in older people living in the community. Cochrane Database Syst Rev 9:CD007146, 2012.
97. Cameron ID, Gillespie LD, Robertson MC, et al: Interventions for preventing falls in older people in care facilities and hospitals. Cochrane Database Syst Rev 12:CD005465, 2012.
98. Braak H, Ghebremedhin E, Rub U, et al: Stages in the development of Parkinson's disease-related pathology. Cell Tissue Res 318:121, 2004.
99. Postuma RB, Gagnon JF, Montplaisir JY: REM sleep behavior disorder: from dreams to neurodegeneration. Neurobiol Dis 46:553, 2012.
100. Postuma RB, Gagnon JF, Vendette M, et al: Quantifying the risk of neurodegenerative disease in idiopathic REM sleep behavior disorder. Neurology 72:1296, 2009.
101. McCarter SJ, Boswell CL, St Louis EK, et al: Treatment outcomes in REM sleep behavior disorder. Sleep Med 14:237, 2013.
102. Hobson DE, Lang AE, Martin WR, et al: Excessive daytime sleepiness and sudden-onset sleep in Parkinson disease: a survey by the Canadian Movement Disorders Group. JAMA 287:455, 2002.
103. Verbaan D, van Rooden SM, Visser M, et al: Nighttime sleep problems and daytime sleepiness in Parkinson's disease. Mov Disord 23:35, 2008.
104. Boddy F, Rowan EN, Lett D, et al: Subjectively reported sleep quality and excessive daytime somnolence in Parkinson's disease with and without dementia, dementia with Lewy bodies and Alzheimer's disease. Int J Geriatr Psychiatry 22:529, 2007.
105. Gjerstad MD, Alves G, Wentzel-Larsen T, et al: Excessive daytime sleepiness in Parkinson disease: is it the drugs or the disease? Neurology 67:853, 2006.
106. Alves G, Wentzel-Larsen T, Larsen JP: Is fatigue an independent and persistent symptom in patients with Parkinson disease? Neurology 63:1908, 2004.
107. Postuma RB, Lang AE, Munhoz RP, et al: Caffeine for treatment of Parkinson disease: a randomized controlled trial. Neurology 79:651, 2012.
108. Seppi K, Weintraub D, Coelho M, et al: The Movement Disorder Society Evidence-Based Medicine Review Update: treatments for the non-motor symptoms of Parkinson's disease. Mov Disord 26(suppl 3):S42, 2011.
109. Moreno-Lopez C, Santamaria J, Salamero M, et al: Excessive daytime sleepiness in multiple system atrophy (SLEEMSA study). Arch Neurol 68:223, 2011.
110. Vetrugno R, Provini F, Cortelli P, et al: Sleep disorders in multiple system atrophy: a correlative videopolysomnographic study. Sleep Med 5:21, 2004.
111. Merlo IM, Occhini A, Pacchetti C, et al: Not paralysis, but dystonia causes stridor in multiple system atrophy. Neurology 58:649, 2002.
112. Silber MH, Levine S: Stridor and death in multiple system atrophy. Mov Disord 15:699, 2000.
113. Iranzo A: Sleep and breathing in multiple system atrophy. Curr Treat Options Neurol 9:347, 2007.
114. Wakabayashi K, Takahashi H, Takeda S, et al: Parkinson's disease: the presence of Lewy bodies in Auerbach's and Meissner's plexuses. Acta Neuropathol 76:217, 1988.
115. Lebouvier T, Neunlist M, Bruley des Varannes S, et al: Colonic biopsies to assess the neuropathology of Parkinson's disease and its relationship with symptoms. PLoS One 5:e12728, 2010.
116. Shannon KM, Keshavarzian A, Mutlu E, et al: Alpha-synuclein in colonic submucosa in early untreated Parkinson's disease. Mov Disord 27:709, 2012.
117. Kaye J, Gage H, Kimber A, et al: Excess burden of constipation in Parkinson's disease: a pilot study. Mov Disord 21:1270, 2006.
118. Sakakibara R, Uchiyama T, Yamanishi T, et al: Genitourinary dysfunction in Parkinson's disease. Mov Disord 25:2, 2010.
119. Sakakibara R, Hattori T, Uchiyama T, et al: Videourodynamic and sphincter motor unit potential analyses in Parkinson's disease and multiple system atrophy. J Neurol Neurosurg Psychiatry 71:600, 2001.
120. Hagglund D: A systematic literature review of incontinence care for persons with dementia: the research evidence. J Clin Nurs 19:303, 2010.

SECTION

XVI

Palliative Care

CHAPTER

62

Care at the End of Life

MICHAEL J. AMINOFF

With the advent of increasingly sophisticated technology and more powerful pharmacologic agents, it has become possible to prolong the last stages of life in patients with severe and irreversible medical disorders, in whom a long-term favorable outcome cannot be achieved. In some instances, the futile use of sophisticated technology to maintain certain bodily functions in individuals with no prospect of useful recovery has involved major financial outlay, an added burden on patients in advanced stages of incurable disease, and unnecessary and prolonged emotional distress to relatives and friends. Indeed, impersonal advances in modern medicine have led to increasing indignity and fear in many individuals as the end of life draws near, and some will die with unrelieved and uncontrolled symptoms.

Neurologists are often required to look after patients at the end of life either because a primary neurologic disorder reaches a terminal phase or because patients with primary medical disorders develop a catastrophic neurologic complication leading to consultation. The ability to recognize the last hours or days of life, that is, to diagnose "dying," is an important clinical skill that is a prerequisite to the provision of appropriate care.[1] Such patients are usually obtunded, able to take only sips of fluids, unable to take oral medications, and unresponsive to modifications in their therapeutic regimen; there may be no obvious reversible precipitant of their deterioration. Patient management is optimized when there is agreement between members of the health-care team that the patient is indeed dying.[1] In this circumstance, it is important to avoid giving conflicting messages to patients and their families about the likely course of events.

PHYSICIAN–PATIENT INTERACTIONS

It is the responsibility of all physicians to provide adequate care for patients who have a terminal disease or are dying. The focus of care changes from attempts to reverse or cure an underlying disease to providing compassionate and sensitive care for patients facing imminent death. Such care may be required for no more than a few hours or for as long as several months, depending on the nature of the underlying disorder. Patients or their surrogates will need to be informed of the severity of their disease, and—depending on the circumstances—this is generally best accomplished gradually and with sensitivity, bearing in mind what they do (and do not) want to know. Patients want hope and reassurance—not necessarily that they will live but that there are options to help their isolation, fear, physical discomfort, and mental distress. Physicians must assume responsibility for helping patients to deal with the bleak uncertainty of the future and to cope with the sense of isolation and dependency that is often experienced with the approach of death. Fears concerning pain or discomfort can often be

Aminoff's Neurology and General Medicine, Fifth Edition.

alleviated by proper explanation, and supportive care by family, friends, and medical attendants may help to diminish otherwise overwhelming feelings of isolation and uncertainty. Some physicians still feel a certain guilt or responsibility for the death of patients, and this colors their approach to patients who are dying. Such attitudes will change only with the wider appreciation that death is but a natural milestone.

With the increasing emphasis on the scientific aspects of modern medicine, the art of the discipline—its human side—is often overlooked. Physicians must be prepared to spend time with their patients to provide support, education, and adequate symptomatic relief and to work with them and their family to enable them to come to terms with events. Unfortunately, however, such discussion and resultant decision-making substantially in advance of death are uncommon. The demands on physicians by patients may be considerable as death approaches. It is especially important for physicians to understand the needs of patients who are unable or unwilling to communicate with them. Patients need to know that they will continue to receive support and care from their physician throughout the process of dying. A cursory glance at patients during the course of a busy ward-round is quite inadequate in this regard. The family, also, may require considerable attention from physicians. This requires a sensitivity to their needs and the ability to communicate fully with them at all times, providing adequate responses to their queries; meeting with them after death has occurred often helps to settle unresolved fears and concerns. The care of terminally ill patients usually requires the cooperation of the entire health-care team, including nursing staff, social workers, physical and occupational therapists, dieticians, and psychotherapists, as well as physicians. The spiritual needs of the family must not be overlooked, and the clergy have an important role in this context.

In many countries, the general public has expressed increasing dissatisfaction with the care received by people who are dying. Fueled by concerns about the quality of end-of-life care, support has grown for the concept that patients with terminal illnesses should have the right to request assistance in dying. The extent to which physicians can assist in this regard is governed by national statutes, and the extent to which physicians choose to become involved in this context is personal and individual. Regardless, many individual physicians support the legalization of medically assisted suicide and voluntary euthanasia,[2] although numerous professional organizations (including the American Academy of Neurology[3]) are opposed to such an approach. Medically assisted suicide involves providing the means for a patient intentionally to kill himself or herself, whereas voluntary euthanasia consists of the deliberate killing of a patient at his or her request. The provision of appropriate palliative care for dying patients would make such radical alternatives unnecessary in many instances. Pain relief, for example, must be adequate even if, as an unintended side effect, the medications used to control pain lead to some shortening of life in consequence.

Ethicists and educators have emphasized patient autonomy in the decision-making process. However, in a study of 8,308 hospitalized patients, 67 percent ultimately preferred to leave medical decisions to their doctor, even though 97 percent wanted their physician to offer them therapeutic choices and consider their opinions.[4] Thus, both patient autonomy and physician beneficence remain important in guiding clinical care. Some patients with advanced medical disease may seek a particular therapeutic intervention that seems unjustified to their physician. Clinicians should behave in a manner that does not conflict with their own beliefs; if differences with patients and their families cannot be resolved by discussion and explanation, it is sometimes worthwhile to transfer patients—with their consent—to the care of another physician. Physicians have the responsibility of withholding treatment when the distress or other adverse effects of therapy cannot be justified by unrealistic hopes of curing or arresting the underlying medical disorder and of withdrawing life-prolonging maneuvers when these have become too burdensome for patients.

Competent adults have the right to refuse medical treatment or to request its discontinuation. Despite this, many patients dying in hospital continue to receive unwanted interventions such as intensive life support that postpone death.[5] Patients' refusals of supportive measures are not necessarily indicative of a wish to die: rather, they often signify simply a wish to do without the burden of life-sustaining medical treatment.[6] The goals of such treatment must constantly be reappraised by patients, relatives, and medical staff. Even routine procedures such as radiographs, blood tests, and respiratory care may become unwelcome and tiresome interruptions during the last days of life, and the need for them must be re-evaluated as the patient's condition deteriorates. When patients do refuse treatment, however, physicians are responsible for ensuring that this is not an impulsive decision but is based on an understanding of the implications of such a choice.

For patients to make informed decisions, it is important that they are properly educated by their physician about their options. They should also be encouraged to use advance directives such as a living will to ensure that their own wishes regarding medical intervention are followed if they later become unable to express their preferences because of physical or mental limitations. A durable power of attorney for health care in the United States gives another person the power to make medical decisions for the patient as necessary. It is important that physicians educate patients about such opportunities and the ability to make advance directives. Clinicians must also properly inform proxy decision-makers about the patient's disorder, therapeutic options, and prognosis. They are generally expected to make decisions based on what the patient would have wished, and this assumes some knowledge of the patient's preferences (the substituted judgment standard). Without such knowledge, the proxy can only balance the benefits of any treatment or course of action against the possible burdens (the best interests standard). When the perceived benefits are greater, consent is provided; if the likely burdens exceed any potential benefit, consent is refused.

However, there is a discrepancy between theoretical ethical concepts and clinical reality. A study of dialysis patients revealed that many would allow their designated surrogate to override their advance directives if this was in their interests. Subjects varied greatly in how much leeway they would give surrogates to override advance directives: "no leeway" was given by 39 percent, "a little leeway" by 19 percent, "a lot of leeway" by 11 percent, and "complete leeway" by 31 percent.[7] Another study found that many elderly or seriously ill hospitalized patients (more than 70%) would not want their stated resuscitation preferences to be followed if they were to lose decision-making capacity but preferred that their family and physician make such decisions for them.[8] It seems that proxy decision-makers have the discretion to assess novel and perhaps unforeseen circumstances, make moral judgments, and sometimes make decisions that differ from the patient's original intent; for example, because the patient's wishes cannot be applied in certain clinical contexts.[9]

When patients do not have the capacity to make clinical decisions and have no designated surrogate, many states allow a next-of-kin surrogate to be appointed. Decisions by both patient-designated and next-of-kin surrogates are prone to error. A systematic literature review and analysis of 16 eligible studies involving 151 hypothetical scenarios and 2,595 surrogate–patient pairs, which collectively analyzed 19,526 patient–surrogate paired responses, showed that surrogates predicted patients' end-of-life treatment preferences with only 68 percent accuracy.[10] Surrogates were least accurate in scenarios involving stroke or dementia. Surprisingly, accuracy was not improved when the patient had designated the surrogate or by prior discussion between patients and surrogates about treatment preferences. Nevertheless, surrogates were more accurate than physicians in predicting patients' treatment preferences.

To better understand the moral obligations of the patient–proxy relationship, Fins and colleagues surveyed 50 patient–proxy pairs and 52 individuals who had been proxies for someone who had died.[9] They used structured vignettes of three separate diseases (one of which was acute stroke), and examined whether respondents believed that proxies should follow explicit instructions and thus act contractually regarding life-sustaining therapy or whether more discretionary (or covenantal) judgments were acceptable. Other variables included the "valence" of initial patient instructions (e.g., "to do nothing" or "to do everything") and the quality of information available to the proxy. They found that the patient–proxy relationship exists on a contractual to covenantal continuum and that disease course, the clarity of prognosis, instructional valence, and quality of patient instructions led to response differences. The use of interpretative or covenantal judgment was desired by patients and proxies when the prognosis was grim, despite initial instructions to pursue more aggressive care. When hopeful feelings modified initial negative instructions, proxies were more uncertain about the propriety of doing nothing. Nonetheless, patients and proxies intended that negative instructions to be left alone should be heeded. Respondents did not adhere to narrow

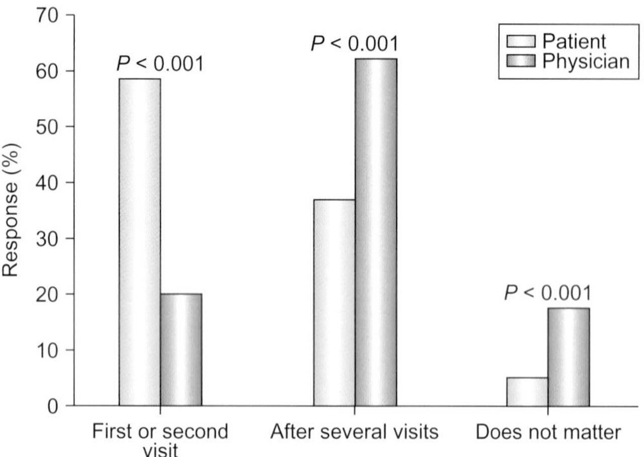

FIGURE 62-1 ■ Patient and physician opinions regarding when advance directives should be discussed. (From Johnston SC, Pfeifer MP, McNutt R, for the End of Life Study Group: The discussion about advance directives. Patient and physician opinions regarding when and how it should be conducted. Arch Intern Med 155:1025, 1995, with permission.)

notions of patient self-determination but made nuanced and contextually informed moral judgments that were not viewed by patients or proxies as violations of the principal's autonomy. Although respondents were better educated than the general public and were restricted to self-identified, English-speaking Americans of European origin (to avoid the possible confounders of race and ethnicity), these data suggest that advance-care planning should consider both the exercise of autonomy and the interpretative function assumed by the proxy.[9]

Studies indicate that patients would like to discuss advance directives earlier than their physicians and before they are "extremely ill" (Fig. 62-1). Most believe that such discussion should occur when they are still healthy.[11] Both patients and clinicians believe that it is the physician who should initiate the discussion (Fig. 62-2), but physicians are often reluctant or fail to do so.[11–13] Many patients believe that others (e.g., a spouse or "significant other," children, or parents) should be brought into the discussion.[11] Most also believe that it should occur before hospitalization and over several visits.

Many healthy subjects consider certain neurologic states to be unacceptable and express the belief that they would not want to remain alive in those circumstances. However, after developing such disability, some patients change their opinion and may experience a better quality of life than previously envisioned. This possibility must be borne in mind when statements made by a patient before their illness are considered.[14]

Decisions about whether to adopt life-sustaining measures often need to be made in a context where the prognosis is uncertain. It is important to note, however, that such decisions can be changed later as the prognosis becomes clearer because no logical distinction exists between withholding and withdrawing life-sustaining measures.[15]

For patients nearing the end of life, decisions have to be made about whether cardiopulmonary resuscitation should be attempted, if the need arises. In patients with terminal diseases, such decisions often bear more on the issue of how a patient will die than on whether death will occur, and it is important for patients and family members to understand this distinction. A decision by a patient (or family members) needs to be made in advance, so that individual wishes can be taken into account in the event that resuscitation is required. In many European countries, physicians take an active role in advising patients and family members about the most appropriate course of action to follow, whereas many physicians in the United States believe that this is an individual decision that is best left to the patient. It is this author's view that the physician—as the most informed person in the health-care team—should be responsible for ensuring that the patient or surrogate is sufficiently well educated about the issues to make informed decisions, guided by suggestions or recommendations when these are requested of the medical staff.

It is often helpful to discuss the possibility of organ donation with dying patients when this is a significant consideration. This makes it easier for family members, who may otherwise have to be approached about the issue shortly after the death of their relative. A variety of ethnic, religious, and cultural factors affect attitudes concerning organ donation, and these must be respected. Physicians must appreciate that patients are not obliged to donate organs and may choose to limit any donation that they make.

PROVISION OF CARE

With their increasing emphasis on surgery and advanced technology, hospitals no longer are able to provide for the long-term care of patients who are dying. By contrast, the needs of the terminally

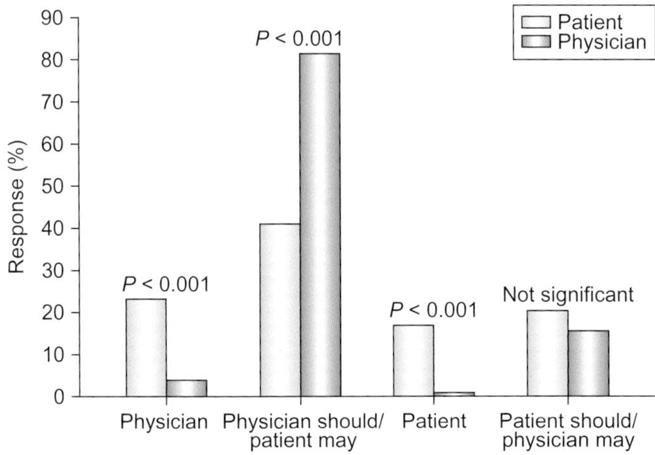

FIGURE 62-2 ■ Patient and physician opinions about who should initiate discussion about advance directives. (From Johnston SC, Pfeifer MP, McNutt R, for the End of Life Study Group: The discussion about advance directives. Patient and physician opinions regarding when and how it should be conducted. Arch Intern Med 155:1025, 1995, with permission.)

ill are often met more fully in the environment of a hospice, where a multidisciplinary team can focus on their care and support, or at home, if an adequate family structure and medical/paramedical support are available. Care for patients in a home environment requires careful education of the family, reduction of probable causes of stress (such as violence, agitation, or incontinence), support of caregivers by ensuring assistance from other ancillary health-care providers, and provision of periodic respite to the family.[16] The interests of patients nevertheless remain the prime concern. When family members appear preoccupied more with their own welfare than that of a severely demented or dying patient, the possibility of patient abuse may require consideration.[16] Abuse of the weak or elderly is becoming an increasing problem and a matter of grave public health concern.

The care of terminally ill patients should be focused on improving the quality of life rather than simply on extending the duration of life. This aspect has in general been neglected until recently and still receives relatively little attention in the clinical literature or medical school curricula. Palliative medicine constitutes an important emerging medical specialty in which the focus is on the quality of life for patients with advanced and progressive disease.[17] The aim is to ensure that patients are as comfortable as possible, even during the process of dying. Curative treatment is not provided for disorders that do not cause discomfort, even if this leads to some shortening of life. Such an approach, traditionally associated with the care of patients with terminal cancer, is also relevant in the management of patients with a number of neurologic and general medical disorders, such as amyotrophic lateral sclerosis, severe cerebrovascular disease, locked-in syndrome, or advanced dementia. The emphasis is on the control of symptoms. Pain is the most common symptom in dying patients.[18] Pain, discomfort, distress, fatigue, dyspnea, anorexia, nausea, vomiting, cognitive disturbances, and affective disorders all require particular care. When the ability of patients to communicate is impaired, it is necessary to infer the presence of distress by such signs as agitation, restlessness, tachypnea, and tachycardia and to initiate treatment accordingly. Many patients fear that any later inability to communicate their distress will lead to unnecessary and increased suffering. The relatives of dying patients frequently complain that signs of distress were ignored in patients unable to communicate their needs verbally. No justification exists for limiting symptomatic measures in such circumstances; overtreatment is preferable to undertreatment.

Opioids have an important role in providing pain relief when nonopioid analgesia is inadequate. Morphine is also particularly useful in relieving dyspnea. The optimal dose is that providing adequate relief. When it is introduced, morphine is best started in an immediate-release formulation. A starting dose of 5 to 10 mg every 4 hours is often adequate, but higher doses may be needed if patients have previously received another opioid, such as dihydrocodeine. A double dose at bedtime may also be helpful. Rescue supplements of morphine are necessary for "breakthrough" pain. The total daily dose of morphine should be titrated upward rapidly (e.g., by 30 to 50%) if pain relief is inadequate.[19] Once pain is controlled, a modified-release preparation of morphine can be used. Side effects of morphine, especially nausea and constipation, may require concomitant treatment. Delirium resulting from opioid treatment may respond to substitution with an alternative opioid. It may be necessary to administer opioids by a nonoral route in patients with severe vomiting or dysphagia, those with intestinal obstruction or malabsorption, or those who are unable to comply with an oral regimen.[15] Subcutaneous infusion of diamorphine may be used for pain control in dying patients.[1] Anxiety, agitation, or delirium may respond to benzodiazepines or neuroleptic agents. In one study of critically ill patients, it was found that large doses of sedatives and analgesics were administered to relieve pain and distress during the withholding or withdrawal of life-supporting measures, but that death was not hastened by such medication.[20] Supportive therapy is important. Attention to the environment may be rewarding. The intensive care unit, with its harsh light, endless noise, monitoring and other equipment, and frequent alarms, is an overwhelming place that provides no respite for dying patients.

Withdrawal of ventilator support is often particularly distressing for both relatives and medical staff,[5] even though this is ethically no different from limiting other therapeutic or supportive measures. Ventilator withdrawal may be accomplished by extubation or by "terminal weaning" (in which ventilator rate, positive end-expiratory pressure, or tidal volume is gradually reduced with the endotracheal tube in place). Regardless of the method used, patient comfort must be ensured, as must the family's perception in this regard. For conscious patients requesting sedation for ventilator withdrawal, Brody and colleagues recommend 2 to 4 mg of midazolam intravenously before withdrawal, and 5 to 10 mg of morphine by intravenous bolus for distress during weaning, followed by continuous infusion (50% of bolus dose per hour); in patients with tolerance to such agents because of prior use, higher doses are needed.[5] Others have used pretreatment with the equivalent of 15 mg per hour of intravenous diazepam or 15 mg per hour of intravenous morphine, increasing the dose as necessary to relieve dyspnea and anxiety, even to the point of unconsciousness if required and requested.[21]

Neuromuscular blocking agents should be discontinued before withdrawal of ventilator support, and indeed probably in all dying patients, to allow verbal communication when this is otherwise possible and to permit signs of distress to be manifest so that appropriate treatment can be provided.[5] The masking of such signs by neuromuscular paralysis serves no useful purpose, and the inability to exhibit signs of distress in this context cannot be taken to imply that such distress is absent.

Attention must be devoted to nutrition, hydration, care of the skin, and sphincter function. The nutrition and hydration of dying patients require careful consideration. The points to consider include whether such support should be provided at all, the manner in which it is best provided, and patients' tolerance of any resulting discomfort, complications, or side effects. There are benefits of withholding nutrition and hydration to shorten life when other treatment is to be discontinued. The artificial provision of nutrition and hydration is a life-sustaining maneuver that does not differ from other maneuvers that supplement or substitute for normal bodily functions. Withdrawal of artificial nutrition and hydration, however, has particular emotional implications for the general public and many clinicians. Such a course therefore demands specific discussion with patients (when communication is possible) and family members, as well as with other members of the health-care team who may be concerned. It is avoided by some clinicians who fear it will add to patients' discomfort.[22] In fact, however, it is unlikely to lead to much additional distress, and by shortening life may actually limit further discomfort. When distress does follow withdrawal of nutrition or hydration, additional symptomatic measures are necessary.[5] Dryness of the mouth is often relieved by ice chips, glycerin swabs, or petroleum jelly lip balm; withdrawal of medication that may be exacerbating this symptom should also be considered. Mouthwashes may relieve poor oral hygiene, and antimonilial therapy is indicated for candidiasis, antiemetics for nausea, and opiates or benzodiazepines for restlessness or pain.[5]

Thus, the focus is on comfort measures, and nonessential medications and interventions (such as blood tests, intravenous fluids, and the like) are discontinued. Relief of pain, agitation, respiratory difficulty, and other distressing symptoms is assured. There must be good communication with the patient, family, and primary medical practitioner, and the plan of care must be explained to them and understood. Attention should also be focused on religious and spiritual needs.

Various systems, such as the Liverpool Care Pathway in the United Kingdom, have been developed to facilitate care practices and monitor their results. The extent to which they improve care is not entirely clear,[23] although some studies do suggest better outcomes,[24] as by improved documentation of care and reduction in average total symptom burden among the dying.[25]

An attempt has been made to determine the effectiveness of multi-component palliative care for residents of care homes for the elderly and to describe the range and quality of outcome measures, based on a review of existing studies.[26] However, only three studies could be included, all conducted in the United States, and they had several potential sources of bias that rendered interpretation difficult. Further studies are therefore needed that focus on standard outcome measures, assess cost-effectiveness, and are less biased.

SPECIAL NEUROLOGIC CIRCUMSTANCES

Palliative care is important for patients with acute stroke, whose needs are often poorly understood. It may also facilitate discussion about such difficult issues as fears of dependence, disability, and death.[27] Symptomatic treatment and comfort measures can improve the quality of life of patients with advanced-stage chronic neurologic diseases such as Parkinson disease. The spouses and other family members of such patients are often exhausted, socially isolated, and without adequate support to help them through bereavement.[28] Bereavement counseling may then help in the transition to a noncaregiver role.[28]

Certain circumstances that are particularly likely to be encountered by neurologists merit brief additional comment here. Difficulties are particularly likely in circumstances in which diagnosis and prognostication are based on purely descriptive aspects of clinical status rather than more objective quantitative laboratory criteria, such as in the management of patients with disorders of consciousness.[29] This requires physicians to be very specific about their limitations in predicting the outcome of certain neurologic catastrophes.

Persistent Vegetative and Minimally Conscious States

The persistent vegetative state is characterized by loss of awareness despite the presence of sleep-wake cycles. It occurs in patients with destruction of the cerebral cortex but preservation of brainstem function. Such patients may survive for prolonged periods if provided with nutrition and fluids. There is general agreement that they do not experience pain or suffering, based on the lack of any behavioral indications of distress and the presence of extensive cortical damage that destroys the substrate of consciousness. Life-prolonging medical treatment can be withdrawn from a patient in a persistent vegetative state when it is clear that this accords with the previously expressed wishes of the patient and the family concurs with the withdrawal of such support. In general, the provision of nutrition and hydration is not to be withheld when the patient's prognosis is uncertain; its withdrawal at a later date is, however, appropriate when it is clear that the patient's condition is hopeless.[30] This usually requires the vegetative state to have persisted for at least 1 month.[30] However, recovery from a vegetative state may take longer than this, depending in part on the underlying etiology.[29] Indeed, a vegetative state is generally required to last for more than 3 months after an anoxic injury or 1 year after a traumatic brain injury before it is considered permanent, and even then a slim chance remains of further recovery with time.[31] Thus, decisions to remove life-supporting measures are commonly made while the likelihood and extent of recovery are uncertain and, consequently, may be influenced by the personal biases of treating medical and nursing staff. It is clearly appropriate in such a context to explain the prognostic dilemma to family members so that decisions are truly informed ones.[29] Management problems may occur when the family is not of one mind about how to proceed. A case in point was that of Terri Schiavo, who was in a postanoxic persistent vegetative state for some 8 years when her husband took legal steps—opposed by her parents—to remove her feeding tube and discontinue life-prolonging measures.[32] The resulting legal struggle continued over several years and involved various levels of the judiciary as well as state and federal legislative interventions, but support was eventually withdrawn and autopsy confirmed the presence of extensive, irreversible brain damage.

The so-called minimally conscious state designates a state in which patients exhibit inconsistent but discernible evidence of consciousness. It is thus quite distinct from the vegetative state, but it remains difficult to define. Some degree of functional recovery of behaviors suggesting self- or environmental awareness has occurred.[33] Such behaviors may, for example, include basic verbalization or context-appropriate gestures (regardless of accuracy), appropriate emotional responses (e.g., smiling or crying) to the linguistic or visual content of emotional but not neutral stimuli, or more simple activities such as purposive behaviors in response to environmental stimuli (e.g., a finger movement or eye blink apparently to command) or pursuit eye movement or sustained ocular fixation in response to moving or prominent stimuli. Improvement from this state is demonstrated by the restoration of consistent functional communication with the patient.

The minimally conscious state may occur in different neurologic contexts in which there has been a loss of cerebral function and may be temporary or permanent. Only limited information is available about the natural history or long-term outlook, and it depends in part on the etiology of the underlying neurologic disorder. Thus, the prognosis is better for those in whom traumatic brain injury was responsible than in other instances.[34] The likelihood of useful functional recovery declines with time, and patients remaining in a minimally conscious state for more than 12 months are likely to remain severely disabled and without a reliable means of communication, although well-publicized clinical exceptions exist. The patient Terry Wallis, for example, was in a post-traumatic minimally conscious state for some 19 years before recovering awareness and fluent speech, but then remained unaware of all that had transpired since his injury.[35] The clinical examination provides only limited help in defining the prognosis[33] and whether imaging and electrophysiologic techniques eventually help in this regard and in decision-making remains to be determined. In the meantime, cultural, religious, and family values will govern the responses of relatives to a patient in a minimally conscious state, and health-care providers must respect these responses and the previously expressed wishes of patients.

In the context of both the persistent vegetative and minimally conscious states, clinicians must be careful about suggesting at an early stage that no hope exists of useful recovery in order to justify decisions to discontinue life-supporting therapy when the evidence is lacking.[29] Instead, a frank discussion of the limited information available and the generally poor (but uncertain) prognosis may be more ethically appropriate and lead to more informed management decisions.

The serial clinical assessment of patients in both the acute and chronic setting will help to detect subtle but important changes that may otherwise pass unnoticed and that may affect management. It will also help to clarify for family members the significance of any changes that they have themselves observed. For example, relatives and friends may assume that eye opening, eye movements, swallowing movements, smiling, and other motor activities represent signs of recovery when they develop in a comatose subject, and it is incumbent on physicians to explain that this is not the case so that realistic expectations can be maintained.

Functional imaging may also come to be important in the assessment of these patients. In minimally conscious patients, activation patterns similar to those of healthy subjects have been described and suggest conscious awareness.[36] In patients diagnosed as being in a vegetative state, changes in positron emission tomography or functional magnetic resonance imaging sometimes reveal cortical activation, for example, in response to face-recognition or speech-perception paradigms,[37] instructions to imagine motor activity,[38] or a familiar voice saying the patient's name.[39] Such findings suggest awareness similar to that in patients in a minimally conscious state and may help to indicate which patients behaviorally classified as in a vegetative state are in fact in a minimally conscious state or are likely to recover clinical signs of awareness, thereby providing a guide to prognosis.[40]

There have been occasional anecdotal cases in the lay media of apparently miraculous recovery from a prolonged vegetative or minimally conscious state. The accuracy of some of these reports is unclear, as is the extent to which any recovery was clinically meaningful. In some instances, imaging studies have raised the possibility of axonal regrowth,[35] but whether this is responsible for any clinical improvement is uncertain.

Reports of arousal after deep brain stimulation of minimally conscious patients are intriguing. In one such instance, bilateral thalamic electrical stimulation was found to modulate behavioral responsiveness in a patient who had been in a minimally conscious state for 6 years after traumatic brain injury.[41] These findings underscore the importance of investigations into the mechanism of recovery and emphasize the need to clarify the role of neuromodulatory interventions in such patients.

Anecdotal reports of arousal and temporary improvement after administration of zolpidem to patients in a persistent vegetative state[42] also require confirmation. In a careful study, Brefel-Courbon and co-workers evaluated the efficacy of zolpidem in a 48-year-old woman who was not in a vegetative state but who had a severe postanoxic encephalopathy causing her to be akinetic and mute.[43] Acute administration of zolpidem led to enhanced arousal and markedly improved motor and cognitive performance. Positron emission tomography showed that cerebral metabolism increased in postrolandic territories and in frontal cortex, and there was drug-induced activation in the anterior cingulate and orbitofrontal cortex. These effects were tentatively attributed to an activation of limbic loops modulating motivational processes.

It appears that in a few patients with abnormalities of arousal or responsiveness, certain interventions may lead to temporary improvement. The systematic evaluation of function in brain-injured patients and of the effects of various manipulations on arousal and prognostication may be rewarding.[44] In the meantime, it is the responsibility of medical and paramedical staff to ensure that anecdotal case reports are not taken out of context and do not result in unrealistic expectations by family and friends attempting to come to terms with the predicament of a patient in a vegetative or minimally conscious state.

De-efferented State

Patients in a "locked-in" or de-efferented state are conscious but quadriplegic and incapable of communication except by eye closure or vertical eye movements. They typically are ventilator dependent. They may be excluded erroneously from clinical decision-making unless the impediment to normal communication is recognized and steps are taken to facilitate other means of communication.

Somewhat surprisingly, in one survey of 44 patients in this state, many had some social interactions, almost half had a positive attitude, and only 12.5 percent reported being depressed.[45] Thus, the quality of life may be acceptable to patients despite severe handicap. Nevertheless, some de-efferented patients may decide on withdrawal from further life support, and clinicians are obligated to respect these decisions when they have been competently made.[46] The withdrawal of support must be accompanied by measures to minimize further pain and distress while the patient succumbs.

Advanced Dementia

Meta-analyses indicate that from 60 years of age, the prevalence of dementia doubles with every 5 years of age.[47] The management of patients with advanced dementia may be especially challenging for neurologists. Cognitive decline and the disintegration of personality do not justify any disregard of and loss of respect for the individual patient. Medical problems require as much attention as in patients who are cognitively intact. This is particularly difficult because demented patients are often unable to cooperate fully, making the recognition and management of such problems more demanding. The care of patients with advanced dementia requires close interaction of clinicians with other family members to improve the quality of life and to find practical solutions for the minor problems that complicate daily life. Depression may enhance an apparent cognitive decline and may even be mistaken for dementia; the possibility of its presence always merits consideration. Patients in the early stages of progressive, dementing disorders should be encouraged to make their preferences known by discussion with family and health-care providers and by written advance directives while they are still competent. In the absence of such written directives, it eventually is necessary to identify a proxy decision-maker to act for the patient.

Linkage of hospital and death report data improves case ascertainment and has increased substantially population mortality estimates in patients with dementia.[47] Patients with advanced dementia are not necessarily terminally ill and may undergo a protracted period during which they are unable to speak or respond to their environment, but decisions about life-sustaining treatment for them are usually made by reference to the same ethical and legal principles as for patients who are dying,[6,48] although there is no unanimity in this regard. In such circumstances, for example, the artificial provision of nutrition and hydration in a demented patient who has lost the ability to eat is best decided based on the previously expressed wishes of the patient or the decision of a surrogate.[6,16] Palliative care is the preferred approach and is often provided in a nursing-home or hospice environment,[41] although not always satisfactorily.[49]

In one study of patients with advanced dementia living in nursing homes, almost 55 percent died over an 18-month period; the probability of death within 6 months was approximately 25 percent.[49] Among those who died, pneumonia occurred in 37 percent, febrile episodes in 32 percent and eating problems in 90 percent in the last 3 months of life. Distressing symptoms were common—dyspnea or pain for at least 5 days per month occurred in 46 and 39 percent, respectively; pressure ulcers in 39 percent; agitation in 54 percent; and aspiration in 41 percent. Such symptoms became more common as the end of life approached. Many patients underwent burdensome interventions of uncertain benefit, such as tube-feeding or parenteral therapy, or hospitalization, within 3 months of death.[49] In many instances, such interventions were not necessitated by the need to reduce physical suffering and were inconsistent with a palliative approach to care.[49] Studies show that despite traditional medical and nursing care, many demented patients—who are unable to communicate their physical or emotional needs—experience increasing amounts of suffering as death approaches, as judged by a quantitative suffering scale.[50]

Ambiguity about the care of severely demented patients is common. Thus, Wray and co-workers found a major difference between the decision to limit care, which usually involved the patient's family, and the decision to provide full care, which involved families less often.[48] The physicians involved in these decisions often thought that less intensive care would have been more appropriate, but nevertheless provided full care because the acute condition was potentially reversible (e.g., with antibiotics). Morrison and Siu compared the care received by patients admitted to a New York hospital for hip fracture or pneumonia and who had either advanced dementia or intact cognition.[51] The demented patients received as many burdensome procedures as the nondemented patients. Moreover, in the group with hip fracture, patients with dementia received significantly fewer morphine sulfate equivalents daily for pain relief than patients with preserved cognition, and only 24 percent received a standing order for any analgesics, even though such patients are often unable to communicate the presence of pain. Even fewer of the demented than nondemented patients had advance directives, and no documentation was found of any discussion about goals of care or decisions to withhold life-sustaining therapies in 90 percent of the patients with severe dementia.

Patients with advanced dementia often have difficulty with eating, and this is particularly distressing for family members and the health-care team. The benefits of tube feeding have been questioned. There is little or no evidence in this population that malnutrition is prevented or that tube feeding is associated with greater comfort, improved functional status, or prolonged survival.[52,53] To the contrary, placement of a tube may increase patient suffering, and tube feeding may be associated with adverse effects such as the increased use of restraints.[52] In many circumstances, hand feeding may be an alternative that should be favored because—although it also may not prevent malnutrition or dehydration—it provides more comfort and intimate care of the patient.[52]

The understanding, knowledge and perceptions of health-care proxies of nursing-home residents with advanced dementia influence the care that patients receive. Because the ability of patients with dementia to communicate declines with time until grossly impaired, proxies and health-care professionals must interpret patient behavior with particular care. When proxies are well informed and have a realistic understanding of the clinical complications expected in advanced dementia, patients are less likely to undergo unnecessary aggressive interventions in the final 3 months of life.[49] Clearly, closer consultation with family members and surrogates is necessary to define a rational treatment and management approach, which can then be followed.

Amyotrophic Lateral Sclerosis

Ganzini and co-workers measured pain, quality of life, suffering, sense of hopelessness, depression, level of disability, desire for life-sustaining medical treatment, and interest in assisted suicide of patients with amyotrophic lateral sclerosis and also asked their caregivers to rate the patients' quality of life, pain, and suffering.[54] Suffering was graded as 4 or more on a 6-point scale by 20 percent of patients and correlated with increasing pain, hopelessness, and level of disability. No relationship was found, however, between ratings of pain, suffering, and quality of life and interest in life-sustaining treatment or physician-assisted suicide. Pain and depression were often unrecognized or inadequately managed by treating physicians.

Nevertheless, others have found that most patients in the dying phase of amyotrophic lateral sclerosis die peacefully and, despite the common fear of suffocation, no patient choked to death.[55] The most frequent symptoms in the last 24 hours were dyspnea, coughing, anxiety, and restlessness. About half the patients died at home. The main palliative measures in use were mechanical ventilation, percutaneous gastrostomy, morphine, and benzodiazepines.

Regardless, early involvement of multidisciplinary palliative care services (such as neurologists and other specialty physicians; nursing staff; physical, occupational, and respiratory therapists; speech pathologist; dietician; medical social worker; and pastoral counselor) in the management of patients and their families, that is, before the terminal phase of illness, would probably improve the quality of life over the course of the disease and help to ensure integrated care by physicians and paramedical personnel with different perspectives.[56]

In patients with amyotrophic lateral sclerosis, ventilatory support should be discussed before the development of respiratory symptoms, and noninvasive ventilation should be considered before tracheostomy.[21] Noninvasive positive pressure ventilation may postpone the need for tracheostomy and mechanical ventilation, and may improve hypoventilatory symptoms, cognitive function, and quality of life.[57] The financial, social, and emotional burden of chronic invasive ventilation must be discussed fully with patients and their families so that informed decisions can be made. Many patients on ventilatory support are able to lead high-quality lives.[13] As the disease progresses, the goal of treatment evolves from optimizing and maximizing function to palliative care. Two of the most common distressing symptoms in advanced cases are dyspnea and mood disorders or anxiety, although recognition of the latter may depend on the instrument used.[58] Specific guidelines for treatment of intermittent or constant symptoms of this sort are available.[21] Pain may also occur and, if non-narcotic analgesics, anti-inflammatory drugs, and antispasticity agents are inadequate, may necessitate opioids. Sialorrhea can be managed by positioning and suction, by pharmacologic means, or with botulinum toxin injected into the parotid and submandibular glands.[59] Low-dose radiation has also been used successfully in this context.[60] Sleep disturbances are frequent and may be helped by treating mood disorders, respiratory inadequacy, bulbar dysfunction (by managing sialorrhea that is leading to choking episodes), and the inability to turn in bed (frequent repositioning; use of a hospital bed and mattress).

The wishes of patients with amyotrophic lateral sclerosis concerning life-sustaining therapy are not stable, and preferences frequently change over time.[61,62] Frequent discussion of options is therefore important, and advance directives for end-of-life care require periodic re-evaluation.

Patients and caregivers will not agree on all issues. Their attitudes to treatment options and their perceptions on quality of life have been examined. In one study, no significant difference was found between patients and caregivers on depression and quality-of-life scores, but patients tended to overestimate the quality of life of their caregivers, whereas caregivers underestimated that of patients.[59] Over half of both groups endorsed the future use of noninvasive mechanical ventilation, but more patients (41%) than caregivers (5%) were uncertain; just 3 percent of patients responded negatively compared to 32 percent of caregivers. Both groups were generally uninterested in invasive ventilation.[63] Spirituality or religion influences the readiness to accept percutaneous endoscopic gastrostomy, noninvasive assisted ventilation, or a tracheotomy, and attitude toward the process of dying.[64] Thus, psychosocial factors, personality traits, and spiritual factors, in addition to symptoms and disability, require consideration and discussion with patients and families throughout the illness.[65]

The incidence and predictors of percutaneous endoscopic gastrostomy have been examined in a group of patients with amyotrophic lateral sclerosis.[66] Patients undergoing percutaneous endoscopic gastrostomy were more likely than otherwise to undergo tracheostomy, more likely to have had a baseline preference for the procedure, and more likely to have initiated health-care proxies early in the disease course. The results imply that use of percutaneous endoscopic gastrostomy is part of a consistently proactive approach to the disease among patients and their supporting family.[66]

CONCLUDING COMMENTS

Physical distress remains common in many patients facing the end of life, but fear of suffering is probably even more common. Greater education of health-care providers about palliative medicine and easier access for patients to hospice programs and related resources will help to improve care for those who are dying. The apprehensions of dying patients may also be diminished by the knowledge that caregivers are fully committed to prevent, limit, or treat any discomfort that might arise. It is not possible to guarantee an "easy" death, but a commitment to provide optimal care is certainly realistic and reassuring. Such care must take into account the wishes of patients and their families.

REFERENCES

1. Ellershaw J, Ward C: Care of the dying patient: the last hours or days of life. BMJ 326:30, 2003.
2. Carver AC, Vickrey BG, Bernat JL, et al: End-of-life care: a survey of US neurologists' attitudes, behavior, and knowledge. Neurology 53:284, 1999.
3. Ethics and Humanities Subcommittee of the American Academy of Neurology: Assisted suicide, euthanasia, and the neurologist. Neurology 50:596, 1998.
4. Chung GS, Lawrence RE, Curlin FA, et al: Predictors of hospitalised patients' preferences for physician-directed medical decision-making. J Med Ethics 38:77, 2012.
5. Brody H, Campbell ML, Faber-Langendoen K, et al: Withdrawing intensive life-sustaining treatment: recommendations for compassionate clinical management. N Engl J Med 336:652, 1997.
6. Bernat JL, Goldstein ML, Viste KM: The neurologist and the dying patient. Neurology 46:598, 1996.
7. Sehgal A, Galbraith A, Chesney M, et al: How strictly do dialysis patients want their advance directives followed? JAMA 267:59, 1992.
8. Puchalski CM, Zhong Z, Jacobs MM, et al: Patients who want their family and physician to make resuscitation decisions for them: observations from SUPPORT and HELP. Study to Understand Prognoses and Preferences for Outcomes and Risks of Treatment. Hospitalized Elderly Longitudinal Project. J Am Geriatr Soc 48(suppl):S84, 2000.
9. Fins JJ, Maltby BS, Friedmann E, et al: Contracts, covenants and advance care planning: an empirical study of the moral obligations of patient and proxy. J Pain Symptom Manage 29:55, 2005.
10. Shalowitz DI, Garrett-Mayer E, Wendler D: The accuracy of surrogate decision makers: a systematic review. Arch Intern Med 166:493, 2006.
11. Johnston SC, Pfeifer MP, McNutt R, for the End of Life Study Group: The discussion about advance directives. Patient and physician opinions regarding when and how it should be conducted. Arch Intern Med 155:1025, 1995.
12. Davidson KW, Hackler C, Caradine DR, et al: Physicians' attitudes on advance directives. JAMA 262:2415, 1989.
13. McDonald ER, Hillel A, Wiedenfeld SA: Evaluation of the psychological status of ventilatory-supported patients with ALS/MND. Palliat Med 10:35, 1996.
14. Cochrane TI: Withdrawing and withholding life-sustaining treatment. Handb Clin Neurol 118:147, 2013.
15. Cochrane TI: Unnecessary time pressure in refusal of life-sustaining therapies: fear of missing the opportunity to die. Am J Bioeth 9:47, 2009.
16. American Academy of Neurology Ethics and Humanities Subcommittee: Ethical issues in the management of the demented patient. Neurology 46:1180, 1996.
17. American Academy of Neurology Ethics and Humanities Subcommittee: Palliative care in neurology. Neurology 46:870, 1996.
18. Foley KM: Competent care for the dying instead of physician-assisted suicide. N Engl J Med 336:54, 1997.
19. Working Group of the Ethical Issues in Medicine Committee of the Royal College of Physicians: Principles of pain control in palliative care for adults. J R Coll Physicians Lond 34:350, 2000.
20. Wilson WC, Smedira NG, Fink C, et al: Ordering and administration of sedatives and analgesics during the withholding and withdrawal of life support from critically ill patients. JAMA 267:949, 1992.
21. Miller RG, Rosenberg JA, Gelinas DF, et al: Practice parameter: the care of the patient with amyotrophic lateral sclerosis. (an evidence-based review.). Muscle Nerve 22:1104, 1999.
22. Solomon MZ, O'Donnell L, Jennings B, et al: Decisions near the end of life: professional views on life-sustaining treatments. Am J Public Health 83:14, 1993.
23. Clark JB, Sheward K, Marshall B, et al: Staff perceptions of end-of-life care following implementation of the Liverpool care pathway for the dying patient in the acute care setting: a New Zealand perspective. J Palliat Med 15:468, 2012.
24. Kinley J, Froggatt K, Bennett MI: The effect of policy on end-of-life care practice within nursing care homes: A systematic review. Palliat Med 27:209, 2013.
25. Veerbeek L, van Zuylen L, Swart SJ, et al: The effect of the Liverpool Care Pathway for the dying: a multi-centre study. Palliat Med 22:145, 2008.
26. Hall S, Kolliakou A, Petkova H, et al: Interventions for improving palliative care for older people living in nursing care homes. Cochrane Database Syst Rev:CD007132, 2011.
27. Burton CR, Payne S, Addington-Hall J, et al: The palliative care needs of acute stroke patients: a prospective study of hospital admissions. Age Ageing 39:554, 2010.
28. Bunting-Perry LK: Palliative care in Parkinson's disease: implications for neuroscience nursing. J Neurosci Nurs 38:106, 2006.
29. Fins JJ: Clinical pragmatism and the care of brain damaged patients: toward a palliative neuroethics for disorders of consciousness. Prog Brain Res 150:565, 2005.
30. American Academy of Neurology: Position of the American Academy of Neurology on certain aspects of the care and management of the persistent vegetative state patient. Neurology 39:125, 1989.
31. Kobylarz EJ, Schiff ND: Functional imaging of severely brain-injured patients: progress, challenges, and limitations. Arch Neurol 61:1357, 2004.

32. Hook CC, Mueller PS: The Terri Schiavo saga: the making of a tragedy and lessons learned. Mayo Clin Proc 80:1449, 2005.
33. Giacino JT, Ashwal S, Childs N, et al: The minimally conscious state: definition and diagnostic criteria. Neurology 58:349, 2002.
34. Giacino JT, Kalmar K: The vegetative and minimally conscious states: a comparison of clinical features and functional outcome. J Head Trauma Rehabil 12:36, 1997.
35. Voss HU, Uluc AM, Dyke JP, et al: Possible axonal regrowth in late recovery from the minimally conscious state. J Clin Invest 116:2005, 2006.
36. Schiff ND, Rodriguez-Moreno D, Kamal A, et al: fMRI reveals large-scale network activation in minimally conscious patients. Neurology 64:514, 2005.
37. Owen AM, Menon DK, Johnsrude IS, et al: Detecting residual cognitive function in persistent vegetative state. Neurocase 8:394, 2002.
38. Owen AM, Coleman MR, Boly M, et al: Detecting awareness in the vegetative state. Science 313:1402, 2006.
39. Di HB, Yu SM, Weng XC, et al: Cerebral response to patient's own name in the vegetative and minimally conscious states. Neurology 68:895, 2007.
40. Bernat JL, Rottenberg DA: Conscious awareness in PVS and MCS: the borderlands of neurology. Neurology 68:885, 2007.
41. Schiff ND, Giacino JT, Kalmar K, et al: Behavioural improvements with thalamic stimulation after severe traumatic brain injury. Nature 448:600, 2007.
42. Clauss R, Nel W: Drug induced arousal from the permanent vegetative state. Neurorehabilitation 21:23, 2006.
43. Brefel-Courbon C, Payoux P, Ory F, et al: Clinical and imaging evidence of zolpidem effect in hypoxic encephalopathy. Ann Neurol 62:102, 2007.
44. Schiff ND, Posner JB: Another "Awakenings". Ann Neurol 62:5, 2007.
45. Leon-Carrion J, van Eeckhout P, Dominguez-Morales M, del R, et al: The locked-in syndrome: a syndrome looking for a therapy. Brain Inj 16:571, 2002.
46. Ethics and Humanities Subcommittee of the American Academy of Neurology: Position statement: certain aspects of the care and management of profoundly and irreversibly paralyzed patients with retained consciousness and cognition. Neurology 43:222, 1993.
47. Zilkens RR, Spilsbury K, Bruce DG, et al: Linkage of hospital and death records increased identification of dementia cases and death rates estimates. Neuroepidemiology 32:61, 2009.
48. Wray N, Brody B, Bayer T, et al: Withholding medical treatment from the severely demented patient: decisional processes and cost implications. Arch Intern Med 148:1980, 1988.
49. Mitchell SL, Teno JM, Kiely DK, et al: The clinical course of advanced dementia. N Engl J Med 361:1529, 2009.
50. Aminoff BZ, Adunsky A: Dying dementia patients: too much suffering, too little palliation. Am J Hosp Palliat Med 22:344, 2005.
51. Morrison RS, Siu AL: Survival in end-stage dementia following acute illness. JAMA 284:47, 2000.
52. Li I: Feeding tubes in patients with severe dementia. Am Fam Physician 65:1605, 2002.
53. Candy B, Sampson EL, Jones L: Enteral tube feeding in older people with advanced dementia: findings from a Cochrane systematic review. Int J Palliat Nurs 15:396, 2009.
54. Ganzini L, Johnston WS, Hoffman WF: Correlates of suffering in amyotrophic lateral sclerosis. Neurology 52:1434, 1999.
55. Neudert C, Oliver D, Wasner M, et al: The course of the terminal phase in patients with amyotrophic lateral sclerosis. J Neurol 248:612, 2001.
56. Blackhall LJ: Amyotrophic lateral sclerosis and palliative care: where we are, and the road ahead. Muscle Nerve 45:311, 2012.
57. Simmons Z: Management strategies for patients with amyotrophic lateral sclerosis from diagnosis through death. Neurologist 11:257, 2005.
58. Wicks P, Abrahams S, Masi D, et al: Prevalence of depression in a 12-month consecutive sample of patients with ALS. Eur J Neurol 14:993, 2007.
59. Verma A, Steele J: Botulinum toxin improves sialorrhea and quality of living in bulbar amyotrophic lateral sclerosis. Muscle Nerve 34:235, 2006.
60. Neppelberg E, Haugen DF, Thorsen L, et al: Radiotherapy reduces sialorrhea in amyotrophic lateral sclerosis. Eur J Neurol 14:1373, 2007.
61. Silverstein MD, Stocking CB, Antel JP: Amyotrophic lateral sclerosis and life-sustaining therapy: patients' desires for information, participation in decision making, and life-sustaining therapy. Mayo Clin Proc 66:906, 1991.
62. Albert SM, Murphy PL, Del Bene ML, et al: A prospective study of preferences and actual treatment choices in ALS. Neurology 53:278, 1999.
63. Trail M, Nelson ND, Van JN, et al: A study comparing patients with amyotrophic lateral sclerosis and their caregivers on measures of quality of life, depression, and their attitudes toward treatment options. J Neurol Sci 209:79, 2003.
64. Murphy PL, Albert SM, Weber CM, et al: Impact of spirituality and religiousness on outcomes in patients with ALS. Neurology 55:1581, 2000.
65. Nelson ND, Trail M, Van JN, et al: Quality of life in patients with amyotrophic lateral sclerosis: perceptions, coping resources, and illness characteristics. J Palliat Med 6:417, 2003.
66. Albert SM, Murphy PL, Del Bene M, et al: Incidence and predictors of PEG placement in ALS/MND. J Neurol Sci 191:115, 2001.

Index

Note: Page numbers followed by "*f*" and "*t*" refers to figures and tables, respectively.

B

C

E

F

G

H

J

K

L

M

N

Q

R

S

T

W

X

Y

Z

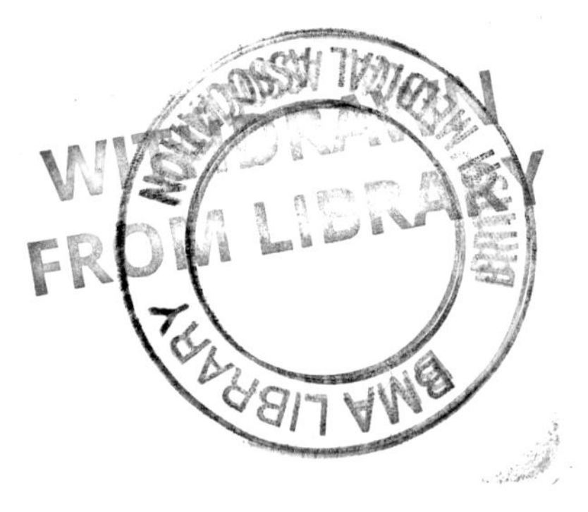